OCCUPATIONAL
and
ENVIRONMENTAL
RESPIRATORY DISEASE

OCCUPATIONAL *and* ENVIRONMENTAL RESPIRATORY DISEASE

Philip Harber, M.D., M.P.H.

Professor of Medicine,
University of California, Los Angeles
Los Angeles, California

Marc B. Schenker, M.D., M.P.H.

Professor of Medicine,
Chairman, Department of Community and International Health;
Director, Center for Occupational and Environmental Health, Davis;
Department of Internal Medicine;
Institute of Toxicology and Environmental Health;
University of California, Davis
School of Medicine,
Davis, California

John R. Balmes, M.D.

Associate Professor,
Chief, Division of Occupational and Environmental Medicine,
Attending Physician, Pulmonary and Critical Care Service,
San Francisco General Hospital,
Department of Medicine,
School of Medicine,
University of California, San Francisco
San Francisco, California

291 illustrations

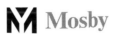

St. Louis Baltimore Boston Carlsbad Chicago Naples New York Philadelphia Portland
London Madrid Mexico City Singapore Sydney Tokyo Toronto Wiesbaden

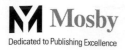

Editor: Laura DeYoung
Developmental Editor: Carolyn A. Malik
Associate Developmental Editor: Jennifer J. Byington
Project Manager: Dana Peick
Designer: Amy Buxton

FIRST EDITION

Printed in the United States of America
Composition by Clarinda Company
Printing/binding by Maple Vail

Mosby–Year Book, Inc.
11830 Westline Industrial Drive
St. Louis, Missouri 63146

Library of Congress Cataloging-in-Publication Data

Occupational and environmental respiratory disease / [edited by]
  Philip Harber, Marc B. Schenker, John R. Balmes.
      p.   cm.
    Includes bibliographical references and index.
    ISBN 0-8016-7728-9 (alk. paper)
    1. Lungs—Diseases.   2. Lungs—Dust diseases.   3. Occupational
diseases.   4. Environmentally induced diseases.   I. Harber, Philip.
II. Schenker, Marc.   III. Balmes, John.
    [DNLM: 1. Respiratory Tract Diseases.   2. Occupational Diseases.
WF   140   015   1995]
RC756.023   1995
616.2—dc20
DNLM/DLC
for Library of Congress   95-14252
                                                  CIP

95 96 97 98 99 / 9 8 7 6 5 4 3 2 1

CONTRIBUTORS

Denise R. Aberle, M.D.
Associate Professor,
School of Medicine,
University of California, Los
    Angeles,
Los Angeles, California

Michael Attfield, Ph.D.
Division of Respiratory Disease
    Studies,
Epidemiological Investigations
    Branch,
Morgantown, West Virginia

John R. Balmes, M.D.
Associate Professor of Medicine,
University of California, San
    Francisco,
San Francisco, California

Scott Barnhart, M.D., M.P.H.
Associate Professor,
Department of Medicine,
University of Washington,
Seattle, Washington

Rebecca Bascom, M.D., M.P.H.
Associate Professor and Director,
Environmental Research Facility,
University of Maryland School of
    Medicine,
Baltimore, Maryland

David V. Bates, M.D.
Professor Emeritus of Medicine,
Department of Health Care and
    Epidemiology,
University of British Columbia,
Vancouver, British Columbia,
Canada

William S. Beckett, M.D., M.P.H.
Associate Professor,
Yale University School of Medicine,
New Haven, Connecticut

Raymond Bégin, M.D.
Professor of Medicine,
Centre Hospital University of
    Sherbrooke,
Sherbrooke, Québec, Canada

Paul D. Blanc, M.D., M.S.P.H.
Associate Professor of Medicine,
University of California, San
    Francisco,
San Francisco, California

Brian A. Boehlecke, M.D., M.S.P.H.
Associate Professor of Medicine,
University of North Carolina,
Chapel Hill, North Carolina

Eddy A. Bresnitz, M.D., M.S.
Director,
Division of Occupational and
    Environmental Health;
Professor,
Medical College of Pennsylvania,
Philadelphia, Pennsylvania

William B. Bunn, M.D., J.D., M.P.H.
Director, Medical Clinic Services,
Mobil Oil Corporation Medical
    Department,
Princeton, New Jersey

Harriet A. Burge, Ph.D.
Associate Professor,
Harvard School of Public Health,
Boston, Massachusetts

Jerrold T. Bushberg, Ph.D.
Director, Nuclear Medicine,
University of California, Davis,
Medical Center,
Sacramento, California

Arch I. Carson, M.D., Ph.D.
Assistant Professor of Occupational
    Medicine and Environmental
    Sciences,
University of Texas,
School of Public Health,
Houston, Texas

André Cartier, M.D.
Sacre-Cœur of Montreal,
Associate Professor,
University of Montreal,
Montréal, Québec, Canada

Robert M. Castellan, M.D., M.P.H.
Chief, Epidemiological Investigations
    Branch,
National Institute for Occupational
    Safety and Health;
Adjunct Associate Professor,
Departments of Medicine and
    Community Medicine,
West Virginia University,
Morgantown, West Virginia

Moira Chan-Yeung, M.B.
Professor of Medicine,
University of British Columbia,
Vancouver General Hospital,
Vancouver, British Columbia, Canada

Jacqueline Karnell Corn, D.A., M.A.
Associate Professor,
Department of Environmental Health
    Sciences,
The Johns Hopkins University,
School of Hygiene and Public Health,
Baltimore, Maryland

Julian Crane, M.D.
Senior Research Fellow,
Department of Medicine,
Wellington School of Medicine,
Wellington South, New Zealand

Gerald S. Davis, M.D.
Professor of Medicine,
Director, Pulmonary Disease
    and Critical Care Medicine,
University of Vermont,
Burlington, Vermont

Roy DeHart, M.D., M.P.H.
Professor and Chair,
Department of Family Medicine,
University of Oklahoma, Health
    Sciences Center,
Oklahoma City, Oklahoma

George L. Delclos, M.D.
Associate Professor of Occupational
    Medicine,
University of Texas,
School of Public Health,
Houston, Texas

Michael A. Dias, M.D.
Research Fellow,
Otolaryngology – Head and Neck
    Surgery,
University of Maryland School of
    Medicine,
Baltimore, Maryland

Fran DuMelle
Deputy Managing Director,
American Lung Association,
Washington, D.C.

Don Enarson, M.D.
Director of Scientific Activities,
International Union Against
    Tuberculosis and Lung Disease,
Paris, France

M. Joseph Fedoruk, M.D., C.I.H.
Assistant Clinical Professor,
University of California, Irvine,
School of Medicine,
Irvine, California

Maureen A. Finnerty, R.N., M.N.
Pulmonary Clinical Nurse Specialist,
University of Southern California,
Los Angeles, California

John R. Froines, Ph.D.
Director, Center for
    Occupational and Environmental
    Health;
Chair, Department of Environmental
    Health Sciences
School of Public Health,
University of California, Los
    Angeles,
Los Angeles, California

Eric Garshick, M.D., M.O.H.
Assistant Professor of Medicine,
Harvard Medical School,
Brockton/West Roxbury Veteran
    Affairs Medical Center,
Brockton, Massachusetts

**Julie Louise Gerberding, M.D.,
Ph.D., M.P.H.**
Assistant Professor of Medicine,
    Epidemiology, and Biostatistics,
University of California, San
    Francisco;
Director, Epidemiology and
    Prevention Interventions Center,
San Francisco General Hospital,
San Francisco, California

Stacy H. Grimes
University of California, Davis
Davis, California

Samuel P. Hammar, M.D.
Clinical Professor of Pathology,
University of Washington,
Director, Diagnostic Specialties,
Bremerton, Washington

John Hankinson, Ph.D.
Division of Respiratory Disease
    Studies,
National Institute of Occupational
    Safety and Health,
Morgantown, West Virginia

John P. Hanrahan, M.D., M.P.H.
Assistant Professor of Medicine,
Channing Laboratory,
Harvard Medical School,
Brigham and Women's Hospital,
Boston, Massachusetts

Philip Harber, M.D., M.P.H.
Professor of Medicine,
University of California, Los
    Angeles,
Los Angeles, California

Eric Michael Hart, M.D.
Assistant Professor,
Department of Radiological Sciences,
School of Medicine,
University of California, Los
    Angeles,
Los Angeles, California

Jeffrey A. Jacobs, M.D., M.P.H
Division of Occupational/
    Environmental Medicine and
    Epidemiology,
University of California, Davis,
Davis, California

**Elizabeth A. Jennison, M.D.,
M.P.H.**
Cincinnati, Ohio

Paul A. Jensen, Ph.D.
National Institute for Occupational
    Safety and Health,
Cincinnati, Ohio

Susan M. Kennedy, Ph.D.
Associate Professor,
Occupational Hygiene Program,
University of British Columbia,
Vancouver, British Columbia, Canada

Michael P. Kenny, J.D.
General Counsel,
State of California Air Resources
    Board,
Sacramento, California

Jana N. Kesavanathan, M.S.
Division of Environmental Health
    Engineering,
The Johns Hopkins University,
School of Hygiene and Public Health,
Baltimore, Maryland

Ellen R. Kessler, M.D., M.P.H.
Medical Director, Personnel Health,
Fairfax Hospital,
Falls Church, Virginia

Kenneth W. Kizer, M.D., M.P.H.
Office of the Undersecretary,
Department of Veteran Affairs,
Washington, D.C.

Leslie M. Krinsk, J.D.
Senior Staff Counsel,
State of California Air Resources
    Board,
Sacramento, California

Gregory J. Kullman, Ph.D.
Division of Respiratory Disease
    Studies,
National Institute for Occupational
    Safety and Health,
Morgantown, West Virginia

William E. Lambert, Ph.D.
Research Assistant Professor,
Epidemiology and Cancer Control
    Program,
Department of Family and
    Community Medicine,
University of New Mexico School of
    Medicine,
Albuquerque, New Mexico

Arthur M. Langer, Ph.D.
Environmental Sciences Laboratory,
Brooklyn College of the City
    University of New York,
Brooklyn, New York

N. LeRoy Lapp, M.D.
Professor,
Pulmonary and Critical Care
    Division,
West Virginia University School of
    Medicine,
Morgantown, West Virginia

Teofile L. Lee-Chiong, M.D.
Senior Research Fellow,
Pulmonary and Critical Care Section,
Yale University School of Medicine,
New Haven, Connecticut

James E. Lockey, M.D., M.S.
Professor and Director,
Occupational and Environmental
    Medicine,
University of Cincinnati Medical
    Center,
Cincinnati, Ohio

Dana Loomis, Ph.D.
Assistant Professor,
Department of Epidemiology,
University of North Carolina,
Chapel Hill, North Carolina

Jean-Luc Malo, M.D.
Chest Physician,
Sacre-Cœur of Montreal;
Associate Professor,
University of Montreal,
Montréal, Québec, Canada

Nicole Massin, M.D.
Institut de la Santé et de la
    Recherche Médicale
Villejuif, France

Richard A. Matthay, M.D.
Professor and Associate Chairman,
Department of Medicine,
Associate Director,
Pulmonary and Critical Care Section,
Yale University School of Medicine,
New Haven, Connecticut

John J. May, M.D.
Director, New York Center for
    Agricultural Medicine and Health;
Head, Division of Pulmonary
    Medicine,
The Mary Imogene Bassett Hospital
Cooperstown, New York;
Associate Clinical Professor of
    Medicine,
Columbia University,
New York, New York

Michael A. McCawley
West Virginia University,
Department of Civil and
    Environmental Engineering,
Morgantown, West Virginia

Melissa McDiarmid, M.D., M.P.H.
Director, Office for Occupational
    Medicine,
Occupational Safety and Health
    Administration,
United States Department of Labor,
Washington, D.C.

Philip R. Morey, Ph.D., C.I.H.
Clayton Environmental Consultants,
Director of Microbiology,
Gettysburg, Pennsylvania

Sean R. Muldoon, M.D., M.P.H.
University of Pittsburgh,
Graduate School of Public Health,
Pittsburgh, Pennsylvania

Lee S. Newman, M.D.
Associate Professor,
University of Colorado,
National Jewish Center for
    Immunology and Respiratory
    Medicine,
Denver, Colorado

Peter J. Nigro, M.D.
Robert Wood Johnson,
University of New Jersey
    School of Medicine and
    Dentistry
Piscataway, New Jersey

Robert P. Nolan, Ph.D.
Environmental Sciences Laboratory,
Brooklyn College of the City
    University of New York,
Brooklyn, New York

Dennis M. O'Brien, Ph.D.
National Institute for Occupational
    Safety and Health,
Cincinnati, Ohio

John E. Parker, M.D.
Division of Respiratory Disease
    Studies,
National Institute for Occupational
    Safety and Health,
Morgantown, West Virginia

Neil Pearce, Ph.D.
Associate Professor,
Department of Medicine,
Wellington School of Medicine,
Wellington South, New Zealand

Edward L. Petsonk, M.D.
Division of Respiratory Disease
    Studies,
National Institute for Occupational
    Safety and Health,
Morgantown, West Virginia

Q.T. Pham, M.D.
Research Director
Institut de la Santé et de la
    Recherche Médicale,
Nancy, France

Kent E. Pinkerton, Ph.D.
Associate Professor,
Institute of Toxicology and
    Environmental Health,
University of California, Davis,
Davis, California

Patricia Quinlan, M.P.H., C.I.H.
University of California, San
    Francisco,
San Francisco, California

Otto G. Raabe, Ph.D.
Professor Emeritus,
Institute of Toxicology and
    Environmental Health,
University of California, Davis,
Davis, California

Anna Rask-Andersen, M.D., Ph.D.
Department of Occupational and
    Environmental Medicine,
University Hospital,
Uppsala, Sweden

Carrie A. Redlich, M.D., M.P.H.
Assistant Professor of Medicine,
Yale University School of Medicine,
New Haven, Connecticut

Kathleen M. Rest, Ph.D., M.P.A.
Assistant Professor,
University of Massachusetts,
Worchester, Massachusetts

Cecile Rose, M.D., M.P.H.
Associate Professor,
University of Colorado,
National Jewish Center for Immunology
    and Respiratory Medicine,
Denver, Colorado

Harriet L. Rubenstein, M.P.H., J.D.
Assistant Professor,
Medical College of Pennsylvania,
Philadelphia, Pennsylvania

Jonathan M. Samet, M.D., M.S.
Professor and Chairman,
Department of Epidemiology,
The Johns Hopkins University,
School of Hygiene and Public Health,
Baltimore, Maryland

Robert Thayer Sataloff, M.D., D.M.A.
Professor of Otolaryngology,
Thomas Jefferson University,
Philadelphia, Pennsylvania;
Adjunct Professor of Otolaryngology,
Georgetown University,
Washington, D.C.

Paul D. Scanlon, M.D.
Assistant Professor,
Director, Pulmonary Function
    Laboratory,
Mayo Medical School,
Rochester, Minnesota

Marc B. Schenker, M.D., M.P.H.
Professor of Medicine,
Chairman, Department of Community
    and International Health;
Department of Internal Medicine,
University of California, Davis,
Davis, California

Noah S. Seixas, Ph.D.
Assistant Professor,
Department of Environmental Health,
University of Washington,
Seattle, Washington

Rashid A. Shaikh
Executive Director,
Health Effects Institute–Asbestos
    Research,
Cambridge, Massachusetts

Bertrand Shapiro, M.D.
Division of Pulmonary and Critical
    Care Medicine,
University of Southern California,
Los Angeles, California

Steven Short, M.D.
Division of Respiratory Disease
    Studies,
National Institute for Occupational
    Safety and Health,
Morgantown, West Virginia

Dennis Shusterman, M.D., M.P.H.
Assistant Professor of Medicine,
University of California, San
    Francisco,
San Francisco, California

Carl Shy, M.D.
Professor and Chair,
Department of Epidemiology,
University of North Carolina,
Chapel Hill, North Carolina

Neal Simonsen, Ph.D.
Department of Epidemiology,
University of North Carolina,
Chapel Hill, North Carolina

Joseph R. Spiegel, M.D.
Associate Professor of Otolaryngology,
Thomas Jefferson University,
Philadelphia, Pennsylvania

Kyle Steenland, Ph.D.
National Institute for Occupational
    Safety and Health,
Cincinnati, Ohio

Michael S. Stulbarg, M.D.
Professor of Medicine,
University of California, San
    Francisco,
San Francisco, California

David L. Swift, Ph.D.
Professor,
Division of Environmental Health
    Engineering,
The Johns Hopkins University,
School of Hygiene and Public Health,
Baltimore, Maryland

Abba I. Terr, M.D.
Clinical Professor of Medicine,
Director,
Allergy Clinic,
Stanford University,
Palo Alto, California

David J. Tollerud, M.D., M.P.H.
Associate Professor,
Department of Environmental
    Occupational Health,
Chief, Occupational and
    Environmental Medicine,
University of Pittsburgh,
Graduate School of Public Health,
Pittsburgh, Pennsylvania

Thomas L. Vaughan, M.D.
Associate Professor,
Department of Epidemiology,
University of Washington and Fred
    Hutchinson Cancer Research
    Center,
Seattle, Washington

Gregory R. Wagner, M.D.
Director, Division of Respiratory
    Disease Studies,
National Institute for Occupational
    Safety and Health,
Morgantown, West Virginia

Virginia Weaver, M.D., M.P.H.
Instructor,
Division of Occupational Health,
Department of Environmental
    Health Sciences,
The Johns Hopkins University,
School of Hygiene and Public
    Health,
Baltimore, Maryland

Scott T. Weiss, M.D., M.P.H.
Associate Professor,
Channing Laboratory,
Harvard Medical School,
Brigham and Women's Hospital,
Boston, Massachusetts

Neil Walton White, M.D.
Specialist Physician,
Respiratory Clinic,
University of Cape Town
Cape Town, Observatory, South
    Africa

Leslie Zimmerman, M.D.
Assistant Professor of Medicine,
University of California, San
    Francisco,
San Francisco, California

This book is dedicated to three generations of women in my family: Jennifer, Jean, and Dora. Their support, insight, and tolerance have contributed immeasurably.

Philip Harber

This book is dedicated to the four wonderful women in my life: my wife and lifetime companion Heath and my three daughters, Yael, Phoebe, and Hilary. They not only tolerate the time I spend on my work, but they give the work raison d'être. *Their astute insights and observations put my work in particular, and occupational and environmental health in general, into a social, political, cultural, aesthetic, and personal context, and I am profoundly grateful to them.*

Marc B. Schenker

I dedicate my contributions to this book to Drs. Herbert Berger and Alvin Tierstein, who inspired me to become a pulmonary physician; Dr. Arthur Frank, who inspired my interest in occupational and environmental health; and to my wife, Dr. Sherry Katz, who correctly opined that I was crazy to take on the additional work involved.

John R. Balmes

FOREWORD

There are many reasons for considering occupational and environmental respiratory diseases separately. Each exposure is the responsibility of a different agency; there are major legal and jurisdictional differences; exposures often involve consideration of different substances. Whereas environmental questions usually involve the general population, occupational risks are primarily contained within specific and well-defined populations. Nevertheless it is instructive to consider the evolution of occupational and environmental respiratory diseases together and to note specific instances in which advance understanding in one area has led to changes in the other.

OCCUPATIONAL HEALTH

The genesis of occupational medicine can be precisely dated to Ramazzini's book *De Morbis Artificum* in 1713. Dr. Samuel Johnson, the great English lexicographer, was 4 years old at the time; many years later Johnson was to propound the first statement of moral responsibility for diseases contracted by workers on behalf of others. In the nineteenth century the torch of social reform was carried by Charles Dickens, and scrotal cancer in chimney sweepers in London was described by Percival Pott. Scientific and systematic study of an occupational hazard may be dated to 1895 when Haldane published the results of his experiments on himself involving the controlled breathing of carbon monoxide. Early in the twentieth century the public was scandalized by phosphorus poisoning in factory workers, and legislative action was taken to prevent the disease. By the 1930s, both silicosis and coal worker's pneumoconiosis were recognized to be significant problems, and by this date worker's compensation legislation was in place in most jurisdictions. Although the potential hazard of asbestos was beginning to be recognized at the time of the outbreak of World War II in 1939, there was no incentive to pay attention to it—if one was in danger of being torpedoed, the long-term risk of disease caused by asbestos insulation below decks would have seemed laughably remote.

From 1950 onward the study of occupational disease, and in particular occupational respiratory disease, accelerated rapidly. By 1972 the risk of asbestos was becoming generally recognized; the consequences of radon exposure in uranium miners were becoming apparent; new substances such as vinyl chloride were found to be hazardous; and, ten years later, the widely dispersed but common problems of occupationally-induced asthma were being generally recognized. Although the field is still plagued by problems of inadequate funding for training and, in some jurisdictions, difficulty of access, by 1990 the field of occupational medicine had become well established, with a major component being occupational lung disease

ENVIRONMENTAL HEALTH

Concern about air pollution stretches back several hundred years in coal-burning countries. Effective action can be dated to the 1946 city ordinance in Pittsburgh and the public concern surrounding the Donora and Meuse Valley episodes. The major London fog in December of 1952, which caused in excess of 4000 deaths, accelerated inquiry and legislation in Britain, and the Industrial West initiated effective controls over the subsequent 20 years. By 1960 the formidable problem of cigarette smoking-induced disease was beginning to be realized, although some years would pass before the magnitude of the adverse health effects attributed to smoking would be recognized. These two environmental exposures and their major effects on respiratory disease have caused environmental lung diseases to be continuing major concern in the general area of environmental health.

By 1980 new environmental problems had been identified. So much lead was being used in gasoline that public exposure had become a justifiable concern. The use of asbestos in public buildings 20 years previous had led to public environmental exposure in schools and libraries; radon had been identified as a problem in some houses in some geologic regions wherein the public could be exposed to levels comparable with those encountered by uranium miners. The careless disposal of chemical wastes from public exposure through a contaminated water supply to a wide spectrum of substances with adverse effects on animals was tested. In addition, new data indicated that new forms of air pollution, leading to the formation of ozone and acid aerosols, were probably affecting the population. Since 1980 the remarkable occurence of "sick building syndrome" and the phenomenon of acquired general chemical sensitivity (not yet understood) have attracted general attention.

Many environmental problems are characterized by exposure of large populations, by difficulty in characterizing the adverse health outcome (which may affect the reproductive or immunologic system), and by the contentious question of deducing low-level risks from earlier higher-level exposures. Whereas in the 1950s pollution was thought to be a problem for an individual city, by the 1970s it was realized that long-range transmission of pollutants was occurring. By the 1980s the implications of emissions on earth in regard to stratospheric chemistry and global earth warming were beginning to be understood. As with occupational medicine, respiratory disease from environmental exposures have remained a major area of research and public concern.

CONVERGENCE OF OCCUPATIONAL AND ENVIRONMENTAL CONCERNS

There has been a remarkable convergence of occupational and environmental concerns in recent years. The case of asbestos is an obvious example. Radon is another. "Sick building syndrome," which may be attributable to exposure to mixtures of volatile organic compound, commonly occurs in offices and, consequently, becomes a disease of occupational origin. Exposure to lead was formerly confined to industrial operatives, but the general uses of lead in gasoline (accompanied by a fivefold increase in the lead content of snow cores in Greenland) has now made it an environmental issue. Fine particulate air pollution has been found to have measurable effects on the general population, which raises interesting issues in relation to occupational dust exposure.

COMMON LESSONS

Although most of the contemporary concern (and almost all of the news coverage) about health care relates to economic issues, a longer perspective suggests that advances in the understanding of occupational and environmental disease, and particularly respiratory diseases, has come to be seen as highly significant compared with the thinking in 1965. In this progress, several important trends are discernible; these are likely to dominate advances for the next few years.

First, it has been learned that careful characterization of individual exposure (by whatever means possible) greatly strengthens epidemiologic studies. Whereas when the agent is powerful (as in the case of cigarette smoke), linear relationships to risk can be obtained by approximate estimates of lifetime smoking habits. In more common circumstances, to demonstrate the increased risk at all, it may be necessary to refine the exposure data. As with all pendulums, this one can swing too far—there is still a great deal of information to be gained in the absence of precise exposure data.

Second, the use of computers has greatly expanded the potential for epidemiologic studies on large populations. This applies not only to industrially exposed cohorts (such as asbestos-exposed insulators or diesel locomotive drivers) but also to the exposed general population (such as the exposure to air pollution of modern urban residents). It is possible to use time-series analyses on populations of several millions of people to relate health outcomes such as hospital admissions to environmental parameters.

Third, there have been major advances in statistical methodology, not only in the use of multiple logistic regression techniques and modelling but also in the automated reading of questionnaires and in the methods of time-series analysis. One report suggests that in the case of panel studies of asthmatics, the use of "neural network analysis" may refine conventional methodology.

These advances have not been paralleled by significant progress in the intractable social problems of worker's compensation, in which diseases such as occupational asthma do not fit into legislation that dealt with silicosis written 60 years previously. Some advances have occurred in the process of setting standards, but enforcement in the individual workplace has remained a Cinderella in most places. That some progress has been achieved in the Industrial West became apparent when the appalling environmental degradation in Eastern Europe was revealed with the collapse of Communist regimes. Working conditions and the common environment in those countries, and in much of the third world, resemble those of Britain in the early days of the industrial revolution.

The most recent economic recession in the West was a powerful threat to further advances in the control and prevention of occupational and environmental respiratory disease. It will be the important responsibility of those who understand what has been achieved in these disciplines since the end of World War II to ensure that such gains are not lost in the future.

This new text embodies advances and typifies the common overlaps between occupational and environmental respiratory diseases. Detailed attention is given to problems that are critical to both areas, such as exposure assessment and the use of common tools of the investigative method. It is hoped that the new knowledge that this text encompasses will act as a foundation for long overdue social and political initiatives to mitigate the existence of a major burden of preventable lung disease.

David V. Bates, M.D.
Professor Emeritus of Medicine,
University of British Columbia,
Vancouver

PREFACE

Occupational and environmental exposures play major roles in causing many forms of respiratory disease. All humans are exposed to potential occupational or environmental toxins such as indoor or ambient air pollutants or unique respiratory toxins occurring in the workplace. No longer are occupational toxin exposures limited to blue-collar jobs in heavy industries such as mining and manufacturing; significant hazards exist in modern industries and office environments. The disorders resulting from these exposures are diverse in nature, ranging from acute lung injury from toxic gas inhalation to subtle effects of environmental pollutants upon persons with asthma. All aspects of the respiratory system, from the nose to the alveoli, can be affected by inhaled environmental agents; therefore this book seeks to address the full range of respiratory effects of environmental exposures. The respiratory system does not distinguish whether an inhaled agent came from a workplace or a community (nonoccupational) source. For this reason, a unitary approach, jointly considering occupational and environmental respiratory disease, is employed in this book. However, exposure assessment methods and control strategies often differ between workplace and community environments, these differences are discussed

There are many perspectives and approaches to understanding occupational and environmental respiratory diseases. These include clinical approaches, focused upon the diagnosis and treatment of disease in an individual patient; environmental monitoring perspectives, emphasizing evaluation of the potential exposures; epidemiologic assessment, evaluating patterns of health and disease in *groups* of persons; biologic considerations of the mechanisms by which environmental agents produce disease; and public policy aspects, emphasizing control by regulation and law.

This book is predicated on the belief that approaches to understanding respiratory disease are intertwined, and all must be integrated to prevent and manage such disorders. There is also a strong emphasis on the relationship between disease and exposure, recognizing that disease prevention is directly related to controlling exposure. However, discussion of fundamental biologically oriented research, without direct clinical or public health implications, has been deemphasized. These topics are covered in more detail in other texts.

Figure 1 suggests a *"user's guide"* for this book. It reflects the organization of the major sections. Section I presents a historical overview of the field. Section II discusses the major approaches employed in the field, presenting the "tools" (e.g., radiology, epidemiology) from a methodologic standpoint. Section III presents methods employed for assessing exposures. Section IV provides an overview of the major disease categories, emphasizing aspects that are common to the disease group regardless of the etiology. For example, the symptoms and treatment of lung cancer are generally similar regardless of the underlying etiology. A clinician faced with an individual patient with a respiratory disease may move from this section of the book to sections dealing with specific exposures causing a disease or group of diseases.

Sections V and VI discuss disorders resulting from exposure to known agents; specifically, Section V includes the interstitial lung diseases, and Section VI covers disorders that primarily affect the airways. In instances where an agent can produce diseases in either category, the agent is discussed in the section appropriate to the major associated disease and is cross-referenced in the other section.

Section VII includes agents that cause upper airway disorders, cancers, and acute toxic effects. This section also discusses classes of agents such as metals, which may lead to diverse categories of disease. Section VIII discusses industries that are associated with the development of occupational and environmental respiratory disease. In some industries the agent is well identified, whereas in others a complex mixture of etiologic agents exists. Diagnosis and control may be based on general characteristics of the industry rather than on controlling a specific agent. Section IX emphasizes respiratory disorders caused by nonoccupational pollutants in both indoor and outdoor environments.

The next several sections discuss systematic approaches to occupational and environmental respiratory diseases. Section X focuses upon person-oriented approaches, and it includes discussions of disability assessment, accommodation, and rehabilitation of individuals with occupational and environmental respiratory diseases and includes organized surveillance methods for the detection and prevention of disease in *groups*. Section XI addresses occupational and environmental respiratory disease from a policy perspective. The legal and regulatory framework in the United States is discussed. Special considerations are presented for the recognition and control of occupational and environmental respiratory disease in developing nations where resources and approaches to the diagnosis and control of disease may be different. The final section deals with control technologies.

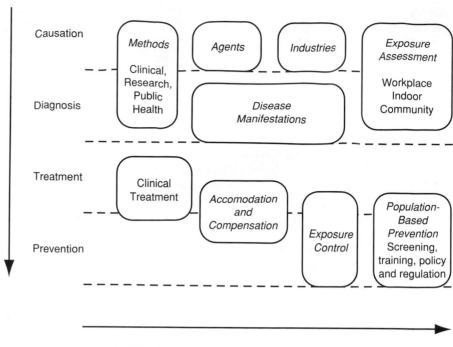

Fig. 1. Occupational and environmental respiratory disease.

Individuals   Populations

Occupational and environmental respiratory disease can be avoided by primary prevention methods that control adverse exogenous exposures. Therefore, assessment of an individual patient should always be accompanied by the questions, "Why did he/she develop this illness?" "Is there an intervention to prevent disease progression?" and "What should be done to prevent this in others?"

As shown in Fig. 1, the book is organized to be used in several ways. For example, the exposure may be known, and the associated diseases requiring control measures may be of interest. Conversely, a clinician with a sick patient in the office may use the general disease category unit as the point of entry. An occupational physician treating a patient with known occupational disease caused by a specific agent may desire more information about methods of confirming the diagnosis, evaluating disease progression, pharmacologic treatment of the disease, or dealing with accommodation and compensation of the injured worker.

Occupational and environmental respiratory disease is a worldwide problem. There are large numbers of cases of disease that still occur, even though these diseases have been known to be preventable for many years. Other diseases are caused by modern industries, and new pollutants and may be particularly common in developed countries at present.

Tobacco use is a major contributor to respiratory disease. In view of the multifactorial etiology of respiratory disease and the interaction of smoking with other exposures, the presence of one factor (smoking) does not preclude the presence of a significant impact of another occupational or environmental exposure or even a synergistic interaction of both factors.

We hope this book will fill the important need for a comprehensive volume providing integrative apporaches to the treatment, prevention, and control of occupational and environmental respiratory disease. The scope is wider than that found in existing textbooks of occupational lung disease. New information about the potentially adverse effects of environmental exposures is included. The often-overlooked upper airway is treated in depth. In addition to the mining and manufacturing industries, which have traditionally received most attention as causes of occupational lung disease, this book includes information about other work settings in which occupational and environmental respiratory disease occurs, such as the health care industry, petroleum industry, office settings, agriculture, semiconductor industries, and others. Indoor air pollution—its health effects, policy implications, and control measures—is covered in detail. Exposure assessment, risk evaluation, hazard communication, and protective measures are also discussed.

The editors gratefully thank the contributors to this book who have shared their expertise. We thank Jill Oversier for her organizational skills as assistant to the editors. We also thank our office staff members who provided invaluable assistance including Ann Lavallee, David Brightman, Fran

Stewart, Laura Peña, Alice Yick, Paul Hsu, Weiling Chen, and Chy Tran. Finally, we thank our developmental editors at Mosby–Year Book, Carolyn Malik and Jennifer J. Byington, without whose perseverance this book might still be in production.

Philip Harber, M.D., M.P.H.
Professor of Medicine,
University of California,
Los Angeles

Marc B. Schenker, M.D., M.P.H.
Professor of Medicine,
University of California,
Davis

John R. Balmes, M.D.
Associate Professor of Medicine,
University of California,
San Francisco

CONTENTS

OCCUPATIONAL
and
ENVIRONMENTAL
RESPIRATORY DISEASE

History of Occupational and Environmental Respiratory Disease

JOHN R. BALMES

Occupational and environmental diseases have been of concern to physicians since at least the time of the ancient Greeks. Chapter 1 places modern regulatory efforts in appropriate historical context using efforts to control silicosis as an example.

Chapter 1

HISTORICAL PERSPECTIVE

Jacqueline Karnell Corn

Effects of industrialization and urbanization
Federal regulation
Air pollution
The Occupational Safety and Health Act
Silicosis
    Nature of the disease
    Early recognition of disease
    Industrialization and silicosis
Gauley Bridge

Occupational and environmental respiratory disease has a long history. Observations of the relationship between health and environment can be traced to Hippocratic writings in which philosophic reasoning and observation led to the idea that ill health resulted from an imbalance between human beings and their environment. *Air, Waters, Places* presented, in a systematic manner, the relationship between environmental factors and disease.[14] Because it would be presumptuous in the space available to portray the history of environmental lung disease in its entirety, this chapter focuses mainly on the twentieth century, when industrial, technologic, scientific, political, and social developments led to interventions that shaped contemporary responses to occupational and environmental respiratory disease.

The first part of this chapter discusses factors that affect reaction to occupational and environmental health (sometimes referred to here as occupational and nonoccupational). It should be noted that many concepts used for the prevention and control of nonoccupational hazards were first developed by physicians, industrial hygienists, and toxicologists to control and prevent *occupational* hazards. The second part presents an historic case study of silicosis, an occupational lung disease. It illustrates changes that have

occurred in how we have defined the disease and in how we have approached the prevention and control of this ever-present occupational lung disease.

EFFECTS OF INDUSTRIALIZATION AND URBANIZATION

The roots of modern efforts to prevent and control risk associated with occupational and nonoccupational exposures reach back to the nineteenth century, when rapid industrialization and urbanization occurred. Evolving definitions and changing understanding of occupational and nonoccupational respiratory diseases were based, in part, on the growing realization that the urbanization and industrialization processes and the growth of technology profoundly affected the health of urban dwellers and factory workers. Changes in the occupational and nonoccupational environment illustrate the increasing complexity of the physical, chemical, biologic, and social bases of environmental health problems.

After World War II, new processes, new chemicals, and new sources of energy presented even more complicated problems with implications for the health of workers and the general public.[1] Both insidious industrial poisonings stemming from chemical substances capable of causing chronic illness and subtle environmental effects created complex and perplexing questions that called for equally complex, and often controversial, answers. At the same time that technology made possible new processes and chemicals, our knowledge base for understanding, defining, discovering, and preventing occupational and nonoccupational respiratory diseases also became more refined. Subtle long-term health effects made solutions to environmental health problems more difficult. The ability to make more accurate and sensitive measurements further complicated the process of surveillance and control.

By the beginning of the twentieth century, the deteriorating urban environment had already caused health problems associated with air pollution, sewage disposal, and the growth of slums. The rapid development of mines and factories led to polluted air, polluted water, and an inordinate number of occupational diseases and accidents. Contact with inhaled gases, vapors, fumes, fibers, and particles caused diseases affecting the lungs and other parts of the respiratory tract.

Social change, technologic developments, scientific observation, and political intervention have all shaped the modern American response to occupational and nonoccupational illness. Technology altered the nature of work and created new hazards. Medical scientists recognized the new hazards, social reformers brought the new dangers to public attention, and legislation attempted to enlarge employer and governmental responsibility. More often, barriers to effective action were political and economic rather than technical and scientific.

Decisions to control the environment are public health decisions that contain elements of value and science. The element of value determines the degree and extent of health a society wants and is willing to pay for. The scientific element determines how much knowledge a society has on which to base its environmental policies. We have learned that science and scientific approaches alone cannot provide solutions. Environmental hazards pose political, social, and economic problems that reach beyond scientific ones. These are further complicated by the perception of *hazard,* which continually alters in response to changing scientific understanding interwoven with social, political, and economic conditions.

By the second decade of the twentieth century, industrial pollution could no longer be ignored. A slow change of attitude in the field of occupational health could also be discerned. Spurred on by increased industrial activity, pressure exerted by the progressive segment of American society, the growth of labor unions, new scientific and technical knowledge, more data relevant to the incidence of occupational diseases, a changing attitude toward governmental responsibility, and social legislation, including workmen's compensation, efforts in occupational medicine and hygiene led to minimal control of some of the more obvious evils of excessive hazards.

FEDERAL REGULATION

Change is painfully slow; but by the mid-1960s, issues associated with environmental and occupational health could no longer be ignored. They became national. The result was establishment of new agencies and new protective regulations. The new laws and regulatory agencies of the 1960s and 1970s defined the federal government's policy toward the environment.

The following is a list of major legislation passed from 1938 to 1986. Note that most of the legislation was passed in the 1970s.

Federal Drug and Cosmetics Act (FDCA), 1938
Federal Insecticide, Fungicide and Rodenticide Act (FIFRA), 1948, 1972, 1975
Federal Hazardous Substances Act (FHSA), 1966

National Environmental Policy Act (NEPA), 1969
Federal Coal Mine Safety and Health Act (MSHA), 1969
Poisonous Packaging Prevention Act (PPPA), 1970
Occupational Safety and Health Act, 1970
Clean Air Act (CAA), 1970, 1977
Federal Water Pollution Control (now Clean Water) Act (FW-PCA), 1972, 1977
Marine Protection Research and Sanctuaries Act (MPRSA), 1972
Consumer Product Safety Act (CPSA), 1972
Federal Environmental Pollution Control Act (FEPCA), 1972
Safe Drinking Water Act (SDWA), 1974, 1979
Toxic Substances Control Act (TSCA), 1976
Surface Mine Control and Reclamation Act (SMCRA), 1977
Uranium Mill Tailings Control Act (UMTCA), 1978
Comprehensive Environmental Response, Compensation and Liability Act (CERCLA), 1980
Superfund Amendments and Re-authorization Act (SARA), 1986
Asbestos Hazard Emergency Response Act (AHERA), 1986

Concern had been triggered by a new awareness of the potential dangers inherent in the technologic and chemical revolutions that occurred after World War II, when new processes, new chemicals, and new sources of energy presented new hazards and augmented old ones that affected the health of workers and the general public. Rapid proliferation of the new hazards generated concern among the scientific community, the press, and public interest groups and placed environmental health (occupational and nonoccupational) on the public agenda. Furthermore, the focus changed from diseases of short duration to the long-term, life-threatening effects of disease. Lower concentrations of chemicals, dusts, and other hazards caused new concern based on the concept that low levels of a dose over a long period could cause disease.

AIR POLLUTION

Although the old problems created by smoke and gases from fossil fuels remained largely uncontrolled, new pollutants with toxic properties adversely affected air quality and public health. Air pollution incidents created a new public awareness that this pollution could cause ill health. Three smog episodes shocked the public into recognition of the problem. The first occurred in 1948 in Donora, Pennsylvania; the second, in 1952 in London; and the third, in 1962, also in London. The episodes resulted in marked increases in morbidity and mortality from respiratory effects. These crises led to increased public concern over the effects of air pollution on human health and the environment. Chemical agents, radioactive materials, and automotive exhaust emissions stimulated concern for health effects caused by airborne materials. Increased awareness that chemicals and motor vehicles could cause air pollution led to the need to understand the health effects of airborne materials from occupational and nonoccupational exposures and the need to limit their potential to induce disease.

THE OCCUPATIONAL SAFETY
AND HEALTH ACT

In 1970 Congress enacted sweeping occupational safety and health legislation. In retrospect the Occupational Safety and Health Act, which was 12 years in the making,[2] was finally passed because of an increasing industrial accident rate and the threat of health hazards on the job. The act requires safe and healthful working conditions for over 65 million employees in an estimated 5 million workplaces. Employers are required to furnish an environment free of recognized hazards and to comply with safety and health standards. A regulatory agency, the Occupational Safety and Health Administration (OSHA), was created to set and enforce standards. The act also created the National Institute for Occupational Safety and Health (NIOSH) to perform research to support regulatory activity.

The impact of the Occupational Safety and Health Act has been great.[3] Occupational safety and health are now well-known issues. Both workers and employers know about occupational hazards, and the scientific community has become involved in the workings of the law, for example, in the process of setting standards. The act also calls for recordkeeping, research, training activities to provide professionals who will implement the act, and education for workers about the hazards associated with work and how to deal with them.

It is not surprising that scientific uncertainties and the lack of information necessary to form a basis for regulatory action opened a Pandora's box full of conflicts, divergent views, and the inability to separate scientific from political inputs.[4] Although many environmental policy decisions are dependent on the capabilities or limitations of science, controversy over goals and how to achieve them often becomes a controlling factor in shaping environmental policies.

The lesson we have learned is that the causes of health hazards, as well as their solutions, are multifaceted and complex. The changes in our approach to occupational and nonoccupational health hazards during the twentieth century have been guided by alterations in philosophic and scientific approaches. We know a great deal about the mechanism of diseases of the lung, and the knowledge gained from science has been applied to creating strategies of prevention. The unsolved problem remains as to how to apply scientific knowledge to nonscience issues for effective social decisions.

SILICOSIS

Silicosis, one of civilization's oldest known occupational respiratory diseases, at various times has been named dust consumption, gannister disease, grinders' asthma, grinders' consumption, grinders' rot, grit consumption, masons' disease, miners' asthma, miners' phthisis, potters' rot, sewer disease, stonemasons' disease, chalicosis, and schistosis.

Knowledge of the association between inhalation of dust and its ill effect on an individual's health has a long history, starting in ancient times with recognition that a connection existed between inhalation of mine dust and the diseases that affected the lungs of miners.[5] In antiquity silicosis affected mainly miners, but the disease became widespread concomitant with the growth of technology and industrial society.

The history of silicosis highlights the present dichotomy between the possession of sufficient technical knowledge to prevent disease and the failure to eradicate it. This gap between awareness of hazards and effective action to eliminate the danger is a recurrent feature of the history of silicosis in particular, and occupational respiratory diseases in general. The problem of controlling or eradicating this severe, irreversible, disabling, but preventable disease now, as in the past, demands medical, technical, social, economic, and political solutions.

Exposure to silica dust and the risk of silicosis continue. In 1974, NIOSH recommended criteria for a standard to protect workers from occupational exposure to the hazard of crystalline silica dust.[6] Currently, although permissible limits for airborne silica in the workplace are contained in regulations promulgated by OSHA and the Mine Safety and Health Administration, there is still no permanent OSHA standard. Permissible limits do not contain provisions for physical examinations, protective equipment, engineering controls, recordkeeping, etc.

In 1980 the U.S. Department of Labor submitted an interim report to Congress on occupational disease. It estimated the number of workers exposed to silica dust and the number of silicosis cases. For example, over 1 million workers were exposed to free silica in metal mining; rock quarrying; glass, ceramic, cement, and brick production; and abrasive blasting. Estimates did not include 700,000 heavy-construction workers, 2.5 million agricultural workers, 600,000 chemical and allied product workers, and others with varying levels of exposure to free silica. It was estimated that 59,000 exposed persons would ultimately suffer from all stages of silicosis.[7] Because of inadequate medical and environmental monitoring and unclear job classifications, the exact percentage of workers exposed to silica and the amount of silica dust are unknown. Tables 1-1, 1-2, and 1-3 indicate, respectively, deaths from silicosis between 1970 and 1986 in men of selected ages, deaths attributed to silicosis between 1968 and 1985 in white men, and compensation data for silicosis from 1979 to 1983.[8]

Nature of the disease

Silicosis, ". . . a condition of massive fibrosis of the lungs marked by shortness of breath and resulting from prolonged inhalation of silica dust,"[9] is one of the pneumoconioses, a group of lung diseases that result from inhalation of excessive amounts of dust in certain occupations. *Silico-*

Table 1-1. Deaths from silicosis for males according to age and selected years

Age (yr)	Number of deaths each year										
	1970	1975	1978	1979	1980	1981	1982	1983	1984	1985	1986
25 and over	351	243	162	220	202	165	176	149	160	138	135
25-64	90	64	50	51	49	44	42	37	34	30	22
65 and over	261	179	112	169	153	121	134	112	126	108	113

From Health United States, 1988, Publ (PHS) 89-1232, Washington, D.C., 1988, U.S. Department of Health and Human Services, Public Health Service, Centers for Disease Control, National Center for Health Statistics.

Table 1-2. Deaths in white men attributed to silicosis (1968-1985)

Mean age at death due to silicosis (yr)	Age 65 or less	States accounting for 61% of silicosis-related deaths
72.9	16%	California
		Colorado
		Kentucky
		Michigan
		New Jersey
		New York
		Ohio
		Pennsylvania
		West Virginia
		Wisconsin

From unpublished data, Mine Health Research Advisory Committee Meeting (summary of work in progress on silicosis surveillance), 1989. Construction was the most frequently listed industry. Mining machine operator was the most frequently listed occupation. Pennsylvania had the most deaths.

sis describes only the condition caused by inhaling uncombined or free silica. Only dust containing free silica can cause silicosis. The disease can develop rapidly, but in general it is chronic and develops slowly. Pulmonary tuberculosis frequently accompanies silicosis and may be present at any stage of the disease. There is also a suspected relationship with cancer; both epidemiologic and experimental data bear on the relationship between silica exposure or silicosis and the development of lung cancer.

The International Agency for Research on Cancer (IARC), in a 1987 monograph entitled *Evaluation of the Carcinogenic Risk of Chemicals to Humans: Silica and Silicates,* came to the following conclusions: "There is *sufficient evidence* for carcinogenicity of crystalline silica to experimental animals. There is *inadequate evidence* for carcinogenicity of amorphous silica to experimental animals. There is *limited evidence* for carcinogenicity of crystalline silica to humans. There is *inadequate evidence* for carcinogenicity of amorphous silica to humans."[10] Obviously, the IARC classification of crystalline free silica as an animal carcinogen is a very controversial subject.

Early recognition of disease

Silicosis has long been associated with the history of mining. From earliest times miners have been exposed to dusts that caused disease. Hippocrates noted the connection between dust and disease in a metal miner who breathed with difficulty and had other symptoms similar to those found in silicosis. Pliny described devices used by miners to prevent inhalation of "fatal dust," and Celsus wrote, "By far the most terrible form of emaciation is that which the Greeks call phthisis. It spreads to the lung. On top of this ulceration occurs and slow fever which at times disappears and at other times reappears."[11] The association among mining, dust, and disease had been made. George Rosen, an historian, noted that little medical interest in miners' diseases existed in antiquity because of the inferior status of miners as servile laborers, illustrating the social indifference with which they were viewed.[5,12]

Few contributions to the subject of occupational dust diseases were made in the sixteenth through eighteenth centuries. Table 1-4 lists the contributions made during this time frame.[12]

Bernardino Ramazzini, a physician considered by many to be the founder of occupational medicine, wrote the following on the subject of stonecutters[13]: "We must not underestimate the maladies that attack stone-cutters, sculptors, quarrymen and other such workers. When they hew and cut marble underground or chisel it to make statues and other objects, they often breathe in the rough, sharp, jagged splinters that glance off; hence, they are usually troubled with cough, and some contract asthmatic affections and become consumptive."

The body of knowledge based on observations of the association between dust and the risk of disease in mining and other dusty occupations continued to grow, but remained severely limited by the lack of understanding of specific dust diseases and the few statistics on morbidity and mortality of workers in dusty trades. Silicosis was still unnamed, inadequately defined, and misunderstood.

Industrialization and silicosis

As industry and mining expanded in the nineteenth century, the incidence of disease caused by dust grew and, not

Table 1-3. Compensation data for silicosis

Men (%)	Over 55 yr (%)	Mean age	States reporting 94% of cases	Industries with most reports	Other industries with high rates
90	70	55	Kentucky Colorado Ohio New York Wisconsin North Carolina	Bituminous coal (161 cases) Gray foundries (71 cases) Steel foundries (56 cases)	Talc Soapstone Pyrophyllite mining Clay refractories Ferro-alloy mining Lead and zinc mining Industrial sand

From unpublished data, Mine Health Research Advisory Committee Meeting (summary of work in progress on silicosis surveillance), 1989.
Data are based on 941 reports of silicosis in 27 states, 1979-1983.
The mean annual incidence for mining was at least double that of nonmining.
Kentucky had the most cases (260, or 28% of the total).

Table 1-4. Recognition of occupational lung disease in the sixteenth through eighteenth centuries

Century	Author	Contribution or observation
16	Agricola	Wrote *De Re Metalica,* an encyclopedic treatise on mining and metal industries, which included a description of ills and accidents that affect miners
16	Paracelsus	Described miners' phthisis
17	Martin Pansa	Wrote *Consilium Peripneumaniaceum*
17	Ursinus	Believed dust inhalation caused peripneumonia
17	Stockhausen	Wrote about miners' phthisis
17	Diemerbroech	Described the effects of miners' work
17	Loehness	Described the effects of miners' work
18	Ramazzini	Wrote *De Morbis Artificum,* a book that contained a section on diseases of stonecutters

surprisingly, received renewed attention from the medical community. It was during the nineteenth century that Visconte (1870) coined the term *silicosis* to denote the pathologic condition of lungs resulting from the inhalation of dust.[14] Interest in pigmented and dusty lungs of miners led to observation and study, and new contributions were made to the study of dust diseases.

Early in the nineteenth century physicians believed that pulmonary pigmentation resulted from two separate entities, either natural black matter or *melanosis,* a term for a diseased lung, characterized by deposition of black matter.

Some physicians attributed the origin of the pigmentation to an external source. Others theorized that alterations of blood and other organic disturbances caused the pigmentation. The attention of physicians to pulmonary pigmentation among coal miners led many to believe that a noxious agent of extraneous origin was inhaled into the lungs.

In 1831 Thackrah began a study of the effects of dusty trades on British workmen's longevity. His important con-

tributions included bringing to light the fact that not all dusts shorten the lives of exposed workers. For example, he noted that although sandstone workers generally died before age 40, there seemed to be no unusual evidence of lung disease in brick and limestone workers.[15] Greenhow investigated potteries, metal trades, cutlery making, as well as tin, copper, coal, and lead mining, and Peacock established the existence of miners' disease as an entity and distinguished it clinically from pulmonary tuberculosis.[16] Thus by the end of the nineteenth century, the effects of dust inhalation on the lungs had been observed and reported, and the significance of occupation as an influence on the occurrence of silicosis had been established. The manner in which silica dust exerted its effect on the lungs, however, remained a matter of conjecture.

Until the twentieth century silicosis was widely misunderstood and inadequately defined. Then a significant increase in workers at risk generated new interest, new information, and new concepts of control and prevention. The rapid industrialization of the twentieth century had caused economic, social, and technologic change. Dangerous conditions in dusty trades, which always existed, grew with the increase in production, new machines, and the larger numbers of workers in mines, factories, quarries, and other dusty industries. New technology, for example, the use of machines in mines, increased production. Mechanization also increased the amount of dust. As the dangerous and unhealthy conditions increased with productivity and the growing number of exposed workers, the problem grew more and more pervasive and created renewed interest in occupational diseases, particularly silicosis.

In the early decades of the twentieth century, German, British, and South African researchers added to the knowledge of the effects of dust on lungs and the disease silicosis. In England in 1902, a governmental commission studied the high mortality rate among tin miners in Cornwall.[17] Haldane, a physiologist and a member of the commission, attributed the illness of the miners to rock dust, which he said injured the lungs. In the same period in England, commissions and factory inspectors intensively investigated the refractories industry, the sandstone industry, potteries, metal grinding, and coal mining, all dusty industries with a high incidence of silicosis. Investigations pointed to free silica as the inciting agent in silicosis. It was also believed to be a factor that increased susceptibility to tuberculosis. As early as 1918 English workers received compensation for disability caused by silicosis and tuberculosis.

The research of the Miners Phthisis Prevention Committee of South Africa found that the essential factor contributing to the development of chronic lung disease among gold miners was the inhalation, over long periods, of dust containing free silica, generated in mining operations. The committee found that the majority of cases of early and intermediate silicosis were free from tuberculosis complications, and that cases of silicosis could reach advanced stages and end in death without tuberculosis. They also found that all mineral dusts were not equally dangerous; the most dangerous dusts were characterized by the presence of uncombined crystalline silica. It was discovered that silica, in order to cause disease, was in a state of minute subdivision as very fine, sharp-edged, and insoluble particles. Seventy percent of silica particles in the lungs were found to be less than 1 μm in diameter. In other words, only quartz dust generated the specific disease silicosis, and the smallest particles, about 1 μm in diameter, were the dangerous ones.[18] In 1912 compensation for silicosis was first introduced in South Africa.

There was little interest in silicosis in the United States until the second decade of the twentieth century. The newly aroused concern was coincident with the progressive movement that sought protective labor legislation and workmen's compensation laws. A series of studies of mining and other dusty occupations, indicated in Table 1-5, revealed that silicosis was a severe health problem in this country.

Laboratory research also extended the knowledge of silicosis, and the use of roentgenologic diagnosis of silicosis was applied. Engineering and chemical methods for dust de-

termination and control were introduced. In 1922 Greenburg and Smith introduced the impinger, a dust-sampling device. The impinger method became the standard dust-sampling method used by the Bureau of Mines and the Public Health Service. Drinker and Hatch,[19] and others also contributed to engineering methods of dust control.

As a result of research and field studies, much was known about silicosis by the 1930s. For example, silicosis had been identified as an industrial disease resulting from the inhalation of silica dust. Its development depended on the amount of free silica in the dust, the concentration of dust in a state of fine division in the air breathed, and the duration of exposure to the dust. Physicians had clinically described the disease and diagnosed it with x-ray films, history of the patient's exposure, nature of exposure, symptoms, and physical examinations. The prevention and control of silicosis by using engineering devices were also understood. Dust-sampling methods existed that could determine the amount of silica, leading to judgments of the severity of the hazard and the adequacy of dust control.

Silicosis had become a preventable but uncontrolled occupational disease because scientific knowledge had not yet been translated into a public policy of prevention and control. Between 1914 and 1930 compensation for occupational disease remained minimal, and up to 1935 not one state that operated under a schedule included silicosis in its list of compensable occupational diseases. In states with "all-inclusive" coverage, the number of awards for silicosis was negligible.[20]

GAULEY BRIDGE

During the Great Depression, as the economic crisis deepened and the number of unemployed grew larger, workers were willing to face any known or unknown danger to receive a paycheck. During these years industry felt little pressure to create hazard-free working conditions. Perhaps the most vivid and tragic illustration of the social situation is the Gauley Bridge incident.

In 1930 to 1931 the New Kanawha Power Company, a

Table 1-5. U.S. studies related to silicosis 1919-1935

Date	Title	Government agency	Author
1917	*Siliceous Dust in Relation to Pulmonary Disease Among Miners in the Joplin District*	U.S. Bureau of Mines, Bulletin 132	Higgins, Lanza, Laney, and Rice
1918	*Mortality from Respiratory Diseases in Dusty Trades*	U.S. Bureau of Labor Statistics, Bulletin 231176	Hoffman
1928	*The Health of Workers in Trades, I. Health of Workers in a Portland Cement Plant Later Studied Sandstone, Pottery and Abrasive Industries*	U.S. Public Health Service, Bulletin 176	Thompson, Brundage, Russell, and Bloomfield
1935	*Anthraco-silicosis Among Hard Coal Miners*	U.S. Public Health Service, Bulletin 221	Sayers, Bloomfield, Dalla Valle, Jones, Dreessen, Brundage, and Britten

subsidiary of Union Carbide, was contracted to drill a tunnel through a mountain at Gauley Bridge, West Virginia, to divert water from the New River to a hydroelectric plant. The subcontractor was Rhinehart-Dennis Company. The men were employed to drill through the rock that had a high silica content. Rhinehart-Dennis employed an estimated 2000 men from Pennsylvania, Georgia, North Carolina, South Carolina, Florida, Kentucky, Alabama, Ohio, and West Virginia (many of them black and unskilled) over a period of 2 years. Four hundred seventy-six men died and eventually 1500 were disabled.[21] The men received low pay, and as the work progressed, the pay dropped even lower. Employees lived in squalid houses and worked under horrendous conditions. Descriptions of the dust are startling. It was so thick in the tunnel that the atmosphere resembled a patch of dense fog. It was estimated on the witness stand in the courtroom in Fayetteville, West Virginia, where lawsuits against the builders of the tunnel were tried, that workmen in the tunnel could see only 10 to 15 feet ahead of them at times. Man after man—drillers, drill helpers, nippers, muckers, dinkey runners, and members of the surveying crew, who were the plaintiff's witnesses—told of the dusty conditions.[22]

In 1936 a subcommittee of the U.S. House of Representatives held hearings on the Gauley Bridge disaster and concluded (1) that there was an utter disregard for all and any of the approved methods of prevention, (2) that dust was allowed to collect in such quantities that it lowered the men's visibility, (3) that the majority of drills were dry, and (4) that no appliances were used on drills to prevent the concentration of dust. The committee stated, "The whole driving of the tunnel was begun, continued, and completed with grave and inhuman disregard for all consideration for the health, lives and future of the employees," and that ". . . such negligence was either willful or the result of inexcusable and indefensible ignorance." The committee also found that silicosis was prevalent in many states where mine and tunnel operations occur and "that silicosis is one of the greatest menaces among occupational diseases and that state laws governing prevention and compensation are totally inadequate."[23] The committee recommended that Congress fund a study of silicosis, but to no avail. Frances Perkins, then Secretary of Labor, convened a series of conferences on silicosis, but they accomplished little. Punitive action was not taken against Rhinehart-Dennis Company, New Kanawha Power Company, or Union Carbide. Indeed, the hearings, conferences, and publicity did not lead to effective action to curtail silicosis. In the case of Gauley Bridge, the failure to protect the tunnel workers by applying established control measures cost workers an inordinately high price.

The New Deal and World War II brought about renewed interest in occupational health. Postwar efforts to provide more salubrious working conditions and to alleviate the dust hazard took the form of continued investigations and research into the problem of silicosis, extension of workers' compensation to cover occupational diseases in many states, and in some states continuation of existing occupational health programs.

In 1950 the U.S. Department of the Interior, Bureau of Mines, reviewed the literature on dusts, with emphasis on the relationship to dust diseases.[24] Efforts to control dust in industry followed the earlier conceived essential principle that there is a systematic dose-response relationship between the severity of exposure to the dust hazard and the degree of response in the individual exposed. As the level of exposure decreases, there is a decrease in the risk of injury. Thus the risk becomes negligible when exposure falls below certain tolerable levels. This concept assumes that harmful agents such as silica dust can be dealt with and that human exposure to this potentially harmful agent can be kept within tolerable limits. Control could then be effected by setting standards for acceptable levels of exposure. A threshold limit value (TLV) was adopted by the American Conference of Governmental Industrial Hygienists. This value was expressed as millions of particles per cubic foot and served as a guideline for compliance before 1970. The

Table 1-6. U.S. studies on silicosis from 1941 to 1964

Date	Title	Source	Author
1941	*The Health of Workers in Dusty Trades—VI. Restudy of a Group of Granite Workers*	Public Health Service, Bulletin 269	Russel
1950	*Review of Literature on Dust*	U.S. Department of Interior, Bureau of Mines, Bulletin 48	Forbes, Davenport, and Morgis
1956	"Some Facts on the Prevalence of Silicosis in the United States"	*Archives of Industrial Health*	Trasko
1957	*Control of Silicosis in Vermont Granite Industry: Progress Report*	Public Health Service, Publication 557	Mosey, Asher, and Trasko
1963	*Silicosis in the Metal Mining Industry, A Reevaluation 1958-1961*	Public Health Service, Publication 1071	Flinn and colleagues
1964	"Twenty-six Years' Experience with Dust Control in the Vermont Granite Industry"	*Industrial Medicine and Surgery*	Ashe and Bergstrom

TLV is currently a highly controversial occupational health concept.

The continuing environmental studies of the granite quarries and sheds of Vermont and of the prevalence of silicosis among workers in the granite industry have furthered understanding of the correlation between granite dust exposure and its health effects. Over the years the incidence of silicosis was reduced as dust controls were introduced and dust concentrations were drastically reduced. Table 1-6 indicates studies on this subject conducted between 1941 and 1964.

Without adequate quantitative description of the incidence of silicosis in the United States, it was impossible to assess and control the hazard. Once again, in the 1970s, Americans learned that accurate statistics reflecting the incidence of silicosis did not exist, and that no one knew the full extent of the silicosis problem. Testimony at hearings before the Subcommittee on Labor and Public Welfare of the U.S. Senate on the Occupational Safety and Health Act of 1970 described the shortcomings of the industrial health efforts in general and showed the need for a comprehensive federal occupational health and safety program.[25] While acknowledging that efforts toward a hazard-free workplace had been made and that achievements had been realized, witnesses also stressed that there was still much to do. They sought provisions for research, collection of needed statistics, a method of recording and accumulating information, and the establishment and enforcement of meaningful standards.

Today, 25 years after the Occupational Safety and Health Act became law, exposure to silica dust and the risk of silicosis continue for many American workers. OSHA still has not promulgated a standard for occupational exposure to crystalline silica. There are still unanswered questions, including the extent of silicosis in the United States. We still do not know some of the fundamental aspects of silicosis. For example, what is the mechanism of the toxic action of silica? Dust suppression methods based on existing knowledge may be inadequate for control in all affected industries. We may need new and more accurate methods of collecting and measuring dust samples. However, even though we have unanswered questions, there is enough information to succeed in controlling silicosis through technology.

The significance of the history of silicosis up to this time is that it highlights the present dichotomy between the possession of sufficient technical knowledge to prevent the disease and the failure to eradicate it. In the past, social, economic, and political aspects of worker protection received little attention. Risks we once judged to be acceptable are now being reevaluated in light of changed social attitudes and scientific knowledge. Public policy toward occupational diseases such as silicosis now centers on the issues of priorities and the basis for setting standards. Until there is consensus to support a legally acceptable permanent standard, promulgation of a legally enforceable standard will be highly controversial, enforcement will be difficult, and silicosis probably will not be eliminated from the roster of occupational diseases.

REFERENCES

1. Corn J: *Protecting the health of workers,* Cincinnati, 1989, American Conference of Governmental Industrial Hygienists.
2. The Bureau of National Affairs: *The Job Safety and Health Act of 1970,* Washington, D.C., 1971.
3. U.S. Congress, Office of Technology Assessment: *Preventing illness and injury in the workplace,* ch 13, Washington, D.C., April 1985.
4. Nelkin D, editor: *Controversy,* ed 2, Beverly Hills, Calif, 1984, Sage.
5. Rosen G: *The history of miners' diseases,* ch 1, New York, 1943, Schuman's.
6. U.S. Department of Health, Education and Welfare: *NIOSH—criteria for a recommended standard for occupational exposure to crystalline silica,* pp 2-13, Washington, D.C., 1974, Public Health Service, Centers for Disease Control.
7. U.S. Department of Labor: *An interim report to Congress on occupational diseases,* Washington, D.C., 1980.
8. Corn J: *Response to occupational health hazards,* pp 126-127, New York, 1992, Van Nostrand Reinhold.
9. Thrush PW, editor: *A dictionary of mining, mineral and related terms,* Washington, D.C., 1968, U.S. Department of Interior.
10. International Agency for Research on Cancer, World Health Organization (WHO): *Evaluation of the carcinogenic risk of chemicals to humans: silica and silicates,* vol 42, Lyons, France, 1987, WHO.
11. Lanza AJ, editor: *Silicosis and asbestosis,* New York, 1938, Oxford University Press.
12. Rosen G: *The history of miners' diseases,* chs 3 and 4, New York, 1943, Schuman's.
13. Ramazzini B: *Diseases of workers,* New York, 1964, Hafner.
14. Hunter D: *Diseases of occupations,* Boston, 1969, Little, Brown.
15. Thackrah CT: *The effects of the principal arts, trades and professions, and the civic states and habits of living on health and longevity,* London, 1831, Longmans.
16. Meiklejon A: History of lung diseases of coal miners in Great Britain; Part I 1800-1875, *Br J Ind Med,*:127-137, 1951.
17. Haldane JBS, Marint JS, and Thomas RA: *Report to the Secretary of State for Home Department on the health of Cornish miners,* London, 1904, His Majesty's Stationery Office.
18. Teleky L: *History of factory and mine hygiene,* New York, 1948, Columbia University Press.
19. Drinker P and Hatch T: *Industrial dust,* New York, 1954, McGraw-Hill.
20. Lanza AJ: In Lanza AJ, editor: Silicosis and asbestosis, p 409, New York, 1938, Oxford University Press.
21. *Hearings before a subcommittee of the Committee on Labor,* House of Representatives, H.J. Res. 449, 74th Congress, Jan 16, 17, 20, 21, 27, 28, 29 and Feb 4, 1936, Washington, D.C., 1936, U.S. Government Printing Office.
22. *Hearings before a subcommittee of the Committee on Labor,* House of Representatives, H.J. Res. 449, 74th Congress, p 4, Washington, D.C., 1936, U.S. Government Printing Office.
23. *Hearings before a subcommittee of the Committee on Labor,* House of Representatives, H.J. Res. 449, 74th Congress, pp 201-202, Washington, D.C., 1936, U.S. Government Printing Office.
24. Forbes JJ, Davenport SJ, and Genevieve GM: *Review of literature on dusts,* U.S. Department of Interior, Bureau of Mines, bull 48, Washington, D.C., 1950, U.S. Government Printing Office.
25. *Hearings before the Subcommittee on Labor of the Committee on Labor and Public Welfare,* U.S. Senate, 90th Congress, Feb 15, June 12, 19, 24, and 28, July 2, Washington, D.C., 1968, U.S. Government Printing Office.

Clinical and Epidemiologic Methods

JOHN R. BALMES

A multidisciplinary approach is often necessary to confirm a diagnosis of an occupational or environmental respiratory disease. The chapters in this section provide outlines of the methods used by experts in each of the key disciplines in their approach to individual cases or at-risk populations. Some chapters will be more relevant to pulmonary physicians than to occupational and environmental medicine physicians, and vice versa. The outline of a comprehensive exposure history, contained in Chapter 3, should be familiar to occupational and environmental medicine physicians, whereas the chapter on physiologic methods covers material that should be basic for pulmonary physicians. The chapters on epidemiologic and immunologic methods will be useful to both groups. In the absence of a standardized methodology for bronchoprovocation with either specific or nonspecific stimuli, the approach described in Chapter 5 by two experienced physicians will allow greater use of these techniques. The increasing application of computed tomographic scanning to the diagnosis of occupational and environmental respiratory disease is discussed in detail in Chapter 7, in addition to the traditional use of chest radiography. The upper airway typically receives a large fraction of the total dose of an inhaled toxin, but is often forgotten by clinicians. Chapter 6, on upper airway diagnostic techniques, will enable its readers to better define the degree of upper airway injury in exposed individuals or populations. Although obtaining a tissue sample is not usually necessary to establish a diagnosis of occupational or environmental respiratory disease, when a biopsy is obtained, it needs to be properly handled and reviewed by a pathologist with specific expertise. Chapter 8 provides a helpful overview of appropriate pathologic methods.

Chapter 2

EPIDEMIOLOGIC METHODS

Neil Pearce
Julian Crane

EPIDEMIOLOGY

Public health is primarily concerned with the prevention of disease in human populations. Epidemiology is the branch of public health that attempts to discover the causes of disease in order to make disease prevention possible. Thus it differs from clinical medicine both in its emphasis on prevention (rather than treatment) and in its focus on populations (rather than individual patients). Thus the epidemiologic approach to a particular disease is intended to identify high-risk subgroups within the population, determine the causes of such excess risks, and determine the effectiveness of subsequent preventive measures. This chapter reviews basic epidemiologic methods, the various types of epidemiologic studies, and the various types of study design issues involved; it is thus intended to assist in the appraisal of epidemiologic studies, rather than in the conduct of actual studies.

Although the epidemiologic approach has been used for more than a century for the study of communicable diseases, epidemiology has grown considerably in scope and sophistication in the last few decades as it has been increasingly applied to the study of chronic diseases, including the well-known studies of tobacco smoking and lung cancer[1,2] and the more recent studies of environmental tobacco smoke and lung cancer.[3]

An early example of the successful application of the epidemiologic approach to respiratory disease was the establishment of the association between asbestos exposure and lung cancer by Sir Richard Doll.[4] At that time, although it had long been known that asbestos workers were at increased risk for diseases such as asbestosis, only 61 cases of lung cancer had been reported since 1935 in persons with asbestosis and the excess risk of lung cancer had not been conclusively established.

Doll followed the course of a group of 113 men who had worked for at least 20 years in "dusty" areas of a large asbestos factory. Among this group there had been 11 deaths due to lung cancer, whereas only 0.8 would have been expected on the basis of national mortality rates (Table 2-1). Doll[4] argued that there were four possible explanations for the findings: (1) that all of the men who died of lung cancer were recorded because of interest in the condition, whereas the records of some other men were omitted, thus underestimating the expected number of deaths; (2) that lung cancer was incorrectly and excessively diagnosed among asbestos workers; (3) that lung cancer was insufficiently diagnosed among the general population; and (4) that the asbestos workers suffered

Table 2-1. Causes of death among male asbestos workers compared with those expected from national mortality rates

Cause of death	No. observed deaths	No. expected deaths	Ratio
Lung cancer	11	0.8	13.8
Other respiratory diseases	20	7.6	2.6
Neoplasms other than in the lung	4	2.3	1.7
All other diseases	4	4.7	0.9
TOTALS	39	15.4	2.5

Adapted from Doll R: Mortality from lung cancer in asbestos workers, *Br J Ind Med* 12:81-86, 1955.

an excess mortality from lung cancer. Doll concluded that explanations 1 through 3 were unlikely and that the fourth explanation was the most reasonable one. This conclusion has been confirmed by numerous subsequent studies.[5]

This example illustrates some of the features of the epidemiologic approach. The key feature of epidemiologic studies is that they are observational rather than experimental. This is a major strength of the epidemiologic approach, because it enables a study to be conducted in a situation in which a randomized trial would be unethical or impractical (because of the large numbers of subjects required); it is also the main limitation of epidemiologic studies, in that the lack of randomization means that the groups being compared may differ with respect to various causes of respiratory disease (other than the main exposure under investigation). Thus epidemiologic studies, in general, experience the same potential problems as randomized controlled trials, but may suffer additional problems of bias because exposure has not been randomly allocated and there may be differences in baseline disease risk between the populations being compared.

SPECIFIC FEATURES OF RESPIRATORY EPIDEMIOLOGY

Respiratory epidemiology includes studies of malignant diseases (e.g., lung cancer) that are usually rapidly fatal, as well as studies of nonmalignant diseases (e.g., asthma) that are not usually life-threatening but may result in considerable morbidity over a lengthy period. Studies of malignant respiratory disease usually involve studying incidence (the number of new cases of disease over a specified period) or mortality (a special case of incidence in which the outcome under study is death rather than disease detection). On the other hand, studies of nonmalignant respiratory disease frequently involve studying prevalence (the number of people who have the disease at a particular time), since it is often difficult to determine the precise date on which each person develops nonmalignant respiratory disease without intensive monitoring.

Nonmalignant respiratory disease epidemiology involves two major facets: the investigation of factors that may cause a "healthy" person to develop respiratory disease and the investigation of factors that affect prognosis in persons who have already developed respiratory disease. These two branches of respiratory disease epidemiology can be referred to, respectively, as population-based studies and patient-based studies.

Another feature of respiratory disease epidemiology is the problem of measuring the prevalence of nonmalignant respiratory disease or related symptoms or conditions of interest such as wheezing or airway hyperresponsiveness (AHR). There are analogous problems with measuring nonmalignant respiratory disease morbidity in patient-based studies, since particular events, such as hospital admissions for respiratory disease, may reflect access to health services and management policies as much as they reflect actual morbidity.

TYPES OF EPIDEMIOLOGIC STUDIES

All epidemiologic studies should be based on a particular population followed over a particular period. Miettinen[6] has termed this study population the "base population" and its experience over time the "study base." The different epidemiologic study designs differ only in the manner in which the study base is defined and the manner in which information is drawn from the study base.[7] In this section we briefly describe the basic study designs and the measures of effect that are involved (these are described in more detail in the section discussing basic data analysis and in the appendix).

Case series

The simplest respiratory epidemiologic study is the case series report. Such reports are of limited value, however, since it is usually unclear how the cases were identified, which study base they represent, whether case ascertainment has been completed, and whether the cases reported actually represent an excess disease occurrence. Furthermore, respiratory disease is relatively common, whereas case series reports have generally been most useful in studies of rare diseases. For example, the occurrence of several cases of lung cancer in a particular factory may not be exceptional, and it is difficult to know whether such cases represent an excess unless a formal epidemiologic study is conducted with an appropriate comparison group. Even if a statistically significant excess of lung cancer is then found to exist, this may represent merely a chance "cluster" rather than a true increase in risk.[8] Nevertheless, case series reports have played a valuable role in indicating the possible role of many environmental causes of respiratory disease, which have then been investigated further in more formal studies.

Incidence studies

The most complete and definitive approach to studying the causes of respiratory disease involves using all of the information from the study base in a cohort study of respiratory disease incidence (also known as a follow-up study). Follow-up may be prospective (which is more expensive and time consuming but may enable better quality data to be collected), or it may be based on historical records, with follow-up occurring up to the present.

For example, in the historical cohort study by Doll,[4] 113 asbestos workers with at least 20 years of exposure were followed over time. Table 2-2 shows the total number of "person-years" for which the 113 men were followed up during the period from 1922 to 1953.

The most common measure of disease occurrence is the incidence rate, which is a measure of disease occurrence per unit of time and has the reciprocal of time as its dimension. In the study by Doll,[4] 11 cases of lung cancer were diagnosed during the follow-up period of 1042.25 person-years. Thus the overall incidence rate was 11/1042.25 = 0.0106 (or 10.6 per 1000 person-years).

The usual aim of conducting a study is to compare the incidence rates in those exposed and those not exposed to a particular factor (e.g., asbestos), and to estimate the rate ratio. This may involve comparing the disease incidence in the study group with some nonexposed external reference population, such as the national population. In the study by Doll,[4] this involved an external comparison with national mortality rates for lung cancer in men. The national rates for each time period and age group were multiplied by the number of person-years in the study for the same time period and age group (Table 2-2), and these were added in order to estimate the "expected" number of lung cancer deaths in the study population. In this instance the observed number of lung cancer deaths was 11, the expected number (on the basis of time- and age-specific national mortality rates) was 0.8, and the standardized mortality ratio (SMR) was 11/0.8 = 13.8 (see Table 2-1).

Alternatively, if the population under study includes both exposed and nonexposed persons, then a direct comparison can be made within this population. Table 2-3 shows examples of external and internal comparisons conducted for a study of lung cancer in asbestos textile workers,[9] adjusted for age and calendar period. Overall, there were 35 deaths caused by lung cancer in the cohort during the 32,362 person-years of follow-up, and the expected number of deaths based on national mortality rates was 10.90, yielding an overall SMR of 3.2. In this cohort information was available on average levels of asbestos exposure in various jobs and departments, and it was therefore possible to estimate the annual exposure for each worker. The cumulative exposure for each worker was therefore estimated over time [this involves following each worker through increasing categories of cumulative exposure, just as workers are fol-

lowed through age groups and calendar periods (Table 2-2)], and for each category of cumulative exposure, the person-years at risk (by age and calendar period), the expected lung cancer deaths, and the observed lung cancer deaths were calculated. This revealed a striking dose-response pattern, with the SMR being close to 1.0 in the lowest exposure category (i.e., the lung cancer death rate in those with low exposure was similar to the national lung cancer death rate), and 14.9 in the highest exposure category (Table 2-3). This analysis was then repeated in an internal comparison, in which each exposure category was compared with the lowest exposure category, while adjusting for age and calendar period. This once again revealed a striking dose-response trend (Table 2-3).

Incidence case-control studies

Cohort studies are the most complete and definitive approach to studying the causes of respiratory disease, since they make use of all of the information in the study base. The study by Doll[4] described above was unusual in that the cohort comprised workers with heavy exposures, and useful information on lung cancer could be obtained despite the small size of the study (although no individual exposure information was available). More generally, cohort studies often require large numbers and may be expensive in terms of time and resources, and the same findings can often be achieved more efficiently by using a case-control design.

The case-control approach developed as a logical progression from daily clinical practice. It starts with a group of patients with a particular disease (the effect) and then attempts to discover the cause. It thus appeared to be quite different from the prospective approach (whether experimental or observational), which starts with exposure to a particular factor (a cause) and follows its effects over time. However, modern epidemiology texts now emphasize that the case-control design proceeds from cause to effect (just as for cohort studies) and is not inherently more prone to bias, or even inherently different.[10] The modern perspective was implicit in some of the earliest case-control studies of smoking and lung cancer conducted by Doll and Hill[11,12] and others. However, this perspective was reinforced with the development of the nested case-control design in the 1970s.[7] This design arose out of large-cohort studies of occupational cancer. Such studies might typically involve 10,000 workers (perhaps 5000 exposed to a particular chemical and 5000 not exposed) who would be followed up for 20 years or more in order to yield sufficient cases of a tumor such as lung cancer. Such studies involved a massive undertaking, particularly since each worker's exposure had to be estimated by combining information from personnel records and industrial hygiene monitoring data.

Eventually, it was realized that such studies could be conducted more efficiently by enumerating the entire

Table 2-2. Number of person-years lived by men with 20 or more years of work in a "dusty area"

Age (yr)	Period					
	1922-1933	1934-1938	1939-1943	1944-1948	1949-1953	Total
30-34	0	0.5	1.5	0	0	2.0
35-39	4.5	2.0	11.0	17.5	9.0	44.0
40-44	9.5	16.0	33.5	48.0	55.0	162.0
45-49	9.5	19.5	50.0	78.5	84.0	241.5
50-54	6.5	25.5	39.5	85.0	96.5	253.0
55-59	12.0	6.0	30.0	52.0	85.5	185.5
60-64	15.0	3.0	5.25	25.5	36.0	84.75
65-69	1.0	13.5	3.0	10.0	21.5	49.0
70-74	0	2.0	9.0	3.0	3.5	17.5
75-79	0	0	1.0	1.5	0.5	3.0
TOTALS	58.0	88.0	183.75	321.0	391.5	1042.25

Adapted from Doll R: Mortality from lung cancer in asbestos workers, *Br J Ind Med* 12:81-86, 1955.

Table 2-3. Lung cancer relative risks using external and internal comparisons

Cumulative exposure (1000 fibers/cc days)	Person-years	Observed mortality	External comparison			Internal comparison	
			Expected mortality	SMR	95% CI	RR	95% CI
<1	13,146	5	3.76	1.3	0.4-3.1	1.0	—
1-9	12,823	10	3.72	2.7	1.3-4.9	1.8	0.6-5.4
10-39	4976	7	2.19	3.2	1.3-6.6	1.9	0.8-4.9
40-99	1270	11	1.10	10.0	5.0-17.9	8.0	2.6-32.0
100+	139	2	0.13	14.9	1.7-53.9	15.9	3.7-64.7

Adapted from Checkoway HA, Pearce NE, and Crawford-Brown DJ: *Research methods in occupational epidemiology,* New York, 1989, Oxford University Press.
CI, Confidence interval; *RR*, rate ratio; *SMR*, Standardized mortality ratio.

cohort but only collecting exposure histories on the *cases* of disease (e.g., cases of lung cancer) and a similar number of randomly sampled *controls* who did not develop the disease.[13] Such a nested case-control study would only involve collecting exposure histories on several hundred workers instead of the entire cohort.

This approach revolutionized the understanding of case-control studies, since it showed that they did not involve an inherently different approach, but could actually be incorporated within cohort studies as a more efficient manner of achieving the same findings. This nested case-control approach only differed from the full-cohort approach in one respect: that cases were compared with a sample of the cohort rather than the complete cohort. All of the other supposed shortcomings of case-control studies did not apply: there was no need for a "rare disease" assumption; there was no greater tendency to bias (provided that the control sample was genuinely random); and causal inference proceeded from cause to effect, just as in a full-cohort study.[10] Furthermore, the case-control approach had several important advantages; in particular, when the outcome under study was rare, it was considerably more efficient. This in-

crease in efficiency usually meant that a much larger study (in terms of the number of cases) could be conducted.

In case-control studies the relative risk measure is the odds ratio, which is the ratio of the odds of exposure in the cases (i.e., the number of patients exposed divided by the number of those not exposed) and the odds of exposure in the controls.

Table 2-4 shows the findings of a nested case-control study, based on the cohort of 1261 white male asbestos workers from one textile manufacturing plant[9] shown in Table 2-3. The case group included all 35 lung cancer deaths generated by the cohort during the period from 1940 to 1975; controls were chosen by sampling from the rest of the cohort, with four controls per case. Cases and controls were classified into the same five cumulative exposure categories as used in Table 2-3. Table 2-4 shows the exposure distribution of cases and controls and the crude odds ratios obtained from comparing each level with the lowest exposure level. For example, when comparing the second level of exposure (1 to 9 units) with the lowest level (less than 1 unit), the odds of exposure in the cases were 10/5, the odds of exposure in the controls were 43/49, and the odds ratio was $(10/5)/(43/49) = 2.28$. The strong exposure-response trend shown in Table 2-4 is similar to that found in the full cohort analysis (see Table 2-3); the one exception is for the highest exposure category (100+ units), in which the small number of cases and controls makes the odds ratio estimates unstable and imprecise.

Prevalence studies

Incidence studies are usually conducted when investigating malignant respiratory disease, since cases can be identified through death registrations or cancer registrations. The situation is more complex when studying nonmalignant respiratory disease, since it is difficult to detect incident cases of disease without intensive follow-up procedures. Thus it is more common to study the *prevalence* of nonmalignant respiratory disease in a particular population. This can be defined as point prevalence, estimated at one point in time, or period prevalence, which denotes the number of cases that existed at any time during some time interval (e.g., 1 year). Respiratory epidemiologic studies usually involve point prevalence, but the definition of disease may still involve specification of a particular time interval (e.g., asthma may be defined as current AHR and occurrence of symptoms during the previous 12 months[14]).

Prevalence studies represent a considerable savings in resources compared with cohort studies, since it is necessary to evaluate disease prevalence at only one point in time, rather than continually searching for incident cases over an extended period. On the other hand, this gain in efficiency is achieved at the cost of some loss of information, since it may be much more difficult to understand the temporal relationship between various exposures and the occurrence of respiratory disease. For example, it is well known that asthma can be provoked by allergies to household pets; however, a prevalence study may find a relatively low current pet ownership rate in children with asthma because the families concerned have identified the animal as a factor in the child's asthma and removed it from the household. This phenomenon can only be identified by collecting detailed information on both past and current pet ownership,[15] and such information may be more difficult to collect historically in a prevalence study than to collect prospectively in an incidence study. A related problem is that it is usually difficult to ascertain, in a prevalence study, at what age disease first occurred, and it is therefore difficult to determine which exposures preceded the development of disease, even when accurate historical exposure information is available.

It can be shown[10] that, in a "steady state" population the prevalence odds are equal to the incidence rate *(I)* times the average disease duration (see the section on basic data analysis). The prevalence odds ratio is thus the basic effect measure in a prevalence study. However, an elevated prevalence odds ratio may reflect the influence of factors that increase the duration of disease, as well as those that increase disease incidence; interpretation of the findings of a preva-

Table 2-4. Exposure distribution of cases and controls: 1000 fiber/cc days

	Asbestos exposure				
	<1	1-9	10-39	40-99	100+
Cases	5	10	7	11	2
Controls	49	43	28	16	4
Odds ratio	1.00	2.28	2.45	6.74	4.90

Derived from Checkoway HA, Pearce NE, and Crawford-Brown DJ: *Research methods in occupational epidemiology,* New York, 1989, Oxford University Press.

Table 2-5. Findings from a prevalence study of asthma and pesticide exposure

	Pesticide exposure			
	Exposed	Nonexposed	Odds ratio	95% CI
Cases (asthmatics)	32	51	1.88	1.20-2.94
Noncases	465	1391		

Adapted from Senthilselvan A, McDuffie HH, and Dosman JA: Association of asthma with use of pesticides, *Am Rev Respir Dis* 146:884-887, 1992.

CI, Confidence interval.

lence study is therefore more difficult for an incidence study.

Table 2-5 shows the findings of a study by Senthilselvan and colleagues,[16] who investigated self-reported asthma and pesticide use in 1939 male farmers in 17 municipalities in Saskatchewan, Canada. Farmers were defined as including every male farmland taxpayer or farmworker; each of the 2375 farmers was visited and 1939 (81.6%) agreed to take part in the study, of whom 83 (4.3%) were found to be asthmatics. Of the 83 asthmatics, 32 (38.6%) reported having used carbamate insecticides, compared with 465 (25.1%) of the 1856 nonasthmatics. Thus the prevalence odds ratio for asthma and exposure to carbamate insecticides was 1.9 [95% confidence interval (CI), 1.2 to 2.9]. The authors concluded that these findings raise the possibility that exposure to agricultural chemicals could be related to lung dysfunction in farmers.

Prevalence case-control studies

Just as an incidence case-control study can be used to obtain the same findings as a full cohort study, a prevalence case-control study can be used to obtain the same findings as a full prevalence study in a more efficient manner. In particular, if obtaining exposure information is difficult or costly (e.g., if it involves lengthy interviews or collection of serum samples), then it may be more efficient to conduct a prevalence case-control study by obtaining exposure information on all of the prevalent *cases* of disease and a sample of *controls* selected at random from the noncases. Sampling on the basis of disease (particularly if the disease is rare) may have advantages in terms of study efficiency.

Suppose that a prevalence case-control study is conducted in the study population, involving all of the 1385 prevalent disease cases and a group of 1385 controls. In this instance there is one main option for selecting controls, namely, to select them from the noncases. In this example a sample of controls will estimate the exposure odds (*b/d*) of the noncases, and the odds ratio obtained in the prevalence case-control study will therefore estimate the prevalence odds ratio in the base population (2.00), which in turn estimates the incidence rate ratio, provided that the average duration of disease is the same in the exposed and nonexposed groups (discussed previously).

As in the case of a full prevalence study, the statistical methods for estimation, testing, and calculating CIs for the prevalence odds ratio in a prevalence case-control study are identical to those for odds ratios in other contexts.

Table 2-6 shows an example from the study by Flatt and associates,[17] who conducted a prevalence case-control study involving 56 asthmatic patients (cases) and 59 nonasthmatic controls in Dunedin, New Zealand, a region with a low dietary selenium intake. The cases of asthma were identified in an outpatient chest clinic and a general practice, whereas controls were selected from a general medical outpatient and blood donor population and from the families of the asthmatic subjects. For each study participant a 10-ml venous blood sample was collected for assay of selenium and glutathione peroxidase in whole blood and plasma. There was a 5.8-fold increased risk of asthma in subjects with the lowest range of whole-blood glutathione peroxidase activity. The authors concluded that the findings were consistent with the hypothesis that low selenium concentrations may have a role in the pathogenesis of asthma in New Zealand.

BIAS IN EPIDEMIOLOGIC STUDIES

Systematic error, or "bias," occurs if there is a difference between what the study is actually estimating and what it is intended to estimate.[18] Systematic error is thus distinguished from random error in that it would be present even with an infinitely large study, whereas random error can be reduced by increasing the study size.

There are many different types of bias, but three general forms have been distinguished[10]: confounding, selection bias, and information bias. In general terms these refer to biases inherent in the study base because of differences in disease risk between the groups being compared (confounding), biases resulting from the manner in which study subjects are selected from the study base (selection bias), and biases resulting from the misclassification of these study subjects with respect to exposure or disease (information bias).

Confounding

Confounding occurs when the exposed and nonexposed groups (in the study base) are not comparable because of inherent differences in background disease risk,[19] usually due to exposure to other risk factors. Similar problems can occur in randomized trials, in that randomization is not always successful and the groups to be compared may have different characteristics (and different baseline disease risks) at the time they enter the study. However, there is more concern about noncomparability in epidemiologic studies because of the absence of randomization.

If no other biases are present, three conditions are necessary for a factor to be a confounder.[10] First, a confounder is a factor that is predictive of the study outcome, for example, respiratory disease (in the absence of the exposure under study). Note that a confounder need not be a genuine cause of respiratory disease, but merely "predictive." Hence, surrogates for causal factors, such as age, may be regarded as potential confounders, even though they are rarely directly causal factors.

Second, a confounder is associated with exposure in the study base (in case-control studies this means that a confounder is associated with exposure among the controls); an association can occur among the cases simply because the study factor and a potential confounder are both risk factors for the disease, but this does not, in itself, cause confounding unless the association also exists in the study base.

Finally, a variable that is intermediate in the causal pathway between exposure and disease is not a confounder. For example, a factor may cause AHR, which may then increase the risk of developing asthma. In this instance AHR would be an intermediate step in the causation of disease, but would not be a confounder.

Confounding can be controlled in the study design, in the analysis, or both. Control at the design stage involves three main methods.[10] The first is randomization, but this is not an option (by definition) in epidemiologic studies.

A second method of control at the design stage is restriction of the study to narrow ranges of values of the potential confounders, for example, by restricting the study to

Table 2-6. Findings from an asthma prevalence case-control study

Whole-blood glutathione activity (Units/g Hg)	Cases	Controls	Odds ratio	95% CI
30+	7	13	1.0	—
25-29	14	19	1.4	0.4-4.5
20-24	15	20	1.6	0.5-5.2
<20	20	7	5.8	1.6-21.2

From Flatt A, Pearce NE, Thomson CD, et al: Reduced selenium status in asthmatic subjects in New Zealand, *Thorax* 45:95-99, 1990.
CI, Confidence interval; *Hg*, hemoglobin.

white women in a particular age group. This approach has some conceptual and computational advantages, but may severely restrict the number of potential study subjects and the informativeness of the study.

A third method of control involves matching study subjects on potential confounders (e.g., matching on age, gender, and ethnicity). This will remove confounding in a cohort study but is not usually done, as it may be very expensive. Matching can also be expensive in case-control studies, and does not remove confounding in this setting but merely facilitates its control in the analysis. Furthermore, matching may actually reduce precision in a case-control study if it is done on a factor that is associated with exposure but is not a risk factor for respiratory disease (and hence not a true confounder).

The most common approach for reducing confounding is *control* in the analysis (although it may be desirable to match on potential confounders in the design to optimize the efficiency of the analysis). This involves stratifying the data into subgroups according to the levels of the confounder(s) and calculating a summary effect estimate that summarizes the information across strata (see appendix).

It is usually not possible to control for more than two or three confounders in a stratified analysis, since finer stratification often leads to many strata containing no exposed or no nonexposed persons (or no cases or no controls). Such strata are uninformative, and hence fine stratification is wasteful of information. This problem can be mitigated, to some extent, by the use of mathematical modeling that allows the simultaneous control of more confounders by "smoothing" the data across confounder strata.[20] These models provide powerful tools when used appropriately, although they are often used inappropriately, and should always be used in combination with the more straightforward methods presented here.[10]

When appropriate information is not available to control confounding directly, it is still desirable to assess its potential strength and direction.

For example, it may be possible to obtain information on a surrogate for the confounder of interest; for example, social class is associated with many lifestyle factors (e.g., smoking) and may therefore be a useful surrogate. Even though confounder control will be imperfect in this situation, it is still possible to examine whether the main effect estimate changes when the surrogate is controlled in the analysis and to assess the strength and direction of the change. For example, if the relative risk actually increases (e.g., from 2.0 to 2.5) or remains stable (e.g., at 2.0) when the analysis is controlled for social class, then it is unlikely that the observed excess risk is due to smoking, since control for social class involves partial control for smoking.

Alternatively, it may be possible to obtain accurate confounder information for a subgroup of participants (cases and noncases) in the study and to assess the effects of confounder control in this subgroup.

A related approach involves obtaining confounder information for a sample of the study base (or a sample of the controls in a case-control study). For example, in a cohort study of asthma in children, it may not be possible to obtain information on humidity levels in the homes of all the children. However, it may be possible to obtain humidity measurements for a sample of the exposed and nonexposed groups to check that the average levels of humidity in the home are similar in the two groups.

Finally, even if it is not possible to obtain confounder information for any study subjects, it may still be possible to estimate how strong the confounding is likely to be by examining particular risk factors. For example, this is often done in studies of occupational causes of lung cancer, in which smoking is a potential confounder, but smoking information is rarely available.[21]

Selection bias

Whereas confounding generally involves biases inherent in the study base, selection bias involves biases arising from the procedures by which the study subjects are chosen from the study base. Thus, selection bias is generally not a problem in cohort studies, since these use all of the information from the study base, but selection bias is of more concern in case-control studies, since these involve sampling from the study base. In particular, selection bias can occur in a case-control study if controls are chosen in a nonrepresentative manner (e.g., if exposed persons were more likely to be selected as controls than nonexposed persons).

Selection bias can sometimes be controlled in the analysis by identifying factors that are related to subject selection and controlling for them as confounders. For example, if white-collar workers are more likely to be selected for (or participate in) a study than manual workers (and white collar work is negatively or positively related to the exposure of interest), this bias can be partially controlled by collecting information on social class and controlling for social class in the analysis as a confounder. Thus, selection bias and confounding can often be viewed as separate aspects of the same phenomenon.

Information bias

Information bias involves misclassification of the study subjects with respect to disease or exposure status. Thus the concept of *information bias* refers to those people actually included in the study (whereas *selection bias* refers to the selection of the study subjects from the study base, and *confounding* generally refers to noncomparability within the study base).

Nondifferential information bias occurs when the likelihood of misclassification of exposure is the same for diseased and nondiseased persons (or when the likelihood of misclassification of disease is the same for exposed and nonexposed persons). Nondifferential misclassification of exposure generally biases the effect estimate toward the null value of 1.0.[22] Hence, nondifferential information bias tends to produce false-negative findings and is of particular concern in studies that find no association between exposure and disease.

Differential information bias occurs when the likelihood of misclassification of exposure is different in diseased and nondiseased persons (or the likelihood of misclassification of disease is different in exposed and nonexposed persons). This can bias the observed effect estimate in either direction, either toward or away from the null value. For example, in a lung cancer case-control study the recall of exposures (e.g., passive smoking) in healthy controls might be different from that of cases with lung cancer. In this situation differential information bias would occur, and it could bias the odds ratio toward or away from the null value, depending on whether cases were more or less likely to recall previous exposures than controls.

Information bias can drastically affect the validity of a study. As a general principle it is important to ensure that the misclassification is nondifferential, by making certain that exposure information is collected in an identical manner in diseased and nondiseased persons (and that disease information is collected in an identical manner in exposed and nonexposed groups). In this situation the bias is in a known direction (toward the null value), and although there may be concern that negative findings may be due to nondifferential information bias, one can at least be confident that any positive findings are not due to information bias. Thus, the aim of data collection is not to collect perfect information, but to collect comparable information in an identical manner from the groups being compared, even if this means ignoring more detailed exposure information if it is not available for both groups. However, it is clearly important to collect information that is as detailed and accurate as possible, within the constraints imposed by the need to ensure that information is collected in an identical manner in the groups being compared.

MEASUREMENT OF EXPOSURE

In studies of the occupational and environmental causes of respiratory disease, the distinction must be made between *exposure* and *dose*. The term *exposure* refers to the presence of a substance (e.g., asbestos, pesticides, or house dust mite feces) in the external environment. The term *dose* refers to the amount of substance that reaches susceptible targets within the body (e.g., the concentration of asbestos fibers in the lungs).

Exposure levels are assessed with reference to the *intensity* of the substance in the environment (e.g., asbestos concentration in the air) and the *duration* of time for which exposure occurs. If an acute effect (e.g., an asthma attack) is under study, then the intensity of exposure may be crucial, and the disease outcome may occur after an exposure of relatively short duration. On the other hand, if a chronic effect (e.g., lung cancer) is under study, then the risk of dis-

ease may be much greater if the duration of exposure is long; furthermore, there may be 20 years or more between the occurrence of exposure and the occurrence of disease.

Exposure assessment methods are discussed in Chapter 11 and thus are considered only briefly here. Two particular issues should be emphasized at this stage, however.

First, data collected for monitoring purposes may be of limited value in epidemiologic studies. For example, industrial hygienists usually concentrate on monitoring areas of the factory where they believe exposures are likely to be highest and choose the workers who are believed to have the heaviest exposures, to ensure compliance with exposure limits. Epidemiologic studies, by contrast, usually require information on "average" levels of exposure, and it may therefore be necessary to conduct a special survey involving random sampling, rather than relying on data collected for monitoring purposes.

Second, epidemiologic studies rarely have optimal exposure data and often rely on relatively crude measurements of exposure. The key issue is not that the exposure data need be perfect, but that they must be of similar quality for the various groups being compared. Provided that this principle is followed, then any bias from misclassification of exposure will be nondifferential (discussed in the previous section) and will tend to produce false-negative findings. Thus, if positive findings do occur, one can be confident that these are not due to inaccuracies in the exposure data; on the other hand, if no association (or only a weak association) is found between exposure and disease, then the possibility of nondifferential information bias should be considered. In general, the aim of exposure assessment is to ensure (1) that the exposure data are of equal quality in the groups being compared and (2) that the data are of the best possible quality given the former restriction. Thus, there is no benefit (and often there are substantial problems) in collecting more detailed exposure information if this is only available for one of the groups being compared (e.g., for cases but not for controls in a case-control study).

For these reasons exposure data in occupational epidemiologic studies may often be based on routine employment records, perhaps in combination with industrial hygiene surveys of typical levels of exposure in various jobs or tasks (Table 2-7). For example, despite obvious limitations, data of this type have been used in discovering all of the known occupational lung carcinogens to date. On the other hand, such information is not available in many environmental epidemiologic studies, and it is usually necessary to conduct a specific survey to determine levels of exposure to environmental factors such as indoor and outdoor air pollution, pollens, indoor humidity, and house dust mites.

Traditionally, exposure to risk factors such as cigarette smoking has been measured using questionnaires, and this approach has a long history of successful use in epidemiology. More recently, it has been argued that the major problem in epidemiology is the lack of adequate exposure data,

Table 2-7. Types of exposure data in occupational epidemiology studies

Type of data	Approximation to dose
1. Quantified personal measurements	Best
2. Quantified job-specific data	↑
3. Ordinally ranked jobs or tasks	
4. Duration of employment in the industry	
5. Ever employed in the industry	Poorest

From Checkoway HA, Pearce NE, and Crawford-Brown DJ: *Research methods in occupational epidemiology,* New York, 1989, Oxford University Press.

and that this situation can be rectified by increasing use of molecular markers of exposure.[23] In fact, there are a number of major limitations of currently available biomarkers of exposures such as cigarette smoking,[24] particularly with regard to historical exposures. Questionnaires have good validity and reproducibility with regard to current exposures[25] and are likely superior to biological markers with respect to historical exposures. Thus, questionnaires will continue to play a major role in exposure assessment in respiratory disease epidemiology.

MEASUREMENT OF RESPIRATORY DISEASE

The identification and diagnosis of respiratory disease are discussed in depth in Chapters 3-9 and so are considered only briefly here. The most important consideration is that the type of information required for epidemiologic studies may be different from that required in clinical practice. As with exposure data the key issue is that information should be of similar quality for the various groups being compared. For example, suppose that the lung cancer incidence in a group of asbestos workers is being compared with national incidence rates; then it would be inappropriate to conduct a pathologic review and reclassification of the cases of the cancer identified in the asbestos workers, since such a reclassification had not been made for the national data and the information would not be comparable. Rather, the cancer cases in the asbestos workers should be classified exactly as they had been in routine national cancer statistics.

Thus, the emphasis must be on the comparability of information across the various groups being compared. This is relatively straightforward when studying malignant respiratory disease; however, the situation is much more difficult when studying nonmalignant respiratory disease. For example, international comparisons of asthma prevalence have been hampered by differences in methods and diagnostic criteria.[26] A problem with such international comparisons is that there may be cultural or language differences between the countries being compared. Although the presence of AHR has been used in working

definitions of current asthma,[14] symptoms are the cornerstone of large-scale epidemiologic surveys of asthma in children.[27]

Questionnaires

Questionnaires on asthma symptoms do not provide data that are adequate in the clinical context; however, they can provide data that are comparable across populations and are readily obtainable using simple, inexpensive methods in epidemiologic studies.

Standard written questionnaires have been the principal instrument for measuring asthma prevalence in community surveys, and in homogeneous populations these have been standardized, validated, and shown to be reproducible. However, in studies of populations speaking different languages and from different cultural backgrounds, standard written questionnaires may not be reliable. This problem has been experienced in studies of the Tokelauan community in New Zealand,[28] in the translation into German of the International Union against Tuberculosis and Lung Disease (IUATLD) questionnaire,[29] since there is no colloquial term for *wheezing* in the German language, and in a recent study in a French-speaking population.[30] In an attempt to minimize these difficulties of comparability of information in large surveys among diverse populations, a video questionnaire involving the audiovisual presentation of clinical signs and symptoms of asthma has been developed.[31,32] It was found[32] that the video questionnaire was at least as valid as, and was significantly more repeatable than, the standard IUATLD written questionnaire in a population for which English was the primary language.

Physiologic measurements

Many of the physiologic measurements are discussed in Chapters 4 and 5 and are mentioned briefly here in relation to epidemiologic methods.

Lung function tests for airway obstruction. Airway obstruction may be measured either preceding a maximal inspiratory maneuver [forced expiratory volume in 1 second (FEV1), forced vital capacity (FVC), or peak expiratory flow rate (PEFR)] or during tidal breathing (airway resistance). Whereas a maximal inspiratory or expiratory maneuver may lead to small, transient changes in airway caliber, the simplicity, standardization, and reproducibility of maximal expiratory maneuvers (particularly FEV1 and FVC) make them the measurement of choice in epidemiologic studies.[33]

Airway hyperresponsiveness. Measurements of AHR in epidemiologic studies of obstructive respiratory disease have been used increasingly in the past decade. They have often been used to help define a group of subjects whose symptomatology, as assessed by questionnaire, suggests asthma. It is important to recognize that these tests are neither wholly sensitive nor specific for asthma. However, a combination of recent symptoms and abnormal AHR is probably the most useful epidemiologic definition of asthma currently available.[14]

In adults abnormal airway responsiveness is found in smokers and in those with chronic obstructive pulmonary disease and in children concerns over the influence of lung size have confounded the interpretation of AHR.[34] In all studies it is important to consider the influence of bronchodilator and antiinflammatory therapy on the results of individual tests.

A wide variety of methodologies, bronchoconstrictors (including physiologic and nonphysiologic agents), and physical methods has been used to induce bronchoconstriction in susceptible individuals. These techniques include exercise, isocapnic hyperventilation, cold/dry air, hypotonic and hypertonic aerosols, pharmacologic agents, allergens, occupational sensitizers, and a variety of experimental challenge agents.[35] In epidemiologic studies challenge with histamine or methacholine has been the most widely used method and has been the best standardized and validated. These agents are generally interchangeable, with methacholine having fewer systemic and local side effects at higher doses than histamine. Aerosols are usually generated by nebulizer and involve either tidal breathing or a discreet dose delivery from a dosimeter. Results are expressed either as a dose (in micromoles) causing a 10% or 20% decrease in FEV1 (PD_{10} or PD_{20}) from the baseline level or, in the case of tidal breathing methods, the concentration required to cause a fall of 10% or 20% (PC_{10} or PC_{20}). These doses are usually calculated by plotting the cumulative dose of bronchoconstrictor delivered to the airways on a log scale against the percentage decrease in FEV1, with extrapolation of the dose-response curve if required. More recently, some investigators have suggested the use of the dose-response slope rather than the PD_{20} or PC_{20}, essentially providing a measure of the percentage decline in FEV1 per mole of methacholine or histamine administered. This technique has the advantage of providing information on a much larger proportion of the population under study rather than simply categorizing individuals as responsive or nonresponsive. In the laboratory setting, under optimal conditions and with patients whose respiratory status is stable, the 95% CI for single measurements of PD_{20} or PC_{20} is less than one twofold dose or concentration difference; in the community setting, where clinical stability and intertechnician variability are less easily controlled, the 95% CI may increase to two to three twofold dose differences.[35]

Recently, concerns have been raised in a number of countries by health and regulatory authorities over the use of methacholine and histamine from laboratory sources that have not been approved for human use. Difficulty in obtaining supplies or gaining the appropriate authority to use these agents has led to a renewed interest in alternative methods for assessing AHR in field studies. A better standardized exercise protocol for use in children has recently been developed (M. Haby, personal communication, 1994)

although exercise challenge suffers from the intrinsic problem of a decreased response with increasing ambient air-water content (above 10 mg/L), leading to the possibility of differential bias in comparative population studies. Challenge with nonisotonic aerosols is also likely to be increasingly considered as an alternative to pharmacologic challenge in field studies of AHR.

BASIC DATA ANALYSIS

In this section we review the most basic methods of statistical analysis for epidemiologic studies of occupational and environmental respiratory disease, using the notation of Table 2-8. We present only the most basic methods of statistical analysis of asthma epidemiologic studies (formulas are included in the appendix), and readers are encouraged to consult standard texts (e.g., Rothman[10]) for a more comprehensive review.

Measures of disease occurrence

As discussed in the section on types of epidemiologic studies, the most complete and definitive approach to environmental epidemiology involves using all of the information from the study base in a cohort study of disease incidence or mortality (also known as a follow-up study). People enter the study in a particular year, and some of them subsequently develop the disease under study; some eventually die of the disease, but others die because of some other cause. However, the information is "censored" since the study cannot last indefinitely; thus follow-up stops at a particular age, by which time some members of the cohort have died and some have been lost to follow-up for other reasons (e.g., emigration). Table 2-9[36] shows the findings of a hypothetical cohort study of 10,000 people who are exposed to a particular risk factor (e.g., radon) and 10,000 people who are not exposed; both groups are followed up for 10 years.

It is important to emphasize that some study participants contribute more information than others. People who die (because of any cause), are lost to follow-up, or emigrate, halfway through a study, stop contributing information. A

Table 2-8. Notation for data for stratum i in studies of disease incidence and prevalence

	Exposed	Nonexposed	Total
Cases	a_i	b_i	M_{1i}
Noncases	c_i	d_i	M_{0i}
Base population	N_{1i}	N_{0i}	T_i
Person-years	Y_{1i}	Y_{0i}	T_i
Incidence rate	I_{1i}	I_{0i}	
Cumulative incidence	CI_{1i}	CI_{0i}	
Odds	O_{1i}	O_{0i}	

related problem is that if a cohort is followed up for long enough, then everyone will eventually die. Thus, the difference between the exposed and nonexposed groups will not be the proportion dying (since everyone died), but when death occurred (in that people exposed to a hazardous substance may die at a younger age than people who are not exposed). Thus it is important to consider the amount of time that each person contributes to the study by using the person-time method.

In this context perhaps the most common measure of disease occurrence is the (person-time) incidence rate (or incidence density[6]), which is a measure of the disease occurrence per unit of time. In the study summarized in Table 2-9, 952 cases of lung cancer were diagnosed in the nonexposed group during the 10 years of follow-up, which involved a total of 95,163 person-years. This is less than the total possible person-time of 100,000 person-years, since people who developed the study disease, died or were lost to follow-up before the end of the 10-year period and therefore stopped contributing person-years at that time. (For simplicity we will ignore the problem of people whose disease disappears and then recurs over time, and we will assume that we are studying the incidence of the first occurrence of disease.) Thus the incidence rate in the nonexposed group (b/Y_0) was $952/95,163 = 0.0100$ (or 1000 per 100,000 person-years).

A second measure of disease occurrence is the cumulative incidence or risk, which is the proportion of study subjects who develop the disease of interest at any time during the follow-up period. Since it is a proportion, it is dimensionless, but it is necessary to specify the period over which it is being measured. In Table 2-9 there were 952 incident cases among the 10,000 people in the nonexposed group, and the cumulative incidence (b/N_0) was therefore $952/10,000 = 0.0952$ over the 10-year follow-up period.

When the disease of interest is rare over the follow-up period (e.g., a cumulative incidence of less than 10%), then the cumulative incidence is approximately equal to the product of the incidence rate times the follow-up period (in the example this product is 0.1000, whereas the cumulative incidence is 0.0952). In this example we have assumed, for simplicity, that no one died or was lost to follow-up during the study period (and therefore stopped contributing person-years to the study). When this assumption is not valid (i.e., when a significant proportion of people have died or have been lost to follow-up), then the cumulative incidence cannot be estimated directly, but must be estimated indirectly from the incidence rate (which takes into account, by the person-years method, the fact that follow-up was not complete for all study subjects).

A third possible measure of disease occurrence is the incidence odds, which is the ratio of the number of subjects who experience the outcome (b) to the number of subjects who do not (d). This measure is rarely used in cohort studies, but it is used to calculate the odds ratio in case-control studies (see the section later on prevalence studies). In Table 2-9 the incidence odds (b/d) is $952/9048 = 0.1052$.

These three measures of disease occurrence involve the same numerator: the number of incident cases of disease (b). They differ in whether their denominators represent person-years at risk (Y_0), persons at risk (N_0), or survivors (d).[36]

Measures of effect

Cohort studies. Corresponding to these three measures of disease occurrence, there are three principal ratio measures of effect that can be used in cohort studies (the details of these are presented in the appendix).

The measure of primary interest is often the *rate ratio* (or incidence density ratio), which is the ratio of the incidence rate in the exposed group (a/Y_1) to that in the nonexposed group (b/Y_0). In the example in Table 2-9, the incidence rates are 0.02 per person-year in the exposed group and 0.01 per person-year in the nonexposed group; the rate ratio is therefore 2.00.

A second commonly used effect measure is the *risk ratio* (or cumulative incidence ratio), which is the ratio of the cumulative incidence in the exposed group (a/N_1) to that in the nonexposed group (b/N_0). In Table 2-9 the cumulative incidence ratio is $0.1813/0.0952 = 1.90$. When the outcome is rare over the follow-up period, the risk ratio is approximately equal to the rate ratio.

A third possible effect measure is the incidence *odds ratio,* which is the ratio of the incidence odds in the exposed group (a/c) to that in the nonexposed group (b/d). In this example the odds ratio is $0.2214/0.1052 = 2.11$. Once again, when the outcome is rare over the study period, the incidence odds ratio is approximately equal to the incidence rate ratio.

The three multiplicative effect measures are sometimes referred to under the generic term *relative risk.* Each involves the ratio of a measure of disease occurrence in the exposed group to that in the nonexposed group. The

Table 2-9. Findings from a hypothetical cohort study of 20,000 persons followed up for 10 years

	Exposed	Nonexposed	Ratio
Cases	1813 (a)	952 (b)	
Noncases	8187 (c)	9048 (d)	
Base population	10,000 (N_1)	10,000 (N_0)	
Person-years	90,635 (Y_1)	95,163 (Y_0)	
Incidence rate	0.0200 (I_1)	0.0100 (I_0)	2.00
Cumulative incidence	0.1813 (CI_1)	0.0952 (CI_0)	1.90
Odds	0.2214 (O_1)	0.1052 (O_0)	2.11

Adapted from Pearce NE: What does the odds ratio estimate in a case-control study?, *Int J Epidemiol* 22:1189-1192, 1993.

various measures of disease occurrence all involve the same numerators (incident cases), but differ in whether their denominators are based on person-years, persons, or survivors (people who do not develop the disease at any time during the follow-up period). They are all approximately equal when the disease is rare during the follow-up period.

Case-control studies. In case-control studies the relative risk measure is the odds ratio.[37] The statistical aspects of the estimation, testing, and calculation of CIs for odds ratios are exactly as presented above in the cohort study context.

Prevalence studies. The prevalence is a proportion, and the statistical methods for calculating a CI for the prevalence are identical to those already presented for calculating a CI for the cumulative incidence (which is also a proportion). However, if we assume that the incidence rate is constant over time, then it can be shown[10] that the prevalence odds are equal to the incidence rate (I) times the average disease duration (D):

$$\frac{P}{1 - P} = ID$$

Thus the prevalence odds is directly proportional to the disease incidence, and the prevalence odds ratio estimates that

$$OR = I_1 D_1 / I_0 D_0$$

An increased prevalence odds ratio may thus reflect the influence of factors that increase the duration of disease, as well as those that increase disease incidence. However, in the special case in which the average durations of disease are the same in the exposed and nonexposed groups (i.e., when exposure has no effect on disease duration), then the prevalence odds ratio reduces to

$$OR = I_1 / I_0$$

That is, under this assumption, the prevalence odds ratio directly estimates the incidence rate ratio. The prevalence odds ratio is thus the basic effect measure in a prevalence study. The statistical methods of the prevalence odds ratio are identical to those for odds ratios in other contexts.

Table 2-10 shows data from a prevalence study of 20,000 people. This is based on the cohort study represented in Table 2-9, with the assumptions that the incidence rate is constant over time, that the average duration of disease is 5 years, and that the population has reached a steady state at which the number of people who "lose" the disease each year (either by recovering or dying) is balanced by the number of new cases generated from the susceptible population in the study base. In the nonexposed group there are 476 people who currently have disease, and 95 (20%) of these lose their disease each year; this is balanced by the 95 people who develop the disease each year (0.0100 of the susceptible population of 9524 people). In this steady-state situation the prevalence odds ratio (2.00) validly estimates the incidence rate ratio.

Table 2-10. Findings from a hypothetical prevalence study of 20,000 persons

	Exposed	Nonexposed	Ratio
Cases	909 (*a*)	476 (*b*)	
Noncases	9091 (*c*)	9524 (*d*)	
Total population	10,000 (N_1)	10,000 (N_2)	
Prevalence	0.0909 (P_1)	0.0476 (P_0)	1.91
Prevalence odds	0.1000 (O_1)	0.0500 (O_0)	2.00

Adapted from Pearce NE: What does the odds ratio estimate in a case-control study?, *Int J Epidemiol* 22:1189-1192, 1993.

Prevalence case-control studies. As in the case of a full prevalence study, the statistical methods for estimation and testing of the prevalence odds ratio in a prevalence case-control study are identical to those for odds ratios in other contexts.

INTERPRETATION OF EPIDEMIOLOGIC EVIDENCE

The first task in interpreting the findings of a study is to assess the likelihood that the study findings represent a real association, or whether they may be the result of various biases (confounding, selection bias, or information bias) or chance. If it is concluded that the observed associations are likely to be real, then attention shifts to more general causal inference, which should be based on all available information, rather than on the findings of a single study. A systematic approach to causal inference was elaborated by Hill[38] and has since been widely used and adapted.

The temporal relationship is crucial; the cause must precede the effect. This is usually self-evident, but difficulties may arise in studies (usually case-control or cross-sectional studies) when measurements of exposure and effect are made at the same time (by questionnaire and blood tests).

An association is plausible if it is consistent with other knowledge. For instance, laboratory experiments may have shown that a particular environmental exposure can cause cancer in laboratory animals, and this would make more plausible the hypothesis that this exposure could cause cancer in humans. However, biologic plausibility is a relative concept; many epidemiologic associations were considered implausible when they were first discovered but were subsequently confirmed in experimental studies. Lack of plausibility may simply reflect a current lack of medical knowledge.

Consistency is demonstrated by several studies giving the same result. This is particularly important when a variety of designs are used in different settings, since the likelihood that all studies are making the same mistake is thereby minimized. However, a lack of consistency does not exclude a causal association, because different exposure levels and other conditions may reduce the impact of exposure in certain studies.

The strength of association is important, in that a strongly elevated relative risk is more likely to be causal than a weak association, which could be influenced by confounding or other biases. However, the fact that an association is weak does not preclude it from being causal; rather, it means that it is more difficult to exclude alternative explanations.

A dose-response relationship occurs when changes in the level of exposure are associated with changes in the prevalence or incidence of the effect. The demonstration of a clear dose-response relationship provides strong evidence for a causal relationship, since it is unlikely that a consistent dose-response relationship would be produced by confounding.

Reversibility is also relevant, in that when the removal of a possible cause results in a reduced disease risk, the likelihood of the association's being causal is strengthened.

In conclusion, it should be stressed that, because of the nonexperimental nature of the discipline, individual epidemiologic studies are invariably imperfect. There is rarely a single definitive study that establishes a particular causal relationship; rather, causality is established by considering all of the available evidence from a variety of studies and populations. This has not prevented epidemiologic studies from making a major contribution to the understanding of occupational and environmental causes of respiratory disease. Thus, despite the need to carefully and cautiously interpret epidemiologic findings, this does not remove the need to ensure that public health action occurs when this is warranted, albeit on the basis of imperfect data. As Bradford-Hill[38] writes,

All scientific work is incomplete—whether it be observational or experimental. All scientific work is liable to be upset or modified by advancing knowledge. That does not confer upon us a freedom to ignore the knowledge that we already have, or to postpone the action that it appears to demand at a given time.

GLOSSARY OF KEY EPIDEMIOLOGIC TERMINOLOGY*

bias deviation of results or inferences from the truth

case-control study a study in which cases of disease are compared with a sample of nondiseased persons with respect to various exposures

cohort study a study in which a particular population (the study population) is followed up over a particular period (the study base) and the disease incidence is compared between exposed and nonexposed persons

confounding a situation in which the measure of effect of an exposure on risk is distorted because of the association of exposure with another factor(s) that influences the outcome under study

incidence the number of instances of illness commencing, or of persons falling ill, in a given period in a specified population

incidence rate the rate at which new events occur in a population

information bias bias arising because of misclassification of either exposure or disease

prevalence the number of instances of a given disease in a given population at a specific time; the prevalence may be expressed as a proportion of the total population, and this measure is sometimes termed the *prevalence rate*

prevalence study a study in which the prevalence of disease is measured at a specific time

rate the frequency of the occurrence of disease (per unit of person-time)

risk the probability that disease will occur (the proportion of people in which it does occur)

selection bias errors caused by systematic differences between those who were selected for a study and those who were not

study base the population-time experience that forms the basis of a study

study population the population on which a study is based

*Adapted from Last JM, editor: *A dictionary of epidemiology,* ed 2, New York, 1988, Oxford University Press.

ACKNOWLEDGMENTS

The authors' work is funded by Senior Research Fellowships of the Health Research Council of New Zealand. This work was conducted in part during the tenure (by N.P.) of a Visiting Scientist Award of the International Agency for Research on Cancer.

APPENDIX
Measures of disease occurrence

The *incidence rate* in the nonexposed group (see Table 2-8) has the form

$$I_0 = \frac{\text{cases}}{\text{person-time}} = \frac{b}{Y_0}$$

This has a standard error (SE) (under the Poisson distribution) of

$$SE(I_0) = \frac{b^{0.5}}{Y_0}$$

and a 95% confidence interval (CI) for the incidence rate is thus

$$I_0 \pm 1.96 \ SE(I_0)$$

The *cumulative incidence* in the nonexposed group has the form

$$CI_0 = \frac{\text{cases}}{\text{persons}} = \frac{b}{N_0}$$

This has an SE (under the binomial distribution) of

$$SE(CI_0) = \frac{[b(N_0 - b)]^{0.5}}{N_0^{1.5}}$$

and a 95% CI for the cumulative incidence is

$$CI_0 \pm 1.96 \ SE(CI_0)$$

Measures of effect

The *rate ratio* (RR) has the form

$$RR = \frac{I_1}{I_0} = \frac{a/Y_1}{b/Y_0}$$

The hypothesis that the RR is significantly different from the null value (1.0) can be tested with the person-time version of the Mantel-Haenszel χ^2 test,[39] which essentially tests whether the observed number of exposed cases differs from the number expected under the null hypothesis that exposure has no effect:

$$\chi^2 = \frac{[\text{Obs(a)} - \text{Exp(a)}]^2}{\text{Var[Exp(a)]}} = \frac{[a - Y_1 M_1/T]^2}{M_1 N_1 N_0/T^2}$$

where M_1, N_1, N_0, and T are as depicted in Table 2-8.

An approximate 95% CI for the RR is then given by[37]

$$RR^{1+1.96/\chi}$$

However, as discussed in the section on bias, we usually stratify the analysis on various risk factors (e.g., age and calendar period) to control for these extraneous risk factors and to obtain an estimate of the effect of exposure that is not confounded by the effects of these other risk factors. This involves stratifying the data into subgroups according to the levels of the confounder(s) and calculating a summary effect estimate by taking a weighted average of the RRs in each stratum.

The Mantel-Haenszel summary RR uses weights of

$$w_i = \frac{b_i Y_{1i}}{T_i}$$

and has the form

$$RR = \frac{\Sigma\, w_i RR_i}{\Sigma\, w_i} = \frac{\Sigma\, a_i Y_{0i}/T_i}{\Sigma\, b_i Y_{1i}/T_i}$$

The hypothesis that the summary RR is significantly different from the null value (1.0) can be tested with the person-time version of the Mantel-Haenszel summary χ^2 test[39]:

$$\chi^2 = \frac{[\Sigma\, \text{Obs(a)} - \Sigma\, \text{Exp(a)}]^2}{\Sigma\, \text{Var[Exp(a)]}} = \frac{[\Sigma\, a_i - \Sigma\, Y_{1i} M_{1i}/T_i]^2}{\Sigma\, M_{1i} N_{1i} N_{0i}/T_i^2}$$

where M_{1i}, N_{1i}, N_{0i}, and T_i are as depicted in Table 2-8.

An approximate 95% CI for the summary RR is then given by

$$RR^{1+1.96/\chi}$$

The *risk ratio* has the form

$$CIR = \frac{CI_1}{CI_0} = \frac{a/N_1}{b/N_0}$$

The hypothesis that the risk ratio is significantly different from the null value (1.0) can be tested with the Mantel-Haenszel χ^2 test[39]:

$$\chi^2 = \frac{[\text{Obs(a)} - \text{Exp(a)}]^2}{\text{Var[Exp(a)]}} = \frac{[a - N_1 M_1/T]^2}{M_1 M_0 N_1 N_0/T^2(T - 1)}$$

where M_1, M_0, N_1, N_0, and T are as depicted in Table 2-8.

An approximate 95% CI for the risk ratio is then given by

$$CIR^{1+1.96/\chi}$$

The Mantel-Haenszel summary risk ratio uses weights of

$$w_i = \frac{b_i N_{1i}}{T_i}$$

and has the form

$$OR = \frac{\Sigma\, w_i OR_i}{\Sigma\, w_i} = \frac{\Sigma\, a_i N_0/T_i}{\Sigma\, b_i N_1/T_i}$$

The hypothesis that the summary cumulative incidence ratio is significantly different from the null value (1.0) can be tested with the Mantel-Haenszel summary χ^2 test[39]:

$$\chi^2 = \frac{[\Sigma\, \text{Obs(a)} - \Sigma\, \text{Exp(a)}]^2}{\Sigma\, \text{Var[Exp(a)]}} = \frac{[\Sigma\, a_i - \Sigma\, N_{1i} M_{1i}/T_i]^2}{\Sigma\, M_{1i} M_{0i} N_{1i} N_{0i}/T_i^2}$$

where M_{1i}, M_{0i}, N_{1i}, N_{0i}, and T_i are as depicted in Table 2-8.

An approximate 95% CI for the summary risk ratio is then given by

$$OR^{1+1.96/\chi}$$

The *odds ratio* (OR) has the form

$$OR = \frac{O_1}{O_0} = \frac{a/c}{b/d} = \frac{ad}{bc}$$

The hypothesis that the OR is significantly different from the null value (1.0) can be tested with the Mantel-Haenszel χ^2 test[39]:

$$\chi^2 = \frac{[\text{Obs(a)} - \text{Exp(a)}]^2}{\text{Var[Exp(a)]}} = \frac{[a - N_1 M_1/T]^2}{M_1 M_0 N_1 N_0/T^2(T - 1)}$$

where M_1, M_0, N_1, N_0, and T are as depicted in Table 2-8.

An approximate 95% CI for the OR is then given by

$$OR^{1+1.96/\chi}$$

The Mantel-Haenszel summary OR uses weights of

$$w_i = \frac{b_i c_i}{T_i}$$

and has the form

$$OR = \frac{\Sigma\, w_i OR_i}{\Sigma\, w_i} = \frac{\Sigma\, a_i d_i/T_i}{\Sigma\, b_i c_i/T_i}$$

The hypothesis that the summary OR is significantly different from the null value (1.0) can be tested with the Mantel-Haenszel summary χ^2 test[39]:

$$\chi^2 = \frac{[\Sigma \, \text{Obs(a)} - \Sigma \, \text{Exp(a)}]^2}{\Sigma \, \text{Var[Exp(a)]}} = \frac{[\Sigma \, a_i - \Sigma \, N_{1i}M_{1i}/T_i]^2}{\Sigma \, M_{1i}M_{0i}N_{1i}N_{0i}/T_i^2}$$

where M_{1i}, M_{0i}, N_{1i}, N_{0i}, and T_i are as depicted in Table 2-8.

An approximate 95% CI for the summary OR is then given by

$$OR^{1 + 1.96/\chi}$$

REFERENCES

1. Doll R and Hill AB: Mortality in relation to smoking: ten years' observations of British doctors, *Br Med J* 1:1399-1410, 1964.
2. Doll R and Peto R: Mortality in relation to smoking: 20 years' observations on male British doctors, *Br Med J* 2:1525-1536, 1976.
3. U.S. Environmental Protection Agency (EPA): *Respiratory health effects of passive smoking: lung cancer and other disorders,* Washington, D.C., 1983, EPA.
4. Doll R: Mortality from lung cancer in asbestos workers, *Br J Ind Med* 12:81-86, 1955.
5. Lee DHK and Selikoff IJ: Historical background to the asbestos problem, *Environ Res* 18:300-314, 1979.
6. Miettinen OS: *Theoretical epidemiology,* New York, 1985, Wiley.
7. Checkoway HA, Pearce NE, and Crawford-Brown DJ: *Research methods in occupational epidemiology,* New York, 1989, Oxford University Press.
8. Schulte PA: Investigation of occupational cancer clusters: theory and practice, *Am J Public Health* 77:52-56, 1987.
9. Dement JM, Harris RL, Symons MJ, et al: Exposures and mortality among chrysotile asbestos workers. Part II: mortality, *Am J Ind Med* 4:421-433, 1983.
10. Rothman KJ: *Modern epidemiology,* Boston, 1986, Little, Brown.
11. Doll R and Hill AB: Smoking and carcinoma of the lung, *Br Med J* 2:739-748, 1950.
12. Doll R and Hill AB: A study of the aetiology of carcinoma of the lung, *Br Med J* 2:1271-1286, 1952.
13. Kupper LL, McMichael AJ, and Spirtas R. A hybrid epidemiologic study design useful in estimating relative risk, *J Am Stat Assoc* 70:524-528, 1975.
14. Toelle BG, Peat JK, Salome CM, et al: Toward a definition of asthma for epidemiology, *Am Rev Respir Dis* 146:633-637, 1992.
15. Brunekreef B, Groot B, and Hoek G: Pets, allergy and respiratory symptoms in children, *Int J Epidemiol* 1:338-342, 1992.
16. Senthilselvan A, McDuffie IIIH, and Dosman JA: Association of asthma with use of pesticides, *Am Rev Respir Dis* 146:884-887, 1992.
17. Flatt A, Pearce NE, Thomson CD, et al: Reduced selenium status in asthmatic subjects in New Zealand, *Thorax* 45:95-99, 1990.
18. Last JM, editor: *A dictionary of epidemiology,* ed 2, New York, 1988, Oxford University Press.
19. Greenland S, Robins JM: Identifiability, exchangeability and epidemiological confounding, *Int J Epidemiol* 15:412-418, 1986.
20. Pearce NE, Checkoway HA, and Dement JM: Exponential models for analyses of time-related factors: illustrated with asbestos textile worker mortality data, *J Occup Med* 30:517-522, 1988.
21. Axelson O: Aspects on confounding in occupational health epidemiology, *Scand J Work Environ Health* 4:85-89, 1978.
22. Copeland KT, Checkoway H, McMichael AJ, et al: Bias due to misclassification in the estimation of relative risk, *Am J Epidemiol* 105:488-495, 1977.
23. Schulte PA: A conceptual and historical framework for molecular epidemiology. In Schulte P and Perera FP, editors: *Molecular epidemiology: principles and practices,* pp 3-44, San Diego, 1993, Academic Press.
24. Armstrong BK, White E, and Saracci R: *Principles of exposure measurement in epidemiology,* New York, 1992, Oxford University Press.
25. Forastiere F, Agabiti N, Dell'orco V, et al: Questionnaire data as predictors of urinary cotinine levels among nonsmoking adolescents, *Arch Environ Health* 48:230-234, 1993.
26. Pearce NE, Weiland S, Keil U, et al: Self-reported prevalence of asthma symptoms in children in Australia, England, Germany and New Zealand: an international comparison using the ISAAC written and video questionnaires, *Eur Respir J* 6:1455-1461, 1993.
27. Anderson HR: Is the prevalence of asthma changing?, *Arch Dis Child* 64:172-175, 1989.
28. Crane J, O'Donnell TV, Prior IAM. Symptoms of asthma, methacholine airway responsiveness and atopy in migrant Tokelauan children, *N Z Med J* 102:36-38, 1989.
29. Burney PGJ, Laitinen LA, Perdrizet S, et al: Validity and repeatability of the IUALTD (1984) bronchial symptoms questionnaire: an international comparison, *Eur Respir J* 2:940-945, 1989.
30. Osterman JW, Armstrong BG, Ledoux E, et al: Comparison of French and English versions of the American Thoracic Society Respiratory Questionnaire in a bilingual working population, *Int J Epidemiol* 20:138-143, 1991.
31. Shaw RA, Crane J, O'Donnell TV, et al: The use of a videotaped questionnaire for studying asthma prevalence: a pilot study amongst New Zealand adolescents, *Aust N Z J Med* 157:311-314, 1992.
32. Shaw RA, Crane J, Pearce NE, et al: Validation of a video questionnaire for assessing asthma prevalence, *Clin Exp Allergy* 22:562-569, 1992.
33. Quanjer PM, Tammeling GJ, Cotes JE, et al: Lung volumes and forced ventilatory flows, *Eur Respir J* 6(suppl 16):4-39, 1993.
34. Le Souef PN: Can measurements of airway responsiveness be standardized in children?, *Eur Respir J* 6:1085-1087, 1993.
35. Sterk PJ, Fabbri LM, Quanjer PM, et al: Airway responsiveness standardized challenge testing with pharmacological physical and sensitizing stimuli, *Eur Respir J* 6(suppl 16):53-83, 1993.
36. Pearce NE: What does the odds ratio estimate in a case-control study?, *Int J Epidemiol* 22:1189-1192, 1993.
37. Miettinen OS: Estimability and estimation in case-referent studies, *Am J Epidemiol* 103:226-235, 1976.
38. Hill AB: The environment and disease: association or causation?, *Proc R Soc Med* 58:295-300, 1965.
39. Mantel N and Haenszel W: Statistical aspects of the analysis of data from retrospective studies of disease, *J Natl Cancer Inst* 22:719-748, 1959.

Chapter 3

HISTORY AND PHYSICAL EXAMINATION

Paul D. Blanc
John R. Balmes

For the clinician in practice, identifying an occupational or environmental risk factor and then assessing its possible causal link to a specific respiratory disorder in an individual patient is a daunting task. This is true for the occupational specialist and all the more true for the pulmonary specialist in general practice. Only rarely are there exceptions, such as a massive, clear-cut exposure followed by an effect that is immediate and unequivocal. One example might be a chlorine release from a transportation mishap in which a railroad worker develops adult respiratory distress syndrome. However, even in this scenario, the treating clinician initially may know only that a toxic release took place but may be unaware of the details of exposure intensity or even the specific substance involved. Moreover, the clinical focus of an evaluation may not be related to the acute response to exposure, but rather may be an assessment of residual signs and symptoms of impairment in follow-up to an exposure that took place at some point in the past.

The presentation of occupationally or environmentally caused illness is rarely pathognomonic, either clinically or pathologically. Rarely is the diagnostician in occupational and environmental medicine provided with laboratory data that establish a specific exposure-linked diagnosis. A clinical presentation of silicosis with small, rounded opacities and eggshell hilar calcification on a chest radiograph, coupled with a lung biopsy demonstrating birefringent particles in silicotic nodules, can be invoked as one of the few exceptions that prove the rule.

Identifying risk factors and then linking occupational or environmental exposures to the respiratory disorder being evaluated is a two-step process. It is pivotal to the initial component to entertain the possibility that such occupational and environmental risk factors play a role in the differential diagnosis as formulated. Although this is axiomatic to occupational and environmental medicine, its importance cannot be overemphasized. After considering this possibility, the clinician must then attempt to elicit the appropriate history and carry out a physical examination in a systematic yet targeted fashion with such risk factors in mind.

The goal of this chapter is to provide an orientation to such a targeted history and physical examination geared toward the practicing clinician evaluating pulmonary conditions that are potentially occupationally or environmentally related. The concept of a targeted approach is important, because standard guidelines for an occupational and environmental assessment are not easily adaptable to general practice. For example, typical recommendations for occupational history-taking delineate a stepwise approach addressing all past employment, usually starting with the present and working backward systematically.[1-5] Formated histories may also emphasize environmental exposures, for example, those linked to hobbies, the neighborhood, or potential household exposures.[6] These structured histories are useful in certain contexts, for example, structured interview schedules in epidemiologic research, lengthy work-ups in a specialty practice setting, or medical-legal evaluations. Realistically, however, the busy clinician will not elicit such an all-encompassing occupational history in most situations.[7–10]

First, we illustrate the key components of focused occupational and environmental history-taking through a series of brief clinical case vignettes. This is followed by a summary outline of a brief, targeted history. Finally, we present a structured approach to the physical examination in occupational and environmental lung disease. We intend this material, taken together, to serve as a basis on which to build more extensive evaluations that may be dictated by a variety of different clinical situations.

ILLUSTRATIVE CASE SCENARIOS
Case 1

A 45-year-old Hispanic man is referred to you from your hospital's nonemergent screening clinic because of complaints of progressive dyspnea of several months' duration with a normal chest radiograph. Simple spirometry demonstrates mild obstruction to airflow with a significant reversible component after inhaled β-agonist. The patient has been in good health, with no previous history of cardiopulmonary disease. Specifically, there is no history of asthma or atopy. The dyspnea is not exertional. There is sometimes a cough, but the patient has not noted any wheezing. There has been no chest pain, fever, weight loss, or other constitutional symptoms. The patient's symptoms occur mostly at night. He does not notice any difference on weekdays as compared with weekends, although when he was off work for a week 2 months ago with muscle sprain he remembers feeling considerably better. There is a 20-year history of smoking a pack of cigarettes a day.

The patient is concerned that his symptoms may be job related because one of his friends at work has recently been told by his doctor that he has asthma. The patient's occupation is that of machine operator. He works on the curing line in a metal drum manufacturing plant. Because the drums are intended for food, they are lined with a special baked coating. The coating is a two-part powder that is sprayed onto the drums and then heat cured. There is considerable dust on the patient's work clothes by the end of the day, although it is not so dusty that the room in which he works is cloudy or dim. If he blows his nose at the end of the day, some dust is present on the tissue paper. No specific respiratory protection is used. The curing oven is open at both ends in a continuous feeding system. This manufacturing process is relatively new, having been introduced into the patient's workplace 1 year ago. The patient has brought with him material safety data sheets (MSDS) that identify the coating as an epoxy formulation comprising primarily solvents and inert components. No respiratory irritants are mentioned. When you contact the epoxy manufacturing company directly, they admit that the product contains trimellitic anhydride (a well-known cause of oc-

cupational asthma), which they did not list on the MSDS because it comprises less than 1% of the product by weight.

What are the salient features of the occupational history in this case of occupational asthma?[11] First and foremost, the patient himself raises the possibility of an occupational or environmental factor in his illness. More often than not, the first person to suspect such a link will be the patient and not the health care provider. To reiterate the point made earlier, including occupational and environmental illness within the differential diagnosis is the critical first step. Assessing potential illness among others also exposed is important.

The description of the work process, and the patient's job duties within it, contains the crucial information. The job title "machine operator" is meaningless from the point of view of an occupational history. All too often, work history-taking begins and ends with the notation of such nonilluminating job titles. It is far better to ask "What do you do?" than "What is your job title?" If faced with a response that is not informative, one can then pursue the issue: "No, I mean what do you *do* exactly?" What the patient does is work in an industrial painting (i.e., coating) operation. By description it is an "open" process, a key factor meaning that few barriers exist between the worker and potential exposure.[12] It is important to remember that even a process that, by description, is routinely a closed system (e.g., a sealed reaction vat in a petrochemical plant) may become an "open process" at times of maintenance, cleanup, or system failure. The patient's simple descriptions of dust levels are not as precise as industrial hygiene measurements, but, nonetheless, they document ample airborne exposure. Other clues to high ambient exposures can be reports of deposit of aerosols or dusts on surfaces (e.g., overhead crossbeams) or even peeling paint secondary to a corrosive atmosphere.

Two other factors are highly suspicious. The first is the introduction of a new process or product in temporal relation to the onset of symptoms. For suspected occupational asthma it may also be useful to pinpoint a temporal link between the workday or workweek and the reported symptoms. As in this case, by the time of presentation, symptoms may not abate with only brief (weekend) work absences, although with a longer removal the pattern may be clearer. Similarly, delayed asthma symptoms, as in this case, may mean that the patient is typically worse when away from the job, for example, when home in the evenings after work.

The second factor that raises the index of suspicion for an occupational etiology is the identification of a two-component chemical product, such as the epoxy paint noted here (epoxy resins, polyurethane paints and coatings, and cyanoacrylate glues would be other examples of common two-part systems).[11] Assessing exposure to two-part products in manufacturing or construction trades is a reasonable screening question. These multicomponent systems must be used rapidly after mixing because they contain reactive chemicals that, in general, may also act as pulmonary irritants or sensitizers. Although in this case the patient provides an MSDS supposedly delineating the risks of the product with which he works, this proves to be misleading. These information sheets are helpful for the data they do contain, but they should not be accepted on face value because of information omitted on proprietary grounds or simply because of inaccuracy.[13]

Case 2

A 25-year-old white woman is admitted to the intensive care unit in the early morning hours after presenting to the emergency department in acute respiratory failure. A chest radiograph and physiologic parameters are consistent with noncardiogenic pulmonary edema. There was no significant prodrome, with rapid progression of dyspnea beginning only a few hours before presentation. The patient takes no prescription or over-the-counter medications, although she had used oral contraceptives until 1 year previously. She is a nonsmoker with no history of drug abuse. There is no significant travel history.

The occupational history is that of bicycle delivery messenger. The day before admission, as well as the previous workweek, were without extraordinary events. The patient's work involves the delivery of documents, primarily to downtown office buildings. She is sometimes caught in traffic behind buses and trucks. She frequently climbs stairs rapidly as part of her job and has done so until now without difficulty. She has not encountered any spills, leaks, or other chemical exposures while at work.

When asked about any recent possible chemical, fume, or dust exposures at work or at home, the patient mentions her vocation. She states that she is employed as a messenger in order to financially support her work as an artist. She works in "mixed media." When asked to elaborate ("What do you do exactly?"), she describes her work as being metal sculpture of found objects. She has recently been welding, using electric arc stick welding, to build a new piece comprised of old automobile carburetors. She acquired the discarded carburetor parts in a 55-gallon drum soaking in "cleaner." The cleaner is described as "not exactly gasoline" but "more than soap and water." She does not thoroughly dry the parts before welding. The drum sits in a corner of her workshop (a small garage next to her house). Because of the cold weather, she has been working with the garage door shut. She last worked on the piece about 8 hours before the onset of her symptoms. She did not notice any irritation at that time.

This case of "occult" pulmonary edema underscores the point that most occupational or environmental pulmonary disease is not pathognomonic. In routine clinical practice a search for likely precipitating factors for pulmonary edema, such as in this case, would only be pursued after pneumonia, congestive heart failure, adult respiratory distress syndrome due to sepsis, and other, more common etiologies had been excluded. Moreover, the occupational history does not identify any obvious risk factors for the clinical presentation described.

The history of "hobby" exposures was elicited in response to a fairly simplistic question soliciting report of any exposures to chemicals, dusts, or fumes at work *or at home*. Exposures outside of the workplace can be critical and should be explored, particularly when a review of potential risks associated with the patient's salaried employment is unrevealing. In this case the patient's vocation was distinct from her paid job and involved a number of potential exposures as an artist. There has been a growing awareness that artists are at risk for exposure to heavy metals, toxic gases, solvents, caustics, hazardous organic chemicals, and dusts in a variety of endeavors, some of the most noteworthy being metal- and woodworking, ceramics, textiles, photography, and printing.[14] Often, household exposures are more intermittent than those of an artist or craftsperson, for example, risks from cleaning chemicals, automobile repair products, garden pesticides, furniture strippers, or other home refurbishing materials.[6]

The exposure history and the clinical presentation strongly suggest a diagnosis of acute lung injury caused by phosgene inhalation. Phosgene can be produced when chlorinated hydrocarbons (e.g., methylene chloride, a common carburetor-cleaning solvent) are heated to high temperatures or exposed to ultraviolet light.[15] De novo toxicants, created in situ as a by-product of other processes or a combination of materials, can be critical exposure factors. The patient will not be able to identify the specific toxin (let alone provide an MSDS for it, since it was not a component of the original starting materials). Key historical clues are any burning or high-temperature activity (welding or flame-cutting is prototypical) or mixing of materials associated with bubbling, heat, or a strong smell (e.g., mixing bathroom tile cleaner with bleach).[16,17]

A final teaching point in this clinical vignette is the relevance of "confined space" as an exposure cofactor. Strictly defined, a confined space is a poorly ventilated enclosure without open windows and with limited egress, for example, manure pits, where hydrogen sulfide gas toxicity is an important risk. For practical purposes, any closed space without directed ventilation may act as a relatively confined space, including, as in this case, a converted garage workshop with its doors shut.[18,19]

Case 3

A 4-year-old white girl is brought by her mother to the pediatrician, who has referred the case for specialty evaluation as possible new-onset allergic asthma. The previously healthy child had an abrupt onset of an illness 3 weeks ago characterized by nausea, vomiting, and headache. The mother assumed that it was a viral syndrome since both she and her other child (aged 8 years) had experienced nausea and malaise at around the same time. However, the child, who has been kept home from day care, also began to complain of a burning sensation in her nose and has been coughing a lot as well. The mother is worried about allergy to formaldehyde, because the house was "done over" last month. This included new rolled fiberglass insulation and double-glazed windows, interior repainting of the family room, shampooing of wall-to-wall carpets (which were not changed), and installation of central air conditioning. The weather has turned quite hot and the air conditioning has been on nearly full-time. The concern about formaldehyde was raised by a friend (who had read about it in a health magazine) after the child's mother complained about a persistent odor in the house.

The work in the house was done by her brother-in-law. She has brought in labels of some of the products used. The paint is a standard latex formulation. There is also a label from a "mildew control" product that was added separately to the paint at the time of application. You note that it states on the label in small print "For commercial exterior use." A call to the regional Poison Control Center identifies its principal component as bis(tributyltin) oxide in a 25% concentration. The center confirms that this organotin mildewcide is a respiratory irritant and that it also causes gastrointestinal distress.[20]

The previous two cases highlighted the occupational and vocational histories. This case illustrates the potential importance of environmental factors and the frequently difficult task of pinpointing specific risks from among a myriad of seemingly mundane exposures. *Environmental* is, of course, not interchangeable with *outdoors*. As this case demonstrates, the indoor air environment also represents a complex mix of substances with potential respiratory effects.[21]

The home refurbishing activities reported in temporal association with a family cluster of symptoms suggest a possible cause-and-effect relationship but certainly does not establish one. The specific question of formaldehyde may be important as a potential indicator of the patient's concerns and belief system. Frequently, an important benefit of a targeted occupational and environmental history may be to reassure the patient that these factors do not appear to have a causal relationship to the symptoms reported. In this case none of the generic home improvements made would be anticipated to be associated with formaldehyde off-gassing. This is in contrast to potential release from sprayed foam insulation (as opposed to fiberglass) or new carpets or upholstery (as opposed to merely cleaning old carpets). Moreover, the severity of the symptoms reported here is inconsistent with low-level exposure to a trace contaminant.[21]

However, key points in the history do raise suspicions of potentially high exposures manifesting a dose-response effect. The use of heavy insulation of walls and windows together with recirculating air can transform homes or offices into the functional equivalent of "confined" spaces.

This has proved important in assessing "sick building syndrome," in which it may be necessary to obtain specific data on the frequency of air exchanges in the space in question. Air conditioning or cooler use may also be important as an actual point source of contamination, for example, in infectious disease outbreaks, hypersensitivity pneumonitis, or "humidifier fever."

The age of the index case is another key historical point. From a dose-response point of view, children easily achieve higher environmental exposures when considered on a per-weight basis and factoring in respiratory rate and body surface area.[6] Moreover, children may spend greater amounts of time in the contaminated environment, as in this case when kept home from day care (likely playing in the family room).

Abnormal smells frequently motivate environmental health assessments and may even induce symptoms via mechanisms that do not represent direct toxicity.[22] Important characteristics of odors include not only their quality (sweet or acrid, for example) but also their persistence. "Olfactory fatigue," the diminished ability to appreciate an odor with ongoing exposure, is a recognized attribute of certain chemical vapors and gases.

Material safety data sheets are not easily accessible outside the workplace. Product labels frequently are. They can be a crucial adjunct when taking a targeted occupational and environmental history. Even cursory examination of product labels may identify use of industrial-strength chemical products brought home for household use or other important potential risk factors, such as inappropriate dilution or, as in this case, misapplication of an outdoor formulation. Whereas the labels on many commercial products have scant information on toxicity, contacting a regional Poison Control Center or the manufacturer (a product information number may appear on the label) can supplement the history and help focus questions in targeted areas.[23]

Case 4

A 16-year-old man has a 2-week history of fever, chills, nonproductive cough, dyspnea, and a 5-lb weight loss. A chest radiograph shows diffuse, nodular infiltrates. When asked whether anyone around him has had similar symptoms or specifically if anyone has had tuberculosis, he denies illness in family or friends but volunteers that his dog Blue (a golden retriever) was also recently ill and had to be taken to the veterinarian. He was told that an x-ray of the dog showed "pneumonia," and the dog was treated with antibiotics. Because of suspicion of fungal disease, both the patient and the dog underwent serologic testing, which demonstrated evidence findings of acute infection with *Histoplasma capsulatum*.

Ten days before the onset of symptoms, the patient had carried out a weekend landscaping job for family friends with a weekend house "down near the river." He had spent most of the day cutting up a large, decayed fallen tree, using a chain saw. There was enough dust to prompt him to wear a bandanna over his nose and mouth. His dog accompanied him on the day of the landscaping job.

Infectious processes may often be "occupational" in etiology.[24] Because the pathogen and its treatment are typically no different in occupational as compared with nonoccupational infectious disease, the occupational history may be inappropriately downplayed. However, there can be important implications for work-related secondary prevention after identification of an index case. In this apparent point-source outbreak of histoplasmosis, secondary prevention of exposure to others is an academic issue, unless, of course, the patient were to report that a friend is about to go finish the landscaping job for him. The link is more straightforward in an outbreak of brucellosis in a slaughterhouse or *Legionella* pneumonia in an office building. Another important role for the occupational history in suspected infectious disease is as a tool to hone the differential diagnosis, much as the "travel history" does (which is de rigueur in such cases). Clearly, an occupational history of laboratory work in a sheep confinement facility elevates the likelihood of Q fever (for which sheep are an important source of infection) high in the differential diagnosis of what would otherwise be a presumed community-acquired pneumonia. Finally, occupational attribution has an implicit impact on case management, including compensation and cost reimbursement, of relevance both to the patient and the health care provider.

The case vignette is consistent with documented reports of concomitant occupational or environmental illness in humans and pets.[25] Small animals often manifest toxic effects that can be important clues to human exposures, particularly in environmental illness. One example would be the cats of Minamata, Japan, where high-fish diets per body weight produced one of the earliest manifestations of organomercurialism among village pets. The abandoned practice of taking canaries down into mines to serve as an early warning of "bad air" is another example. Interspecies differences in sensitivity to toxins can also make pets or other animals harbingers of effects that may only later become apparent among humans similarly exposed.

Although simple screening questions may elicit exposure to chemicals or mineral dusts, organic materials may escape attention. Nonetheless, naturally occurring plant- and animal-derived materials are causally related to a number of acute and chronic lung responses and should not be ignored. For instance, the exposure history in this vignette (although not the clinical course) could have as easily been associated with organic dust toxic syndrome, a brief, flu-like illness that would invariably be attributed to a viral syndrome without identification of a history of heavy acute inhalational exposure to wood chip or other thermophilic bacterially contaminated material.[26]

A final teaching point of this vignette is that persons neither under age 18 nor over age 65 should be considered as being beyond the likelihood of labor force participation in terms of etiology.[27,28] Not only do a significant proportion of minors work, but moreover, their occupations are frequently in relatively dangerous trades. Often, as in this case, the employment may be casual, poorly supervised, noninsured, and difficult to monitor.

Case 5

A 63-year-old African-American male school administrator has recently moved to the area after taking advantage of an early retirement plan. He complains of cough and wheezing, with mild dyspnea. All of his symptoms are much worse since moving. He was hoping that the climate change from the relocation would be to his advantage, since every winter for the past few years he has had "chest colds" that lasted for several weeks. His most troubling symptom during those episodes was a nonproductive cough, although he did occasionally wheeze. His doctor at one point gave him an inhaler that he used briefly but he was never told he had asthma or any other chronic lung disease. His medical history is significant for borderline hypertension controlled with diet. He had briefly been on a "water pill" in the past but specifically denies β-blocker use or any other current prescription medication. Asked about over-the-counter formulations, he does admit to buying a Bronkaid inhaler a few weeks ago, which seems to help his symptoms, especially at night.

The patient has no drug allergies but is allergic to cats. There is a family history of hypertension and asthma. The patient had smoked one-half pack of cigarettes per day for 12 years but discontinued use 17 years previously. The review of symptoms is positive only for bilateral mild to moderate hearing loss, for which the patient reports that he has been tested and has been told that a hearing aid would not help.

The occupational history is that of being a teacher (of mathematics) and later an administrator throughout his career. He studied "on the GI bill"; his military service during the Korean War was in the artillery corps. Asked about his living environment, he describes in some detail the loft space he has acquired in a trendy industrial area. All of the renovations were completed before his moving in. None of the rooms is carpeted, there is minimal house dust, he has no pets, he sleeps on a tatami mat, and the house is a "cigarette smoke-free and drug-free" environment. He does have one complaint about the loft. He says the rumbling of the trucks from the Portland cement factory across the street is quite irritating, particularly at night.

The patient's convincing history of asthma that initially was mild but is now worsening invites a number of questions ruling out potential exacerbating factors. These questions would typically cover medication effects, common environmental allergens (e.g., cats and house dust mites), and lifestyle. No less so, possible environmental chemical exposures, especially air pollutants, should also be considered in relation to relevant lung processes. Although, in general, the principal contributor to ambient air pollution is the automobile, point-source pollution is also important. In this case sulfur dioxide, a major by-product of Portland cement manufacture (as it is in metal smelting and petrochemical refining), is known to affect persons with nonspecific airway hyperresponsiveness at exposure levels one order of magnitude lower than would produce such effects in the rest of the population.[29] Just because an alternative (nonoccupational and nonenvironmental) etiology of a condition is established, a targeted occupational and environmental history does not become irrelevant. Occupational or environmental factors that may worsen underlying conditions should be addressed as a part of tertiary prevention of disease progression and disability. Workers' compensation systems often recognize work-related exacerbations of preexisting conditions.[11]

In this case the occupational history, within the clinical context of the patient's chief complaint, is unrevealing. Basic information is still pertinent: clarifying that the patient was a teacher of mathematics and not, for example, a biology teacher, for whom frequent laboratory animal contact might have been a cause of asthma. For practical purposes detailed elaborations of the occupational history after a few such screening questions will not provide further illumination. Even with an apparently innocuous occupational history, as this case vignette illustrates, it is useful to specifically assess military service. Often, the patient will ignore military service as being outside of any work history unless directly asked.[5] The hearing deficit noted in the review of systems, although unrelated to the pulmonary chief complaint, may quite likely be noise-induced hearing loss as a sequela of artillery exposure. A related screening question, addressed to men or women of an age having been employed during World War II, should be whether there is any history of shipyard work. On both the Pacific and Atlantic coasts hundreds of thousands of men and women were employed in shipyards during that period, with nearly ubiquitous asbestos exposure. As with military service, brief employment in the remote past may be associated with long-term illness but may easily be skipped over by the patient without specific prompting.

Case 6

The patient is a 45-year-old Korean-American with progressive dyspnea over several months. He has few other symptoms, has no weight loss, and was previously in good health. There is a 20-year pack-a-day smoking history. After a chest radiograph demonstrates diffuse alveolar infiltrates, he is admitted to the hospital for further evaluation and treatment. The work-up includes a bronchoscopy with a transbronchial biopsy revealing periodic acid–Schiff-positive material filling the alveoli, consistent with a diagnosis of pulmonary alveolar proteinosis (PAP).

The occupational history is that of construction painter for the past 19 years. Specifically, the patient is an iron and bridge worker, painting outdoor metal (steel) structures. The materials are oil based and frequently "marine" paints. He does both high-pressure spray painting and hand-held brush painting, depending on the job.

He does wear a mask when painting. It is a screw-in cartridge-type mask covering the nose and mouth. He has not changed the cartridges in at least 1 year. He does have direct skin contact with the paints, especially when tending to the "pot" when spray painting. Sometimes he feels "a little drunk" from the work. He denies exposure to asbestos or silica. He has never had a blood lead test. No uniforms are provided by the employer; the crew typically eats and smokes at the work site.

He works for a small (eight-employee) subcontracting company owned by a friend of his cousin. It is not unionized. He does not know whether there is a safety and health committee in his company. He has heard of OSHA (the Occupational Safety and Health Administration) but does not remember anyone ever taking air samples at a work site where he was employed.

Going back over the patient's work, you ask him to describe in a step-by-step manner how the job gets done, starting with preparation of metal structures for a paint job, mixing of the paint, setting up of the paint pot for spraying, location of the compressor for the pressure gun, the painting itself, and clean-up afterward. From this description you learn that on a job that lasted several months and ended approximately 6 months ago, the structure required extensive sandblasting before painting. The sandblaster (employed by another subcontractor) had a full air-supplied respirator with a hood over his head. The job was fraught with disagreements between the painters and the sandblaster. The sand was always blowing over and getting in the way of the painting work (the patient could often feel it hitting against his face). At the same time, the sandblaster complained that their paint spray compressor gave him a headache.

The diagnosis of PAP is one of a handful of uncommon pulmonary conditions for which occupational or environmental causes have been clearly established in what would otherwise be labeled an "idiopathic" condition. In PAP heavy exposure to dust, particularly free crystalline silica, appears to play a causal role in a significant number of cases.[30]

Despite this association, the initial occupational history does not suggest a suspect dust, although overexposure to solvent-containing paints (and possibly lead) is strongly indicated. The patient has frequent skin contact with the materials and sometimes feels drunk from them, suggesting heavy solvent contamination.[31] Overall hygiene is poor, including the absence of uniform changes and separate eating areas. Smoking on the job site potentially allows volatilization of toxic materials if they contaminate the cigarette.[32] The lack of unionization and poor awareness of safety and health issues are typical of workplaces with small numbers of employees, particularly in subcontracting arrangements.[33] Taken together, all of this information points to a high potential risk and yet does not identify an exposure relevant to the diagnosis at hand. Indeed, when asked directly, the patient denies silica exposure.

To clarify the work history, taking a "work station" approach that goes through the entire work process from starting material to finished product can serve as a powerful focus in history taking.[12] The work station approach applies not merely to manufacturing but to service and white-collar occupations as well. Using this technique, one can learn about nearby work stations and potential exposures they may entail. In this case, despite the patient's high-exposure activities in painting, it is the sandblasting work station from which the causal silica exposure has arisen. The patient denied exposure to "silica," but a more generic question of "sand" might have yielded the correct response. Similarly, it may be useful to ask about exposure both to asbestos and to generic "insulation material."

This case also demonstrates that respiratory "protection" depends on a number of factors. The reported regular use of a cartridge-type face mask could reassure the history taker that appropriate respiratory protection was in place. However, the lack of maintenance with filter replacement indicates that the mask was likely to be ineffectual. It may also be useful to verify that the cartridge used, even if changed frequently, is of a type appropriate to the exposure in question.[1] History of formal respirator fit testing (i.e., properly determining that there is a tight seal of the mask against the face) is, unfortunately, quite uncommon, although it is required by certain OSHA regulations. The most salient point is that the respiratory protection reported for the painter was clearly inappropriate for sandblasting exposure, which is why the sandblaster used an air-supplied (positive-pressure) respirator. Even with that level of protection, it is important to clarify where the air *intake* is located—for example, near a gasoline-powered compressor, where carbon monoxide fumes might be entrained (such fumes may have accounted for the sandblaster's headaches).

CORE COMPONENTS OF THE OCCUPATIONAL AND ENVIRONMENTAL EXPOSURE HISTORY

These six case scenarios touch on the core aspects of an occupational and environmental history focused on respiratory disease. The box presents a brief outline of the key features of such a targeted history. The primary components include: understanding the job process, not just noting the job title; addressing potential off-the-job environmental exposures, including those from nonsalaried vocations, household work, and the ambient air; assessing the degree of exposure, even if indirectly, without the benefit of industrial hygiene monitoring; evaluating temporal and dose-response associations between exposure and illness; delineating protective measures used; gauging general hygienic conditions;

and finally, ruling out certain specific exposures of particular importance.

PHYSICAL EXAMINATION

Few occupational or environmental diseases present specific clinical findings. Children with lead intoxication may have a dark line along their gums, and adults with overexposure to phenoxy herbicides may have chloracne, but occupational and environmental respiratory diseases are not characterized by such pathognomonic features. It is difficult to distinguish byssinosis from chronic bronchitis caused by cigarette smoking, asbestosis from idiopathic pulmonary fibrosis, or chronic beryllium disease from sarcoidosis on the basis of clinical presentation alone. Only in the context of the exposure history will the correct diagnosis be made.

The physician suspecting the presence of occupational or environmental respiratory disease should, nonetheless, perform a complete physical examination rather than focus narrowly on possible findings suggested by the exposure history. Relevant non–exposure-related disease may otherwise be missed. For example, careful auscultation of the heart may reveal evidence of valvular heart disease that turns out to be a more important cause of the patient's dyspnea and exercise intolerance than his or her past asbestos exposure. The general appearance should be noted, especially for evidence of respiratory distress and chronic debilitating disease, such as end-stage lung disease or cancer. If the patient comes to the examination straight from work, it is wise to look for evidence of the level of workplace exposure, such as dust on the face and clothes or flash burns from welding. Tobacco-stained fingers and the presence of a cigarette pack in a shirt pocket are telling clues that a patient who claims that he or she has quit smoking is not telling the truth. The degree of difficulty breathing while speaking long sentences and walking on level ground or climbing steps can be helpful in determining the level of respiratory impairment. Hoarseness may be a sign of laryngeal inflammation or tumor. Involuntary coughing during the examination suggests that respiratory tract irritation is persistent. In addition to respiratory rate, blood pressure and pulse should be measured as signs of possible cardiovascular disease.

The head, eye, ear, nose, and throat examination can provide important evidence of mucosal inflammation when exposure to water-soluble respiratory tract irritants has occurred. Conjunctival erythema, sinus tenderness, nasal mucosal erythema and edema, rhinorrhea, and pharyngeal erythema are all signs consistent with irritant-induced injury. The presence of facial burns, either thermal or chemical, increases the probability of lower respiratory tract injury. Nasal ulcers can be caused by excessive exposure to chromium salts, and nasal polyps are a sign of allergic rhinitis, which may be occupational in origin. When a history of long-term occupational exposure to wood dust, formaldehyde, nickel compounds, or asbestos has been elicited,

---

Taking an occupational and environmental history: key questions in a targeted interview

Job and job process

What is your job title? What exactly do you do? What gets made (done) in your workplace? Take me, step by step, through the work process from starting material or first step to the finished product.

Describe the equipment you work with. Is there any power equipment around you? (If so, how is that equipment powered?)

Is the process a closed system or an open system? (If closed, is it opened at certain times for sampling, for mixing, or from leaks?)

Who does maintenance and how often? Where are you at those times?

What other work stations are near your work station?

Exposure levels

Do you see dust or mist in the air at your work site? Can you see nearby clearly?

Is there a strong smell or taste? (If so, does it then go away?)

Are surfaces dusty or damp? Is paint peeling, discolored, or damp?

Do you blow dust out from your nose or cough it up by day's end? Do you have direct skin contact with the materials you use?

Do you work in a room without windows or other general ventilation?

Is there any special ventilation, air conditioning, suction, fan, or laboratory fume hood? (If so, where does the ventilation air come from? Is the airflow or air exchange known? Are filters changed and checked?)

Is your work in a space originally designed for its current use?

Has anyone ever come to your job site and carried out any kind of air monitoring or sampling for a specific exposure or substance?

General hygiene

How many employees are there at your workplace? Does anyone else have symptoms on the job? (If so, which jobs?)

Do you eat in the workplace? Does anyone smoke in the workplace?

Are you provided with a uniform? (If so, is it left there?)

Is your job unionized? Is there a health and safety committee?

Did you ever receive specific chemical safety training?

Temporal aspects

Are your symptoms different on the first day of your workweek. . . at the end of the first shift. . . at the end of the workweek. . . at the end of the shift when you go home . . . days off. . . vacation?

Has there been any change in the job process, the product, or your duties?

Respiratory precautions

Is any kind of mask available or provided to you? (If so, how often and under what circumstances do you wear it? What kind of mask: Disposable paper? Screw-in cartridge? Type? When is it changed? Air-supplied? Where is the air supply intake located?)

Were you ever specially tested to see whether you could wear a mask?

Environmental factors

Does anyone else at home have similar symptoms? Do you own pets or livestock? Has there been any recent construction or refurbishing, either at home or at work?

Do you do any crafts or artwork? Do you have any hobbies or second vocations? Do you do any unusual or heavy maintenance, auto repair, or gardening? Does anyone bring home dusty or contaminated work clothes?

Do you live or work near any specific air pollution sources?

How is your home heated and cooled? (If so, are there any problems with these systems?)

Specific exposures

Were you ever around asbestos. . . insulation material. . . heat-resistant material? (If so, was it dusty, or did you disturb it?)

Have you ever worked around silica. . . sand. . . abrasives. . . sandblasting. . . mining, quarrying, or crushing? Have you ever done blasting work? Have you ever used two-part glues, coatings, or products that had to be mixed just before they "set" or hardened? Have you ever used polyurethane or epoxy? Have you ever used solvents or degreasers? (If so, did you get dizzy or "drunk"?) Have you ever done construction or shipyard work? Ever had any military exposures?

Are there any dusts, fumes, or other exposures at work or at home that I haven't asked about that you think might be important?

---

the examination should be directed toward the possibility of head and neck tumors.

The examination of the chest in patients with suspected occupational and environmental lung disease need be no different than in patients with other types of lung disease. The examination should include inspection, percussion, and auscultation. Hyperexpansion of the chest suggests the presence of emphysema, which is much more likely to be caused by cigarette smoking than by occupational exposures. Chest percussion may provide evidence of lobar consolidation, a pleural effusion, or a large tumor mass. The character of adventitious breath sounds should be described during both resting tidal breathing and slow, deep breaths. The relative duration of inspiration and expiration should be noted,[34] although a recent study documented the relatively low specificity of prolonged expiration as a sign of airway obstruction.[35] Any wheezing, rhonchi, or crackles should be described as to intensity, location, and phase of the respiratory cycle. The presence of wheezing, rhonchi, crackles, or pleural rubs upon chest auscultation is presumptive evidence of respiratory tract disease.

Wheezing is produced by turbulent flow through an airway(s). Wheezing heard only during inspiration suggests upper airway obstruction and should prompt a more thorough examination of the neck for evidence of stridor. Expiratory wheezing usually indicates intrathoracic bronchoconstriction. Unilateral expiratory wheezing in a patient with exposure to a lung carcinogen is a finding that warrants further work-up for an obstructing tumor. It is difficult to assess the severity of bronchoconstriction on the basis of physical examination findings alone, although wheezing heard during both inspiration and expiration is evidence of more severe bronchoconstriction (because the caliber of the intrathoracic airways is normally greater during inspiration, when the lungs expand because of the negative intrapleural pressure generated). One study demonstrated that chest auscultation for wheezing, even with maximal forced exhalation, is neither a sensitive nor specific test for the detection of asthma in patients with normal or near-normal baseline spirometry.[36] Another study showed that pulmonary physicians were not much better than chance alone at predicting the results of methacholine inhalation challenge tests based on history and physical findings.[37]

It is important to recognize the relative lack of sensitivity and specificity of historical features and physical findings when evaluating patients with possible occupational asthma away from the workplace. On the other hand, wheezing heard only after a certain exposure at work should be considered a sign of potential occupational asthma. Auscultation of rhonchi suggests the presence of increased airway secretions and is thus a sign of bronchitis. Because airway inflammation (i.e., bronchitis) is a key feature of asthma, rhonchi can be a presenting sign of this disease.

Inspiratory rales, or crackles, are thought to be generated from the explosive equalization of gas pressure between two areas of the lung when a closed small airway between them is suddenly opened.[38] The presence of crackles is usually a sign of abnormal lung parenchyma. Atelectasis, pneumonia, noninfectious inflammation, interstitial fibrosis, and left ventricular failure are all causes of crackles. The sound quality of crackles is thought to be a clue to the type of disease process. For example, late-inspiratory, "fine," "dry," or "Velcro-like" crackles heard posterolaterally at the lung bases are supposed to indicate the presence of interstitial lung disease.[39] It is important, however, to check for their persistence following coughing before recording this finding as evidence of interstitial lung disease.[39] Unfortunately, persistent crackles are often a late finding in interstitial lung disease, suggesting that fibrosis has already developed.[39] The original British exposure standard for asbestos was based on auscultation of inspiratory crackles, and Murphy et al. have demonstrated a reasonable degree of correlation between electronic stethoscope-derived data on the intensity of such crackles and chest radiographic evidence of asbestosis.[40] Although specific data are lacking, it is likely that the sensitivity of chest auscultation for diagnosing asbestosis is low. There are data, however, that suggest that crackles may occur before asbestosis is detected on chest radiographs,[41] and crackles appear to be more common in asbestosis than in other types of interstitial lung disease.[42] In a case of mild hypersensitivity pneumonitis, intermittent crackles may be the only abnormal physical finding, so that with an appropriate exposure history, this observation should suggest further evaluation.

The so-called "coarse" or "wet" crackles of pulmonary edema are supposed to sound different than those of interstitial fibrosis, but most physicians are not able to reproducibly distinguish wet from dry crackles.[43] Therefore, examination of the cardiovascular system for evidence of left ventricular failure is important whenever crackles are heard. Of course, noncardiogenic pulmonary edema as a result of toxic inhalation injury (e.g., oxides of nitrogen or phosgene) is another potential cause of wet crackles. Flooded alveoli produce the same kind of crackling sound whether the source of the alveolar fluid is elevated hydrostatic pressure or injury to the alveolar-capillary membrane.

A pleural rub can occur with asbestos-related pleural fibrosis, and the signs of a pleural effusion (increased dullness to percussion, decreased breath sounds, and egophony at the level of the air-fluid interface) can be caused by a benign asbestos effusion, lung cancer, or mesothelioma.

The examining physician should look for evidence of pulmonary hypertension, cor pulmonale, and right ventricular failure when chronic obstructive or interstitial lung disease is suspected. The buccal mucosa, lips, and nail beds should be inspected for cyanosis. Because occupational exposures are much more likely to contribute to chronic bronchitis than to emphysema, a classic "blue bloater" appearance is more likely to be seen in an affected worker than the "pink puffer" appearance of pure emphysema. The presence or absence of clubbing of the fingers and toes should also be noted. Clubbing may be caused by interstitial lung disease and, when present, is an indicator of relatively severe disease. Since clubbing does not usually occur with hypersensitivity pneumonitis or with pneumoconioses other than asbestosis, its presence in a patient with interstitial lung disease tends to exclude these diagnoses. Although the American Thoracic Society guidelines for the diagnosis of asbestosis include clubbing as one of the clinical criteria that supports the diagnosis,[44] the prevalence of clubbing in asbestosis is only about 20% with low-grade radiographic disease.[45] Because clubbing is not typically caused by chronic obstructive lung disease, its presence in a smoker means that lung cancer must be included in the list of differential diagnostic possibilities.

The physical examination may be helpful if abnormal, but one should remember that it is relatively insensitive for detection of mild respiratory tract injury. Pulmonary function and chest imaging studies may have greater sensitivity. In general, the physical examination is probably more useful for the detection of signs of nonrespiratory organ system dysfunction that could be contributing to disability, such as left ventricular failure, than in characterizing the level of respiratory impairment. An exception would be when there is evidence of end-stage disease, such as cyanosis or right ventricular failure.

SUMMARY

The linkage between an occupational or environmental risk factor and a specific respiratory disorder is often difficult to establish because the presentation of occupationally or environmentally caused illness is rarely pathognomonic. It is first necessary to have a high index of suspicion that occupational or environmental risk factors may be playing a role in a patient's illness. A careful but targeted history may then provide appropriate evidence to support the diagnosis of an exposure-related respiratory disorder. The approach to such a history, outlined in the box earlier, will allow occupational or environmental respiratory disease to be ruled in or out in most cases. Finally, a thorough physical examination is essential, not only to confirm the suspected diagnosis but to exclude non–exposure-related or even extrapulmonary etiologies.

REFERENCES

1. Occupational and Environmental Health Committee of the American Lung Association of San Diego: Taking the occupational history, *Ann Intern Med* 99:641-651, 1983.
2. Goldman RH and Peters JM: The occupational and environmental health history, *JAMA* 246:2831-2836, 1981.
3. Landrigan PJ and Baker DB: Using the occupational history to pinpoint the diagnosis, *Geriatrics* 46:61-67, 1991.
4. Perry GF: Occupational health history: an often neglected part of medical education, *Ind Med* 84:402-404, 1991.
5. Becker CE: Key elements of the occupational history for the general physician, *West J Med* 137:581-582, 1982.
6. Agency for Toxic Substances and Disease Registry: Obtaining an exposure history, *Am Fam Physician* 48:483-491, 1993.
7. American College of Physicians: *The role of the internist in occupational medicine: a position paper of the American College of Physicians*, Philadelphia, 1984, American College of Physicians.
8. Schwartz DA, Wakefield DS, Fieselmann JF, et al: The occupational history in the primary care setting, *Am J Med* 90:315-319, 1991.
9. Landrigan PJ and Baker DB: The recognition and control of occupational disease, *JAMA* 266:676-680, 1991.
10. Institute of Medicine, Division of Health Promotion and Disease Prevention: *Role of the primary care physician in occupational environmental medicine*, Washington, D.C., 1988, National Academy Press.
11. Bernstein IL, Chan-Yeung M, Malo J-L, et al, editors: *Asthma in the workplace*, New York, 1993, Dekker.
12. Burgess WA: *Recognition of health hazards in industry: a review of materials and processes*, New York, 1981, Wiley.
13. Lerman SE: Material Safety Data Sheets: caveat emptor, *Arch Intern Med* 150:981-984, 1990.
14. McCann M: *Artist beware: the hazards and precautions in working with art and craft materials*, New York, 1979, Watson-Guptill.
15. Snyder RW, Mishel HS, and Christensen GC: Pulmonary toxicity following exposure to methylene chloride and its combustion product, phosgene, *Chest* 101:860-861, 1992.
16. Shusterman DJ and Peterson JE, editors: De novo toxicants: combustion toxicology, mixing incompatibilities, and environmental activation of toxic agents, *Occup Med: State Art Rev* 8(3), 1993.
17. Centers for Disease Control: Chlorine gas toxicity from mixture of bleach with other cleaning products—California, *Morbid Mortal Week Rep* 40:619-621, 627-629, 1991.
18. National Institute for Occupational Safety and Health (NIOSH): *Criteria for a recommended standard: working in confined spaces*, Department of Health and Human Services (NIOSH) Pub No 80-106, Morgantown, WVa, 1979, NIOSH.
19. Greenberg SR: The confined space: a review of a recently discerned medical entity, *Am J Forens Med Pathol* 10:31-36, 1989.
20. Centers for Disease Control: Acute effect of indoor exposure to paint containing bis(tributyltin) oxide—Wisconsin, 1991, *Morbid Mortal Week Rep* 40:280-281, 1991.
21. Samet JM and Spengler JD, editors: *Indoor air pollution: a health perspective*, Baltimore, 1991, Johns Hopkins University Press.
22. Shusterman DJ and Sheedy JE: Occupational and environmental disorders of the special senses, *Occup Med: State Art Rev* 7:515-542, 1992.
23. Blanc PD, Maizlish N, Hiatt P, et al: Occupational illness and the Poison Control Center: referral patterns and service needs, *West J Med* 152:181-184, 1990.
24. Cohen R: Occupational infections. In LaDou J, editor: *Occupational medicine*, pp 170-181, Norwalk, Conn, 1990, Appleton & Lange.
25. Davies SF and Colbert RL: Concurrent human and canine histoplasmosis from cutting decayed wood, *Ann Intern Med* 113:252-253, 1990.
26. Von Essen S, Robbins RA, Thompson AB, et al: Organic dust toxic syndrome: an acute febrile reaction distinct from hypersensitivity pneumonitis, *Clin Toxicol* 28:389-420, 1990.
27. Belville R, Pollack SH, Godbold JH, et al: Occupational injuries among working adolescents in New York State, *JAMA* 269:2754-2759, 1993.
28. Blanc PD, Katz P, and Yelin E: Mortality risk among elderly workers, *Am J Ind Med* 26:543-547, 1994.
29. Centers for Disease Control: Sulfur dioxide exposure in Portland cement plants, *Morbid Mortal Week Rep* 33:195-196, 1984.
30. Blanc PD and Golden JA: Unusual occupationally-related disorders of the lung: case reports and a literature review, *Occup Med: State Art Rev* 7:403-422, 1992.
31. Grandjean P, Berlin A, Gilbert M, et al: Preventing percutaneous absorption of industrial chemicals: the "skin" denotation, *Am J Ind Med* 14:97-107, 1988.
32. Centers for Disease Control: Polymer-fume fever associated with cigarette smoking and the use of tetrafluoroethylene—Mississippi, *Morbid Mortal Week Rep* 36:515-516, 521-522, 1987.
33. Blanc PD, Galbo MS, Balmes JR, et al: Occupational factors in work-related inhalations: inferences for prevention strategy, *Am J Ind Med* 25:783-791, 1994.
34. Macdonald JB, Cole TJ, and Seaton A: Forced expiratory time—its reliability as a lung function test, *Thorax* 30:554-559, 1975.
35. Kern DG and Patel SR: Auscultated forced expiratory time as a clinical and epidemiologic test of airway obstruction, *Chest* 100:636-639, 1991.
36. King DK, Taylor Thompson B, and Johnson DC: Wheezing on maximal forced exhalation in the diagnosis of atypical asthma: lack of sensitivity and specificity, *Ann Intern Med* 110:451-455, 1989.
37. Dales RE, Nunes F, Partyka D, et al: Clinical prediction of airways hyperresponsiveness, *Chest* 93:984-986, 1988.

38. Forgacs P: The functional basis of pulmonary sounds, *Chest* 73:399-405, 1978.

39. Nath AR, Capel LH: Inspiratory crackles and mechanical events of breathing, *Thorax* 29:695-698, 1974.

40. Murphy RLH, Gaensler EA, Holford S, et al: Crackles in the early detection of asbestosis, *Am Rev Respir Dis* 129:375-379, 1984.

41. Shirai F, Kudoh S, Shibuya A, et al: Crackles in asbestos workers: auscultation and lung sound analysis, *Br J Dis Chest* 75:386-396, 1981.

42. Epler GR, Carrington CB, and Gaensler EA: Crackles (rales) in the interstitial pulmonary diseases, *Chest* 73:333-339, 1978.

43. Hudson LD, Conn RD, Matsubara RS, et al: Rales: diagnostic uselessness of qualitative adjectives, *Am Rev Respir Dis* 113(4, part 2):187, 1976.

44. American Thoracic Society: The diagnosis of nonmalignant disease related to asbestos, *Am Rev Respir Dis* 134:363-368, 1986.

45. Huuskonen MS: Clinical features, mortality, and survival of patients with asbestosis, *Scand J Work Environ Health* 4:265-274, 1978.

Chapter 4

PHYSIOLOGIC METHODS

Paul D. Scanlon
John Hankinson

Physiologic methods for the assessment of occupational and environmental diseases provide objective measurements to correlate with clinical assessments and other laboratory studies. Many of these are common and familiar tests used daily in the clinical practice of primary care medicine as well as occupational and pulmonary medicine. In the evaluation of occupational and environmental respiratory disorders, issues of cost control, large-population screening, and quality control are more critical issues than in general medical practice. This chapter reviews methods for physiologic measurements with an emphasis on spirometry, the most commonly used test of respiratory function.

HISTORY

After the introduction of the clinical use of auscultation by Laennec in the early nineteenth century, the next major advance in the quantitative assessment of respiratory disorders was made by Hutchinson, who, in 1848, published his studies on using a water displacement volume spirometer to measure the vital capacity of a large number of English subjects. In his treatise he described the relationships between vital capacity (VC) and body size, sex, and disease states.[1]

There was little change in the clinical application of spirometry for the next 80 years, during which tuberculosis remained the most important pulmonary disease. During the 1940s and 1950s tuberculosis prevalence declined, and the epidemic of chronic obstructive pulmonary disease (COPD) related to tobacco smoking began. This added to the established population of asthmatics and prompted the development and clinical use of time-based spirometric measurements. After World War II the development of newer physiologic techniques for evaluation of obstructive airways disorders promoted a deeper understanding of lung mechanics and the physiologic basis of airflow obstruction.

In the 1960s and 1970s inflammation and fibrosis of the terminal bronchiole were observed to be the earliest histologic abnormalities in cigarette smokers who may develop COPD. A search for sensitive methods to identify "early small airways disease" led to development of an array of tests, including different measurements from flow and volume tracings from the forced vital capacity (FVC) maneuver and other more specialized techniques.[2,3]

In 1979 the American Thoracic Society (ATS) published its first standards paper for spirometry testing, the so-called "Snowbird standard."[4] At that time there was a great deal of variation in the quality of instrumentation and many instruments that did not meet any minimal standard of performance. A performance evaluation of spirometers in 1980 found that no flow-based spirometer, and only 8 of 12 volume-based spirometers, performed to standards.[5] With the publication of the revised spirometry standards paper in 1987,[6] the equipment design and performance specifications were better defined. A review in 1990, using more modern, computerized spirometers, was also disappointing, in that only 57% of spirometers performed adequately when tested against 24 standard waveforms specified by the ATS.[7] Frequent software errors (25%) were thought to be responsible for some of the poor performances.[8]

In recent years computerized, automated spirometers have been developed, which are compact and simple to use. Some have standardized quality control procedures, high-quality reporting capabilities, and long-term data storage capability. These are needed to make testing for occupational or environmental disease a helpful clinical tool. The current debate over allocation of health care resources highlights the importance of cost effectiveness in both the health care setting and the occupational setting. Although the best devices and procedures may be complex, computerization can make these procedures efficient and cost effective.

SPIROMETRY
Instrumentation

To perform spirometry, the device used must be able to measure either expiratory airflow or volume of expired air, as a function of time. Since flow is the first time derivative of volume and, conversely, volume is the time-based integral of flow, automated spirometers can measure one and derive the other by simple electronic or digital differentiation or integration. In the majority of clinical testing sites in the United States, the cost of technician time is sufficient to justify an automated computerized or microprocessor-controlled spirometer to save the techni-

cian time in making measurements and hand calculations from tracings of FVC maneuvers.

Volume spirometers. All volume spirometers collect exhaled gas and measure the volume displaced within the spirometer as a function of time. The simplest volume spirometers have a mechanical linkage between the air collection reservoir and a recording device, which generates a volume-time tracing. More sophisticated devices can record volume as a function of time with a microprocessor or microcomputer. This signal can be differentiated to obtain flow. Analysis can then be performed with either a volume-time or flow-volume curve (Fig. 4-1). Advantages of a volume spirometer include a greater degree of certainty (with some devices) of the volume collected, simplicity of design, and ease of maintenance with some models. Disadvantages include insensitivity to rapid flow transients (peak flow may be underestimated), difficulty in cleaning some models, and large size and weight, which limit portability.

Flow spirometers. A great variety of flow-measuring devices have been used in recent years, including pneumotachographs, other resistor-type flow-measuring devices, heated wire flow elements (sometimes called mass flow elements), turbine devices, and others. Virtually all flow-based spirometers use a microprocessor or microcomputer to translate signals of the flow-measuring device into a linearized flow signal, which is then integrated to obtain volume. The advantages of flow spirometers include light weight (and therefore portability); inexpensive, disposable flow elements for some; ease of cleaning for others; and sensitivity to rapid flow transients. Whether a volume- or flow-based spirometer is chosen, the best spirometers have comparable accuracy and precision.

Disadvantages of flow-based spirometers include: (1) *Errors in volume measurement if flows exceed calibrated linear flow ranges.* Many flow elements are nonlinear at high flows. If the microprocessor does not take nonlinearities into account, significant errors can occur in peak flow, forced expiratory volume in the first second of the FVC maneuver (FEV1), and VC. (2) *Errors in VC if zero flow is not correctly determined* (e.g., an error of 25 ml/sec in the zero flow signal will result in a 250-ml error in VC for a 10-second maneuver). (3) *Software errors in calculation or maneuver error detection.* Since we are dependent on microprocessor or microcomputer software, errors can be subtle and difficult to detect. A recent review of commercially available spirometers found many with performance deficiencies, 25% of which were attributed to software problems.[8] (4) *Loss of data.* The absence of a mechanical linkage for hard-copy recording on some devices can lead to loss of data if computers malfunction or technicians inadvertently delete data. (5) *Calibration errors.* Failure to calibrate spirometers on a regular basis and to check results can lead to systematic bias in data.

Equipment specifications. Performance requirements for spirometers of either type were described in the 1987

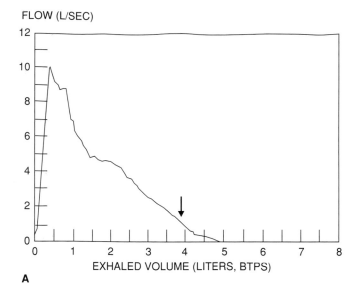

FLOW (L/SEC)

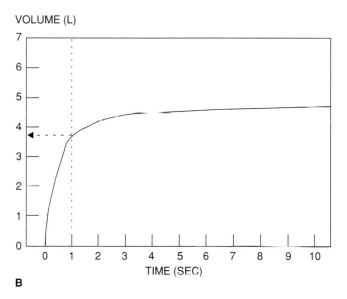

VOLUME (L)

TIME (SEC)

B

Fig. 4-1. A, Flow-volume and **B,** volume-time curves representing a single forced vital capacity maneuver. The flow-volume curve typically has a roughly triangular shape. By convention total lung capacity is shown at left. At any given lung volume, flow has a maximal achievable value. The shape of the flow-volume curve for any individual should be very reproducible, including irregularities or "bumps." The volume-time tracing provides less quality control information, but can be generated by a simple mechanical linkage with noncomputerized equipment. Volume is adjusted to body temperature and pressure, saturated (BTPS). (Adapted from Enright PL and Hyatt RE: Office spirometry: a practical guide to the selection and use of spirometer, Philadelphia, 1987, Lea & Febiger.)

spirometry standards.[6] A series of 24 standardized waveforms have been developed that can be used for testing spirometers' compliance with equipment standards.[7] Data displays have likewise been standardized. At least one independent laboratory performs equipment validation stud

ies to assess conformity with ATS standards for equipment performance.[8] Some spirometer manufacturers use an internal equipment performance evaluation program to ensure equipment performance.

Procedures

The FVC maneuver, a maximal expiratory effort beginning at total lung capacity (TLC) and ending at residual volume, is the basis for most spirometry tests. Human lungs have a maximal achievable flow at lung volumes below about 75% of TLC. As a result the effort required to perform reproducible maneuvers is not great; therefore, most well-coached subjects can perform acceptable and reproducible maneuvers, even patients with serious respiratory disorders. Variations in the FVC maneuver may be caused by variation in maximal expiratory flow rates and lung volumes, as well as variations in depth of inspiration, force of expiration, and depth of expiration.

Measurements

FVC. The most basic measurement from the FVC maneuver is the FVC itself. The amount of air collected in the volume spirometer, or the amount of air calculated from the integration of flow over time, is adjusted to allow for the fact that air is warm and humid while in the lungs but colder and sometimes dry in the spirometer. The volume is therefore lower in the spirometer. The ideal gas laws are applied to calculate the volume as it was while the air was in the lungs (BTPS correction). A variety of strategies have been developed to determine the instantaneous temperature and humidity of the air as it is measured.[9,10]

Hutchinson observed in 1848 that the VC is reduced in subjects with lung disease.[1] It is still the simplest and one of the best measurements to quantify the degree of respiratory impairment, particularly in restrictive disorders.

FEV1. The FEV1 is the most reproducible measurement used in pulmonary function testing. In the presence of airflow obstruction, the amount of air exhaled in the first second is reduced. The FEV1 is used to quantify the degree or severity of obstruction.[11] FEV1 is a strong predictor of total mortality and mortality caused by respiratory and cardiac disorders.[12]

FEV1/FVC or FEV1/VC ratio. The ratio of the FEV1 to the FVC or VC is used as an indicator of the presence of airflow obstruction. When flow is reduced, the fraction of the VC exhaled in the first second is reduced. Typically, 70% to 80% of the VC is exhaled in the first second of an FVC maneuver (this value is lower in older subjects). This can be reduced to 30% or less in patients with severe airflow obstruction. Because of gas trapping, VC is often reduced in subjects with severe obstruction. As a result the quantitative relationship between the FEV1/FVC ratio and the severity of obstruction is poor. Therefore it is recommended that the FEV1/FVC ratio be used only to indicate the presence of obstruction, not to quantify the severity of obstruction. Because FVC is often lower than the slow VC, some authors recommend using the VC rather than the FVC in the denominator. The FEV1/VC ratio is commonly used in Europe and is sometimes known as the Tiffeneau-Votchal index. In North America most predicted values are determined using the FEV1/FVC ratio.[13]

FEF25–75% (forced expiratory flow from 25% to 75% of vital capacity). A number of studies have attempted to detect mild airways obstruction in cigarette smokers and in workers exposed to substances that can cause obstruction. The quest for the "Holy Grail" never succeeded. Likewise, the search for the best indicator of small airways disease has not been productive. Among the measurements identified as having a high positive rate in patients with mild airflow obstruction, the FEF25-75 was once thought to be one of the most sensitive, as well as the least expensive and easiest to do. Unfortunately, it is not very reproducible, and although it is fairly sensitive for mild airflow obstruction, it is nonspecific. It has not been shown to correlate well with the histologic presence of small airways disease.[3,13]

Maximal expiratory flow, or peak flow. Maximal expiratory (or peak) flow is discussed later in this chapter.

Other measurements. A great variety of other measurements from the FVC maneuver have been used, including FEV3, FEV6, FEF75-85, FEF25, FEF50, FEF75, and others. It is not recommended that these be used, since no standards exist for comparisons. They provide no information that is not also provided by the measurements described previously plus the flow-volume curve, or volume-time tracing. A long array of these measurements can clutter pulmonary function test reports to the point that they can be mind-numbing to those who do not use them regularly. For the sake of simplicity and for better communication with our colleagues, we recommend keeping reports as simple as possible.

Several authors have argued that FVC should be terminated after 7 or 10 seconds (FEV7 or FEV10) to improve uniformity of end-of-test determination. Although there are reasonable arguments for these ideas, they require further evaluation and have not yet been generally accepted.[9]

Sources of variation in lung function

The process of interpreting test results involves determination of the significance of the test result for the test subject. An attempt is made to determine how well the result represents the subject and to compare the result with a reference or normal value. Variation of the test result from a predicted value may be due to the presence of disease; however, it may also be due to another unwelcome source of variation.[13,14] There are a number of technical sources of variation that can be controlled with optimal testing system design. Instrument performance can be ensured with sound initial system design, careful individual instrument evaluation, regular calibration, careful maintenance, and continued monitoring of equipment performance. Technician performance can vary with training, aptitude, and experience, but can be improved with a careful quality control feedback system.[15] Environmental conditions can affect test results if extreme or if not properly considered in making calculations.[6]

Intraindividual sources of variability include comprehension, motivation and effort, body position, and temporal timing of testing (circadian and menstrual cycle variability have been demonstrated). The most important interindividual sources of variability and the factors used as predictors of normal values for spirometry include height, age, sex, and race.[13]

Height. Height is a powerful predictor of spirometric measurements. Most equations for predicting spirometric variables vary in direct proportion to height. Seated height or arm span are sometimes used as a surrogate for standing height. Stated height is not accurate enough, so virtually all research studies and most clinical laboratories use measured standing height for obtaining predicted values. Because predicted equations are derived from normal populations, extremes of height are not well represented and comparisons with predicted values at extremes of height or age must be made with caution. Weight is a relatively poor predictor of lung function, producing rather small effect at high and low extremes.[16]

Age. Spirometry variables increase during childhood and adolescence. Maximal spirometric values, as a function of lung growth, are reached in the late teens or early 20s. Lung function is thought to be relatively stable until the mid to late 30s, at which point there is a gradual but accelerating decline in lung function.[17] FEV1 and FVC both decline by approximately 25 to 30 ml/yr after age 35 to 40 and more rapidly in older persons. These "normal" changes with age must be taken into account when evaluating the longitudinal change in lung function (see the section on analysis of trends).

Sex. Men of a given height and age have slightly greater lung volumes and maximal flows than women. Most equations for predicted values use separate equations for men and women.

Race. Most published equations for calculating predicted values have been derived from groups of white North American or European subjects. Far fewer studies have been done with African, Asian, or Native American subjects. Even less is known about the effect of mixed ancestry on pulmonary function. The current practice in most laboratories is to use predicted equations derived from white populations. For descendants of African or Asian natives (but not Native Americans), predicted values are adjusted with a "race correction" or "ethnic correction" factor, which is a multiplier between 0.85 and 0.90. This adjusts for the slightly smaller lung volumes (for a given height) of individuals in these populations, compared with the populations from which the standards were derived. Many subjects have mixed ancestry. There is no published recommendation for choosing predicted values for these subjects. In the absence of a better recommendation, most laboratories use race as stated or as reported on income tax forms or on the government census.

Other sources. Other between-subject variations that are predictive of pulmonary function, but for which predicted values are not adjusted, include personal exposure history, including cigarette smoking and occupational exposure; personal health history; socioeconomic factors; and presence of airways hyperresponsiveness and atopy. All of these have significant effects but are related to disease processes, not normal variations.

A normal population sample will have a range of variation distributed around predicted values. This range of variation is not just a simple percentage variation (i.e., 80% of the predicted value is not always the lower limit of normal). Young and tall normal subjects have less scatter around the normal value than do shorter and older normal subjects.[18] There are additional subject-to-subject, day-to-day, and test-to-test variations. Month-to-month variation, with an excellent testing technique, can be less than 6%.[15] Day-to-day variation for an individual subject is approximately 200 to 250 ml for both FEV1 and FVC (K.C. Beck and P.D. Scanlon, unpublished data 1991). Note that these variations are much larger than the average annual declines in FEV1 and FVC.

Testing quality control

Proper spirometry technique is essential for obtaining useful data in any testing program. The basic specifications for performance of spirometry are in the 1987 ATS spirometry standardization paper.[6] The paper includes specifications for equipment performance, FVC maneuver performance, measurements, and acceptability and reproducibility criteria.

A thorough quality control program can provide better reproducibility of measurements in long-term repeated testing.[15] This will allow much greater confidence in the significance of changes over time. A thorough quality control program includes (1) selection of high-quality equipment; (2) careful training and monitoring of technicians to ensure that tests are performed according to strict standards; (3) regularly scheduled (preferably daily) calibration using a calibration syringe; (4) a regular program of "biologic quality control" using healthy subjects, usually technicians, who are tested repeatedly to ensure that the global function of the equipment (over and above calibration syringe or other simple calibration) is stable; (5) careful instruction of the test subject, demonstrating the maneuver; (6) vigorous encouragement of maximal effort; (7) performance of multiple efforts until acceptable and reproducible maneuvers are performed (see Table 4-1); (8) selection and reporting of the best effort performed, along with an

Table 4-1. Acceptability and reproducibility criteria[6]

Acceptability: technician's observations of each forced vital capacity (FVC) maneuver
1. Maximal inspiration at start
2. Maximal expiratory effort with no hesitation or false start
   Extrapolated volume <5% of FVC or <100 ml
3. No cough or discontinuity of effort in the first second
4. No obstruction of airflow by mouthpiece, tongue, teeth, or glottis
5. Satisfactory end of effort
   Plateau on volume-time curve with <40 ml exhaled over the last 2 seconds
   Usually at least 6 seconds, often longer
6. No leak (e.g., from nose, lips, mouthpiece, hose, or spirometer)

Reproducibility

Largest and second largest FVC within 5% or 100 ml
Largest and second largest forced expiratory volume in 1 second (FEV1) within 5% or 100 ml

Reporting

A testing session may consist of three to eight acceptable efforts.
Failure to meet acceptability and reproducibility criteria should be noted. The largest FEV1 and the largest FVC from all acceptable maneuvers should be reported.

Adapted from American Thoracic Society: Standardization of spirometry—1987 update, *Am Rev Respir Dis* 136;1285-1298, 1987.

indication of the quality of effort; (9) posttest review of the quality of results with feedback to the performing technician; (10) interpretation of the test by a qualified physician; and (11) long-term secure storage of data for future comparison.

Test interpretation

Interpretation of spirometry results is generally performed by a physician, usually a pulmonary disease specialist or allergist. There are few statutory regulations regarding qualifications of the interpreter. The ATS has published a position paper on the qualifications and responsibilities of the director of the pulmonary function laboratory.[19] The most important qualifications are a strong background in pulmonary physiology and medical instrumentation and experience in clinical and laboratory evaluation of patients with respiratory disorders.

The first step in interpreting pulmonary function data is assessment of the reliability of the data. A strong quality control program will have objective information to inform the interpreter about subject cooperation, level of understanding, degree of effort, any unusual testing conditions, and pertinent or necessary clinical information for correlation.

The next step is comparison of the data with the normal reference or predicted value for the subject.[13] Predicted values are derived from populations of subjects thought to rep resent the spectrum of normal lung function. Current or former smokers are usually excluded from such populations. The data from the test subject must be compared with the predicted values using the question— Are the predicted values representative of what would be expected to be normal for the test subject? For test subjects who are at the extremes of height or age, the predictive equations may not represent truly normal values as well as for subjects of average height and age. Many predictive equations behave poorly in extreme value ranges. Many ethnic groups are not well studied, and their lung function may vary significantly from values established with European and North American studies. Genetic diversity is greater among African- Americans than with any other ethnic group. To use a single multiplier as a "race correction factor" is simplistic at best. We also have difficulty in determining what is normal for subjects who are not measurable or proportioned normally, such as patients whose height is affected by spinal deformity, those who cannot stand, and others. Use of arm span or seated height as a surrogate for standing height introduces another variable into consideration.

The upper or lower limit of the normal range is not a simple multiplier. A simplistic categorization includes 20% above and 20% below the normal value as the normal range. This is clearly incorrect, since there is a wider range of normal in the elderly and in short subjects than in those who are young or tall. A $\pm 20\%$ range will misclassify some abnormal subjects in the latter group and some normal subjects in the former group.[13,20]

In comparing predicted values with test data, we generally look for one of the common ventilatory defects: obstruction or restriction. An obstructive defect may be considered a "disproportionate reduction of maximal airflow from the lung with respect to the maximal volume (VC) that can be displaced from the lung."[13] The flow-volume curve in obstructive disorders typically has a scooped-out shape, concave downward at volumes below maximal flow. Other, less common disorders, such as a tracheal obstructive lesion, can cause a reduction in all flows so that the flow-volume curve has a plateau (Fig. 4-2). In most cases of obstruction, the FEV1/FVC ratio will be reduced. Most interpretive strategies look first at the flow-volume curve and the FEV1/FVC ratio for evidence of obstruction. If the shape of the curve and a low FEV1/FVC ratio support that judgment, the degree of obstruction is quantified on the basis of the degree of reduction in the FEV1 compared with the predicted value.[11,13]

In older subjects it is common to see concavity of the flow-volume curve at low lung volumes with very low flows near residual volume, despite a normal FEV1/FVC ratio. Some interpreters consider this finding, or a relatively low FEF25-75, indicative of small airways disease. This practice is not recommended since these findings are nonspecific and have not been shown to correlate with progres-

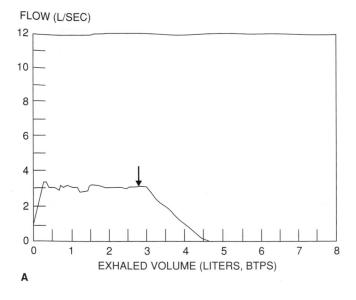

A

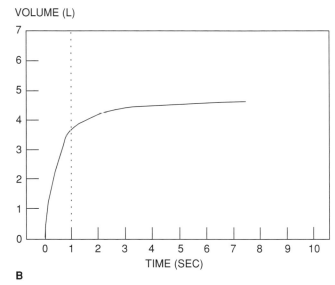

B

Fig. 4-2. A, Flow–volume curve from a patient with tracheal obstruction. **B,** The plateau indicates central airway expiratory flow limitation. This can occur from intrathoracic pathology (e.g., a tracheal tumor, stenosis, or stricture) or from extrathoracic pathology (e.g., subglottic stenosis, an obstructing goiter or tumor, or vocal cord obstruction). This degree of flow limitation cannot occur if only one main stem bronchus is obstructed. Volume is adjusted to body temperature and pressure, saturated (BTPS). (Adapted from Enright PL and Hyatt RE: Office spirometry: a practical guide to the selection and use of spirometer, Philadelphia, 1987, Lea & Febiger.)

sion to more serious impairment. This topic is discussed earlier in this chapter, under FEF25–75%.

A restrictive defect is present when there is reduction in lung volumes. This may be due to a reduction in TLC or to a nonobstructive increase in residual volume resulting in a reduced VC (in patients with a neuromuscular restrictive disorder). The degree of restriction is quantified by the reduction in VC compared with the predicted value. Although some authorities argue that the severity of restriction should be based on the degree of reduction in TLC,[13] this can lead to confusing interpretation of severe impairment due to neuromuscular weakness or chest wall deformity in patients with a normal or near-normal TLC. As many as 11% of patients tested in a clinical laboratory may have a normal TLC and FEV1/FVC ratio with a low VC.[21] This nonspecific pattern can be seen in patients with neuromuscular weakness, obesity, congestive heart failure, borderline restriction or obstruction, or poor effort.

Analysis of trends: cross-sectional versus longitudinal

When pulmonary function is measured at regular intervals, the resulting data must be looked at using a method other than simply comparing results with predicted values each year. A subject who began at 80% of the predicted value and remained stable is likely much better off than one who started at 120% of the predicted value and declined to 85% over 5 years of observation. Many ways of looking at trends in lung function have been proposed, including (1) monitoring the percentage of the predicted value for a drop below a critical threshold (e.g., 80%, or the 5th percentile); (2) evaluation of the annual change in values such as FEV1, expressed in milliliters per year or percentage[13]; and (3) use of percentile curves, as used for monitoring growth in children.[16]

After age 35 to 40 the annual rate of decline in FEV1 in adults is about 25 to 30 ml. The decline in FVC is similar.

There is an acceleration in the rate of decline with age. In cross-sectional studies the annual rate of decline may be more or less than in cohorts followed up longitudinally. A greater rate of decline in longitudinal studies may be attributed to survivor effects: the tendency of subjects with the lowest lung function to die or be lost to follow-up. A greater rate of decline in cross-sectional studies may be due to cohort effect: older groups may have worse underlying lung function and therefore appear to have a more rapid decline. Various epidemiologic studies have evaluated the cross-sectional and longitudinal decline of lung function over intervals of time (less than 15 years). Whether the short- to intermediate-term rate of decline can be projected to anticipate lung function much later in life remains controversial. In evaluating long-term trends in lung function, the most common statistical approach is to evaluate the linear regression of lung function over time. This does not take into account signal events that produce a sudden change in function or a change in the rate of decline of lung function. Other methods, such as percentile curves, may be helpful, but the large magnitude of random fluctuation in lung function makes interpretation difficult. Other factors, such as learning effect, can confound interpretation of periodic monitoring data.[22]

The ATS has recommended that a greater than 15% change from year to year be considered significant.[13] For example, in Figure 4-3 an individual starts with an FEV1 equal to the predicted value of 4.00 L (age 34). Eleven years later his level has dropped to 2.90 L (age 45). The value at

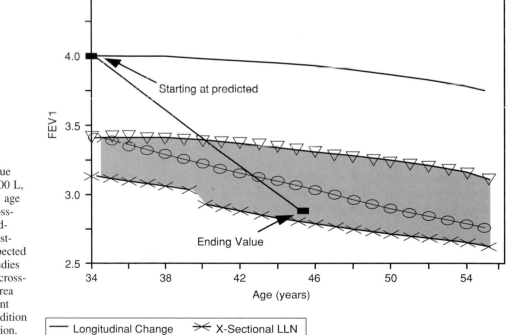

Fig. 4-3. Example of longitudinal change in FEV1 with the initial value starting at the predicted amount (4.00 L, age 34) and decreasing to 2.90 L at age 45. Comparisons are made with cross-sectional reference value and age adjusted 15% change limits. Age adjustments were performed using an expected longitudinal change from cohort studies ($\triangledown$)[23] and a 30-ml/yr change from cross-sectional studies ($\bigcirc$). The shaded area represents values at which significant changes in FEV1 occur with the addition of a 15% longitudinal change criterion. LLN, lower limit of normal; LAD, longitudinal age adjustment.

age 45 would still be above the lower limit of normal based on a cross-sectional reference value. However, the value at age 45 represents a greater than 15% change whether a longitudinal age adjustment[23] or a 30-ml/yr age adjustment is used. As can be seen in Fig. 4-3, longitudinal comparison may offer increased sensitivity over cross-sectional comparisons alone, particularly for those individuals whose initial values are at or above the predicted value.[24]

Often the most important function of the interpreting physician is to alert the clinician that a change has occurred for which clinical correlation is needed to determine the appropriate course of action or plan for continued monitoring.

Clinical uses of spirometry

Routine screening. Routine screening spirometry has been recommended for workers exposed to respiratory hazards. This was established for cotton workers by the Occupational Safety and Health Administration (OSHA) in the cotton dust standard in 1974.[25] Standards have been developed for workers exposed to asbestos and certain other occupational exposures.[26] These standards have in common the requirement that exposed workers be offered annual screening spirometry as part of an ongoing health-screening program. Screening spirometry may be performed at the work site or in the medical testing setting. Because of the large volume of testing required for a large number of workers, the cost of testing, quality control, and long-term data storage have become important issues (as discussed later in this chapter). The ATS has published an official statement on surveillance for respiratory hazards in the occupational setting and a more recent review is available.[27,28]

Diagnostic studies. For workers or patients who develop respiratory symptoms, diagnostic spirometry may be performed. Certain patterns of abnormality are known to correlate with specific disease entities (see the section on test interpretation). These laboratory results are incorporated as part of the diagnostic evaluation by the clinician. Follow-up studies may be performed to assess the response to therapy or to assess long-term trends during the course of a chronic illness.

Bronchodilator studies. Performance of spirometry before and after inhalation of a bronchodilator has been used to assess reversibility of airways obstruction. Interpretation of bronchodilator response is confounded by the test-to-test variability of bronchodilator response. Some patients will have differing responses to a bronchodilator on a day-to-day basis. The presence of bronchodilator responsiveness correlates with the degree of airway hyperresponsiveness as measured by methacholine challenge, but the correlation is loose. An acute response to the bronchodilator has been said to correlate with the clinical response to both bronchodilators and corticosteroid therapy in asthma and COPD. Several problems arise in evaluating the acute response to the bronchodilator in pulmonary function testing. First, the lack

of an acute bronchodilator response does not rule out the presence of airway hyperresponsiveness[29] and also does not preclude a beneficial clinical response to bronchodilator therapy. Second, there is a great deal of controversy over what constitutes a significant bronchodilator response. By this do we mean *clinically significant, statistically significant,* or *physiologically significant?* Determining the presence of a "significant response" can be done on the basis of changes in the flow-volume curve, a subjective judgment, plus the magnitude of the change in FEV1 expressed as a percentage increase (12%, by several authorities) or an absolute volume (greater than a 200-ml increase in FEV1). These issues were discussed in the 1991 ATS statement on lung function interpretation.[13]

Any of a variety of bronchodilator agents may be used. For purposes of convenience, most laboratories use inhaled β-agonists from metered-dose inhalers. Albuterol may be the most commonly used. It is safe and effective, with a minimal incidence of tachycardia, palpitations, tremor, and other minor side effects. The proper metered-dose inhaler technique can be problematic. The use of a large-volume spacer device is recommended. Some laboratories use inhaled isoproterenol, which has less selectivity for the β_2-receptor and may have more cardiac side effects. It is used primarily because of its more rapid onset of action, saving time in the laboratory. Commercially available preparations of isoproterenol use an alcohol carrier, which may be irritating to the airways and may cause paradoxical bronchospasm in some patients.[30] The same sort of paradoxical bronchospasm has been observed with other β-adrenergic agonists as well.[31]

Preshift and postshift testing. In the occupational setting significant changes can occur which affect spirometry because of either airflow obstruction or pulmonary restriction. These can occur over a period as short as a work shift. Testing before and after exposure can demonstrate a significant physiologic change that may then be traced to occupational exposures.

Quality control is of paramount importance in performing comparative measurements. Conditions of measurements must be closely comparable. The fact of diurnal variability in bronchomotor tone must be kept in mind to avoid overinterpreting small changes in spirometry results. Spirometry is not effort independent, so if quality of effort is not comparable, comparisons may not be valid. Comparisons of preshift and postshift measurements have been studied extensively in the cotton industry and have been used in the occupational setting with exposure to sensitizers such as toluene diisocyanate, sawmill wood dust, animal proteins, platinum salts, and other exposures.

One limitation of preshift and postshift spirometry is that some workers may develop a delayed response after spirometry measurements have been made. For this reason some have advocated the use of serial measurements of peak expiratory flow using a portable peak flow meter.

Measurements of "small airways disease." In the 1970s many studies were done seeking physiologic methods to detect "small airways disease," the earliest or mildest histologic changes observed in smokers who may later develop obstructive airways disease. It was known that lung function declines more rapidly in smokers than in nonsmokers.[32-34] Some studies showed a dose-response relationship, with heavier smokers' function deteriorating more rapidly than that of light smokers and a less rapid decline in those who quit smoking.[35] Furthermore, morphometric studies showed a relationship between inflammatory changes in small (<2-mm) airways and functional changes on sensitive tests.[36,37] A variety of tests were developed or adapted for the purpose of detecting small airways disease. It was argued that the FEV1 was insensitive. The FEF25-75 and other measures of flow at low lung volumes were used. Other tests tried include the single breath nitrogen test, spirometry using mixtures of helium with oxygen, plethysmographic measurements of lung volumes, static lung compliance, and frequency–dependent changes in dynamic lung compliance. Most of these measurements were found to be sensitive but highly variable, poorly reproducible, and often misleading.[2] With the exception of spirometric measurements, the cost of instrumentation and level of expertise required to perform these measurements made them impractical for epidemiologic studies or screening in the occupational setting.

The FEF25-75 was found to distinguish smokers from nonsmokers in large groups, but the degree of variability of measurement made it impractical for clinical use.[38,39] For clinical measurements it is sensitive but it is nonspecific, is not reproducible from one measurement to the next, and correlates poorly with bronchodilator responsiveness. For these reasons it has fallen out of favor to the point that, in some laboratories and in some COPD research studies,[15] it is not used.

Indications. Spirometry is useful in the clinical setting for evaluations of patients with respiratory symptoms such as dyspnea on exertion, cough, chest tightness, and wheezing. It can be used as a screening tool for cigarette smokers, one third of whom develop airways obstruction. It can be used as a regular follow-up tool for the clinical evaluation of patients with COPD, asthma, and other obstructive or restrictive disorders. It is often recommended for presurgical evaluation, particularly before upper abdominal or thoracic surgery.[40-42]

Annual screening spirometry is recommended for workers who are exposed to hazardous respiratory agents or who use respiratory protective equipment. Effective respiratory protection should prevent respiratory effects of hazardous exposures; however, inadvertent exposure is common, and many workers smoke cigarettes or have other medical causes of accelerated decline in lung function. As part of a worker protection program, annual screening spirometry can detect a rapid decline in lung function before workers become symptomatic or impaired.

Employer testing programs

The approach to pulmonary function testing by an employer may depend on organizational size and resources. The benefits to the worker are of paramount importance. The future fiscal health of the employer is also important. Prevention of disability is far less costly than compensation for long-term disability. Large corporations with a medical department and trained personnel can more easily establish a thorough testing program. Smaller companies must more carefully review available testing services in light of limited worker health budgets. The value of an effective health promotion program is an investment or insurance against future health care and disability costs.

The design of the employer health program requires overall supervision by the corporate medical director or by the human resources director with medical consultative input. Spirometry programs should be integrated into the overall health program when possible. In addition, information from the medical screening program should be used for primary prevention: control of exposure when abnormalities are detected.

Technician training

The most commonly accepted form of technician training for spirometry in the occupational setting is the National Institute for Occupational Safety and Health (NIOSH)-certified course, a 2-day course in spirometry technique and measurements that was established as part of the OSHA cotton dust standard[25] and remains the standard for industrial spirometry technician training. NIOSH courses are offered in many locations around the country. The quality of courses varies, so investigation of the sponsoring organization is worthwhile before committing to an NIOSH course. A typical NIOSH course emphasizes training in spirometry techniques, including maneuver acceptability and reproducibility criteria, calibration, standards for data display, quality control, calculations, recordkeeping, and interpretation. It also includes discussions of occupational obstructive airways diseases and restrictive diseases, lung cancer, asbestosis, byssinosis, and other occupational respiratory disorders.

The ATS has published a position paper on pulmonary function laboratory personnel qualifications.[43] Certifying written examinations are administered annually, by the National Board of Respiratory Care, for competency in pulmonary function testing. After successful completion of the levels of examination, a technician may be awarded credentials as a certified pulmonary function technologist or a registered pulmonary function technologist.

Equipment maintenance

A regular preventive maintenance program is recommended for all equipment. A regular cleaning program should follow appropriate practices of hygiene. Equipment problems should be addressed by a well-qualified technician, and a log should be kept of equipment problems and service performed. Regular, scheduled preventive maintenance for equipment should likewise be performed. This may be available with a service contract from the manufacturer or from an independent service agent.

Data storage

Long-term data storage can be a substantial burden for occupational clinics. Asbestos surveillance requires retention of records for 30 years or more. Other medicolegal requirements for data retention can be equally burdensome. From the standpoint of day-to-day operations, it is most prudent to plan on keeping records permanently. For this reason it is critical that records be both compact and secure. Printed reports on paper are the most commonly used "permanent record." We recommend low acid content, high-quality paper. The value of a compact record becomes rapidly apparent as data accumulates. A five-drawer file cabinet can hold approximately 20,000 pages of reports. A busy laboratory can easily fill one or more in 1 year.

Magnetic storage media or optical disks are convenient for data storage, since they require less space than paper files. However, it is critical that these forms of data storage have adequate back-up in the event of equipment failure or other cause of data loss. There are some legal jurisdictions in which electromagnetic data storage is not accepted for permanent storage of medical data because it can be so readily altered or lost.

Summary

Spirometry is the most basic and most valuable test for clinical assessment of workers at risk for respiratory disorders. A carefully organized system for test performance and interpretation can provide reliable information. To minimize costly false-positive results, an organized quality control program is recommended.

PEAK FLOW MEASUREMENTS

The use of peak flow meters has become increasingly common in recent years for assessment and management of asthma. This use has increased further since the publication of the National Asthma Education Program's *Guidelines for the Diagnosis and Management of Asthma.*[44] Peak flow meters are mainly used for evaluating asthma but may also be useful for evaluating other obstructive airways disorders in the occupational setting. Many manufacturers produce inexpensive ($20 to $25) peak flow meters that have been shown to be reliable in short-term testing.

Asthmatics who are being followed up for daily trends in asthma control can keep a regular log of peak flows measured two or more times daily. Space should be allowed for comments on symptoms and medications. Similar peak flow records can be kept for workers with other respiratory problems related to work exposure. With such a log, patients can better follow their own clinical course and seek help if their flow declines below a threshold.

Figure 4-4 shows the results of self-administered portable peak flow meter measurements conducted by a worker over a 15-day period. To facilitate comparisons and detection of trends, measurements are expressed as a percentage of the mean value for the 15-day period. In Figure 4-4 on the 11th day, the worker exhibited a significant drop in peak expiratory flow. A greater than 20% change in peak flow is usually considered significant. The decrease in peak flow on the 11th day is followed by a slow return to normal over the next several days. As shown in the figure, peak flow trend analysis can be particularly useful in detecting a relationship to environmental exposures when coupled with symptoms, use of medications, and work activities.

Peak flow is effort dependent and may vary considerably, especially if subjects are not well trained to be consistent. This can make interpretation difficult since the subject is not blinded to the results. A series of caveats has been developed for evaluating peak flow measurements.[45-47]

Comparative studies between peak flow and FEV1 in asthmatics have found peak flow to have greater within-subject variability and may underestimate the degree of impairment in subjects with severe obstruction.[48,49] Some patients with severe airways obstruction can have normal or near-normal peak flow, and likewise peak flow can be reduced for reasons other than airways obstruction. Some studies have found good correlation between FEV1 and peak flow, however.[50,51]

The devices are not indestructible. Often their accuracy is impaired because of wetness or accumulated dust or other grime. There is no inexpensive calibration method available, and no feature for direct recording of the data. Long-term reliability of peak flow meters has not been established, and routine periodic replacement of peak flow meters is therefore advisable.[52]

OTHER METHODS

A great variety of other methods for pulmonary function evaluation exists. Although these may be very helpful in the clinical evaluation of pulmonary disease, none has been shown to be beneficial as a screening tool, even in industries with specific associated disorders of gas exchange (e.g., beryllium processing). Because these tests are rarely used for screening and because most equipment required for such tests is expensive, they are rarely performed in the occupational health setting. More commonly, they are performed in a hospital or outpatient clinic under the guidance of a pulmonary physician as part of a clinical evaluation for symptomatic respiratory disorders.

Since these techniques are not routinely used in the occupational setting, they are not discussed here in great detail. Further references are included, or the reader can refer to a general text of pulmonary function testing.[53-59]

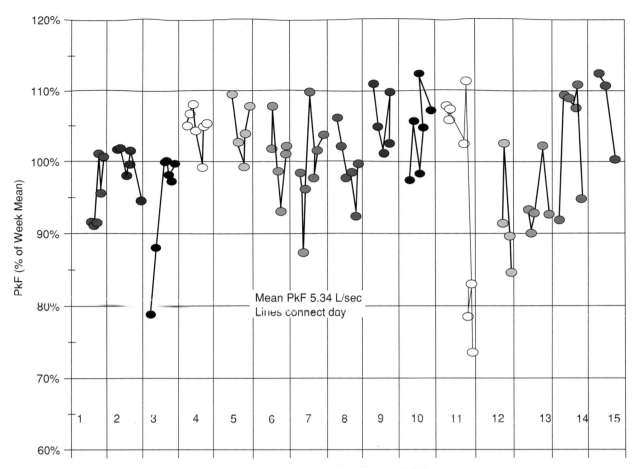

Fig. 4-4. Self-administered portable peak flow (PkF) measurement conducted by a worker over a 15 day period. Measurements are expressed as a percentage of the mean value for the 15-day period. On the 11th day the worker exhibited a significant drop in peak expiratory flow. A greater than 20% change in peak flow is considered significant. The decrease in peak flow is followed by a return to normal over the next several days. Peak flow trend analysis can be useful in detecting a relationship to environmental exposures, when coupled with symptoms, use of medications, and work activities. (Adapted from Hankinson JL and Wagner GR: Occupational Medicine: State of the Art Reviews, Philadelphia, 1993, Hanley & Belfus.)

Measurement of "absolute" lung volumes

Spirometry can determine the volume of air exchanged into and out of the lungs during respiratory maneuvers, but there is an unaccounted for volume of air present in the lungs at the end of a maximal expiratory effort. This "residual volume" cannot be measured with a spirometer but must be measured with other techniques. These techniques estimate the amount of air present in the lungs at a given lung volume, usually either TLC, functional residual capacity (or end-expiratory lung volume), or residual volume. There are three common general techniques for measuring lung volumes: gas dilution techniques, body plethysmography, and radiographic techniques.

Gas dilution techniques: helium dilution and nitrogen washout. In the helium or other inert gas dilution technique inert gas of known volume and concentration is held in a reservoir. The subject breathes the gas mixture repeatedly

until equilibrium is achieved. Oxygen consumption and carbon dioxide production must be considered. The final concentration of the gas can be used to calculate the volume of the lungs using a simple algebraic relationship.[60,61]

The open-circuit nitrogen washout technique also uses the concept of conservation of mass. The concentration of nitrogen in the lungs is measured at the beginning of the test. The subject breathes from a source of pure oxygen. All exhaled gas is collected into a reservoir. The final reservoir volume and nitrogen concentration can be used to calculate back to determine the original lung volume.[60,62]

Body plethysmography. A body plethysmograph is a closed chamber in which the subject sits. The technique used for measuring lung volume requires alternating Valsalva's and Müller's maneuvers against a closed valve, usually at functional residual capacity. The relationship between changes in mouth pressure and the pressure in the plethysmograph are a function of lung volume. The calculation is simple and rapid using either analog techniques or a digital computer. With proper calibration and quality control this technique is the most reliable for measurement of lung volume in patients with airflow obstruction. It is not quite as commonly used as the other techniques because the equipment is more expensive and requires more space in the laboratory. However, laboratories equipped with plethysmographs can not only obtain more accurate information, but they can test more rapidly. In addition, measurement of airways resistance is often done along with measurement of plethysmographic lung volume with little additional time required for the measurement.[61,63]

Radiographic techniques. There are several techniques for determining TLC from a chest radiograph.[64,65] Each depends on the radiograph's being taken reliably at TLC, perhaps an act of faith when the usual instructions ("Take a deep breath and *hold* it!") provide little in the way of quality control. Using a careful technique for obtaining films, there is a good correlation between radiographic techniques and other methods. The principal utility for radiographic methods is the ability to obtain retrospective data from films obtained for other reasons.[66]

Gas transfer studies

Spirometry and measurement of lung volumes evaluate the first step in respiration: the bulk transfer of gas from the environment to the lungs. The next step in respiration is the absorption and excretion of gas between the alveoli and the pulmonary capillaries. This is most commonly evaluated with the diffusing capacity measurement, oximetry, or arterial blood gas measurements.

Diffusing capacity. The diffusing capacity is a measure of the efficiency of gas transfer into the lungs. This is a function of the surface area and efficiency of the alveolar membrane, as well as the pulmonary capillary bed. In modeling the diffusing capacity, it is often expressed like an electrical conductance, the inverse of resistance. Like its electrical analog, it can be broken down into components:

$$1/D_L = 1/D_M + 1/\theta V_c$$

where D_L is the diffusing capacity, D_m is the diffusing capacity of the pulmonary membrane, (which may be further broken down to D_t and D_p, the tissue and plasma components, respectively), θ is the reaction rate of hemoglobin with carbon monoxide (CO), and V_c is the capillary blood volume.

If any of the above components changes, it can affect the DLCO. The most common disorders to cause a reduction in DLCO are those of the pulmonary parenchyma or vasculature. Patients with emphysema have lost gas-exchanging surface and capillary space. Patients with asthma may have comparable obstruction but normal gas exchange within the lungs because of the intact lung parenchyma.

The technique for measurement of diffusing capacity, by the single-breath technique, has been standardized in North America since the publication of an official statement by the ATS in 1987.[67] The diffusing capacity technique requires careful attention to technique and quality control. Comparability of diffusing capacity results between laboratories has been shown to be poor.[68] With the establishment of standards for test performance, equipment manufacturers have developed greater uniformity in their methods, yet there remains considerable variability among both laboratories and manufacturers. It is recommended that results from automated equipment be examined carefully with manual calculation of results from raw data.[69] Some laboratories monitor equipment performance on a regular schedule by performing biologic quality control tests on the same subjects (technicians) to ensure that equipment performance is stable over time.

To measure diffusing capacity by the single-breath technique, a mixture of gas with a small concentration of carbon monoxide and helium is inhaled and held for a defined period (usually about 10 seconds). When gas is exhaled, the initial dead-space gas is discarded. The following "alveolar sample" is thought to represent a well-mixed, representative sample of alveolar gas. The helium concentration in the exhaled gas is a function of lung volume. The change in carbon monoxide is a function of both lung volume and absorption within the lungs. From these concentrations the ratio DLCO/VA can be determined, as well as alveolar volume (VA). The product of these two measurements is the diffusing capacity. It is common practice in Europe to use DLCO/VA as the primary indicator of disease. In North America DLCO is more often used. The correlation with severity of disease in restrictive disorders may be better using DLCO, supporting the North American practice.[70]

A number of issues, such as the method for calculation of breath-hold time, volume of the discarded dead-space sample, and volume of the alveolar sample, remain unstandardized.[67] Whatever method is chosen for these options, consistency of practice is recommended. Other techniques exist for the measurement of diffusing capacity, including the steady-state exercise technique, the rebreathing technique, and the morphometric technique. These techniques have merits but are not commonly used in the clinical setting.[69]

A number of confounding factors must be considered in interpreting measurements of DLCO. Confounding factors include variations in hemoglobin, carboxyhemoglobin, altitude, and body position. Adjustment can be made for the first three of these.[69]

There is no consensus regarding indications for measurement of DLCO. It has been advocated as a "valuable screening test and a sensitive indicator of occupational-related interstitial lung disease."[71] However, utility and cost effectiveness have not been clearly shown in prospective studies. Possible indications include restrictive disorders, obstructive disorders, cardiovascular disorders, and other causes of gas-exchange impairment, as well as disability evaluation.

DLCO is typically abnormal in restrictive disorders as a result of interstitial diseases.[72,73] It has been used both for diagnosis and for long-term follow-up of disease. It may be helpful in discriminating between restriction caused by parenchymal disorders and that caused by chest wall abnormalities.

DLCO has been used to distinguish emphysema from other forms of obstructive airways disease and may be equal or superior to measurement of lung compliance.[74] DLCO is also typically reduced in cystic fibrosis.[75] A variety of cardiovascular disorders can cause a reduction in DLCO, including thromboembolism, fat embolism, pulmonary hypertension, and pulmonary edema.[69]

DLCO may be increased in a variety of conditions, including obesity, asthma, polycythemia, pulmonary hemorrhage, exercise, and increased pulmonary capillary blood volume (e.g., due to left-to-right intracardiac shunt).

Oximetry. Noninvasive oximeters have been developed in recent years as a simple and inexpensive technique for measuring arterial oxygen saturation.[76] The technique relies on the relative absorbance of oxyhemoglobin versus reduced hemoglobin for red and near-infrared light. This allows determination of the proportion of oxygenated to deoxygenated hemoglobin. Pulse oximetry measures the change in absorption caused by the pulsation during the cardiac cycle. This effectively subtracts out absorbance by tissue and venous blood, allowing the oximeter to calculate the oxygenation of pulsatile or arterial blood. Correlation with arterial oxygen saturation as measured by other techniques is good; however, false-positive results occur, and the correlation with arterial saturation is poor below approximately 70%. Since pulse oximeters use only two wavelengths of light, they cannot distinguish the presence of other forms of hemoglobin, such as carboxyhemoglobin, methemoglobin, or sulfhemoglobin. Pulse oximeters are not confounded by differences in skin pigmentation.[77] Fingernail polish, particularly darker colors, can interfere with pulse oximetry.[78]

Pulse oximeters have been promoted in recent years as "the fifth vital sign." Indeed, their use for real-time monitoring of oxygenation in potentially unstable patients has been widely accepted. They have been used in pulmonary function laboratories as a supplement to measurement of diffusing capacity and as a substitute for some measurements of arterial blood gases. Oximeters may be helpful in screening for mild gas-exchange abnormalities. Clinical studies of efficacy and cost effectiveness have not yet been done. The accuracy of pulse oximeters is estimated to be within 3% to 5% of the measured oxygen saturation of arterial blood between 70% and 100%.[76]

Other noninvasive measures of gas exchange include transcutaneous measurement of oxygen tension or carbon dioxide tension and end-tidal sampling of expired gases. These methods may be helpful in the critical care setting. They are still under development and have not been shown to be useful in the outpatient setting.[76]

Arterial blood gases. Arterial blood gas measurement is the most accurate means of assessing levels of oxygen, carbon dioxide, and hydrogen ion in the blood. It requires arterial puncture or cannulation and therefore is not suitable as a screening technique. Its greatest use is in the hospital inpatient setting or in the evaluation of patients with severe respiratory disorders. A fuller discussion of the utility, procedure, and interpretation of arterial blood gas testing is available in standard pulmonary function texts.[79]

Problems with instrumentation and procedural quality control have been addressed in recent years by improved standardization of methodologies and equipment. The Clinical Laboratories Improvement Amendments of 1988 set minimum standards for laboratory practices and quality control.

Cardiopulmonary exercise testing

The use of cardiopulmonary exercise testing (CPX) has evolved in recent years to the point that it is now common. The physiology of exercise in patients with lung disease is well understood.[80-83] However, this modality of testing lags behind spirometry and other tests since there are not yet standards for test performance,[84] quality control,[8] or interpretation of results.[85]

For the evaluation of occupational respiratory disorders, the use of CPX must be divided into studies done to gain physiologic understanding of disease and studies done to evaluate impairment for the individual worker. Most of the studies done to evaluate specific disease states have been done with asbestosis, silicosis, and coal worker's pneumoconiosis. This chapter does not discuss these studies in detail.[86] For evaluation of workers with respiratory impairments, often workers whose respiratory symptoms are more severe than would be expected from other tests such as spirometry, CPX may be a useful next line for evaluation.[87-91] As with other forms of evaluation, CPX can be used to assist in determining degree of impairment; however, the determination of disability, which affects the worker's life and work potential, is an administrative decision in which the physician's role is merely advisory.

Monitoring data during the test and evaluating results after the test can be daunting. Computerized systems are available that make the complexity of the task seem less. However, when problems arise, and they always do, complex systems can be difficult to trouble-shoot.

The major variables monitored include expiratory or inspiratory airflow, exhaled oxygen and carbon dioxide, the ECG, oxygen saturation, workload, and blood pressure. Under some circumstances it is helpful to measure arterial blood gases, blood lactate, and cardiac output.

Airflow can be measured by any of the means described

in the section on spirometry. Because expired air totals hundreds of liters in a typical study, flow-measuring devices are preferred.

Exhaled oxygen and carbon dioxide can be measured with zirconium oxide and infrared analyzers, respectively, or by a mass spectrometer. The time lag in sampling a constantly changing signal must be carefully considered in calculating results. Oxygen consumption and carbon dioxide production results can be grossly inaccurate if these are not properly done. Regular comparison with a "gold standard" is recommended. Some laboratories calculate these values from collected mixed exhaled gases to compare with the automated system.

Performance and interpretation of the ECG have been standardized.[92] Joint laboratory direction with, or consultative access to, a cardiologist is helpful for assistance in interpretation of arrhythmias and other ECG changes during or after exercise.

Pulse oximetry is useful for monitoring during exercise tests. Falsely low values have been reported, presumably due to poor tissue perfusion. Falsely high values have also been observed.[93]

Workload is read directly from the cycle ergometer, treadmill, or other exercise device. It must be kept in mind that nominal workloads may be imprecise, and also that transition from one workload to the next is not instantaneous. In fact, test subjects often do not attain a true "steady state," especially at high workloads. It should also be remembered that work efficiency is variable among patients; that is, the same workload may require different amounts of metabolic work for different patients. This is especially true among elderly subjects and those with certain conditions such as Parkinson's disease.

Blood pressure can be measured either indirectly or directly. It must be remembered that the two techniques are different. Results should therefore be interpreted with caution.[94] It is often helpful to monitor blood pressure immediately after exercise for patients who complain of postexercise dizziness. Peripheral vasodilatation with decreased venous return after exercise can cause an abrupt drop in blood pressure. Subjects should be coached to "cool down" gradually, not stop suddenly.

Arterial blood gas measurement from an arterial cannula can help in evaluating gas exchange during exercise, particularly for subjects in whom pulse oximetry may be inaccurate. This requires expertise and equipment not available in every laboratory. Additional benefits of an arterial cannula include continuous monitoring of blood pressure and ability to measure the lactate concentration of arterial blood. Lactate concentrations correlate with the degree of anaerobic metabolism.

Measurement of cardiac output by rebreathing either carbon dioxide or acetylene can help in evaluating subjects with suspected or known cardiac disease.

A variety of protocols have been developed for performing exercise studies.[81] Each has its advocates, advantages, and disadvantages. Whatever protocols are chosen, it is recommended that a limited number be used. Some laboratories vary protocols depending on the anticipated work capacity of test subjects. Comparison of one test with another is easier and more reliable if the same protocol is used from test to test. There is debate over whether and when to perform maximal or submaximal exercise studies for disability evaluations.[86]

A number of interpretive strategies have been developed. Many laboratories use a modification of the interpretive schema of Wasserman et al.[81] or some other relatively simple algorithm.[85] At this point the large number of variables measured yields almost limitless possibilities for results and interpretation. There is currently no adequate substitute for expertise in exercise physiology and experience.

It should be obvious that limited exercise tolerance is a greater handicap in some professions than in others. A stevedore or an underground miner requires a greater aerobic capacity than a clerical worker. Knowledge of the metabolic requirements of a worker's job is helpful in interpreting the significance of the degree of impairment.

Grading of the degree of impairment can follow any of several standards for interpretation. The ATS recommends a $\dot{V}O_2max$ lower than 15 ml/kg/min or a job whose work requirements are greater than 30% to 40% of the subject's $\dot{V}O_2max$, or a $\dot{V}O_2max$ fewer than 3 standard deviations below the predicted value.[11]

Specialized measurements

Some specialized laboratories and research laboratories have facilities for making more detailed assessment of respiratory mechanics or gas exchange. Such techniques include measurement of lung recoil (pressure-volume curve), transdiaphragmatic pressure, and the multiple inert gas technique for assessment of ventilation-perfusion relationships. These have not been shown to be useful in the clinical or occupational setting in any consistent manner. Special circumstances may occasionally indicate their usefulness.

SUMMARY

This chapter has reviewed some of the physiologic methods available for evaluation of workers at risk for respiratory disorders. Spirometry is the cornerstone of respiratory evaluation. Other measurements are generally decided on an ad hoc basis. The principal indications for making measurements are for occupational disease surveillance, evaluation of symptoms for diagnosis, and quantification of the severity of disease, particularly disabling disease.

REFERENCES

1. Hutchinson J: On the capacity of the lungs and on the respiratory function, with a view of establishing a precise and easy method of detecting disease by the spirometer, *Med Chir Trans (Lond)* 29:137-252, 1848.
2. Hayes GB and Christiani DC: Measures of small airways disease as

predictors of chronic obstructive pulmonary disease, *Occup Med: State Art Rev* 8:375-395, 1993.

3. Wright JL, Cagle P, Churg A, et al: Diseases of the small airways (state of the art), *Am Rev Respir Dis* 146:240-262, 1992.

4. Gardner RM, chairman: ATS statement—Snowbird workshop on standardization of spirometry, *Am Rev Respir Dis* 119:831-838, 1979.

5. Gardner RM, Hankinson JL, and West BJ: Evaluating commercially available spirometers, *Am Rev Respir Dis* 121:73-82, 1980.

6. American Thoracic Society: Standardization of spirometry—1987 update, *Am Rev Respir Dis* 136:1285-1298, 1987.

7. Hankinson JL and Gardner RM: Standard waveforms for spirometer testing, *Am Rev Respir Dis* 126:362-364, 1982.

8. Nelson SB, Gardner RM, Crapo RO, et al: Performance evaluation of contemporary spirometers, *Chest* 97:288-297, 1990.

9. Hankinson JL: Instrumentation for spirometry, *Occup Med: State Art Rev* 8:397-407, 1993.

10. Hankinson JL, Viola JO, Petsonk EL, et al: BTPS correction for ceramic flow sensors, *Chest* 105:1481–1486, 1994.

11. American Thoracic Society: Evaluation of impairment/disability secondary to respiratory disorders, *Am Rev Respir Dis* 133:1205-1209, 1986.

12. Speizer FE, Fay ME, Dockery DW, et al: Chronic obstructive pulmonary disease mortality in six U.S. cities, *Am Rev Respir Dis* 140:S49-S55, 1989.

13. American Thoracic Society: Lung function testing: selection of reference values and interpretative strategies, *Am Rev Respir Dis* 144:1202-1218, 1991.

14. Becklake MR and White N: Sources of variation in spirometric measurements, *Occup Med: State Art Rev* 8:241–264, 1993.

15. Enright PL, Johnson LR, Connett JE, et al: Spirometry in the Lung Health Study. 1. Methods and quality control, *Am Rev Respir Dis* 143:1215-1223, 1991.

16. Dockery DW, Ware JH, Ferris BG Jr, et al: Distribution of forced expiratory volume in one second and forced vital capacity in healthy, white, adult never-smokers in six U.S. cities, *Am Rev Respir Dis* 131:511-520, 1985.

17. Buist AS: Evaluation of lung function: concepts of normality. In Simmons DH, editor: *Current pulmonology*, vol 4, pp 141-165, New York, 1982, Wiley.

18. Miller MR and Pincock AC: Predicted values: how should we use them?, *Thorax* 43:265-267, 1988.

19. George RB, Cheney FW Jr, Kanner RE, et al: The ATS Respiratory Care Committee position on the director of the pulmonary function laboratory, *ATS News* 4:6, 1978.

20. Dockery DW: Percentile curves for evaluation of repeated measures of lung function, *Occup Med: State Art Rev* 8:323-338, 1993.

21. Beck KC, Offord KP, and Scanlon PD: Comparison of four methods for calculating diffusing capacity by the single breath method, *Chest* 105:594–600, 1994.

22. Vollmer WM: Reconciling cross-sectional with longitudinal observations on annual decline, *Occup Med: State Art Rev* 8:339-351, 1993.

23. Burrows B, Lebowitz MD, Camilli AE, et al: Longitudinal changes in forced expiratory volume in one second in adults: methodologic considerations and findings in healthy nonsmokers, *Am Rev Respir Dis* 133:960-974, 1986.

24. Hankinson JL and Wagner GR: Medical screening using periodic spirometry for detection of chronic lung disease, *Occup Med: State Art Rev* 8, 1993.

25. U.S. Department of Labor: Occupational exposure to cotton dust: final mandatory occupational safety and health standard. Appendix D: pulmonary function standards, *Fed Regist* 43:122, 1974.

26. U.S. Department of Health and Human Services (DHHS), National Institute for Occupational Safety and Health, Centers for Disease Control: 37(S-7) DHHS Pub No 88-8017, Washington, D.C., 1988.

27. American Thoracic Society: ATS statement—surveillance for respiratory hazards in the occupational setting, *Am Rev Respir Dis* 126:952-956, 1982.

28. Balmes JR: Medical surveillance for pulmonary endpoints, *Occup Med: State Art Rev* 5:499-513, 1990.

29. Tashkin DP, Altose MD, Bleecker ER, et al: The Lung Health Study: airway responsiveness to inhaled methacholine in smokers with mild to moderate airflow limitation, *Am Rev Respir Dis* 145:301-310, 1992.

30. Travtlein J, Allegra J, Field J, et al: Paradoxical bronchospasm after inhalation of isoproterenol, *Chest* 70:711-714, 1976.

31. Nicklas RA: Paradoxical bronchospasm associated with the use of inhaled beta agonists, *J Allergy Clin Immunol* 85:959-964, 1990.

32. Fletcher C and Peto R: The natural history of chronic airflow obstruction, *Br Med J* 1:1645-1648, 1977.

33. Sorlie P, Lakatos E, Kannel WB, et al: Influence of cigarette smoking on lung function at baseline and at follow-up in 14 years: the Framingham Study, *J Chronic Dis* 40:849-856, 1987.

34. Camilli AE, Burrows B, Knudson RJ, et al: Longitudinal changes in forced expiratory volume in one second in adults: effects of smoking and smoking cessation, *Am Rev Respir Dis* 135:794-799, 1987.

35. Xu X, Dockery DW, Ware JH, et al: Effects of cigarette smoking on rate of loss of pulmonary function in adults: a longitudinal assessment, *Am Rev Respir Dis* 146:1345-1348, 1991.

36. Niewohner DE, Kleinerman J, and Rice DB: Pathologic changes in the peripheral airways of young cigarette smokers, *N Engl J Med* 291:755-758, 1974.

37. Cosio M, Ghezzo MSC, Hogg MD, et al: The relationships between structural changes in small airways and pulmonary function tests, *N Engl J Med* 298:1277-1281, 1977.

38. Black LF, Offord K, and Hyatt RE: Variability in the maximal expiratory flow volume curve in asymptomatic smokers and nonsmokers, *Am Rev Respir Dis* 110:282-292, 1974.

39. Knudson RJ, Slatin RC, Lebowitz MD, et al: The maximal expiratory flow-volume curve: normal standards, variability, and effects of age, *Am Rev Respir Dis* 113:587-600, 1976.

40. Zibrak JD, O'Donnell CR, and Marton K: Indications for pulmonary function testing, *Am Coll Chest Physicians* 112:763-771, 1990.

41. American College of Physicians: Preoperative pulmonary function testing, *Ann Intern Med* 112:793-794, 1990.

42. Dunn WF and Scanlon PD: Preoperative pulmonary function testing for patients with lung cancer, *Mayo Clin Proc* 68:1-7, 1993.

43. American Thoracic Society: Pulmonary function laboratory personnel qualifications, *Am Rev Respir Dis* 134:623-624, 1986.

44. National Asthma Education Program: *Expert panel report. Guidelines for the diagnosis and management of asthma*, Bethesda, Md, Pub No 91-3042, 1991, National Institutes of Health.

45. Eisen EA, Wegman DH, and Kriebel D: Application of peak expiratory flow in epidemiologic studies of occupation, *Occup Med: State Art Rev* 8:265-277, 1993.

46. Burge PS: Use of serial measurements of peak flow in the diagnosis of occupational asthma, *Occup Med: State Art Rev* 8:279-294, 1993.

47. Dahlqvist M, Eisen EA, Wegman DH, et al: Reproducibility of peak expiratory flow measurements, *Occup Med: State Art Rev* 8:295-302, 1993.

48. Vaughan MT, Weber RW, Tipton WR, et al: Comparison of PEFR and FEV1 in patients with varying degrees of airway obstruction. Effect of modest altitude, *Chest* 95:558-562, 1989.

49. Meltzer AA, Smolensky MH, D'Alonzo GE, et al: An assessment of peak expiratory flow as a surrogate measurement of FEV1 in stable asthmatic children, *Chest* 96:329-333, 1989.

50. Henry RL, Mellis CM, South RT, et al: Comparison of peak expiratory flow rate and forced expiratory volume in one second in histamine challenge studies in children, *Br J Dis Chest* 76:167-170, 1982.

51. Nowak RM, Pensler MI, Sarkar DD, et al: Comparison of peak expiratory flow and FEV1 admission criteria for acute bronchial asthma, *Ann Emerg Med* 11:25-30, 1982.

52. Shapiro SM, Hendler JM, Ogirala RG, et al: An evaluation of the accuracy of Assess and MiniWright peak flowmeters, *Chest* 99:358-362, 1991.

53. Taylor AE, Rehder K, Hyatt RE, et al: *Clinical respiratory physiology,* Philadelphia, 1989, Saunders.

54. Sackner MA, editor: *Diagnostic techniques in pulmonary disease. Part I. Lung biology in health and disease,* vol 16, New York, 1980, Dekker.

55. Miller A, editor: *Pulmonary function tests in clinical and occupational lung disease,* Orlando, Fla, 1986, Grune & Stratton.

56. Clausen JL, editor: *Pulmonary function testing guidelines and controversies. Equipment, methods, and normal values,* New York, 1982, Grune & Stratton.

57. Bates DV: *Respiratory function in disease,* ed 3, Philadelphia, 1989, Saunders.

58. Intermountain Thoracic Society: *Clinical pulmonary function testing. A manual of uniform laboratory procedures,* ed 2, Salt Lake City, UT, 1984, Intermountain Thoracic Society.

59. Mahler DA, editor: Pulmonary function testing. *Clin Chest Med* 10(2), 1989.

60. Tisi GM: *Pulmonary physiology in clinical medicine,* ed 2, Baltimore, 1983, Williams & Wilkins.

61. Zarins LP: Closed circuit helium dilution method of lung volume measurement. In Clausen JL and Zarins LP, editors: *Pulmonary function testing: guidelines and controversies,* pp 129-140, New York, 1982, Academic.

62. Jalowayski AA and Dawson A: Measurement of lung volume: the multiple breath nitrogen method. In Clausen JL and Zarins LP, editors: *Pulmonary function testing: guidelines and controversies,* pp 115-127, New York, 1982, Academic.

63. DuBois AB, Botelho SY, Bedell GN, et al: A rapid plethysmographic method for measuring thoracic gas volume: a comparison with a nitrogen washout method for measuring functional residual capacity in normal subjects, *J Clin Invest* 35:322-326, 1956.

64. Harris TR, Pratt PC, and Kilburn KH: Total lung capacity measured by roentgenograms, *Am J Med* 50:756-763, 1971.

65. Barnhard HJ, Pierce JA, Joyce JW, et al: Roentgenographic determination of total lung capacity, *Am J Med* 28:51-60, 1960.

66. Ries AL: Measurement of lung volumes, *Clin Chest Med* 10:177-186, 1989.

67. American Thoracic Society: Single breath carbon monoxide diffusing capacity (transfer factor): recommendations for a standard technique, *Am Rev Respir Dis* 136:1299-1307, 1987.

68. Crapo RO and Gardner RM, chairmen: Single breath carbon monoxide diffusing capacity (transfer factor): recommendations for a standard technique, *Am Rev Respir Dis* 136:1299-1307, 1987.

69. Crapo RO and Forster RE II: Carbon monoxide diffusing capacity, *Clin Chest Med* 10:187-198, 1989.

70. Kanengiser LC, Rapoport DM, Epstein H, et al: Volume adjustment of mechanics and diffusion in interstitial lung disease. Lack of clinical relevance, *Chest* 96:1036-1042, 1989.

71. Make B, Miller A, Epler G, et al: Single breath diffusing capacity in the industrial setting, *Chest* 82:351-356, 1982.

72. Watters LC, King TE, Schwarz MI, et al: A clinical, radiographic, and physiologic scoring system for the longitudinal assessment of patients with idiopathic pulmonary fibrosis, *Am Rev Respir Dis* 133:97-103, 1986.

73. Winterbauer RH and Hutchinson JF: Use of pulmonary function tests in the management of sarcoidosis, *Chest* 78:640-647, 1980.

74. Morrison NJ, Abboud RT, Ramadan F, et al: Comparison of single breath carbon monoxide diffusing capacity and pressure-volume curves in detecting emphysema, *Am Rev Respir Dis* 139:1179-1187, 1989.

75. Cotton DJ, Graham BL, Min JT, et al: Reduction of the single breath CO diffusing capacity in cystic fibrosis, *Chest* 87:217-222, 1985.

76. Wiedemann HP and McCarthy K: Noninvasive monitoring of oxygen and carbon dioxide, *Clin Chest Med* 10:239-254, 1989.

77. Mendelson Y, Kent JC, Shahnarian A, et al: Evaluation of the datascope ACCUSAT pulse oximeter in healthy adults, *J Clin Monit* 4:59-63, 1988.

78. Rubin AS: Nail polish can affect pulse oximeter saturation, *Anesthesiology* 68:825, 1988.

79. Hansen JE: Arterial blood gases, *Clin Chest Med* 10:227-237, 1989.

80. Jones NL: *Clinical exercise testing,* ed 3, Philadelphia, 1988, WB Saunders.

81. Wasserman K, Hansen JE, Sue DY, et al: *Principles of exercise testing and interpretation,* Philadelphia, 1987, Lea & Febiger.

82. Weber KT and Janicki JS: *Cardiopulmonary exercise testing. Physiologic principles and clinical applications,* Philadelphia, 1986, WB Saunders.

83. Loke J, guest editor: Exercise: physiology and clinical applications, *Clin Chest Med* 5(1), 1984.

84. Staats BA, Grinton SF, Mottram CD, et al: Quality control in exercise testing, *Prog Pediatr Cardiol* 2:11-17, 1993.

85. Eschenbacher WL and Mannina A: An algorithm for the interpretation of cardiopulmonary exercise tests, *Chest* 97:263-267, 1990.

86. Wiedemann HP, Gee JBL, Balmes JR, et al: Exercise testing in occupational lung diseases, *Clin Chest Med* 5:157-171, 1984.

87. Oren A, Sue DY, Hansen JE, et al: The role of exercise testing in impairment evaluation, *Am Rev Respir Dis* 135:230-235, 1987.

88. Pearle J: Exercise performance and functional impairment in asbestos-exposed workers, *Chest* 80:701-705, 1981.

89. Epler GR, Saber FA, and Gaensler EA: Determination of severe impairment (disability) in interstitial lung disease, *Am Rev Respir Dis* 121:647-659, 1980.

90. Howard J, Mohsenifar Z, Brown HV, et al: Role of exercise testing in assessing functional respiratory impairment due to asbestos exposure, *JOM, J Occup Med* 24:685-689, 1982.

91. Agostoni P, Smith DD, Schoene RB, et al: Evaluation of breathlessness in asbestos workers. Results of exercise testing, *Am Rev Respir Dis* 135:812-816, 1987.

92. American Heart Association Subcommittee on Rehabilitation, Target Activity Group: Standards for adult exercise testing laboratories, *Circulation* 59:421A-430A, 1979.

93. Hansen JE and Casaburi R: Validity of ear oximetry in clinical exercises testing, *Chest* 91:333-337, 1987.

94. Rasmussen PH, Staats BA, Driscoll DJ, et al: Direct and indirect blood pressure during exercise, *Chest* 87:743-748, 1985.

Chapter 5

BRONCHOPROVOCATION TESTING

Jean-Luc Malo
André Cartier

Inhalation challenges with nonspecific pharmacologic agents were first introduced for humans in the 1940s.[1] Allergenic extracts such as pollens and house dust were also used for human challenges following the pioneering experiences of Charles Blackley.[2] Based on the work of these early researchers,[3-7] Jack Pepys in the 1970s suggested challenging humans with occupational agents. He summarized the historical background for the tests in a recent review.[8]

Before showing that a given subject experiences a reduction in airway caliber after being exposed to an occupational agent, it is important to document whether he or she also reacts to a nonspecific, nonallergenic agent. The authors therefore first cover the use of nonallergenic agents, more specifically pharmacologic agents.

ASSESSMENT OF AIRWAY RESPONSIVENESS USING NONALLERGENIC (PHARMACOLOGIC) AGENTS
Background

Behavior of nonspecific airway responsiveness after exposure to common allergens and occupational agents. Tiffeneau was the first to suspect that both nonallergic airway responsiveness and the degree of immunologic reactivity contribute to the way in which human airways react when exposed to common allergens.[9] This inverse relationship—that is, the higher the degree of airway responsiveness, the lower the level of immediate immunoglobulin E (IgE)-type immunologic reactivity required for causing an asthmatic reaction—was later confirmed in two works by a Canadian group.[10,11] The magnitude of the immediate reduction in airway caliber following exposure to a common allergen can therefore be predicted by determining nonallergic airway responsiveness and immunologic reactivity by skin testing.

Exposure to allergens can trigger nonallergic airway responsiveness to pharmacologic agents. This has been shown by natural exposure during the pollen season.[12-14] Conversely, removal from exposure to common inhalants (e.g., house dust or mites) can reduce airway hyperresponsiveness.[15,16] An increase in airway responsiveness has also been demonstrated after exposure in the laboratory to common allergens.[17] Increases in airway responsiveness are more likely to occur after late reactions as opposed to isolated immediate reactions.[17,18] Although increases in airway responsiveness have been demonstrated after exposure to occupational agents, the changes occur not only after late reactions but also, in approximately one third of workers, after apparently isolated immediate reactions.[19] Changes in airway responsiveness can occur after exposure to occupational agents at work and in the laboratory.[20-22] This information can be used as a diagnostic means in the same way changes in airway caliber are.

Airway responsiveness as a reflection of bronchial inflammation. There is a relationship between bronchial inflammation, a key feature of asthma,[23] and airway responsiveness. Although the relationship is far from consistent,[24] generally speaking, the greater the response to inhaled methacholine or histamine, the more pronounced the bronchial inflammation.

Aims

Screening for occupational asthma. It is often necessary to screen for occupational asthma in high-risk workplaces; however, this assessment in the prevention of occupational respiratory conditions is rarely practiced, unlike screening for pneumoconiosis, in which chest radiographs at regular intervals are routine in high-risk workplaces. Prevention programs for occupational asthma should be based on exposure reduction and early case recognition. Preemployment assessment in workplaces where known occupational sensitizers are used should include testing for methacholine responsiveness. The presence of increased responsiveness should not be used, however, to exclude subjects, as this characteristic is not a predisposing factor in the development of occupational asthma.[25] Responsiveness to methacholine (or histamine) should be reassessed serially at work and in the case of a worker reporting respiratory symptoms suggestive of asthma. Provided that the offending agent is present as usual in the workplace and that the worker has been exposed long enough (a period of 2 weeks, for example), the absence of airway hyperresponsiveness virtually excludes asthma and occupational asthma (Fig. 5-1). On the other hand, the presence of airway hyperresponsiveness may indicate the presence of asthma or other respiratory diseases. Indeed, airway hyperresponsiveness is not unique to asthma, as reviewed elsewhere.[26] Significant increases in airway responsiveness as compared with the preemployment value suggest the possibility of occupational asthma. Workers showing such an increase should be referred for further investigation (Peak expiratory flow rate [PEFR] monitoring and/or specific inhalation tests). The other screening tools are questionnaire and immunologic tests aimed at evaluating type I, IgE-mediated reactivity. Questionnaires are sensitive tools but they are not specific,[27] although the combination of a "positive" questionnaire and increased airway responsiveness seems to improve specificity.[28] Skin tests or specific IgE counts can be used in the case of high–molecular weight agents (mostly protein-derived antigens) for which the mechanism of sensitization is IgE dependent. A combination of increased airway responsiveness and immediate skin reactivity to a high–molecular weight agent makes the diagnosis of occupational asthma likely (~80% chance)[29] (Fig. 5-1).

Diagnosing occupational asthma. As presented in Chapter 3, the clinical history is a sensitive but nonspecific tool in identifying cases of occupational asthma.[30] The best means of confirming work-related asthma is serial monitoring of PEFRs or specific inhalation challenges in a hospital laboratory or at the workplace, the latter being considered the "gold standard."[31] Combining several PEFRs with changes in airway responsiveness at work as compared with a period away from work does not seem to add to the specificity and sensitivity of PEFR alone in the diagnosis of occupational asthma,[32,33] although in individual case reports changes in airway responsiveness after a period at work are useful in making the diagnosis[21] and can be more sensitive than changes in airway caliber.[34]

It is essential to determine the level of *nonspecific* airway responsiveness before assessing *specific* airway responsiveness to an occupational agent. The level of nonspecific airway responsiveness is a good guide when conducting specific challenges. The dose to be administered

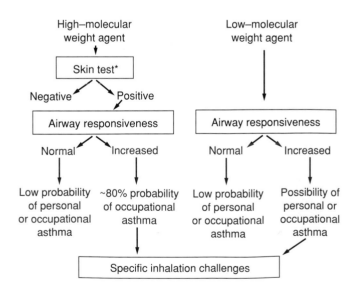

*It is important to make sure that the right agent, the one normally encountered in the workplace, is used for skin testing.

Fig. 5-1. Proposed screening for occupational asthma according to the nature of the occupational agent (high– as opposed to low–molecular weight agent).

should be lower in the presence of more pronounced airway responsiveness to methacholine, as the specific responsiveness to the offending agent is related to the level of nonspecific responsiveness[35,36] as reviewed elsewhere.[37]

For high–molecular weight agents that can be aerosolized, the initial dose likely to cause a significant immediate reduction in airway caliber [i.e., a 20% fall in the forced expiratory volume in 1 second (FEV1)] is determined by two criteria: the concentration of methacholine causing a 20% fall in FEV1 (PC20) and the dose of allergen inducing a wheal reaction on skin prick testing. A close inverse relationship was found between these two variables in the case of common allergens,[10] as originally suspected by Tiffeneau.[9] In the case of low–molecular weight agents, which often cause isolated late[31] or atypical[38] asthmatic reactions, it has been our experience that workers with a PC20 value below 0.25 mg/ml should not be exposed to isocyanates for longer than 1 minute on the first day (see "Dose delivery" on page 60).

Exposure to occupational agents not only can induce changes in airway caliber but also can increase airway responsiveness. As discussed previously, this increase is more common after a late asthmatic reaction than after an isolated immediate reaction,[17] although increased airway responsiveness can occur after the latter.[19] Moreover, exposure to an occupational agent can, on occasion, induce significant changes in airway responsiveness without concomitant changes in airway caliber. Changes in airway responsiveness are often more sensitive and occur earlier than can be detected by airway caliber alone[34] and suggest that the dose of the occupational agent be increased to achieve changes in airway caliber. Even then, some workers will demonstrate changes in airway responsiveness without showing any changes in airway caliber; this, from the authors' point of view, still indicates the presence of occupational asthma.

Assessment of permanent disability after removal from exposure. It was thought for a while that occupational asthma could be "cured" after removal from exposure to the offending agent. In 1977 Chan-Yeung's group demonstrated a persistence of symptoms, a need for medication, airway obstruction, and hyperresponsiveness after removal from the offending agent in some individuals with occupational asthma to western red cedar.[39] The same group subsequently confirmed its initial findings.[40] In general, individuals with occupational asthma will be left with symptoms of mild to moderate asthma with enhanced airway responsiveness.[41] Only a minority will be affected with permanent airway obstruction. Several studies have shown that the longer the exposure in general, the longer the exposure after the onset of symptoms, and the more severe the asthma at the time of diagnosis (before ending exposure), the more likely it is that the symptoms, airway obstruction, and hyperresponsiveness will persist.[41] Although all of these studies were retrospective (airway caliber and responsiveness were not assessed at the time of employment

nor before the onset of symptoms), some may question the findings. One recent prospective study showed that airway hyperresponsiveness was not present at the time of employment in four workers exposed to western red cedar who later developed occupational asthma. The presence of airway hyperresponsiveness is therefore not a necessary predisposing factor in the development of occupational asthma.[25]

Because occupational asthma causes permanent impairment or disability, it was suggested that subjects be assessed after removal from exposure for medicolegal purposes, using criteria such as the level of airway obstruction and hyperresponsiveness, as well as the need for medication.[42] These criteria have been used in Quebec since 1985.[43] A recent statement by the American Thoracic Society (ATS) suggests assessing permanent impairment and disability 2 years after removal from exposure because a plateau of improvement is generally reached at that point.[44] The ATS criteria also include the level of airway responsiveness.[45]

Increased airway responsiveness in other types of occupational respiratory conditions. Besides occupational asthma, which occurs after a variable duration of exposure to a potential "sensitizing" agent at work, a variant known as reactive airways dysfunction syndrome has also been described.[46,47] This syndrome occurs after exposure to an irritant agent, such as chlorine or ammonia. Affected individuals begin developing symptoms in the minutes or hours following the inhalational event. They can be left with permanent symptoms similar to asthma as well as with increased airway hyperresponsiveness.[48,49] The response of these patients to bronchodilator therapy is usually less pronounced than in those with occupational asthma involving a latency period.[50] Increased airway responsiveness is also found in some grain handlers and is related to changes in airway caliber during a work shift; it can predispose subjects to the development of a nonspecific obstructive disease.[51] Exposure to cotton dust can also increase the level of airway hyperresponsiveness.[52]

Methodology and strategy

Assessing airway responsiveness is now a standard test not only in the hospital setting but also in field studies for assessing the prevalence of asthma[53,54] and occupational asthma in high-risk workplaces.[28,29,55,57] The test is harmless, provided that a standardized methodology is used,[58,59] and suggested safety regulations are observed.[60] The methodology can be abbreviated for epidemiologic surveys. Pharmacologic agents, particularly methacholine, which has fewer side effects than histamine,[61] should be given preference over other means of assessing airway responsiveness because a dose-response curve can be easily generated; this is not the case for exercise or hyperventilation.

If testing for nonspecific airway hyperresponsiveness is to be used for screening purposes, it is necessary that the workers to be screened are actually exposed to the potential offending agent. When assessment of PC20 is combined with PEFR monitoring to determine a diagnosis of occupational asthma, nonspecific airway responsiveness should then be assessed during periods at work and away from work (Fig. 5-2).

As a guideline for specific inhalation challenges, PC20 should first be assessed on a control day. In the case of a positive reaction to the specific agent in terms of FEV1, PC20 should be reassessed when FEV1, has returned to the baseline value ($\pm 10\%$). If the results show an increase in airway responsiveness, the subject should be treated until the PC20 returns to the baseline level. In the case of a negative specific challenge, PC20 should be reassessed at the end of the testing period. If there is significant enhancement of airway responsiveness, provisions should be made to increase the duration of exposure to the putative agent in a repeat laboratory challenge or to return the subject to work before a repeat challenge (Fig. 5-2).

ASSESSMENT OF AIRWAY RESPONSIVENESS TO SPECIFIC AGENTS: SPECIFIC INHALATION CHALLENGES
Definitions, aims, and indications

Laboratory and workplace inhalation challenges can be defined as tests in which workers are asked to inhale occupational agents in a nonirritant dose-response manner. Occupational agents can exist in the form of particles, gases, or aerosols. The environment should be controlled in such a way that a dose-response curve can be generated. Work-

ers should not be exposed to irritant levels. In the laboratory set-up the usual working environment should be reproduced in such a way that the inhaled dose of the causal agent is below the recommended threshold limit value–short-term exposure limit (TLV-STEL).

The aim of the test is to document the occurrence of a reduction in airway caliber and/or increase in airway responsiveness after exposure to the offending agent in the laboratory or workplace.

Specific inhalation challenges should be considered to determine that the asthma is caused by the workplace. This has considerable medical and medicolegal implications, however. Leaving a worker exposed to a causal agent at work can result in permanent impairment or disability and progressive worsening of the disease.[62] A case has been reported of a worker who died after going back to work although he had been informed he had occupational asthma.[63] A diagnosis of occupational asthma also has considerable personal and social consequences. The quality of life of workers with occupational asthma is less satisfactory than that of control asthmatic patients.[64] From a social point of view, workers with occupational asthma may suffer financial prejudice.[65] It has been estimated that a single case of occupational asthma costs the Quebec Workers' Compensation Board $50,000. For all of these reasons it is of the utmost importance that a diagnosis of occupational asthma be confirmed or rejected in a convincing manner. Exposing a worker to the product he or she normally encounters at work in a controlled laboratory set-up is an appropriate and

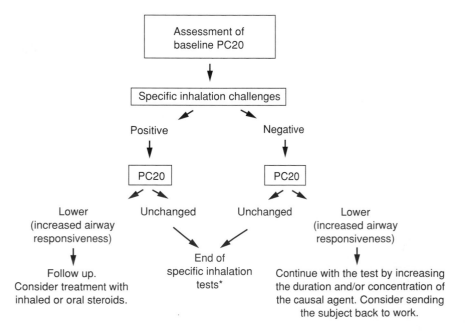

* It is important to send the subject back to the workplace with the provision that peak expiratory flow rates (PEFR) are monitored and PC20 is assessed after 2 weeks at work. If there are significant changes in PEFR or if PC20 decreases (increase in airway responsiveness), specific inhalation challenges should be repeated in the laboratory or at the workplace.

Fig. 5-2. Use of nonspecific airway responsiveness in the investigation of occupational asthma by specific inhalation challenges.

ethical method of establishing the diagnosis of occupational asthma.

If a worker is exposed to an agent that is known to cause occupational asthma, either specific inhalation challenge, if a center is available, or PEFR monitoring should be considered. If the agent has never been reported as causing occupational asthma, specific inhalation challenge is clearly indicated. A decision tree for the investigation of occupational asthma is shown in Fig. 5-3.[66,67]

Recommendations for carrying out these tests have been made by a special committee of the American Academy of Allergy and Clinical Immunology[68] and, more recently, by a committee appointed by the European Respiratory Society.[60]

Safety precautions

Laboratory challenges should be carried out in a specialized hospital center with trained personnel. They can be done on an outpatient basis. The worker comes in at 7:30 or 8:00 AM and leaves at 4:00 or 5:00 PM. The baseline FEV1 should be at least 2 L. The potential risk is negligible if they are well conducted with consideration of the worker's history, initial spirometry, and level of PC20, and a dose-response approach is used. The threat of severe bronchospastic reaction, which is negligible if the tests follow the recommended procedure, is related to immediate reactions, that is, a reduction in airway caliber occurring during or immediately after ending exposure. A physician should be in the laboratory when exposure takes place and in the hospital where he or she can rapidly be reached for the hours following end of exposure. Although late reactions are of considerable interest in the pathophysiology of asthma, there is ample time to treat and reverse them with an oral steroid because they develop slowly. Moreover, contrary to a commonly held belief, late asthmatic reactions are often readily reversible with an inhaled β_2-adrenergic agent.[19] In the rare case when the response to a bronchodilator at the end of the day is insufficient (i.e., the FEV1 has not returned to within 10% of the preexposure value), the worker should be kept in the hospital for further observation, and the asthmatic reaction should be treated accordingly with bronchodilators and steroids. An intravenous catheter should be installed on the first day of exposure to the possible causal agent if the PC20 is no higher than 0.25 mg/ml or the history points to severe bronchospastic reactions. Oxygen, an inhaled bronchodila-

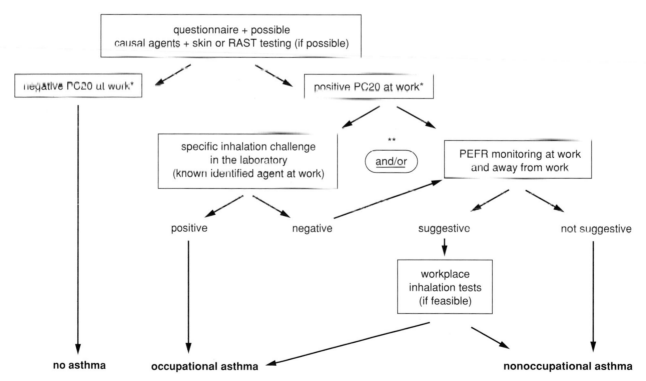

*Assessed at the end of a working day and after a minimal period of 2 weeks at work.

**The choice depends on the facilities of the investigation center.

Fig. 5-3. Decision tree for the investigation of occupational asthma. RAST, radioallergosorbent test. (Adapted from Bernstein DI: Clinical assessment and management of occupational asthma. In Bernstein IL, Chan-Yeung M, Malo J-L, et al, editors: *Asthma in the workplace,* pp 103-123, New York, 1993, Marcel Dekker, Inc.)

tor solution, aminophylline, and steroid solutions, as well as the equipment necessary for intubation, should be available.

Sequence of testing

The testing sequence is illustrated in Fig. 5-4. On the morning of the test inhaled β_2-adrenergic agents and theophyline derivatives should be withheld for the generally recommended intervals.[58,59] Antiinflammatory preparations should not be stopped during the course of the test to ensure that the asthmatic status remains stable. The total daily dose should remain the same, but the morning dose should be skipped so as not to block possible nonimmediate asthmatic reaction following exposure to the causal agent.

The point of a first day of nonexposure is to ensure that the FEV1 is relatively stable (i.e., within a ±10% change) throughout the day. The PC20 is assessed at the end of the day. On the second day the worker is exposed to a control product. It has been the authors' experience that exposing workers for 30 minutes or so to the control product is sufficient. The selected product can be a control dry aerosol (lactose, wood dust) if the causal agent is in dry aerosol form or a diluent in the case of isocyanates (isocyanates are normally mixed with diluents). On the third and subsequent day (more if required) the worker is exposed to the offending agent in a dose-dependent fashion (see "Dose delivery" on this page.) In the case of high–molecular weight agents for which the mechanism of reaction is IgE dependent, exposure to the causal agent can be done in one day because the expected reaction is either immediate or dual (i.e., im-

mediate and late). Exposure should be increased to up to 2 hours until a reduction in FEV1 is observed or, if there is no reaction, until the total duration of exposure is 2 hours (see "Functional assessment" on page 63). For low–molecular weight agents, which can often cause isolated late reactions, it is preferable to increase the duration of exposure on different days until a reaction occurs or until the total exposure time is 2 hours. Longer durations of exposure can be considered in rare instances, for example, when changes in PC20 without changes in airway caliber are detected at the end of the period of exposure (on the last day) or if returning the worker back to his or her job results in the reappearance of symptoms and changes in PEFR.

Dose delivery

Most agents that cause asthma via an IgE-dependent mechanism and induce isolated immediate or dual asthmatic reactions are water soluble. The dose that causes an immediate reaction (a 20% fall in FEV1 generally 10 to 30 minutes after the end of exposure) can be determined by assessing immediate skin reactivity and PC20 as for common allergens.[10] As for occupational agents that exist in dry aerosols (powder or dust) or vapors, it was initially suggested that they be generated in challenge rooms in a manner mimicking workplace exposure (Fig. 5-5). These agents can be tipped from one tray to another in a challenge room that is well ventilated and protected against contamination of the laboratory and sensitization of the personnel. The concentration of the particles is not usually assessed by this method, although it could be by

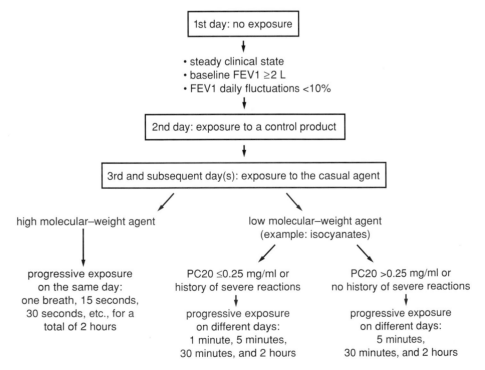

Fig. 5-4. Scheme for the investigation of occupational asthma through specific inhalation challenges.

using personal samplers close to the subject's mouth. In the case of isocyanates, concentrations should be monitored with, for example, the MDA-7100 monitor (MDA Scientific, Glenview, Illinois). Toluene diisocyanate is highly volatile, and depositing it into a small cup results in measurable concentrations in the air. Hexamethylene diisocyanate (HDI) must be aerosolized with the diluent (1:3 concentration) using a commercial nebulizer. Diphenylmethane diisocyanate (MDI) must be heated in a metal cup to approximately 80°C.

There are pitfalls to this approach, however. When subjects tip dust or powders from one tray to another, the concentrations of particles are not assessed and can be high at times, above the recommended TLV-STEL. The exposure can result in immediate nonspecific irritant reactions. The temporal pattern of such reactions cannot be distinguished from those that occur after exposure to nonsensitizing agents, such as pharmacologic products or hyperventilation. This intense exposure can also result in severe bronchospastic reactions.[69] With isocyanates it is difficult to obtain steady concentrations, particularly for the new types, such as HDI, which should be aerosolized, and MDI, which must be heated. Finally, using challenge rooms can result in exposing personnel to the offending agent, which puts them at risk of sensitization.

Models of small, closed-circuit challenge rooms have been developed for exposing subjects to isocyanates.[70,71] Recent improvements make exposure to steady and low concentrations of particles and isocyanates possible.[72-74] With the new apparatus the total dose administered can be adjusted by modifying either the concentration or the duration of exposure (Figs. 5-6 and 5-7). It is known that the

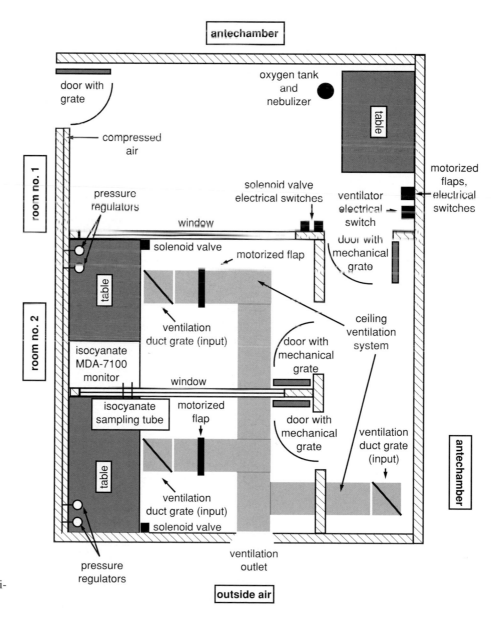

Fig. 5-5. Challenge rooms as originally proposed by J. Pepys and as present at the Department of Chest Medicine, Hôpital du Sacré-Cœur, Montreal.

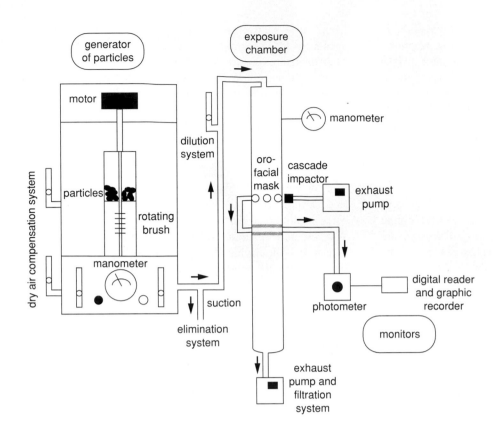

Fig. 5-6. Closed-circuit apparatus for inhalation challenges with particles. (Adapted from Cloutier Y and Malo J-L: Technical update on an exposure system for particles in the diagnosis of occupational asthma, *Eur Respir J* 5:887-890, 1992.)

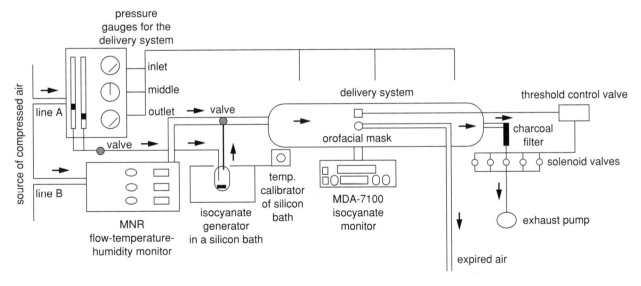

Fig. 5-7. Closed-circuit apparatus for inhalation challenges with isocyanates. (Adapted from Vandenplas O, Malo J-L, Cartier A, et al: Closed-circuit methodology for inhalation challenge test with isocyanates, *Am Rev Respir Dis* 145:582-587, 1992.)

total dose, more than the concentration or the duration alone, is the main determinant of the reaction.[75] Using the apparatus, changes in FEV1 between 20% and 30% can be obtained progressively by increasing the concentration, the duration of exposure, or both. We have now validated the use of the particle generator on more than 50 subjects referred for investigation of occupational asthma.[74] As for isocyanates, these compounds are generated in gas form. We have observed cases of occupational asthma caused by the prepolymers of isocyanates and not to the polymers.[76,77]

These prepolymers can be generated in aerosol form. Modifications to the isocyanate generator are under way to make it possible to generate isocyanates either as a gas or as an aerosol.

It has been the authors' experience that workers who do not demonstrate a reduction in airway caliber after a progressive exposure for a total of 2 hours are unlikely to suffer significant airway obstruction if they are sent back to work. Assessing airway responsiveness to methacholine after exposure allows for the decision to increase the duration of exposure (to 4 hours, for example) if a significant fall in PC20 (increase in airway responsiveness) occurs after the 2-hour exposure.

Functional assessment

FEV1 is still regarded as the gold standard for assessing airway caliber. It has the advantage of being easy for both the technician and the subject to perform. It also requires only portable and relatively inexpensive instruments. From a physiologic point of view it reflects the presence of large and small airway obstruction. However, the test is effort dependent and requires cooperation on the part of the subject. It is also influenced by volume history (i.e., the inspiratory maneuver from tidal volume breathing to total lung capacity), which can provoke bronchodilatation in a situation of induced bronchoconstriction. Forced expiratory maneuvers can cause bronchoconstriction in subjects with enhanced airway responsiveness. Other tests have also been proposed. Peak expiratory flow rates are less sensitive than FEV1 in detecting airway obstruction, especially during late reactions, which are common after exposure to occupational agents.[78] Flow rates derived from the lower half of the expiratory flow-volume curve and those in the middle half of forced vital capacity have poor reproducibility, and the interpretation of what constitutes a significant change is open to question. Tests not requiring maximum inspiratory breathing maneuvers for assessing airway resistance or conductance in a body plethysmograph or using the recently introduced oscillometry methodology have been proposed as well. However, their relative advantage of not being affected by breathing maneuvers is counterbalanced by the fact that they have a less satisfactory reproducibility in a challenge situation.[79] They also require more expensive equipment.

FEV1 should be assessed before exposure, serially after each exposure interval, every 10 minutes for 1 hour, every 30 minutes for 2 hours, and hourly for a total of 8 hours after the end of exposure. PC20 should be assessed on a control day and after the end of exposure (see "Sequence of testing" on page 60). Oral temperature should be assessed hourly and white blood cell counts, before exposure and at the end of exposure days or the following morning, should be taken to exclude the possibility of hypersensitivity pneumonitis.

Interpretation of results

A significant reaction is defined as a pattern of changes in FEV1 reaching a maximum fall of at least 20% over the baseline value in the absence of significant (less than 10%) changes in FEV1 on a control day (demonstrating a stable asthmatic condition) and after exposure to a control product (no irritant reaction). An isolated fall in FEV1 that reaches 20% or more should not be interpreted as a positive reaction unless there is a time pattern showing some reduction in FEV1 (i.e., a 10% to 20% change) before or after this assessment.

Patterns of reactions

Besides the classic immediate, late, and dual reactions, atypical reactions have been described.[38] Atypical reactions are more common after exposure to low–molecular weight agents, especially isocyanates.

Special considerations

Specific inhalation challenges in the case of hypersensitivity pneumonitis. Hypersensitivity pneumonitis can often induce a state of airway hyperresponsiveness, particularly in the acute phase of the disease. In these cases it is not generally necessary to consider specific inhalation challenges for confirming the diagnosis, other means (e.g., history, precipitins, and/or lung function tests) are sufficiently suggestive. Isocyanates and other low–molecular weight agents can cause a hypersensitivity pneumonitislike reaction, with chills, fever, myalgia, peripheral leukocytosis with a predominance of neutrophils and an influx of neutrophils and lymphocytes in the bronchoalveolar lavage.[37,80] In this instance it might be necessary to confirm the diagnosis with specific inhalation challenges. It is our habit to record oral temperatures hourly and white blood cell counts before exposure and at the end of exposure days for all types of occupational challenges in case a significant "alveolar" reaction occurs. Forced vital capacity should also be assessed before exposure and as needed in the case of changes in oral temperature. Although there might be changes in diffusing capacity and the chest radiograph, these are much less sensitive and specific than oral temperature, white blood cell counts, and forced vital capacity in detecting a "positive" alveolar response.[81]

Workplace challenge tests. If specific challenges cannot be carried out in the laboratory because the facilities are not available and if the pattern of PEFR recording is dubious, provisions should be made for conducting challenges at the workplace. After making sure that spirometry is stable during a control day without exposure at the hospital laboratory, a technician then records FEV1 serially at the workplace after progressive intervals of exposure. Although the test has the advantage of reflecting what normally occurs at the workplace, it is at times difficult to exclude nonspecific irritant reactions.

Specific inhalation challenges as a research tool. Specific inhalation challenges can lead to useful observations concerning the pathophysiology of asthma. Fabbri et al. have shown that both neutrophils and eosinophils are involved in late asthmatic reactions caused by isocyanates, as demonstrated by bronchoalveolar lavage at different time intervals after exposure.[82] Lam et al. have demonstrated an increase in eosinophils in bronchoalveolar lavage after late asthmatic reactions caused by plicatic acid.[83] This work should be extended so as to compare the pathophysiology of asthma induced by high– and low–molecular weight agents using bronchoalveolar lavage and biopsies during late reactions and serially thereafter.

REASONS FOR FALSE-POSITIVE OR FALSE-NEGATIVE TESTS

False-positive immediate reactions can occur under two circumstances: (1) the worker has very "twitchy" airways with greatly enhanced airway responsiveness, or (2) the worker has been exposed to irritant concentrations of the causal agent. It can be difficult to distinguish the bronchospastic reaction, which can be nonspecific, from those occurring after inhaling pharmacologic agents or after hyperventilation. False-positive late reactions can occur if the subject is not in a steady asthmatic state. This problem can be avoided by making sure that FEV1 monitoring on the first and second days in the sequence of testing shows a stable functional state and by repeating the tests on other days by reexposing the subject to the control and causal agents if necessary.

False-negative tests can result if the wrong agent is used. For example, all isocyanates are not equivalent in terms of inducing asthmatic reactions, although there is some cross-reactivity.[84] Some workers can react to the prepolymers but not to the monomers.[76,77] Therefore, if a specific inhalation challenge is negative, it is the authors' habit to send the worker back to his or her job with serial PEFR monitoring. If this shows evidence of possible occupational asthma, specific inhalation challenges with serial monitoring of FEV1 should be carried out in the workplace, coupled with a thorough environmental inquiry to get information on all products that can cause asthma.

CONCLUSION

A diagnosis of occupationally caused asthma of the sensitizer type should not rely solely on evidence obtained from a questionnaire, immunologic sensitization, or the presence of airway responsiveness. The diagnosis can be confirmed with an experimental design by exposing workers to a control product and an occupational agent in a standardized manner. Peak expiratory flow rate monitoring for periods at work and off work is an alternative approach. Specific challenges are sometimes necessary because of the significant medical and social consequences of rejecting or confirming a diagnosis of occupational asthma. The tests are also useful in furthering our understanding of the pathophysiology of asthma induced by high– and low–molecular weight agents.

REFERENCES

1. Dautrebande L and Philippot E: Crise d'asthme expérimental par aérosols de carbaminoylcholine chez l'homme traitée par dispersat de phénylaminopropane, *Presse Med* 49:942-946, 1941.
2. Blackley CH: Experimental researches on the causes and nature of *Catarrhus aestivus*. (After 1873 original manuscript,) pp 80-81, London, 1959, Dawson's of Pall Mall.
3. Dominjon-Monnier F, Carton J, Guibert L, et al: Épreuves ventilatoires aux extraits de moisissures atmosphériques, *Rev Fr Mal Respir* 2:191-202, 1962.
4. Colldahl H: A study of provocation test on patients with bronchial asthma, *Acta Allergol* 5:133-142, 1952.
5. Pepys J, Riddell RW, Citron KM, et al: Clinical and immunologic significance of *Aspergillus fumigatus* in the sputum, *Am Rev Respir Dis* 80:167-180, 1959.
6. Pepys J and Jenkins PA: Precipitin (F.L.H.) test in farmer's lung, *Thorax* 20:21-35, 1965.
7. Hargreave FE, Pepys J, Longbottom JL, et al: Bird breeder's (fancier's) lung, *Lancet* 1:445-449, 1966.
8. Pepys J: Historical aspects of occupational asthma. In Bernstein IL, Chan-Yeung M, Malo J-L, et al, editors: *Asthma in the workplace*, pp 5-27, New York, 1993, Dekker.
9. Tiffeneau R: Hypersensibilité cholinergo-histaminique pulmonaire de l'asthmatique. Relation avec l'hypersensibilité allergénique pulmonaire, *Allergy* 5:187-221, 1958.
10. Cockcroft DW, Murdock KY, Kirby J, et al: Prediction of airway responsiveness to allergen from skin sensitivity to allergen and airway responsiveness to histamine, *Am Rev Respir Dis* 135:264-267, 1987.
11. Cockcroft DW, Ruffin RE, Frith PA, et al: Determinants of allergen-induced asthma: dose of allergen, circulating IgE antibody concentration, and bronchial responsiveness to inhaled histamine, *Am Rev Respir Dis* 120:1053-1058, 1979.
12. Altounyan REC: Changes in histamine and atropine responsiveness as a guide to diagnosis and evaluation of therapy in obstructive airways disease. In Pepys J and Franckland AW, editors: *Disodium cromoglycate in allergic airways disease*, p 47, London, 1970, Butterworth.
13. Boulet LP, Cartier A, Thomson NC, et al: Asthma and increases in nonallergic bronchial responsiveness from seasonal pollen exposure, *J Allergy Clin Immunol* 71:399-406, 1983.
14. Sotomayor H, Badier M, Vervloet D, et al: Seasonal increase of carbachol airway responsiveness in patients allergic to grass pollen, *Am Rev Respir Dis* 130:56-58, 1984.
15. Boner AL, Niero E, Antolini I, et al: Pulmonary function and bronchial hyperreactivity in asthmatic children with house dust mite allergy during prolonged stay in the Italian Alps (Misurina, 1756 m.), *Ann Allergy* 54:42-45, 1985.
16. Platts-Mills TAE, Mitchell EB, Nock P, et al: Reduction of bronchial hyperreactivity during prolonged allergen avoidance, *Lancet* 675-678, 1982.
17. Cartier A, Thomson NC, Frith PA, et al: Allergen-induced increase in bronchial responsiveness to histamine: relationship to the late asthmatic response and change in airway caliber, *J Allergy Clin Immunol* 70:170-177, 1982.
18. Malo J-L and Cartier A: Late asthmatic reactions. In Weiss EB and Stein M, editors: *Bronchial asthma*, pp 135-146, Boston, 1993, Little, Brown.
19. Malo J-L, Ghezzo H, L'Archevêque J, et al: Late asthmatic reactions to occupational sensitizing agents: frequency of changes in nonspecific bronchial responsiveness and of response to inhaled β_2-adrenergic agent, *J Allergy Clin Immunol* 85:834-842, 1990.
20. Cockcroft DW, Cartier A, Jones G, et al: Asthma caused by occupa-

tional exposure to a furan-based binder system, *J Allergy Clin Immunol* 66:458-463, 1980.

21. Cartier A, Pineau L, and Malo J-L: Monitoring of maximum expiratory peak flow rates and histamine inhalation tests in the investigation of occupational asthma, *Clin Allergy* 14:193-196, 1984.

22. Cartier A, Malo J-L, Forest F, et al: Occupational asthma in snow crab–processing workers, *J Allergy Clin Immunol* 74:261-269, 1984.

23. O'Byrne PM: *Asthma as an inflammatory disease,* New York, 1990, Dekker.

24. Bousquet J, Chanez P, Lacoste J-Y, et al: Eosinophilic inflammation in asthma, *N Engl J Med* 323:1033-1039, 1990.

25. Chan-Yeung M and Desjardins A: Bronchial hyperresponsiveness and level of exposure in occupational asthma due to western red cedar. Serial observations before and after development of symptoms, *Am Rev Respir Dis* 146:1606-1609, 1992.

26. Woolcock AJ: What is bronchial hyperresponsiveness from the clinical standpoint. In Page CP and Gardiner PJ, editors: *Airway hyperresponsiveness: is it really important for asthma,* pp 1-9, Oxford, England, 1993, Blackwell Scientific.

27. Malo J-L and Chan-Yeung M: Population surveys of occupational asthma. In Bernstein IL, Chan-Yeung M, Malo J-L, et al, editors: *Asthma in the workplace,* pp 145-170, New York, 1993, Dekker.

28. Malo J-L and Cartier A: Occupational asthma in workers of a pharmaceutical company processing spiramycin, *Thorax* 43:371-377, 1988.

29. Malo J-L, Cartier A, L'Archevêque J, et al: Prevalence of occupational asthma and immunologic sensitization to psyllium among health personnel in chronic care hospitals, *Am Rev Respir Dis* 142:1359-1366, 1990.

30. Malo J-L, Ghezzo H, L'Archevêque J, et al: Is the clinical history a satisfactory means of diagnosing occupational asthma?, *Am Rev Respir Dis* 143:528-532, 1991.

31. Pepys J and Hutchcroft BJ: Bronchial provocation tests in etiologic diagnosis and analysis of asthma, *Am Rev Respir Dis* 112:829-859, 1975.

32. Côté J, Kennedy S, and Chan-Yeung M: Sensitivity and specificity of PC 20 and peak expiratory flow rate in cedar asthma, *J Allergy Clin Immunol* 85:592-598, 1990.

33. Perrin B, Lagier F, L'Archevêque J, et al: Occupational asthma: validity of monitoring of peak expiratory flow rates and non-allergic bronchial responsiveness as compared to specific inhalation challenge, *Eur Respir J* 5:40-48, 1992.

34. Cartier A, L'Archevêque J, and Malo J-L: Exposure to a sensitizing occupational agent can cause a long lasting increase in bronchial responsiveness to histamine in the absence of significant changes in airway caliber, *J Allergy Clin Immunol* 78:1185-1189, 1986.

35. Burge PS: Non-specific bronchial hyper-reactivity in workers exposed to toluene di-isocyanate, diphenyl methane di-isocyanate and colophony, *Eur J Respir Dis* 63(suppl 123):91-96, 1982.

36. Lam S, Tan F, Chan G, et al: Relationship between types of asthmatic reaction, nonspecific bronchial reactivity, and specific IgE antibodies in patients with red cedar asthma, *J Allergy Clin Immunol* 72:134-139, 1983.

37. Vandenplas O, Malo J-L, Saetta M, et al: Occupational asthma and extrinsic alveolitis due to isocyanates: current status and perspectives, *Br J Ind Med* 50:213-228, 1993.

38. Perrin B, Cartier A, Ghezzo H, et al: Reassessment of the temporal patterns of bronchial obstruction after exposure to occupational sensitizing agents, *J Allergy Clin Immunol* 87:630-639, 1991.

39. Chan-Yeung M: Fate of occupational asthma. A follow-up study of patients with occupational asthma due to western red cedar *(Thuja plicata), Am Rev Respir Dis* 116:1023-1029, 1977.

40. Chan-Yeung M, Lam S, and Koener S: Clinical features and natural history of occupational asthma due to western red cedar *(Thuja plicata), Am J Med* 72:411-415, 1982.

41. Chan-Yeung M and Malo J-L: Natural history of occupational asthma. In Bernstein IL, Chan-Yeung M, Malo J-L, et al, editors: *Asthma in the workplace,* pp 299-322, New York, 1993, Dekker.

42. Chan-Yeung M: Evaluation of impairment/disability in patients with occupational asthma, *Am Rev Respir Dis* 135:950-951, 1987.

43. Malo J-L: Compensation for occupational asthma in Quebec, *Chest* 98:236S-239S, 1990.

44. Malo J-L, Cartier A, Ghezzo H, et al: Patterns of improvement on spirometry, bronchial hyperresponsiveness, and specific IgE antibody levels after cessation of exposure in occupational asthma caused by snow-crab processing, *Am Rev Respir Dis* 138:807-812, 1988.

45. American Thoracic Society: Guidelines for the evaluation of impairment/disability in patients with asthma, *Am Rev Respir Dis* 147:1056-1061, 1993.

46. Brooks SM, Weiss MA, and Bernstein IL: Reactive airways dysfunction syndrome (RADS). Persistent asthma syndrome after high level irritant exposures, *Chest* 88:376-384, 1985.

47. Brooks SM and Bernstein IL: Reactive airways dysfunction syndrome or irritant-induced asthma. In Bernstein IL, Chan-Yeung M, Malo J-L, et al, editors: *Asthma in the workplace,* pp 533-549, New York, 1993, Dekker.

48. Courteau JP, Cushman R, Bouchard F, et al: A survey of construction workers repeatedly exposed to chlorine in a pulpmill over a 3-6 month-period. I. Exposure and symptomatology, *Occup Environ Med* 51:219-224, 1994.

49. Bhérer L, Cushman R, Courteau JP, et al: A survey of construction workers repeatedly exposed to chlorine over a 3-6 month-period in a pulpmill. II. Follow-up of affected workers with questionnaire, spirometry and assessment of bronchial responsiveness 18 to 24 months after exposure ended, *Occup Environ Med* 51:225-228, 1994

50. Gautrin D, Boulet LP, Boutet M, et al: Is reactive airways dysfunction syndrome (RADS) a variant of occupational asthma?, *J Allergy Clin Immunol* 93:12-22, 1994.

51. Chan-Yeung M, Kennedy S, and Enarson D: Grain dust–induced lung diseases. In Bernstein IL, Chan-Yeung M, Malo J-L, et al, editors: *Asthma in the workplace,* pp 577-594, New York, 1993, Dekker.

52. Merchant JA and Bernstein IL: Cotton and other textile dusts. In Bernstein IL, Chan-Yeung M, Malo J-L, et al, editors: *Asthma in the workplace,* pp 551-576, New York, 1993, Dekker.

53. Burney PGI, Britton JR, Chinn S, et al: Descriptive epidemiology of bronchial reactivity in an adult population: results from a community study, *Thorax* 42:38-44, 1987.

54. Woolcock AJ, Peat JK, Salome CM, et al: Prevalence of bronchial hyperresponsiveness and asthma in a rural adult population, *Thorax* 42:361-368, 1987.

55. Bardy JD, Malo J-L, Séguin P, et al: Occupational asthma and IgE sensitization in a pharmaceutical company processing psyllium, *Am Rev Respir Dis* 135:1033-1038, 1987.

56. Séguin P, Allard A, Cartier A, et al: Prevalence of occupational asthma in spray painters exposed to several types of isocyanates, including polymethylene polyphenylisocyanates. *J Occup Med* 29:340-344, 1987.

57. Malo J-L, Cartier A, L'Archevêque J, et al: Prevalence of occupational asthma and immunological sensitization to guar gum among employees at a carpet-manufacturing plant, *J Allergy Clin Immunol* 86:562-569, 1990.

58. Chai H, Farr RS, Froehlich LA, et al: Standardization of bronchial inhalation challenge procedures, *J Allergy Clin Immunol* 56:323-327, 1975.

59. Cockcroft DW, Killian DN, Mellon JJA, et al: Bronchial reactivity to inhaled histamine: a method and clinical survey, *Clin Allergy* 7:235-243, 1977.

60. Sterk PJ, Fabbri LM, Quanjer PH, et al: Airway responsiveness. Standardized challenge testing with pharmacological, physical and sensitizing stimuli in adults. Report of working party standardization of lung function tests, European Community for Steel and Coal. Official

statement of the European Respiratory Society, *Eur Respir J* 6(suppl 16):53-83, 1993.

61. Juniper EF, Frith PA, Dunnett C, et al: Reproducibility and comparison of responses to inhaled histamine and methacholine, *Thorax* 33:705-710, 1978.

62. Côté J, Kennedy S, and Chan-Yeung M: Outcome of patients with cedar asthma with continuous exposure, *Am Rev Respir Dis* 141:373-376, 1990.

63. Fabbri LM, Danieli D, Crescioli S, et al: Fatal asthma in a subject sensitized to toluene diisocyanate, *Am Rev Respir Dis* 137:1494-1498, 1988.

64. Malo J-L, Dewitte JD, Cartier A, et al: Quality of life of subjects with occupational asthma, *J Allergy Clin Immunol* 91:1121-1127, 1993.

65. Gannon PFG, Weir DC, Robertson AS, et al: Health, employment, and financial outcomes in workers with occupational asthma, *Br J Ind Med* 50:491-496, 1993.

66. Bernstein DI: Clinical assessment and management of occupational asthma. In Bernstein IL, Chan-Yeung M, Malo J-L, et al, editors: *Asthma in the workplace*, pp 103-123, New York, 1993, Dekker.

67. Malo J-L: The case for confirming occupational asthma: why, how much, how far?, *J Allergy Clin Immunol* 91:967-970, 1993.

68. Cartier A, Bernstein IL, Burge PS, et al: Guidelines for bronchoprovocation on the investigation of occupational asthma. Report of the Subcommittee on Bronchoprovocation for Occupational Asthma, *J Allergy Clin Immunol* 84:823-829, 1989.

69. Cartier A, Malo J-L, and Dolovich J: Occupational asthma in nurses handling psyllium, *Clin Allergy* 17:1-6, 1987.

70. Butcher BT, Karr RM, O'Neil CE, et al: Inhalation challenge and pharmacologic studies of toluene diisocyanate (TDI)–sensitive workers, *J Allergy Clin Immunol* 64:146-152, 1979.

71. Gerblich AA, Horowitz J, Chester EH, et al: A proposed standardized method for bronchoprovocation tests in toluene diisocyanate–induced asthma, *J Allergy Clin Immunol* 64:658-661, 1979.

72. Cloutier Y, Lagier F, Lemieux R, et al: New methodology for specific inhalation challenges with occupational agents in powder form, *Eur Respir J* 2:769-777, 1989.

73. Vandenplas O, Malo J-L, Cartier A, et al: Closed-circuit methodology for inhalation challenge test with isocyanates, *Am Rev Respir Dis* 145:582-587, 1992.

74. Cloutier Y, Lagier F, Cartier A, et al: Validation of an exposure system to particles for the diagnosis of occupational asthma, *Chest* 102:402-407, 1992.

75. Vandenplas O, Cartier A, Ghezzo H, et al: Response to isocyanates: effect of concentration, duration of exposure, and dose, *Am Rev Respir Dis* 147:1287-1290, 1993.

76. Vandenplas O, Cartier A, Lesage J, et al: Prepolymers of hexamethylene diisocyanate (HDI) as a cause of occupational asthma, *J Allergy Clin Immunol* 91:850-861, 1993.

77. Vandenplas O, Cartier A, Lesage J, et al: Occupational asthma caused by a prepolymer but not the monomer of toluene diisocyanate (TDI), *J Allergy Clin Immunol* 89:1183-1188, 1992.

78. Bérubé D, Cartier A, L'Archevêque J, et al: Comparison of peak expiratory flow rate and FEV 1 in assessing bronchomotor tone after challenges with occupational sensitizers, *Chest* 99:831-836, 1991.

79. Dehaut P, Rachiele A, Martin RR, et al: Histamine dose-response curves in asthma: reproducibility and sensitivity of different indices to assess response, *Thorax* 38:516-522, 1983.

80. Vandenplas O, Malo J-L, Dugas M, et al: Hypersensitivity pneumonitis-like reaction among workers exposed to diphenylmethane diisocyanate (MDI), *Am Rev Respir Dis* 147:338-346, 1993.

81. Hendrick DJ, Marshall R, Faux JA, et al: Positive "alveolar" responses to antigen inhalation provocation tests: their validity and recognition, *Thorax* 35:415-427, 1980.

82. Fabbri LM, Boschetto P, Zocca E, et al: Bronchoalveolar neutrophilia during late asthmatic reactions induced by toluene diisocyanate, *Am Rev Respir Dis* 136:36-42, 1987.

83. Lam S, LeRiche J, Phillips D, et al: Cellular and protein changes in bronchial lavage fluid after late asthmatic reaction in patients with red cedar asthma, *J Allergy Clin Immunol* 80:44-50, 1987.

84. O'Brien IM, Harries MG, Burge PS, et al: Toluene di-isocyanate–induced asthma. I. Reactions to TDI, MDI, HDI and histamine, *Clin Allergy* 9:1-6, 1979.

Chapter 6

UPPER AIRWAY DIAGNOSTIC METHODS

Michael A. Dias
Dennis Shusterman
Jana N. Kesavanathan
David L. Swift
Rebecca Bascom

A diverse group of occupational and environmental agents may cause upper airway symptoms and disease. The intent of this chapter is to provide a background of the anatomy and physiology of the upper airway, followed by a discussion of methods for the clinician and researcher to use in understanding upper airway symptoms and diseases.

The upper airway serves disparate functions. It serves as a filter, removing material from the inspired airstream including infectious, allergenic, or toxic particles, and vapors. It serves in mucosal defense, sensing, identifying, metabolizing, or removing a diverse range of xenobiotics. It contributes to the function of the special senses including vision, hearing, olfaction, and taste. It contributes to communication through phonation. The upper airway serves as a conduit for the transport of 10,000 to 20,000 L of air daily to the lung and warms and humidifies the inhaled air. Taken together, these functions help protect the body from adverse effects of the external environment, but they make the upper airway a target of occupational and environmental exposures. Adverse health effects of the upper airway can impinge on the ability of the worker to do a range of common functions in and out of the workplace.

In the clinical setting a systematic approach is needed to evaluate the upper airway with the degree of complexity of the evaluation determined by the presenting complaint. A questionnaire can be used to obtain an initial overview of medical, environmental, and occupational aspects of the history, however, patients should be allowed the opportunity to describe their chief complaint to the clinician. Examination of the upper airway is an often neglected part of the physical examination but may demonstrate facial tenderness, changes in mucosal appearance, or the presence of nasal discharge or nasal passage obstruction. Treatment of upper airway pathology is often instituted based on a history and nonspecialist visualization of the nasal passages.[1,2] Efficacy of treatment and confirmation of the diagnosis typically are based on relief of symptoms.

Although methods are available to characterize many of the functions of the upper airway, diagnosis and clinical management of upper airway complaints continue to rely heavily on the clinical history. In the lower airway, physiologic function of the lung can be quantified with standardized spirometry,[3] followed longitudinally, and compared with well-documented reference values.[3] In contrast, generally accepted, standardized screening tests of upper airway function do not exist.

Direct visualization of the upper airway is possible using a wide-bore otoscope, nasal specula, or fiberoptic rhinoscope. Radiologic evaluation was originally performed with plain sinus films or tomograms, however, improved imaging is now possible with computerized tomography (CT), spiral CT, or magnetic resonance imaging (MRI). These technologies demonstrate the patient's nasal, ostiomeatal, and paranasal anatomy, as well as gross anatomic variations, masses, and sequelae of disease processes.

Objective measures of upper airway structure and function have been developed that have some utility in the clinical setting and are often used in epidemiologic research or controlled human exposure studies. These techniques include rhinomanometry, nasal peak flow measurements, acoustic rhinometry and nasal compliance, tympanomanometry, assessment of mucosal blood flow, nasal provocation with agents such as methacholine or histamine, quantitation of mucociliary clearance, sampling of surface fluid or tissue for evidence of inflammation or cell injury, and measurement of nasal transepithelial potential difference or trigeminal evoked potentials. Nasal provocation to document IgE-allergic disease to specific antigens is used in some countries as part of compensation evaluations. Serial evaluation of nasal peak flow may be performed with protocols analogous to those recommended for occupational lower airway diseases.[4]

Documentation of the patient's allergic status through skin testing or serologic testing is often needed, and assessment of immune competence may be indicated. Systemic diseases such as sarcoidosis or Wegener's granulomatosis or inherited disorders such as cystic fibrosis or Kartagener's syndrome may affect the upper respiratory tract, and the decision to search for these possibilities should be guided by the clinical history.

ANATOMY AND PHYSIOLOGY

An understanding of the anatomy of the upper respiratory tract is useful in understanding and assessing diagnostic methods. Factors influencing the physiologic characteristics of the nose and the ability of the nose to filter and remove xenobiotics are the nasal passage shape and size, the presence of vibrissae, the path and characteristics of air flow, and the characteristics of the nasal mucosa including the epithelium, vasculature, innervation, mucosal response mechanisms, and mucociliary apparatus.

The dimensions of the nostril can be described by the "nasal index" (the ratio between the nostril width and length).[5] Average racial differences in the nasal index have been documented: the Negroid nasal index is greater than 0.85, the Asian nasal index approximates 0.75, and the Caucasian nasal index is less than 0.65. In fact, heterogeneity exists within racial groups, and recent research has used the nasal index as the basis for characterizing subjects, rather than racial groups. The nostril shape tends to alter the fractional deposition of inhaled particles in the nose with a trend toward increased penetration of particles in the lungs of subjects with round nostrils.[6] Fractional deposition is unrelated to nasal resistance, age, gender, or minimum nasal cross-sectional area, however, there is a close correlation between the fractional deposition in the two nasal passages of a single subject despite varying unilateral nasal resistance.[6] Vibrissae are coarse hairs at the vestibular entrance, which filter coarse particles. Additionally, nerve receptors in the hair follicle will discharge with exposure to certain stimuli to produce itching and sneezing.

Figure 6-1, *A* and *B* shows the nasal passage anatomy in the sagittal and coronal views. The medial wall of each nasal passage is a vertical barrier called the septum. The lateral wall of the nasal passage contains the inferior, middle, and superior turbinates, three scroll-like structures that project medially toward the septum (Fig. 6-1, *A*). The presence of these structures facilitates conditioning and humidification of inspired air as well as particle deposition and pollutant removal by creating turbulent air flow.

The frontal, maxillary, ethmoid, and sphenoid sinuses are air-filled structures that connect to the nasal cavity through the ostiomeatal complex (Fig. 6-1, *B*). The complex is the natural drainage site of the ciliary system within the anterior ethmoidal and maxillary sinuses. It has been hypothesized that obstruction of the ostiomeatal complex may predispose patients to allergic or irritant rhinitis and chronic sinusitis. The ostiomeatal complex is considered a key area in the pathophysiology of sinus disease, and obstruction at this location is present in the majority of cases of sinusitis.[2] The ostia (connections between the sinuses and the nasal passage) are lateral to the middle turbinate. The ostia open into the infundibulum (a funnel-shaped space), which then opens into the hiatus semilunaris portion of the nasal passage. As depicted in Fig. 6-1, mucosal thickening in this area, shifting of the middle turbinate to a more lateral position, or septal deviation can cause obstruction in the ostiomeatal complex.

Nasal airflow can be understood in terms of bulk flow and mass and heat transfer, two aspects of the discipline of fluid mechanics.[7] Nasal airflow resistance is calculated by

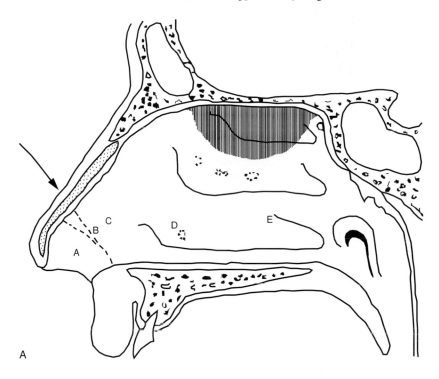

A

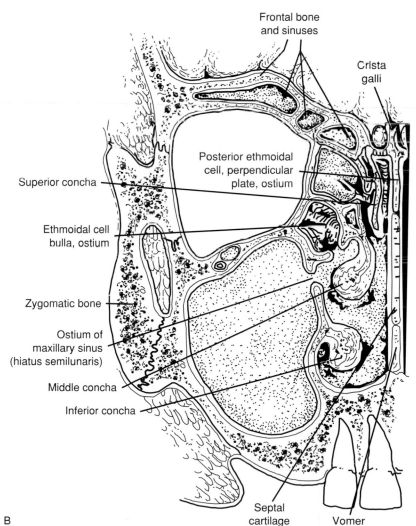

Frontal bone
and sinuses

Crista
galli

Superior concha

Posterior ethmoidal
cell, perpendicular
plate, ostium

Ethmoidal cell
bulla, ostium

Zygomatic bone

Ostium of
maxillary sinus
(hiatus semilunaris)

Middle concha

Inferior concha

Septal
cartilage

Vomer

B

Fig. 6-1. A, Sagittal view of structures of the upper airway. **B,** Coronal view of the structures of the upper airway. (Adapted from Mygind N, Pedersen M, and Nielsen MH: Morphology of the upper airway epithelium. In Proctor DF and Andersen I, editors: *The nose. Upper airway physiology and the atmospheric environment, Ch. 4.* New York, 1982, Elsevier Biomedical.)

measuring airflow rates in relation to drops in pressure along the nasal airway. The airflow rates in the nasal passage vary in direction, velocity, and pattern of flow (Fig. 6-2). The narrowest portion of the nasal passage is located 2 to 3 cm distal to the nasal antrum, at the beginning of the inferior turbinate. Airflow is laminar entering the nostril, then rapidly increases in linear velocity at the nasal valve, a narrow area of constriction in the anterior nose.[8] Airflow is turbulent beyond the nasal valve, enabling effective conditioning of the air. The nasal flow limiting segment is toxicologically important as the site of greatest inspiratory flow velocity and generally is the site of the greatest pollutant deposition. The anatomic site of the flow-limiting segment has been thought to be either the anterior portion of the inferior turbinate or the nasal septum just upstream to the turbinate. A large fraction of the total airflow passes through the middle and lower meatuses (i.e., inferior to the middle and inferior turbinates).[7] In addition to the common structures that alter airflow patterns in most individuals, anatomic differences and pathologic lesions may alter or halt airflow on the affected side. In a Canadian study the bilateral nasal resistance showed racial differences: the average was 0.13 ± 0.05 Pa/cm^3/sec among the Negroid subjects, 0.15 ± 0.05 among Asian subjects, and 0.18 ± 0.05 among Caucasian subjects.[9] Interracial differences in nasal resistance were not altered with administration of a decongestant, supporting the role of the nasal antrum in determining nasal resistance.

Humidification and warming of inspired air with evaporation of water vapor from the nasal mucosa is an example of mass and heat transfer. The respiratory heat exchange equation indicates the importance of evaporation as a source of heat transfer from the airway surface. The presence or absence of cold-induced rhinitis in healthy normal subjects appears to be related to the ability to maintain an isosmolar environment at the nasal airway surface when inspiring cold air.[10,11]

The nasal epithelium changes dramatically between the nostril and the pharynx.[12] The anterior entrance to the nose, called the vestibule, is lined with keratinized squamous epithelium and can be visualized by the clinician with a nasal speculum. The epithelium then transitions to a nonkeratinized squamous epithelium, then to a cuboidal epithelium with some microvilli, and then to a pseudostratified columnar epithelium similar to the lower airway. The pseudostratified columnar epithelium consists of basal cells, mucous cells, and ciliated cells with submucosal glands present below the basement membrane.

Blood supply

The blood supply to the nose consists of a parallel system of vascular plexuses.[13] Deep helical arteries deliver blood, warmed to core temperatures, to a superficial, subepithelial capillary plexus that assists in conditioning and humidifiying inspired air. Veins draining the superficial plexus feed the deep cushion veins, which comprise the spongy nasal erectile tissue known as the cavernous plexus. This cavernous plexus is also fed by arteriovenous anastomoses arising from the helical arteries. Nasal vasculature may influence the size of the lumen of the nasal passages by engorgement of the cavernous plexus, which is located on the inferior and anterior aspect of the inferior turbinates, as well as the middle turbinates and septum. Resistance and capacitance vessels at either end of the cavernous plexus enable a rapid changing of the blood volume within the plexus and hence control nasal patency.

Innervation

There are three chemosensory systems in the upper aerodigestive tract: smell (olfaction), taste (gustation), and the common chemical sense (irritation). These are anatomically distinct sensory systems,[14] but each may contribute to the perception of flavor or other sensations that derive from mixed inputs. The cerebral cortical areas for these three sys

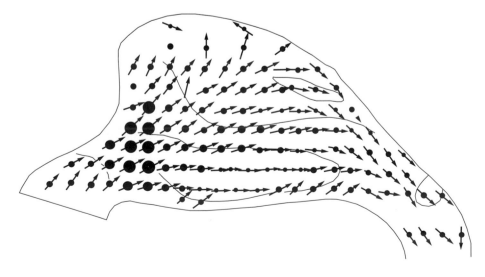

Fig. 6-2. Patterns of air flow in the upper airway. (Adapted from Swift D and Proctor D: Access of air to the respiratory tract. In Brian JD, Proctor DF, and Reid LM, editors: *Respiratory defense mechanisms.* New York, 1977, by courtesy of Marcel Dekker, Inc.)

tems are small but interact with the ventral forebrain (the limbic system), providing "affective and motivational aspects" to taste, smell, and chemical irritation.[14]

The receptors for smell are the neuroepithelial cells located on the superior part of the nasal septum and the superior and middle turbinates. Each of the olfactory chemoreceptive cells has an average life span of 50 days and are primary neurons, projecting directly to the brain via the first cranial nerve.[14] Stimulus transduction is thought to occur at the cilia, which project from the olfactory knobs. The receptors for taste are the 50 or more cells of each taste bud, each cell having a life span of 10 days.[14] Stimulus transduction is thought to be mediated by proteinaceous receptor molecules or ion channels in the microvilli or taste receptor cells. These receptor cells then synapse with primary sensory neurons that carry action potentials to three sensory ganglia: the geniculate (VII), petrosal (IX), and nodose (X).

The chemoreceptors for the common chemical sense are free nerve endings in the mucosa and are not regenerated in adults.[14] Nerve endings can be found throughout the nose in the epithelium, in blood vessels, and in glands and are most concentrated in the posterior portion of the nasal cavity.[15] The membranes of these nerve endings are specialized for chemoreception, and airborne chemicals can activate the sensory irritant receptor by two different mechanisms: physical adsorption and chemical reaction.[16] Physi-

cal adsorption is thought to occur with alkanes, alkylbenzenes, alcohols, ketones, and ethers. The alkylbenzenes activate the receptors via a benzene-binding site and the alcohols activate the receptor via a hydrogen bond. Capsaicin is also believed to be physically adsorbed to the receptor. Due to the high potency of this substance, it is believed that it fits extremely well into a receptive site. Substances that activate the receptor through chemical reactions generally are more potent than substances only physically adsorbed to the receptor. An example is sulfur dioxide, which is thought to break a disulfide bond in the receptor, thereby activating the receptor. Many substances activate the receptor by a chemical reaction with a nucleophilic group. Formaldehyde, acrolein, and related substances, and chlorobenzylidene malononitriles and related substances all are believed to react with a thiol group in the receptor. Oxidizing agents such as chlorine and ozone may oxidize the thiol group and thereby activate the receptor. The thiol group might also be involved in the acid–base reactions responsible for the receptor activation process of amines. Other nucleophilic groups (HO- or NH_2 groups) may be involved in the binding of isocyanates and some of the aldehydes.[16]

The nerve supply of the lateral wall of the nose is shown in Fig. 6-3.[2] The majority of the nasal passage contains nerves comprised of sensory, parasympathetic, and sympathetic fibers (Fig. 6-4).[13] Sensory nerve stimulation will re-

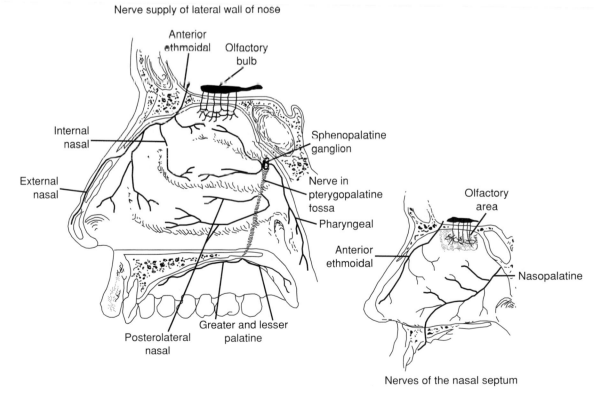

Fig. 6-3. Nerve supply of the lateral wall of the nose. (From Cummings C et al, editors: *Otolaryngology—head and neck surgery,* St. Louis, 1993, C.V. Mosby.)

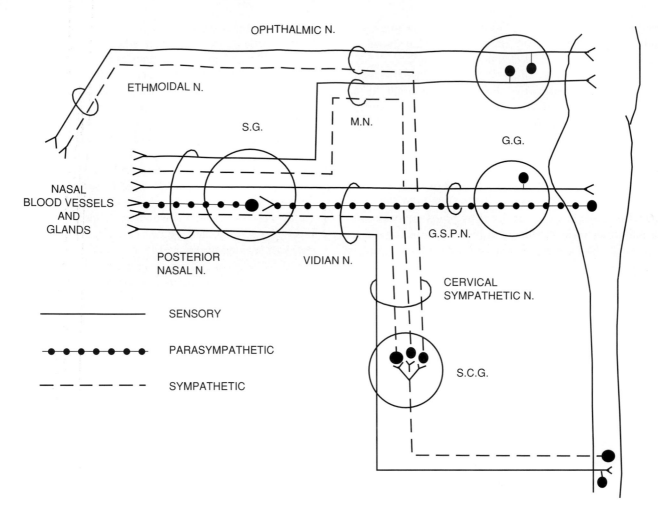

Fig. 6-4. Innervation of the upper respiratory tract. (Adapted from Eccles R: Neurologic and pharmacologic considerations. In Proctor DF and Andersen I, editors: *The nose, Ch. 8.* New York, 1982, Elsevier Biomedical.)

sult in a local axonal reflex, which will cause local events such as vasoconstriction and an inflammatory response. Neuropeptide receptors have recently been localized in the human nose and the biologic effects of the neuropeptides are throught to be related to the presence, density, and activity of receptors.[17,18] Trigeminal nerve receptors, as well as receptors associated with autonomic nerve endings, initiate events such as sneezing, the nasopulmonary reflex, nasal congestion associated with cold, and others. Sympathetic nerves release neuropeptide Y and norepinephrine, potent vasoconstrictors that act to decompress the nasal mucosa and produce nasal patency.[19]

Mucosal response mechanisms

Physiologic increases in nasal resistance are associated with pathologic changes in vessels and glands with congestion of the vascular plexus, transudation and edema, and mucus secretion.[20] Anatomic and pharmacologic studies have identified three main acute mucosal response mechanisms in the nose. The first mechanism is activation of cen-

tral cholinergic reflexes leading to the release of acetylcholine from the parasympathetic nerves with secondary release of lysozyme, lactoferrin, and secretory IgA.[21] The second mechanism is activation of the sensory axon reflex (such as by irritants, mucosal injury, or mast cell products) leading to the release of the neuropeptides, substance P,[22] calcitonin gene-related peptide (CGRP),[23] neurokinin A, and gastrin releasing peptide[24] from the c-fiber neurons.[25] Secondary markers of activation of these neurons are under investigation. The third mucosal response mechanism is through local mast cell activation, typically through the cross-linking of mast cell surface-bound IgE by antigen. Local release of mast cell-derived mediators including histamine,[26] tryptase, leukotriene C_4,[27] and prostaglandin D_2 result in vascular extravasation with increases in albumin, IgG, and nonsecretory IgA.[28] Kinins are generated in vivo following nasal challenge with allergen.[29]

Mediators released by antigen–antibody reactions and viral infections will disrupt nasal function in three main ways.[20] First, mediators such as histamine, bradykinin, and leukotrienes will act directly on blood vessels and submucosal glands, causing mucosal thickening and secretion. Second, the same mediators will excite terminals of sensory nervous receptors in the nose, setting up axon reflexes with release of neuropeptides from other branches of the nervous receptors. Neurokinins, such as substance P, will augment vasodilatation and transudation and may modulate the secretions from submucosal glands. Third, the same sensory receptors when stimulated will set up central nervous reflex actions. The responses include sneezing and nasal irritation (both prominent features of rhinitis), reflex nasal vasodilatation and mucus secretion, and actions on the lower airways. The relative importance of these three mechanisms is difficult to assess in man.

The effect of irritants on nasal function in the human nose is less well characterized. Some irritants (e.g., ozone) increase transudation of plasma proteins and cause an influx of inflammatory cells.[30,31] Others, such as environmental tobacco smoke and capsaicin, do not increase plasma protein transudation and cause variable effects on glandular stimulation.[32,33] The mechanism of regulation of irritant effects is not well understood.

Xenobiotic metabolism

The presence of enzymes with recognized capacity for xenobiotic metabolism or their activity have been increasingly demonstrated, primarily in the nose of animals.[34,35,36] Their role in enhancing or preventing local or distant tissue injury is largely unexplored in the human nose.

Metabolic processes involving cytochrome P-450, alcohol dehydrogenase, monoamine oxygenase, or the aldehyde dehydrogenase systems have not been found to be involved in bioactivations that influence the sensory irritation responses.[16] Clear conclusions cannot yet be reached on the role of hydrolytic enzymes or the glutathione system.[16]

Mucociliary apparatus

The nasal mucociliary apparatus produces a bidirectional removal of particles that deposit in the nasal passage: particles deposited in the anterior 2 cm of the nose move toward the nasal vestibule to be removed by sneezing or wiping.[37] Particles deposited distal to this zone are cleared in a posterior direction, then are coughed up or swallowed. The mucociliary apparatus is a complex multicomponent system that has been likened to a "river or series of streams."[38] The airway surface fluid is present as two distinct phases: a more viscous superficial layer (epiphase) floating on a less viscous fluid (hypophase or periciliary phase). The exact sources and control mechanisms involved in the regulation of the hypophase are unknown but are thought to involve the movement of water, which is in turn influenced by ion transport.[38,39] Surface secretions are propelled along the airway surface by the action of cilia, and regional differences have been noted in the density, length, and beat frequency of cilia in animal studies.[38] Mucus flow rates have been

considered to be related more to the nature of surface secretions than to local ciliary activity.[38] The type and distribution of epithelial cells, including those with microvilli, the permeability of blood vessels, neural function, and the secretion of mucoserous cells may also potentially affect the functioning of the mucociliary apparatus.

CLINICAL EVALUATION

The initial evaluation of the patient with upper airway complaints consists of a history and physical examination (Table 6-1). A careful history often indicates a likely etiology. In many instances, such as with an evident etiology or mild symptoms of brief duration, empiric treatment is initiated.

At the initial visit, the clinician should consider whether symptoms indicate a need for early evaluation or modification of the work environment. New onset of work-related nasal irritation may indicate malfunctioning of local ventilation, for example. Requests for evaluation by an industrial hygienist can be initiated as discussed elsewhere (See Section III: Exposure Assessment Methods).

General history

The purpose of the upper airway history is to establish the presence and nature of the upper respiratory symptoms, to gauge their severity, to determine the effect of the symptoms on the ability of the individual to perform the central duties of their position, and to identify environmental or occupational exposures leading to or exacerbating upper respiratory inflammation.

Clinical evaluation should identify the presence or absence of cardinal symptoms and their duration, temporal associations, and associated symptoms. The patient should be asked about sneezing, nose blowing, runny nose (rhinorrhea) including color and character of discharge, nasal congestion, nasal drying, nasal itching, bleeding (epistaxis), watery eyes or tearing (epiphora), difficulty or changes in olfactory function (smelling), facial pain, headaches, hoarseness, or difficulty breathing. Patients should be asked whether they had childhood respiratory troubles[1] and whether they were raised with household smokers.[40] A careful allergy history should be obtained; local allergists are typically knowledgeable about the pattern of indoor and outdoor allergens in the community. Seasonal symptoms in the spring and fall have been correlated with skin test reactivity to seasonal outdoor allergens trees (spring) or weeds (fall),[41] but skin test reactivity typically does not correlate significantly with a history of chronic rhinitis. Patients with perennial allergic rhinitis (e.g., caused by cats or dust mites) may not recognize exposure–response relationships, or chonic rhinitis may be due to a nonallergic cause. A history may be revealing only after physical examination findings stimulate renewed interest in an allergic etiology. An estimate of symptom variation by month is useful to identify background seasonal symptom patterns. A retrospective

Table 6-1. Components of upper airway symptom evaluation

History

1. Symptoms (symptom diary)

Nature	Nasal itching, sneezing, nose blowing, runny nose (color and character of discharge), postnasal drip, nasal congestion, asymmetric nasal blockage, nasal drying, burning or irritation, bleeding (epistaxis), watery eyes or tearing, difficulty or changes in olfactory function, facial pain, and headaches, hoarseness, coughing
Timing	Seasonal, perennial, episodic, weekends, vacations
Severity	0–3 scale (absent, mild, moderate, severe); number and length of attacks, boxes of tissue used
Precipitants	Specific environments, odors, exposures
History	Childhood respiratory troubles, childhood seasonal symptoms, childhood otorhinolaryngologic surgery (e.g. tonsillectomy, "ear tubes"), nasal trauma or fracture

2. Environmental

Home	Age, structure, dampness, insulation type(s), heating and air conditioning, carpets, renovations or remodeling, environmental tobacco smoke, roaches, rodents, dust, visible mold, history of leaks or standing water (have allergy reduction measures been taken such as carpet removal, encasement of mattress and pillow)
Pets	Dogs, cats, birds, guinea pigs

3. Occupational

	Type of work and length at past and present jobs, materials used, known exposures
	Industrial hygiene sampling results, material safety data sheets information, workplace layout, process description
	Other employee problems

4. Hobbies

Materials	Solvents, finishes, pesticides, herbicides, exotic plants, prints, glues, epoxies, paints, lubricants
Activities	Grinding, spraying, gluing, soldering, welding, cleaning

5. Habits and medications

Habits	Tobacco smoke, cocaine, over-the-counter decongestant sprays
Medications	Prescription drugs, nasal decongestants

Physical Examination

1. Ears

	Erythema, tympanic light reflex, mobility, air-fluid levels

2. Nasal mucosa

Color	Red, pale, bluish
Exudate	Amount and nature
Abnormal features	Swelling, polyps, septal deviation, ulcers, pigmentation

3. Pharynx

	As with nasal mucosa, plus tonsils and dentition; audible clearing of pharyngeal and laryngeal secretions

4. Sinuses

	Localized tenderness, ostia or posterior pharyngeal prurulence

5. Neck

	Thyroid, lymphadenopathy, muscle trigger points

6. Lungs

	Spontaneous cough, I/E ratio, A/P diameter, accessory muscles, percussion, wheezes, crackles, rhonchi, e-to-a changes

7. Neurologic

	Cranial nerves, posterior fossa signs (cerebellum, gait)

seasonal diary for the year preceding the onset of symptoms may help to identify specific causative allergens (Table 6-2).

Sometimes the presenting history is of recurrent upper airway infections or a "decreased resistance to infections." In this instance, a detailed history of antecedent patterns of acute upper respiratory illness and their evaluation and management is needed. A detailed history of childhood respiratory troubles and their management is needed in this instance as well as a fertility history in adults. A search for immunodeficiency states (e.g., IgA deficiency) or inherited defects in mucociliary function (e.g., cystic fibrosis or Kartagener's syndrome) may be indicated when the history indicates a chronic process.

The history should also focus on symptoms such as paroxysmal cough or nocturnal dyspnea, which may suggest gastroesophageal reflux, asthma, or chronic sinus disease. Other symptoms suggestive of asthma or reactive airways include episodic chest discomfort and exercise or nocturnal dyspnea or wheezing. Evaluation of the lower airways is discussed in further detail in Chapters 3, 4, 5, and 13.

Environmental and occupational history

The purpose of the environmental history is to understand the likely exposures in the home environment to allergens,[42] other bioaerosols, infectious agents, volatile organic compounds (VOCs), or other irritants. An environ-

Table 6-2. Example of a seasonal symptom diary

Think back over the previous year; then rate the presence and severity of EACH of the following three upper respiratory symptoms for each month of the previous year: (1) congestion, (2) runny nose, and (3) sneezing. Rate the severity of the problem according to the following scale: 0 = no symptoms, 1 = mild symptoms, 2 = moderate symptoms, 3 = severe symptoms. Enter one of these numbers for EACH problem for EACH month during the year.

THIS PAST YEAR
CONGESTION

Jan	Feb	Mar	Apr	May	June	July	Aug	Sept	Oct	Nov	Dec
---	---	---	---	---	---	---	---	---	---	---	---

RUNNY NOSE

Jan	Feb	Mar	Apr	May	June	July	Aug	Sept	Oct	Nov	Dec
---	---	---	---	---	---	---	---	---	---	---	---

SNEEZING

Jan	Feb	Mar	Apr	May	June	July	Aug	Sept	Oct	Nov	Dec
---	---	---	---	---	---	---	---	---	---	---	---

PREVIOUS YEAR
(The year before your current problem began)
CONGESTION

Jan	Feb	Mar	Apr	May	June	July	Aug	Sept	Oct	Nov	Dec
---	---	---	---	---	---	---	---	---	---	---	---

RUNNY NOSE

Jan	Feb	Mar	Apr	May	June	July	Aug	Sept	Oct	Nov	Dec
---	---	---	---	---	---	---	---	---	---	---	---

SNEEZING

Jan	Feb	Mar	Apr	May	June	July	Aug	Sept	Oct	Nov	Dec
---	---	---	---	---	---	---	---	---	---	---	---

mental history should also be taken of other sites if patients have lived at more than one location since the onset of their illness or spend significant time in another home, such as a vacation home or a relative's home. The history should include a description of the home: its age, structure, the presence of damp basements, type of insulation, heating and air-conditioning systems and their maintenance, and whether wall-to-wall carpets are present. In addition, a history of major or recent renovations to the home and the presence of pets including cats, dogs, and birds or infestation of cockroaches or rodents should be noted. Hobbyrooms or workrooms should be identified, and the specific nature of the activity and materials used as well as ventilation should be discussed. Episodic problems such as roof leaks, pipe breakage, or basement flooding should be identified. The frequency and severity of the problems and adequacy of their solution should be noted. Tasks that patients may omit mentioning include household chores (including those in small spaces with poor ventilation) and the use of cleaning agents with strong irritant potential.

A typical chronological occupational history should be obtained including episodic tasks such as daily or weekly cleaning or troubleshooting, which involve higher exposure than do routine tasks. Attention should be paid to whether the worker identifies the presence of chemicals at the workplace because of odor or sentinel symptoms (e.g., nasal irritation).[43]

The history taker should be familiar with common substances that affect the upper respiratory tract and should

Table 6-3. Upper airway sensitizers

Protein allergens
  Trees*
  Grasses*
  Weeds*
  Dust mites*
  Cockroach*
  Cat*
  Latex
  Laboratory animals
  Guar gum (galactomannans)
  Psyllium
  Coffee beans
  Grain mites
  Grain dusts
  Flour dusts
Low-molecular-weight chemicals
  Western red cedar (pilcatic acid)
  Trimellitic anhydride
  Phthalic anhydride
  Diisocyanates

*More detailed information about the identity of environmental allergens in a community may be obtained by consulting a local allergist. The list of agents causing occupational asthma (Appendix B) should be consulted for other possible causative agents.

have access to a more complete list and seek to obtain material safety data sheets from the workplace. For example, researchers, biologists, and students are exposed to allergenic animal proteins, health care students may be exposed to phenol-formaldehyde vapors, and health care workers

Table 6-4. Upper airway irritants*

At levels <1 ppm

Acrolein
Antimony oxide
Arsenic
Azinphos-methyl
Barium compounds
Benzene (NIOSH Ca)
Benzoyl peroxide
Bromine
Bromoform
tert-Butyl chromate
Cadmium
Calcium oxide
Camphor
Chlorine
Chlorine dioxide
Chlorine difluoride
Chlorobenzylidene malonixide
bis-Cholromethyl other
Chromic acid and chromates
Copper dusts, mists and fumes
Cotton dust
Dematon
Diazomethane
1,2-Dibromo-3-chloropropane (NIOSH Ca)
Dibutyl phthalate
3,3'-Dichlorobenzidine
1,3-Dichloro-5, 5-dimethylhydantoin
Dichlorvos
Diglycidyl ether (NIOSH Ca)
Dimethylphthalate
Dimethyl sulfate (NIOSH Ca)
Dinitrobenzene
Di-sec octyl phthalate (NIOSH Ca)
Dioxane (NIOSH Ca)
Diphenyl
2-Ethoxyethylacetate
Ethylene dibromide (NIOSH Ca)
Ethyleneimine (NIOSH Ca)
Ethylene oxide
Ethyl mercaptan
Ferbam
Ferrovanadium dust
Fluorine and Fluorides
Formaldehyde
Hafnium
Hydrazine (NIOSH Ca)
Iodine
Ketene
Lindane
Maleic anhydride
Manganese compounds
Methylene bisphenyl diisocyanate
Methyl hydrazine (NIOSH Ca)
Methyl isocyanate
Molybdenum
2-Nitropropane
Oxalic acid
Oxygen difluoride
Ozone
Paraquat
Parathion
Pentachlorophanol

Perchlorometylmercaptan
Phosgene
Phosphoric acid
Phosphorus
Phosphorus pentachloride
Phosphorus pentasulfide
Phosphorus trichloride
Pindone
Platinum
Selenium
Sulfur pentafluoride
Terphenyls
Thiram
Organotins
Toluene 2, 4-diisocyanate
Tributyl phosphate
2,4,6-Trinitrotoluene
Vanadium pentoxide
Zinc chloride
Zirconium compounds

At levels 1–9 ppm

Acetic acid
Acetylene tetrabromide
Acrylonitrile (NIOSH Ca)
Allyl alcohol
Allyl chloride
Allyl glycidyl ether
Benzyl cholride
Boron oxide
Boron trifluoride
Butylamine
Chloroacetaldahyde
Crotonaldehyde
Dibutylphosphate
p-Dichlorobenzene (NIOSH Ca)
Dichloroethylether (NIOSH Ca)
Ethanolamine
Ethylacrylate (NIOSH Ca)
Ethylene chlorohydrin
N-Ethylmorpholine
Formic acid
Furfural (NIOSH D)
N-Hexanone
Hydrogen bromide
Hydrogen chloride
Hydrogen fluoride
Hydrogen peroxide
Hydrogen selenide
Isophorone
Isopropylamine (D)
Magnesium oxide
Nitric oxide
Nitrous oxide
Perchlorylfluoride
Phenol
Phenylether
Phenylether-biphenyl mixture
Phenyl glicidyl ether
Phthalic anhydride
Sulfur dioxide
Sulfur monochloride

Continued.

Table 6-4. Upper airway irritants*—cont'd.

Sulfuryl fluoride
Tetranitromethane

At levels 10–49 ppm

Acetic acid
Ammonia
2-Butoxyethanol
β-Chloroprane (NIOSH Ca)
Cyclohexanone
Diethylamine
2-Diethylaminoethanol
Diisobutylketone
Dimethylamine
Furfuryl alcohol
Glycidol
Hydrogen sulfide
Messityl oxide
Methyl acrylate
Methylamine
Methylcellosolve acetate
5-Methyl-3-heptanone
Morpholine
Propylane oxide
Tetrachloroethylene (perchloroethylene) (NIOSH Ca)
1,1,2-Trichloroethane (NIOSH Ca)
Trichloroethylene (NIOSH Ca)
1,2,3-Trichloropropane
Triethylamine (NIOSH Ca)

At levels 50–99 ppm

n-Butyl alcohol
Chlorobenzene (NIOSH D)
Cumene
Cyclohexanol
Cyclopentadiene
Diacetone alcohol
o-Dichlorobenzene
Ethylbutylketone
n-Hexane
Hexone
sec-Hexyl acetate
Isobutyl alcohol
Isopropyl glycidyl ether
Methylcyclohexanol
Methylcyclohexanone
Methyl styrene
Octane
Petroleum distillates
Mineral spirits
Styrene

At levels 100–199 ppm

Acetaldehyde (NIOSH Ca)
n-Amyl acetate
sec-Amyl acetate

n-Butyl acetate
Dibromodifluoromethane
Dipropyleneglycolmonomethyl ether
Ethylbenzene
Ethylformate
Isoamylacetate
Isoamylalcohol
Isobutyl acetate
Methyl (n-amyl ketone)
Methyl formate
Methyl methacrylate
Naptha
n-Pentane
2-Pentanone
Turpentine
Vinyl toluene
Xylenes

At levels ≥200 ppm

1,3-Butadiene (NIOSH Ca)
2-Butanone
sec-Butyl acetate
tert-Butyl acetate
Chlorobromomethane
Cyclohexane
Dichloroethylene
Dichlorotetrafluoroethane
Ethylacetate
Ethyl bromide (NIOSH D)
Ethyl ether (NIOSH D)
Fluorotrichloromethane
Isopropylacetate (NIOSH D)
Isopropyl alcohol
Isopropyl ether
Methyl acetate
Methyl acetylene
Methylal
Methylcyclohexane
N-Propyl acetate
N-Propyl alcohol
Tetrahydrofuran

Other

Tobacco dust (tobacco factory)
Carbonless copy paper
Grain dust

*Note: this list is primarily drawn from the *NIOSH Pocket Guide to Chemical Hazards* (June 1990) and includes all substances listed as causing "irritation, laryngeal, mucous membrane, pharyngeal, or respiratory." Compounds are grouped by the exposure limits (see text for explanation). NIOSH Ca means the substance should be considered a possible carcinogen. See Acheson for additional discussion of upper airway carcinogens. NIOSH D indicates substances for which NIOSH has questioned whether the permissible exposure limits were adequate to protect workers from recognized health hazards.

may be exposed to latex allergen. Although the patient may not be a smoker, occupations such as bartender, waiter, busperson, disk-jockey, as well as others may predispose the patient to significant environmental tobacco smoke. Upper airway sensitizers are listed in Table 6-3 and upper airway irritants in Table 6-4.

Self-described irritant sensitivity is common in a healthy working population,[44] but it is useful for the clinician to determine if the degree of irritant sensitivity is stable, its impact on the patient's perceived health, and whether the patient's health or activities are disrupted by the symptoms. The patient should be asked to indicate the types of exposures that precipitate symptoms, and whether activities of daily living are altered by the encounters. The clinician may wish to ask the patient about symptoms[45,46] associated with exposures such as environmental tobacco smoke,[32] perfumes,[47] and cleaning materials. Seasonal exacerbations in irritant sensitivitiy should be noted. For example, one patient reported that "each year, when the trees bloom, I can't stand my wife's perfume." The examiner can also ask about cold-induced rhinitis.[10]

A more complete daily symptom diary may provide clues to environmental precipitants and document particular patterns of reaction (Table 6-5). The diary should encompass 2 weeks of usual activities and should include cardinal symptoms identified in the initial history. Rough quantification helps to indicate patterns and can be recorded as severity of the symptom on a zero to three scale, the number and length of sneezing attacks, and number of tissues used during an episode of rhinorrhea.

Physical examination

The clinician may begin the physical examination while taking the history by observing the patient for signs of upper airway disease, such as rhinorrhea, sniffling, sneezing, clearing of the throat, nasal voice, hoarseness, or cough.

The examination should be done in a systematic fashion so that thoroughness is ensured. The patient's face should be inspected for swelling or asymmetry. An otoscopic examination should include removal of any external auditory canal debris as necessary to visualize the tympanic membranes. The ears are examined and tympanic membranes inspected for erythema or fluid by insufflation and then by asking the patient to forcefully blow against pinched-closed nose while observing the light reflex. Any retraction of the tympanic membrane will make the membrane look tightly adherent to the middle ear contents and the malleus will be particulary prominent. Retraction is often accompanied by fluid in the middle ear with negative middle ear pressures, nonequalization of middle ear and external enviornmental pressures, and eustachian tube dysfunction. Patients may be asked about the quality of voices they hear, since patients with eustachian tube dysfunction often report that sounds are muffled.

Most otolaryngologists visualize the nose with a speculum. Optimal examining conditions include brilliant illumination with a head mirror or a head lamp. As many physicians will not have these instruments available in an office setting, an otoscope with a large-bore speculum or handheld illumination source is generally used. Although somewhat crude, this minimum inspection is strongly advised as part of the screening evaluation for upper airway symptoms. The mucosa is inspected for thickening or atrophy, discoloration (pale, bluish, red), bogginess; the presence, color, and thickness of secretions; for hypertrophy of turbinate mucosa, enlarged turbinates, any masses such as polyps or malignancies, ulcerations in mucosa, septal ulcers, perfora-

Table 6-5. Daily symptom diary

Enter the presence and severity of each of the following symptoms; rate the severity of the problem according to the following scale: 0 = no symptoms, 1 = mild symptoms, 2 = moderate symptoms, 3 = severe symptoms.

Over the next 2 weeks, enter one of these numbers for each problem three times daily: (1) in the morning before going to work, (2) at the end of each work-shift, while at work; (3) before bed, at home. Record the date, specific location and time, as well as symptom score. Note any additional symptoms or specific symptom triggers.

Date	Day	Place	Time	Nasal congestion	Runny nose	Headache	Nose irritation	Other

tions (holes), or deviations. A nasal swab can be obtained at the time of the inspection, spread on a slide, and allowed to air dry for later staining.

In healthy patients without uncontrolled hypertension, arrhythmias, or ischemic heart disease, repeat inspection should be performed after the application of topical α-adrenergic vasoconstrictor agents such as pseudoephedrine or phenylephrine. Decongestion allows improved visualization of the nasal passages, but does not allow detailed visualization of the ostiomeatal complex or definite exclusion of sinus disease. In cases of clinical uncertainty, fiberoptic rhinoscopy may be performed by experienced clinicians or appropriate consultants (see below).

The oral mucosa is visualized with particular attention to the presence and nature of secretions descending from the nasopharynx, one of the most sensitive signs of draining sinuses. Cobblestoning of the posterior pharynx suggests lymphoid tissue hypertrophy. This may be indicative of any process in the head and neck that mounts an immunologic response. Mucosa affected by irritants or allergies may mount such a response, particularly when associated with subsequent chronic bacterial infection of the sinuses. Chronic sinusitis caused by anatomic obstruction or other local processes such as viral pharyngitis may be associated with cobblestoning.

Visualization of the larynx and lower pharynx may be useful to evaluate symptoms such as hoarseness, episodic respiratory distress, stridor, dyspnea, "laryngospasm," dysphagia (difficulty swallowing), and scratchy or itchy throat. Abnormalities may be seen that are due to irritant exposure, to allergic pharyngitis, to gastroesophageal reflux, or to chronic sinusitis with subsequent irritating purulent laryngopharyngeal drainage. This exam may be done by a specialist with mirrors and/or a flexible fiberoptic laryngoscope. As with asthma, the physical examination of patients with upper airway symptoms may be normal despite the history of episodic respiratory distress. Functional abnormalities may be visualized or may be demonstrable with flow volume loops only during a symptomatic episode. Additionally, the larynx and pharynx may be appreciated by the trained eye during the entrance and exit portion of bronchoscopy. This type of exam may serve to demonstrate a continuity of irritant effects along the entire respiratory tract or to show localization of effects to particular portions of the airway.

The neck is palpated for adenopathy, and the thyroid is palpated for tenderness, nodules, or enlargement. Sinuses are palpated by applying gentle pressure over the maxillary sinuses below the orbits, the frontal sinuses over the eyebrows, and the ethmoids over the bridge of the nose. Maxillary tenderness may indicate dental disease and is an insensitive sign of maxillary sinusitis. Frontal tenderness is more commonly found in frontal sinusitis because of concomitant osteitis.

A neurologic examination pertinent to the upper aerodigestive tract includes evaluation of the extraocular movements, all three branches of the facial nerve, hearing (Rinne and Weber tests), determination of an intact gag reflex, and normal cerebellar function and gait.

VISUALIZING OR IMAGING THE UPPER AIRWAY
Endoscopic rhinoscopy

Fiberoptic endoscopic rhinoscopy is an outpatient procedure[48] that is performed under local anesthesia to evaluate refractory complaints, and, increasingly, in the initial evaluation of nasal complaints. Color atlases are available to orient clinicians interested in the procedure,[49] and professional societies offer training at annual meetings. Rhinoscopy allows identification of smaller polyps, sinusitis (through purulence at the ostia),[48] septal deviation, posterior nasopharyngeal lesions, and lesions of the larynx. It is the authors' recommendation that its use should be reserved for difficult cases (e.g., sinusitis that does not resolve with first line therapy, persistent hoarseness) and in consultation with an otolaryngologist, allergist, or other experienced operator.[49] A referral to an allergist is appropriate for extensive diagnostic evaluation for IgE allergies or for consideration of immunotherapy. A referral to an otolaryngologist is appropriate when treatment of a condition of the sinuses or nasal passages responds poorly to standard management and allergic disease has been excluded or unsuccessfully treated. Additionally, any unusual findings on anterior rhinoscopy such as large polyps, other masses, severe nasal septal deviation, or very enlarged turbinates warrant otolaryngologic referral.

Rigid laryngoscopy

Rigid laryngoscopy, performed by otolaryngologists under general anesthesia, is used to search for and remove foreign objects located in the upper aerodigestive tract, to perform examinations in patients suspected of malignancy, and to provide airway control and access for surgical procedures.

Radiologic evaluation

Clinicians interested in occupational and environmental medicine will primarily seek to uncover evidence of sinusitis or lesions responsible for persistent symptoms of obstruction. Nasal cancer has been associated with occupational and environmental exposures[50] but is a much less common disease. The radiologic evaluation of the upper respiratory tract has altered markedly since the advent of CT and MRI.[51] These techniques have typically replaced plain sinus films. Plain films are now primarily obtained in the acute evaluation of trauma, and tomograms are used only occasionally to evaluate tracheal stenosis. A sinus series of x-rays usually will uncover maxillary[52] or frontal sinusitis but may miss ethmoid or sphenoid disease. Excellent references allow the clinician to become familiar with the cross-sectional anatomy of the upper respiratory tract, knowledge necessary to understand CT scan images.[51]

Computerized tomography of the sinuses, although sensitive in establishing the diagnosis of sinusitis, does not qualify for cost-effective inclusion in the initial workup of sinus problems. Scans are typically obtained at the completion of a course of antibiotics, when fixed lesions are distinguishable from reversible effects of acute inflammation. The normal ostiomeatal complex is best seen in the coronal noncontrast CT scan. Imaging should include fine cuts in coronal and axial planes of the paranasal sinuses. Contrast is generally not necessary unless complications of sinusitis or maligancy are suspected. The MRI is superior to the CT scan in distinguishing between tumor and sinus secretions in an opacified sinus. Computerized tomography of the sinuses should typically be reserved for situations where other approaches, including rhinoscopy, prove unilluminating and almost always after referral of problematic cases for specialist consultation.

The sinonasal region can be divided radiographically into three regions: the sinuses, the ostiomeatal complex, and the nasal cavity. The frontal, maxillary, ethmoid, and sphenoid sinuses are typically air-filled structures lined with a thin mucosa. The normal sinus drainage is from the maxillary sinus, up through the infundibulum and maxillary sinus ostium into the middle meatus.[51] Abnormalities of the sinus contents that are demonstrable by CT or MRI include mucosal thickening indicative of chronic sinusitis, retention cysts or polyps, air fluid levels indicative of acute sinusitis, intubation or trauma, or complete opacification, indicative of a mucocele, trauma, or acute or chronic sinusitis.[51] Examination of the bony walls of the sinuses may also indicate pathologic processes. The anterior wall of the frontal and maxillary sinuses may range from 1 to 3 mm thick, but the posterior wall is typically thinner. Abnormalities of the bony walls that are demonstrable by CT or MRI include bony thickening and sclerosis (indicative of chronic sinusitis or sclerosis), fractures, remodeling (indicating a slowly expanding mucocele or neoplasm), or destruction (indicating a malignancy or invasive infection such as mucormycosis).

PHYSIOLOGIC STUDIES
Acoustic rhinometry

Acoustic rhinometry is a quick, practical tool for use in clinical applications. A spark generator produces an acoustic click, which travels past a microphone and is directed into the nasal passages via a conduit. The click is reflected by various intranasal contours and the microphone receives the reflected sounds. A computer program analyzes the direct and reflected sounds and produces a graph of cross-sectional area for the nasal passage as a function of distance, from the vestibule to the nasaopharynx. The acoustic

tracing has been validated both by CT scan and water displacement techniques[53] and has excellent reproducibility, particularly in the anterior half of the tracing. Acoustic rhinometry has been used to demonstrate fixed nasal lesions such as septal deviations,[53] as well as alterations in cross-sectional area induced by environmental stimuli or pharmacologic agents.[54,55,56]

Rhinomanometry

The nose is one of the most important components of resistance to airflow, contributing 30% to 50% of total inspiratory resistance.[57] Rhinomanometry provides an objective and reproducible[58] measure of nasal patency by describing the pressure-flow characteristics of the nose.[8] Rhinomanometry has become practical and affordable, largely because of transducers, microcircuitry, and computer software. A limitation of the technique is that "patience and persuasion are required to coach each patient in the suitable positioning of the tongue and soft palate to maintain patency of both oropharyngeal and nasopharyngeal orifices while breathing through the nose."[8] Success rates of 85%, with patients using a face mask technique, are reported by the most experienced laboratories.[8,58]

The International Committee on Standardization of Rhinomanometry[59] recommends that "nasal patency be expressed as a ratio between concurrent measurements of transnasal pressure and flow of respiratory air in a patient breathing exclusively through the nose while seated at rest in a comfortable environment."[8] It further recommends that resistance (R_n) be expressed in SI units as $Pa/cm^3/sec$ (or $kPa/L/sec$), which closely approximates the more familiar cm $H_2O/L/sec$. Nasal airway resistance (NAR_n) is usually measured at an arbitrary transnasal pressure, typically 75 to 150 Pa (0.75 to 1.5 cm H_2O).

Pressure–volume measurements of the nasal passage can be made using one of several techniques. Advantages and limitations of each technique are presented in detail in an excellent review.[8] Rhinomanometry performed with a pressure tap in the oral cavity (or oropharynx) and a face mask is called "posterior" rhinomanometry; net bilateral resistance to airflow is measured in this manner. Figure 6-5 shows a schematic of the apparatus and a typical nasal resistance tracing. "Unilateral posterior" rhinomanometry can also be performed by taping one nostril shut during measurements. Rhinomanometry performed with a pressure tap inserted into a sealed nostril is called "anterior" rhinomanometry. Nasal plethysmography is performed in a few research centers and can be performed with a high rate of success, even in pediatric populations.[8] A noninvasive technique has been reported that uses oscillating nasal airflow delivered through the mouth under conditions of nasal patency and occlusion;[60] however, it has not yet been compared in the clinical setting with more traditional measures.

Measured nasal resistance correlates resonably well with

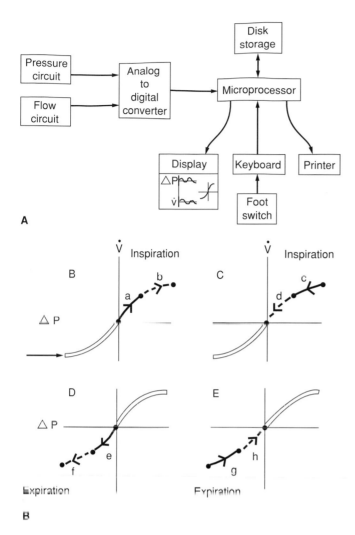

Fig. 6-5. A, Schematic diagram of the apparatus for posterior rhinomanometry. **B,** An example of a tracing of nasal airway resistance. (From Cummings C et al, editors: *Otolaryngology—head and neck surgery,* St. Louis, 1993, C.V. Mosby.)

the results of a rhinoscopic evaluation but correlates less well with the subjective assessment of severity of chronic nasal obstruction.[61] Posterior rhinomanometry correlated to a moderate degree ($r=0.47$) with subjective assessment of nasal patency.[62] In a series of 500 measurements performed with anterior rhinomanometry, there was no correlation between nasal resistance and subjective assessment of "nasal obstruction."[63] Using anterior rhinomanometry to study 974 subjects, McCaffrey et al. found that moderate to severe subjective symptoms of nasal obstruction occurred primarily above 3 cm H_2O/L/sec.[64] James et al. did not find a similar separation in the subjects they studied.[58]

In 100 normal adult subjects in England, the mean NAR was 0.31 Pa/cm³/sec (range 0.13 to 0.84); in 56 subjects in New Mexico, studies on each of 2 days, the mean NAR was 1.46 cm H_2O/L/sec (range 0.3 to 5.41) on day 1 and 1.61 ± 1.54 (range 0.24 to 9.62) on day 2. In 96% of the individu-

als, the difference in NAR between test day 1 and 2 was within 2 standard deviation of the mean. In contrast, the between subject variability was large, accounting for 75% of the total variance.[58] Analysis of data after eight individuals had been tested indicated that 65% of the mean NAR values were estimated to within ± 0.4 cm H_2O/L/sec when five tracings were obtained. The author's laboratory typically obtains five tracings to determine a single resistance value.

In most laboratories, posterior rhinomanometry shows less variation than does anterior rhinomanometry.[65] Repeated posterior nasal resistance measurements of healthy individuals with resting, untreated noses show a coefficient of variation of less than 20% and less variation in decongested noses. One laboratory did publish coefficients of variation for anterior rhinomanometry of 12% and for posterior rhinomanometry of 16%.[66] Posterior rhinomanometry can be repeated after decongestants, helping to separate fixed lesions (e.g., deviated septum) from vascular congestion.

A limitation of rhinomanometry has been that resistance values are commonly determined by structures in the anterior nasal passage, and structures in the mid and posterior nasal passsages typically do not influence nasal resistance, although they may alter the sensation of obstruction.[63] The maximum inspiratory flow maneuver, a variation of rhinomanometry, was used to assess posterior changes[67]; however, it was cumbersome and is rapidly being supplanted by acoustic rhinometry.

Nasal peak flow meters have been used in some epidemiologic studies. These measures may provide confirmation of congestive symptoms and document their possible association with workplace exposures. Both inspiratory and expiratory nasal peak flows have been recorded; the inspiratory flow measurement has a hygienic advantage since it reduces the risk of nasal secretions obstructing the meter. Nasal peak flow meters have also been used in clinical evaluations during workplace challenges.[68]

Nasal compliance

Nasal compliance, the change in nasal volume per unit pressure, has been hypothesized to be an important determinant of the transition from nasal to oronasal breathing. Nasal compliance was not measurable because of the technical inability to perform rapid measurements of nasal volume, until the advent of acoustic rhinometry (see above). Early studies have shown that anterior nasal compliance is greater than posterior compliance and that vasoconstrictors will reduce midnasal compliance, whereas the induction of congestion and edema will not alter compliance.[69] Pulmonary compliance, defined as the change in thoracic volume per unit pressure, has been useful in the evolution of certain lung diseases because data are available about the range of normal values. Comparable data are not available for nasal compliance measurements.

Nasal mucociliary clearance

The largest component of the normal nasal mucociliary clearance apparatus moves mucus-imbedded particulate matter (and dissolved gaseous pollutants) from the anterior nares posteriorly to the nasopharynx, oropharynx, and hypopharynx, where they are cleared either by swallowing or expectoration. Intact mucociliary function depends on the anatomic continuity of the airway, anatomic and motor properties of nasal cilia, and rheologic (or flow) properties of secreted nasal mucus.[69a] Congenital or acquired defects in anatomy (e.g., septal deviation, polyposis), ciliary structure and function (primary ciliary dyskinesia), and mucus formation (cystic fibrosis) can all disrupt nasal mucociliary function.[70-73] There is also both in vitro and in vivo evidence that mucociliary function is disrupted by such environmental insults as viral infection (the common cold), antigenic challenge ("hay fever"), and irritant inhalants (cigarette smoke).[70-74] Unfortunately for those who would apply these techniques to the environmental sciences, controversy exists regarding the optimal methods and interpretation of mucociliary function tests.

One component of the assessment of the nasal mucociliary apparatus is the observation of ciliary beat frequency in vitro. This method is often employed as a screening step (prior to electron microscopic examination of biopsy specimens) in the diagnosis of disorders involving ultrastructural abnormalities of cilia (e.g., Kartagener's syndrome). Specimens are typically obtained either by scraping or biopsy of the inferior turbinate; ciliary beat frequency so determined is normally in the 9 to 15 Hz range.[72,75] In addition to frequency, trained observers can note the degree of spatial coordination of adjacent ciliary units, an important component of intact function. Although ciliary beat frequency is a relatively objective and reproducible measure, its relationship to particle clearance and clinical symptoms is less constant. Ciliary beat frequency can be altered by experimental conditions (e.g., cooling); therefore, considerable attention to detail is needed if looking for subtle changes induced by environmental agents.

The saccharin test has been used as a screening device for nasal mucociliary dysfunction. In this procedure, a small drop of saccharin solution is placed on the anterior portion of the inferior turbinate, and the time interval before the subject "tastes" the saccharin is recorded. A prolonged test—defined as greater than 30 minutes—indicates impaired mucociliary function.[76-78] This test is noninvasive, carries negligible risk, and is intrinsically related to the physiologic endpoint of interest. The major drawback of the saccharin test lies in its lack of cross-test validity (see below). A second drawback is that the saccharin test measures mucociliary clearance in only a small surface area of the nose.

Various methods have been devised to validate (or cross-validate) measures of nasal mucociliary function. Stanley and colleagues[79] found a tight correlation between saccharin clearance times in the right and left nostrils, measured on separate occasions. Moriarty et al.[80] found significantly slower mean ciliary beat frequencies and saccharin clearance times among otolaryngology clinic patients compared with normal controls, but found no systematic relationship between saccharin clearance time and ciliary beat frequency within the patient group. Katz and co-workers[75] compared nasal ciliary beat frequency with *tracheal* mucociliary clearance rates in nonatopic nonsmokers but found no systematic relationship. In sum, the various techniques for evaluating nasal mucociliary function involve substantial trade-offs in terms of invasiveness, reliability, and validity, such that it is difficult at this time to specify a "gold standard."

Another method of documenting mucociliary clearance involves tracking, radiographically, the movement of objects placed in the nasal cavity, typically on the superior surface of the inferior turbinate. The object in question may be a radioopaque disk or spherule (in which case imaging is by serial plain films), or a radiotagged particle that is tracked with a gamma camera.[76] An advantage of this set of techniques is the close approximation of the experimental measure to the physiologic endpoint of interest; a limitation is the exposure of patients (or experimental subjects) to small doses of ionizing radiation.

Mucous rheology

Characteristics of mucus, such as viscoelastic properties, can be determined on samples that have been obtained from subjects or patients. Comparable methods, used in rats, showed that exposure to urban air pollution resulted in a more rigid mucus, a change that would impair mucociliary clearance.[81]

Nasal mucosal blood flow measurement

Changes in nasal mucosal blood flow are significant physiologically, since engorgement of submucosal venous capacitance vessels produces reversible thickening of the mucosa and a consequent decrease in airway cross-sectional area and increase in airway resistance.[20] The latter physiologic change is experienced subjectively as nasal congestion. Both invasive and noninvasive measures have been employed to measure this parameter. Whereas nasal mucosal blood flow changes have been documented experimentally after pharmacologic and antigenic challenge,[82-84] they have not been studied directly after environmental stimuli. Nevertheless, indirect evidence indicates that blood flow alterations may underlie environmentally induced nasal airway resistance changes (e.g., after exposure to environmental tobacco smoke.[85]

Mucosal blood flow measurements have traditionally employed invasive techniques (e.g., injection of radioactive tracers). One such method is known as the xenon washout technique. This method, which has been used in both experimental animals and humans, requires the injection of a radioactive tracer (^{133}Xe) into the nasal submucosa, with the decay of gamma activity ("washout") being taken as a measure of mucosal blood flow. Given its invasiveness, radiologic hazard (however small) and potential for variability in the anatomic placement of the injected radionuclide, this test is not destined to become a widely used clinical measure.

A relatively recent development—laser Doppler flowmetry—enables investigators to noninvasively measure flow rate (per unit volume of tissue), mean red blood cell (RBC) velocity, and tissue blood volume percent. The technique works on the principle that coherent light reflected from moving blood elements is shifted in frequency relative to incident (and reflected) light.[84,86] A drawback of this technique is the requirement that a fiberoptic probe remain in relatively constant approximation to the mucosa, severely restricting an experimental subject's movement during provocation testing. Consistent with this limitation, provocation tests to date have focused on rapidly acting (pharmacologic or antigenic) stimuli. Notwithstanding these limitations, this technique could be adapted for irritant inhalation challenge tests in the future, particularly with such rapidly acting agents as environmental tobacco smoke.

Interestingly, different investigators have found varied effects of antigen challenge on nasal mucosal blood flow (i.e., increases or decreases) using the xenon washout technique.[87,88] Similarly, xenon washout and laser Doppler flowmetry (below) appear to have distinct sensitivities to

blood flow changes induced by different topical vasoconstrictors, leading at least one investigator to speculate that the two techniques reflect blood flow in different parts of the vascular bed.[89]

Transepithelial potential difference

Functioning, healthy upper airway mucosa generates a potential difference between its lumen and the submucosa. The potential is lumen negative and is variable in magnitude in the nasal cavity. As different potentials are associated with different types of nasal lining and competency of the mucosa, this technique may be used to identify mucosa that generates no potential or an unusual potential, currently used to identify cystic fibrosis patients.[90]

A schematic of the apparatus is shown in Fig. 6-6. A subdermal needle placed in the hand or forearm is an isoelectric probe that serves as a submucosal electrode. A lumen electrode is placed intranasally, and a voltmeter measures the difference in potential between the two. Salt bridges serve as biologic electrodes.

Trigeminal evoked potentials

Neurotoxicologists have long been interested in measuring trigeminal evoked potentials (i.e., the speed and quality of impulse transmission from the nasal epithelial

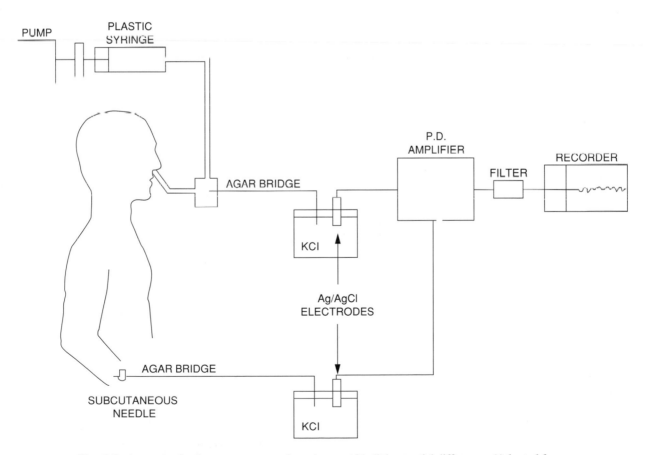

Fig. 6-6. Apparatus for the measurement of nasal transepithelial potential difference. (Adapted from Guyton AC, editor: *Textbook of medical physiology,* 7th ed., Philadelphia, 1986, Saunders.)

surface to the cerebral cortex), but technical difficulties impaired progress. A key to evoked potentials is the ability to deliver a sharp stimulus that can be time-linked to the cortical recordings. Recently developed and validated methods use a brief pulse of carbon dioxide delivered to the nasal epithelial surface. With this apparatus, the magnitude of the perceived intensity of the stimulus is correlated with the magnitude of the cortical recording.[91,92]

Olfactory function

Although most nasal pathology caused by occupational or industrial exposures has not been documented to impair olfaction, many agents have not been tested for their potential to cause olfactory impairment. Various research centers have developed panels of olfactory stimulants to present to patients in a systematic manner to test olfactory threshold, as well as olfactory discrimination. Olfactory evoked potential (OEP)[93] recording and contigent negative variation (CNV) are techniques that measure very small changes in voltage along the olfactory neuronal circuit as it ascends to the brain. Olfactory evoked potential recording determines the voltage changes at various locations on the scalp, which reflect action potentials in the olfactory circuit. These changes are triggered by a suprathreshold olfactory stimulus. Contingent negative variation is a negative voltage developing at the vertex after discrimination of one of two smells while the patient is expecting a second stimulus. Contingent negative variation requires attention and some cooperation, whereas OEPs do not. Of these two techniques, parosmia can be evaluated only with CNV. Hyposmia and anosmia may be detected by both techniques, but OEPs may still be undetectable with hyposmia. Additionally, CNV may be less variable in assessing anosmia.

Pulmonary function

Since an exposure causing upper respiratory symptoms may also be delivered to the lungs, it is critical to establish baseline pulmonary function studies. For protein allergens, spirometry and 2 weeks of peak flow tracings are usually sufficient.[4] For prolonged upper respiratory symptoms associated with significant exposure to irritants or low-molecular-weight sensitizers, a complete set of pulmonary function studies including spirometry and diffusing capacity, is advised. If the evaluation suggests concomitant lower respiratory tract disease, further workup should proceed as described in Chapters 3, 4, 5, 13, 14, and 16.

TESTS CHARACTERIZING NASAL AIRWAY BIOLOGY

A variety of biologic indexes may be examined by the use of various well-established sampling methods such as nasal scrapes or swabs obtained with a curette or probe, nasal spritz, nasal discs, nasal biopsy, nasal lavage, nasal cultures, and collection of nasal mucus. Indexes include the enumeration and characterization of structural cells in the nasal mucosa, inflammatory cells entering the nasal mucosa, and the presence and quantity of a variety of proteins and mediators at the airway surface.

Nasal scrape or swab

The purpose of the nasal swab is to identify the characteristics of cells present at the nasal airway surface. This can have diagnostic utility in the evaluation of rhinitis. Samples of nasal mucosa can be obtained with a curette such as the Rhinoprobe™, or a swab such as a Calge™ swab. Eosinophils are characteristic of allergic diseases or, in the case of negative skin tests, the NARES syndrome. Neutrophils are more commonly seen with infections or irritant exposures. Increased metachromatic cells (basophils or mast cells) have been observed in allergic patients during periods of seasonal exposure. For example, nasal mucosal cytology by scraping has been used successfully in studies of residents exposed to formaldehyde insulation to detect squamous metaplasia.[94] The Rhinoprobe™ is inserted in the nasal passage and gently pulled along the medial surface of the inferior turbinate.[1] The swab is inserted approximately 3 cm and gently pulled along the septum of the nasal cavity below the inferior or middle turbinate. Once off of the mucosa, the swab is rotated and a second pull made, up to a total of five passes. One sample from each nostril is rolled onto two glass slides, air dried, and stained. Commonly available stains such as Wright stain or Diff Quik™ will identify neutrophils and eosinophils on one slide, whereas the Alcian blue stain allows identification of basophils on the other.

Nasal disc

The technique of placing a paper disk on the nasal mucosal surface has been used to quantify the weight of secretions on the surface and to collect secretions for analysis. An advantage of the technique is that serial disks can be applied (as with a nasal methacholine disk challenge).[95] Furthermore the nasonasal reflex can be studied by performing an ipsilateral challenge and comparing the response on the ipsilateral and contralateral side.[96]

Nasal lavage

Nasal lavage has been performed in research settings to define the inflammatory response to specific agents. The lavage is performed by having subjects close the palate with the Valsava maneuver and extend the neck 45° while 2.5 to 5 ml of saline (37°C) is instilled in each nostril. After 10 seconds, subjects flex the neck and expel the contents into a basin. The volume of liquid is quantified and the lavage fluid analyzed for total and differential cell counts and for the concentration of mediators and proteins, such as albumin, kinins, TAME-esterase activity, histamine, fibrinogen, interleukin-8, lactoferrin, secretory IgA, calcitonin gene-related peptide, neurokinin A, and other markers of nasal activity. Similar to nasal swab, the presence of inflammatory cells in the absence of infection raises the possibility of a reaction to airborne allergens or irritants. Besides pharmacologic markers, a variety of inflammatory cell types can be examined by nasal lavage.[97]

Nasal spritz

Investigators have recently modified the techniques to collect nasal surface secretions. This technique has the advantage of collecting more concentrated samples and of being performed without inserting catheters into the nose. The spritz is performed by having seated subjects place a metered nasal dispenser in the nasal passage and actuate the dispense five times, following each actuation with a sniff. At the end of the five actuations, the subject blows the secretions into a specimen cup that is held below the nose throughout the procedure. This series is repeated eight times, resulting in a total of 4.0 ml delivered to the nasal passage and a return of approximately 3.6 ml. Earlier techniques used a combinations of spritzes combined with suctioning of secretions with a catheter placed on the floor of the nasal passage.[21]

Nasal biopsy

Nasal biopsy rarely provides additional information in the clinical setting unless physical exam identifies specific lesions. Nasal biopsies showing an increased population of basophils and mast cells have been described in patients with vasomotor rhinitis.

Cultures

If the physical exam indicates a pharyngitis, cultures of the throat may be taken. Nasal cultures are not indicated routinely. Correlation of nasal swab culture with organisms in the ipsilateral maxillary sinus organisms is fair; however, correlation with contralateral maxillary sinus culture results is poor. When purulence is seen exiting the middle meatus (under the middle turbinate), the yield of nasal swab culture becomes satisfactory. Although nasal swab cultures may assist in antibiotic selection and in organization of epidemiologic data, the culture results in most cases should not alter therapy that is based on a full clinical evaluation. Recently, the hypothesis has been proposed that chronic sinusitis may be due to allergy to constituents of "normal respiratory flora." As yet there is

Table 6-6. Work-up for upper airway symptoms

History	Physical	Procedures	Dx
Seasonal symptoms Asthma, eczema Cat, rodents, roach exposure Stuffed furniture, carpets Air conditioning and forced air heat Damp basements or crawl space	Boggy, pale or blue mucosa Clear discharge	+ Eos swab + MultiRAST + Skin tests + Wheezes + Ag provocation	Allergic rhinitis (IgE)
Work-related onset LMW chemical exposure Exposure-related symptoms		+ Eos swab − IgE/RAST/skin tests + Serology + Provocation	LMW allergic rhinitis

Irritant exposures
  ETS
  New carpets
  Roofing fumes
+ atopy
No seasonal pattern
	Dry mucosa or a clear discharge
	Erythematous mucosa ± erosions
		+ PMN swab
		− IgE/RAST/skin tests
		(+ provocation)
			Irritant rhinitis

Multiple VOC triggers Perennial symptoms	Clear discharge Blue or red mucosa ±congestion	− IgE/RAST/skin tests + MeCh challenge + Basos swab	"Vasomotor rhinitis"
	±Polyps	+ Eos swab − Skin tests	NARES syndrome
Localized headache Prurulent discharge	Localized tenderness Prurulence of ostia/pharynx	+ PMN swab + CT scan (+ endoscopy)	Sinusitis

CT, computerized tomography; *ETS,* environmental tobacco smoke; *LMW,* low-molecular weight; *PMN,* polymorphonuclear cell; *RAST,* radioallergosorbent test; *VOC,* volatile organic compound.

insufficient information to advise on the clinical relevance of this hypothesis.

ASSESSMENT OF ATOPIC STATUS

If the history is suggestive of IgE-mediated allergies, or if medicolegal considerations make it essential to confirm or exclude allergy, a referral may be made for allergy skin testing. The allergist will typically perform a screening skin test battery, including locally relevant seasonal allergens (trees, grasses, weeds, and some fungi) and common perennial allergens (dust mites, cat, dog, cockroach, rodent, some molds, and fungi). A suspicion of allergy to a specific substance should be communicated to the allergist so that appropriate skin testing can be performed. There are many antigens available for skin testing that are not used in the screening skin tests typically performed by consulting allergists. The presence of skin test reactivity simply indicates that the subject has IgE antibody against the antigen. Diagnosis of allergic disease requires a congruence of the clinical history and skin test reactivity.

A multiallergen radioallergosorbent test (RAST) is a serologic screening test that identifies the presence or absence of specific IgE antibody against a group of common allergens. The advantage of the test is that it has a reasonable sensitivity. The major limitation is that specific allergens are not identified, and clinical correlation is not possible. A total serum IgE is useful if it is very low since allergic disease is distinctly uncommon in the presence of a very low total IgE level. However, allergic disease may certainly occur in the presence of a normal total serum IgE.

If a patient previously had allergy skin testing, a copy of the results should be obtained for review. If skin tests did not include the suspected antigen, additional testing is indicated. If skin tests were previously negative, but symptoms are strong and increase in the middle of a known allergy season, retesting may be warranted at the time of seasonal symptoms. Skin tests are appropriate when exposure is to protein allergens that cause IgE-mediated reactions. An etiologic role for other agents, such as formaldehyde or cigarette smoke, remains best established by a combination of symptom-diary, environmental sampling, and occasionally blinded provocation testing.

RESPONSE TO INTRANASAL CHALLENGE

Nasal reactivity can be assessed using methacholine or histamine challenge. A variety of techniques have been employed. In the experimental setting, nasal reactivity shows increases following antigen challenge. An increase in secretions has also been demonstrated following methacholine challenge in subjects with vasomotor rhinitis when compared with unaffected subjects. However, this test has primarily been used in a research setting. A new method for methacholine challange utilizing impregnated paper disks obviates the need for mist inhalation, making the procedure considerably safer, more comfortable, and more convenient.

Specific challenge

Nasal challenge with antigen is used in some clinical settings to establish a diagnosis of nasal allergy. The use of provocation with other agents (e.g., cold air, ozone, environmental tobacco smoke) may demonstrate specific hyperresponsiveness, but its use has been limited to a few centers and it remains a research tool. The issue of acute upper respiratory tract responses to low-level airborne chemical exposures, particularly involving indoor air pollutants, has generated considerable interest. Symptomatic endpoints include nasal irritation, rhinorrhea, nasal congestion, sneezing, and throat irritation. Several relatively noninvasive measures of upper airway function hold promise for objectively documenting such symptoms in humans. These techniques include rhinomanometry, nasal lavage, nasal mucosal blood flow measurement, and measurements of mucociliary clearance. Volunteers exposed to ozone or to levels of volatile organic compounds (VOCs) typical of so-called "sick buildings," and office workers using carbonless copy paper, may show nasal inflammatory responses and/or increases in nasal airway resistance. Individuals who give a history of rhinitis with environmental tobacco smoke (ETS) exposure show significantly greater increases in nasal airway resistance after brief high levels of tobacco smoke than do ETS-insensitive individuals. Possible mechanisms of upper airway reactivity include allergy, chemical injury, and neurogenic inflammation. Preexisting allergy appears to modulate the threshold for trigeminal irritant chemoreceptors and the magnitude of neurogenic response.

MEDICAL MONITORING

When workers are potentially exposed to agents that may potentially harm the upper airway, an assessment of the upper airway is a necessary part of a monitoring program. The components of the surveillance may range from direct inspection of the nasal mucosa for ulcers (e.g., with exposure to hexavalent chromium dust) to identification of symptom patterns using an interview or questionnaire. Incorporation of medical monitoring in a surveillance program is useful to reduce the risk of upper airway disease and to identify and control exposure to agents that could cause lower respiratory tract disease. For episodic clinical evaluations (i.e., those prompted by the occurrence of symptoms), diagnostic evaluation of the upper airway should be undertaken in the presence of either upper and lower airway complaints.

CONCLUSION

Through a complete history and physical examination combined with appropriate use of various laboratory tests, a patient's upper respiratory status may be thoroughly assessed (Table 6-6). Additionally, as therapeutic options are applied, their efficacy and progression of pathology may be monitored. Familiarity with the tools of an upper respiratory evaluation is necessary for the clinician treating patients with occupational and environmental respiratory diseases.

REFERENCES

1. Meltzer EO, Schatz M, and Zeiger RS: Allergic and nonallergic rhinitis. In: Middleton E Jr, Reed CE, Ellis EF, Adkinson NF Jr, Yunginger JW, editors, *Allergy principles and practice, pp 1253-1289, Washington DC, 1988, C. V. Mosby.*

2. Cummings C, et al, editors: *Otolaryngology—head & neck surgery,* St. Louis, 1993, C. V. Mosby.

3. Standardization of spirometry—1987 update. Official statement of the American Thoracic Society. *Am Rev Respir Dis* 136:1285-1298, 1987.

4. American College of Chest Physicians: Occupational airways disease: a consensus statement. *Chest* 1995(in press).

5. Matory WE Jr: Non-Caucasian rhinoplasty: a 16-year experience, *Plast Reconstr Surg* 72:239-251, 1986.

6. Keysavanathan J: Effect of nostril shape on particle deposition and removal, unpublished data, 1994.

7. Scherer P, Hahn I, and Mozell M: The biophysics of nasal airflow, *Otolaryngol Clin North Am* 22:265-278, 1989.

8. Cole P: Rhinomanometry 1988: practice and trends, *Laryngoscope* 99:311-315, 1989.

9. Ohki M, Naito K, and Cole P: Dimensions and resistances of the human nose: racial differences, *Laryngoscope* 101:276-278, 1991.

10. Togias AG, Naclerio RM, Proud D, Fish JE, Franklin N, Adkinson J, Kagey-Sobotka A, Norman PS, and Lichtenstein LM. Nasal challenge with cold, dry air results in release of inflammatory mediators: possible mast cell involvement, *J Clin Invest* 76:1375-1381, 1985.

11. Togias AG, Proud D, Lichtenstein LM, Kagey-Sobotka A, Kenneth G, Adams I, Norman PS, and Naclerio RM: The osmolality of nasal secretions increases during the response to inhalation of cold dry air, *Am J Respir Crit Care Med* (in press).

12. Mygind N, Pedersen M, and Nielsen MH: Ch. 4. Morphology of the upper airway epithelium. In Proctor DF and Andersen I, editors: *The nose. Upper airway physiology and the atmospheric environment,* pp 71-97, New York, 1992, Elsevier Biomedical.

13. Cauna N: Ch. 3. Blood and nerve supply of the nasal lining. In Proctor DF and Andersen I, editors: *The nose. Upper airway physiology and the atmospheric environment,* pp 45-69, New York, 1982, Elsevier Biomedical Press.

14. Frank M and Rabin M: Chemosensory neuroanatomy and physiology, *Ear Nose Throat J* 68:291-292, 294, 296, 1989.

15. Silver WL: The common chemical sense. In Finger TE and Silver WL, editors: *Neurobiology of taste and smell,* pp 65-87, New York, 1987, John Wiley.

16. Nielsen GD: Mechanisms of activation of the sensory irritant receptor by airborne chemicals, *CRC Crit Rev Toxicol* 21:183-208, 1991.

17. Baraniuk J: Sensory, parasympathetic, and sympathetic neural influences in the nasal mucosa, *J Allergy Clin Immunol* 90:1045-1050, 1992.

18. Baraniuk J: Neural control of human nasal secretion, *Pulmon Pharmacol* 4:20-31, 1991.

19. Baraniuk J, Silver P, Kaliner M, and Barnes P: Neuropeptide Y is a vasoconstrictor in human nasal mucosa, *J Appl Physiol* 73:1867-1872, 1992.

20. Widdicombe J: Nasal pathophysiology, *Respir Med* 84 Suppl A:3-9; discussion 9-10, 1990.

21. Raphael GD, Druce HM, Baraniuk JN, and Kaliner MA: Pathophysiology of rhinitis. 1. Assessment of the sources of protein in methacholine-induced nasal secretions, *Am Rev Respir Dis* 138:413-420, 1988.

22. Baraniuk JN, Lundgren JD, Okayama M, Goff J, Mullol J, Merida M, Shelhamer JH, and Kaliner MA: Substance P and neurokinin A in human nasal mucosa, *Am J Respir Cell Mol Biol* 4:228-236, 1991.

23. Baraniuk JN, Lundgren JD, Goff J, Mullol J, Castellino S, Merida M, Shelhamer JH, and Kaliner MA: Calcitonin gene-related peptide in human nasal mucosa. *Am J Physiol (Lung Mol Cell Physiol)* 258:L81-L88, 1990.

24. Baraniuk J, Lundgren J, Goff J, Peden D, Merida M, Shelhamer J, and Kaliner M: Gastrin-releasing peptide in human nasal mucosa, *J Clin Invest* 85:998-1005, 1990.

25. Baraniuk JN and Kaliner M: Neuropeptides and nasal secretion, *Am J Physiol (Lung Cell Mol Physiol)* 261:L223-L235, 1991.

26. Naclerio RM, Meier HL, Kagey-Sobotka A, Adkinson NF, Meyers DA, Norman PS, and Lichtenstein LM: Mediator release after nasal airway challenge with allergen, *Am Rev Respir Dis* 128:597-602, 1983.

27. Creticos PS, Peters SP, Adkinson NF, Naclerio RM, Hayes EC, Norman PS, and Lichtenstein LM: Peptide leukotriene release after antigen challenge in patients sensitive to ragweed, *New Engl J Med* 310:1626-1630, 1984.

28. Raphael GD, Meredith SD, Baraniuk JN, Druce HM, Banks SM, and Kaliner MA: The pathophysiology of rhinitis. II. Assessment of the sources of protein in histamine-induced nasal secretions, *Am Rev Respir Dis* 139:791-800, 1989.

29. Proud D, Togias A, Naclerio RM, Crush SA, Norman PS, and Lichtenstein LM: Kinins are generated in vivo following nasal airway challenge of allergic individuals with allergen, *J Clin Invest* 72:1678-1685, 1983.

30. Bascom R, Naclerio R, Fitzgerald T, Kagey-Sobotka A, and Proud D: Effect of ozone inhalation on the response to nasal challenge with antigen of allergic subjects, *Am Rev Respir Dis* 142:594-601, 1990.

31. Graham DE and Koren HS: Biomarkers of inflammation in ozone-exposed humans. Comparison of the nasal and bronchalveolar lavage, *Am Rev Respir Dis* 142:152-156, 1990.

32. Bascom R, Kulle T, Kagey-Sobotka A, and Proud D: Upper respiratory tract environmental tobacco smoke sensitivity, *Am Rev Respir Dis* 143:1304-1311, 1991.

33. Bascom R, Kagey-Sobotka A, and Proud D: Effect of intranasal capsaicin on symptoms and mediator release, *J Pharmacol Exp Ther* 259:1323-1327, 1991.

34. Brittebo EB, Castonguay A, Rafter JJ, Kowalski B, Ahlman M, and Brandt I: 13. Metabolism of xenobiotics and steriod hormones in the nasal mucosa, In Barrow CS, editor: *Toxicology of the nasal passages,* pp 211-234, Washington, 1986, Hemisphere.

35. Dahl AR: 16. Possible consequences of cytochrome P-450-dependent monooxygenases in nasal tissues, In Barrow CS, editor: *Toxicology of the nasal passages,* pp 345-372, Washington, D. C., 1986, Hemisphere.

36. Dahl AR and Hadley WM: Nasal cavity enzymes involved in xenobiotic metabolism: effects on the toxicity of inhalants, *Crit Rev Toxicol* 21:345-372, 1991.

37. Proctor DF: Measurement of mucociliary activity in man, *Ann Otol Rhinol Laryngol* 78:518-531, 1969.

38. Morgan KT, Patterson DL, and Gross EA: 8. Responses of the nasal mucociliary apparatus to airborne irritants, In Barrow CS, editor: *Toxicology of the nasal passages,* pp 123-133, Washington, 1986, Hemisphere.

39. Boucher R: Mechanisms of pollutant-induced airways toxicity, *Clin Chest Med* 2:377-392, 1981.

40. Weiss S, Tager I, Schenker M, and Speizer F: State of the art: the health effects of involuntary smoking, *Am Rev Respir Dis* 128:933-942, 1983.

41. Gergen PJ and Turkeltaub PC: The association of allergen skin test reactivity and respiratory disease among whites in the US population. Data from the second National Health and Nutrition Examination Survey, 1976-1980, *Arch Int Med* 151:487-492, 1991.

42. Pope AM, Patterson R, and Burge H, ed: *Indoor allergens. Assessing and controlling adverse health effects.* Committee on the Health Effects of Indoor Allergens, Division of Health Promotion and Disease Prevention, Institute of Medicine, p 308, Washington, D.C., 1993, National Academy Press.

43. Kennedy S, Enarson D, Janssen R, and Chan-Yeung M: Lung health consequences of reported accidental chlorine gas exposures among pulpmill workers, *Am Rev Respir Dis* 143:74-79, 1991.

44. Environmental Protection Agency: Indoor air quality and work environment study: EPA healdquarters' buildings Volume 1: Employee survey. November 1989.

45. Cullen MR: The worker with multiple chemical sensitivities: an overview. In Cullen MR, editor: *Workers with multiple chemical sensitivities,* pp 655-662, Philadelphia, 1987, Hanley & Belfus.

46. Bascom R: Differential responsiveness to irritant mixtures: possible mechanisms, *Ann NY Acad Sci* 641:225-247, 1992.

47. Shim C and Williams MH: Effect of odors in asthma, *Am J Med* 80:18-22, 1986.

48. Castellanos J and Axelrod D: Flexible fiberoptic rhinoscopy in the diagnosis of sinusitis, *J Allergy Clin Immunol* 83:91-94, 1989.

49. Shaw JD and Lancer JM: *A color atlas of fiberoptic endoscopy of the upper respiratory tract,* p 81, Ipswich, England, 1987, W. S. Cowell.

50. Acheson ED: 9. Epidemiology of nasal cancer, In Barrow CS, editor: *Toxicology of the nasal passages,* pp 135-141, Washington D.C., 1986, Hemisphere.

51. Dalley RW and Robertson WD: Chapter 2. Diagnostic imaging of the head and neck, In Cummings CW and Krause CJ, editors: *Otolaryngology— head and neck surgery,* pp 13-71, St. Louis, 1993, Mosby–Year Book.

52. Axelsson A and Runze U: Comparison of subjective and radiological findings during the course of acute maxillary sinusitis, *Ann Otol Rhinol Laryngol* 92:75-77, 1983.

53. Hilberg O, Jackson AC, Swift DL, and Pedersen OF: Acoustic rhinometry: evaluation of nasal cavity geometry by acoustic reflection, *J Appl Physiol* 66:295-303, 1989.

54. Yamagiwa M, Hilberg O, Pedersen O, and Lundqvist G: Evaluation of the effect of localized skin cooling on nasal airway volume by acoustic rhinometry, *Am Rev Respir Dis* 141:1050-1054, 1990.

55. Swift DL, Nadarajah J, Fitzgerald TK, Permutt T, and Bascom R: Acoustic rhinometry as a tool for human inhalation toxicology studies. Proceedings of the meeting of the American Industrial Hygiene Association, 1992.

56. Bascom R, Fitzgerald TK, Permutt T, Sauder L, Nadarajah J, and Swift DL: Response to environmental tobacco smoke: dose-response studies and the effect on acoustic rhinometry, *Am Rev Respir Dis* 145:A92, 1992.

57. Geurkink N: Nasal anatomy, physiology, and function, *J Allergy Clin Immunol* 72:123-128, 1983.

58. James D, Stidley C, Mermier C, Lambert W, Chick T, and Samet J: Sources of variability in posterior rhinomanometry, *Ann Otol Rhinol Laryngol* 102:631-638, 1993.

59. Clement PR: Committee report on standardization of rhinomanometry, *Rhinology* 22:151-155, 1984.

60. Tawfik B, Sullivan K, and Chang H: A new method to measure nasal impedance in spontaneously breathing adults, *J Appl Physiol* 71:9-15, 1991.

61. Naito K, Cole P, and Chaban R: Nasal resistance, sensation of obstruction and rhinoscopic findings compared, *Am J Rhinol* 2:65-69, 1988.

62. Gleeson M, Youlton L, Shelton D, Siodlak M, Eiser N, and Wengraf C: Assessment of nasal patency: comparison of four methods, *Clin Otolaryngol* 11:99-107, 1986.

63. Jones A, Willatt D, and Durham L: Nasal airflow: resistance and sensation, *J Laryngol Otol* 103:909-911, 1989.

64. McCaffrey TV and Kern EB: Clinical evaluation of nasal obstruction, *Arch Otolaryngol* 105:542-545, 1979.

65. Dvoracek JE, Hills A, and Rossing RG: Comparison of sequential anterior and posterior rhinomanometry, *J Allergy Clin Immunol* 76:577-582, 1985.

66. Shelton D and Eiser N: Evaluation of active anterior and posterior rhinomanometry in normal subjects, *Clin Otolaryngol* 17:178-182, 1992.

67. Bridger GP and Proctor DF: Maximum nasal inspiratory flow and nasal resistance, *Ann Otol* 79:481-488, 1970.

68. Ahman M: Nasal peak flow rate records in work related nasal blockage, *Acta Otolaryngol (Stockh)* 112:839-844, 1992.

69. Keysavanathan JN, Bascom R, and Swift DL: Nasal compliance studies, *J Appl Physiol* 1994 (in revision).

69a. Wanner A: Clinical aspects of mucociliary transport, Am Rev Respir Dis 116:73-125, 1977.

70. Afzelius BA: Disorders of ciliary motility, *Hosp Pract* 21:73-80, 1986.

71. Mygind N, Pedersen M, and Nielsen MH: Primary and secondary ciliary dyskinesia, *Acta Otolaryngol* 95:688-694, 1983.

72. Rossman CM, Lee R, Forrest JB, and Newhouse MT: Nasal ciliary ultrastructure and function in patients with primary ciliary dyskinesia compared with that in normal subjects and in subjects with various respiratory diseases, *Am Rev Respir Dis* 129:161-167, 1984.

73. Wanner A: Allergic mucociliary dysfunction, *J Allergy Clin Immunol* 72:347-350, 1983.

74. Sakakura Y: Changes of mucociliary function during colds, *Eur J Respir Dis Suppl* 128 (Pt 1):348-354, 1983.

75. Katz I, Zwas T, Baum G, Aharonson E, and Belfer B: Ciliary beat frequency and mucociliary clearance. What is the relationship? *Chest* 92:491-493, 1987.

76. Andersen I and Proctor D: Measurement of nasal mucociliary clearance, *Eur J Respir Dis Suppl* 127:37-40, 1983.

77. Corbo G, Foresi A, Bonfitto P, Mugnano A, Agabiti N, and Cole P: Measurement of nasal mucociliary clearance, *Arch Dis Child* 64:546-550, 1989.

78. Stanley P, MacWilliam L, Greenstone M, Mackay I, and Cole P: Efficacy of a saccharin test for screening to detect abnormal mucociliary clearance, *Br J Dis Chest* 78:62-65, 1984.

79. Stanley P, Wilson R, Greenstone M, MacWilliam L, and Cole P: Effect of cigarette smoking on nasal mucociliary clearance and ciliary beat frequency, *Thorax* 41:519-523, 1986.

80. Moriarty B, Robson A, Smallman L, and Drake-Lee A: Nasal mucociliary function: comparison of saccharin clearance with ciliary beat frequency, *Rhinology* 29:173-179, 1991.

81. Saldiva P, King M, Delmonte V, Macchione M, Parada M, Daliberto M, Sakae R, Criado P, Silveira P, and Zin W: Respiratory alterations due to urban air pollution: an experimental study in rats, *Environ Res* 57:19-33, 1992.

82. Rangi S, Sample S, Serwonska M, Lenahan G, and Goetzl E: Mediation of prolonged increases in nasal mucosal blood flow by calcitonin gene-related peptide (CGRP), *J Clin Immunol* 10:304-310, 1990.

83. Juliusson S and Bende M: Allergic reaction of the human nasal mucosa studied with laser Doppler flowmetry, *Clin Allergy* 17:301-305, 1987.

84. Druce HM, Bonner RF, Patow C, Choo P, Summers RJ, and Kaliner MA: Response of nasal blood flow to neurohormones as measured by laser-Doppler velcimetry, *J Appl Physiol* 57:1276-1283, 1984.

85. Bascom R and Fitzgerald TK: A vasoconstrictor partially alters the nasal response to sidestream tobacco smoke, *Ann J Respir Crit Care Med* 149:A391, 1994.

86. Olsson P, Bende M, and Ohlin P: The laser Doppler flowmeter for measuring microcirculation in human nasal mucosa, *Acta Otolaryngol (Stockh)* 99:133-139, 1985.

87. Druce H: Measurement of nasal mucosal blood flow [editorial], *J Allergy Clin Immunol* 81:505-508, 1988.

88. Holmberg K, Bake B, and Pipkorn U: Reflex activation in allergen-induced nasal mucosal vascular reactions, *Acta Otolaryngol (Stockh)* 108:130-135, 1989.

89. Olsson P: A comparison between the ^{133}Xe washout and laser Doppler techniques for estimation of nasal mucosal blood flow in humans, *Acta Otolaryngol (Stockh)* 102:106-112, 1986.

90. Knowles M, Gatzy J, and Boucher R: Increased bioelectric potential difference across respiratory epithelia in cystic fibrosis, *N Engl J Med* 305:1489-1496, 1981.

91. Thurauf N, Friedel I, Hummel C, and Kobal G: The mucosal potential elicited by noxious chemical stimuli with CO_2 in rats: is it a peripheral nociceptive event? *Neurosc Lett* 128:297-300, 1991.

92. Hummel T, Gruber M, Pauli E, and Kobal G: Chemo-somatosensory event-related potentials in response to repetitive painful chemical stimulation of the nasal mucosa, *Electroencephelogr Clin Neurophysiol 92:426-432, 1994.*

93. Kobal G and Hummel T: Olfatory evoked potentials in humans. In Getchell TV, Doty RL, Bartoshuk LM, and Snow Jr. JB, editors: *Smell and taste in health and disease, pp 255-275, New York, 1991, Raven.*

94. Broder I, Corey P, Cole P, and Lipa M: Comparison of the health of occupants and characteristics of houses among control homes and homes insulated with urea formaldehyde foam. II. Initial health and house variables and exposure-response relationships, *Environ Res* 45:156-178, 1988.

95. Baroody FM, Majchel AM, Roecker MM, Rosko PJ, Zegarelli EC, Wood CC, and Naclerio RM: Ipratropium bromide (Natrovent nasal spray) reduces the nasal response to methacholine, *J Allergy Clin Immunol* 89:1065-1075, 1992.

96. Baroody F and Naclerio R: Response of the nasal mucosa to histamine or mechacholine challenge: use of a quantitative method to examine the modulatory effects of atropine and ipratropium bromide, *J Allergy Clin Immunol* 90:1051-1054, 1992.

97. Bascom R, Pipkorn U, Lichtenstein LM, and Naclerio RM: The influx of inflammatory cells into nasal washings during the late response to antigen challenge. Effect of systemic steroid pretreatment, *Am Rev Respir Dis* 138:406-412, 1988.

Chapter 7

RADIOLOGIC METHODS

Eric Michael Hart
Denise R. Aberle

This chapter reviews the imaging features of the major chest diseases caused by occupational and environmental dust exposures. Emphasis is placed on conventional chest radiography and computerized tomography (CT), including high-resolution CT (HRCT). Where appropriate, important considerations of imaging technique are introduced.

IMAGING METHODS
Chest radiography

The term *pneumoconiosis* (*pneumo* = lung, *konis* = dust) was first introduced in the nineteenth century in reference to the inhalation of inorganic particulate dusts and its pathologic consequences. The chest radiograph is an important tool for the epidemiologic study of the pneumoconioses, in detecting the effects of dust exposure, as well as assessing disease progression. In addition, the chest radiograph has become central to the clinical assessment of exposed persons.[1] The International Labour Office (ILO) 1980 *Classification of Radiographs of the Pneumoconioses* is the most recent classification that provides a standardized nomenclature for purposes of codifying the appearances and extent of radiographic change caused by pneumoconiosis.[2,3] The ILO classification consists of a glossary of descriptive terms and a set of 22 standard radiographs illustrative of the pleural and parenchymal changes of the pneumoconioses. The system, based on the posteroanterior radiograph, is purely descriptive[4] and makes no attempt to correlate radiographic observation with pathology. Its strength is in providing a systematic and reproducible means to describe changes caused by the pneumoconioses. Although not comprehensive, a brief description of the ILO classification of terms follows.

Pulmonary parenchymal opacities

In the ILO scheme parenchymal opacities are classified according to size, shape, profusion (concentration), and extent (Fig. 7-1). There are two major size categories of lung opacities: small opacities, measuring from barely visible to 10-mm diameter, and large opacities, which measure greater than 10-mm diameter. Small opacities are subcategorized according to shape, which may be rounded or irregular (reticular or linear). Further subclassification is based on size. Small rounded opacities *p, q,* and *r* represent size ranges of up to 1.5 mm, 1.5 to 3 mm, and 3 to 10 mm in diameter, respectively. Similar size classifications pertain to the small irregular opacities *s, t,* and *u*. When scoring the chest radiograph according to the ILO classification, two letters are used to record the size and shape of lung opacities, allow-

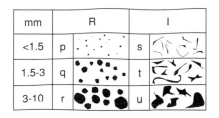

mm		R		I
<1.5	p		s	
1.5-3	q		t	
3-10	r		u	

Fig. 7-1. Diagrammatic representation of the International Labour Office (ILO) classification system for small pulmonary opacities. (Modified from Guidelines for the use of ILO international classification of radiographs of pneumoconioses, *Occupational safety and health series* No 22, revised 1980, Geneva, 1980, ILO.)

ing the reader to indicate both the predominant and secondary opacities (e.g., *p/s*).

The profusion of small opacities reflects their concentration and is determined by reference to the standard ILO radiographs. There are four major categories of profusion.

Category 0: small opacities absent or less profuse than in category 1

Category 1: small opacities present but few in number; normal lung markings usually visible

Category 2: numerous small opacities; normal lung markings usually partly obscured

Category 3: very numerous small opacities; normal lung markings totally obscured

A 12-point profusion scale has been adopted, which recognizes a continuum of changes and permits greater accuracy Two numbers are required to code profusion, the first representing the category of profusion chosen and the second representing an alternative category seriously considered. The 12-point scale is as follows:

0/−	0/0	0/1
1/0	1/1	1/2
2/1	2/2	2/3
3/2	3/3	3/+

The extent of opacities is recorded as the zones in which opacities are identified. For purposes of classification, each lung is divided into upper, middle, and lower zones. If only small opacities are present in silicosis, coal worker's pneumoconiosis (CWP), or silicate pneumoconioses other than asbestosis, the term *simple pneumoconiosis* is often used.

Opacities 10 mm or more in diameter are described as large opacities. There are three categories of large opacities based on size.

Category A: an opacity with a diameter of 10 to 50 mm or multiple opacities, each at least 10 mm in diameter, with combined diameters that total no more than 50 mm

Category B: an opacity of 50 mm or more in diameter or multiple opacities with combined diameters that do not exceed the area of the right upper lung zone

Category C: the combined area of large opacities is more than the area of the right upper lung zone

Large opacities are seen only in silicosis, CWP, and silicate pneumoconioses other than asbestosis. If large opacities are present, the term *complicated pneumoconiosis* is often used.

Pleural abnormalities

Pleural abnormalities such as those that occur in occupational asbestos exposure are also coded in the ILO classification according to type, location, thickness, extent, and presence or absence of calcification. Pleural thickening may be either focal (circumscribed plaques) or diffuse. The sites of involvement are recorded for each hemithorax as chest wall, diaphragm, or costophrenic angle. Pleural thickening seen en face is distinguished from that seen in profile, which is further categorized according to thickness, as measured from the inner line of the bony chest wall to the margin of the lung-pleura interface: category A has a maximum width of 5 mm, category B ranges in width from 5 to 10 mm, and category C is greater than 10 mm in width. The extent of pleural thickening, defined as the maximum length or the sum of involvement whether seen en face or in profile, is divided into extent 1, representing up to one quarter of the length of the lateral chest wall; extent 2, between one-quarter and one-half the length of the lateral chest wall; and extent 3, greater than one-half the length of the lateral chest wall. There are provisions for recording the presence, site, and extent of pleural calcification. Pleural effusions are also recorded.

Other designations and image quality considerations

A number of radiographic observations are coded in the ILO scheme, including changes suggestive of emphysema, cor pulmonale, cavities, cancers, and several other abnormalities. The ILO guidelines also provide for the recording of image quality on a four-point scale and define recommendations for good radiographic technique, including the use of high-kilovoltage technique (110 to 150 kVp), appropriate grids (100 lines or more per inch, with a grid ratio of 10:1), good screen-film contact, and small focal spot size (0.6 to 1.2 mm).

Chest radiographic scoring considerations

Because of the importance of the ILO classification system as an epidemiologic tool, a number of recommendations have been put forth to minimize reader variability in chest radiographic scoring. Among them is strict attention to radiographic technique, formal chest radiographic interpretation only by experienced readers, inclusion of additional radiographic projections such as oblique views, scoring of all radiographs in known temporal sequence, and the practice of side-by-side (multiple-observer) reading in lieu of independent reading. Although these have been shown in various trials to minimize reader variability, their implementation has not been standardized.

In the United States a certification process for readers using the ILO classification system has been developed under the auspices of the National Institute for Occupational Safety and Health (NIOSH). Because of what was perceived to be excessive variability in the interpretation of films for the U.S. Department of Labor's Black Lung Benefits Program, a certification examination was developed. The purpose of the examination was to identify a pool of ILO readers for the Black Lung Program and for NIOSH-sponsored epidemiologic research. The certification examination requires ILO classification of 125 films in 8 hours. Certification is for 4 years, and the recertification examination requires classification of 50 films in 3 hours. By NIOSH parlance, an A reader has taken the American College of Radiology (ACR) pneumoconiosis course but has not passed the NIOSH certification examination. A B reader has taken the ACR course and passed the examination. A C reading involves a panel of B readers. Although the purpose of the NIOSH certification process was as described above, the use of B readers in medicolegal settings other than the Black Lung Program has increased markedly over time.

ASBESTOS-RELATED DISEASE

Asbestos is the generic term for a group of naturally occurring fibrous silicates that share several properties, including heat resistance.[5] They are broadly classified into two mineralogic groups, the serpentines and the amphiboles, based on chemical structure and physical nature. This separation is of biologic importance in that fiber characteristics appear to influence deposition patterns and the propensity to cause certain diseases. Chrysotile, the principal serpentine fiber, accounts for more than 90% of asbestos used in the United States.[6] The fibers are slender, tend to curl, and may dissolve slowly. Crocidolite, an amphibole, is a thicker, relatively straight fiber that is extremely stable in the lungs and is highly associated with malignant mesothelioma.[6,7] Benign and malignant diseases of both the pleura and the pulmonary parenchyma are the most prevalent pathologic consequences of asbestos exposure.[5,8]

Asbestosis

The term *asbestosis* refers specifically to interstitial fibrosis resulting from asbestos fiber inhalation. The histologic diagnosis is made when interstitial fibrosis is observed in conjunction with asbestos bodies, the iron-protein–coated fiber.[9] The fibrosis is initially subpleural and basilar and is situated around the respiratory bronchioles. With advanced disease the adjacent lung parenchyma is involved. In clinical practice the diagnosis is established in the context of known occupational exposure and from a combination of physical, physiologic, and radiographic abnormalities.[1,10]

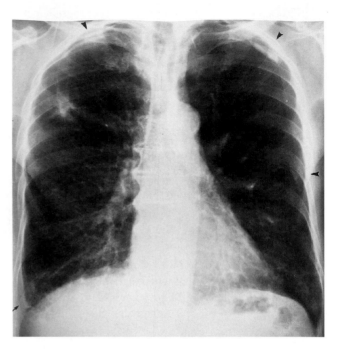

Fig. 7-2. Early asbestosis on the frontal chest radiograph. Fine irregular reticulation is present at both lung bases. The radiograph also demonstrates costal pleural thickening *(arrow)* and costal pleural plaques *(arrowheads)*. The small right pneumothorax resulted from needle aspiration of the spiculated right upper lobe adenocarcinoma.

Most cases of asbestosis occur after exposure to high dust concentrations over many years.[11,12] A dose-effect relationship is present[11,13] and latencies of 20 years or greater are common between exposure and the onset of symptoms.

On conventional chest radiographs, early changes consist of small irregular opacities or fine linear reticulation,[11,12,14] predominating at the lung bases (Fig. 7-2). Rockoff et al. observed isolated visceral pleural thickening on chest radiographs in a small group of asbestos workers.[15] This was found on pathologic correlation to represent mild subpleural interstitial fibrosis, suggesting that visceral pleural thickening identifies interstitial fibrosis that is otherwise radiographically occult.

With progressive fibrosis the reticulation becomes more coarse and irregular and will be observed in the middle and upper lung zones as well. The hemidiaphragmatic borders and cardiac silhouette become poorly outlined and "shaggy." Honeycombing characterizes advanced, end-stage interstitial fibrosis. The findings are nonspecific and can be seen in other conditions of basilar interstitial fibrosis, including usual interstitial pneumonitis and fibrosing alveolitis associated with the collagen vascular diseases. A well-documented exposure history or the presence of associated pleural changes supports the diagnosis of asbestosis (Fig. 7-3).

Although the ILO system was designed to be used as an epidemiologic tool, it has become a routine part of the diagnostic algorithm for asbestos-exposed individuals. In some schemes, ILO radiographic abnormalities are essential to the clinical diagnosis of asbestosis.[1] Studies have shown that lung fibrosis may be present histologically in the absence of ILO profusion abnormalities in 10% to 20% of persons with asbestosis.[13,16-20] Moreover, there is considerable inter- and intraobserver variability in the determination of parenchymal profusion scores.[21-24] The greatest variation occurs with the lowest, most nearly normal pro-

fusion categories of small opacities. These discrepancies can influence the basic distinction between individuals with no disease and those with minimal, potentially compensable disease and therefore may have significant epidemiologic and medicolegal implications.

Data on the effects of cigarette smoking on ILO radiographic interpretation are somewhat controversial. When chest radiographs of hospitalized patients were scored with the ILO classification system, there was a high prevalence of small opacities in presumably "normal" individuals, of whom one half had a history of smoking.[25] However, other large population studies indicate that fewer than 1% of the chest radiographs of smoking non–asbestos-exposed persons are interpreted as abnormal using the ILO system.[26] Cigarette smoking does appear to influence radiographic interpretation in workers with asbestos exposure, by significantly increasing the likelihood that irregular opacities will be found.[27-33] Moreover, the progression of asbestosis is probably greater in cigarette smokers.[34] Animal studies suggest that this combined cigarette smoke–asbestos effect results from smoke-induced alterations in fiber clearance and from increased bronchiolar inflammation and fibrosis.[35,36]

Computerized tomography and high-resolution computerized tomography

The limitations of chest radiographic diagnosis have contributed to the application of newer technologies to the diagnosis of asbestosis, particularly conventional CT and HRCT. Conventional CT is generally performed with subjects in the supine position using 10-mm slice thickness (collimation). In early trials interstitial fibrosis was described as areas of hazy increased opacity, coarse reticulonodular patterns, or honeycombing (Fig. 7-4), frequently

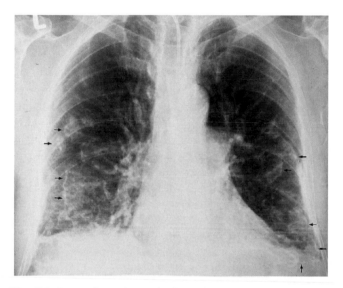

Fig. 7-3. Late asbestosis on the frontal chest radiograph. Coarse irregular interstitial reticulation is greatest at the lung bases but is also present in the midlung zones. Extensive bilateral calcific costal and diaphragmatic pleural plaques are present *(arrows)*, which partially obscure the underlying lung disease.

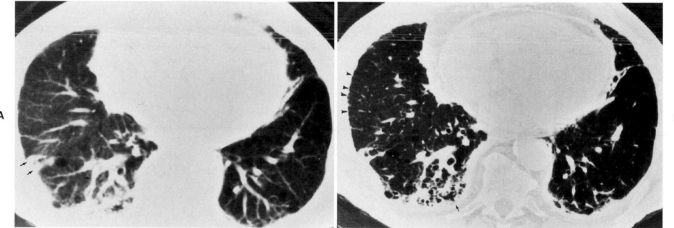

Fig. 7-4. A, A conventional (10-mm collimation) CT section demonstrates thick parenchymal bands in the right lower lobe *(arrows)*. Coarse, nearly coalescent opacities involve the dependent posterior right base. **B,** A high-resolution (1.5-mm collimation) CT section at the same level demonstrates discrete "honeycombing" posteriorly *(arrow)*. In addition, subtle subpleural short lines and visceral pleural serration are seen laterally *(arrowheads)*.

in association with a loss of the normal gravity-dependent perfusion.[37,38] Lung attenuation measurements have been proposed as an alternative to morphologic description.[29,39] In one study lung density on CT was significantly greater in asbestos-exposed workers than in nonexposed controls. Lung density measurements correlated inversely with static lung volumes. The authors suggested that increased lung density on CT reflects lung fibrosis or a decrease in lung volume caused by interstitial fibrosis. Inspiratory volumes during scanning and other factors have a dramatic effect on lung density measurements, which limits the practical utility of this method for diagnosis.

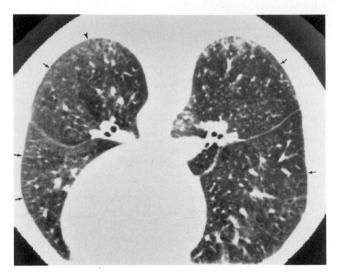

Fig. 7-5. A prone high-resolution CT section in early asbestosis demonstrates thickened interlobular septa (short lines, *arrows*) and centrilobular nodules (diffuse dotlike opacities, *arrowhead*) in the subpleural parenchyma bilaterally.

High-resolution CT is a modification that uses thin-collimation (1 to 2 mm) and high spatial frequency reconstruction algorithms that sharpen interstitial interfaces. These technical modifications reduce volume-averaging artifacts seen with conventional CT and effectively increase spatial resolution to that of macroscopic Gough sections.[40] High-resolution CT protocols typically include five to eight scans spaced through the mid to lower thorax, corresponding to the usual distribution of both pleural and parenchymal asbestos-related changes.[41] Additional scans through the upper lobes are often acquired to assess for the presence and severity of centrilobular emphysema, which commonly occurs in cigarette-smoking workers. Imaging is performed in the prone position or with subjects both prone and supine, so that the subpleural lung of the lower lobes is seen to best advantage and normal gravity-related changes in blood volume and ventilation can be distinguished from fixed structural abnormalities of the parenchyma.[41-43]

A number of findings have been described in the lungs of asbestos workers on HRCT. Limited radiologic-pathologic correlation studies indicate that these findings reflect peripheral interstitial fibrosis of the subpleural interstitium, the centrilobular interstitium that surrounds the small airways, and the interlobular septa.[44-46] The earliest changes occur in the subpleural lung, usually within 1 cm of the pleural surface, and consist of short lines, small linear arcades, and dotlike opacities (Fig. 7-5). Fibrosis of the visceral pleura may be reflected by subtle serration at the lung-pleura interface. Parenchymal bands are nontapering linear opacities measuring from 2 to 5 cm in length that extend from the lung to the pleura (Fig. 7-6). These bands usually occur in relation to sites of asbestos-related pleural thickening and have been shown to correspond to dense

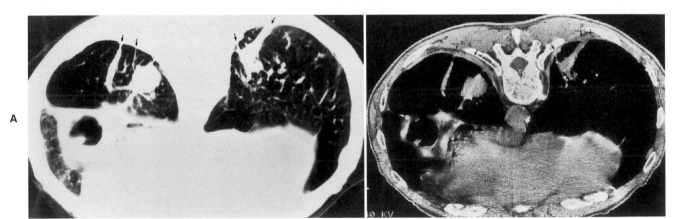

Fig. 7-6. A, A prone high-resolution CT section in advanced asbestosis demonstrates coarse parenchymal bands bilaterally at the lung bases *(arrows).* **B,** On soft-tissue windows at the same level, the association of the parenchymal bands with sites of pleural thickening is evident *(arrows).* The mass at the left base represents an area of round atelectasis, better appreciated on other images (not shown).

sheets of fibrosis along connective tissue septa and the bronchovascular sheaths.[44,47] They have also been postulated to correspond to potential future sites of round atelectasis. Curvilinear subpleural lines, curvilinear opacities within 1 cm of the pleura and paralleling the pleural surface, have been correlated with peribronchiolar and alveolar fibroses.[44,48] This finding also occurs in subjects without known interstitial disease[49] and is sometimes reversible when subjects are positioned prone. When curvilinear subpleural lines occur in conjunction with other parenchymal abnormalities, such as short lines and subpleural centrilobular dots, they are more likely to reflect fibrosis. Honeycombing, seen as tiny (1- to 3-mm-diameter) circular holes with discrete margins, is visible in advanced fibrosis and is indistinguishable in macroscopic appearance from other conditions of end-stage lung fibrosis (Fig. 7-7).

In a small prospective study using HRCT, 29 workers with the clinical diagnosis of asbestosis were compared with age-similar individuals without asbestos exposure or known interstitial lung disease. High-resolution CT was found to be more sensitive than conventional CT in the detection of pleural and parenchymal fibroses.[43] In workers with asbestosis, subpleural interstitial abnormalities were commonly seen in combination and at multiple sites. Some of these features were also observed in the control subjects but usually as isolated findings. Similar findings have been reported by others.[50]

Controversies in the use of high-resolution computerized tomography

In clinical trials HRCT has been found to be more sensitive than chest radiography in detecting asbestos-related interstitial abnormalities.[43,45,47,51-54] In one study of 100 asbestos-exposed workers, individual interstitial features on HRCT were shown to correlate with chest radiographic profusion scores, asbestos-related pleural thickening, and latency from initial exposure; very small correlations were also observed with decreases in both forced vital capacity and diffusing capacity.[55] Other investigators have observed similar correlations between HRCT abnormalities and functional indicators of lung restriction.[51] In another clinical study of 169 asbestos workers, HRCT scans defined a functionally distinct subgroup with significantly decreased forced vital capacity, decreased diffusing capacity, and worse dyspnea scores relative to workers with normal or near-normal HRCT scans.[54] These studies support the growing consensus that HRCT detects early disease preceding appreciable alterations in chest radiographic morphology and function.

The use of HRCT is a controversial addition to the imaging strategy of the asbestos-related diseases. Because of its greater sensitivity, HRCT has the potential to substantially alter existing clinical definitions of disease by identifying abnormalities not detectable with conventional radiographic and pulmonary function tests. The specificity of HRCT has been challenged on several grounds.[56] The parenchymal features described on HRCT in asbestosis are not histospecific and occur in other conditions of fibrosing alveolitis, including usual interstitial pneumonitis and the fibrosing alveolitis associated with some of the connective tissue diseases. However, most would agree that it is reasonable to ascribe HRCT abnormalities to asbestosis when they are observed in the context of substantial asbestos exposure and when associated with typical asbestos-related pleural disease. Central to the controversy surrounding the use of HRCT is the fact that there are relatively few data on pathologic correlation, particularly in subjects with early or minimal interstitial fibrosis. Although there have been few studies correlating chest radiographic ILO features with pathologic findings, the greater sensitivity of HRCT relative to projectional chest radiography has imposed more rigorous standards of pathologic proof. Given the rarity of

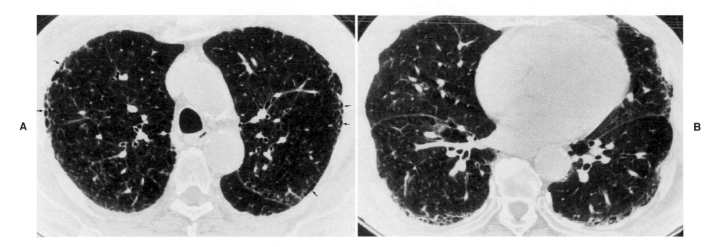

Fig. 7-7. **A,** A supine high-resolution CT section demonstrates patchy subpleural "honeycombing" *(arrows)* secondary to asbestosis. **B,** At a lower level bilateral calcific pleural plaques are also well depicted.

open lung biopsy in the assessment of asbestos-related diseases, pathologic correlation will likely be realized over several years, with data extracted from autopsy material or from asbestos-exposed individuals undergoing cancer resections.

The issue of the specificity of HRCT is important because most asbestos-exposed workers are at risk for respiratory impairment on the basis of both asbestos exposure and cigarette smoking. Historically, cigarette smoking has been associated with progressive airflow obstruction and air trapping, whereas asbestosis is considered a restrictive process associated with reduced vital capacity. Recently, some investigators have challenged this conventional wisdom on the grounds that asbestosis, independent of cigarette smoking, produces peribronchiolar fibrosis that can lead to small airways obstruction and air trapping. Preliminary data suggest that the HRCT features of asbestosis are not correlated with cigarette smoking[51,54,55]; moreover, the HRCT appearances of emphysema and asbestosis are readily distinguishable.

Another potential limitation of HRCT is the lack of a standardized interpretation scheme similar to the ILO classification for chest radiographs. Interestingly, most studies report that, because of the clarity of detail on HRCT, abnormalities are more consistently recognized, and there is less observer variability relative to chest radiographic interpretation, despite the absence of an ILO-like scoring system.[51] Recently, standards for detecting and quantitating asbestos-related changes on HRCT have been described.[57-59] The adoption of these standardized schemes will be important in further reducing reader variability and

in validating the relationship between HRCT abnormalities and known clinical, functional, and pathologic indices of interstitial fibrosis. Moreover, a standardized nomenclature will strengthen the use of HRCT as an epidemiologic tool for comparison between different study populations and may serve to enhance our understanding of the respective contributions of interstitial fibrosis and emphysema to respiratory impairment in smoking asbestos-exposed workers.

Rounded atelectasis

The term *round atelectasis* (also called *folded lung, pleuroma,* and *pulmonary pseudotumor*) is used to describe atelectasis of the peripheral lung resulting from underlying pleural adhesions and fibrosis.[60-63] Although not specific to asbestos, a history of exposure is frequently present.[60,62,64] Radiographically, round atelectasis consists of a tumorlike mass with adjacent thickened pleura or pleural effusion. The mass is generally round or lentiform and is associated with volume loss in the affected lobe. Bronchovascular structures often sweep into the margins of the mass, resulting in the so-called "comet tail" appearance[42,65,66] (Fig. 7-8). These observations, combined with the invariate association of the mass with pleural disease, are necessary to distinguish round atelectasis from lung neoplasms, which also occur with high frequency in asbestos-exposed persons. Because of its cross-sectional perspective, round atelectasis is seen to best advantage with CT. On CT, the morphologic features previously described should be sought. In addition, moderate homogeneous contrast enhancement of the atelectatic lung is typical, although occasionally peripheral lung

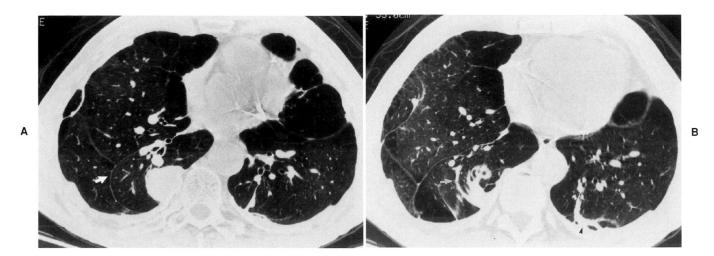

Fig. 7-8. Round atelectasis in a patient with severe diffuse calcific pleural thickening. **A,** A high-resolution CT section through the midthorax demonstrates severe right lower lobe volume loss with arcuate posterior displacement of the major fissure *(arrow).* Parenchymal bands are present in both hemithoraces, in contact with underlying sites of calcific pleural disease. **B,** A high-resolution CT section at a lower level demonstrates sweeping of the bronchovascular structures into the lesion *(arrow),* the "comet tail" sign. A thick parenchymal band is present in the posterior left base *(arrowhead),* in contact with an underlying site of calcific pleural disease.

neoplasms demonstrate similar enhancement characteristics.

The initiating event in the development of round atelectasis is injury to the pleura, which results in an inflammatory reaction and subsequent fibrosis of the visceral pleura. In the process of fibrosis, there is contraction of the subjacent lung, resulting in buckling and collapse. In anecdotal reports, pleurectomy has resulted in relaxation of the atelectatic lung. The involved lung may or may not exhibit interstitial fibrosis.

The prevalence of rounded atelectasis is unknown, although with the increasing use of CT in asbestos-exposed persons, peripheral atelectasis is seen with high frequency. A number of variants of round atelectasis have also been described on CT. In some cases a discrete mass is not present, and only single or multiple fibrous bands radiate from the parenchyma to pleural thickening or fibrosis. This phenomenon has been termed "crow's feet"[61,65] (Fig. 7-9). In most instances the CT appearances of round atelectasis and its variant forms are characteristic enough to preclude further evaluation. In equivocal situations percutaneous lung needle aspiration may be helpful in confirming the benign nature of the mass.

Asbestos-related lung cancer

An association between asbestos exposure and lung cancer is well documented,[8,16] and there is a dose-response re-

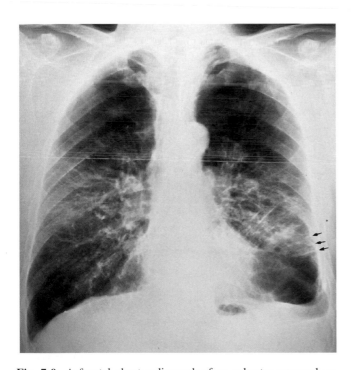

Fig. 7-9. A frontal chest radiograph of an asbestos-exposed patient. Multiple fibrous bands extend to the thickened lateral costal pleural surface *(arrows).* This has been termed "crow's feet" and represents a tethered lung related to pleural fibrosis. In addition, there is severe bilateral upper lobe emphysema.

lationship at occupational exposure levels. All histologic types are observed; the tumors demonstrate no predilection for any given location, occurring with nearly equal frequency in the upper and lower lobes.[8] In many asbestos-exposed individuals significant asbestos-related pleural or parenchymal fibrosis has the potential to obscure focal lung lesions on chest radiographs. The frequency of chest radiographically occult lung masses is unknown, although Lynch et al.[65] reported a 10% incidence of unsuspected benign and malignant masses on CT in a small group of heavily exposed workers. Given the high risk of lung cancer among cigarette-smoking asbestos workers, aggressive surveillance strategies that include conventional CT may be necessary to improve detection rates.

Asbestos-related pleural disease

Circumscribed pleural plaques and diffuse pleural thickening account for more than 90% of asbestos-induced pleural abnormalities, and their prevalence is expected to increase over the next two decades.[67] Benign exudative effusions are also known to occur but are frequently clinically unrecognized. There is also a strong causal relationship between asbestos exposure and malignant mesothelioma.

Circumscribed plaques are the most common manifestation of asbestos exposure and are considered a radiologic hallmark.[11] Plaques are usually first identified 20 or more years following initial exposure.[68] Their development and progression are most closely related to latency from initial exposure and not to total inhaled fiber burden; in fact, plaques are associated with remote nonoccupational exposures.

Circumscribed plaques typically involve the parietal pleura, although they have rarely been observed on the visceral pleural surfaces of the fissures.[15,69-71] Circumscribed plaques are presumed to result from an inflammatory response of the pleura to small fibers that have migrated to the pleura from the respiratory tract. On chest radiographs pleural plaques appear as focal plaquelike areas of soft-tissue or calcific thickening viewed in profile or en face and are most numerous along the lower costal and diaphragmatic pleural surfaces.[12,14,72] Occasionally, focal plaques may have a nodular character, making their distinction from lung nodules difficult. Circumscribed plaques are usually bilateral, symmetric, and most prominent between the sixth and ninth lateral ribs[14,72]; the lung apices and costophrenic angles are usually spared. With CT the posterior costal and paraspinous regions are frequently involved, although these areas are poorly visualized on standard frontal or lateral projection chest radiographs.

In the absence of calcification, the chest radiographic detection of plaques is dependent on their thickness. Autopsy studies suggest high false-negative detection rates on chest radiographs.[73] Furthermore, normal extrapleural soft tissues such as the musculature or extrapleural fat may be confused with plaques, resulting in high false-positive rates of up to

20% in some series.[74] The inclusion of oblique views has been suggested as a means of increasing the detection of pleural disease. However, in a recent study the accuracy of pleural assessment using oblique chest radiographs was compared with that of HRCT in a small cohort of asbestos-exposed subjects. Considering HRCT as the standard of reference, the positive predictive value of oblique views was less than 30%, primarily because extrapleural fat was confused with pleural disease in a high proportion of cases.[75]

Because of greater contrast resolution (hence, a greater ability to discriminate different soft-tissue densities) and the axial imaging display, CT is the most accurate radiographic method for detecting pleural plaques.[14,38,43,76] Limited HRCT protocols afford a relatively limited sample of the thorax, but have been found to detect pleural plaques with an accuracy roughly equivalent to that of conventional CT.[55] On HRCT subtle pleural thickening appears as a focal or discrete line, frequently separated from the underlying rib and extrapleural soft tissues by a thin layer of fat

(Fig. 7-10). In the paraspinous regions the intercostal blood vessels are prominent and may be confused with pleural thickening. For these reasons focal pleural plaques are most reliably identified on HRCT if the thickening is observed on multiple levels, the thickened pleura indents the subjacent lung, extrapleural fat separates the pleura from the normal extrapleural soft tissues, or there is dystrophic calcification of the pleural plaque.[77] Pleural plaques are not unique to asbestos exposure, having been reported with prior tuberculosis, empyema, and hemothorax; however, in these conditions plaques tend to be unilateral.

Diffuse pleural thickening

Diffuse pleural thickening is a less common manifestation of asbestos exposure than are circumscribed plaques. The etiology of diffuse pleural thickening is debatable, although in most cases it is thought to represent the fibrous residual of prior benign exudative pleural effusion or confluent circumscribed plaques.[11,16,67,78] Despite modifications of the 1980 ILO classification for chest radiographs, diffuse pleural thickening is variably defined, usually as a smooth uninterrupted pleural opacity extending over at least one fourth the length of the chest wall. Obliteration of the costophrenic angle may or may not be present.

On CT diffuse pleural thickening often appears as a continuous sheet of fibrous or partially calcified pleural thickening measuring up to 1 cm in thickness (Fig. 7-11). There is normally a fibrous symphysis of the parietal and visceral pleural surfaces. The posterior and lateral costal surfaces are invariably involved, but it is not unusual to see thickening of all costal surfaces at a given cross-sectional level. Sparing of the mediastinal pleura helps to distinguish diffuse

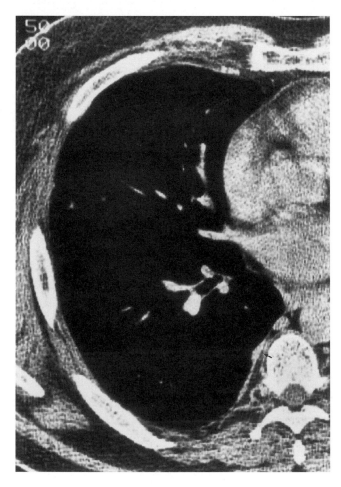

Fig. 7-10. A coned high-resolution CT section through the mid right hemithorax demonstrates subtle right paraspinous pleural thickening *(arrow)*. The plaque projects into the subjacent lung and is separated from the extrapleural soft tissues by underlying fat.

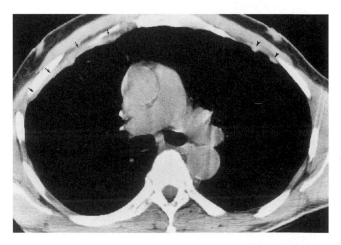

Fig. 7-11. A conventional CT section through the midthorax demonstrates diffuse pleural thickening in the anterolateral right hemithorax *(arrows)*. On other images (not shown) the plaque extended approximately 12 cm in the cephalocaudal direction and contained scattered dystrophic calcifications. Two small noncalcified circumscribed plaques involve the left lateral costal pleura *(arrowheads)*.

pleural thickening from malignant disease of the pleura, particularly malignant mesothelioma.[41] Increased extrapleural fat is frequently observed internal to the bony chest wall, presumably drawn inward in the course of pleural contraction and cicatrization.[41] Moreover, there is invariably some abnormality of the immediately subjacent pulmonary interstitium.

Benign asbestos-related pleural effusions

Benign exudative effusion is the only asbestos-related process seen within the first 10 years of onset of exposure,[79] but has also been observed after long latencies of up to 30 years.[80] The prevalence of benign effusions is estimated at 3% to 7%, although, because many affected individuals are asymptomatic, these estimates may be conservative. Radiographically, benign exudative effusions are nonspecific; the diagnosis is presumptive in an individual with known dust exposure in whom other causes of effusion, particularly malignant mesothelioma, have been excluded.[69,74] The natural history of benign asbestos effusions is one of chronicity with frequent recurrences, the development of contralateral effusions, and occasional evolution to diffuse pleural thickening.

Malignant mesothelioma

Malignant mesothelioma is an uncommon neoplasm of the pleura or the peritoneum with strong causal association with asbestos exposure.[9,16] The neoplasm typically develops after a long latency of 30 years or more and has been reported with relatively trivial exposures, including environmental and household exposures. In a majority of cases, other pleural or parenchymal manifestations of asbestos exposure are lacking.[9,16,41,81]

On chest radiographs malignant mesothelioma typically appears as diffuse nodular thickening of the pleura (Fig. 7-12). All pleural surfaces are involved, and the tumor often extends into the fissures. The involved hemithorax generally shows volume loss despite a large tumor volume; there is encasement of the underlying lung and fixation or ipsilateral shift of the mediastinum. In the absence of other radiographic manifestations of asbestos exposure, such as contralateral plaques, the appearance may be impossible to distinguish from that of diffuse pleural carcinomatosis.[11,41]

Computerized tomography is considered to be an imperfect but necessary tool for staging and is more accurate than chest radiography for defining the extent of the tumor, the invasion of extrapleural sites, and the status of the underlying lung.[82] It is the principal staging device in those centers in which aggressive multimodality therapy or radical surgical approaches are treatment considerations.[82-85] On CT the appearance of malignant mesothelioma can vary from that of pleural effusion to bulky lobulated soft-tissue thickening involving the costal, fissural, and mediastinal pleural surfaces. Malignant mesothelioma generally spreads

by contiguous extension into the contralateral hemithorax or the chest wall or below the diaphragm. Hematogenous metastases are less common, but have been reported to the lung, bone, liver, and thoracic or abdominal lymph nodes.[8] The use of CT to stage malignant mesothelioma has increased the frequency with which metastases to the lung are observed.[86] Although more accurate than chest radiography, CT is not without limitations, and does not consistently define mediastinal lymph node involvement or extrapleural extension that would preclude surgical resection.

Imaging considerations

The chest radiograph is the mainstay in the initial assessment of asbestos-exposed individuals and provides an inexpensive and rapid appraisal of the presence of asbestos-related diseases. Because of its greater contrast resolution and transaxial image display, CT has extended our sensitivity and precision in investigating both pleural and parenchymal processes. Imaging strategies that incorporate CT should ideally address issues of differential diagnosis, alter the management or habits of the individual, stimulate modifications in the work environment, or further our understanding of asbestos-induced diseases. Given the large number of asbestos-exposed persons who will undergo screening over the coming decades, the additional information gained from advanced imaging procedures must be balanced by the potential additional time and expense involved.

Conventional CT in which the whole thorax is systematically surveyed may be an important adjunct to the chest radiograph in the following settings: (1) to clarify the presence of asbestos-related pleural thickening, particularly in distinguishing pleural disease from normal extrapleural soft tissues; (2) to clarify morphology or identify optimal sites for biopsy of suspicious lung or pleural disease; (3) to stage and determine the tumor extent of malignant neoplasms such as lung cancer or malignant mesothelioma; and (4) to improve the detection of focal neoplasms that may be obscured by extensive pleural or parenchymal fibrosis.

Limited HRCT examinations are roughly competitive in time and cost with four-view chest radiographic examinations. It is generally appreciated that HRCT is the most sensitive radiographic indicator of interstitial abnormality and often detects changes despite a normal chest radiograph. The application of HRCT as a routine screening procedure is controversial. This issue will likely be resolved as we gain greater understanding of the specificity of HRCT and establish guidelines for standardizing technique and interpretation. At present, limited HRCT scans can supplement the assessment of asbestos-exposed subjects in whom there are equivocal changes on chest radiographs, unexplained symptoms or abnormalities of pulmonary function, or confounding variables such as cigarette smoke exposure that could contribute to respiratory impairment. In persons with sig-

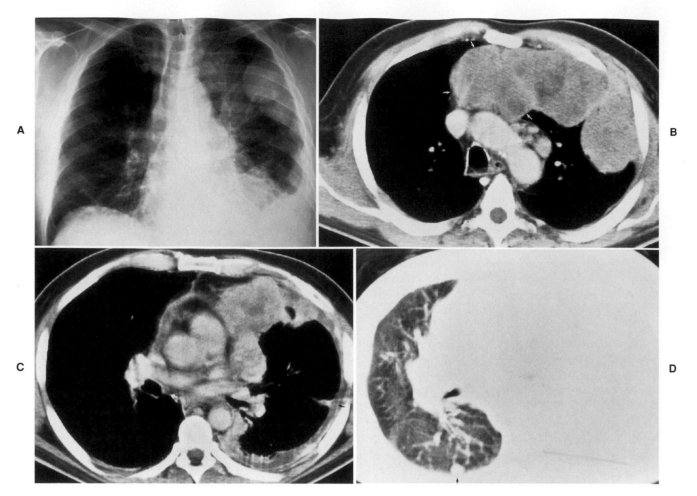

Fig 7-12. Malignant mesothelioma. **A,** A frontal chest radiograph demonstrates diffuse lobulated pleural thickening in the left hemithorax. **B,** A conventional CT section through the upper thorax demonstrates a bulky soft tissue mass extending into the mediastinum *(arrows),* with internal areas of low attenuation suggesting necrosis. **C,** At a lower level the pleural mass is seen to extend circumferentially to involve the mediastinal pleura. There is also extension into the major fissure *(arrow),* and a small pleural effusion is present posteriorly. Despite the large tumor burden, there is ipsilateral volume loss, best appreciated in relation to the normal volume of the right hemithorax. **D,** A preterminal repeat CT section demonstrates obliteration of the left lung by the massive mesothelioma. Additionally, hematogenous metastasis to the contralateral right lower lobe *(arrow)* is now identified.

nificant pleural disease, HRCT scans may be critical in documenting the presence of asbestosis that is otherwise radiographically occult.

SILICOSIS AND COAL WORKER'S PNEUMOCONIOSIS

Silicosis refers to lung disease resulting from the inhalation of free crystalline silica. Pathologically, the disease results in chronic fibrosis of the pulmonary parenchyma and may progress even in the absence of further dust exposure.[87] The diagnosis of silicosis is generally made in the context of documented exposure in conjunction with typical chest radiographic changes. Silicosis has three principal radiographic forms: simple (nodular) silicosis, complicated silicosis, and acute silicoproteinosis.

Simple (nodular) silicosis is usually first appreciated on chest radiographs after a latency of 20 years or more and appears as small rounded opacities (silicotic nodules), with or without calcification,[87] that predominate in the middle and upper lung zones (Fig. 7-13). In the ILO classification system these lesions correspond to the round opacities $p, q,$ and $r.$[88] Silicotic nodules consist of a concentric fibrous laminar core with a dust-laden periphery, usually centered in the peribronchiolar, perivascular, interlobular septal, and subpleural interstitium.[89] Parenchymal nodularity is often accompanied by hilar and mediastinal adenopathy. Eggshell or rim calcification of the enlarged lymph nodes is highly suggestive of silicosis but has also been described in sarcoidosis, tuberculosis, irradiated lymphomas, and amyloidosis (Fig. 7-14).

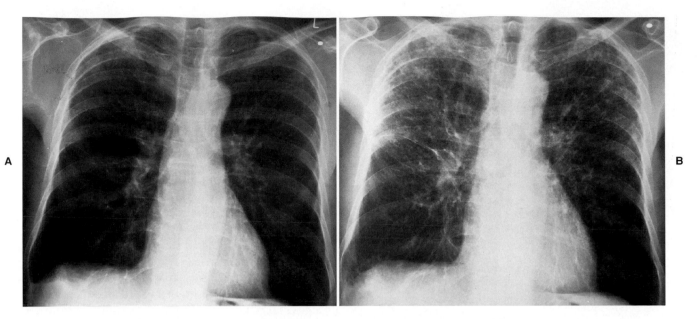

Fig. 7-13. A, A frontal chest radiograph in early silicosis. Small rounded opacities are present in the apices bilaterally. **B,** A repeat frontal chest radiograph 1 year later demonstrates a dramatic increase in the profusion of upper lobe nodules.

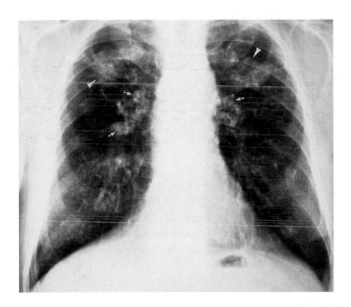

Fig. 7-14. A frontal chest radiograph demonstrates eggshell calcifications in the hila bilaterally *(arrows)* in a patient with silicosis. Also present are bilateral upper lobe conglomerate masses of progressive massive fibrosis *(arrowheads)*. There is significant associated bilateral upper lobe volume loss, with superior hilar retraction.

Conglomeration of nodules may occur to cause complicated silicosis (i.e., when nodules greater than 1 cm in diameter are present). Histologically, conglomerate lesions represent fused whorled silicotic nodules. When large masses are present, the term *progressive massive fibrosis*

(PMF) is used (Fig. 7-14). The lesions of PMF may occupy entire lobes and can cross the fissures to involve adjacent lobes; the lung peripheral to the PMF lesion is usually emphysematous. The lesions of PMF may cavitate on the basis of ischemic necrosis. Because individuals with silicosis are at increased risk for tuberculosis, the development of cavitation in PMF lesions should prompt a search for mycobacterial infection.

On CT the earliest lesions of simple silicosis appear as small nodular or binary branching structures (Fig. 7-15). These lesions, in both silicosis and coal worker's pneumoconiosis (CWP), have been classified on CT according to size as *micronodules* measuring less than ≤7 mm diameter and macronodules (or simply *nodules*) ranging from 8- to 20-mm diameter.[90] They are randomly distributed throughout the lung, but are often best seen in the subpleural regions, where, because of their increased concentration, they can be distinguished from normal blood vessels. Limited studies with CT-pathologic correlation have identified the earliest lesions as sites of peribronchiolar fibrosis at the level of the respiratory bronchioles[91]; the lesions are often radiographically indistinguishable from the earliest lesions of cigarette smoke–induced respiratory bronchiolitis. As the silicotic nodules increase in size, they become recognizable as discrete nodules[90] and are frequently more numerous in the right upper lobe region. Fine irregular reticular interstitial radiopacities have also been noted[92] but are not a constant feature in all series.[93]

As with the chest radiograph, there is no significant correlation between pulmonary function tests and the extent of

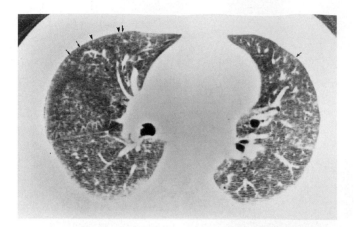

Fig. 7-15. HRCT section through the midthorax of a worker with silicosis demonstrates an increase in centrilobular binary branching structures *(arrows)* and fine micronodules *(arrowheads)*. These are the earliest CT changes in both silicosis and CWP.

nodular profusion on CT in subjects with simple silicosis. However, in workers with silicosis, significant correlations have been observed between CT estimates of emphysema and both decreased diffusing capacity and measures of airflow obstruction.[93]

On CT the lesions of PMF appear as irregularly marginated masses, often with calcification, that converge on the hila and result in emphysematous spaces peripherally. In contrast to chest radiography in which ischemic necrosis is appreciated only as cavitation, necrosis on CT may result in either central liquefaction or cavitation and is commonly observed in PMF lesions greater than 4 cm in diameter.[90] With cross-sectional imaging PMF lesions have been observed to occur most commonly in the upper or midlung zones; they exhibit a posterior predominance and are more common in the right lung.[90,93]

Acute silicoproteinosis refers to a rare but fulminant respiratory complication of intense exposure to respirable silica, usually in the context of sandblasting, silica flour manufacture, or other jobs in which there is heavy exposure to fine particulate silica.[89] Unlike classic silicosis, the disease is manifest within 6 months to 3 years of initial exposure and usually culminates in severe respiratory impairment and death. Pathologically, acute silicoproteinosis resembles idiopathic pulmonary alveolar proteinosis in which there is diffuse air space filling with a lipid-protein material that stains positive with periodic acid-Schiff stain. The chest radiograph demonstrates diffuse multifocal ground glass and air space consolidations.[90]

Coal worker's pneumoconiosis

Inhalational exposure to pure coal dust is responsible for CWP.[94] There are two primary clinical and radiographic patterns of CWP: simple (nodular) and complicated pneumoconioses (PMF).[3] Although CWP may be radiographically indistinguishable from silicosis, there are distinct his-

topathologic features that enable their discrimination. The essential defining lesion of simple nodular CWP is the coal dust macule, most numerous in the upper and midlungs.[94] The macule is composed of coal dust laden macrophages within the walls of respiratory bronchioles and adjacent alveoli, with variable amounts of collagen and reticulin in the matrix. A zone of emphysema surrounding the macule, focal emphysema, is an integral aspect of the lesion. Focal emphysema occurs independently of the cigarette-smoking habit, although smokers show much more extensive centrilobular emphysema as well. Coal dust nodules represent a more fibrous parenchymal lesion; they usually occur in combination with macules and tend to cluster to produce progressive massive fibrosis.[94] Calcification within the nodules of CWP is uncommon relative to that seen with silicosis and infectious granulomatous disease.

Complicated pneumoconiosis, in which large conglomerate lesions develop, is of two etiologic and pathologic types.[92,94-96] Lesions with irregular borders that are associated with peripheral lung distortion represent fusion of small fibrotic nodules and indicate a high ash content in the lungs. These masses resemble the conglomerate masses of complicated silicosis but lack their whorled pattern. Lesions with more regular borders and unassociated with peripheral lung distortion appear to represent progressive enlargement of a single nodule and occur in lungs with high carbon content and little ash.

Simple CWP, as with nodular silicosis, appears on chest radiography as diffuse small nodular opacities, most prevalent in the upper lungs. Focal emphysema is not normally visible, although centrilobular emphysema may be evident in smokers. In patients with more severe lung involvement, the size and number of nodules increase. The lesions of PMF first appear in the posterior aspects of the upper lobes and are observed on a background of simple nodular CWP. Large opacities, defined on chest radiographs as larger than 1-cm diameter, frequently have irregular borders, tend to involve the middle and upper zones of the lung, and produce considerable volume loss of the affected lobe. Cavitation can occur and may be difficult to distinguish from tuberculosis.

Computerized tomography may be complementary to chest radiography in CWP. However, the terminology used for ILO chest radiographic interpretation is insufficient for CT description. The most suitable terminology for CT analysis of the nodular pneumoconioses has been borrowed from pathology classification schemes for CWP. The following CT definitions have emerged: *micronodules,* appearing as round or binary branching structures measuring 7 mm in diameter or less; *nodules,* measuring from 8 to 20 mm in diameter; and *masses* of PMF, identified as lesions larger than 20-mm diameter. The former two criteria define simple CWP; the latter defines complicated CWP. Because of the upper thoracic distribution of CWP, limited CT imaging protocols should be primarily directed to the upper thorax and hila. Both conventional (10-mm thick) and high-resolution (1- to 2-mm thick) techniques have merits with respect to the depiction of nodular pneumoconioses.[92] Conventional CT can benefit from summation effects and identify micronodules of high attenuation as clusters easily distinguishable from normal intrapulmonary vessels. Conversely, low-attenuation lesions, including focal emphysema and some micronodules, may require HRCT for detection because they are obscured by volume-averaging effects with conventional collimation. CT imaging strategies for nodular pneumoconiosis generally incorporate some combination of conventional and high-resolution techniques directed primarily to the middle and upper thorax.

Parenchymal micronodules are an almost constant CT feature in workers with simple CWP and can be detected despite normal chest radiographs.[90] With minimal lung involvement the micronodules are few in number, are exclusive to the upper lung zones, and exhibit a right-sided and posterior predominance. With more advanced disease the micronodules increase in size and profusion bilaterally and are readily apparent on conventional or thin-section CT images. Micronodules are usually randomly distributed throughout the lung, may occasionally exhibit a definite centrilobular distribution, and are often first appreciated in the subpleural lung, where they are most easily distinguished from normal vessels. On CT, linear opacities or plaques, resulting from the coalescence of subpleural micronodules, have been termed *pseudoplaques*.[90] Micronodules have been shown to correspond with coal dust macules, nodules, and areas of irregular fibrosis surrounding the respiratory bronchioles.[91,97] In the subpleural parenchyma these micronodules often identify subpleural lymph nodes or localized visceral pleural thickening.[97]

The CT appearances of PMF mirror the two pathologic types just described. Those with irregular borders and associated with gross lung distortion often occur in relation to focal increases in extrapleural fat, indicating cicatricial fibrosis and contraction of the lesions. The second form, in which there is no surrounding lung distortion, may be confused with lung neoplasm. With CT a topographic tendency has been observed with PMF in the upper and posterior portions of the lung, specifically the posterior segment of the upper lobes or the superior segment of the lower lobes.[97,98] When greater than 4 cm in diameter, these lesions frequently undergo ischemic necrosis and may exhibit central liquefaction or cavitation. The topography and morphology of lesions on CT may be helpful in distinguishing PMF from a complicating neoplasm. However, CT never provides complete accuracy in discriminating benign and malignant processes. Image-guided lung needle aspiration may be indicated in equivocal or suspicious cases. Tuberculosis and aspergillus superinfection can occur in the lesions of PMF, frequently in the context of hemoptysis.

Rheumatoid pneumoconiosis

Rheumatoid pneumoconiosis, or Caplan's syndrome, is a rare condition characterized by the concomitant presence of rheumatoid arthritis and CWP or, less commonly, silicosis.[94] The disease is characterized by the presence of large necrobiotic (rheumatoid) nodules superimposed on a background of simple CWP or silicosis.[6,92] Pulmonary nodules generally develop at the time of joint disease, but may appear both before and after the onset of arthritis. The underlying lungs may show minimal evidence of pneumoconiosis. The necrobiotic nodules are typically well circumscribed, measure 0.5 to 5 cm in diameter, are evenly distributed, and may enlarge rapidly. Necrobiotic nodules may calcify or cavitate and are radiographically indistinguishable from the lesions of tuberculosis and other infective granulomata.[92]

HYPERSENSITIVITY PNEUMONITIS (EXTRINSIC ALLERGIC ALVEOLITIS)

Occupational or environmental exposure to dusts containing a wide variety of organic antigens can result in the clinical entity known as hypersensitivity pneumonitis.[99,100] Acute, subacute, and chronic forms of hypersensitivity pneumonitis are recognized both clinically and radiographically. It is important to note, however, that all three forms may coexist to greater or lesser degrees in an individual at any given time.

In the acute stage of hypersensitivity pneumonitis, the chest radiograph is frequently normal.[101,102] In fact, hypersensitivity pneumonitis may be the most common diffuse interstitial lung disease exhibiting a normal chest radiograph.[100] Hodgson et al. recently analyzed the results of previously published reports of hypersensitivity pneumonitis and found a significant decline in the chest radiographic detection of the disease between 1950 and 1980.[103] The reason for this is not known; although, clearly, patients may be symptomatic despite normal chest radiographs.

When present, acute abnormalities usually consist of finely granular or nodular opacities having a miliary or ground glass appearance (Fig. 7-16).[99,104-106] These opacities usually predominate in the lower or middle and lower lung zones.[107] Very early, within hours of the onset of symptoms, there may be generalized ground glass opacification or air space consolidation, which evolves to a more granular or micronodular pattern over several days.[108] Others have observed acinar opacities[109] and diffuse or focal linear interstitial patterns in the acute stages of allergic alveolitis.[102] Other radiographic findings, such as pleural thickening or effusion, adenopathy, calcifications, or cavities, are rare.[102,104,105] McLoud et al. modified the ILO classification scheme in an effort to enhance the radiographic description of diffuse lung disease. These investigators included a third category for small reticulonodular opacities (*x*, *y*, and *z*) that correspond in size to the opacities of *p*, *q*,

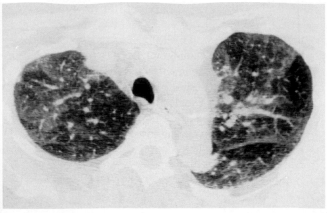

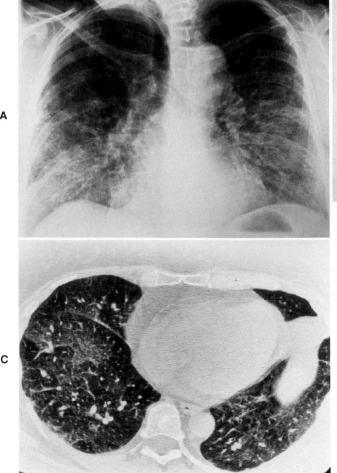

Fig. 7-16. Acute hypersensitivity pneumonitis. **A,** Frontal chest radiograph in a worker exposed to birds. Hazy, primarily ground glass opacity is present in the middle and lower lung zones bilaterally. High-resolution CT sections through the upper, **B,** and lower, **C,** thorax demonstrate relatively diffuse ground glass opacity throughout the lungs with subtle centrilobular prominence. The patient was removed from environmental exposure and treated with corticosteroids for acute hypersensitivity pneumonitis. Subsequent chest radiographs (not shown) showed dramatic clearing of the radiographic opacities.

and *r.* In their study 55% of patients with hypersensitivity pneumonitis had these reticulonodular markings.[110] In the absence of continued exposure, chest radiographic findings of acute hypersensitivity pneumonitis typically resolve over several weeks to months.[99,102,105,106]

With chronic hypersensitivity pneumonitis, interstitial fibrosis develops and is usually more prominent in the upper lobes.[99,107] Peribronchiolar thickening, linear fibrosis, granular opacity, and mixed interstitial patterns have been described.[111] Progressive upper lobe contraction occurs because of cicatricial atelectasis, and honeycombing may be seen.[112] Radiographic findings may simulate tuberculosis or sarcoidosis late in the disease.[100] The subacute stage of hypersensitivity pneumonitis shares features of both the acute and chronic stages. The distribution of disease varies, potentially representing differences in the disease continuum; in most patients the midzones are the most affected.[99,112] Radiographic features include reticulation, tiny nodules, and patchy ground glass opacity.[111]

Radiographic abnormalities do have significant correlations with pulmonary function abnormalities and cellular differential at bronchoalveolar lavage. In one study in which chest radiographs were scored according to the ILO classification, radiographic severity was negatively correlated with diffusing capacity of carbon monoxide and total lung capacity and positively correlated with lavage lymphocytosis.[113]

Computerized tomographic scans during the acute stage show patchy air space consolidations and small (1- to 3-mm) opacities throughout the lungs.[114] In some patients the nodules have a distinct centrilobular location, which parallels pathologic observations of peribronchiolar granuloma formation.[115] In some series, ground glass opacification has been the predominant initial finding and is usually relatively uniform in distribution.[108] Linear opacities and small nodules have also been described. Nakata et al.[116] demonstrated HRCT findings of widespread miliary nodules in a study of eight patients with Japanese summer-type hypersensitivity pneumonitis. In two patients ground glass opacity was also observed. They correlated the HRCT findings with alveolar wall granulomata on pathologic specimens. With recovery, air space consolidations may resolve, leaving residual ground glass opacity not seen on chest radiographs. In the chronic stage, linear opacities predominate (Fig. 7-17). The role of CT in the diagnosis of hypersensitivity pneumonitis has yet to be determined. Cross-sectional im-

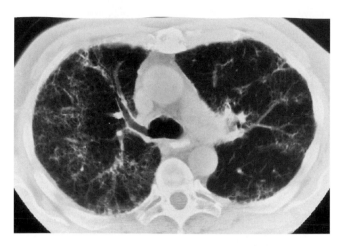

Fig. 7-17. Chronic hypersensitivity pneumonitis. A conventional CT section through the midthorax in a patient with chronic hypersensitivity pneumonitis demonstrates diffuse linear reticulation. Although patchy in distribution, both the central and subpleural parenchyma are affected. Findings are those of pulmonary fibrosis.

aging better assesses the character, distribution, and extent of abnormalities and may reveal parenchymal abnormalities despite normal chest radiographs.[111,114] Nonetheless, CT, including HRCT, may be normal in affected patients.[108,116] Moreover, in studies of diffuse infiltrative lung disease, diagnostic accuracy on CT is least consistent with hypersensitivity pneumonitis.[117] Computerized tomography may make a contribution in those patients undergoing biopsy and may prove to be important in assessing the response of the disease to therapy.

BERYLLIOSIS

Berylliosis results from the inhalation of various forms of the light metal beryllium, which has important uses in many industries. In the past, two forms of the disease were encountered. Acute toxic beryllium pneumonitis is almost never seen today as a result of industrial safeguards. It was the result of short-term, high-level airborne exposure. Radiographically, the picture was that of a diffuse chemical pneumonitis, with widespread parenchymal opacification. If the patient recovered from the acute episode, the radiograph typically normalized following recovery[118] with approximately 15% of patients progressing to chronic beryllium disease.[119]

Chronic beryllium disease, which continues to be a potential industrial problem,[120,121] is a systemic granulomatous disease with predominant pulmonary manifestations. The most common radiographic findings are small parenchymal opacities involving all pulmonary segments.[120] The opacities may be rounded or reticular[120,122-124] and may calcify microscopically or macroscopically over time.[123,125] Mild hilar adenopathy is frequently present,[123] typically to a lesser degree than that seen in sarcoidosis, and may calcify. The small opacities tend to become more visible over

time; however, they may regress with the use of steroid therapy.[120,122,123] Disease progression may lead to the formation of conglomerate masses and interstitial fibrosis. Volume loss occurs, with formation of bullae and cicatrical emphysema.[120,123] Spontaneous pneumothorax has been reported in the older literature.[120] Areas of linear scarring may develop, and pleural thickening (frequently bilateral) has been noted, generally in the middle and upper lung zones in patients with advanced disease.[122,123] Computerized tomographic findings have been less well described, but one recent study generally confirmed those findings seen on chest radiography.[126]

CHEMICAL PNEUMONITIS

Chemical pneumonitis results from the inhalation of a wide variety of toxic agents. Pathologically, several reactions are seen, depending on the nature of the inhaled agent. Radiographically, several patterns are also evident, again depending on the nature of what is inhaled. Commonly, radiography demonstrates a nonspecific generalized opacification of the lung fields consistent with pulmonary edema. Other appearances may be seen, however, and the reader is referred to the recent article on the subject by White and Templeton[127] for additional information.

SUMMARY

It has been the authors' intent in this chapter to give the reader an appreciation of the variety of radiographic appearances that may be seen in the major occupational and environmental lung diseases. Radiography is a central tool for the diagnosis of many occupational lung diseases. Despite limitations, the standard chest radiograph is widely available, relatively inexpensive, and of low radiation risk; as such, it remains the cornerstone of the imaging algorithm of the pneumoconioses. With the appropriate indications, CT, both conventional and high resolution, complements the chest radiographic assessment of exposed individuals. These advanced imaging procedures have been shown to provide greater sensitivity and precision in defining both parenchymal and pleural diseases. Ultimately, the accurate assessment of the occupational lung diseases requires a synthesis of all available clinical, functional, and radiologic data.

REFERENCES

1. American Thoracic Society: Statement on diagnosis of nonmalignant diseases related to asbestos, *Am Rev Respir Dis* 134:363-368, 1986.
2. Guidelines for the use of ILO international classification of radiographs of pneumoconioses, *Occupational safety and health series* No 22, revised 1980, Geneva, 1980, ILO.
3. Sargent EN: The pneumoconioses. In Taveras JM and Ferrucci JT, editors: *Radiology: diagnosis-imaging-intervention,* Philadelphia, 1991, JB Lippincott.
4. Batra P and Brown K: Radiology in prevention and surveillance of occupational lung disease, *Occup Med: State Art Rev* 6:81-100, 1991.
5. Churg A: Nonneoplastic diseases caused by asbestos. In Churg A and

Green FHY, editors: *Pathology of occupational lung disease,* New York, 1988, Igaku-Shoin Medical Publishers.

6. McLoud TC: Occupational lung disease, *Radiol Clin North Am* 29:931-941, 1991.

7. Chen W and Mottet NK: Malignant mesothelioma with minimal asbestos exposure, *Hum Pathol* 9:253-258, 1978.

8. Churg A: Neoplastic asbestos-induced diseases. In Churg A and Green FHY, editors: *Pathology of occupational lung disease,* New York, 1988, Igaku-Shoin Medical Publishers.

9. Craighead JE: The pathology of asbestos-associated disease of the lungs and pleural cavities: diagnostic criteria and proposed grading schema. Report of the Pneumoconiosis Committee of the College of American Pathologists and the National Institute for Occupational Safety and Health, *Arch Pathol Lab Med* 106:544-596, 1982.

10. Gamsu G, Aberle DR, and Lynch D: Computed tomography in the diagnosis of asbestos-related thoracic disease, *J Thorac Imaging* 4:61-67, 1989.

11. McLoud TC: Conventional radiography in the diagnosis of asbestos-related disease, *Radiol Clin North Am* 30:1177-1189, 1992.

12. McLoud TC: Diffuse infiltrative lung disease. In Putman CE, editor: *Pulmonary diagnosis, imaging and other techniques,* New York, 1981, Appleton-Century-Crofts.

13. Casey KR, Rom WN, and Moatamed F: Asbestos-related diseases, *Clin Chest Med* 2:179-202, 1981.

14. McLoud TC: Asbestos-related diseases: the role of imaging techniques, *Postgrad Radiol* 9:65-74, 1989.

15. Rockoff SD, Kagen E, Schwartz A, et al: Visceral pleural thickening in asbestos exposure: the occurrence and implications of thickened interlobar fissures, *J Thorac Imaging* 2:58-66, 1987.

16. Becklake MR: Asbestos-related diseases of the lung and other organs: their epidemiology and implications for clinical practice, *Am Rev Respir Dis* 114:187-227, 1976.

17. Epler GR, McLoud TC, Gaensler EA, et al: Normal chest roentgenograms in chronic diffuse infiltrative lung disease, *N Engl J Med* 298:934-939, 1978.

18. Gaensler EA and Carrington CB: Open biopsy for chronic diffuse infiltrative lung disease: clinical, roentgenographic, and physiologic correlations in 502 patients, *Ann Thorac Surg* 30:411-426, 1980.

19. Gaensler EA, Carrington CB, Coutu RE, et al: Pathological, physiological, and radiological correlations in the pneumoconioses, *Ann NY Acad Sci* 200:574-607, 1972.

20. Kipen HM, Lilas R, Suzuki Y, et al: Pulmonary fibrosis in asbestos insulation workers with lung cancer: a radiological and histopathological evaluation, *Br J Ind Med* 44:96-100, 1987.

21. Preger L: ILO U/C international classification of radiographs of the pneumoconioses. In Preger L, editor: *Asbestos-related disease,* New York, 1978, Grune & Stratton.

22. Rockoff SD and Schwartz A: Roentgenographic underestimation of early asbestosis by international labor organization classification: analysis of data and probabilities, *Chest* 93:1088-1091, 1988.

23. Rossiter CE: Initial repeatability trials of the UICC/Cincinnati classification of the radiographic appearance of pneumoconiosis, *Br J Ind Med* 29:407-419, 1972.

24. Rossiter CE, Browne K, and Gibson JC: International classification trial of AIA set of 100 radiographs of asbestos workers, *Br J Ind Med* 45:538-543, 1988.

25. Epstein DM, Miller WT, Bresnitz EA, et al: Application of ILO classification to a population without industrial exposure: findings to be differentiated from pneumoconiosis, *AJR* 142:53-58, 1984.

26. Blanc PD and Gamsu G: The effect of cigarette smoking on the detection of small radiographic opacities in inorganic dust diseases, *J Thorac Imaging* 3:51-56, 1988.

27. Barnhart S, Thornquist M, Omenn GS, et al: The degree of roentgenographic parenchymal opacities attributed to smoking among asbestos-exposed subjects, *Am Rev Respir Dis* 141:1102-1108, 1990.

28. Blanc PD, Golden JA, Gamsu G, et al: Asbestos exposure–cigarette smoking interactions among shipyard workers, *JAMA* 259:370-373, 1988.

29. Delclos GL, Wilson RK, and Bradley BL: Influence of smoking on radiographic profusion and pleural changes in asbestos-exposed subjects, *J Occup Med* 32:577-581, 1990.

30. Ducatman AM, Withers BF, and Yang WN: Smoking and roentgenographic opacities in US Navy asbestos workers, *Chest* 97:810-813, 1990.

31. Kilburn KH, Lilis R, Anderson HA, et al: Interaction of asbestos, age, and cigarette smoking in producing radiographic evidence of diffuse pulmonary fibrosis, *Am J Med* 80:377-381, 1986.

32. Kraut A, Bodbold J, and Lilis R: Effect of tobacco smoking on the presence of asbestosis at postmortem and on the reading of irregular opacities on roentgenograms in asbestos-exposed workers, *Am Rev Respir Dis* 139:1567-1568, 1989. Letter.

33. Lilis R, Selikoff IJ, Lerman Y, et al: Asbestosis: interstitial pulmonary fibrosis and pleural fibrosis in a cohort of asbestos insulation workers: influence of cigarette smoking, *Am J Ind Med* 10:459-470, 1986.

34. Sluis-Cremer GK and Hnizdo E: Progression of irregular opacities in asbestos miners, *Br J Ind Med* 46:846-852, 1989.

35. Churg A, Tron V, and Wright JL: Effects of cigarette smoke exposure on retention of asbestos fibers in various morphologic compartments of the guinea pig lung, *Am J Pathol* 129:385-393, 1987.

36. Hobson J, Gilks B, Wright J, et al: Direct enhancement by cigarette smoke of asbestos fiber penetration and asbestos-induced epithelial proliferation in rat tracheal explants, *JNCI* 80:518-521, 1988.

37. Katz D and Kreel L: Computed tomography in pulmonary asbestosis, *Clin Radiol* 30:207-213, 1979.

38. Kreel L: Computed tomography in the evaluation of pulmonary asbestosis: preliminary experiences with the EMI general purpose scanner, *Acta Radiol (Stockh)* 17:405-412, 1976.

39. Eterovic D, Dujic Z, Tocilj J, et al: High-resolution pulmonary computed tomography scans quantified by analysis of density distribution: application to asbestosis, *Br J Ind Med* 50:514-519, 1993.

40. Meziane MA, Hruban RH, Zerhouni EA, et al: High-resolution CT of the lung parenchyma with pathologic correlation, *Radiographics* 8:27-54, 1988.

41. Aberle DR and Balmes J: Computed tomography of asbestos-related pulmonary parenchymal and pleural diseases, *Clin Chest Med* 12:115-131, 1991.

42. Aberle DR: High-resolution computed tomography of asbestos-related diseases, *Semin Roentgenol* 26:118-131, 1991.

43. Aberle DR, Gamsu G, Ray CS, et al: Asbestos-related pleural and parenchymal fibrosis: detection with high-resolution CT, *Radiology* 166:729-734, 1988.

44. Akira M, Yamamoto S, Yokoyama K, et al: Asbestosis: high-resolution CT–pathologic correlation, *Radiology* 176:389-394, 1990.

45. Akira M, Yokoyama K, Yamamoto S, et al: Early asbestosis: evaluation with high-resolution CT, *Radiology* 178:409-416, 1991.

46. Murata K, Khan A, and Herman PG: Pulmonary parenchymal disease: evaluation with high-resolution CT, *Radiology* 170:629-635, 1989.

47. Lynch DA, Gamsu G, and Aberle DR: Conventional and high-resolution computed tomography in the diagnosis of asbestos-related diseases, *Radiographics* 9:523-551, 1989.

48. Yoshimura H, Hatakeyama M, Otsuji H, et al: Pulmonary asbestosis: CT study of subpleural curvilinear shadow, *Radiology* 158:653-658, 1986.

49. Pilate I, Marcelis S, Timmerman H, et al: Pulmonary asbestos: CT study of subpleural curvilinear shadow, *Radiology* 164:584, 1987. Letter.

50. Friedman AC, Fiel SB, Fisher MS, et al: Asbestos-related pleural disease and asbestosis: a comparison of CT and chest radiography, *AJR* 150:269-275, 1988.

51. Bégin R, Ostiguy G, Filion R, et al: Computed tomography in the early detection of asbestosis, *Br J Ind Med* 50:689-698, 1993.

52. Dujic Z, Tocilj J, and Saric M: Early detection of interstitial lung disease in asbestos-exposed non-smoking workers by mid-expiratory flow rate and high-resolution computed tomography, *Br J Ind Med* 48:663-664, 1991.

53. Klaas VE: A diagnostic approach to asbestosis, utilizing clinical criteria, high-resolution computed tomography, and gallium scanning, *Am J Ind Med* 23:801-809, 1993.

54. Staples CA, Gamsu G, Ray CS, et al: High-resolution computed tomography and lung function in asbestos-exposed workers with normal chest radiographs, *Am Rev Respir Dis* 139:1502-1508, 1989.

55. Aberle DR, Gamsu G, and Ray CS: High-resolution CT of benign asbestos-related diseases: clinical and radiographic correlation, *AJR* 151:883-891, 1988.

56. McLoud TC: The use of CT in the examination of asbestos-exposed persons, *Radiology* 169:862-863, 1988. Editorial.

57. Al Jarad N, Wilkinson P, Pearson MC, et al: A new high-resolution computed tomography scoring system for pulmonary fibrosis, pleural disease, and emphysema in patients with asbestos-related disease, *Br J Ind Med* 49:73-84, 1992.

58. Julien PJ, Sider L, Silverman JM, et al: Use of newly developed standardized form for interpretation of high-resolution CT in screening for pneumoconiosis, *Radiology (P)* 181:117, 1991.

59. Preteux F, Remy-Jardin M, and Hel-Or Y: Pattern recognition and estimation of micronodular profusion on pulmonary CT images, *Radiology (P)* 177:307, 1990.

60. Hanke R and Kretzschmar R: Round atelectasis, *Semin Roentgenol* 15:174-182, 1980.

61. Hillerdahl G: Asbestos-related pleural disease, *Semin Respir Med* 9:65-74, 1987.

62. Hillerdahl G: Rounded atelectasis: clinical experience with 74 patients, *Chest* 95:836-841, 1989.

63. Menzies R and Fraser R: Round atelectasis: pathologic and pathogenetic features, *Am J Surg Pathol* 11:674-681, 1987.

64. Tylen U and Nilsson U: Computed tomography in pulmonary pseudotumors and their relation to asbestos exposure, *J Comput Assist Tomogr* 6:229-237, 1982.

65. Lynch DA, Gamsu G, Ray CS, et al: Asbestos-related focal lung masses: manifestations on conventional and high-resolution CT scans, *Radiology* 169:603-607, 1988.

66. Schneider HJ, Felson B, and Gonzalez LL: Rounded atelectasis, *AJR* 134:225-232, 1980.

67. Oliver LC, Eisen EA, Green RE, et al: Asbestos-related pleural plaques and lung function, *Am J Ind Med* 14:649-656, 1988.

68. Albelda SM, Epstein DM, Gefter WB, et al: Pleural thickening: its significance and relationship to asbestos dust exposure, *Am Rev Respir Dis* 126:621-624, 1982.

69. Gefter WB and Conant EF: Issues and controversies in the plain-film diagnosis of asbestos-related disorders in the chest, *J Thorac Imaging* 3:11-28, 1988.

70. Sargent EN, Felton JS, and Barnes LT: Calcified interlobar pleural plaques: visceral pleural involvement due to asbestos, *Radiology* 140:634, 1981.

71. Solomon A, Sluis-Cremer GK, and Goldstein B: Visceral pleural plaque formation in asbestosis, *Environ Res* 19:258-264, 1979.

72. Sargent EN, Gordonson J, and Jacobson G: Bilateral pleural thickening: a manifestation of asbestos dust exposure, *AJR* 131:579-585, 1978.

73. Hourihane D, Lessof L, and Richardson PC: Hyaline and calcified pleural plaques as an index of exposure to asbestos: a study of radiological and pathological features of 100 cases with a consideration of epidemiology, *Br Med J* 1:1069-1074, 1966.

74. Gefter WB, Epstein DM, and Miller WT: Radiographic evaluation of asbestos-related chest disorders, *CRC Crit Rev Diagn Imaging* 21:133-181, 1984.

75. Ameille J, Brochard P, Brechot JM, et al: Pleural thickening: a comparison of oblique chest radiographs and high-resolution computed tomography in subjects exposed to low levels of asbestos pollution, *Int Arch Occup Environ Health* 64:545-548, 1993.

76. Kreel L: Computed tomography of the lung and pleura, *Semin Roentgenol* 13:213-225, 1978.

77. Im JG, Webb WR, Rosen A, et al: Costal pleura: appearances at high-resolution CT, *Radiology* 171:125-131, 1989.

78. McLoud TC, Woods BO, Carrington CB, et al: Diffuse pleural thickening in an asbestos-exposed population: prevalence and causes, *AJR* 144:9-18, 1985.

79. Epler GR, McLoud TC, and Gaensler EA: Prevalence and incidence of benign asbestos pleural effusion in a working population, *JAMA* 247:617-622, 1982.

80. Hillerdahl G and Ozesmi M: Benign asbestos pleural effusion: 73 exudates in 60 patients, *Eur J Respir Dis* 71:113-121, 1987.

81. Lilis R, Ribak J, Suzuki Y, et al: Non-malignant chest x-ray changes in patients with mesothelioma in a large cohort of asbestos insulation workers, *Br J Ind Med* 44:402-406, 1987.

82. Rusch VW, Godwin JD, and Shuman WP: The role of computed tomography scanning in the initial assessment and the follow-up of malignant pleural mesothelioma, *J Thorac Cardiovasc Surg* 96:171-177, 1988.

83. DaValle MJ, Faber LP, Kittle CF, et al: Extrapleural pneumonectomy for diffuse, malignant mesothelioma, *Ann Thorac Surg* 42:612-618, 1986.

84. Strankinga WFM, Sperber M, Kaiser MC, et al: Accuracy of diagnostic procedures in the initial evaluation and follow-up of mesothelioma patients, *Respiration* 51:179-187, 1987.

85. Weissman LB and Antman KH: Incidence, presentation and promising new treatments for malignant mesothelioma, *Oncology* 3:67-72, 1989.

86. Wechsler RJ, Steiner RM, and Conant EF: Occupationally induced neoplasms of the lung and pleura, *Radiol Clin North Am* 30:1245-1268, 1992.

87. Stark P, Jacobson F, and Shaffer K: Standard imaging in silicosis and coal worker's pneumoconiosis, *Radiol Clin North Am* 30:1147-1154, 1992.

88. Greening RR and Heslep JH: The roentgenology of silicosis, *Semin Roentgenol* 2:265-275, 1967.

89. Gibbs AR and Wagner JC: Diseases due to silica. In: Churg A and Green FHY, editors: *Pathology of occupational lung disease*, New York, 1988, Igaku-Shoin Medical Publishers.

90. Remy-Jardin M, Degreef JM, Beuscart R, et al: Coal worker's pneumoconiosis: CT assessment in exposed workers and correlation with radiographic findings, *Radiology* 177:363-371, 1990.

91. Akira M, Higashihara T, Yokoyama K, et al: Radiographic type p pneumoconiosis: high-resolution CT, *Radiology* 171:117-123, 1989.

92. Remy-Jardin M, Remy J, Farre I, et al: Computed tomographic evaluation of silicosis and coal worker's pneumoconiosis, *Radiol Clin North Am* 30:1155-1176, 1992.

93. Bergin CJ, Muller NL, Vedal S, et al: CT in silicosis: correlation with plain films and pulmonary function tests, *AJR* 146:477-483, 1986.

94. Green FHY: Coal worker's pneumoconiosis and pneumoconiosis due to other carbonaceous dusts. In Churg A and Green FHY, editors: *Pathology of occupational lung disease*, New York, 1988, Igaku-Shoin Medical Publishers.

95. Corrin B: Occupational diseases of the lungs. In *The lungs*, London, 1991, Churchill Livingstone.

96. Davis JMG, Chapman JS, Collings P, et al: Variations in the histological patterns of the lesions of coal workers' pneumoconiosis in Britain and their relationship to lung dust content, *Am Rev Respir Dis* 128:118-124, 1983.

97. Remy-Jardin M, Beuscart R, Sault MC, et al: Subpleural micronodules in diffuse infiltrative lung diseases: evaluation with thin section CT scans, *Radiology* 177:133-139, 1990.

98. Lyons JP and Campbell H: Relation between progressive massive fibrosis, emphysema, and pulmonary dysfunction in coal worker's pneumoconiosis, *Br J Ind Med* 38:125-129, 1981.

99. Gurney JW: Hypersensitivity pneumonitis, *Radiol Clin North Am* 30:1219-1230, 1992.

100. Hargreave F, Hinson KF, Reid L, et al: The radiologic appearances of allergic alveolitis due to bird sensitivity (bird fancier's lung), *Clin Radiol* 23:1-10, 1972.

101. Fink J, Schleuter D, Sosman A, et al: Clinical survey of pigeon breeders, *Chest* 62:277-281, 1972.

102. Unger GF, Scanlon GT, Fink JN, et al: A radiologic approach to hypersensitivity pneumonias, *Radiol Clin North Am* 11:339-356, 1973.

103. Hodgson MJ, Parkinson DK, and Karpf M: Chest x-rays in hypersensitivity pneumonitis: a metaanalysis of secular trend, *Am J Ind Med* 16:45-53, 1989.

104. Dickie HA and Rankin J: Farmer's lung: an acute granulomatous interstitial pneumonitis occurring in agricultural workers, *JAMA* 167:1069-1076, 1958.

105. Mindell HJ: Roentgen findings in farmer's lung, *Radiology* 97:341-346, 1970.

106. Seal RME, Hapke EJ, Thomas GO, et al: The pathology of the acute and chronic stages of farmer's lung, *Thorax* 23:469-489, 1968.

107. Cook PG, Wells IP, and McGavin CR: The distribution of pulmonary shadowing in farmer's lung, *Clin Radiol* 39:21-27, 1988.

108. Hansell DM and Moskovic E: High-resolution computed tomography in extrinsic allergic alveolitis, *Clin Radiol* 43:8-12, 1991.

109. Fraser RG and Paré JAP: Extrinsic allergic alveolitis, *Semin Roentgenol* 10:31-42, 1975.

110. McLoud TC, Carrington CB, and Gaensler EA: Diffuse interstitial lung disease: a new scheme for description, *Radiology* 149:353-363, 1983.

111. Buschman DL, Gamsu G, Waldron JA Jr, et al: Chronic hypersensitivity pneumonitis: use of CT in diagnosis, *AJR* 159:957-960, 1992.

112. Adler BD, Padley SPG, Muller NL, et al: Chronic hypersensitivity pneumonitis: high-resolution CT and radiographic features in 16 patients, *Radiology* 185:91-95, 1992.

113. Cormier Y, Bélanger J, Tardif A, et al: Relationships between radiographic change, pulmonary function, and bronchoalveolar lavage fluid lymphocytes in farmer's lung disease, *Thorax* 41:28-33, 1986.

114. Silver SF, Muller NL, Miller RR, et al: Hypersensitivity pneumonitis: evaluation with CT, *Radiology* 173:441-445, 1989.

115. Lynch DA, Rose CS, Way D, et al: Hypersensitivity pneumonitis: sensitivity of high-resolution CT in a population-based study, *AJR* 159:469-472, 1992.

116. Nakata H, Egashira K, Tsuda T, et al: High-resolution computed tomography of Japanese summer-type hypersensitivity pneumonitis, *Clin Imaging* 15:185-190, 1991.

117. Mathieson JR, Mayo JR, Staples CA, et al: Chronic diffuse infiltrative lung disease: comparison of diagnostic accuracy of CT and chest radiography, *Radiology* 171:111-116, 1989.

118. Parkes WR: Beryllium disease. In *Occupational lung disorders,* ed 2, London, 1982, Butterworth.

119. Ridenour PK and Preuss OP: Acute pulmonary beryllium disease. In Rossman MD, Preuss OP, and Powers MB, editors: *Beryllium: biomedical and environment aspects,* Baltimore, 1981, Williams & Wilkins.

120. Aronchik JM: Chronic beryllium disease, *Radiol Clin North Am* 30:1209-1217, 1992.

121. Kanarek DJ, Wainer RA, Chamberlin RI, et al: Respiratory illness in a population exposed to beryllium, *Am Rev Respir Dis* 108:1295-1302, 1973.

122. Aronchik JM, Rossman MD, and Miller WT: Chronic beryllium disease: diagnosis, radiologic findings, and correlation with pulmonary function tests, *Radiology* 163:677-682, 1987.

123. Stoeckle JD, Hardy HL, and Weber AL: Chronic beryllium disease: long-term follow-up of 60 cases and selective review of the literature, *Am J Med* 46:545-561, 1969.

124. Weber AL, Stoeckle JD, and Hardy HL: Roentgenologic patterns in long-standing beryllium disease: report of 8 cases, *AJR* 93:879-890, 1965.

125. Sargent EN: Radiological aspects of chronic beryllium disease. In Rossman MD, Preuss OP, and Powers MB, editors: *Beryllium: biomedical and environment aspects,* Baltimore, 1981, Williams & Wilkins.

126. Harris KM, McConnochie K, and Adams H: The computed tomographic appearances in chronic berylliosis, *Clin Radiol* 47:26-31, 1993.

127. White CS and Templeton PA: Chemical pneumonitis, *Radiol Clin North Am* 30:1231-1243, 1992.

Chapter 8

PATHOLOGIC METHODS

Samuel P. Hammar

A variety of pathologic methods are available to evaluate occupational- and environmental-related lung diseases. In many instances, several pathologic methods can be applied to a given case. Each case has to be evaluated on its own merits to determine what pathologic methods are indicated to answer the questions posed. In most cases, the type of tissue specimen pathologists receive dictates what method of pathologic evaluation is used. For example, if both lungs are obtained at necropsy, several methods can be employed to evaluate the disease processes. If a transbronchial lung biopsy specimen is obtained, only light microscopic examination might be applicable, although many of the methodologies described below can be applied to small tissue specimens and to fluid samples.

MACROSCOPIC EVALUATION OF LUNG SPECIMENS

Macroscopic evaluation of lung tissue can be extremely important in recognizing various diseases caused by occupational and environmental agents. Macroscopic examination is most important in situations where a sizable portion of lung tissue is available for examination, such as both lungs obtained at autopsy, lobectomy specimens, pneumonectomy specimens, and occasionally segmentectomy and wedge biopsy type of specimens. In general, transbronchial biopsy specimens provide samples of tissue ranging from 1 to 3 mm in greatest dimension, and little information can be obtained by macroscopic examination.

There are a variety of occupational and environmental-induced lung diseases that have fairly characteristic macroscopic patterns:

1. Diffuse malignant mesothelioma is a neoplasm that can be documented to be caused by asbestos in at least 80% of cases. Diffuse malignant mesothelioma is characterized by a rind of grayish-white to grayish-tan tumor that encases the lung, usually obliterating the pleural cavity (Fig. 8-1).[1]
2. Centrilobular emphysema caused by cigarette smoke is characterized by the irregular destruction of tissue within the secondary lobule of the lung,[2,3] with the predominant disease occurring in the upper portion of the upper lobe (Fig. 8-2).
3. Panlobular emphysema, such as that causally related to Ritalin abuse,[4] has an appearance similar to panlobular emphysema associated with α_1-antitrypsin deficiency (Fig. 8-3).
4. Diffuse pleural fibrosis caused by asbestos is characterized by thickening of the visceral and parietal layers of the pleura,[5] with frequent fusion, which can form a rind around the lung measuring as much as 1 cm in thickness and is occasionally confused with a diffuse malignant mesothelioma (Figs. 8-4, 8-5).
5. Hyaline pleural plaques caused by asbestos most frequently involve the diaphragmatic parietal pleura and

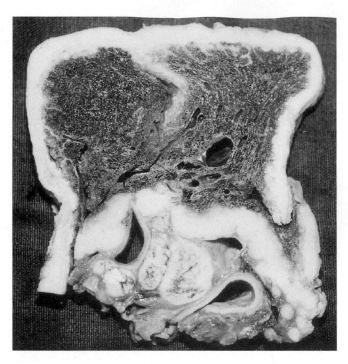

Fig. 8-1. Diffuse malignant mesotheliomas characteristically show a rind of grayish-white to tan tumor that encases the lung.

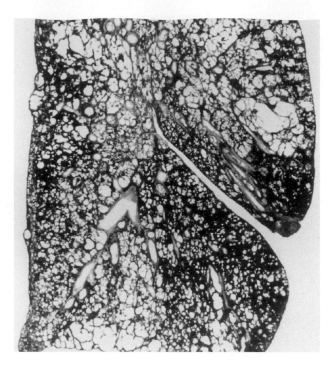

Fig. 8-3. Panlobular emphysema, which has recently been associated with Ritalin abuse, is characterized by diffuse uniform destruction of parenchymal lung tissue.

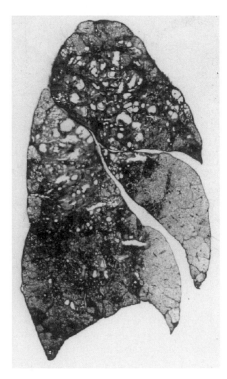

Fig. 8-2. Centrilobular emphysema, most cases of which are caused by cigarette smoke, characteristically involves the upper portion of the upper lobe and shows irregular destruction of tissue within the secondary lobules.

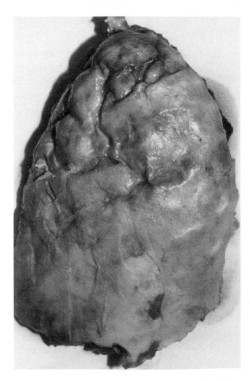

Fig. 8-4. This lung, from a patient who was occupationally exposed to asbestos, shows diffuse pleural fibrosis.

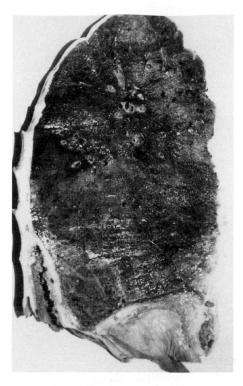

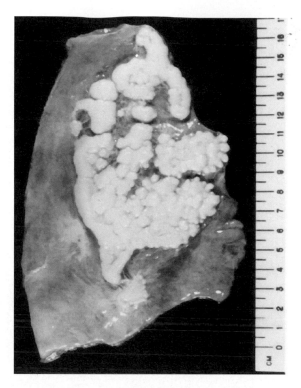

Fig. 8-5. The sectioned lung in Fig. 8-4 shows a rind of thickened pleural tissue surrounding the lung tissue. The thickened pleura can sometimes be confused with diffuse malignant mesothelioma.

Fig. 8-6. This hyaline pleural plaque is on the diaphragmatic surface of a person occupationally exposed to asbestos. Pleural plaques are often calcified and are composed of dense hypocellular connective tissue.

consist of raised white to whitish-yellow, firm, often-calcified, dense fibrous tissue[6] (Fig. 8-6).

6. Primary lung cancers, whether caused by asbestos, chloromethyl ether, arsenic, or many other environmental and occupational agents, have no characteristic features that distinguish them from those that occur without any obvious cause or those that are caused by cigarette smoke. There is some evidence that lung cancers associated with asbestos occur more frequently in the lower lobes,[7] whereas those that are caused by cigarette smoke occur more frequently in the upper lobes, although this is not a constant finding.[8] There is one type of rare primary lung cancer referred to as pseudomesotheliomatous carcinoma that macroscopically looks identical to mesothelioma (Fig. 8-7) and appears to be caused by asbestos in many cases.[9,10]

LIGHT MICROSCOPIC EVALUATION OF LUNG TISSUE

Light microscopic evaluation of lung tissue is important in every disease process and is the most commonly used technique to evaluate lung diseases. There are a variety of environmental and occupational lung diseases that have fairly specific histologic features.

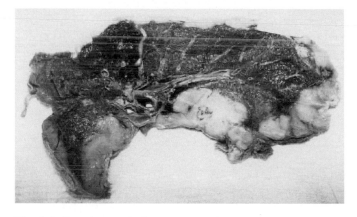

Fig. 8-7. Pseudomesotheliomatous carcinoma is a primary carcinoma of the lung that grows in a pleural distribution and forms a rind around the lung. Macroscopically it is identical to mesothelioma.

Diffuse malignant mesothelioma

Diffuse malignant mesotheliomas can be categorized histologically into four major categories (box), although this is a marked oversimplification of the entire spectrum of these neoplasms.[11,12] As published by this author and by others,[11,13] the more sections taken of a mesothelioma, the more histologic patterns are identified. In general, the epithelial pattern is the most frequent, and the tubulopapillary subtype of the epithelial pattern is perhaps the best known

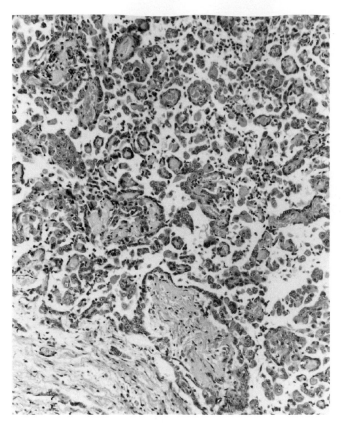

Fig. 8-8. This histologic type of mesothelioma is referred to as tubulopapillary and is the most frequent microscopic form of mesothelioma (×125).

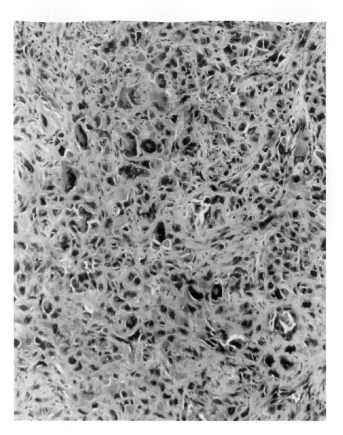

Fig. 8-9. Some mesotheliomas are composed of large anaplastic cells and can be confused with anaplastic carcinomas of the lung (H&E, ×550).

Major histologic types of mesothelioma

Epithelial
Sarcomatoid (sarcomatous, malignant fibrous)
Biphasic
Desmoplastic

---

histologic type of malignant mesothelioma (Fig. 8-8). However, a wide variety of histologic patterns of mesothelioma exist, including an anaplastic cell type, and even a giant cell type (Fig. 8-9).

Primary carcinoma of the lung

Certain histologic types of lung cancer have been implicated as being associated with a variety of environmental and occupational agents. However, some of the initial studies suggesting a specific cell type with specific environmental and occupational agent have not withstood the test of time.[14] For example, asbestos was initially stated to most frequently cause adenocarcinomas that usually occurred in the lower lobes; in 1985, Churg[15] published a study reviewing the types of lung cancer caused by asbestos versus those that did not occur in occupationally asbestos-exposed persons and found no significant difference in cell types. Cigarette smoke has most frequently been implicated in causing squamous cell carcinoma and small cell undifferentiated carcinoma, although the other major cell types, adenocarcinoma and large cell undifferentiated carcinoma, are frequently caused by cigarette smoke.[16] Squamous cell carcinoma has been most frequently associated with arsenic exposure, although in many of these studies, adequate controls were not present.[14] The same is true for beryllium, with which small cell undifferentiated carcinoma and adenocarcinoma have been stated to be associated. Nickel has been associated with squamous cell carcinomas most frequently, as has exposure to chromate, although in both situations the majority of individuals who developed these cancers were cigarette smokers. Bischloromethyl ether has been associated with small cell undifferentiated carcinoma of the lung,[17] although the total number of cases is relatively small. Adenocarcinoma and large cell undifferentiated carcinoma appear to be the major types of cancer that occur in workers who are exposed to vinyl chloride.[18] Those exposed to radon gas (radon daughters) are stated to most frequently develop small cell undifferentiated carcinoma,[19-21] although some studies evaluating the histopathologic type of lung cancer have shown a difference between the diagnosis made by the hospital pathologists and a panel of reviewing pathologists.[22]

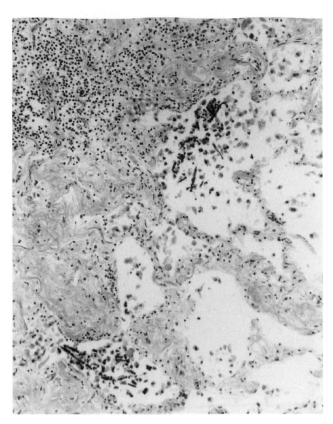

Fig. 8-10. Grade 4 asbestosis is characterized by diffuse interstitial pulmonary fibrosis with honeycombing in association with asbestos bodies (H&E, ×330)

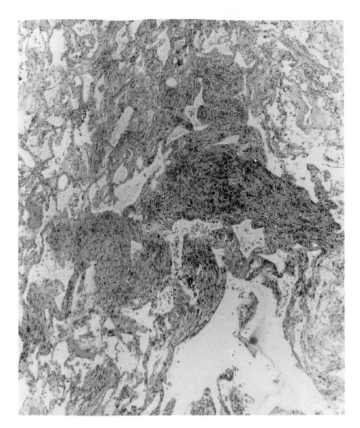

Fig. 8-11. Grade 1 asbestosis is characterized by peribronchiolar fibrosis in association with asbestos bodies (H&E, ×75).

Pathologic grades of asbestosis

Grade 0. No fibrosis

Grade 1: Peribronchiolar fibrosis involving at least one respiratory bronchiole

Grade 2: Peribronchiolar fibrosis plus fibrosis of adjacent alveolar ducts of two or more layers of alveoli

Grade 3: Coalescence of fibrotic change of all lung tissue between at least two adjacent bronchioles

Grade 4: Diffuse fibrosis with honeycombing

Asbestosis

The criterion for the most basic histologic diagnosis of asbestosis is the identification of fibrosis in association with two or more asbestos bodies. Asbestosis has been graded on the degree of severity of fibrosis as grades 1 through 4 (box), with 4 being the most severe and representing end-stage pulmonary fibrosis with honeycombing (Fig. 8-10), and grade 1 fibrosis (Fig. 8-11) representing peribronchiolar fibrosis. As pointed out by Churg and colleagues,[23,24] there are other dusts besides asbestos that can cause peribronchiolar fibrosis, and perhaps a better name for the scarring occurring in this location associated with a variety of mineral dusts is mixed-dust pneumoconiosis. As described by Wright et al.[25] it is not proven that grade 1 asbestosis

progresses to grade 4 asbestosis, although most studies strongly suggest that grade 1 asbestosis is the earliest lesion caused by asbestos.[26,27] Grade 4 asbestosis is different from end-stage idiopathic pulmonary fibrosis only in that asbestos bodies are identified in areas of fibrosis in grade 4 asbestosis, whereas they are not present in cases of idiopathic pulmonary fibrosis. Even this criterion, however, is not absolute, since there are cases reported of asbestosis in which asbestos bodies are not observed in histologic sections of lung tissue, but an elevated concentration of asbestos fibers capable of causing asbestosis is identified in lung tissue[28,29] (Fig. 8-12). Roggli[30] reported that the severity of asbestosis and asbestos exposure is best correlated with total number of asbestos fibers in the lung, and the combined asbestos body and asbestos fiber concentration in lung tissue, rather than asbestos body concentration. A convenient "rule" for the practicing pathologist is that the identification of one asbestos body on casual inspection (not using mechanical stage) of a 2 × 2 cm, hematoxylin and eosin-stained or iron-stained section is equivalent to an asbestos body concentration of approximately 1000 asbestos bodies per gram of wet lung tissue by digestion technique. The ratio of asbestos bodies to asbestos fibers in lung tissue is highly variable and, in this author's experience, ranges from 1:50 to greater than 1:100,000.

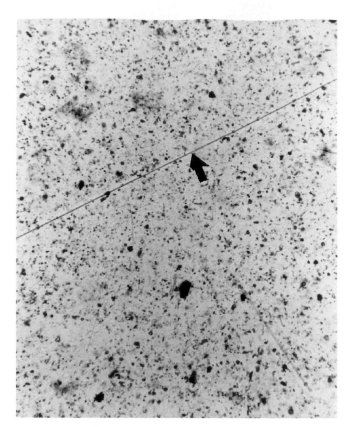

Fig. 8-12. In some cases of asbestosis, asbestos bodies are not easily identified in lung tissue. In such cases, the diagnosis of asbestosis is identified by showing an increased number of uncoated asbestos fibers (arrow), as demonstrated by this filter preparation ($\times$550).

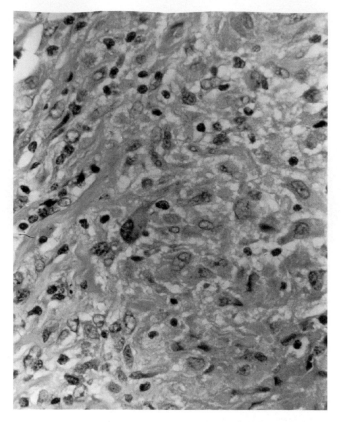

Fig. 8-13. The cellular phase of silicosis is characterized by an infiltrate of macrophages that are usually present in a peribronchiolar location in the upper lobes ($\times$330).

Silicosis

Silicosis is characterized by the presence of palpable silicotic nodules composed of dense fibrotic connective tissue ranging from a few millimeters to several centimeters in greatest dimension.[31] Silicosis has a propensity to involve the upper lobes and progress from a cellular stage, in which predominantly macrophages are seen (Fig. 8-13), to a fibrotic stage, in which there are nodules of relatively hypocellular connective tissue.

Silicotic nodules are characterized by a concentric arrangement of hyalinized collagen, relatively little dust pigmentation, and a peripheral border of mononuclear cells, primarily macrophages and some plasma cells (Fig. 8-14). The whorled appearance of a typical silicotic nodule has been described as that of an "onion skin." Silica particles can be demonstrated in variable amounts in the center and periphery of nodules by their birefringence under polarized light, but they are not present in the hyalinized collagenous areas.

Silicotic nodules are proliferative lesions and tend to coalesce into conglomerate masses. When such masses are greater than 1 cm in diameter on chest radiographs, the term complicated silicosis is often used. When the masses grow to large size, distorting the normal architecture of the lungs, the term progressive massive fibrosis (PMF) is used. With PMF, there may be necrosis, cavitation can occur, and vascular structures and bronchi may be obliterated. Hilar lymph nodes may contain silicotic nodules and fibrosis. Nodules in the lungs and lymph nodes may calcify. The latter gives a radiographic appearance that has been described as "eggshell calcification."

Other pneumoconioses

Several other mineral-induced lung diseases occur, including coal worker's pneumoconiosis, talcosis, kaolin pneumoconiosis, berylliosis, welder's pneumoconiosis, hematite miner's lung disease, stannosis, baritosis, dental technician's pneumoconiosis, fly ash lung disease, and volcanic ash lung disease.[32] Many of these have fairly distinct histologic features (Table 8-1), although some do not.

A variety of abnormalities are found in the lungs of coal workers and depend on the type of inhaled dust, the occupation in a given mine, the duration of exposure to the dust, the latent period, and other factors such as cigarette smok-

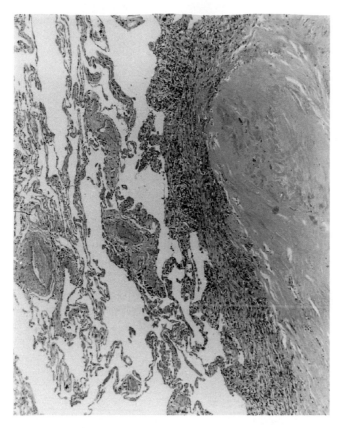

Fig. 8-14. Silicotic nodule (arrow) is composed of round to elliptical masses of dense, relatively hypocellular connective tissue (H&E, ×125).

Table 8-1. Histologic features of several common pneumoconioses

Disease	Mineral dust	Pathologic features
Coal worker pneumoconiosis	Coal dust	Black macules; micronodules, macronodules, progressive massive fibrosis; Caplan lesion
Berylliosis	Beryllium	Congestion, edema, alveolar damage; lymphocyte-plasma cell interstitial inflammatory cell infiltrate with noncaseating granulomata
Kaolin pneumoconioses	Kaolinite	Macules and nodules composed of dust-laden macrophages with minimal fibrosis
Talcosis	Talc	Foreign body granulomata; diffuse interstitial fibrosis
Hard metal lung disease	Cobalt	Giant cell interstitial pneumonitis; lymphocyte-plasma cell interstitial infiltrate

ing. Coal dust consists of a variety of substances, including amorphous, noncrystalline carbon in association with variable amounts of crystalline silica (quartz), mica, kaolin, and other silicates. The quartz content of coal dust is important in determining the pathologic response to the dust. The characteristic lesion in coal worker pneumoconiosis is referred to as the "coal dust macule," and consists of 1 to 4 mm in diameter macular black areas that are distributed throughout the lung. These macules, in association with a relatively diffuse increase in black pigmentation of the lung, are responsible for the term "black lung" disease. The macular lesions are more frequent in the upper lobes and occur along the secondary lobular septa, as well as subpleurally. The macules themselves are not palpable, and when one identifies palpable lesions in a coal worker's lung, they are usually the result of changes induced by silica and are directly related to the concentration of silica in the inhaled dust. The silica, in association with carbon, gives rise to lesions referred to as anthracosilicosis, and these are generally in the distribution that one observes in silicosis. Clinically, these nodular lesions of coal worker pneumoconiosis have been classified similarly to those of silicosis with nodules >1 cm in diameter on chest radiographs indicating the presence of complicated pneumoconiosis and masses

≥2 cm in diameter indicating the presence of PMF. Pathologists have also described nodular lesions in CWP as *micronodules* if ≤7mm in diameter, *macronodules* if 8-20 mm in diameter, and PMF if >20 mm in diameter. The lesions of PMF resemble those of silicosis, most frequently involve the upper lobes, and can extend across fissures to involve adjacent lobes. Necrosis and cavitation can occur; vascular structures and bronchi can be obliterated. Histologically, the simple coal worker's macule consists of dust-laden macrophages located at the respiratory bronchiole level, extending into the alveolar ducts. These dust-containing macrophages are sometimes but not always associated with an increase in reticulin and collagen fibers, as well as fibroblasts. Centrilobular emphysema, so-called "focal emphysema," may be seen in the lungs of coal workers with little evidence of fibrosis. How much fibrosis is found appears to relate to the silica content of the coal.

Caplan lesions are seen in the lungs of some coal miners who also have rheumatoid arthritis. These lesions appear as giant silicotic nodules greater than 4 cm in diameter, with smooth borders and concentric internal laminations. These nodules show palisading of macrophages at the periphery, with focal areas of necrosis, as occur in rheumatoid nodules in other sites. Caplan lesions are thought to represent a combination of silicotic nodules and rheumatoid nodules.

Talcosis is a type of pneumoconiosis caused by talc, a high grade type of magnesium silicate. Talc is often contaminated with quartz and amphibole asbestos, specifically tremolite and anthophyllite. In tissue sections, talc particles appear as brightly birefringent needle-shaped particles, 0.5

to 10.0 μm in length, that represent the talc, viewed on edge. Inhalation of talc usually results from occupational exposure, although talc can also reach the lung through embolization caused by intravenous injection of crushed tablets, such as the common drug Ritalin. The changes in the lungs of persons exposed to talc vary and are generally seen in those who are exposed to the highest concentrations of talc. Hyaline pleural plaques occur in some individuals, presumably from contamination of talc with asbestos. Talc causes small palpable nodules and, in some instances, diffuse interstitial fibrosis or even progressive massive fibrosis. The fibrotic nodules are not as well defined as silicotic nodules but are formed in response to the silicate component of talc. Nonnecrotizing foreign body granulomata similar to those seen in sarcoid are observed in some individuals, and talc can usually be identified in these granulomata. Diffuse interstitial fibrosis with birefringent talc also occurs. In those persons who inject crushed talc-containing tablets, the granulomata occur in association with and within blood vessels.

Kaolinite is a hydrated aluminum silicate, a member of the group of sheet silicates. It is the major component of kaolin (china clay). In addition to occupational exposure, cigarette smoking is a potential source of exposure. Kaolinite has been identified on tobacco leaves, in cigarette smoke, and in pulmonary macrophages where it appears as tiny crystals. In vitro, kaolinite is cytotoxic for peritoneal and alveolar macrophages, causing the release of cytoplasmic enzymes, such as elastase. Pneumoconiosis caused by kaolinite has been reported in kaolin miners and millers. The most common changes identified in the lung are numerous gray-brown firm nodules, ranging from 5 mm to 12 cm in diameter. The nodules are similar to those seen in coal worker pneumoconiosis, with golden-brown particulates present in a peribronchiolar distribution. The larger nodular lesions are caused by association of the dust-containing macrophages with varying amounts of collagen.

Beryllium is a lightweight metal that has many industrial uses and is derived from the mineral beryl, which is beryllium aluminum silicate. Berylliosis is the term used for pulmonary disease caused by beryllium and occurs in both an acute and a chronic form. In acute berylliosis, the lungs are characteristically heavy and congested, and microscopically show congestion, edema, and in some instances acute alveolar damage. Chronic berylliosis is a diffuse interstitial disease with a lymphocyte-plasma cell infiltrate and noncaseating granulomata. This type of histologic picture can be difficult to distinguish pathologically from sarcoidosis and hypersensitivity pneumonitis.

Persons exposed to tungsten carbide, or "hard metal," can develop interstitial fibrosis or obstructive airway disease. Tungsten carbide is produced by heating tungsten and carbon in the presence of a binder, cobalt. Hard-metal pneumoconiosis is characterized by a giant cell interstitial pneumonitis with numerous multinucleate histiocytic giant cells, with some features resembling hypersensitivity pneumonitis or desquamative interstitial pneumonitis. Cobalt is thought to be the injurious agent in hard metal lung disease. Hard metal pneumoconiosis is differentiated from hypersensitivity pneumonitis and idiopathic pulmonary fibrosis by the finding of the giant cell pattern, which is essentially pathognomonic of this condition.

Some lung diseases classified as pneumoconioses are caused by inhalation of metal fumes. Fumes are fine particles, less than 1 μm in dimension, and act more like gases than particulate matter. Shaver's disease, or bauxite lung disease, is caused by metal fumes generated in the production of corundum, an alumina abrasive.[32]

The fumes consist of aluminum oxide, amorphous silica, ferric oxide, small amounts of titanium oxide, and other substances. The histologic changes in bauxite lung disease are somewhat nonspecific and consist of diffuse interstitial fibrosis in association with aggregates of black dust particles. Cadmium oxide fumes may caused emphysematous changes in the lung associated with a lymphocytic inflammatory cell infiltrate and perivascular fibrosis.[33] Mercury vapor has been reported to cause pulmonary edema and acute diffuse alveolar damage.[33]

Organic dust-induced diseases

The inhalation of organic dusts can result in several different types of diseases, including hypersensitivity pneumonitis, organic dust toxic syndrome (pulmonary mycotoxicosis), and byssinosis. Hypersensitivity pneumonitis is a disease most frequently caused by a variety of organic antigens. The characteristic histologic pattern seen in hypersensitivity pneumonitis is a diffuse lymphocytic-plasma cell interstitial inflammatory cell infiltrate (Fig. 8-15) with varying numbers of small nonnecrotizing granulomata that are often present in a bronchial distribution.[34] Recently, asbestos was reported as producing a pattern that resembles hypersensitivity pneumonitis.[35]

Exposure to certain organic dusts causes a syndrome characterized by fever, myalgias, chest tightness, dyspnea, cough, and headache, and is referred to as pulmonary mycotoxicosis or organic dust syndrome.[36,37] The pathologic changes seen in organic dust toxic syndrome are nonspecific but include alveolar damage with intraalveolar exudates, in various stages of organization, and obliterative bronchiolitis.[38]

Byssinosis is an obstructive lung disease associated with the inhalation of cotton dust. The mechanism of injury is uncertain, and the histologic changes are nonspecific, consisting of mucus gland hyperplasia in the large bronchi and goblet cell metaplasia in the bronchioles. So-called "byssinosis bodies" have been observed in a minority of individuals with byssinosis, but there is no evidence that these have diagnostic or pathogenetic significance. The byssinosis body is thought to be composed of cellulose fibers that caused an inflammatory reaction with resulting calcification

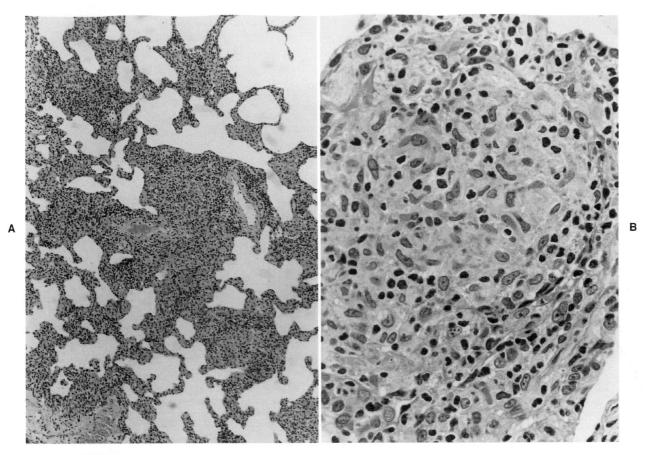

Fig. 8-15. A,B, This section of lung tissue shows a diffuse interstitial inflammatory cell infiltrate of lymphocytes and plasma cells in association with small nonnecrotizing granulomata. This histologic pattern is characteristic of hypersensitivity pneumonitis (H&E; **A,** ×5; **B,** ×330).

and ferruginization. Histologically, it measures up to 200 μm in greatest dimension, being hematoxyphilic and coated with golden-brown hemosiderin.

Pulmonary histiocytosis X (pulmonary eosinophilic granuloma—Langerhans cell granulomatosis)

Pulmonary histiocytosis X is a disease occurring almost exclusively in persons who are heavy cigarette smokers. This unusual disease is characterized by the accumulation of Langerhans cells in a peribronchiolar location and surrounding alveolar parenchyma in association with varying numbers of inflammatory cells, including eosinophils, neutrophils, lymphocytes, and plasma cells (Fig. 8-16).[39] Langerhans cells have hyperconvoluted nuclei and, as seen by electron microscopy, contain Langerhans cell granules (Fig. 8-17) in their cytoplasm that are most frequently in the region of the Golgi apparatus and may often be attached to the cell membrane.

Respiratory bronchiolitis and desquamative interstitial pneumonitis

Respiratory bronchiolitis and desquamative interstitial pneumonitis are pulmonary diseases that also occur almost

exclusively in cigarette smokers.[40,41] Respiratory bronchiolitis is characterized histologically by mild peribronchiolar and alveolar duct fibrosis with alveolar macrophages within the lumen of the respiratory bronchioles and within alveoli (Fig. 8-18). Desquamative interstitial pneumonitis is characterized by accumulation of alveolar macrophages (usually smoker's macrophages) within alveolar spaces and bronchioles, in association with mild interstitial fibrosis, lymphoid nodules, and a fair number of eosinophils (Fig. 8-19).

Asthma

Asthma can be induced by occupational and environmental agents and has a fairly distinctive histologic pattern, characterized by sloughing of respiratory epithelium with varying numbers of eosinophils and degenerating respiratory columnar epithelial cells and mucus within the lumens of the bronchi and bronchioles. The histologic pattern is further characterized by marked thickening of the basement membranes separating the respiratory epithelium from the underlying lamina propria, hyperplasia of the mucus-secreting glands in the lamina propria, and an increased thickness of the muscular wall (Fig. 8-20). Charcot-Leyden crystals, which are formed from the

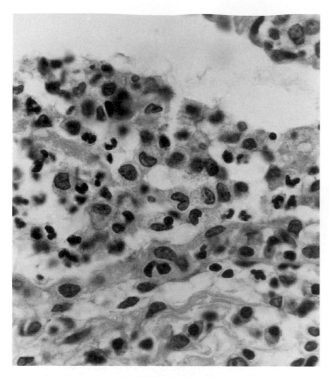

Fig. 8-16. Pulmonary histiocytosis X, also known as pulmonary eosinophilic granuloma and Langerhans cell granulomatosis, is a disease occurring almost exclusively in cigarette smokers and is characterized in the cellular phase by the nodular accumulation of Langerhans cells admixed with eosinophils, lymphocytes, and plasma cells (H&E, ×330).

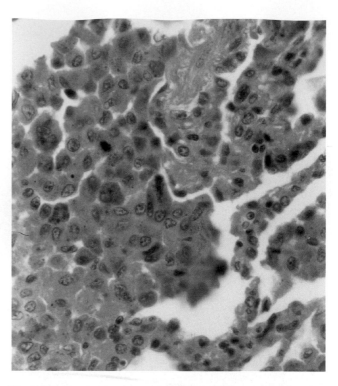

Fig. 8-18. Respiratory bronchiolitis, a condition caused by cigarette smoke, is characterized by mild peribronchiolar and perialveolar duct fibrosis with accumulation of macrophages within the lumens of these structures (H&E, ×330).

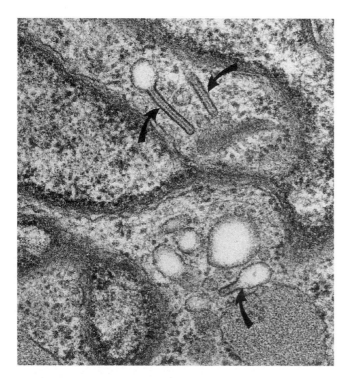

Fig. 8-17. Ultrastructurally, Langerhans cells contain unique rod and racket-shaped pentalaminar structures referred to as Langerhans cell granules (arrows) (×42,000).

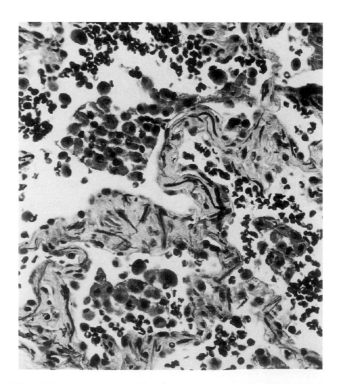

Fig. 8-19. Desquamative interstitial pneumonitis is caused by cigarette smoke in most cases and is characterized by the accumulation of alveolar macrophages (cigarette smoker's macrophages) in alveolar spaces with mild interstitial fibrosis, focal lymphoid follicles, and associated eosinophils (H&E, ×125).

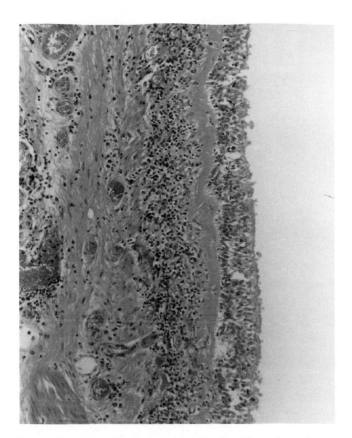

Fig. 8-20. Asthma is characterized by sloughing of respiratory epithelium into the lumens of bronchi, thickening of the basement membrane separating the respiratory epithelium from the lamina propria, hypertrophy of the smooth muscle wall, and a mixed inflammatory cell infiltrate rich in eosinophils. In this case there was minimal sloughing of the respiratory epithelium (H&E, ×125).

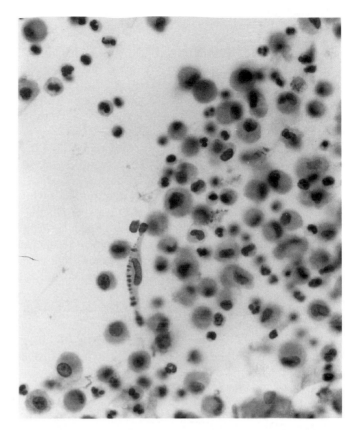

Fig. 8-21. This cytocentrifuge preparation of bronchoalveolar lavage fluid contained easily recognized ferruginous body (arrow), characteristic of asbestos body (H&E, ×330).

granules of eosinophils, and Curschmann spirals, which are composed of mucus, can be seen in histologic sections, as well as in cytologic preparations of sputum and bronchial washings.

CYTOLOGIC EVALUATION OF PULMONARY SPECIMENS

Cytology is a technique that is helpful in a variety of lung diseases, including those caused by occupational and environmental agents. Mineral fibers, such as asbestos, sheet silicates, and titanium coated with iron and protein (ferruginous bodies), can be identified in samples of sputum, bronchial washings, and bronchoalveolar lavage fluid (Fig. 8-21). Correlations have been made, for example, between the number of asbestos bodies in sputum cytology specimens and the number of asbestos bodies found in lung tissue.[42] Likewise, studies have been published correlating the concentration of asbestos bodies in bronchoalveolar lavage fluid and the concentration in lung tissue.[43] The same has also been done for asbestos fibers.[44] Other occupational and environmental lung disease–associated structures can be identified in cytologic preparations of sputum, bronchial washings, and bronchoalveolar lavage fluid. These include

hemosiderin-laden macrophages, cigarette smokers macrophages, Charcot Leyden crystals, Curschmann spirals, and Creola bodies.

Cytologic evaluation of pulmonary specimens is most frequently used to identify neoplastic cells. In most instances, identification of neoplastic cells has no implication to any specific environmental or occupational agent. However, if one were to identify a malignant cell in a cytologic preparation of sputum or bronchial washings and in the same specimen identify an asbestos body, it could be said with a relatively high degree of certainty that there would be a concentration of asbestos in the lung tissue great enough to cause the cancer. Cytologic evaluation of pleural fluid is sometimes useful in identifying mesothelioma caused by asbestos. In most instances, ancillary techniques such as electron microscopy and immunohistochemistry would have to be used to prove that the neoplastic cells were of mesothelial origin.

IMMUNOHISTOCHEMICAL EVALUATION OF LUNG TISSUE SPECIMENS

Immunohistochemistry is used most frequently by pathologists to accurately classify malignant neoplasms. A wide spectrum of commercially available polyclonal and monoclonal antibodies is available to perform these techniques. The use of these antibodies is based on the premise that certain neoplastic cells contain or express certain antigens that are specific for a given neoplasm, which can be recognized using an avidin–biotin immunoperoxidase technique.[45] For example, well- to moderately well-differentiated epithelial mesotheliomas have an immunophenotype that is relatively specific and is significantly different in most instances from pulmonary adenocarcinomas (Fig. 8-22) and other adenocarcinomas.[46] The differentiation of epithelial mesothelioma from pulmonary adenocarcinoma is more important from a legal point of view than a medical point of view, in that a tumor involving the pleural cavity is associated with a grave prognosis with no adequate therapy. Other examples of neoplastic pulmonary disease in which immunohistochemical techniques are used would be to differentiate lymphoma from carcinoma and to subtype lymphomas as to their B cell or T cell differentiation.

Antibodies against various antigens can also be helpful in evaluating nonneoplastic conditions. For example, the type of lymphocyte involved in such diseases as hypersensitivity pneumonitis and sarcoidosis can be determined. One can also evaluate the types of lymphocytes infiltrating neoplasms, and whether histiocytes are present, by using spe-

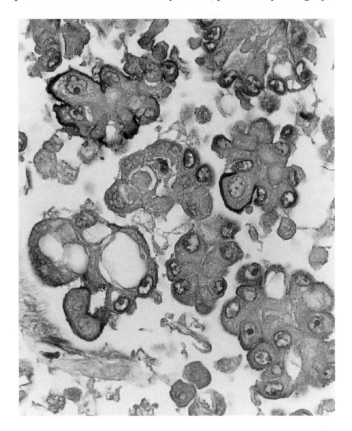

Fig. 8-22. These neoplastic epithelial mesothelial cells showed intense cell membrane staining for epithelial membrane antigen and human milk fat globule protein-2 (arrows, black), findings highly suggestive of an epithelial mesothelioma (×500).

cific monoclonal antibodies against lymphocyte subtypes and macrophages. Such studies are often more useful in helping to understand the pathogenesis of a given disease process than they are in diagnosing it. Antibodies have also been developed against the various molecular species of collagen, and one can evaluate the progression or the pathogenesis of scarring in such conditions as asbestosis, silicosis, and drug-induced fibrosis.

ELECTRON MICROSCOPIC (ULTRASTRUCTURAL) EVALUATION OF LUNG TISSUE SPECIMENS

Electron microscopic (EM) evaluation can be done on virtually any type of pulmonary specimen. This includes pleural fluid, sputum, bronchial washings, bronchoalveolar lavage specimens, and tissue samples. This is possible because ultrastructural evaluation requires a small specimen for evaluation. Ultrastructural examination is extremely valuable in classifying neoplasms. One of the most frequent uses of EM is to differentiate asbestos-induced mesotheliomas from pulmonary adenocarcinomas. Epithelial mesotheliomas have a distinct ultrastructural appearance, the most important feature of which is long, thin, branching, sinuous microvilli arising from the cell surface (Fig. 8-23). These microvilli are not covered by a fuzzy glycocalyx as seen in pulmonary adenocarcinomas (Fig. 8-24), and there are other features such as large desmosomes, intracellular glycogen, and perinuclear bundles of tonofilaments that are more common in epithelial mesotheliomas than they are in pulmonary adenocarcinomas or other types of adenocarcinomas.

Transmission and scanning electron microscopy have been used extensively to understand the normal structure of the lung and have been used in correlating structure with function. One of the most dramatic scanning EM features is the pleural surface, which shows the long microvilli arising from the mesothelial cells. Analytical instruments can be attached to scanning and transmission electron microscopes that make it possible to analyze certain substances identified in lung tissue, pleural fluid, and bronchoalveolar lavage fluid, for their elemental composition. This technique is commonly used for the quantitation of asbestos fibers in lung samples from persons suspected of having asbestos-induced lung disease. Other mineral fibers can also be detected using this technique.

SPECIALIZED METHODS FOR ANALYSIS OF LUNG TISSUE

A variety of special methods are available to analyze lung tissue, some of which are relatively simple and others of which require sophisticated equipment and technology. Many of the special analyses are directed toward the determination of mineral dust content in lung tissue. The techniques for identification of inorganic minerals in lung

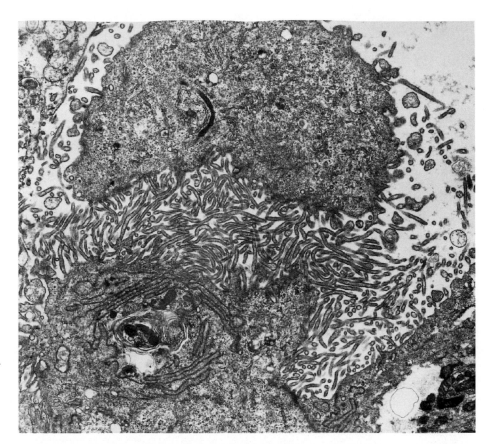

Fig. 8-23. These neoplastic epithelial mesothelial cells have long, thin, sinuous, branching microvilli arising from the cell surface. These microvilli usually have length:width ratios greater than 50 and have a smooth surface (×16,000).

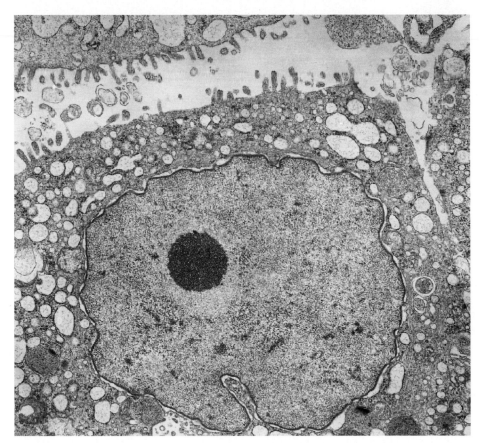

Fig. 8-24. In contrast to neoplastic epithelial type mesothelial cells, these neoplastic pulmonary adenocarcinoma cells are surfaced by relatively short and straight microvilli that are covered by a fuzzy glycocalyx (×16,000).

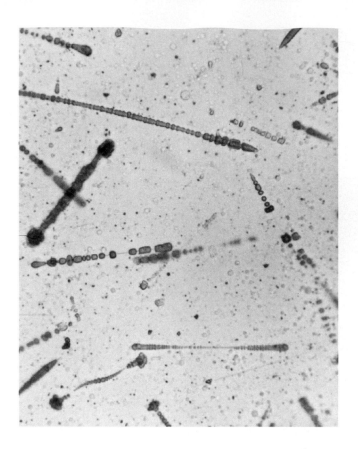

Fig. 8-25. This filter preparation made from a 5-g sample of peripheral lung tissue shows numerous asbestos bodies, indicative of occupational exposure to asbestos (×330).

Table 8-2. Techniques for identification of inorganic materials in lung tissue

Technique	Materials identified	Application
Energy-dispersive x-ray analysis (EDXA)	Elements of inorganic compounds (anatomic number ≥11)	Identification of elements in inorganic particles (e.g., asbestos)
Selected-area electron diffraction (SAED)	Crystallographic structure of an individual particle	Identification of silicates and other inorganic particulates
X-Ray diffraction	Crystallographic structure of an individual particle	Kaolinite, talc, mica, etc.
Electron energy-loss spectrometry	Elemental composition of inorganic particles, atomic number <11	Identification of beryllium and other light elements

tissue are listed in Table 8-2. For lung tissue to be analyzed for mineral content, it has to be treated in a way to destroy the organic part of the specimen. There are a variety of methods to prepare tissue for analytical evaluation, although the most commonly used method in the United States is to digest the tissue in commercial bleach, the active component of which is 5.25% sodium hypochlorite.[47,48] This digestion technique is commonly used for quantitating asbestos bodies and asbestos fibers, after recovering the residue of digested lung tissue with equal volumes of 50% ethyl alcohol and chloroform and extracting the mineral with 0.22-μm pore diameter Millipore filter. The asbestos bodies and fibers are trapped in the filter. The filter is processed, cleared in xylene, mounted on a glass slide, and dried. The asbestos bodies are easily

seen, and can be counted (Figs. 8-25 and 8-26), resulting in a determination of the number of asbestos bodies per gram of wet or dry lung tissue.

Small portions of the filter can be mounted on a supported (coated) nickel grid for electron microscopic evaluation. Asbestos and most other mineral compounds are identified by energy-dispersive x-ray analysis (Fig. 8-27A) and x-ray diffraction (Fig. 8-27B). These techniques are time consuming and expensive, but they provide critical information concerning the exact type of mineral compounds in lung tissue.

SUMMARY

This chapter has discussed pathologic methods used in the evaluation of occupational and environmental lung dis-

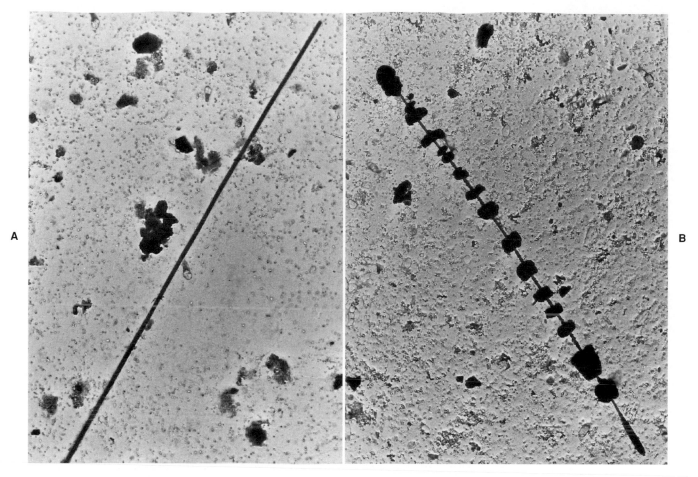

Fig. 8-26. Uncoated amosite fiber (**A**) and an asbestos body formed on an amosite fiber (**B**) (×3000) (Courtesy of Ronald F. Dodson.)

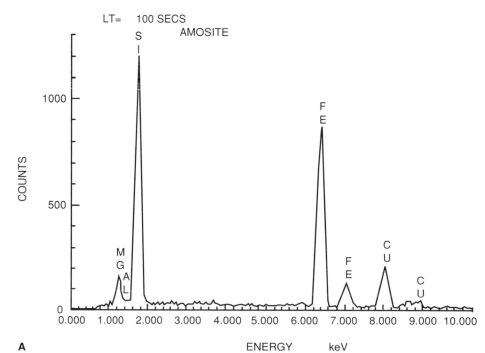

Fig. 8-27. A, Energy-dispersive x-ray analysis spectrum of amosite fiber. Note iron peaks. *Continued.* **A**

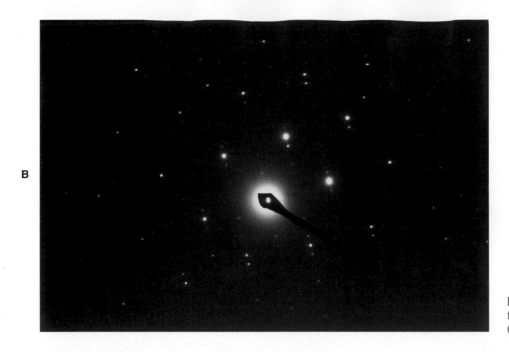

Fig. 8-27. Continued. **B,** X-Ray diffraction pattern of amosite fiber. (Courtesy of Ronald F. Dodson.)

ease. Many of these methods are routinely used in pathology laboratories, whereas others are more complicated and are used in certain situations and specialized laboratories.

Each case of lung disease thought to have an occupational or environmental basis must be evaluated on its own merits, and the appropriate pathologic studies must be performed on the tissues that are most helpful in answering the questions posed.

REFERENCES

1. Henderson DW, Shilkin KB, Whitaker D, Attwood HD, Constance TJ, Steele RH, and Leppard PJ: The pathology of malignant mesothelioma, including immunohistology and ultrastructure. In Henderson DW, Shilkin KB, Langlois SLP, Whitaker D, editors, *Malignant mesothelioma,* pp 69-139, New York, 1992, Hemisphere.
2. Pratt PC: Emphysema and chronic airways disease. In Dail DH and Hammar SP, editors, *Pulmonary pathology,* ed 2, pp 847-865, New York, 1994, Springer-Verlag.
3. Ciba Guest Symposium Report: Terminology, definitions, and classification of chronic pulmonary emphysema and related conditions, *Thorax* 14:286-299, 1959.
4. Schmidt RA, Glenny RW, Godwin JD, Hampson NB, and Reichenbach DD: Panlobular emphysema in young intravenous Ritalin abusers, *Am Rev Respir Dis* 143:649-656, 1991.
5. Schwartz DA: New developments in asbestos-induced pleural disease, *Chest* 99:191-198, 1991.
6. Hourihane DO, Lessof L, and Richardson PC: Hyaline and calcified pleural plaques as an index of exposure to asbestos; a study of radiological and pathological features of 100 cases, with consideration of the epidemiology, *Br Med J* 1:1069-1074, 1966.
7. Weiss W: Lobe of origin in the attribution of lung cancer to asbestos, *Br J Ind Med* 45:544-547, 1988.
8. Auerbach O, Garfinkel L, Parks VR, Conston A, Galdi V, and Joubert L: Histologic type of lung cancer and asbestos exposure, *Cancer* 54:3017-3021, 1984.
9. Koss M, Travis W, Moran C, and Hochholzer L: Pseudomesotheliomatous adenocarcinomas: a reappraisal, *Semin Diagn Pathol* 9:117-123, 1992.
10. Robb JA, Hammar SP, and Yokoo H: Pseudomesotheliomatous lung carcinoma: a rare asbestos-related malignancy readily separable from epithelial pleural mesothelioma, *Hum Pathol* (in press).
11. Hammar SP: Pleural diseases, In Dail DH and Hammar SP, editors: *Pulmonary pathology,* ed 2, pp 1463-1580, New York, 1994, Springer-Verlag.
12. McCaughey WTE: Criteria for the diagnosis of diffuse mesothelial tumors, *Ann NY Acad Sci* 132:603-613, 1965.
13. van Gelder T, Hoogsteden HC, Vandenbroucke JP, Van der Kwast TH, Flanteydt HT: The influence of the diagnostic techinque on the histopathological diagnosis in malignant mesothelioma, *Virch Arch A Pathol Anat* 418:315-317, 1991.
14. Ives JC, Buffler PA, and Greenberg SD: Environmental associations and histopathologic patterns of carcinoma of the lung: the challenge and dilemma in epidemiologic studies, *Am Rev Respir Dis* 128:195-209, 1983.
15. Churg A: Lung cancer cell type and asbestos exposure, *JAMA* 253:2984-2985, 1985.
16. Zang EA and Wynder EL: Cumulative tar exposure: a new index for estimating lung cancer risk among cigarette smokers, *Cancer* 70:69-76, 1992.
17. Figueroa WG, Raszkowski R, and Weiss W: Lung cancer in chloromethyl methyl ether workers, *N Engl J Med* 288:1096-1097, 1973.
18. Waxweiler FEJ, Smith AH, Falk H, and Tyroler HA: Excess lung cancer risk in a synthetic chemicals plant, *Environ Health Perspect* 41:159-165, 1981.
19. Radford EP: Radon daughters in the induction of lung cancer in underground miners, In Peto R and Schneiderman M, editors: *Quantification of occupational cancer,* pp 151-163, Cold Spring Harbor, New York, 1981, Cold Spring Laboratory.
20. Samet JM, Kutvirt DM, Waxweiler RJ, and Key CR: Uranium mining and lung cancer in Navajo men, *N Engl J Med* 310:1481-1484, 1984.
21. Radford EP and St Clair Renard KG: Lung cancer in Swedish iron miners exposed to low doses of radon daughters, *N Engl J Med* 310:1481-1484, 1984.
22. Watkin SW: Temporal demographic and epidemiologic variation in histologic subtypes of lung cancer: a literature review, *Lung Cancer* 69-81, 1989.

23. Churg A and Wright JL: Small airway lesions in patients exposed to non-asbestos mineral dusts, *Hum Pathol* 14:688-693, 1983.

24. Churg A: Non-neoplastic diseases caused by asbestos, In Churg A and Green FHY, editors: *Pathology of occupational lung diseases,* pp 253-277, New York, 1988, Igaku-Shoin.

25. Wright JL, Cagle P, Churg A, Colby TV, and Myers J: Diseases of the small airways, *Am Rev Respir Dis* 146:240-262, 1992.

26. Bellis D, Andrion A, Desedime L, et al: Minimal pathologic changes of the lung and asbestos exposure, *Hum Pathol* 20:102-106, 1989.

27. Roggli VL: Pathology of human asbestosis; a critical review, *Adv Pathol* 2:31-60, 1989.

28. Warnock ML and Worley G: Asbestos bodies or fibers and the diagnosis of asbestosis, *Environ Res* 44:29-44, 1987.

29. Dodson RF, Williams MG, O'Sullivan MF, Corn CJ, Greenberg SD, and Hurst GA: A comparison of ferruginous body and uncoated fiber content in the lungs of former asbestos workers, *Am Rev Respir Dis* 132:143-147, 1985.

30. Roggli VL: Asbestosis. In Roggli VL, Greenberg SD, and Pratt PC, editors: *Pathology of asbestos-associated diseases,* pp 77-108, Boston, 1992, Little-Brown.

31. Kleinerman J: The pathology of some familiar pneumoconioses, *Semin Roentgenol* 2:244-264, 1967.

32. Roggli VL and Shelburne JD: Pneumoconioses, mineral and vegetable, In Dail DH and Hammar SP, editors: *Pulmonary pathology,* 2nd ed, pp 867-900, New York, 1994, Springer-Verlag.

33. Spencer H: The pneumoconioses and other occupational lung diseases. In Spencer H, editor: *Pathology of the lung,* ed 4, vol 1, pp 413-510, Oxford, 1985, Pergamon.

34. Hammar SP: Extrinsic allergic alveolitis. In Dail DH and Hammar SP, editors: *Pulmonary pathology,* ed 2, pp 597-614, New York, 1994, Springer-Verlag.

35. Rom WN and Travis WD: Lymphocyte-macrophage alveolitis in non-smoking individuals occupationally exposed to asbestos, *Chest* 101:779-786, 1992.

36. May JJ, Stallones L, Darrow D, and Pratt DS: Organic dust toxicity (pulmonary mycotoxicosis) associated with silo unloading, *Thorax* 41:919-923, 1986.

37. Brinton WT, Vastbinder EE, Greene JW, Marx JJ Jr, Hutcheson RH, and Schaffner W: An outbreak of organic dust toxic syndrome in a college fraternity, *JAMA* 258:1210-1212, 1987.

38. Lecours R, Laviolette M, and Cormier Y: Bronchoalveolar lavage in pulmonary mycotoxicosis (organic dust toxic syndrome), *Thorax* 41:924-926, 1986.

39. Hammar SP: Pulmonary histiocytosis X, In Dail DH and Hammar SP, editors: *Pulmonary pathology,* ed 2, pp 567-596, New York, 1994, Springer-Verlag.

40. Myers JL: Respiratory bronchiolitis with interstitial lung disease, *Semin Respir Med* 13:134-139, 1991.

41. Carrington CB, Gaensler EA, Coutu RF, Fitzgerald MX, and Gupta RG: Natural history and treated course of usual and desquamative interstitial pneumonia, *N Engl J Med* 298:801-809, 1978.

42. Roggli VL, Greenberg SD, McCarty JW, et al: Comparison of sputa and lung asbestos body count in former asbestos workers, *Am Rev Respir Dis* 122:941, 1980.

43. DeVuyst P, Dumortier P, Moulin E, et al: Asbestos bodies in bronchoalveolar lavage reflect lung asbestos body concentrations, *Env Respir J* 1:362-367, 1988.

44. Dodson RF, Garcia JGN, O'Sullivan M, et al: The usefulness of bronchoalveolar lavage in identifying past occupational exposure to asbestos; a light and electron microscopic study, *Am J Ind Med* 19:619-628, 1991.

45. DeLellis RA and Dayal Y: Principles of immunohistochemistry as applied to the surgical pathology of neoplasms, In Azar HA, editor: *Pathology of human neoplasms,* pp 131-181, New York, 1988, Raven.

46. Hammar SP: Mesothelioma, In Sheppard MN, editor: *Practical pulmonary pathology,* Kent, Edward Arnold (in press).

47. Smith MJ and Naylor B: A method for extracting ferruginous bodies from sputum and pulmonary tissue, *Am J Clin Pathol* 58:250-254, 1972.

48. Churg A, Sakoda N, and Warnock ML: A simple method for preparing ferruginous bodies for electron microscopic examination, *Am J Clin Pathol* 68:513-517, 1977.

Chapter 9

IMMUNOLOGIC METHODS

Abba I. Terr

The immune system functions at the interface between the body and the environment. Therefore, the practitioner interested in occupational and environmental respiratory diseases benefits from a solid knowledge base of the immune system, including its normal function, its role in diseases, the spectrum of immune dysfunction and pathology, and relevant diagnostic testing procedures. This chapter will present a brief outline of the anatomy and function of the immune system, the immune response and the inflammatory response, immunopathology, principles of diagnostic methods, and the applications of immunologic methods to the diagnosis of occupational and environmental respiratory diseases.

The diagnosis of immunologic disease should proceed in an orderly fashion by the sequential use of the medical and environmental history, physical examination, and then selected laboratory tests. Selection of tests is based on information from the history and physical examination. Because so many individual immune cells and their products (immunoglobulins, antibodies, cytokines, and inflammatory mediators) can now be detected and quantitated accurately and usually with great precision, it is tempting to use the laboratory as a substitute for the clinical examination, but it is rarely if ever appropriate to rely on test results alone to make a clinical diagnosis.

In the practice of occupational and environmental medicine, the use of immunologic diagnostic methods is most often helpful when occupational allergy is suspected. Appropriate immunologic testing may also be indicated to rule out the presence of nonoccupational diseases, such as infection, autoimmunity, and immune deficiency. In workplace-related or other environmental diseases caused by a direct irritation or toxicity from an environmental chemical, immunologic tests cannot identify the causative agent, but the laboratory may be helpful to distinguish these from allergic reactions, especially when the allergen is airborne and the target tissue is the respiratory mucosa.

There is increasing interest in the potential toxicity of many environmental chemicals on the human immune system. In this emerging area it is critical to avoid the mistake of interpreting the laboratory's "reference range" for the various constituents of the immune system as a formula to separate normal from abnormal or health from disease. Some tests, such as the total serum immunoglobulin levels, have reasonably well-established ranges, whereas others, particularly blood lymphocyte subset counts based on flow cytometry and monoclonal antibodies to cell membrane markers, are yet to be standardized in large numbers of normals. The total numbers and percentage distribution of circulating cells, especially lymphocytes, fluctuate considerably under normal physiologic conditions, and they may be influenced by age, smoking, stress, drugs, and diurnal variations.[1] Serum levels of immunoglobulins may reflect racial and geographic factors and—in the case of IgE—genetic factors as well. In general, immune cells and their products function in tissues and not in the circulation, so that blood concentrations do not directly reflect their function or their participation in tissue pathology. The blood and lymph serve as conduits for transporting cells and antibodies from organs of production or reservoir to other organs and tissues where they are needed.

It should be noted also that well-established normal reference ranges for immune system components in blood may be quite wide. For example, lymphocytes make up 20% to 40% of total white blood cell (WBC) count, and the latter in turn ranges from 4000 to 11,000 cells per μl. Serum IgG ranges from 800 to 1800 mg/dl. Therefore, observed values slightly above or below these limits do not necessarily indicate pathologic conditions, nor do results within these ranges necessarily ensure the absence of disease.

OVERVIEW OF THE IMMUNE SYSTEM

The immune system responds to the host's environment by recognizing and responding to the chemical nature of environmental molecules, referred to as antigens. In contrast, the nervous system responds to external physical stimuli, and the endocrine system responds to internal chemicals to maintain physiologic homeostasis.

Immunologic recognition has two cardinal characteristics: exquisite specificity and the ability to distinguish self from nonself. Immunologic specificity derives from the fact that every individual has a large number of immunologically competent lymphocyte clones, each of which provides a single recognition specificity. The complete repertoire of specificities is present before antigen exposure. Self and nonself distinction is thought to occur principally in the thymus through clonal deletion of those cells possessing the ability to recognize the chemical structure of native molecules of the host (i.e., self).

The function of the immune system that is the most obvious and critically important is the acquisition of immunity to infectious microorganisms and their toxins. Rejection of tissue and organ grafts is immunologically mediated. A role for the immune system in protection against cancer by recognizing and destroying mutant cells (immune surveillance) has been postulated but not yet generally accepted as proven.

Anatomically, the immune system consists of a heterogeneous combination of mobile cells. These are located in the blood and lymphatic circulation and in virtually all tissues. Some components of the immune system reside in nonimmunologic organs, such as the Peyer's patches in the intestine and Kuppfer cells in the liver. Other organs are entirely immunologic in function, e.g., the thymus, lymph nodes, and spleen. The cell types that carry out the functions of immunity are the mononuclear phagocytes, lymphocytes, plasma cells, neutrophils, eosinophils, basophils, and mast cells. The bone marrow stem cell is the ultimate precursor of all of these functioning cellular elements.

Lymphocytes may be seen between airway epithelial cells and in the lamina propria below the epithelium. Outside the airway epithelium, there are often aggregates of lymphocytes, so-called bronchus-associated lymphoid tissue (BALT). The presence of lymphocytes along the airways is probably adaptive to the continuous challenge of the respiratory tract by inhaled immunologic stimuli.

The immune response

The acquiring of a state of immunity following exposure to an antigen is called the immune response. It has been well described, especially for its role in handling protein antigens. Nucleic acids, carbohydrates, and simple organic and inorganic compounds can also be antigenic and induce an immune response, but these usually require prior conjugation of the molecule to a host carrier protein. Antigen recognition begins with antigen uptake, processing, and presentation by specialized cells known as antigen-presenting cells (APC). Depending on the nature and location of the antigen, any of the mononuclear phagocytes (tissue macrophage, circulating monocyte, skin Langerhans cell, and liver Kuppfer cell) or the B lymphocyte can function as APC. Processing consists of ingestion and proteolytic degradation of the protein antigen to peptide fragments. Some of these peptides bind to intracellular proteins that are coded for by genes of the major histocompatibility complex (MHC). The peptide–MHC protein complex is then transported to the cell surface, a process known as antigen presentation.

The antigenic peptide–MHC protein complex presented on the APC surface membrane then interacts with the helper T lymphocyte (T_H cell), which has a T cell receptor (TCR) that has specific recognition of both the peptide and the MHC gene product.[2] This brings the APC and the T_H cell into direct contact, which in addition to the antigen–MHC–TCR trimolecular complex also involves contact by other nonspecific cell surface receptors and their ligands. The next step of the immune response is the activation of the T_H cell through the secretion of cytokines.[3] The APC secretes interleukin-1 (IL-1), which promotes expression by the APC of adhesion molecules that enhance cell–cell binding and IL-2 by the T_H cell. The expression of IL-2 and other cytokines by the T_H cell results in clonal cell proliferation and stimulation of other lymphocyte classes.

There are two different classes of MHC molecules that can be recognized by T_H cells. MHC Class I proteins

Table 9-1. Structure and function of the five immunoglobulin classes

	IgG	IgA	IgM	IgD	IgE
Serum concentration (mg/dl)	1200	250	150	3	0.0001
Molecular weight	150,000	160,000 400,000*	900,000	180,000	190,000
Number of subunits	1	1,2†	5	1	1
Complement activating	Yes	No‡	Strong	No	No
Mast cell activating	No	No	No	No	Yes
Crosses placenta	Yes	No	No	No	No

*Secretory IgA dimer with secretory piece.
†Monomer in circulation; dimer in secretions.
‡Activates the alternative complement pathway.

present antigenic peptides to T cells that express the CD8 cell marker and are generally cytotoxic. Almost all somatic cells can express MHC Class I, so that intracellular antigens, such as viruses, are immunologically eliminated by lysis of the infected cell. MHC Class II proteins are expressed only on monocytes and B lymphocytes, and they present antigenic peptides to T cells that bear the CD4 marker. Immune responses resulting from this pathway involve soluble antigens and antibody or cell-mediated effector mechanisms.

CD8 T lymphocytes become activated to function in immunologically specific cytotoxicity and are then known as cytotoxic T cells (T_C cells). The TCR on the T_C cell makes contact with the antigenic peptide presented in the context of MHC Class I protein on the APC. An additional signal to achieve cytotoxic activity by the T_C cell comes from IL-2 secreted by activated T_H cells. The result is lysis of the cell that contains the antigen intracellularly, such as a virally infected cell.

As noted above, T_H cell activation results in cell proliferation, producing a clone of cells with identical antigenic specificity, some of which become long-lived memory cells, whereas the rest carry out their helper function on B cells and effector T cells. The clonal expansion of memory cells means that reexposure at a later encounter with the same (or cross-reacting) antigen results in a more rapid and quantitatively greater response, called an anamnestic response.

B lymphocytes recognize soluble antigen through specific antibodylike surface molecules. When contact with antigen occurs, the B cell becomes activated, but optimal activation requires contact with the activated T_H cell and certain cytokines.[4] The B cell then proliferates into a clone of daughter cells; some become long-lived memory cells, whereas others differentiate into specific antibody-secreting plasma cells. The antibody molecule contains the antigenic specificity, and by functioning outside the cell in the circulation and in tissues and interstitial fluid spaces, antibody-mediated immunity increases the extent and versatility of the immune response.

Table 9-2. Structure and functions of IgG subclasses

	IgG1	IgG2	IgG3	IgG4
Percent of total IgG	70	20	7	3
Complement activating	Slight	Slight	Yes	No
Crosses placenta	Yes	Slight	Yes	Yes

Antibody-mediated immunity, often referred to as humoral immunity, is made even more versatile by the heterogeneity of the molecules that carry out antibody function (i.e., the immunoglobulins). There are five immunoglobulin classes with differing structures and biological functions (Table 9-1). The largest class, IgG, consists of four subclasses with further diversity of function (Table 9-2). The most efficient subclass for generating antibodies to protein antigens is IgG1, and for antibodies to carbohydrate antigens it is IgG2. Complement fixation ability is greatest with antibodies of the IgG3 subclass. IgA antibodies are uniquely adapted to survive in gastrointestinal and respiratory secretions. IgA antibodies exist in mucosal secretions as IgA dimers complexed with a nonimmunoglobulin protein known as the secretory component. IgM antibodies are large pentamers with high efficiency for activating the complement system. IgE antibodies have strong affinity for mast cells and basophils, whereby reaction with antigen liberates chemical mediators that are especially effective for the destruction of pathogenic helminths. They are also notable for mediating allergic reactions.

T_H cell clones exhibit two distinct patterns of cytokine release leading to two different types of immune responses. Those that secrete primarily IL-2 and interferon gamma (IFN-γ) are known as T_H1 cells. These cytokines lead to cell-mediated immune responses and also favor IgM and IgG2 antibody production by B cells. Those that secrete a pattern of cytokines dominated by IL-4 and IL-5 are known as T_H2 cells, and these cytokines lead to a predominantly IgE antibody response and an eosinophilic inflammation.

Effector mechanisms

The immune response outlined above in brief form is the afferent portion of the process by which protective immunity to microbial pathogens and other functions of the immune system are achieved. It consists of specific antigen recognition and the recruitment of an arsenal of sensitized cells and antibodies. In the case of a soluble protein antigen such as a bacterial toxin, simple binding of the toxin by antibody may be sufficient to neutralize and eliminate it from the host. Immune elimination of intracellular or extracellular microbes or multicellular pathogens requires one of two additional immune-generated effector mechanisms, cytotoxicity and inflammation.

Cytotoxicity. Acquired immune-mediated cytotoxicity is accomplished through either cellular or humoral mechanisms. An example of cellular cytotoxicity involves the specifically sensitized activated CD8 T lymphocyte (T_C cell), which, as discussed above, comes in contact with the cell containing the antigen and destroys the cell by secreting cytotoxins and by stimulating the target cell to undergo programmed cell death, called apoptosis. An example of humoral cytotoxicity involves IgG or IgM antibodies that are capable of activating the complement system through its classical pathway, proceeding through the terminal complement components, C5–9, known as the membrane attack complex (MAC). The MAC causes osmotic lysis of the target cell by producing pores in the cell surface for entry of extracellular fluid.[5]

Inflammation. Immune-mediated inflammation also proceeds through a number of diverse pathways. Cell-mediated inflammation (CMI) is triggered by sensitized CD4 lymphocytes, called effector lymphocytes. In the presence of antigen the cell elaborates chemotactic cytokines that recruit various mononuclear phagocytes, including monocytes, lymphocytes, and plasma cells, resulting in a granulomatous focus of inflammation. The granuloma containing multinucleated giant cells is the histologic hallmark of this form of inflammation and is characteristic of tuberculosis, fungal infections, and other chronic infections. It is also the mechanism for the typical form of allograft rejection and for the pathogenesis of allergic contact dermatitis. Another mechanism of inflammation involves IgE antibodies, which coat the surfaces of mast cells and basophils by attaching to a high affinity receptor for IgE on these cells. Contact of antigens with their corresponding cell-bound IgE antibodies activates the cell to generate and release a number of potent chemical mediators of inflammation (box, top of column two). The effect is to cause localized stimulation of mucosal secretory glands, contraction of visceral smooth muscle, and chemotaxis of eosinophils, which in turn releases and activates toxic products. This form of inflammation is thought to be especially effective in immobilizing and expelling multicellular infecting organisms such as helminths and appears to be an important factor in the pathogenesis of asthma. Still another example of

---

Mediators of allergic inflammation

Mast cell-associated mediators

Histamine
Platelet-activating factor (PAF)
Tryptase
Heparin
Arachidonic acid metabolites
Leukotrienes (e.g., LTB_4, LTC_4)
Prostaglandins (e.g., PGD_2)

Eosinophil-associated mediators

Eosinophil cationic protein (ECP)
Major basic protein (MBP)
Eosinophil peroxidase (EPO)
Eosinophil-derived neurotoxin (EDN)

Cytokines

From T_H2 cells
Interleukin-3 (IL-3)
IL-4
IL-5
Granulocyte colony-stimulating factor

---

antibody-mediated inflammation involves IgG and IgM antibodies and their ability to activate complement, as discussed above. In addition to the cytolytic process of the terminal components in the MAC, other components, especially C5 and C3, when activated, generate degradation products with chemotactic properties that attract neutrophils. C3 is opsonic, coating the surface of bacteria for more efficient interaction with antibody. These inflammatory activities of complement are important in acquired immunity to extracellular bacterial infections.

Immune response regulation

A major focus of immunologic research in recent years has been the elucidation of an array of mechanisms for internal regulation of the immune response. Much of this work has identified a series of cytokines, endogenous molecules produced by each of the cells involved in immunity. Cytokines are secreted locally to act on other cells (paracrine) or on the cell of origin (autocrine) to enhance, suppress, or otherwise alter cell–cell interaction. These molecules are ligands for corresponding receptors on the target cells. Unlike endocrine hormones, cytokines perform their function in the immediate vicinity of their release, and so detection of their presence or concentration in plasma or serum does not usually reflect their functional activity. Depending on their particular function, they are referred to generically as cytokines, or more descriptively as interleukins, interferons, adhesion molecules, growth factors, colony-stimulating factors, or tumor necrosis factor. They are mostly proteins, and some of them have been purified, sequenced, and synthesized by techniques of genetic engineering. Individual cytokines have multiple activities, often overlapping those of other cytokines, and sometimes variable, depending on the target cell.

IMMUNOPATHOLOGY

The above discussion is an overview of how the immune system functions normally. Like any other organ system, it can itself become diseased. It is subject to a variety of congenital and acquired forms of deficiency. It can be the target of infection, neoplasm, or injury. Two unique types of disease—allergy and autoimmunity—arise from excessive or inappropriate immune responses. This section will outline briefly the current knowledge of immunopathology of these diseases.

Immunodeficiency diseases

A number of disorders of immune deficiency have been described and characterized. They may be congenital or acquired in origin, and the extent of deficiency may be partial or complete in extent. There are laboratory methods for accurately identifying the defect in the majority of cases. Clinically, immunodeficiency is marked by an unusual propensity to infection, and the nature and extent of these infections can often provide important clues to the nature of the defect. Certain congenital immunodeficiencies are associated with failures or anomalies in other organ systems because of the nature of the embryologic anomaly. Since the normal immune response includes numerous pathways and considerable redundancy, partial deficiencies can exist with little or no infectious complications; on the other hand, complete or profound defects are incompatible with life if untreated. It is important to bear in mind that recurrent or recalcitrant infections may also arise from anatomic or epidemiologic factors, rather than from immunologic failure.

The currently established immune system deficiency disorders encompass defects in the normal functioning of cells of the immune response (antigen presenting cells, T cells, B cells), inflammatory cells (neutrophils), and inflammatory mediators (complement components). In the future, specific syndromes will undoubtedly be recognized as arising from deficient functioning of many of the cytokines and other soluble factors that have recently been discovered.

Immunodeficiency disorders can involve either or both cellular or antibody-mediated immunity. Most of the inherited deficiency diseases listed in Table 9-3 are rare, and many of them are recognized in infants and children. Acquired deficiencies of immunity and inflammation overall are more common and involve all age groups. These conditions are primarily attributed to the widespread current use of certain therapeutic agents—immunosuppressant and antiinflammatory drugs—and to the human immunodeficiency virus. The possibility of immunotoxicity by a number of occupational and environmental chemicals has been suggested in recent years. Animal toxicologic research has demonstrated immunologic effects of some organic chemicals under certain experimental protocols using specific animal species or strains,[12] but definitive evidence of similar human immunotoxicity from environmental chemicals at this time is speculative.

Table 9-3. Principal immune system deficiency disorders

Disorder	Immune deficiency
Severe combined immunodeficiency (SCID)	No cellular or antibody-mediated immunity
Ataxia telangiectasia	Combined partial cellular and immunoglobulin deficiencies
Nezelof's syndrome	Combined partial cellular and immunoglobulin deficiencies
Wiskott-Aldrich syndrome	Combined partial cellular and immunoglobulin deficiencies
Congenital absence of adenosine deaminase or nucleoside phosphorylase	Combined partial cellular and immunoglobulin deficiencies
X-linked agammaglobulinemia	No antibody-mediated immunity
Selective IgA deficiency	No IgA
Common variable immunodeficiency	Partial B cell deficiency
DiGeorge syndrome	Partial T cell deficiency
Chronic granulomatous disease	Decreased neutrophil respiratory burst
Complement component deficiency	Dysfunctional complement activation

Allergy

Allergy (hypersensitivity) refers to a group of diseases in which a normal or expected immune response to an otherwise innocuous environmental antigen results in a localized or systemic inflammatory response. The antigen is called an allergen in this case, and it usually consists of nonpathogenic components of the environment, such as plant pollens, fungal spores, organic dust materials, airborne animal emanations, arthropod or acarid products, foods, and drugs. The resulting immune-generated inflammation, however, is pathogenic, because it causes anatomic and physiologic disturbances in the target tissues. Exposure to allergens may be through inhalation, ingestion, skin contact, or injection.

Allergic diseases are multiple, and the most useful classification scheme is by the particular immune pathway involved (box, top left, page 131).[13] The atopic diseases and allergic contact dermatitis are very common, whereas others are uncommon to rare. Allergy is diagnosed primarily by history and confirmatory physical findings, and the specific allergens causing disease in each case are identified by laboratory or in vivo tests that indicate the presence of the relevant immune response (e.g., IgE or T cell mediated)

Classification of allergic diseases

IgE antibody-induced release of mast cell mediators

ATOPY
  Allergic rhinitis
  Allergic asthma
  Atopic dermatitis
ANAPHYLAXIS
  Systemic anaphylaxis
  Urticaria/angioedema

IgG or IgM antibody-induced, immune complex-activated, complement-mediated generation of inflammatory mediators

  Arthus reaction
  Serum sickness
  Acute hypersensitivity pneumonitis

Effector T cell-induced inflammation

  Allergic contact dermatitis
  Chronic hypersensitivity pneumonitis

Types of autoimmune diseases

Postinfectious organ or tissue pathology
Organ or cell-specific disease caused by the autoantibody
Multisystem disease with circulating non–organ-specific autoantibodies

---

to the suspected allergen. Allergy usually occurs in only a portion of the exposed population, probably because of genetically determined factors that control various immune response pathways. For example, atopic persons generate IgE antibodies readily to allergens in numerous inhaled organic materials, and this tendency is familial. Allergic disease is treated by avoidance of the allergen, drugs that inhibit the relevant inflammatory responses, and desensitization in the case of IgE allergics.

The particular diseases caused by allergy—for example, asthma, contact dermatitis, and urticaria—can also occur in the absence of detectable allergy. The underlying nonallergic causes of these diseases are obscure. In some cases exacerbations of these diseases may be traced to an exposure to a nonallergenic environmental irritant. For example, some asthmatics experience acute attacks from inhalation of irritant dusts, mists, vapors, or fumes. Nonallergic irritant contact dermatitis is also common.

Allergy is a significant cause of occupational disease. Work-related allergic contact dermatitis and asthma are special risks in certain occupations. Hypersensitivity pneumonitis is a relatively rare condition that involves either an immune complex-mediated or a cell-mediated form of allergy, depending upon the phase of illness; a number of cases have involved occupational allergens.

Autoimmune diseases

Although it is now well accepted that antibodies and T cell clones with immunologic specificity for self-antigens exist normally, such autoantibodies and autoreactive T cells were originally discovered in connection with certain diseases. The category of autoimmune diseases comprises a long list of conditions characterized by unusually high titers of one or more autoantibodies in the serum and chronic noninfectious inflammation. In a significant number of these diseases, a particular HLA haplotype has been found to be a risk factor for the disease. The autoimmune diseases can be classified into three types, based on the relationships of the autoantibody and clinical disease or pathology (box above).

Pathogenic autoimmunity was first recognized as the mechanism for poststreptococcal carditis and poststreptococcal nephritis. In these cases, the existence of valvular heart disease or nephritis as a late noninfectious sequela of streptococcal pharyngitis was discovered by epidemiologic research, and later the existence of circulating autoantibodies to cardiac or renal antigens, respectively, led to the concept that the host response to a bacterial antigen and not the microbe itself was responsible for these diseases. The discovery of streptococcal antigens that cross-react with antigens of human origin is consistent with one theory of autoimmune pathogenesis, molecular mimicry.[14]

Several diseases exist in which there is clear evidence that a circulating autoantibody to a particular self-antigen is directly pathogenic, because the disease results from a failure of the organ containing the antigen to function properly (top box, page 132). A prime example is myasthenis gravis, in which the autoantibody to the acetylcholine receptor blocks transmission of acetylcholine released from nerve endings to receptors on striated muscle.[15] Antibodies to red cell antigens cause complement-dependent cell lysis in the various autoimmune hemolytic anemias.[16] In Goodpasture's syndrome, antiglomerular basement membrane antibodies cause glomerulitis and cross-react with antigens in the alveolus, causing diffuse alveolar hemorrhage as well.[17]

The third group of autoimmune diseases includes a number of related and overlapping multisystemic syndromes that feature remitting periods of inflammatory activity involving joints and periarticular tissues, blood vessels, skin, and other organs (bottom box, page 132). This group of diseases is commonly called the connective tissue diseases. The immune system involvement in their inflammatory processes is suggested by the frequent occurrence of complement consumption during active periods and the presence of circulating immune complexes. However, the circulating autoantibodies that characterize these conditions are not specific to the involved organs, but rather to antigens present in the nucleus or cytoplasm of most cells. Many of these diseases feature antinuclear antibodies (ANA). The laboratory detection of ANA has depended on tissue immunofluorescence, in which antibodies in the patient's serum

Organ-specific autoimmune diseases

Disease	Auto-antibody Target
Myasthenia gravis	Acetylcholine receptor
Multiple sclerosis	Myelin basic protein
Autoimmune thyroiditis	Various thyroid antigens
Graves' disease	Various thyroid antigens
Type I diabetes	Islet cell antigens; insulin
Autoimmune hemolytic anemia	Various blood group antigens
Autoimmune neutropenia	Various neutrophil antigens
Autoimmune thrombocytopenia	Various thrombocyte antigens
Autoimmune adrenalitis	Adrenal cell microsomes
Pernicious anemia	Parietal cell antigen
Bullous pemphigoid	Basement membrane zone antigen
Pemphigus vulgaris	Keratinocyte antigen

Principal multisystem inflammatory diseases associated with circulating autoantibodies

Systemic lupus erythematosus
Rheumatoid arthritis
Progressive systemic sclerosis
Sjögren's syndrome
Mixed connective tissue disease
Undifferentiated connective tissue disease
Polymyositis/dermatomyositis

overlaying a tissue slice or culture cell layer on a microscope slide are detected visually by a technician using fluorescence microscopy.[18] Different antibodies to various cellular components are judged by location and pattern. Antibody titers are determined by the serum dilutions at which fluorescence is still visible. Thus, the technique is highly dependent on the quality of the tissue substrate, a subjective interpretation of the presence or absence of microscopic fluorescence, and quality control by the laboratory. This methodology is gradually being supplanted by more reproducible immunochemical assays.[19] The rheumatoid factor that occurs in the serum of most patients with rheumatoid arthritis is an antibody to human immunoglobulin. In general, several different autoantibodies are associated with each clinically defined disease entity, although a particular one or combination of several may be characteristic of a particular disease. Thus, these autoantibodies are useful markers for diagnosis, but their role in the disease process, if any, is not currently established.

Immune system malignancies

Each mature cell type involved in the immune and inflammatory responses derives from the same ultimate pre-

cursor, the bone marrow hematopoietic stem cell. Neoplastic transformation can arise at any stage of differentiation, presumably because of a genetic mutation that interferes with the normal maturation process. Immune system malignancies—lymphomas and leukemias—can thus be classified by cell of origin (Table 9-4). Cell membrane proteins expressed at various stages of cell differentiation, identified by the CD marker designation described above, can be detected by specific monoclonal antibodies.[20]

Immune system infections

Although the immune system serves its most notable purpose in protecting its host from exogenous infections, the cells that participate in immunity can themselves become infected. To date, known infections of immunocytes are limited to certain viruses: human immunodeficiency virus (HIV), Epstein-Barr virus (EBV), and the human T cell lymphotropic viruses (HTLV-1 and HTLV-2). HIV infection of the CD4 T lymphocyte results in slow but progressive depletion of this cell population.[21] Because the CD4 cell is central in the normal immune response, loss of these cells results in the opportunistic infections that would otherwise have been prevented by cell-mediated immunity (CMI) or immunologic cytotoxicity. The EBV is a B cell tropic virus, and infection by this virus takes place in a large majority of the general population during childhood, usually resulting in an asymptomatic or mild transient illness and leaving lifelong circulating antibodies and immunity to reinfection without any impairment in immunologic function.[22,23] Infection during adolescence or early adulthood is more likely to produce the typical syndrome of infectious mononucleosis. Although this illness may be symptomatic and incapacitating, it is generally self limited. The disease may result in a lifelong carrier state with viral shedding, but it also produces permanent immunity to reinfection and no immune system compromise. The EBV much less commonly causes certain malignancies, such as Burkitt's lymphoma and nasopharyngeal carcinoma. EBV infection of patients with cellular immunodeficiency may result in a neoplastic lymphoproliferative syndrome. HTLV-1 has been identified as the causal agent of adult T cell leukemia.[24] HTLV-2 has not yet been confirmed as the cause of any disease.

IMMUNOLOGIC METHODS

The clinical laboratory devoted to diagnostic immunology testing is a highly specialized facility that uses some of the latest techniques of molecular biochemistry along with well-established immunologic methods such as the precipitin reaction and complement fixation. The exquisite specificity of antibodies to recognize antigens is the basis of tests for (1) assessing the capacity of the immune system to function, (2) diagnosis and prognosis of immune system diseases, and (3) diagnosis and prognosis of nonimmunologic diseases (e.g., quantitating hormones or drugs in

Table 9-4. Immune system malignancies by cell type of origin with representative examples

Cell of origin	Malignancy
Stem cell	Stem cell leukemia
T lymphocyte	Acute T cell leukemia
	Chronic T cell leukemia
	Non-Hodgkin's lymphoma (some)
	Sezary syndrome
B lymphocyte	Acute B cell leukemia
	Chronic B cell leukemia
Plasma cell	Multiple myeloma
	Waldenstrom's macroglobulinemia
NK cell	NK cell leukemia
Monocyte	Monocytic leukemia
	Hodgkin's disease (most)
	Histiocytoses
Inflammatory cells	Neutrophilic leukemia
	Eosinophilic leukemia
	Basophilic leukemia

blood or other body specimens). New methods and measurements are being constantly transferred from the research bench to the clinical laboratory. The sheer number, range, and dynamic nature of the diagnostic immunology armamentarium require the clinician to select carefully those tests indicated by the patient's clinical examination and interpret the results in that context.

It is not possible here to describe individual tests and their methodology in detail. Reference manuals are available for this purpose.[25-28] Instead, categories and examples of tests and their main clinical applications are presented in the following classification: (1) quantitation of the immune system components, (2) antigen-specific immune response tests, and (3) functional assays.

Quantitation of immune system components

The cells involved in the immune response and inflammation can be identified and microscopically quantitated by standard methods of histopathology and cytopathology using appropriate stains. The functional subgroups that comprise many of these cell types are identified through their cell surface molecules. Cells engaged in the immune response secrete soluble molecules such as immunoglobulins and cytokines that are identified by a specific antibody. The wide array of inflammatory mediators are identified by various methods depending on their chemical structure and concentration.

Cellular enumeration. Laboratory confirmation of immune deficiency usually requires a panel of tests to assess both quantitation of the cellular components of immunity and the adequacy for specific immune responses. During each stage of maturation of the immunocompetent cell (lymphocyte) from its origin in the primitive stem cell, through activation by antigen and differentiation along T

cell or B cell lineage to the mature helper or inducer, cytotoxic or suppressor, or effector T cell and antibody-secreting plasma cell, these cell markers become expressed on the cell surface membrane where they can be detected while earlier markers disappear. Thus, any individual cell can in theory be "typed" by its clusters of differentiation (CD) markers that are present at each maturational stage. Many CD markers found on lymphocytes are expressed as well on the monocyte or macrophage and inflammatory cells and also on cells of other organs.

The total lymphocyte compartment of blood (or bone marrow, lymph nodes, or dimercaprol [BAL] fluid) and the proportions of the various lymphocyte subsets are quantitated by flow cytometry using fluorescent-labeled monoclonal antibodies to specific CD cell surface molecules.[29] These molecules are expressed on the cell surface membrane during stages of lymphocyte differentiation as they become functionally active. In practice, flow cytometric analysis separates cells by size into lymphocyte, monocyte, and granulocyte compartments and identifies the percentage of cells in each compartment that reacts to a labeled monoclonal antibody specific for a limited panel of those CD markers of clinical importance (as well as monoclonal antibodies that identify other surface proteins of interest, such as HLA gene products and surface immunoglobulins). Currently, more than 100 CD markers can be detected, but the clinical significance and the "normal" ranges for these measurements in blood samples have not yet been rigorously established. Identifying and quantitating the cells in blood or other body fluids for one or more of these cell markers is widely used as a research tool, but application to clinical diagnosis is limited to certain immunodeficiency diseases and immunologic malignancies.

Congenital T cell immunodeficiencies have varying degrees of reduction in the expected numbers of peripheral blood lymphocytes bearing the various T cell CD markers. Nevertheless, quantitation of absolute numbers of CD4 lymphocytes in the blood is an established procedure for monitoring the course of HIV infection. Since this cell is the one that is targeted and destroyed by the virus, progressive loss of CD4 cells results in susceptibility to opportunistic infections in the acquired immunodeficiency syndrome (AIDS).[21]

As discussed above, leukemias and lymphomas are neoplastic monoclonal proliferations of lymphocytes. Flow cytometry can be used to "type" the neoplastic cell, although the analysis may require bone marrow or lymph node tissue. The neoplasm typing displays its pattern of CD markers indicating the cell lineage (T cell, B cell, NK cell, or macrophage) and the stage of cell differentiation arrest at which the genetic mutation occurred. This information is useful for prognosis and selection of therapy when combined with the clinical examination and histopathology. Flow cytometric analysis with cell typing by appropriate monoclonal antibodies to CD (and other) markers is employed using a sample of blood, bone marrow, lymph node, or tumor tissue.

Measurements of the products of immune and inflammatory cells

In addition to quantifying immunocompetent and inflammatory cells, the numerous soluble products of these cells can also be measured. Although clinically useful in some situations, these measurements do not directly indicate immunologic specificity. Some immune system neoplasms synthesize and secrete soluble products that appear in the serum or urine. Examples include monoclonal immunoglobulins and Bence-Jones protein in the monoclonal gammopathies and β_2-microglobulin in some lymphomas. Their detection can further assist diagnosis and in some cases prognosis as well.[30,31]

Immunoglobulins. The serum concentrations of each of the five classes of immunoglobulin are usually stable over time in adults, and age-related "normal" concentration ranges are fairly well established. IgG, IgA, and IgM serum concentrations are measured by precipitation with class-specific antiserum, and the resulting complex is assayed by radioimmunodiffusion (RID) in gel or by nephelometry.[32] Subclass-specific antibody reagents to the four IgG subclasses and two IgA subclasses are assayed similarly. These tests are usually definitive in the diagnosis of the various antibody deficiency diseases, although testing for specific antibody responses, discussed below, may also be desirable, especially in patients with selective IgG subclass deficiency. Since no clinical syndrome or disease has yet been identified with an IgD abnormality, its serum concentration is currently not of interest. Serum IgE concentration in both health and disease is in the nanogram per milliliter range, necessitating special methodology. This is accomplished by a two-site recognition assay, such as radioimmunoassay (RIA) or enzyme-linked immunosorbent assay (ELISA).[33] These methods require a highly specific heterologous antihuman IgE antibody and a labeled antiserum to that antibody. No defined IgE deficiency disease is currently known, and in fact some healthy individuals have no detectable IgE levels by current test methods. The mean level of total (nonallergen specific) serum IgE is significantly higher in the atopic than in the nonatopic population, and some patients with atopic dermatitis have levels more than 100-fold higher than the upper limit of the nonatopic range. Nevertheless, many atopic patients—even some with numerous specific IgE antibodies—fall within the normal range of total serum IgE. The test, therefore, is not a useful screening tool for allergy. One exception is allergic bronchopulmonary aspergillosis. Total serum IgE is almost always high during disease activity, and it falls during remission. Only a small fraction of the total IgE is *Aspergillus*-specific antibody.

Polyclonal increases in serum IgG, and sometimes IgA and IgM as well, accompany a large number of chronic infections, sarcoidosis, and connective tissue diseases. A monoclonal excess of immunoglobulin, often detected as a spike on the serum protein electrophoresis, occurs in multiple myeloma and Waldenstrom's macroglobulinemia. The monoclonal immunoglobulin can be typed by RID or immunoelectrophoresis using antisera to a panel of each of the immunoglobulin classes and subclasses (i.e., heavy chain-specific) and the κ and λ light chain types.

Cytokines. The immune response is primarily a cellular phenomenon, involving maturation, activation, and differentiation, as well as cell-to-cell interactions. All of these processes are initiated, facilitated, and regulated by an array of cytokines. Since cytokines act locally on cells in tissues, blood levels of cytokines are extremely low and do not generally reflect their potent influence on cells. At this time, blood or serum cytokine concentrations are not diagnostic for disease. A possible exception is the elevated levels of certain cytokines in some immune system neoplasms, although cytokine measurements in these cases may be confirmatory rather than diagnostic.

Mediators of inflammation. A spectrum of proinflammatory mediators is synthesized, activated, and/or released when antigen exposure occurs in the immunized state. These mediators are diverse in their chemical structure. They are essential in eradicating or limiting infections, but they also mediate the adverse tissue effects of allergy and autoimmunity.

The complement components and their regulatory inhibitors are proteins that circulate at substantial concentrations that are measured immunochemically by RID or nephelometry with specific antibody reagents or functionally by an in vitro hemolytic assay. These tests are indicated where there is clinical suspicion of a deficiency of specific complement components. These conditions are frequently associated with a connective tissue disease. Total complement hemolytic activity or levels of C3 or C4 will often be low during periods of active inflammation in systemic lupus or other autoimmune diseases.[34] Other diseases that may be responsible for pathologic complement consumption secondary to immune complex formation include certain acute and subacute infections and serum sickness. Paradoxically, clinical activity of the connective tissue diseases and acute infections may also elevate the serum levels of complement components, because of enhanced hepatic synthesis as part of the acute phase response.[35]

Among the recognized mediators of IgE allergic diseases, shown in the box on page 129, only histamine and tryptase are currently available for assay. The clinical utility of measuring these mediators in vivo is limited by the fact that their release is focal, and histamine is rapidly metabolized. Immediately following an episode of systemic anaphylaxis, the histamine level in plasma rises and is maximal at 5 minutes after its release, and it returns to baseline within minutes. Tryptase serum concentration is maximal at about 1 hour after release, and it may continue to be elevated for up to 24 hours.

Specific immune responses

The laboratory detection of specific immune responses by either antibody or the effector T lymphocyte is the basic tool of both immunologic science and clinical diagnostic immunology. The sheer number and variety of tests that document the antigen specificity of immunity, autoimmunity, and allergy preclude a detailed description of methodology here. Emphasis instead will be placed on the principles of test selection based on the information needed for clinical diagnosis.

Specific in vitro tests

Tests for specific antibodies. For diagnosis, it is important to select the test that is appropriate to the particular diagnosis under consideration. In diagnosing the presence of infection or allergy, evidence of an immune response to a specific antigen of the infectious microbe or allergen is sought. A negative test result in this case would usually rule out that cause, but a positive test indicates only that there was exposure and response. Other information is needed to prove etiology. In the case of infection, the presence of IgM antibodies or a rising antibody titer with time would be consistent with acute and not remote exposure to the organism, and in the case of allergy the specific test result would need to be correlated with the clinical and environmental history. Furthermore, the test method must detect the appropriate type of immune response; for example, IgE antibodies would be sought for atopy, delayed-type hypersensitivity (DTH) for allergic contact dermatitis, and CMI for tuberculosis.

In the diagnosis of autoimmune diseases, certain combinations of antibodies with specificity to particular autoantigens have been shown to correlate with clinical syndromes. In many cases the autoantibodies detected by these tests are not known to be pathogenic for any of the clinical disease manifestations, although they nevertheless serve as markers of the disease. Therefore negative test results do not negate a clinical diagnosis.

Tests for specific cell-mediated immunity. Testing for the ability to generate competent CMI or DTH is usually accomplished by skin testing with a standard panel of antigens, often referred to as "recall antigens," from commonly encountered microbes. Almost all persons with adequately functioning CMI will respond positively to one or more of these antigens, so that absent responses to all of them suggest cellular immune deficiency. Details of the testing procedure are described above.

In vitro testing of antigen-specific CMI is accomplished by incubating the patient's peripheral blood mononuclear cells with antigen, which will result in activation and proliferation of specifically sensitized lymphocytes. Lymphocyte proliferation is quantitated by measuring the incorporation of [^{3}H]thymidine into the cells. The same procedure using a lectin mitogen, such as phytohemagglutinin (PHA) or concanavalin A (Con A) in place of antigen, measures the capacity of lymphocytes to respond nonspecifically (i.e., nonantigenically). These testing procedures are semiquantitative at best and must be performed with proper controls.

Specific in vivo tests

Skin tests for antibody responses. Skin testing can detect several different immune response pathways, depending on (1) the route of exposure of the antigen to the skin—topical, epicutaneous, or intracutaneous; (2) the timing and gross appearance of the resulting skin inflammation; and (3) the histopathology of the skin test lesion. The test antigen is usually given in the form of an aqueous extract, and the concentration used for testing varies with the testing method. Skin testing is used diagnostically for both allergic and infectious diseases. In either case a positive skin test result indicates only that a specific immune response to the particular antigen tested exists in the patient. Other clinical information in the context of the skin test result is needed to determine whether an allergic or infectious disease is currently present.

The absence of an immune response as determined by skin testing can be helpful in the diagnosis of certain types of immunodeficiencies. This particular situation requires independent knowledge that the patient with a current negative skin test result had previously reacted positively or that significant exposure to the antigen had occurred. The state of immunodeficiency determined in this way by skin testing is known as anergy, and the deficiency applies only to the particular immune pathway tested, usually T cell–mediated immunity.

Skin testing for IgE antibody-mediated diseases is accomplished by one of two methods.[13,36] Prick (epicutaneous) testing is performed by lightly pricking the skin through a drop of concentrated extract solution on the skin. Intracutaneous (intradermal) testing consists of the injection of 0.005 to 0.02 ml diluted sterilized antigen extract into the skin. To minimize the chance of a systemic reaction to the testing, a sequential prick-intradermal or serial titration intradermal protocol is usually followed. Negative (diluent) and positive (histamine or histamine-liberator) control skin test sites should be included to ensure accuracy of results. The test is read at 15 to 20 minutes for an "immediate" reaction of erythema and whealing at the test site, which typically is extremely pruritic. A positive result is graded as 1+ (erythema) to 4+ (erythema and a wheal with pseudopods). A cutaneous "late phase" reaction may or may not occur approximately 8 hours later. This reaction consists of erythema, tenderness, and diffuse erythema without pruritus, but there is no standardized system of grading the late phase reaction, and its diagnostic significance in the skin is currently unknown. The IgE-mediated test is inhibited by antihistaminic drugs.

The immediate wheal-and-erythema skin test is used routinely in the diagnostic detection of allergens causing atopic allergy (pollens, fungi, dusts, mites, animals) and anaphylaxis (drugs, insect venoms), but it has not played a significant role in specific diagnosis of infectious diseases.

Skin testing for detection of immune complex-mediated diseases caused by complement-activating IgG or IgM antibodies is known as the Arthus reaction. The method consists of injecting 0.10 ml antigen extract intracutaneously, and a positive result is the appearance at 24 hours of tender induration. In theory, the test would be appropriate for the diagnosis of the causative allergen in serum sickness or other diseases in which immune-complex vasculitis is believed to be involved in pathogenesis, but in practice it is rarely necessary, and the test procedure has not been standardized.

Skin tests for cell-mediated immunity. Skin testing for CMI or DTH may be accomplished by one of two methods. The intracutaneous method consists of the injection of 0.10 ml sterilized diluted antigen extract, and the result is read in approximately 48 hours for the presence of tender induration greater than 10 ml in diameter determined by palpation. An alternative procedure is a multiple prick test method that yields a positive result of at least 2 ml diameter induration.[37] The latter is best suited to large-scale epidemiologic surveys because of its simplicity, but it has had limited validation.

Intracutaneous skin testing is useful clinically in the diagnosis of certain bacterial and fungal infections, such as tuberculosis, histoplasmosis, and coccidiodomycosis. A positive test result indicates that the patient has been exposed by infection to the organism at some undetermined time in the past, since persistence of such evidence of an immune response is potentially lifelong. Therefore, the clinical significance to the patient's current infectious status with regard to that specific organism requires other clinical information.

For the determination of a state of CMI anergy, a panel of several commonly encountered antigens that typically induce CMI in most persons is applied by either the intracutaneous or multiple-prick method. The antigens used for this purpose are shown in Table 9-5. A positive test to any one antigen indicates that the person has functional CMI. If all tests are unreactive, the patient is considered to be anergic and therefore immunologically deficient in T cell function, unless by chance that individual had never encountered any of these specific antigens at any time in the past.

The second method of CMI or DTH testing is the skin patch test in which the test antigen is applied topically to the skin surface. Contact of the antigen to the skin is secured for 48 hours by taping the patch to the skin. After removal of the patch the skin site is inspected and sometimes reinspected for up to an additional 48 hours for the presence of erythema, papules, and vesicles denoting varying degrees of a positive test result, usually graded from 1+ to 3+.

Patch testing is used routinely in the diagnosis of the allergen causing allergic contact dermatitis. The most common allergens causing this disease are listed (box). The list constitutes the standard "routine" patch test set used in clinical practice in North America. Contact dermatitis is the most frequent cause of industrial skin disease. It is important to

Table 9-5. Skin test antigen panel commonly used to test for intact CMI, with concentrations for testing

Antigen	Amount injected in 0.1 ml
Tetanus toxoid	0.5 Lf
Diphtheria toxoid	3.0 Lf
Tuberculin	5 TU
Mumps	20 CFU
Trichophytin	1:50 concentration
Candida albicans	1:50 concentration
Coccidioidin*	1:100 concentration
Histoplasmin*	1:100 concentration

*For use in geographic areas where infection is endemic.

Common North American contact allergens and concentrations used for patch testing

Benzocaine 5%	Formaldehyde 1%
Mercaptobenzothiazole 1%	Ethylenediamine dihydrochloride 1%
Colophony 20%	Epoxy resin 1%
p-Phenylenediamine 1%	Quaternium-15 2%
Imidazolidinyl urea 2%	p-tert-Butylphenol formaldehyde 1%
Cinnamic aldehyde 1%	Mercapto mix 1%
Lanolin alcohol 30%	Black rubber mix 0.6%
Carba mix 3%	Potassium dichromate 0.25%
Neomycin sulfate 20%	Balsam of Peru 25%
Thiuram mix 1%	Nickel sulfate 2.5%

distinguish irritant from allergic contact dermatitis. Irritant contact dermatitis is a disease caused by damage to the skin from the physical or chemical property of an environmental agent when it contacts the skin. Allergic contact dermatitis is an immunologic disease mediated by the patient's DTH acquired from a prior contact with the same or cross-reacting allergen. Many contact allergens, especially those encountered in the workplace, are primary skin irritants as well, so the concentration of allergen used in patch testing is critical to separate an irritant from a specific allergic response, since these cannot be differentiated by either gross or microscopic appearance of the skin patch test response. For each chemical allergen, the threshold concentration of skin irritation must be determined by field testing a panel of "normal" control subjects. The concentration of the chemical in the allergen patch test is significantly lower than the threshold for irritation but high enough to elicit a positive result in known allergic patients.

Both intradermal and patch tests for cell-mediated immunity are inhibited by systemic corticosteroid drugs, but not by antihistamines.

Functional assays

The laboratory can be used to assess the capacity of the immune system to generate specific antibodies. Various aspects of the humoral immune response (i.e., the B cell pathway) can be examined using a panel of test procedures to determine (1) the existence of antibodies from prior antigenic exposure, (2) the anamnestic response to a booster antigenic challenge, and (3) the primary antibody response to an antigen to which there had been no prior experience.

The simplest way to measure preexisting antibodies is the standard blood bank test for blood group antibodies in serum, since all immunologically competent persons routinely and continuously synthesize antibodies to those ABO blood group antigens that they lack on their own erythrocytes. The test of course cannot be used for persons of AB blood type, but only about 4% of the population have this blood type.

Persons who have previously been immunized with tetanus or diphtheria toxoid or pneumococcal vaccine should have detectable circulating serum antibodies if they are immunologically competent, unless they had been immunized in the remote past so that the current antibody level is below the limit of detection. Serum antibody testing before and after booster immunization with tetanus or diphtheria toxoid should reveal a substantial rise in antibody titer. Booster pneumococcal vaccine immunization is not recommended because of the risk of adverse reactions.

On special occasions it may be desirable to show whether a patient currently can mount a primary immune response. The bacteriophage ΦX-174 has been shown to be safe for this purpose. It is a potent antigen that almost all patients would not have encountered by prior natural exposure.[38]

REFERENCES

1. Burton RC, Ferguson P, Gray M et al: Effects of age, gender, and cigarette smoking on human immunoregulatory T-cell subsets: establishment of normal ranges and comparison with patients with cancer and multiple sclerosis, *Diagn Immunol* 1:216, 1983.
2. Kronenberg M, Siu G, Hood LE et al: The molecular genetics of the T-cell antigen receptor and T-cell antigen recognition, *Annu Rev Immunol* 4:529, 1986.
3. Oppenheim JJ, Rossio JL, and Bearing AJK, editors: *Clinical applications of cytokines,* New York, 1993, Oxford University Press.
4. Kishimoto T and Hirano T: Molecular regulation of B lymphocyte response, *Annu Rev Immunol* 6:485, 1988.
5. Kinoshita T: Biology of complement: the overture, *Immunol Today* 10:17, 1993.
6. Huston DP, Kavanaugh AF, Rohane PW, et al: Immunoglobulin deficiency syndromes and therapy, *J Allergy Clin Immunol* 87:1, 1991.
7. Markert ML: Purine nucleoside phosphorylase deficiency, *Immunodef Rev* 3:45, 1991.
8. Buckley RH: Immunodeficiency diseases, *JAMA* 268:2797, 1992.
9. Rosen F, Cooper M, and Wedgwood R: The primary immunodeficiencies: part 1, *N Engl J Med* 311:235, 1984.
10. Rosen F, Cooper M, and Wedgwood R: The primary immunodeficiencies: part 2, *N Engl J Med* 311:300, 1984.
11. Frank MM: Detection of complement in relation to disease, *J Allergy Clin Immunol* 89:641, 1992.
12. Gibson CG, Hubbard R, and Parke DV: *Immunotoxicology,* London, 1983, Academic Press.
13. Terr AI: Mechanisms of hypersensitivity, In Stites DP, Terr AI, and Parslow T, editors: *Basic and clinical immunology,* ed. 8, Ch. 24, pp 315-326, Norwalk, CT, 1994, Appleton and Lange.
14. Steinberg AD: Mechanisms of disordered immune regulation, In Stites DP, Terr AI, and Parslow T, editors: *Basic and clinical immunology,* ed. 8, Ch. 30, pp 380-388, Norwalk, CT, 1994, Appleton and Lange.
15. Protti MP, Manfredi AA, Horton RM et al: Myasthenis gravis: recognition of a human autoantigen at the molecular level, *Immunol Today* 14:363, 1993.
16. Sokol RJ, Hewitt S, and Stamps BK: Autoimmune haemolysis: an 18-year study of 865 cases referred to a regional transfusion centre, *Br Med J* 282:2023, 1981.
17. Donaghy M, Rees AJ: Cigarette smoking and lung hemorrhage in glomerulonephritis caused by autoantibodies to glomerular basement membrane, *Lancet* 1:1390-1392, 1983.
18. Tan EM: Relationship of nuclear staining patterns with precipitating antibodies in systemic lupus erythematosus, *J Lab Clin Med* 70:800, 1967.
19. Pisetsky DS: Antinuclear antibodies, *Immunol Allergy Clin North Am* 14:371, 1994.
20. Borrowitz MJ: Immunophenotyping of acute leukemia by flow cytometry, *Clin Immunol Newslett* 13:54, 1993.
21. Phillips AN, Lee CA, Elford J et al: Serial CD lymphocyte counts and development of AIDS, *Lancet* 337:389, 1991.
22. Okano M, Thiele GM, Davis JR et al: Epstein-Barr virus and human diseases: recent advances in diagnosis, *Clin Microbiol Rev* 1:300, 1988.
23. Straus SE, Cohen JI, Tosato G et al: NIH Conference, Epstein-Barr infections: biology, pathogenesis, and management, *Ann Intern Med* 118:45, 1993.
24. Okochi K and Sato H: Adult T-cell leukemia virus, blood donors and transfusion: experience in Japan. In Dodd RY, Barker LF, editors: *Infection, immunity and blood transfusion,* New York, 1985, Alan R Liss.
25. *Manual of clinical laboratory immunology,* ed 4, Washington, DC, 1992, American Society of Microbiology.
26. Stites DP, Terr AI, and Parslow T, editors: *Basic and clinical immunology,* ed 8, Norwalk, CT, 1994, Appleton and Lange.

27. Huston DP editor: Diagnostic laboratory immunology, *Immunol Allergy Clin* 14:2, 1994.

28. Coligan KE, Kruisbeek AM, Margulies DH et al: *Current protocols in immunology,* New York, 1992, Greene Publishing and Wiley-Interscience.

29. Knapp W, Dorken B, Rieber P et al: CD antigens 1989, *Blood* 74:1448, 1989.

30. Bataille R, Durie BGM, and Grenier J: Serum β_2-microglobulin and survival duration in multiple myeloma: a simple reliable marker for staging, *Br J Haematol* 55:439, 1983.

31. Dimopoulos MA, Cabanillas F, Lee JJ et al: Prognostic role of β_2-microglobulin in Hodgkin's disease, *J Clin Oncol* 11:1108, 1993.

32. Hamilton RG: Human immunoglobulins, In Rose N editor: *Handbook of human immunology,* Boca Raton, FL, 1994, CRC Press.

33. Rodgers RPC: Clinical laboratory methods for detection of antigens and antibodies, In Stites DP, Terr AI, and Parslow T, editors: *Basic and clinical immunology,* ed. 8, Ch. 12, Norwalk, CT, 1994, Appleton and Lange.

34. Lloyd W and Schur PH: Immune complexes, complement and anti-DNA in exacerbations of systemic lupus erythematosus (SLE), *Medicine* 60:208, 1981.

35. Kushner I: C-reactive protein and the acute-phase response, *Hosp Pract* 25:13, 1990.

36. Norman PS: Skin testing, In *Manual of clinical laboratory immunology,* ed 4, Ch. 100, Washington, DC, 1992, American Society of Microbiology.

37. Kniker WT, Lesourd BM, McBryde JL et al: Cell-mediated immunity assessed by Multitest CMI testing in infants and preschool children, *Am J Dis Child* 139:840, 1985.

38. Pyun KH, Ochs HD, Wedgwood RJ et al: Human antibody responses to bacteriophage ΦX-174: sequential induction of IgM and IgG antibody, *Clin Immunol Immunopathol* 51:252, 1992.

Exposure Assessment Methods

PHILIP HARBER

Exposure assessment is critical for determining the risk of occupational and environmental respiratory disease, for establishment of a diagnosis in an individual patient, and for identifying sites requiring additional effort to control exposures. This section describes methods for assessing *exposures* in several settings: *workplace* ("occupational"), *community* (also commonly called "environmental"), and the *"indoor"* environment (commonly referring to home or office exposures to agents such as bioaerosols not primarily associated with heavy industry or to levels lower than those typically found in manufacturing or mining settings). Methods range from qualitative worksite walk-through visits to quantitative determination of exposure levels. In addition to these methods of direct environmental assessment, valuable indirect information can be obtained from approaches such as epidemiologic surveys or clinical interviews of workers and patients. Furthermore, biologic specimens may be analyzed chemically or mineralogically to assess past exposures. Qualitative or quantitative methods must be carefully chosen to be appropriate for the information needed.

Although this section discusses methods of determining exposures, Section XII includes discussion of exposure control methodologies.

Chapter 10

SITE VISITS

PART I

Worksite Evaluations

Elizabeth A. Jennison
Gregory J. Kullman
John E. Parker

> Preparation for the worksite evaluation
> Walk-through evaluation
> In-depth worksite evaluations
> After the worksite evaluation
> Limitations of site visits
> Summary

There are many reasons to conduct worksite evaluations. Evaluations may be part of the activities of physicians, nurses, engineers, epidemiologists, industrial hygienists, and others who conduct health and safety work for companies, unions, public health entities, or regulatory bodies. Worksite evaluations may be conducted to ensure compliance with appropriate Occupational Safety and Health Administration (OSHA) and Mine Safety and Health Administration (MSHA) standards. Evaluations may be conducted as part of the educational process for students of industrial hygiene, safety engineering, occupational health medicine, and nursing. Evaluations are sometimes done to assess the effectiveness of control technology used to reduce worker exposures. Several large U.S. research projects have used worksite evaluations as a means of collecting data about occupational exposures, including the National Occupational Hazard Survey (NOHS),[1] the National Occupational Exposure Survey (NOES),[1] and the National Occupational Health Survey of Mining (NOHSM),[2] all conducted by the U.S. National Institute for Occupational Safety and Health

(NIOSH). The investigation of specific health complaints is often a justification for workplace evaluations. This part focuses on overall assessment of worksites whereas Part II emphasizes assessment as a part of the evaluation of a specific patient with suspected occupational lung disease. In this chapter, evaluations conducted by consultants who survey worksites in response to occupational health and safety concerns are presented. These evaluations may be brief walk-through surveys or more in-depth investigations, which include environmental and medical testing.

PREPARATION FOR THE WORKSITE EVALUATION

The consultants should gather as much information as possible about the worksite before the site visit. Worksite evaluations may include combinations of review of existing records, medical testing, and environmental measurements. They may include several phases: previsit preparation, walk-through evaluation, in-depth evaluation, and follow-up. Information may be available from workers, union representatives, or management. The state or local health departments and the area offices of regulatory agencies such as OSHA, MSHA, and the U.S. Environmental Protection Agency (EPA) may be able to provide information about previous inspections and citations at the facility. There are references that describe common industrial processes and potential exposure problems.[3] A search of the NIOSHTIC database[4] may yield information as to whether NIOSH has conducted any health hazard evaluations at this or similar facilities.

The consultants should also review the literature relating to the known health effects of any materials or processes used. They should also be alert to the possibility that exposure to a known hazard is occurring in a previously unrecognized setting or that a known hazard is causing previously unrecognized adverse health effects. As an example, silicosis was described recently in a railroad maintenance-of-way worker, an occupation not recognized previously as being at risk from this well-known hazard.[5] Lack of published information about adverse health effects caused by a substance should not preclude further investigation of health concerns at the worksite. The list of known occupational hazards continues to expand. This is especially true in the study of occupational asthma, where estimates of the number of agents identified as inducing asthma has risen from around 200 in 1980[6] to over 270[7] in 1993.

Once a date has been set for the initial site visit, it is important to clarify who will be participating in the site visit. For the opening conference or meeting, in addition to the investigators, key attendees generally include the plant manager, an individual responsible for plant health and safety, and at least one worker representative familiar with the worksite. Other attendees may include plant nurses, physicians, industrial hygienists, plant engineers, as well as corporate health and safety personnel. It is important to keep the walk-through group to a manageable size; usually six to eight individuals is the maximum size that can reasonably be accommodated on a walk-through. The participation of both labor and management in all phases of the survey helps to ensure that the investigators receive a balanced perspective on all potential health and safety issues. All survey participants should adhere to plant safety and health regulations during the survey; investigators may be required to obtain and use certain types of clothing and personal protective equipment. This practice not only provides personal protection for the investigators, but emphasizes that health and safety standards apply to everyone in the workplace, from management to employees to consultants. Health or safety training may be required for entry into certain plant areas or workplaces such as coal mines.

WALK-THROUGH EVALUATION

The main objective of the walk-through evaluation is to become familiar with the workplace, its operations and processes, and the potential for occupational health and safety problems. From a medical standpoint, the purposes of the initial site visit are to determine whether there are adverse health effects that merit further study and to obtain the information necessary to direct the development of such study.

Investigators from NIOSH have considerable experience in performing worksite evaluations for respiratory disease. The general methods employed are described.

Company medical records are often a valuable source of information. Medical records are generally confidential. Consultants should not review them unless they have legal authority to do so. Logs of injury and illness reports should be reviewed; in the United States, these are recorded by companies on the OSHA 200 logs. If the investigation has been prompted by worker illness or injury, it is important to note whether these inciting events are reported on the OSHA 200 log. If they are not, this suggests possible deficiencies in company recordkeeping practices, since any injury or illness serious enough to require medical treatment, lost work days, or temporary job reassignment is recordable.[8] A review of the injuries or illnesses by specific department or job category may highlight problem areas. If

available, logs from a company nurse, physician, or first aid center will give additional information and are likely to include illnesses and injuries that were not considered to be reportable. Some companies keep records of "near miss" events. A review of these records can yield further information about breakdowns in the health and safety system.

When permitted, the consultant should attempt to review the medical records from all workers who have sought medical consultation relating to the occupational conditions under investigation. Companies may allow consulting physicians to review medical records that their employees have submitted in support of workers' compensation claims. This information can be supplemented by obtaining information directly from the workers' physicians provided that the workers have given written authorization for the release of medical information. All such information should be viewed as confidential and not be released in any manner allowing identification of individuals.

It is also important to review any surveillance data maintained by the company. OSHA standards mandate both medical and environmental surveillance for workers exposed to a number of toxic and hazardous substances including lead,[9] cotton dust,[10] asbestos,[11] and noise.[12] For testing that is not done for regulatory compliance, there may be appropriate performance standards. For example, is spirometry performed and interpreted according to American Thoracic Society criteria?[13,14]

The physician also should review what medical screening data are being collected and why. Historically, there has been poor correlation between the potential hazards observed in a workplace and the screening that workers received; for example, 28% of workers exposed to dust had chest radiographs as compared with 25% overall in industry.[15] Many companies collect screening data that have been shown to have little effect on predicting or preventing an adverse outcome. For example, companies may require lumbar spine films for workers who will be involved in heavy lifting, even though these have been shown to be a poor predictor of back injury.[16] Likewise, routine chest radiographs performed as screening for lung cancer have little value,[17] although such studies are required for workers exposed to asbestos.[17] The occupational physician may be able to work with the company's occupational health and safety personnel to design a medical screening and surveillance system that will appropriately serve both the workers and the company.

The company's hazard communication program is another source of information available to investigators. To comply with U.S. federal regulations, companies are required to develop a written program to inform workers of occupational safety and health problems at the worksite.[18] This program can be a resource to investigators by identifying recognized exposure hazards in the workplace. Compliance with this program requires the development of an inventory of hazardous materials at the worksite; material safety data sheets (MSDS) must be maintained for each material. The MSDS provide a description of the chemical nature of the material, as well as the recognized health and safety hazards associated with product use.

Many companies have written programs describing the use of personal protective equipment (PPE). This may include respiratory protection, hearing protection, eye protection, a work clothes program, and others. Some of these programs are required by federal law such as the use of PPE to control worker exposures to respiratory hazards during asbestos removal.[11] Respirators must be used only as a part of a formal respiratory protection program with written provisions for worker training, respirator selection, fit testing, and maintenance.[19,20] These programs can provide additional information on potential exposure hazards and control practices in the workplace.

Although the review of company programs and policies is important, inspection of the workplace and plant processes is the purpose of the walk-through survey. This usually is best accomplished by following the process from the entry of raw materials into the plant until the point where the finished product leaves the facility. Although this may require several moves between different areas or levels of the plant, it allows investigators who are unfamiliar with the process to visualize the flow of materials through the plant. The company may have process flow charts that can help the investigator during the course of the walk-through. The investigator may find it helpful to carry a small tape recorder, a camera, or video device to record information during the course of the walk-through.

On the initial site visit, it is useful to talk with employees about any work-related health problems they may have experienced. These interviews should be brief and informal and, above all, confidential. Initial questions should be open-ended, rather than directed at specific symptoms or complaints. For example, a good starting point might be to ask, "Do you have any health problems that you feel are related to your work?" A positive response can be followed up with more specific questions about the nature, duration, timing, and frequency of symptoms, as well as their association with work activities. Some assessment of symptom severity is useful, such as asking whether the individual has ever had to seek first aid or medical attention or has ever had to leave work early because of symptoms.

A useful strategy for interviews is to begin with several workers selected at random from each work area. Although the initial interviewees may not report any work-related symptoms, they may be aware of other workers who are symptomatic. The symptomatic workers are interviewed next. These symptomatic workers frequently know of other symptomatic workers who may be willing to be interviewed. Since employees may have fears about being identified as a complainer, it is prudent to intersperse these interviews of specific individuals with random interviews. It is also helpful to ask workers whether they know of any individuals who left employment with this company for health-related reasons.

The review of plant operations provides the opportunity to observe work activities by job category and department along with the potential for exposure. Observation of work activities may help identify workers at increased risk for exposure and, potentially, health problems. It may be important to review plant operations during different shifts to determine if significant shift differences exist. Conversations with union representatives, management, and other workers can help determine if the plant operations observed during the survey are typical. It is important to observe whether PPE is being used in an appropriate manner and as described in company programs. There may be discrepancies between the written programs and the actual workplace practices that will help the investigator to identify potential problem areas. Eating and smoking within production areas may increase exposures; the occurrence of these activities should be noted during the walk-through. The plant tour also provides a chance to observe the types of engineering controls used for different plant processes. Engineering blueprints may be available to describe system layout and design specifications.

The walk-through survey may provide the opportunity for some limited environmental monitoring to help identify potential workplace contaminants, worker exposure, and potential sources or exposure areas in the plant. This type of monitoring is generally best suited to direct reading sampling equipment. Smoke tubes are a convenient means of observing airflow patterns related to plant operations or ventilation systems; velocity meters can be used to obtain more exact information on plant ventilation.[21] Short-term indicator tubes provide a means to rapidly assess concentration of a number of gases and vapors in the workplace.[22] Other types of direct reading sampling meters are available to assess airborne chemical contaminants such as carbon monoxide, oxides of nitrogen, acid gases, and combustible hydrocarbons.[22] For example, NIOSH investigators used a photoionization meter during a walk-through investigation of health complaints related to gasoline odors in an office building; the use of direct reading sampling equipment during the preliminary survey helped to identify the sources of contaminant entry and to direct subsequent sampling during a more in-depth survey.[23] There are also direct reading samplers that can measure concentrations of airborne particulates. The number of direct reading sampling instruments applicable for use during walk-through surveys continues to expand.[22]

The investigators should consider the possibility that two or more adverse health effects exist concurrently; NIOSH investigations have documented concurrent health hazards caused by lead, noise, and hydrogen chloride in a company that produces lead-lined metal tanks,[24] and hazards caused by respirable silica, noise, and products of diesel combustion in an underground metal mine.[25] There may be more than one route of exposure to a given toxin; workers can be exposed to lead through inhalation or ingestion[26] or to organic solvents via inhalation and skin absorption.[27] In one work setting, the lungs may be both a target organ and a route of exposure for systemic toxicity, as in sandblasters who are at risk for both silicosis and lead poisoning if they use silica sand for the abrasive blasting of lead-based paints.

IN-DEPTH WORKSITE EVALUATIONS

The decision to pursue an in-depth survey, whether medical, environmental, or both, should be based on the findings of the walk-through evaluation. If industrial hygiene data demonstrate significant exposures or the potential for overexposure, it may be worthwhile to pursue a systematic study looking for known effects of the agents in question, even if the initial site visit does not confirm adverse health effects. This is particularly true for exposures to agents whose health effects include long periods with asymptomatic changes and conditions that may benefit from early detection.[28] If the initial survey indicates that a potential health hazard exists for which control methods are well described, it may be appropriate to make recommendations without further study. Compliance with existing governmental regulations should be recommended. When the OSHA or MSHA standards for the agents involved are not totally protective (for example, for isocyanates) or there are no established standards, employers may be reluctant to follow recommendations, especially if the workplace is in compliance with the appropriate standards. In these circumstances it is often important to demonstrate the presence of an adverse health effect and its relationship to the workplace before making recommendations. As an example, NIOSH investigations have demonstrated IgE-mediated occupational asthma associated with exposure to egg proteins, for which there are no applicable exposure recommendations or standards.[27]

Once the decision has been made to proceed with an in-depth medical survey, the investigating physician should enlist the assistance of other scientific and support personnel as necessary. This may include technicians to perform and process medical tests and occupational epidemiologists and statisticians to assist in the design and analysis of study questionnaires. Individuals with special expertise may be called on as needed; for example, veterinarians may be of assistance in identifying and implementing control measures for infectious agents of animal origin, such as Q-fever[29] or brucellosis.[30]

It may be appropriate to involve appropriate officials from local or state health departments, especially if the investigation involves an infectious agent such as tuberculosis. Most states require the reporting of at least a few occupational conditions[31]; occupational physicians should familiarize themselves with the reporting requirements for their region and report conditions to the appropriate agencies. In many cases, these data are reported without individual identifiers.

In addition to the investigating physician, medical participants in the investigation may include company occu-

pational health nurses and physicians, as well as company occupational health and safety personnel. The level of interaction between the investigating physician and company medical personnel is dictated by the nature of the investigation. If the investigating physician is a consultant to company medical personnel, the investigation may be a true collaboration. If the investigating physician is acting on behalf of a union or other entity, the nature of his or her interaction with company medical personnel will vary accordingly. In this situation the investigating physician should act independently from company medical personnel. Company medical personnel should not be present during employee interviews or examinations, and individual employee records may not be released to the company medical departments unless the employee has signed an appropriate medical release. Of course, company medical personnel should receive a full summary report of the investigating physicians' findings. The investigator should be sure that the information contained in the final report is insufficient to allow specific test or survey results to be attributed to individual workers.

The physician should choose appropriate screening tests based on the expected adverse health effects associated with a given occupational exposure. For example, isocyanates frequently induce late asthmatic reactions, which occur after the individual has left the worksite. Thus isocyanate asthma may be identified by serial peak flow monitoring in addition to cross-shift spirometry.[6] The physician should also be alert for minor symptoms that may be experienced by many individuals and that may be a marker for exposures that could cause more serious disease in a few individuals. For example, a recent study found that immediate onset symptoms of rhinitis and eye irritation related to organic dusts were common among a Scandinavian farming population, with a prevalence of 40% to 50%; asthma, a much more serious consequence of organic dust exposure, had a prevalence of 2% to 3% among a similar population.[32]

If feasible, all current employees should be invited to participate in the medical survey. If the size of the workplace precludes this, it may be necessary to use some form of representative sampling or preliminary screening to limit the size of the study population. One technique is to use a brief questionnaire to identify symptomatic individuals and to conduct further evaluations on all symptomatic and some subset of the asymptomatic workers. The study population should include workers on all shifts since there tends to be a strong association between shift and job tenure. This may require the medical survey to span several shifts over the better part of a week, especially if testing requires cross-shift or cross-week evaluations. Participation is generally highest if the company will allow testing to occur during an employee's normal working hours or will pay overtime wages for preshift or postshift testing. It may be necessary to schedule a variety of night and weekend hours to accommodate all workers.

All study participants should give informed consent before participating in any formal medical interviews or testing. The consent forms should identify the nature, purpose, and risks of the tests involved, describe the confidentiality policy of the investigators, and provide the name and telephone number of the individual responsible for conducting the study. A signed copy of the consent form should be retained in the investigator's files. Participants should receive a copy of this form to retain for their own reference.

All individuals who undergo medical testing as part of a workplace evaluation should receive the results of their personal medical tests in a timely and confidential fashion. This is often in the form of a letter sent to the employee's home address. The report should contain a brief description of the tests performed, the individual's results, and an explanation of the significance of the results. To the extent possible, this should be written in language that the worker will be able to understand. A telephone number should be provided so that individuals who have questions about their test results can contact the examiner. Individuals should be able to obtain copies of their test results or radiographs or have these sent to their physician.

If there is concern that workers may have left the work environment for health reasons, whether voluntarily or involuntarily, additional information may be obtained by contacting previous employees. The company may be willing to supply names and addresses of former employees, but information on individuals not receiving benefits may be inaccurate. This information may also be obtained from union locals or from current employees. Newspaper advertisements may be useful, especially if one is trying to reach individuals who have been away from the company for a number of years. Even if former employees are to be interviewed by telephone, it is desirable that they first receive a letter describing the study and telling them to expect a telephone call. Individuals who receive their first contact by telephone may be unwilling to participate in the study since they have no basis for assuming that the caller is conducting a legitimate investigation.

The in-depth medical survey is frequently complemented by a thorough environmental assessment; the nature of the survey and the occupational health issues involved will determine the scope of this assessment. As with the medical component, the development of an in-depth environmental evaluation of the worksite is based on information collected during the walk-through survey. In-depth environmental surveys, like their medical counterparts, are typically larger and require more detailed planning and increased resources than do walk-through surveys. Presurvey planning and preparation are important to success and should include the development of an environmental survey protocol.

In planning the in-depth survey, consideration should be given to the selection of environmental analyses as well as the sampling and analytical methods that will be used.[33] Some sampling or analytical methods may be inappropri-

ate in certain work environments; for instance, sampling equipment that is not explosionproof should not be operated in areas with the potential for fire and explosions. A sampling plan of the plant areas or processes to be included in the survey should be developed to ensure that the survey results are representative. The methods of sampling are also an important consideration. Personal sampling is generally regarded as the most appropriate means of measuring worker exposure. Area sampling may be more appropriate in some instances, such as to identify point sources or to assess specific operations or controls. The sampling period or interval is another consideration in planning the in-depth survey. Short-term or "grab" samples may be appropriate to measure certain analytes, for instance, those with ceiling or short-term exposure limits (STELs). Time-weighted average (TWA) measures may be the more appropriate measure for other analytes or operations where exposure is incurred over a longer interval or where existing standards reference TWAs. The opportunity to collect real time exposure monitoring data now exists for many analytes, providing the opportunity to obtain both instantaneous and TWA exposure results. The survey plan should address the potential for exposure differences caused by the work shift and season. Detailed information about sampling methods is provided in Chapter 11.

Although it is difficult to conduct in-depth medical surveys without advance scheduling, in some circumstances it may be desirable to conduct environmental sampling without giving the company advance notice. Advance notice may provide an opportunity for temporary hazard amelioration resulting in atypical plant conditions and worker exposures during the survey. The environmental assessment should be carefully integrated with other survey components (e.g., medical or epidemiologic) to ensure that the overall survey objectives are met. This would include a careful coordination of sampling periods and survey participants when medical outcomes are evaluated relative to employee exposure.

The decision to embark on an in-depth evaluation of a worksite should not be made lightly. Both medical and environmental evaluations involve commitments of personnel, financial resources, and time, which may be beyond the capacities of a single investigator or a small consulting firm. A number of resources in the United States, including state and federal OSHA consulting services, are available to provide assistance and information to investigators. Information about these resources is contained in Appendix A.

AFTER THE WORKSITE EVALUATION

A well-written and thoughtful report completes the workplace investigation. This generally starts with a description of why the investigation was performed, followed by a description of the process and materials involved. If the report is to be distributed to individuals outside the company or prepared for publication, trade secret information should be protected by discussing production processes in general terms and only to the extent necessary. Methodology for both the industrial hygiene and medical components is described, including a description of the pertinent equipment and procedures. Company records or programs that were reviewed, such as the Hazard Communication Program, OSHA 200 logs and medical surveillance data, should be described and discussed. The report should include a brief review of the known toxicities of the materials or processes involved and evaluation criteria (pertinent OSHA standards, NIOSH, and ACGIH criteria). A section on medical results would include summary information from worker interviews or questionnaires and medical testing. The environmental results section should provide sampling data from environmental monitoring referenced to appropriate concentration or exposure units. The occupational standards and exposure guidelines should be presented to permit interpretation of the sampling results. The conclusions and recommendations complete the body of the report and are followed by appropriate figures, tables, appendixes, and references. The report should be distributed to both company and worker representatives.

The investigators may play a role in the continuing health and safety of the workplace that extends beyond the scope of this single investigation. For example, the physician may help the company design an ongoing medical surveillance system. Such a system should be based on an assessment of hazards encountered by the employees, the potential end-organ toxicities associated with these exposures, and the selection of appropriate screening tests to look for these end-organ effects.[27] A priori decisions should determine what constitutes an abnormal test result and what actions are appropriate for each level of abnormality. The industrial hygienist could provide assistance in selecting appropriate control technology, identifying qualified contractors for the installation of the control technology, or for follow-up evaluations to measure the effectiveness of the controls.

LIMITATIONS OF SITE VISITS

The majority of workplace studies conducted by consultants will be cross-sectional studies. Although relatively easy to conduct, these studies have two main limitations. First, cross-sectional studies cannot determine whether the exposure preceded the disease or whether any association between the two is spurious. This is of less importance if the industry being studied is one in which there is little or no job mobility and in which current exposures are reasonable surrogates for past exposure. The second limitation of cross-sectional studies is that they measure disease prevalence rather than incidence. Since prevalence is a factor of disease incidence and duration, cross-sectional studies are best suited for studying diseases of long duration but of low enough severity that affected individuals remain in the workplace. Cross-sectional studies are also useful for studying acute effects, especially those that are self-limited and nondisabling. Other study designs such as cohort studies and case-control studies may be more appropriate for investigating certain conditions. The reader is referred to Chapter 2 and to standard texts of occupational epidemiology for further information about these study designs.[34]

Proper attention to study design can reduce, but not completely resolve, sources of bias that may affect study results. Evaluating prior employees can reduce the selection bias associated with testing only the "survivor population" of individuals who can tolerate workplace exposures. Enlisting the cooperation of both management and employees can maximize the participation of current employees. This can reduce the selection bias associated with studying a volunteer cohort, but it can never overcome the statistical power limitations imposed by a small workforce. This may limit the ability of the study to detect a difference between exposed and unexposed individuals, even if such a difference exists.

The investigator should take care not to allow his or her own knowledge of the exposures to bias the interpretation of test or questionnaire results toward detecting adverse health effects. As an example, radiographs being read for the presence of pneumoconiosis should be reviewed without knowledge of the individual's exposure status. If the investigator cannot review test results in a blinded fashion, these results should be reviewed by an independent reader.

SUMMARY

The worksite evaluation is an important tool in the collection of data to evaluate occupational health problems. The occupational medicine literature contains many references to the role of the "astute clinician" in establishing disease–toxin connections in the workplace.[35] A well-planned and executed worksite evaluation can provide considerable intellectual satisfaction to the investigator while contributing to the occupational health and safety of the affected workforce.

REFERENCES

1. Sundin DS and Frazier TM: Hazard surveillance at NIOSH, *Am J Public Health* 79(suppl.):32-37, 1989.
2. CDC (Centers for Disease Control and Prevention): The national occupational health survey of mining, *MMWR* 35(2 SS):17ss-22ss, 1986.
3. Burgess WA: *Recognition of health hazards in industry.* New York, 1981, John Wiley.
4. NIOSH: *NIOSHTIC database,* Cincinnati, OH, 1994, U.S. Department of Health and Human Services, Public Health Service, Centers for Disease Control and Prevention, National Institute for Occupational Safety and Health, Division of Standards Development and Technology Transfer, Technical Information Branch.
5. NIOSH: *Hazard evaluation and technical assistance report: Norfolk Southern Railway Company,* Cincinnati, OH, 1993, U.S. Department of Health and Human Services, Public Health Service, Centers for Disease Control and Prevention, National Institute for Occupational Safety and Health, NIOSH Report No HHE 90-341-228.
6. Newman Taylor AJ: Occupational asthma (editorial), *Thorax* 35:241-245, 1980.

7. Chan-Yeung M and Malo JL: Table of the major inducers of occupational asthma. In Bernstein IL, Chang-Yeung M, Malo JL, and Bernstein DI, editors: *Asthma in the workplace,* pp 595-623, New York, 1993, Marcel Dekker.

8. CFR: *Code of Federal Regulations,* Washington, DC, U.S. Government Printing Office, Office of the Federal Register. 29 CFR Part 1904—Recording and reporting occupational injuries and illnesses.

9. CFR: *Code of Federal Regulations,* Washington, DC, U.S. Government Printing Office, Office of the Federal Register. 1910.1025, lead.

10. CFR: *Code of Federal Regulations,* Washington, DC, U.S. Government Printing Office, Office of the Federal Register. 29 CFR 1910.1043, cotton dust.

11. CFR: *Code of Federal Regulations,* Washington, DC, U.S. Government Printing Office, Office of the Federal Register. 29 CFR 1910.1101, asbestos.

12. CFR: *Code of Federal Regulations,* Washington, DC, U.S. Government Printing Office, Office of the Federal Register. 1910.95, occupational noise exposure.

13. American Thoracic Society: Standardization of spirometry—1987 update, *Am Rev Respir Dis* 136:1285-1298, 1987.

14. American Thoracic Society official statement: Lung function testing: selection of reference values and interpretative strategies, *Am Rev Respir Dis* 144.1202-1218, 1991.

15. Halperin WE and Frazier TM: Surveillance for the effects of workplace exposure, *Annu Rev Public Health* 6:419-432, 1985.

16. U.S. Preventive Services Task Force: *Guide to clinical preventive services: an assessment of the effectiveness of 169 interventions,* pp 67-70, 245-249, Report of the U.S. Preventive Services Task Force, Baltimore, MD, 1989, Williams & Wilkins.

17. Cone JE and Rosenberg J: Medical surveillance and biomonitoring for occupational cancer endpoints. In Rempel D, editor: *Occupational medicine: state of the art reviews,* vol 5, no. 3—*Medical surveillance in the workplace,* pp 563-582, Philadelphia, 1990, Hanley & Belfus.

18. CFR: *Code of Federal Regulations,* Washington, DC, U.S. Government Printing Office, Office of the Federal Register. 1910.1200, hazard communication.

19. CFR: *Code of Federal Regulations,* Washington, DC, U.S. Government Printing Office, Office of the Federal Register. 1910.134, respiratory protection.

20. NIOSH: *NIOSH recommendations for occupational safety and health,* Cincinnati, OH, 1992, U.S. Department of Health and Human Services, Public Health Service, Centers for Disease Control, National Institute for Occupational Safety and Health, DHHS (NIOSH) Pub No 92-100.

21. ACGIH: *Industrial ventilation,* ed 20, Cincinnati, OH, 1988, American Conference of Governmental Industrial Hygienists.

22. ACGIH: *Air sampling instruments for evaluation of atmospheric contaminants,* ed 7, Cincinnati, OH, 1989, American Conference of Governmental Industrial Hygienists.

23. Kullman GJ and Hill RA: Indoor air quality affected by abandoned gasoline tanks, *Appl Occup Environ Hyg* 5(1):36-37, 1990.

24. NIOSH: *Hazard evaluation and technical assistance report: New England Lead Burning Co. (NELCO), Eaton Metals, Salt Lake City, Utah,* Cincinnati, OH, 1991, U.S. Department of Health and Human Services, Public Health Service, Centers for Disease Control and Prevention, National Institute for Occupational Safety and Health, NIOSH Report No 91-290-2131.

25. NIOSH: *Hazard evaluation and technical assistance report: ASARCO—Troy Unit Mine, Troy, MT,* Cincinnati, OH, 1992, U.S. Department of Health and Human Services, Public Health Service, Centers for Disease Control and Prevention, National Institute for Occupational Safety and Health, NIOSH Report No HHE 88-104-2207.

26. NIOSH: *Hazard evaluation and technical assistance report: Seaway Painting, Inc., Annapolis, MD,* Cincinnati, OH, 1991, U.S. Department of Health and Human Services, Public Health Service, Centers for Disease Control and Prevention, National Institute for Occupational Safety and Health, NIOSH Report No HHE 91-209-2249.

27. NIOSH: *Hazard evaluation and technical assistance report: Estherville Foods, Inc., Estherville, Iowa,* Cincinnati, OH, 1988, U.S. Department of Health and Human Services, Public Health Service, Centers for Disease Control, National Institute for Occupational Safety and Health, NIOSH Report No HETA 86-447-1919.

28. Matte TD, Fine L, Meinhardt TJ, and Baker EL: Guidelines for medical screen in the workplace. In Rempel D, editor: *Occupational medicine: state of the art reviews—vol 5, no 3, Medical surveillance in the workplace,* pp 439-456, Philadelphia, 1990, Hanley & Belfus.

29. NIOSH: *Hazard evaluation and technical assistance report: M-I Drilling Fluids, Greybull, WY,* Cincinnati, OH, 1993, U.S. Department of Health and Human Services, Public Health Service, Centers for Disease Control and Prevention, National Institute for Occupational Safety and Health, NIOSH Report No HETA 92-361.

30. CDC (Centers for Disease Control and Prevention): Brucellosis outbreak at a pork processing plant—North Carolina, 1992, *MMWR* 43(7):113-116, 1994.

31. Freund E, Seligman PJ, Chorba TL, Safford SK, Drachman JG, and Hull HF: Mandatory reporting of occupational diseases by clinicians, *JAMA* 262(21):3041-3044, 1989.

32. Malmberg P: Health effects of organic dust exposure in dairy farmers, *Am J Ind Med* 17:7-15, 1990.

33. NIOSH: *Occupational exposure sampling strategy manual,* Cincinnati, OH, 1977, U.S. Department of Health, Education, and Welfare, Public Health Service, Centers for Disease Control, National Institute for Occupational Safety and Health, DHEW (NIOSH) Pub No 77-173.

34. Checkoway H, Pearce N, and Crawford-Brown DJ: *Research methods in occupational epidemiology,* New York, 1989, Oxford University Press.

35. Fleming LE, Ducatman AM, and Shalat SL: Disease clusters: a central and ongoing role in occupational health, *J Occup Med* 33(7):818-825, 1989.

Part **II**

The Worksite Evaluation for Patients

Patricia Quinlan
Philip Harber

The worksite visit
Adequacy of controls
Postsite visit

A worksite evaluation is occasionally required in conjunction with the medical evaluation of a specific single patient. Such a single patient-oriented evaluation can provide very useful information to clinicians for determining the work relatedness of a patient's symptoms. This may help with the differential diagnosis or may be related to the determina-

---

Steps in worksite visit for evaluation of patients

Previsit

Review industry and processes
Interview patient
Define scope and purpose of visit

Visit

Meet plant personnel
Walk through entire plant
Detailed review of patient's work area
Air monitoring

Evaluate adequacy of controls

Engineering (enclosure, process isolation, ventilation)
Administrative
Personal protective equipment

Postvisit

Review results with patient
Report (as appropriate) to employer, health authorities
Prepare recommendations and report

Physical state of agents

Dust: A suspension of solid particles in air

Mist: A suspension of liquid droplets in air

Gas: A gas phase contaminant

Vapor: A gas phase contaminant that is primarily liquid at room temperature

Fume: A solid suspension resulting from condensation of products of combustion

Fiber: A solid particle whose length:diameter ratio is high (typically 10:1, although certain regulations employ a 3:1 ratio for definition)

Aerosol: A suspension of particles in air

---

tion of compensability for workers' compensation purposes (see Chapter 53). In addition, a worksite visit may be needed to determine whether a worker with respiratory disease can safely work and whether special accommodations for the individual worker need to be implemented so that he or she may be able to work (see Chapter 52). University-based occupational health clinics often incorporate worksite visits as a didactic tool in conjunction with clinic-based teaching. Finally, a worksite visit may be used to observe the patient and other workers at their tasks, to determine the hazards to which the patient and others may be exposed, to ascertain if any monitoring has been or should be conducted, and to determine the effectiveness, or lack thereof, of any controls in place. This may suggest that there are other workers at risk.

Before conducting the worksite evaluation, the industrial hygienist and health practitioners often familiarize themselves with the industry and processes to be surveyed. Company brochures may have descriptions of the industry, the processes, and the products or services produced. Useful information may also be obtained from reference books describing various work processes and common health and safety hazards associated with the industry in question.[1-3] The patient is often the best source of information. For example, he or she may describe specific tasks performed as a molder for a local nonferrous foundry, making aluminum, brass, and bronze castings for various industries. The practitioner can then research the industry in various textbooks, such as Burgess's *Recognition of Health Hazards in Industry,* to obtain a description of the foundry industry, the terminology used (e.g., coremaking, molding, shakeout, and

finishing), a discussion of the various elements in the alloys (e.g., copper, zinc, and lead in brass and bronze alloys), and potential exposures one may find in this industry (heavy metals, silica, phenolic binders, etc.).[4]

Patients should be asked about chemicals used by both themselves and other workers. Reference books or computer databases, such as Medline, Toxline, or Toxnet, contain information on the toxic effects of these chemicals.[5-7] The NIOSH-Tic database is available on CD-ROM.[8] In addition to published articles, this database also contains the results of NIOSH Health Hazard Evaluations (HHEs) of various industries and may provide valuable information on health effects associated with particular exposures.

If the patient knows only the brand name of the products, the practitioners may request that the patient ask his or her employer for the material safety data sheets (MSDS) for the product(s) that are of concern. Although not always complete, the MSDS are required in the United States to list the hazardous ingredients (if >1% or >0.1% for carcinogens), the acute and chronic health effects, information regarding reactivity, explosiveness, and fire precautions, disposal information, and information regarding the use of personal protective equipment and proper ventilation. More information regarding the product may be obtained by the practitioners from the regional Poison Control Center or directly from the manufacturer's toxicologist. The practitioner may find when contacting the manufacturer that the actual ingredients that are causing the patient's symptoms may not have been listed on the MSDS because they either constituted less than 1% of the product or the information on the chemicals was not disclosed because of trade secrets. Before visiting the worksite, the patient should be interviewed in detail. In addition, the purpose and scope of the worksite visit should be defined in advance. The physical state, as well as the chemical identity, should be ascertained. The accompanying box describes these common terms.

THE WORKSITE VISIT

The worksite visit usually begins with a meeting with plant personnel. Information collected may include the results of past medical and environmental monitoring, a review of MSDS, a review of the Occupational Safety and Health Administration (OSHA) 200 log for previous years, job descriptions for the employee, results of previous OSHA investigations, medical reports from other physicians, and any other useful information.

For manufacturing operations, the industrial hygienist attempts to follow the production process, from raw ma-terials to finished products. The worksite survey will start at the loading dock, looking at warning labels and packaging of the raw materials, and then follow all the materials through the production process, noting all the chemicals in use in each area. Special emphasis is given to the area in which the patient works. However, it is advisable to review the entire work process since exposures generated elsewhere in the plant may affect the patient. Areas through which the patient walks should be reviewed. In addition to regular operations, potential exposures to the patient during shutdown or maintenance periods should be assessed. Each process should be observed while in action to determine how the employees are handling the products. It is important to note what intermediate products and by products are formed, as these may be the source of the health complaints. For example, on a site visit to a pesticide manufacturing plant, an industrial hygienist determined, based on where the individual worked on the line, that the source of his problem was a by-product produced during manufacture of the pesticide and not a reaction to the fairly inert final product. Incompatible operations in close proximity to each other should be noted. For instance, arc welding operations placed too close to a vapor degreaser containing chlorinated hydrocarbon solvents that are not properly vented may allow formation of phosgene gas.

The worksite visitors should also look at areas such as the office areas of manufacturing operations, break rooms, eating areas, bathrooms, and change rooms. Hazardous materials storage and disposal areas are also inspected for potential leaks and offgassing of hazardous materials. Maintenance operations are also inspected as there may be a greater potential during these operations than during normal operation. For example, at an auto assembly plant, it was determined that the maintenance operators cleaning the paint spray booths had the potential for much greater exposure to the solvents from the paints than spray painters.

Housekeeping practices are also noted, as these may also produce hazardous exposures. To the extent possible, the specific patient should be assessed, since interpersonal differences in work habits exist. For example, dry sweeping of silica containing clay in a ceramics studio of a local art school generated a significant exposure to the silica. Hydroblasting or steamcleaning may also generate contaminants.

Industrial hygienists may measure exposures with monitoring devices such as detector tubes and pumps or other direct reading instruments. Such short-term testing may be supplemented with follow-up testing for a longer period of time. Exposures may vary dramatically over the course of a day, week, or month. Therefore, it is important for the industrial hygienist to know when obtaining measurements on a site visit, or evaluating measurements taken before the visit, what the actual operating conditions are (were) on the day of sampling. It is important to determine if the workload and potential exposure are (were) lighter than normal, heavier than normal, or average. Often the greatest potential exposure of concern occurs on the swing or night shift. Monitoring during the day shift may not adequately represent the exposure of a patient who is on the other shift.

The monitoring results are compared with relevant standards, such as ACGIH threshold limit values (TLVs) or OSHA permissible exposure limits (PELs).[9,10] Often the results indicate that the levels for suspect contaminants are within the legally allowable limits. However, unusually susceptible patients may develop symptoms at these levels.

ADEQUACY OF CONTROLS

The worksite visit should also evaluate the effectiveness of methods taken to control exposure to hazards. These include engineering controls, such as enclosure of materials, isolation of processes, or ventilation; administrative controls, such as rotation of workers; and personal protective equipment, such as respirators and protective clothing. The adequacy of these measures for specific patients should be evaluated. Relatively simple methods may provide an approximate indication of the adequacy of these controls.

Local exhaust ventilation systems, such as lab fume hoods or portable exhaust ventilation for welding operations, can be evaluated with smoke tubes. Observing the direction of the smoke and how fast it is exhausted will give an indication of the effectiveness, or lack thereof, of the system. The site visitor may examine the exhaust system, checking for holes or improper modification to the ductwork, the positioning of the exhaust ducts, the frequency of filter changes, and the presence or absence of dusts on the surfaces near the exhaust system. On one site visit to a jewelry studio, an industrial hygienist noted the satin buffing wheel was not properly exhausted. There was an abundance of visible dust within the small enclosure for the machine and the filters were quite dirty. Moreover, the air was being recirculated through the filters and back into the room, rather than to the outside. Correcting this problem led to a substantial reduction in the dust generated during this operation.

For general dilution ventilation systems, such as heating, ventilating, and air-conditioning (HVAC) systems in buildings, additional parameters must be checked. It should be determined where the intake and exhaust are for the system, whether there is possible entrainment of contaminants from outside sources, and whether the system is adequate for the number of occupants and activities in the building, and the frequency of maintenance of the system should be evaluated.

Finally, personal protective equipment should be evaluated while in use. The industrial hygienist should review the appropriateness of the equipment selected for the specific hazards. For worksites requiring the use of respirators, the entire respiratory protection program for the patient should be assessed. Documentation of the training, medical clearance, and fit testing of the worker should be examined, as should the procedures for selection, cleaning, storage, and maintenance of the respirators. Frequently, visits to workplaces reveal that the workers are wearing improper cartridges for the particular hazard of concern, the respirators are being worn improperly, or the respirators are stored in the open, allowing dirt and vapors to accumulate on them.

Conversation with the workers will reveal that they do not like to wear them because they are uncomfortable and they find it difficult to communicate with their co-workers. For example, during a visit to an autobody shop, a spray painter stated he was wearing his organic vapor cartridge respirator (which was not sufficient to protect him from the isocyanates in the polyurethane paints) because it was more comfortable than the recommended air-supplied respirator that the owner had purchased. The air supplied by the compressor was very hot and uncomfortable for the worker. The owner was advised to purchase an inexpensive device that would cool the air supply and make the equipment more acceptable to the workers to wear.

POSTSITE VISIT

After completion of the site visit, the information should be reviewed with the patient. This can ensure that the relevant chemicals, processes, and areas were assessed. In addition, the patient and his or her physicians can benefit from the information.

Based on the visit, recommendations can be made about the likely work relatedness of the patient's illness, methods to decrease the exposure to the patient, and measures to control exposures to co-workers.

Increasingly, there is close association between clinicians and industrial hygienists in evaluating individual patients and using clinically detected index cases to facilitate more general preventive actions.[11]

REFERENCES

1. International Labor Organization: *Encyclopedia of occupational health and safety,* vol 1 and 2, 3rd rev ed, Geneva, 1983, ILO.
2. Cralley L and Cralley Lewis: *Industrial hygiene aspects of plant operations,* vol 1-3, New York, 1982, Macmillan.
3. Grayson Martin, editor: *Kirk-Othmer concise encyclopedia of chemical technology,* New York, 1985, Wiley Interscience.
4. Burgess William A: *Recognition of health hazards in industry,* New York, 1981, Wiley Interscience.
5. Lewis Richard J: *Sax's dangerous properties of industrial materials,* ed 8, vol 1-3, New York, 1992, Van Nostrand Reinhold.
6. Hathaway G, Proctor N, Hughes J, and Fischman M: *Chemical hazards of the workplace,* New York, 1991, Van Nostrand Reinhold.
7. National Library of Medicine: Medline, Toxline, Toxnet, 8600 Rockville Pike, Bethesda, MD 20894, (301)496-1131.
8. CCOHS, NIOSH Tic on CCInfoDisc, 250 Main Street East, Hamilton, Ontario, L8N 1H6, 1-800-668-4284.
9. ACGIH: *Threshold limit values for chemical substances and physical agents,* 6500 Glenway Ave., Cincinnati, OH, 1994, American Conference of Governmental Industrial Hygienists.
10. CFR: *Code of Federal Regulations,* Washington, DC, US Government Printing Office, Office of the Federal Register. 29 CFR Part 1910.1000 to end.
11. Harber P, Levin M, Lew Weinberg J, and Oversier J: The industrial hygienist as a clinical consultant, *Am J Ind Med* 26:339-347, 1994.

Chapter 11

ENVIRONMENTAL MONITORING

PART I

Workplace

Noah S. Seixas

Occupational and environmental health practice is unique among specialties of medicine or public health largely as a result of the major role played by exposure assessment. In the context of a diagnostic evaluation, or as part of a large epidemiologic study, exposure assessment is an integral part of understanding the health effects and designing an appropriate preventive response. Exposure assessment and health evaluation need to be seen as two pieces of a whole; information about exposure is required to fully evaluate the health endpoints, and information about health effects is required to design an appropriate exposure assessment study. Part I of this chapter explores methods used for exposure assessment for occupational and environmental respiratory disease studies and attempts to maintain the link between the methods used and the outcome being considered. General principles are emphasized. Parts II and III discuss ways in which sampling of bioaerosols and nonoccupational exposures have unique aspects.

Although many of the concepts and methods discussed in this chapter are relevant to any occupational or environmental hazard, assessment of airborne gases, vapors, or particulates that may be *inhaled* are the focus. Other exposure assessment methods such as dermal exposure evaluation and biological monitoring for absorbed materials are not considered. For information on biological monitoring, the reader is directed to Chapter 51 on surveillance, and for dermal exposure assessment to Fenske.[1] Chapter 10 focuses upon the worksite walk-through survey as a tool for exposure assessment.

EXPOSURE AND DOSE

Whether for an individual case evaluation or a large-scale epidemiologic study, the underlying goal of exposure assessment is to define and quantify an individual's (or group's) *dose* of a specific agent. Dose may be defined as *the total amount of a toxicologically relevant material reaching the target site over a specific time period.*[2,3] Thus, dose includes four dimensions: the qualitative *identity* of the agent (toxicologically relevant material), the quantity or *concentration* of the substance (total amount), the *form* of the agent (reaching the target site), and the *time course* of the agent's presence (over a specific time period).

Because dose relates to a specific target site (generally an internal organ) and is defined over time, direct measurement of dose is generally impossible. As a result, surrogate measures of dose are substituted. In particular, exposure (meaning the presence of a substance in the immediate external environment of the individual) is substituted for dose and must therefore be defined along the same four dimensions of *identity, concentration, form,* and *time.* Each one of these dimensions needs to be considered when developing an exposure assessment methodology. To the degree that these four aspects can be defined and measured well, exposure substitutes well for dose.

However, since there are inevitably errors introduced both in the definition of the relevant parameters of exposure and in their actual measurement, exposure always contains some degree of error. The *accuracy* of exposure assessments includes both *bias* and *precision.*[4] (Note that the word accuracy is used here to include both aspects of error, which differs from its use in certain fields to represent only bias.) *Bias* is a systematic error in which the measured value is higher or lower on average than the true value. A biased assessment of exposure can lead the evaluator toward either a false sense of security or an overestimate of hazard. *Precision,* or degree to which a measurement yields the same value repeatedly, also greatly affects the interpretation of an exposure assessment. Imprecise (highly variable) measurements or assessment strategies yield uncertain conclusions. In the context of exposure–response analyses of epidemiologic data, imprecision also biases any observed relationship toward the null, that is, toward a conclusion that there is no effect of the exposure.[5] The degree to which these errors are controlled, that is, the degree of accuracy including both precision and lack of bias, determines the success of the exposure assessment. Thus, exposure assessment methods can be described in terms of the potential errors they introduce.

The following discussion of exposure assessment methods takes place in the context of the errors inherent in the definitions used to define exposure and the methodologies used to measure or estimate exposure. Although this approach stresses the errors associated with exposure assessment methods, it should not be interpreted as questioning the validity or importance of exposure evaluations; rather, understanding potential sources of error is a necessary step in fully appreciating the power inherent in quantifying occupational and environmental exposures.

First, general principles of exposure assessment are dis|cussed; then, specific measurement methods are broadly described. General principles of exposure assessment are explored first by considering the effects of substituting exposure for dose in the four identified dimensions of exposure: identity, concentration, form, and time. Second, sources of variability in exposure assessments, primarily sampling and analytic uncertainty and environmental variability, are explored for their implications on exposure assessment strategies.

GENERAL PRINCIPLES AND SOURCES OF ERROR IN EXPOSURE ASSESSMENT

Identifying exposure agents

Identification of etiologic agents in population-based studies. Specific identification of an etiologic agent among many potential candidates may be the goal of an exposure assessment. This may be the case for studies in complex environments in which many potentially hazardous agents are present, or especially in an industry-wide or population-based study of a specific outcome (e.g., lung cancer, in which an etiologic agent is sought).

Direct interviews of workers can provide information that is useful in clinical evaluations; interview methods are discussed in Chapter 3. In research studies, interviews concerning past exposures provide only rudimentary exposure information. Interviews are clearly possible only where the study subjects, or their next of kin, are alive and available for questioning. The information obtained is limited by the subjects' knowledge of their exposures (sometimes only obscure trade names are known), and their ability to recall specific aspects of working conditions over a long period of time.[6-8] Furthermore, in case-control studies, a serious source of information bias may be introduced by the cases being more able to recall certain exposures than controls because of heightened concern or awareness about their health.[9]

Some of the potential bias inherent in subject interviews for research studies may be controlled through the use of independent sources of information structured into a job exposure matrix (JEM). A JEM involves defining all possible jobs for the cohort (whether in a plant, an industry, or across a population), and identifying all possible exposure agents in each job.[10] JEMs may also frequently contain a time dimension since the substances used in a particular job may vary over time. Information on the presence of specific agents in each cell of the matrix may be obtained from interviews with experienced industrial hygienists and plant personnel, or through a systematic survey of hazards in industry such as the National Occupational Hazard Survey, which was conducted by the National Institute for Occupational Safety and Health (NIOSH) in the mid-1980s.[11] The study subjects' work histories (which locate the individual in location and time) are then matched to the JEM, and a list of the agents to which each subject was exposed can be developed.

The JEM methodology is attractive for its simplicity and objectivity but is limited by its lack of specificity.[12] Although JEMs identify potential exposures by job category, the results represent only an increased probability that a particular study subject was actually exposed. JEMs may therefore be useful for hypothesis-generating studies, or for identifying clusters of relatively high hazard agents; the errors inherent in the method give the study low power to detect more subtle hazards. The specificity of a JEM may be significantly increased through refining the exposure assignments for each subject with intensive interviews conducted by industrial hygienists or chemists.[13] Within a plant or industry, jobs can be much more specifically defined and characterized through the use of plant records, such as engineering plans and product inventories, and interviews with long-term employees who may be familiar with specific processes. In these ways, exposure information derived by a JEM can be maximized, but may still be inadequate to detect etiologic agents with mild effects; under most circumstances, a JEM approach cannot be used to quantitate exposure levels.

Specific agent identification for measurement strategy. Identification of a specific agent can also be important in studies in which the hazard is only crudely identified. For instance, if asbestos is the agent of interest, the specific mineral type and fiber dimensions should be specified before a measurement technique can be chosen. To the degree that information is available to specify the exact agent responsible for the outcome of interest, the measurement strategy can be highly specific. Often, however, there is only partial information about the particular agent responsible for the hazard, and the measurement technique must balance the need to be specific and reduce errors with the need to measure a quantity that will adequately represent the (unidentified) etiologic agent. For instance, in a study of the acute respiratory effects of exposure to "machining fluids" in metal machining and grinding operations, the specific etiologic agent for observed changes in pulmonary function, among the many organic, inorganic, metallic, biocidal, and biological constituents of the fluids, was not known before designing the measurement strategy.[14] Thus, the measurement technique chosen was for "total particulate," a relatively nonspecific measure. The validity of using such a measure is based on the assumption that total particulate would be reasonably well correlated with the specific component of fluid giving rise to any observed outcomes. The degree to which this assumption is true determines the usefulness of the measurement strategy in identifying an exposure–response relationship for machining fluids.

Surrogate exposure markers. In the machining fluid case above, one might call total particulate a surrogate, or marker of the true etiologic agent. In other situations a surrogate exposure measurement strategy might be adopted for agents that are difficult or expensive to measure.[15] The multitude of polycyclic aromatic hydrocarbons in environmental tobacco smoke (ETS) would be a reasonable set of compounds to measure in studying the lung cancer in populations exposed to ETS. However, measurement of these compounds is difficult and very expensive. One strategy to evaluate individual exposures to ETS is to use a specific marker of ETS that correlates well with the more toxicologically relevant constituents. Vapor phase nicotine, although not itself the carcinogen, provides such a marker since it is specific to tobacco smoke (there are few other sources of nicotine exposure), it is relatively simple and inexpensive to measure, and it is highly correlated with ETS particulate measurements. Thus, in a study of lung cancer and exposure to diesel fume, nicotine exposure was measured as a marker of carcinogenic particulate exposure from tobacco and could be quantified separately from the other potentially carcinogenic diesel fume particulates.[16] Although the use of a surrogate overcomes some logistical problems, it also entails the introduction of some error into the exposure assessment. The trade-off between the degree of error introduced by the surrogate and its greater feasibility of measurement depends on the specific exposure assessment problem at hand.

Concentration

Quantification of the concentration of agents in air has traditionally been given most attention by industrial hygienists. Concentration is expressed as the quantity of the agent per unit volume of air. For agents in a gaseous state at ambient temperatures (including substances that do not condense at room temperature and vapors of volatile liquids) the common units of exposure are parts per million by volume (ppm). Before the 1960s, solid aerosols were quantified by microscopic particle counts. Thus, the units of exposure were a number of particles per unit volume, such as millions of particles per cubic foot (mppcf). However, during the 1960s the technology for gravimetric determination of aerosols was developed at the same time as epidemiologic results began to show the greater relevance of the total mass of an aerosol deposited, rather than the number of particles.[17] Thus, since the late 1960s, solids and liquids dispersed in air (aerosols, or particulate exposures) have generally been quantified as the mass per volume, such as milligrams per cubic meter (mg/m^3). For certain agents, units are still given as counts per volume. For instance fibers are quantified as the number of fibers (of specified dimensions) per cubic centimeter.

Both the process of collecting contaminants from air and conducting the laboratory analysis of the sample may entail significant errors including those due to pump calibration and timing, interferences, sample losses or contamination during transit or storage, inaccurate standards, and chemical reactions.[18] To control such biases, standard methods that have been tested repeatedly under stated conditions and published should be used.[19] By using standard methods the degree of both bias and precision in the method itself is known. For instance, most NIOSH methods have minimal bias and a coefficient of variation for sampling and analysis of less than 10% (depending on the type of analyte). These errors, of course, apply only under ideal conditions where no gross errors are made in the procedures and the work is conducted by a well-qualified industrial hygienist.

If measurements taken with different methods or by different personnel are combined or compared, large errors may occur. This problem is of particular concern for the measurement of aerosols where the methods employed (and even the units of exposure) have changed over time. For instance, in a historical reconstruction of exposure in an asbestos textile plant, Dement et al.[20] used measurements taken during the 1950s and 1960s with an impinger and on a membrane filter in the late 1960s and 1970s. The two methods differ dramatically in their collection efficiency and by their definition of a fiber. In the earlier data, the method specified counting all visible (by light microscope) particles and the data were quantified as mppcf. In later years, phase contrast microscopy was used on membrane filter samples to count fibers >5 μm in length with an aspect ratio >3 and the data were expressed as fibers per cubic centimeter. Thus, the two assessment methods were entirely different, although they were both designed to measure the degree of hazard from exposure to asbestos aerosols. Since the size of the fibers is highly variable, there was no exact way to convert from one of these methods to the other. Instead, using side-by-side measurements taken prior to the abandonment of the old method, an empirical solution was found to make the older data consistent with the modern information.

Spatial gradients: area and personal measurement. Another important aspect of the measurement of exposure concentration is spatial gradients. Prior to the development of small light-weight and battery-operated air sampling pumps most exposure measurements were conducted with the use of stationary or hand-held instruments located close to the study subject. Because of the importance of the distance between the worker and the source of the air contamination, such "area" samples may provide highly biased representations of the actual exposure delivered to the workers.[21] Area samples have been shown to be valid only where the source is either distant from the worker for a majority of the exposure time or generated diffusely throughout the workspace, yielding relatively uniform exposure concentrations in space.[22] Thus stationary monitors will be relatively unbiased for exposures such as indoor air contaminants generated by carpeting throughout the work area, whereas personal monitors are particularly important where a machine that a worker operates is the primary point source of exposure.

Nevertheless, in certain applications where the technology for personal sampling is not available, stationary monitors are still the method of choice. For instance, where direct-reading instruments with a high degree of chemical specificity and rapid or continuous monitoring are required, such as for highly reactive gases in semiconductor manufacturing, stationary multiport sampling locations feeding a highly specific analytic instrument may be used.[23] For cotton dust, which contains a large quantity of large and very long fibers that must be separated from the more toxicologically relevant particulate, no personal monitoring device is available. Thus, exposure assessment for cotton dust still relies on large stationary "vertical elutriators" set up in close

proximity to the work station, and assignment of individual exposure, or dose, potentially involves a significant bias.[24]

Even with the use of personal monitors, high spatial gradients of exposure may affect the accuracy of a personal exposure measurement. Air currents around a worker's body create downwind "wake zones" in which contaminants may reach very high levels, depending on the direction and speed of the cross-draft, the orientation of the worker, and the placement of the exposure source. Depending on the placement of the exposure monitor on the body, these non-uniformities in concentration may introduce large biases in the exposure data.[25]

Form

Closely related to the issue of identity is the importance of the specific form in which the agent exists in air and how this determines its bioavailability or potential to reach the target organ. Airborne chemicals may exist as individual molecules mixed in air (e.g., as gases or vapors, or in aerosol [particulate] form).

Deposition and absorption of gases and vapors by the respiratory tract are determined primarily by the agent's solubility in water. Highly hygroscopic agents such as ammonia are absorbed rapidly by the mucosa of the nasal and oral passages with little gas penetrating to the lung tissues. Less water-soluble gases such as ozone partially pass through the upper airways to be absorbed more completely in the deep lung.

Aerosols include dust (created by mechanical action on solids), mists (liquid droplets), and fumes (solids created by heating to vaporization and condensed in air to form very small particles). Deposition of aerosols in the respiratory tract is determined by the particle size distribution, as discussed below.

Some agents may be present as both aerosol and vapor form, and the relative proportions of each, help determine both the target site dose and the appropriate sampling methods. For instance, exposure to polyisocyanate systems may occur as both particulate and vapor. Each molecule in vapor form would be expected to contribute to the effect of the isocyanate on the lung airways. However, when in aerosol form, some portion of the reactive sites may have polymerized, or be enveloped within the particle by the time the agent is deposited in the respiratory tract yielding a lesser degree of hazard on a weight basis. Methods for isocyanate quantification have attempted to overcome this potential limitation by measuring the chemical in vapor and aerosol form simultaneously, and by quantifying the concentration on the basis of available reactive sites rather than by weight.[26]

Particle deposition and penetration. For particulate respiratory hazards, size is a major determinant of penetration into the respiratory tract and deposition in different areas of the system. For practical purposes the respiratory tract is divided into three anatomic and functional regions:

the head and airways region (HAR) including the nasal passages, mouth, and oropharynx; the tracheobronchial region (TBR) including the larynx, main and segmental bronchi, and terminal bronchioles; and the gas-exchange region (GER) consisting of the respiratory bronchioles and alveoli.[27,28] The three major divisions of the respiratory tract can be distinguished on the basis of anatomy (especially their diameter), physiology, and primary defense mechanisms. As a result of the differences, region-specific effects may also be identified; the deposition of an agent in one portion of the respiratory tract may represent a different type or degree of hazard than if the same agent were deposited elsewhere. Exposure evaluation must consider the potential deposition sites of the airborne particles to reduce the possible errors associated with the measurement.[29]

The classic application of site-specific health hazard evaluation is in the evaluation of pneumoconiosis-producing dusts such as silica. Silica deposited in the HAR or ciliated airways of the TBR would be rapidly cleared and produces little risk of pneumoconiosis. However, the smaller particles that penetrate to and deposit in the GER may eventually lead to the development of silicosis. Therefore, exposure assessment of silica dust relevant to the production of silicosis involves sampling only the relatively small "respirable" dust fraction that penetrates to the GER.

Aerosol penetration and deposition in the respiratory tract are determined primarily by the particle's inertia and, for smaller particles, diffusion, both of which are strongly dependent on the particle's size.[30] To account for differences in shape and density, sizing is generally done on the basis of "aerodynamic diameter," that is, the diameter of a spherical particle of uniform density (i.e., water droplet) with the same settling velocity as the particle being sized. Thus, by using aerodynamic diameter, particle deposition in the respiratory tract can be represented as a function of size. Several models have been developed to represent the efficiency of particulate deposition in different regions of the respiratory tract. A recent one based on data from numerous published studies of aerosol deposition is given in Fig. 11-1-1.[31] Although the model can be used to predict deposition, there is wide inter- and intraindividual variability because of individual morphology, breathing rates, nose versus mouth breathing, disease status, etc.[32]

Although particle *deposition* is the most valid representation of particulate dose to the respiratory tract, designing simple instruments to collect particulates conforming to these models has proved elusive. As a result, simpler models for particulate *penetration* into the respiratory tract regions have been developed along with practical sampling devices that sample in close conformance to the models. The American Conference of Governmental Industrial Hygienists (ACGIH)[33] current definitions for particle size-selective sampling based on particulate penetration into the respiratory tract (inhalable) or to the TBR (thoracic) or GER

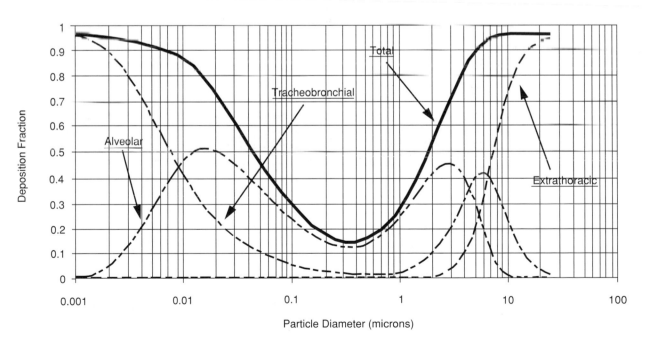

Fig. 11-1-1. Estimated deposition fraction by aerodynamic particle size as predicted by the model presented by Stahlhofen et al.[31] Fractions of inhaled particulate depositing in the whole respiratory tract (Total), extrathoracic (HAR), tracheobronchial (TBR), and alveolar (GER) regions are provided. Fractions are calculated assuming mouth breathing with functional residual capacity = 2200 cm^3, breathing rate = 15 breaths/min, and tidal volume = 1450 cm^3. (Generated with assistance from P. Hewett, NIOSH, Morgantown, WV.)

(respirable) regions are given in Table 11-1-1 and shown in Fig. 11-1-2. Note that the definitions of thoracic and respirable fractions are given as fractions of inhalable particulate, not of total airborne particulate. These definitions reflect recent revisions that conform with an international standard supported by the European Economic Community and the International Standards Organization. Although the definitions are slightly revised from earlier ACGIH definitions, there is little practical implication for the revisions and the same sampling devices may be used.[34]

Although sampling according to penetration definitions may be more practical, they imply some error in comparison with the more valid deposition models. Comparison of the ACGIH penetration definitions for respirable and thoracic mass fractions to the Stahlhofen deposition model pre-

dictions for comparable regions and under the same assumptions is shown in Fig. 11-1-3. The divergence between penetration and deposition models for either region is pronounced. An analysis of the differences between these curves has demonstrated that significant biases could result in the use of penetration curves for epidemiologic analysis instead of the more toxicologically valid deposition models.[35] This theoretical observation was confirmed in a study of lead absorption, in which modeling dose on the basis of deposition provided significant improvements over the simpler penetration models.[36]

Time-related factors

The temporal aspects of dose are typically represented in exposure measures as linear functions, that is, concen-

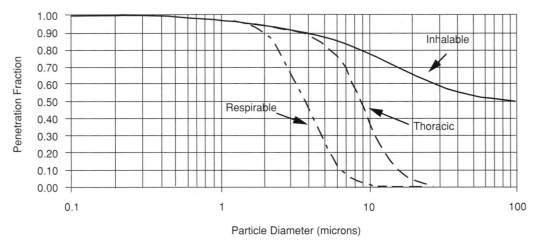

Fig. 11-1-2. Current particle size-specific sampling definitions based on penetration into the respiratory tract.[33]

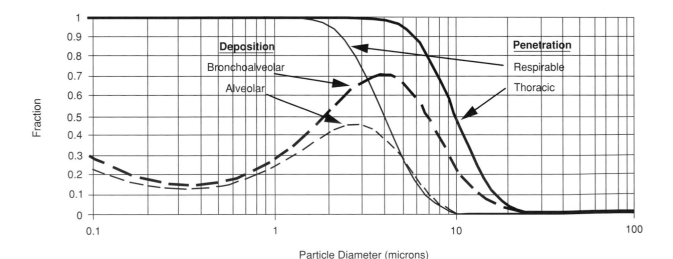

Fig. 11-1-3. Comparison of particulate penetration and deposition in the alveolar (respirable) and bronchoalveolar (thoracic) regions of the respiratory tract. Penetration curves are those defined by the American Conference of Governmental Industrial Hygienists[33] and deposition is estimated from Stahlhofen et al.[31] Both curves represent fractions of the inhaled particulate.

tration is simply summed or averaged over the total exposure time. The most common expression for exposure is thus the average concentration across a typical workday and is expressed as an 8-hour time-weighted average (TWA). For toxicants with potential acute effects, an 8-hour average may be insufficient for controlling the effects, and an average exposure over a shorter duration, usually 15 minutes, is used.

For the epidemiology of chronic toxicants, exposure has frequently been represented as "years worked," or a similar simple expression of time of exposure without reference to concentration. Use of these surrogates of exposure may be necessary in situations where there is incomplete or unreli-

Table 11-1-1. Particle size fraction penetration fractions as defined by ACGIH

Particle diameter (μm)	Penetration (%)
Inhalable fraction	
0	100
1	97
2	94
5	87
10	77
20	65
30	58
40	54.5
50	52.5
100	50
Thoracic fraction	
0	100
2	94
4	89
6	80.5
8	67
10	50
12	35
14	23
16	15
18	9.5
20	6
25	2
Respirable fraction	
0	100
1	97
2	91
3	74
4	50
5	30
6	17
7	9
8	5
10	1

ACGIH. *1993-1994 Threshold limit values for chemical substances and physical agents and biological exposure indices,* Cincinnati, 1993, American Council of Governmental Industrial Hygienists.

able information on historical exposure levels. Where exposure information is more complete, a measure comparable with the TWA, cumulative exposure (the sum of the products of duration and concentration over a series of exposure periods), is the usual representation of exposure. Under assumptions of linear toxicokinetics, and chronic processes, it has been clearly demonstrated that cumulative exposure is directly proportional to toxicologically effective dose,[37] and so it is not surprising that these exposure metrics have proved quite effective in many situations.

However, the assumptions inherent in use of the TWA and cumulative exposure should be carefully examined before they are adopted.[38] These dose metrics assume that both duration and concentration are appropriately summarized on a linear scale; that is, twice the exposure concentration or duration of exposure represents twice the dose. There are numerous biological processes that make this an inappropriate assumption for many toxicants. For instance, using a simple pharmacokinetic model to translate exposure to dose, Smith[39] demonstrated that for relatively insoluble particles, the inhibition of dust clearance from the lungs at high dose rates (e.g., concentrations) results in a nonlinear translation of exposure into tissue dose. Short high exposures result in a larger tissue dose than would be represented by simple cumulative exposure. Conversely, the saturation of an activating enzyme (e.g., the oxidation of hexane to its toxic ketone metabolites) results in lower doses than would be predicted by cumulative exposure when high exposure levels occur. These two examples clearly demonstrate how nonlinearities in the toxicokinetics of inhalation hazards may result in significant errors in the representation of dose by linear functions of time such as the TWA or cumulative exposure.

The assumptions underlying the use of cumulative exposure and of the TWA also imply that the time at which the exposure occurs is irrelevant to the outcome. For instance, exposures that occurred 20 years ago are considered to have the same importance to a disease as do exposures within the last year. On the scale of the TWA, this would suggest that exposures at the beginning of the work shift have the same importance as do those occurring in the last minutes prior to leaving work, or that high peak exposures occurring within a short period of time have the same effect as peaks distributed across the workday with a recovery period after each. Although these assumptions may be correct under some circumstances, they may be the source of large errors for some biological processes.

For instance, chronic exposure to crystalline silica has generally been represented by cumulative exposure. However, once silica is deposited in the lung a large portion of it remains in place exerting its toxic properties indefinitely. Thus, exposure to silica many years ago has more importance to the development of silicosis than recent exposure. To accommodate this concept, Jahr[40] proposed a model of silicosis that weights the exposure concentration by the residence time in the lung, thus incorporating the appropriate toxicologic model into the representation of exposure by weighting earlier exposures more heavily than those more recently received. For acute respiratory irritants such as ozone, the respiratory tract responds to exposures on the scale of minutes to a few hours. Thus, exposures occurring several hours previous to the measurement of outcome (e.g., at the end of a work shift) may contribute little to the observed response.[41]

Another way in which time of exposure can be considered is by the use of exposure windows, or latency periods.[42] Given sufficient knowledge concerning the natural history of the disease, relevant periods of exposure may be defined and only exposure within that period considered. For instance, for lung cancer arising from asbestos exposure, only exposure occurring 10 to 15 years prior to the recognition of disease might be included in the exposure metric. In an epidemiologic study of a disease for which specific knowledge of the appropriate latency period is missing, the dose–response relationship may be observed in a series of "moving exposure windows (in time)" to find the period of exposure most significantly related to the outcome of interest.[43]

Given the many unknowns concerning the appropriate characterization of duration, concentration, and time of exposure in a dose metric, the use of cumulative exposure for chronic hazards, and the 8-hour TWA for a typical work shift are reasonable approximations, or surrogates, for a true dose metric. However, for substances for which a considerable amount is known about the toxicokinetics and mechanism of action, more accurate dose metrics may be developed.[44] If little is known or assumed about the agent's mechanism of damage, a flexible dose metric that allows for varying contributions of duration, concentration, and time of exposure may also be used.[45] However, the flexibility of this approach requires that it be applied only in relatively large epidemiologic data sets for which highly specific exposure data are available.

Thus, time-related aspects of the representation of dose form a basic part of an exposure assessment. Use of simple 8-hour TWAs, or simple cumulative exposure, may serve general exposure assessment well but depends on the validity of the assumptions implied for each specific application. As a result, the use of these simple metrics may introduce a substantial degree of error in the true representation of dose for a particular exposure history and a particular agent. As knowledge about the mechanism of action of particular agents is accumulated, improved models to express dose can be constructed.

SOURCES AND EFFECTS OF EXPOSURE VARIABILITY

As discussed in the introduction, both bias and precision are important to the accurate assessment of exposure or dose. Exposure variability is important because it introduces

uncertainty in either an individual measurement of concentration or uncertainty in the estimation of parameters of an exposure distribution such as the mean. In addition, uncertainty or random errors in exposure assessments for epidemiology studies will generally cause an underestimation of any underlying exposure–response relationship, thus reducing the power of the study and providing biased estimates of exposure-related risks.[5]

The two primary sources of variability in exposure measurements, sampling and analytic variability, and environmental variability are discussed on page 159. In addition, for estimating dose from exposure, variability in individual characteristics such as body size, metabolism and work (breathing) rate, respiratory tract morphology, and use of personal protective equipment may introduce considerable variability into the assessment of dose.

It should be noted that under some circumstances, the biases in exposure assessment discussed above may become sources of imprecision as well. For instance, if a respirable dust sampler conforming to the ACGIH definition of alveolar penetration is used to estimate deposited particulate dose to the lung tissues, any particular sample may be biased, but taken on many individuals working in variable conditions, the bias may be highly variable, and therefore produce imprecision in the average measure of respiratory dose, as well as bias. Thus, what appears to be a systematic error may also imply variability.

Sampling and analytic variability

Random errors in a single exposure measurement may come about as a result of errors both in the sampling procedure (including pump flow calibration, timing, etc.) and in analysis (e.g., weighing errors and instability in the measuring device). Total sampling and analysis variability is usually expressed as the method's coefficient of variation (CV), which is calculated as the standard deviation divided by the mean of a set of replicate samples taken in the same environment.

The precision of sampling and analysis varies greatly with the type of measurement. For instance, in the absence of an interlaboratory quality control program, the CV for asbestos sampling and analysis using currently recommended NIOSH practices may be as great as 45% (Method #7400). Direct-reading detector tubes may measure with a CV of about 25%, although some methods, for instance, total dust weighed on a membrane filter, may be as precise as 5% CV.[21,46] Frequently the CV cited in the documentation for a standard method is the best that might be expected since it is generally estimated by highly motivated laboratory personnel working under ideal conditions. Application of the method by minimally trained individuals in field conditions may result in considerably higher uncertainty.[47] The CV is also generally estimated for concentrations near the permissible exposure limit (PEL) and may be substantially larger at lower levels.

Environmental variability

Random processes in work rate, contaminant generation, and air movement result in highly variable workplace concentrations of contaminants. As a result of this variability, individual samples on a particular worker or on a particular day are insufficient to characterize one's usual, or long-term exposure. In some studies, for instance those looking at acute respiratory changes over a work shift, an individual measurement on the study subject on the day that the testing is conducted is the appropriate exposure quantity. However, if one attempts to characterize exposure more generally, over many individuals in a workplace, or over time, many more samples are required and a sampling strategy designed to estimate parameters of the exposure distribution as precisely as possible is needed.

It has been repeatedly observed that exposure data sets, whether as measurements of a group of individuals on one day, of one individual over time, or of short-term averages within a single workday, approximately conform to the lognormal distribution.[48,49] Parameters of the lognormal distribution have thus been widely used for describing environmental exposure data. The lognormal distribution is recognizable by its rightward skewness, indicating that most values are at the lower end of the distribution but a small fraction of the data may reach very high levels (see Fig. 11-1-4). If lognormally distributed data are transformed by taking their logarithms, the resulting distribution is normal or gaussian. This property allows for the application of a variety of statistical models that rely on normally distributed data to environmental data.

The lognormal distribution can be simply described with two parameters, the geometric mean (GM), and the geometric standard deviation (GSD). The GM is the location parameter, or descriptor for the central tendency of the distribution, whereas the GSD is a measure of the spread, or variability of the data. The arithmetic mean (AM) may also be calculated and used to indicate the expected value of the distribution. The importance of the GSD is illustrated in Fig. 11-1-4 for two distributions with the same GM. The larger

the GSD, the larger is the skewness of the distribution, and as a result, the larger is the spread between the GM and the AM. The GM and GSD can be calculated from the data directly by transforming it first (taking the logarithm) and then making the usual calculations of mean and standard deviation (box) or by plotting the data on log-probability paper. (Procedures for plotting and interpreting log-probability plots are given in Leidel et al.,[21] Appendix J.) The advantages of the plotting procedure are that it facilitates an examination of the distributional assumptions, readily allows calculation of a variety of distribution parameters such as quantiles, and provides a method for dealing with censored information (e.g., data lower than the lower limit of detection).

Although the GM is a useful descriptor of most exposure concentration data, under most circumstances the AM is a more relevant parameter for describing the toxicologically significant exposure or dose[37] or describing exposure for most epidemiologic analyses.[50] The AM can be calculated in the usual way (sum of the n measured

---

Calculation of the geometric mean (GM) and geometric standard deviation (GSD)

$$GM = \exp\left(\sum_{i=1}^{n} y_i / n\right)$$

$$GSD = \exp\left[\frac{\sqrt{\sum_{i=1}^{n} (y_i - \bar{y})^2}}{n-1}\right]$$

where $y_i = \log_e(x_i)$, and the x_i represent the $i = 1$ to n measured concentrations.

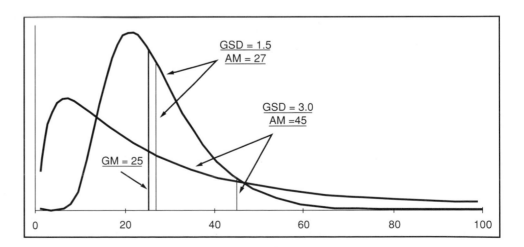

Fig. 11-1-4. The lognormal model represented for two distributions, each with geometric mean equal to 25.

concentrations divided by n). However, this simple method does not produce the most accurate estimate. Minimum variance unbiased methods of calculating the AM and its standard error are presented by Attfield and Hewett[51] and Armstrong.[52]

Exposure groups. For epidemiologic analysis or risk assessment, in which there are limited exposure data for each individual, the AM is frequently calculated on all data observed on individuals within a homogeneous exposure group (HEG), or exposure zone, and then used to represent the expected exposure received by each member of the group. The HEG has been defined as individuals engaged in similar work, with similar exposure potential and controls.[53] The use of HEGs has also become a primary method for prospective exposure monitoring strategies.[54]

The use of HEGs implies that there is some method by which the groups can be accurately identified. For epidemiologic analysis, crude categories such as Department or Job Title are frequently used; for prospective strategies, observation of work tasks and exposure potential may be employed. The ability of even trained individuals to divide individuals into "homogeneously exposed" groups through subjective observation is uncertain.[49] A considerable overlap in concentration distributions was observed when a group of hygienists was asked to categorize a small set of jobs in several plants[55] and similar limitations to subjective exposure estimation have been observed by others.[56,57]

In addition, application of a group mean to all individuals within the group implies that each individual within the group has the same average exposure, and therefore risk. By using analysis of variance techniques, the total variance of an exposure data distribution can be divided into inter- and intraindividual components of variance.[49] The division of total variance into these components allows the investigator to consider the degree to which individuals' long-term means vary, and can therefore consider different risks to individuals within a similarly exposed group. Kromhout et al.[58] and Rappaport et al.[59] have examined a large number of data sets to consider the degree to which the reported HEGs were truly homogeneous. They found that individual mean exposures (interindividual variability) were highly divergent in most of the data sets. For instance, there was greater than 10-fold range of mean exposures between the 2.5th and 97.5th percentile for 30% of 165 predefined groups. Although these findings point out that individual exposures do vary substantially even within seemingly homogeneous groups, grouping still provides the only feasible method of historical exposure estimation for many epidemiologic studies and also has some advantageous statistical properties.[50,60]

Interpreting variability. Although for most applications, estimation of the mean exposure is the most important aspect of the exposure distribution, in some circumstances the variability may be important. In evaluating compliance with occupational health standards, the coefficient of variation of the sampling and analytic method should be taken into account. For instance, if a method has a CV of 10%, an analytic result must be 117% of the standard in order to be 95% confident that the true exposure exceeds the standard (one-sided confidence limit).[21] Rappaport[61] has explored some of the limitations of this simple method for determining compliance with an exposure standard, and regulatory compliance issues are discussed further in Chapters 55 and 56.

Exposure variability may also be an important indicator of hazard for substances exhibiting acutely irritant or toxic properties. While an 8 hour TWA may be very low, a short-term excursion of an acutely toxic material such as an asphyxiant or irritant like chlorine gas must be accounted for. Thus, exposure limits for acutely toxic materials are provided as short-term (e.g., 15-minute average concentrations). More precise definitions of appropriate averaging times for some acute hazards have been developed.[62]

Furthermore, under some circumstances, exposure variability may affect dose for chronic hazards. Rappaport demonstrated that substances with long elimination half-times from the body, burden rises with exposure, whereas for substances with short elimination half-times, no such build-up of burden is seen.[63] Using this analysis, it is suggested that day-to-day variability is unimportant to the quantification of dose for chronic hazards with elimination half-times greater than about 40 days. Thus, for typical chronic hazards such as fibrogenic dusts and heavy metals, which have long elimination half-times, day-to-day exposure variability is much less important than the mean exposure over an extended period of time. However, for substances with relatively short elimination half-times, but for which the kinetics of dose to damage are nonlinear,[39] the degree of variability and the mean exposure may contribute to the overall effective dose.

Summary: variability

The two major types of variability in exposure measurements, sampling and analytic errors, and environmental variability may be summarized by comparing the importance of the errors with an exposure assessment. For an individual measurement, such as required on an individual study day for the assessment of acute cross-shift changes, environmental variability is irrelevant since only the particular exposure measurement, not the distribution from which that measurement arises, is of interest. The same is true of an OSHA compliance measurement, which is interpreted only by whether the individual measurement exceeds (by a statistically valid margin of error) the specified air concentration standard. However, for characterizing probabilities of individuals exceeding a standard, or estimating an average exposure to a group or individual over time, the environmental variability is far more important than the sampling and analytic errors. Nicas et al.[64] calculated the percent contribution of sampling an analytic error to total error given various degrees of the two types of error. They demonstrated that even with a CV of as much as ±25%, the analytic variability contributes less than 20% to the total variability of a measurement when environmental variability is moderate (GSD ≥ 2).

Thus, depending on the purpose of the exposure assessment, both sampling and analytical errors, and environmental variability may contribute to the uncertainty in a measurement or an estimate of average exposure. Under most circumstances, when the measurements are used to represent a parameter of an exposure distribution such as the mean, environmental variability is a much more important source of random error in exposure assessment and a large number of measurements may be required to estimate the relevant exposure distribution parameters with sufficient accuracy.

MEASUREMENT TECHNIQUES
General

There are many techniques employed in making the actual measurements of particular exposures. A number of comprehensive sources can be consulted for detailed information on industrial hygiene sampling and analytic methods.[18,19,65] Here, techniques for air contaminant measurement are broadly described. Measurement of airborne contaminants generally involves the quantitative transfer of contaminant from air to a device for determination of the amount of contaminant.[66] Contaminant collection may be by active or passive means. Active collection involves use of an air mover or pump to pull contaminated air through a collection device that separates the intended contaminant from air and stores it for later analysis. Passive collection utilizes diffusion of the contaminants from air onto the surface of a collection medium and is therefore useful only for gases and vapors and not collection of aerosols. In each case, the concentration is calculated as the total amount of the contaminant collected divided by the air volume sampled. Thus, the sampling time and the sampling (or flow) rate of the sampler must be accurately measured. A third type of measurement system, direct-reading instruments, avoids the collection step and directly measures the concentration of contaminant with an analytic detector exposed directly to the atmosphere.

Active and passive sampling

Active sampling is the most commonly used and most flexible system and is depicted in Fig. 11-1-5. The components of the system include an air mover or sampling pump, a flow regulator and/or meter, which is sometimes incorporated into the sampling pump, and a sample collection device. For particulate sampling, a preselector or specialized inlet is also sometimes included.

A wide variety of different types of air sampling pumps have been developed for monitoring air contaminants.[67] For personal exposure monitoring, for which size, weight, and power source determine the pump's utility, battery-operated air movers weighing less than about a kilogram have been developed that will maintain constant air flows for greater than 10 hours from about 0.001 L/min up to about 5 L/min. Feedback systems have recently been added to these pumps that allow them to maintain preset flow rates as resistance to flow increases with contaminant collection. For area, or ambient air pollution measurements, for which high flow rates over longer periods of time are required, stationary air pumps are used.

The flow rate of the system may be regulated, by passing the air through a precalibrated "critical orifice," or metered by a flow meter such as a rotameter. More commonly, a primary standard such as a spirometer or bubble meter is used to calibrate the flow of the pump prior to sampling.[30] Because changes in flow resistance may occur as a result of build-up of contaminant on the sampling device (e.g., filter), calibration should be done with all components of the sampling train in place. Calibration generally is done at least once before and after a sampling period, even if "constant flow" sampling pumps are employed.

A second type of mass transfer device, called passive monitors or dosimeters, has more recently been developed to avoid both the expense and errors associated with the use of air sampling pumps. Passive monitors use diffusion and/or permeation through a membrane as the mechanism for collecting contaminant from the air into the collection media such as activated charcoal or an absorbent solution. Because they work by molecular diffusion, passive monitors are not useful for aerosols but are only for gases and vapors. The sampling rate for passive monitors is determined by the geometry of the instrument and the diffusion

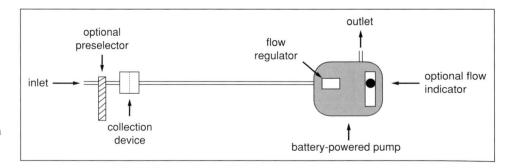

Fig. 11-1-5. Schematic of a typical active sampling train showing the sampling inlet, contaminant collection device, flow regulator/indicator, and air moving pump.

coefficient for the contaminant through air. Because these parameters may be quite variable, empirical calibration of the sampling rate is generally preferred to theoretical values. Other sources of error include temperature, pressure, and humidity effects, under- or oversampling of short-term peak concentrations, and low or high air movement across the sampler's surface. Despite these potential errors, diffusive samplers generally compare well with active sampling methods for accuracy and precision, at least for those compounds for which they have been tested.[68,69]

Contaminant collection

A wide variety of contaminant collection media are available and should be specifically suited to the contaminant to be collected. Gases and vapors are collected generally by adsorption onto a solid surface, or by absorption into a liquid solution (for detailed information, see Brown and Woebkenberg).[68] For some special problems, gases may be collected in gas sampling bottles or bags. Solid sorbents such as activated charcoal are commonly used packed in a glass sampling tube. In addition to high efficiency and capacity for collecting contaminant out of the air, the sorbent must retain the contaminant effectively, and also allow efficient desorption for analysis. As air is drawn through the tube and past the sorbent, contaminant adsorbs to the surface until the sorbent becomes saturated. Sampling times and volumes must be limited to avoid "breakthrough" of the contaminant out the back end of the tube due to saturation of most of the sorbent material. A variety of sorbents are available and may be chosen based on the particular contaminant or mixture of agents to be sampled. Activated charcoal is generally an efficient sorbent for nonpolar compounds organic vapors. Silica gel may be used for more polar compounds such as amines, although it also collects water vapor and therefore has a limited capacity in certain environments. Several other more specialized sorbent systems have also been developed.

Particulates are collected most frequently by filtration but, using the inertial properties of particles, are also collected by impaction or impingement.[70] Many different types of filters are available and must be selected for a particular application based on requirements of sampling rate, size, and shape of the particulate being collected, as well as the presence of other contaminants and the analytic method to be employed. In addition to the filter, the filter holder or cassette must be designed to allow efficient and even flow of air across the filter surface without interfering with collection. A detailed description of available filters and selection criteria is available.[32]

Particle size-specific sampling methods. Particle size is a major determinant of particles' penetration to and deposition in specific functional regions of the respiratory tract, and sampling devices that sample aerosols likely to effect the specific regions may greatly enhance the specificity of an exposure assessment. The inlet to the sampling train may be a significant source of error, or may be specifically designed as a preselector, allowing only the relevant particles to be collected. Until recently, common practice has been to sample for "total particulate" with the 37-mm filter cassette with either an open- or closed-face configuration and assume that all particulate suspended in air was sampled proportionately, and that all airborne particulate would be inhaled. In recent years, these assumptions have been challenged and the importance of determining the "inhalable" dust fraction as opposed to the "total" particulate has been recognized.[71] It has been clearly shown that the 37-mm cassette in either configuration does not sample total particulate, nor does it conform to the "inhalable" particulate curve.[72] A new sampler has now been developed and made commercially available that samples in close conformance to the inhalable particulate definition under many cross-draft directions and velocities.[73] Although the 37-mm cassette is still commonly used for industrial hygiene monitoring, the new sampler should slowly gain acceptance as a new standard method.

The standard method for sampling according to the respirable particulate curve, using a 10-mm nylon cyclone operated at 1.7 L/min, does correspond well to the respirable dust penetration definition.[74] Unfortunately, only stationary sampling methods for tracheobronchial or thoracic (tracheobronchial and respirable) dust fractions have been developed.[75] However, with increased attention paid to the potential importance of particle size selective sampling and to the importance of occupational diseases of the airways, practical personal sampling devices should soon be available.

An alternative approach to particle size selective sampling is to characterize the whole particle size distribution. The most common particle size spectrometer is the multistage cascade impactor, which collects an increasingly small particle size fraction on each of several impaction devices arranged sequentially.[76] A variety of such instruments are available and are designed to obtain precise particle size information by avoiding inlet and internal losses of material as the aerosol passes through the device. Most of the instruments available are relatively large, stationary devices but an 8-stage personal cascade impactor is commercially available and has found relatively wide use.[77] A variety of direct-reading particle size spectrometers are also available and are discussed in detail elsewhere.[78] With information on the entire particle size distribution, one may estimate exposures to any of the regional penetration, or deposition fractions. However, characterizing the distribution has numerous errors associated with it. Use of a multistage impactor requires multiple analytic measurements (one for each stage) that must be conducted for a single sample, thus the potential errors involved are multiplied.

Direct-reading instruments

Direct-reading instruments differ from the sampling and analytic procedures described above in that the instrumental detector that quantitatively responds to the presence of an agent in air is sufficiently portable to bring to the exposure measurement site, and it is sufficiently fast and simple to use that the analytic result is obtained either instantaneously, or within a period of minutes. Some instruments such as electrochemical cells may be small enough to be worn as personal monitors, sometimes including an alarm to warn of dangerously high concentrations to acutely toxic materials. Other instruments such as infrared analyzers are only transportable, to be used as hand-held or area monitors.

In general, direct-reading instruments are adaptations of laboratory analytic methods to practical field applications. The clear advantages of such instruments are that the results are available immediately; coupled to a strip-chart or data-logging recorder, near real-time time distributions of exposure may be obtained. With real-time measurements of exposure variability, especially as instruments become available for *personal* real-time measurements, the importance of peak exposures to acute hazards, and toxicokinetic modeling of tissue dose will be much more readily addressed through epidemiologic research. Some recent advances in this area have begun to be made.[79] Real-time monitoring has also been effectively used in conjunction with video monitoring of work processes to demonstrate the sources of exposure potential in particular work processes.[80] However, in trade-off for the advantages of real-time monitors, the miniaturization and simplification of laboratory analytic instruments often entail a loss of chemical specificity, sensitivity, accuracy, and precision. A wide variety of instruments are available differing greatly in size, cost, and applicability. Only the general types of instruments available are reviewed here.

Colorimetric indicators. Direct-reading colorimetric indicators take on a variety of forms but are most commonly used as a chemically impregnated solid packed in a glass tube.[81] A small volume of air is drawn through the tube and the specific air contaminant reacts with the reagent to form a visible color or stain. The color change, or length of stain can be read as a concentration of contaminant in air. Because of the remarkable simplicity and economy of this method, colorimetric tubes have been widely applied and over 400 specific tubes are now available. Colorimetric tubes are generally used as grab samples, taken over a period of a few minutes at most by drawing a known volume of air through the tube with a calibrated hand-held piston-type pump. Long-term tubes have been developed for a limited number of compounds, which allow air to be drawn continuously over, for instance, 8 hours by a low flow battery-operated personal sampling pump.

Three aspects of colorimetric indicators are of particular concern. First, the chemical reaction of the reagent may not be highly specific, and chemically related compounds may therefore interfere either positively or negatively with the intended analyte. Thus, detector tubes may be best used either in an atmosphere in which either a single agent or a small number of well-known agents are present, or as a screening device to determine the possible presence of an agent for subsequent analysis by a more specific technique. Second, detector tubes have relatively low precision. Although the targeted coefficient of variation is $\pm 25\%$, few tubes reach this level and results are generally thought to be reliable only within 50%. Finally, the limit of detection is limited for most tubes, which are designed to be most accurate for concentrations around the ACGIH threshold limit value (TLV). It should also be noted that many direct-reading tubes have a very limited shelf-life after which the reliability may degrade considerably. In summary, despite the attractive economy and simplicity of direct-reading colorimetric indicator tubes, proper use and interpretation of the results require appropriately trained personnel.

Direct-reading instruments for gas and vapor detection. A very large number of direct-reading instruments using a wide variety of technologies are available for monitoring gases and vapors. The general classes and applications of the instruments are given in Table 11-1-2, and thorough discussion of the instruments may be found elsewhere.[82,83] A variety of highly nonspecific detectors including combustible gas, photoionization, and flame ionization detectors are widely used to detect organic vapors in air. As a result of their responsiveness to most organic species,

Table 11-1-2. Types of direct-reading instruments

Instrument	Typical analyses	Measurement technique	Range (ppm)
Chemiluminescence	NO_2, NO, O_3	Light emission	0.1-10^4
Combustible gas detectors	Combustible gases and vapors	Electrical resistance of heated filament	%LEL
Electrochemical cells	CO, NO, NO_2, H_2S	Chemical oxidation/reduction	1-3000
Flame ionization detectors	Organic vapors	Conductivity of hydrogen flame	0.1-10^5
Infrared spectrometers	Organic and inorganics	IR absorbance	Variable by gas
Metal oxide detectors	H_2S, CO	Electrical resistance	1-50
Photoionization detectors	Organics	Conductivity in UV, UV light field	0.2-2000
Portable gas chromatographs	Organics and inorganics	Gas/solid separation, variable detection	0.1-10^4

Adapted from Herrick et al. Measurement of vapors and gases. In Rappaport SM and Smith TJ, editors: *Exposure assessment for epidemiology and hazard control,* pp 21-40, Chelsea, 1991, Lewis Publishers.

these detectors are generally poor for quantification of exposure levels but may be very useful for qualitative applications such as leak detection and alarm systems. Instruments with the capability of separating agents in air or identifying spectra from specific compounds have also been developed. Ultraviolet, infrared, and visible light spectrometers measuring absorption or emission of light at speci fied wavelengths are commonly used to detect and quantify specific gases with known absorption wavelengths, or to identify gases that may be present in mixtures. As a result of interference by water vapor, carbon dioxide, or mixtures of agents in air, the specificity and reliability of measurements made with these instruments may be significantly poorer than those made with laboratory-based systems. Portable gas chromatographs have been developed to separate multiple species from air and provide quantitation relatively quickly. As a result of their miniaturization and shortening of the separation column, resolution and quantification are significantly less than are obtained with laboratory gas chromatography (GC). Finally, a series of chemical-specific electrochemical or electromagnetic detectors such as chemiluminescence, electrochemical cells, and metal oxide sensors are available for a limited but important set of specific agents.

Direct-reading instruments for particulate detection.
A number of direct-reading instruments for particulate monitoring have been developed. Detailed discussion of direct-reading instruments for particulate exposures may be found elsewhere.[78,84] Most instruments rely on optical properties of the aerosol suspended in air, especially light scattering or light attenuation. As a result of the size dependence of light scattering, the instruments are designed to provide quantitation in specified particle-size ranges. Calibration of light-scattering instruments should be conducted with the aerosol being measured to account for differences in response due to the particular aerosol's particle size and optical properties. A few instruments have been developed based on other principles. Aerosol may be deposited on an oscillating crystal by an electrostatic precipitator. The change in frequency of oscillation is proportional to the deposited mass. Another approach is the impaction of aerosol onto a surface that is placed between a source of β radiation and a detector. Attenuation of the β particles is proportional to the mass of deposited aerosol. Although numerous approaches to direct-reading instrumentation for particulate exposures have been developed, problems with particle-size specificity, reliability, and expense have generally prohibited their wide application to exposure monitoring. In addition, only a few instruments have been sufficiently miniaturized to be used as personal monitors.

CONCLUSION

Exposure assessment is frequently inappropriately identified as a purely technical task involving the use of advancing technologies for measuring airborne agents. However, if the task is appropriately identified as an integral component of an occupational or environmental health assessment, the various sources of potential errors may be identified and the task becomes one of interplay between clinical, epidemiologic, toxicologic, and technical measurement problems and solutions. A wide variety of potential errors, both systematic and random, have been identified. The relative importance of any one particular type of error can be judged or quantified only within a particular exposure assessment problem. Nevertheless, the success of an exposure assessment for a health evaluation, whether it be clinical or epidemiologic in nature, will depend on how well each of these potential sources of error and uncertainty is identified, controlled, or ultimately accounted for in the data analysis. With sufficient attention given to exposure assessment, our ability to prevent or limit disease will be greatly enhanced.

REFERENCES

1. Fenske RA: Dermal exposure assessment techniques, *Ann Occup Hyg* 37:687-706, 1993.
2. Hatch TF: Significant dimensions of the dose-response relationship, *Arch Environ Health* 16:214, 1968.
3. Checkoway H, Pearce NE, and Crawford-Brown DJ: *Research methods in occupational epidemiology,* New York, 1989, Oxford University Press.
4. Hornung RW: Statistical evaluation of exposure assessment strategies, *Appl Occup Environ Hyg* 6:516-520, 1989.
5. Thomas D, Stram D, and Dwyer J: Exposure measurement error: influence on exposure-disease relationships and methods of correction, *Annu Rev Publ Health* 14:69-93, 1993.
6. Armstrong BK, White E, and Saracci R: *Principles of exposure measurement in epidemiology,* Oxford, 1992, Oxford University Press.
7. Fidler AT, Baker EL, and Letz RE: Estimation of long term exposure to mixed solvents from questionnaire data: a tool for epidemiological investigations, *Br J Ind Med* 44:133-141, 1987.
8. Rosenstock L, Logerfo J, Heyer NJ, and Carter WB: Development and validation of a self-administered occupational health history questionnaire, *J Occup Med* 26:50-54, 1984. Snedecor GW and Cochran WG: Statistical Methods, ed 7, pp 171-172, Ames, 1984, Iowa University Press.
9. Axelson O: The case-referent study—some comments on its structure, merits and limitations, *Scand J Work Environ Health* 11:207-213, 1985.
10. Acheson ED: What are job exposure matrices? In Medical Research Council, Environmental Epidemiology Unit. Job exposure matrices: Proceedings of a conference held in April 1982 at the University of Southampton, Southampton, 1983, pp 1-4.
11. Sieber WK, Sundin DS, Frazier RM, and Robinson CF: Development, use and availability of a job exposure matrix based on the National Occupational Hazard Survey, *Am J Indus Med* 20(2):163-174, 1991.
12. Plato N and Steineck G: Methodology and utility of a job-exposure matrix, *Am J Ind Med* 23:491-502, 1993.
13. Gerin M, Siemiatycki J, Kemper H, and Begin D: Obtaining occupational exposure histories in epidemiological case-control studies, *J Occup Med* 27:420-426, 1985.
14. Robins T: Respiratory effects of machining fluid aerosols. Grant proposal submitted to the UAW/GM Occupational Advisory Board, Ann Arbor, MI, 1990, University of Michigan, School of Public Health.
15. Hammond SK: The use of markers to measure exposures to complex mixtures. In Rappaport SM and Smith TJ, editors: *Exposure assessment for epidemiology and hazard control,* pp 53-66, Chelsea, 1991, Lewis Publishers.

16. Woskie SR, Smith TJ, Hammond SK, et al: Estimation of the diesel exhaust exposures of railroad workers; I. Current exposures, *Am Rev Respir Dis* 135:1242-1248, 1987.

17. Jacobsen M, Walton WH, and Rogan JM: The relation between pneumoconiosis and dust-exposure in British coal mines. In Walton, WH editor: *Inhaled particles III*, Old Woking, Surrey, Unwin Brothers.

18. Lodge JP: Methods of air sampling and analysis, ed 3, Chelsea, 1989, Lewis Publishers.

19. NIOSH: *NIOSH manual of analytical methods*, ed 3, National Institute for Occupational Safety and Health Pub No DHHS(NIOSH)84-100, Washington, DC, 1984, U.S. Government Publications Office.

20. Dement JM, Harris RL, Symons MJ, and Shy CM: Exposures and mortality among chrysotile asbestos workers. Part 1: Exposure estimates, *Am J Ind Med* 4:399-419, 1983.

21. Leidel NA, Busch KA, and Lynch JR: *Occupational exposure sampling strategy manual,* NIOSH Pub No 77-173, National Institute for Occupational Safety and Health, Washington, DC, 1977, U.S. Government Printing Office.

22. Norwood SK: Estimating employee exposures from continuous air monitoring data, doctoral dissertation, 1984, University of Oklahoma.

23. Perry WH: Sequential and tape samplers—unattended sampling. In *Air sampling Instruments for evaluation of atmospheric contaminants,* pp 291-303, Cincinnati, 1989, American Conference of Governmental Industrial Hygienists.

24. Neefus JD, Lumsden JC, and Jones MT: Cotton dust sampling, II—verticle elutration, *Am Ind Hyg Assoc J* 38:394-400, 1977.

25. Flanagan ME: Air sampling at the lapel and ear as representative of the breathing zone, master's thesis, University of Washington, 1993, Department of Environmental Health.

26. Dharmarajan V and Weill H: Physical state of airborne p,p′-diphenylmethane diisocyanate (MDI) and its measurement, *Am Ind Hyg Assoc J* 39:737-744, 1978.

27. Lippman M: Size-selective health hazard sampling. In *Air sampling instruments for evaluation of atmospheric contaminants,* ed 7, pp 163-198, Cincinnati, 1989, American Conference of Governmental Industrial Hygienists.

28. Phalen RF: Airway anatomy and physiology. In *Particle size-selective sampling in the workplace: Report of the ACGIH technical committee on air sampling procedures,* pp 15-26, Cincinnati, 1985, American Conference of Governmental Industrial Hygienists.

29. Stewart BO, Lioy PJ and Phalen RF: Use of size-selection in establishing TLVs. In *Particle size-selective sampling in the workplace: Report of the ACGIH Technical committee on air sampling procedures,* pp 65-76, Cincinnati, 1985, American Conference of Governmental Industrial Hygienists.

30. Lippman M: Calibration of air sampling instruments. In Hering SV, editor: *Air sampling instruments for evaluation of atmospheric contaminants,* pp 73-110, Cincinnati, 1989, American Conference of Governmental Industrial Hygienists.

31. Stahlhofen W, Rudolf G, and James AC: Intercomparison of experimental regional aerosol deposition data, *J Aerosol Med* 2:285-308, 1989.

32. Lippman M: Sampling aerosols by filtration. In Hering SV, editor: *Air sampling instruments for evaluation of atmospheric contaminants.* pp 305-336, Cincinnati, 1989, American Conference of Governmental Industrial Hygienists.

33. ACGIH: *1993–1994 Threshold limit values for chemical substances and physical agents and biological exposure indices,* Cincinnati, 1993, American Conference of Governmental Industrial Hygienists.

34. Soderholm SC: Why change ACGIH's definition of respirable dust? *Appl Occup Environ Hyg* 6:248-250, 1991.

35. Hewett P: Limitations in the use of particle size-selective sampling criteria in occupational epidemiology, *Appl Occup Environ Hyg* 6:290-300, 1991.

36. Hodgkins D, Robins TG, Hinkamp DL, Schork MA, Levine SP, and Krebs WH: The effect of airborne lead particle size on worker blood-lead levels: an empirical study of battery workers, *J Occup Med* 33:1265-1273, 1991.

37. Rappaport SM: Biological considerations in assessing exposures to genotoxic and carcinogenic agents, *Int Arch Occup Environ Health* 65:S29-S35, 1993.

38. Atherley G: A critical review of time-weighted average as an index of exposure and dose, and of its key elements, *Am Ind Hyg Assoc J* 46:481-487, 1985.

39. Smith TJ: Occupational exposure and dose over time: limitations of cumulative exposure, *Am J Ind Med* 21:35-51, 1991.

40. Jahr J: Dose-response basis for setting a quartz threshold limit value, *Arch Environ Health* 29:338-340, 1974.

41. Kriebel D and Smith TJ: A nonlinear pharmacologic model of the acute effects of ozone on the human lungs, *Environ Res* 51:120-146, 1990.

42. Checkoway H, Pearce N, Hickey JLS, and Dement JM: Latency analysis in occupational epidemiology, *Arch Environ Health* 45:95-100, 1990.

43. Finkelstein MM: Use of time windows to investigate lung cancer latency intervals at an Ontario steel plant, *Am J Ind Med* 19:229-235, 1991.

44. Smith TJ: Exposure assessment for occupational epidemiology, *Am J Ind Med* 12:249-268, 1987.

45. Seixas NS, Robins TG, and Becker M: A novel approach to the characterization of cumulative exposure for the study of chronic occupational disease, *Am J Epidemiol* 137:463-471, 1993.

46. NIOSH: NIOSH manual of analytic methods, ed 3 (and supplements). NIOSH Publ 84-100, Washington, D.C., 1984, USGPO.

47. National Bureau of Standards: *An evaluation of the accuracy of the coal mine dust sampling program administered by the Department of the Interior,* Washington DC, 1975, NBS, U.S. Government Printing Office.

48. Leidel NA, Busch KA, and Crouse WE: Exposure measurement action level and occupational environmental variability, USDHEW, NIOSH Pub No 76-131, Washington DC, 1975, U.S. Government Printing Office.

49. Rappaport SM: Assessment of long-term exposure to toxic substances in air, *Ann Occup Hyg* 35:61-121, 1991.

50. Seixas N, Robins TG, and Moulton L: The use of geometric and arithmetic mean exposures in occupational epidemiology, *Am J Ind Med* 14:467-477, 1988.

51. Attfield MA and Hewett P: Exact expressions for the bias and variance of estimators of the mean of a lognormal distribution, *Am Ind Hyg Assoc J* 53:432-435, 1992.

52. Armstrong BG: Confidence intervals for arithmetic means of lognormally distributed exposures, *Am Ind Hyg Assoc J* 53:481-485, 1992.

53. Corn M and Esmen NA: Workplace exposure zones for classification of employee exposures to physical and chemical agents, *Am Ind Hyg Assoc J* 40:47-57, 1979.

54. Hawkins NC, Norwood SK, and Rock JC: *A strategy for occupational exposure assessment,* Akron, OH, 1991, American Industrial Hygiene Association.

55. Kromhout H, Oostendorp Y, Heederik D, and Boleij JSM: Agreement between qualitative exposure estimates and quantitative exposure measurements, *Am J Ind Med* 12:551-562, 1987.

56. Hawkins NC and Evans JS: Subjective estimation of toluene exposures: a calibration study of industrial hygienists, *Appl Ind Hyg J* 4:61-68, 1989.

57. Teschke K, Hertzman C, Dimich-Ward H, Ostry A, Blair J, and Hershler R: A comparison of exposure estimates by worker raters and industrial hygienists, *Scand J Work Environ Health* 15:424-429, 1989.

58. Kromhout H, Symanski E, and Rappaport SM: A comprehensive evaluation of within- and between-workers components of occupational exposure to chemical agents, *Ann Occup Hyg* 37:253-270, 1993.

59. Rappaport SM, Kromhout H, and Symanski E: Variation of exposure between workers in homogeneous exposure groups, *Am Ind Hyg Assoc J* 54:654-662, 1993.

60. Seixas NS and Sheppard E: Maximizing bias and precision in exposure assessment. Paper presented to the American Industrial Hygiene Conference and Exposition, Anaheim, CA, May 23, 1994.

61. Rappaport SM: The rules of the game: an analysis of OSHA's enforcement strategy, *Am J Ind Med* 6:291-303, 1984.

62. Lippman M: Assessing relevant exposures to airborne irritants. In Rappaport SM and Smith TJ, editors: *Exposure assessment for epidemiology and hazard control*, pp 77-96, Chelsea, 1991, Lewis Publishers.

63. Rappaport SM: Smoothing of exposure variability at the receptor: implications for health standards, *Ann Occup Hyg* 29:201-214, 1985.

64. Nicas M, Simmons BP, and Spear RC: Environmental versus analytical variability in exposure measurements, *Am Ind Hyg Assoc J* 52:553-557, 1991.

65. Hering SV: *Air sampling instruments for evaluation of atmospheric contaminants,* Cincinnati, 1989, American Conference of Governmental Industrial Hygienists.

66. First MW: Air sampling and analysis for contaminants: an overview. In Hering SV, editor: *Air sampling instruments for evaluation of atmospheric contaminants,* Cincinnati, 1989, American Conference of Governmental Industrial Hygienists.

67. Rubow KL and Furtado VC: Air movers and samplers. In Hering SV, editor: *Air sampling instruments for evaluation of atmospheric contaminants,* pp 241-274, Cincinnati, 1989, American Conference of Governmental Industrial Hygienists.

68. Brown RH and Woebkenberg ML: Gas and vapor sample collectors. In Hering SV, editor: *Air sampling instruments for evaluation of atmospheric contaminants,* pp 421-448, Cincinnati, 1989, American Conference of Governmental Industrial Hygienists.

69. Mulik JD and Lewis RG: Recent developments in passive sampling devices. In *Recent advances in air sampling,* pp 117-132, Chelsea, 1989, Lewis Publishers.

70. Hering SV: Inertial and Gravitation collectors. In *Air sampling Instruments for evaluation of atmospheric contaminants,* pp 337-386, Cincinnati, 1989, American Conference of Governmental Industrial Hygienists.

71. Vincent JH and Mark K: The measurement of aerosols in relation to risk assessment. In Rappaport SM and Smith TJ, editors: *Exposure assessment for epidemiology and hazard control,* pp 41-52, Chelsea, 1991, Lewis Publishers.

72. Buchan RM, Soderhom SC, and Tillery MI: Aerosol sampling efficiency of 37 mm filter cassettes, *Am Ind Hyg Assoc J* 47:825-831, 1986.

73. Mark D and Vincent JH: A new personal sampler for airborne total dust in workplaces, *Ann Occup Hyg* 30:89-102, 1986.

74. John W: Sampler efficiencies: respirable mass fraction. In *Particle size-selective sampling in the workplace: Report of the ACGIH technical committee on air sampling procedures,* pp 61-64, Cincinnati, 1985, American Conference of Governmental Industrial Hygienists.

75. John W: Sampler efficiencies: thoracic mass fraction. In *Particle size-selective sampling in the workplace: Report of the ACGIH technical committee on air sampling procedures,* pp 55-59, Cincinnati, 1985, American Conference on Governmental Industrial Hygienists.

76. Lodge JP and Chan TL: *Cascade impactor sampling and analysis,* Akron, 1986, American Conference of Governmental Industrial Hygienists.

77. Rubow KL, Marple VA, Olin J, and McCawley MJ: A personal cascade impactor: Design, evaluation and calibration, *Am Ind Hyg Assoc J* 48:532-538, 1987.

78. Swift DL: Direct-reading instruments for analyzing airborne particles. In Hering SV, editor: *Air sampling instruments for evaluation of atmospheric contaminants,* pp 477-506, Cincinnati, 1989, American Conference of Governmental Industrial Hygienists.

79. Wegman DH, Eisen EA, Woskie SR, and Hu X: Measuring exposure for the epidemiologic study of acute effects, *Am J Ind Med* 21:77-89, 1992.

80. Gressel MG and Heitbrink WA, editors: Analyzing workplace exposures using direct reading instruments and video exposure monitoring techniques. US DHHS (NIOSH) Pub No 92-104, Washington DC, 1992, U.S. Government Printing Office.

81. Saltzman BE and Caplan P: Detector tubes, direct-reading passive badges and dosimeter tubes. In Hering SV, editor: *Air sampling instruments for evaluation of atmospheric contaminants,* pp 449-476, Cincinnati, 1989, American Conference of Governmental Industrial Hygienists.

82. Herrick RF, Kennedy ER, and Woebkenberg ML: Measurement of vapors and gases. In Rappaport SM and Smith TJ, editors: *Exposure assessment for epidemiology and hazard control,* pp 21-40, Chelsea, 1991, Lewis Publishers.

83. Nader JS, Lauderdale JF, and McCammon CS: Direct-reading instruments for analyzing airborne gases and vapors. In *Air sampling instruments for evaluation of atmospheric contaminants,* pp 507-558, Cincinnati, 1989, American Conference of Governmental Industrial Hygienists.

84. Baron PA: Modern real-time aerosol samplers. In *Advances in air sampling,* pp 205-224, Chelsea, 1989, Lewis Publishers.

PART II

Community

Harriet A. Burge

The agents and diseases
Approaches to exposure assessment
    Biomarkers
    Observation and sampling of reservoirs
    Air sampling
Sources of error (bias)
    Identity of the agent
    Concentration
    Form of the agent
    Exposure groups
Sources of variability
Measurement techniques for biological aerosols
Conclusions

THE AGENTS AND DISEASES

Bioaerosols are airborne particles that are derived from living organisms. Examples of some kinds of aerosols and the diseases they cause are summarized in Table 11-2-1. As noted, infections involve invasion of the host by a living organism.[1,2] Allergens induce the formation of circulating antibodies of the immunoglobulin E (IgE) class in genetically susceptible people, causing asthma and allergic rhinitis.[3] Other antigens induce the production of immunoglobulin G (IgG) and cell-mediated immune responses producing hypersensitivity pneumonitis (HP) (also called allergic

Table 11-2-1. A summary of diseases caused by bioaerosols

Disease type	Examples	Agents	Mechanism
Infections	Chicken pox Tuberculosis Aspergillosis	Viruses Bacteria Fungi	Growth in the host
Hypersensitivity	Hay fever Asthma HP	Glycoproteins from pollen, fungi, mites, mammals, etc.	Antigen/antibody, cellular immune responses
Toxicoses	Lung cancer, ODTS, immune suppression	Toxins from fungi, bacteria	Direct toxic effects as for nonbiological toxins

HP, Hypersensitivity pneumonitis; *ODTS,* organic dust toxic syndrome.

alveoli tis). Biological toxins produce direct effects on the host that are similar to those produced by other kinds of toxins.[4]

The risk of any of these diseases is related both to exposure and (for infections and hypersensitivity conditions) to specific risk factors within the hosts. Although a single organism can cause an infection, the risk of all the bioaerosol-associated diseases is related to the number of organisms or the amount of a specific agent that penetrates the airway. It appears likely that threshold doses exist for some agents. In addition, it is extremely important to remember that no hypersensitivity response (i.e., symptom) occurs on the first exposure to the agent and that sensitizing exposures always occurred in the past relative to current symptoms.

Host susceptibility factors for infectious disease include the absence of specific immunity (either naturally acquired through the disease process or artificially through immunization), and the overall status of the immune system. Only genetically susceptible people are likely to produce specific IgE antibodies, and hence develop allergic rhinitis or asthma. Host factors that control cell-mediated responses are less clear. As far as is known, there are no predisposing factors that make a host particularly sensitive to biological toxins.

The effects of each of these kinds of agents can be modified by coexposure to other agents. For example, it appears that exposure to diesel exhaust increases the risk of development of sensitization to pollen allergens.[5] Failure to account for these kinds of effects probably introduces bias into most studies of bioaerosols and disease. For example, aflatoxin exposure might be expected to increase the risk of lung cancer in heavily exposed populations. However, aflatoxin requires conversion in the lung to its active form, and coexposures with cytotoxins that prevent this conversion would obscure actual risk associated with aflatoxin exposure in environments where the cytotoxin is not present.

APPROACHES TO EXPOSURE ASSESSMENT

Bioaerosol sampling has and continues to focus on culture of viable agents and microscopy of recognizable par-

ticles. Exposure to and dose of infectious agents, allergens/antigens, and toxins are inferred from these data. However, air sampling and culture/microscopy are not necessarily the best approach to exposure assessment. Representative air samples are difficult to collect, and culture and microscopy are highly selective methods for sample analysis. There are other approaches to both sampling and sample analysis that may more accurately estimate exposure.

Biomarkers

Cases of specific infectious disease are, essentially, biomarkers of exposure to the agent. An additional biomarker for infectious disease is the specific antibody produced as a result of infection. Antibody measures ("seroconversion") can be used to document the extent of the population exposed to an infectious dose. For example, exposure to *Mycobacterium tuberculosis* may result in no effect, reproduction and the stimulation of antibodies without disease, or active tuberculosis. Since environmental monitoring is extremely difficult for this organism, seroconversion and the presence of disease are usually used to document exposure.[6]

Specific antibodies can also be used to document exposure to allergens. In the case of asthma and hay fever, allergen-specific IgE is produced as a part of the disease process.[7] The specific IgG antibodies produced during the development of hypersensitivity pneumonitis may not be associated directly with the disease, but they do indicate that exposure has occurred.[8] Note that the term "specific" is crucial. You have to decide which antigen(s) might have caused the disease before you can do the test, and negative results may only mean that the incorrect antigen was chosen. Antibodies can also be used as specific antigen markers in assays of environmental samples (see below and page 168).

Observation and sampling of reservoirs

The visual observation of reservoirs known to support and disseminate disease-causing organisms is often sufficient evidence for exposure. The visible presence of fungus growth (mold, mildew), bacterial slimes, or stagnant or recirculating water reservoirs, pets, or cockroaches, can be used as indicators for potential exposure. In problem-solving investigations, these observations can lead to recommendations and remediation without further sampling. Visual sampling has been used in epidemiologic studies to document the relationship between the presence of fungus growth or conditions known to be conducive to such growth (dampness) and the incidence of asthma.[9,10] If one must know the kinds of organisms present to make connections with existing disease, then bulk samples can be collected and analyzed. Bulk sampling of carpet dust, for example, is usually used as a surrogate measure of exposure to dust mite allergens.[11]

Air sampling

Representative air sampling for bioaerosols is a significant challenge because of the many uncontrollable errors that are inherent in the process. Some of these errors are caused by factors within the aerosol-producing populations, others by limitations of sample collection approaches, and many by variables associated with sample analysis. Before beginning an air sampling study, the following steps are essential:

1. *Clearly define the aerosol of interest with respect to the health outcome(s) to be studied.* For example, to study the potential for infection with *Aspergillus fumigatus* during surgery, only culturable *A. fumigatus* spores are of interest. On the other hand, to study asthma related to fungus exposure, fungus *antigens* are of interest, and these can be associated with any kind of fungus spore, living or dead, as well as with spore fragments and fungus metabolites that have been excreted into the environment.
2. *Decide on a sample collection mode.* The *most* important factor to consider in making this choice is the sample analysis method to be used. Some factors to consider are summarized in Table 11-2-2. Two often neglected factors in sampler selection are the length of time over which the sample can be collected and the total volume of air to be collected. These factors must be balanced against the constraints of the analytical process.
3. *Develop a sample collection protocol.* A sample must be collected that is representative of exposure. This includes minimizing variance as discussed below, providing appropriate controls, sampling in areas and at times where exposures are likely to be occurring, and, finally, remaining within budgetary constraints. In general, the collection of large amounts of air over long periods is most likely to be representative of exposure. However, high sampling rates indoors can change aerosol concentrations, and long (many hours) sampling times may obscure important peaks in concentration.

SOURCES OF ERROR (BIAS)
Identity of the agent

Many agents can cause bioaerosol-related disease, and significant bias can be introduced into studies where exposure assessment is restricted to familiar and easily sampled agents. Microscopic identification of bioaerosol particles is limited to the largest and most distinctive, and culture is highly selective for organisms with broad nutritional requirements.[12] This is why pollen and *Alternaria* are so well known as aeroallergens. Both are readily identified microscopically, and *Alternaria* grows well in culture. This approach results in large classes of fungi being ignored because they are difficult to resolve, too abundant to count, and impossible to culture and identify.

Concentration

Concentration biases related to particle collection efficiency of samplers are the same for biological as for other aerosols. Systematic bias is always introduced when using cultural analysis for bioaerosols since all culture media are selective, and many agents do not have to be alive to cause disease. Microscopy is selective in the same sense—all particles carrying specific allergens or toxins are not recognizable. Another source for counting bias using microscopy is the fact that bioaerosols are often present in low concentration relative to other particles, and that masking can occur. Counting accuracy is directly related to the biological/nonbiological particle ratio.

Finally, concentration bias is readily introduced by failing to recognize the discontinuity of bioaerosol sources and the often cyclic release patterns from such sources. Even where spatial discontinuities are recognized, sampling strategies can inadvertently be designed to either overestimate or underestimate airborne concentrations of some agents unless release is random. For example, if an organism contaminating a central ventilation system undergoes a major burst of growth during a weekend when the system is not operated, failure to sample before and during system startup on Monday morning is likely to seriously underestimate exposure.

Form of the agent

Failure to recognize the form that disease-causing agents take in aerosols and the particle size that is required to cause disease is another source of bias. For example, some infectious particles must penetrate the lower airway to cause disease (e.g., *Mycobacterium tuberculosis*).[13] Many common colds, on the other hand, require virus deposition in the upper airway, so that large particles are important.[14] Large allergen-carrying particles may be more effective than small. Consider the fact that pollens are nearly always larger than 10 μm, and that house dust mite allergen is borne in a 20-μm particle.[15] On the other hand, it appears that antigens must be respirable to cause HP.[16]

Table 11-2-2. Sampling and analysis characteristics for bioaerosols

Aerosol type	Particle size (μm)	Analytic method	Characteristics
Viable particles	0.5–50	Culture	Protect viability, prevent overloading
Bacteria	0.5–10		
Fungi	2.0–50		
Countable particles	0.5–50	Microscopy	Optical quality, prevent overloading, sufficient concentration
Fungus spores	2.0–50		
Bacteria	0.5–5		
Assayable particles	0.1–50		Elutability, sufficient concentration
Antigens	0.1–50	Immunoassay	
Endotoxin	0.1–50	Bioassay	
Mycotoxins	0.1–10	Chemistry/immunoassay	

Exposure groups

As has been previously noted, some specific susceptibility is required for many bioaerosol-related diseases. Although understanding the rate of these diseases in general populations is important, evaluating the role of specific agents in causing disease requires that studies be conducted on sensitive populations.

SOURCES OF VARIABILITY

Because bioaerosol sources are discontinuous and release effector agents into the air sporadically, environmental variability is inevitably large, and usually far exceeds both sample collection and analytical variability. Sound sampling strategies for biological aerosols that minimize variability rely on a thorough knowledge of the sources and factors affecting dispersion.

Factors affecting sample collection variability are similar to those for other kinds of aerosols. However, most kinds of bioaerosol analysis carry an inherent variability that makes aerosol collection variability insignificant. For cultural sampling, one common and often unavoidable source of variability is introduced by having too few colonies on a culture plate. Variance between side-by-side Andersen culture plate samples decreases with increasing counts on the plates. However, too many colonies allow crowding and inhibition between colonies, thus underestimating total recoveries. Similar concentration-based variability occurs with microscopic analysis.

MEASUREMENT TECHNIQUES FOR BIOLOGICAL AEROSOLS

Samplers that are commonly used for biological aerosols are clearly described by Macher et al.[17] in the ACGIH Air Sampling Instruments Manual. In general, all of the available samplers collect particle size fractions that are appropriate for most bioaerosols with the exception of the rotating arm impactors, which are useful only for particles exceeding about 15 μm. Note that any aerosol sampler could be used for a bioaerosol, providing the sample collection mode is compatible with the analytical method to be used,

again emphasizing the point that samplers should be chosen primarily to be compatible with the desired analytical method.

Available samplers fall into four categories: culture plate devices, spore traps, filtration, and liquid collectors (impingers, electrostatic precipitators). The culture plate samplers all are specifically designed to collect culturable aerosols, although they have been used (following extraction of the collection medium) for antigen assays and could similarly be used for other "assayable" agents. The Andersen culture plate sampler (the original Andersen design with 400 holes) remains the most efficient particle collection device. However, the slit impactors, the new Burkard sieve plate impactor, and the Spiral Air Systems device all collect a broad range of culturable aerosols efficiently. The centrifugal sampler appears to undersample, although this error may be due to faulty estimates of the amount of air actually collected by the device.[18] Available spore traps are similar in design to the culture-plate slit samplers and collect particles with similar efficiency. The primary factor to consider when using filtration for biological aerosols is the ease with which the agent(s) can be removed from the filter medium. At this point, smooth-surfaced polycarbonate filters appear to be the material of choice for endotoxin,[19] and similar smooth-surface materials (which limit surface area for adhesion) work well for fungus spores and bacteria. The liquid collection devices require either that particles have a hydrophilic surface or that a detergent solution be used. This is limiting for most fungus spores.

No direct-reading instruments are currently available that will measure concentrations of any biological aerosol. Direct particle counters may be useful in occupational settings where a single kind of bioaerosol is the major component of "dust" aerosols (e.g., in fermentation industries where fungi are used to mass-produce specific metabolites). However, in nearly all other environments, nonbiological particles will far exceed biologicals in concentration, making the relatively small changes in bioaerosol concentrations imperceptible to the instrument.

CONCLUSIONS

In conclusion, the most important point to remember regarding bioaerosols is that the term represents many disparate kinds of aerosols and that assessment of exposure (including sample collection, analysis, extrapolation of dose, and risk assessment) is specific to the individual kind of aerosol. Any exposure assessment study must be designed either to be agent-specific, or must be broad enough so that unknown agents are equally represented in the sampling and analysis plan.

REFERENCES

1. Burge HA: Indoor air and infectious disease. In Cone JE and Hodgson MJ, editors: *Problem buildings: building-associated illness and the sick building syndrome. State of the art reviews. Occup Med* 4(4):713-721, 1989.
2. Burge HA: Risks associated with indoor infectious aerosols, *Toxicol Indust Health* 6(2):263-273, 1990.
3. Roitt I, Brostoff J, and Male D: *Immunology,* ed 3, St. Louis, MO, 1993, Mosby.
4. Cole RJ: *Modern methods in the analysis and structural elucidation of mycotoxins.* New York, 1986, Academic Press.
5. Takafuji S, Suzuki S, Koizumi K, Tadokoro K, Miyamoto T, Ikemori R, and Muranaka M: Diesel exhaust particulates inoculated by the intranasal route have an adjuvant activity for IgE production in mice. *J Allergy Clin Immunol* 79:639-645, 1987.
6. Kent DC et al: Tuberculin conversion: the iceberg of tuberculosis pathogenesis, *Arch Environ Health* 14:580, 1967b.
7. Barbee RA, Brown GB, Kaltenborn WS, and Halonen M: Allergen skin test reactivity in a community population sample: correlation with age, histamine skin reaction and total serum immunoglobulin E. *J Allergy Clin Immunol* 68:15, 1981.
8. Burrell R and Rylander R: A critical review of the role of precipitins in hypersensitivity pneumonitis, *Eur J Respir Dis* 62:332-343, 1981.
9. Strachan DP and Sanders CH: Damp housing and childhood asthma, respiratory effects of indoor temperature and relative humidity, *J Epidemiol Commun Health* 43:7-14, 1989.
10. Waegemaekers M, Van Wageningen N, Brunekreef B, and Boleij JS: Respiratory symptoms in damp homes. A pilot study, *Allergy* 44(3):192-198, 1989.
11. Chapman MD, Heymann PW, Wilkins SR, Brown MJ, and Platts Mills TAE: Monoclonal immunoassays for the major dust mite *(Dermatophagoides)* allergens, *Der p* I and *Der f* I, and quantitative analysis of the allergen content of mite and house dust extracts, *J Allergy Clin Immun* 80:184-194, 1987.
12. Muilenberg ML: Aeroallergen assessment by microscopy and culture, *Immunol Allergy Clin N Am* 9(2):245, 1989.
13. Wells WF, Radcliffe HL, and Crumb C: On mechanics of droplet nuclei infection: quantitative experimental airborne infection in rabbits, *Am J Hyg* 47:11-28, 1948.
14. Dick EC, Jennings LC, Mink KA et al: Aerosol transmission of rhinovirus colds, *J Infect Dis* 156:442, 1987.
15. Swanson MC, Campbell AR, Klauck MJ, and Reed CE: Correlations between levels of mite and cat allergens in settled and airborne dust, *J Allergy Clin Immunol* 83(4):776-783, 1989.
16. Fink J: Hypersensitivity pneumonitis, *J Allergy Clin Immunol* 74:1, 1984.
17. Macher JM, Chatigny MA, and Burge HA: Sampling airborne microorganisms and aeroallergens, In Hering SV, editor: *Air sampling instruments,* ed 8, Cincinnati, 1995, American Conference of Governmental Industrial Hygienists, in press.
18. Macher JM and First MW: Reuter centrifugal air sampler: measurement of effective airflow rate and collection efficiency, *Appl Environ Microbiol* 45:1960-1962, 1983.
19. Milton DK, Gere RJ, Feldman HA, and Greaves IA: Endotoxin measurement: aerosol sampling and application of a new Limulus method, *Am Ind Hyg Assoc J* 51(6):331-337, 1990.

PART III

Exposure Assessment in the Ambient Environment

Michael A. McCawley

TEAM AND THE APPROACHES

The major differences between exposure assessment methods developed for the occupational environment and those developed for the ambient environment arise due to the unbounded nature of the community exposure and the relative importance of routes of exposure other than the respiratory system. In the occupational environment, the job and job tasks can be used to help define exposure. In the community environment, area of residence has been used in a manner comparable with the job. This has led, historically, to exposure assessment schemes in the nonoccupational environment that are *source based*, attempting to assign exposure on the basis of an average ambient concentration. In turn, the average ambient concentration is assumed to be the result of the strength of a source or sources of the ambient pollutant at a specific location.

Alternatively, a *risk-based* strategy has been proposed that attempts to apportion sources, including indoor air pollutants, to individuals. The two approaches are similar to the approaches in the industrial environment of area and personal sampling. *Total Human Exposure* (THE), the term coined to encompass the risk-based or personal exposure assessment strategies,[1] indicates a change in direction toward more personal sampling. *Total Exposure Assessment Methodology* (TEAM) employ both personal sampling and biological markers to determine individual dose as part of a THE assessment.[2-4] Although the THE approach can provide useful information to correlate response with exposure, there is a drawback. The drawback in a risk-based approach is the effort that must be expended to monitor the exposure of a large population. Because of temporal[5] and spatial variability,[6] it is not clear that personal sampling of a very small percentage of a population over short time periods will provide sufficient information to determine the average exposure or the variability in exposure of the population. If the purpose of the exposure assessment is to ensure that adequate protection is being provided to the population in general, a source-based strategy may still provide the best information.

Source-based exposure assessments require information from air models, which in turn may rely on meteorologic and topographic information. The information from the air models yields concentration isopleths and allows source apportionment. As the final check, area monitoring stations yield either time-weighted concentrations or continuous data. Because of the cost of purchasing and maintaining the monitors it is not uncommon for tens to hundreds of square kilometers to be represented by a single monitoring site. The ability of the monitoring station to represent the effect of local sources is therefore less than that of distant sources, since the distant sources will more likely be uniformly mixed throughout the area. As long as one understands the shortcomings of the various approaches, it is still possible to work with the data they provide.

AIR POLLUTION MODELS

There are three basic classes of models. *dispersion models,*[7] *box models,*[8] and *receptor models.*[9,10] Dispersion and box models use the known output of sources to predict the downwind concentration from the source. Receptor models, conversely, use the characteristics of the downwind concentration to apportion the concentration from the various contributing sources. The receptor models have been used where either trace elements or particular compounds allow a source to be uniquely identified or *fingerprinted.* Thus sources of both particles[11-13] and volatile organic compounds[14,15] have been studied.

The difference between the dispersion and box models lies in the underlying assumption concerning the movement of the contaminant away from the source. The dispersion model assumes no build-up of contaminant within the volume being modeled. The concentration is inversely proportional to the wind speed, however. Therefore at low wind speeds the model tends to overpredict the downwind concentration. The box model, on the other hand, allows for some build-up and is not necessarily affected by low wind speeds. The information required to use the box model to reasonably predict the concentration on a volume scale the size of a human makes the approach almost unusable. That is why the evaluation of most industrial site air pollution impacts is done using the dispersion model modified for various situations.

The receptor model is a statistical model using a least squares regression technique with known tracer compounds to identify the contribution of various sources. This technique may also be useful in determining whether all sources impacting on a given site have been identified.

MEASUREMENT TECHNIQUES

In general, measurement techniques for ambient air monitoring are similar to those used in the occupational environment. The thoracic fraction of airborne particulate has its equivalent, for example, in the PM-10 sampler used for ambient particle sampling.[16,17] In fact, one of the primary concerns in ambient particle sampling is the effect of high wind speed on the sampling characteristics of the PM-10, with special emphasis given to inlet design.[18,19]

One area of difference is remote sensing. Remote sensing is useful in ambient air for sampling inaccessible locations or detecting fugitive emissions. The techniques used for remote sensing also allow short sample duration, simultaneous measurement of multiple contaminants, and no worries about sample integrity or sampling loss. As well, the remotely sensed contaminant concentrations can be combined with meteorologic data to yield information on emission rates for an area.[20] Fourier transform infrared (FTIR) spectroscopy and differential optical absorption spectroscopy (DOAS) are both commercially available means of doing the remote sensing.

Secondary pollutants

Another difference is the concern over the formation and subsequent detection of secondary pollutants. In the presence of sunlight, emitted contaminants can undergo chemical transformation. The chemical smog so frequently associated with Los Angeles air, though actually ubiquitous in most urban areas, is the result of complex photochemical interactions of nitrogen oxides, hydrocarbons, and particulate as well as water vapor.[21,22] Once formed, these secondary species and the primary species from which they have evolved can be transported by weather systems in the atmosphere over continental distances. For example, the haze in the eastern United States appears to be due to sulfate particulate, generated photochemically and dispersed over may hundreds of kilometers.[23] Contaminant levels of these species will be independent of local activity in most cases, making exposure assessment more complicated.

Ambient air quality standards

There are actually three separate sets of standards used to control atmospheric contamination. *Source,* or emission standards, regulate the amount of material a source is allowed to release into the atmosphere. *Prevention of significant deterioration* (PSD) standards are used in conjunction with air model to limit the potential impact a new source will have on existing air quality in a region. Finally, *ambient air quality standards* are used in conjunction with am-

Table 11-3-1. U.S. national ambient air quality standards (40 CFR Part 50)

Pollutant	Primary standard ($\mu g/m^3$)	Averaging time
Sulfur dioxide	80	1 yr
	365	24 hr
Nitrogen dioxide	100	1 yr
Carbon monoxide	10,000	8 hr
	40,000	1 hr
Ozone	235	1 hr
PM-10 (particulate)	50	1 yr
	150	24 hr
Lead	1.5	¼ yr

bient air sampling to protect both health and property. For protecting health, primary standard levels are set with various averaging times depending on the action of the pollutant. By regulation, one exceedance per year of any of the averaging time values is allowed. Table 11-3-1 gives the values and averaging times for the federally regulated ambient air contaminants in the United States. The regulatory basis for air pollution control in the United States is discussed in detail in Chapter 55.

CONCLUSIONS

The trend toward more personal sampling for ambient exposures is a clear indication of the difficulty in assigning personal exposure from ambient area data. The sources of variation include spatial and temporal differences in air concentration, the effect of indoor activity to increase exposure in some cases while decreasing it in others, and a level of uncertainty in predicting the impact from local or distant sources on a particular area. These sources of variability are in addition to those mentioned for the occupational environment. Area monitoring, on the other hand, is probably the best way to ensure that regional compliance is being maintained. Although this is not an assurance that any single individual is overexposed, it is probably a better indicator of population exposure. If the health of individuals is being monitored, personal sampling would appear to be the best alternative, but to draw conclusions about a large population, area monitoring and source characterization cannot be neglected.

REFERENCES

1. Ott WR: Total human exposure: basic concepts, EPA field studies and future research needs, *J Air Waste Manage Assoc* 40:966-975, 1990.
2. Wallace LA: *The total exposure assessment methodology (TEAM) study: summary and analysis,* vol 1, EPA 600/6-87/002a, Washington, DC, 1987, U.S. Environmental Protection Agency.
3. Wallace LA, Pellizzari ED, Hartwell TD, Whitmore R, Zelon H, Perritt R, and Sheldon L: The California TEAM study: breath concentrations and personal exposures to 26 volatile compounds in air and drinking water of 188 residents of Los Angeles, Antioch, and Pittsburg, CA, *Atmos Environ* 22:2141-2163, 1988.
4. Levin A, Fratt DB, Leonard A, Bruins RJF, and Fradkin L: Comparative analysis of health risk assessments for municipal waste combustors, *J Air Waste Manage Assoc* 41:20-31, 1991.
5. Aceves M and Grimalt JO: Seasonally dependent size distributions of aliphatic and polycyclic aromatic hydrocarbons in urban aerosols from densely populated areas, *Environ Sci Technol* 27:2896-2908, 1993.
6. Hewitt CN: Spatial variations in nitrogen dioxide concentrations in an urban area, *Atmos Environ* 25B:429-434, 1991.
7. Turner BB: *Workbook of atmospheric dispersion estimates,* U.S. Department of Health Education and Welfare, Cincinnati, OH, 1970, National Air Pollution Control Administration.
8. Stern AC, Boubel RW, Turner DB, and Fox DL: *Fundamentals of air pollution,* ed 2, Orlando, 1984, Academic Press.
9. Cooper JA and Watson JG: Receptor oriented methods of air particulate source apportionment, *J Air Pollut Control Assoc* 30:1116-1125, 1980.
10. Gordon GE: Receptor models, *Environ Sci Technol* 22:1132-1142, 1988.
11. Kneip TJ, Mallon RP, and Kleinman MT: The impact of changing air quality on multiple regression models for coarse and fine particle fractions, *Atmos Environ* 17:299-304, 1983.
12. Thurston GD and Spengler JD: A quantitative assessment of source contributions to inhalable particulate matter in metropolitan Boston, *Atmos Environ* 19:9-25, 1985.
13. Morandi MT, Daisey JM, and Lioy PJ: Development of a modified factor analysis/multiple regression model to apportion suspended particulate matter in a complex urban airshed, *Atmos Environ* 21:1821-1831, 1987.
14. Nelson PF, Quigley SM, and Smith MY: Sources of atmospheric hydrocarbons in Sydney: a quantitative determination using source reconciliation techniques, *Atmos Environ* 17:439-449, 1983.
15. Scheff PA and Kleos M: Source-receptor analysis of volatile hydrocarbons, *J Environ Eng* 113:994-1005, 1987.
16. EPA: *Air quality criteria for particulate matter and sulfur oxides,* Research Triangle Park, NC, 1982, U.S. Environmental Protection Agency.
17. McFarland AR and Ortiz CA: A 10μm outpoint ambient aerosol sampling inlet, *Atmos Environ* 16:2959-2965, 1982.
18. Rodes CE, Holland DM, Purdue LJ, and Rehme KA: A field comparison of PM inlets at four locations, *J Air Pollut Control Assoc* 35:345-354, 1985.
19. Wedding JB and Weigand MA: The Wedding ambient aerosol sampling inlet ($D_{50} = 10\mu m$) for the high volume sampler, *Atmos Environ* 19:535-538, 1985.
20. Grant WB, Kagan RH, and McClenny WA: Optical remote measurement of toxic gases, *J Air Waste Manage Assoc* 42:18-30, 1992.
21. Calvert JC: Test of the theory of ozone generation in Los Angles atmosphere, *Environ Sci Technol* 10:248-255, 1976.
22. Kelly NA: Ozone precursor relationships in the Detroit metropolitan area derived from captive air irradiation and an empirical photochemical model, *J Air Pollut Control Assoc* 35:27-34, 1985.
23. Lippmann M and Schlesinger RB: *Chemical contamination in the human environment,* p 134, New York, 1979, Oxford University Press.

Chapter 12

MINERALOGY

Robert P. Nolan
Arthur M. Langer

Minerals are defined as naturally occurring inorganic substances that possess a defined range of elemental composition, have a set of characteristic properties, and are crystalline.[1,2] Substances that are inorganic, noncrystalline, and somewhat variable in composition, such as diatomaceous earth and volcanic glasses, are referred to as mineraloids. Organic bitumens fall into this latter category as well.

This chapter reviews general principles of mineral characteristics and methods of identification. We also discuss several specific minerals in detail to illustrate the importance of mineralogy in understanding respiratory health effects.

More than 3500 minerals have been described in the literature, but exposure to only a relative few has been recognized as causing disease in humans or has produced adverse effects in experimental animals. For humans the common route of exposure comes about through the inhalation of dust (i.e., suspensions of fine mineral particulates carried as aerosols into the lungs during inspiration). The aerosol may be composed of a single mineral type, but exposure to complex mineral mixtures is far more common. Therefore, much of the observed human health effects have been associated with exposure to mixtures of minerals crushed to fine respirable powders during mining, milling, industrial processing, product manufacturing, and use. It is noted that some minerals with little or no industrial importance, such as the fibrous zeolite and erionite, have been linked to human disease in the environmental setting.[3]

Mineral types defined

A single mineral type is characterized by a particular crystal structure and often a range of elemental composition. A crystal structure defines a highly ordered spatial arrangement of atoms or molecules repeated over long distances three dimensionally. The elements of the crystal structure can be described almost entirely by a small number of atoms (usually fewer than 100) contained in a parallelepiped, defined as the unit cell.[4] The entire crystal is thus formed through periodic repetition in three dimensions of the atomic matter, contained within the volume of the unit-cell. These two characteristics, structure and elemental composition, basically define a mineral. Even though large single crystals can be meters in size, the physicochemical characteristics required to identify the mineral type are on the order of tens of angstroms ($\sim 10^{-8}$ m).

Mineral varieties and habits

Even small chemical variation in minerals may give rise to differences in color or some physical property that typifies the species. As an example, quartz constitutes the varietal minerals called amethyst, cat's eye, tiger's eye, and aventurine, as well as the massive varieties called chalcedony, flint, agate, onyx, and jasper, among others. Small differences in crystal growth conditions or the presence of trace metals can account for the color differences in these varieties. Grinders, polishers, and cutters exposed to dusts generated from these varieties are all exposed to the same substance: quartz.

In addition to the chemical variation of mineral types, the physical form in which it occurs in nature may vary as well. Some minerals can occur in several different common forms, referred to as mineral habits. For example, the amphibole mineral grunerite may develop in nature as a massive, morphologically formless, rock-forming silicate; as prism-shaped crystals (prismatic); or, under appropriate conditions, as long flexible fibers. Grunerite having this asbestiform habit is called amosite asbestos.[4,5]

A mineral type can also form in nature with two distinctly different crystal structures but have the same chemical composition. This polymorphism is usually the result of local variation in temperature or pressure. Often, the two distinct forms are given different mineral names. The crystalline silica minerals, all SiO_2 in composition, are a good example of this.

Physicochemical properties giving rise to biologic activity

Three physicochemical properties of the constituent particulates are important for health hazard evaluation of minerals: morphology, surface properties, and durability in tissue.[6]

There are seven polymorphs of SiO_2, all having distinct crystal structures. These are quartz, cristobalite, tridymite, moganite, melanophlogite, coesite, and stishovite. There are three polymorphs within the serpentine mineral group—antigorite, lizardite, and chrysotile—the latter an asbestos mineral (Table 12-1).

The morphology of a mineral particle, which includes size and shape, determines respirability. Generally, at least one dimension must be less than 5 μm for a particle to be considered respirable, although particles less than 1 μm have been more commonly associated with disease. For those particles with a fibrous morphology, particular importance is associated with length and diameter. Fibers greater than 100 μm in length are respirable as long as the diameter is less than 5 μm. Fibers having lengths of at least 8 μm and diameters of 0.25 μm or less, referred to as the Stanton dimensions, are thought to be particularly dangerous in terms of carcinogenesis.[7,8]

If surface properties impart some of a mineral's biologic activity, then the surface area and the mass of dust are of importance. Therefore, exposure to a given mineral (e.g., quartz) may produce a range of health hazards depending on factors beyond mineral name. This concept has been studied in detail for quartz,[9,10] the titanium dioxide polymorphs,[11] and the fibrous clay palygorskite, each derived from a different geologic locale.[12]

It is widely held that the greater the residence time in tissues, the greater the effect exerted by a toxic particle.[13]

Methods of identification

A mineral may be identified on the basis of its crystal structure and elemental composition. This has led to the development of a wide array of methodologies to determine these properties (see reference 14 for a recent review). Two of the most commonly used methods for mineral analysis are continuous scan x-ray diffraction and polarized light microscopy.[15,16] When used together, these two methods are generally adequate to identify the major mineral components present in most bulk powders.

For a mineral to produce a pneumoconiosis, the particles must be small enough to penetrate the lung defenses and come to lodge in the target tissue. Therefore, it is important to characterize size, concentration, and type of minerals present in the fine dust fraction. Respirable particles can

Table 12-1. Mineralogy of regulated asbestos fiber types

Commercial name	Mineral name	Mineral group	Chemical formula
Amosite	Grunerite	Amphibole	$(Fe^{2+},Mg)_7[Si_8O_{22}](OH)_2$
Anthophyllite	Anthophyllite*	Amphibole	$(Mg,Fe^{2+})_7[Si_8O_{22}](OH)_2$
Chrysotile	Chrysotile*	Serpentine	$Mg_3[Si_2O_5](OH)_4$
Crocidolite	Riebeckite	Amphibole	$Na_2Fe_2^{3+}(Fe^{2+},Mg)_3[Si_8O_{22}](OH)_2$
Tremolite	Tremolite*	Amphibole	$Ca_2Mg_5[Si_8O_{22}](OH)_2$
Actinolite	Actinolite*	Amphibole	$Ca_2(Mg,Fe^{2+})_5[Si_8O_{22}](OH)_2$

*These minerals do not have separate names for their asbestos analogs. Mineralogists now refer to amosite as *grunerite asbestos* and crocidolite as *riebeckite asbestos*. Note that grunerite is an end member of the iron-magnesium series cummingtonite-grunerite (see Table 12-2). Amosite is occasionally referred to as cummingtonite-grunerite asbestos.

be collected on a membrane filter or separated from a tissue specimen. However, these particles may be present in mass concentrations too low to obtain an interpretable x-ray diffraction pattern. The use of light optical methods is also limited because the very small particles cannot be resolved. Such samples, especially dusts recovered from lung tissues, may best be analyzed by using a transmission electron microscope equipped with an energy-dispersive x-ray spectrometer.[17] Under certain conditions transmission electron microscopy allows the analyst to determine the elemental composition and crystallographic characteristics (by electron diffraction) of fine particles. Identification, again, relies on morphology, structure, and chemistry. The application of mineralogy to the study of health effects is illustrated here by several examples: asbestos, zeolites, palygorskite, synthetic organic fibers, silica polymorphs, talc, and the polymorphs of titanium dioxide.

NATURALLY OCCURRING AND MAN-MADE FIBERS
Regulated asbestos minerals

Five of the six minerals regulated in the United States as asbestos are part of an important group of rock-forming silicates referred to as amphiboles (Table 12-1). This mineral group accounts for approximately 5% by volume of the earth's crust.[18] A small amount of three of these amphiboles—amosite, anthophyllite, and crocidolite—occurs as asbestos in deposits of commercial importance. Actinolite and tremolite complete the group of five U.S.-regulated asbestos amphiboles, although commercially important deposits of these two minerals are rare.

Amphiboles. All amphiboles are characterized by double chains of linked silica tetrahedra that lie parallel to the *c* axis, almost always in the direction of crystal elongation. Amphiboles crystallize in either the orthorhombic

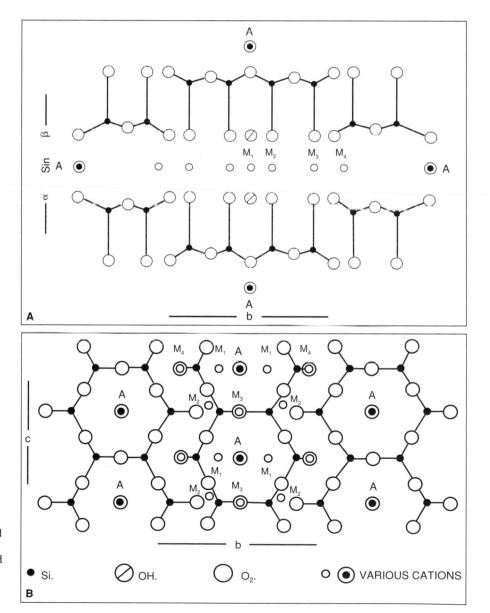

Fig. 12-1. The crystal structure of amphiboles: schematic 001 and 100 projections of the structure of monoclinic amphiboles. **A,** Projected normal to the *c* axis; **B,** Projected normal to a sin β. (Adapted from Pooley FD: Asbestos mineralogy. In Antman K and Aisner J, editors: *Asbestos-related malignancy,* Orlando, Fla, 1987, Grune & Stratton.)

(a ≠ b ≠ c and α = β = γ = 90°) or monoclinic *(a ≠ b ≠ c* and α = γ = 90°, while β ≠ 90°) crystal systems. Between the facing silica double chains are four dissimilar octahedral sites with seven atomic positions (Fig. 12-1). These sites can accommodate cations of different sizes. Therefore, the amphibole group has complex and far-ranging elemental compositions. The amphibole group is made up of 27 separate mineral types with a large number of varietal species based on 23 chemical prefixes.[19,20]

Because crystal structures of the different amphiboles are similar, a knowledge of the elemental composition is often required to assign a mineral name to a given specimen. The chemical prefixes mentioned are necessary because of occasional and marked changes in the concentration of a particular cation. Continuous substitution of cations in a structure produces a solid solution. The replacement of the magnesium in tremolite by ferrous iron (which has virtually the same ionic radius in sixfold coordination) produces a change in mineral designation. Tremolite becomes actinolite when the ratio of Mg to Mg + Fe is between 0.5 and 0.9.

In 1978 an effort was made to simplify the number of mineral names used to describe the chemically diverse amphibole group. Recommendations were made that the names used to describe two of the commercially important amphibole asbestos minerals, amosite and crocidolite, be changed. *Amosite* (an acronym for *asbestos mines of South Africa*) and *crocidolite* (meaning "woolly rock") were recommended for abandonment, and the formal mineral names, *grunerite asbestos* and *riebeckite asbestos,* were to be used instead.[19,20]

Crystal structure. The modern understanding of amphiboles began in 1916 with the determination of the elemental composition of tremolite $[Ca_2Mg_5Si_8O_{22}(OH)_2]$ and some of the characteristics of the crystal structure.[21,22] With the development of x-ray structure analysis by 1930, Warren[21] was able to determine that tremolite was monoclinic, with two unit chemical formulas in the unit cell (Z = 2). As the crystal structures of a number of monoclinic and orthorhombic amphiboles of diverse elemental composition were elucidated, the structures were found to be remarkably similar (Table 12-2). The salient structural features are the following:

- Silica tetrahedra form a double chain with the repeating unit having the composition $Si_4O_{11}^{6-}$. This unit repeats approximately every 5.3 Å in the *c* direction. There are eight silicon atoms in the tetrahedral sites (T sites) per formula unit. In some amphiboles aluminum can partly replace silicon.
- The silica chain structure is four octahedra wide. These octahedra form four crystallographically distinct cation sites and are referred to as M_1, M_2, M_3, and M_4. Within these four octahedral sites lie seven cations per formula unit: $2M_1$, $2M_2$, $1M_3$, and $2M_4$. The octahedra can have corners that are not shared with the silica tetrahedra. These corners are occupied by hydroxyl groups, al-

Table 12-2. Physicochemical characteristics of the regulated amphibole asbestos minerals

	Anthophyllite	Cummingtonite-grunerite (amosite)	Tremolite-actinolite	Riebeckite (crocidolite)
Formula	$(Mg,Fe)_7Si_8O_{22}(OH)_2$	$(Fe,Mg)_7Si_8O_{22}(OH)_2$	$Ca_2(Mg,Fe)Si_8O_{22}(OH)_2$	$Na_2Fe_2^{3+}(Fe^{2+},Mg)_3[Si_8O_{22}](OH)$
Crystal system	Orthorhombic	Monoclinic	Monoclinic	Monoclinic
a	18.56	9.51	9.86	9.73
b	18.01	18.19	18.11	18.06
c	5.28	5.33	5.34	5.33
β		101.83°	105.00°	103.30°
Z	4	2	2	2
Space group	*P2/nma*	*C2/m*	*C2/m*	*C2/m*
Indices of refraction				
α	1.60*	1.644	1.608	1.693
β	1.62	1.657	1.618	1.701
γ	1.674	1.674	1.674	1.709
Density (g/cm³)	2.9-3.2	2.9-3.2	3.0-3.3	3.38-3.41

*The indices of refraction range according to chemistry. Substitution of, for example, iron for magnesium produces a corresponding increase in values. The range in density changes accordingly as well.

Table 12-3. Bulk chemical analyses of the regulated asbestos minerals*

	Amosite (grunerite asbestos)	Anthophyllite	Crocidolite (riebeckite asbestos)	Tremolite	Actinolite	Chrysotile
SiO_2	49.70	57.20	50.90	55.10	53.80	41.80
Al_2O_3	0.40	—	—	1.14	1.20	0.11
Fe_2O_3	0.03	0.13	16.85	0.32	1.90	0.68
FeO	39.70	10.12	20.50	2.00	25.30	0.05
MnO	0.22	—	0.05	0.10	0.40	0.04
MgO	6.44	29.21	1.06	25.65	4.30	42.82
CaO	1.04	1.02	1.45	11.45	10.20	0.10
K_2O	0.63	—	0.20	0.29	0.40	0.01
Na_2O	0.09	—	6.20	0.14	0.10	0.03
H_2O^+	1.83	2.18	2.37	3.52	2.60	14.04
H_2O^-	0.09	0.28	0.22	0.16	—	0.28
CO_2	0.09	—	0.20	0.06	0.20	0.01
TOTALS	100.26	100.14	100.00	99.93	100.40	99.97

*Amosite, Transvaal, Republic of South Africa; anthophyllite, Paakkila, Finland; crocidolite, Cape Province, Republic of South Africa; tremolite, Pakistan; actinolite, Cape Province; chrysotile, New York.

though rarely another anion (Cl^- or F^-) can substitute for OH.

- Between the double chains, within the sixfold rings of linked silica tetrahedra, there is an additional row of sites referred to as the A sites. These sites can be occupied by large cations (e.g., sodium or potassium only) to the extent required to balance the charge. These sites are never fully occupied in the amphibole asbestos minerals.

Chemical composition. The M_1, M_2, and M_3 octahedral sites form a chain consisting of five cations per formula unit, which are between facing sixfold rings of silica tetrahedra (Fig. 12-1). These octahedral chains are linked by the large M_4 cations. Additional large ions, A ions, can be found in the A structural site. The general formula for all amphibole compositions is

$$A_{0-1}(M_4)_2(M_1)_2(M_2)_2(M_3)_1T_8O_{22}(OH)_2$$

where $A = Na^+$ and K^+ in 10- to 12-fold coordination. $M_4 = Ca^{2+}$, Na^+, Mn^{2+}, Fe^{2+}, Mg^{2+}, and Li^+ in six- or eight-fold coordination. M_1, M_2, and $M_3 = Mg^{2+}$, Fe^{2+}, Mn^{2+}, Fe^{3+}, Al^{3+}, and Ti^{4+} in sixfold coordination. $T = Si^{4+}$ and Al^{3+} in the tetrahedral sites forming the double chains.

Complete substitution can occur between Na^+ and Ca^{2+} and between Mg^{2+} and Fe^{2+} or Mn^{2+}. Limited substitution can occur between Fe^{3+} and Al^{3+}. A more limited substitution occurs in the T sites between Al^{3+} and Si^{4+}; this rarely occurs in amphibole asbestos[23] (Table 12-3). In the earlier literature the designations *W, X,* and *Y* were used to describe the (A), (M_4), and (M_1, M_2, and M_3) sites, respectively.

Serpentines. Serpentines contain two sheets: one of $(Si_2O_5)^{2n-}$ and the other a nonsilicate sheet of

Table 12-4. Worldwide production of chrysotile asbestos, 1990 to 1993 (in metric tons)

	1990	1992	1993*
Russia	2,593,000	ND	ND
Canada	685,627	585,000	ND
Brazil	232,332	233,000	230,000
China	191,800	240,000	240,000
Zimbabwe	165,085	140,000	140,000
South Africa	154,000	124,000	124,000
Greece	65,953	ND	ND
Swaziland	26,000	ND	ND
India	25,950	ND	ND
United States	20,000	16,000	15,000
Yugoslavia	20,000	ND	ND
Columbia	10,500	ND	ND
Others	18,526		
TOTALS	4,209,773	1,338,000	749,000

Data are from the U.S. Bureau of Mines, Washington, D.C., and the Asbestos Institute, Montreal.
*Estimates.
ND, No data available.

$[Mg_3O_2(OH)_4]_n^{2n+}$. The most important member of the group is chrysotile, which is the sixth mineral regulated under the U.S. asbestos standard. This is the type of asbestos that has been used most commonly in commerce and represents the only form of asbestos still of commercial importance (Table 12-4). There is currently no amosite production worldwide, whereas crocidolite production is approximately 16,000 tons/yr. The crocidolite produced is almost exclusively used as a component in high-pressure cement pipe in eastern Mediterranean regions. Two other important magnesium silicates—lizardite and antigorite—form part of the serpentine group.[24]

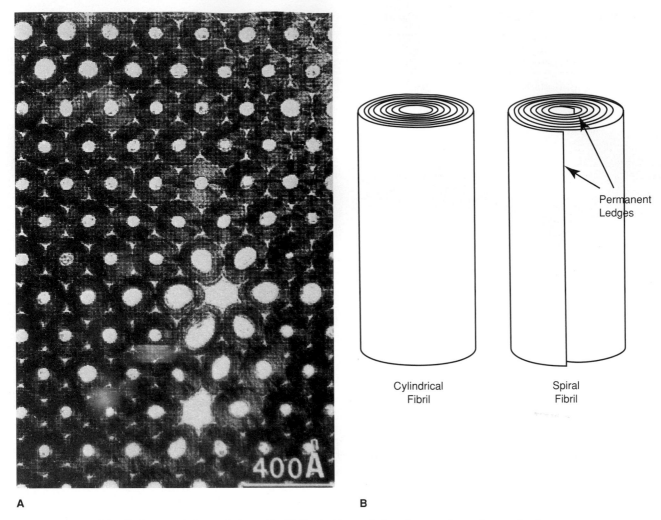

A

B

Fig. 12-2. Morphology of chrysotile fibrils. **A,** Transmission electron photomicrograph of a cross-section of chrysotile fibrils. (Adapted from Baronnet A: Polytypism and stacking disorder. In Bureck PR, editor: *Minerals and reactions at the atomic scale: transmission electron microscopy,* reviews in mineralogy, vol 27, Washington, DC, 1992, Mineralogical Society of America.) **B,** Schematic representation of the cylindrical and spiral fibril. (Adapted from Veblen DR and Wylie AG: Mineralogy of amphiboles and 1:1 layer silicates. In: Guthrie GD and Mossman BT, editors: *Health effects of mineral dusts,* reviews in mineralogy, vol 28, Washington, DC, 1993, Mineralogical Society of America.)

These three magnesium silicates form part of a larger group of layered silicates—the phyllosilicates—which include kaolin, talc, vermiculite, and micas, among many others.[25] The serpentine group is less diverse in its elemental composition than the amphiboles, but its members are structurally more complex. Lizardite and chrysotile can have identical elemental composition, whereas antigorite chemically differs slightly but systematically from them.[26,27,28]

These three common serpentine minerals, which include chrysotile (Fig. 12-2), arise because of the different means by which the unit chemical layers are structurally accommodated. The three minerals all consist of two component layers, a tetrahedral $(Si_2O_5)^{2n-}$ sheet and an octahedral $(Mg[OH]_2)$ sheet. The basic units of the tetra-

hedral sheet are six-membered rings, having pseudohexagonal or trigonal symmetry. These rings are similar to those found in amphibole double chains. The amphibole chains differ in that the growth is restricted to a single direction to form chains, whereas in the serpentines growth extends in two directions to form an infinite sheet. The octahedral sheet is formed by magnesium octahedrally coordinated with oxygen and hydroxyl groups and is similar to that found in brucite. The dimensions of the two sheets differ. Attention is generally focused on the *b* axis of the octahedral sheet, which is larger than the same axial direction in the tetrahedral sheet (9.45 Å compared with 9.15 Å). The three different serpentine minerals arise from the three structural solutions that compensate for the mismatch.[24,26]

Erionite and other zeolites

Chemistry, structure, and morphology. The zeolite group of minerals are framework aluminosilicates [a mineral has a three-dimensional framework structure through the linking of $(Si,Al)O_4$ tetrahedral to four like tetrahedra] and were first described by Cronstedt, a Swedish mineralogist, in 1756. The name *zeolite* is also derived from the Greek meaning "stone that boils," an attribution to the fact that water is released from the mineral when it is heated. The ability to absorb water into channels formed by the aluminosilicate framework is a fundamental property of all zeolite minerals. The water in the channels can be driven off by heating and reabsorbed from the atmosphere as the temperature is reduced. The large internal surface area makes zeolites useful for catalysis, for ion exchange, and as molecular sieves. These minerals can occur in platy, equant, or fibrous forms.

The general formula for the framework of all the naturally occurring zeolites is $(Al_mSi_{n-m}O_{2n})^{m-}$. The negative charge in natural zeolite is balanced by loosely bound extra-framework alkali and alkaline cations. Usually, these are potassium, sodium, and calcium and less frequently lithium, magnesium, strontium, and barium are found. The general formula for natural zeolite is:

$$(Li,Na,K)_a (Mg,Ca,Si,Ba)_d[Al_{(a+2d)}Si_{n\ (a+2d)}O_{2n}]mH_2O$$

The portion of the generic formula in the brackets represents the atoms of the framework, whereas the notation outside the brackets represents the extra-framework alkali and alkaline earth cations and water.

The name *erionite* is derived from the Greek for "woolly." It was proposed in 1898 by Eakle to describe a fibrous mineral occurring in the seams of rhyolite tuffs in Durkee, Oregon. Erionite is one of approximately 48 known naturally occurring zeolites.[29,30]

The chemical formula for erionite is $NaK_2MgCa_{1.5}[Al_8Si_{28}O_{72}] \cdot 28H_2O$. The erionite framework is characterized by the presence of three types of cavities—those formed by double sixfold rings, the cancrinite cages, and the erionite cages (Fig. 12-3). The AlO_4^{5-} and SiO_4^{4-} tetrahedra are linked to each other in the framework to form the interconnected cages and channels. The double sixfold rings are empty, and the extra-framework cations and water molecules are found in the cancrinite and erionite cages. In hydrated erionite the potassium is in the cancrinite cage, although, as the framework is dehydrated, internal exchange with calcium occurs. In the hydrated crystal, calcium, as well as sodium and magnesium, are present in several sites within the erionite cage.

Human health effects and exposure. The study of erionite illustrates the critical role of mineralogic considerations in evaluating respiratory effects. In the early 1970s a survey to identify and treat rural cases of tuberculosis was undertaken in a mountainous region on the central Anatolian plateau in Turkey called Cappadocia. Chest radiographs showed pleural fibrosis and calcification that resembled healed tuberculosis scars but also demonstrated bilateral pleural thickening, which is not normally associated with tuberculosis. Interviews revealed histories of recurrent benign pleural effusions (known to be associated with asbestos exposure).[31,32]

One case of malignant pleural mesothelioma (see reference 31 for a review) was found. This raised interest because previously mesothelioma had been considered as a signal tumor for asbestos exposure.[33] Subsequent study showed that between 1970 and 1974, in the small Cappadocian village of Karain (population 575), 24 of the 56 total deaths were the result of malignant mesothelioma. No asbestos-exposed cohort had ever experienced such a high mesothelioma mortality. A follow-up study of this population through 1987 reported 62 mesothelioma deaths of about 175 deaths in the village. The study was extended to other towns in the Cappadocian region. In all, 94 mesotheliomas were discovered over approximately 17 years among a total population of about 5000.

The Anatolian plateau is made up of geologically recent volcanic ash deposits called tuffs. The tuffaceous sediments are largely unconsolidated and are easily worked with hand tools. The inhabitants of these villages sometimes carved their homes or other structures out of the soft tuff outcroppings or cut them into dimension stone for use in building. Mineralogic analysis of the Cappadocian soils and rocks indicates that the tuffs, which were originally volcanic glasses, feldspars, and other silicate minerals, had been altered by ground water to montmorillonite and zeolite minerals. The assemblage of zeolites includes clinoptilolite, chabazite, and erionite. The erionite occurs, morphologically, as a fine fiber. Erionite fiber was found in the lung tissues of patients who died of mesothelioma.[34,35]

Environmental exposure to erionite probably began at birth. Analysis of outdoor air samples by transmission electron microscopy has confirmed the presence of low concentrations of erionite fibers in the air of the villages studied (Table 12-5). However, the levels found do not necessarily represent past exposures, nor do they indicate that individuals in the village did not experience higher fiber exposures during certain activities (see references 31 and 36 for a discussion).

Experimental animal studies of erionite. A number of animal studies were initiated to verify the hypothesis that the mineralogically identified erionite fiber was the agent causing the malignant mesotheliomas observed in the Cappadocian region of Turkey. The most important of the animal studies was an inhalation study in rats (for recent reviews see references 37 and 38). Although erionite produced 27 mesotheliomas in 28 rats, the positive control, crocidolite, produced no mesotheliomas in 28 rats.[39] The erionite and crocidolite were reported to be indistinguishable on the basis of morphology. The Stanton hypothesis, which states that tumorigenicity of a fiber is related to its physical dimensions, was not supported by this study. In this particular instance, fiber dimension does not provide any insight for prognosticating the relative mesotheliomagenic potency of these mineral fibers.[40]

Palygorskite

Palygorskite is a naturally fibrous clay mineral.[3,12,24] As discussed here, studies of palygorskite carcinogenicity illustrate that mineralogic considerations, such as geographic origin, very much affect the degree of risk. The name *palygorskite* originates from the Palygorsk mountain range in the Urals (Novgorod, Russia), where the mineral was first reported in 1861. *Attapulgite,* a synonym for *palygorskite,* originates from the discovery of the same mineral in Attapulgus, Georgia, in the southeastern United States, in 1935. Its structure consists of two facing amphibolelike double chains of tetrahedra aligned parallel to the *c* axis that are linked by octahedrally coordinated cations. These chains are

referred to as ribbons and impart the fiber with structural elements of both chain and layer silicates.

The two chains contribute four silica tetrahedra each to the unit cell structure. Adjacent ribbons share the common oxygen edges of the outermost tetrahedra; the tetrahedra in adjacent ribbons point in opposite directions, and only their bases fall within a common plane. The chemical formula for palygorskite is $(Mg,Al)_4Si_8O_{20}(OH)_2 \cdot 8H_2O$ (Table 12-6). Another fibrous clay, sepiolite, is included for comparison.[3,24]

Aluminum may substitute for silica in the tetrahedral site, expressed as $(Si^{4+}_{8-x} Al_x)$. The octahedral sites created by two facing silica tetrahedra chains generally contain magnesium but other divalent cations, especially Fe^{2+}, may be found as well. Insufficient oxygens (eight of which form the apices of the inwardly facing tetrahedra) are present to complete the octahedral configuration of the ribbons; thus six hydroxyl groups are required to complete the sixfold co-

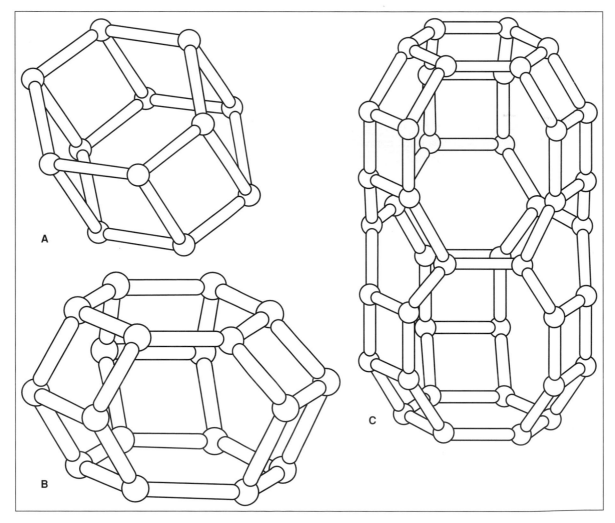

Fig. 12-3. Schematic representation of the three framework cages found in erionite: **A,** the double sixfold ring; **B,** the cancrinite cage; and **C,** the erionite cage. (Adapted from Gottardi G and Galli E: *Natural zeolites,* Berlin, 1985, Springer-Verlag.)

ordination and satisfy the valence requirements. On average only four of the octahedral cation sites are occupied. The octahedral sites are thought to take on some dioctahedral character—substitution of Si with trivalent cations such as Al^{3+} or Fe^{3+} so that only two thirds of the sites are filled. Reports indicate that some specimens contain almost equal concentrations of Mg^{2+} and Al^{3+}.

Additionally, internal channels, approximately 4×5 Å in cross-section, are created by the structural configuration.

Table 12-5. Fiber concentration and mineral content of outdoor air samples collected from Turkish villages

Village	Concentration (No. of fibers/ml)*	Description of fibers and other major particles present
Karain	0.002-0.010	80% Zeolite + calcium oxide and calcium sulfate (gypsum?)
Sarihidir	0.001-0.029	60% Zeolite + calcite, quartz, volcanic glass, tremolite, and chrysotile fibers
Tuzköy	0.005-0.025	85% Zeolites and quartz + volcanic glass and aluminum silicate
Karlik†	0.002-0.006	20% Erionite + calcium oxide and calcium sulfate (gypsum?)

Data are from references 31 and 36.
*Determined by transmission electron microscopy of 150 samples. The fibers counted were >5 μm
†Considered a "control" village.

Two water molecules, commonly referred to as zeolitic water, are accommodated within each side channel so that four are contained within each unit cell. Further sites exist that may be occupied by calcium, and potassium is a common minor constituent assumed to be bound at the base of the silicate chain in the structural channel.

Experimental animal studies of the carcinogenicity of palygorskite. Experimental studies of palygorskite carcinogenicity illustrate the importance of the mineralogic characteristics of the materials tested. The studies have been limited to naturally occurring specimens from different geologic locales. None of the palygorskites or sepiolites modified industrially—for example, by heating to enhance absorption—have been evaluated. The naturally occurring specimens from different geologic locales produce a range of activities in the experimental carcinogenesis studies.

Table 12-7 summarizes the frequency of tumor production and the characteristics of the specimens used. By intraperitoneal injection specimens from Attapulgus (United States) and Mormoiron, France, produced few tumors, but one from Torrejon, Spain, induced a tumor rate of 40%. A different sample from the same Torrejon geologic locale produced 35% tumors by intrapleural injection, whereas a different specimen from Mormoiron yielded none. Chrysotile specimens with size distributions comparable with those of the three specimens from Attapulgus have produced tumors in experimental animals.[12]

The International Agency for Research on Cancer (IARC) currently classifies the animal experimental data for palygorskite as limited.[3] Animal experimental studies show variable carcinogenicity for palygorskite, depending on the specimen's geologic origin. The IARC classification would

Table 12-6. Physicochemical characteristics of the fibrous clays palygorskite and sepiolite

	Palygorskite	Sepiolite
Formula	$(Mg,Al)_4Si_8O_{20}(OH)_2 8H_2O$	$(Mg,Fe)_8Si_{12}O_{30}(OH)_4 4H_2O$
Crystal system	Monoclinic/orthorhombic	Orthorhombic
a	~5.21	~5.28
b	~17.9	~26.95
c	~12.7	~13.37
β	90°, 96°, or 107°	
Z	2	2
Space group	Pnmb, A2/m, P2/a, Pn	Pnan
Indices of refraction		
α	1.50-1.52	1.51
β	1.54-1.56	1.52
γ	1.55	1.53
Density	2.2	~2
(g/cm³)		

Table 12-7. Characteristics of palygorskite fibers used in animal experimental models

Geologic origin	Route of administration*	Dose	Fiber length distribution (μm)	% Mesotheliomas
Attapulgus, Georgia	Surgical implant on pledget	40 mg	0.01-1.0 (52.3%), >1.0-4.0 (47.3%), >4.0 (0.5%)	6.9%
	Surgical implant	40 mg	0.01-1.0 (62.2%), >1.0-4.0 (37.8%)	6.9%
	Intraperitoneal injection	60 mg	>5.0 (0.021%)	3.6%
Torrejon, Spain	Intraperitoneal injection	10 mg	>5.0 (1.03%)	40.0%
Lebrija, Spain	Intraperitoneal injection	60 mg	>5.0 (0.024%)	3.5%
Mormoiron, France	Intraperitoneal injection	60 mg	>5.0 (0.0067%)	3.5%
Torrejon	Intrapleural injection	NR*	Length >6.0 μm; diameter <0.5 μm (0.54%), <0.2 μm (0.054%)	35.0%
Lebrija	Intrapleural injection	NR*	Length >6.0 μm; diameters all <2.0 μm	5.0%
Leicester, England	Intrapleural injection	NR	Diameter <0.5 μm (19.0%), <0.2 μm (18.1%)	93.8%
Lebrija	Inhalation	10 mg/cm	—	2.5%
Leicester	Inhalation	10 mg/cm	Diameter <0.5 μm (0.0%),† <0.2 μm (100.0%)†	7.5%
Mormoiron	Intrapleural injection	20 mg	Mean length 0.77 μm	0%

*See data in reference 12. *NR,* Not Reported.
†Recovered from lung tissue.

be better served if some notation of the range of activities depending on fiber size distribution and surface characteristics were made.

Synthetic organic fibers

The adverse health effects associated with exposure to the commercial asbestos minerals have resulted in the development of a large market for asbestos substitutes. Among the substitutes are synthetic organic fibers such as carbon/graphite, aramid, and polyolefin.

Recently, the International Programme on Chemical Safety reviewed the potential for adverse health effects for humans from inhalation exposure to synthetic organic fibers.[41] The only available chronic study of respirable aramid fibers in rats caused fibrosis (at least 25 fibers per milliliter) and lung neoplasms (100 fibers or more per milliliter). The lack of human data concerning the health effects of these fibers led to the recommendation that exposure to respirable and biopersistent synthetic fibers "should be controlled to the same degree as that required for asbestos until data supporting a lesser degree of control become available."[41]

NONFIBROUS MINERALS
Silica polymorphs

The physicochemical characteristics of the silica polymorphs, quartz, tridymite, and cristobalite, are shown in

Table 12-8. Physicochemical characteristics of three polymorphs of crystalline silica

	α-Quartz	α-Tridymite	α-Cristobalite
Formula	SiO_2	SiO_2	SiO_2
System	Trigonal	Orthorhombic	Tetragonal
a	4.913 Å	9.9 Å	4.97 Å
b	—	17.1 Å	—
c	5.405 Å	16.3 Å	6.93 Å
Z	3	64	4
Space group	$P3_121$ (right), $P3_221$ (left)		P422
Indices of refraction	$\epsilon = 1.553$ $\omega = 1.544$	$\alpha = 1.478$ $\beta = 1.479$ $\gamma = 1.481$	$\epsilon = 1.482$ $\omega = 1.489$
Density (g/cm³)	2.65	2.28	2.33

Table 12-8. Quartz is the third most common mineral in the earth's crust; therefore human exposure is unavoidable.[18] The polymorphs of silica have been reviewed,[42,43] and this discussion focuses on dose and polymorph type. The hazard presented by the inhalation of the dusts generated from

the different silica polymorphs cannot be evaluated by knowing its airborne mass concentration alone. Evaluation of the disease risk associated with a given exposure should include a determination of the properties of the dust that are known to affect its pathogenic activity.

The physicochemical properties of the silica polymorphs are important for defining dose. These have been illustrated using damage to the erythrocyte membrane as a model. A quartz specimen's ability to lyse the erythrocyte membrane is a rapid in vitro assay that may be used to quantitatively evaluate specific physicochemical properties of quartz thought to impart its fibrogenic activity. By controlling for other variables, defined characteristics may be tested in each challenge dust.

Effects of particle size distribution and density on membranolytic activity. The membranolytic activity of a given mass concentration of quartz dust will vary depending on the particle size distribution of the dust. Activity may be quantitated in the hemolysis assay by determining the mass concentration of a given quartz specimen required to lyse 50% of the erythrocytes in a suspension containing 1.8×10^8 cells per milliliter.[9,10] This is called the HC_{50}, which is expressed as the mass of quartz in milligrams per milliliter of erythrocyte suspension, that induces a 50% cell lysis.

Even a population of quartz particles as fine as a silica flour can have a wide distribution of particle sizes. One method for separating size classes is by sedimentation in water. The size distribution may be calculated using the Stokes equation. Silica flour (quartz), unfractionated, yields an HC_{50} value of 2.83 ± 0.23 mg/ml. By size fractionation, using Stokes' equation, the 1.0-μm and 20.0 μm Stokes diameter size fractions show values of 0.3 ± 0.0 mg/ml and 12.2 ± 1.8 mg/ml, respectively. This represents a 40-fold difference in hemolytic potency. This in vitro assay does not discriminate against nonrespirable particles. Although the 5-μm Stokes fraction contained a large number of particles in the respirable size range, its activity was 24-fold *lower* than that of the 1-μm size fraction.[10] These values represent differences in the activity of respirable size dust. The silica standard in the United States is based on mass rather than particle size. Two populations of people exposed to similar masses of quartz may experience very different health effects caused by differences in particle size distribution.

Injection of different flints (principally quartz) into the lungs of rats has shown that the finer-sized flint particles caused more fibrosis, at both constant mass and constant surface area (see reference 42 for a review). The activity of finely crushed crystalline silica and the range of silicosis pathology produced vary as a function of particle size. This is not always appreciated and is not reflected in the current U.S. silica standard.

The different silica polymorphs have different densities, that is, mass per unit of volume. Quartz, cristobalite, and tridymite have densities of 2.65, 2.33, and 2.26 g/cm³, respectively. The dose of powder used in experimental mod-

els is most often given on the basis of mass, which is easily determined. When King and colleagues[44,45] injected 50 mg of tridymite, cristobalite, and quartz, of *similar* size distribution, into rats to evaluate the action of the different polymorphs of crystalline silica, they did not normalize the particle number per unit mass of dust on the basis of density. The experimental results showed the order of fibrogenic response to be tridymite > cristobalite > quartz. However, this also follows the same order of surface area and particle number per unit mass of dust based on density. Did King and colleagues observe differences in the activity of the individual silica polymorphs or the influence of surface area *and* particle number?

Effects of surface properties on membranolytic activity. The quartz surface can exist in at least two physicochemically distinct states, one of which is not membranolytically active. The active quartz surface can be inactivated by reaction with, for example, hydrofluoric acid or potassium hydroxide. Chemically etched quartz has been correlated with changes in activity in vivo as well, using a rat model. The surface can also be inactivated by reaction with chloromethylsilanes, which render quartz hydrophobic.[46] Mechanical grinding of the surface, followed by hydration, has inactivated several quartz varieties. These inactivated quartz particles are indistinguishable from active quartz on the basis of optical and chemical properties, and continuous-scan x-ray diffraction characteristics are identical as well. These methods characterize the quartz on the basis of gross structure but are generally insensitive to alterations in surface structure.

Receptors on the erythrocyte membrane are able to recognize characteristics of the mineral's surface structure that can vary independently from the internal structure. Inactivated surfaces may be manipulated to recover activity. For example, crushed quartz or acid-treated quartz, both of which are inactive, may be heated past 575°C to produce an active dust.

There is a recognition event that occurs between the silica surface and the erythrocyte membrane. This interaction has been the subject of much research. The pathologic activity of the quartz surface is most commonly attributed to the hydrogen-bonding character of its surface. The best evidence for this is the strong interaction between the quartz surface and the hydrogen-bonding polymer, 2-polyvinylpyridine-*N*-oxide (2-PVPNO). When the 2-PVPNO polymer has a molecular weight greater than 50,000, it can antagonize the effect of quartz in many in vivo and in vitro models. The quartz specimens that have been rendered inactive by chemical attack, or mechanical manipulation, do not always lose the ability to bind 2-PVPNO, even though their membranolytic activity has been reduced to nil. Much of the inhibitory activity of this polymer can be related to stearic properties, and therefore the importance of the hydrogen bonding site may be only an epiphenomenon.

Surface charge has been shown to affect the membranolytic activity of quartz.[9] Blocking the ionized silanol group with a metal cation such as Al^{3+} or Fe^{3+} inhibits the membranolytic activity of the surface. This isoelectric surface retains its hydrogen bonding character, although its membranolytic activity is lost. Hydrogen bonding alone is not enough to impart membranolytic activity. The ionized silanol group must be available for interaction with the membrane.

Talc

The mineral talc is a phyllosilicate with the ideal composition $Mg_3Si_4O_{10}(OH)_2$. It consists of a compositional layer that offsets obliquely in the stacking c direction. This lowers the unit cell symmetry to triclinic, although the gross morphology remains pseudohexagonal.[47]

Compositions can vary by the substitution of iron in the octahedral site for magnesium (up to 1.22 of the 3 Mg sites). The 2:1 layers in talc are stacked with no interlayer cation. The bonds between the layers are weak, imparting to the mineral the lowest hardness on the Mohs scale. The ease of glide of adjacent planes imparts a slippery feel to the mineral.

In 1986 IARC reviewed the experimental animal studies in which the talc was evaluated and found "inadequate evidence for the carcinogenicity of talc to experimental animals."[3] Since then a preliminary report on a National Toxicology Program inhalation study of talc in rats and mice has become available.[48] Although the talc produced no tumors in the male or female mice, the male and female rats developed neoplasms of the adrenal glands, and among the highest exposed female rats, lung neoplasms occurred. Health effects are discussed in Chapters 21 and 22.

Titanium dioxide

The four titanium dioxide polymorphs that have been identified in nature are rutile, anatase, brookite, and $TiO_2(B)$.[11,43] Brookite and $TiO_2(B)$ are unimportant in terms of human exposure. Rutile and anatase are formed under a wide range of physicochemical conditions and are present throughout several geologic provenances. Although common in nature, industrially used titanium dioxide is mostly the product of chemical synthesis. In 1985 the United States produced 800,000 tons of synthetic titanium dioxide. Virtually all of the titanium dioxide produced is in the respirable size range. The material is used in many consumer products, including paint pigment, food items, and cosmetics.

The TiO_2 polymorphs, rutile and anatase, are composed of titanium atoms octahedrally coordinated by six oxygen atoms, each of the oxygens occupying a corner of a regular octahedron. In turn, every oxygen atom is coordinated with three titanium atoms occupying the approximate corners of an equilateral triangle. In rutile two opposite edges of each TiO_2 octahedron are shared with other octahedra, whereas in anatase the shared edges at the top and bottom of the octahedra are at right angles to each other. The octahedral bond angles and distances differ among the polymorphs so the sharing of edges increases from two in rutile to four in anatase. For the two commercially important polymorphs, rutile and anatase, the position of the octahedra in the lattice and the number of octahedra in the unit cell differ (see Table 12-9 and Fig.12-4). Anatase contains four TiO_2 molecules per unit cell, whereas rutile contains two.

The small variation in the structures of rutile and anatase leads to different cleavage and twin planes along which separation tends to occur. Therefore one would assume that, for anatase and rutile, the density of surface hydroxyl groups and their isoelectric points, would differ regardless of whether the crystals were grown to similar sizes or reduced in size from larger particles.

Experimental animal studies. The occurrence of interstitial fibrosis, bronchoalveolar adenomas, and squamous cell carcinomas in rats exposed to high concentrations of synthetic rutile by inhalation has been reported.[49,50] Previously, low biologic activity was attributed to the two titanium dioxide polymorphs: rutile and anatase. To emphasize how inert rutile and anatase have been considered, these materials were often used as control or "sham" dusts against which the activity of other mineral particles are compared.[51] Although both titanium dioxide polymorphs have occasionally been found to have in vitro properties consistent with a biologically active particulate, both are generally considered to be inert.[11]

CONCLUSIONS

Mineralogy is an integral part of the health hazard evaluation of human exposure to fine particles.[2] Often, the clinical features and pathology of a particular disease

Table 12-9. Comparison of the physical and chemical properties of two titanium dioxide polymorphs

	Rutile	**Anatase**
Formula	TiO_2	TiO_2
System	Tetragonal	Tetragonal
a	4.59	3.78
b	—	—
c	2.96	9.50
Z	2	4
Space group	$P4_2/mnm$	$I4_1/amd$
Indices of refraction	$\epsilon = 2.899\text{-}2.901$ $\omega = 2.613\text{-}2.665$	$\epsilon = 2.488$ $\omega = 2.501$
Density (g/cm^3)	4.13	3.79

provide little or no evidence of the agent responsible for its origin. With the development and application of modern analytic transmission electron microscope, complex analysis of fine mineral particles in the air and human tissues have become possible.[17] For example, the clinical features of a mesothelioma caused by erionite or crocidolite asbestos are indistinguishable. Yet with the use of mineralogy and the described analytical methods, the type and quantity of fiber present in the lung tissue can be determined and the agent involved in the etiology of the tumor can be identified.

Once an agent is associated with a disease, the environment in which the exposure occurred can be characterized so the source of the agent can be determined. For example,

for erionite, a fibrous zeolite, analysis of the concentration and types of fiber present in the air can further assist in establishing dose and the association between the observed mesothelioma and erionite. Tumors in experimental animals exposed to an erionite sample selected to have mineralogic characteristics similar to those associated with the pulmonary neoplasm in humans establish the etiology.

If a specific mineral is found to cause a particular disease, other environments can be evaluated for similar risks. Will an individual who is exposed to erionite in a different geologic locale, for example, riding a trail bike over a dried lake bed that contains erionite, experience a similar risk? Here again mineralogy plays an important role. A single mineral can exist with a wide range of physicochemical properties that affect its ability to induce disease. These properties must be defined using the science developed for this purpose: mineralogy.

ACKNOWLEDGMENT

We thank Dr. Malcolm Ross for his excellent critique and comments.

REFERENCES

1. Klein C and Hurlbut CS: *Manual of mineralogy,* ed 21. New York, 1993, John Wiley & Sons.
2. Guthrie GD and Mossman BT, editors: *Health effects of mineral dusts,* reviews in mineralogy, vol 28, Washington, DC, 1993, Mineralogical Society of America.
3. International Agency for Research on Cancer (IARC): Evaluation of the carcinogenic risk of chemicals to humans. In: *Silica and some silicates,* vol 42, Lyon, France, 1987, IARC.
4. Veblen DR and Wylie AG: Mineralogy of amphiboles and 1:1 layer silicates. In: Guthrie GD and Mossman BT, editors: *Health effects of mineral dusts,* reviews in mineralogy, vol 28, Washington, DC, 1993, Mineralogical Society of America.
5. Langer AM, Nolan RP, and Addison J: Distinguishing between amphibole asbestos fibers and elongate cleavage fragments of their non-masbestos analogues. In Brown RC, Hoskins JA, and Johnson NF, editors: *Mechanisms of fibre carcinogenesis,* New York, 1991, Plenum Press.
6. Brown RC, Hoskins JA, and Johnson NF, editors: *Mechanisms of fibre carcinogenesis,* New York, 1991, Plenum Press.
7. Stanton MF, Layard M, Tegeris A, et al: Relationship of particle dimensions to carcinogenicity of amphibole asbestoses and other fibrous minerals, *JNCI* 67:965-975, 1981.
8. Harington JS: Fibre carcinogenesis: epidemiological observations and the Stanton hypothesis, *JNCI* 57:977-989, 1981.
9. Nolan RP, Langer AM, Harington JS, et al: Quartz hemolysis related to its surface functionalities, *Environ Res* 26:503-520, 1981.
10. Nolan RP, Langer AM, Eskenazi RA, et al: Membranolytic activities of quartz standards, *Toxicol In Vitro* 1:239-245, 1987.
11. Nolan RP, Langer AM, Weisman I, et al: Surface character and membranolytic activity of rutile and anatase: two titanium dioxide polymorphs, *Br J Ind Med* 44:687-698, 1987.
12. Nolan RP, Langer AM, and Herson GB: Characteristics of palygorskite specimens from different geological locales for health hazard evaluation, *Br J Ind Med* 48:463-475, 1991.
13. Biopersistence of respirable synthetic fibres and minerals, *Environ Health Perspect* 102:Suppl 5, 1994.
14. Guthrie GD: Mineral Characterization in biological studies. In Guthrie GD and Mossman BT, editors: *Health effects of mineral dusts,* vol 28, Washington, DC, 1993, Mineralogical Society of America.

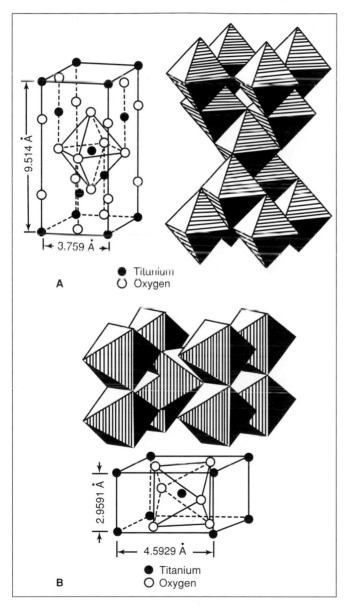

Fig. 12-4. Crystal structure of, **A,** rutile and, **B,** anatase. (Adapted from Nolan RP, Langer AM, Weisman I, et al: Surface character and membranolytic activity of rutile and anatase: two titanium dioxide polymorphs, *Br J Ind Med* 44:687-698, 1987.)

15. Bish DL and Post JE, editors: *Modern powder diffraction,* reviews in Mineralogy, vol 20. Washington, DC, 1989, Mineralogical Society of America.

16. Nesse WD: *Introduction to optical mineralogy,* ed 2, New York, 1991, Oxford University Press.

17. Kohyama N, Kyono H, Yokoyama K, et al: Evaluation of low-level asbestos exposure by transbronchial lung biopsy with analytical electron microscopy, *J Electron Microsc* 42:315-327, 1993.

18. Liebau F: *Structural chemistry of silicates,* Berlin, 1985, Springer-Verlag.

19. Whittaker EJW: Mineralogy, chemistry and crystallography of amphibole asbestos. In Ledoux RL, editor: *Short course in mineralogical techniques of asbestos determination,* Quebec, 1979, Mineralogical Association of Canada.

20. Leake BE: Nomenclature of amphiboles, *Am Mineral* 63:1023-1052, 1978.

21. Pooley FD: Asbestos mineralogy. In Antman K and Aisner J, editors: *Asbestos-related malignancy,* Orlando, Fla, 1987, Grune & Stratton.

22. Skinner HCW, Ross M, and Frondel C: *Asbestos and other fibrous minerals,* New York, 1988, Oxford University Press.

23. Dorling M and Zussman J: Characteristics of asbestiform and nonasbestiform calcic amphiboles, *Lithos* 20:469-489, 1987.

24. Brindley GW and Brown G, editors: *Crystal structures of clay minerals and their x-ray identification,* London, 1980, Mineralogical Society.

25. Bignon J, editor: *Health related effects of phyllosilicates,* Berlin, 1990, Springer-Verlag.

26. Wicks FJ: Mineralogy, chemistry and crystallography of chrysotile. In Ledoux RL, editor: *Short course in mineralogical techniques of asbestos determination,* Quebec, 1979, Mineralogical Association of Canada.

27. Langer AM and Nolan RP: The properties of chrysotile asbestos as determinants of biological activity. In Wagner JC, editor: *The biological effects of chrysotile. Accomplishments in oncology,* Philadelphia, 1987, JB Lippincott.

28. Baronnet A: Polytypism and stacking disorder. In Bureck PR, editor: *Minerals and reactions at the atomic scale: transmission electron microscopy,* reviews in mineralogy, vol 27, Washington, DC, 1992, Mineralogical Society of America.

29. Gottardi G and Galli E: *Natural zeolites,* Berlin, 1985, Springer-Verlag.

30. Tschernich RW: *Zeolites of the world,* Phoenix, 1992, Geoscience.

31. Baris YI: Fibrous zeolite (erionite)—related diseases in Turkey, *Am J Ind Med* 19:374-378, 1991.

32. Ross M, Nolan RP, Langer AM, et al: Health effects of mineral dusts other than asbestos. In Guthrie GD and Mossman BT, editors: *Health effects of mineral dusts,* reviews in mineralogy, vol 28, Washington, DC, 1993, Mineralogical Society of America.

33. Wagner JC and Pooley FD: Mineral fibres and mesothelioma, *Thorax* 41:161-166, 1986.

34. Pooley FD: Evaluation of fiber samples taken from the vicinity of two villages in Turkey. In Lemen R and Dement J, editors: *Dusts and disease,* Park Forest South, Ill, 1979, Pathotox.

35. Sébastien P, Gaudichet A, Bignon J, et al: Zeolite bodies in human lungs from Turkey, *Lab Invest* 44:420-425, 1981.

36. Simonato L, Baris YI, Saracci R, et al: Relation of environment erionite fibres to risk of respiratory cancer. In: Bignon J, Peto J, and Saracci R, editors: *Nonoccupational exposure to mineral fibres,* International Agency for Research on Cancer (IARC) Pub No 90. Lyon, France, 1989, IARC.

37. Guthrie GD: Biological effects of inhaled minerals, *Am Mineral* 77:225-243, 1992.

38. Johnson NF: The limitation of inhalation, intratracheal and intracaclonic routes of administration for identifying hazardous fibrous minerals. In Warheit DB, editor: *Fiber toxicology,* San Diego, 1993, Academic Press.

39. Wagner JC, Skidmore JW, Hill RJ, et al: Erionite exposure and mesothelioma in rats, *Br J Cancer* 51:727-730, 1985.

40. Nolan RP and Langer AM: Limitations of the Stanton hypothesis. In Guthrie GD and Mossman BT, editors: *Health effects of mineral dusts,* reviews in mineralogy, vol 28, Washington, DC, 1993, Mineralogical Society of America.

41. International Programme on Chemical Safety: *Selected synthetic organic fibres,* environmental health criteria No 151, Geneva, 1993, World Health Organization.

42. Langer AM: Crystal faces and cleavage planes in quartz as templates in biological processes, *Q Rev Biophys* 11:543-575, 1980.

43. Heany PJ and Banfield JA: Structure and chemistry of silica, metal oxides, and phosphates. In: Guthrie GD and Mossman BT, editors: *Health effects of mineral dusts,* reviews in mineralogy, vol 28, Washington, DC, 1993, Mineralogical Society of America.

44. King EJ, Mohanty GP, Harrison CV, et al: The action of different forms of pure silica on the lungs of rats, *Br J Ind Med* 10:9-17, 1953.

45. Zaidi SH, King EJ, Harrison CV, et al: Fibrogenic activity of different forms of free silica, *Arch Ind Health* 15:112-121, 1956.

46. Nolan RP, Langer AM, and Foster KW: Particle size and chemically-induced variability in membranolytic activity of quartz: preliminary observations. In Beck EG and Bignon J: *In vitro effects of minerals,* Berlin, 1985, Springer-Verlag.

47. Ross M, Smith WL, and Ashton WH: Triclinic talc and associated amphiboles from Gouverneur mining district, New York, *Am Mineral* 53:496-506, 1968.

48. National Toxicology Program: *Technical report on the toxicology and carcinogenesis studies of talc,* No 421, Research Triangle Park, NC, 1992, National Institutes of Health.

49. Lee KP, Trochimowicz HJ, and Reinhardt CF: Transmigration of titanium dioxide (TiO$_2$) particles in rats after inhalation exposure, *Exp Mol Pathol* 42:331-343, 1985.

50. Lee KP, Trochimowicz HJ, and Reinhardt CF: Pulmonary response of rats exposed to titanium dioxide (TiO$_2$) by inhalation for two years, *Toxicol Appl Pharmacol* 79:179-192, 1985.

51. Ferin J and Oberdörster G: Biological effects and toxicity assessment of titanium dioxides: anatase and rutile, *Am Ind Hyg Assoc J* 46:69-72, 1985.

Section **IV**

General Disease Categories

JOHN R. BALMES

For virtually every respiratory disease there are occupational or environmental exposures that can cause or contribute to it. This section is primarily designed to provide occupational and environmental physicians with essential pathophysiologic and clinical information about the major categories of respiratory disease. Pulmonary physicians, however, will find that the chapters on inhalation fevers, hypersensitivity pneumonitis, and upper airway cancers provide clinically relevant material with which they are less than familiar. The chapters in this section do not discuss occupational or environmental etiologies in any depth. Sections V through IX are designed to provide such discussion.

Chapter 13

ASTHMA

John R. Balmes

Asthma is a disease that eludes easy definition. An expert panel in the United States recently developed a consensus definition that included the following characteristics: "airway obstruction that is reversible (but not completely so in some patients) either spontaneously or with treatment; airway inflammation; and increased airway responsiveness to a variety of stimuli."[1] Asthma is usually distinguished from chronic obstructive pulmonary disease (COPD), (i.e., chronic bronchitis and emphysema) by the reversibility of airway obstruction in the former, but there may be a component of reversible obstruction in COPD as well. Because it is now recognized that airway inflammation (i.e., bronchitis) is a key feature of asthma and that severe persistent asthma may have a component of fixed obstruction, there is the potential for considerable overlap between asthma and chronic bronchitis. The term *asthmatic bronchitis* has been used by clinicians to describe patients with chronic productive cough and chronic airflow limitation who also have improvement in expiratory flow rates after inhaled β-agonist bronchodilator administration. Another term, *reactive airways disease,* is used by some physicians to avoid the potential stigmatizing effect of the asthma label, especially in children. *Reactive airways dysfunction syndrome* (RADS)

was coined to refer to persistent asthma after high-level irritant exposure,[2] but *irritant-induced asthma* works just as well. To prevent unnecessary confusion, the use of terms other than *asthma* should be avoided.

EPIDEMIOLOGY

The National Center for Health Statistics has estimated that 11 million people in the United States have asthma.[3] The prevalence of asthma in the general population has been increasing dramatically in recent years—at least 30% over the past decade.[4] A similar increase in asthma prevalence has been occurring in other countries as well.[5] Although some of the increase may be the result of a change in diagnostic classification and increased reporting, a true increase in disease prevalence is likely. The causes of this increase are currently unknown, but environmental pollution is one potential contributory factor.

In addition to the increased prevalence of asthma, there has also been an increase in morbidity and mortality as a result of the disease. From 1970 to 1987, the hospital discharge rate for asthma in the United States increased by 30%.[6] During this period the death rate from asthma was also rising with a 30% increase between 1980 and 1987 alone.[4] Although most groups in the population appear to be affected by increased asthma morbidity and mortality, the young black population has been affected the most. Over the past decade black patients were more than twice as likely to be hospitalized for asthma than white patients. The asthma death rate for all ages is currently almost threefold higher among the black population, but the death rate is approximately five times higher for black clients between ages 15 and 44 than for white clients of the same age group.[7]

Asthma is usually managed in the outpatient setting. It has been estimated that 1% of all ambulatory care visits in the United States have asthma as the primary diagnosis.[6]

ETIOLOGY

Allergy is associated with asthma. Up to 80% of patients with asthma have positive immediate reactions to skin-prick testing with a battery of common aeroallergens,[8] although this percentage probably overrepresents the importance of allergy in asthma. Whereas allergy clearly plays a primary role in childhood asthma, many adults with asthma do not appear to be sensitized to specific aeroallergens. This observation provides the basis for the traditional characterization of the disease by two major types—extrinsic asthma (with sensitization to specific aeroallergens) and intrinsic asthma (without specific sensitization).

There is a genetic component to the risk of developing asthma. Children with one asthmatic parent have an increased risk of developing the disease themselves, and when both parents are asthmatic, the risk is even higher. A parental history of atopy also increases the risk. Up to 40% of the population is atopic; however, many sensitized people do not develop asthma or asymptomatic airway hyperresponsiveness.[9] Thus allergy alone does not explain the development of persistent asthma, although continuous or recurrent exposure to allergen may serve to sustain asthma in a genetically susceptible subpopulation.

Exposure to environmental tobacco smoke is now well established as a risk factor for the development of asthma in childhood. The evidence supporting this assertion is discussed in Chapter 47.

It is likely that viral respiratory tract infections play an important contributory role in the development of asthma. Lower respiratory viral infections cause airway epithelial injury and inflammation that may initiate the asthmatic disease process, although the specific process(es) by which this occurs is not well understood. An increase in nonspecific airway responsiveness can be a consequence of viral respiratory tract infections even in nonasthmatic people, and such infections frequently exacerbate preexisting asthma.[10] Airway remodeling and increased sensitivity of afferent neuroreceptors in the airway mucosa are two possible mechanisms by which virally induced injury and inflammation may induce asthma. Other possible mechanisms are the generation of specific immunoglobulin E (IgE) antibodies to viral proteins and the increased access of aeroallergens to subepithelial T lymphocytes and mast cells in the wake of a virally induced increase in airway epithelial permeability.

Exposure to chemical irritants can precipitate asthma and may do so by producing airway inflammation (i.e., chemical bronchitis), which may then have many of the same effects described for virally induced inflammation. Most individuals who develop severe viral or chemical bronchitis do not even proceed to develop asthma, so predisposing host factors are clearly required. In the author's experience a history of allergy, a family history of asthma, or cigarette smoking are often present in patients who develop persistent asthma after viral infections or chemical inhalation injury. Presumably, specific markers of genetic risk of asthma will be available in the future.

In contrast to childhood asthma, which usually has an allergic basis, adult-onset asthma may occur in a patient without any history or evidence of allergies. The term *intrinsic asthma* has been used to refer to adult-onset asthma in which specific allergies do not appear to play a role. Although the distinction between intrinsic and extrinsic asthmas is not always clear, there may be important differences in the pathogenesis of these two broad types of asthma. Occupational asthma associated with sensitization to a high-molecular-weight protein provides a model of extrinsic asthma, and it seems reasonable to postulate that asthma that develops after high-level irritant exposure (i.e., RADS) is a model of intrinsic asthma. Because adult-onset asthma is more often of the intrinsic type, the possibility of occupational and environmental exposure to irritants should always be considered.

Once asthma has developed, exacerbations can be precipitated by multiple factors (see box). Because people with asthma have nonspecific airway hyperresponsiveness, at least during periods of exacerbation, exposure to irritants at relatively low concentrations may aggravate the underlying condition.

PATHOPHYSIOLOGY

Over the past decade airway inflammation has emerged as the paramount feature of asthma. It has long been known from autopsy studies of patients that die from status asthmaticus that airway inflammation is present in such patients. In recent years, however, the use of fiberoptic bronchoscopy to obtain bronchoalveolar lavage and bronchial-mucosal biopsy specimens has allowed the study of patients with less severe asthma.[11-15] Airway inflammation is clearly present in these patients as well. Asthmatic airways are characterized by (1) infiltration with inflammatory cells, especially eosinophils, (2) edema, and (3) loss of epithelial integrity. Airflow obstruction in asthma is believed to be the result of changes associated with airway inflammation. Airway inflammation is also believed to play an important role in the genesis of airway hyperresponsiveness in asthma.[16]

Asthma precipitating or aggravating factors

Exposure to environmental allergens
Exposure to environmental irritants (e.g., environmental tobacco smoke or outdoor air pollutants)
Exposure to occupational allergens or irritants
Viral respiratory tract infections
Exercise
Exposure to cold air
Drugs (e.g., aspirin, other nonsteroidal antiinflammatory drugs, or β-blockers)
Food additives (e.g., tartrazine or sulfites)
Emotional stress
Environmental change (e.g., new home or change in work process)
Pregnancy

Much of the research on mechanisms that mediate airway inflammation in asthma has focused on allergen-induced responses. In previously sensitized individuals inhalation of aeroallergens allows interaction of these allergens with airway cells (mast cells and alveolar macrophages) that have specific antibodies (usually IgE) on the cell surface. This interaction initiates a series of redundant amplifying events that lead to airway inflammation. These events include mast cell secretion of mediators, lymphocyte activation, and eosinophil recruitment to the airways. The generation and release of various cytokines from alveolar macrophages, mast cells, sensitized lymphocytes, and bronchial epithelial cells are central to the inflammatory process. Cytokine networking, with both enhancing and inhibitory feedback loops, is responsible for inflammatory cell targeting to the bronchial epithelium, activation of infiltrating cells, and potential amplification of epithelial injury. Adhesion molecules also appear to play a critical role in the amplification of the inflammatory process. The expression of various adhesion molecules is upregulated during the inflammatory cascade, and these molecules are essential for cell movement, cell attachment to the extracellular matrix and other cells, and possibly cell activation.

Inhalation of allergen in a specifically sensitized patient with asthma will trigger rapid-onset but self-limited bronchoconstriction, called the early response (Fig. 13-1). In 30% to 50% of extrinsic asthmatic subjects undergoing an allergen inhalation challenge, a delayed reaction will occur 4 to 8 hours later, called the late response.[17] The late response is characterized by persistent airflow obstruction, airway inflammation, and airway hyperresponsiveness.[18] Mast cell degranulation and release of mediators such as histamine are believed to be responsible for the immediate response.[19] The role of the mast cell in the genesis of the late response is more controversial, but the release of chemoattractant substances such as leukotrienes and cytokines

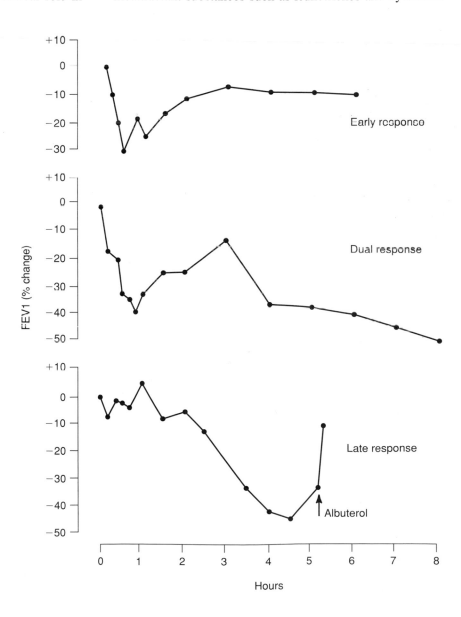

Fig. 13-1. Potential responses to inhalation of allergen in sensitized people with asthma.

(i.e., interleukins IL-3, IL-4, and IL-5) may be involved in the influx of neutrophils and eosinophils into the airway epithelium, which is a key feature of this response.[20] The infiltration of the airway wall with eosinophils is also a key feature of the late response.[14,21] The eosinophil can release proteins (e.g., major basic protein, eosinophilic cationic protein, eosinophilic peroxidase, or eosinophil-derived neurotoxin), lipid mediators, oxygen radicals, and enzymes that can cause epithelial injury. There is increasing evidence that lymphocytes, especially a subset of CD4$^+$ lymphocytes known as TH$_2$ cells, are involved in the release of cytokines that may activate both mast cells (IL-3 and IL-4) and eosinophils (IL-5).[22] The number of TH$_2$ cells in the airway epithelium appears to be higher in patients with allergy-related asthma and may be responsible for the maintenance of chronic airway inflammation.[23]

Although the mechanisms by which airway inflammation occurs in intrinsic asthma are not well understood, neurogenic pathways may be involved.[24] The axonal reflex involving C-fiber stimulation and the release of neuropeptides have been implicated in models of irritant-induced airway inflammation. Of course, with high-level irritant exposure, direct chemical injury may lead to an inflammatory response. The important question is what causes or allows this response to persist in susceptible individuals.

As the allergen or irritant-induced airway inflammatory process proceeds, mucosal edema, mucus secretion, and vascular and epithelial permeability all increase, leading to a reduction of the caliber of the airway lumen and resultant airflow obstruction (Fig. 13-2). The development of airflow obstruction in patients with asthma is a marker of the severity of the disease. With mild asthma there may be no obvious evidence of obstruction, but nonspecific airway hyperresponsiveness is likely to be present. With more severe asthma there is increased airway responsiveness and airflow obstruction is evident.

Airway hyperresponsiveness

Several hypotheses have been advanced to explain how airway hyperresponsiveness develops in asthma (Fig. 13-3). The primary abnormality suggested to be responsible for airway hyperresponsiveness has included airway inflammation, alterations in autonomic neural control of bronchial smooth muscle tone, and intrinsic changes of bronchial smooth muscle function. Although each of these mechanisms may play a role, airway inflammation is currently believed to be the key factor. In several studies of patients with asthma, the degree of inflammation on bronchial biopsy specimens has been found to correlate with the level of airway responsiveness.[12,25] There is also evidence to suggest that altered cellular responses and increased levels of inflammatory mediators are associated with airway hyperresponsiveness.[15,19] Moreover, therapeutic interventions that result in decreased airway inflammation also appear to diminish airway responsiveness.[26]

Bronchial biopsy studies in patients with asthma have also demonstrated changes consistent with airway epithelial injury that range from the loss of some ciliated cells to almost complete denudation of the epithelium.[11,12] These changes would be expected to lead to increased epithelial permeability to inhaled allergens, inhaled irritants, and inflammatory mediators present in the airway lumen. In ad-

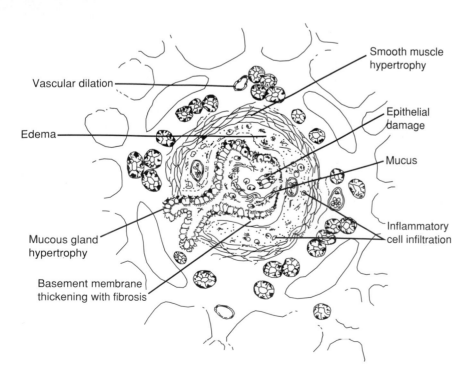

Vascular dilation

Edema

Mucous gland hypertrophy

Basement membrane thickening with fibrosis

Smooth muscle hypertrophy

Epithelial damage

Mucus

Inflammatory cell infiltration

Fig. 13-2. Morphologic changes in asthma. (Adapted from National Asthma Education Program Expert Panel: *Guidelines for the diagnosis and management of asthma*, NIH Pub No 91-3042A, Bethesda, Md, 1991, National Heart, Lung and Blood Institute.)

dition, increased transudation of fluid into the airway lumen and decreased mucociliary clearance of respiratory tract secretions would result. There is mounting evidence that the bronchial epithelium plays an important role in cytokine and mediator release and regulation.[27]

In addition to the role of neurogenic inflammation already mentioned, neural mechanisms may be involved in mediating the airway hyperresponsiveness of asthma. It has been suggested that changes in the parasympathetic control of airway function are responsible for the increased responsiveness to cholinergic substances that characterizes asthma.[28] Increased parasympathetic tone and reflex bronchoconstriction may occur as consequences of either heightened cholinergic sensitivity or changes in muscarinic receptor function. It is doubtful, however, that altered parasympathetic control is the sole mechanism responsible for bronchospasm produced by inhaled irritants.

Abnormalities of bronchial smooth muscle may have a role in the airway hyperresponsiveness of asthma. Patients with severe asthma have hypertrophy of bronchial smooth muscle. There is evidence that smooth muscle hypertrophy and abnormal contractility may be a result of stimulation by inflammatory cell-derived growth factors and mediators.[29]

Airflow obstruction itself has been proposed as a major determinant of airway hyperresponsiveness. Because airflow decreases exponentially as the radius of the airway lumen becomes smaller, baseline airflow obstruction in asthmatic patients can contribute to measured airway hyperresponsiveness. This is not the primary cause, however, because airway hyperresponsiveness is usually still present in asthmatic patients when their pulmonary function is normal during asymptomatic periods between exacerbations.

Exacerbations of asthma

Patients with asthma typically develop acute episodes characterized by respiratory symptoms (e.g., dyspnea, chest tightness, cough, or wheezing) and airflow obstruction. Narrowing of the airways in asthmatic patients can be caused

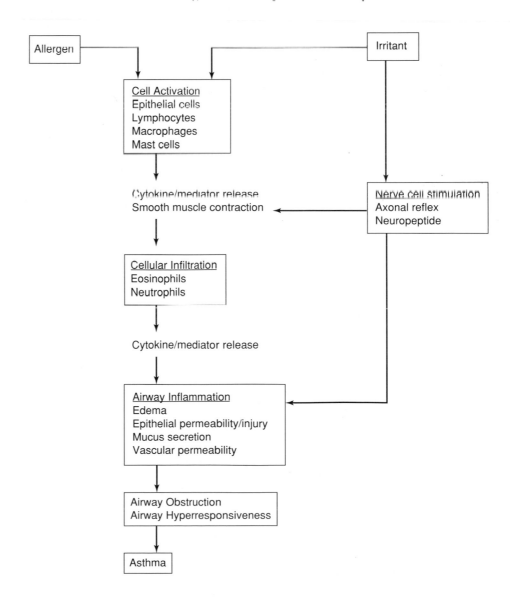

Fig. 13-3. Proposed pathways in the pathogenesis of asthma.

by several mechanisms, including bronchial smooth muscle contraction, mucosal edema, and mucus plugging. Early closure of narrowed small airways leads to air trapping and hyperinflation. While this process progresses, the asthmatic patient's tidal breathing occurs at lung volumes increasingly closer to total lung capacity. Breathing at high lung volumes allows asthmatic patients to keep their airways open and to permit gas exchange to occur. Accessory muscles of respiration are used to maintain the lungs in a hyperinflated state.

The use of accessory muscles of respiration and the degree of hyperinflation are better predictors of the severity of an acute exacerbation of asthma than either the level of dyspnea or wheezing.[30] Severity of an asthma attack is best assessed by objective measures of pulmonary function. Peak expiratory flow (PEF) and forced expiratory volume in 1 second (FEV1) are decreased because of airflow obstruction during expiration, and forced vital capacity is decreased because of hyperinflation. Intrapleural pressure becomes more negative than normal during inspiration because of hyperinflation, and the phenomenon of "auto-PEEP" (positive end-expiratory pressure) occurs during expiration. These changes are reflected in the systemic blood pressure as pulsus paradoxus, a greater than normal fall in systolic pressure during each inspiration. The presence of pulsus paradoxus is another relatively reliable sign of the severity of an asthma attack and suggests that the FEV1 is reduced to below 50% of the normal value.[31]

Abnormal gas exchange is another important feature of severe asthma exacerbations. Hypoxemia occurs as a consequence of ventilation-perfusion mismatching. In response, alveolar ventilation may initially be increased so that arterial $PaCO_2$ is often reduced early during an acute attack. As airflow obstruction becomes more severe and the patient tires, alveolar hypoventilation may develop and the $PaCO_2$ may rise. A $PaCO_2$ even in the normal range during an acute exacerbation of asthma is a sign of impending respiratory failure. It has been shown that the FEV1 will be reduced to below 25% of the normal value when hypercapnia is present during an acute attack of asthma.[32]

DIAGNOSIS

A key feature of the history in patients with asthma is the generally episodic nature of respiratory symptoms. The most common symptoms are cough (productive or nonproductive), wheezing, chest tightness, and shortness of breath. These symptoms are typically provoked by certain trigger factors, such as exposure to allergen or viral respiratory tract infections. Nonspecific airway hyperresponsiveness to a variety of stimuli, such as exercise, cold air, and irritants, is also characteristic of asthma, and simple questions about the effects of such stimuli should be asked. Thus both the pattern of symptoms (i.e., seasonal or perennial, daytime or nocturnal, workdays or weekends) and specific precipitating or aggravating factors (see box in the section on etiol-

ogy) should be elicited in the history. Inquiry should be made about allergies and conditions known to be associated with asthma, such as rhinitis, sinusitis, nasal polyps, and atopic dermatitis. Previous respiratory illness other than asthma, current or past cigarette smoking, and any family history of allergies or asthma should be noted. If a patient has already been diagnosed with asthma, the age of onset, the overall course (including emergency room visits, hospitalizations, and endotracheal intubations), the results of previous evaluations (including specific allergen testing), the response to treatment, and present management should be discussed. Severity of asthma is indicated by the frequency of attacks, frequency of need for medication, level of exercise tolerance, recent hospitalization for asthma treatment, and presence of nocturnal symptoms.

The patient's home, work, and recreational environments should be addressed with regard to potential exposures to precipitating or aggravating factors. For the home, questions should be asked about the age of the home, heating and cooling sources, use of a wood-burning stove or fireplace, carpeting, humidifier use, pets, environmental tobacco smoke, and how the house is cleaned. A complete chronological occupational history is desirable, since previous jobs may have involved sensitizing or irritant exposures. More detailed understanding is needed of the patient's job at the time of onset of his or her respiratory illness and of all the processes at the workplace. The potential for avocational exposure to sensitizing or irritant agents should be explored as well. The impact of asthma on the patient's home, work, and recreational life should be assessed, as well as the impact on his or her family. It is also important to ascertain the level of the patient's and family's knowledge about asthma.

The physical examination of a patient suspected of having asthma who is not experiencing an acute exacerbation should be focused on the upper and lower respiratory tract. As noted, rhinitis or sinusitis frequently coexist with asthma, whether the asthma is sensitizer or irritant induced. Thus the nasal mucous membranes and the pharynx should be inspected and the sinuses should be palpated. The presence of nasal polyps should be noted. Auscultation of the chest during quiet breathing and forced exhalation should be performed, with notation of wheezes, rhonchi, or crackles. Examination of the cardiovascular system should be performed to rule out a nonrespiratory cause of the patient's symptoms. The skin should be inspected for evidence of eczematous dermatitis that can accompany allergy-related asthma. The extremities should be inspected for clubbing, cyanosis, and edema. Examination of other organ systems should be guided by the patient's history.

It is important to recognize that the physical examination of a patient with asthma is often normal when the patient is not experiencing an exacerbation. Equally important, the severity of asthma cannot be adequately gauged from the patient's history and physical examination. Objective confirmation of the diagnosis and severity of asthma is necessary.

Objective evaluation of asthma should begin with the first visit. Spirometry should be performed before and after inhaled β-agonist bronchodilator administration to look for reversible airflow limitation at the time of the initial assessment. A 12% improvement or better in FEV1, with an absolute value increase of at least 200 ml after bronchodilation, is considered evidence of the reversibility of airflow limitation.[33] Spirometry should be performed using equipment and techniques that meet the criteria of the American Thoracic Society.[34]

If spirometry shows no airflow limitation and asthma is suspected, a methacholine or histamine challenge test to look for nonspecific airway hyperresponsiveness is indicated. When the baseline FEV1 is below 70% of the predicted value, response to inhaled bronchodilator rather than measurement of airway responsiveness is the appropriate test to establish the diagnosis of asthma.[35] It is imperative that standardized methods be used in the performance of nonspecific challenge tests. The results should be expressed as the provocative concentration to cause a decline in FEV1 of 20% (PC_{20}). Airway hyperresponsiveness is present when the PC_{20} is no higher than 8 mg/ml methacholine.[35]

The serial measurement of PEF is useful in assessing the severity or level of control of asthma. Measurements should be made at least four times per day.[36] Patients must be trained in peak flow measurement. A minimum of three forced expiratory maneuvers should be recorded, and the two best readings should be within 20 L/min of each other or else further readings should be taken. The best PEF rate should be recorded and used for analysis. A diurnal variability of 20% or more in PEF is supportive evidence for the diagnosis of asthma.[36]

Additional tests that should be considered and performed, when appropriate, include the following: complete blood cell count (primarily to look for eosinophilia), chest radiography, sputum and/or nasal secretion cell differential count (again, to look for eosinophilia), complete pulmonary function testing (to rule out other causes of airflow obstruction), sinus x-ray films, and tests to confirm the presence of gastroesophageal reflux. Determination of the presence of specific IgE antibodies to common aeroallergens by skin-prick testing may be useful, given the high prevalence of specific allergy among patients with asthma and the benefits of limiting exposure to known allergens as part of effective asthma management. In vitro laboratory tests for specific IgE antibodies may be used in place of skin-prick tests but often have lesser sensitivity and greater cost.

Most people with asthma have nonspecific airway hyperresponsiveness that leads to exercise-induced asthma (EIA). A history of respiratory symptoms or lack of endurance during or after exercise suggests EIA. Exercise testing should not be done routinely in the diagnostic work-up of asthma. However, when doubt exists about the presence of EIA, an exercise challenge can establish the presence of this condition. Spirometry is performed before and after exercise; if a patient has at least a 15% decline in FEV1 from the baseline level after exercise, then EIA is present.[1]

TREATMENT

Because asthma is a chronic condition with acute exacerbations, treatment requires continuous efforts to control symptoms, prevent exacerbations, and reduce persistent airway inflammation. Prevention of exacerbations involves avoidance of trigger factors and, for many patients, regular medication use. The increased awareness of the importance of airway inflammation in the pathogenesis of asthma has led to a greater emphasis on the role of antiinflammatory medications. Patients who have recurring symptoms, frequent nocturnal symptoms, and poor exercise tolerance will often benefit from more aggressive treatment with antiinflammatory medications. If an acute exacerbation does begin, early intervention with systemic corticosteroids may prevent severe airflow obstruction.

Effective management of asthma depends on both pharmacologic and nonpharmacologic measures. Prevention, or at least reduction, of exposure to the causative or aggravating agent(s) in the home and work environments, patient education about the condition, a step-care approach to pharmacologic therapy, and objective measures to monitor the severity of disease and response to therapeutic interventions (including serial monitoring of PEF) are all important components of an asthma management strategy. The goals of asthma management include the following: maintain normal activity levels (including exercise); maintain "normal" (or near-normal) pulmonary function; prevent chronic and troublesome symptoms (e.g., coughing or breathlessness at night, in the early morning, or after exercise); prevent recurrent exacerbations of asthma; and avoid adverse effects from asthma medications.[1] With some patients it may take several months to achieve these goals.

Avoidance of aeroallergens and irritants, in both indoor and outdoor environments, is a key principle of effective asthma management. House dust contains multiple potential allergens, including those from mites, molds, pets, and cockroaches. Exposure to mite allergen can be reduced by decreasing humidity in the house, removing carpets, keeping the house clean (but having the patient refrain from dusting or vacuum cleaning), frequently washing pillowcases and bedding, and encasing mattresses. Exposure to indoor molds can be reduced by decreasing humidity, ventilating adequately, and cleaning bathrooms, kitchens, and basements. Pets should be kept outdoors. If cockroaches infest the home, appropriate control measures should be taken. Air conditioning is, in general, beneficial to asthmatic patients because it allows windows to remain closed and tends to reduce indoor humidity. Although controlling the sources of allergens is preferable, the use of indoor air-cleaning devices, especially those with high efficiency particulate air-purifying (HEPA) filters, can sometimes help reduce exposure to airborne allergens. In cases of occupational asthma caused by sensitizer agents, complete elimination of workplace exposure is the goal. Avoidance of environmental tobacco smoke, wood smoke, and irritant chemicals, in both the home and the workplace, is essential. Remaining indoors, preferably in an air-conditioned environment, on days when the pollen count, mold count, or pollution index is high in the outdoor air will also help to decrease exposure to agents that may precipitate or aggravate asthma.

Avoidance of exposure to allergen should always be the primary method of management of allergy-related asthma. However, when avoidance is not possible and appropriate medication fails to control allergy-related asthma, allergy immunotherapy (hyposensitization) may have a role. Injections of allergen extract have been shown to reduce asthmatic symptoms in several double-blind studies of exposures to house dust, cat, grass pollen, and alternaria allergens.[37-40] Decreased skin or airway reactivity to allergen has also been demonstrated after specific immunotherapy.[38-41] Evaluation for, and administration of, allergy immunotherapy should be done only under the supervision of physicians who have had appropriate training.

Health education is a critical tool in the management of asthma.[1,42,43] Patient education on asthma should begin at the time of diagnosis and be integrated with follow-up care. An asthma management strategy should be established between the patient and the health care provider, and the patient should be encouraged to understand asthma and to learn and practice the skills necessary to manage his or her disease. The essentials of patient education on asthma include the following: (1) key points about the symptoms and signs of asthma; (2) characteristic airway changes in asthma (inflammation, bronchospasm, or excessive and thick mucus); (3) asthma triggers and how to avoid them; (4) appropriate medications, how they work, and potential adverse effects; (5) demonstration of the correct use of metered-dose inhalers (MDIs); (6) criteria for premedicating to prevent the onset of symptoms and initiating treatment after the onset of symptoms; (7) indications for seeking emergency care; and (8) optimal use of serial PEF monitoring.

Appropriate medications for the treatment of asthma include inhaled β_2-agonist bronchodilators, inhaled corticosteroids, cromolyn sodium, nedocromil, theophylline, ipratropium bromide, and oral corticosteroids. A step-care approach (see box) to the use of these medications has been recommended.[1] The key to rational pharmacologic therapy of asthma is recognition of the importance of treatment and prevention of airway inflammation, in addition to reversal of acute bronchoconstriction.

Inhaled corticosteroids have become the mainstay of the management of asthmatic adults with more than mild intermittent symptoms.[44-46] Systemic adverse effects are infrequent with long-term high-dose regimens, and such regi-

---

Step-care approach to pharmacologic treatment of asthma

Step 1: Inhaled β-agonist as needed
Step 2: Inhaled β-agonist as needed and either an inhaled corticosteroid or cromolyn sodium/nedocromil
Step 3: Step 2 plus either theophylline or ipratropium bromide
Step 4: Addition of an oral corticosteroid

---

mens reduce the need for chronic use of oral steroids, which can have significant adverse effects.[47] Local adverse effects of corticosteroids from MDIs include oropharyngeal candidiasis, dysphonia, and coughing resulting from aerosol-induced upper airway irritation.[48] These adverse effects can be reduced by the use of a spacer device that reduces large-particle deposition and by rinsing the mouth after inhaling the aerosol. Nonsteroidal antiinflammatory drugs for asthma, such as cromolyn sodium and nedocromil, produce only minimal side effects.[49,50] The exact mechanisms of action of these drugs are not completely understood, but there is some evidence for inhibition of mediator release from mast cells. If administered before exposure, cromolyn sodium can inhibit both immediate and late-phase allergen-induced responses, as well as responses to cold air, exercise, and sulfur dioxide. There is no way to reliably predict whether a patient will respond to cromolyn sodium or nedocromil; a 4- to 6-week trial may be required to determine efficacy.

β_2-agonists relax airway smooth muscle and may have some effect on mediator release from mast cells.[51] The newer drugs in this class are more β_2 selective and have a more prolonged duration of action, although some β_1 cardiac activity remains. Inhalation of β_2-agonists is preferable to oral administration because of a more rapid onset, similar duration of action, and less adverse effects. Inhaled β_2-agonists are available in both MDIs and dry-powder inhalers. Medications in this class are the treatment of choice for acute bronchoconstriction[52] and for the prevention of EIA. Concern has been raised recently about the possible role of β_2-agonists in death because of asthma.[53] Cardiac arrhythmias and myocardial ischemia can occur from either drug-induced hypokalemia or direct stimulation of the myocardium.[54] However, these complications of β_2-agonist therapy are rare, usually occurring only in elderly patients with preexisting cardiac disease.[55,56] Most deaths from asthma appear to be related to severe irreversible airflow obstruction and mucus plugging of the airways. An association between increased use of inhaled β_2-agonist therapy and asthma mortality has been reported.[57] One explanation that has been offered for this observation is that symptomatic relief from inhaled β_2-agonist therapy may cause asthmatic patients to avoid seeking appropriate care for severe acute exacerbations that require treatment of airway inflammation. Another study reported that the regular use, as opposed to the as-needed use, of inhaled β_2-agonists was associated with decreased control of asthma.[58] The mechanism of the decreased control is unclear, although slight increases in airway responsiveness during inhaled β_2-agonist therapy have been described.[46] Tolerance as a result of down-regulation of β-adrenergic receptors during chronic therapy is another possible explanation,[59] although most of the evidence suggests that significant tolerance to inhaled β_2-agonists does not usually develop in patients with asthma.[60]

Theophylline is an orally administered drug that has bronchodilator and other effects beneficial to the treatment of asthma.[61] The precise mechanism by which theophylline causes bronchodilation is not clear. In the past theophylline was considered a first-line medication for the control of asthma. Because of a relatively high rate of adverse effects and a narrow toxic-therapeutic window in terms of serum levels, theophylline is currently a step 3 medication.[1] A steady-state serum concentration of 10 to 20 μg/ml has been shown to produce an optimal bronchodilator effect.[61] There is a linear relationship between serum concentration and bronchodilator effect in the range of 5 to 15 μg/ml, and severe toxicity is not usually associated with concentrations below 15 μg/ml.[62] Severe toxic effects include seizures and cardiac arrhythmias, although gastrointestinal symptoms and stimulation of the central nervous system are the most commonly reported side effects. The adverse effects of theophylline are similar to those of caffeine, a related methyl xanthine, but can usually be minimized by appropriate dosing and monitoring of the serum concentration. Because of its long duration of action when given as a sustained-release product, theophylline is useful in the control of nocturnal asthma.[63]

Inhaled anticholinergic medications can produce bronchodilation in asthmatic patients by blocking postganglionic efferent vagal pathways, thereby reducing airway smooth muscle tone. These agents also inhibit reflex bronchoconstriction caused by inhaled irritants. Atropine is the prototype drug of this class but causes systemic side effects because it is readily absorbed through the respiratory tract. Ipratropium bromide is an atropine derivative that is not readily absorbed through the respiratory tract and thus does not cause systemic effects.[64] Ipratropium bromide has been shown to be an effective treatment for status asthmaticus when given in combination with β_2-adrenergic agents.[65] Although the regular use of ipratropium bromide has been shown to have a role in the management of COPD,[66] the benefits of its regular use in asthma are less clearly established.

All step 1 medications for asthma are available in MDIs. The advantage of this mode of therapy is that high concentrations of drug can be delivered directly into the airways so that systemic side effects are minimized.[67] When the correct technique is used, MDIs can deliver medication as well as a nebulized aerosol. Because it may be hard for some patients to learn how to coordinate activation of an MDI with inhalation of the drug, patient training and periodic observation of MDI technique are essential. The use of certain spacer devices can reduce the difficulty of activation-inhalation coordination. In addition, spacer devices reduce deposition of drug in the mouth and the pharynx (larger particles fall out in the spacer) and reduce rapid initial particle velocity so that less throat irritation and cough occur. Dry-powder inhalers, which require a different technique than MDIs, are becoming more widely available, primarily because chlorofluorocarbons (CFCs or freons) are not used as propellants in these inhalers.[68] Atmospheric contamination with CFCs has led to depletion of stratospheric ozone, and the commercial use of these compounds is being phased out.[68,69]

Treatment of associated rhinitis and sinusitis can lead to more effective control of asthma.[1] Treatment of the upper airway should include efforts to reduce nasal obstruction, control nasal secretions, and treat bacterial sinus infections. Nasal corticosteroids can both treat and prevent nasal inflammation. Cromolyn sodium nasal spray may have some effect by inhibiting the response to allergen. Oral and topical decongestants can reduce nasal obstruction by decreasing mucosal edema as a result of vasoconstriction. Antihistamines can decrease nasal secretions. Appropriate antibiotic therapy should be administered whenever there is evidence of sinus infection, such as grossly purulent nasal discharge.

Management of gastroesophageal reflux, if present, can also lead to improved control of asthma.[1]

The presence of EIA is important to consider when advising patients about work and recreational activities. Exercise-induced asthma can be prevented by premedication with inhaled β-agonist bronchodilators or cromolyn sodium.[1] Patients with asthma should be encouraged to exercise to stay physically fit. Their asthma must be effectively managed so that they are able to do so.

The management of acute severe exacerbations of asthma is beyond the scope of this chapter, but several published guidelines are available.[1,70]

PROGNOSIS AND NATURAL HISTORY

As previously noted, the natural history of asthma is one of periodic exacerbations and remissions. Effective management should reduce the frequency of the former and prolong the duration of the latter. Some investigators have postulated that sensitization and continued exposure to house dust mites are the main factors responsible for the development of persistent asthma in childhood.[71] Some children with asthma "outgrow" the disease as they get older, but others do not.[72] In general, children with episodic and mild persistent asthma have a good prognosis, but those with more severe asthma continue to have some degree of airway hyperresponsiveness and will be at risk for developing acute exacerbations as adults. Asthma can begin in adult life, often because of exposure to sensitizing or irritant agents at the workplace. The percentage of adult patients with asthma who had asthma as children is unknown. However, there is evidence that the greater the severity of asthma in childhood, the greater the severity of the disease as an adult.[73] Adults with more severe asthma also tend to be more atopic.[74]

A major concern regarding patients with severe asthma is whether they will develop chronic irreversible airflow obstruction, presumably caused by airway remodeling as a consequence of chronic or recurrent airway inflammation. Although this question requires further study, there are data that suggest that the development of chronic airflow obstruction is related to the severity and duration of the disease.[75-77] There is also evidence that children with asthma tend to have lower values for FEV1 than children without asthma.[78]

SUMMARY

Asthma is a disease characterized by reversible airway obstruction, airway inflammation, and increased airway responsiveness to a variety of stimuli. The prevalence of asthma appears to be increasing in a number of countries, and in the United States both morbidity and mortality as a result of asthma appear to be increasing as well. It is likely that asthma is a multifactorial disease in most patients. Although there is clearly a strong genetic component, exposure to aeroallergens, environmental tobacco smoke, viral respiratory tract infections, and chemical irritants are other factors that have been associated with the development of asthma. Airway inflammation has emerged as the paramount feature of asthma. Asthma is a complex disease process that involves multiple interactions among inflammatory, airway epithelial, nerve, and smooth muscle cells. Mast cell- and eosinophil cell-derived products, cytokines, and adhesion molecules are also involved in the process. The release of inflammatory mediators from mast cells, macrophages, and airway epithelial cells appears to cause the targeted migration and activation of neutrophils and eosinophils, which, in turn, produce alterations in epithelial integrity, autonomic neural control, mucociliary function, and smooth muscle responsiveness. T lymphocytes may play an important role in the maintenance of chronic airway inflammation in asthma. Much more is understood about the mechanisms of allergy-related asthma than about those responsible for irritant-induced asthma. As the allergen- or irritant-induced airway inflammatory process proceeds, mucosal edema, mucus secretion, and vascular and epithelial permeability all increase, leading to a reduction of the caliber of the airway lumen and resultant airflow obstruction. The level of airway hyperresponsiveness in asthma appears to be associated with the degree of airway inflammation present. Acute exacerbations of asthma are triggered by a number of factors and can be potentially life-threatening when severe bronchospasm, mucus plugging, hyperinflation, and gas-exchange abnormalities occur.

A key to the diagnosis of asthma is the generally episodic nature of respiratory symptoms. Confirmation of the diagnosis and assessment of the severity of asthma, by objective testing, are necessary. Because asthma is a chronic condition with acute exacerbations, treatment requires continuous efforts to control symptoms, prevent exacerbations, and reduce persistent airway inflammation. Effective management of asthma depends on both pharmacologic and nonpharmacologic measures. Prevention, or at least a reduction, of exposure to the causative or aggravating agent(s) in the home and work environments, patient education on asthma, a step-care approach to pharmacologic therapy, and objective measures to monitor the severity of disease and response to therapeutic interventions (including serial monitoring of PEF) are all important components of an asthma management strategy.

REFERENCES

1. National Asthma Education Program Expert Panel: *Guidelines for the diagnosis and management of asthma,* NIH Pub No 91-3042A, Bethesda, Md, 1991, National Heart, Lung and Blood Institute.
2. Brooks SM, Weiss MA, and Bernstein IL: Reactive airways dysfunction syndrome (RADS), *Chest* 88:376-383, 1985.
3. *1989 national health interview survey,* Hyattsville, Md, 1990, National Center for Health Statistics, Centers for Disease Control.
4. Centers for Disease Control: Asthma—United States, 1980-1987, *Morbid Mortal Weekly Rep* 39:493-497, 1990.
5. Buist AS and Vollmer WM: Reflections on the rise in asthma morbidity and mortality, *JAMA* 264:1719-1720, 1990.
6. Bryant E and Shimizu I: *Sample design, sampling variance, and estimation procedures for the National Ambulatory Medical Care Survey,* Vital and Health Statistics, ser 2, No 108, DHHS Pub No (PHS) 88-1382, Washington, DC, 1988, National Center for Health Statistics, US Government Printing Office.
7. Weiss KB and Wagener DK: Changing patterns of asthma mortality: identifying target populations at high risk, *JAMA* 264:1683-1687, 1990.
8. Nelson HS: The atopic diseases, *Ann Allergy* 55:441-447, 1985.
9. Witt C, Stuckey MS, Woolcock AJ, et al: Positive allergy prick tests associated with bronchial histamine responsiveness in an unselected population, *J Allergy Clin Immunol* 77:698-702, 1986.
10. Empey DW, Laitinen LA, Jacobs L, et al: Mechanisms of bronchial hyperreactivity in normal subjects after upper respiratory tract infection, *Am Rev Respir Dis* 113:131-139, 1976.
11. Djukanovic R, Roche WR, Wilson JW, et al: Mucosal inflammation in asthma, *Am Rev Respir Dis* 142:434-457, 1990.
12. Laitinen LA, Heino M, Laitinen A, et al: Damage of the airway epithelium and bronchial reactivity in patients with asthma, *Am Rev Respir Dis* 131:599-606, 1985.
13. Beasley R, Roche WR, Roberts JA, et al: Cellular events in the bronchi in mild asthma and after bronchial provocation, *Am Rev Respir Dis* 139:806-817, 1989.
14. Djukanovic R, Wilson J, Britten K, et al: Quantitation of mast cells and eosinophils in the bronchial mucosa of symptomatic atopic individuals and healthy control subjects using immunohistochemistry, *Am Rev Respir Dis* 142:863-871, 1990.
15. Wardlaw AJ, Dunnette S, Gleich GJ, et al: Eosinophils and mast cells in bronchoalveolar lavage in subjects with mild asthma, *Am Rev Respir Dis* 137:62-69, 1988.

16. Holgate ST, Beasley R, and Twentyman OP: The pathogenesis and significance of bronchial hyperresponsiveness in airways disease, *Clin Sci* 73:561-572, 1987.

17. O'Byrne PM, Dolovich J, and Hargreave FE: Late asthmatic responses, *Am Rev Respir Dis* 134:740-751, 1987.

18. Cartier A, Thompson NC, Frith PA, et al: Allergen-induced increase in bronchial responsiveness to histamine: relationship to the late asthmatic response and change in airway caliber, *J Allergy Clin Immunol* 70:170-177, 1982.

19. Liu MC, Bleecker ER, Lichtenstein LM, et al: Evidence for elevated levels of histamine, prostaglandin D_2, and other bronchoconstricting prostaglandins in the airways of subjects with mild asthma, *Am Rev Respir Dis* 142:126-132, 1990.

20. Kelly J: Cytokines of the lung, *Am Rev Respir Dis* 141:765-788, 1990.

21. Metzger WJ, Zavala D, Richerson HB, et al: Local allergen challenge and bronchoalveolar lavage of allergic asthmatic lungs, *Am Rev Respir Dis* 135:433-440, 1987.

22. Robinson DS, Hamid Q, Ying S, et al: Predominant TH-2 like bronchoalveolar T cell population in atopic asthma, *N Engl J Med* 326:298-304, 1992.

23. Ollerenshaw S and Woolcock AJ: Characteristic of inflammation in biopsies from large airways of subjects with asthma and subjects with chronic airflow limitation, *Am Rev Respir Dis* 145:922-927, 1992.

24. Kowalski ML, Diddier A, and Kaliner MA: Neurogenic inflammation in the airways, *Am Rev Respir Dis* 140:101-109, 1989.

25. Bousquet J, Chanez P, Lacoste JY, et al: Eosinophilic inflammation in asthma, *N Engl J Med* 323:1033-1039, 1990.

26. Cockroft DW: Airway hyperresponsiveness: therapeutic implications, *Ann Allergy* 59:405-414, 1987.

27. Vanhoutte PM: Epithelium-derived relaxing factor(s) and bronchial reactivity, *J Allergy Clin Immunol* 83:855-861, 1989.

28. Bleecker ER: Cholinergic and neurogenic mechanisms in obstructive airways disease, *Am J Med* 81:93-102, 1986.

29. Hallahan AR, Armour CL, and Black JL: Products of neutrophils and eosinophils increase the responsiveness of human isolated bronchial tissue, *Eur Respir J* 3:554-558, 1990.

30. McFadden ER, Kiser R, and deGroot WJ: Acute bronchial asthma: relations between clinical and physiologic manifestations, *N Engl J Med* 288:221-225, 1973.

31. Rebuck AS and Read J: Assessment and management of severe asthma, *Am J Med* 51:788-790, 1971.

32. McFadden ER and Lyons HA: Arterial blood gas tension in asthma, *N Engl J Med* 278:1027-1032, 1968.

33. American Thoracic Society: Lung function testing: selection of reference values and interpretational strategies, *Am Rev Respir Dis* 144:1202-1218, 1991.

34. American Thoracic Society: Standardization of spirometry—1987, *Am Rev Respir Dis* 136:1285-1288, 1987.

35. American Thoracic Society: Guidelines for the evaluation of impairment/disability in patients with asthma, *Am Rev Respir Dis* 147:1056-1061, 1993.

36. Malo JL, Cote J, Cartier A, et al: How many times per day should peak expiratory flow rates (PEFR) be assessed when investigating occupational asthma? *Thorax* 48:1211-1217, 1993.

37. Reid MJ, Moss RB, and Hsu Y-P: Seasonal asthma in northern California: allergy causes and efficacy of immunotherapy, *J Allergy Clin Immunol* 78:590-600, 1986.

38. Aas K: Controlled trial of hyposensitization to house dust, *Acta Paediatr Scand* 60:264-268, 1971.

39. Ohman JL Jr, Findlay SR, and Leiterman KM: Immunotherapy in cat-induced asthma: double-blind trial with evaluation of in vivo and in vitro response, *J Allergy Clin Immunol* 74:230-239,1984.

40. Horst M, Hejjaoui A, Horst V, et al: Double-blind, placebo-controlled rush immunotherapy with a standardized alternaria extract, *J Allergy Clin Immunol* 85:460-472, 1990.

41. Van Bever HP and Stevens WJ: Suppression of the late asthmatic reaction by hyposensitization in asthmatic children to house-dust mites (*Dermatophagoides pteronyssinus*), *Clin Exp Allergy* 19:399-404, 1989.

42. Feldman CH, Clark NM, and Evans D: The role of health education in medical management in asthma, *Clin Rev Allergy* 5:195-205, 1987.

43. Clark NC: Asthma self-management education: research and implications for clinical practice, *Chest* 95:1110-1113, 1989.

44. Juniper EF, Kline PA, Vanzielehgem MA, et al: Effect of long-term treatment with an inhaled corticosteroid on airway hyperresponsiveness and clinical asthma in nonsteroid-dependent asthmatics, *Am Rev Respir Dis* 142:632-636, 1990.

45. Bel EH, Timmers MC, Hermans J, et al: The long-term effects of nedocromil sodium and beclomethasone diproprionate on bronchial responsiveness to methacholine in nonatopic asthmatic subjects, *Am Rev Respir Dis* 141:21-28, 1990.

46. Kraan J, Koeter GH, Mark W, et al: Changes in bronchial hyperreactivity induced by 4 weeks of treatment with anti-asthmatic drugs in patients with allergic asthma: a comparison between budesonide and terbutaline, *J Allergy Clin Immunol* 76:628-636, 1985.

47. Salmeron S, Guerin JC, Godard P, et al: High doses of inhaled corticosteroids in unstable chronic asthma, *Am Rev Respir Dis* 140:167-171, 1989.

48. Toogood JH: Complications of topical steroid therapy for asthma, *Am Rev Respir Dis* 141:S89-S96, 1990.

49. Petty TL, Rollins DR, Christopher K, et al: Cromolyn sodium is effective in adult chronic asthmatics, *Am Rev Respir Dis* 139:694-701, 1989.

50. North American Tilade Group: A double-blind multicenter group comparative study of the efficacy and safety of nedocromil sodium in the management of asthma, *Chest* 97:1299-1306, 1990.

51. Nelson HS: Adrenergic therapy of bronchial asthma, *J Allergy Clin Immunol* 77:771-785, 1986.

52. Rossing TH, Fanta CH, Goldstein DH, et al: Emergency therapy of asthma: comparison of the acute effects of parenteral and inhaled sympathomimetics and infused aminophylline, *Am Rev Respir Dis* 122:365-371, 1980.

53. Burrows B and Lebowitz MD: The β-agonist dilemma, *N Engl J Med* 326:560-561, 1992.

54. Crane J, Burgess C, and Beasley R: Cardiovascular and hypokalemic effects of inhaled salbutamol, fenoterol, and isoprenaline, *Thorax* 44:136-140, 1989.

55. Neville E, Corris PA, Vivian J, et al: Nebulized salbutamol and angina, *Br Med J* 285:796-797, 1982.

56. Higgins RM, Cookson W, Lane DJ, et al: Cardiac arrhythmias caused by nebulized beta-agonist therapy, *Lancet* 2:863-864, 1987.

57. Spitzer WO, Suissa S, Ernst P, et al: The use of β-agonists and the risk of death and near death from asthma. *N Engl J Med* 326:501-506, 1992.

58. Sears MR, Taylor DR, Print CG, et al: Regular inhaled beta-agonist treatment in bronchial asthma, *Lancet* 336:1391-1396, 1990.

59. Tashkin DP, Conolly ME, and Deutsch RI: Subsensitization of beta-adrenoreceptors in airways and lymphocytes of healthy and asthmatic subjects, *Am Rev Respir Dis* 125:185-193, 1982.

60. Repsher LH, Anderson JA, and Bush RK: Assessment of tachyphylaxis following prolonged therapy of asthma with inhaled albuterol aerosol, *Chest* 85:34-38, 1984.

61. Ellis EF: Theophylline toxicity, *J Allergy Clin Immunol* 76:297-301, 1985.

62. Tsiu SJ, Self TH, and Burns R: Theophylline toxicity: update, *Ann Allergy* 64:241-257, 1990.

63. Arkinstall WW, Arkins ME, Harrison D, et al: Once-daily sustained-release theophylline reduces diurnal variation spirometry and symptomatology in adult asthmatics, *Am Rev Respir Dis* 135:316-321, 1987.

64. Gross NJ: Ipratropium bromide, *N Engl J Med* 319:486-494, 1988.

65. Storms WW, Bodman SF, Nathan RA, et al: Use of ipratropium bromide in asthma, *Am J Med* 81:61-66, 1986.

66. Tashkin DP, Ashutosh K, Bleecker ER, et al: Comparison of the anticholinergic bronchodilator ipratropium bromide with metaproterenol in chronic obstructive pulmonary disease, *Am J Med* 81:81-90, 1986.

67. Newhouse MT and Dolovich MB: Control of asthma by aerosols, *N Engl J Med* 315:870-874, 1986.

68. Newman SP: Metered dose pressurized aerosols and the ozone layer, *Eur Respir J* 3:495-497, 1990.

69. Balmes JR: The environmental impact of chlorofluorocarbon use in metered dose inhalers, *Chest* 100:1101-1102, 1991.

70. British Thoracic Society: Guidelines for the management of asthma in adults: 2. Acute severe asthma, *Br Med J* 301:797-800, 1990.

71. Platts-Mills TAE and deWeck WA: Dust-mite allergens and asthma—a worldwide problem: report of the international workshop, *J Allergy Clin Immunol* 83:416-427, 1989.

72. Blair H: Natural history of childhood asthma: 20-year follow-up, *Arch Dis Child* 52:613-619, 1977.

73. Williams H and McNicol KN: Prevalence, natural history, and relationship of wheezy bronchitis and asthma in children: an epidemiological study, *Br Med J* 4:321-325, 1969.

74. Martin AJ, Landau LI, and Phelan PD: Natural history of allergy in asthmatic children followed to adult life, *Med J Aust* 2:470-474, 1981.

75. Martin AJ, Landau LI, and Phelan PD: Lung function in young adults who had asthma in childhood, *Am Rev Respir Dis* 122:609-616, 1980.

76. Brown PJ, Greville HW, and Finucane KE: Asthma and irreversible airflow obstruction, *Thorax* 39:131-136, 1984.

77. Connolly CK, Chan NS, and Prescott RJ: The relationship between age and duration of asthma and the presence of persistent obstruction in asthma, *Postgrad Med J* 64:422-425, 1988.

78. Weiss S, Toteson T, Segal M, et al: Effects of asthma on pulmonary function in children, *Am Rev Respir Dis* 145:58-64, 1992.

Chapter 14

HYPERSENSITIVITY PNEUMONITIS

Cecile Rose

Hypersensitivity pneumonitis (HP), also known as extrinsic allergic alveolitis, constitutes a spectrum of granulomatous, interstitial, bronchiolar, and alveolar lung diseases resulting from repeated inhalation of and sensitization to a wide variety of organic dusts and low-molecular-weight chemical antigens. Previously considered a rare disease, increasing recognition of the ubiquity of environmental antigens and earlier diagnosis have led to the understanding that the illness is more common than was earlier thought.

The nature of the inhaled antigen, the circumstances of exposure, and the immunologic reactivity of the host all contribute to the risk for HP. Disease is characterized initially by a lymphocytic alveolitis and granulomatous pneumonitis, with improvement or complete reversibility if antigen exposure is terminated early. Continued antigen exposure may lead to progressive interstitial fibrosis. No single historical or clinical feature is diagnostic of HP. Rather, diagnosis relies on a strong index of suspicion and a constellation of clinical findings. When the diagnosis is suspected, the clinician must undertake appropriate clinical assessment and environmental intervention to prevent progressive, irreversible lung damage.

CAUSATIVE ANTIGENS

The list of agents that cause HP is lengthy, and new etiologies and exposure circumstances continue to appear. Most particulate antigens are of respirable size and deposit in the alveoli; some (e.g., *Alternaria* spores) are deposited in airways and then solubilized. Intrinsic properties of the antigens capable of causing HP include their nondigestibility by alveolar macrophages and their ability to fix complement, and act as adjuvants, thereby enhancing lung immune responses and activating inflammatory cells.[1] The three major categories of antigens causing HP are microbial agents, animal proteins, and low-molecular-weight chemicals (Table 14-1). At least 28 different drugs have been shown to cause hypersensitivity reactions in the lungs,[2] but a discussion of these is beyond the scope of this chapter.

Microbial agents

Microbial organisms, including bacteria, fungi, and amoebae, are the most commonly recognized causes of HP. Microbial contaminants are environmentally ubiquitous and probably cause many more cases of HP than are recognized clinically. Warm, moist environments often provide ideal circumstances for the amplification and

Table 14-1. Major antigen categories and common examples of agents causing hypersensitivity pneumonitis

Antigen	Exposure	Syndrome
Bacteria		
Thermophilic bacteria		Farmer's lung
Faenia rectivirgula	Contaminated hay	Bagassosis
Thermoactinomyces vulgaris	Contaminated compost	Mushroom worker's lung
Thermoactinomyces sacchari	Mushroom compost	Humidifier lung
Thermoactinomyces candidus	Heated water reservoirs	Air conditioner lung
Nonthermophilic bacteria		
Bacillus subtilis and *B. cereus*	Water	Humidifier lung
	Detergent	Washing powder lung
Klebsiella oxytoca	Water	Humidifier lung
Fungi		
Aspergillus spp.	Moldy hay	Farmer's lung
	Water	Ventilation pneumonitis
Aspergillus clavatus	Barley	Malt worker's lung
Penicillium casei and *P. roqueforti*	Cheese	Cheese washer's lung
Penicillium frequentans	Cork dust	Wood pulp worker's lung
Alternaria spp.	Wood pulp	Maple bark stripper's lung
Cryptostroma corticale	Wood bark	Sequoiosis
Graphium spp., *Aureobasidium pullulans*	Wood dust	Dry rot lung
Merulius lacrymans	Rotten wood	Suberosis
Aureobasidium pullulans	Water	Humdifier lung
Cladosporium spp.	Hot tub mists	Hot tub HP
Trichosporon cutaneum	Damp wood and mats	Japanese summer-type HP
Amoebae		
Naegleria gruberi, Acanthamoeba polyphaga, and *Acanthamoeba castellani*	Contaminated water	Humidifier lung
Animal proteins		
Avian proteins	Bird droppings and feathers	Bird-breeder's lung
Urine, sera, and pelts	Rats and gerbils	Animal-handler's lung
Wheat weevil (*Sitophilus granarius*)	Infested flour	Wheat weevil lung
Chemicals		
Toluene diisocyanate	Paints and resins	Isocyanate HP
Diphenylmethane diisocyanate	Polyurethane foams	
Hexamethylene diisocyanate		
Trimellitic anhydride (TMA)	Plastics, resins, and paints	TMA-HP
Copper sulfate	Bordeaux mixture	Vineyard-sprayer's lung
Sodium diazobenzene sulfate	Chromatography reagent	Pauli's reagent alveolitis
Pyrethrum	Pesticide	Pyrethrum HP

proliferation of microbial antigens which, if disseminated into an occupied space, can cause sensitizing lung disease when inhaled.

Bacteria. Thermophilic actinomycetes including *Faenia rectivirgula* (formerly *Micropolyspora faeni*), *Thermoactinomyces vulgaris, T. sacharii, T. viridis,* and *T. candidus* are causally associated with the prototypical example of HP, farmer's lung, first described by Campbell in 1932.[3] These bacteria thrive at 56°C to 60°C temperatures and under moist conditions, secreting enzymes that cause decay of vegetable matter such as hay, sugar cane, and mushroom compost.[4-6] They are often found contaminating ventilation and humidification systems in which temperatures reach 60°C and stagnant water is present.[7]

Nonthermophilic bacteria used in detergent powders and contaminating humidifiers can also cause HP.[8,9] An outbreak of *Bacillus subtilis* alveolitis occurred in six family members exposed during home renovation to contaminated wood dust from bathroom flooring.[10] The gram-negative bacterium *Klebsiella oxytoca* can cause humidifier lung.[11] In addition to the bacteria themselves, endotoxins contained in the cell walls of gram-negative bacteria stimulate the cytokines tumor necrosis factor α (TNF-α) and interleukin-1 (IL-1) and may act as adjuvants, enhancing the inflammatory events leading to alveolitis and granuloma formation.[12]

Fungi. Fungi are nonmotile, eukaryotic organisms that have rigid cell walls, lack chlorophyll, and reproduce by means of spores, most of which are designed for airborne transport (disseminators). Fungal spores germinate to produce morphologically diverse forms, including molds and yeasts. Molds are branching hyphal filaments; yeasts are round, oval, or elongated single cells that reproduce mostly by budding and form moist or mucoid colonies. The cell walls of fungi contain polysaccharides (including glucan and chitin) and glycoproteins. Many components of fungi are capable of becoming airborne and acting as antigen sources, including fungal spores, mycelial fragments, metabolites and partially degraded substrates, and fungal toxins.[13]

Fungal spore content in air comes mainly from species adapted to using wind energy for dispersal. The particular species and concentration in air at any given time depend on prevailing winds, temperature, seasonal climatologic factors, circadian patterns of sunlight and darkness, degree of precipitation, availability of substrates, and extent of substrate and atmospheric moisture content. Several studies in the United States have shown that *Cladosporium* spp., *Alternaria* spp., and basidiospores are the most common atmospheric spores.[14] Atmospheric mold counts in Canada found *Alternaria* spp., *Cladosporium* spp., and yeasts to be the most numerous molds, with the peak season occurring between July and October. The indoor pattern of fungal spores reflects both the outdoor spore composition and indoor fungal flora dominated by the small, spored Deuteromycetes spp., including *Penicillium* spp., *Aspergillus* spp., *Rhizopus* spp., *Mucor* spp., and yeasts. Among the interior sites for mold growth are garbage containers, food storage areas, wallpaper, upholstery, and areas of increased moisture, such as shower curtains, window moldings, drip pans, window air conditioners, damp basements, and emissions from cool-mist vaporizers.[15-22] Saunas, hot tubs, and even tap water may also become contaminated with microorganisms capable of causing hypersensitivity lung disease.[23-25]

Domestic fungal exposure associated with decaying wood and damp walls in inner city dwellings is the most common cause of HP in Australia.[26] Multiple fungal species were identified in the homes of individuals with disease, including *Serpula lacrymans*, *Geotrichum candidum*, *Penicillium* spp., *Alternaria tenuis*, *Fusarium solani*, and *Aspergillus* spp., suggesting that sensitizing microbial exposures may be complex mixtures and that disease may not always be attributable to a single, well-defined antigen.

Many fungal species have been causally associated with hypersensitivity lung diseases in a wide variety of occupational and environmental circumstances. The respirable conidia of *Aspergillus* spp. are ubiquitous in nature and are commonly found in water, soil, and organic debris. A variety of *Aspergillus* spp. have been associated with HP in soy sauce brewers, bird hobbyists, farmers, and compost, sawmill, mushroom, greenhouse, tobacco, cane mill, grain, and brewery workers.[27-31] *Penicillium* spp. are common contaminants of indoor environments and have been associated with HP in cork workers (*Penicillium frequentans*), cheese workers (*P. casei* and *P. roqueforti*), laboratory workers, farmers, and tree cutters.[32-34] *Alternaria* spp., *Cladosporium* spp., *Aureobasidium* spp., and many other fungal species can cause HP. For example, mixed fungal contaminants in wood dust, bark, and chips have caused HP in sawmill workers, tree cutters, and other wood handlers.[35-43]

Amoebae. Free-living amoebae can ingest gram-negative bacteria and dissolved organic material, protecting bacteria such as *Legionella* spp. from environmental stresses. The amoebae *Naegleria gruberi* and *Acanthamoeba castellani* have been implicated in HP from exposure to contaminated humidifiers,[44] but their precise etiologic role awaits further clarification.

Animal proteins

Particulates from a variety of animal sources can cause HP when inhaled. Hypersensitivity pneumonitis from exposure to avian antigens, referred to as bird-breeder's or bird-fancier's lung, was first described by Plessner in 1960.[45] Avian antigens have been demonstrated in the feathers, droppings, and sera of turkeys, chickens, geese, ducks, parakeets, parrots, budgerigars, pigeons, doves, lovebirds, and canaries and are highly immunogenic.[46,47] Highest exposures are associated with cleaning out bird lofts, cages, and coops. Bird-breeder's lung is the most common form of HP in Great Britain, where approximately 12% of the general population keep budgerigars as pets.[48]

Animal handlers, such as laboratory workers, are at risk for HP from exposure to inhaled animal proteins (including those from rats and gerbils) in pelts, sera, and excreta.[49,50] Inhalation of grain infested with the wheat weevil *Sitophilus granarius* can cause a form of HP known as miller's lung.[51] Japanese sericulturists engaged in silk production can develop HP from exposure to larval secretions and cocoon particulates.[52] Mollusk shells cut and polished to make nacre (mother-of-pearl) buttons caused HP in two production workers.[53] An obsolete form of HP, snuff-taker's lung, resulted from sensitization to the bovine and porcine proteins contained in pituitary snuff used in the past to treat diabetes insipidus.[54]

Chemical sensitizers

The chemical-induced forms of HP are generally less well recognized than are classic microbial and animal protein-induced cases, but many of the inorganic antigens that cause disease are common in industry.

Isocyanates are widely used for large-scale production of polyurethane polymers used in the manufacture of flexible and rigid foams, elastomers, adhesives, and surface coatings. Several isocyanates, including toluene diisocyanate (TDI), diphenylmethane diisocyanate (MDI), and hexamethylene diisocyanate (HDI), can cause HP in addition to the more common occupational asthma associated with their exposure.[55-58] Specific immunoglobulin G (IgG) antibodies to isocyanates have been detected in the serum and bronchoalveolar lavage (BAL)of affected workers.[59,60] T-lymphocyte suppressor cell-predominant alveolitis was detected in five symptomatic workers who underwent BAL, indicating a role for cell-mediated immunity.[61]

Trimellitic anhydride, used in plastics, paints, and resins and as a curing agent for epoxy resins, has been associated with an HP-like syndrome often accompanied by anemia.[62,63] Trimellitic anhydride appears to act as a hapten, combining with endogenous proteins to create new antigenic determinants capable of eliciting IgE or IgG responses.[64]

Rare case reports of HP have been described from exposure to the pesticide pyrethrum, from Pauli's reagent (sodium diazobenzene sulfate) used in chromatography, and from copper sulfate used in Bordeaux mixture to spray vineyards.[65-67]

OCCUPATIONAL AND ENVIRONMENTAL EXPOSURE RISKS

Although acute symptoms are often attributed to intense, intermittent antigen exposure and chronic forms of HP are thought to result from lower-level, more prolonged exposure, the limited available environmental exposure data provide little insight into dose-response relationships. Understanding of these relationships is further complicated by the fact that the latency period between exposure to an environmental antigen and onset of HP may vary from a few weeks to years.

Environmental risk factors, including antigen concentration, duration of exposure before onset of symptoms, frequency and intermittency of exposure, particle size, antigen solubility, use of respiratory protection, and variability in work practices may influence disease prevalence, latency, and severity. Farmer's lung shows both seasonal and geographic variations in incidence. Disease is most common in late winter, when stored hay is used to feed cattle, and in regions with heavy rainfall and harsh winter conditions, when feed is likely to become damp and therefore an ideal substrate for microbial proliferation. A longitudinal study of pigeon breeders showed a seasonal variation in specific antibody levels among subjects with pigeon-breeder's disease, with a peak in antibody production during late summer, when maximum avian exposure was associated with the sporting season.[68]

Indirect and apparently trivial antigen exposure may be important. Hypersensitivity pneumonitis developed in two wives of pigeon hobbyists, one exposed to her husband's dusty coveralls and the other to a room adjacent to the pigeons.[69] A duvet containing goose feathers was a source of avian antigen causing HP, and down comforters and pillows can be similar exposure risks.[70] Feathers used for making fishing lures have also been associated with cases of HP.[71]

Summer-type HP due to the imperfect yeast *Trichosporon cutaneum* is the most prevalent form of HP in Japan.[72,73] Illness is characterized by recurrent sea-

sonal symptoms, familial occurrence of cases, and symptom provocation upon occupancy of homes containing *Trichosporon*-contaminated damp, decayed wood, and woven straw tatami mats. Removal of damaged and colonized areas, disinfection, and elimination of conditions leading to seasonal mold contamination are effective in preventing disease recurrence.[74]

HOST RISK FACTORS

Although many people are exposed to environmental antigens associated with HP and some develop serum antibodies, fewer manifest disease. This suggests that unique host susceptibility or resistance influences individual responses to inhaled antigen. Studies of human leukocyte antigen (HLA) haplotypes in patients with HP have shown no clear association of disease with a specific histocompatibility locus. No significant association between HLA-A, -B, or -C locus antigens and farmer's lung disease was found in a study of 100 farmers with disease, compared with normal farmers with and without precipitating antibodies.[75] A similar lack of association with HLA haplotypes is described for budgerigar-fancier's disease.[76,77]

A number of studies have shown that HP occurs more frequently in nonsmokers than in smokers; the mechanism for this effect is not known.[78,79]

Pregnancy and delivery appear to trigger symptoms and overt illness in women with pigeon-breeder's lung, but the associated hormonal and immunologic changes are not understood.[80]

Typically associated with occupational antigenic exposures, HP does occur in infants and children, and diagnosis is often elusive. A 5-year-old boy developed a recurrent flu-like illness that progressed to severe respiratory failure over 3 months.[81] Open-lung biopsy showed multiple granulomata associated with a diffuse interstitial mononuclear cell infiltrate. A detailed history revealed that the boy's father had arranged a comfortable bed of hay so that the child could rest in the barn during chores; that year the hay was very moldy and ventilation in the barn was poor. Treatment with corticosteroids and avoidance of the barn resulted in complete clinical resolution. A 10-month-old infant developed wheezing and tachypnea that progressed over 2 months to severe respiratory failure requiring mechanical ventilation.[82] Open-lung biopsy showed histologic findings of HP. Serum precipitins were positive to *Penicillium* spp. Environmental sampling in the home revealed predominantly *Penicillium* species, the source of which was unclear. Removal of the child from the home and repeated courses of corticosteroids resulted in slow resolution of the child's clinical abnormalities over 14 months. Avian proteins are the most common antigen associated with HP in the pediatric population. In an initial study of five children with pigeon-breeder's lung, Stiehm et al. noted that children are more likely to present with the subacute or chronic form of HP than with acute illness.[83]

IMMUNOPATHOGENESIS

Hypersensitivity pneumonitis is characterized by the presence of activated T lymphocytes in BAL and an interstitial mononuclear cell infiltrate. The pathogenesis of HP involves (1) repeated antigen exposure, (2) immunologic sensitization of the host to the antigen, and (3) immune-mediated damage to the lung. The immune inflammation resulting in the lymphocytic alveolitis and granulomatous pneumonitis appears to involve a combination of immune complex-mediated, humoral, and, most importantly, cell-mediated immune reactions to inhaled antigen.

Animal models support the importance of cell-mediated immunity in HP. Lymphoid cells passively transferred from sensitized rabbits to unexposed, nonsensitized animals result in disease similar to human HP when animals are subsequently exposed to antigen via inhalation.[84] A similar response occurs using passively transferred T lymphocytes that have been activated in vitro with either mitogen or antigen.[85] Several studies demonstrate that peripheral blood and lung lymphocytes from individuals with HP can undergo blastogenic transformation and generate cytokines when exposed in vitro to antigen.[86-88]

The cellular and humoral events that characterize HP have been examined with BAL. Within the first 48 hours after exposure of a sensitized host to the antigen, there is an immediate influx of neutrophils,[89] probably stimulated by formation of intraairway immune complexes, activation of the alternative complement pathway, or endotoxin effects of the inhaled antigen.[90-93] Several days later the local immune response shifts to a T lymphocyte-predominant alveolitis, often with 60% to 70% lymphocytes.[94] Mast cell numbers are increased in BAL following antigen exposure, returning to the normal range within 1 to 3 months after removal from exposure.[95] A mild neutrophilia (8% to 10%) is often found.[96]

Examination of the BAL lymphocyte subpopulations in patients with symptomatic HP reveals activated T lymphocytes, often with a predominance of CD8[+] cells having suppressor/cytotoxic functions.[97] Helper/suppressor ratios are usually less than 1.[98] Both cellular redistribution from peripheral blood to the lungs and in situ lymphocyte proliferation contribute to the increased number of lung T cells.[99] Natural killer cells are also increased in BAL from patients with HP compared with nonsmokers and those with sarcoidosis.[100,101]

A number of investigators have shown that CD4[+]/CD8[+] ratios vary widely in patients with HP, with some having normal or increased numbers of CD4[+] cells.[102,103] A CD4[+]-predominant BAL lymphocytosis has been described in patients with the fibrotic stage of HP.[104] Smoking also affects the cellular phenotypes seen in HP.[105] In a follow-up study of patients with farmer's lung who remained in the agricultural environment but without further exposure to specific antigens at work, Trentin et al. described a recovery of CD4[+] cells, a decrease in CD8[+] cells, and an increase in the CD4[+]/CD8[+] ratio to the normal range 6 months after initial observation.[106]

A BAL lymphocytosis can occur in asymptomatic pigeon breeders and farmers.[107] None of these subjects had developed symptomatic HP at the time of follow-up 2 to 3 years later.[108] There appears to be little correlation between BAL findings and other clinical abnormalities, including radiographic changes, pulmonary function, and the presence of precipitating antibody.

Macrophages play a pivotal role in disease pathogenesis by processing and presenting antigen to T-helper lymphocytes in the early phases of the immune response.[109] The alveolar macrophage and its products are also important in the early inflammatory events of granulomatous lung diseases. Early activation of alveolar macrophages by specific antigen–antibody complexes, with release of proinflammatory cytokines such as TNF-α, IL-1, and macrophage-derived lipoxygenase products, sets the stage for the development of HP.[1,110] Macrophage-derived factors with chemotactic activity for lymphocytes (including IL-1 and IL-8) probably contribute to the influx of CD8[+] cells specifically sensitized to antigen in the lungs of affected individuals. The accumulation of inflammatory and immune effector cells and the release of fibronectin and vitronectin by activated alveolar macrophages are associated with remodeling of the interstitial matrix and with the lung fibrosis seen in later stages or in the more chronic form of HP.[111]

Many of the particulate antigens capable of causing HP are potent immunologic adjuvants.[112] *Faenia rectivirgula*, a thermophilic actinomycete capable of causing farmer's lung disease, induces the release of the proinflammatory cytokines IL-1 and TNF-α from human macrophages.[113] Both IL-1 and TNF-α induce fever and inflammation and are important mediators of tissue destruction and remodeling.

PATHOLOGY

The histopathology of HP is distinctive, but it is not pathognomonic, and histologic features vary depending on the stage of illness at the time of biopsy.[114] The typical histologic triad of disease includes cellular bronchiolitis, interstitial mononuclear cell infiltrates, and small, scattered granulomas (Fig. 14-1).[115]

In acute HP there is a patchy infiltrate of the alveolar walls with mononuclear cells (predominantly lymphocytes and plasma cells) in a bronchocentric distribution, usually with accompanying epithelioid granulomas. Neutrophils and eosinophils are uncommon, as is generalized vasculitis. Mild interstitial fibrosis may be seen. In a study of 60 patients with acute farmer's lung disease, Reyes et al. found interstitial pneumonitis in all patients, characterized by a patchy infiltrate of the alveolar walls, mainly by lymphocytes, along with plasma cells and occasional polymorphonuclear leukocytes and eosinophils.[116] Granulomas were found in 70%, and foreign body material (demonstrable by

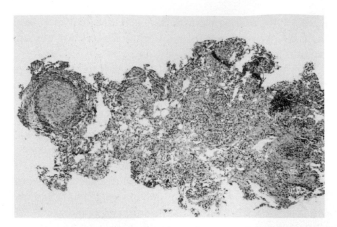

Fig. 14-1. Photomicrograph (×10) of a hematoxylin- and eosin-stained transbronchial lung biopsy from a patient with hypersensitivity pneumonitis. A discrete, nonnecrotizing interstitial granuloma is present at right. To the left is a mononuclear cell interstitial pneumonitis containing ill-defined macrophage aggregates.

polarized light) appeared in 60% of the biopsies. Fifty percent were found to have bronchiolitis obliterans.

The subacute and chronic forms of HP are characterized by infiltration of the interstitium with lymphocytes, plasma cells, and macrophages. Lymphocytes may form germinal centers, and there are often scattered, small, poorly formed, noncaseating interstitial granulomas. Histologic abnormalities are centered around respiratory bronchioles, and bronchiolar inflammation and obstruction (bronchiolitis obliterans) are common. Large histiocytes with foamy cytoplasm are seen in the alveoli and the interstitium.[117] Interstitial fibrosis with honeycombing is found late in disease, by which time the granulomatous phase may have resolved.

EPIDEMIOLOGY

Most of the population-based studies of HP focus on the prevalence of illness among agricultural workers.[118] Using a questionnaire survey, Grant et al. found the prevalence of farmer's lung in three agricultural areas in Scotland to range from 2.3% to 8.6%.[119] A questionnaire survey of western Wyoming dairy and cattle ranchers elicited a history typical of acute farmer's lung disease in 3% of those surveyed.[120] A study of Wisconsin farmers described a disease prevalence of 9% to 12% in adult males exposed to moldy hay.[121] A cross-sectional respiratory morbidity survey of mushroom farm workers found that 20% of the heavily exposed workers reported symptoms consistent with mushroom worker's lung.[29] In Finland, data on clinically confirmed farmer's lung showed a mean annual incidence rate of 44 per 100,000 persons in farming.[122]

The prevalence of HP among bird hobbyists is estimated to range between 0.5% and 21% and probably varies depending on bird type and circumstance of exposure.[123]

Using specific inhalation challenge, Vandenplas et al. detected MDI-induced HP in 8 (4.8%) of 167 workers employed in a wood chipboard manufacturing plant.[124] Affected subjects were identified through workers' compensation claims, undoubtedly underestimating the actual prevalence of HP in the plant. Interestingly, only 1 of the 8 cases worked continuously near the source of MDI, indicating that intermittent exposures can lead to illness.

Reports of HP outbreaks in microbially contaminated office buildings have described widely varying attack rates, in some reports affecting up to 70% of exposed individuals.[125,126] A history of respiratory and systemic symptoms is often the most sensitive screening parameter when investigating populations exposed to common antigen sources of illness. Measurement of pulmonary function before and after exposure may be of value for case finding in these circumstances.[127] It is clear that disease prevalence and attack rates will vary significantly depending not only on the case definition chosen but on exposure variables and host risk factors that are poorly understood.

CLINICAL FEATURES
Signs and symptoms

A clinical history suggesting a temporal relationship between symptoms and certain activities is often the first clue to the diagnosis of HP. The history should include a chronology of current and previous occupations, with a description of job processes and exposures. The environmental history should explore exposure to pets and other domestic animals; hobbies and recreational activities such as gardening and lawn care; circumstances in the home, such as the use of humidifiers, cool-mist vaporizers, and air conditioners; leaking or flooding in the basement or the attic; previous water damage to carpets and furnishings; and visible mold or mildew contamination in bathrooms or other rooms in the home (see box).

The classification of HP into distinct acute, subacute, and chronic forms can be misleading, as the clinical findings frequently overlap and all three forms may coexist in one individual. Nevertheless, the varying presentations are associated with different clinical findings. Acute illness typically begins 4 to 12 hours after exposure, with the patient describing both respiratory and constitutional symptoms of cough, dyspnea, chest tightness, fevers, chills, malaise, and myalgias. Symptoms may be accompanied by physical findings of fever, tachypnea, tachycardia, and crepitant rales. Peripheral blood leukocytosis with neutrophilia and lymphopenia is often present. Eosinophilia is unusual.

The subacute and chronic presentations of illness often require a high degree of clinical evidence to confirm the diagnosis and initiate appropriate management. Exertional dyspnea and cough are the predominant symptoms, and patients frequently report sputum production, fatigue, anorexia, and weight loss. Physical examination may be normal or may reveal basilar crackles. Wheezing occurs in some patients, probably reflecting antigen-mediated inflammatory effects on the airways. Cyanosis and right ventricu-

Necessary components of the clinical history in patients with suspected or confirmed hypersensitivity pneumonitis

Occupational history

- Chronology of current and previous occupations
- Description of job processes and specific work practices (e.g., maintenance work in a bird-contaminated loft or regular dry sweeping in a barn)
- List of specific chemical and dust exposures
- Review of Material Safety Data Sheets (MSDS) for the presence of known sensitizers
- Improvement in symptoms away from work or an increase in symptoms with specific workplace exposures (although this history is often not present)
- Presence of persistent respiratory and/or constitutional symptoms in exposed coworkers

Environmental and home history

- Pets and other domestic animals (especially birds)
- Hobbies and recreational activities (especially those involving chemicals, feathers, or organic dusts)
- Presence of humidifiers, dehumidifiers, swamp coolers, or cool-mist vaporizers
- Indoor venting of the clothes dryer (usually for heat)
- Use of hot tubs or saunas
- Leaking or flooding in the basement or the attic
- Water damage to carpets or furnishings
- Visible mold or mildew contamination in the home
- Feathers in pillows, comforters, or clothing

lar failure may be evident with severe fibrotic disease. Clubbing occurred in approximately half of the patients in a case series of pigeon-breeder's disease and is associated with a poorer prognostic outcome.[128] Clubbing is unusual in other forms of HP.

Precipitating antibodies

The finding of specific precipitating antibodies in the serum of a patient with suspected HP indicates exposure sufficient to generate a humoral immunologic response and may be a helpful diagnostic clue. Precipitins appear to have no role in disease pathogenesis but serve as markers of antigen exposure and are often found in individuals without clinically evident disease.[129] Serum precipitins are found in 3% to 30% of asymptomatic farmers and in up to 50% of asymptomatic pigeon breeders.[130,131] The prevalence of positive tests in asymptomatic individuals fluctuates over time, with subjects testing variably positive or negative at different times.[132]

Specific precipitating antibodies frequently are not demonstrable in patients with HP. False-negative results may occur because of poorly standardized antigens or the wrong choice of antigen. For example, there is little cross-reactivity between different *Penicillium* species, limiting the usefulness of a commercial antigen preparation that may contain a different species than the relevant environmental fungal exposure. The antibody response in some patients may be too meager to give a precipitin reaction using the traditional Ouchterlony double-immunodiffusion technique. More sensitive assays for specific IgG, such as enzyme-linked immunosorbent assay (ELISA), may lead to confusion because of decreased specificity. Serum precipitins may disappear over variable periods after exposure ceases, adding to the difficulty of antigen-specific diagnosis.[133] In some cases disease may not be a reaction to one organism alone but a cumulative reaction to a number of airborne antigens unlikely to be reflected in available laboratory antigen panels.

Other laboratory studies

Mild elevations in erythrocyte sedimentation rate, C-reactive protein, and immunoglobulins of IgG, IgM, or IgA isotype are occasionally evident, reflecting acute or chronic inflammation. Serum angiotensin-converting enzyme concentrations may rarely be increased in patients with recurrent acute symptoms.[134] Antinuclear antibodies and other autoantibodies are rarely detected.

Pulmonary function tests

Pulmonary function abnormalities in acute HP are classically restrictive, with a decrease in forced vital capacity, forced expiratory volume in 1 second, total lung capacity, and diffusion capacity. Hypoxemia is often present, and an exercise-induced fall in oxygen tension is an early sign of functional impairment. Four to 6 weeks may be required for complete resolution of these acute abnormalities following removal from exposure.[135]

Either restrictive or obstructive defects in pulmonary function occur in chronic HP, and a combined restrictive and obstructive pattern is common. In 1965 Pepys and Jenkins reported that 10% of 205 farmer's lung patients showed obstruction alone rather than restriction.[136] Decreased diffusion capacity is also commonly observed. Gas-exchange abnormalities, particularly with exercise, may be marked. Nonspecific airway hyperresponsiveness as determined by methacholine inhalation challenge has been described in 22% to 60% of patients with HP.[137,138]

Chest imaging

The chest radiograph in the acute form of disease may be normal but typically reveals small, scattered, 1- to 3-mm nodules, often with a lower-lobe predominance. Diffuse, patchy infiltrates or a ground glass appearance may be present. In one study, 4% of acute cases of farmer's lung had normal radiographic films and another 40% to 45% had minimal changes that might easily be overlooked. The extent of radiographic abnormality correlated poorly with the severity of symptoms or functional impairment.[139] Radio-

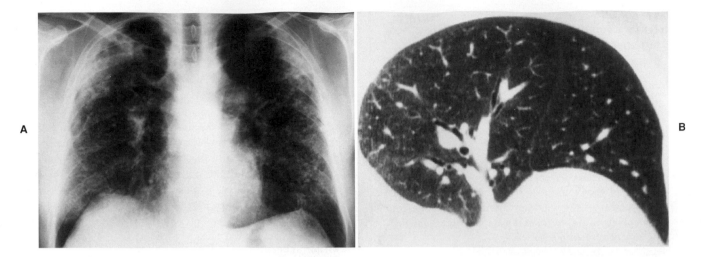

Fig. 14-2. A, This posteroanterior chest radiograph of a patient with chronic hypersensitivity pneumonitis demonstrates several typical findings, including linear interstitial markings most prominent in the periphery and the upper lung zones, emphysematous changes, and diminished lung volumes. **B,** This high-resolution (1.5-mm thin section) computerized tomographic image of the lung of a patient with subacute hypersensitivity pneumonitis shows subtle, diffuse nodular densities.

graphic abnormalities in acute illness regress or resolve over 4 to 6 weeks if further exposure is avoided.

In chronic HP linear interstitial markings become more distinct and are often most prominent in the periphery or upper lung zones on a plain chest radiograph (Fig. 14-2A). There may be progressive loss of lung volume. Pleural abnormalities, hilar adenopathy, calcification, and atelectasis are rarely described.

The computerized tomographic (CT) appearance of HP is variable, and the high-resolution CT scan may be normal if disease is diagnosed early.[140] In subacute HP the predominant pattern on high-resolution CT scanning is poorly defined centrilobular micronodules, most often with concurrent ground glass attenuation (Fig. 14-2B).[141-143] These findings probably reflect a cellular bronchiolitis, noncaseating granulomas, and active alveolitis. Either patchy or diffuse ground glass attenuation was observed in 52% of subacute and 71% of chronic forms of bird-breeder's HP.[144] Honeycombing was seen in only 50% of the patients with chronic disease, a number of whom also had concurrent micronodules and/or ground glass attenuation, suggesting subacute changes superimposed on chronic disease. Emphysematous changes were observed in patients with subacute or chronic disease, most of whom were nonsmokers. Other CT features of HP include patchy air space opacification and reticular densities with a central distribution.[145] Pretracheal lymph nodes may be enlarged, but hilar adenopathy is rare.[146]

Inhalation challenge

The use of inhalation challenge in the diagnosis of HP is limited by the lack of standardized antigens and techniques. Inhalation of an aerosolized antigen suspected to be causative is helpful only when acute symptoms and

clinical abnormalities are part of the disease presentation and are likely to occur within hours after exposure.[147] In some patients with acute symptoms, exposure to the suspect environment with postexposure monitoring of symptoms, temperature, leukocyte count, spirometry, and chest radiograph may be preferable to laboratory challenge. Interpretation of results is often difficult, and routine inhalation challenge is not recommended in most patients with suspected HP.[148]

Bronchoalveolar lavage

Bronchoalveolar lavage appears to play a useful role in the evaluation of patients with HP.[149] Typically, a marked lavage lymphocytosis without eosinophilia or neutrophilia is found. The total white blood cell count is increased, often up to fivefold of that of controls. The absolute number of macrophages is similar to that of controls, although their percentage in lavage is reduced due to the high number of lymphocytes. Mast cells have been reported to be increased in symptomatic patients with HP.[150] Concentrations of IgG, IgM, and IgA antibodies are typically increased in BAL in subjects with HP (although smoking may mitigate this effect), as are total protein and albumin.[151,152] The lavage cellular profile may vary considerably depending on the stage of illness and the time interval between BAL and the last antigen exposure.[106] The BAL lymphocytosis may persist for years following removal from exposure and despite improvement in other clinical parameters, limiting its utility as a tool to follow the course and progression of disease.[153]

Lung biopsy

Lung biopsy may be indicated in patients without sufficient clinical criteria for definitive diagnosis or to rule out other diseases requiring different treatment. Transbronchial biopsies are often sufficient but may sample unrepresentative areas, and open-lung biopsy is occasionally required. Special stains and cultures are helpful to distinguish HP from infectious granulomatous conditions such as fungal diseases and tuberculosis. Hypersensitivity pneumonitis differs from sarcoidosis in the finding of inflammatory infiltrates at interstitial sites distant from granulomas, whereas in sarcoidosis such infiltrates are found generally in and around the granulomas.[114,148] Given the substantial overlap in the histologic appearance of these granulomatous processes, pathology without clinical correlation is usually insufficient for diagnosis.

DIAGNOSTIC CRITERIA

Efforts to standardize reporting have led to the development of diagnostic criteria for HP. Terho proposed major and minor criteria for farmer's lung; the diagnosis is considered confirmed if the patient fulfills all of the major criteria and at least two additional criteria and if other diseases with similar clinical findings have been ruled out.[154] A negative chest film is allowed if the biopsy is positive. The major criteria include (1) exposure to offending antigens revealed by history, by environmental measurements, or by the presence of antigen-specific IgG antibodies; (2) symptoms compatible with HP appearing several hours after exposure; and (3) an abnormal chest x-ray. Additional criteria include basilar crepitant rales, decreased diffusing capacity, decreased oxygen tension or saturation at rest or with exercise, abnormal histology compatible with HP, and a positive provocation test by either work exposure or controlled inhalation challenge.

Stringent diagnostic criteria may underestimate milder cases of HP in which the chest radiograph is normal or in which symptoms are subtle or insidious. Hodgson et al. showed a decline in the sensitivity of the chest radiograph for diagnosis of HP from 1950 to 1980.[155] Chest x-rays were also less likely to be abnormal when a population-based approach to diagnosis was undertaken.

The diagnosis of HP in a patient may have considerable public health importance, since others exposed to the same environment are likely to be affected. Because exposure is part of the case definition for disease, absent or inadequate occupational and environmental history-taking probably results in underrecognition of disease. The likelihood that unrecognized HP is quite common is based on several other factors as well: (1) the signs and symptoms of illness are nonspecific and mimic those of many other diseases, such as asthma, influenza, viral pneumonia, and sarcoidosis (see box); (2) early disease may be accompanied by a normal chest radiograph and resting pulmonary function; (3) the antigens that cause HP proliferate in common environmental niches, particularly in areas where water damage creates circumstances in which microbial contaminants are amplified and disseminated; and (4) precipitating antibodies are often difficult to measure and may disappear after exposure

---

Differential diagnosis of hypersensitivity pneumonitis (HP)

Inhalation fevers (acute respiratory and systemic symptoms following exposure)

Humidifier fever
Organic dust toxic syndrome
Metal fume fever
Pontiac fever (nonpneumonic legionellosis)

Granulomatous disorders (histology compatible with HP)

Sarcoidosis
Beryllium disease
Drug-induced pneumonitis
Granuloma–vasculitis syndromes
Lymphatoid granulomatosis
Eosinophilic granuloma

Immunologic diseases (often similiar respiratory symptoms and serologic and/or radiographic findings)

Asthma
Collagen–vascular diseases
Allergic bronchopulmonary aspergillosis
Eosinophilic pneumonias

Infections (fever and respiratory symptoms)

Viral and mycoplasma pneumonias
Psittacosis
Fungal infections
Mycobacterial infections

Fibrosing lung diseases (findings similar to chronic HP)

Idiopathic pulmonary fibrosis
Bronchiolitis obliterans from other causes
Inorganic dust pneumoconioses

---

ceases, so that a patient with fibrotic lung disease from previous episodes of HP may not be recognized as such.[156]

NATURAL HISTORY AND PROGNOSIS

The clinical course of HP is variable, but if illness is recognized early, the prognosis for recovery is usually quite good.[157]

In acute forms of HP, fever, chills, and cough symptoms usually disappear within days after exposure ceases. Malaise, fatigue, and dyspnea may persist for several weeks. There is usually rapid improvement in lung vital capacity and diffusion capacity in the first 2 weeks after an acute attack, but mild abnormalities in pulmonary function often persist for several months. Generally, single acute episodes are self-limited. Occasionally, disease may progress despite removal from exposure. Continued symptoms and progressive lung impairment have been reported after recurrent acute attacks and even after a single severe attack.[158,159]

The chronic form of HP, having insidious symptoms and more subtle clinical abnormalities than the acute form, is probably recognized later in the course of illness and may have a poorer prognosis. Symptomatic pigeon breeders followed for 18 years showed a fourfold average rate of decline in pulmonary function compared with the expected rate.[160] Four children and five adults with chronic avian HP were followed from 6 months to 10 years after treatment with corticosteroids and reduction or elimination of exposure.[161] Five were completely asymptomatic, two had improved but persistent symptoms, and one had progressive symptoms. Seven of eight who had follow-up chest radiographs had resolution of interstitial infiltrates. Spirometry was obtained in seven patients, one of whom had severe restrictive abnormalities; in the three who had diffusing capacity measured at follow-up, only one was normal. The patient with progressive symptoms, honeycombing on chest film, and restrictive pulmonary function ultimately died of HP following unsuccessful lung transplantation. Precipitating antibodies remained positive in all patients tested. Overall, long-term mortality for patients with chronic illness ranges from 3% to 10%.[162]

No single functional or biochemical marker exists to predict the probability of developing pulmonary fibrosis in an individual patient. The BAL lymphocytosis may persist for years following removal from exposure and despite clinical recovery. Age at diagnosis, duration of antigen exposure after onset of symptoms, and total years of exposure before diagnosis seem to have predictive value in the likelihood of recovery from pigeon-breeder's lung disease.[163] Pigeon breeders with HP were more likely to improve or recover completely if they had been in contact with birds for less than 2 years. Neither the form of clinical presentation (acute versus chronic) nor the degree of lung function abnormality at the time of diagnosis was related to recovery in another study of pigeon-breeder's disease.[164] Rather, younger age at diagnosis (27 years versus 42 years) and exposure to antigen for less than 6 months after symptom onset were associated with complete recovery.

TREATMENT AND PREVENTION

An accelerated decline in lung function with continued antigen exposure has been demonstrated for most forms of HP. Thus, early diagnosis and avoidance of antigen exposure are the mainstays of treatment. Avoidance is usually accomplished by removing the affected individual from the antigen-containing environment. In some circumstances this approach is simple and adequate for recovery. However, the social consequences and economic disruption to the affected individual may preclude strict abstinence from exposure. A 6-year follow-up study of affected farmers revealed that 50% to 60% remained on the farm[133]; by 15 years as many as 70% had returned to farming.[165] In such cases regular follow-up of pulmonary function, radiography, and symptoms is essential to detect clinical deterioration and direct efforts to minimize antigen exposure.

Continued antigen exposure may not lead to clinical deterioration in some cases.[166] Bourke et al. found that 18 of 21 pigeon breeders with acute pigeon-breeder's lung had continued regular exposure to pigeons 10 years after diagnosis, although many used improved ventilation and respiratory protection; only 6 of these reported continued respiratory symptoms.[167] This phenomenon has been demonstrated in several animal models of disease, in which repeated antigen inhalation in sensitized animals results in resolution rather than progression of the pulmonary inflammatory response.[168] This modulation of the inflammatory response is not well understood. As yet, no markers are available to predict the resolution or progression of disease.

Avoidance of exposure by eliminating the offending antigen from the environment may be difficult. In five homes followed serially after bird removal, antigen levels measured by inhibition ELISA declined gradually despite extensive environmental control measures, with high levels still detectable at 18 months in one home.[169] Significant amounts of bird antigens can be found in homes without pet birds if wild bird excrement is heavily deposited outside the house and tracked in on shoes.

An outbreak of HP traced to fungal contamination of an open water-spray ventilation system was controlled by extensive cleaning of the system and corresponding work areas and replacement of the system with a dry (closed-coil) ventilation system.[170] In another large outbreak of HP due to microbial contamination of a chilled water air-conditioning system, a variety of cleaning and water treatment measures were used to reduce antigen concentration. A solid-phase radioimmunoassay method using antiserum from affected workers was used thereafter to assess levels of airborne antigen and monitor the efficacy of control measures.[171]

Strategies recommended to reduce the prevalence of farmer's lung disease include efficient drying of hay and cereals before storage, use of mechanical feeding systems, and better ventilation of farm buildings.[119,172] Education of individuals in at-risk occupations in antigen avoidance and early symptom recognition may also be helpful.[173]

The efficacy of various types of respirators in preventing antigen sensitization and disease progression once sensitization has occurred is unknown. Helmet-type powered air-purifying respirators (PAPRs) have been used to prevent episodic exposure in individuals with previous acute episodes of farmer's lung.[174] Respiratory protection has been examined in bird breeders with HP, many of whom are reluctant to abandon their at-risk hobby. Serial measurements of pigeon-specific IgG antibodies were obtained in 22 pigeon fanciers with HP who had ongoing exposure, 13 of whom wore a PAPR, and 9 of whom refused respiratory protection.[175] Serum antibody levels declined by 65% over 14 months in those wearing respirators compared with no decline in antibody levels in those without respirators; no data were reported on changes in symptoms or pulmonary function in the two groups. Prolonged wearing of respiratory protection is limited by the fact that most respirators are hot and cumbersome. Dust respirators offer substantial, but in some cases incomplete, protection against organic dusts[176] and are not recommended once sensitization has occurred.

Indoor microbial contamination is often related to problems with control of moisture. Source, dilution, and administrative controls are used to reduce these indoor contaminants.[177] Source control includes preventing leaking and flooding, removing stagnant water sources, eliminating aerosol humidifiers and vaporizers, and maintaining indoor relative humidity below 70%. Dilution of contaminants can be effected by increasing the amount of outdoor air in a building, and high-efficiency filters can be added to the ventilation system to clean recirculated air. Complete elimination of indoor allergens is probably impossible, and it is often necessary to relocate immunologically sensitized individuals once hypersensitivity lung disease has occurred.

Personal spore sampling with Burkard personal volumetric air samplers and indirect immunofluorescence testing for spore-specific IgG have been used to assess individual mold sensitization and air quality control.[178] However, quantitative bioaerosol sampling for microbial antigens is often difficult to interpret. A negative result should not be used to disprove disease or exposure. Settle plates are unreliable in assessing indoor microbial contaminants.

The effect of corticosteroids on the long-term course of various forms of HP has not been adequately investigated. There are many anecdotal reports of the beneficial effects of steroids in acute attacks, but controlled clinical trials are lacking. In cases in which pulmonary function abnormalities are minor and spontaneous recovery is likely with removal from exposure, steroids are probably unnecessary. In one study 36 patients, most having suffered only one acute attack of farmer's lung disease, were randomly assigned to receive prednisolone or a placebo for 2 months.[179] The steroid-treated group showed more rapid improvement in physiologic abnormalities (particularly diffusing capacity) at 1-month follow-up, but no differences were found between the treated and untreated groups 5 years later. Interestingly, the group treated with steroids suffered more frequent recurrences of symptomatic farmer's lung during the 5-year follow-up period, although this finding did not reach statistical significance. In a study of pigeon breeders with HP, there were no significant clinical outcome differences between patients who were treated with steroids and those who were not; the mean time for improvement or normalization of pulmonary function after treatment and removal from exposure was 3.4 months.[164]

In cases in which disease is progressive despite other measures, an empiric trial of steroids (1 mg/kg/day of prednisone) is indicated, with monitoring of pulmonary function 4 weeks after initiation of treatment. If there is objective improvement, a gradual taper to minimum sustaining doses should follow; otherwise, the steroid regimen should be tapered and discontinued.[180] Monkare showed that 12 weeks of steroid treatment did not produce better results than 4 weeks in patients with farmer's lung disease.[181]

Inhaled steroids and β-agonists may be helpful in patients with HP manifested by symptoms of chest tightness and cough and with airflow limitation on pulmonary function. A 12-year-old boy with allergic alveolitis due to bird antigen was treated with 5 days of oral prednisolone followed by nebulized budesonide for 3 months; the investigators suggest that inhaled nebulized budesonide penetrates to the peripheral airways in the same manner as the antigen itself.[182] There are as yet no data from controlled clinical trials on the efficacy of inhaled steroids in the treatment of HP.

REFERENCES

1. Salvaggio JE and Millhollon B: Induction and modulation of pulmonary inflammation by organic dusts: cytokines, immune complexes and 'all those things,' *Clin Exp Allergy* 22:731-233, 1992. Editorial.
2. Akoun GM, Cadranel JL, Rosenow EC 3rd, et al: Bronchoalveolar lavage cell data in drug-induced pneumonitis, *Allerg Immunol* 23(6):245-252, 1991.
3. Campbell JM: Acute symptoms following work with hay, *Br Med J* 2:1143-1144, 1932.
4. Dickie HA and Rankin J: Farmer's lung: an acute granulomatous interstitial pneumonitis occurring in agricultural workers, *JAMA* 167:1069-1076, 1958.
5. Pepys J, Jenkins PA, Festenstein GN, et al: Farmer's lung: thermophilic actinomycetes as a source of "farmer's lung hay" antigen, *Lancet* 18:182-196, 1963.
6. Buechner H, Prevatt A, Thompson J, et al: Bagassosis: review with further historical data, studies of pulmonary function, and results of adrenal steroid therapy, *Am J Med* 25:234-247, 1958.
7. Banaszak EF, Thiede WH, and Fink JN: Hypersensitivity pneumonitis due to contamination of an air conditioner, *N Engl J Med* 283:271-276, 1970.
8. Franz T, McMurrain K, Brooks S, et al: Clinical, immunologic, and physiologic observations in factory workers exposed to *B. subtilis* enzyme dust, *J Allergy* 47:170-178, 1971.
9. Kohler P, Gross G, Salvaggio J, et al: Humidifier lung: hypersensitivity pneumonitis related to thermotolerant bacterial aerosols, *Chest* 69(suppl):294-305, 1976.
10. Johnson CL, Bernstein IL, Gallagher JS, et al: Familial hypersensitivity pneumonitis induced by *Bacillus subtilis*, *Am Rev Respir Dis* 122:339-348, 1980.
11. Kane GC, Marx JJ, and Prince DS: Hypersensitivity pneumonitis secondary to *Klebsiella oxytoca*. A new cause of humidifier lung, *Chest* 104:627-629, 1993.
12. Brade H, Brade L, Schade U, et al: Structure, endotoxicity, immunogenicity and antigenicity of bacterial lipopolysaccharides (endotoxins, O-antigens). In Levin J et al, editors: *Bacterial endotoxins: pathophysiological effects, clinical significance, and pharmacological control*, pp 17-45, New York, Alan R. Liss.
13. Burge HA: Airborne allergenic fungi: classification, nomenclature, and distribution, *Immunol Allergy Clin North Am* 92:307-319, 1989.
14. Fernandez-Caldas E and Fox RW: Environmental control of indoor air pollution, *Clin Allergy* 76:935-952, 1992.
15. Volpe BT, Sulavik SB, Tran P, et al: Hypersensitivity pneumonitis associated with a portable home humidifier, *Conn Med* 55:571-573, 1991.
16. Reynolds SJ, Streifel AJ, and McJilton CE: Elevated airborne concentrations of fungi in residential and office environments, *Am Ind Hyg Assoc J* 51:601-604, 1990.

17. Siersted HC and Gravesen S: Extrinsic allergic alveolitis after exposure to the yeast *Rhodotorula rubra, Allergy* 48:298-299, 1993.

18. Hodges GR, Fink JN, and Schlueter DP: Hypersensitivity pneumonitis caused by a contaminated cool-mist vaporizer, *Ann Intern Med* 80:501-504, 1974.

19. Burke GW, Carrington CB, Strauss R, et al: Allergic alveolitis caused by home humidifiers, *JAMA* 238:2705-2708, 1977.

20. Robertson AS, Burge PS, Wieland GA, et al: Extrinsic allergic alveolitis caused by a cold water humidifier, *Thorax* 42:32-37, 1987.

21. Baur X, Richter G, Pethran A, et al: Increased prevalence of IgG-induced sensitization and hypersensitivity pneumonitis (humidifier lung) in nonsmokers exposed to aerosols of a contaminated air conditioner, *Respiration* 59:211-214, 1992.

22. Fink JN, Banaszak EF, Barboriak JJ, et al: Interstitial lung disease due to contamination of forced air systems, *Ann Intern Med* 84:406-413, 1976.

23. Metzger WJ, Patterson R, Fink J, et al: Sauna-takers disease: hypersensitivity pneumonitis due to contaminated water in a home sauna, *JAMA* 236:2209-2211, 1976.

24. Jacobs RL, Thorner RE, Holcomb JR, et al: Hypersensitivity pneumonitis caused by *Cladosporium* in an enclosed hot-tub area, *Ann Intern Med* 105:204-206, 1986.

25. Muittari A, Kuusisto P, Virtanen P, et al: An epidemic of extrinsic allergic alveolitis caused by tap water, *Clin Allergy* 10:77-90, 1980.

26. Bryant DH and Rogers P: Allergic alveolitis due to wood-rot fungi, *Allergy Proc* 12:89-94, 1991.

27. Meeker DP, Gephardt GN, Cordasco EM Jr, et al: Hypersensitivity pneumonitis versus invasive pulmonary aspergillosis: two cases with unusual pathologic findings and review of the literature, *Am Rev Respir Dis* 143:431-436, 1991.

28. Tsuchiya Y, Shimokata K, Ohara H, et al: Hypersensitivity pneumonitis in a soy sauce brewer caused by *Aspergillus oryzae, J Allergy Clin Immunol* 91:688-689, 1993.

29. Sanderson W, Kullman G, Sastre J, et al. Outbreak of hypersensitivity pneumonitis among mushroom farm workers, *Am J Ind Med* 22:859-872, 1992.

30. Riddle HF, Channel S, and Blyth W: Allergic alveolitis in a malt-worker, *Thorax* 23:271-280, 1968.

31. Yoshida K, Neda A, Yamasaki H, et al: Hypersensitivity pneumonitis resulting from *Aspergillus fumigatus* in a greenhouse, *Arch Environ Health* 48:260-262, 1993.

32. Schlueter D: Cheesewasher's disease: a new occupational hazard?, *Ann Intern Med* 78:606-613, 1973.

33. Avila R and Lacey J: The role of *Penicillium frequentans* in suberosis (respiratory disease in workers in the cork industry), *Clin Allergy* 4:109-117, 1974.

34. Fergusson RJ, Milne LJR, and Crompton GK: *Penicillium* allergic alveolitis: faulty installation of central heating, *Thorax* 39:294-298, 1984.

35. Van Assendelft AHW, Raitio M, and Turkia V: Fuel chip-induced hypersensitivity pneumonitis caused by *Penicillium* species, *Chest* 87:394-396, 1985.

36. Cohen H, Merrigan T, Kosek J, et al: Sequoiosis, *Am J Med* 43:785-794, 1967.

37. Dykewicz MS, Laufer P, Patterson R, et al: Woodman's disease: hypersensitivity pneumonitis from cutting live trees, *J Allergy Clin Immunol* 81:455-460, 1988.

38. Emanuel DA, Wenzel FJ, and Lawton BR: Pneumonitis due to *Cryptostroma corticale* (maple-bark disease), *N Engl J Med* 274:1413-1418, 1966.

39. Sosman AJ, Schlueter DP, Fink JN, et al: Hypersensitivity to wood dust, *N Engl J Med* 281:977-980, 1969.

40. Cohen H, Merigan T, Kosek J, et al: A granulomatous pneumonitis associated with redwood sawdust inhalation, *Am J Med* 43:785-794, 1967.

41. Belin L: Clinical and immunological data on "wood trimmer's disease" in Sweden, *Eur J Respir Dis* 107(suppl):169-176, 1980.

42. O'Brien I, Bull J, Creamer B, et al. Asthma and extrinsic allergic alveolitis due to *Merulius lacrymans, Clin Allergy* 8:535-542, 1978.

43. Enarson DS and Chan-Yeung M: Characterization of health effects of wood dust exposures, *Am J Ind Med* 17:33-38, 1990.

44. Edwards JH, Griffiths AJ, and Mullins J: Protozoa as sources of antigen in humidifier fever, *Nature* 264:438-439, 1976.

45. Plessner MM: Une maladie des trieurs de plumes: la fièvre du canard, *Arch Mal Prof Med Trav Secur Soc* 21:67-69, 1960.

46. Fink J, Sosman A, Barboriak J, et al: Pigeon breeder's disease: a clinical study of a hypersensitivity pneumonitis, *Ann Intern Med* 68:1205-1219, 1968.

47. Moore VL, Fink JN, Barboriak JJ, et al: Immunologic events in pigeon breeder's disease, *J Allergy Clin Immunol* 53:319-328, 1974.

48. Boyd G, McSharry C, Banham S, et al: A current view of pigeon fancier's lung, *Clin Allergy* 12:53-59, 1982.

49. Carrol KB, Pepys J, Longbottom J, et al: Extrinsic allergic alveolitis due to rat serum proteins, *Clin Allergy* 5:443-456, 1975.

50. Pimental JC: Furrier's lung, *Thorax* 25:387-398, 1970.

51. Lunn J and Hughes D: Pulmonary hypersensitivity to the grain weevil *(Sitophilus granarius), Br J Ind Med* 24:158-161, 1967.

52. Nakazawa T and Umegae Y: Sericulturist's lung disease: hypersensitivity pneumonitis related to silk production, *Thorax* 45:233-234, 1990.

53. Orriols R, Manresa JM, Aliaga JL, et al: Mollusk shell hypersensitivity pneumonitis, *Ann Intern Med* 113:80-81, 1990.

54. Harper K, Burrell R, Lapp J, et al: Allergic alveolitis due to pituitary snuff, *Ann Intern Med* 73:581-584, 1970.

55. Vandenplas O, Malo JL, Saetta M, et al: Occupational asthma and extrinsic alveolitis due to isocyanates: current status and perspectives, *Br J Ind Med* 50:213-228, 1993.

56. Zeiss CR, Kanellakes TM, Bellone JD, et al: Immunoglobulin E-mediated asthma and hypersensitivity pneumonitis with precipitating anti-hapten antibodies due to diphenylmethane diisocyanate (MDI) exposure, *J Allergy Clin Immunol* 65:346-352, 1980.

57. Malo JL and Zeiss CR: Occupational hypersensitivity pneumonitis after exposure to diphenylmethane diisocyanate, *Am Rev Respir Dis* 125:113-116, 1982.

58. Yoshizawa Y, Ohtsuka M, Noguchi K, et al: Hypersensitivity pneumonitis induced by toluene diisocyanate: sequelae of continuous exposure, *Ann Intern Med* 110:31-34, 1989.

59. Selden AI, Belin L, and Wass U: Isocyanate exposure and hypersensitivity pneumonitis—report of a probable case and prevalence of specific immunoglobulin G antibodies among exposed individuals, *Scand J Work Environ Health* 15:234-237, 1989.

60. Walker CL, Grammer LC, Shaughnessy MA, et al: Diphenylmethane diisocyanate hypersensitivity pneumonitis: a serologic evaluation, *J Occup Med* 31:315-319, 1989.

61. Bascom R, Kennedy TP, Levitz D, et al: Specific bronchoalveolar lavage IgG antibody in hypersensitivity pneumonitis from diphenylmethane diisocyanate, *Am Rev Respir Dis* 131:463-465, 1985.

62. Patterson R, Zeiss C, and Pruzansky J: Immunology and immunopathology of trimellitic anhydride pulmonary reactions, *J Allergy Clin Immunol* 70:19-23, 1982.

63. Patterson R, Addington W, Banner AS, et al: Antihapten antibodies in workers exposed to trimellitic anhydride fumes: a potential immunopathogenetic mechanism for the trimellitic anhydride pulmonary disease–anemia syndrome, *Am Rev Resp Dis* 120:1259-1267, 1979.

64. Zeiss CR, Levitz D, Chacon R, et al: Quantitation and new antigenic determinant specificity of antibodies induced by inhalation of trimellitic anhydride in man, *Int Arch Allergy Appl Immunol* 61:380-388, 1980.

65. Carlson JE and Villaveces JW: Hypersensitivity pneumonitis due to pyrethrum, *JAMA* 237:1718-1719, 1977.

66. Evans W and Seaton A: Hypersensitivity pneumonitis in a technician using Pauli's reagent, *Thorax* 34:767-770, 1979.

67. Pimental J and Marques S: Vineyard sprayer's lung: a new occupational disease, *Thorax* 24:678-683, 1969.

68. McSharry C, Lynch PP, Banham SW, et al: Seasonal variation of antibody levels among pigeon fanciers, *Clin Allergy* 13:293-299, 1983.

69. Riley DJ and Saldana M: Pigeon breeder's lung: subacute course and the importance of indirect exposure, *Am Rev Respir Dis* 107:456-460, 1973.

70. Haitjema TJ, vanVelsenBlad H, and vandenBosch JM: Extrinsic allergic alveolitis caused by goose feathers in a duvet, *Thorax* 47:990-991, 1992.

71. Kim KT, Dalton JW, and Klaustermeyer WB: Subacute hypersensitivity pneumonitis to feathers presenting with weight loss and dyspnea, *Ann Allergy* 71:19-23, 1993.

72. Kawai T, Tamura M, and Murao M: Summer-type hypersensitivity pneumonitis: a unique disease in Japan, *Chest* 85:311-317, 1984.

73. Ando M, Arima K, Yoneda R, et al: Japanese summer-type hypersensitivity pneumonitis, *Am Rev Respir Dis* 144:765-769, 1991.

74. Yoshida K, Ando M, Sakata T, et al: Prevention of summer-type hypersensitivity pneumonitis: effect of elimination of *Trichosporon cutaneum* from the patients' homes, *Arch Environ Health* 44:317-322, 1989.

75. Flaherty DK, Braun SR, Marx JJ, et al: Serologically detectable HLA-A, -B and -C loci antigens in farmer's lung disease, *Am Rev Respir Dis* 122:437-446, 1980.

76. Muers MF, Faux JA, Ting A, et al: HLA-A, -B, -C and HLA-DR antigens in extrinsic allergic alveolitis (budgerigar fancier's lung disease), *Clin Allergy* 12:47-53, 1982.

77. Rodey CF, Fink J, Koethe S, et al: A study of HLA-A, -B, -C and -DR specificities in pigeon breeder's disease, *Am Rev Respir Dis* 119:755-759, 1979.

78. Boyd G, Madkour M, Middleton S, et al: Effect of smoking on circulating antibody levels to avian protein in pigeon breeders disease, *Thorax* 32:651-662, 1977.

79. Warren C: Extrinsic allergic alveolitis: a disease commoner in nonsmokers, *Thorax* 32:567-573, 1977.

80. Selman Lama M, Chapela R, Salas J, et al: Hypersensitivity pneumonitis: clinical approach and an integral concept about its pathogenesis: a Mexican point of view. In Lama MS and Barrios R, editors: *Interstitial pulmonary diseases: selected topics,* pp 171-195, Boca Raton, Fla, 1991, CRC Press.

81. Bureau MA, Fecteau C, Patriquin H, et al: Farmer's lung in early childhood, *Am Rev Respir Dis* 119:671-675, 1979.

82. Eisenberg JD, Montanero A, and Lee RG: Hypersensitivity pneumonitis in an infant, *Pediatr Pulmonol* 12:186-190, 1992.

83. Stiehm ER, Reed CE, and Tooley WH: Pigeon breeder's lung in children, *Pediatrics* 39:904-915, 1967.

84. Bice DE, Salvaggio JE, and Hoffman ED: Passive transfer of experimental hypersensitivity pneumonitis with lymphoid cells in the rabbit, *J Allergy Clin Immunol* 58:250-262, 1976.

85. Schuyler M, Subramanyan S, and Hassan MO: Experimental hypersensitivity pneumonitis: transfer with cultured cells, *J Lab Clin Med* 109:623-630, 1987.

86. Hansen PJ and Penny R: Pigeon-breeder's disease: study of the cell-mediated immune response to pigeon antigens by the lymphocyte culture technique, *Int Arch Allergy Appl Immunol* 47:498-507, 1974.

87. Schatz M, Patterson R, Fink J, et al: Pigeon breeder's disease. II. Pigeon antigen induced proliferation of lymphocytes from symptomatic and asymptomatic subjects, *Clin Allergy* 6:7-17, 1976.

88. Mornex JF, Cordier G, Pages J, et al: Activated lung lymphocytes in hypersensitivity pneumonitis, *J Allergy Clin Immunol* 74:719-728, 1984.

89. Fournier E, Tonnel AB, Gosset PH, et al: Early neutrophil alveolitis after antigen inhalation in hypersensitivity pneumonitis, *Chest* 88:563-566, 1985.

90. Tanoue M, Yoshizawa Y, Sata T, et al: The role of complement-derived chemotactic factors in lung injury induced by preformed immune complexes, *Int Arch Allergy Appl Immunol* 101:47-51, 1993.

91. Yoshizawa Y, Nomura A, Ohdama S, et al: The significance of complement activation in the pathogenesis of hypersensitivity pneumonitis: sequential changes of complement components and chemotactic activities in bronchoalveolar lavage fluids, *Int Arch Allergy Appl Immunol* 87:417-423, 1988.

92. Yoshizawa Y, Ohdama S, Tanoue M, et al: Analysis of bronchoalveolar lavage cells and fluids in patients with hypersensitivity pneumonitis: possible role of chemotactic factors in the pathogenesis of the disease, *Int Arch Allergy Appl Immunol* 80:376-382, 1986.

93. Rylander R and Haglind P: Airborne endotoxins and humidifier disease, *Clin Allergy* 14:109-112, 1984.

94. Salvaggio JE and deShazo RD: Pathogenesis of hypersensitivity pneumonitis, *Chest* 89:190-193, 1986.

95. Bjermer L, Engstrom-Laurent A, Lundgren R, et al: Bronchoalveolar mastocytosis in farmer's lung is related to the disease activity, *Arch Intern Med* 148:1362-1365, 1988.

96. Haslam P, Dewar A, Butchers P, et al: Mast cells, atypical lymphocytes and neutrophils in bronchoalveolar lavage in extrinsic allergic alveolitis, *Am Rev Respir Dis* 135:35-47, 1987.

97. Leatherman JW, Michael AF, Schwartz BA, et al: Lung T cells in hypersensitivity pneumonitis, *Ann Intern Med* 100:390-392, 1984.

98. Semenzato G, Agostini C, Zambello R, et al: Lung T cells in hypersensitivity pneumonitis: phenotypic and functional analyses, *J Immunol* 137:1164-1172, 1986.

99. Semenzato G, Zambello R, Trentin L, et al: Cellular immunity in sarcoidosis and hypersensitivity pneumonitis, *Chest* 103(suppl):139-143, 1993.

100. Denis M, Bedard M, Laviolette M, et al: A study of monokine release and natural killer activity in the bronchoalveolar lavage of subjects with farmer's lung, *Am Rev Respir Dis* 147:934-939, 1993.

101. Costabel U, Bross KJ, Ruhle KH, et al: Ia-like antigens on T-cells and their subpopulations in pulmonary sarcoidosis and in hypersensitivity pneumonitis: analysis of bronchoalveolar and blood lymphocytes, *Am Rev Respir Dis* 131:337-342, 1985.

102. Cormier Y, Belanger J, and Laviolette M: Prognostic significance of bronchoalveolar lymphocytosis in farmer's lung, *Am Rev Respir Dis* 135:692-695, 1987.

103. Brummond W, Kurup VP, Resnick A, et al: Immunologic response to *Faenia rectivirgula (Micropolyspora faeni)* in a dairy farm family, *J Allergy Clin Immunol* 82:190-195, 1988.

104. Muryama J, Yoshizawa Y, Ohtsuka M, et al: Lung fibrosis in hypersensitivity pneumonitis, *Chest* 104:38-43, 1993.

105. Ando M, Konishi K, Yoneda R, et al: Difference in the phenotypes of bronchoalveolar lavage lymphocytes in patients with summer-type hypersensitivity pneumonitis, farmer's lung, ventilation pneumonitis and bird fancier's lung: report of a nationwide epidemiologic study in Japan, *J Allergy Clin Immunol* 87:1002-1009, 1991.

106. Trentin L, Marcer G, Chilosi M, et al: Longitudinal study of alveolitis in hypersensitivity pneumonitis patients: an immunological evaluation, *J Allergy Clin Immunol* 82:577-585, 1988.

107. Cormier Y, Belanger J, Beaudoin J, et al: Abnormal bronchoalveolar lavage in asymptomatic dairy farmers: study of lymphocytes, *Am Rev Respir Dis* 130:1046-1049, 1984.

108. Cormier Y, Belanger J, and Laviolette M: Persistent bronchoalveolar lymphocytosis in asymptomatic farmers, *Am Rev Respir Dis* 133:843-847, 1986.

109. Stankus RP, Cashner FM, and Salvaggio JE: Bronchopulmonary macrophage activation in the pathogenesis of hypersensitivity pneumonitis, *J Immunol* 120:685-688, 1978.

110. Fink JN: The alveolar macrophage and hypersensitivity pneumonitis, *J Lab Clin Med* 117:435-436, 1991. Editorial.

111. Teschler H, Thompson AB, Pohl WR, et al: Bronchoalveolar lavage procollagen-III–peptide in recent onset hypersensitivity pneumonitis: correlation with extracellular matrix components, *Eur Respir J* 6:709-714, 1993.

112. Bice DE, Salvaggio JE, Hoffman ED, et al: Adjuvant properties of *Micropolyspora faeni, J Allergy Clin Immunol* 55:267-274, 1976.

113. Denis M, Cormier Y, Tardif J, et al: Hypersensitivity pneumonitis: whole *Micropolyspora faeni* or antigens thereof stimulate the release of proinflammatory cytokines from macrophages, *Am J Respir Cell Biol* 5:198-203, 1991.

114. Colby TV and Coleman A: Histological diffferential diagnosis of extrinsic allergic alveolitis, *Prog Surg Pathol* 10:11-26, 1989.

115. Coleman A and Colby T: Histologic diagnosis of extrinsic allergic alveolitis, *Am J Surg Pathol* 12:514-518, 1988.

116. Reyes CN, Wenzel FJ, Lawton BR, et al: The pulmonary pathology of farmer's lung disease, *Chest* 81:142-146, 1982.

117. Sutinen S, Reijula K, Huhti E, et al: Extrinsic allergic bronchioalveolitis: serology and biopsy findings, *Eur J Resp Dis* 64:271-282, 1983.

118. Pether JVS and Greatorex FB: Farmer's lung disease in Somerset, *Br J Ind Med* 33:265-268, 1976.

119. Grant IWB, Blyth W, Wardrop VE, et al: Prevalence of farmer's lung in Scotland: a pilot survey, *Br Med J* 1:530-534, 1972.

120. Madsen D, Klock LE, Wenzel FJ, et al: The prevalence of farmer's lung in an agricultural population, *Am Rev Respir Dis* 113:171-174, 1976.

121. Marx JJ, Guernsey J, Emanuel DA, et al: Cohort studies of immunologic lung disease among Wisconsin dairy farmers, *Am J Ind Med* 18:263-268, 1990.

122. Terho EO, Heinonen OP, and Lammi S: Incidence of clinically confirmed farmer's lung disease in Finland, *Am J Ind Med* 10:330, 1986.

123. Christensen LT, Schmidt CD, and Robbins L: Pigeon breeder's disease—a prevalence study and review, *Clin Allergy* 5:417-430, 1975.

124. Vandenplas O, Malo JL, Dugas M, et al: Hypersensitivity pneumonitis-like reaction among workers exposed to diphenylmethane diisocyanate (MDI), *Am Rev Respir Dis* 147:338-346, 1993.

125. Kreiss K and Hodgson MJ: Building-associated epidemics. In Walsh PJ, Dudney CS, and Copenhave ED, editors: *Indoor air quality,* pp 87-108, Boca Raton, Fla, 1984, CRC Press.

126. Hodgson MJ, Morey PR, Simon JS, et al: An outbreak of recurrent acute and chronic hypersensitivity pneumonitis in office workers, *Am J Epidemiol* 125:631-638, 1987.

127. Arnow PM, Fink JN, Schlueter DP, et al: Early detection of hypersensitivity pneumonitis in office workers, *Am J Med* 64:236-242, 1978.

128. Sansores R, Salas J, Chapela R, et al: Clubbing in hypersensitivity pneumonitis: its prevalence and possible prognostic role, *Arch Intern Med* 150:1849-1851, 1990.

129. Burrell R and Rylander R: A critical review of the role of precipitins in hypersensitivity pneumonitis, *Eur J Respir Dis* 62:332-343, 1981.

130. Roberts RC, Wenzel FJ, and Emanuel DA: Precipitating antibodies in a midwest dairy farming population toward the antigens associated with farmer's lung disease, *J Allergy Clin Immunol* 62:518-524, 1976.

131. McSharry C, Banham SW, Lynch PP, et al: Antibody measurement in extrinsic allergic alveolitis, *Eur J Respir Dis* 65:259-265, 1984.

132. Cormier Y and Belanger J: The fluctuant nature of precipitating antibodies in dairy farmers, *Thorax* 44:469-473, 1989.

133. Barbee RA, Callies Q, Dickie HA, et al: The long-term prognosis in farmer's lung, *Am Rev Respir Dis* 97:223-231, 1968.

134. Huls G, Lindemann H, and Velcovsky HG: Angiotensin converting enzyme (ACE) in the follow-up control of children and adolescents with allergic alveolitis, *Monatsschr Kinderheilkd* 137:158-161, 1989.

135. Cormier Y and Belanger J: Long-term physiologic outcome after acute farmer's lung, *Chest* 87:796-800, 1985.

136. Pepys J and Jenkins PA: Precipitin (FLH) test in farmer's lung, *Thorax* 20:21-35, 1935.

137. Warren CPW, Tse KS, and Cherniack RM: Mechanical properties of the lung in extrinsic allergic alveolitis, *Thorax* 33:315-321, 1978.

138. Freedman PM and Ault B: Bronchial hyperreactivity to methacholine in farmer's lung disease, *J Allergy Clin Immunol* 67:59-63, 1981.

139. Monkare S, Ikonen M, and Haahtela T: Radiologic findings in farmer's lung: prognosis and correlation to lung function, *Chest* 84:460-466, 1985.

140. Lynch DA, Rose CS, Way D, et al: Hypersensitivity pneumonitis: sensitivity of high-resolution CT in a population-based study, *Am J Roentgenol* 159:469-472, 1992.

141. Buschman DL, Gamsu G, Waldron JA, et al: Chronic hypersensitivity pneumonitis: use of CT in diagnosis, *Am J Roentgenol* 159:957-960, 1992.

142. Hansell DM and Kerr IH: The role of high resolution computed tomography in the diagnosis of interstitial lung disease, *Thorax* 46:77-84, 1991.

143. Akira M, Kita N, Higashihara T, et al: Summer-type hypersensitivity pneumonitis: comparison of high-resolution CT and plain radiographic findings, *Am J Roentgenol* 158:1223-1228, 1992.

144. Remy-Jardin M, Remy J, Wallaert B, et al: Subacute and chronic bird breeder hypersensitivity pneumonitis: sequential evaluation with CT and correlation with lung function tests and bronchoalveolar lavage, *Radiology* 189:111-118, 1993.

145. Bergin CJ and Muller NL: CT in the diagnosis of interstitial lung disease, *Am J Radiat* 145:505-510, 1985.

146. Hansell DM and Moskovic E: High resolution computed tomography in extrinsic allergic alveolitis, *Clin Radiol* 43:8-12, 1991.

147. Hendrick DJ, Marshall R, Faux JA, et al: Positive "alveolar" responses to antigen inhalation provocation tests: their validity and recognition, *Thorax* 35:415-427, 1980.

148. Richerson HB, Bernstein IL, Fink JN, et al: Guidelines for the clinical evaluation of hypersensitivity pneumonitis, *J Allergy Clin Immunol* 84:839-844, 1989.

149. Drent M, Mulder PGH, Wagenaar SS, et al: Differences in BAL fluid variables in interstitial lung diseases evaluated by discriminant analysis, *Eur Respir J* 6:803-810, 1993.

150. Laviolette M, Cormier Y, Loiseau A, et al: Bronchoalveolar mast cells in normal farmers and subjects with farmer's lung: diagnostic, prognostic, and physiologic significance, *Am Rev Respir Dis* 144:855-860, 1991.

151. Patterson R, Wang JLF, Fink JN, et al: IgA and IgG antibody activities of serum and bronchoalveolar fluid from symptomatic and asymptomatic pigeon breeders, *Am Rev Respir Dis* 120:1113-1118, 1979.

152. Calvanico NJ, Ambegaonkar SP, Schlueter DP, et al: Immunoglobulin levels in bronchoalveolar lavage fluid from pigeon breeders, *J Lab Clin Med* 96:129-140, 1980.

153. Cormier Y, Belanger J, and Laviolette M: Prognostic significance of bronchoalveolar lymphocytosis in farmer's lung, *Am Rev Respir Dis* 135:692-695, 1987.

154. Terho EO: Diagnostic criteria for farmer's lung disease, *Am J Ind Med* 10:329, 1986.

155. Hodgson MJ, Parkinson DK, and Karpf M: Chest x-rays in hypersensitivity pneumonitis: a metaanalysis of secular trend, *Am J Ind Med* 16:45-53, 1989.

156. Rose C and King TE Jr: Controversies in hypersensitivity pneumonitis, *Am Rev Respir Dis* 145:1-2, 1992. Editorial.

157. Monkare S and Haahtela T: Farmer's lung—a 5 year follow up of eighty six patients, *Clin Allergy* 17:143-151, 1987.

158. Chasse M, Blanchette G, and Malo JL: Farmer's lung presenting as respiratory failure and homogeneous consolidation, *Chest* 90:783-784, 1986.

159. Greenberger PA, Pien LC, Patterson R, et al: End-stage lung and ultimately fatal disease in a bird fancier, *Am J Med* 86:119-122, 1989.

160. Schmidt CD, Jensen RL, Christensen LT, et al: Longitudinal pulmonary function changes in pigeon breeders, *Chest* 93:359-363, 1988.

161. Grammer LC, Roberts M, Lerner C, et al: Clinical and serologic follow-up of four children and five adults with bird-fancier's lung, *J Allergy Clin Immunol* 85:655-660, 1990.

162. Pitcher WD: Southwestern internal medicine conference: hypersensitivity pneumonitis, *Am J Med Sci* 300:251-266, 1990.

163. Allen DH, Williams GV, and Woolcock AJ:. Bird breeder's hypersensitivity pneumonitis: progress studies of lung function after cessation of exposure to the provoking antigen, *Am Rev Respir Dis* 114:555-566, 1976.

164. DeGracia J, Morell F, Bofill JM, et al: Time of exposure as a prognostic factor in avian hypersensitivity pneumonitis, *Respir Med* 83:139-143, 1989.

165. Braun SR, doPico GA, Tsiatis A, et al: Farmer's lung disease: long-term clinical and physiologic outcome, *Am Rev Respir Dis* 119:185-191, 1979.

166. Cuthbert OD and Gordon MF: Ten year follow up of farmers with farmer's lung, *Br J Ind Med* 40:173-176, 1983.

167. Bourke SJ, Banham SW, Carter R, et al: Longitudinal course of extrinsic allergic alveolitis in pigeon breeders, *Thorax* 44:415-418, 1989.

168. Richerson HB, Richards DW, Swanson PA, et al: Antigen-specific desensitization in a rabbit model of acute hypersensitivity pneumonitis, *J Allergy Clin Immunol* 68:226-234, 1981.

169. Craig TJ: Bird antigen persistence in the home environment after removal of the bird, *Ann Allergy* 69:510-512, 1992.

170. Woodard ED, Friedlander B, Lesher RJ, et al: Outbreak of hypersensitivity pneumonitis in an industrial setting, *JAMA* 259:1965-1969, 1988.

171. Reed CE, Swanson BA, Lopez M, et al: Measurement of IgG antibody and airborne antigen to control an industrial outbreak of hypersensitivity pneumonitis, *J Occup Med* 25:207-210, 1983.

172. Zejda JE, McDuffie HH, and Dosman JA: Epidemiology of health and safety risks in agriculture and related industries. Practical applications for rural physicians, *West J Med* 158:56-63, 1993.

173. Clark S: Report on prevention and control, *Am J Ind Med* 10:267-273, 1986.

174. Nuutinen J, Terho EO, Husman K, et al: Protective value of powered dust respirator helmet for farmers with farmer's lung, *Eur J Respir Dis* 152:212-220, 1987.

175. Anderson K, Walker A, and Boyd G: The long-term effect of a positive pressure respirator on the specific antibody response in pigeon breeders, *Clin Exp Allergy* 19:45-49, 1988.

176. Hendrick D, Marshall R, Faux J, et al: Protective value of dust respirators in extrinsic allergic alveolitis: clinical assessment using inhalation provocation tests, *Thorax* 36:917-921, 1981.

177. Macher JM: Inquiries received by the California indoor air quality program on biological contaminants in buildings, *Adv Aerobiol* pp 275-278 1987.

178. Zwick H, Popp W, Braun O, et al. Personal spore sampling and indirect immunofluorescent test for exploration of hypersensitivity pneumonitis due to mould spores, *Allergy* 46:277-283, 1991.

179. Kokkarinen JI, Tukiainen HO, and Terho EO: Effect of corticosteroid treatment on the recovery of pulmonary function in farmer's lung, *Am Rev Respir Dis* 145:3-5, 1992.

180. Shellito JE: Hypersensitivity pneumonitis, *Semin Respir Med* 12:196-203, 1991.

181. Monkare S: Influence of corticosteroid treatment on the course of farmer's lung, *Eur J Respir Dis* 64:283-293, 1983.

182. Carlsen KH, Leegaard J, Lund OD, et al: Allergic alveolitis in a 12-year-old boy: treatment with budesonide nebulizing solution, *Pediatr Pulmonol* 12:257-259, 1992.

Chapter 15

PULMONARY FIBROSIS AND INTERSTITIAL LUNG DISEASES

Carrie A. Redlich

The interstitial lung diseases are a group of heterogeneous lung diseases that diffusely involve the lung parenchyma with chronic alveolitis and fibrosis.[1] Although it is called interstitial, the disease process usually also involves the alveolar and capillary endothelia. These processes eventually lead to loss of functional gas exchange units and respiratory impairment. Pulmonary fibrosis can result from a vast array of exogenous exposures and disease processes (see boxes). Airway involvement in most fibrotic interstitial disorders has traditionally been felt to be minimal or related to concomitant cigarette smoking. However, more recent studies have demonstrated that certain exposures, such as asbestos, in the absence of substantial exposure to cigarette smoke, can result in peribronchial fibrosis and some degree of airflow obstruction[2,3] (see Chapter 27). This chapter provides an overview of interstitial lung diseases caused by occupational and environmental exposures as well as their etiology, pathogenesis, clinical presentation, evaluation, and management. The more common diseases, such as asbestosis, silicosis, and coal worker's pneumoconiosis, are dealt with in greater detail in subsequent chapters. The term *pneumoconiosis* has traditionally been defined as the accumulation of dust in the lungs and the resulting tissue reaction. Although originally used to describe inorganic dust-induced diseases such as asbestosis or silicosis, *pneumoconiosis* is also used more to describe diseases resulting from the inhalation of organic material such as fungi or other substances that may not accumulate in the lungs, such as cobalt or various chemicals. This chapter focuses primarily on the processes of interstitial fibrosis due to inorganic dust diseases. Fibrosis may also occur as part of other pulmonary processes, such as hypersensitivity pneumonitis or asthma, or following acute inhalational injuries, and is discussed separately in those respective chapters.

ETIOLOGY AND EPIDEMIOLOGY

There is a large number of occupational and nonoccupational causes of pulmonary interstitial fibrosis, summarized in the boxes. The prevalence of all interstitial lung diseases in the United States has been estimated to be approximately 20 to 40 per 100,000 of the population and has been reported in 15% of the patients seen by pulmonary physicians.[4] A recent population-based study suggested that the prevalence of this disease may be higher and that these dis-

More common causes of occupational interstitial lung diseases

Free silica

Silicates

Fibrous—asbestos
Mixed dust

Coal

Metals

Beryllium
Hard metal—cobalt

Less common causes of occupational interstitial lung diseases

Silicates

Talc
Kaolin
Diatomaceous earth
Man-made vitreous fibers (MMVF)
Mica

Hydrocarbon-containing sedimentary rocks

Graphite
Oil shale

Metals

Tin
Aluminum
Antimony
Barium
Iron
Titanium

Irritant gases, fumes, vapors

Sequelae of toxic pneumonitis

Plastics

Polyvinylchloride
Toluene diisocyanate

Organic dusts

Bacteria
Fungi
Animal proteins
Plant proteins

Paraquat

Most common causes of nonoccupational interstitial lung disease

Unknown etiology

Idiopathic
Sarcoidosis
Bronchiolitis obliterans organizing pneumonia (BOOP)

Collagen vascular diseases

Rheumatoid arthritis
Progressive systemic sclerosis
Systemic lupus erythematosus
Mixed connective tissue disease

Pulmonary granulomatoses

Wegener's granulomatosis
Bronchocentric granulomatosis

Vasculitides

Churg–Strauss syndrome

Lymphoproliferative disorders

Lymphomatoid granulomatosis

Inherited disorders

Tuberous sclerosis
Neurofibromatosis
Cystic fibrosis

Drugs and treatment (selected examples)

Antibiotics (nitrofurantoin, penicillins, and sulfasalazine)
Cardiac drugs (hydralazine, procainamide, and amiodarone)
Antineoplastic agents (bleomycin, busulfan, methotrexate, cyclophosphamide, and nitrosureas)
Antiinflammatory agents (gold salts and penicillamine)
Central nervous system drugs (diphenylhydantoin)
Radiation
Oxygen
Bone marrow transplantation
Miscellaneous
    Intravenous use of illicit drugs
    Mineral oil
    Silicone
    Penicillamine

Infections

Viruses
Mycobacteria
Fungi

Other

Aspiration
Pulmonary edema
Pulmonary hemorrhage

eases may go unrecognized.[5] This study found a prevalence of 80.9 per 100,000 in men and 67.2 per 100,000 in women.[5]

The most common nonoccupational cause of interstitial lung disease is idiopathic pulmonary fibrosis, which has been estimated to account for 25% to 40% or more of all cases.[5,6] Some of these cases may have an occupational or environmental origin that has gone unrecognized. The other major nonoccupational causes of interstitial lung disease are listed in the third box.

The overall incidence or prevalence of occupational and environmental interstitial lung diseases in the United States is unknown, but varies significantly among different exposed populations. Surveillance data have been incomplete due to the lack of a mandatory national reporting system. The U.S. Bureau of Labor Statistics reported approximately 2600 occupational illnesses due to dust exposure in 1989, based on voluntary reporting.[7] Such figures are believed to significantly underestimate the prevalence of occupational disorders. A population-based registry of patients estimated the prevalence of occupational and environmental interstitial lung diseases to be 20.8/100,000 among men and 0.6/100,000 among women.[5] Hospital discharge data can be used to monitor trends in occupational diseases but do not determine the true incidence of disease. For example, data from New Jersey showed an age-adjusted average annual discharge rate of 19.3 cases of asbestosis in white men per 100,000 of the population from 1979 to 1986 and a 20% annual increase in asbestosis for white men during this time.[8] Such an increase could represent a true increase in the incidence of asbestosis or heightened awareness of the disease leading to more frequent diagnoses.

Most of the data available on the prevalence of occupational interstitial lung diseases are based on studies of occupational cohorts. Variable disease prevalences among selected populations of workers exposed to the same agent, such as asbestos, have been reported, likely due to differences in the exact type, intensity, and duration of exposure; differing criteria for case ascertainment; and host susceptibility factors. For certain agents, such as asbestos or silica, there is a general linear dose–response relationship, but for others, such as beryllium or cobalt, the relationship is much less clear (discussed in Chapter 29).

Historically, interstitial lung disease was most common in patients who had inhaled mineral dusts such as silica, asbestos, and coal. With improved industrial hygiene and reduced mining, production, and use of these agents in the United States, heavy exposure to these dusts has declined overall. For example, the effects of improved controls have lowered the prevalence of silicosis among underground coal miners.[9] However, several recent reports demonstrate that high levels of exposure still exist in the United States, frequently in small, uncontrolled workplaces, which can result in miniepidemics of disease. For example, outbreaks of silicosis in sandblasters, foundry workers, and pottery

workers have recently been reported.[10,11] Even with overall improved control measures, the prevalences of these diseases still remain high in many exposed populations because of the latency between exposure and disease and persistent inadequate exposure controls in certain industries. Asbestos-related lung diseases remain the dominant occupational lung disease seen in occupational medicine clinics.[12] Although accurate data are limited, the incidence and prevalence of pneumoconioses in developing countries are high and appear to be increasing.[13] Worldwide, silicosis probably remains the most common occupational interstitial lung disease. Fibrotic lung diseases due to agents that appear to involve immune-mediated mechanisms and that have less clear dose–response relationships, such as those caused by beryllium or hard metal, are more difficult to control because disease may occur at lower exposure levels and in a more sporadic fashion.

Nonoccupational environmental exposure to dusts such as asbestos and silica can result in detectable disease that is usually mild and of unclear clinical significance. A high incidence of silicosis was recently reported among inhabitants of Himalayan villages who were exposed to frequent storms of dust containing silica.[14] A higher incidence of presumed asbestos-induced pleural abnormalities has been found in locations where asbestos occurs naturally.[15] Isolated cases have been reported of pneumoconiosis related to accidental or intentional overexposures in the home setting, such as silicosis following inhalation of a domestic cleaning powder containing silica.[16]

The fibrogenic potential of inorganic dusts varies considerably, with silica and asbestos having greater fibrogenic potential than coal dust or more benign agents such as iron or man-made vitreous fibers. Most inorganic dusts, such as coal, asbestos, or silica, require prolonged exposure for at least 6 months, usually years, at relatively high levels in order for significant pulmonary disease to develop. However, disease can occur following shorter, more intense exposures.[17] The response to agents such as beryllium is much more idiosyncratic, and disease has been reported to occur after much lower exposures.[18]

PATHOPHYSIOLOGY
Anatomy and pathology

The lung interstitium is made up of the alveolar and peribronchovascular interstitia. The alveolar interstitium is the tiny space across which gas exchange occurs. Following lung injury, cellular infiltration and edema distort the normally thin alveolar wall. Epithelial and endothelial cell injury and alveolar collapse also occur following lung injury. Proliferation of mesenchymal cells and accumulation of connective tissue products, primarily collagen, can follow, resulting in increased lung matrix and a scarred, fibrotic interstitium. Fibroblasts also proliferate within the alveolar space, resulting in intraalveolar fibrosis. The alveolo–capillary units become less distinguishable, and end-stage lung injury with massive, fibrotic changes and honeycombing is seen. The initial epithelial injury, accumulation of inflammatory cells, and edema can be reversible, but as the fibrosis and structural deformity progress the changes become irreversible. Although the term *diffuse* is used, the pathologic changes seen in interstitial lung disease can be irregular and variable.

Despite multiple causative agents, most agents result in one or more common pathologic patterns of interstitial lung disease, such as nodular fibrosis, diffuse fibrosis, bronchiolitis obliterans, granulomas, or fibrotic mass lesions.[19] The most common histologic patterns seen in occupational interstitial lung disorders and representative causative agents are listed in Table 15-1. Once the lung reaches end-stage scarring, classification is much more difficult. Patients frequently come to biopsy late in the course of their disease, thus histologic analysis can be very nonspecific and diagnostically of little significance.

Physiology

Functionally, the abnormally thickened and scarred interstitium results in restricted lung volumes, decreased pulmonary diffusing capacity for carbon monoxide (DLCO), and stiff nondistensible lungs with increased elastic recoil.[1,6] Certain exposures that classically cause restrictive disease, such as asbestos, may also result in some small airways disease and mild obstructive changes.[2,3,20] Exposures such as cobalt can cause both interstitial fibrosis and significant occupational asthma, either independently or with both processes occurring simultaneously in the same patient.[21] Other exposures may result in minimal, if any, detectable functional changes. For example, simple nodular fibrosis seen in silicosis may be associated with only minor physiologic changes, since these nodular lesions may be isolated and have little effect on overall lung compliance or gas exchange. Metals such as iron, tin, barium, and antimony produce dense opacities on radiography but usually no functional impairment.

PATHOGENESIS: MECHANISMS OF INFLAMMATION AND FIBROSIS

Although multiple exogenous agents can initiate an inflammatory alveolitis and result in interstitial lung disease, it is likely that the underlying pathogenetic mechanisms that mediate the development and progression of pulmonary fibrosis are similar.[1,22-24] An overview, by necessity simplified, of the processes involved in the pathogenesis of interstitial lung diseases is presented here. These processes most likely involve complex interactions between a number of different lung cell types and mediators. A more comprehensive review of the pathogenesis of specific diseases, such as asbestosis, silicosis, or chronic beryllium disease, is provided in subsequent chapters. Our current knowledge concerning these processes is based primarily on in vitro studies, in vivo animal work, and clinical studies using

Table 15-1. Common histologic patterns found in interstitial lung disorders

Pathologic response	Example of causative occupational/environmental agent
Bronchiolitis obliterans	Fumes and gases
Macules	Coal, iron, tin, graphite, and aluminum
Nodular fibrosis	Coal, silica, and mixed dust
Diffuse fibrosis	Asbestos, talc, mica, hard metal, and aluminum
Fibrotic mass lesions	Coal and silica
Granulomatous disease	Beryllium and organic dusts
Emphysema	Cigarettes and coal

bronchoalveolar lavage or lung tissue specimens. Individual chapters in this volume discuss the pathologic mechanisms of specific agents such as asbestos or silica in greater detail. The basic underlying theme is that various exposures can cause lung injury and initiate a chronic inflammatory process that may either progress to interstitial fibrosis or result in successful repair (Fig. 15-1).

Deposition and clearance of inorganic dusts

In order for an exposure to cause interstitial lung disease, the agent must overcome the various host defense mechanisms of the lungs and reach the lower respiratory tract. The lungs are highly efficient at removing particulate material. Major determinants of the extent and site of deposition of particles include the size and shape of the particle, minute ventilation, lung anatomy, pattern of breathing, and preexisting lung disease. Two major mechanisms by which organic dust particles impacted on the airway epithelial surface can be cleared are (1) airway reflexes of cough and bronchoconstriction and (2) mucociliary clearance, or *escalator,* a complex system by which substances are moved toward the pharynx.[6] Clearance of particles may be modified by the presence of other exposures, such as cigarettes, air pollutants, medications, and underlying lung disease.

Most particulates that reach the terminal bronchioles and alveolar surface are ingested by alveolar macrophages. These macrophages can move proximally by mucociliary clearance or can transport the particles to regional lymph nodes. Exactly how effective these different mechanisms are at clearing particles in humans is not clear and likely varies depending on the particle type and other factors. It has been estimated that 98% to 99% of deposited coal dust is cleared from the lungs.[25]

Lung injury

The fibrogenic potential of a given exposure is dependent on various factors including its ability to reach the lower respiratory tract; the extent of exposure, durability, and various chemical and physical properties of the agent; and individual host susceptibility factors.

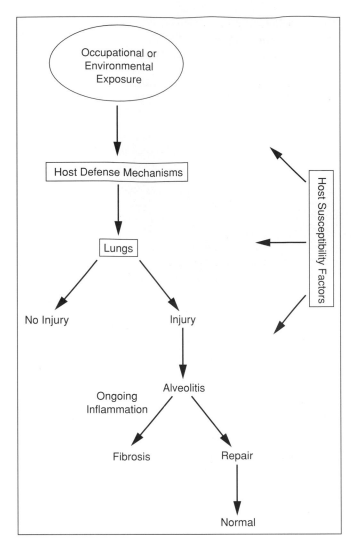

Fig. 15-1. Schematic presentation of relationships between environmental exposures, lung injury, lung inflammation, and host susceptibility factors.

The causative agent may directly injure the airway epithelium and interstitium and activate pulmonary cells, primarily macrophages, to release factors such as oxidants, cytokines, or other mediators. These mediators either directly cause lung injury or initiate and perpetuate the inflammatory response.[6,22,24,26-28] The resulting alveolitis can resolve with restoration of normal lung architecture and function or, it has been postulated, progress to chronic lung scarring with fibrosis. Epithelial cell injury, basement membrane damage, and migration of fibroblasts into the alveoli resulting in airspace fibrosis is believed to play an important role in lung fibrosis.[22] Alveolar collapse following lung injury is also felt to be a significant component of the fibrotic process.[22] However, it remains unclear whether alveolar wall injury is required for the development of fibrosis. Why, under certain circumstances, the lung host defense system and repair mechanisms are able to handle the exogenous exposures without permanent injury and scarring, yet under other circumstances ongoing inflammation and fibrosis ensue, is not well understood. The severity and extent of the epithelial injury and alveolitis may be important determinants of the extent and pattern of fibrosis.[22]

Influx, proliferation, and activation of inflammatory cells

The macrophage is believed to be a major effector cell in defense of the integrity of the lower respiratory tract following mineral dust exposure and likely plays a central role in the pathogenesis of occupational interstitial fibrotic disorders. In vivo and in vitro studies have demonstrated that alveolar macrophages can ingest particulates such as silica, asbestos, and coal dust, and become injured or activated.[28,29] These macrophages can release various cytokines and other mediators (see next section) that can directly injure the lung parenchyma and epithelial cells or recruit additional inflammatory and mesenchymal cells. Increased vascular permeability and fibrin deposition are believed to play an important role in the pathogenesis of pulmonary fibrosis.[22]

The alveolitis found in patients exposed to asbestos, silica, and coal is dominated by alveolar macrophages. However, increased numbers of neutrophils and lymphocytes, are also found.[6,28] Certain patterns of inflammatory cells are more common with certain interstitial lung diseases. A neutrophil alveolitis can be seen in asbestosis and idiopathic pulmonary fibrosis, whereas granulomatous disorders such as sarcoidosis and chronic beryllium disease are characterized by increased CD4$^+$ (helper) T lymphocytes.[6] Increased neutrophil alveolitis has been associated with the progression of certain interstitial lung diseases, such as asbestosis,[30,31] which is consistent with the neutrophil's ability to produce reactive oxygen species, proteases, and other toxic substances.

Role of chemoattractants, cytokines, and adhesion molecules

A number of different cytokines and growth factors have been implicated in the pathogenesis of occupational interstitial fibrotic diseases, based on both in vitro work and in vivo animal and human studies. Alveolar macrophages from patients with interstitial lung injury or following various in vitro or in vivo exposures can release increased amounts of a number of mediators, including platelet-derived growth factor (PDGF), alveolar macrophage-derived growth factor, interleukin-1 (IL-1), IL-2, IL-6, IL-8, transforming growth factor β (TGF-β), leukotriene B_4, tumor necrosis factor (TNF), interferon-γ, and monocyte chemotactic protein 1 (MCP-1).[9,24,28,32-38] Different agents, such as silica or asbestos, result in the release of different patterns of cytokines and other mediators, including fibronectin and arachidonic acid metabolites, which differentially regulate various cells in the lungs, including the recruitment and/or activation of monocytes, endothelial cells, mast cells, fibroblasts, neutrophils, and T and B lymphocytes. Such mediators also modulate matrix production and degradation, and the production of various other cytokines and growth factors.

In addition to macrophages, a number of other cell types in the lung, including epithelial cells, endothelial cells, lymphocytes, neutrophils, and fibroblasts, can produce various cytokines and other mediators to form complex regulatory networks.[24,34] Such networks likely mediate the processes that both stimulate and inhibit inflammatory and fibrotic responses in the lungs. Many of these cytokines can interact in a synergistic fashion to cause a greater inflammatory response. For example, activated macrophages release MCP-1, which can result in the accumulation of more macrophages; IL-1 and TNF interact in regulating multiple functions, including superoxide, collagen, and granulocyte accumulation.[34] Interleukin-1, TNF, and other mediators result in endothelial cell activation with altered expression of adhesion molecules such as intercellular adhesion molecule (ICAM-1) and E-selectin, which are involved in leukocyte binding and entry into the interstitium.[24] It is believed that dysregulated or exaggerated production of certain cytokines and mediators may lead to ongoing injury, inflammation, and fibrosis rather than normal healing.[22,24]

Role of oxidants and antioxidants

The generation of reactive oxygen species is also believed to play an important role in the pathogenesis of occupational interstitial lung disorders such as asbestosis and silicosis.[39,40] Asbestos and silica can generate reactive oxygen species directly or indirectly by activation of macrophages and other inflammatory cells.[40,41] Alveolar macrophages recovered from humans or animals exposed in vivo to asbestos, silica, or coal exhibit enhanced release of reactive oxygen species such as superoxide anion and hydrogen peroxide.[28,40,42] Such oxidants can injure or alter the function of epithelial, endothelial, and fibroblast cells. Epithelial and endothelial cells in particular are sensitive to oxidant injury. The lungs contain various antioxidant defense systems, including antioxidant enzymes such as superoxide dismutase, catalase, and glutathione reductase, and glutathione, the major nonenzymatic antioxidant present in the lung. Recent studies have shown that the presence of iron may potentiate the toxicity of particles such as asbestos or silica by enhancing their ability to generate reactive oxygen species.[40] Likewise, antioxidants and iron chelators can inhibit such oxidant-induced toxicity.[40,43]

Lung repair and fibrosis

Following lung injury, it is believed either that the inflammation can resolve and the lungs repair themselves or that persistent inflammation and fibrosis may result in interstitial lung disease.[1] Restoration of the epithelial surface and basement membrane, if injured, is also felt to be a key factor in the repair process.[22] The factors that determine whether repair or fibrosis will predominate in a given situation are poorly understood.

Epithelial cell and basement membrane damage can result in fibroblast migration into the alveolar space, proliferation, and activation.[1,22] The TGF-β, PDGF, and other mediators released by macrophages, fibroblasts, epithelial, or other cell types in the lungs result in the proliferation and activation of mesenchymal cells.[22]

Fibroblast proliferation and increased production of matrix molecules such as collagen can lead to both interstitial and intraalveolar fibrosis. As fibrosis progresses, extensive remodeling in the lungs occurs, with progressive loss of alveolocapillary units, honeycomb lung, permanent scarring, and functional impairment.

Recent studies suggest that endothelial, epithelial, and fibroblast programmed cell death can occur at the air–lung interface following lung injury,[44,45] and may be an important aspect of the remodeling process. The alteration or dysregulation of processes such as programmed cell death, mesenchymal proliferation, and reepithelialization may result in abnormal repair and fibrosis rather than restoration of the normal lung architecture.[22,44]

Host determinants susceptibility

Clinical and epidemiologic studies have demonstrated marked individual variability in the response to a given exposure, especially with disorders that are likely to be idiosyncratic or immune mediated, such as chronic beryllium disease or hard metal disease, as compared with those that are more direct toxic responses, such as asbestosis. There undoubtedly are individual susceptibility factors, both inherited and acquired, that modify the risk of developing interstitial lung disease, but such factors remain poorly understood. Several studies have demonstrated that cigarette smoke may potentiate the effects of exposure to inorganic dusts such as silica and asbestos on the lungs, resulting in reduced lung function and greater abnormalities on chest radiography.[46,47] Rodent studies have demonstrated synergistic effects of cigarettes and mineral fibers on the production of certain cytokines, such as TNF.[48] A recent study has found that inherited glutathione-S-transferase deficiency may be associated with an increased risk for developing asbestosis.[49] Certain MHC class II genes (HLA-DR, -DQ, and -DP) are associated with susceptibility to autoimmune disease and have been investigated as possible susceptibility genes to chronic beryllium disease and other pneumoconioses. A strong association between the HLA-DPB1 Glu[69] phenotype and chronic beryllium disease has recently been demonstrated.[50] The relationship between HLA antigens and risk for asbestos-related pulmonary disease has also been investigated, but no strong associations have been found.[51] Dietary factors such as vitamin A, β-carotene, and vitamin E may also be host determinants of susceptibility to lung injury.

Many of the cytokines and other mediators identified in patients with interstitial lung diseases may prove to be sensitive and specific biomarkers of early disease activity or may provide important prognostic information. Such findings may also lead to new and improved therapeutic approaches. However, despite significant advances in understanding the pathogenetic mechanisms underlying lung injury, inflammation, and interstitial fibrosis, this information has unfortunately, to date, resulted in few major advances in the treatment of patients with occupational interstitial lung disease.

CLINICAL PRESENTATION AND EVALUATION

The clinical presentation and natural history of interstitial fibrotic disorders can be quite variable depending on the agent and the circumstances. The patient typically has a history of progressive dyspnea on exertion over a period of months to years, although occasionally there can be a more rapid progression. Acute exacerbations with spontaneous remissions are more suggestive of another etiology, such as asthma. It is helpful to document the patient's current and past levels of activity and any symptoms that limit the patient: fatigue, chest pain, dyspnea, or others. Cough (either productive or nonproductive) is also a common symptom. Chest pain, shortness of breath at rest, and wheezing are less common and may suggest another diagnosis. Systemic complaints such as weight loss and fever can occur, more commonly with beryllium disease or hard metal disease. A careful review of systems, especially for symptoms of possible connective tissue disorders or gastroesophageal reflux, is important.

History

As with most occupational diseases, a careful medical and occupational history is key to the diagnosis of occupational and environmental fibrotic lung disorders. With the less common disorders, such as hard metal disease, a high index of suspicion is critical. Although there is a long list of known causes of pulmonary fibrosis (see boxes), a careful history will usually eliminate most possibilities. History of pulmonary infections, collagen vascular disorders, cancer chemotherapy, or radiation therapy should be determined. Use of medications, including chemotherapeutic agents, antibiotics, and cardiac medications, as well as intravenous drug use, should be determined and their timing should be carefully assessed. Risk factors for acquired immunodeficiency syndrome (AIDS) should also be determined.

Several aspects of the occupational and environmental history are critical. As most interstitial lung diseases are chronic in nature and may have a latency of up to 20 or more years, it is important to obtain a history of all potentially relevant past jobs, including military duty. Job title, job description, details of the production process, levels of dust, use of respiratory protection, and the presence of ventilation should all be evaluated. The timing, duration, and intensity of any relevant exposures are important to assess, in determining whether sufficient exposure occurred to cause the disease. Because of the chronicity of most occupational interstitial lung diseases and the long latency between exposure and disease, useful industrial hygiene data are rarely available to help assess the degree of exposure. Epidemiologic data on the prevalence of disease in similarly exposed workers can be helpful in evaluating an individual patient. The onset of exposure is frequently important because of the characteristic latencies between first exposure and disease manifestation (e.g., for interstitial fibrosis secondary to asbestos exposure, the latency is usually 20 or more years). A shorter latency should suggest another diagnostic possibility.

In addition to a careful occupational history, a careful environmental exposure history should also be obtained, including information on hobbies, pets, and changes in housing or heating and ventilation systems. Smoking history is important, both for diagnostic and management purposes. A careful smoking history is important for interpreting pulmonary function tests (discussed later) and advising the patient on reducing the risk of further lung disease, especially lung cancer.

Physical examination

The physical examination can be quite variable and surprisingly unrevealing, even in advanced disease. Fine basilar end-inspiratory crackles or rales are the classical finding in pulmonary fibrosis, but may be absent. Digital clubbing is most common with asbestosis or idiopathic pulmonary disease, but is frequently absent. Resting tachypnea and tachycardia may be present with more advanced disease. Cardiac manifestations of end-stage pulmonary fibrosis, such as pulmonary hypertension and cor pulmonale, may be evident. The physical examination is also helpful in ruling out nonoccupational causes of pulmonary fibrosis, such as connective tissue diseases, systemic vasculitides, or sarcoidosis. Skin, eye, and joint evaluation are particularly helpful.

DIAGNOSIS AND WORK-UP
Chest radiography

Chest radiography is the most important diagnostic test for occupational fibrotic disorders. It is critical that radiographs of high technical quality be obtained. The chest radiograph can be unique or highly suggestive of an occupational interstitial lung disorder and is frequently sufficient, along with an appropriate exposure history, to establish a diagnosis. Silicosis, coal worker's pneumoconiosis, asbestosis with pleural disease, and other pneumoconioses all have characteristic radiographic findings strongly suggestive of the specific occupational diagnosis.[6] For example, the findings of small rounded opacities, progressive massive fibrotic lesions in the upper lung zones, and "eggshell" calcification of the hilar lymph nodes are highly suggestive of silicosis. Similarly, the findings of bilateral pleural plaques and diffuse small irregular linear opacities in the lower lung zones are highly suggestive of asbestosis. However, chest radiographic findings can also be nonspecific, as with asbestosis without pleural plaques, hard metal disease, or beryllium disease. Chest radiographs can also be normal in approximately 10% to 20% or more of patients with symptomatic interstitial lung disease.[52] For example, 15% to 20% or more of patients with pathologic evidence of pleural disease or asbestosis may have normal-appearing chest radiographs.[53]

An international uniform classification system, under the auspices of the International Labor Organization (ILO), has designed a system for evaluating chest radiographs for epidemiologic studies, clinical evaluation, and screening.[54] The system classifies radiographic opacities according to the shape, size, extent, and concentration of opacities. Pleural changes are also graded according to site, pleural thickening, and pleural calcification. The ILO system is described in Chapter 7.

Computerized tomography

Much has been written about the role of computerized tomography (CT) scanning in the evaluation of patients with occupational interstitial lung disease, primarily asbestosis. Conventional CT scanning (8- to 10-mm-thick slices) and high-resolution CT (HRCT) scanning (1- to 3-mm-thick slices) can be used to better evaluate pleural and parenchymal abnormalities. Conventional CT scanning is more sensitive than chest radiography for the diagnosis of pleural disease and is helpful in distinguishing subpleural fat from pleural fibrosis. It is most useful for evaluating focal pulmonary masses.

The HRCT scanning technique enables improved visualization of the lung parenchyma, such as thickened and irregular interfaces, linear abnormalities, nodular abnormalities, cysts, and airspace opacification. In addition, HRCT can identify parenchymal abnormalities not evident on standard radiographs and is being increasingly used in the evaluation of patients with asbestosis and other interstitial lung diseases.[55] The HRCT scan has also been used experimentally to demonstrate an association between pleural fibrosis and restrictive lung function, the volume of pleural fibrosis identified on an HRCT scan being inversely associated with total lung capacity.[56] Interstitial lung abnormalities found using HRCT scanning have been associated with reduced lung volumes, abnormal gas exchange, and ILO profusion scores.[53,57]

However, the clinical significance and usefulness of HRCT scanning, in most patients, remains unclear. In the majority of cases in which the diagnosis of an occupational interstitial lung disease is clear on the basis of the chest radiograph and the patient's history, HRCT scanning is not indicated. Unexplained dyspnea or abnormal physiology (e.g., restrictive lung function, abnormal gas exchange, or abnormal response to exercise) should raise suspicion for interstitial lung disease. In patients with suspected interstitial lung disease but a normal chest radiograph, HRCT may be helpful in identifying parenchymal abnormalities. The specific features and distribution of the HRCT changes may occasionally be suggestive of a specific cause and help narrow the differential diagnosis. In two retrospective studies HRCT was found to have greater diagnostic accuracy than chest radiography for the diagnosis of specific interstitial lung diseases such as asbestosis, silicosis, and lymphangitic carcinomatosis.[3,58] However, it should be remembered that although HRCT may provide interesting additional information, in most cases HRCT is not required for the diagnosis or management of patients with occupational interstitial lung disease and can be an unnecessary expense. Although conventional CT scanning is helpful in evaluating focal pulmonary masses, such as pseudotumors (rounded atelectasis) caused by asbestos, and is helpful in differentiating between pleural fat and fibrosis, it should not be ordered routinely.

Gallium scanning

Abnormal uptake of the radioactive nuclide gallium-67 occurs with acute and chronic inflammation and with certain malignancies. Many patients with interstitial fibrosis have abnormal gallium uptake. However, such findings are not particularly sensitive or specific and are difficult to quantify. Thus gallium scanning is not recommended in the routine evaluation of patients with interstitial fibrosis.

Pulmonary function tests

Resting lung function testing is the most important tool for assessing functional respiratory status. Physiologic testing in diffuse fibrotic diseases typically shows a restrictive pattern with reduced lung volumes and decreased DLCO capacity. Vital capacity, residual volume, functional residual capacity, and total lung capacity are reduced. Air flow rates and the ratio of forced expiratory volume in 1 second to forced vital capacity (FEV1/FVC) ratio are preserved. The DLCO is usually reduced because of ventilation–perfusion mismatching. The findings on physiologic testing are generally not specific for a particular etiology but are important for evaluating dyspnea and assessing the degree of pulmonary impairment.

Although interstitial lung disorders traditionally are thought of as having pure restrictive defects, a mixed pattern of obstructive and restrictive defects can also be seen. Mixed obstructive and restrictive defects have usually been attributed to concomitant smoking, but more recent studies have clearly demonstrated that asbestos itself can cause airflow obstruction.[3] Mixed obstructive and restrictive defects can result in underestimating the degree of restriction present, making total lung capacity an insensitive measure of functional impairment.[59] In a given patient chest radiographic findings, lung volumes, and DLCO may or may not be correlated in assessing the extent of disease and functional impairment.

Arterial blood gases may be normal or may show varying degrees of hypoxemia, depending on the severity of disease. Patients with interstitial lung disease have a tendency to hyperventilate, resulting in a reduced $PaCO_2$ and respiratory alkalosis. Patients with more severe disease should be evaluated for hypoxemia both at rest and with exertion.

Cardiopulmonary exercise testing

Cardiopulmonary exercise testing is being used increasingly to assess functional impairment and disease progression in patients with interstitial occupational lung disorders. Exercise testing can help distinguish among cardiac, pulmonary, and deconditioning causes of dyspnea.[60] In patients with significant interstitial lung disease, exercise results in an increase in the alveolar–arterial oxygen gradient, P(A − a)o_2 difference, and arterial hypoxemia. Exercise results in increased ventilation–perfusion mismatching with increased calculated dead space, and the V_D/V_T ratio rises rather than falls, as occurs normally with exercise. Cardiopulmonary exercise testing is helpful in evaluating a select group of patients with dyspnea and normal pulmonary function tests, or dyspnea that appears out of proportion to the changes in lung function.[60] However, in most patients exercise testing adds little to their evaluation or management, and its usefulness is primarily for determination of the degree of impairment. Cardiopulmonary exercise testing is not helpful in determining the specific cause of interstitial lung disease.

Bronchoscopy

Although the diagnosis of occupational interstitial lung disease can usually be made on the basis of the occupational history, chest radiography, and pulmonary function testing, under certain circumstances bronchoscopy with transbronchial biopsy and bronchoalveolar lavage may be helpful diagnostically and is variably performed if the diagnosis is unclear on initial evaluation. Bronchoscopy with transbronchial lung biopsy and bronchoalveolar lavage are relatively noninvasive means of sampling, respectively, the lung parenchyma and the cellular contents and products of the distal alveolar space. Much has been written about the usefulness (and lack thereof) of bronchoscopy and bronchoalveolar lavage in the diagnosis and management of patients with interstitial lung disease.[6,61]

Transbronchial biopsies yield small tissue samples that may be adequate to diagnose the presence of interstitial fibrosis in general and occasionally shed light on the etiology. Transbronchial biopsies are most helpful in diagnosing granulomatous interstitial processes such as sarcoidosis, beryllium disease, and hypersensitivity pneumonitis or a diffuse malignant process. Sufficient tissue is not obtained to perform extensive analyses for dust content, and the histologic results may be misleading for nongranulomatous forms of interstitial lung disease.

Although not routinely performed in many institutions, under certain circumstances bronchoalveolar lavage can be diagnostically helpful. The predominance of lymphocytes on bronchoalveolar lavage suggests certain diagnoses, such as sarcoidosis, hypersensitivity pneumonitis, lymphangitic carcinoma, and beryllium disease, but is not itself diagnostic.[6,61] The diagnosis of beryllium disease can be established with the finding of a positive lymphocyte transformation test in the bronchoalveolar lavage of exposed patients. Characteristic multinucleated giant cells may be seen on bronchoalveolar lavage or transbronchial biopsy in patients with hard metal disease. Unfortunately, only a few other interstitial lung diseases, all quite uncommon, such as alveolar cell carcinoma or eosinophilic pneumonia, can be diagnosed on the basis of bronchoalveolar lavage findings.

Cells obtained from bronchoalveolar lavage contain dust particles that reflect current and possibly past exposures. Such particles can be identified and counted. For example, uncoated asbestos fibers and asbestos bodies (asbestos particles coated with iron) have been quantitated from bronchoalveolar lavage fluid. However, it is unclear how well such assays correlate with other measures of exposure or with the presence or extent of disease.[62,63] At present, such assays have little practical clinical utility and are rarely used clinically.

Bronchoalveolar lavage has also been advocated as useful for predicting disease activity and outcome and possibly response to treatment. However, none of these uses currently has proven clinical utility. The presence of a neutrophilic alveolitis in bronchoalveolar lavage fluid may represent more active ongoing inflammation and an increased likelihood of disease progression. In asbestos-exposed workers increased neutrophils, lymphocytes, and fibronectin in bronchoalveolar lavage fluid have been associated with reduced lung function and/or progressive loss of lung function.[28,64]

Lung biopsy

Although usually not needed to make a diagnosis of occupational interstitial lung disease, when there is no clear etiology, open lung biopsy provides the most definitive means for diagnosis and can also diagnose nonoccupational causes of interstitial lung disease, such as malignancy, pulmonary vascular disease, infection, or bronchiolitis obliterans. Open lung biopsy can obtain a more adequate sample of tissue for histologic and mineralogic (qualitative and quantitative) analyses. In general, open lung biopsy is a safe procedure with a low rate of morbidity, even in compromised patients, and should be considered in the work-up of any patient with interstitial lung disease of unclear origin.

To establish a diagnosis, histopathologic changes should be consistent with the known disease and the suspected causative dusts or particles can, in most cases, be detectable in the lungs. The various methods used to analyze the dust content of tissue are discussed in Chapters 8 and 12. Briefly, light microscopic evaluation with polarization is widely available and can provide a qualitative assessment of the presence of dust particles and ferruginous bodies but cannot identify the specific dust particles or enable quantification.

A number of bulk and microanalytic techniques are available that enable more definitive identification and quantification of minerals and dusts.[19] Bulk analysis techniques (such as x-ray fluorescence or x-ray diffraction) usually involve digestion or destruction of the tissue and are useful for quantifying individual elements but not as good at identifying specific minerals such as different silicates. Microanalytic techniques such as scanning electron microscopy and energy dispersion x-ray spectroscopy can be used to identify and quantify specific minerals in sections or tissue digests. Certain methods are better for certain substances, such as scanning electron microscopy for asbestos fibers. If a patient with interstitial lung disease of unclear etiology in whom an occupational or environmental cause is being considered undergoes open lung biopsy, more extensive particle analysis should be considered if light microscopic histologic examination is not diagnostic. There are some serious limitations that should be remembered. Only particulates that are insoluble, retained in tissue, and at sufficient concentration will be detected. These analytic methods can be tedious, and there can be significant differences in results from different laboratories. In addition, a positive finding indicates some degree of exposure but not necessarily disease.

Laboratory tests

Various laboratory test abnormalities have been reported with occupational interstitial lung diseases such as asbestosis or silicosis, including abnormal serum immunoglobulin levels, rheumatoid factor, antinuclear antibodies, sedimentation rate, and serum–immune complexes. Such findings are generally nonspecific but may help establish a diagnosis of a connective tissue disorder. Such testing should be reserved for cases in which there is diagnostic uncertainty or a connective tissue disorder is being considered. Peripheral blood lymphocyte blast transformation in response to beryllium is one of the few specific laboratory assays available. Serum precipitins to specific antigens can help confirm a diagnosis of hypersensitivity pneumonitis to that antigen, but a positive finding indicates exposure, not disease, and a negative finding does not rule out the disease.

Natural history, prognosis, and complications

Most occupational interstitial lung diseases currently diagnosed in the United States progress relatively slowly over months to years or may stabilize with minimal further progression. However, progression to end-stage lung disease and death can occur. Occasionally, as with some cases of acute silicosis, progressive massive fibrosis attributable to coal dust, chronic beryllium disease, or rare cases of asbestosis, the course can be more aggressive. In patients with immune-mediated or idiosyncratic disorders such as hypersensitivity pneumonitis or chronic beryllium disease, improvement following removal from the offending agent can also occur. In general, adequate studies have not been done to compare the natural histories of occupational with other forms of interstitial lung disease. In recent years increased screening of patients for asbestosis, silicosis, and other occupational interstitial lung diseases has resulted in more early and mild cases being brought to medical attention and thus the impression that such diseases generally have a more benign course.

Attempts have been made to determine the degree of disease activity, namely, the degree of inflammation or alveolitis, with the hope that disease activity could help determine prognosis and guide effective therapy. Various bronchoalveolar lavage parameters, including macrophage, lymphocyte, and polymorphonuclear cell counts, certain cytokines, and other mediators, have been studied as possible markers of disease activity or response to therapy. Although these studies have provided valuable information on the pathogenesis of the alveolitis present in these diseases, to date they are of little help in managing an individual patient. Gallium scanning has also been investigated as a way to stage patients with interstitial lung disease, but the findings are difficult to quantify and remain nonspecific.

The major complications of interstitial fibrosis are (1) progressive loss of pulmonary function with eventual right heart failure and (2) an increased risk of lung cancer, especially among workers exposed to asbestos.[65,66] Nonpulmonary complications can also occur, such as immune-mediated disorders or renal disease with silicosis.

Management and treatment

The management and treatment of most occupational and environmental interstitial lung disorders are similar. Determination of the presence and severity of impairment can be used to guide management and follow disease progression. Most helpful is conventional pulmonary function testing with DLCO. Further exposure to the causative or suspected agent should be eliminated or minimized. Most occupational interstitial lung diseases, such as asbestosis or silicosis, persist and may progress after exposure has ceased. Exposure to other fibrogenic exposures and cigarettes should be minimized.

As with most interstitial lung diseases, in general there are few, if any, proven therapeutic interventions. Corticosteroid and cytotoxic agents have been tried in patients with various occupational interstitial fibrotic disorders but have no proven efficacy. If airways disease is present, a trial of standard bronchodilator therapy and inhaled steroids should be given. Other possible contributing factors, such as congestive heart failure, should be treated. Patients with more severe disease should be closely monitored for hypoxemia at rest or with exertion, and if present, treated with supplemental oxygen. Influenza and pneumococcal pneumonia vaccines are indicated as preventive measures. Purified protein derivative (PPD) screening in patients with silicosis is recommended because of their particularly increased risk for developing active tuberculosis. Regular follow-up with annual chest radiographs and spirometry is generally recommended, although medical monitoring has not been proven to reduce mortality.

REFERENCES

1. Crystal RG, Ferrans VJ, and Basset F: Biologic basis of pulmonary fibrosis. In Crystal RG and West JB, editors: *Lung injury,* New York, 1992, Raven.

2. Churg A, Wright JL, Wiggs B, et al: Small airways disease and mineral dust exposure, *Am Rev Respir Dis* 131:139-143, 1985.

3. Griffith DE, Garcia JG, Dodson RF, et al: Airflow obstruction in non-smoking, asbestos- and mixed dust-exposed workers, *Lung* 171:213-224, 1993.

4. Crystal RG: Interstitial lung disease. In Wyngaarden JB, Smith LH, and Bennett J, editors: *Textbook of medicine,* Philadelphia, 1992, WB Saunders.

5. Coultas DB, Zumwalt RE, Black WC, and Sobonya RE: The epidemiology of interstitial lung diseases, *Am J Respir Crit Care Med* 150:967-972, 1994.

6. Schwarz MI and King TE Jr, editors: *Interstitial lung disease,* ed 2, St. Louis, 1993, Mosby–Year Book.

7. Althouse RB, Castellan RM, and Wagner GR: Pneumoconioses in the United States: highlights of surveillance data for NIOSH and other federal sources, *Occup Med: State Art Rev* 7:197-208, 1992.

8. Henneberger PK and Stanbury MJ: Patterns of asbestosis in New Jersey, *Am J Ind Med* 21:687-697, 1992.

9. Atfield M and Castellan R: Epidemiological data on U.S. coal miners' pneumoconiosis, 1960 to 1988, *Am J Publ Health* 82:964-970, 1992.

10. Nugent K, Perrotta D, Dodson RF, et al: A cluster of silicosis in sandblasters, *Am Rev Respir Dis* 142(part 1):1466, 1990. Letter.

11. Valiante DJ, Richards TB, and Kinsley KB: Silicosis surveillance in New Jersey: targeting workplaces using occupational disease and exposure surveillance data, *Am J Ind Med* 21:517-526, 1991.

12. Cullen MR, Cherniack MG, and Rosenstock L: Medical progress: occupational medicine, *N Engl J Med* 322(part 1):594-601, 322(part 2):675-683, 1990.

13. van Sprundel MP: Pneumoconioses: the situation in developing countries, *Exp Lung Res* 16:5-13, 1990. Review.

14. Norboo T, Angchuk PT, Yahya M, et al: Silicosis in a Himalayan village population: role of environmental dust, *Thorax* 46:341-343, 1991.

15. Navratil M and Trippe F: Prevalence of pleural calcification in persons exposed to asbestos dust and in the general population in the same district, *Environ Res* 5:210-216, 1972.

16. Dumontet C, Biron F, Vitrey D, et al: Acute silicosis due to inhalation of a domestic product, *Am Rev Respir Dis* 143(part 1):880-882, 1991.

17. Talcott JA, Thurber WA, Kantor AF, et al: Asbestos-associated diseases in a cohort of cigarette-filter workers, *N Engl J Med* 321:1220-1223, 1989.

18. Cullen MR, Kominsky JR, Milton D, et al: Chronic beryllium disease in a precious metal refinery. Clinical epidemiologic and immunologic evidence for continuing risk from exposure to low level beryllium fume, *Am Rev Respir Dis* 135:201-208, 1987.

19. Churg A and Green FHY, editors: *Pathology of occupational lung disease,* New York, 1988, Igaku-Shoin.

20. Wright JL and Churg A: Severe diffuse small airways abnormalities in long-term chrysotile asbestos miners, *Br J Ind Med* 42:556-559, 1985.

21. Cugell DW, Morgan WKC, Perkins G, et al: The respiratory effects of cobalt, *Arch Intern Med* 150:177-183, 1990.

22. Crouch E: Pathobiology of pulmonary fibrosis, *Am J Physiol* 259:L159-L184, 1990.

23. Davis GS and Calhoun WJ: Occupational and environmental causes of interstitial lung disease. In Schwarz MI and King TE Jr, editors: *Interstitial lung disease,* ed 2, St. Louis, 1993, Mosby–Year Book.

24. Rochester CL and Elias JA: Cytokines and cytokine networking in the pathogenesis of interstitial and fibrotic lung disorders, *Semin Respir Med* 14:389-416, 1993.

25. Gerrity TR and Garrard CS: A mathematical model of particle retention in the airspaces of human lungs, *Br J Ind Med* 40:121-130, 1983.

26. Lapp NL and Castranova V: How silicosis and coal workers' pneumoconiosis develop—a cellular assessment, *Occup Med: State Art Rev* 8:35-56, 1993.

27. Rom WN, Bitterman PB, Rennard SI, et al: Characterization of the lower respiratory tract inflammation of non-smoking individuals with interstitial lung disease associated with chronic inhalation of inorganic dusts, *Am Rev Respir Dis* 136:1429-1434, 1987.

28. Rom WN, Travis WD, and Brody AR: Cellular and molecular basis of the asbestos-related diseases, *Am Rev Respir Dis* 143:408-422, 1991.

29. Spurzem JR, Saltini C, Rom W, et al: Mechanisms of macrophage accumulation in the lungs of asbestos-exposed subjects, *Am Rev Respir Dis* 136:276-280, 1987.

30. Rom WN: Accelerated loss of lung function and alveolitis in a longitudinal study of non-smoking individuals with occupational exposure to asbestos, *Am J Ind Med* 21:835-844, 1992.

31. Schwartz DA, Davis CS, Merchant JA, et al: Longitudinal changes in lung function among asbestos-exposed workers, *Am Rev Respir Dis* 150:1243-1249, 1994.

32. Antoniades HN, et al: Platelet-derived growth in idiopathic pulmonary fibrosis, *J Clin Invest* 86:1055-1064, 1990.

33. Car BD, Meleoni F, Luisetti M, et al: Elevated IL-8 and MCP-1 in the bronchoalveolar lavage fluid of patients with idiopathic pulmonary fibrosis and pulmonary sarcoidosis, *Am J Respir Crit Care Med* 14:655-659, 1994.

34. Elias JA and Zitnik RJ: Cytokine–cytokine interactions in the context of cytokine networking, *Am J Respir Cell Mol Biol* 7:365-367, 1992.

35. Kline JN, Schwartz DA, Monick MM, et al: Relative release of interleukin-1 beta and interleukin-1 receptor antagonist by alveolar macrophages. A study in asbestos-induced lung disease, sarcoidosis, and idiopathic pulmonary fibrosis, *Chest* 104:47-53, 1993.

36. Martinet Y, Rom WN, Grotendorst GR, et al: Exaggerated spontaneous release of platelet-derived growth factor by alveolar macrophages from patients with idiopathic pulmonary fibrosis, *N Engl J Med* 317:202-209, 1987.

37. Nagaoka I, Trapnell BC, and Crystal RG: Upregulation of platelet-derived growth factor-A and -B gene expression in alveolar macrophages of individuals and idiopathic pulmonary fibrosis, *J Clin Invest* 85:2023-2027, 1990.

38. Piguet PF, et al: Requirement of tumour necrosis factor for development of silica-induced pulmonary fibrosis, *Nature* 344:245-247, 1990.

39. Crystal RG: Oxidants and respiratory tract epithelial injury: pathogenesis and strategies for therapeutic intervention, *Am J Med* 91:395-445, 1991.

40. Mossman BT and Gee JBL: Pulmonary reactions and mechanisms of toxicity of inhaled fibers In Gardner DE, editor: *Toxicology of the lung,* ed 3, pp 371-387, New York, 1993, Raven Press.

41. Janssen YM, Marsh JP, Absher MP, et al: Expression of antioxidant enzymes in rat lungs after inhalation of asbestos or silica, *J Biol Chem* 267:10625-10630, 1992.

42. Cantin A, Dubois F, and Begin R: Lung exposure to mineral dusts enhances capacity of lung inflammatory cells to release superoxide, *J Leukocyte Biol* 43:299-303, 1988.

43. Mossman BT, Marsh JP, Sesko A, et al: Inhibition of lung injury, inflammation, and interstitial pulmonary fibrosis by polyethylene-glycol–conjugated catalase in a rapid inhalation model of asbestosis, *Am Rev Respir Dis* 141:1266-1271, 1990.

44. Bitterman PB, Polunovsky VA, and Ingbar DH: Repair after acute lung injury, *Chest* 105:118S-121S, 1994.

45. Polunovsky VA, Chen B, Henke C, et al: Role of mesenchymal cell death in lung remodeling after injury, *J Clin Invest* 92:388-397, 1993.

46. Hnizdo E, Baskind E, and Sluis-Cremer GK: Combined effect of silica dust exposure and tobacco smoking on the prevalence of respiratory impairments among gold miners, *Scand J Work Environ Health* 16:411-422, 1990.

47. Kilburn KH and Warshaw RH: Severity of pulmonary asbestosis as classified by International Labour Organisation profusion of irregular opacities in 8749 asbestos-exposed American workers. Those who never smoked compared with those who ever smoked, *Arch Intern Med* 152:325-327, 1992.

48. Morimoto Y, et al: Synergistic effects of mineral fibres and cigarette smoke on the production of tumour necrosis factor by alveolar macrophages of rats, *Br J Ind Med* 50:955-960, 1993.

49. Kelsey KT, Smith CM, Wiencke JK, et al: Inherited glutathione-S-transferase deficiency is a risk factor for pulmonary asbestosis, *Am Assoc Cancer Res* 35:A1749, 1994.

50. Richeldi L, Sorrentio R, and Saltini C: HLA-DPB1 glutamate 69: a genetic marker of beryllium disease, *Science* 262:242-244, 1993.

51. Shih JF, Hunninghake GW, Goeken NE, et al: The relationship between HLA-A, B, DQ, and DR antigens and asbestos-induced lung disease, *Chest* 104:26-31, 1993.

52. Epler GR, et al: Normal chest roentgenograms in chronic diffuse infiltrative lung disease, *N Engl J Med* 27:934-939, 1978.

53. Aberle DR: High-resolution computed tomography of asbestos-related diseases, *Semin Roentgenol* 26:118-131, 1991.

54. International Labor Organization: Guidelines for the use of ILO international classification of radiographs of pneumoconioses, *Occup Safety Health Ser* 22 (rev), 1980.

55. Begin R, et al: Computed tomography in the early detection of asbestosis, *Br J Ind Med* 50:689-698, 1993.

56. Schwartz DA, Galvin JR, Yagla SJ, et al: Restrictive lung function and asbestos-induced pleural fibrosis. A quantitative approach, *J Clin Invest* 91:2685-2692, 1993.

57. Staples CA, Gamsu G, Ray CS, et al: High resolution computed tomography and lung function in asbestos-exposed workers with normal chest radiographs, *Am Rev Respir Dis* 139:1502-1508, 1989.

58. Mathieson JR, Mayo JR, Staples CA, et al: Chronic diffuse infiltrative lung disease: comparison of diagnostic accuracy of CT and chest radiography, *Radiology* 171:111-116, 1989.

59. Barnhart S, Hudson LD, Mason SE, et al: Total lung capacity. An insensitive measure of impairment in patients with asbestosis and chronic obstructive pulmonary disease?, *Chest* 93:299-302, 1988.

60. Neuberg GW, Friedman SH, Weiss MB, et al: Cardiopulmonary exercise testing. The clinical value of gas exchange data, *Arch Intern Med* 148:2221-2226, 1988.

61. Daniele RP, et al: Bronchoalveolar lavage: role in the pathogenesis, diagnosis, and management of interstitial lung disease, *Ann Intern Med* 102:93-108, 1985.

62. Schwartz DA, Galvin JR, Burmeister LF, et al: The clinical utility and reliability of asbestos bodies in bronchoalveolar fluid, *Am Rev Respir Dis* 144:684-688, 1991.

63. Teschler H, Freidrichs KH, Hoheisel GB, et al: Asbestos fibers in bronchoalveolar lavage and lung tissue of former asbestos workers, *Am J Respir Crit Care Med* 149:641-645, 1994.

64. Schwartz DA, Galvin JR, Frees KL, et al: Clinical relevance of cellular mediators of inflammation in workers exposed to asbestos, *Am Rev Respir Dis* 148:68-74, 1993.

65. Berry G: Mortality of workers certified by pneumoconiosis medical panels as having asbestosis, *Br J Ind Med* 38:130-137, 1981.

66. Nicholson WJ, Perkel G, and Selikoff IJ: Occupational exposure to asbestosis: population at risk and projected mortality, 1980-2030, *Am J Ind Med* 3:259-311, 1982.

Chapter 16

CHRONIC OBSTRUCTIVE PULMONARY DISEASE

Michael S. Stulbarg
Leslie Zimmerman

The term *chronic obstructive pulmonary disease* (COPD) refers to a spectrum of chronic respiratory diseases characterized by airflow limitation in association with cough, sputum production, dyspnea, wheezing, or chest discomfort (e.g., pain or tightness). The disease may be present by physiologic criteria well before its clinical presentation. The term *COPD* is often used loosely to apply to patients who may have exclusively or predominantly emphysema, chronic bronchitis, or asthma. The disadvantage of lumping these disease states is that pathophysiologic mechanisms and therapeutic responses may be quite different.

Emphysema is usually defined pathologically by destruction of airspaces with loss of airway support and hyperinflation or a decrease in the pulmonary vascular bed with loss of diffusing capacity, and it is often associated with weight loss. Emphysema is due primarily to destruction of the lung parenchyma by an excess of proteolytic enzymes caused by either excessive recruitment of polymorphonuclear leukocytes (e.g., by damage caused by cigarette smoke) or a deficiency of proteinase inhibitors (e.g., in α_1-antitrypsin deficiency).

Chronic bronchitis is usually defined clinically by cough and sputum production persisting for at least 3 months of the year and for at least 2 years. It may occur as simple chronic bronchitis with mucorrhea alone or as chronic obstructive bronchitis with mucorrhea in combination with airflow limitation. Pathologically, chronic bronchitis is characterized by thickening of the bronchial walls with edema and cellular infiltration, smooth muscle hypertrophy, and glandular hypertrophy. At the time of autopsy, airways are variably filled with mucus, inflammatory cells, and bacteria. Chronic bronchitis must be distinguished from chronic sinusitis, cystic fibrosis (CF), and bronchiectasis. Chronic sinusitis can present with chronic expectoration of secretions that have "dripped" into the oropharynx, whether because of chronic infection, irritation, or allergic reactions in the nose and sinuses. It may occur alone or in concert with lower airway disease. Bronchiectasis, characterized by dilation of the bronchi, may be focal or diffuse and is usually the result of prior bacterial or mycobacterial infection. It is often suspected in the presence of large amounts of daily expectoration and dilated airways on plain chest radiographs, but establishment of the diagnosis usually requires special visualizing techniques. Computerized tomography (CT) scans, especially with high-resolution techniques, have largely replaced bronchograms for this diagnosis. The clinical importance of proper diagnosis is that bronchiectasis may require more prolonged antibiotic therapy and, when localized, may be amenable to surgical resection. Distinction from CF is usually not difficult because CF occurs in much younger patients, usually nonsmokers, and is diagnosable by specific tests (e.g., sweat chloride testing or genetic screening).

As much of the medical literature fails to distinguish adequately the predominant pathophysiologic abnormalities, the term *COPD* will be understood here to include patients with ill-defined and varying degrees of chronic bronchitis, emphysema, and airway hyperresponsiveness.

EPIDEMIOLOGY
Prevalence

The prevalence of COPD has been estimated to be at least 5% in the U.S. population.[1-3] In the Tecumseh Study of over 9000 adults, 14% of men and 8% of women had COPD.[4] In the SPRINT study of postmyocardial infarction patients in the United States, the estimated prevalence of COPD was somewhat lower, at 7%.[5] Using the spirometric criterion of a ratio of forced expiratory volume in 1 second to forced vital capacity (FEV_1/FVC) of less than 0.75, Sherrill et al. reported that COPD increased in prevalence from 5% to 25% from the fourth through the eighth decades of life (Fig. 16-1).[2]

Symptoms possibly due to COPD occur even more frequently. Sherrill's group found that 20% to 40% of men and 8% to 20% of women in the United States reported production of phlegm.[2] Lebowitz described wheezing in 8% to 18% of American men but did not have adequate data regarding symptoms in women.[6]

Trend data from the National Center for Health Data Systems suggest that the prevalence and mortality of COPD in U.S. men has peaked and may actually be decreasing, es-

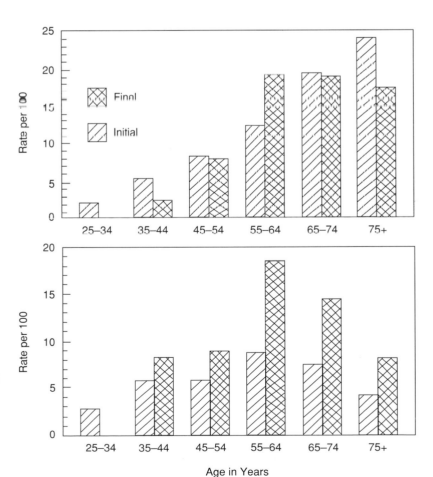

Fig. 16-1. Cumulative prevalence rates of physician-confirmed COPD in male (*top*) and female (*bottom*) patients with an FEV_1/FVC ratio of less than 75%. The prevalence rates of COPD significantly increased over time (from the initial Tucson epidemiologic survey in 1972 to a later "final" survey in 1985) among women of most age groups but only among men aged 55 to 64 years. (Adapted from Sherrill DL, Lebowitz MD, and Burrows B: Epidemiology of chronic obstructive pulmonary diseases, *Clin Chest Med* 11:375-387, 1990.)

pecially in younger men. Even though the prevalence of COPD in U.S. women is lower than that in men, the trend is not decreasing, likely reflecting current smoking habits. Because of these mixed trends, the overall prevalence of COPD continues to increase slowly.

Morbidity and mortality

Chronic obstructive pulmonary disease is a major cause of morbidity and mortality in the United States. Patients with COPD are more likely to report their health as poor, spend more days in the hospital, and lose more days from work.[7] This disease becomes a more serious health problem with age, especially in men, as measured by the frequency of office visits and hospitalizations.[7]

Chronic obstructive pulmonary disease is cited as the underlying cause of 3% of deaths in the United States,[8] making it the fifth leading cause.[9] Comparing the leading causes of death in this country from 1980 to 1986, there has been a yearly increase of 2.8% and 1.0% in age-adjusted death rates for COPD and lung cancer, respectively.[2,10] This is in contrast to decreasing death rates for heart disease and strokes in the same time period.[2,10] Moreover, COPD-related deaths may be underrepresented because of multiple-cause coding of death in COPD patients.[2] Kuller et al. estimated from the multiple risk factor intervention trial (MRFIT) study[11] that COPD death rates measure only about one third of all deaths that include a COPD diagnosis on the death certificate. Age and baseline FEV1, especially postbronchodilator FEV1, which reflects more fixed

airway obstruction, appear to be the best predictors of mortality from COPD (Fig. 16-2).[12]

Changes in the international coding of chronic airways disease have made country-to-country comparisons difficult,[13] and mortality is likely better estimated than morbidity. In Canada mortality from both emphysema and chronic bronchitis, after rising since the mid-1950s, has leveled off in men but continues to increase in women.[14] In other developed countries COPD appears to cause fewer than 10% of deaths, but there is no sign of decreasing mortality.[13] Until smoking is curbed around the world, it is likely that the incidence of COPD will continue to rise.

Causes

Cigarettes. The 1964 Surgeon General's report[15] established the connection between smoking and COPD and demonstrated a dose–response relationship between degree of smoking and likelihood of chronic lung disease. Cigarette smoking remains the most important cause of COPD and accounts for 80% to 90% of COPD deaths.[16]

Data from the National Health Interview Surveys[17,18] showed that smoking prevalence declined at a linear rate from 1974 to 1984. In 1986 smoking prevalence was 29.5% for U.S. men and 23.8% for U.S. women, substantially lower than the 1964 rates of 52.9% and 31.5% for men and women, respectively.[19] During this time approximately 1.3 million smokers quit, while 1 million persons, primarily teenagers and preteens, initiated smoking. Although smoking prevalence is decreasing in both men and women, the

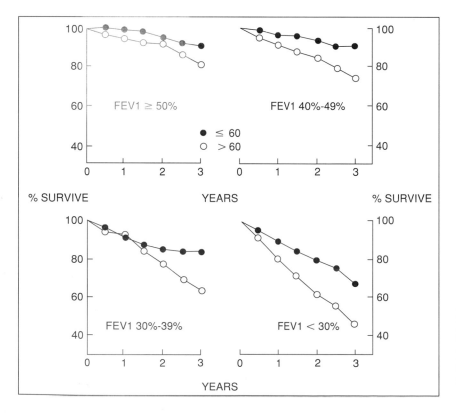

Fig. 16-2. Survival among patients in the IPPB Trial ($n = 4$), segregated according to baseline FEV1 and the median age of 60 years. (Adapted from Anthonisen NR: Prognosis in chronic obstructive pulmonary disease: results from multicenter trials, *Am Rev Respir Dis* 140:95S-99S, 1989.)

rate of decline is slower in women, and among less-educated young women, smoking prevalence is actually increasing.[17,18] In teenagers as a group, the previously steady decline in smoking initiation has plateaued.[19] Currently, lower educational status is a stronger predictor of smoking than is age, race, or gender.[18] Although cigarette sales have fallen by 1.8% per year since 1982, the mortality from COPD has not, perhaps reflecting residual risk in former smokers (Figs. 16-3 and 16-4).[19]

Low-tar cigarettes may be less hazardous with respect to the development of COPD and its severity.[20] However, smokers are addicted to the nicotine and are likely to compensate by smoking more cigarettes, puffing deeper or occluding ventilation holes in the filter tips with fingers and lips when smoking lower-tar cigarettes.[21,22] Overall, the benefits of switching from high- to low-tar cigarettes appear to be small, whereas the benefits of quitting are great.[20]

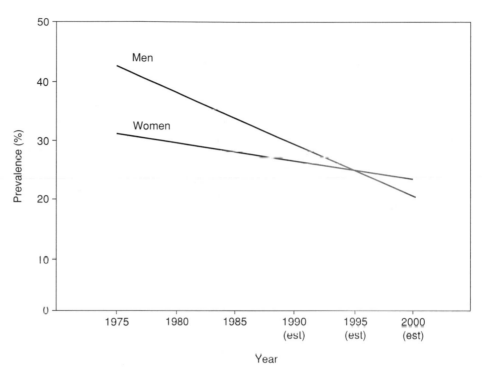

Fig. 16-3. Smoking prevalences for men and women with projections to the year 2000. Lines were computed via linear regression based on observed values from National Health Interview Surveys by the National Center for Health Statistics in 1974, 1976, 1978 through 1980, 1983, and 1985. Slopes (the percentage point change per year) are -0.91 ± 0.06 for men and -0.33 ± 0.06 for women. est, Estimate. (Adapted from Pierce JP, Fiore MC, Novotny TE, et al: Trends in cigarette smoking in the United States: projections to the year 2000, *JAMA* 261:49-55, 1989.)

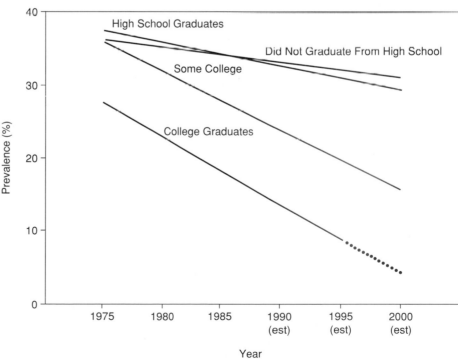

Fig. 16-4. Smoking prevalences by educational status with projections to the year 2000. Lines were computed via linear regression based on observed values from National Health Interview Surveys by the National Center for Health Statistics in 1974, 1976, 1978 through 1980, 1983, and 1985. Slopes (the percentage point change per year) are 0.19 $\pm$ 0.03 for persons who did not graduate from high school, -0.30 ± 0.07 for high school graduates, -0.78 ± 0.09 for persons with some college, and -0.91 ± 0.13 for college graduates. est, Estimate. (Adapted from Pierce JP, Fiore MC, Novotny TE, et al: Trends in cigarette smoking in the United States: projections to the year 2000, *JAMA* 261:49-55, 1989.)

Passive smoking. Passive, or involuntary, smoking is the exposure of nonsmokers to tobacco smoke, generally in an enclosed setting. Mainstream smoke is that which is drawn through the cigarette into the smoker's lungs and exhaled; sidestream smoke is that from the burning end of the cigarette. Eighty-five percent of smoke in a closed setting is from sidestream smoke, which generally has a higher concentration of tars, nicotine, carcinogens, and carbon monoxide than does mainstream smoke.[23] Exposure to involuntary smoke may be appreciable: for example, in 1983, 63% of nonsmokers reported some daily exposure, 35% reported exposure of greater than 10 hours/week,[24] and 70% of children in U.S. homes lived where there was at least one smoker.[25] The 1986 Surgeon General's report on passive smoking reported that nonsmokers with spouses who smoked had an increased risk of lung cancer.[26] It has been more difficult to establish a link between exposure to involuntary smoking and development of COPD.[27,28] Nonsmokers over age 40 who had a spouse who smoked had a statistically lower forced expiratory flowrate (FEF25-75) than those married to nonsmokers.[29] Nonsmokers exposed to smoke in the workplace had decreased FEV1 and FEF25-75, similar to the decreased levels seen in light smokers.[23] The physiologic and clinical importance of this is unknown.

Young children exposed to passive smoking in the home have consistently shown increased risk in the frequency and severity of acute respiratory infections,[16,29,30] but the significance of these findings in the later development of COPD is unclear. Active smoking is a much greater risk factor for COPD than is involuntary childhood exposure in the home. Unfortunately, children of parents who smoke are more likely to become smokers themselves.[30]

Air pollution. Outdoor air pollution consists of variable amounts of suspended particles or smoke, water-soluble materials, gases such as nitrogen and sulfur oxides, ozone, and derivatives from reactive hydrocarbons from motor exhaust.[31,32] In the urban United States the highest concentration of air pollutants occurs in the summer, and exposure to this pollution can cause short-term changes in lung function and acute respiratory symptoms.[32] Those with established COPD clearly can have worsening of symptoms during periods of heavy pollution.[33] It remains controversial whether chronic exposure to levels of outdoor pollutants found in developed countries can cause COPD in the absence of smoking, but most authors have concluded that the contribution is minor compared with that of smoking.[31,32,34] Exceptions have included those cities heavily polluted by the burning of coal, in which chronic bronchitis may be increased.[32,34]

Indoor pollution in most developed countries consists mostly of elevated levels of nitrogen dioxide, primarily from cooling and heating with natural gas or kerosene, but this does not appear to play a role in the development of COPD.[35] In contrast, in developing countries indoor air pollution from the burning of biomass (e.g., coal, wood, or animal dung) in poorly or unvented settings may be a significant contributor to COPD in adults and acute respiratory infections in children.[35-38]

Occupational exposures. It has been difficult to quantify the role of occupational exposures in the development of COPD because the effect of smoking is so strong. However, in 1985 the Surgeon General's report[39] concluded that smoking and occupational exposure to coal, cement, grain, welding, and sulfur dioxide are usually additive for symptoms of chronic cough and phlegm production. See Chapter 27 for further discussion of the risk of COPD from occupational exposures.

Host factors

α_1-**antitrypsin deficiency.** In 1963 Laurell and Eriksson discovered that severe deficiency of a protein, α_1-antitrypsin or α_1-antiprotease inhibitor, was associated with the premature development of emphysema.[40] This protein blocks the action of neutrophil elastase and presumably the destruction of lung elastin fibers induced by it.[41,42] Homozygous deficiency of this protein is the only host factor known unequivocally to cause emphysema; deficiency of this protein does not lead to the development of chronic bronchitis. Imbalance of lung proteases and antiproteases is a proposed, though still controversial, mechanism for all forms of emphysema.[42] For example, cigarette smoking may cause neutrophil chemotaxis into the lungs as well as inactivate protective α_1-antiprotease inhibitor.[41-43]

Homozygous deficiency is rare, affecting 1 in 4000 in North America.[44] Not all individuals with homozygous deficiency develop emphysema,[2] but those who also smoke have a greatly increased risk of developing severe and even fatal pan-lobular emphysema before age 35.[44] Homozygous deficiency accounts for about 0.1% of COPD cases in the United States.[8]

Although heterozygosity for this deficiency is common (up to 3% of the population),[45] an association between this genotype and impaired lung function (after controlling for smoking and age) has not been established.[45,46]

Host "susceptibility." Lung function normally declines by about 25 to 30 ml/yr in adults after the age of 30.[47] Whereas smokers as a group have increased rates of decline in FEV1, peak expiratory flow rates, and diffusing capacity for carbon monoxide (DLCO) that are correlated with amount of smoking, there is considerable variation.[27,28] Heavy smokers, as measured by total pack-years, generally have more impairment of lung function.[11,48]

Although smoking is the most important risk factor for COPD, only 10% to 15% of smokers can be expected to develop COPD (Fig. 16-5).[49] The reason for this variable "susceptibility" remains obscure. One theory, dubbed the "Dutch hypothesis,"[50-53] suggests that individuals with increased nonspecific airway hyperresponsiveness (i.e., to methacholine) have more rapid decline in FEV1 with smoking. However, it is unclear whether smoking-induced hy-

Fig 16-5. Risks for various men if they smoke. Differences between these lines illustrate the effects that smoking, and stopping smoking, can have on the FEV1 of a man who is liable to develop COPD if he smokes. †, Death, the underlying cause of which is irreversible COPD, whether the immediate cause of death is repiratory failure, pneumonia, cor pulmonale, or aggravation of other heart disease by respiratory insufficiency. This shows the rate of loss of FEV1 for one particular susceptible smoker; other susceptible smokers will have different rates of loss, thus reaching "disability" at different ages. (Adapted from Fletcher C and Peto R: The natural history of chronic airflow obstruction, *Br Med J* 1:1645-1648, 1977.)

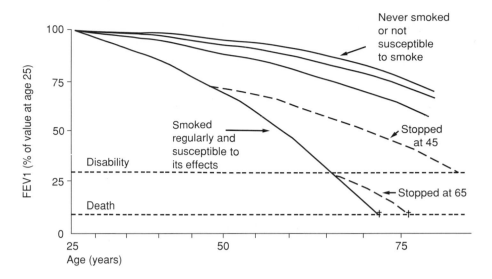

perresponsiveness accelerates the decline in FEV1 or whether rapid FEV1 decline and airway hyperresponsiveness are two independent outcomes of smoking.

DIAGNOSIS
History

Although many patients can be categorized as having predominantly chronic bronchitis or predominantly emphysema, the majority of individuals with COPD have a combination of both. The diagnosis of chronic bronchitis is made clinically from a history of chronic productive cough persistent for several months over a period of at least 2 years. Once the disease is established, a patient with chronic bronchitis usually has several exacerbations per year, typified by an increase in sputum production, onset or exacerbation of wheezing, or both. As the process worsens, the patient becomes the classic "blue bloater" with more frequent exacerbations, persistent wheezing, signs of right ventricular failure, emergency room visits, or hospital admissions and, in some the need for chronic home oxygen therapy. Patients with a predominantly emphysematous process, the "pink puffers," have a slower onset of dyspnea without productive cough. They typically have fewer complaints of wheezing and note less improvement with bronchodilator use (more fixed airway obstruction).[8,54]

Physical examination

Early in the course of COPD, there may be no abnormal findings on physical examination. A gradual increase in the size of the thoracic cage and a decrease in diaphragmatic excursion may be quite subtle. Use of pursed lips while exhaling and leaning forward with the arms supported are important clues to the presence of COPD. A forced expiratory time greater than 6 seconds is moderately good in predicting airflow limitation on subsequent spirometry.[55]

The chronic bronchitic patient is likely to be overweight, plethoric, and coughing. Scattered rhonchi may be replaced by persistent wheezing, often with "wet," or productive, coughs. As the disease progresses, cyanosis and findings of right ventricular failure, including ankle edema, hepatomegaly, ascites, and elevated jugular venous pressure, may predominate. In contrast, the patient with emphysema is usually thin, or even cachectic. Just the effort of undressing or climbing onto the examination table may be sufficient to elicit pursed-lips breathing or the use of accessory muscles of respiration. Chest examination is likely to reveal decreased breath sounds with little wheezing, except during forced expiration.[56] Cyanosis and signs of right ventricular failure occur only in the terminal stages of emphysema.[8]

Laboratory studies

Early in the course of COPD, laboratory values will be within normal limits. The exception, of course, is the patient with homozygous α_1-antitrypsin deficiency in whom levels of this protective protein will be very low. This test should be ordered in patients with onset of emphysema at an unusually young age, typical radiographic findings of basilar rather than apical bullous emphysema, or family history of emphysema.[8]

As COPD progresses, especially in the patient with predominant bronchitis, the onset of polycythemia suggests periodic or persistent hypoxemia. Elevated serum bicarbonate levels may reflect a chronic compensatory metabolic alkalosis from chronic respiratory failure with elevated $Paco_2$. Either polycythemia or an elevated serum bicarbonate level should prompt investigation of arterial blood gases. A substantially elevated leukocyte count in the patient with an exacerbation of COPD may suggest pneumonia.

Examination of the sputum is often helpful in the management of an acute exacerbation of chronic bronchitis. Purulence and bacterial species adequate to guide antibiotic therapy can be identified on Gram's stain. Sputum culture is less helpful because of the fastidiousness of some organisms (e.g., *Haemophilus influenzae, Streptococcus pneumoniae*) or because of overgrowth by oral flora. However, cultures are useful when the patient fails to respond to routine antibiotics or when there is suspicion of *Staphylococcus aureus* or gram-negative rod infection.[57]

Although the role of allergy in the progression of COPD is uncertain, this question is often raised by patients. Establishment of a historical relationship between environmental exposure and exacerbations of disease will usually suffice, especially if there is a personal or family history of atopy. Under certain circumstances, skin testing, especially for house dust mites, has been reported to be useful in indicating the need for environmental controls.[58]

Chest imaging

Except for the diagnosis of complications or comorbid problems (e.g., pneumonia, lung cancer, enlarging bullae, congestive heart failure, or bronchiectasis), chest radiographs are remarkably insensitive for estimation of the severity of COPD. Bronchial wall thickening, which may suggest chronic bronchitis, is both insensitive and nonspecific. "Overinflation" (increased anteroposterior diameter, increased retrosternal airspace, flat diaphragms, and increased radiolucency) is the most reliable indicator of emphysema, but accuracy in diagnosis ranges only from 65% to 80%.[59] Although most patients with severe emphysema can be recognized, only half of those with mild to moderate disease are detected.[59] Conventional CT scanning is superior to chest radiographs in detecting mild to moderate disease, with accuracy approaching 90%.[59] High-resolution CT scanning is more sensitive, detecting emphysema even in patients with low diffusing capacity but normal spirometry results.[60] However, CT scanning correlates poorly with functional evaluation using FEV1 and the FEV1/FVC ratio.[61]

During COPD exacerbations a chest radiograph adds additional important information in fewer than 5% of the cases, unless there is historical or laboratory evidence to suggest pneumonia or pulmonary edema.

Pulmonary function tests

Whereas COPD may be strongly suspected from the history and chest examination, pulmonary function testing is critical to confirm the diagnosis.[62] Simple spirometry (i.e., FVC and FEV1) may suffice to demonstrate airflow limitation with a decrease in the ratio of FEV1/FVC. Complete reversibility of airflow limitation with inhaled bronchodilators is more suggestive of asthma than COPD. A reduction only in the maximal midexpiratory flow rates (FEF25-75 or maximal mid-expiratory flow rate [MMEF]) may be the earliest physiological sign of COPD but is usually not associated with symptoms of dyspnea or exercise limitation. Unfortunately, spirometry is often not ordered even in patients at high risk for COPD. In a recent study of primary care practitioners presented with a case scenario involving a 52-year-old smoker with persistent cough, 38% ordered spirometry if the history included "chronic bronchitis" but only 5% did so if it did not.[63] In contrast, 80% ordered chest x-rays and 50% ordered sputum cultures, studies much less likely to give a specific diagnosis.

Measurement of lung volumes and diffusing capacity are important additional studies in the assessment of the patient with suspected COPD. Lung volumes [total lung capacity (TLC) and residual volume (RV)] may be measured by helium dilution or by body plethysmography. An increase in these volumes, especially in the ratio of RV/TLC, is common in COPD. A decrease in these volumes in the presence of airflow limitation raises the specter of combined restrictive and obstructive disease, as might be seen in smoking asbestos workers. Diffusing capacity is a measure of the interface between the alveolar wall and the capillary and is reduced in patients with emphysema but not in chronic bronchitis. A reduction in diffusing capacity in the presence of airflow limitation is strong evidence of emphysema.

Exercise testing

Chronic obstructive pulmonary disease limits exercise capacity in a number of ways: (1) mechanical limitation, (2) abnormal gas exchange, (3) altered cardiac function, (4) respiratory muscle dysfunction, (5) nutritional factors, and (6) symptoms, especially dyspnea. Exercise testing is not helpful for the diagnosis of COPD. However, cardiopulmonary exercise testing is a safe way to measure exercise performance and may clarify which of the above factors are limiting. It is also useful in diagnosing patients whose dyspnea seems out of proportion to the severity of their airflow limitation, in assessing the response to therapy or the need for supplemental oxygen, and in preoperative evaluation before lung resection.[64] Although simple timed walk tests give some information about exercise capacity, testing by treadmill or cycle ergometry with measurement of expired gases, oxygen saturation of hemoglobin, and heart rate provides information about ventilatory and cardiac function during exercise. Echocardiography during supine exercise may identify the earliest stage of pulmonary hypertension.[65,66] Patients with COPD may be unable to boost cardiac output during exercise because of right ventricular dysfunction, resulting in premature lactic acidosis and dyspnea or fatigue. This can be detected by radionuclide ventriculography.[67]

TREATMENT

Treatment of COPD is a complex affair that may require the skills of a management team including physicians, nurses, dietitians, physical therapists, and respiratory therapists.[68] Although physicians tend to focus on drug treatment, attention to other modalities may impact more on the patient's quality of life.

Prevention and prophylaxis

Smoking cessation. The health benefits of smoking cessation are vast and the risk of cigarette-related morbidity and mortality decreases with each year of abstinence.[69] The risk from coronary heart disease, peripheral vascular disease, and stroke drops quickly with cessation, approaching that of nonsmokers within 5 to 10 years.[69,70] Lung cancer risk overall is highest in the heaviest smoker, as measured both by total pack-years and by number of cigarettes smoked per day. Lung cancer risk also declines with abstinence but never appears to equal the nonsmokers' risk level, even 20 to 30 years after quitting.[69,70] Respiratory symptoms of cough, phlegm production, and wheezing decrease quite quickly (within 3 months) after quitting.[71] There is also a decrease in the rate of decline of lung function that may prevent or delay the onset of COPD in susceptible smokers.[49] Once COPD is well established, smoking cessation may not necessarily improve dyspnea.[70]

Spontaneous quit rates are lower than 1% per year,[21] despite estimates that 30% to 70% of smokers wish to stop smoking. Even minimal physician intervention appears to increase the quit rate to 5%[21] and appears to be as cost effective as other common preventive medical practices such as treating hypertension.[72] Surprisingly, only 30% to 70% of smokers have been advised to stop smoking by their physicians.

Nicotine is the constituent of cigarettes and other tobacco products that causes dependence. In about 80% of smokers, abstinence results in a withdrawal syndrome of restlessness, anxiety, irritability, and intense craving for cigarette smoking which peaks in 24 to 48 hours and lasts 1 to 2 weeks; the psychologic addiction to smoking can last months to years.[21] Although most smokers who quit do so without formal programs, pharmacologic intervention with nicotine gum or patch with counseling increases long-term success rates to the range of 15% to 30%.[73,74] Nicotine replacement therapy with physician counseling alone (no formal smoking cessation clinic) has a lower long-term success rate of 9%.[21] Nicotine gum or patch use in the smoker who does not wish to quit does not appear to be at all effective.[21]

Changing the work environment. If an individual with established COPD has a "dusty" occupation (e.g., mining or foundry work), it may be advisable to remove the patient from that environment. The impact on the patient's career must be weighed against the severity of pulmonary symptoms or decrements in pulmonary function.

Vaccinations. Influenza vaccination reduces the frequency of exacerbations of COPD with their attendant morbidity and mortality.[75,76] Amantadine may be given during an influenza outbreak to those who failed to receive vaccination. Although the value of pneumococcal vaccination in COPD patients has not been universally accepted,[77] the Centers for Disease Control and Prevention (CDC) has reported that it is safe and effective.[78]

Reducing or liquefying secretions

Despite the widespread use of cough syrups and expectorants, there is remarkably little evidence that they are effective in patients with COPD and they are not frequently prescribed for these patients. However, a recent national cooperative study did conclude that iodinated glycerol is helpful in reducing respiratory symptoms and easing expectoration.[79]

Treatment of infection

The proper role of antibiotics in the treatment of COPD remains controversial. Although several studies showed no improvement after treatment of exacerbations with an antibiotic,[80,81] one well-controlled study by Anthonisen and coworkers did show some benefit.[82] They studied 372 exacerbations in 173 patients and found that treatment with doxycycline, amoxicillin, or trimethoprim–sulfamethoxasole produced clinical improvement in 68% of acute exacerbations versus 55% in those treated with a placebo. Unfortunately, because of the difficulty in obtaining uncontaminated sputum and doing proper Gram's staining, it is usually easier to prescribe antibiotics than to determine whether a patient actually has a *bacterial* exacerbation of his COPD. Thus it has become accepted practice to prescribe broad-spectrum antibiotics (e.g., ampicillin, amoxicillin, trimethoprim–sulfamethoxasole, tetracycline, or doxycycline) empirically for 7 to 14 days for COPD patients with increased cough and change in character of sputum (e.g., more tenacious, darker, or larger volume), even in the absence of fever, leukocytosis, or pulmonary infiltrates. Newer antibiotics (e.g., ciprofloxacin[83] and cefuroxime[84]) are effective but have not been shown to be superior to the older and much less expensive agents except in the treatment of resistant organisms (e.g., *Pseudomonas*).

If the patient fails to improve or requires hospitalization, sputum culture and Gram's stain should be obtained, looking for resistant strains (e.g., some strains of *H. influenzae*) or more serious organisms (e.g., *S. aureus, Pseudomonas,* or other gram-negative rods), and broad-spectrum parenteral antibiotics should be initiated. Once the patient begins to improve, treatment can usually be completed with oral agents on an outpatient basis. Gram-negative "infection" may respond to one of the newer oral agents mentioned or may require prolonged intravenous antibiotics. Failure to improve with antibiotics suggests the need to look for malignancy or for unusual organisms (e.g., fungi or mycobacteria).

Bronchodilatation

Inhaled bronchodilators. Although the reversibility of airflow limitation in COPD is to a lesser degree than in asthma, bronchodilatation remains a critical part of the therapy of COPD. Inhalation therapy is preferred to oral therapy because of the speed of onset, convenience, and reduction in side effects. Most patients will exhibit at least a 10% increase in FEV1 with maximal inhaled bronchodilator therapy, and some will improve by 20% or more, but the response to inhaled agents is heterogeneous. Inhaled anticholinergic therapy, is generally at least as effective as β-agonist therapy, with fewer side effects, and should be considered first-line therapy in COPD patients.[68] Many patients require greater than the usual recommended dose of bronchodilator to achieve maximal bronchodilatation and this can be established by individual dose–response curves. Even if there is no immediate reversibility on spirometric testing, patients should be given an empiric trial of bronchodilators for use at home, as response may be delayed or may be limited to more symptomatic periods. If documentation of reversibility is desirable, body plethysmographic measurement of airway resistance is more sensitive.[85]

Inhaled β-agonists (e.g., albuterol, metaproterenol, or pirbuterol) remain popular agents for bronchodilatation in COPD. In standard doses side effects are few and bronchodilatation is rapid. Increasing doses of β-agonists will result in improved bronchodilatation in patients with COPD but only at the expense of side effects such as tremors and headaches.[86,87] Because of this variability in response and side effects, it is important to titrate the dose for the individual patient.

The most significant recent change in bronchodilator therapy is the addition of inhaled ipratropium bromide, an anticholinergic agent that, unlike atropine, does not cause cardiac or central nervous system side effects.[88] Its only drawback is its slower onset of action, requiring 30 minutes or more for peak effect. In COPD, in contrast to asthma, standard doses of ipratropium usually produce greater bronchodilatation than do β-adrenergic agents,[89,90] and tachyphylaxis does not occur, at least over the first 3 months of treatment.[90] In one dose–response study increasing doses of ipratropium produced significantly greater improvement than did the standard dose of two puffs (40 μg).[91] The standard dose produced 73% of the improvement seen with maximal doses. Ipratropium has also been shown to improve dyspnea and exercise tolerance in this patient population.[92] In addition, ipratropium may increase the magnitude as well as the duration of response to a β-agonist, suggesting an important role for combined therapy.[93,94]

Medication delivery. The key to the use of inhaled bronchodilators is adequate delivery of the medication to the lower airways by nebulizers or metered-dose inhalers (MDIs). Intermittent positive-pressure breathing equipment was previously thought superior to MDIs or simple nebulizers for drug delivery, but a national multicenter trial showed no advantages to this approach[95] and positive pressure may cause pneumothoraces. Although some patients prefer nebulizers for drug delivery, the bulk of available evidence suggests that MDIs are equally effective at a lower cost and without the risk of nosocomial infection.[96]

Although MDIs represent an efficient, multidose, portable, safe, and cost-effective way to deliver inhaled medications, many patients do not use this equipment correctly, and many health care providers do not know how to instruct them.[97,98] The most common problems are (1) inability to coordinate actuation with inhalation; (2) poor compliance, with both overuse and underuse; (3) failure to shake the canister before actuation; and (4) an empty canister. These problems may be solved with adequate instruction, the addition of spacers or holding chambers, or the use of a breath-activated device.[99] Inspiration should be slow, approximately 0.5 L/sec, and the breath should be held for 5 to 10 seconds at the end of inspiration with a delay of 1 to 5 minutes between puffs. Spacers decrease oropharyngeal deposition and improve lung delivery of a radiolabeled aerosol. In one study the fraction of an inhaled dose rose from 6.5% without instruction to 11.2% with correct technique and to 14.8% with addition of a spacer.[100] Use of the spacer device with the MDI decreased oropharyngeal deposition of the drug from about 80% of the dose to 9.5%, a particular advantage with inhaled steroids.

Theophylline

Although theophylline has been a mainstay in the treatment of COPD for many years, the potential for serious side effects, combined with increased appreciation of the efficacy of inhaled bronchodilators, has led many physicians to abandon its use. Despite variability in study design and results, there is still evidence that theophylline alone or in combination with inhaled therapy may benefit some patients with COPD.[101] It may be particularly useful for patients with nocturnal or early morning symptoms. More recent studies suggest that theophylline may have therapeutic efficacy apart from its bronchodilator effect by improving respiratory muscle contractility, decreasing muscle fatigue, and decreasing dyspnea.[102,103] If theophylline is to be used, treatment should begin with low doses (e.g., 200 to 400 mg/day) and increase slowly. Awareness of possible cardiovascular, gastrointestinal, and central nervous system side effects, combined with monitoring of blood theophylline levels, should prevent serious toxicity, which usually occurs only at blood levels in excess of 20 μg/ml.

Cost effectiveness of treatment is an issue of increasing importance. A recent retrospective study of 600 COPD patients receiving theophylline or ipratropium bromide evaluated the total costs and cost effectiveness of these two agents in three different health care settings and found substantial clinical advantages and cost savings with ipratropium.[104]

Corticosteroids

Although the supporting data are limited, corticosteroids are widely used in the management of COPD in both the inpatient and outpatient settings.[105] In one study of patients with acute exacerbations of COPD, intravenous methylprednisolone (0.5 mg/kg every 6 hours) produced superior improvement in spirometry at the end of 3 days of treatment.[106] If patients are sick enough to be admitted to the hospital, methylprednisolone is generally used, 0.5 to 1.0 mg/kg intravenously every 6 hours. A response is usually seen within 72 hours, after which steroid therapy is completely tapered within 2 to 3 weeks.

In the stable but persistently symptomatic patient, there is a limited place for steroid therapy.[107] The subgroup of patients who may respond is not usually evident from clinical or pulmonary function data, although acute responsiveness to bronchodilators is of some predictive value.[108] A trial of oral corticosteroids, usually in the range of 30 to 40 mg of prednisone daily for 2 to 3 weeks, for patients persistently limited by their disease is frequently recommended. Justification of continuing treatment should include clear-cut subjective and objective improvement, and the dosage should be as low as tolerable, preferably on alternate days. The euphorigenic and stimulatory effects of steroids may make tapering or discontinuation of them difficult, although patient education about side effects and the symptoms of steroid withdrawal will facilitate the process.

Although most side effects of steroid therapy are minor (e.g., weight gain, insomnia, and irritability), serious (e.g., compression fractures, ischemic hip necrosis, and diabetes) and even life-threatening complications (e.g., gastrointestinal bleeding and serious infections) do occur. Wiest and colleagues described life-threatening infections in seven elderly patients with COPD receiving high-dose corticosteroids for 5 months to 10 years.[109] Women may be at especially increased risk for side effects.[110]

Inhaled corticosteroids are a potentially useful alternative to oral steroids, although their role in the treatment of COPD remains uncertain. A recent 4-year prospective Dutch study of 56 patients (28 with asthma and 28 with COPD) concluded that inhaled steroids were useful in both groups in improving peak expiratory flow rate, respiratory symptoms, and the number of exacerbations per year, although the results in the patients with COPD were less impressive.[111] Airway hyperresponsiveness measured with methacholine improved in the asthmatic but not the COPD patients.

α_1-antitrypsin

Recombinant α_1-antitrypsin is now available for replacement therapy in patients with established homozygous deficiency. The drug is extremely expensive, must be given parenterally, and is not of proven value for any other subgroups of COPD patients.

Treatment of complications

Major complications of COPD include (1) hypoxemia, (2) cor pulmonale, (3) respiratory failure, (4) pneumothorax, (5) pneumonia, (6) lung cancer, and (7) the overall impact of the disease on functional status and quality of life.

Respiratory failure occurs when the patient is no longer able to maintain adequate ventilation to sustain life. This may occur gradually but usually occurs following a specific complication such as acute bronchitis, pneumonia, or pneumothorax. Pneumonia and pneumothorax are treated as in any other patient population, although their significance is more grave in the patient with underlying COPD. In a recent study patients with COPD represented 48% of a group of 92 nonimmunosuppressed patients with severe community-acquired pneumonia.[112] Lung cancer is increased in patients with COPD but this is discussed elsewhere (see Chapter 18). The other complications are dealt with specifically here.

Hypoxemia. Oxygen therapy may decrease pulmonary hypertension, cardiac arrhythmias, frequency of hospitalization, and mortality in COPD patients with severe chronic hypoxemia.[113-115] The primary goal of oxygen supplementation is to reverse chronic tissue hypoxia by maintaining O_2 saturation at greater than 90% (corresponding to a Pao_2 of 60 to 80 mm Hg), although it may reduce dyspnea as well. A minimum of 12 to 15 hr/day of oxygen therapy can ameliorate polycythemia and pulmonary hypertension,[113] but continuous therapy is more effective. The 2-year mortality for a group receiving nocturnal oxygen for an average of 12 hr/day was double that of a group receiving "continuous" oxygen for about 20 hr/day.[113]

Oxygen may be provided as a compressed gas, as a liquid, or via an O_2 concentrator. Oxygen is usually given nasally, but patients with high flow requirements or nasal irritation or who find oxygen aesthetically unacceptable may benefit from direct transtracheal delivery of oxygen via a percutaneous catheter.[116] Guidelines for initiating long-term therapy are a resting Pao_2 persistently below 55 mm Hg when the patient is free of an exacerbation or 56 to 59 mm Hg if polycythemia (hematocrit, over 55) or cor pulmonale is present. Treatment of exercise-induced desaturation with oxygen supplementation is often recommended, although its value has not been established.[115] A recent study showed that the severity of oxygen desaturation during walking was not related to either walking distance or levels of breathlessness,[117] emphasizing the need for careful consideration before treating a laboratory observation such as desaturation, particularly with a therapy as expensive and inconvenient as portable oxygen.

The issue of oxygen supplementation during air travel for patients not on chronic oxygen therapy is frequently raised because airplanes are pressurized only to an altitude of 5000 to 8000 feet. This can result in substantial hypoxemia. Although a few hours of hypoxemia is unlikely to be harmful in patients with borderline Pao_2 values at rest, it may be best to provide oxygen for sojourns at high altitude or during airplane travel.[118]

An alternative approach to hypoxemia is to stimulate ventilation with medications. Medroxyprogesterone acetate has been shown to improve arterial blood gases, but not symptoms or exercise tolerance.[119] Almitrine, a respiratory stimulant not yet available in this country, has been studied as an alternative to home oxygen therapy in patients with hypoxemia and hypercapnia. In one multicenter trial it increased the mean Pao_2 from 57 to 67 mm Hg and decreased the frequency of hospitalizations and episodes of right ventricular failure.[120] Others have found similar improvement in Pao_2, but its use is often limited by side effects including paresthesias, weight loss, and dyspnea.[120-122]

Pulmonary hypertension and cor pulmonale. Whereas the diagnosis of cor pulmonale previously required overt signs of right ventricular failure by examination or electrocardiogram, it may now be made noninvasively with echocardiography.[123] Two-dimensional echocardiography is more sensitive than physical examination or plain chest radiographs. In some cases technical factors may make adequate visualization of the chambers impossible, necessitating either transesophageal echocardiography or cardiac catheterization.

Pharmacologic treatment of cor pulmonale may supplement oxygen therapy, but it is not widely used. Calcium channel blockers may decrease pulmonary vascular resistance and improve cor pulmonale,[124] but they may do this in part by restoring perfusion to poorly ventilated areas. This may result in significant hypoxemia due to increasing venous admixture.[125] If such treatment is under consideration, arterial blood gases, as well as systemic blood pressure, should be closely monitored.

Pulmonary rehabilitation. As COPD worsens, patients become progressively less active. Afraid of dyspnea, they may choose to avoid physical activities that elicit it. This leads to a vicious cycle of reduced activity, deconditioning, and fear and anxiety, which may result in excessive disability. Pulmonary rehabilitation programs have addressed this cycle with a multidimensional approach drawing from medical, nursing, physical therapy, respiratory therapy, nutritional, and psychologic expertise. Utilizing varying combinations of education, psychosocial support, aerobic exercise training, inspiratory muscle training, and relaxation training, these programs have been able temporarily to improve substantially patients' exercise performance as well as their quality of life. Even patients with mild disease may demonstrate significant improvement in endurance, psychologic parameters, ability to work, and consumption of medical care after pulmonary rehabilitation even with no improvement in pulmonary function.[126,127]

Since dyspnea is related to the strength of inspiratory muscles, some investigators have studied whether strengthening the muscles of inspiration results in less dyspnea and better functional status.[128] Unfortunately, most of the results have been variable and unpredictable. However, one small sham-controlled study of inspiratory muscle training 15 minutes twice daily for 8 weeks did show substantial improvement both in inspiratory muscle strength and in dyspnea with activities of daily living.[129] Whether this approach should be more widely applied, particularly in rehabilitation programs, remains unknown.

Reduction in fear and anxiety may be critical elements of all pulmonary rehabilitation programs.[130] Listening to a taped relaxation message has been shown to induce relaxation and improve dyspnea.[131] It appears that exercise training per se may reduce fear and anxiety as well.[132] The authors' preliminary results suggest that exercise training is the key element of such programs and that increased attention to this aspect of pulmonary rehabilitation is justified.

Despite the enthusiasm with which pulmonary rehabilitation is recommended, evidence that it causes long-term improvement in physical competence, respiratory symptoms, well-being, emotional state, level of depression, everyday coping skills, and general activity and independence is limited. For example, a recent report of an intensive 3-week rehabilitation program described striking short-term benefits that disappeared by the end of 6 months.[133] Rather than abandon pulmonary rehabilitation, such results emphasize the need for identifying the best strategies to achieve long-term changes in physical activity and quality of life. It is likely that some sort of maintenance program will help achieve these long-term goals. However, COPD is generally progressive, and there is no evidence that pulmonary rehabilitation will improve pulmonary function tests or change the poor long-term prognosis for this disease.

Resting the muscles of inspiration is an intuitively appealing therapeutic approach for the COPD patient. It was presumed that ventilatory muscle fatigue was a major contributor to dyspnea and that resting the muscles of inspiration at night with nocturnal ventilatory assistance would reduce dyspnea and improve exercise capacity during the day. However, the value of this approach remains controversial. One randomized trial comparing 3 weeks of in-hospital rehabilitation alone with rehabilitation plus nocturnal negative-pressure ventilation (with an Emerson Pulmowrap, Cambridge, MA) showed no advantage of the nocturnally assisted ventilation either for measures of transdiaphragmatic pressure or for patients' reported well-being.[134] There may still be a place for partial ventilatory assistance in the COPD patient with respiratory failure, but its place appears to be quite limited.

Nutrition. Maintenance of weight is a problem for many patients (up to 70%) with COPD. Loss of greater than 15% of ideal body weight is suggestive of significant malnutrition, and weight loss is associated with decreased longevity.[135] The malnutrition itself significantly decreases diaphragmatic and limb muscle mass, contributing to dyspnea and the fatigue of respiratory muscles.

Proposed explanations for weight loss in this patient population have included inadequate dietary intake, a hypermetabolic state due to the excess work of breathing, impaired gastrointestinal function (including peptic ulcer disease), and an adaptive mechanism to decrease oxygen consumption.[136-138] Most malnourished COPD patients consume at least as many calories (and sometimes more) as those who are not malnourished.[139-142] Although the caloric intake may appear to be adequate, some patients may lose weight because energy requirements still exceed intake, with the basal metabolic rate 25% to 60% higher than expected. The "adaptive" theory, that energy expenditure is minimized by a decrease in total body mass by weight loss, does not appear to be true in the malnourished COPD patient. These patients continue to burn excess calories despite the weight loss. Interestingly, the emphysematous patient with hyperinflation, flattened diaphragms, and presumably respiratory muscles at poor mechanical advantage is much more likely to lose weight than the chronic bronchitic patient.[140]

Many groups have studied "refeeding" of malnourished COPD patients. The results of these studies can be summarized as follows: short-term refeeding can increase body weight, increase fat stores, improve subjective sense of well-being and dyspnea, increase exercise tolerance, and improve respiratory muscle strength as assessed by force generation at the mouth or across the diaphragm. Generally, refeeding is accomplished by the addition of dietary supplements to the regular diet and patients are often able to tolerate 250 to 1000 extra calories per day. Attempts at refeeding with supplements may be defeated by a reduction in routine meal intake. No study has shown an improvement in spirometry with calorie replenishment. Although there have been case reports of worsening CO_2 retention and even respiratory failure with high carbohydrate loads, controlled trials with an intent to increase calories have not shown significant changes in baseline $Paco_2$.

Management of end-stage chronic obstructive pulmonary disease.

Lung transplantation. Lung transplantation is now an established treatment for end-stage COPD.[143] Most centers are currently doing only single-lung transplants except in patients with chronic purulent bronchitis (e.g., bronchiectasis or CF) in whom there is concern that the remaining lung would contaminate the new one.

Pharmacologic treatment of dyspnea. Patients with COPD initially develop dyspnea only with strenuous exercise, but as the disease progresses, dyspnea, and its counterpart, fatigue, may occur with less provocation. In theterminal stages of the disease, dyspnea may occur with activities of daily living such as dressing or eating. Although aggressive use of inhaled medications and oxygen therapy may help greatly, in many patients they are inadequate. In such cases it is still incumbent on the physician to relieve the patient's symptoms (e.g., dyspnea) and the distress associated with them. Teaching breathing and relaxation strategies, providing physical assistance with the tasks of daily living (e.g., arranging for visiting nurses), and finding a supervised living environment may all help. If all of these prove inadequate, a physician may need to provide palliation of symptoms. Long-acting oral opiates given orally or by skin patch may significantly reduce patients' symptoms and the distress associated with them. The risk of respiratory depression is justified by the need to provide symptom relief. Obviously, such treatment should not be offered until all standard therapies have been exhausted. The patient and his family should be informed about the goals and risks of therapy and the decision to forgo resuscitation should have been clearly discussed. The dose chosen should be as low as possible to provide symptom relief and minimize risks. Constipation and urinary retention may need to be addressed. Assistance with this palliative approach may be obtained from local hospice organizations whose workers are specially trained to help patients deal with the terminal phase of their disease.

REFERENCES

1. Lebowitz M, Knudson R, and Burrows B: Tucson epidemiologic study of obstructive lung diseases. 1. Methodology and prevalence of disease, *Am J Epidemiol* 102:137-152, 1975.
2. Sherrill DL, Lebowitz MD, and Burrows B: Epidemiology of chronic obstructive pulmonary disease, *Clin Chest Med* 11:375-387, 1990.
3. Burrows B, Knudson RJ, Cline MG, et al: Quantitative relationships between cigarette smoking and ventilatory function, *Am Rev Respir Dis* 115:195-205, 1977.
4. Higgins MW, Keller JB, and Metzner HL: Smoking, socioeconomic status and chronic respiratory disease, *Am J Respir Dis* 116:403-410, 1977.
5. Behar S, Panosh A, Reicher-Reiss H, et al: Prevalence and prognosis of chronic obstructive pulmonary disease among 5,839 consecutive patients with acute myocardial infarction. SPRINT Study Group, *Am J Med* 93:637-641, 1992.
6. Lebowitz M: Occupational exposures in relation to symptomatology and lung function in a community population, *Environ Res* 44:59-67, 1977.
7. Woolcock AJ: Epidemiology of chronic airway disease, *Chest* 96:S302-S306, 1989.
8. Snider GL: Chronic bronchitis and emphysema. In Murray JF and Nadel JA, editors: *Textbook of respiratory medicine,* pp 1075-1090, Philadelphia, 1988, WB Saunders.
9. Feinleib M, Rosenberg HM, Collins JG, et al: Trends in COPD mortality in the United States, *Am Rev Respir Dis* 140:S9-S18, 1989.
10. Standards for the diagnosis and care of patients with chronic obstructive pulmonary disease (COPD) and asthma. [This official statement of the American Thoracic Society was adopted by the ATS Board of Directors], November 1986, *Am Rev Respir Dis* 136:225-244, 1987.
11. Kuller LH, Ockene JK, Townsend M, et al: The epidemiology and pulmonary function and COPD mortality in the multiple risk factor intervention trial. *Am Rev Respir Dis* 140:S76-S81, 1989.
12. Anthonisen NR: Prognosis in chronic obstructive pulmonary disease: results from multicenter clinical trials, *Am Rev Respir Dis* 140:S95-S99, 1989.
13. Thom TJ: International comparisons in COPD mortality, *Am Rev Respir Dis* 140:S27-S34, 1989.
14. Manfreda J, Mao Y, and Litven W: Morbidity and mortality from chronic obstructive pulmonary disease, *Am Rev Respir Dis* 140:S19-S26, 1989.
15. *Smoking and health: a report of the Advisory Committee to the Sur-*

geon General of the Public Health Service, Washington, DC, 1964, US Department of Health, Education, and Welfare.

16. *The health consequences of smoking. Chronic obstructive lung disease: a report of the Surgeon General,* Washington, DC, 1984, US Department of Health, Education, and Welfare.

17. Pierce JP, Fiore MC, Novotny TE, et al: Trends in cigarette smoking in the United States: projections to the year 2000, *JAMA* 261:61-65, 1989.

18. Pierce JP, Fiore MC, Novotny TE, et al: Trends in cigarette smoking in the United States: education differences are increasing, *JAMA* 261:56-60, 1989.

19. Davis RM and Novotny TE: Changes in risk factors: the epidemiology of cigarette smoking and its impact on chronic obstructive pulmonary disease, *Am Rev Respir Dis* 140:S82-S84, 1989.

20. Kaufman DW, Palmer RJ, Rosenberg L, et al: Tar content of cigarettes in relation to lung cancer, *Am J Epidemiol* 129:703-711, 1989.

21. Benowitz NL: Pharmacologic aspects of cigarette smoking and nicotine addiction, *N Engl J Med* 319:1318-1330, 1988.

22. Benowitz NL: Health and public policy implications of the "low yield" cigarette, *N Engl J Med* 320:1619-1621, 1989.

23. Fielding JE and Phenow MS: Health effects of involuntary smoking, *N Engl J Med* 319:1452-1460, 1988.

24. Friedman GD, Petitti DB, and Bawol RD: Prevalence and correlates of passive smoking, *Am J Public Health* 73:401-405, 1983.

25. Weiss ST: Passive smoking and lung cancer: what is the risk?, *Am Rev Respir Dis* 133:1-3, 1986.

26. *The health consequences of involuntary smoking: a report of the Surgeon General,* Washington, DC, 1986, Department of Health and Human Services.

27. Crofton J and Masironi R: Chronic airways disease: the smoking component, *Chest* 96:S349-S355, 1989.

28. Crofton J and Bjartveit K: Smoking as a risk factor for chronic airways disease, *Chest* 96:S307-S312, 1989.

29. Kauffman F, Tessier JF, and Oriol P: Adult passive smoking in the home environment: a risk factor for chronic airflow limitation, *Am J Epidemiol* 117:269-280, 1983.

30. Colley JRT and Miller DL: Acute respiratory infections, *Chest* 96:S355-S360, 1989.

31. Higgins M: Chronic airways disease in the United States; trends and determinants, *Chest* 96:S328-S334, 1989.

32. Waller RE: Atmospheric pollution, *Chest* 96:S363-S368, 1989.

33. Sunyer J, Saez M, Murillo C, et al: Air pollution and emergency room admissions for chronic obstructive pulmonary disease: a 5 year study, *Am J Epidemiol* 137:701-705, 1993.

34. Buist AS: Smoking and other risk factors. In Murray JF and Nadel JA, editors: *Textbook of respiratory medicine,* vol 1, pp 1011-1012, Philadelphia, 1988, WB Saunders.

35. Spengler JD and Sexton K: Indoor air pollution: a public health perspective, *Science* 221:9-17, 1983.

36. Boleij JS and Brunekreef B: Domestic pollution as a factor causing respiratory health effects, *Chest* 96:S368-S372, 1989.

37. Koning H: *Biomass fuel combustion and health,* WHO Int Doc EFP/84.64, Geneva, 1984, World Health Organization.

38. Chretien J: Pollution (atmospheric, domestic, and occupational) as a risk factor for chronic airways disease, *Chest* 96:S316-S317, 1989.

39. *Cancer and chronic lung disease in the workplace: a report of the Surgeon General,* Rockville, MD, 1985, US Department of Health and Human Services.

40. Laurell CB and Eriksson S: The electrophoretic alpha-1-globulin pattern of serum in alpha-1-antitrypsin deficiency, *Scand J Clin Lab Invest* 1:132-140, 1963.

41. Wewers MD and Gadel JE: The protease theory of emphysema, *Ann Intern Med* 107:761-763, 1987.

42. Snider GL, Lucey EC, and Stone PJ: State of the art: animal models of emphysema, *Am Rev Respir Dis* 133:149-169, 1986.

43. Janoff A and Carp H: Possible mechanisms of emphysema in smokers: cigarette smoke condensate suppresses proteinase inhibition *in vitro, Am Rev Respir Dis* 116:65-72, 1977.

44. Larsson C: Natural history and life expectancy in severe alpha-1 antitrypsin deficiency, *Acta Med Scand* 204:345-351, 1978.

45. McDonough DJ, Nathan SP, Knudson RJ, et al: Assessment of alpha-1 antitrypsin deficiency: heterozygosity as a risk factor in the etiology of emphysema, *J Clin Invest* 63:299-309, 1979.

46. Buist AS, Sexton GJ, Azzam AMH, et al: Pulmonary function in heterozygotes for alpha-1-antitrypsin deficiency: a case control study, *Am Rev Respir Dis* 120:759-766, 1979.

47. Tager IB, Segal MR, Speizer FE, et al: The natural history of forced expiratory volumes: effect of cigarette smoking and respiratory symptoms, *Am Rev Respir Dis* 138:837-849, 1988.

48. Gori GB and Lynch CJ: Towards less hazardous cigarettes: current advances, *JAMA* 240:1255-1259, 1978.

49. Fletcher C and Peto R: The natural history of chronic airflow obstruction, *Br Med J* 1:1645-1648, 1977.

50. Orie NG and Sluiter HG, editors: *Bronchitis, an international symposium,* Assen, the Netherlands, 1961, Charles C Thomas/Royal Vangorcum.

51. Tashkin DP, Altose MD, Bleeker ER, et al: The Lung Health Study: airway responsiveness to inhaled methacholine in smokers with mild to moderate airflow limitation, *Am Rev Respir Dis* 145:301-310, 1992.

52. Kanner RE: The relationship between airways responsiveness and chronic airflow limitation, *Chest* 86:54-57, 1984.

53. Frew AJ, Kennedy SM, and Chan-Yeung M: Methacholine responsiveness, smoking, and atopy as risk factors for accelerated FEV1 decline in male working populations, *Am Rev Respir Dis* 146:878-883, 1992.

54. Thurlbeck WM, Henderson JA, Fraser RG, et al: Chronic obstructive lung disease: a comparison between clinical, roentgenologic, functional and morphological criteria in chronic bronchitis, emphysema, asthma, and bronchiectasis, *Medicine* 49:81-145, 1970.

55. Schapira RM, Schapira MM, Funahashi A, et al: The value of the forced expiratory time in the physical diagnosis of obstructive airways disease, *JAMA* 270:731-736, 1993.

56. Badgett RG, Tanaka DJ, Hunt DK, et al: Can moderate chronic obstructive pulmonary disease be diagnosed by historical and physical findings alone?, *Am J Med* 94:188-196, 1993.

57. Chodosh S: Treatment of acute exacerbations of chronic bronchitis: state of the art, *Am J Med* 91(suppl 6A):87-92, 1991.

58. Brand PL, Kerstjens HA, Jansen HM, et al: Interpretation of skin tests to house dust mite and relationship to other allergy parameters in patients with asthma and chronic obstructive pulmonary disease. The Dutch CNSLD Study Group, *J Allergy Clin Immunol* 91:560-570, 1993.

59. Sanders C: The radiographic diagnosis of emphysema, *Radiol Clin North Am* 29:1019-1030, 1991.

60. Klein JS, Gamsu G, Webb WR, et al: High-resolution CT diagnosis of emphysema in symptomatic patients with normal chest radiographs and isolated low diffusion capacity, *Radiology* 182:817-821, 1992.

61. Gelb AF, Schein M, Kuei J, et al: Limited contribution of emphysema in advanced chronic obstructive pulmonary disease, *Am Rev Respir Dis* 147:1157-1161, 1993.

62. Bass H: Pulmonary function studies: aid to diagnosis for dyspnea, *Prog Cardiovasc Dis* 14:621-631, 1972.

63. Kesten S and Chapman KR: Physician perceptions and management of COPD, *Chest* 104:254-258, 1993.

64. Epstein SK and Celli BR: Cardiopulmonary exercise testing in patients with chronic obstructive pulmonary disease, *Cleveland Clin J Med* 60:119-128, 1993.

65. Himelman RB, Stulbarg MS, Kircher B, et al: Non-invasive evaluation of pulmonary pressure with exercise by Doppler echocar-

diography in chronic pulmonary disease, *Circulation* 79:863-871, 1989.

66. Burghuber OC, Brunner CH, Schenk P, et al: Pulsed Doppler echocardiography to assess pulmonary artery hypertension in chronic obstructive pulmonary disease, *Monaldi Arch Chest Dis* 48:121-125, 1993.

67. Oliver RM, Fleming JS, and Waller DG: Right ventricular function at rest and during exercise in chronic obstructive pulmonary disease. Comparison of two radionuclide techniques, *Chest* 103:74-80, 1993.

68. Ferguson GT and Cherniack RM: Management of chronic obstructive pulmonary disease, *N Engl J Med* 328:1017-1022, 1993.

69. *The benefits of smoking cessation: a report of the Surgeon General,* Rockville, MD, 1990, Department of Health and Human Services.

70. Samet JM: Health benefits of smoking cessation, *Clin Chest Med* 12:669-679, 1991.

71. Buist AS, Sexton GJ, Nagy JM, et al: The effect of smoking cessation and modification on lung function, *Am Rev Respir Dis* 114:115-120, 1976.

72. Cummings SR, Rubin SM, and Oster G: The cost-effectiveness of counseling smokers to quit, *JAMA* 261:75-79, 1989.

73. Tonnesen P, Fryd V, Hansen M, et al: Effect of nicotine chewing gum in combination with group counseling on the cessation of smoking, *N Engl J Med* 318:15-18, 1988.

74. Tonnesen P, Norregaard J, Simonsen K, et al: A double-blind trial of a 16-hour transdermal nicotine patch in smoking cessation, *N Engl J Med* 325:311-315, 1991.

75. Centers for Disease Control: Prevention and control of influenza (parts I and II), *Morbid Mortal Weekly Rep* 37:361-364 and 369-373, 1988.

76. Marine WN: Influenza prevention: the key to reduction in morbidity and mortality from acute respiratory disease (ARD), *Am Rev Respir Dis* 136:546-547, 1987.

77. Simberkoff MS, Cross AP, Al-Imbrahim M, et al: Efficacy of pneumococcal vaccine in high risk patients. Results of a Veterans Administration cooperative study, *New Engl J Med* 315:1318-1327, 1986.

78. Centers for Disease Control: Pneumococcal polysaccharide vaccine, *Morbid Mortal Weekly Report* 38:64-68 and 73-76, 1989.

79. Petty TL: The National Mucolytic Study. Results of a randomized, double-blind, placebo-controlled study of iodinated glycerol in chronic obstructive bronchitis [see comments], *Chest* 97:75-83, 1990.

80. Nicotra M, Rivera M, and Awe R: Antibiotic therapy of acute exacerbations of chronic bronchitis. A controlled study using tetracycline, *Ann Intern Med* 97:18-21, 1982.

81. Pines A, Rafat H, Plucinski K, et al: Antibiotic regimens in severe and acute purulent exacerbations of chronic bronchitis, *Br Med J* 2:735-738, 1968.

82. Anthonisen N, Manfreda J, Warren C, et al: Antibiotic therapy in exacerbations of chronic obstructive pulmonary disease, *Ann Intern Med* 106:196-204, 1987.

83. Davies B, Maesen F, and Baur C: Ciprofloxacin in the treatment of acute exacerbations of chronic bronchitis, *Eur J Clin Microbiol* 5:226-231, 1986.

84. Davies B, Maesen F, and Teengs J: Cefuroxime axetil in acute purulent exacerbations of chronic bronchitis, *Infection* 15:253-256, 1987.

85. Gimeno F, Postma DS, and van Altena R: Plethysmographic parameters in the assessment of reversibility of airways obstruction in patients with clinical emphysema, *Chest* 104:467-470, 1993.

86. Jenkins SC and Moxham J: High dose salbutamol in chronic bronchitis: comparison of 400 micrograms, 1 mg, 1.6 mg, 2 mg and placebo delivered by Rotahaler, *Br J Dis Chest* 81:242-247, 1987.

87. Vathenen AS, Britton JR, Ebden P, et al: High-dose inhaled albuterol in severe chronic airflow limitation, *Am Rev Respir Dis* 138:850-855, 1988.

88. Chapman KR: Anticholinergic bronchodilators for adult obstructive airways disease, *Am J Med* 91:13S-16S, 1991.

89. Braun SR, McKenzie WN, Copeland C, et al: A comparison of the effect of ipratropium and albuterol in the treatment of chronic obstructive airway disease, *Arch Intern Med* 149:544-547, 1989. (Published erratum appears in *Arch Intern Med* 150:1242, 1990.)

90. Tashkin DP, Ashutosh K, Bleecker ER, et al: Comparison of the anticholinergic bronchodilator ipratropium bromide with metaproterenol in chronic obstructive pulmonary disease. A 90-day multi-center study, *Am J Med* 81:81-90, 1986.

91. Gross NJ, Petty TL, Friedman M, et al: Dose response to ipratropium as a nebulized solution in patients with chronic obstructive pulmonary disease. A three-center study [see comments], *Am Rev Respir Dis* 139:1188-1191, 1989.

92. Teramoto S, Fukuchi Y, and Orimo H: Effects of inhaled anticholinergic drug on dyspnea and gas exchange during exercise in patients with chronic obstructive pulmonary disease, *Chest* 103:1774-1782, 1993.

93. Imhof E, Elsasser S, Karrer W, et al: Comparison of bronchodilator effects of fenoterol/ipratropium bromide and salbutamol in patients with chronic obstructive lung disease, *Respiration* 60:84-88, 1993.

94. Chan C, Brown I, Kelly C, et al: Bronchodilator responses to nebulised ipratropium and salbutamol singly and in combination in chronic bronchitis, *Br J Clin Pharmacol* 17:103-105, 1984.

95. IPPB Trial Group: Intermittent positive pressure breathing therapy of chronic obstructive pulmonary disease, *Ann Intern Med* 99:612-620, 1983.

96. Mestitz H, Copland JM, and McDonald CF: Comparison of outpatient nebulized vs metered dose inhaler terbutaline in chronic airflow obstruction [see comments], *Chest* 96:1237-1240, 1989.

97. Interiano B and Guntupalli KK: Metered-dose inhalers. Do health care providers know what to teach?, *Arch Intern Med* 153:81-85, 1993.

98. Aerosol consensus statement, *Chest* 100:1106-1109, 1991.

99. Newman SP, Weisz AW, Talaee N, et al: Improvement of drug delivery with a breath actuated pressurised aerosol for patients with poor inhaler technique, *Thorax* 46:712-716, 1991.

100. Newman SP, Woodman G, Clarke SW, et al: Effect of InspirEase on the deposition of metered-dose aerosols in the human respiratory tract, *Chest* 89:551-556, 1986.

101. Vaz FC and Miller MA: Review of the clinical efficacy of theophylline in the treatment of chronic obstructive pulmonary disease, *Am Rev Respir Dis* 147:S40-S47, 1993.

102. Mahler DA, Matthay RA, Snyder PE, et al: Sustained-release theophylline reduces dyspnea in nonreversible obstructive airway disease, *Am Rev Respir Dis* 131:22-25, 1985.

103. Murciano D, Auclair MH, Pariente R, et al: A randomized, controlled trial of theophylline in patients with severe chronic obstructive pulmonary disease, *N Engl J Med* 320:1521-1525, 1989.

104. Jubran A, Gross N, Ramsdell J, et al: Comparative cost-effectiveness analysis of theophylline and ipratropium bromide in chronic obstructive pulmonary disease. A three-center study, *Chest* 103:678-684, 1993.

105. Eliasson O, Hoffman J, Trueb D, et al: Corticosteroids in COPD: a clinical trial and reassessment of the literature, *Chest* 89:484-490, 1986.

106. Albert RK, Martin TR, and Lewis SW: Controlled trial of methylprednisolone in patients with chronic bronchitis and acute respiratory insufficiency, *Ann Intern Med* 92:753, 1980.

107. Mendella LA, Manfreda J, Warren CPW, et al: Steroid response in stable obstructive pulmonary disease, *Ann Intern Med* 96:17-21, 1982.

108. Koyama H, Nishimura K, Mio T, et al: Response to oral corticosteroid in patients with chronic obstructive pulmonary disease, *Intern Med* 31:1179-1184, 1992.

109. Wiest PM, Flanigan T, Salata RA, et al: Serious infectious complications of corticosteroid therapy for chronic obstructive pulmonary disease, *Chest* 95:1180-1184, 1989.

110. Strom K: Survival of patients with chronic obstructive pulmonary disease receiving long-term domiciliary oxygen therapy, *Am Rev Respir Dis* 147:585-591, 1993.

111. Dompeling E, van Schayck CP, van Grunsven PM, et al: Slowing the deterioration of asthma and chronic obstructive pulmonary disease observed during bronchodilator therapy by adding inhaled corticosteroids. A 4-year prospective study, *Ann Intern Med* 118:770-778, 1993.

112. Torres A, Serra BJ, Ferrer A, et al: Severe community-acquired pneumonia. Epidemiology and prognostic factors, *Am Rev Respir Dis* 144:312-318, 1991.

113. Nocturnal Oxygen Therapy Trial Group: Continuous or nocturnal oxygen therapy in hypoxemic chronic obstructive lung disease: a clinical trial, *Ann Intern Med* 93:391-398, 1980.

114. Long term domiciliary oxygen therapy in chronic hypoxic cor pulmonale complicating chronic bronchitis and emphysema. Report of the Medical Research Council Working Party, *Lancet* 1:681-686, 1981.

115. Tiep BL: Long-term home oxygen therapy, *Clin Chest Med* 11:505-521, 1990.

116. Christopher KL, Spofford BT, Petrun MD, et al: A program for transtracheal oxygen delivery. Assessment of safety and efficacy, *Ann Intern Med* 107:802-808, 1987.

117. Mak VH, Bugler JR, Roberts CM, et al: Effect of arterial oxygen desaturation on six minute walk distance, perceived effort, and perceived breathlessness in patients with airflow limitation, *Thorax* 48:33-38, 1993.

118. Dillard TA, Rosenberg AP, and Berg BW: Hypoxemia during altitude exposure. A meta-analysis of chronic obstructive pulmonary disease, *Chest* 103:422-425, 1993.

119. Al Damluji S: The effect of ventilatory stimulation with medroxyprogesterone on exercise performance and the sensation of dyspnoea in hypercapnic chronic bronchitis, *Br J Dis Chest* 80:273-279, 1986.

120. Voisin C, Howard P, and Ansquer JC. Almitrine bismesylate: a long-term placebo-controlled double-blind study in COAD—Vectarion International Multicentre Study Group, *Bull Eur Physiopathol Respir* 23:169s-182s, 1987.

121. Watanabe S, Kanner RE, Cutillo AG, et al: Long-term effect of almitrine bismesylate in patients with hypoxemic chronic obstructive pulmonary disease, *Am Rev Respir Dis* 140:1269-1273, 1989.

122. Evans TW, Tweney J, Waterhouse JC, et al: Almitrine bismesylate and oxygen therapy in hypoxic cor pulmonale, *Thorax* 45:16-21, 1990.

123. Machraoui A, von Dryander S, Hinrichsen M, et al: Two-dimensional echocardiographic assessment of right cardiac pressure overload in patients with chronic obstructive airway disease, *Respiration* 60:65-73, 1993.

124. Sajkov D, McEvoy RD, Cowie RJ, et al: Felodipine improves pulmonary hemodynamics in chronic obstructive pulmonary disease, *Chest* 103:1354-1361, 1993.

125. Kalra L and Bone MF: Effect of nifedipine on physiologic shunting and oxygenation in chronic obstructive pulmonary disease, *Am J Med* 94:419-423, 1993.

126. Carter R, Nicotra B, Blevins W, et al: Altered exercise gas exchange and cardiac function in patients with mild chronic obstructive pulmonary disease, *Chest* 103:745-750, 1993.

127. Cox NJ, Hendricks JC, Binkhorst RA, et al: A pulmonary rehabilitation program for patients with asthma and mild chronic obstructive pulmonary diseases (COPD), *Lung* 171:235-244, 1993.

128. Gimenez M: Exercise training in patients with chronic airways obstruction, *Eur Respir J* (suppl) 2:611s-617s, 1989.

129. Harver A, Mahler DA, and Daubenspeck JA: Targeted inspiratory muscle training improves respiratory muscle function and reduces dyspnea in patients with chronic obstructive pulmonary disease, *Ann Intern Med* 111:117-124, 1989.

130. Levine S, Weiser P, and Gillen J: Evaluation of a ventilatory muscle endurance training program in the rehabilitation of patients with chronic obstructive pulmonary disease, *Am Rev Respir Dis* 133:400-406, 1986.

131. Gift AG, Moore T, and Soeken K: Relaxation to reduce dyspnea and anxiety in COPD patients, *Nurs Res* 41:242-246, 1992.

132. Carrieri-Kohlman V, Douglas M, Gormley J, et al: Exercise may result in greater decreases in anxiety and distress associated with dyspnea than in dyspnea intensity or perceived work of breathing, *Am Rev Respir Dis* 145:A765, 1992.

133. Ojanen M, Lahdensuo A, Laitinen J, et al: Psychosocial changes in patients participating in a chronic obstructive pulmonary disease rehabilitation program, *Respiration* 60:96-102, 1993.

134. Celli B, Lee H, Criner G, et al: Controlled trial of external negative pressure ventilation in patients with severe chronic airflow obstruction, *Am Rev Respir Dis* 140:1251-1256, 1989.

135. Hoch D, Murray D, Blalock J, et al: Nutritional status as an index of morbidity in chronic airflow limitation, *Chest* 85(Suppl):66-67, 1984.

136. Wilson DO, Rogers RM, Pennock BE, et al: Nutritional intervention in malnourished emphysema patients, *Am Rev Respir Dis* 131(part 2):61, 1985.

137. Browning RJ and Olsen AM: The functional gastrointestinal disorders of pulmonary emphysema, *Mayo Clin Proc* 36:537-543, 1961.

138. Weber JM and Gregg L: The coincidence of benign gastric ulcer and chronic pulmonary disease, *Ann Intern Med* 42:1026-1030, 1955.

139. Hofford JM, Milakofsky L, Vogel WH, et al: The nutritional status in advanced emphysema associated with chronic bronchitis: a study of amino acids and catecholamine levels, *Am Rev Respir Dis* 141:902-908, 1990.

140. Openbrier D, Irwin M, Rogers RM, et al: Nutritional status and lung function in patients with emphysema and chronic bronchitis, *Chest* 83:17-22, 1983.

141. Hunter AMB, Carey MA, and Larsh HW: The nutritional status of patients with chronic obstructive pulmonary disease, *Am Rev Respir Dis* 124:376-378, 1981.

142. Lewis MI, Belman MJ, and Dorr-Uyemura L: Nutritional supplementation in ambulatory patients with chronic obstructive pulmonary disease, *Am Rev Respir Dis* 135:1062-1068, 1987.

143. Egan TM, Westerman JH, Lambert CJ, et al: Isolated lung transplantation for end-stage lung disease: a viable therapy, *Ann Thorac Surg* 53:590-595, 1992.

Chapter 17

INHALATION FEVER

Anna Rask-Andersen

Inhalation fever is an acute, febrile, noninfectious, flulike, short-term reaction that can be produced by inhalation of a number of unrelated agents. The symptoms are influenza-like and dominated by fever and chills. It is often associated with myalgias, cough, headache, and chest discomfort. The condition is of a benign nature and is self-limiting, and no sequelae have been reported. A polymorphonuclear leukocytosis is common, as is tolerance to the causative agent after repeated exposure. No treatment is required if the exposure is terminated. The condition is quite common.

Causative agents of inhalation fever may be classified into three groups: metals, combustion products of polymers and highly reactive chemicals used in polymer production, and bioaerosols such as organic dusts and humidifier mist. There are striking similarities between the febrile conditions described after these exposures despite their different nature; therefore the term *inhalation fever* has been proposed as an embracing term for all febrile reactions to inhalation of noxious substances.

The purpose of this chapter is to give an overview of the inhalation fevers caused by different exposures.

HISTORICAL NOTES

The hazardous effects of inhalation of organic dust was reported as early as 1555 in Olaus Magnus' masterpiece *Historia de Gentibus Septentrionalibus,* a history of the Northern peoples.[1] In the chapter entitled "Threshing during the Winter Time" Magnus described how the dust may damage the vital organs of the threshers. Bernardino Ramazzini reported symptoms from the respiratory tract in flax and hemp carders, as well as in sifters and measurers of grain, although the symptom *fever* was not specifically mentioned.[2] This reference is often cited incorrectly in terms of date, since the second edition of 1713 was translated to English in 1940.[3] In the second edition Ramazzini had added twelve chapters, but the chapters on organic dust problems were already included in the first edition of *De Morbis Artificum* published in 1700.

Ramazzini also described diseases after exposure to metals such as lead and mercury poisoning, but he did not mention any condition resembling metal fume fever. Usually, the first report of metal fume fever (called brass-founders' ague) among brass founders exposed to zinc oxide is attributed to Thackrah in 1832.[4] Some authors cite Patissier (often misspelled as *Potissier*) in 1822 as providing the earliest description of metal fume fever, but the symptoms he reported were colic and pain after zinc oxide inhalation.[5] The first extensive modern review in the English language on metal fume fever was by Drinker in 1922.[6]

Febrile illnesses are also well known after exposure to dust in the textile industry, in which natural fibers are used. The so-called mill fever, Monday morning fever, or gin fever follows the exposure to dusty cotton in cotton mill workers, while engaged in the initial stages of cotton processing. Identical illnesses occur in workers inhaling jute, soft hemp, kapok, and flax dust.[7] The latter is called heckling fever. In 1942 Neal et al. reported on an acute illness among rural mattress makers using low-grade stained cotton.[8] They showed that the condition was caused by inhalation of gram-negative, rod-shaped bacteria.

Another account of a febrile syndrome after exposure to organic dust was published in 1959 by Plessner, who described *la fièvre de canard* (duck fever).[9] Workers were affected by fever after cleaning feathers to produce down. However, this report in French did not achieve much attention in the English-speaking world. Exposure to bird proteins in bird droppings may also cause inhalation fever. In 1959 humidifier fever was also reported for the first time.[10] Over the years a number of other exposures to bioaerosols have also been reported to cause febrile syndromes, such as exposure to mold dust in farming and sawmills, grain dust in grain elevators, and endotoxin in sewage handling, garbage plants, and swine confinement buildings.[11]

In 1951 it was reported that inhalation of fumes from Teflon (a thermoplastic) heated at high temperatures produced symptoms closely resembling those of metal fume fever.[12] Subsequently, febrile syndromes have also been reported after exposure to isocyanates and trimellitic anhydrides.[13,14]

TERMINOLOGY

The terminology of this field has been very confusing. Earlier, the names mentioned above, as well as a variety of other names, such as spelter shakes, brass-founders' ague, metal fume fever, polymer fever, and organic dust toxic syndrome, were used to describe inhalation fever—colorful names that give a hint of the exposure and environment causing these illnesses.

The terminology of the febrile conditions that inhalation of different organic dusts may cause has been especially confusing. The respiratory problems of farmers and especially farmer's lung (the hypersensitivity pneumonitis of farmers) achieved a growing interest during the second half of the 1970s. Several research groups realized that there were cases of illnesses caused by inhalation of mold dust that did not fit into the general pattern of hypersensitivity pneumonitis. This condition was called precipitin-negative farmer's lung, pulmonary mycotoxicosis, or silo-unloader's syndrome.[15-17] Following a symposium held in 1985 to attempt to decrease the confusion, it was proposed to call the febrile attacks caused by inhalation of organic dust the *organic dust toxic syndrome.*[18] Unfortunately, some researchers started to use the name, *toxic organic dust syndrome,* proposed during the meeting. The term *organic dust toxic syndrome* has been criticized as being "clumsy and ugly."[19] Ugly or not, it was definitely a step forward to have a name for these febrile illnesses, although the term can be a little hard to remember. Another disadvantage is that it is not logical to use the term for humidifier fever, since this is caused by mist, not by dust.

There is a striking resemblance between the febrile syndromes caused by inhalation of different agents. Independently of the exposure, the symptoms and signs, as well as the course and duration of the illnesses, are almost identical. Even bronchoalveolar lavage (BAL) findings are similar in febrile reactions caused by different exposures. Therefore *inhalation fever* has been proposed as a unifying term for febrile reactions to the inhalation of noxious substances. The term *inhalation fever* was originally used in a 1978 editorial in *The Lancet* as a heading to describe the febrile and constitutional symptoms of metal fume fever, byssinosis, and humidifier fever, but no one paid further attention to the term until it was recently revived.[20,21] *Inhalation fever* should perhaps become the preferred term, with *organic dust toxic syndrome* being omitted in favor of it. If one wants to be more specific about the exposure causing a specific type of inhalation fever, combinations such as *organic dust inhalation fever* could be used. *Metal fume fever, polymer fume fever,* and *humidifier fever* are so established that there is probably no need to add the word *inhalation* to these names.

The term *inhalation fever* has the advantage of being easy to understand even by people who are not experts in the field. If exposed workers see a physician during the acute stage of their illness, they often see a general practitioner and not a specialist in pulmonary or occupational medicine. It is important to differentiate inhalation fever from other conditions that require specific treatment. It is also of importance not to give unnecessary treatment to patients with inhalation fever. Thus the terminology must be simple and allow no room for mistakes.

There is a risk of unnecessary treatment with oral corticosteroids in cases of inhalation fever. For example, a 48-year-old farmer had a febrile attack after working with moldy hay. He had had the condition several times before. This time he was treated in an emergency room with high doses of cortisone. The therapy went on for months until it was discovered that he had developed an abscess with 1.5 L of pus in his thigh with osteitis that required surgery and a deep venous thrombosis. These complications are especially depressing because they developed unnecessarily, since the patient received the cortisone treatment for a benign condition that would have resolved spontaneously without treatment in, at most, 3 days.

Inhalation fever after inhalation of bioaerosols has probably frequently been misdiagnosed as hypersensitivity pneumonitis both in single cases and in epidemiologic studies. This could explain some of the high prevalences of farmer's lung reported in the 1970s that other groups have not been able to confirm.[22-24]

There have been critical voices against the term *inhalation fever.*[25] Some workers do not have fever after exposure to fumes or dust; they report only some frozenness and tiredness after these exposures. However, fever is an important symptom that clearly demonstrates that the worker has reacted to the exposure. There are milder reactions without fever after dust exposure though. Workers react, for example, with changes in the amounts of inflammatory cells in the BAL, but this is a different condition than the febrile syndromes. In a study of experimental welding operations in volunteers, fever and myalgia occurred only with the heaviest exposure, but even "subclinical" welding fume exposure was associated with a significant inflammatory cellular response in the lungs.[26] In a study of volunteers weighing pigs, an inflammatory response was also shown in all exposed individuals, although only some developed a febrile reaction.[27] However, fever and chills are the key symptoms in *inhalation fever*. Incidentally, the condition has been recognized by workers for years and it has actually already been called *fever* by the affected workers (e.g., mill fever or grain fever).[11] Today many researchers agree that inhalation fever is a distinct clinical entity.

Most cases of disease after mold dust exposure in farmers are possible to classify as either hypersensitivity pneumonitis or inhalation fever.[24,28-30] In our studies there were only a few cases that did not fit into these categories. Recently, Cormier et al. reported such a case with recurrent bouts of acute febrile episodes over at least eight winters of work in a dairy barn with no massive exposure to organic dust.[31] They suggested the name farmer's fever for such cases. There is a risk of adding more to the confusion by introducing a term for the transitional condition between *inhalation fever* and *hypersensitivity pneumonitis* that does not seem to be very common.

The disadvantage of the term *inhalation fever* is that it gives no hint of the mechanisms involved in the condition. However, most of these mechanisms are still unknown and are the subject of hypotheses and speculations. The term *toxic alveolitis* relates more about pathogenesis and is suitable since the lungs are the target organs in inhalation fever.[25,32] A major disadvantage of *toxic alveolitis*, however, is that the term could easily be confused with the European term for hypersensitivity pneumonitis, *allergic alveolitis*. An alternative to *toxic alveolitis* is *toxic pneumonitis* (or *toxic pneumonia*), since the disease process is not limited to the alveoli, but this term is already in use as a synonym for toxic pulmonary edema or chemical pneumonitis after very high-exposure inhalation of irritant gases such as nitrogen dioxide, cadmium fumes, and zinc chloride.[33,34]

To conclude, *inhalation fever* is possibly the best term to describe this condition for practical use and is used throughout this review.

EXPOSURE

Inhalation fever has been reported in a variety of environments after exposure and inhalation of a high level of different substances. Causative agents of inhalation fever may be classified into three groups:

1. Metals
2. Combustion products of polymers and highly reactive chemicals used in polymer production
3. Bioaerosols such as organic dusts and humidifier mist

Metals (Table 17-1)

Metal fume fever is caused by inhalation of high concentrations of metal fumes, most frequently, but not exclusively, zinc oxide (Fig. 17-1).[32,35,36] It is often stated that in addition to zinc a number of other metal oxides (e.g., magnesium, copper, cadmium, chromium, antimony, tin, and iron) can and do commonly cause metal fume fever.[35,36] However, in many reports the metallic fume to which workers were exposed contained several metals and it was uncertain which constituent(s) was responsible for the reactions observed. Only zinc, copper, and magnesium have been proven to cause reactions in a highly pure form.[32,37] Workers at occupational risk for metal fume fever are those involved in brazing, bronzing, copper rolling, brass foundering, galvanizing, manganese bronze welding, and welding of zinc or galvanized iron.[32,36]

Zinc oxide, the most frequent cause of metal fume fever, is formed when zinc or one of its alloys is heated to an oxidizing atmosphere near its boiling point of 907°C. This heating results in the formation of zinc oxide particles, which range in size from 0.2 to 1 μm and may subsequently be inhaled.[38] Larger particles are too large to penetrate down to the alveoli and remain there.[6,39] It is often stated in reviews that sources of zinc oxide associated with metal fume fever are almost exclusively in the form of freshly generated fume, that is, fine particulate matter suspended in air.[32] However, there have been several reports of metal

Table 17-1. Metals

Exposure	Name
Metal fume	**Metal fume fever**
Zinc oxide during work such as manufacturing brass or welding	Brass (founders') ague[4]
	Brass chills[38]
	Brass fever
	Brazier's disease[38]
	Foundry ague
	Foundry fever[38]
	Foundry shakes
	Galvanized shakes[112]
	Galvanizer's poisoning[38]
	Galvo[38]
	Metal malaria[112]
	Monday (morning) fever[113]
	Smelter's chills[114]
	Spelter shakes[41]
	The smothers[115]
	Welder's ague[116]
	Zinc ague[41]
	Zinc chills[38]
	Zinc (fume) fever[112,113]
Copper dust	Copper fever[40]
Magnesium	No specific name

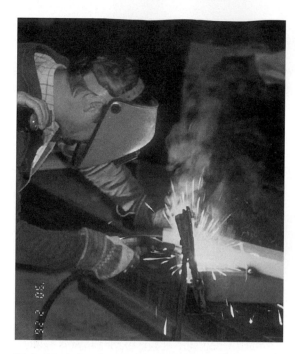

Fig. 17-1. Inhalation of zinc oxide in welding fumes generated during the welding of zinc-containing materials (e.g., stainless steel or galvanized iron) is the most common cause of metal fume fever.

fume fever after exposure to "mature" zinc oxide dust manufactured from a smeltering process but handled hours or days after production.[32] Cases of metal fume fever also occur after exposure to copper dust.[40,41]

In nonoccupational settings exposure to zinc chloride (ZnCl) aerosol from screening smoke bombs used in military survival and disaster training drills may cause symptoms initially resembling those of metal fume fever.[42] With heavy exposure to ZnCl, severe pulmonary damage and even risk of death may occur.[43] This is a response distinct from inhalation fever. Unfortunately, since it is misleading, some authors use the term *serious metal fume fever* to describe this condition and *mild metal fume fever* for *metal fume fever* proper.[44]

Combustion products of polymers and highly reactive chemicals used in polymer production (Table 17-2)

Teflon is a well-known plastic material introduced in the beginning of the 1940s. The most widely used Teflon material is polytetrafluoroethylene (PTFE), a polymer of the gas tetrafluoroethylene. The material is chemically inert, even to temperatures up to 300°C. If the material is heated above this temperature, a fume with Teflon pyrolysis products is produced. If this fume is inhaled, it may induce polymer fume fever.[12] The degradation products of Teflon vary in quantity and type according to the temperature. Above temperatures of 560°C, the nature of the fumes changes to include more toxic products that have been known to produce delayed pulmonary edema.[45]

Table 17-2. Combustion products of polymers and highly reactive chemicals used in polymer production

Exposure	Name
Polymer fume [fume from heated Teflon or polytetrafluoroethylene (PTFE)]	Polymer fume fever[12]
Isocyanate fume	Hypersensitivity pneumonitis-like reaction[81]
Trimellitic anhydride dust or fumes	Late respiratory systemic syndrome[13]

In the original report of two cases of polymer fume fever, PTFE had been heated in ovens in research laboratories.[12] In an in-flight toxic hazard incident in an aircraft, polymer fume fever was reported in half of the 35 passengers. Pyrolysis products from Teflon-impregnated asbestos tape wrappings on the exhaust manifold of the power unit were the cause of the syndrome.[46] Polymer fume fever has also been reported from a variety of other circumstances, such as extruding machines, high-speed machining of components, welding of metal coated with PTFE or attached to PTFE resin blocks, ironing clothes sprayed with a polymer–starch mixture for prolonged periods, and smoking cigarettes contaminated with the polymer either by direct contact or by particles suspended in the workplace atmosphere (Fig. 17-2).[12,47-51]

There have also been reports of inhalation fever and hypersensitivity pneumonitis after exposure to isocyanates, for example, after the inhalation of fumes emitted during pyrolysis of polyurethane driving belts welded by a special process.[14,52] These reactions have been reported after exposure to toluene diisocyanate (TDI), diphenylmethane diisocyanate (MDI), or hexamethylene diisocyanate (HDI).[53] In one report a car spray-painter experienced three episodes of chill, dyspnea, and chest pain followed by general malaise, fever, sweating, headache, and nonrotatory vertigo. He had been exposed to acrylic lacquer containing HDI.[53] In another report a patient engaged in bathtub refinishing showed episodes of recurrent "influenza-like" symptoms of cough, dyspnea, myalgia, malaise, and fever to 40°C.[54] In a case report from Sweden, a carpenter who was spray-painting furniture with a varnish containing isocyanates had repeated attacks of fever, chills, general malaise, headache, and arthralgia some hours after exposure.[55]

Trimellitic anhydride is a low-molecular-weight, highly reactive chemical widely used in the manufacture of plastics, epoxy resin coatings, and paints. Four clinical syndromes have been reported as being induced by the inhalation of trimellitic anhydride dust or fumes.[13] One of these is the *late respiratory systemic syndrome,* characterized by cough, wheezing, dyspnea, mucus production, and systemic symptoms of malaise, chills, myalgias, and arthralgias occurring 4 to 12 hours after exposure.

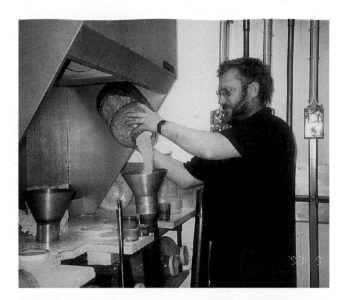

Fig. 17-2. Inhalation of pyrolysis products from the plastic material Teflon [polytetrafluoroethylene (PTFE)] may induce polymer fume fever. This worker is loading Teflon in a tube for a machine making heat-resistant electric cables. Smokers are especially at risk if smoking cigarettes contaminated with the polymer either by direct contact or by particles suspended in the workplace atmosphere.

Bioaerosols such as organic dusts and humidifier mist
(Table 17-3)

An aerosol is a suspension of solid or soluble particles in gas and in a bioaerosol these particles are of a biologic origin. Inhalation fever has been reported in a variety of environments where workers are at risk for exposure to bioaerosols.[10,16,17,29,56 58] There has been no report of specific organisms being more prone to cause inhalation fever than others, as has been reported in hypersensitivity pneumonitis. Probably a number of organisms cause inhalation fever. All the exposures that can cause hypersensitivity pneumonitis can also cause inhalation fever, such as moldy hay, moldy straw, moldy grain, and moldy wood, all known to cause hypersensitivity pneumonitis.

Inhalation fever in farming is frequently associated with one specific job done on a single occasion, such as moving moldy corn, cleaning silos or granaries, or shoveling moldy grain or moldy hay. These jobs are of a limited duration, but the exposure is often extreme. A concentration of up to 10^{10} spores per cubic meter has been observed in worst-case measurements of dust causing inhalation fever.[102] In hypersensitivity pneumonitis, the exposure to mold dust is also high, even if it is less high than in inhalation fever (in the range of 10^9 spores per cubic meter). The exposure is often repeated for weeks during work tasks the farmer performs every day, for example, the distribution of moldy straw as bedding. Moldy grain was the most common cause of inhalation fever in Swedish farmers.

Table 17-3. Bioaerosols such as organic dusts and mists

Exposure	Name
Mist	
Mist from humidifiers contaminated with microorganisms	*Befeuchterfieber* (humidifier fever)[10]
	Monday morning fever[117]
Contaminated tap water	Bath water fever[70]
Steam from water in a sauna bucket	Sauna-taker's disease[71]
Organic dust	**Organic dust toxic syndrome (ODTS)**[18]
Moldy silage	Precipitin test-negative farmer's lung[15]
	Atypical farmer's lung[118]
	Pulmonary mycotoxicosis[16]
	Silo-unloader's syndrome[17]
Stained cotton	Mattress-maker's fever[8]
Work in the cotton textile industry	Cardroom fever[7]
	Factory fever[7]
	Gin fever
	Monday fever[104]
	Mill fever[104]
	Weaver's cough[104]
Flax dust	Heckling fever
Hemp dust	Hemp fever[119]
Jute dust	Mill fever
Grain dust in grain elevators	Grain fever[11]
Working with moldy grain, hay, or straw in farming (e.g., shoveling grain)	No specific name
Sewage sludge	No specific name
Moldy wood chips	No specific name
Work with moldy board in the trimming department of sawmills	Wood-trimmer's disease[57]
Mold dust from composts (e.g., for mushroom cultivation)	No specific name
Moldy oranges	No specific name
Work with moldy books in a museum	No specific name
Work in animal confinement buildings	No specific name
Plucking a duck	*La fièvre de canard* (duck fever)[9]
Probably all other exposures that might cause hypersensitivity pneumonitis	No specific name for the febrile conditions (although there are names for many of the different types of hypersensitivity pneumonitis)

Several authors have reported inhalation fever after work with moldy silage during the opening of "capped" silos (Fig. 17-3).[16,17] Moldy silage has not been associated with hypersensitivity pneumonitis, perhaps because uncapping of silos is a job that is done on a single occasion and not repeated for days or even weeks.

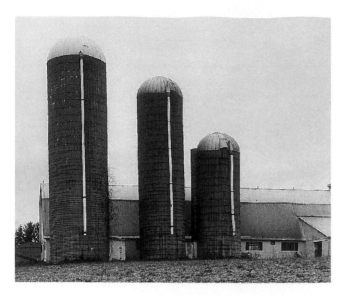

Fig. 17-3. Inhalation fever caused by work with moldy silage during the opening of "capped" silos has been studied by several groups. Dr. John J. May and coworkers, who provided the figure, called the condition *silo-unloader's syndrome* to differentiate it from *silo-filler's disease,* the chemical pneumonitis caused by inhalation of nitrous compounds in silos.[17]

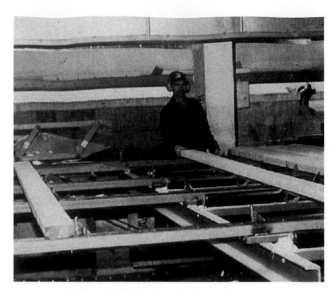

Fig. 17-4. The artificial drying of sawn timber in kilns at sawmills may cause problems because of the favorable conditions inside the kilns for growth of thermotolerant and thermophilic fungi. When the dried contaminated wood is handled in the trimming department, the workers may be exposed to mold dust. Many cases of inhalation fever as well as a few cases of hypersensitivity pneumonitis have been reported in wood trimmers.[62] (Courtesy of Lundström, Department of Wood Biology, Swedish University of Agricultural Sciences, Uppsala.)

In Sweden forest areas often form part of the farm estates. Many farmers use wood chips for heating purposes. If these are stored under damp conditions, there can be substantial mold growth. There have been several reports of both hypersensitivity pneumonitis and inhalation fever caused by moldy wood chips.[29,59] In the United States employees at a municipal golf course became ill with inhalation fever after manually unloading a trailer full of moldy wood chips.[60] There is also a potential risk for exposure to moldy wood chips in the paper pulp industry.[61]

In Scandinavian sawmills there are also problems with mold growing on wood. Earlier, the sawn timber was dried outside in timber yards in Swedish sawmills. To speed up the process, drying in kilns was introduced some decades ago. The temperatures in these kilns are ideal for the growth of thermotolerant and thermophilic fungi, and to prevent mold growth, chemicals were sprayed all over the board. However, the use of chemicals was banned in the 1970s because of cancer risk. When the dried mold-contaminated wood was handled in the trimming department, the workers might have been exposed to mold dust. Both cases of inhalation fever and hypersensitivity pneumonitis have been reported in wood trimmers (Fig. 17-4).[56,62] In North America the timber is also dried in kilns but at a higher temperature. The microorganisms are then killed and there are no problems with mold. If higher temperatures are used when drying Scandinavian timber, it can crackle and become warped.

Grain fever—flulike feverish episodes in the evening after handling grain—is a familiar condition in grain elevator workers and in harbor workers who load and unload grain from ships.[11,63,64] Usually, these grains have not been visibly moldy, although some reports have pointed out the increased probability of grain fever after exposure to moldy grain.[11] From swine confinement buildings there have been reports of flulike complaints after exposure to dust that does not appear to be moldy (Fig. 17-5).[65] In the mill fever appearing in workers in the cardrooms in the cotton industry, there has been no report of mold dust exposure. Increasing evidence from studies of cotton dust exposures suggests that inhaled lipopolysaccharides (endotoxins) arising from gram-negative microorganisms may well play a role in mill fever.[66,67] Febrile attacks in those who work in swine confinement buildings and in sewage workers are also believed to be caused by endotoxin.[57,65] In a Danish waste-sorting plant inhalation fever was suspected in 3 of 15 employees. Measurements showed high levels of bacteria and endotoxin in the air.[58] It has been shown that exposure levels of endotoxin at a level between 1 and 2 $\mu g/m^3$ cause fever.[68] Much lower concentrations of exposure are required to cause bronchoconstriction, dry cough, and upper airway symptoms.

Humidifier mist is another example of an exposure that can cause both inhalation fever and hypersensitivity pneumonitis. The associated illnesses are termed *humidifier fever* and *humidifier lung,* respectively.[69] In humidifier fever, several different microorganisms have been suspected as causative agents, especially thermophilic actino-

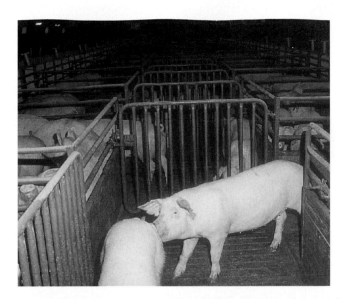

Fig. 17-5. Inhalation fever and a variety of respiratory symptoms have been reported in workers in animal confinement buildings.

mycetes, flavobacteria, aspergilli, and other fungi, as well as algae.[69]

During the late 1970s an outbreak in southern Sweden of repeated symptoms typical of inhalation fever, starting 4 hours after a hot bath, involved 56 persons, nearly all of whom lived in an area supplied with water from the same source.[70] The causal agent, which was never identified, was found to enter the body by inhalation. Similar symptoms have also been reported after a sauna or bath in 100 people living in a small community in Finland.[71] The water source of the community was a small lake and it was found that the water was contaminated with several bacteria, fungi, and algae. Water inhalation provocation tests produced the same kinds of symptoms.

There have been several accounts of inhalation fever symptoms from nonoccupational and unusual exposures. Some examples include (1) several cases of inhalation fever after very dusty work following removal of double flooring during the remodeling of old houses, (2) a baker who cleaned a leavening oven that hadn't been cleaned for 6 months and was full of black moldy flour, (3) mushroom workers changing the compost material on which the mushrooms are cultivated, and (4) a 40-year-old man who was removing paint with a hot-air gun.[72]

EPIDEMIOLOGY

Inhalation fever is probably a common condition involving many different exposures. Only in the last decade has there been interest in the epidemiology of inhalation fever after organic dust exposure. The previous lack of interest is probably because of the limited duration and relatively nonserious nature of inhalation fever and because tolerance to repeated exposure often occurs.[37] However, even though fever tolerance develops, the exposure might still be harm-

ful. Other reactions induced by exposure to fumes and dusts might remain, resulting in a higher than expected frequency of chronic respiratory disorders in populations with these kinds of exposures. Inhalation fever indicates that working conditions are bad. The association of inhalation fever and chronic respiratory diseases must be studied further and persons at risk for developing chronic respiratory disorders should be identified.

There are difficulties in studying inhalation fever since no test is available to detect earlier episodes of this condition. Investigators must rely on questionnaire information, seeking a history of work-related febrile illness, often years in the past. In the Swedish studies of inhalation fever in farmers and wood trimmers, a key question was used: Have you had attacks of fever and chills in relation to your work that do not seem to be caused by common cold or influenza?[24] If the subject answers Yes to this question, he is asked to answer a number of attendant questions on symptoms, exposure, time relation, severity, and duration. This question has a very high sensitivity; the specificity is lower, but can be increased by interviews. Other Scandinavian researchers have had good results with similar key questions. A Scandinavian work group is trying to evaluate and standardize a questionnaire for diagnosing respiratory diseases caused by inhalation of organic dusts. One surprising finding in our studies of farmers was that the incidence of inhalation fever increased over the years and was highest during the last couple of years, probably due to memory lapses, which illustrates that the information sometimes is remote.[29]

It should be pointed out that hypersensitivity pneumonitis cannot be diagnosed on questionnaires alone, since proper diagnosis is based on a combination of clinical, radiologic, and functional findings together with an evaluation of the exposure. Questionnaires are suitable for screening to detect suspected cases. If the patient has met with a physician, medical records should be collected and evaluated. If the patient has not sought medical care, it is impossible to diagnose hypersensitivity pneumonitis retrospectively.

Another difficulty in studying the epidemiology of inhalation fever is that doses and exposure differ greatly because of the complexity of the occupational environments in which this group of conditions occurs.[37] There is also variability in the content of fumes and dusts. It appears that if the exposure is high enough, all individuals are affected by inhalation fever, illustrated by the clustering of cases.[17,46,73]

Inhalation fever after organic dust exposure may affect all age groups, including children, who have been exposed while working with their parents.[74] Since metal and polymer fumes are occupational exposures, there have been no reports of these disorders in children. Grain fever was more common in nonsmokers in a study of 1200 farmers and farmers' wives in Manitoba, Canada.[75] Polymer fume fever is more common in smokers because of the exposure by contaminated cigarettes.[47,49]

Some individuals develop inhalation fever only once, whereas others have recurrent attacks. Of 80 farmers with inhalation fever, 44% had one episode; the remaining had two attacks or more, often several years apart.[29] In the studies of doPico et al., a few grain workers reported over 100 episodes of grain fever during their work life.[76] In our Swedish studies of farmers and wood trimmers, there were also some workers who reported a similar frequency of attacks.[29]

Symptoms of metal fume fever have been noted to be worse in the winter. The reported increased incidence in the winter months could well be explained, for example, by welders seeking to combat low environmental temperatures by closing windows and access to doors, thus depriving the workplace of necessary natural ventilation and reducing mechanical ventilation that draws in the winter chill. Under such circumstances the concentration of freshly formed metallic oxides in the workplace could be expected to rise, and consequently there would be an increased incidence of metal fume fever.

Exposure to zinc oxide is a common exposure in industry, but accurate population-based surveillance data documenting the incidence of metal fume fever do not exist.[32] One estimate suggests that 1500 to 2500 cases of metal fume fever occur annually in the United States.[32] In shipyard welders 20% had chills and fever occasionally, whereas 5% had frequent episodes.[77] In a study of 530 welders, 22% reported a history of metal fume fever.[78] Among welders over the age of 30, almost 40% had experienced metal fume fever. Welding galvanized steel, particularly in an enclosed environment, was the most common cause. In a study of workers exposed to copper dust, all exposed individuals suffered symptoms.[40]

It is not known how commonly febrile reactions occur in isocyanate exposed workers. A hypersensitivity pneumonitis type of reaction has been reported but only in a few isolated cases, except for 9 cases from a wood chipboard factory where metered-dose inhaler (MDI) was used as a binding agent.[79] These 9 workers of 167 had filed a claim with the workers' compensation board. The 9 workers had experienced respiratory symptoms associated with an intense systemic malaise characterized by myalgia, chills, headaches, and nausea appearing 1 to 6 hours after the beginning of a work shift. Eight of these workers participated in a challenge study with MDI and all developed symptoms. The authors believed that 8 of 167 workers (4.8%) is an underestimated rate of response. A thorough medical survey of all the workers employed at the plant could not be conducted because the plant shut down a short time after the 8 subjects were investigated. In this study the systemic symptoms were so severe that affected subjects had to stop working shortly after they started to experience symptoms. It is therefore conceivable that they could have been missed

in cross-sectional surveys. Other authors have also stated that the phenomenon may not be very rare, the reaction is late, and its association with isocyanate exposure is not well known. The cause may thus be easily overlooked.[55]

In the few available studies of trimellitic anhydride, it seems that inhalation feverlike reactions are quite common. In a study of workers involved in the manufacture of trimellitic anhydride, 6 of 61 workers observed over a 4-year period developed late respiratory systemic syndrome.[13]

In an "epidemic" of polymer fume fever, 36 of 61 employees were affected over a 90-day period in a large industrial plant.[47] A new parting compound containing PTFE had been introduced. The majority of cases resulted from the smoking of cigarettes that were contaminated with a fine dust of this material. In a report of polymer fume fever from an aircraft, 39 of 40 personnel on board, including passengers and aircrew, had been affected by symptoms to some degree, although only approximately 50% had the typical fume fever syndrome.[46] Even four persons who collected air samples on two occasions during the following investigation developed typical flulike reactions approximately 3 hours after exposure. Later, six volunteers who were exposed to the fume developed a typical reaction of inhalation fever. In a study of 77 workers in a small PTFE-fabricating plant, 86% had experienced febrile reactions at some time and 18% reported multiple episodes.[80] A prevalence of 47% was observed in workers processing PTFE.[81]

Although cases of hypersensitivity pneumonitis occur almost exclusively during the indoor feeding season for cattle, inhalation fever may affect farmers at any time of the year, depending on work task. However, in a Swedish study of farmers, inhalation fever was most common in the fall, when farmers were cleaning bins for the new crop.[29] Inhalation fever after silo unloading also was most common in the fall in a study from upstate New York.[17]

The clustering effect has been noted by several authors reporting cases of inhalation fever after work in silos with moldy silage.[16,17,29] In contrast, farmer's lung often affects only one person on a farm, even if other individuals are exposed. In the largest outbreak of organic dust toxic syndrome ever reported, 55 of 67 exposed persons (82%) fell ill after a mean latency period of 9.4 hours after a hay party at a college fraternity.[73] For this special event baled straw was spread on the floor in a poorly ventilated basement room. A thick airborne dust was present at the start of the party and as the party progressed, it was no longer possible to see across the room.

Inhalation fever after organic dust exposure is common in farmers. In two Swedish studies 19% and 6%, respectively, of Swedish farmers had experienced febrile attacks.[24,30] It was concluded that approximately every tenth Swedish farmer had experienced inhalation fever (cumulated incidence). Similar figures (13% to 15%) have also been reported from Finland.[82] In Canada flulike symptoms occurred in 15% of the farmers studied.[83] The prevalence of acute febrile episodes in swine growers is 10% to 30%.[65]

On the contrary, in the two Swedish studies, as well as in other Finnish studies, the yearly incidence of hypersensitivity pneumonitis was low, ranging from 0.2 to 0.4 per 1000 in the farming population.[23,24] Surprisingly, in a Scottish study from the 1970s, the prevalence of hypersensitivity pneumonitis was much higher: 2.3% to 8.6%.[22] However, the diagnosis of hypersensitivity pneumonitis was based only on questionnaires in many of the cases in the latter study. It is unknown how many of the cases actually fulfilled more specific diagnostic criteria for hypersensitivity pneumonitis including chest x-ray abnormalities and decreased pulmonary function.[84]

Even for hypersensitivity pneumonitis caused by bird protein, the prevalence varies from one series to another. As early as 1959 duck fever was reported, but otherwise there did not seem to be much distinction between febrile illnesses and hypersensitivity pneumonitis caused by this exposure.[9] Some authors probably have included cases of inhalation fever in their series of pigeon-breeder's disease. For example, in a recent questionnaire study from the Canary Islands, the diagnostic criteria for hypersensitivity pneumonitis were "one or more delayed respiratory symptoms such as cough or breathlessness and at least one systemic symptom such as fever, chills, and arthromyalgias occurring at least at three different occasions, 6 to 8 hours after exposure."[85] These criteria are insufficient to diagnose hypersensitivity pneumonitis without chest x-ray changes and decreased pulmonary function.[84] In the Canary Islands study 8% were reported to have hypersensitivity pneumonitis, but we do not know how many of these cases were actually hypersensitivity pneumonitis and how many were inhalation fever. Probably, if the situation is similar to that in farmers, the majority of these cases were inhalation fever and only a minor fraction was true hypersensitivity pneumonitis.

Actually, the symptoms of inhalation fever are very similar to what was described by Fuller[121] in 1953 as *phase one* or as called by others later *acute farmer's lung*. "The acute attack is characteristically rapid in onset, with rise in temperature on the evening of the day of exposure. The fever lasts for only 2 or 3 days and is accompanied by an irritating cough. A few rhonchi and crepitations may be heard. Frontal headache, lassitude, and marked anorexia are usually present and can persist for several days after the chest symptoms have disappeared. A chest radiograph may show nothing abnormal after a single exposure." This description might be the explanation for the fact that cases of inhalation fever after organic dust exposure have been incorrectly diagnosed as acute hypersensitivity pneumonitis in several studies. Thus a prevalence of hypersensitivity pneumonitis in Scottish farmers of 2% to 8% in reality could have been incidences of inhalation fever after organic dust exposure,

which would be consistent with the Swedish and Finnish findings.[22-24]

When the dried mold-contaminated wood is handled in the trimming department of sawmills, the workers could be exposed to mold dust. In a survey in 1976 to 1978, 10% to 20% of the wood trimmers had experienced wood-trimmer's disease.[56] It is unknown how many cases of wood-trimmer's disease would be reclassified as hypersensitivity pneumonitis or inhalation fever using modern diagnostic criteria.[84] In a questionnaire study 22% of the workers in the trimming departments had experienced febrile attacks that they thought were connected to their work.[62] Febrile attacks were diagnosed by a questionnaire used in earlier studies in farmers.[24] A similar questionnaire was sent to working male controls aged 19 to 65 years, randomly selected from the Swedish population. Three percent of the controls had experienced febrile attacks. Among the controls with febrile illnesses, there were some farmers and some welders who probably had had typical inhalation fever. The others might have given an incorrect answer to the question.

Published reports vary about how frequently grain fever occurs, probably because of differences in definitions, and difficulties in measurement, and differences in exposure. Grain fever was reported by 33% of grain scoopers, whereas 1.4% of grain elevator workers in Thunder Bay, Ontario, Canada, reported grain fever.[86,87]

Mill fever in the cotton industry is common, especially among new employees. Prevalences of 6% to 7% have been reported.[88,89] In a study in a cottonseed oil mill, prevalences in new workers ranging from 10% to 50% were reported.[90]

MECHANISMS

Despite the fact that inhalation fever is common, the exact mechanisms involved in its pathogenesis are unknown. The fact that the exact etiologic agents in inhalation fever are often also unclear helps to explain why it is hard to clarify the mechanisms involved in pathogenesis. It is also obvious that inhalation fever is caused by a number of different agents. Many hypotheses about pathogenesis have been suggested, involving interleukins (ILs), tumor necrosis factor (TNF), the activation of macrophages, immune complexes, and complement.[32,35,37,41,91,92]

Since even nonsensitized individuals not previously exposed to the agents are affected by inhalation fever, no allergy mechanisms are involved. Precipitins to thermophiles are usually negative in organic dust inhalation fever and there is no evidence that antibodies are involved in the mechanisms of the condition.[16,17,29]

In the 1970s the term *pulmonary mycotoxicosis* was used for inhalation fever occurring after uncapping silos, but it has not been possible to identify any significant mycotoxin concentrations in dust causing this syndrome.[93,94] Endotoxin has been found in the cotton industry, as well as in swine and poultry confinement buildings, but a Swedish study found no dose–response relationship between endotoxin levels in dust causing inhalation fever in farmers.[95] Neither could any endotoxin be found in the trimming department of sawmills. Only three kinds of mold grow in this environment: *Aspergillus fumigatus, Rhizopus rhizopodoformis,* and *Paecillomyses variotii.*

It has been shown by several groups that the pathogenesis of inhalation fever involves the induction of a peripheral blood leukocytosis and airway neutrophilia.[16,94,96] Recently, 23 volunteers were studied with BAL after experimental welding exposure. Tumor necrosis factor, IL-6, and IL-8 in BAL fluid supernatant concentrations increased in a time- and exposure-dependent fashion after zinc oxide welding fume exposure. The authors concluded that the time course of increased cytokines, their correlations with one another and with polymorphonuclear leukocytes in the BAL fluid, and the consistency of their findings with the known kinetics and actions of these cytokines support the hypothesis that a network of cytokines released by stimulated macrophages resident in the lungs is involved in the pathogenesis of metal fume fever. Tumor necrosis factor (TNF) is considered to be a probable key factor in the pathophysiology of metal fume fever because of its strong exposure response at 3 hours after exposure, a time at which neither IL-6 nor IL-8 exhibits a statistically significant relationship to the airborne concentration of welding fume. A peak increase of TNF in BAL fluid 3 hours after exposure of guinea pigs has been reported in an animal model of mill fever, another type of inhalation fever.[97]

According to the hypothesis, alveolar macrophages respond initially to a stimulus by secreting TNF and/or IL-1. These cytokines then act in an autocrine or paracrine fashion, leading to IL-6 and IL-8 release by macrophages, epithelial cells, or fibroblasts, triggering an inflammatory response involving neutrophils, macrophages, and lymphocytes.[98]

Recently, an animal model of organic dust toxic syndrome was developed in the guinea pig. Animals were exposed to airborne cotton dust for 6 hours; a febrile response occurred by 5 hours and lasted for several hours. Concurrent with this response was a change in pulmonary function, which consisted of rapid shallow breathing with airflow limitation during exhalation. As in metal fume fever, evaluation of BAL indicated a neutrophilic inflammation of the lung and increased amounts of tumor necrosis factor (TNF).[97]

In an epidemic of acute fever, respiratory tract symptoms, and muscle pain starting 4 hours after a hot bath involving 56 persons, the mean C-reactive protein value was 54 mg/L (reference value, <3 mg/L).[70] Since IL-6 initiates the production of acute phase reactants in the liver, these findings support that mechanisms similar to those in the experimental metal fume fever mentioned above could be involved, especially since there have also been reports of increased C-reactive proteins in metal

fever.[99] These findings and the finding in the above animal model indicate that inhalation fever after exposure to bioaerosols probably involves mechanisms similar to those in metal fume fever.

In a study of acute phase reactants in rabbits exposed to an aerosol of fungal spores, haptoglobin analysis was compared with depressions in arterial oxygen tension (Pa_{O_2}) following challenge. It was found in three experiments that none of seven rabbits with an augmented haptoglobin level before challenge demonstrated a decreased Pa_{O_2} after aerosol challenge. Perhaps this finding could explain some of the mechanisms in the development of tolerance.[100]

It is puzzling that such a variety of exposures might cause a syndrome so similar in symptomatology, course, development of tolerance, laboratory results, and BAL findings. The findings mentioned indicate that inhalation fever is caused by an acute pulmonary inflammatory cellular response involving a network of cytokines. Do the responses to different dusts involve different mechanisms with the same final result, or is inhalation fever a nonspecific pyrexial reaction after inhalation of noxious substances? Much research remains to be done in this field.

CLINICAL ASPECTS
Symptoms

During the actual exposure there might be some preliminary symptoms with irritation in the throat and a dry irritation cough. The constitutional symptoms come on after a latent interval approximately 4 to 8 hours after the original exposure, usually in the late afternoon or early evening. The symptoms are dominated by fever and shivering. The fever has a gradual increase, followed in most cases by a shivering attack and sweating. Temperatures as high as 41°C have been reported. The fever and chills often accompany additional symptoms such as myalgia, headache, general malaise, cough, and chest discomfort.[12,32,35,36,91,92,101] Some patients have a feeling of irritation or oppression retrosternally. Severe dyspnea is not common. Instead, some people experience a sense of discomfort in the chest, especially upon taking a deep breath.[29] These respiratory symptoms, as well as the other additional symptoms, do not occur in all cases. The severity of the condition varies significantly. Perhaps there is some kind of threshold in the extent of the exposure that must be overcome to induce fever. The symptoms resolve 24 to 48 hours after termination of exposure, followed by complete recovery.

There are some differences in the reported symptoms in the different kinds of inhalation fever. In metal fume fever thirst and a metallic taste in the mouth have been reported.[32] Most swallowed metals are direct irritants to the gastrointestinal tract, and this is thought to be the cause of the nausea.[42] Nausea may occur in organic dust inhalation fever but seems to be more common in metal fume fever, as is abdominal pain.[29]

Clustering

As described earlier, all exposed workers develop inhalation fever if the exposure is high enough. This has been shown clearly in several reports of silo unloading.[16,17,29,102] As mentioned, the biggest cluster ever reported was from a hay party where 55 party attenders fell ill due to inhalation fever.[73] Thus several exposed persons with the same symptoms might show up at the emergency room within a relatively short period.

Tolerance, or tachyphylaxis

The reaction includes an unexplained tolerance effect in which symptoms lessen with repeated daily exposure but are much worse upon return to work after a break, such as after a weekend. Thus the condition has been called "Monday morning fever"; such an effect has been described in metal fume fever, mill fever, and humidifier fever and in sawmill workers affected by fever.[69,103,104] Actually, wood trimmers feeling ill on Mondays have been accused of having hangovers after the weekend. The phenomenon of tachyphylaxis was also clearly demonstrated during identification of the responsible agent of polymer fume fever, when a volunteer exposed for the second time was markedly less affected than five other volunteers.[46] This person had suffered from inhalation fever after the first exposure 1 day before.

There has been speculation that primarily new employees in swine confinement buildings experience episodes of inhalation fever.[27] There have been similar reports from the grain industry in North America.[76] Swedish researchers were actually warned about the danger of the work by swine confinement workers when the researchers, as volunteers, were weighing pigs. Subsequently, the project leader himself fell ill with typical inhalation fever, providing an excellent opportunity to study BAL and airway responsiveness in inhalation fever.[92]

Physical examination

Physical signs are notable for their evanescence or complete absence.[29,32,36] However, if the patient has high fever, there might be an increased pulse rate and possibly respiratory rate. Physical examination usually reveals little that is abnormal, except that crackles can be heard in some cases.[16,17,29,32]

Blood tests, pulmonary function tests, airway hyperresponsiveness, bronchoalveolar lavage, and lung biopsy

An increased sedimentation rate, as well as leukocytosis with an increased number of segmented white blood cells, is common.[29,32,36,101] In a case report of inhalation fever after exposure to a varnish containing isocyanates, it could be demonstrated that the peak of the fever and the leukocytosis occurred simultaneously.[55] Farmer's lung precipitins are usually negative in organic dust inhalation fever.[16,17,29,101] However, precipitins to wood mold antigens are often positive in workers in the trimming departments of sawmills, even in workers who had never had inhalation fever.[56,105] A positive precipitin test is thus a sign of exposure, not disease.

In two cases of metal fume fever, an associated elevation of the serum zinc concentration has been reported.[106] In another study of metal fume fever, the blood zinc level was normal when measured shortly after an attack.[78] Even subnormal serum zinc concentrations have been reported in zinc fume fever.[107]

In a patient affected by metal fume fever after burning zinc wire, the serum lactate dehydrogenase (LDH) level was 620 Berger–Broida U/ml (normal range, 100 to 300 Berger–Broida U/ml). The test for C-reactive protein gave a positive result in a dilution of 1:50. In another case of zinc fume fever with elevated LDH, it was possible to construct an LDH zymogram demonstrating an elevation in the level of pulmonary isoenzyme.[108] Lactate dehydrogenase has not been measured in the other inhalation fevers, but it is of interest that LDH was also elevated in Swedish farmers with hypersensitivity pneumonitis.[28] Often, an acute exacerbation after an especially high mold dust exposure brought farmers with hypersensitivity pneumonitis to the hospital. One may speculate that some of these farmers had an attack of inhalation fever superimposed on their hypersensitivity pneumonitis and that the increase in LDH is expressive of this.

There is no association between atopy and inhalation fever.[75] The moldy material that causes inhalation fever gives rise to dense clouds of dust. One would expect instead that subjects with atopy and allergic asthma would be less likely to develop inhalation fever. Because of airway hyperresponsiveness, they are unable to tolerate either the high levels of mold dust or the metal fume levels required to induce inhalation fever.

The chest radiograph, blood gases, and pulmonary function tests are usually normal.[32,101] In some cases, however, there may be transient changes that, in principle, return to normal within 24 hours.[16,17,29,94] Inhalation fever after exposure to isocyanates differs in that transient decreases of the pulmonary function seem to be more common than in the other types of inhalation fever. Decreases in lung volumes as well as in diffusing capacity (DLCO) and Pao_2 have been reported, but most subjects fail to show interstitial infiltrates and a restrictive breathing pattern.[79] In the case report of isocyanate inhalation fever mentioned earlier, repeated spirometry was performed during the acute stage.[55] An approximately 30% decrease in both the vital capacity (VC) and the forced expiratory volume in 1 second (FEV1) was measured starting after the exposure, with a maximum after 10 hours. After 24 hours the VC was still 10% below the value before the exposure.

In eight subjects inhalation challenges with MDI induced significant falls in both FEV1 and forced vital capacity

(FVC) associated with a rise in body temperature and an increase in blood neutrophils, but only two developed a frank obstructive pattern and one had a significant restrictive breathing defect.[79] Also, a significant decline in DLCO was demonstrated in three of eight subjects 8 to 24 hours postchallenge. Comparison of methacholine PC_{20} (concentration of methacholine producing a 20% fall in FEV1) values before and after reactions induced by the MDI resin did not reveal any significant change. Postchallenge chest radiographs did not show significant interstitial infiltrates.

In a bathtub refinisher the entire complex of symptoms and decreases in FEV1, FVC, DLCO, and Pao_2 was measured after challenge with a catalyst containing TDI.[54] All variables with the exception of Pao_2 returned to normal values within 24 hours. In other studies of isocyanate exposure, it has been shown that the decreases in pulmonary function returned to almost normal values in 12 to 24 hours.[54,55]

Perhaps such transient decreases in pulmonary function would be seen in more cases if repeat spirometries were done. Many patients are not evaluated until the spirometry has returned to normal. It is also possible that patients might have decreased lung volumes even if the volumes are within the predicted values. Usually, it is not known what the lung volumes were *before* the exposure, and the patient's original lung volume might be over 100% of the predicted value.

Vogelmeier and coworkers described a particularly severe case of metal fume fever in a German welder, with recurrent episodic illness associated with welding zinc-coated materials.[99] Three to 6 hours after an experimental challenge he experienced a 40% decrease in inspiratory vital capacity, a 60% fall in single-breath DLCO, and a 10% fall in Pao_2, even though the chest radiograph and chest examination were unchanged. During this time blood zinc levels were elevated, whereas cadmium levels were normal. These changes in lung function had almost resolved at 24 hours after exposure, but at that time the total cell count on BAL was increased approximately ten-fold at 9.4×10^7 cells per cubic millimeter, with a polymorphonuclear leukocytosis. In metal fume fever induced under laboratory conditions, decreases of various degrees in DLCO have been seen at 20 and 72 hours after challenge.[26,99]

Moreover, in the study mentioned earlier of volunteers weighing pigs, one of six subjects developed typical inhalation fever.[27] Two experienced malaise, drowsiness, and a fainting sensation but temperature changes of less than 1°C. Airway responsiveness increased in all subjects within 6 hours (more than three doubling steps' difference in a methacholine test compared with preexposure values). In another study in which farmers with organic dust inhalation fever were interviewed, it was quite common for the farmers to report an increased general sensitivity to dust after the febrile attack.[29] This could be an expression of increased airway responsiveness after the febrile attack. Other researchers have had similar impressions, but in a study

from upstate New York increased airway hyperresponsiveness was not found in a follow-up study of 10 farmers.[109]

Bronchoalveolar lavage was recently studied in volunteers after experimental welding exposure.[26] Polymorphonuclear leukocytes increased 9% in BAL at 6 hours and 37% in BAL at 22 hours after welding. The count of polymorphonuclear leukocytes in peripheral blood increased in parallel with the count in BAL fluid. The same group also studied cytokines in metal fume fever and detected TNF, IL-6, and IL-8 in BAL fluid.

Bronchoalveolar lavage performed 24 hours after challenge with MDI in two subjects with inhalation fever revealed an increase in lymphocytes and neutrophils.[79] Bronchoalveolar lavage during the acute stage of organic dust inhalation fever showed an increase in the percentage of neutrophils without any increase in lymphocytes, and a normal concentration of the immunoglobins.[94,96] Bronchoalveolar lavage performed 1 week after the acute illness showed a lymphocyte-dominated infiltration in one patient.[110]

There is one report in the literature of an individual with a severe case of inhalation fever after organic dust exposure who developed pulmonary edema associated with massive fungal inhalation in an orange storehouse.[111] Bronchoalveolar lavage showed 96% alveolar macrophages, 3% lymphocytes, and 1% neutrophils. A transbronchial lung biopsy in the same patient disclosed a hyperemic tracheobronchial tree but almost nothing abnormal in the alveoli and the interstitium. Lung biopsy in two farmers with severe inhalation fever revealed a multifocal process with exudates, neutrophils, and histiocytes in the bronchiole, alveoli, and interstitium and large numbers of fungal spores. Species of mesophilic and thermophilic actinomycetes and of *Aspergillus* and *Penicillium* fungi were recorded in the BAL fluid.[94]

DIFFERENTIAL DIAGNOSIS

A thorough occupational history is important for the diagnosis. Inhalation fever is an exclusion diagnosis made on clinical grounds with no specific test currently available. People who are unaware of the hazard sometimes think that they are developing a cold or influenza and tend to attribute their symptom to this, especially as the illness may not start until they have finished work and returned home. The rapid recovery tends to confirm their belief. Hence it is not uncommon for employees not to seek assistance until they have had more than one attack. Probably a lot of cases of inhalation fever go undiagnosed. In a Swedish study most of the farmers were familiar with the benign nature of inhalation fever and did not seek medical care.[29] If they did, they sometimes knew more about the condition than their physicians.

Differential diagnoses are hypersensitivity pneumonitis and infectious diseases (e.g., virus infections such as influenza). In hypersensitivity pneumonitis, but usually not in organic dust inhalation fever, there are decreased blood gases, chest x-ray changes, and decreased pulmonary function according to the modern diagnostic criteria of Terho[84] (see Table 17-4). As evident after the presentation of the clinical picture in inhalation fever, there is some overlap between inhalation fever and hypersensitivity pneumonitis. Perhaps a time criterion should be added to the diagnostic criteria for hypersensitivity pneumonitis. Hypersensitivity pneumonitis is a severe lung disease lasting for weeks or months.

Symptoms after exposure to cadmium and mercury fume can initially be similar to inhalation fever but are very important to distinguish, since such exposure can cause severe lung damage and intoxication.[32]

TREATMENT, PROGNOSIS, AND PREVENTION

Inhalation fever is of a benign nature, self-limiting, and of short duration. No specific treatment is required. If exposure stops, the symptoms subside spontaneously in 12 to 48 hours.[16,17,29,32,36,55,91,92] The patient should be removed immediately from contact with the causative exposure, placed at rest in bed if needed, and treated symptomatically.

Analgesics and fever-decreasing agents give symptomatic relief. Milk has been used to alleviate gastrointestinal symptoms of nausea, vomiting, and abdominal pain by interfering with the interaction of the heavy metal oxide and gastric hydrochloric acid.[38] The administration of oxygen in severe cases has also been recommended.[12]

There are no reported sequelae in inhalation fever. In Finland farmers' wives who had experienced inhalation fever experienced more chronic bronchitis than others (K. Husman, personal communication, 1993). Extensive investigations have revealed no effects in respiratory function, gas exchange, or exercise capacity in farmers who have experienced inhalation fever, in some cases repeated attacks.[30] Neither does grain fever lead to fibrosis or permanent disability.[11] In an 8-week follow-up with BAL, there was no evidence of ongoing or persistent inflammation in subjects having had metal fume fever.[26]

Earlier, when the differences between hypersensitivity pneumonitis and inhalation fever were not yet realized, workers had unnecessarily been forced to change occupations because of attacks of fever, but we know now that

Table 17-4. Differences between inhalation fever, hypersensitivity pneumonitis, and toxic pneumonia

	Inhalation fever	Hypersensitivity pneumonitis (allergic alveolitis)	Chemical toxic pneumonitis (chemical alveolitis, or toxic or chemical pulmonary edema)
Exposure	Metal fumes Polymer fumes Bioaerosols	Bioaerosols Isocyanates	Irritant gases (e.g., NH_3, Cl_2, NO_2, O_3, and $COCl_2$) Irritant metal fumes (e.g., Be, Cd, Hg, $Ni[CO]_4$, and $ZnCl_2$)
Type of exposure	Heavy exposure during an hour, or half-hour on a single occasion	Repeated exposure 15-30 minutes daily for several weeks	Heavy exposure
Onset after exposure	4-8 hours	4-8 hours	Immediate or after a symptom-free period of 24 hours or longer
Dominating symptoms	Fever and chills with flulike symptoms	Dyspnea, cough, fatigue, bouts of fever and chills	Dyspnea, cough
Clustering	Common	Seldom	Common
Clinical findings	Usually normal	Crackles (dyspnea, cyanosis)	Crackles, often wheezes (cyanosis, tachypnea, tachycardia)
Precipitins	Usually negative	Usually positive	Negative
Chest radiographs	Usually normal or minor transient changes	Nodular or patchy infiltrates	Diffuse edema or miliary pattern
Pulmonary function tests	Normal or transient minor changes	Restriction, DLCO ↓	Restriction, DLCO ↓
Blood gases	Normal, minor decrease	Pao_2 ↓	Pao_2 ↓
Bronchoalveolar lavage	Neutrophils ↑, macrophages ↑	Lymphocytes ↑, CD_4/CD_8 ratio ↓, macrophages ↑, mast cells ↑	?
Biopsy	Alveolitis (only a few cases in the literature)	Mononuclear alveolitis, granulomas	Edema, hyaline membranes, bronchiolitis
Duration	12 hours to 3 days	Weeks, months	Weeks
Prognosis	No sequelae known at this time	Risk of chronic decreased pulmonary function	Risk of chronic decreased pulmonary function and asthma

After doPico,[120] Von Essen et al.,[91] Pratt and May,[17] and Rosenstock and Cullen.[34]

there is no need to do this because of inhalation fever. Instead, good working practice is important to avoid further episodes. Inhalation of toxic fumes can be prevented by adequate exhaust ventilation and the application of local exhaust ventilation to the fume source. In farming the development of mold should be avoided by using proper farming methods. However, due to climatic conditions and weather variations, some instances of mold growth are unavoidable even if the equipment is adequate. New techniques might also introduce new risks. If a worker is forced to handle moldy material or work in toxic fumes, he should use a respirator to avoid unnecessary illness. Education about the danger of inhaling mold dust or toxic fumes is also important in preventing disease.

CONCLUSION

Inhalation fever is an acute, short-term, noninfectious, flulike febrile reaction caused by inhalation of noxious substances in a variety of environments. In principle, inhalation fever can be caused by substances originating from metals, polymers, or organic dust. Clustering of cases is not uncommon. Physical examination usually reveals nothing abnormal. An increased sedimentation rate and polymorphonuclear leukocytosis are common. In organic dust inhalation fever precipitins to mold or bacteria are often absent. In general, chest x-ray and pulmonary function are normal. The condition has no reported sequelae. The histopathology and BAL findings differ from those of hypersensitivity pneumonitis and other conditions. Recent studies of pathogenesis indicate that inhalation fever is caused by an acute pulmonary inflammatory cellular response involving a network of cytokines. Patients are often seen by general practitioners, and it is important to remember this in the differential diagnosis of workers with unclear fever. Clinically, it is important to differentiate inhalation fever from other diseases because the treatment and prognosis differ. Inhalation fever can be prevented by having adequate ventilation, using good working practice, and wearing respirators when needed.

REFERENCES

1. Magnus O: *Historia de gentibus septentrionalibus,* Rome, 1555.
2. Ramazzini B: *De morbis artificum.* Modena, Italy, 1700.
3. Ramazzini B: *De morbis artificum.* (*Diseases of workers: the Latin text of 1713 revised with translation and notes by Wilmer Cave Wright.* Chicago, 1940, University of Chicago Press.)
4. Thackrah CT: *The effects of arts, trades, and professions, and of civic states and habits of living on health and longevity,* ed 2, pp 101-102, London, 1832, Longman, Rees, Orme, Brown, Green, and Longman.
5. Patissier P: Baillière JB, editor: *Traité des maladies des artisans, et de celles qui resultent des diverses professions d'après Ramazzini,* pp 32-34, Paris, 1822.
6. Drinker P: Certain aspects of the problem of zinc toxicity, *J Ind Hyg* 4:177-197, 1922.
7. Parkes WR: In: *Occupational lung disorders,* ed 2, p 435, London, 1982, Butterworths.
8. Neal P, Schneiter R, and Cominita P: Report on acute illness among rural mattress-workers using low grade, stained cotton, *JAMA* 119:1074-1082, 1942.
9. Plessner MM: Une maladie des trieurs de plumes: la fièvre de canard, *Arch Mal Prof Med Trav Secur Soc* 21:67-69, 1959.
10. Pestalozzi C: Febrile gruppenerkrankungen in einer modellschreinerei durch inhalation von mit schimmelpilzen kontaminiertem befeuchterwasser ("Befeuchterfieber"), *Schweiz Med Wochenschr* 89:710-713, 1959.
11. Manfreda J and Warren CPW: The effects of grain dust on health, *Rev Environ Health* 4(3):240-267, 1984.
12. Harris DK: Polymer-fume fever, *Lancet* 261:1008-1015, 1951.
13. Zeiss CR, Wolkonsky P, and Chacon R: Syndromes in workers exposed to trimellitic anhydride, *Ann Intern Med* 98:8-12, 1983.
14. Lob M: Fièvre au diphénylméthane-diisocyanate (MDI), *Schweiz Med Wochenschr* 18:647-649, 1972.
15. Edwards JH, Baker JT, and Davies BH: Precipitin test negative farmer's lung-activation of the alternative pathway of complement by moldy hay dusts, *Clin Allergy* 4:379-388, 1974.
16. Emanuel DA, Wenzel FJ, and Lawton BR: Pulmonary mycotoxicosis, *Chest* 67:293-297, 1975.
17. Pratt DS and May JJ. Feed-associated respiratory illness in farmers, *Arch Environ Health* 39:43-48, 1984.
18. doPico G: Health effects of organic dusts in the farm environment, *Am J Ind Med* 10:261-265, 1986.
19. Waldron HA: In: *Lecture notes on occupational medicine,* ed 4, p 101, Oxford, England, 1990, Blackwell Scientific Publications.
20. Inhalation fevers, *Lancet* 1:249-250, 1978. Editorial.
21. Rask-Andersen A and Pratt DS: Inhalation fever: a proposed unifying term for febrile reactions to inhalation of noxious substances, *Br J Ind Med* 49:40, 1992.
22. Grant IW, Blyth W, Wardrop VE, et al: Prevalence of farmer's lung in Scotland, *Br Med J* 1:530-634, 1972.
23. Terho EO, Heinonen OP, and Lammi S: Incidence of clinically confirmed farmer's lung in Finland, *Am J Ind Med* 10:330, 1986.
24. Malmberg P, Rask-Andersen A, Höglund S, et al: Incidence of organic dust toxic syndrome and allergic alveolitis in Swedish farmers, *Int Arch Allergy Appl Immunol* 87:47-54, 1988.
25. Rylander R and Malmberg P: Non-infectious fever: inhalation fever or toxic alveolitis?, *Br J Ind Med* 49:296, 1992. Letter; comment.
26. Blanc P, Wong H, Bernstein MS, et al: An experimental human model of metal fume fever, *Ann Intern Med* 114:930-936, 1991.
27. Malmberg P and Larsson K: Acute exposure to swine dust causes bronchial hyperresponsiveness in healthy subjects, *Eur Respir J* 6:400-404, 1993.
28. Rask-Andersen A: Allergic alveolitis in Swedish farmers, *Upsala J Med Sci* 94:271-285, 1989.
29. Rask-Andersen A: Organic dust toxic syndrome among farmers, *Br J Ind Med* 46:233-238, 1989.
30. Malmberg P, Rask-Andersen A, Palmgren U, et al: Exposure to microorganisms, febrile and airway-obstructive symptoms, immune status and lung function of Swedish farmers, *Scand J Work Environ Health* 11:287-293, 1985.
31. Cormier Y, Fournier M, and Laviolette M: Farmer's fever; systemic manifestation of farmer's lung without lung involvement, *Chest* 103:632-634, 1993.
32. Blanc P and Boushey HA: The lung in metal fume fever, *Semin Respir Med* 14:212-225, 1993.
33. Malmberg P and Larsson K: Toxic airway inflammation from inhaled organic particles, *J Aerosol Sci* 23(suppl 1):S535-S538, 1992.
34. Rosenstock L and Cullen MR: Toxic pneumonitis or pulmonary edema. In Dyson J, editor: *Clinical occupational medicine,* pp 28-31, Philadelphia, 1986, WB Saunders.
35. Nemery B: Metal toxicity and the respiratory tract, *Eur Respir J* 3:202-219, 1990.

36. Mueller EJ and Seger DL: Metal fume fever: a review, *J Emerg Med* 2:271-274, 1985.

37. Taylor G: Acute systemic effects of inhaled occupational agents. In Merchant JA, editor: *Occupational respiratory diseases,* pp 607-625, Washington, DC, 1986, US Department of Health and Human Services.

38. Papp JP: Metal fume fever, *Postgrad Med* 43:160-163, 1968.

39. McMillan G: Metal fume fever, *Occup Health* 38:148-149, 1986.

40. Gleason RP: Exposure to copper dust, *Am Ind Hyg Assoc J* 29:461-462, 1968.

41. McCord CP: Metal fume fever as an immunological disease, *Ind Med Surg* 29:101-107, 1960.

42. Schenker MR, Speizer FE, and Taylor JO: Acute upper respiratory symptoms resulting from exposure of zinc chloride aerosol, *Environ Res* 25:317-324, 1981.

43. Evans EH: Casualties following exposure to zinc chloride smoke, *Lancet* 249:368-370, 1945.

44. Maj BWB: Two types of metal fume fever: mild vs. serious, *Mil Med* 155:372-377, 1990.

45. Robbins JJ and Ware RL: Pulmonary edema from Teflon fumes: report of a case, *N Engl J Med* 271:360-361, 1964.

46. Nuttal JB, Kelly RJ, Smith BS, et al: Inflight toxic reactions resulting from fluorocarbon resin pyrolysis, *Aerospace Med* 35:676-683, 1964.

47. Lewis CE and Kerby GR: An epidemic of polymer fume fever, *JAMA* 191:103-106, 1965.

48. Evans EA: Pulmonary edema from polytetrafluoroethylene (PTFE), *JOM, J Occup Med* 15:599-601, 1973.

49. Wegman DH and Peters JM: Polymer fume fever and cigarette smoking, *Ann Intern Med* 81:55-57, 1974.

50. Williams N and Smith FK: Polymer-fume fever: an elusive diagnosis, *JAMA* 219 (12):1587-1589, 1972.

51. Sherwood RJ: *Hazards of fluon (polyfluoroetylen) Trans Assoc Ind Med Off* 5:10, 1955.

52. Brugsch HG and Elkins HB: Toluene diisocyanate (TDI) toxicity, *N Engl J Med* 268:353-357, 1963.

53. Selden AI, Belin L, and Wass U: Isocyanate exposure and hypersensitivity pneumonitis—report of a probable case and prevalence of specific immunoglobulin G antibodies among exposed individuals, *Scand J Work Environ Health* 15:234-237, 1989.

54. Fink JN and Schlueter DP: Bathtub refinisher's lung: an unusual response to toluene diisocyanate, *Am Rev Respir Dis* 118:955-959, 1978.

55. Nielsen J, Sangö C, Winroth G, et al: Systemic reactions associated with polyisocyanate exposure, *Scand J Work Environ Health* 11:51-54, 1985.

56. Belin L: Clinical and immunological data on "wood trimmers disease" in Sweden, *Eur J Respir Dis* 107s:169-179, 1980.

57. Lundholm M and Rylander R: Work related symptoms among sewage workers, *Br J Ind Med* 40:325-329, 1983.

58. Malmros P, Sigsgaard T, and Bach B: Occupational health problems due to garbage sorting, *Waste Manage Res* 10:227-234, 1992.

59. Rask-Andersen A: Allergic alveolitis in Swedish farmers. *Upsala J Med Sci* 94:271-285, 1989.

60. Acute respiratory illness following occupational exposure to wood chips, *Morbid Mortal Weekly Rep* 35:483-484, 489-490, 1986.

61. Kryda M, Emanuel DA, Marx JJ, et al: Hypersensitivity pneumonitis due to *Aspergillus fumigatus* in papermill workers. In Dosman JA and Cockcroft DW, editors: *Principles of health and safety in agriculture,* p 80, Boca Raton, Fla, 1989, CRC Press.

62. Rask-Andersen A, Land CJ, Enlund K, et al: Inhalation fever and respiratory symptoms in the trimming department of Swedish sawmills, *Am J Ind Med* 25:65-67, 1994.

63. Cockcroft AE, McDermott M, Edwards JH, et al: Grain exposure—symptoms and lung function, *Eur J Respir Dis* 64:189-196, 1983.

64. Warren CPW, Cherniack RM, and Tse KS: Hypersensitivity reactions to grain dust, *J Allergy Clin Immunol* 53:139-149, 1974.

65. Donham KJ: Health effects from work in swine confinement buildings, *Am J Ind Med* 17:17-25, 1990.

66. Castellan RM, Olenchock S, Hankinson J, et al: Acute bronchoconstriction induced by cotton dust: dose-related responses to endotoxin and other dust factors, *Ann Intern Med* 101:157-163, 1984.

67. Rylander R and Haglind P: Relation between FEV1, changes over the work shift and cotton/endotoxin levels. In Wakelyn PJ and Jacobs RR, editors: *Proceedings of the seventh Cotton Dust Research Conference,* pp 17-18, Memphis, 1983, National Cotton Council.

68. Rylander R, Jacobs RR: *Organic dusts: exposure, effects, and prevention,* Chelsea, Mich, 1994, Lewis Publishers.

69. Baur X, Behr J, Dewair M, et al: Humidifier lung and humidifier fever, *Lung* 166:113-124, 1988.

70. Atterholm I, Ganrot-Norlin K, Hallberg T, et al: Unexplained acute fever after a hot bath, *Lancet* 2:684-686, 1977.

71. Muittari A, Kuusisto P, and Virtanen P: An epidemic of extrinsic allergic alveolitis caused by tap water, *Clin Allergy* 10:77-99, 1980.

72. Blomqvist A: *Chills of hot air pistol,* pp 297-298, Örebro, Sweden, 1986, Newsletter from the Department of Occupational Medicine, Örebro Medical Center.

73. Brinton WT, Vastbinder EE, Greene JW, et al: An outbreak of organic dust toxic syndrome in a college fraternity, *JAMA* 258:1210-1212, 1987.

74. Gatzemeier U: Akute exogen-allergische alveolitis—6 fälle nach verladen verschimmelter gerste, *Prax Pneumol* 35:400-402, 1981.

75. Manfreda J, Holford-Stevens V, Cheang M, et al: Acute symptoms following exposure to grain dust in farming, *Environ Health Perspect* 66:73-80, 1986.

76. doPico G, Reddan W, Tsiatis A, et al: Epidemiologic study of clinical and physiologic parameters in grain handlers of northern United States, *Am Rev Respir Dis* 130:759-765, 1984.

77. Brodie J: Welding fumes and gases: their effects on the health of the worker, *Calif West Med* 59:13-18, 1943.

78. Ross DS: Welders' metal fume fever, *J Soc Occup Med* 24:125-129, 1974.

79. Vandenplas O, Malo J, Dugas M, et al: Hypersensitivity pneumonitis-like reaction among workers exposed to piphenylmethane diisocyanate (MDI), *Am Rev Respir Dis* 147:338-346, 1993.

80. Polakoff PL, Busch KA, and Okawa MT: Urinary fluoride levels in polytetrafluoroethylene fabricators, *Ann Ind Hyg Assoc* 35:99-106, 1974.

81. Adams WGF: Polymer fume fever due to inhalation of fumes from polytetrafluoroethylene, *Trans Assoc Ind Med Off* 13:20-21, 1963.

82. Husman K, Terho EO, Notkola V, et al: Organic dust toxic syndrome among Finnish farmers, *Am J Ind Med* 17:79-80, 1990.

83. Warren CPW, Holford-Stevens V, and Manfreda J: Respiratory disorders among Canadian farmers, *Eur J Respir Dis* 154s:10-14, 1987.

84. Terho EO: Diagnostic criteria for farmer's lung disease, *Am J Ind Med* 10:329, 1986.

85. Rodriguez de Castro MD, Carillo T, Castillo R, et al: Relationships between characteristics of exposure to pigeon antigens, *Chest* 103:1059-1063, 1993.

86. Kleinfeld M: Comparative clinical and pulmonary function study of grain handlers and bakers, *Ann NY Acad Sci* 221:86-96, 1974.

87. Broder I, Mintz S, Hutcheon M, et al: Comparison of respiratory diseases in grain elevator workers and civic outside workers of Thunder Bay, Canada, *Am Rev Respir Dis* 119:193-203, 1979.

88. Schilling RS: Byssinosis in cotton and other textile workers, *Lancet* 271 (6937):261-265, 1956.

89. Werner GCH: De la bronchiolite oedemateuse allergique. Essai statistique sur l'asthme des poussières textiles végétales, *Arch Mal Prof Méd Trav Secur Soc* 16:27-45, 1955.

90. Ritter WL and Nussbaum MA: Occupational illnesses in cotton industries, *Miss Doctor* 22:96-99, 1944.

91. von Essen S, Robbins RA, Thompson AB, et al: Organic dust toxic syndrome: an acute febrile reaction to organic dust exposure distinct from hypersensitivity pneumonitis, *J Toxicol Clin Toxicol* 28:389-420, 1990.

92. Malmberg P and Rask-Andersen A: Organic dust toxic syndrome, *Semin Respir Med* 14:38-48, 1993.

93. May JJ, Pratt DS, Stallones L, et al: A study of dust generated during silo opening and its physiologic effects on workers. In Dosman JA and Cockcroft DW, editors: *Principles of health and safety in agriculture,* pp 76-79, Boca Raton, Fla, 1989, CRC Press.

94. Emanuel DA, Marx JJ, Ault BJ, et al: Organic dust toxic syndrome (pulmonary mycotoxicosis)—a review of the experience in central Wisconsin. In Dosman JA and Cockcroft DW, editors: *Principles of health and safety in agriculture,* pp 72-75, Boca Raton, Fla, 1989, CRC Press.

95. Rask-Andersen A, Malmberg P, and Lundholm M: Endotoxin levels in farming: absence of symptoms despite high exposure levels, *Br J Ind Med* 46:412-416, 1989.

96. Lecours R, Laviolette M, and Cormier Y: Bronchoalveolar lavage in pulmonary mycotoxicosis (organic dust toxic syndrome), *Thorax* 41:924-926, 1986.

97. Griffiths Johnson DA, Ryan L, and Karol MH: Development of an animal model for organic dust toxic syndrome, *Inhalation Toxicol* 3:405-417, 1991.

98. Blanc PD, Boushey HA, Wong H, et al: Cytokines in metal fume fever, *Am Rev Respir Dis* 147:134-138, 1993.

99. Vogelmeier C, Konig G, Benze K, et al: Pulmonary involvement in zinc fume fever, *Chest* 92:946-948, 1987.

100. Baseler MW and Burrell R: Acute-phase reactants in experimental inhalation lung disease, *Proc Soc Exp Biol Med* 168:49-55, 1981.

101. May JJ, Stallones L, Darrow D, et al: Organic dust toxicity (pulmonary mycotoxicosis) associated with silo unloading, *Thorax* 41:919-923, 1986.

102. Malmberg P, Rask-Andersen A, Rosenhall L: Exposure to microorganisms associated with allergic alveolitis and febrile reactions to mold dust in farmers. *Chest* 103:1202-1209, 1993

103. Drinker P, Thomson RM, and Finn JL: Metal fume fever: II. Resistance acquired by inhalation of zinc oxide on two successive days, *J Ind Hyg* 9:98-105, 1927.

104. Merchant JA: Agricultural exposures to organic dusts, *Occup Med: State Art Rev* 2:409-425, 1987.

105. Eduard W: *Assessment of mould spore exposure and relations to symptoms in wood trimmers,* The Hague, 1993, Cip-Gegevens Koninklijke Bibliotheek.

106. Noel NE and Ruthman JC: Elevated serum zinc levels in metal fume fever, *Am J Emerg Med* 6:609-610, 1988.

107. Ulvik RJ: Subnormal serum zinc concentration in a patient with zinc fever, *J Soc Occup Med* 33:187-189, 1983.

108. Fishburn CW and Zenz C: Metal fume fever: a report of a case, *JOM, J Occup Med* 11:142-144, 1969.

109. May JJ, Marvel LH, Pratt DS, et al: Organic dust toxic syndrome: a follow-up study, *Am J Ind Med* 17:111-113, 1990.

110. Raymenants E, Demedts M, and Nemery B: Bronchoalveolar lavage findings in a patient with the organic dust toxic syndrome, *Thorax* 45:713-714, 1990.

111. Yoshida K, Ando M, and Araki S: Acute pulmonary edema in a storehouse of moldy oranges: a severe case of the organic dust toxic syndrome, *Arch Environ Health* 44:382-384, 1989.

112. Sferlazza SJ and Becket WS: The respiratory health of welders, *Am Rev Respir Dis* 143:1134-1148, 1991.

113. Anseline P: Zinc-fume fever, *Med J Aust* 2:316-318, 1972.

114. Anthony JS, Zamel N, and Aberman A: Abnormalities in pulmonary function after brief exposure to toxic metal fumes, *Can Med Assoc J* 119:586-588, 1978.

115. Parkes WR: In: *Occupational lung disorders,* ed 2, p 454, London, 1982, Butterworths.

116. Dula DJ: Metal fume fever, *J Am Coll Emerg Phys* 7:448-450, 1978.

117. Edwards JH: Humidifier fever, *Thorax* 32:653-663, 1977.

118. Jones A: Farmer's lung: an overview and prospectus, *Ann Am Conf Gov Ind Hyg* 2:171-181, 1982.

119. Morgan WMKC and Seaton A: *Occupational lung diseases,* p 286, Philadelphia, 1975, WB Saunders.

120. doPico GA: Hazardous exposure and lung disease among farm workers, *Clin Chest Med* 13:311-328, 1992.

121. Fuller CJ: Farmer's lung: a review of present knowledge, *Thorax* 8:59-64, 1953.

Chapter 18

LUNG CANCER

Teofile L. Lee-Chiong
Richard A. Matthay

Lung cancer was relatively rare in the United States before the 1930s, when the incidence increased markedly in men; a similar increase in women occurred in the 1960s (Figs. 18-1 and 18-2).[1] Lung cancer now accounts for 17% of all cases of cancer in men and 12% of those in women in this country, ranking behind only prostate cancer in men and breast and colorectal cancer in women.[1] Mortality due to lung cancer in women is actually greater than that due to breast cancer. Bronchogenic carcinoma causes approximately 34% of all cancer deaths in men and 22% of those in women (Fig. 18-3).[1] More than 137,000 people died of lung cancer in the United States in 1989, and in 1993 lung cancer diagnosis was projected in 170,000 patients, with a death estimate of 149,000.[1] One half of cases occur in patients age 65 or older, with a peak in incidence at about age 75.[2] Lung cancer mortality in men appears to be declining, likely because of a decrease in the prevalence of cigarette smoking.[3] Women have not quit smoking at the same rate as men; therefore, a decline in mortality in women will not be evident until after the year 2010.[4]

Occupational exposure has been estimated to account for about 10% of all pulmonary malignancies.[5] In certain populations in which the prevalence of smoking is low, hazardous occupations may be causally associated with most lung cancers.

This chapter discusses the etiology, epidemiology, natural history, clinical features, pathology, screening, diagnosis, staging, treatment, and prognosis of lung cancer. Mentioned briefly are specific agents causing lung cancer and industries associated with lung cancer (see Chapter 34 for a more detailed discussion). Upper airway cancers are reviewed in detail in Chapter 19, and agents associated with upper airway cancers are discussed in Chapter 35. Mesotheliomas are discussed in Chapter 20, Part I.

ETIOLOGY AND EPIDEMIOLOGY
Tobacco smoking

Cigarette smoking is the most common cause of lung cancer in the general population,[6] being directly related to 80% to 90% of all cases of lung cancer.[6] Approximately 50 million Americans smoke (28% of men and 32% of women).[4] On average, cigarette smokers have a 10-fold increased risk of lung cancer,[7] and heavy smokers have a 15- to 25-fold increased risk.[7] The main possible carcinogens

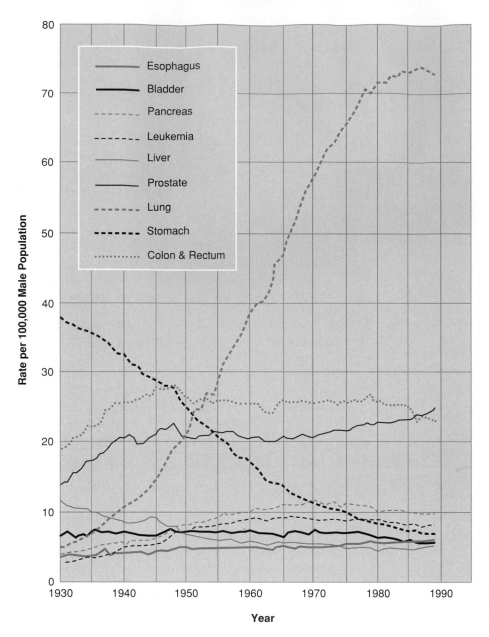

Fig. 18-1. Age-adjusted male cancer death rates for selected sites in the United States, from 1930 to 1989 (age-adjusted to the 1970 U.S. standard population). (From Boring CC, Squires TS, and Tong T: Cancer statistics, 1993, *CA* 43:7-26, 1993. With permission.)

in tobacco smoke are tobacco-specific nitrosamine and polycyclic aromatic hydrocarbons.[8,9] Factors related to the development of lung cancer in smokers include the age at which they start smoking, the amount of tar in each cigarette, how deeply they inhale, and how many cigarettes they smoke each day.[6,10]

There is also evidence that "passive smoking," or the exposure to sidestream smoke, increases the risk of lung cancer for nonsmokers.[11-14] Undiluted sidestream smoke contains higher levels of carcinogens and other toxins than does mainstream smoke.[15] An estimated 500 to 5000 lung cancer deaths per year in the United States may be related to passive exposure to tobacco smoke.[16]

Encouraging current smokers to quit, and young persons not to start, appears to be the most effective way to reduce the incidence of lung cancer.[17] Lung cancer risk declines

progressively after a smoker quits, and the risk for ex-smokers who have not smoked for 10 to 20 years approaches that of lifelong nonsmokers.[17] Furthermore, because smoking may act synergistically with industrial carcinogens, reducing smoking rates further reduces the incidence of occupational lung cancers as well.

Occupational exposure

Exposure to industrial compounds is a major cause of lung cancer. The incidence of occupational lung cancer varies with the extent of industrialization and environmental exposure.[18] Vineis and associates[19] estimate that the percentage of occupational lung cancers ranges from 3% to 17% in different areas of the United States. The percentage of lung cancer attributable to a specific cause will vary with the prevalence exposure, the associated risk for the expo-

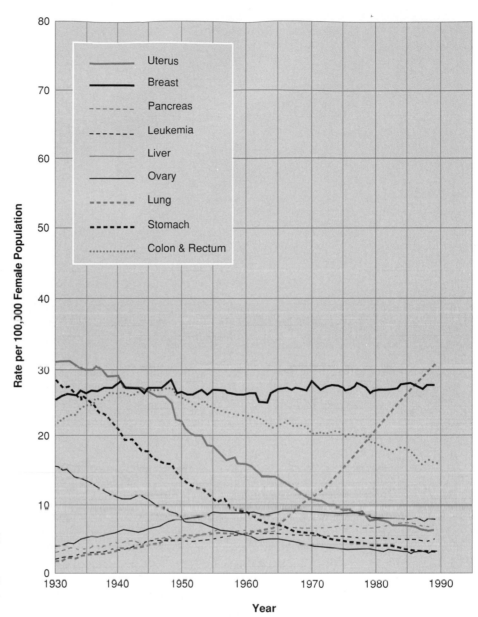

Fig. 18-2. Age-adjusted female cancer death rates for selected sites in the United States, from 1930 to 1989 (age-adjusted to the 1970 U.S. standard population). (From Boring CC, Squires TS, and Tong T: Cancer statistics, 1993, *CA* 43:7-26, 1993. With permission.)

sure, and other factors. In addition, because of the multifactorial etiology of lung cancer and the interaction of different exposures (e.g., asbestos and smoking), the total attributable risk may be greater than 100%. Occupational exposures associated with an increased risk of lung cancer are discussed in detail in Chapter 34.

Diet

Various vitamins and nutrients modify the risk of lung cancer. A prospective study of the incidence of lung cancer among 2080 Western Electric Company employees showed that dietary β-carotene was protective against lung cancer.[20] A diet rich in β-carotene reduces the incidence of lung cancer by an estimated 50%.[21] A trial of oral β-carotene and retinyl palmitate in populations at increased risk is under way, and results are expected in 1999.[22] Retinol (vitamin

A) may modify cancer risk by promoting cellular differentiation.[23] The antineoplastic effects of carotenoids may relate to their ability to serve as antioxidants, removing oxygen-free radicals.[24] Like vitamin A, vitamin C has been shown in some studies to offer protection against lung cancer.[25] Phenethyl isothiocyanate, found in watercress, is believed to inhibit the carcinogenic tobacco-specific nitrosamine.[26] Although questions persist about the relationship between dietary fat and cholesterol and lung cancer risk, no clear consensus is presently available.[27]

Heredity

The risk of lung cancer varies in individuals with similar exposures to tobacco and occupational carcinogens, a differential susceptibility that may be affected by variations in inherited predisposition to carcinogenesis. Relatives of

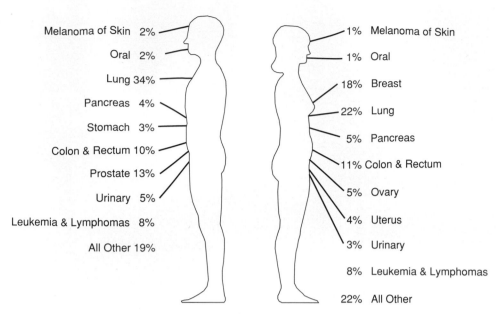

Fig. 18-3. Estimated cancer deaths by site and by sex, 1993. (From Boring CC, Squires TS, and Tong T: Cancer statistics, 1993, *CA* 43:7-26, 1993. With permission.)

patients with lung cancer have an increased risk of developing lung cancer.[28] Moreover, various investigators have detected an association between lung carcinomas and certain genetic abnormalities, including loss of deoxyribonucleic acid (DNA) sequences on the short arm of chromosome 3 or 11; amplification of the oncogenes c-*myc*, N-*myc*, L-*myc*, K-*ras*, H-*ras*, and N-*ras;* and the presence of a 4-debrisoquin hydroxylase phenotype.[7] Mutations of *myc* and retinoblastoma genes and deletion of the short arm of chromosome 3 are usually associated with small cell lung cancers.[29] Non-small cell subtypes predominate in patients with *ras* mutations.[29] Moreover, the presence of the *ras* oncogene appears to predict a worse outcome for some patients with adenocarcinoma.[30]

An enhanced risk of lung cancer was reported by Ayesh and associates[31] among extensive metabolizers of debrisoquin sulfate, an antihypertensive medication. Debrisoquin is hydroxylated by the cytochrome P-450 enzyme, CYP2D6, the activity of which can be measured by calculating the ratio of debrisoquin to the hydroxylated form in the urine after an oral dose of the medication.[31] Aryl hydrocarbon hydroxylase, another enzyme involved in the cytochrome P-450 system, converts the polycyclic hydrocarbons in cigarette smoke into highly carcinogenic epoxides.[32] There is a higher degree of inducibility of this enzyme in the lymphocytes of patients with lung cancer. It is likewise under investigation as a potential factor in carcinogenesis.[32]

NATURAL HISTORY AND CLINICAL FEATURES

Lung tumors undergo three growth phases. Almost three quarters of the natural history of a tumor occurs during its first, or undetectable, phase.[33] This is followed by a pre-clinical phase, during which the tumor may be detected by sputum examination or becomes large enough to be radiographically evident. Many tumors invade adjacent structures and distant sites before entering the third, or clinical, phase. About 95% of patients with lung cancer are symptomatic at the time of diagnosis.[7] Patients with central tumors may present with cough, wheezing, hemoptysis, or dyspnea.[34] Cough and chest wall pain may develop in patients with peripheral tumors.[34] No clinical manifestation of lung cancer is pathognomonic for any subtype. Symptoms may result from the tumor itself or from intrathoracic extension.[35] For example, involvement of the left recurrent laryngeal nerve characteristically produces hoarseness; pleural effusion, pleural plaques, pneumothorax, or chest pain may develop with pleural involvement and dysphagia may occur with esophageal extension. When mediastinal lymph nodes or right-sided tumors compress the superior vena cava, the patient may have edema over the face, neck, and arms, with venous distention, the so-called superior vena cava syndrome. Apical tumors, most commonly squamous cell carcinomas, may involve the cervical and first thoracic nerves and result in Pancoast's superior sulcus tumor syndrome, with destruction of the first and second ribs, development of shoulder and arm pain along the distribution of the ulnar nerve, and Horner's syndrome (ptosis, miosis, and ipsilateral anhidrosis).

Lung tumors may metastasize to virtually any organ by hematogenous or lymphatic routes. The central nervous system, bone, liver, and adrenal glands are the most commonly involved sites.[34]

Paraneoplastic syndromes include a constellation of clinical symptoms appearing in certain malignant diseases but not directly associated with local tumor growth and extension or metastatic involvement. Mechanisms proposed to explain these phenomena include the aberrant release of hormones and polypeptides by derepressed malignant cells or autoimmune processes involving tumor cells.[36] Tumor necrosis factor and interleukin-1 may play a role in the genesis of fever, cachexia, and weakness.[36] Patients with small cell carcinoma may develop Cushing's syndrome, and patients with Cushingoid features should be screened by either an overnight 1-mg dexamethasone suppression test or a 24-hour urinary excretion of free cortisol. Abnormal results should prompt further investigation. Typically, the high corticotropin and cortisol levels produced by ectopic Cushing's syndrome from lung cancer are not suppressed by high-dose dexamethasone.[36]

The syndrome of inappropriate secretion of antidiuretic hormone (SIADH) is most frequently seen in patients with small cell lung cancer.[7] Hyponatremia resulting from SIADH should be suspected in any patient with lung cancer and unexplained confusion, seizure, lethargy, or coma.

The Eaton–Lambert syndrome, also seen most commonly in small cell cancers, is believed to be the result of antibodies to calcium channels that suppress the presynaptic release of acetylcholine.[36] Affected patients may complain of proximal muscle weakness, hyporeflexia, and autonomic dysfunction. Electromyography demonstrates facilitation of muscle strength after contraction or nerve stimulation.

Hypercalcemia is most commonly noted with squamous cell carcinomas.[37] The humoral agent responsible for hypercalcemia, a parathyroid hormone related peptide that shares many of the actions of parathyroid hormone, has been identified.[38] It augments reabsorption of calcium by the kidneys, enhances excretion of phosphorus and urinary cyclic adenosine monophosphate by the kidneys, and augments skeletal resorption.[39] In addition, the action of prostaglandins and direct metastatic bone involvement may contribute to hypercalcemia, leading to symptoms of weakness, confusion, nausea, vomiting, and abdominal pain.[36]

Hypertrophic pulmonary osteoarthropathy occurs equally in patients with squamous cell or large cell carcinoma and adenocarcinoma of the lung but rarely in patients with small cell lung cancers.[7] Many affected patients have clubbing, as well as symmetric painful joints with periostitis and radiographic features of periostal thickening of long bones.[36]

Other paraneoplastic syndromes in patients with lung cancer include polymyositis, subacute cerebellar degeneration, nonbacterial thrombotic endocarditis, migratory thrombophlebitis, disseminated intravascular coagulation, anemia, and leukoerythroblastosis.[34]

PATHOLOGY

The four major histologic types of lung cancer and their approximate incidences are adenocarcinoma (33% to 35%), squamous cell carcinoma (30% to 32%), small cell carcinoma (20% to 25%) and large cell carcinoma (15% to 18%).[7] Adenocarcinoma has overtaken squamous cell cancer as the most common histologic type. Less commonly encountered types are adenosquamous tumors, cylindroma, mucoepidermoid tumors, and carcinoid tumors.[40] Squamous cell carcinoma, adenocarcinoma, and large cell cancers are referred to collectively as non-small cell cancers to distinguish them from small cell lung cancers, which have a unique natural history, clinical behavior, staging, and treatment.

Squamous cell carcinoma

Squamous cell carcinomas of the lungs typically develop in the lumen of large central airways from chronically damaged epithelial cells. These lesions tend to cavitate, invade adjacent structures, and grow centrally toward the main stem bronchus, leading to atelectasis, hemoptysis, and post-obstructive pneumonitis.[33] Pleural effusion may develop after nodal or thoracic duct invasion. Microscopic examination shows keratinization, pearl formation, intercellular bridges, and desmosomes. The cells have a low nucleus/cytoplasm ratio and few nucleoli (Fig. 18-4).

Adenocarcinoma

Adenocarcinoma is often first detected as a peripheral mass on the chest radiograph.[33] These lesions form acino-tubular structures, and most contain mucin-filled cytoplasmic vacuolations displacing the nucleus (Fig. 18-5). They tend to metastasize early, involving the central nervous system, liver, adrenal glands, and bone.[39]

Large cell carcinoma

Like adenocarcinoma, large cell cancers arise peripherally.[44] Microscopic examination shows abundant cytoplasm and enlarged hyperchromatic nuclei with prominent nucleoli and a low nucleus/cytoplasm ratio (Fig. 18-6). Diagnosis is determined by the histologic absence of features suggestive of adenocarcinoma and squamous cell carcinoma.[41] There are two subtypes of large cell carcinoma: giant cell and clear cell. The giant cell variety contains multinucleated cells and is aggressive; patients frequently have presenting symptoms of gastrointestinal metastasis.[41] Clear cell tumors have small cells with cytoplasmic glycogen.[41]

Small cell carcinoma

Three quarters of small cell carcinomas are situated proximally in the central airways and often present as submucosal endobronchial lesions.[7] Microscopic examination shows characteristic finely stippled nuclear chromatin and scanty cytoplasm (Fig. 18-7).[42] Small cell tumors progress more rapidly than non-small cell tumors, metastasize more frequently, and respond better to chemotherapy and radiation therapy. At the time of diagnosis, most small cell tumors extend beyond the confines of a hemithorax. They

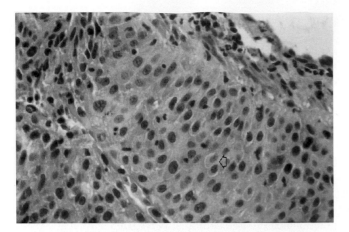

Fig. 18-4. Squamous cell carcinomas have large polygonal cells with prominent irregular nuclei. Note the arrow pointing at a cellular bridge, the light microscopic equivalent of a desmosome.

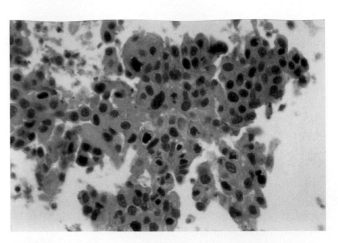

Fig. 18-6. Large cell carcinomas typically have very large irregular nuclei and abundant cytoplasm. Cells vary greatly in size and shape.

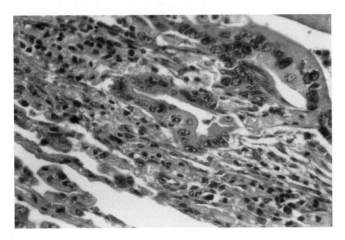

Fig. 18-5. Histologic section of adenocarcinoma showing well-defined glands composed of cells with large irregular hyperchromatic nuclei.

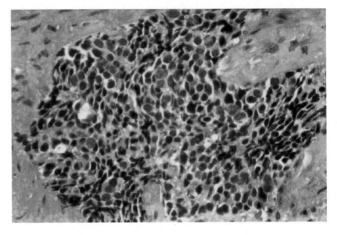

Fig. 18-7. Small cell carcinomas have cells about the size of lymphocytes with scanty cytoplasm.

typically metastasize to bone, bone marrow, liver, and brain and often cause superior vena caval obstruction and recurrent laryngeal nerve palsy.[43] Small cell cancers may cause various paraneoplastic syndromes, notably SIADH, Cushing's syndrome, the Eaton–Lambert syndrome, and cancer-associated retinopathy.[36,44]

Rare pulmonary neoplasms

Miller and Allen,[40] reviewing the histopathologic records of 10,134 patients with lung cancer at the Mayo Clinic during an 11-year period from 1980 through 1990, discovered 80 unusual pulmonary neoplasms. Non-Hodgkin's lymphoma was the most frequently encountered histologic type, followed closely by carcinosarcoma and mucoepidermoid carcinoma.[40] Solitary peripheral pulmonary lymphomas are usually cured by resection, and prognosis is therefore excellent. Carcinosarcomas are highly malignant, and prognosis is poor.[40]

Cell type and environmental exposure

In smokers the risk for squamous and small cell lung carcinomas is 20 to 25 times higher than for nonsmokers.[43] In contrast, the risk for adenocarcinoma is only three times as high for smokers than for nonsmokers.[43]

Using information obtained from the 1970 Finland census and the Finnish Cancer Registry from 1971 to 1980, Sankila and associates[45] noted a high association between farming, mining, and quarrying and small cell carcinoma. Servicemen, repairmen, and welders had an increased risk of epidermoid carcinoma. Vallyathan and associates[46] studied 171 coal miners with lung cancer and found no difference in the incidence of histologic types compared with that of smokers in the general population. Squamous cell carcinoma was the most common, followed by adenocarcinoma, small cell carcinoma, and large cell carcinoma.

Adenocarcinomas have been considered the most common type of lung cancer in asbestos-exposed workers, but

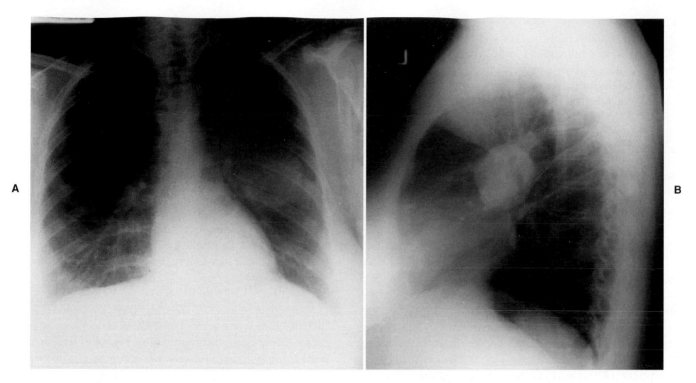

Fig. 18-8. A and **B,** Chest radiograph showing a round 5-cm mass located in the left upper lobe abutting and displacing the major fissure. No calcifications nor involvement of the pleura or ribs is seen.

Churg,[47] in a review of 471 cases of lung cancer in workers exposed to asbestos, found that squamous cell and small cell carcinomas were more common, accounting for 43% and 28%, respectively, of the cases. Adenocarcinomas accounted for only 19%, and large cell carcinomas were the least common, occurring in only 10% of the cases. Furthermore, no significant difference was found in the incidence of adenocarcinomas and large cell carcinomas between asbestos-exposed and nonexposed controls.

SCREENING

Screening for lung cancer with chest radiography and cytologic analysis of sputum is controversial, with proponents reporting a survival advantage and improved surgical results for patients diagnosed by mass screening.[48] Some advocates claim that screening may reduce mortality by almost 28%.[49] However, the American Cancer Society recommends that chest radiography and sputum cytology not be used for screening.[50] A National Cancer Institute study of lung cancer screening conducted at the Memorial Sloan–Kettering Cancer Center, Johns Hopkins University Hospital, and the Mayo Clinic, including more than 30,000 men with increased risk of lung cancer, concluded that screening is not cost effective.[51-53]

Screening workers employed in increased-risk occupations with chest radiography and cytologic analysis of sputum is being advocated by some to improve prognosis through early detection. Although it is not clear whether screening for occupational lung cancer will lead to improved outcome, screening programs for high-risk smokers have not improved outcome from lung cancer.[54]

DIAGNOSIS
Chest radiography

The chest radiograph is more sensitive than cytologic analysis of sputum for detecting lung cancer (Fig. 18-8A and B).[55] Central tumors may appear on the chest radiograph as abnormal hilar contours or postobstructive atelectasis.[55] Peripheral tumors larger than 2 to 3 mm in diameter may be detectable radiographically, but most peripheral tumors are 1 cm or larger at the time of diagnosis. Conventional chest radiography has an accuracy of 70% to 88% in the detection of lung cancer.[56] Although it is difficult to determine whether a mass on the chest radiograph is benign or malignant, malignant lesions have certain characteristic features, including a spiculated or poorly defined margin, eccentric calcification, a doubling time of less than 18 months, and a size larger than 3 cm.[57] Homogeneous, ringlike, or popcornlike calcification favors benignity.[7] Squamous cell and small cell carcinomas are typically central, whereas large cell carcinoma and adenocarcinomas tend to be peripheral.[33] Tumors arising in the apical segments of the upper lobes may be difficult to detect radiographically because of the overlying bony structures.

The lungs are a frequent site of metastasis of tumors from the breast, head and neck, colon, and genitourinary tract, including the prostate.[58] The radiographic patterns of pulmonary metastatic lesions include multiple bilateral peripheral nodules, reticulonodular infiltrates, masses with or without cavitation, mediastinal adenopathy, and pleural effusions.[58] Metastatic adenocarcinoma of the breast, stomach, and pancreas are suggested by a lymphangitic pattern on the chest radiograph.[58] Colorectal and renal cancers, as well as melanomas and sarcomas, often manifest as large "cannonball" tumors.[58]

Chest computerized tomographic scanning and magnetic resonance imaging

Once a lung tumor is detected on the chest radiograph, a chest computerized tomographic (CT) scan may be obtained for further evaluation (Fig. 18-9). The CT scan is useful for evaluating endobronchial structures, the pulmonary hila, the mediastinum, and the chest wall, and can be used to guide transcutaneous needle biopsies. Furthermore, the chest CT scan is routinely extended below the diaphragm to visualize the intraabdominal structures, including the liver and the adrenal glands. In general, chest CT scanning is more readily available, costs less, and offers better spatial resolution than magnetic resonance imaging (MRI).[57]

The MRI technique, however, does not emit ionizing radiation and can image over several planes. In addition to the horizontal or transaxial plane that can be obtained from CT scanning, MRI may image nonaxial planes including sagittal cuts. The latter is particularly helpful in visualizing superior sulcus tumors. This method is also sensitive to flow and does not, therefore, require the use of intravenous contrast media to detect vascular structures, making it useful

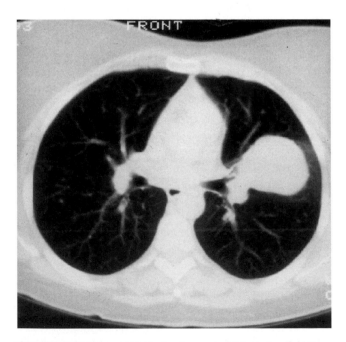

Fig. 18-9. A chest computerized tomographic scan showing a round left upper lobe mass.

for evaluating possible tumor involvement of the superior vena cava.[57]

Magnetic resonance imaging is more sensitive than CT for (1) differentiating postobstructive atelectasis from the tumor mass; (2) determining tumor extension to the chest wall, heart, and major vessels; (3) documenting metastatic involvement of the brain; and (4) distinguishing posttherapy scar formation from recurrence of the tumor.[56]

A solitary pulmonary nodule can be evaluated by CT using a reference phantom.[59] Lesions that are more dense than the phantom and contain more than 10% calcium are likely benign, but lesions that contain less than 10% calcium should be investigated further. Phantom scanning is not recommended in patients with gastrointestinal or genitourinary mucinous carcinomas and integumentary sarcomas, which may develop calcium-rich metastatic lesions.[59]

Obtaining tissue samples

Pathologic diagnosis of lung cancer is essential for therapy. Tumor tissue can be obtained by cytologic examination of sputum, fiberoptic bronchoscopy, transthoracic needle biopsy, pleural biopsy, mediastinoscopy, or mediastinotomy to confirm the diagnosis of lung cancer.

Sputum cytology. Cytologic examination of three sputum specimens has a reported sensitivity rate of 80% for central tumors and 50% for peripheral ones.[33] The diagnostic yield may be improved by inducing sputum production with an ultrasonic nebulizer.[60] Cell morphology in sputum is more apparent in a fresh specimen; therefore, morning sputum samples, either spontaneously produced from a deep cough or induced, are collected and examined microscopically before being fixed in 95% ethyl alcohol.[61] In an alternative method, the Saccomanno technique, the sputum is immediately fixed with 50% ethyl alcohol and 2% polyethylene glycol. This method, however, provides inferior morphologic detail and is less sensitive for detecting small cell carcinoma.[62]

The diagnostic yield of sputum examination is higher for central and upper lobes and large (T_3) lesions and lower for peripheral, lower lobe, and small (T_1) tumors.[61,63,64] The diagnostic yield of sputum examination is highest for squamous cell carcinomas and lowest for adenocarcinoma,[65,66] with the yield for small cell and large cell carcinomas being intermediate. The concordance between sputum cytologic examination and tissue histologic diagnosis is highest for the centrally located tumors and squamous or small cell lesions and lowest for large cell subtypes.[67,68]

Cytologic examination of sputum has a high specificity for lung cancer but a low sensitivity, and therefore a high false-negative rate.[69-71] False-negative results may be caused by total bronchial occlusion, inflammation within the tumor, and sloughing of necrotic cells by large tumors.[66,69,72] The use of monoclonal antibodies, DNA image cytometry, and quantitative cytology may improve the diagnostic yield of sputum examination.[73-75]

Bronchoscopy. Flexible fiberoptic bronchoscopy is one of the most useful invasive procedures in the initial evaluation of a suspected lung cancer. With bronchoscopy, endobronchial lesions to the level of the subsegmental divisions of the bronchial tree can be directly seen; bronchoscopy is therefore the preferred method for evaluating proximal lesions.[76] Specimens for cytologic and histologic analyses can be obtained by forceps biopsy, brush biopsy, bronchial washing, or transbronchial needle biopsy. The diagnostic yield from forceps biopsy ranges from 55% to 85% for central lesions and from 15% to 46% for peripheral lesions. For central tumors bronchial brushing and washing are as accurate as forceps biopsy, with the yield ranging from 62% to 78%. For peripheral lesions the diagnostic yield falls to 29% to 50% for brushing and 42% to 46% for bronchial washing.[76]

Transbronchial needle aspiration is increasingly used in staging malignant disease of hilar and mediastinal lymph nodes and in diagnosing tumors presenting as either submucosal lesions or extrinsic masses adjacent to the bronchial tree.[77] Overall, transbronchial needle aspiration has a diagnostic yield as high as 97% for central tumors when used with forceps biopsy and bronchial washing and brushing.[78] Pneumothorax, the most common complication, occurs in only 0.5% of patients, and significant hemorrhage is rare.[76]

The recent introduction of the analysis of tumor markers in bronchoalveolar lavage fluid[76] and fluorescence bronchoscopy,[79] wherein the patient inhales fluorescein and bronchoscopy is performed with an ultraviolet light source, may further increase diagnostic yield.

Flexible fiberoptic bronchoscopy is safe in experienced hands. Minor complications (including hypoxemia, bleeding less than 50 ml, and cardiac arrhythmias) were noted in 10% or fewer patients by 80% of the respondents in a recent American College of Chest Physicians survey.[80] Major complications are even more rare.

Transthoracic needle biopsy. Because bronchoscopy has an unacceptably low yield for small peripheral lesions, particularly tumors less than 2.0 cm in diameter, transthoracic needle biopsy is the diagnostic procedure of choice for these lesions. It is also useful in diagnosing focal lung metastases and hilar and mediastinal masses.[81] With fluoroscopic or CT guidance, percutaneous transthoracic needle biopsy has a sensitivity rate of over 90% in the diagnosis of lung cancer.[81,82] Fluoroscopy is often used because of its greater availability and simplicity, but small peripheral lesions can be seen better with CT guidance.[83] The CT scan is also used for transthoracic needle biopsies of hilar, mediastinal, and thoracic inlet lesions; for lesions obstructing the superior vena cava; and in patients with chronic obstructive pulmonary disease (COPD).[83,84]

Pneumothorax, which is the main complication of transthoracic needle aspiration, occurs significantly more often (1) in patients with underlying COPD,[85] (2) when multiple biopsies are obtained from deep lung lesions, and (3) in elderly patients.[86,87] The incidence of pneumothorax is 7% in patients without COPD and 46% in those with COPD.[85] Other complications include hemoptysis and air embolism.[88] Transthoracic needle aspiration is contraindicated in patients with a coagulopathy, in uncooperative patients, and in patients with suspected vascular lesions or hydatid cysts.[88]

Other procedures. In patients with lung cancer and a pleural effusion, a diagnostic thoracentesis may be useful. Percutaneous needle biopsy of the pleura may improve the yield further.[89,90] Thoracoscopically guided biopsy of the pleural and peripheral parenchymal lesions under direct vision is being increasingly used.

STAGING

Accurate staging of lung cancer is also essential for therapy. The new international staging system published in 1986 replaced the 1979 classification developed by the American Joint Committee for Cancer Staging and End Results Reporting.[91-93] Both systems characterize the primary tumor (T), regional lymph nodes (N), and distant metastases (M), and are used for all types of non-small cell lung cancer (Table 18-1). Small cell cancer is staged as either limited or extensive (Table 18-2). Limited disease is confined to one hemithorax, the mediastinum, or the ipsilateral supraclavicular space; extensive disease extends beyond the confines of the hemithorax and the adjacent lymph nodes, or either recurs after radiotherapy or induces a malignant pleural effusion.[91] The TNM classification may be combined into six clinical stages, each with its own management options and expected survival rates (Table 18-3). Stage 0 is carcinoma in situ. Stage I comprises lesions contained in the lungs and includes T_1 or T_2 tumors without the involvement of regional lymph nodes or distant metastases. Clinical stage I disease has the best prognosis, with 5-year postoperative survival rates between 40% and 60%.[94] Clinical stage II includes disease involving the peribronchial and ipsilateral hilar lymph nodes (N_2). Patients with clinical stage II disease are candidates for resection, but the 5-year survival rate is only 20% to 40%.[94] Clinical stage IIIa includes lesions that extend to the pericardium, chest wall, or mediastinal pleura or the presence of ipsilateral lymph nodes.[91] Stage IIIa also includes lesions within 2 cm of the main carina but are not involving it. Surgical resection remains an option for selected patients with clinical stage IIIa disease, but 5-year survival, despite surgical resection, is less than 20%.[94]

Clinical stage IIIb tumors involve the vertebrae, heart and great vessels, esophagus, trachea, carina, contralateral mediastinal and hilar lymph nodes, and scalene and supraclavicular nodes or have induced a malignant pleural effusion.[91] The 5-year survival rate is less than 5%, and patients with stage IIIb disease are not considered candidates for surgical resection.[94] Stage IV consists of extrathoracic meta-

Table 18-1. Classifications and stages of non-small cell lung cancer

Primary tumor (T)

T_X Tumor proven by the presence of malignant cells in bronchopulmonary secretions but not visualized roentgenographically or bronchoscopically, or any tumor that cannot be assessed, as in a retreatment staging

T_0 No evidence of primary tumor

T_{IS} Carcinoma in situ

T_1 A tumor that is 3 cm or less in greatest dimension, surrounded by lung or visceral pleura, and without evidence of invasion proximal to a lobar bronchus at bronchoscopy*

T_2 A tumor more than 3 cm in greatest dimension or a tumor of any size that either invades the visceral pleura or has associated atelectasis or obstructive pneumonitis extending to the hilar region. At bronchoscopy the proximal extent of demonstrable tumor must be within a lobar bronchus or at least 2.0 cm distal to the carina. Any associated atelectasis or obstructive pneumonitis must involve less than an entire lung

T_3 A tumor of any size with direct extension into the chest wall (including superior sulcus tumors), the diaphragm, or the mediastinal pleura or pericardium without involving the heart, great vessels, trachea, esophagus, or vertebral body, or a tumor in the main bronchus within 2 cm of the carina without involving the carina

T_4 A tumor of any size with invasion of the mediastinum or involving the heart, great vessels, trachea, esophagus, vertebral body, or carina or the presence of malignant pleural effusion†

Nodal involvement (N)

N_0 No demonstrable metastasis to regional lymph nodes

N_1 Metastasis to lymph nodes in the peribronchial or ipsilateral hilar region, or both, including direct extension

N_2 Metastasis to ipsilateral mediastinal and subcarinal lymph nodes

N_3 Metastasis to contralateral mediastinal lymph nodes, contralateral hilar lymph nodes, or ipsilateral or contralateral scalene or supraclavicular lymph nodes

Distant metastasis (M)

M_0 No (known) distant metastasis

M_1 Distant metastasis present—specify site(s)

From Mountain CF: A new international staging system for lung cancer, *Chest* 89(suppl):225S-233S, 1986. With permission.

*The uncommon superficial tumor of any size with its invasive component limited to the bronchial wall that may extend proximal to the main bronchus is classified as T_1.

†Most pleural effusions associated with lung cancer are due to tumor. There are, however, a few patients in whom results of cytopathologic examination of pleural fluid (on more than one specimen) are negative for tumor; the fluid is nonbloody and is not an exudate. In such cases in which these elements and clinical judgment dictate that the effusion is not related to the tumor, the patient should be staged T_1, T_2, or T_3, excluding effusion *as a staging element*.

Table 18-2. Definition of limited and extensive stage for patients with small cell lung cancer

Stage	Percentage
Limited: Disease confined to one hemithorax with or without ipsilateral or contralateral mediastinal or supraclavicular lymph node metastasis, and with or without ipsilateral pleural effusions independent of cytology	30%-40%
Extensive: Any disease at sites beyond the definition of limited disease	60%-70%

Adapted from Stahel RA, Ginsberg R, Havemann K, et al: Staging and prognostic factors in small cell lung cancer: a consensus report, *Lung Cancer* 5:119, 1989. With permission.

Table 18-3. Stage grouping of TNM subsets in the new system of lung cancer staging

Occult carcinoma	T_X	N_0	M_0
Stage 0	T_{IS}	Carcinoma in situ	Carcinoma in situ
Stage I	T_1	N_0	M_0
	T_2	N_0	M_0
Stage II	T_1	N_1	M_0
	T_2	N_1	M_0
Stage IIIa	T_3	N_0	M_0
	T_3	N_1	M_0
	T_{1-3}	N_2	M_0
Stage IIIb	Any T	N_3	M_0
	T_4	Any N	M_0
Stage IV	Any T	Any N	M_1

From Mountain CF: A new international staging system for lung cancer, *Chest* 89(suppl):225S-233S, 1986. With permission.

static disease, and affected patients have a dismal prognosis (Fig. 18-10).

Only 20% to 25% of patients with non-small cell lung cancer have resectable disease.[95] Therefore staging often documents regional or distant involvement, which obviates curative resection. Small cell cancers metastasize widely early in their natural history, and staging often shows silent metastatic disease; however, in non-small cell lung cancer staging rarely reveals extension in asymptomatic patients.[96]

Staging starts with a comprehensive laboratory study, including a complete blood cell count, measurement of serum electrolytes and calcium, and liver function tests. Imaging modalities that are used for staging include chest and brain CT scans and radionuclide scans of the bone, liver, and spleen. Bone, brain, liver, and spleen scans are recommended only when symptoms or signs suggest other organ involvement in patients with non-small cell lung cancers. On the other hand, these scans, along with bone marrow biopsies, are routinely performed to detect metastasis in patients with small cell lung cancer.[97]

The chest CT scan is routinely used to evaluate mediastinal disease. Unless obvious heavy mediastinal involve-

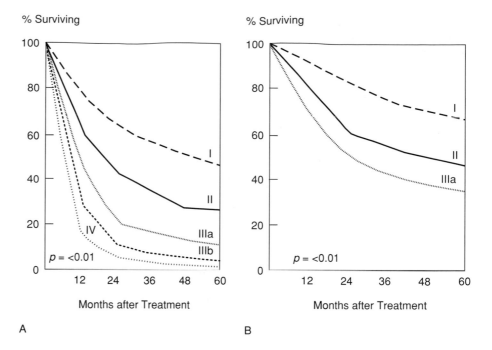

% Surviving

% Surviving

Fig. 18-10. Cumulative proportion of patients with non-small cell lung cancer expected to survive 5 years or more according to (**A**) clinical and (**B**) surgical pathologic stages, operative deaths excluded (1975 to 1982 collected series). (From Mountain CF: Lung cancer staging classification, *Clin Chest Med* 14:43-53, 1993. With permission.)

A

B

Months after Treatment

Months after Treatment

ment is detected on initial chest radiographs, the chest CT scan is indicated in all patients being considered for surgery.[95] Most surgeons proceed at once to thoracotomy in patients with lymph nodes smaller than 1 cm, reserving preoperative mediastinoscopy and mediastinotomy for patients with nodes larger than 1 cm.[98] The chest CT scan, however, cannot usually differentiate benign from malignant lymphadenopathy. Lymph nodes smaller than 1.0 cm contain malignant cells 7% of the time, and larger nodes may be tumor free.[95] There is incidence of occult metastatic involvement in patients with multiple small nodes, and therefore preoperative mediastinoscopy may be undertaken even if the nodes are smaller than 1 cm.[95] The MRI method adds little to information gleaned from the chest CT scan and is rarely used in the evaluation of mediastinal involvement.[95]

Mediastinoscopy and mediastinotomy are among the invasive procedures used to obtain specimens from the mediastinal lymph nodes. Anterior mediastinoscopy or mediastinotomy consisting of a limited parasternal thoracotomy (the Chamberlain procedure) is necessary to sample lymph nodes involving the anterior mediastinal region. The superior mediastinum may be reached by cervical mediastinoscopy. The diagnostic yield of mediastinoscopy is highest for small cell and large cell carcinomas.[7] Mediastinoscopy is contraindicated if the patient has had prior mediastinal irradiation or tracheotomy.

Biopsies of the adrenal glands, liver, and supraclavicular or other lymph nodes should be obtained if imaging studies suggest metastatic involvement. If a biopsy specimen is positive, the tumor is unresectable, and nonsurgical treatment must be considered.

TREATMENT
Surgery

Surgery is the primary curative treatment for non-small cell bronchogenic carcinoma, but, as previously stated, only 20% to 25% of affected patients are candidates for surgery.[95]

Patients with moderate to severe pulmonary hypertension, hypercapnia [carbon dioxide tension ($Paco_2$), >45 mm Hg] or severe hypoxemia breathing room air [arterial oxygen tension (Pao_2), <50 mm Hg], recent myocardial infarction, severe heart failure, and uncontrolled arrhythmia are high surgical risks.[7,95]

The cardiopulmonary system is routinely evaluated to determine whether a patient will tolerate surgery; the evaluation commonly includes pulmonary function testing, measurement of arterial blood gases, and an electrocardiogram.[95] An electrocardiogram is adequate for most patients, but those with arrhythmias, angina, previous myocardial infarction, congestive heart failure, or an abnormal electrocardiogram should undergo cardiac stress testing.[95]

Pulmonary function testing may help determine surgical risk and predict postoperative outcome. The surgical risk of pneumonectomy is acceptable if the patient's forced vital capacity (FVC) and forced expiratory volume in 1 second (FEV1) are at least 80% of predicted values.[99] If the patient's preoperative FEV1 is below 80% of the predicted value, a quantitative ventilation–perfusion lung scan, using either xenon 133 or krypton-81m radiospirometry and technetium-99m–labeled macroaggregated albumin, may be done to determine the postoperative residual lung function.[99-101] The predicted postoperative FEV1 is calculated by multiplying the preoperative FEV1 by the per centage of remaining lung assessed by the ventilation–perfusion lung scan; a projected postoperative FEV1 over 40% of that predicted in an asymptomatic patient is acceptable, whereas a projected FEV1 less than 30% of the predicted value predicts a poor outcome. Other variables associated with high mortality and morbidity are a calculated postoperative diffusing capacity for carbon monoxide less than 40% of that predicted and exercise-induced arterial desaturation of more than 2%.[99] Smith and associates[102] performed preoperative exercise testing on 22 patients and found that patients rarely develop postthoracotomy complications if the maximal oxygen consumption was greater than 20 ml/kg/min, whereas all patients with maximal oxygen consumption less than 10 ml/kg/min developed complications.

The goal of surgery is to remove all tumor-involved tissue while preserving as much normal lung parenchyma as possible. Lobectomy is the procedure of choice for patients with tumors confined to a lobe without regional nodal involvement.[103] Complications of lobectomy, which include arrhythmias, persistent air space between the remaining lung and the chest wall, atelectasis, and hemothorax, are rare, and the 30-day mortality rate is only 3%.[95,103] Less extensive procedures, such as segmentectomy or wedge resection, may be done for small peripheral tumors ($T_1N_0M_0$), particularly in patients with reduced lung function. However, patients who undergo these less extensive procedures have a higher recurrence rate than those who undergo lobectomy.[104] More extensive local disease may require a bilobectomy or a pneumonectomy. Pneumonectomy has a higher mortality and rate of complications, which include cardiac arrhythmias, bronchopleural fistula, and delayed pulmonary hypertension.[103]

Surgery is the treatment of choice for patients with stage I or II and for a select group of patients with stage IIIa (T_3N_0) non-small cell lung carcinoma.[95] Surgery is not indicated in patients with stage IIIb or IV disease. Patients with stage IIIa disease often have distant metastases, and therefore adjuvant chemotherapy and radiotherapy are often used, although adjuvant therapy has not been shown to improve survival.[105-107]

The role of surgery for small cell lung cancer is undefined, and trials are under way to evaluate primary surgical therapy followed by adjuvant chemotherapy, with or without radiation therapy, and to evaluate adjuvant surgery after subtotal eradication of the lesion by chemotherapy.[108,109]

The in-hospital postoperative mortality rate in patients who undergo resection ranged from 3.7% for a segmental resection, to 4.2% for lobectomy, to 11.6% for pneumonectomy in a community hospital.[110] Postoperative mortality is lower in academic and referral centers.[110] Patients with completely resected lung cancer most commonly die of cardiovascular diseases, COPD, or new cancers, either a second primary lung tumor or a tumor involving other organ(s).[111]

Survival for patients with resected non-small cell cancers depends principally on the stage of the disease. The outlook is best for patients with radiographically occult carcinomas who have a median survival after surgery of about 9 years.[112] Burt and Martini[112] have not seen any case of recurrence of the original tumor after resection of a radiographically occult lung cancer on long-term follow-up. However, up to 45% of the patients in their series developed new carcinomas, mostly involving the airways. They therefore recommend continued follow-up of patients with resected radiographically occult tumors once or twice annually to detect possible new cancers.

The 5-year survival rate ranges from 60% to 80% for surgical stage I cancers.[94] Patients with $T_1N_0M_0$ lesions at the time of surgery have a 5-year survival rate of 80% to 83%, whereas patients with $T_2N_0M_0$ tumors have a survival rate of 62% to 65%.[112] Because cancer recurs or a new primary tumor develops in a large percentage of patients, periodic evaluation, including chest radiography, is recommended every 3 months during the first year, every 4 months during the second year, and every 6 months thereafter.[112]

The 5-year survival falls to between 40% and 60% for surgical stage II patients and below 40% for those with surgical stage IIIa cancers.[94] Recurrence is a major problem with stage II lesions. Martini and associates[113] observed an 11% local and regional recurrence rate and 39% distant recurrence. Recurrence tends to be distant for adenocarcinomas and local for squamous cell cancers.[113]

Patients with surgical stage IIIb with invasion of mediastinal structures have an overall survival of only 7% after 5 years.[112] The average survival rate for patients with stage IV non-small cell cancers with solitary brain metastasis ranges from less than 1 month to 6 months from the onset of symptoms.[114,115]

Small cell carcinoma has a poorer prognosis than non-small cell cancers. The 2-year survival rate is 12% to 21% for limited and 1% to 4% for extensive small cell cancer (Fig. 18-11).[43] Aside from disease stage, other features may be prognostically significant. A poor initial performance status, male gender, increased serum lactate dehydrogenase concentration, and the presence of skeletal and hepatic metastases negatively influence the outcome of small cell cancer patients.[116] The increased serum lactate dehydrogenase may result from a large tumor burden.

Initial performance status is also an important prognostic factor for inoperable non-small cell carcinomas. Histologic characteristics of the tumor have been shown to influence the survival rate among operable non-small cell cancers.

Chemotherapy

Non-small cell lung cancer. Chemotherapy has not shown clear benefit for non-small cell carcinoma at any stage. Although various agents have been shown to induce

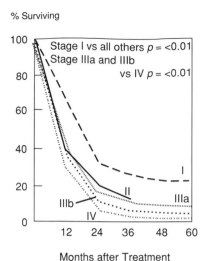

% Surviving

Stage I vs all others *p* = <0.01
Stage IIIa and IIIb
vs IV *p* = <0.01

Months after Treatment

Fig. 18-11. Cumulative proportion of patients with small cell lung cancer expected to survive 5 years or more according to clinical stage. (From Mountain CF: Prognostic implications of the international staging system for lung cancer, *Semin Oncol* 15:236, 1988. With permission.)

remission, the response is usually partial and short-lived.[33] Trials of combination chemotherapy have been disappointing, and no clear consensus has emerged.[33] Furthermore, adjuvant chemotherapy after surgical resection of stage I, II, and IIIa disease has not significantly improved either disease-free or overall survival.[107]

Small cell lung cancer. On the other hand, chemotherapy traditionally has been considered the primary therapy for small cell carcinoma.[33] Before the introduction of nitrogen mustard in the 1940s, the median survival for patients with small cell lung cancers was 10 weeks. With combination chemotherapy the median survival has increased from 5 to 14 months.[117] Overall response rates to chemotherapy are 80% for limited disease and 60% for extensive disease.[2] The 2-year survival rate is 12% to 21% for limited disease and 1% to 4% for extensive disease.[2] Frequently used regimens include vincristine, Adriamycin (doxorubicin), and cyclophosphamide (VAC); lomustine (CCNU), methotrexate, and cyclophosphamide (CMC); and etoposide and cisplatin (EP).[116] Therapy with VAC or EP may induce a complete response rate of over 50% in limited disease and 20% in extensive disease.[116,118] Patients with limited disease have a median survival of over 14 months and a 2-year cancer-free survival rate of 20% to 25% with these regimens.[116] Although patients with extensive disease rarely achieve 2-year cancer-free survival despite chemotherapy, their median survival may be increased to over 7 months.[116]

Radiation therapy

Radiation therapy, or radiotherapy, may be considered for patients with potentially resectable, localized non-small cell cancer who have an unacceptably high surgical risk because of coexisting illnesses or for patients who refuse surgery.[33] Although postoperative radiation therapy after complete resection of stage II and IIIa lung cancers does not improve survival, it may diminish the incidence of local recurrent disease.[119,120] It has also been used after incomplete resection of non-small cell cancers, either alone or in combination with chemotherapy. Radiation therapy is usually offered to patients with residual cancer at the margin of resection.[119] Prophylactic cranial irradiation in stage II non-small cell carcinoma is routinely offered in some centers and is reported to delay the development of metastatic lesions but has not been shown to improve outcome.[121]

In patients with small cell lung cancer, radiotherapy has been used alone or combined with chemotherapy. With radiotherapy the overall response rate is about 75%.[116,122,123] Radiotherapy combined with chemotherapy for limited small cell lung cancer results in approximately a 5% additional survival at 2 and 3 years over combination chemotherapy alone.[116] However, toxicity and mortality are increased in patients who receive combined radiotherapy and chemotherapy.[116]

For patients with extensive small lung cell cancers, radiotherapy is used for palliation of cranial, skeletal, or orbital metastasis. Hemoptysis and local pain from bony metastasis also may be alleviated by radiation therapy. Chest radiotherapy does not improve survival in patients with extensive small cell lung cancer and has no therapeutic role.[107,116]

When radiation is used with curative intent, either a continuous or split-course schedule may be chosen. Patients are offered 50 to 60 Gy of megavoltage therapy in 200-cGy fractions given 5 days each week for 5 to 6 weeks or in two courses several weeks apart.[107]

Small cell carcinomas are the most radiosensitive and may be eradicated following treatment with 35 to 40 Gy.[7] Squamous cell carcinoma and adenocarcinoma are less radiosensitive than small cell cancer, and large cell tumors are the least radiosensitive.

The primary complication of thoracic irradiation is acute pneumonitis, which often occurs 1 to 3 months after therapy. It may present as dyspnea and nonproductive cough. The chest radiograph characteristically demonstrates a sharply outlined infiltrate matching the radiation port. Most patients improve over several weeks. Subacute radiation fibrosis may also occur several months after radiation therapy. Depending on the organ situated within the radiation port and the dose administered, patients may develop esophagitis, spinal cord toxicity, central nervous system dysfunction (e.g., memory loss, optic atrophy, or dysphonia), and cardiomyopathies.[33]

Supportive care

Chemotherapy may cause nausea, anorexia, and mucositis, and the treated patient's nutritional status must be closely monitored. Moreover, patients treated with cytotoxic drugs may become myelosuppressed and neutropenic, and therefore prone to infection. Granulocyte–macrophage colony-stimulating factor therapy has been shown to shorten the duration of neutropenia.[124] Fever should prompt a thorough search for possible infection, which, if present, must be promptly and aggressively treated.

Cancer pain may be managed in a stepwise fashion, with nonsteroidal antiinflammatory agents as first-line drugs. Narcotic medications must be considered for refractory pain. Corticosteroids and antidepressants may also alleviate some cancer pain.[2,43]

The clinician must always be alert for the development of a treatable paraneoplastic syndrome. Hyponatremia from SIADH may be managed by simply limiting water intake, often in combination with a loop diuretic to enhance the excretion of free water. Demeclocycline and lithium carbonate are additional therapeutic options. Elevated serum calcium may be corrected by forced saline diuresis or therapy with biphosphonates, gallium nitrate calcitonin, or mithramycin.[36] Adrenal inhibitors (aminoglutethimide and metyrapone), bilateral adrenalectomy, or adrenal arterial embolization may offer significant relief to patients with Cushing's syndrome.[36]

Patients with Eaton–Lambert syndrome may respond to therapy with corticosteroids, azathioprine, or cholinesterases, or to 3,4-diaminopyridine, which facilitates presynaptic acetylcholine release.[36]

Psychosocial issues, caregiver stress, financial difficulties, and other patient concerns should be identified and managed. Often, the only way such varied difficulties can be properly addressed is with a team approach involving the patient's physician(s), social workers, dietitians, nurses, pharmacists, financial planners, and legal advisors working closely with the patient and the patient's family.

CONCLUSION

Lung cancer is a major worldwide health problem. Although tobacco smoking is by far its most common cause, occupational exposure to carcinogens results in a substantial number of lung cancers. As the prevalence of cigarette smoking continues to decrease and as more new substances are introduced into the workplace, the proportion of occupational lung carcinomas is expected to increase. Until newer, more effective screening and treatment strategies are discovered, the major measures available to reduce the death rate from lung cancer are to encourage smoking prevention and cessation and to decrease workplace exposure to known carcinogens. Once lung cancer is suspected, a deliberate and thorough evaluation must be undertaken. This invariably includes obtaining tissue samples for cytologic and histologic confirmation. Proper staging is crucial in choosing the most appropriate therapeutic modality and in predicting survival.

ACKNOWLEDGMENTS

We wish to thank Dr. Eric Hyson, Dr. Marc Eisenberg, Dr. J. Bernard L. Gee, Dr. Matthew Bushey, William Coffey, Leslye Stein, and Grace Zamudio.

REFERENCES

1. Boring CC, Squires TS, and Tong T: Cancer statistics, 1993, *CA* 43:7-26, 1993.
2. O'Rourke MA and Crawford J: Lung cancer in the elderly, *Compr Ther* 14:47-54, 1988.
3. US Department of Health and Human Services: *The health consequences of smoking: cancer and chronic lung disease in the workplace. A report of the Surgeon General*, Office on Smoking and Health Pub No 85-50207, Washington, DC, 1985, US Department of Health and Human Services.
4. Garfinkel L and Silverberg E: Lung cancer and smoking trends in the United States over the past 25 years, *CA* 41:137-145, 1991.
5. Doll R and Peto R: The causes of cancer: quantitative estimates of avoidable risks of cancer in the United States today, *JNCI* 66:1191-1308, 1981.
6. Loeb L, Einster VL, Warner KE, et al: Smoking and lung cancer: an overview, *Cancer Res* 44:5940-5948, 1984.
7. Matthay RA and Carter DC: Lung neoplasms. In George RB, Light RW, Matthay MA, et al, editors: *Chest medicine: essentials of pulmonary and critical care medicine*, ed 2, pp 353-379, Baltimore, 1990, Williams & Wilkins.
8. Gazdar AF, Carney DN, and Minna JD: The biology of non-small cell lung cancer, *Semin Oncol* 10:3-19, 1983.
9. Preston-Martin S: Evaluation of the evidence that tobacco-specific nitrosamine (TSNA) causes cancer in humans, *Crit Rev Toxicol* 21:295-298, 1991.
10. US Department of Health and Human Services: *The health consequences of smoking: cancer. A report of the Surgeon General*, Pub No 82-50179, Washington, DC, 1982, US Department of Health and Human Services.
11. US Department of Health and Human Services, Centers for Disease Control: *Health consequences of involuntary smoking: a report of the Surgeon General*, No. CDC 87-8398, Washington, DC, 1986, US Government Printing Office.
12. Miller GH: The impact of passive smoking: cancer deaths among nonsmoking women, *Cancer Detect Prev* 14:497-503, 1990.
13. National Research Council, Committee on Passive Smoking: *Environmental tobacco smoke: measuring exposures and assessing health effects*, Washington, DC, 1986, National Academy Press.
14. Sandler DP, Everson RB, and Wilcox AJ: Passive smoking in adulthood and cancer risk, *Am J Epidemiol* 121:37-48, 1985.
15. Davila DG and Williams DE: The etiology of lung cancer, *Mayo Clin Proc* 68:170-182, 1993.
16. US Environmental Protection Agency: *Health effects of passive smoking: assessment of lung cancer in adults and respiratory disorders in children*, Rep No 6000690006A, Washington, DC, 1990, US Environmental Protection Agency.
17. Wynder EL: The etiology, epidemiology and prevention of lung cancer, *Semin Respir Med* 3:135-139, 1982.
18. Whitesell PL and Drage CW: Occupational lung cancer, *Mayo Clin Proc* 68:183-188, 1993.
19. Vineis P, Thomas T, Hayes RB, et al: Proportion of lung cancers in males, due to occupation in different areas of the US, *Int J Cancer* 42:851-856, 1988.
20. Shekelle RB, Lepper M, Liu S, et al: Dietary vitamin A and risk of cancer in the Western Electric Study, *Lancet* 28:1185-1190, 1981.
21. Fontham ETH: Protective dietary factors and lung cancer, *Int J Epidemiol* 19(suppl 1):S32-S42, 1990.
22. Omenn GS, Goodman G, Grizzle J, et al: CARET, the beta-carotene

and retinol efficacy trial to prevent lung cancer in asbestos-exposed workers and in smokers, *Anticancer Drugs* 2:79-86, 1991.

23. Sporn MB and Roberts AB: Role of retinoids in differentiation and carcinogenesis, *Cancer Res* 43:3034-3040, 1983.

24. Burton GW and Ingold KU: β-Carotene: an unusual type of lipid antioxidant, *Science* 224:569-573, 1984.

25. Block G: Vitamin C and cancer prevention: the epidemiologic evidence, *Am J Clin Nutr* 53:270S-282S, 1991.

26. Chung FL, Morse MA, and Eklind KI: New potential chemopreventive agents for lung carcinogenesis of tobacco-specific nitrosamine, *Cancer Res* 52:2719s-2722s, 1992.

27. Knekt P, Seppanen R, Jarvinen R, et al: Dietary cholesterol, fatty acids, and the risk of lung cancer among men, *Nutr Cancer* 16:267-275, 1991.

28. Tokuhata GK and Lilienfeld AM: Familial aggregation of lung cancer in humans, *JNCI* 30:289-312, 1963.

29. Viallet J and Minna JD: Dominant oncogenes and tumor suppressor genes in the pathogenesis of lung cancer, *Am J Respir Cell Mol Biol* 2:225-232, 1990.

30. Slebos RJC, Kibbelaar RE, Dalesio O, et al: K-*ras* oncogene activation as a prognostic marker in adenocarcinoma of the lung, *N Engl J Med* 323:561-565, 1990.

31. Ayesh R, Idle JR, Ritchie JC, et al: Metabolic oxidation phenotypes as markers for susceptibility to lung cancer, *Nature* 312:169-170, 1984.

32. Frank AL: The epidemiology and etiology of lung cancer, *Clin Chest Med* 3:219-228, 1982.

33. Carr DT and Holoye PY: Bronchogenic carcinoma. In Murray JF and Nadel JA, editors: *Textbook of respiratory medicine,* pp 1174-1250, Philadelphia, 1988, WB Saunders.

34. Ihde DC and Minna JD: Non-small cell lung cancer. Part I: biology, diagnosis, and staging, *Curr Probl Cancer* 15(2):63-104, 1991.

35. Patel AM and Peters SG: Clinical manifestations of lung cancer, *Mayo Clin Proc* 68:273-277, 1993.

36. Patel AM, Davila DG, and Peters SG: Paraneoplastic syndromes associated with lung cancer, *Mayo Clin Proc* 68:278-287, 1993.

37. Bender RA and Hansen H: Hypercalcemia in bronchogenic carcinoma: a prospective study of 200 patients, *Ann Intern Med* 80:205-208, 1974.

38. Broadus AE, Mangin M, Ikeda K, et al: Humoral hypercalcemia of cancer: identification of a novel parathyroid hormone-like peptide, *N Engl J Med* 319:556-563, 1988.

39. Yates AJP, Gutierrez GE, Smolens P, et al: Effects of a synthetic peptide of a parathyroid hormone-related protein on calcium homeostasis, renal tubular calcium reabsorption, and bone metabolism in vivo and in vitro in rodents, *J Clin Invest* 81:932-938, 1988.

40. Miller DL and Allen MS: Rare pulmonary neoplasms, *Mayo Clin Proc* 68:492-498, 1993.

41. Yesner R and Carter D: Pathogenesis and pathology [of lung cancer], *Clin Chest Med* 14:17-30, 1993.

42. Hirsch FR, Matthews MJ, Aisner S, et al: Histopathologic classification of small cell lung cancer: changing concepts and terminology, *Cancer* 62:973-977, 1988.

43. O'Rourke MA and Crawford J: Lung cancer in the elderly, *Clin Geriatr Med* 3:595-623, 1987.

44. Thirkill CE, Fitzgerald P, Sergoff RC, et al: Cancer-associated retinopathy (CAR syndrome) with antibodies reacting with retinal optic nerve and cancer cells, *N Engl J Med* 321:1589-1594, 1989.

45. Sankila RJ, Karjalainen ES, Oksanen HM, et al: Relationship between occupation and lung cancer as analyzed by age and histologic type, *Cancer* 65:1651-1656, 1990.

46. Vallyathan V, Green FH, Rodman NR, et al: Lung carcinoma by histologic type in coal miners, *Arch Pathol Lab Med* 109:419-423, 1985.

47. Churg A: Lung cancer cell type and asbestos exposure, *JAMA* 253:2984-2985, 1985.

48. Shimizu N, Ando A, Teramoto S, et al: Outcome of patients with lung cancer detected via mass screening as compared to those presenting with symptoms, *J Surg Oncol* 50:7-11, 1992.

49. Sobue T, Suzuki T, and Naruke T: Efficacy of lung cancer screening: comparison of results from a case-control study and a survival analysis. The Japanese Lung Cancer Screening Research Group, *Jpn J Cancer Res* 83:424-430, 1992.

50. Eddy DM: Guidelines for the cancer-related checkup: recommendations and rationale, *Cancer J Clin* 30:194-240, 1980.

51. Flehinger BJ, Melamed MR, Zaman MB, et al: Early lung cancer detection: results of the initial (prevalence) radiologic and cytologic screening in the Memorial Sloan–Kettering Study, *Am Rev Respir Dis* 130:555-560, 1984.

52. Fontana RS, Sanderson DR, Taylor WF, et al: Early lung cancer detection: results of the initial (prevalence) radiologic and cytologic screening in the Mayo Clinic Study, *Am Rev Respir Dis* 130:561-565, 1984.

53. Frost JK, Ball WC Jr, Levin ML, et al: Early lung cancer detection: results of the initial (prevalence) radiologic and cytologic screening in the Johns Hopkins Study, *Am Rev Respir Dis* 130:549-554, 1984.

54. US Preventive Services Task Force: Screening for lung cancer. In *Guide to clinical preventive services. An assessment of the effectiveness of 169 interventions,* p 67, Baltimore, 1989, Williams & Wilkins.

55. Bragg DG: Imaging in primary lung cancer: the roles of detection, staging and follow-up, *Semin Ultrasound CT MR* 10:453-466, 1989.

56. Karsell PR and McDougall JC: Diagnostic tests for lung cancer, *Mayo Clin Proc* 68:288-296, 1993.

57. White CS and Templeton PA: Radiologic manifestations of bronchogenic cancer, *Clin Chest Med* 14:55-68, 1993.

58. Whitesell PL and Peters SG: Pulmonary manifestations of extrathoracic malignant lesions, *Mayo Clin Proc* 68:483-491, 1993.

59. Huston J III and Muhm JR: Solitary pulmonary nodules: evaluation with a CT reference phantom, *Radiology* 170:653-656, 1989.

60. Khajotia RR, Mohn A, Pokieser L, et al: Induced sputum and cytological diagnosis of lung cancer, *Lancet* 338:976-977, 1991.

61. Mehta AC, Lee FYW, and Marty JJ: Sputum cytology, *Clin Chest Med* 14:69-86, 1993.

62. Saccomanno G, Saunders RP, Ellis H, et al: Concentration of carcinoma or atypical cells in sputum, *Acta Cytol* 7:305-310, 1963.

63. Risse EKJ, van't Hof MA, and Vooijs PG: Relationship between patient characteristics and the sputum cytologic diagnosis of lung cancer, *Acta Cytol* 31:159-165, 1987.

64. Umiker WO, DeWeese MS, and Lawrence GH: Diagnosis of lung cancer by bronchoscopic biopsy, scalene lymph node biopsy and cytology smears. A report of 42 histologically proven cases, *Surgery* 41:705-713, 1957.

65. Koss LG, Melamed MR, and Goodner JT: Pulmonary cytology: a brief survey of diagnostic results from July 1st, 1954 until December 31st, 1960, *Acta Cytol* 8:104-113, 1964.

66. Rosa UW, Prolla JC, and Gastal ES: Cytology in diagnosis of cancer affecting the lung, *Chest* 63:203-207, 1973.

67. Ng ABP and Horak GC: Factors significant in the diagnostic accuracy of lung cytology in bronchial washing and sputum samples: II. Sputum samples, *Acta Cytol* 27:397-402, 1983.

68. Truong LD, Underwood RD, Greenberg SD, et al: Diagnosis and typing of cell carcinomas by cytopathologic methods: a review of 108 cases, *Acta Cytol* 29:379-384, 1985.

69. Farber SM: Clinical appraisal of pulmonary cytology, *JAMA* 175:345-348, 1961.

70. Farber SM, McGrath AK Jr, Benioff MA, et al: Evaluation of cytological diagnosis of lung cancer, *JAMA* 144:1-4, 1950.

71. Spjut HJ, Fier DJ, and Ackerman LV: Exfoliative cytology and pulmonary cancer, *J Thorac Surg* 30:90-107, 1955.

72. Dobray GS: The evaluation of cytology in the early diagnosis of pulmonary carcinoma, *Acta Cytol* 14:95-103, 1970.

73. Auffermann W and Bocking A: Early detection of precancerous lesions in dysplasias of the lung by rapid DNA image cytometry, *Anal Quant Cytol Histol* 7:218-226, 1985.

74. Koprowska I and Zipfel SA: The potential usefulness of monoclonal antibodies in the determination of histologic types of lung cancer in cytologic preparations, *Acta Cytol* 32:675-679, 1988.

75. Saito Y, Imai T, Nagamoto N, et al: A quantitative cytologic study of sputum in early squamous cell bronchogenic carcinoma, *Anal Quant Cytol Histol* 10:365-370, 1988.

76. Arroliga AC and Matthay RA: The role of bronchoscopy in lung cancer, *Clin Chest Med* 14:87-98, 1993.

77. Schenk DA, Bower JH, Bryan CL, et al: Transbronchial needle aspiration staging of bronchogenic carcinoma, *Am Rev Respir Dis* 134:146-148, 1986.

78. Shure D and Fedullo PF: The role of transcarinal needle aspiration in the staging of bronchogenic carcinoma, *Chest* 86:693-696, 1984.

79. Hurzeler D: Ultraviolet–fluorescence bronchoscopy in early detection of bronchogenic carcinoma, *Ann Otolaryngol* 87:528-532, 1978.

80. Prakash U, BS, Offord KB, and Stubbs SE: Bronchoscopy in North America: the ACCP survey, *Chest* 100:1668-1675, 1991.

81. Khouri NF, Stitik FP, Erosan YS, et al: Transthoracic needle aspiration biopsy of benign and malignant lung lesions, *AJR* 144:281-288, 1985.

82. Wescott JL: Direct percutaneous needle aspiration of localized pulmonary lesions: results in 422 patients, *Radiology* 137:31-35, 1980.

83. Gobien RP, Stanley JH, Vujic I, et al: Thoracic biopsy: CT guidance of thin-needle aspiration, *AJR* 142:827-830, 1984.

84. van Sonnenberg E, Casola G, Ho M, et al: Difficult thoracic lesions: CT-guided experience in 150 cases, *Radiology* 167:457-461, 1988.

85. Fish GD, Stanley JH, Miller KS, et al: Post-biopsy pneumothorax: estimating the risk by chest radiography and pulmonary function tests, *AJR* 150:71-74, 1988.

86. Poe RH, Kallay MC, Wicks CM, et al: Predicting risk of pneumothorax in needle biopsy of the lung, *Chest* 85:232-235, 1984.

87. Sinner WN: Complications of percutaneous transthoracic needle aspiration biopsy, *Acta Radiol* 17:813-828, 1976.

88. Weisbrod GL: Transthoracic percutaneous lung biopsy, *Radiol Clin North Am* 28:647-655, 1990.

89. Canti G: The role of cytology in diagnosis. In Bates M, editor: *Bronchial carcinoma: an integrated approach to diagnosis and management,* pp 61-75, Berlin, 1984, Springer-Verlag.

90. Edmondstone WM: Investigation of pleural effusion: comparison between fiberoptic thoracoscopy, needle biopsy and cytology, *Respir Med* 84:23-26, 1990.

91. American Joint Committee on Cancer: Lung. In Beahrs OH, Hensen DE, Hutter RVP, et al, editors: *Manual for staging of cancer,* pp 115-121, Philadelphia, 1988, JB Lippincott.

92. *Staging of lung cancer,* Chicago, 1979, American Joint Committee for Cancer Staging and End Results Reporting.

93. Mountain CF: Value of the new TNM staging system for lung cancer, *Chest* 96:47S-49S, 1989.

94. Mountain CF: Lung cancer staging classification, *Clin Chest Med* 14:43-53, 1993.

95. Shields TW: Surgical therapy for carcinoma of the lung, *Clin Chest Med* 14:121-148, 1993.

96. Quinn DL, Ostrov LB, Porter DK, et al: Staging of non-small cell bronchogenic carcinoma: relationship of the clinical evaluation to organ scans, *Chest* 89:270-275, 1986.

97. Carney DN and Minna JD: Small cell cancer of the lung, *Clin Chest Med* 3:389-398, 1992.

98. Ikezoe J, Kadowaki K, Morimoto S, et al: Mediastinal lymph node metastases from non-small cell bronchogenic carcinoma: reevaluation with CT, *J Comput Assist Tomogr* 14:340-344, 1990.

99. Marko J, Mullan BP, Hillman DR, et al: Preoperative assessment as a predictor of mortality and morbidity after lung resection, *Am Rev Respir Dis* 139:902-910, 1989.

100. Olsen GN, Block AJ, and Tobias JA: Prediction of post-pneumonectomy pulmonary function using quantitative macroaggregate lung scanning, *Chest* 66:13-16, 1974.

101. Wernly JA, De Meester TR, Kirchner PT, et al: Clinical value of quantitative ventilation–perfusion lung scans in the surgical management of bronchial carcinoma, *J Thorac Cardiovasc Surg* 80:533-543, 1980.

102. Smith TP, Kinasewitz GT, Tucker WY, et al: Exercise capacity as a predictor of post-thoracotomy morbidity, *Am Rev Respir Dis* 129:730-734, 1984.

103. Ginsberg RJ, Hill LD, Eagan RT, et al: Modern thirty-day operative mortality for surgical resections in lung cancer. *J Thorac Cardiovasc Surg* 86:654-658, 1983.

104. Ginsberg RJ and Rubenstein LV: Patients with T1N0 non-small cell lung cancer, *Lung Cancer* 7(suppl):83, 1991. Abstract 304.

105. Holmes EC and Gail M for the Lung Cancer Study Group: Surgical adjuvant therapy for stage II and stage III adenocarcinoma and large-cell undifferentiated carcinoma, *J Clin Oncol* 4:710-715, 1986.

106. Lung Cancer Study Group: The benefit of adjuvant treatment for resected locally advanced non-small cell lung cancer, *J Clin Oncol* 6:9-17, 1988.

107. Murren JR and Buzaid AC: Chemotherapy and radiation for the treatment of non-small cell lung cancer. A critical review, *Clin Chest Med* 14:161-172, 1993.

108. Karrer K and Shields T (ISC Lung Cancer Study Group): The importance of complete resection in the multimodality treatment of SCLC, *Lung Cancer* 7(suppl):71, 1991. Abstract 254.

109. Meyer JA, Comis RL, Ginsberg SJ, et al: Selective surgical resection in small cell carcinoma of the lung, *J Thorac Cardiovasc Surg* 77:243-248, 1979.

110. Romano PS and Mark DH: Patient and hospital characteristics related to in-hospital mortality after lung cancer resection, *Chest* 101:1332-1337, 1992.

111. Read RC, Yoder G, and Schaefer RC: Survival after conservative resection for T1N0M0 non-small cell lung cancer, *Ann Thorac Surg* 49:391-400, 1990.

112. Burt M and Martini N: Surgical treatment of lung carcinoma. In Baue AE, Geha AS, Hammond GL, et al, editors: *Glenn's thoracic and cardiovascular surgery,* pp 355-373, Norwalk, Conn, 1991, Appleton & Lange.

113. Martini N, Flehinger BJ, Nagasaki F, et al: Prognostic significance of N_1 disease in carcinoma of the lung, *J Thorac Cardiovasc Surg* 86:646-653, 1983.

114. Knights EM Jr: Metastatic tumors of the brain and their relation to primary and secondary pulmonary cancer, *Cancer* 7:259-264, 1954.

115. Richard P and McKissock W: Intracranial metastases, *Br Med J* 1:15-18, 1963.

116. Johnson BE: Management of small cell lung cancer, *Clin Chest Med* 14:173-188, 1993.

117. Spiro SG: Chemotherapy of small cell lung cancer, *Clin Oncol* 4:105-120, 1985.

118. Aisner J, Alberto P, Bitran J, et al: Role of chemotherapy in small cell lung cancer: a consensus report of the International Association for the Study of Lung Cancer Workshop, *Cancer Treat Rep* 67:37-43, 1983.

119. Shaw EG, Bonner JA, Foote RL, et al: Role of radiation therapy in the management of lung cancer, *Mayo Clin Proc* 68:593-602, 1993.

120. Lung Cancer Study Group: Effects of postoperative mediastinal radiation on completely resected stage II and stage III epidermoid cancer of the lung, *N Engl J Med* 315:1377-1381, 1986.

121. Russell AH, Pajak TE, Selim HM, et al: Prophylactic cranial irradiation for lung cancer patients at high risk for development of cerebral metastasis: results of a prospective randomized trial conducted by

the Radiation Therapy Oncology Group, *Int J Radiat Oncol Biol Phys* 21:637-643, 1991.

122. Ochs JJ, Tester WJ, Cohen MH, et al: Salvage radiation therapy for intrathoracic small cell carcinoma of the lung progressing on combination chemotherapy, *Cancer Treat Rep* 67:1123-1126, 1983.

123. Salazar OM, Yee GJ, and Slawson RG: Radiation therapy for chest recurrences following induction chemotherapy in small cell lung cancer, *Int J Radiat Oncol Biol Phys* 21:645-650, 1991.

124. Drings P and Fisher JR: Biology and clinical use of GM-CSF in lung cancer, *Lung* 168:1059s-1068s, 1990.

Chapter 19

CANCERS OF THE HEAD AND NECK

Joseph R. Spiegel
Robert Thayer Sataloff

Malignant neoplasms of the head and neck are a diverse group of tumors in both anatomic site of origin and histologic cell type. They are considered together because of the complex and profound functional and cosmetic deformities that can result from these cancers and their subsequent treatment. Additionally, the epidemiology of head and neck cancers reveals many relationships to occupational and environmental influences, particularly toxic or carcinogenic exposure that may affect the upper aerodigestive tract (see Table 19-1). Agents associated with upper airway cancers are discussed in detail in Chapter 35.

As the reader will note throughout this chapter, most tumors that arise in the head and neck can be treated with acceptable functional and cosmetic results if they are diagnosed when they are small and at an early stage of invasion. Larger, more advanced tumors can often be successfully treated, with a high percentage of long-term survivors. However, the treatment often results in severe secondary deficits. Since occupational and en-vironmental exposures are a significant factor in the development of many of these cancers, it is important to define the subset of individuals who are at risk so that adequate preventive and screening programs can bedeveloped.

EPIDEMIOLOGY

Primary malignant neoplasms of the head and neck account for 5% of new cancers each year in the United States, excluding skin cancer. In 1992 there were approximately 42,800 new cases in this country with 11,600 deaths, and the worldwide incidence is estimated at 500,000 new cases annually.[1,2] The male-female ratio is between 3:1 and 4:1, but the percentage of females has risen steadily during the last 30 years. Most lesions occur in patients who are over age 40, but in certain specific types of cancer, younger age groups may be at significant risk. Approximately 80% of primary head and neck cancers are squamous cell carcinomas, arising from the mucosal lining of the upper aerodigestive tract.[3] In patients with squamous cell carcinoma, the number who will be found to have a second primary malignancy at the time their initial head and neck cancer is diagnosed has been reported to be as high as 17%.[4] The remainder of the nonepidermoid neoplasms includes thyroid cancers, salivary neoplasms, lymphomas, and more rare tumor types.

Most of this chapter is devoted to a discussion of the specific epidemiologic factors, evaluation, staging, and treatment options for tumors that arise from each specific defined anatomic site in the head and neck. The more uncommon neoplasms are considered separately because they affect the head and neck as an entire region.

Table 19-1. Basic characteristics of head and neck cancer

Location	Most prominent symptom	Risk factor exposure	Risk of cervical metastases
Nose and sinus	Mass	Nickel or wood	Moderate
Nasopharynx	Neck mass or SOM	EBV	High
Oral cavity	Pain	Tobacco or EtOH	Moderate
Oropharynx	Dysphagia	Tobacco or EtOH	High
Larynx	Hoarseness	Tobacco	Glottic, low; supraglottic, high
Hypopharynx	Dysphagia	Tobacco or EtOH	High
Salivary glands	Mass	Radiation	High grade, high; others, low

SOM, Serous otitis media; *EBV,* Epstein–Barr virus; *EtOH,* alcohol.

EVALUATION

In addition to the usual comprehensive medical history, special attention must be paid to specific symptoms frequently seen in the presentation of patients with head and neck cancer. Hoarseness and sore throat are common, everyday complaints for many people. However, when they persist for more than 2 to 3 weeks in a patient with other risk factors, a complete evaluation is indicated. Dysphagia, dyspnea, nonhealing ulcers, persistently painful mucosal lesions, hemoptysis, and the presence of a neck mass may be associated symptoms as well. Of course, any history of treatment for head and neck cancer, or any other malignancy, must raise suspicions about the possibility of a new or recurrent tumor.

The patient must be questioned about all potential risk factors. The social history regarding tobacco, alcohol, or illicit drug use and the details of any extended medical treatment must be obtained. The patient should be asked about all potential occupational or environmental exposures, including dusts, chemicals, ionizing radiation, and solar radiation, and whether any protection against these exposures was used. Possible carcinogenic exposures in the patient's distant past are often quite significant. If necessary, the patient may be asked to obtain records on previous employment or on medical treatment in childhood (e.g., radiation for acne).

Nutritional and psychosocial status must be established to determine prognosis and the potential for different treatment options. Many patients who develop head and neck cancer are malnourished because of the secondary effects of the tumor on swallowing and digestion, the effects of alcoholism, or a poor daily diet. Treatment may be delayed or significantly limited in patients with malnutrition, whereas those who are in good general medical condition often benefit from immediate, aggressive, multimodality therapy. Measurements of the patient's height and weight and an assessment of general physical strength may be adequate. Serum levels of protein, albumin, electrolytes, and liver enzymes are helpful in patients whose nutritional status remains questionable.

An adequate physical examination includes a thorough inspection of the skin, soft tissues, and mucosal surfaces of the head and neck, as well as an assessment of neurologic and muscular function. With the advent of easily obtained flexible fiberoptic endoscopy, a comprehensive evaluation can be provided in the office setting of most otolaryngologists (head and neck surgeons).[5] Palpation of the structures in the oral cavity and the oropharynx, with particular attention to the tongue base and tonsils, will often yield the suspicion of a tumor mass that would otherwise be unsuspected by inspection alone. Occasionally, patients will require endoscopy under general anesthesia for persistent symptoms that are difficult to evaluate because of anatomic restrictions or marked mucosal inflammatory changes. Endoscopy (nasopharyngoscopy, direct laryngoscopy, bronchoscopy, and esophagoscopy) under local or general anesthesia is usually the final step in evaluation, and it is used to obtain biopsies of suspicious tissues not easily obtained in the office setting.

Radiologic evaluation is rarely essential in the initial evaluation, but it can be critical in determining the extent of a primary lesion, involvement of adjacent bony structures, and the presence of regional metastases. In patients who are being evaluated for possible recurrent head and neck cancer, radiologic evaluation is more often used as a primary tool. Computerized tomographic (CT) scanning with intravenous contrast remains the best single study for evaluating head and neck cancers because of its ability to define the soft-tissue extent of most tumors, as well as any adjacent bony and vascular structures. Magnetic resonance imaging (MRI) provides much better resolution of soft-tissue structures, and it has become especially useful in defining tumors in the deep musculature of the tongue and in evaluating the potential for central nervous system involvement in tumors that affect the bony skull base. When mandibular involvement is suspected in tumors of the oral cavity, panorex imaging of the lower jaw, nuclear bone scans, and special CT techniques are often used.[6]

TREATMENT

Treatment protocols specific to tumors arising at the different anatomic sites must be considered separately. In general, almost all head and neck cancers are treated with complete surgical excision, radiation therapy, or a combination of these two modalities (Fig. 19-1). The choice of surgery is often limited by the patient's general physical condition and the presence of coexistent systemic disease (e.g., diabetes mellitus, chronic obstructive pulmonary disease, or coronary artery disease). The functional and cosmetic deformities that can result from the excision of affected tissue must be considered individually for each patient. Radiation therapy is often as effective as surgical excision in the local control of small, early lesions. However, its effectiveness as a single modality is limited in more advanced cancer, and long-term complications such as reduced salivary function and tissue atrophy must also be considered. Additionally, radiation therapy requires a high degree of patient cooperation, as most treatment courses last at least 6 to 7 weeks, and it often requires ongoing medical attention.

Chemotherapy has long been used in palliative protocols for patients who have had tumor recurrence after failed initial treatment with surgery and/or radiation. Over the past decade a multitude of trials using chemotherapy in a neoadjuvant role have been evaluated. Cisplatin is the most effective drug, with initial complete response rates as high as 50% to 75% in squamous cell carcinoma of many head and neck sites. As yet, no such chemotherapy protocol is curative, and when combined with traditional radiation and surgery, there has been no demonstrated statistical advantage in long-term survival. However, it appears that selected patient groups may benefit from neoadjuvant chemotherapy by sparing them the need for aggressive extirpative surgery after a complete chemotherapeutic response. Neoadjuvant chemotherapy protocols for laryngeal cancer, described as "organ-sparing protocols," have now been developed. Clinical research continues in hopes of determining additional uses for neoadjuvant chemotherapy and the potential for long-term adjuvant protocols to prevent the late recurrence of local, regional, and distant disease.[7]

Rehabilitation should be planned at the time initial treatment is discussed. When surgery is one of the primary modalities, reconstruction of functional and cosmetic deformities is provided at the time of the initial surgery whenever possible. Prosthetics are fabricated to replace portions or all of the maxilla, mandible, or palate when they are resected. Often, these prosthetics can be implanted immediately to minimize functional deficits postoperatively. When surgical excision, radiation therapy, or the tumor itself affects vocal communication, this is discussed with the patient preoperatively, and rehabilitation to facilitate vocal communication postoperatively is initiated as soon as possible. Swallowing function can also be severely affected, and nutrition is planned by alternative methods (e.g., enteral tube feedings or parenteral nutrition), whereas rehabilitation occurs in the posttreatment period.

CANCERS OF THE UPPER AERODIGESTIVE TRACT
Cancer of the neck

Discovery of a neck mass is often the initial sign of a head and neck malignancy. When head and neck cancers spread to the cervical nodes, defining the extent and nature of the regional metastases is usually the most critical factor in determining prognosis and treatment options. Lymphoma commonly presents with cervical adenopathy, and often, enlarged cervical lymph nodes are the only manifestation of the disease.

Each side of the neck is divided into anterior and posterior triangles by the sternocleidomastoid muscle. The anterior triangle is further subdivided into submandibular, submental, superior carotid, and inferior carotid triangles. Most head and neck areas have primary and/or secondary lymphatic drainage patterns to the deep lymphatic chains: anteriorly along the internal jugular vein and posteriorly along the spinal accessory nerve. The internal jugular system is divided into upper, middle, and lower lymph node groups. The posterior spinal accessory chain is divided into upper and lower groups. There are approximately 75 lymph nodes on each side of the neck.

Often, the initial presentation of a head and neck neoplasm is the finding of a painless, perhaps enlarging, neck mass.[8] As a general rule, patients who are over 40 years

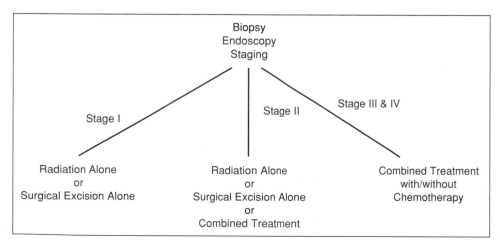

Fig. 19-1. Basic algorithm for the treatment of head and neck cancer.

old are evaluated with the primary suspicion that the neck mass is malignant, whereas those under age 40 are more likely to have a neck mass of inflammatory origin. Patients with risk factors such as cigarette smoking, high alcohol intake, and occupational or environmental carcinogenic exposures are also regarded with a much higher degree of suspicion for malignancy. Commonly, the initial examination of the head and neck reveals the primary tumor on a mucosal surface in the head or neck, and subsequent planning is based on staging and treatment protocols for this primary site. When no primary site is identified, a radiologic evaluation including chest x-ray, barium swallow, CT scanning of the paranasal sinuses (and often of the chest, mediastinum, and abdomen) is carried out in order to look for an occult primary site. When the radiologic evaluation is negative, panendoscopy under general anesthesia is carried out, and in the absence of an obvious primary site, random biopsies of the nasopharynx, tongue base, and tonsils are often necessary. When all such evaluation fails to determine a primary cancer, surgical excision of the neck mass is necessary.

Before an open biopsy is planned, fine needle aspiration (FNA) with cytologic evaluation can provide histologic diagnosis of the neck mass in most cases. This information can be used to guide the search for a primary tumor site. For example, discovery of a thyroid neoplasm on FNA will significantly limit the required evaluation and consideration of treatment protocols. Additionally, a high suspicion of lymphoma on FNA would probably lead to a much earlier open excisional biopsy of the neck mass to provide a direct tissue examination.[9–11] When squamous cell carcinoma is suspected or diagnosed in the neck mass, yet no primary site is identified, excisional biopsy should be carried out, with a plan for radical neck dissection if malignancy is confirmed. Delayed treatment after open biopsy of an epidermoid cancer may reduce ultimate long-term survival rates.[12,13] Cancer of the neck with an unknown primary site is treated by surgical excision (usually by selective or radical neck dissection), followed by full-course radiation therapy to both neck fields and to the sites of most likely occult primary cancer (the nasopharynx, oropharynx, and tongue base).[14]

Staging of metastatic cancer to the cervical lymph nodes is based on the number of involved nodes and their size. Staging is determined on the basis of the physical examination at the time of initial presentation (*clinical staging*). However, *radiologic stage* and *pathologic stage* are terms that are also used when different staging is obtained on a given patient based on radiologic or histopathologic findings. A description of staging for neck disease and for other anatomic sites can be found in the box.

Metastatic squamous cell carcinoma to the cervical lymph nodes can be cured by radiation therapy when the involved lymph node is relatively small (usually less than 3 cm) and when it has not spread beyond the lymph node capsule.[15] If the lymph node is large, if multiple enlarged nodes are present, if extracapsular spread is suspected, or,

in most cases, when surgery is the mode of treatment chosen for the primary site, surgical excision of the affected lymph node tissue is suggested.[16] Radical neck dissection, as originally described by Crile in 1906, was the original, and for many years the standard, surgical procedure.[17] In a radical neck dissection both the anterior and posterior cervical lymph node chains are removed with all of their enveloping fascial compartments, the internal jugular vein, the sternocleidomastoid muscle, the spinal accessory nerve, and the submandibular gland.[18] Over the past 20 years various modifications of the radical neck dissection method have been developed, so that today selective neck dissections are planned based on the lymph nodes at risk and on the extent of disease present in the neck on an individual basis. The most selective dissection can spare all of the vital components while removing only the lymph nodes and the fascial components. Selective neck dissections are usually reserved for patients with N_0 or N_1 disease.[19–21]

Controversy continues regarding the treatment of the N_0 neck. Patients with a greater than 20% risk of occult cervical metastases (those not noted on clinical examination or radiologically but subsequently proven pathologically) will benefit from prophylactic treatment.[22,23] Surgery and radiation therapy are equally efficacious in treatment of the N_0 neck. Thus treatment protocols that include prophylactic modified radical neck dissection are usually based on whether there is an advantage to treating the primary site surgically.[24–26]

Cancer of the nasal cavity and the paranasal sinuses

The paranasal sinuses are paired, mucosally lined, air-filled cavities that are outgrowths of the nose and connected to the nasal cavity through their natural ostia. They are lined with respiratory mucosa. Anteriorly, the nasal vestibule is lined with skin, and squamous metaplasia is common. Lymphatic drainage is primarily to the parapharyngeal and retropharyngeal lymph nodes, with secondary drainage to the internal jugular chain. Neoplasms involving the vestibule of the nose can drain through the superficial skin lymphatics to periparotid and facial lymph nodes and, subsequently, to the deep jugular system.

The nose and the paranasal sinuses account for 3% of all upper aerodigestive tract carcinomas. In the United States they occur at a frequency of 0.3 to 1.0 per 1 million of the population. The peak incidence is between age 50 and 79, and these carcinomas are rare in the younger population.[27] Fifty-nine percent of these tumors are found in the maxillary sinus; 24%, in the nasal cavity; 16%, in the ethmoid sinuses; and 1%, in the frontal and sphenoid sinuses. Approximately 80% of these malignancies arise from the mucosal surface, the great majority being squamous cell carcinoma.[28] Epidermoid tumors that arise anteriorly in the nasal cavity tend to be well differentiated, whereas those arising in the posterior nasal cavity, ethmoid sinuses, and maxillary sinuses are generally poorly differentiated. These

Staging of head and neck tumors

Cancer of the neck

N_0:	No clinically positive node
N_1:	A single clinically positive node homolateral to the primary tumor and 3 cm or less in greatest diameter
N_{2a}:	A single clinically positive homolateral node larger than 3 cm but less than 6 cm in greatest diameter
N_{2b}:	Multiple clinically positive homolateral nodes with none larger than 6 cm in greatest diameter
N_{3a}:	Multiple clinically positive homolateral nodes with at least one larger than 6 cm in greatest diameter
N_{3b}:	Bilateral clinically positive nodes
N_{3c}:	Only contralateral clinically positive nodes

Cancer of the maxillary sinus

T_x:	Cannot be assessed
T_0:	No evidence of a primary tumor
T_1:	Tumor confined to the inferior antrum without bone erosion
T_2:	Tumor confined to the superior antrum without bone erosion of the inferior or medial walls
T_3:	Extensive tumor involving the skin of the cheek, the orbit, the anterior ethmoids, or the pterygoid muscles
T_4:	Massive tumor involving the cribriform plate, the posterior ethmoids, the sphenoid, nasopharynx, pterygoid plates, or the base of the skull

Cancer of the nasopharynx

T_{1s}:	Carcinoma in situ
T_1:	Tumor is confined to one site, or no tumor is visible but random biopsy is positive
T_2:	Tumor involves two sites (posterosuperior and lateral walls)
T_3:	Tumor has extended to the oropharynx or the nasal cavity
T_4:	Tumor has invaded the skull or a cranial nerve

Cancer of the oral cavity

T_1:	Tumor less than 2 cm in greatest diameter
T_2:	Tumor larger than 2 cm but less than 4 cm in greatest diameter
T_3:	Tumor more than 4 cm in greatest diameter
T_4:	Massive tumor with involvement of the mandible pterygoid muscles, the antrum, the root of the tongue, or the skin

Cancer of the oropharynx

T_{1s}:	Carcinoma in situ
T_1:	Lesion of 2 cm or less in greatest diameter
T_2:	Lesion larger than 2 cm but less than 4 cm in greatest diameter
T_3:	Lesion larger than 4 cm in greatest diameter
T_4:	Lesion larger than 4 cm, with invasion of bone, soft tissues of the neck, or the root of the tongue

Cancer of the hypopharynx

T_{1s}:	Carcinoma in situ
T_1:	Carcinoma confined to the site of origin
T_2:	Extension of the tumor to an adjacent site without fixation of the hemilarynx (vocal fold)
T_3:	Extension of the tumor to an adjacent site with fixation of the hemilarynx
T_4:	Massive tumor with invasion of bone, cartilage, or the soft tissues of the neck

Cancer of the larynx

T_{1s}:	Carcinoma in situ
T_1:	Tumor confined to the site of origin
T_2:	Tumor spread to an adjacent laryngeal site
T_3:	Tumor confined to the larynx with fixation of the hemilarynx
T_4:	Tumor with cartilage destruction or extension beyond the larynx

Malignant melanoma (Breslow's)

T_1:	Up to 0.75 mm depth of skin invasion
T_2:	0.76 to 1.5 mm
T_3:	1.51 to 3.0 mm
T_4:	More than 3.0 mm

cancers are usually locally invasive, but nodal metastases are unusual. When regional metastases occur, they tend to appear late in the course of disease.[29] Approximately 10% to 14% of nose and sinus malignancies are adenocarcinomas, including adenoid cystic carcinoma (a tumor of minor salivary gland origin).[30,31] The remaining malignancies are sarcomas, melanomas, and other much more rare cancers.[32] Inverted papilloma is a benign, locally invasive lesion that must be treated aggressively because of a 12% to 15% incidence of associated squamous cell carcinoma.[33,34]

Up to 44% of all carcinomas of the nose and the paranasal sinuses are attributable to occupational exposures.[27,35] These include nickel, chromium, isopropyl oils, volatile hydrocarbons, and organic fibers found in the woodworking, shoe-making, and textile industries. Squamous cell carcinoma, usually primary to the maxillary sinus, has been associated with work in the nickel-refining industry and with high exposures to chromates.[36–39] Adenocarcinoma, usually primary to the ethmoid sinus, has been associated with the furniture making, textile, and shoe-making industries.[40–49] Human papillomavirus has been linked to the development of sinonasal cancer as a cofactor.[50] Chronic sinusitis and inhalant allergies have also been implicated in the development of nasal and sinus cancer, but substantiating evidence has yet to be provided. Until recently, cigarette smoking was not directly associated with the development of cancer of the nose and the paranasal sinuses. However, a study evaluating the incidence of these tumors in workers in the lumber and woodworking industry has shown that the statistical risk associated with tobacco use may be as great as that of the occupational exposure itself.[51] Further investigation is certainly warranted to determine whether the link between tobacco use and cancer of the nose and paranasal sinuses is in any way comparable with that found in other head and neck sites.

Tumors in this area present with symptoms of nasal obstruction, epistaxis, facial pain, or dental pain. More advanced tumors may present with cranial nerve deficits, proptosis, trismus, or a mass involving the facial tissues, palate, or maxillary alveolus. The extent of the disease can be partially determined by physical examination, but CT scanning of the area is necessary in all cases. An MRI scan is particularly valuable when involvement of the skull base is suspected. Arteriography is rarely needed, except in cases with intracranial extension. Many staging systems have been developed, but the currently accepted system has only limited usefulness in determining prognosis and therapeutic options (see box).

Early-stage tumors (T_1 and T_2) of the paranasal sinuses are usually treated with surgical excision, since even small tumors may have early bony invasion that could limit the effectiveness of radiation therapy. Surgical excision can usually be accomplished by partial maxillectomy and ethmoidectomy, although total maxillectomy is sometimes required.[52] In more advanced tumors (T_3 and T_4), radical surgery is necessary.[29,53] Most patients with large tumors are treated with adjuvant radiation therapy and possibly chemotherapy, but the evidence that this additional treatment has any impact on survival is inconclusive.[54,55] The decision is usually determined by the patient's physical condition at the time of presentation and by the suspicion of tumor extension to the orbital and intracranial structures. When these cancers are proven to extend to or involve the skull base and the dura, combined craniofacial resection can be successfully accomplished in selected cases.[56] Prophylactic treatment of the cervical lymph nodes is not necessary, even in extensive tumors. However, clinically apparent cervical metastases are treated with radical neck dissection and/or radiation therapy, depending on the chosen treatment at the primary site.

The overall cure rate of carcinoma of the nose and the paranasal sinuses is 30% to 35%. Five-year survival rates range from as high as 70% in T_1 and T_2 lesions to 15% to 20% in T_3 and T_4 lesions.[57,58] In selected patients with extensive disease who successfully undergo craniofacial resection and radiation therapy, survival rates as high as 50% to 70% have been realized.[56]

Cancer of the nasopharynx

The nasopharynx is the most cephalad portion of the pharynx. It is bounded on its roof by the sphenoid bones and posteriorly by the atlas. The lateral walls contain the eustachian tube orifices, and the nasal choanae are at the anterior margin. The inferior limit is the free margin of the soft palate. The lymphatic drainage of the nasopharynx is to the lateral retropharyngeal nodes, high jugular nodes, and upper spinal accessory nodes.

Eighty-five percent of nasopharyngeal tumors are epithelial, and 7.5% are lymphomas. The epidemiology of epidermoid cancer at this site is different than at most other sites in the head or neck. There is no association with tobacco use, alcohol use, or other environmental factors. The population tends to be younger, with bimodal peaks between age 30 and 69.[59] There is a high incidence of nasopharyngeal carcinoma among southern Chinese, especially those from the Kwantung province,[60] and there is a significant association of elevated Epstein–Barr virus titers in people suffering from this tumor. Most patients will have elevated titers at the time of initial presentation, and titers can be followed as a prognostic sign for recurrent disease. However, elevated titers are not found in all patients.[61,62]

Nasopharyngeal carcinoma presents either with serous otitis media secondary to eustachian tube obstruction or with cervical adenopathy in over 50% of patients. Nasal obstruction and epistaxis are also common symptoms. Headache, diplopia, facial numbness, trismus, ptosis, and hoarseness may also be present. At the time of presentation, 60% to 70% of patients have cervical metastasis clinically, and 15% to 17% have some cranial nerve involvement.[63,64]

Diagnosis is usually suspected by endoscopic examination and confirmed with biopsy. Evaluation is completed with CT and MRI scanning and, as previously stated, Epstein–Barr virus titers. The staging system that is available is not helpful at present, but it is beginning to be used to help determine which patients may benefit from surgical excision after radiation therapy.

The primary mode of treatment in nasopharyngeal carcinoma is radiation therapy. In all cases both cervical fields are treated, with the nasopharynx receiving a potentially curative dose. Five-year survival rates are reported in the 40% to 50% range for patients without cervical metastasis, and approximately 20% in those with nodal disease at the time of presentation.[59,64] Surgical excision has been attempted in patients with persistent disease after radiation therapy, but the impact of this aggressive treatment on ultimate survival has yet to be determined.[65]

Cancer of the oral cavity

The oral cavity extends from the lips anteriorly to the faucial arches posteriorly. It includes the lips, buccal mucosa, gingiva, retromolar trigones, hard palate, anterior two thirds of the tongue, and the floor of the mouth. The lymphatic drainage is primarily to the submental and submandibular nodes and secondarily to the deep jugular system.

Cancers of the oral cavity are almost exclusively squamous cell carcinoma, but an occasional tumor of minor salivary origin is encountered. There is a high association with smoking or the use of smokeless tobacco.[66,67] Ninety percent of patients are heavy cigarette smokers or snuff dippers. Additionally, areas of chronic irritation of the oral mucosa that arise from poorly fitting dentures or the tip of a pipe or cigar can lead to the development of precancerous and cancerous lesions. Sun exposure is a primary etiologic factor in carcinoma of the lips, especially of the lower lip. Herpes virus type I is currently under investigation as a potential etiologic cofactor.

Patients often complain of a painful or nonhealing ulcer of the oral mucosa with or without bleeding. Loose teeth, odynophagia, otalgia, and cervical adenopathy are also common presenting signs and symptoms. The lip is the most common site for oral cavity carcinoma, followed by the oral tongue and the floor of the mouth.

Initial evaluation and biopsy are usually easily carried out in an office setting. Any suspected involvement of the maxilla or the mandible must be evaluated before treatment options can be considered. The CT scan is used in all cases of extensive disease, and the MRI scan is useful in determining soft-tissue extension in the deep tissues of the tongue. Mandibular involvement can be further assessed by nuclear bone scanning and by panorex x-ray technique.

Cervical metastases are common, even in patients with small primary lesions. Involved nodes are found in up to 50% of patients with squamous cell carcinoma of the anterior tongue (30% occult) and in as many as 58% of patients with cancer of the floor of the mouth (12% occult). Cervical metastases are uncommon in cancer of the lip and buccal mucosa.[23]

Tumors of the oral cavity are staged by size (see box). Carcinomas of the tongue can be difficult to stage by physical examination alone, and often, examination under general anesthesia and MRI scanning are necessary to determine the true volume of tumor and the extent of invasion through the tongue musculature.

Stage I tumors of the oral cavity can be treated by either surgical excision or radiation therapy. When the surgery will result in minimal functional or cosmetic deformity, excision is usually preferred.[68] Stage II and larger lesions are most often treated by a combination of surgery and postoperative radiation therapy.[69] Brachytherapy with radiation implants is often necessary to deliver a curative dose without extensive mandibular radiation exposure that could lead to osteoradionecrosis. Surgery usually involves en bloc resection of the primary tumor and selective or radical neck dissection. When there is no mandibular involvement, this can be accomplished as a "pull-through" procedure or with a mandibular osteotomy. When the bone is involved, mandibular resection is combined with the en bloc soft-tumor excision, in what has traditionally been termed a "commando" procedure. Reconstruction of the osseous and soft-tissue defect is considered at the time of surgical resection or as a delayed second procedure after the completion of postoperative radiation therapy. The use of vascularized free flaps has greatly advanced the ability to provide aggressive immediate reconstruction of the mandible and adjacent soft tissues and to improve the early and extended posttreatment quality of life.[70,71]

The overall 5-year survival rate for all patients with oral cavity cancers is approximately 65%. Five-year survival rates for those with early-stage lip cancers are as high as 90%. However, despite the ability to provide more aggressive surgery and radiation therapy, overall 5-year survival for those with advanced oral cavity tumors (T_3 and T_4) remains between 15% and 40%.[68,69,72]

Cancer of the oropharynx

The oropharynx extends from the free edge of the soft palate superiorly to the tip of the epiglottis inferiorly and from the anterior tonsillar pillars anteriorly to the posterior pharyngeal wall posteriorly. It contains the soft palate, tonsillar fossae, and faucial tonsils; the lateral and posterior pharyngeal walls; and the base of the tongue. Tumors of the oropharynx have access to extend laterally to the parapharyngeal space that contains the glossopharyngeal, lingual, and inferior alveolar nerves; the pterygoid muscles; the internal maxillary artery; and the contents of the carotid sheath. They can also extend inferiorly to involve the preepiglottic space and thus gain access to the laryngeal structures and a plethora of deep lymphatic channels. Primary lymphatic drainage of the oropharynx is to the jugulodigastric (tonsillar) nodes of the middle jugular chain. Tumors of the soft palate, lateral wall, and tongue base can also spread to the retropharyngeal and parapharyngeal nodes. Lesions that extend to the retromolar trigone anteriorly can drain primarily to the submaxillary nodes.

Squamous cell carcinoma predominates in oropharyngeal cancer, with occasional lymphomas found primary to the lymphatic tissue of Waldeyer's ring. Heavy use of tobacco and alcohol are common in patients with oropharyngeal cancer.[73] Exposure to ionizing radiation, malnutrition, and immune system defects have also been implicated in the development of oropharyngeal cancer, but the effects of these factors have not been substantiated.

The most common presenting symptom in oropharyngeal cancer is a sore throat. There is frequently ipsilateral otalgia secondary to referred pain through the tympanic branch of the glossopharyngeal nerve. Extensive lesions restrict tongue motion, resulting in a "hot potato voice." Odynophagia and bleeding from an ulceration may also be noted. Patients will often have symptoms late in the course of their disease, and they are commonly malnourished because of the effects of long-term dysphagia and alcoholism.

Metastases to the cervical lymph nodes are found in 76% of patients with carcinoma of the tongue base and in 60% of patients with carcinoma of the tonsil. The rate of occult metastases with clinically N_0 necks is greater than 20%.[23,73]

Primary oropharyngeal tumors are usually suspected on an initial comprehensive examination of the head and neck. Small tumors can be difficult to visualize, and thus palpation of the tongue base and tonsils is required. A CT scan is necessary in most cases, and it will help define suspected involvement of the parapharyngeal and preepiglottic spaces. As previously stated, MRI scanning can be particularly helpful in defining the extent of involvement of the tongue musculature. Staging is by size of the primary tumor, and it is similar to that of the oral cavity (see box).

T_1 and T_2 tumors of the oropharynx are usually treated with primary radiation therapy. The rate of control of small tumors with radiation is close to that of surgical excision, and radiation therapy is as effective as surgery in the prophylactic treatment of N_0 necks bilaterally. In advanced T_3 and T_4 lesions combined surgery with postoperative radiation therapy is recommended.[74] The surgery involves en bloc resection of the primary tumor and ipsilateral neck dissection. In tumors of the tongue base, prophylactic treatment of the contralateral neck, with either selected neck dissection or postoperative radiation, is required. Mandibulotomy or partial mandibulectomy is often necessary,[74] and a laryngectomy may also be necessary when a total glossectomy is performed or when there is involvement of the preepiglottic space. Reconstruction of the soft-tissue defect after total glossectomy is possible with regional, distant, or microvascular free flaps. However, functional reconstruction of the tongue is difficult at best. Organ-sparing protocols using neoadjuvant chemotherapy, comparable to those that have been successful with laryngeal cancer, are currently under investigation.

Overall survival in patients with oropharyngeal cancer is poor because such a high percentage present late in the course of disease. Five-year survival rates range from 63% for patients with T_1 tumors down to 21% for those with T_4 disease. For patients with tumors of the palatal arch, 5-year survival rates can be as high as 77% for T_1, but they drop to 20% for T_4 disease. The presence of cervical metastasis is the single worst prognostic sign, with 5-year survival rates ranging from 75% in those patients with N_0 disease down to 25% in those with N_1 disease at the time of initial presentation.[73,75]

Cancer of the hypopharynx and the cervical esophagus

The hypopharynx extends from the pharyngoepiglottic folds superiorly to the inferior border of the cricoid cartilage inferiorly, excluding the larynx. It includes the structures of the pyriform sinuses, the postcricoid area of the larynx, and the posterior pharyngeal wall. Tumors arising in the hypopharynx frequently extend inferiorly to the cervical esophagus. There is a rich lymphatic network. The pyriform sinuses drain primarily to the jugulodigastric and middle jugular lymph nodes. The posterior pharyngeal wall drains primarily to the retropharyngeal nodes and secondarily to the middle jugular chain. Lower hypopharyngeal and cervical esophageal mucosae drain to the paratracheal and lower jugular nodes, and more inferior esophageal regions may drain to mediastinal nodes.

Ninety-five percent of cancers of the hypopharynx and the cervical esophagus are epidermoid carcinomas. Sixty percent to 75% arise in the pyriform sinuses, 10% to 25% arise on the posterior pharyngeal wall, and the remaining 5% to 20% arise in the postcricoid region. There is a high association with tobacco and alcohol use, with almost every patient having a substantial history of exposure to both substances. There is a heavy predominance of males to females.[76–78]

The presenting triad of deep throat pain, referred otalgia, and dysphagia is found in more than 50% of patients. Hoarseness and airway obstruction are found in patients with laryngeal involvement. Small postcricoid tumors may present with an irritative sore throat or simply a foreign body sensation deep in the throat that leads to frequent throat clearing. Patients with persistent symptoms and elevated risk due to substance abuse should be evaluated aggressively, and they often require endoscopy under general anesthesia to visualize the postcricoid region. A barium swallow is helpful in defining potential lesions in the hypopharynx and the cervical esophagus. Computerized tomographic scanning is used to determine the extent of disease after the diagnosis is made. Staging is determined by involvement of adjacent sites and the extent of laryngeal involvement (see box).

Cervical metastases are very common in cancers of these sites. Involved nodes are found in 65% to 75% of patients with carcinoma of the hypopharynx. Seventy-five percent of patients with pyriform sinus primary sites (41% occult) and 83% of patients with tumors of the posterior and lateral pharyngeal walls (66% occult) have nodal disease at the time of presentation.[77,79] Prophylactic treatment of the N_0 neck must therefore be considered in patients with any stage of primary tumor of the hypopharynx and the cervical esophagus.

Unfortunately, tumors of the hypopharynx and the cervical esophagus are not commonly recognized when they are small. When diagnosed, the primary tumor can be treated by either primary radiation therapy or surgical excision. Surgery for small tumors can be accomplished via various pharyngotomy approaches. The more common extensive T_3 and T_4 lesions of these sites are treated by laryngopharyngectomy and postoperative radiation therapy.[76–78] Partial soft-tissue defects can be reconstructed primarily or with the use of local, regional, and distant soft-tissue flaps. Circumferential defects are best reconstructed by a gastric "pull-up" procedure (especially useful in patients in whom a total esophagectomy is indicated), and in selected patients reconstruction with a colon interposition or a free jejunal graft can be considered.[80,81]

Prognosis is poor in primary cancers of these anatomic sites because of the potential for extensive submucosal spread and the high incidence of cervical metastases. The overall 5-year survival rate is approximately 30%, and it rises to 50% in patients who are candidates for conservative surgical resections.[76–78]

Cancer of the larynx

The larynx has three anatomical divisions. The *supraglottis* extends from the tip of the epiglottis superiorly to include the epiglottis, aryepiglottic folds, false vocal folds, and the roof of the laryngeal ventricle. The *glottis* extends from the depth of the laryngeal ventricle laterally to 1 cm below the free margin of the true vocal folds, and it includes both vocal folds and the anterior and posterior commissures. The *subglottis* extends from 1 cm below the free margin of the true vocal folds to the inferior border of the cricoid cartilage.

The supraglottis has a rich lymphatic network that crosses the midline and drains primarily to the middle jugular lymph nodes. The glottis has poorly developed, sparse lymphatics. The subglottis drains through the cricothyroid membrane to the prelaryngeal (delphian) nodes, paratracheal lymph nodes, and inferior deep jugular chains.

Other than cancer of the skin and lips, the larynx is the most common primary site for cancers of the head and neck. It is estimated that there are approximately 12,000 new cases annually in the United States, resulting in an estimated 3700 deaths.[82] Over 90% of patients with laryngeal cancer have a significant history of cigarette smoking, and tobacco

has shown to exert a dose-dependent relationship in the development of laryngeal cancer.[83] Heavy alcohol consumption is common in this patient population, and it appears to exert a synergistic effect with tobacco in the development of supraglottic cancers.[84,85] Occupational exposures to nickel, mustard gas, pesticides, wood dust, and asbestos have also been implicated as potential contributors in the development of laryngeal cancers.[86–90] Recently, human papillomavirus has been found in association with laryngeal carcinoma.[91,92]

Between 95% and 98% of tumors are squamous cell carcinomas. Verrucous carcinoma is a variant of squamous cell carcinoma that is well differentiated and locally invasive but almost never involves cervical metastases.

The most common presenting symptom is hoarseness. All patients with persistent hoarseness and a significant history of cigarette smoking require expert laryngeal examination. Stridor, cough, hemoptysis, dysphagia, and aspiration are also signs and symptoms of laryngeal cancer. The presence of a neck mass is rare in patients with glottic carcinoma, but it is much more common in patients with tumors involving the supraglottic larynx. Cervical metastases are found in as many as 50% of patients with T_2 and higher stages of disease of the supraglottis (20% occult).[93]

Initial diagnosis is made by indirect or fiberoptic laryngoscopy, and in small mucosal lesions strobovideolaryngoscopy is helpful. Operative direct laryngoscopy and biopsy are required for confirmation in almost all cases. The CT scan is used to determine the extent of laryngeal involvement and the presence of occult cervical metastases. The MRI scan may be helpful in determining the extent of soft-tissue involvement in some tumors, and a barium swallow can be helpful in determining hypopharyngeal extension. Staging is determined by the extension of the tumor to adjacent sites and by laryngeal function (see box).

T_1 and T_2 laryngeal tumors are most often treated with primary radiation therapy because of the functional deficits to voice and swallowing that can result from surgical excision. Long-term control rates at the primary site are about equal with both modalities in T_1 cancers, and they are only slightly worse with radiation therapy in T_2 lesions. T_2 and larger lesions of the supraglottis require prophylactic treatment of N_0 necks because of the risk of occult metastases. Surgical treatment of small lesions of the supraglottic larynx can be accomplished by endoscopic laser excision or supraglottic laryngectomy (excision of all of the laryngeal tissues superior to the vocal folds). Successful postoperative rehabilitation after these procedures is dependent on a cooperative patient with adequate pulmonary function. Small glottic lesions can be treated surgically by removal of the affected membranous vocal fold, either endoscopically (usually using laser techniques) or by external surgery via a laryngofissure. Surgical excision of small laryngeal lesions is often chosen for patients who are poor candidates for radiation therapy because of difficult positioning, poor compliance, or prior radiotherapy to the head and neck.[94]

T_3 and T_4 lesions of the larynx are treated by combined surgery and postoperative radiation therapy. Most of these lesions will require total laryngectomy or laryngopharyngectomy. Voice is restored with an electrolarynx or the use of an indwelling tracheoesophageal valve. In selected cases partial laryngectomy techniques can be used to accomplish total resection, but these patients often have extended swallowing difficulties, and long-term or permanent tracheotomy may be necessary. With this in mind, protocols have been developed using neoadjuvant chemotherapy. Chemotherapy protocols based on cisplatin are used, and patients who attain a complete response can often be treated successfully with full-course radiation therapy, thereby avoiding the need for laryngectomy.[95]

Verrucous carcinoma is treated surgically in all cases. Conservative laryngectomy techniques are used when possible, and there is no need for prophylactic treatment of cervical metastases. Radiotherapy should be avoided because of the risk of anaplastic transformation.[96]

Prognosis for laryngeal carcinoma is generally better than with epidermoid carcinoma of other head and neck sites. This is probably because many of these lesions are found early in their course, since primary lesions of the vocal folds cause hoarseness even when they are quite small. Five-year survival rates in T_1 carcinomas are as high as 90% to 95% with radiation or surgery, and they range from 75% to 85% with T_2 lesions. Cure rates as high as 65% to 75% have been reported in T_3 lesions treated with combined surgery and radiation therapy, but survival rates for T_4 lesions remain in the 25% to 30% range. The presence of cervical metastases is still an ominous prognostic sign, with 5-year survival rates reduced by as much as 50% in patients with nodal involvement compared to patients with N_0 staging.[97,98]

OTHER HEAD AND NECK CANCERS
Cancer of the salivary glands

The major salivary glands include the paired parotid glands, submandibular glands, and sublingual glands. There are hundreds of minor salivary glands in the palate, oral cavity mucosa, and tongue. They are also occasionally found in the mucosal lining of the nose, paranasal sinuses, and pharynx.

Salivary gland tumors are rare, accounting for only 3% of all head and neck neoplasms.[99] The majority of salivary gland tumors arise in the parotid gland, of which 80% are benign. Fifty percent of tumors arising in the submandibular gland are malignant, as are 80% of those arising in the sublingual and minor salivary glands. The most common malignant neoplasm is mucoepidermoid carcinoma, which has both low- and high-grade variations.[100] High-grade mucoepidermoid carcinoma is similar to squamous cell carci-

noma, and it has a high incidence of cervical metastases. Adenoid cystic carcinoma is the next most common malignant histologic type in the parotid gland, but it is the most common malignancy in the submandibular and minor salivary glands.[101] It is a locally aggressive tumor with a tendency for perineural invasion, and it commonly involves and follows the track of adjacent cranial nerves. Lymph node metastases are rare in adenoid cystic carcinoma. Adenocarcinoma and squamous cell carcinoma can be highly malignant primary cancers of the salivary glands, but they are uncommon.

The only etiologic factor specifically linked to the development of salivary gland cancer is exposure to ionizing radiation. In the population of survivors of the Hiroshima and Nagasaki atomic explosions, there has been an increased incidence of benign and malignant salivary neoplasms after latency periods of 20 to 30 years, and, although rare, cases have been seen long after other forms of radiation exposure.[102,103] However, salivary neoplasms have occurred at a much less frequent rate than have postradiation thyroid neoplasms.

Salivary gland neoplasms almost always present as an enlarging, painless mass. Associated cranial nerve deficits are an ominous sign for malignancy. After salivary masses have been discovered upon physical examination, they are usually evaluated by CT and, occasionally, by MRI. Diagnosis can be suggested by FNA, but incisional biopsy is rarely possible because of the risk of spreading tumor and damaging closely adjacent anatomic structures. Thus, in most cases salivary neoplasms, benign or malignant, are usually treated by complete surgical excision. In cases of high-grade mucoepidermoid carcinoma, poorly differentiated adenocarcinoma, and squamous cell carcinoma, treatment of the cervical lymph nodes at risk is necessary. Five-year survival rates are excellent in low-grade malignancies, but they are usually less than 50% in high-grade cancers. Adenoid cystic carcinomas often have a long clinical course, with late recurrences noted as long as 20 years after the time of primary resection.

Cancer of the thyroid gland

The thyroid gland consists of two lobes on either side of the upper trachea, with a small tissue isthmus bridging the midline just below the level of the cricoid cartilage. Thyroid neoplasms can involve the recurrent laryngeal nerve and trachea, and often, they can grow inferiorly into the anterior mediastinum.

Thyroid nodules are common, but the incidence of cancer is estimated at only 12,000 new cases in the United States annually. A patient is considered to be at greatest risk for thyroid carcinoma if there is a single nodule that is determined to be nonfunctional on radioactive uptake scanning. Carcinomas can arise from multinodular goiters, but this presentation is uncommon. A cancerous nodule would be more likely in a patient under age 25, and risk increases steadily after age 45. The risk of cancer is also slightly higher in men.[104]

A specific association has been noted between the history of radiation exposure in childhood and the subsequent development of thyroid neoplasms. From the early 1920s through the mid-1960s, radiation therapy was used for a variety of medical and nonmedical purposes that have since been abandoned. These included treatment for an enlarged thymus gland, enlarged tonsils, acne, and recurrent upper respiratory infections. Large recall studies of patients who were irradiated in this fashion show an incidence of carcinoma of 7% to 9%, with an average latency period of 10 to 20 years and even as long as 30 years. The incidence of benign lesions was also increased, with nodules found in 27% of all patients who were screened. Thus the history of such childhood irradiation greatly increases the risk of benign or malignant thyroid neoplasm, and it is perhaps the single most important historical factor when evaluating a patient with a suspicious thyroid lesion.[105–107]

After physical examination has raised the suspicion of a thyroid nodule, the nature and extent of the lesion are determined by radionucleotide scanning and ultrasound. A CT scan can also be useful in determining the size and extent of the lesion and the presence of any enlarged cervical lymph nodes. Initial histologic determination is best made by FNA. When a thyroid nodule is large enough to be aspirated, an experienced cytologist can make an accurate diagnosis in most cases.[108]

Sixty percent to 65% of thyroid cancer are papillary carcinomas, and most of these are well differentiated. Thirty percent of malignant neoplasms are follicular, and the remainder are either medullary or anaplastic tumors. Mixed papillary–follicular types are also reported. Papillary carcinomas are often multifocal, although the clinical significance of additional microscopic primary tumors within the gland is controversial. Lymph node metastases in papillary carcinoma are not uncommon, but in most cases they do not significantly affect survival. Follicular neoplasms are usually unifocal, and cervical metastases are rare. Medullary carcinoma can be very aggressive locally, and cervical and distant metastases are frequently found. Medullary carcinomas are often linked to multiple endocrine neoplasm syndromes. Anaplastic carcinomas are rare, rapidly enlarging aggressive lesions with an exceedingly poor prognosis. Lymphomas can occur primarily in the thyroid gland, but they are usually seen as part of a systemic disease process.[109]

Thyroid carcinoma is treated by surgical excision. The choice of thyroid lobectomy or total thyroidectomy is controversial. Despite the increased surgical risk, total thyroidectomy is preferred in most cases. Radioactive iodine is used to ablate remaining thyroid tissue, as well as diagnose and treat any residual or late-recurring tumor. Involved lymph nodes are removed selectively in patients with papillary carcinoma; and radical or selective neck dissections are necessary only in cases of medullary carcinoma.[110]

Well-differentiated thyroid carcinoma rarely results in death, except in patients with distant metastases at the time of presentation or in those who develop direct invasion of the laryngotracheal structures.[111,112] However, the mortality rate in these patients is significant. In patients who are over age 50 with distant metastases, a mortality rate of 30% has been reported.

Malignant melanoma

Malignant melanoma accounts for 1% of all human neoplasms. Twenty percent to 30% of melanomas arise in the head and neck, and they tend to be more aggressive than primary lesions of the trunk and extremities.[113] Melanomas occur primarily in caucasians. They are most common between ages 40 and 79, and they are rare in children. The etiology of melanoma has been significantly related to sun exposure, but in many cases there is no definite etiologic factor. The incidence of melanoma is rising rapidly. The current risk is 1 in 128 and it is projected to be 1 in 90 by the year 2000.[114]

Melanomas may arise from junctional nevi or with no underlying lesion. Pathologic variations include lentigo maligna melanoma, superficial spreading melanoma, and nodular melanoma. Staging is based on the depth of invasion through the cutaneous tissues (see box). Melanoma can also arise from the mucosal surfaces of the head and neck, and it has been reported as a primary tumor in the nasal cavity, paranasal sinuses, oral cavity, and pharynx.[115] The staging system that was developed for cutaneous melanoma is not useful in mucosal primary lesions.

The treatment for melanoma is wide surgical excision. Neck dissection is performed for clinically positive lymph nodes, and it is occasionally performed electively in patients with T_3 and T_4 tumors because of the prognostic implications of occult cervical metastases. Radiation therapy and chemotherapy are reserved for palliative treatment.

The prognosis of melanoma is related to the depth of invasion and the presence of lymphatic metastases. Five-year survival rates for T_1 lesions are as high as 90%, and usually less than 10% for T_4 lesions. N_0 lesions have a 5-year survival rate of greater than 90%, but the presence of a lymph node metastasis reduces 5-year survival to less than 10%.[113] The prognosis for all mucosal melanomas is extremely poor.[115]

Lymphoma

Eighty percent of all malignant lymphomas arise from lymph nodes, and many present in the head and neck. Sixty-five percent to 70% of patients with Hodgkin's lymphoma have cervical lymph node involvement. Extranodal presentations (e.g., Waldeyer's ring, salivary gland involvement, or thyroid involvement) are rare in Hodgkin's disease, but they occur in 20% of non-Hodgkin's lymphoma cases.

There have been no specific etiologic factors linked to Hodgkin's disease. Non-Hodgkin's lymphoma has been found to be related to chemical exposure, specifically in patients with a history of occupational exposure to pesticides. Increased levels of non-Hodgkin's lymphoma have been found in crop dusters and in farmers exposed to such chemicals.

Non-Hodgkin's lymphomas are a group of diseases that are divided histologically into favorable and unfavorable types. Favorable types include well-differentiated lymphocytic, follicular, and nodular lymphomas. Unfavorable types include diffuse poorly differentiated lymphocytic, diffuse histiocytic, diffuse undifferentiated, and nodular histiocytic, and immunoblastic lymphomas. Hodgkin's disease is also subdivided, with lymphocyte-predominant and nodular sclerosing types being favorable, mixed cellular types carrying a guarded prognosis, and lymphocyte-depleting types being unfavorable.[116]

The most common presenting symptom of lymphoma in the head and neck is a single enlarged cervical lymph node. Most enlarged nodes involved in lymphoma are described as firm and rubbery. Non-Hodgkin's lymphoma typically involves upper cervical lymph nodes, whereas Hodgkin's disease can be discovered anywhere throughout the cervical chain. The most common site of extranodal involvement of non-Hodgkin's lymphoma is in the head and neck, particularly in Waldeyer's ring. Other sites of involvement include the nasal cavity, paranasal sinuses, orbit, salivary glands, and thyroid gland. Forty percent of patients with lymphoma have systemic symptoms of fever, sweats, weight loss, and malaise. The presence of these symptoms, young age (less than 40 years), and the absence of traditional risk factors of epidermoid carcinoma may increase the index of suspicion for lymphoma. Diagnosis is confirmed by excisional biopsy of the involved lymph node or extranodal tissue.

Staging is determined by the involvement of other nodal sites, the involvement of extranodal organs (spleen and bone marrow), and the presence of systemic symptoms (stage B symptoms).

Stage I and II lesions limited to the head and neck may be considered for treatment with radiation therapy alone. However, in higher-stage tumors or in patients with an unfavorable histologic type or systemic systems, chemotherapy is used as the primary treatment. Radiation therapy is occasionally used with chemotherapy in aggressive tumors.

In Hodgkin's disease stage I and II tumors have 5-year relapse-free rates of 80% to 90%. Rates as low as 30% have been reported in stage IV lesions. Cure rates for non-Hodgkin's lymphoma range from 50% to 70% in stage I and II lesions, with 5-year survival rates universally less than 40% in patients with unfavorable histology or extensive disease.

Unusual tumors

Chemodectomas are also called paragangliomas or glomus tumors. They arise from chemoreceptor tissue and are most common in the head and neck. They are benign in most cases, with only a 2% to 6% rate of malignancy, but they have the propensity for extensive local invasion. They may also occur synchronously at multiple sites. These tumors can arise from the carotid body (carotid body tumors), the ganglion nodosum of the vagus nerve (glomus vagale tumors), the jugular bulb (glomus jugulare tumors), and the middle ear (glomus tympanicum tumors). They have also been reported as primary tumors in the orbit, nose, nasopharynx, and larynx, probably as a result of ectatic chemoreceptor tissue. Chemodectomas usually present either as painless masses or because of the cranial nerve deficits that arise from their progressive growth. They are usually highly vascular lesions. Evaluation must include arteriography, as well as CT and MRI scanning. Biopsy should be performed only under controlled circumstances because of the risk of life-threatening hemorrhage. The choice of treatment is surgical excision, when it can be accomplished with minimal morbidity. However, in cases in which surgical excision cannot be attempted safely, radiation therapy has been shown to retard tumor growth and provide long periods of symptom-free survival. Some slow-growing tumors may be watched expectantly without treatment in selected cases.[117–119]

Esthesioneuroblastoma is a primary neurogenic malignancy of the olfactory epithelium. It presents as a nasal mass, and it commonly leads to epistaxis and anosmia. Involvement of the cribriform plate must be considered in all cases. Histologic diagnosis can be difficult, and it often requires electron microscopy and immunohistochemical staining. These tumors are best treated by complete surgical excision, and they almost always require a combined intracranial and transfacial approach. Local recurrence rates are as high as 50%, but regional and distal metastases are uncommon. Five-year survival rates are approximately 50%.[120]

Other soft-tissue tumors, including osteogenic sarcoma, Ewing's sarcoma, angiosarcoma, chondrosarcoma, hemangiopericytoma, rhabdomyosarcoma, ameloblastoma, and chordoma have all been reported in the head and neck, but these tumors are exceedingly rare. Osteogenic sarcoma and soft-tissue sarcoma have been reported in prior radiation fields 7 to 25 years after initial treatment, and they are believed to occasionally occur as a sequela of ionizing radiation. Osteogenic sarcoma has been noted particularly as a long-term complication of radiation treatment for retinoblastoma in childhood. With the exception of ameloblastoma, which is a benign tumor of the odontogenic apparatus, all soft-tissue sarcomas of the head and neck carry an extremely poor prognosis.

SUMMARY

Cancer of the head and neck can be a devastating disease because of the functional and cosmetic deficits that arise from the tumor invasion and subsequent treatment. However, when these tumors are diagnosed early in their course, they can often be treated successfully with minimal long-term sequelae. Many of the most common cancers of the upper aerodigestive tract are associated with the common risk factors of tobacco and alcohol use, and specific tumor sites such as the nose and the paranasal sinuses have been linked to occupationally related exposures that are carcinogenic. Understanding the potential etiologic factors involved in the development of head and neck cancer will assist in the development of successful prevention and surveillance programs for patients who are at risk.

REFERENCES

1. Boring CC, Squires TS, and Tong T: Cancer statistics, 1992, *CA* 42:19-38, 1992.
2. Parkin DM, Laara E, and Muir CS: Estimates of the worldwide frequency of sixteen major cancers in 1980, *Int J Cancer* 41:184-197, 1988.
3. Zarbo RJ and Crissman JD: The surgical pathology of head and neck cancer, *Semin Oncol* 15:10-19, 1988.
4. Lippman SM and Hong WK: Second malignant tumors in head and neck squamous cell carcinoma: the overshadowing threat for patients with early stage disease, *Int J Radiat Oncol Biol Phys* 17:691-694, 1989.
5. Bastian RW, Kaniff T, Collins SL, et al: Indirect videolaryngoscopy versus direct laryngoscopy for larynx and pharynx cancer staging, *Ann Otol Rhinol Laryngol* 98:693-698, 1989.
6. Castelijins JA: Diagnostic radiology of head and neck oncology, *Curr Opin Oncol* 3:512-518, 1991.
7. Dimery IW and Hong WK: Overview of combined modality therapies for head and neck cancer, *JNCI* 85:95-111, 1993.
8. Martin H and Romieu C: The diagnostic significance of a "lump in the neck," *Postgrad Med* 11:491-500, 1952.
9. Baatenburg de Jong RJ, Rongen RJ, Verwoerd CDA, et al: Ultrasound-guided fine-needle aspiration biopsy of neck nodes, *Arch Otolaryngol* 117:402-404, 1991.
10. Schwartz R, Chan NH, and MacFarlane JK: Fine needle aspiration cytology in the evaluation of head and neck masses, *Am J Surg* 159:482-487, 1990.
11. Weinberger MS, Rosenberg WW, Meurer WT, et al: Fine-needle aspiration of parotid gland lesions, *Head Neck* 14:483-485, 1992.
12. Ellis ER, Mendenhall WM, Rao V, et al: Incisional or excisional neck-node biopsy before definitive radiotherapy, alone or followed by neck dissection, *Head Neck* 13:177-183, 1991.
13. McGuirt WF and McCabe BF: Significance of node biopsy before definitive treatment of cervical metastatic carcinoma, *Laryngoscope* 88:594-597, 1978.
14. Wang RC, Goepfert H, Barber AE, et al: Unknown primary squamous cell carcinoma metastatic to the neck, *Arch Otolaryngol* 116:1388-1393, 1990.
15. Wizenberg MJ, Bloedorn FG, Weiner S, et al: Treatment of lymph node metastases in head and neck cancer, *Cancer* 29:1455-1462, 1972.
16. Jesse RH and Fletcher GH: Treatment of the neck in patients with squamous cell carcinoma of the head and neck, *Cancer* 39:868-872, 1977.
17. Crile GW: Excision of cancer of the head and neck: with special reference to the plan of dissection based on one hundred and thirty-two operations, *JAMA* 47:1780–1785, 1906.
18. Beahrs OH: Surgical anatomy and technique of radical neck dissection, *Surg Clin North Am* 57:663-700, 1977.
19. Gavilan C and Gavilan J: Five-year results of functional neck dissection for cancer of the larynx, *Arch Otolaryngol* 115:1193-1196, 1989.
20. Khafif RA, Gelbfish GA, Asase DK, et al: Modified radical neck dissection in cancer of the mouth, pharynx and larynx, *Head Neck* 12:476-482, 1990.
21. Lingeman RE, Stephens R, Helmus C, et al: Neck dissection: radical or conservative, *Ann Otol* 86:737-744, 1977.
22. Lee JG and Krause CJ: Radical neck dissection: elective neck dissection for pharyngeal and laryngeal cancers, *Ann Otol* 101:656-659, 1975.
23. Lindberg R: Distribution of cervical lymph node metastases from squamous cell carcinoma of the upper respiratory and digestive tracts, *Cancer* 29:1446-1449, 1972.
24. Mendenhall WM, Million RR, and Cassisi NJ: Elective neck irradiation in squamous cell carcinoma of the head and neck, *Head Neck* 3:15-20, 1980.
25. Ogura JH, Biller HF, and Wette R: Elective neck dissection for pharyngeal and laryngeal cancers, *Ann Otol* 80:646-651, 1971.
26. Suarez C, Llorente JL, Nunez F, et al: Neck dissection with or without postoperative radiotherapy in supraglottic carcinomas, *Head Neck* 109:3-9, 1993.
27. Roush GC: Epidemiology of cancer of the nose and paranasal sinuses, *Head Neck* 2:3-11, 1979.
28. Robin PE, Powell DJ, and Stansbie JM: Carcinoma of the nasal cavity and paranasal sinuses: incidence and preservation of different histologic types, *Clin Otolaryngol* 4:431-456, 1979.
29. Robin PE and Powell DJ: Treatment of carcinoma of the nasal cavity and paranasal sinuses, *Clin Otolaryngol* 6:401-411, 1988.
30. Alessi DM, Trapp TK, Yao YS, et al: Nonsalivary sinonasal adenocarcinoma, *Arch Otolaryngol* 114:996-999, 1988.
31. Goepfert H, Luna M, Lindberg R, et al: Malignant salivary gland tumors of the paranasal sinuses and nasal cavity, *Arch Otolaryngol* 109:662-668, 1983.
32. Kraus DH, Roberts JK, Medendorp SV, et al: Nonsquamous cell malignancies of the paranasal sinuses, *Ann Otol* 99:5-11, 1990.
33. Myers EN, Schramm VL, and Barnes EL: Management of inverted papilloma of the nose and paranasal sinuses, *Laryngoscope* 91:2071-2084, 1981.
34. Vrabec DP: The inverted schneiderian papilloma: a 25-year study, *Laryngoscope* 104:582-605, 1994.
35. Osguthorpe JD and Weisman RA: Medial maxillectomy for lateral nasal wall neoplasms, *Arch Otolaryngol* 117:751-756, 1991.
36. Doll R, Morgan LG, and Speizer FE: Cancers of the lung and nasal sinuses in nickel workers, *Br J Cancer* 24:623-632, 1970.
37. Grandjean P, Anderson O, and Nielsen GD: Carcinogenicity of occupational nickel exposures: an evaluation of the epidemiological evidence, *Am J Ind Med* 13:193-209, 1988.
38. Costa M: Molecular mechanisms of nickel carcinogenesis, *Annu Rev Pharmacol Toxicol* 31:321-337, 1991.
39. Sunderman WJ: A review of the carcinogenicities of nickel, chromium and arsenic compounds in man and animals, *Prev Med* 5:279-294, 1976.
40. Ironside P and Matthews J: Adenocarcinoma of the nose and paranasal sinuses in woodworkers in the state of Victoria, Australia, *Cancer* 36:1115-1121, 1975.
41. Brinton LA, Blot WJ, Stone BJ, et al: A death certificate analysis of nasal cancer among furniture workers in North Carolina, *Cancer Res* 37:3473-3474, 1977.
42. Cecchi F, Buiatti E, Kriebel D, et al: Adenocarcinoma of the nose and paranasal sinuses in shoemakers and woodworkers in the province of Florence, Italy (1963-77), *Br J Ind Med* 37:222-225, 1980.
43. Roush GC, Meigs JW, Kelly J, et al: Sinonasal cancer and occupation: a cancer–control study, *Am J Epidemiology* 111:183-193, 1980.
44. Gerhardsson MR, Norell SE, Kiviranta HJ, et al: Respiratory cancers in furniture workers, *Br J Med* 42:403-405, 1985.
45. Imbus HR and Dyson WL: A review of nasal cancer in furniture manufacturing and woodworking in North Carolina, the United States, and other countries, *JOM, J Occup Med* 29:734-740, 1987.
46. Viren JR and Imbus HR: Case–control study of nasal cancer in workers employed in wood-related industries, *JOM, J Occup Med* 31:35-40, 1989.

47. Shimizu H, Hozawa J, Saito H, et al: Chronic sinusitis and wood-working as risk factors for cancer of the maxillary sinus in Northeast Japan, *Laryngoscope* 99:58-61, 1989.

48. Luce D, Leclerc A, Morcet JF, et al: Occupational risk factors for sinonasal cancer: a case–control study in France, *Am J Ind Med* 21:163-175, 1992.

49. Comba P, Battista G, Belli S, et al: A case–control study of cancer of the nose and paranasal sinuses and occupational exposures, *Am J Ind Med* 22:511-520, 1992.

50. Kashima HK, Kessis T, Hruban RH, et al: Human papillomavirus in sinonasal papillomas and squamous cell carcinoma, *Laryngoscope* 102:973-980, 1992.

51. Elwood JM: Wood exposure and smoking: association with cancer of the nasal cavity and paranasal sinuses in British Columbia, *Can Med Assoc J* 124:1573-1577, 1981.

52. Osguthorpe JD: Sinus neoplasia, *Arch Otolaryngol* 120:19-25, 1994.

53. Lyons BM and Donald PJ: Radical surgery for nasal cavity and paranasal sinus tumors, *Otolaryngol Clin North Am* 24:1499-1521, 1991.

54. LoRusso P, Tapazoglou E, Kish JA, et al: Chemotherapy for paranasal sinus carcinoma, *Cancer* 62:1-5, 1988.

55. Stern SJ, Goepfert H, Clayman G, et al: Squamous cell carcinoma of the maxillary sinus, *Arch Otolaryngol* 119:964-969, 1993.

56. Shah JP, Kraus DH, Arbit E, et al: Craniofacial resection for tumors involving the anterior skull base, *Otolaryngol Head Neck Surg* 106:387-393, 1992.

57. Nunez F, Suarez C, Alvarez I, et al: Sino-nasal adenocarcinoma: epidemiological and clinico-pathological study of 34 cases, *J Otolaryngol* 22:86-90, 1993.

58. St-Pierre S and Baker SR: Squamous cell carcinoma of the maxillary sinus: analysis of 66 cases, *Head Neck Surg* 5:508-513, 1983.

59. Baker SR and Wolfe RA: Prognostic factors of nasopharyngeal malignancy, *Cancer* 49:163-169, 1982.

60. Buell P: Nasopharynx cancer in Chinese in California, *Br J Cancer* 19:459-463, 1965.

61. Feinmesser R, Miyazaki I, Cheung R, et al: Diagnosis of nasopharyngeal carcinoma by DNA amplification of tissue obtained by fine-needle aspiration, *N Engl J Med* 326:17-21, 1992.

62. Henle G and Henle W: Epstein–Barr virus-specific IgA antibodies as an outstanding feature of nasopharyngeal carcinoma, *Int J Cancer* 17:1-7, 1976.

63. Baker SR: Malignant tumors of the nasopharynx, *J Surg Oncol* 17:23-32, 1981.

64. Johansin LV, Mestre M, and Overgaard J: Carcinoma of the nasopharynx: analysis of treatment in 167 consecutively admitted patients, *Head Neck* 14:200-207, 1992.

65. Fisch U, Fagun P, and Valvania A: The infratemporal fossa approach for the lateral skull base, *Otolaryngol Clin North Am* 17:513-552, 1984.

66. Stockwell HG and Lyman GH: Impact of smoking and smokeless tobacco on the risk of cancer of the head and neck, *Head Neck* 9:104-110, 1986.

67. Wray A and McGuirt F: Smokeless tobacco usage associated with oral carcinoma, *Arch Otolaryngol* 119:923-933, 1993.

68. Rodgers LW, Stringer SP, Mendenhall WM, et al: Management of squamous cell carcinoma of the floor of the mouth, *Head Neck* 15:16-19, 1993.

69. Cole DA, Patel PM, Matar JR, et al: Floor of mouth cancer, *Arch Otolaryngol* 120:260-263, 1994.

70. Gehanno P, Guedon C, Barry B, et al: Advanced carcinoma of the tongue: total glossectomy without total laryngectomy. Review of 80 cases, *Laryngoscope* 102:1369-1371, 1992.

71. Salibian AH, Allison GR, Rappaport I, et al: Total and subtotal glossectomy: function after microvascular reconstruction, *Plast Reconstr Surg* 85:513-524, 1990.

72. Leipzig B, Cummings CW, Johnson JT, et al: Carcinoma of the anterior tongue, *Ann Otol* 91:94-97, 1982.

73. Mizono GS, Diaz RF, Fu KK, et al: Carcinoma of the tonsillar region, *Laryngoscope* 96:240-244, 1986.

74. Christopoulos E, Carrau R, Segas J, et al: Transmandibular approaches to the oral cavity and oropharynx, *Arch Otolaryngol* 118:1164-1167, 1992.

75. Spiro JD and Spiro RH: Carcinoma of the tonsillar fossa: an update, *Arch Otolaryngol Head Neck Surg* 115:1186-1189, 1989.

76. Carpenter RJ, DeSanto LW, et al: Cancer of the hypopharynx: analysis of treatment in 162 patients, *Arch Otolaryngol* 102:716-721, 1976.

77. Ho CM, Lam KH, Wei WI, et al: Squamous cell carcinoma of the hypopharynx—analysis of treatment results, *Head Neck* 15:405-412, 1993.

78. Shah JP, Shaha AR, Spiro RH, et al: Carcinoma of the hypopharynx, *Am J Surg* 132:439-443, 1976.

79. Driscoll WG, Nagaorsky MJ, Cantrell RW, et al: Carcinoma of the pyriform sinus: analysis of 102 cases, *Laryngoscope* 93:556-560, 1983.

80. Guillamondegui OM, Geoffray B, and McKenna RJ: Total reconstruction of the hypopharynx and cervical esophagus, *Am J Surg* 150:422-426, 1985.

81. McDonough JJ and Gluckman JL: Microvascular reconstruction of the pharyngoesophagus with free jejunal graft, *Microsurgery* 9:116-127, 1988.

82. Silverberg E and Lubera JA: Cancer statistics, *CA* 38:5-22, 1988.

83. Auerbach O, Hammond EC, and Garfinkel L: Histologic changes in the larynx in relation to smoking habits, *Cancer* 25:92-104, 1970.

84. Flanders WD and Rothman KJ: Interaction of alcohol and tobacco in laryngeal cancer, *Am J Epidemiol* 115:371-379, 1982.

85. Maier H, Gewelke U, Dietz A, et al: Risk factors of cancer of the larynx: results of the Heidelberg case–control study, *Head Neck* 107:577-582, 1992.

86. Burch JD, Howe GR, Miller AB, et al: Tobacco, alcohol, asbestos, and nickel in the etiology of cancer of the larynx: a case control study, *JNCI* 67:1219-1224, 1981.

87. Parnes SM: Asbestos and cancer of the larynx. is there a relationship?, *Laryngoscope* 100:254-261, 1990.

88. Pedersen E, Hogetveit AC, and Andersen A: Cancer of respiratory organs among workers at a nickel refinery in Norway, *Int J Cancer* 12:32-41, 1973.

89. Stell PM and McGill T: Asbestos and laryngeal carcinoma, *Lancet* 2:416-417, 1973.

90. Wynder EL, Covey LS, Mabuchi K, et al: Environmental factors in cancer of the larynx: a second look, *Cancer* 38:1591-1601, 1976.

91. Brandwein MS, Nuovo GJ, and Biller H: Analysis of prevalence of human papillomavirus in laryngeal carcinomas, *Ann Otol Rhinol Laryngol* 102:309-313, 1993.

92. Simon M, Kahn T, Schneider A, et al: Laryngeal carcinoma in a 12-year-old child: association with human papillovirus 18 and 33, *Arch Otolaryngol* 120:277-282, 1994.

93. Bocca E: Supraglottic cancer, *Laryngoscope* 88:1318-1326, 1974.

94. Olsen KD, Thomas JV, DeSanto LW, et al: Indications and results of cordectomy for early glottic carcinoma, *Otolaryngol Head Neck Surg* 108:277-282, 1993.

95. Wolf GT, et al: Induction chemotherapy plus radiation compared with surgery plus radiation in patients with advanced laryngeal cancer, *N Engl J Med* 324:1685-1690, 1991.

96. Hagen P, Lyons GD, and Haindel C: Verrucous carcinoma of the larynx: role of human papillomavirus, radiation and surgery, *Laryngoscope* 103:253-257, 1993.

97. Kaplan MJ, Johns ME, Clark DA, et al: Glottic carcinoma—the roles of surgery and irradiation, *Cancer* 53:2641-2648, 1984.

98. Mendenhall WM, Parsons JT, Stringer SP, et al: Carcinoma of the supraglottic larynx: a basis for comparing the results of radiation therapy and surgery, *Head Neck* 12:204-209, 1990.

99. American Cancer Society: *Other facts and figures*, pp 62-66, New York, 1979, American Cancer Society.

100. Kane WJ, McCaffrey TV, Olsen KD, et al: Primary parotid malignancies, *Arch Otolaryngol* 116:1055-1060, 1990.

101. Weber RS, Byers RM, Petit B, et al: Submandibular gland tumors, *Arch Otolaryngol* 116:1055-1060, 1990.

102. Belsky JL, Tachikawa K, Cihak RW, et al: Salivary gland tumors in atomic bomb survivors. Hiroshima-Nagasaki, *JAMA* 219:864-868, 1972.

103. Ju DMC: Salivary gland tumors occurring after radiation of the head and neck area, *Am J Surg* 116:518-523, 1968.

104. Peake RI: Clinical evaluation of thyroid tumors. In Thawley SE and Panje WR, editors: *Comprehensive management of head and neck tumors,* pp 1580-1598, Philadelphia, 1987, WB Saunders.

105. Hempelmann LH, Hall WJ, Phillips M, et al: Neoplasms in persons treated with x-rays in infancy: fourth survey in 20 years, *JNCI* 55:519-530, 1975.

106. Schneider AB, Favus MJ, Stachura ME, et al: Incidence, prevalence and characteristics of radiation-induced thyroid tumors, *Am J Med* 64:243-252, 1978.

107. Witt TR, Meng RL, Economou SG, et al: The approach to the irradiated thyroid, *Surg Clin North Am* 59:45-63, 1979.

108. Cohen JP and Cho HT: The role of needle aspiration biopsy in the selection of patients for thyroidectomy, *Laryngoscope* 98:35-39, 1988.

109. Schwartz MR: Pathology of the thyroid and parathyroid glands, *Otolaryngol Clin North Am* 23:175-215, 1990.

110. Lando MJ, Hoover LA, and Zuckerbraun L: Surgical strategy in thyroid disease, *Arch Otolaryngol* 116:1378-1383, 1990.

111. Lydiatt DD, Markin RS, and Ogren FP: Tracheal invasion by thyroid carcinoma, *ENT J* 69:145-148, 1990.

112. McConahey WM, Nay ID, Woolner LB, et al: Papillary thyroid cancer treated at the Mayo Clinic, 1946 through 1970: initial manifestations, pathologic findings, therapy, and outcome, *Mayo Clinic Proc* 61:978-996, 1986.

113. Fisher SR: Cutaneous malignant melanoma of the head and neck, *Laryngoscope* 99:822-836, 1989.

114. Seigler HF: Immunobiology and immunotherapy of neoplastic disease; melanoma; soft tissue sarcomas; tumor markers. In Sabiston DC, editor: *Textbook of surgery: the biological basis of modern surgical practice,* Philadelphia, 1991, WB Saunders.

115. Berthelsen A, Andersen AP, Jensen S, et al: Melanomas of the mucosa of the upper respiratory passages, *Cancer* 54:907-912, 1984.

116. McClatchey KD and Schnitzer B: Pathology of lymphorecticular disorders. In Thawley SE and Panje WR, editors: *Comprehensive management of head and neck tumors,* Philadelphia, 1987, WB Saunders.

117. Brown JS: Glomus jugulare tumors revisited: a ten year statistical follow-up of 231 cases, *Laryngoscope* 95:284-288, 1985.

118. Springate SC and Weichselbaum RR: Radiation or surgery for chemodectoma of the temporal bone: a review of local control and complications, *Head Neck Surg* 12:303-307, 1990.

119. van der Mey AGL, Fruns JHM, Cornelisse CJ, et al: Does intervention improve the natural course of glomus tumors?, *Ann Otol Rhinol Laryngol* 101:635-642, 1992.

120. Cantrell RW, Ghorayeb BY, and Fitz-Hugh GS: Esthesioneuroblastoma: diagnosis and treatment, *Ann Otol Rhinol Laryngol* 86:760-765, 1977.

Agents Causing Interstitial Disease

PHILIP HARBER

Agents and the diseases they produce are discussed in Sections V through VIII (agents causing interstitial disease, agents causing airway disease, agents causing other respiratory disease, industries associated with respiratory disease). Where an agent can lead to several different forms of disease, it is discussed in the section that is most commonly relevant. For example, coal dust, which classically causes an interstitial disorder, also affects airway function. Readers should therefore consult other sections as appropriate.

Radiographic methods are critically important for the recognition and classification of interstitial lung diseases. The term "simple pneumoconiosis" is applied when the radiograph shows small rounded opacities (less than 10 mm), whereas "complicated pneumoconiosis" applies when larger opacities are present. The term "progressive massive fibrosis" is used to describe the advanced stage's clinical, radiographic, and pathologic findings. "Pleural fibrosis" is a term that encompasses both circumscribed "pleural plaques" and diffuse pleural thickening.

Chapter 20

ASBESTOS

Raymond Bégin
Jonathan M. Samet
Rashid A. Shaikh

PART I

Asbestos-related diseases

Raymond Bégin

Asbestos and its associated health effects have received considerable attention due to the ubiquitous nature of exposure and the diverse nature of health effects. Effects of occupational exposures at relatively high levels have been studied for many years, and there is increasing interest in the effects of lower level and intermittent exposures. However, despite major strides over the past 15 years in controlling exposures, there are still many persons who have had prolonged and/or high levels of exposures in the past. Therefore, there will be a significant burden of asbestos-related diseases in the foreseeable future.

There are many perspectives on asbestos disease, ranging from prevention to compensation. This chapter provides an overview of the effects of exposure and discusses the mechanisms of asbestos-related disease. Part I includes an overview of asbestos and its use, a discussion of asbestos-related diseases, including biologic mechanisms, pathology, and radiology, and clinical manifestations and course. Part II discusses asbestos in buildings, including health risk, risk assessment models, methods of assessment and management of buildings with asbestos, public policy implications, and risk associated with low level exposures.

Additional relevant information is found in several other chapters; the following chapters deal explicitly with aspects of asbestos-related health effects:

Chapter 7, Radiologic Methods, discusses the Interna

tional Labor Office (ILO) system, which provides a standardized method of interpreting radiographs for preumoccuioses, and application of computerized tomographic (CT) scan methods.

Chapter 8, Pathologic Methods, discusses asbestos-related diseases.

Chapter 12, Mineralogy, characterizes asbestos as a mineral and discusses the mineralogic characteristics related to the mechanism of biologic effects.

Chapter 15, Pulmonary Fibrosis and Interstitial Lung Diseases, discusses the diagnosis and management of interstitial lung disorders.

Chapter 51, Screening and Surveillance, discusses methods for routine periodic evaluation of asbestos-exposed persons.

OVERVIEW

From the beginning of the twentieth century, several diseases have been associated with asbestos exposure. Some have a definite association, whereas others initially considered to be associated with asbestos exposure were afterward proven not to be. The following diseases are unequivocally recognized as asbestos-related diseases:

1. *Asbestosis* is an interstitial fibrosis of the lung parenchyma.
2. *Benign asbestos pleurisy,* also called benign pleural effusion, is an exudative and transient inflammation of the pleura.
3. *Pleural plaques* are accumulations of collagen fibers forming hyalin masses that are avascular, acellular and circumscribed, usually limited to the parietal pleura.
4. *Diffuse pleural thickening (pachypleuritis)* are accumulations of collagen fibers forming hyalin masses that are avascular, acellular, and diffuse, affecting the parietal and visceral pleura, occasionally invading the interlobular spaces of the lung parenchyma. This local association has been called "crow's feet" and is not to be confounded with asbestosis.
5. *Rounded atelectasis* is an effect of asbestos-induced pleural disease that is caused by the scarring of the pleura and adjacent lung tissue, with retraction of the scar tissue and partial collapse of adjacent lung tissue.
6. *Malignant mesothelioma* is a malignant tumor of the mesothelium of the pleura that is rapidly invading and usually fatal within 12 to 24 months after clinical diagnosis.
7. *Bronchogenic carcinoma* is a malignant bronchopulmonary tumor similar to that associated with cigarette smoking or with other lung carcinogen exposures. The increased incidence of this tumor is universally accepted in association with asbestosis, but its relation to asbestos exposure remains controversial in the absence of asbestosis in smokers. It is important to re-

member that the vast majority of lung tumors seen in asbestos workers are bronchogenic tumors originating from the large airways and that few of these lesions are carcinoma based on scars. The multiplicative effect of asbestos exposure and cigarette usage is well recognized in several large studies.

8. *Benign nodules* in the lung parenchyma are occasionally seen in asbestos workers. They can be benign lymphoid nodules, scars of localized fibrosis, or more strikingly, rounded atelectasis.

The diseases that have not been accepted unequivocally as related to asbestos exposure will not be discussed here, and interested readers are referred to exhaustive reviews of the literature.[1-7] The possibility of a relationship between asbestos and laryngeal cancer is discussed in Chapter 19.

HISTORY

Asbestos, from the greek ασβεστοζ (inextinguishable), has been known since antiquity. It was used for wicks of torches in temples. From about the year 2500 BC, asbestos-based pottery was produced. In the time of the Pharaohs, Herod noticed that linens made of asbestos were used to incinerate bodies. The Romans extracted asbestos from near the actual mine of Balangero. Charlemagne stunned his guests by throwing his asbestos-made tablecloth in a fire to clean it. Asbestos was the Salamander wool of alchemists.[3]

Asbestos use remained on a small scale, primarily related to crafts, until the discoveries of the vast asbestos strata of Québec and Russia at the end of the nineteenth century. In Québec, mine exploration started by 1878 at Asbestos, a small township named for its product, and chrysotile, the white asbestos, has been produced since. In Russia, commercial production started in 1885. The crocidolite blue asbestos was initially produced in 1880, whereas amosite and anthophyllite were commercially available from the time of World War I.

The world production af asbestos increased slowly at the beginning of the twentieth century; by 1930 a total amount of 5×10^9 kg had been produced. Rapid acceleration of production in subsequent years resulted in a yearly production of 5×10^9 kg, responding to the demand for asbestos use in some 3000 applications.

Twenty years after the start of industrial use of asbestos in Europe, Auribeault[7a] in 1906 described 50 cases of pulmonary fibrosis in the asbestos textile factory of Cordé-sur Noireau in Normandy, France. In England, Murray[8] described the first case of asbestosis in a 30-year-old asbestos worker, the last survivor of a group of 10 employed in the same workshop. Also in 1906 Marchand[9] described the asbestos bodies. After 1926, it became accepted that asbestos was toxic for the pleura, the lung, and the airways.

The problem of public health and hygiene that industrial use of asbestos creates became clear in the 1950s. In 1955,

Jacob and Bohling reported on calcified pleural plaques[10]; in 1960, Wagner et al.[11] described 33 cases of malignant mesothelioma, of which 28 involved exposure to crocidolite asbestos from the Cape in South Africa. In the following years, animal experimentation confirmed the fibrosing and carcinogenic potential of all types of asbestos fibers.

In the 1960s and 1970s, the large epidemiologic studies of several American and European teams confirmed the clinical observations and quantified the magnitude of the industrial hygiene problems involved with the commercialization of asbestos fibers. These investigations were presented at international conferences in New York in 1964, 1979, and 1990,[12-14] at the International Agency for Research on Cancer (IARC) in 1972 and 1979,[15] in Montréal in 1980,[16] in Cardiff, Wales in 1986 (on the biological effects of chrysotile),[17] and in Paris in 1991 (on malignant mesothelioma).[18]

In the 1980s, studies on the biological mechanisms of asbestos-related diseases were initiated in several laboratories around the world.[19-21] These studies have increased our understanding of the pathogenesis of the disease processes.

ASBESTOS: MINERALOGY

The term asbestos refers to a family of naturally occurring, flexible, fibrous hydrous silicate minerals that is relatively indestructible and heat resistant.

For the mineralogist, the term asbestos is part of the morphologic terminology used to describe a property known in mineralogy as "crystal habit." It is used to describe the fibrous aspect in which some minerals crystallize: the asbestiform aspect. The characteristics of this "crystal habit" are a very accentuated fibrous aspect, with high ratios of length to breadth (aspect ratio), flexibility, and similarity to organic fibers. It is also characterized by the small diameter of elementary units (elementary fibrils) that can be associated longitudinally to form bundles of fibers that aggregate in hairlike bundles, or in less oriented aggregates, due to variations in mineral content and different habits of the component crystals. Other common forms of crystallization are tabular, equant, prismatic, and acicular.

Although more than 30 minerals can crystallize in an asbestiform habit, only six have been of industrial use: chrysotile, crocidolite, amosite, anthophyllite, tremolite, and actinolite. In general terms, only these six minerals are referred to as asbestos fibers. Chrysotile is classified as a serpentine mineral because of its layered silicate structure, and the other five asbestes are classified as amphibole minerals because of their chained silicate structure. These six minerals can also crystallize in other nonasbestiform structures, in which case other terminology is used to describe the minerals, except for anthophyllite, tremolite, and actinolite (Table 20-I-1).

A basic understanding of the structure-related terminology of these minerals is of interest to understand the com-

Table 20-1-1. Classification of asbestos minerals

Asbestiform	Nonasbestiform	Chemical formula
Chrysotile	Antigorite, Lizardite	$Mg_3(Si_2O_5)(OH)_4$
Crocidolite	Riebeckite	$Na_2Fe_5(Si_8O_{22})(OH)_2$
Amosite	Cummingtonite-Grunerite	$(Fe,Mg)_7(Si_8O_{22})(OH)_2$
Anthophyllite	Anthophyllite	$(Mg,Fe)_7(Si_8O_{22})(OH)_2$
Tremolite	Tremolite	$Ca_2Mg_5(Si_8O_{22})(OH)_2$
Actinolite	Actinolite	$Ca_2(Mg,Fe)_5(Si_8O_{22})(OH)_2$

plexities of some of the laws and practices regulating industrial hygiene, as the relative toxicity of these minerals has been linked to their morphology and physicochemical properties.

In early studies of the toxicity of asbestos dusts, the generic term asbestos was used and led to the general class of asbestos-related diseases. Then, all asbestiform minerals were considered equally toxic and only one industrial hygiene standard was in common use. Later, as toxicity was recognized as being greater for the amphiboles, different standards were applied. The debate on the relative toxicity of different forms and structures of asbestos minerals remains open, particularly for the tremolite asbestos, which can have the full spectrum of crystal structure but for which the relative toxicity is not fully understood.

Overall, it should be remembered that whereas asbestos-related diseases have been reported in association with exposure to all types of asbestos fibers, the incidence of various diseases and the intensity of the pathological processes will vary with the different types of fibers.

Chrysotile

Chrysotile fibers result from a peculiar hydrothermic transformation (serpentinization) of ultrabasic rocks (dunites, pyroxenites, and peridonites). Chrysotile is a mineral of the serpentine group, which also includes lizardite and antigorite.

Its name comes from the greek κηρυσοσ (gold) and τιλοσ (fiber). Chrysotile fibers are relatively translucent with a silk sparkle. Depending on the mine of origin, they may have more or less flexibility. The elementary fibrils of chrysotile have an average diameter of 0.03 μm and they are grouped to form an open core cylinder. These tubes are composed of layers of intertwined fibrils, which form an onion-peel apparent structure around the core. Each tube is approximately 200 Å in diameter; the tubes are grouped in slivers of 0.1 mm^2 that contain some 20×10^6 tubular fibrils, in relative parallel orientation.

The major mineral ore deposits in commercial use are presented in Table 20-1-2. Chrysotile fibers are found within veins of serpentine minerals. The direction of the fibers is usually perpendicular to the main direction of the vein but at times is along the main direction of the vein. In the latter case, the fibers can be very long (up to 1 m),

Table 20-1-2. Major deposit sites of asbestos in the world

Chrysotile	Canada (Québec, British Colombia, Yukon, Newfoundland, Ontario), Russia (Oural, Sibéria), Zimbabwe, Botswana, Swaziland, Australia, Cyprus, China, Brazil, USA (Vermont, Arizona, California)
Crocidolite	South Africa, Bolivia, Australia
Amosite	South Africa, India
Anthophyllite	Finland, USA, South Africa, Bulgaria
Tremolite	Italy, South Africa, Pakistan, Korea
Actinolite	Taiwan, South Africa

rough, and friable, thus of less commercial value. Occasionally, chrysotile fibers can be found dispersed and oriented in all directions in the matrix of serpentines as in the Coalinga mine of California, where the fibers are generally shorter and of lower commercial quality.

Other serpentine minerals such as magnetite, brucite, olivine, and tremolite can be found in association with chrysotile. Chrysotile fibers can also be found in other minerals, such as talc, nickel, iron, and mica. Leveling of serpentine grounds can also be the source of chrysotile pollution in the environment.

Chrysotile is of commercial interest because of its mechanical properties of resistance to heat and traction, flexibility, adsorbancy, chemical resistance to alkalines, and its ease of spinning for textile products. It has weak resistance to acid, resists other chemicals well, and resists heat over 100°C. Chrysotile loses its structure above 575°C.

Amphiboles

The amphibole asbestos group contains several minerals, similar in structure but distinct in chemical composition. The asbestiform structure of the five asbestos amphiboles differs slightly from that of chrysotile.

The amphibole fibers are more rigid; they do not form cylindrical structure but run parallel to the chain of silicate tetrahedra. This chain-like structure is stacked lightly, which results in good cleavage of the amphiboles. Because of their rigidity, amphiboles form fewer aggregates than chrysotile. Fibers are more readily seen in aerosols and their handling is reputed to generate more fiber dust. Amphiboles resist acid and heat better.

The major amphibole ore deposits in commercial exploitation are presented in Table 20-1-2.

Crocidolite is a sodium iron silicate, as is amosite, formed in thermally metamorphosed banded ironstones. Crocidolite is often referred to as blue asbestos, and has been mined in South Africa, Australia, and Bolivia. It is not as harsh as amosite and has been used in spinning and insulation. It is reputed to be the most dangerous form because of its strong association with mesothelioma.

Amosite, an amphibole mined only in the Transsval area of South Africa, is an iron magnesium silicate, brownish in color; it has the longest fibers, but its harshness renders it unsuitable for spinning; it has been used mainly as heat insulation material.

Anthophyllite is a white amphibole and a magnesium silicate containing various quantities of iron. It occurs in fibrous masses with short fiber bundles. It was mined and used in Finland up to 1970.

Tremolite is a white amphibole and a green-yellow calcium and magnesium silicate that is mined in relatively pure form in Italy and Japan. It is a common contaminant of most chrysotile mines.

Specialized references can be consulted for further details.[22,23] In addition, general aspects of mineralogy are discussed in Chapter 12.

PRODUCTION AND USES OF ASBESTOS

The world production of asbestos since the early mining in the late nineteenth century increased until about 1975 to 1980.

The development of an asbestos production mine usually starts with an open pit operation in which mechanical shovels and bulldozers work to break down the materials and load trucks or trainwagons for transportation of the raw materials to a processing mill. As opposed to the traditional underground mining process, open pit operations account for 70% of the total production of asbestos.

Then the raw material is further processed by fragmenting, sorting, and screening operations to concentrate the desired asbestos material and eliminate the undesired ore rocks. The milling process permits further concentration of the fiber materials, elimination of undesired mineral components, drying of the asbestos material, removal of grit and dust, and finally the separation of the asbestos fibers into classified samples for various commercial grades.

At present, chrysotile represents 95% of the world production, and the main market for the fibrous mineral is the production of asbestos cement. Chrysotile is produced mainly in Russia, Canada, Swaziland, and Zimbabwe, with minor production plants in California, Australia, Cyprus, Italy, Brazil, and China. Amosite was produced uniquely in South Africa. Crocidolite is produced in South Africa, Australia (now ceased), and Bolivia. Anthophyllite was produced only in Finland.

The asbestos fibers are valued for their mechanical properties, their fire resistance and insulation properties, and their chemical stability.

The material is used in secondary industries in over 3000 applications, of which the major are:

1. Asbestos cement products, including pipes, shingles, clapboards, flat sheets, corrugated sheets, and molded sheets for the building construction industry
2. Vinyl asbestos floor tile

3. Asbestos paper for use in insulation and filtering products
4. Friction materials for brake linings and clutch facings
5. Asbestos textile products such as wisk, yarn, tape felt tubing cord, and rope
6. Spray products for decorative, acoustical, thermal, and fireproofing purposes.

The major end users of the past have been in the building construction industry, the shipbuilding industry, and the automobile and railroad equipment industry, where much of the insulation and friction materials are now made of non-asbestos replacement fiber materials.

The longest asbestos fibers are used mainly in the textile and insulation industries, the intermediate fibers are used in asbestos cement and friction and filter production, and the shortest fibers are used in the vinyl-asbestos tile industry and as an admixture to outdoor paints. The mill tailings of the mining process were used in road construction and for the extraction of magnesium.

ASBESTOS FIBERS IN ENVIRONMENT AND IN HUMAN TISSUES

In industrial settings, the control of asbestos dust exposure has proven to be the most effective mode of disease prevention. The current U.S. Occupational Safety and Health Administration (OSHA) standard is 0.1 fiber/cm^3 of workplace air. In the past, asbestos exposure in the workplace may have been over 100 fibers/cm^3 for some cases and was commonly between 5 and 20 fibers/cm^3.

To enforce the legislation, methods for airborne dust sampling and examination were developed. For the fibrous minerals, air sampling is collected over time with membrane filter methods, and the collected dust is precipitated for examination with light microscope with or without previous incineration to remove organic matter. Magnification is up to 500×; by means of a graticule in one of the eyepieces, the dimensions of fibers can be evaluated and counts can be made in random fields. This method is suited for rapid screening, recognizing readily the fibers of length > 5 μm and width > 0.1 μm. However, many of the chrysotile fibers will not be seen by this optical method.

Transmission electron microscopy (TEM) can magnify up to 100,000× but may overlook the bigger fibers. Although preparation of specimens is more time consuming and expensive, TEM results coupled with those of optical microscopy give a more complete picture of air contamination. The TEM method can use additional technologies such as electron diffraction, electron microprobe, and x-ray spectrometry for specific identification of the fibers and particles under the microscope. The TEM method has been a tool of significant use in assessing environmental air pollution in the neighborhood of asbestos mills, plants, and factories.

For occasional clinical diagnosis, worker's compensation, and medicolegal purposes, the determination of asbestos fibers in biological samples may be used to document past exposures to asbestos. In that context, analyses of human tissues are an adjunctive method to the usual clinical methods of diagnosis of asbestos-related diseases. Laboratory methods in optical and electron microscopy are available in specialized laboratories,[24–26] where samples are first separated by filtration and observed under the microscope.

Observation under optical microscopy permits the visualization and count of ferruginous bodies, the ferritin–protein-coated fibers, which may or may not be asbestos fiber, and the fibers longer than 5 μm and larger than 0.1 μm. This method is widely used by pathologists for usual routine lung pathology and after tissue digestion using phase contrast, sputum cytology, and lung lavage cytology, which may provide a set of fundamental indices of asbestos exposure. The limitations of optical microscopy are the same here as for air sample analyses.

Asbestos fibers and other fibrous particles can be coated by macrophages with an iron–protein coat with formation of beadlike structures on the fibers. These are rarely found on fibers shorter than 10 μm length. They are associated more with amphiboles than chrysotile, possibly because of the greater dissolution and breakdown of chrysotile. The asbestos bodies can be found in virtually anyone in the population as long as appropriate methods are used. In cases of asbestos-related diseases, the asbestos bodies can usually be found in the lung parenchyma, but asbestos bodies may often not be seen in cases of asbestosis employing the usual light microscopy of the clinical pathologist in cases of chrysotile exposure only. However, in such cases, electron microscopy coupled with tissue digestion reveals the fibers and associated asbestos bodies.[24–26]

Asbestos bodies in lung tissue samples

The following values are useful for interpreting the significance of asbestos body and fiber counts in samples of human tissue. It is important to recognize that these values are derived from many different laboratories, and there is significant interlaboratory variation.

1. Sputum cytology samples:
   a. Normal control populations have no asbestos bodies (AB).
   b. Any AB seen constitutes an index of significant exposure.
2. Lung lavage samples:
   a. Normals have less than 1 AB/ml of lavage effluent.
   b. More than 1 AB/ml suggests lung tissue AB >1/mg, which corresponds to a nonsignificant exposure.
3. Lung tissue samples:
   a. Normal white-collar workers without exposure have <0.1 AB/mg.

b. Normal blue-collar workers without exposure have <0.5 AB/mg.

c. Normal blue-collar workers with minimal exposure have >0.5 AB/mg and <2 AB/mg.

d. Patients with pleural plaques have approximately 1.7 AB/mg.

e. Patients with mesothelioma have AB from within the range of normals to the range of patients with asbestosis.

f. Long-term asbestos workers with grade 0 asbestosis have up to 1300 AB/mg.

g. Long-term asbestos workers with grade 1 asbestosis have about 8000 AB/mg.

h. Long-term asbestos workers with grade 2 asbestosis have about 74,000 AB/mg.

Asbestos fibers by optical microscopy in lung tissue

1. The general population has <250 fibers/mg tissue.

2. Exposed persons with grade 0 asbestosis have 2400 fibers/mg.

3. Persons with grade 1 asbestosis have 8000 to 19,000 fibers/mg.

4. Persons with grade 2 asbestosis have 14,000 to 200,000 fibers/mg.

Asbestos fibers by transmission electron microscopy on lung tissue

1. The general population has <1000 fibers/mg, average 2 to 300 fibers/mg (90% of which are <5 μm length) and <100 fibers of >5 μm length, 70% of which are chrysotile and none of which is the amphibole amosite or crocidolite.

2. Residents of mining towns such as Thetford Mines, Québec may have 10 times the level of the general population without disease.

3. Patients with pleural plaques have 100 to 5000 fibers/mg.

4. Patients with mesothelioma have fibers from within the range of normals to the range of patients with asbestosis.

5. Asbestos workers with grade 0 asbestosis have about 2000 to 19,000 fibers/mg; workers with grade 1 asbestosis have about 135,000 fibers/mg; and workers with grade 2 asbestosis have about 1,370,000 fibers/mg.

Finally it is established that uncoated fibers always outnumber coated fibers (ABs), particularly for chrysotile fibers in the general population.

Deposition and clearance of asbestos

For nonfibrous minerals, it is well recognized that only rare particles of diameter >10 μm will reach the lung beyond the upper airways, and most particles deposited in the alveoli are of diameter <5 μm. However, these considerations do not apply to the fibrous minerals such as asbestos. Fiber deposition in the lung is largely ruled by the fiber diameter, the fiber length having a relatively less important effect. Thus fibers with a length of 200 to 300 μm can be found in the lung if the diameter is <3 μm. Typical fiber lengths in asbestos bodies are 20 μm to 50 μm, and many fibers of <5 μm length can also be found.

In animal experiments, it has been clearly shown that the fibers are primarily deposited in the bifurcations of the conducting airways and in the alveolar parenchyma. The deposition of inhaled fibers is diffuse through the lung and extends to the subpleural lung tissue, where concentration may be markedly elevated at times.

Clearance of asbestos fibers from the lung occurs by a variety of pathways, including the mucociliary escalator system, the translocation in the interstitium to the lymphatic system, and the dissolution, degradation, defibrillation, and breakdown of the fiber materials originally inhaled. The short fibers are cleared more readily from the lung so that over time the overall mean length of fibers appears to increase. In a similar way, the chrysotile fibers are cleared more rapidly than the amphiboles.

These considerations are of interest in relation to assessing the effects of fiber type, size, and length-to-width ratio in the pathogenesis of the asbestos-related diseases to be discussed later.

PATHOGENESIS AND BIOLOGICAL MECHANISMS OF ASBESTOS EFFECT

The fundamental effects of asbestos fibers in biological tissues[19–21] are related to the toxicity of the fibers in inducing fibrosis and cancers of the lung and pleural space.

In the fibrosing processes, the disease starts as an inflammatory reaction that evolves in a fibrosing repair process, leaving permanent scars. These can be more or less limiting, depending on the site of the lesion and its extent.

In the cancer processes,[31] the disease starts as a multistep process in which the deoxyribonucleic acid (DNA) of the target cells suffers increasing amounts of damage— genetic mutations—through a variety of molecular injuries. Ultimately, through exposure to carcinogens over time, the affected cells form increasingly damaged tissue reflecting the increasing damage to the DNA of those cells, which then become a tumor cell proliferating over time to a clinically detected disease.

In experiments done in vitro, asbestos fibers can cause cell membrane damage, which, if severe enough, will cause cell death, gene mutation, chromosomal aberration, aneuploidies, and cell transformation. Asbestos fibers may also lead to lung macrophage production of various growth factors for fibroflasts and other cells participating in the pathogenesis of asbestos-related diseases.

The mechanisms of pathogenesis are not completely

understood, but the general schematics are already developed.[3,21]

Pathogenicity of asbestos fibers: type, dimensions, durability, and chemical composition

The dose, the fiber type, the fiber dimension, the durability of the fiber, and the surface chemical functionalities will influence toxicity, carcinogenicity, and fibrogenicity to variable degrees. The dose–response relationship has been well documented epidemiologically and experimentally for the majority of asbestos-related diseases. Several experimental studies in animals and studies in vitro of cell cultures have clearly documented that all types of asbestos fibers can reproduce experimentally all accepted asbestos-related diseases, asbestosis, bronchogenic carcinoma, and mesothelioma.

Studies in vitro and in animal experiments have documented that the toxicity of asbestos fibers is related to the fibrous nature of the mineral, as seen by the absence of toxicity of pulverized asbestos or of nonfibrous analogs of asbestos.

The diameter of the asbestos fibers is also of importance in the pathogenesis. Fibers with diameter >3 μm do not penetrate in the lower lung, but those <3 μm will penetrate cell membranes and be translocated to the interstitium of the lung and the pleural spaces to cause the asbestos diseases.

Length of fibers is also important in the pathogenesis. The shortest fibers of length <3 μm are phagocytosed or translocated to the lymphatics to be drained to the pleural spaces, whereas fibers longer than 5 μm are incompletely phagocytosed, will stay in the tissues longer, and will initiate and sustain the cascade of cellular and molecular events described in the pathogenesis of asbestos-related diseases.

It is often noted that crocidolite fibers are more toxic than chrysotile. The usual explanation relates to the slower clearance of crocidolite when expressed per unit of mineral mass. However, if the distribution of length for each fiber type and the rapid clearance of the shorter fibers are taken into account, the toxicity is comparable for the same number of fibers of the same length.[28]

The fiber type, size, and aspect ratio influence these diseases in different ways. The amphiboles are generally recognized to be about 10 times more carcinogenic than chrysotile for the mesothelium, which is particularly well documented for crocidolite. Amphiboles are also more prone to induce pleural fibrosis than is chrysotile. Lung fibrosis, however, is equally affected by both types of asbestos fibers. Although there is incomplete agreement on the subject of the relative toxicity of short asbestos fibers, it is generally believed that the short fibers (<5 μm) have limited to no capacity to induce any of the accepted asbestos-associated diseases. The length-to-diameter ratio also has a defined influence, at least for the induction of mesothelioma, as the effect increases with decreasing diameter and increasing length of the asbestos fibers.

The composition of asbestos fibers can influence their toxicity. The relative solubility of chrysotile will attenuate its toxicity, whereas its "splitability" (multiplication effect) will enhance toxicity.

Surface properties as well as electrical charge will also influence the toxicity of asbestos fibers. It is well recognized that interactions between solid particles and molecules in the biologic milieu are regulated by the reactivity of the surface of the solids. Surface breakdown of the bonds between atoms at the surface of the solids leads to unstable atoms with residual charges as a function of their nature and environment. These surface atoms constitute the active sites, and the activity of the mineral will be related in part to the nature, strength, and density of these surface sites.

The surface activity of a particle, whether it is globular or fibrous, may result in modification of the prior equilibrium favoring adsorption, and/or the genesis of new chemical species such as free radicals. The adsorption of carcinogens such as benzene or polycyclic aromatic hydrocarbons (PAH) is well recognized to enhance the carcinogenicity of asbestos; similarly, the catalytic action of chrysotile can liberate free radicals, molecules of established toxicity for cells. The surface properties of fibers have been well studied in carcinogenicity and, in recent years, the relative importance of these surface properties has also been addressed for their fibrogenic effect.

INTERNATIONAL CLASSIFICATION OF RADIOGRAPHS OF PNEUMOCONIOSES AS APPLIED TO ASBESTOS-RELATED DISEASES

The International Labor Office (ILO) is an organization that has promoted international conferences and discussions and published guidelines on ways to classify the chest radiographs. It has facilitated the development of an international classification of radiographs of pneumoconioses.[29] The goal of the classification is to code the abnormalities in a simple and reproducible manner. The ILO system provides a standard set of reference chest radiographs, which are used in the classification of the radiographs. The system is described in detail in Chapter 7.

Abnormalities of lung parenchyma

The profusion (number) of opacities is based on the viewers' assessment of the concentration of opacities compared with standard radiographs provided by the ILO. This classification recognizes the existence of a continuum of change, from no opacity to the most advanced category. The scores can be converted to a linear scale of 0 to 10 (12 grades) as follows: ILO grade 0/- (clearly normal) and 0/0 (normal after a good look) = 0 on the linear scale; ILO grades 0/1 = 1, 1/0 = 2, 1/1 = 3, 1/2 = 4, 2/1 = 5, 2/2 = 6, 2/3 = 7, 3/2 = 8, 3/3 = 9, and 3/4 = 10.

To group patients with similar diseases, four categories are defined on the basis of the same profusion scores:

1. Category 0 = profusion scores 0/-, 0/0, and 0/1.
2. Category 1 = profusion scores 1/0, 1/1, and 1/2.
3. Category 2 = profusion scores 2/1, 2/2, and 2/3.
4. Category 3 = profusion scores 3/2, 3/3, and 3/4.

The profusion of opacities is graded to take into account the six usual lung zones, upper, middle, and lower left and right zones, on the chest radiograph, with emphasis on the zones that have abnormalities, in comparison with the reference films.

The shape and size of small opacities are also recorded. The classification recognizes two kinds of shape: rounded and irregular or reticular. The letters p, q, and r are used for rounded opacities and the letters s, t, and u denote the presence of small irregular opacities. For opacities of diameter <1.5 mm, the letter p or s is used, for opacities of diameter 1.5 mm to ≤3 mm, the letter q or t is used, and for opacities of diameter >3 mm to ≤10 mm, the letter r or u is used.

The grouping of opacities or confluence is classified as coalescence (AX) when the confluence is of diameter <10 mm and as large opacity when >10 mm. A large opacity is of category A when its greater diameter is >10 mm and/or <50 mm or when the sum of several opacities of individual diameter >10 mm does not exceed 50 mm. A large opacity is of category B when one or more opacities is larger or more numerous than those in category A and when the combined area does not exceed the equivalent of the right upper zone (one-third of the right hemithorax). A large opacity is of category C when one or more opacities is of individual diameter >10 mm and when the combined area exceeds the equivalent of the right upper lobe.

Pleural abnormalities: classification by the International Labor Office system

The ILO provides a standard method for classifying radiographs of pneumoconioses. This section describes its application to pleural abnormalities, which may result from asbestos exposure.

Pleural thickenings are classified for site (chest wall, diaphragm, costophrenic angle), width, and extent. The classification also recognizes two types of thickenings, circumscribed (plaques) and diffuse (pachypleuritis).

The width between chest wall and the innermost margin of the thickening is classified as *a* for maximal thickness of <5 mm, *b* for thickness >5 mm up to 10 mm, and *c* for thickness >10 mm. For pleural thickening seen face on, the presence is recorded but thickness is not measured.

The extent is defined in terms of the maximal length of pleural thickening or as the sum of maximum lengths of separate plaques. Grade 1 is for extent equivalent to up to one quarter of the projection of the lateral chest wall, grade 2 is for extent exceeding one quarter and less than one half

of the projection of the lateral chest wall, and grade 3 is for extent exceeding one half of the projection of the lateral chest wall.

The abnormalities of diaphragm and costophenic angle obliterations are recorded as present or absent, left and/or right.

Pleural calcifications are recorded for site and extent. Site can be chest wall, diaphragm, or other. Extent is of grade 1 for calcifications of greatest length (individually or as the sum of many) up to about 20 mm. Extent of grade 2 is for one or the sum of calcifications of maximal length >20 mm and <100 mm. Extent is of grade 3 for one or the sum of calcifications of maximal length >100 mm.

This brief summary of the ILO classification of radiographs is incomplete, but provides an initial rapid understanding of the classification, which is presented in detail in the ILO guideline document.[29]

ASBESTOSIS

Asbestosis is interstitial fibrosis caused by inhalation of asbestos fiber.

Mechanisms of asbestos lung injury leading to asbestosis

The initial injury. The first injuries associated with asbestos dust inhalation occur almost immediately after exposure and arise at the alveolar duct bifurcations, where the terminal bronchioles divide into individual alveolar spaces of the lung. The events arise after only a 1-hour exposure to asbestos in animal experiments. Most of the deposited fibers are found at the first and second bifurcations of the alveolar ducts. The first detectable structural cellular response is the active uptake of fibers by type I epithelial cells. It occurs during the first hour of exposure and likely continues as long as fibers are in the alveolar space. This event is significant in that the fibers piercing the alveolar wall appear to initiate a tissue response and provide the major route for asbestos fibers to reach the lung interstitium. The fibers piercing the alveolar wall damage the wall and constitute the initial injury, leading in many instances to cell death.

Within 48 hours after the 1-hour exposure to asbestos, increased numbers of alveolar macrophages accumulate at the alveolar duct bifurcations. The percentage of bifurcations with clusters of macrophages increases from virtually none in the control animals to over 90% by 48 hours postexposure. The macrophages are activated by the presence of asbestos. Furthermore, a threefold increase in the number of fibroblasts is observed at these sites.

Whereas one such exposure may not cause asbestosis in all cases, chronic exposure causes this lesion to progress. There is first a localized peribronchiolar fibrosing alveolitis, followed by diffuse fibrotic scarring, the basic pathologic finding of asbestosis. Any increase in asbestos dose exposure amplifies the cellular responses. This brief exposure produced the fundamental lesion of asbestosis, defined by the American College of Pathologists as grade 1.[4]

The initial injury starts a cascade of events. Following asbestos inhalation, macrophages quickly flood the site of the injury. Macrophages release various substances when exposed to asbestos, but not in the presence of inert materials. In contrast to asbestos dust, inert dusts can be phagocytosed by the alveolar macrophage but will not initiate the cascade of events resulting in production of fibrosis with scar tissue deposition.[19-21]

Following the early lung events, the cells from animals exposed to asbestos stimulate the proliferation of fibroblasts twofold to threefold above control. Thus, asbestos causes the macrophages to release molecules that cause the fibroblasts to proliferate and produce fibrotic scar tissue. The more macrophages called to the area, the more fibroblasts will in turn be recruited; the more the fibroblasts will be caused to proliferate by the macrophage-derived substances, the more fibrotic scar tissue will be formed. While this scarring phenomena starts out as a local lesion, over time this process progressively gets more and more diffuse.

Cytokines are extracellular molecules secreted by effector cells that have the capacity to change the function of adjacent cells. The cytokines act primarly at the local level and do not reach the primary target cells through systemic circulation, as opposed to endocrine hormones.

Macrophages and fibroblasts interact in the lungs. Analysis of the components of the lung lavage fluids has permitted determination of what is stimulating the fibroblasts and whether that was responsible for the generation of fibrotic scar tissue.

Fibronectin is a glycoprotein produced by the macrophage; fibronectin is capable of recruiting fibroblasts to the site of injury and initiating the proliferation of fibroblast. In the lavage fluids, fibronectin increased significantly only in the asbestos-exposed animals.[29a] Levels of procollagen 3 (indicating new production of collagen or scar tissue) in the lavage were increased significantly when a fibrotic process is in the early phase and evolved to a Grade 1 asbestosis.

In asbestos workers without clinically evident disease, levels of fibronectin and procollagen 3 in lavage were comparable with controls, but these levels are significantly elevated in those with asbestos-associated alveolitis (subclinical asbestosis) or clinical asbestosis. In contrast, the substances produced by macrophages in early asbestos-induced lung scarring lesions are not observed after exposure to inert materials.

Thus, the asbestos fibrosing alveolitis is characterized by an excessive macrophage accumulation at site of dust deposition, macrophage-derived chemoattraction of fibroblasts at the site of asbestos deposition, and exaggerated fibroblast growth activities, in part induced by the activated macrophages producing increased amounts of fibronectin. In addition to fibronectin, alveolar macrophages recovered from patients with asbestosis release exaggerated quantities of growth factors, including platelet-derived growth factor (PDGF), insulin like growth factor (IGF-1), and fibroblast growth factor (FGF), signaling proteins that have been regrouped as cytokines.[20,21]

PDGF, IGF-1, and *FGF* are cytokines produced by macrophages to attract fibroblasts to sites of injury and upregulate the proliferative activity of the fibroblasts at the site of disease. The recruitment and proliferation of fibroblasts lead to the formation of scar tissue. All growth factors, fibronectin, PDGF, IGF-1, and FGF interact synergistically in a complex cascade of events to cause the fibroblasts to proliferate and to form scar tissue, irreversibly altering the structure and function of the lung.

The damage to the initially injured area is further aggravated by the asbestos-activated macrophages releasing toxic substances known as oxygen-free radicals, damaging tissues through direct cytotoxicity and peroxidation of cell membranes, which will further sustain the inflammatory process.[30,31]

An additional source of tissue destructive substances comes from the release by the macrophage of *plasminogen activator*,[32] which converts plasminogen to plasmin. Plasmin is a protease that can degrade the interstitial matrix glycoproteins, thus furthering tissue destruction.

Persistence of process: What causes these substances to be released by macrophages and the process to continue? Asbestos fibers are cytotoxic for the cells in direct contact, but much of the adverse effect of asbestos is caused by the fibers being longer than macrophages; such long fibers cannot be completely phagocytosed (Fig. 20-1-1). The long thin asbestos fibers will cause these substances to be released by macrophages. The durability and the mobility of the long fibers in the distal lung will contribute to sustaining the disease process. Furthermore, the natural physical tendency of chrysotile asbestos fibers to split longitudinally multiplies this effect and causes it to continue even after exposure has ceased. Although asbestos fiber coating, with the formation of asbestos bodies, can reduce the toxicity of a given fiber, more than 85% of all fibers in the lung tissue remain uncoated.[25] Thus, the continuous asbestos exposure, the durability and mobility of long asbestos fibers, and/or the longitudinal splitting of fibers are central to the progression of the disease process from localized lesions (Fig. 20-1-2) to diffuse fibrosis (Fig. 20-1-3), through sustained release of the various fibrosis-producing and tissue-damaging substances.

After exposure has ceased, the inflammatory process will spread from the initial peribronchiolar tissue to produce a diffuse interstitial fibrosis (Fig. 20-1-3) because the long fibers persist in the lung, move throughout the lung interstitium, and split along their longitudinal axes. Thus, the effects of incomplete phagocytosis, mobility, and splitting of long asbestos fibers in the lung produce a condition similar to what would exist if the person was continuously inhal-

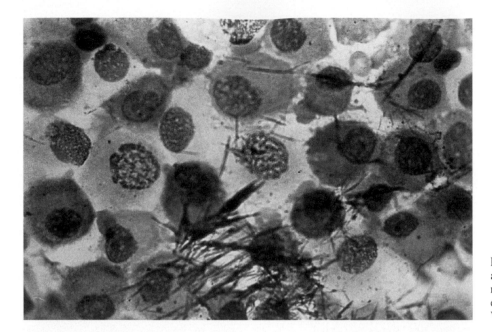

Fig. 20-1-1. Cytospin of a lung lavage in an asbestos worker showing several fibers, many of these of length greater than the average macrophage diameter (8 μm); Wright–Giemsa; magnification × 1000.

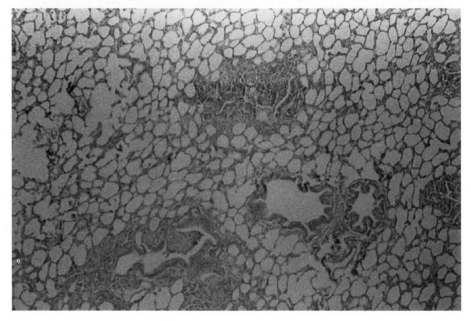

Fig. 20-1-2. Asbestosis grade 1 seen in a sheep as peribronchiolar inflammation and fibrosis limited to some of the surroundings of some of the peripheral airways (hematoxylin–eosin; × 40).

ing the asbestos dust. Any additional external asbestos exposure will further serve to increase the lung fiber burden, increasing the amount and extent of injury, and furthering the progression of the disease.[33]

Thus, the initial injury is characterized by damage to the alveolar wall epithelium, incomplete phagocytosis by alveolar and interstitial macrophages, and release of fibronectin, PDGF, IGF-1, FGF, as well as proinflammatory and cytotoxic agents such as free oxygen radicals and plasminogen activator. These substances interact and cause fibroblasts to be recruited to the site of injury, to proliferate, and to lay down collagen, altering the normal alveolar epithelial architecture and causing irreversible damage and loss of the alveolar space and surrounding interstitium.

The early lesions of asbestosis in animals and humans. Research studies in animals and humans have shown that changes occur relatively soon after exposure. This section will describe these early lesions, and the next will describe the transition from these early changes to clinically diagnosable asbestosis.

The sheep model of asbestosis has been repeatedly documented to parallel human asbestosis and has been particularly useful for correlating the cellular and clinical events.[19] Figure 20-1-2 shows scarring in and around a bronchiole from a sheep exposed to a single dose of asbestos and sacrificed 8 months after exposure. Because of the relative lack of sensitivity of clinical tools, this lesion cannot usually be recognized by routine pulmonary function tests or chest ra-

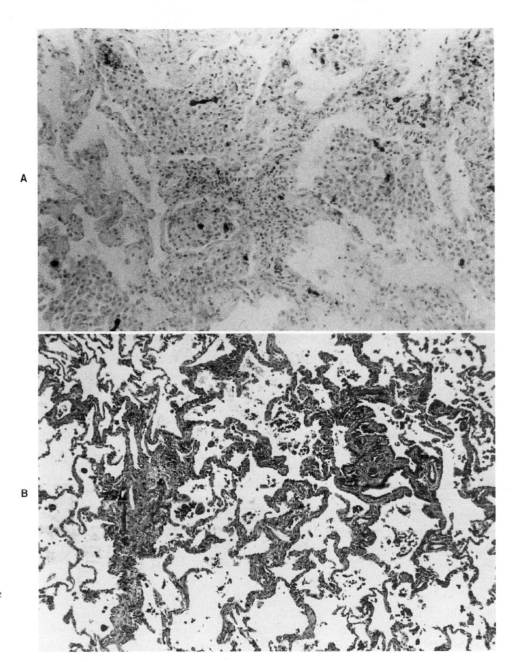

Fig. 20-1-3. A, Asbestosis in a more inflammatory stage with cellular infiltration and asbestos ferruginous bodies (hematoxylin–eosin; × 160). **B,** Asbestosis in a more fibrotic stage with fibrosis around the peripheral airways and extension of the fibrosis in the interstitium between airways (hematoxylin-eosin; × 40).

diograph. Only when these lesions cover some 25% to 50% of the airways of the lung will there be a measurable change in pulmonary function. Similarly, only when the peribronchiolar process becomes sufficiently diffuse and extends between the airways (Fig. 20-1-3, grade 2 or more pathologic asbestosis), will it become detectable by radiographic methods. Such early lesions have been reported in asbestos-exposed individuals with minimal functional impairment as judged by standard clinical diagnostic tools.

Similarly, studies in subjects suspected of interstitial lung diseases also demonstrated the presence of these early lesions. Mildly symptomatic subjects complaining of shortness of breath with normal chest radiographs had pathologic evidence of fibrosis. Such lesions are not visible yet in the chest radiograph because they are not sufficiently widespread.

Progression from early lesions to clinically evident asbestosis. The chronic and progressive nature of asbestosis[19–21,29a,34,35] from the initial subclinical lesion to clinical asbestosis has been documented by means of lung lavage, electron microscopy, thin section computerized tomography (CT) scan, and ^{67}Ga lung uptake, showing that the inflammation and injury produced by exposure to asbestos fibers are continuous from the time of exposure, through the latent or subclinical phase, to the development of clinical disease identifiable by the classic methods of chest radiographic changes and pulmonary functional impairment.

The lung lavage studies discussed earlier have shown lavage changes at time of subclinical disease. Computerized tomography with thin slice image studies have shown significant abnormalities in the presence of normal radiography on 20% to 35% of long-term asbestos workers without clinical asbestosis. Similarly, ^{67}Ga scans are abnormal in a substantial portion of asbestos workers without clinical asbestosis.

[67]Ga is a radioactive element that serves as a specific marker for lung inflammation because it is taken up only by activated macrophages. By using this technique, which is much more sensitive and specific than a standard chest x-ray examination, lung inflammation and injury were detected well before clinical disease became apparent, without having to directly examine the human lung by opening the chest surgically or at autopsy. This correlation between ^{67}Ga uptake and the disease process was further confirmed through lung biopsies performed on human cases.

Thus, ^{67}Ga uptake in asbestos workers is a useful indicator of early (subclinical) lung injury and confirms the presence of the injury long before it can be recognized by traditional chest radiography. As reported,[34] 12 of the 16 subjects who initially had a positive ^{67}Ga scan but did not have clinical asbestosis at that time, did progress to "full blown" clinical asbestosis over a 4-year period. This represents a 75% progression rate. These results demonstrate that before the time of clinical manifestation of the disease through ordinary clinical tests, the disease process is ongoing and that the processes of inflammation and ongoing injury to cells is continuing.

Clinical latency is defined as a state of seeming inactivity, occurring between the instant of stimulation and that of response. The time between exposure to a substance and the clinical manifestation of the disease during which there is an ongoing disease process is typically known as the latency period. The concept of latency is not uniquely related to asbestos exposure. Latency is well known in many diseases, such as in cases of cancer caused by chemicals and radiation and in radiation-exposure fibrosis. Standard medical texts recognize that during this seemingly inactive period, there is ongoing disease and injury on a subclinical level. During the latency period, there is a progressively increasing inflammation, involving greater numbers of macrophages, fibroblasts, and scar tissue formation. This eventually progresses to clinically recognizable asbestosis.

After clinical recognition of asbestosis, the disease is often chronic and progressive.[36] Viallat et al. studied a population of asbestos workers in a Corsican township.[36] The workers were employed at the same plant when the plant closed in 1965. After the plant closed, none of the individuals studied had any further exposure to asbestos dust. Their Table 2 shows that in 1965, almost 80% of the workers had no radiographic evidence of disease, whereas in 1979, despite no further exposure, only 34% had no radiographic evidence of disease. It is observed that 65% had radiographic evidence in 1979. Overall, the authors calculated a progression rate of 46%. Other studies have also documented disease progression after asbestosis is recognized and exposure ceased in animals and in humans. The progression rate at present appears to be closer to 20%, as intensity of exposure has decreased with better industrial hygiene practices and methods of recognition of clinical disease has improved.

The best explanation for the progression in these former workers is the persistence of a substantial lung burden of asbestos in their lungs for years after exposure ceased, which resulted in ongoing inflammation, as well as longitudinal splitting or translocation of asbestos fibers, provoking continual unsuccessful phagocytosis, inflammation, and fibrosis.

Susceptibility to asbestosis

It is recognized that when exposure to a toxic substance is well in excess of the tolerance level, the disease will appear in all exposed subjects, as was the case in the British workshop where Murray[8] described his first cases of asbestosis. That situation can be easily reproduced experimentally. In recent years, it is rare to see such situations. Most often one finds a fraction of the workforce that develops one of the asbestos-related diseases, although apparently not exposed to higher levels than other workers in similar situations.[2,29,34,37,38] This phenomena is related to factors of individual susceptibility.

Recently, these factors have been studied on the basis of immunology, pulmonary structure, and clearance capacity. Human immunohistocompatibility studies have been unable to find an immunologic marker of the HLA system that can be associated as a susceptibility factor.[39] However, some characteristics of the large airways have been linked to the susceptibility factor[38] and these could influence the alveolar clearance of the asbestos dust from the lung.

In humans it is not possible to measure directly the lung clearance of inhaled asbestos dusts and to relate that to the development of asbestosis. However, several independent observations suggest that the capacity of clearance of the lung is linked to the risk of disease.[40]

1. Lung tissue fiber burden has been found to be higher in asbestos workers than in the general population.
2. Asbestos workers with disease limited to the airways have twice the lung fiber burden of workers without the airway disease.
3. Asbestos workers with airway disease only have 50% of the lung fiber burden of patients with asbestosis. This has been reproduced experimentally.
4. Analyses of lung lavage fiber content of workers with asbestosis were also found to be significantly higher than values found in exposed workers without asbestosis.

In that regard, studies in the sheep model have been partlicularly useful, documenting the higher level of fiber retention in the animals with asbestosis than in those without the disease after comparable exposures.[40] The longer fibers were particularly associated with this effect. Thus, the individual clearance capacity appears to play a critical role in individual susceptibility to develop disease.

Tolerance threshold. The relative risk of developing asbestosis for an asbestos worker increases in proportion to the asbestos fiber dust level in the workplace. Recent reports suggested a 1% risk of developing clinically recognizable asbestosis after an exposure to a cumulative dose of 10 fiber-year per cubic meter of air. This contributed to lowering the current threshold limit value (TLV) (level of exposure) to less than 1 fiber per cubic centimeter of air, given the normal 30 to 40 years of work for most asbestos workers.

Dose–response relationships for asbestosis. In asbestos-exposed individuals, those with grade 1 asbestosis have a higher retention of fibers in their lung tissues than those without asbestosis. Also, workers with a more advanced form of asbestosis have more fiber retention. Furthermore, epidemiologic studies have repeatedly documented the relation between cumulative exposure dose and the higher incidence of asbestosis in primary or secondary industries.[2-15,17]

The dose–response relationship is also valid for the other asbestos-related diseases, particularly for primary lung cancer, but to a lesser degree for the mesothelioma, where many of the exposures have been often of low level and of short duration.

Pathology of asbestosis

Exposure of the lung to asbestos dust can initiate one of the following reactions[19]:

1. *A transient inflammatory reaction without lesions, with rapid clearance of the inhaled fibers.* This is the most frequent situation of subjects exposed very occasionally or to very low doses of fibers. Such subjects may never develop asbestosis or other asbestos-related diseases. This situation is also seen in a large portion of long-term asbestos workers who have no detectable changes related to their asbestos exposure. Experimentally, this type of transient tissue reaction occurring without histopathologic lesion (or loss of integrity) has been reproduced in animals.[41]
2. *A low retention reaction.* Here, the asbestos exposed subject seems to possess particularly effective clearance mechanisms; this occurs in subjects with low susceptibility to asbestos. The biological reaction in the lung is limited to the site of deposition of fibers at the bifurcation of peripheral bronchioles. The fibers at the bifurcation initiate macrophage attraction to the site, an inflammatory reaction that evolves to fibrotic

scar limited to the distal airway. This type of lesion has been seen in humans and in animal models.
3. *A high retention reaction.* This reaction is seen in the most susceptible subjects, who retain the most fibers in their lung. The tissue reaction is the most intense and causes a dense accumulation of inflammatory cells, activated macrophages, and neutrophils. A significant fibrosing alveolitis is constituted (Fig. 20-1-3).

   The secretory activities of macrophages and neutrophils are intensified. The cascade of biological events described earlier is activated. This excessive secretory activity of macrophages and neutrophils at the site of fiber deposition is sustained by the weak clearance of the longest fibers and by the multiplicative effect of fiber bundles breaking down into fibrils.

   This high retention reaction initiates asbestosis. It is well recognized in both humans and in animal models.

Pathologically, asbestosis is generally defined as fibrosis of the lung associated with retention of asbestos bodies recognized by optical microscopy or of significant amounts of asbestos fibers as seen by TEM. This general definition has been modified by a committee of the College of American Pathologists. The definition of asbestosis now recognizes the severity and the extension of the fibrotic process.[4,25]

Macroscopically, the lung's gross features vary depending on the severity of the disease process. Early, the visceral pleura loses its transparency and parenchyma has gray streaks of fibrous tissues in the interlobur and interlobular septa with invasion of the lung tissue. In a later phase of disease, the pleural surface has a nodular aspect, quite similar to liver cirrhosis, and the lung parenchyma is characterized by loss of volume, scars, and cyst formations, usually particularly prominent in the lower zones.

The College of American Pathologists has defined four grades of severity of asbestosis; these are now commonly used as reference in the grading of the pathology of asbestosis[4]:

Grade 1. Fibrosis involving the wall of at least one respiratory bronchiole with or without extension into the septa of the immediately adjacent layer of alveoli; there is no fibrosis in more distant alveoli. This is the asbestos airway disease defined by Churg and Green.[25]

Grade 2. Fibrosis as in grade 1, plus involvement of alveolar ducts or two or more layers of adjacent alveoli; there still must be a zone of nonfibrotic alveolar septa between adjacent bronchioles (Fig. 20-I-3).

Grade 3. Fibrosis as in grade 2, but with coalescence of fibrotic change such that all alveoli between at least two adjacent bronchi have thickened, fibrotic septa; some alveoli may be obliterated completely.

Grade 4. Fibrosis as in grade 3, but with formation of new spaces of a size larger than alveoli, ranging up to 1 cm; this lesion has been termed honeycombing. Spaces may or may not be lined by epithelium.

The pathologic description also includes three extension grades based on the proportion of respiratory bronchioles involved by the disease process. Three grades of extension are defined as follows:

Grade A. Only occasional bronchioles are involved; most show no lesion.

Grade B. More than occasional involvement is seen, but less than half of all bronchioles are involved.

Grade C. More than half of all bronchioles are involved.

This approach at pathologic description of disease process is complete, precise, and has been useful in correlation studies of other parameters of disease severity such as radiographs and lung function tests.

Clinical manifestations

The symptoms and physical signs of asbestosis are quite similar to those of other interstitial lung fibrosis, that is dyspnea, dry cough, and nonspecific thoracic malaise. The general clinical manifestations of interstitial disease are discussed in Chapter 15.

Dyspnea on exertion is the usual presenting symptom, which worsens as the disease progresses and is associated with loss of lung function. Nonproductive cough and chest pain are usually present only in some cases, late in the evolution of disease. When cough is productive, it should be considered as likely due to a complication such as bronchitis or pneumonia. The chest tightness and pains of patients with asbestosis are attributed to muscle pain appearing only when dyspnea becomes severe. Hemoptysis is not a usual complaint in asbestosis and should be investigated.

The symptoms of asbestosis may occur during the working years or following exposure cessation, as disease may become clinically apparent only after retirement.

Fine crisp nonmobile crepitations are the most important physical findings in asbestosis. Early in the course of the disease they can be heard in the lower lateral lung fields in the late inspiratory phase. As disease progresses the rales are audible in the lower posterior lung fields, in increasing number in middle and late inspiratory phase. In severe disease, rales have a crisper higher tonality and are audible during all inspiratory phases and in all auscultatory fields of the thorax. Rales provide a good physical sign for early detection of disease when present, as they often precede the changes in lung volumes and airflow parameters. In most cases, however, the rales appear at the time of early changes in lung function and chest radiography. Other adventitious sounds are usually absent.

Finger clubbing can be present in some cases but does not necessarily relate to severity of asbestosis. Cyanosis and reduced chest expansion are late manifestations of the disease.

Lung function tests usually reveal a restrictive change associated with mild end expiratory airflow limitation. The restrictive pattern progresses as the disease worsens, but the airflow obstruction does not worsen as rigidity of the lungs enhances the airflow conductance of the peripheral airways. This, however, causes added work of breathing.

Lung lavage analyses have well documented the inflammatory and fibrosing activity that precedes the clinical and radiographic manifestations of asbestosis and persists during the evolution of the disease.

The evolution of asbestosis has changed significantly since the original observation by Murray[8] of 10 cases of asbestosis mortality before age 30. Currently, with improved industrial hygiene and early disease recognition at time of minimally abnormal chest radiograph (ILO category 1 abnomalities), only 20% of cases so recognized will progress in the following years. It is currently not possible to predict accurately which cases of early asbestosis will progress, and therefore the disease should be considered as potentially progressive and should be followed medically.

Radiology of asbestosis

The radiologic tools used in the diagnosis of asbestos-related disorders are the posteroanterior (PA) and lateral chest radiograph, the oblique chest films, and the computerized axial tomography of the chest in conventional and high resolution modes (CT scan). A comparison of conventional (CCT) and high resolution CT scan (HRCT) techniques is presented in Table 20-1-3.

The plain standard high kilovoltage PA and lateral chest radiographs are adequate for basic radiologic information. The use of oblique films facilitates recognition of pleural changes and pleural-based abnormalities.

On standard chest radiograph asbestosis is usually manifested as diffuse reticulonodular infiltrates at the lung bases.[2,5,22,42] Early in the disease process, the abnormalities of the lung parenchyma are seen in the lower two thirds of the lung fields as fine increases in markings and thickening of the vascular markings (Fig. 20-1-4); later the in-

Table 20-1-3. Comparison of CT scan techniques for examination of asbestos workers

Technical aspects	HRCT	CCT
Slice thickness (mm)	1–2	10
Algorithm	os	standard
Current (mA)	170	140
Voltage (kV)	120	12
Scanning time (sec)	2	2
Matrix	512 × 512	512 × 512
Visual fields (cm)	20–24	30–40

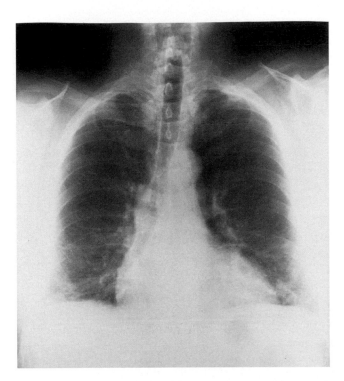

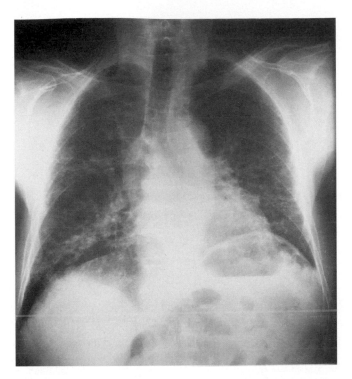

Fig. 20-1-4. Chest radiograph of an asbestos worker showing abnormalities of the lung parenchyma in the lower two thirds of the lung fields as fine increases and thickenings in the vascular markings. There is also a peripheral reticulation of the lung fields and some degree of bilateral pleural thickening. In older patients with cardiomegaly, as in this case, the condition is often confounded with congestive heart failure, at time of initial visit to the physician.

Fig. 20-1-5. Chest radiograph of an asbestos worker showing more advanced abnormalities of the lung parenchyma. The coarse reticulation is diffuse and of higher density and the cardiac silhouette is beginning to be ill-defined.

filtrations become more clearly reticular, better defined in the peripheral lung, and extend more diffusely in other lung fields (Fig. 20-1-5). The images of asbestosis do not have the clarity of silicotic nodules and can mimic chronic congestion of the lung secondary to left heart failure. In the advanced stage of asbestosis, the radiographic images have the appearance of honeycombing, with coarse infiltration associated with severe tissue destruction and distortion. All the infiltrates of asbestosis are nonspecific and can be seen in other lung diseases. When the lung changes are accompanied by pleural manifestations of asbestos exposure, the diagnosis of asbestosis is more likely (Fig. 20-1-6). However, several cases of asbestosis documented pathologically have no pleural changes on either the chest radiograph or HRCT.

The small nodular opacities, septal lines, coarse or fine linear opacities, ground glass appearance, and honeycombing are all part of possible changes seen in asbestosis solely or in association with other processes. Lung volumes are normal or reduced. Progressive massive fibrosis with confluence of masses of fibrotic tissues as seen in other pneumoconioses is possible although less frequently seen, so that any focal mass should be fully investigated for possible tumor origin.

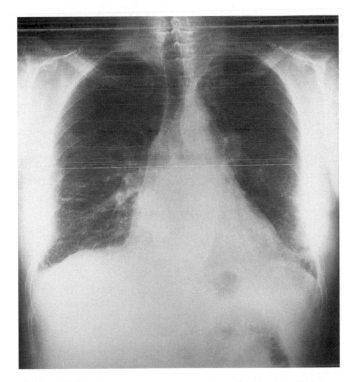

Fig. 20-1-6. Chest radiograph of an asbestos worker showing typical changes of asbestosis, with bilateral interstitial reticular infiltrates and bilateral pleural thickenings. This image is almost diagnostic of asbestosis.

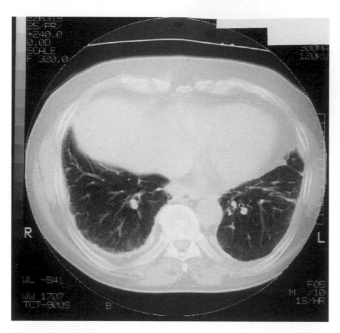

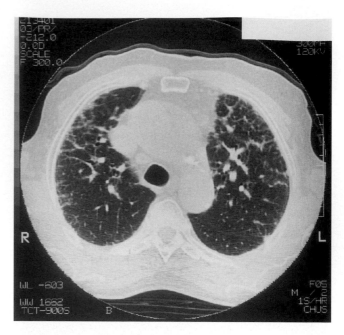

Fig. 20-1-7. CT scan of an asbestos worker with asbestosis and bilateral diffuse pleural thickening. In this window of the lower lung field, there are nondependent subpleural densities, thickening of the interlobar and interlobular septa in the periphery of the lung, and parenchymal bands extending from the pleural surface in the parenchyma. In addition, pleural thickening and calcifications are seen in both lungs fields, more marked in the right field.

Fig. 20-1-8. CT scan of an asbestos worker with asbestosis and bilateral diffuse pleural thickening. Here, the pleural thickening is less intense but the diffuse interstitial abnormalities are more prominent and early honeycombing can be seen in the anterior areas, bilaterally.

The use of the CT scan is not justified in the periodic examination of asbestos-exposed workers, but the CT scan has a definite place in the clinical investigation and improved definition of pleural changes and pleural-based abnormalities and in the early detection of interstitial lung fibrosis not clearly seen on the chest radiograph. In cases of suspected lung cancer or mesothelioma, CT scan allows a better definition of extension of disease, orientation of diagnostic or therapeutic interventions, and follow-up of the disease.

The HRCT can often detect discrete abnormalities of the lung interstitium adjacent to the pleural plaques or thickenings. Furthermore, HRCT permits a better appreciation of emphysematous changes in the lung and can help to differentiate the contribution of these changes and those of early asbestosis in borderline difficult cases.[20,35,43]

The findings of HRCT are not pathopneumonic for the diagnosis of asbestosis but are relatively characteristic when the following are bilaterally seen on the HRCT:

1. Thickening of the interlobar and interlobular septa in the periphery of the lung (Fig. 20-1-7)
2. Parenchymal bands entending from the pleural surface in the parenchyma (Fig. 20-1-7 and 20-1-8)
3. Honeycombing, small cystic zones of lung destruction with thick walls, mostly located in posterior areas and in the nondependent areas of the lung (Fig. 20-1-9)

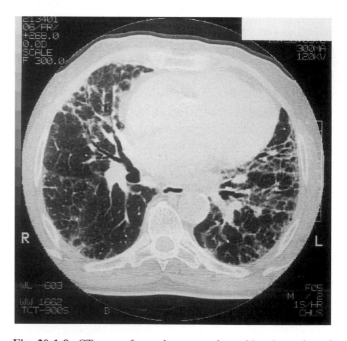

Fig. 20-1-9. CT scan of an asbestos worker with asbestosis and bilateral minimal pleural thickening. The honeycombing is prominent in the left lung field, and parenchymal changes of reticular nature are well appreciated.

4. Curvilinear lines in nondependent areas, parallel to the pleural surface but located at 1 cm from the latter, which appear to correspond either to lung fibrosis that precede the honeycombing aspect or to areas of atelectasis due to local mechanical changes asso-

ciated with adjacent pleural changes, or to an inflammatory component of the disease process

5. Nondependent subpleural densities that are a nonspecific indicator of interstitial lung disease (Fig. 20-1-9)

Although HRCT can recognize subtle changes of early interstitial lung disease often not visible on the chest radiograph, there is currently no technique of imaging that is quite as sensitive as the histopathologic examination of the lung, which recognizes the disease process originating within hours after asbestos fiber deposition in the lung.[21] Even if the pathologic changes leading to lung fibrosis can be recognized experimentally within days after asbestos exposure, in the present human work conditions, it usually takes at least 10 or more years before changes can be seen on the chest radiograph (thus, the notion of latency, the time between initiation of the disease process and the clinical manifestation of the disease).

Generally, the pulmonary abnormalities seen on chest radiograph or HRCT cannot be attributed definitely to asbestosis without the concurrent presence of characteristic pleural plaques and a history of significant asbestos exposure.

Early detection of asbestosis

Pulmonary fibrosis secondary to asbestos dust inhalation is the end-stage of a long inflammatory process initiated by retention of biologically active mineral matter. Early in the tissue reaction, one finds macrophage accumulation and activation in the lung periphery. The chronicity of this process brings the development and organization of a fibrosing peribronchiolar alveolitis, the fundamental lesion of asbestosis. Later, the process extends in adjacent interstitium and progresses to a diffuse fibrosing alveolitis, the lesion recognizable on standard chest radiography.

To use appropriately the various clinical tools available for early recognition, the clinician must know the sensitivity and specificity of each.

Crackling rales. The finding of end-inspiratory rales in axillary lung fields in an asbestos worker constitutes an early indicator of asbestosis. This finding is easily obtained and correlates well with the radiographic findings and lung function changes. In asbestos workers recognized as having asbestosis, rales are usually present. However, in exposed workers not yet recognized as having asbestosis, rales constitute the only abnormality in less than 5% of cases.[29a]

Chest radiograph. The standard PA chest radiograph is the main tool in the detection of pneumoconioses. However, it is well documented that in at least 10% of symptomatic subjects with biopsy proven interstitial lung disease, the chest radiograph is normal, and in asbestos workers, similar observations have been reported.

Computerized tomographic scan of the thorax. The investigation of asbestos workers at risk of asbestosis with conventional 10 mm slice CT scans did not show more abnormalities than the standard chest radiograph, but permitted a better appreciation of the pleural changes. With the newer generation of CT scan and thin 2 mm slices, the clarity and precision have improved significantly and have permitted increased sensitivity of the CT scan. The CT scan with thin slices has now been documented to detect early interstitial lung disease in 10% to 20% of symptomatic asbestos workers with normal radiographs.[20,35,43]

[67]Gallium lung scan. The ^{67}Ga lung scan has been used in clinical practice for over 20 years to detect occult tumors and infections and more recently to quantify lung inflammation. In the latter conditions, the degree of ^{67}Ga lung uptake has been correlated with pathologic changes.

In asbestosis, ^{67}Ga lung scan permits the detection of the inflammatory activity as seen pathologically and progresses to radiographically recognized asbestosis in 75% of cases.[29a,34] [67]Ga lung scan is not a first line method of disease detection but it recognizes the inflammatory activity of early asbestosis, which does not necessarily require withdrawal of the subject from work. The interest in ^{67}Ga lung scans has decreased in recent years, largely due to the improvement in CT scans.

Bronchoalveolar lavage. In the investigation of diffuse interstitial lung diseases, bronchoalveolar lavage (BAL) provides new information on the effector cells and biochemical molecules regulating the disease process. The search for an infectious agent is very effective with BAL and is often the major indication for its application.

In the investigation of workers at risk of asbestosis, BAL is of interest to:

1. eliminate other causes of abnormality such as silicosis, sarcoidosis, and tuberculosis;
2. document the specific mineral dust exposure;
3. support other clinical data suggestive of an alveolitis;
4. study the biologic mechanisms of the disease.

The work of independent laboratories has shown that asbestos workers develop a macrophagic and neutrophilic fibrosing alveolitis that precedes the radiographic recognition of asbestosis.[19,21]

Pulmonary function tests. Abnormalities in the traditional lung function tests such as determination of lung volumes and diffusion capacity will appear at about the same time as the change in the plain chest radiograph.[2,3,5,29a] However, the measurement of the lung pressure–volume curve as an early indicator of asbestosis is correlated with changes in the ^{67}Ga lung scan, BAL, and lung biopsies,[29a,34] demonstrating that these early alterations were associated with the peribronchiolar fibrosing alveolitis. Attempts to detect this lesion with the flow-volume forced maximal expiration curves has not been supported by studies in lifetime nonsmokers.[39]

Chapter 51, Surveillance and Screening, helps define criteria for utilizing testing procedures in exposed populations.

The criteria for diagnosis of asbestosis have been the object of several task force reports such as that of the American Thoracic Society,[42] the Canadian Thoracic Society,[44] and other individual efforts.[45]

Briefly, most agree that histopathologic material is the best and most sensitive and specific method of diagnosis of asbestosis, when the pathologic examination is coupled with mineralogic assessment (see Chapter 12).

In the absence of pathologic material, which is usually the clinical situation, the diagnosis of asbestosis is a judgment based on consideration of:

1. a reliable and significant history of exposure;
2. an appropriate time interval between exposure and detection;
3. radiographic evidence of diffuse lung fibrosis on chest radiograph or CT scan;
4. a restrictive pattern of lung function;
5. bilateral fixed inspiratory crackling rales;
6. clubbing of fingers or toes.

In general, it is suggested that criteria 1 and 3 are essential and the others are confirmatory. The level of abnormalities of the radiologic images needed for the diagnosis of asbestosis is debated, some authors requiring an ILO grade 1/1 and others accepting an ILO grade 1/0. The author of this chapter is of the opinion that asbestosis can be clinically diagnosed by an abnormal chest radiograph or CT scan suggestive of a diffuse interstitial lung disease in association with a significant history of asbestos exposure.

Course and complications of asbestosis

The outcome of patients with asbestosis is currently much better than the first cases of Murray,[8] all of whom were dead before age 30. Although life expectancy after diagnosis of asbestosis remains shorter than normal, only 20% to 40% of cases will have a progression of their disease. A significant contributing cause of increased mortality in patients with asbestosis remains the high incidence of lung carcinoma. As in other fibrotic lung diseases, intercurrent bronchopulmonary infections are frequent and should be treated promptly.

There is now experimental evidence that cessation of exposure reduces the rate of progression.[33] The deterrent effect of immunosuppressor therapy is well documented in animals, but corticosteroid use remains unsuccessful in anecdotal clinical trials.

End-stage respiratory insufficiency and failure are still seen occasionally in the disease. General concepts about the treatment of interstitial lung disease are presented in Chapter 15.

Treatment

Medical interventions in cases of asbestosis occur at time of initial diagnosis and assessment of impairment, in the follow-up of the patient with asbestosis, in the treatement of intercurring respiratory infections complicationg the disease, and in the treatment of hypoxemia and right heart failure, which may occur as late complications. Other modalities of support and prevention of complications to relieve cough symptoms or prevent viral or pneumococcal infections are indicated.

There is currently no documentation of benefit from use of steroids or immunosuppressor therapy in asbestosis. The latter form of treatment has even been shown to worsen experimental asbestosis.

BENIGN PLEURISY

The pathogenesis of benign asbestos pleurisy is largely unknown.[46,47] Nonetheless, a few considerations should be given. The clearance of inhaled asbestos fibers is in part through the lung lymphatics to the interstitium, the pleural cavities, and the lymph nodes.[48] Direct contact of asbestos fibers with the pleura appears as an initial event. Recently, an animal model has been developed, and the role of chemotactic factors for neutrophils and other inflammatory cells has been stressed.[14]

The inflammatory and exudative nonspecific inflammatory reaction of benign pleurisy is characterized on the basis of observations of cellularity of pleural fluid and rare biopsies. An inflammatory reaction with fibrin deposition is seen, accompanied by reaction of mesothelial cells, giving the impression of pseudoorganization.[25]

This pleurisy, most often transient, can leave scars such as pleural thickenings in the costophrenic angles , occasionally an adhesive fibrothorax, or diffuse pleural thickening (pachypleuritis).

Benign pleurisy is defined by[49]

1. asbestos exposure,
2. radiographic or thoracenthesis confirmation of effusion,
3. absence of other causes of effusion, and
4. absence of tumor in follow-up of at least 3 years.

This definition is somewhat arbitrary but nonetheless practical. Many of the cases of asbestos benign pleurisy are asymptomatic and found at periodic radiograph as in the case in Fig. 20-1-10. These cases can have shortness of breath and chest pain. The pleural fluid is usually an exudate with or without blood staining.

The benign pleurisy of asbestos exposure is asymptomatic in 66% of cases and is recurrent in some 28% of cases. At times, it may be associated with acute chest pain (in 17% of cases) with or without fever. It may occur with or without associated asbestosis.

According to Epler et al.,[49] benign pleurisy is the most frequent abnormality seen in asbestos workers with less

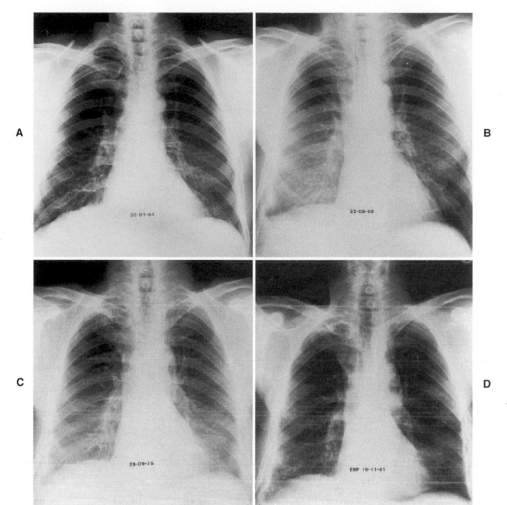

Fig. 20-1-10. Periodic chest radiograph from an asymptomatic asbestos miner. **A,** The oldest film of 1964 is normal. **B,** On the film of 1968, there is the appearance of a pleural effusion and thickening in the right lower field. **C,** On the film of 1975, the right lower field changes are persistent and there is the appearance of similar changes in the left lower field. **D,** On the film of 1981, there is bilateral thickening of the pleura, involving the lower half of the pleura and the costodiaphragmatic angles, which constitute bilateral pachypleuritis.

than 20 years of exposure. Incidence in the exposed population is approximately 3%, with a positive dose–response relationship and a very low tolerance threshold. It can even be seen in the white-collar workers of the asbestos industries. The latency period is usually less than 20 years and it is often the first manifestation of asbestos-related diseases. It is not a precursor of other diseases.

Most benign asbestos pleurisy has less than 500 ml of effusion. The pleural fluid is exudative and often has hemorragic features. On physical examination, findings are those of pleural effusion, with dullness to percussion and pleuritic rub at auscultation. Lung function testing shows a restrictive pattern, which is proportional to the severity of the disease (effusion + pain). Evolution is spontaneously favorable with complete resolution of the effusion. This effusion can leave scars as pleural plaques or pachypleuritis.

Pleural effusions are often indicative of malignant pleural or pulmonary neoplasia. All subjects with a significant exposure to asbestos who are being evaluated because of

pleural effusion should be considered as having a tumor unless proven otherwise. Pleural effusion, however, can be benign. Epler et al.[49] documented that benign pleural effusion is the most frequent of asbestos-related disorders in the first 20 years following initial asbestos exposure and is usually the only one to be seen in the first 10 years. The average latency time can be longer, at times overlapping that of mesothelioma. The diagnosis of benign pleurisy is by exclusion.

Radiographically, the effusion presents as blunting of costophrenic angles (Fig. 20-1-10). The fluid is usually of minimal volume, can be mobilized on lateral decubitus films, and is transient as opposed to that of malignant tumors. Benign pleurisy can often lead to chronic pleural changes. HRCT can be of help to exclude an early mesothelioma, which would have pleural nodularities.

Benign pleurisy follows one of several courses: complete spontaneous painless regression, painful regression with minimal or no pleural scar, one or many recurrences of the effusion, and, in a few cases, evolution to diffuse pleural thickening (pachypleuritis) and/or rounded atelectasis. It is not a precursor of mesothelioma.

Medical interventions are at time of initial diagnosis, where thoracenthesis and pleural biopsy may be needed for exclusion of other causes of pleural effusion. Treatment is to relieve symptoms. Follow-up for at least 3 years is imperative.

PLEURAL PLAQUES

Pleural plaques are focal irregular thickenings of the parietal pleura in the submesothelial portion, in reality extrapleural.[2,3] They can also be seen adjacent to visceral pleura, particularly in the interlobar fissures, which is uncommon.

Pleural plaques are the most frequent manifestation of asbestos exposure, and asbestos exposure is the most frequent cause of pleural plaques. Usually, pleural plaques are considered a good indicator of asbestos exposure. The development and progression of pleural plaques appear to be in direct relation with amphibole exposure, as chrysotile has limited tendency to produce plaques. Latency time for the production of plaques is on the average 30 years with a range of 3 to 57 years.

Pathogenesis

The pathogenesis of pleural plaques has been reviewed and well summarized by Hillerdal,[46] who recognizes two pathogenic theories: the direct effect of fibers reaching the pleural space and an indirect effect not requiring the presence of fibers in the pleural space. The latter theory is in part supported by the association of smoking and asbestos pleural plaques. The direct contact theory is the most plausible. It recognizes the plaques as a local reaction to the fibers reaching the pleural space, which is well documented as a preferential means of clearance of the short fibers.[48] This latter study has particularly well documented that the short and thin fibers were found in the pleural space after inhalation. It is likely that transport is via the lymphatics and that the additional contributions of gravity and respiratory motions are relevant.

The thin and pointed nature of the fibers found in the pleural space would facilitate penetration in the tissues and the scratching of the pleural tissues, the initiation of inflammatory and hemorrhagic reaction organizing to produce the pleural plaques. The latter mechanical theory is partly based on the observation of Epler et al.[49] who reported on 44 subjects who developed pleural plaques following transient pleural effusions. Churg and Green[25] described the occasional transformation of a chronic inflammatory and cellular pleural reaction into an acellular plaque.

Pathology

Pleural plaques are lesions of hyalin fibrosis mainly located in the submesothelial layers of the parietal pleura at the level of the costal margins, the diaphragms, and paraspinal areas. They can be found in the pericardium and less often in other mediastinal pleura. Visceral pleural plaques are less frequently seen but can extend in the interlobar fissures.

Microscopically, plaques are composed of layers of virtually acellular collagen, the surface being covered with a thin layer of mesothelial cells. Calcification is of a dystrophic nature and is often found in plaques. These pleural plaques, although typical of asbestos exposure, are not specific for the exposure. Generally, there is no asbestos body or fiber in the plaques.

Clinical manifestations

Pleural plaques are asymptomatic in the absence of obliteration of the costophrenic angles and/or associated asbestosis. They have a latency period between initial exposure and radiographic recognition of some 20 years. Asbestos-related pleural plaques are usually seen in both hemithoraces, altough to variable extent. The plaques in the retrocardiac area are not easily seen on chest radiograph as in Fig. 20-1-11. They have limited progression and are often found in the absence of asbestosis.

Radiography

Plaques are avascular bands of collagen and 35% have some dystrophic calcification not necessarily seen on standard radiograph. Calcification mainly affects the parietal plaques and is characteristically located along the diaphragm and the posterolateral chest wall. Calcification also can be found in paravertebral areas, which is rarely seen on PA film.

Early, plaques are thin, linear, with sharp margins; early detection depends on thickness of the plaques and optimal radiographic technique. They appear as rounded discrete opacities raising from the parietal pleura. Plaques can have a smooth or uneven surface and may be of gray to white color. Oblique films of the chest increase the radiographic visibility of plaques by 50% over the standard PA and lateral chest films. With time, the margins of the plaques become more rounded and better defined. Plaques rarely occupy more than four intercostal spaces.

The CT scan can recognize plaques much earlier and at a less well-defined stage than the chest radiograph (Fig. 20-1-11). Paravertebral and pericardiac plaques in particularly are better seen by CT. The diaphragmatic plaques that were not always well appreciated with conventional CT are better visualized with multiple thin slices of HRCT. CT scans can clearly differentiate plaques from extrapleural fat pads, which can be difficult to define on the plain chest radiograph. Furthermore in the presence of extensive and calcified pleura plaques, CT scanning permits a clearer appreciation of the lung parenchyma than does the plain radiograph.

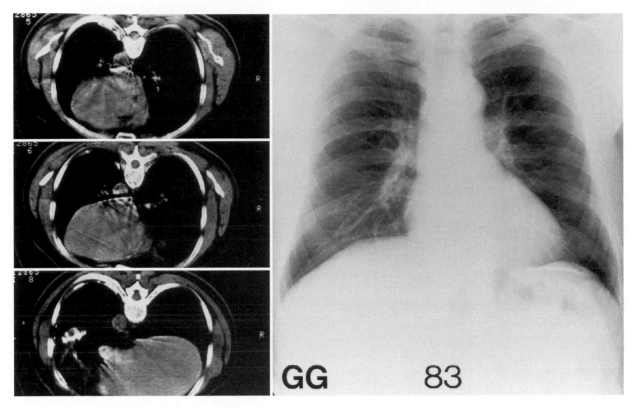

Fig. 20-1-11. CT scan selected views and chest radiograph of an asbestos worker. The chest film shows normal parenchyma and a calcified diaphragmatic plaque. On the CT scan the diaphragmatic calcified plaque is equally appreciated and, in addition, plaques are also present in the left posterior retrocardiac area, which cannot be appreciated on the plain chest film.

Significance

Pleural plaques in asbestos workers are of interest largely for their recognition as markers of exposure. In the majority of cases the pleural plaques do not significantly affect lung function. Nonetheless, several recent studies have shown that the CT scan can permit a better appreciation of pleural changes than the chest radiograph. Pleural plaques usually do not take up the [67]Ga.

Pleural plaques are common in asbestos-exposed individuals. In the past, they were felt to be simply "markers of exposures." The presence of plaques (particularly if bilateral) indicated a high probability that asbestos exposure occurred, but the plaques per se do not lead to physiologic impairments.

Some newer data, however, suggest that plaques have physiologic effects. Rosenstock et al.,[50] Schwartz et al.,[51] Beurbeau et al.,[52] and others have shown statistical associations between pleural plaques and decrements in lung function as determined by spirometry. The former two studies showed relationships with forced vital capacity (FVC), whereas Beurbeau et al. found that reductions of both forced expiratory volume in one second (FEV1) and FVC were statistically associated with the presence of plaques. In general, these associations have been found in persons with no radiographic evidence of fibrosis and in those with interstitial abnormality.

Some radiographic (computerized axial tomography [CAT]) studies suggest that pleural changes may be associated with radiographic (CT scan) evidencing subpleural parenchymal fibrosis. Thus, both structural and physiologic data are quoted to support the contention that pleural plaques can lead to impairment. Oliver et al.[53] found that abnormality of diffusion capacity was not associated with plaques. However, the relationships may be confounded by diffuse pleural thickening. This disorder is clearly associated with restrictive functional effects, and, therefore, inclusion of some diffuse pleural thickening cases in a group of pleural plaque subjects might lead to the statistical finding of a relationship between pleural disease and physiologic effect. Futhermore, the subpleural fibrosis occasionally seen in association with plaques may represent a different process than the fibrosis of asbestos, which extends from a peribronchiolar origin. Finally, because the plaque-pulmonary function test relationships are based on statistical associations, there is a possiblity of confounding by exposure. That is, higher cumulative exposures increase both the probability of developing plaque and the chance of decreased lung function.

Pleural plaques have a tendency to enlarge and calcify with time. They may also become confluent. It has been suggested that mesothelioma may develop at the edge of such plaques. Medical intervention here is limited to recognition of the nature and cause of pleural plaques.

DIFFUSE PLEURAL THICKENING (PACHYPLEURITIS)

Whereas the pleural plaques are pathologies of parietal pleura mainly, diffuse pleural thickening or fibrosis, also called pachypleuritis, is a disease of the visceral pleura. The pathogenic mechanisms differentiating the pachypleuritis from the circumscribed pleural plaques are not defined and the fundamental irritative mechanism of pleural tissue remains likely. In the case of pachypleuritis, the effect may come from fibers deposited in the parenchymal subpleural areas, thus the strong association of the diffuse pleural fibrosis with associated interstitial lung fibrosis.[47] The mechanisms causing pleural fibrosis to extend in the interlobular spaces of the lung are unknown.

Mechanism

Diffuse pachypleuritis can result from three phenomena: (1) the confluence of large pleural plaques in 10% to 20% of cases, (2) the extension of subpleural fibrosis to the visceral pleura, resulting in a diffuse pleural thickening in 10% to 30% of cases, and (3) the scar of an exudative benign pleurisy producing a diffuse pleural thickening that can extend to the interlobar and interlobular fissures. The latter is the most frequent and often causes significant restriction of lung expansion, even in the absence of interstitial lung fibrosis.[47]

The diffuse nature of the pachypleuritis produces the symptom of dyspnea on exertion, which is often present and relates to significant loss of lung function. Dry cough may also be an accompanying symptom.

These diffuse fibrotic thickenings of visceral pleura are not specific to asbestos exposure and can be associated with old inflammatory reaction from tuberculosis, thoracic surgery, hemorrhagic chest trauma, or drug reaction.

The development of pachypleuritis, contrary to pleural plaques, often follows pleural effusions (Fig. 20-1-12) and is likely initiated by the accumulation of fibers in the subpleural zones of the lung.[49] They can be large enough to cause shortness of breath and dry cough. Because of the relative thinness of the fibrosis of the pleura, it cannot be detected easily on physical examination. Diffuse pachypleuritis can be limited to one side or involve both sides and can restrict lung functions but can rarely produce respiratory insufficiency by extrapulmonary restriction.

Most often, asbestos-related diffuse pleural thickening (pachypleuritis) is associated with diffuse interstitial fibrosis. It can extend to the interlobar and interlobular spaces and, less frequently, the pleural fibrosis will produce a retracted fibrotic mass, a pseudotumor, with a pleural basis (the so-called rounded atelectasis). The fibrotic process imposes a torsion and a compression of the lung parenchyma, with the radiologic appearance of crow's paw and pseudotumor at a more advanced stage. These radiologic manifestations of asbestos-related diseases can be totally asymptomatic and have to be differentiated from long tumors. Pachypleuritis often progresses and should be clinically followed. In rare instances it can progress to respiratory failure and death.

On the plain chest radiograph, pachypleuritis or diffuse pleural thickening is a continuous pleural opacity, of smooth surface and extending on more than 25% of the pleural surface, usually with blunting of the costodiaphragmatic-

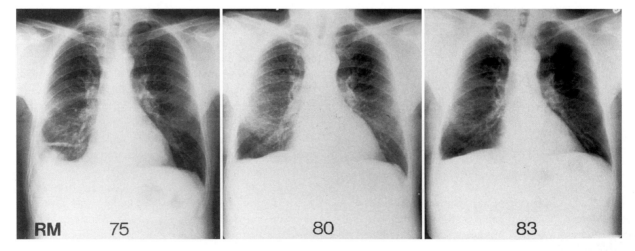

Fig. 20-1-12. Asbestos worker referred in 1975 for acute pleuritic right chest pain. The chest film of 1975 (left panel) shows blunting of the right costodiaphragmatic angle, with some adjacent atelectasis changes. The diagnosis on the exudative effusion was that of an asbestos pleural effusion, which resolved spontaneously, leaving some thickening of the pleura in the lateral wall and costodiaphragmatic angle, which is consistent with a small pachypleuritis, best seen on the 1983 film.

angle, with or without blunting of the costophrenic angle. In over 30% cases, patients recall a history of asbestos benign pleuritis. Other causes are confluence of pleural plaques in 25% cases, malignant pleural effusion, chest trauma, pleural infection, or a combination of the above (33%), and finally the extension of parenchymal fibrosis to the visceral and parietal pleura (10%). The extension of pachypleuritis in two or more fields bilaterally constitutes the best predictor of an asbestos exposure origin of the pachypleuritis. By CT scan, pachypleuritis is defined as a pleural thickening >5 cm wide, >8 cm in length, and >3 mm in thickness.

Pachypleuritis affects mainly visceral pleura (Fig. 20-1-4), in posterior and posterolateral areas of the lower zones. Because of this location, CT scan facilitates its diagnosis. Pachypleuritis can be complicated by extension of the fibrosis in the interlobar and interlobular fissures to form the "crow's paw" and rounded atelectasis images (Fig. 20-1-13).

Clinical manifestations

Pachypleuritis or diffuse pleural thickening is a less specific indicator of asbestos exposure, and early recognition is of interest only as the process can alter lung function. The findings must be differentiated from pleural fat, and CT scan is particularly useful for that. Pachypleuritis can be definitively recognized histopathologically. In most cases it may be identified on the chest radiograph or CT scan as diffuse pleural thickening, unilaterally or bilaterally.

Asbestos pachypleuritis can restrict lung function modestly if limited in degree. If it is extensive and bilateral, lung function effects can be severe to the point of causing respiratory insufficiency and failure in some cases.

As pachypleuritis often has another etiology than asbestos exposure, elimination of the other causes is part of the initial medical assessment. Furthermore, there should be evaluation of functional impairment, which may lead to consideration of compensation for loss of lung function.

ROUNDED ATELECTASIS

This effect of asbestos-induced pleural disease is caused by the scarring of the pleura and adjacent lung tissue, with retraction of the scar tissue and partial collapse of adjacent lung tissue. It is relatively uncommon, and the specific mechanisms causing this pleuropulmonary process are not known beyond those causing the pleural disease.

This condition is relatively uncommon and its existence has been more often recognized with the advent of the CT scan. It is due to scarring of the parietal and visceral pleura with thickening of the interlobar fissure and adjacent lung tissue with retraction of the scar and collapse of the associated lung tissue.

Rounded atelectasis, also called pseudotumor (Fig. 20-1-14), is usually asymptomatic and is detected on chest radiograph as a pleural-based opacity suspected of tumor origin in most cases. Occasionally chest pain in the area may be the presenting symptom. In the past, these preudo

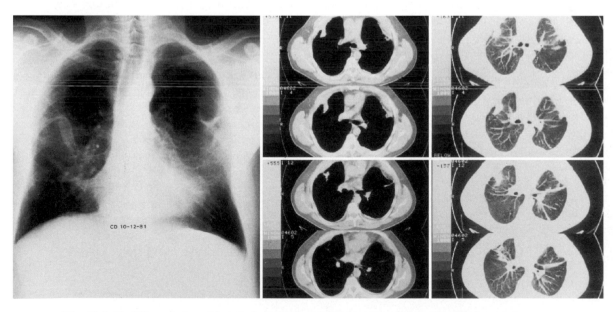

Fig. 20-1-13. Bilateral pleural-based changes in an asbestos worker. Pleural thickening can be seen bilaterally and, in addition, the invasion of the interlobar fissure leads to the formation of bilateral rounded atelectasis or pseudotumors.

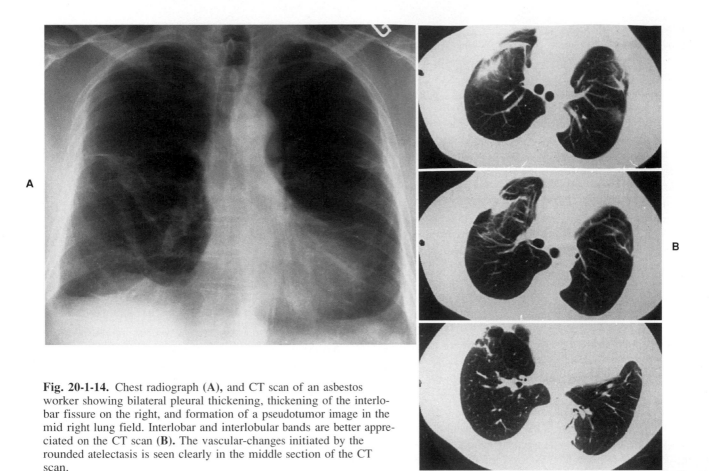

Fig. 20-1-14. Chest radiograph **(A)**, and CT scan of an asbestos worker showing bilateral pleural thickening, thickening of the interlobar fissure on the right, and formation of a pseudotumor image in the mid right lung field. Interlobar and interlobular bands are better appreciated on the CT scan **(B)**. The vascular-changes initiated by the rounded atelectasis is seen clearly in the middle section of the CT scan.

tumors were often resected, but with the CT scan, the true nature of the rounded atelectasis can be recognized without surgery.

Extension of the visceral pleural fibrosis in the interlobar and interlobular fissures often occurs late, sometimes many years after cessation of exposure. It can progress through retraction of the scar tissue to cause a torsion of the adjacent lung tissue, giving rise to the rounded atelectasis lesion, folded lung, or Bleskovsky's syndrome (Fig. 20-1-13), also called a pseudotumor, mimicking a carcinoma or a confluence of the pneumoconiosis. The characteristic aspect of a comet's tail arising from the middle part of the mass can be better appreciated on the oblique chest radiograph or on the CT scan. The curling of the bronchovascular markings toward the center of the mass from the hilum gives the appearance of a comet's tail.

The diagnosis of rounded atelectasis can be made from the radiologic images and usually has the following characteristics:

1. Round lesion of 2 to 7 cm in diameter
2. Pleural-based location
3. Curvilinear shadows extending toward the hilum (comet's tail)
4. Intrapulmonary location (acute angle between pleura and lesion)
5. Pleural thickening adjacent to lesion
6. Thickening of interlobar fissure
7. Separated from diaphragm by lung tissue
8. Low rate of progression (as opposed to tumors)

This is usually a late condition occurring long after pleural changes have been noted. Recognition of this condition can be suspected on the chest radiograph, particularly with the oblique films.

The diagnosis of rounded atelectasis used to be done on histopathologic material until the CT scan provided images that are quite specific for the condition, as detailed in the radiology section.

The recognition of the entity as such is often a clinical problem that necessitates use of CT scan, bronchoscopy, and transthoracic needle aspiration biopsy to eliminate the tumoral nature of the radiographic opacity.

LUNG CARCINOMA

The current knowledge of the pathogenesis of asbestos-related cancers is not completely understood and the subject of controversies.[1] Some investigators consider asbestos as a tumor promoter as opposed to an initiator, on the basis of weak activity in standard tests for carcinogenicity (mutagenicity, production of chromosomal abnormalities). As a tumor promoter, the fibers would have the effect of increasing the susceptibility of the lung to other carcinogens. Others consider asbestos as a tumor initiator in view of the experimental evidence of excess of lung cancers in animals not exposed to carcinogens other than asbestos and the human excess of lung tumor in lifetime non-smokers.

An additional point of debate is the necessity of participation of fibrosing activity in the genesis of lung carcinoma. This position is supported by the findings in several large epidemiologic studies showing excess lung cancers only in the most heavily exposed workers, who also have a higher incidence of radiographic opacities suggestive of asbestosis. However, opposite views consider that bronchogenic carcinoma are found in lifetime nonsmoking asbestos workers and that these lesions can be produced in animals in the absence of fibrosis.

The tenfold increased risk of lung cancer in smokers appears to be potentiated to fiftyfold in smokers who also work with asbestos. The fiber type of asbestos exposure is not significant; each of the asbestos fiber types causes lung carcinoma.

Other risk factors in the workplace such as contaminant metals, ionizing radiation, and other chemicals such as benzopyrene and polycyclic aromatic hydrocarbon (PAH) may also contribute to the added risk in the initiation and promotion of lung cancer in asbestos workers.

Some biologic and epidemiologic data suggest that the risk of excess lung cancer is concentrated in individuals with fibrosis (asbestosis). Epidemiologic studies showed the increased risk of cancer was limited to subjects with prior abnormal chest radiographs (ILO category ≥1/0).[54] In addition, a pathology study showed that all cases of lung cancer studied in a cohort of asbestos insulators had fibrosis demonstrable on a pathologic specimen[55] and another showed very strong associations.[56] Biologic mechanistic considerations also show that profibrotic mediators may also lead to carcinogenicity.[57]

Pathology

The pathology of the asbestos-related cancers is not distinct in type, nature, or location within the lung from those associated only with cigarette smoking. The type distribution is approximately 35% epidermoid, 25% small (oat cell), 30% adenocarcinoma, and 10% large cell carcinoma. This distribution is not distinct from that of populations not exposed to asbestos. The existence of asbestos-related lung cancers in the absence of asbestosis is a debated issue that is further complicated by the smoking risk factor often present.

Clinical aspects

The clinical presentation of asbestos-related lung tumors is indistinguishable from that of the lung tumors caused by other carcinogens, except for the possible association of symptoms of associated asbestosis when present. Clinical manifestations of lung cancer are discussed in Chapter 18.

Cough, chest pain, dyspnea, hemoptysis, recurrent bouts of pneumonia, and localized wheezing are the major symptoms that bring patients to medical attention, but several cases are asymptomatic at the time of initial discovery of a suspect lung lesion. Other manifestations of carcinoma of the lung such as rib pain due to local extension or metastasis, shoulder–arm pain due to a Pancoast tumor, pressure symptoms due to expansion of the lesion in the vicinity of the superior vena cava, and systemic symptoms such as arthritic pain due to osteoarthropathy, loss of weight, migrating phlebitis, effects of hypercalcemia, and other paraneoplastic manifestations can all be seen in asbestos-related lung cancers.

The radiographic manifestations of asbestos lung carcinoma are not distinct from those of lung cancers associated with other carcinogens except that other changes in the pleuropulmonary images as noted above may be present that help in recognizing the possible association. Chapters 7 and 18, discussing radiology and lung tumors, provide further details.

In the asbestos workers, the best hope for early detection of lung tumor is achieved through annual medical visits, sputum cytology, and chest radiographs in workers with more than 20 years of exposure. Chapter 51, which discusses screening methods, indicates that it is still uncertain whether such lung cancer screening techniques are currently of use.

The diagnosis of lung carcinoma rests on histopathologic grounds on cytology or tissue samples. The histologic abnormalities are not specific for asbestos exposure-related cancers.

In asbestos-exposed workers, in the absence of diffuse pleural thickening or asbestosis, the tumor has generally the same course and prognosis as those not associated with asbestos exposure. In the presence of diffuse pleural thickening or asbestosis, the carcinoma is poorly resectable and carries a bad prognosis with the usual complications of lung carcinoma. Chapter 18 discusses lung cancer in more detail.

MALIGNANT MESOTHELIOMA

With an incidence of one to two cases per million in the general population of North America, malignant mesothelioma is considered relatively rare. The clear association of asbestos with mesothelioma has been established initially by Wagner and associates[11,18] and confirmed repeatedly since. After the gathering of careful occupational and environmental exposure history and mineralogic analysis of lung tissues, it is overwhelmingly clear that the majority of cases of mesothelioma are found in subjects exposed to asbestos fibers. Even in cases of mesothelioma in women, which is 2 to 10 times less common than in men, tissue analysis for mineral fibers revealed that 98% of 117 cases in the U.K. had amphibole counts in the lungs greater than controls. In general, the amphiboles are considered, in part due to their relative durability, to be the cause of most cases, but pure chrysotile cases have also been seen although to a lesser degree.[58] In some cases, the near equal number of the two types of fibers in the lung tissue makes it impossible to establish a causal relationship for either of the fiber types.

In animal studies,[59] the process starts after fiber injection in the pleura by the formation of a granulomatous lesion with subsequent deposition of acellular dense collagen, which coalesces and is surrounded by a layer of mesenchyma cells and a surface of normal mesothelium. Later neoplastic transformation with extensive surface growth occurs, with differentiation into mesenchymal and epithelial cells. All asbestos fiber types have produced mesothelioma. Asbestos acts as an initiator and a promoter and thus is considered as a complete carcinogen at least in the induction of mesothelioma in animals.

The rationale for the greater propensity of amphibole to induce more mesotheliomas in humans has been related to its geometric properties (greater diameter, rigidity) favoring deeper penetration and its resistance to degradation, favoring its persistence in lung tissue. It is not established whether fibers that initiate the mesothelial tumor need to be translocated to the pleural space or could act from nearby subpleural lung parenchyma on direct contact with the mesothelial cells or via the cytokine network.

The exposure dose appears to be of some importance as the tumors are often found in cases with asbestosis; however, many cases occur in the absence of lung fibrosis and in subjects with short exposures. The chemical functionalities of the surface appear to have no effects. It is universally accepted that mesothelioma has no association with cigarette smoke exposure.

The sites of presentation of mesothelioma can be in the pleural, pericardial, or abdominal cavities, the latter being more often seen in the cases with high amphibole exposure. The rationale for these preferences is totally unknown.

Mesothelioma shows an apparent period of 20 to 50 years of dormancy (also called latency) of the process in humans. This is unexplained but not unique, as other cancers also have similar dormancy periods after exposure.

Pathology

In the early stage, the mesothelioma appears as multiple small grayish nodules on the visceral and parietal pleura that evolve to coalesce and form larger masses of tumor. They are often accompanied by pleural effusion. Tumor will develop by direct extension, forming large masses of tumor tissue invading the adjacent structures, including chest wall, interlobar fissure, lung parenchyma, mediastinum, pericardium, diaphragm, esophagus, large vessels of the mediastinum, contralateral pleura, and the peritoneal cavity. Death is usually caused by restriction of one or more of these vital structures.

Malignant mesothelioma is of peritoneal origin in less than 25% of cases, usually in association with amphibole exposure. Gross appearance of the tumor is quite similar and invasion involves primarily the abdominal structures.

Histopathology

Malignant mesotheliomas have a variety of histologic presentations classified as epithelial in about 50% of cases, sarcomatoid in 16% of cases, and mixed in 34% of cases. The epithelial type expresses one or more growth patterns such as tubular, papillar, microcystic, and solid, which are often mixed within the tumor with some variation from area to area. The sarcomatoid type has spindle-shaped cells with elongated cells; nuclear pleomorphism and mitosis are common. In the mixed form, epithelial and sarcomatous forms are present in variable portions.

Histochemistry

Malignant mesotheliomas elaborate acid mucosubstances rich in hyaluronic acid, which can provide a histochemical profile distinct from that of adenocarcinoma, a tumor often considered in differential diagnosis. Malignant mesotheliomas are usually periodic acid–Schiff-diastase (PAS-D) and Mucicarmine negative and hyaloronidase-alcian blue positive, whereas adenocarcinomas are PAS-D and Mucicarmine positive, but hyaloronidase-alcian blue negative.

The carcinoembryonic antigen (CEA) is negative in 90% of cases of malignant mesothelioma (and when positive it is very weak) and positive in 90% of cases of adenocarcinoma. Cytokeratin immunochemical staining is usually positive and the pattern of staining is distinct from that of adenocarcinoma, being more diffuse in the mesothelioma and exhibiting a predominantly peripheral location in the adenocarcinoma. Vimentin is usually negative in both types of tumors, but may be positive in 20% of cases of mesothelioma.

The pathological diagnosis of malignant mesothelioma can be difficult, and expertise of an interested pathologist is often necessary for final conclusion on one given case.

Clinical aspects

The incidence of malignant mesothelioma is on the order of one case per million adults in the absence of asbestos exposure and increases to its highest levels in crocidolite-exposed workers. For the North American general population, the incidence rate is estimated at between 2.5 and 13 cases per year per million adult males. In the asbestos-exposed populations, the rates can be fivefold to twentyfold higher,[58] with a gradient of 10 to 1 for crocidolite to chrysotile exposures.[20]

The chief complaint is usually chest pain, dull and aching in nature, occasionally elicited by inspiration. It is persistent and requires progressively higher doses of analgesics. Cough and dyspnea are also frequent, largely due to large pleural effusions. Weight loss, fever, and general malaise are often present at least in the late phase of the deadly disease. The symptoms of osteoarthropathy are very unusual. Shortness of breath is usually progressively worse as the tumor extends within the chest, to encase the lung and infiltrate the mediastinal structures.

The radiologic findings in malignant mesothelioma are the following: solid pleural abnormalities, most often as diffuse circumscribed thickening with irregular nodulated surface (Fig. 20-1-15), multiple pleural nodules or masses or plaque like opacities, and pleural effusion. As the disease progresses there may be involvement of the lung parenchyma, reduction in the size of the involved hemithorax, mediastinal and/or hilar invasion, pericardial thickening and/or effusion, abdominal extension, and chest wall invasion. Most of these changes can be appreciated on plain chest radiograph, but the CT scan adds precision and clarity to the observations. There is no method of early recognition of mesothelioma at present. The majority of patients with mesothelioma have chest pain as the earliest reason for seeking medical consultation.

Open thoracotomy biopsy is usually needed for estab-lishing a firm diagnosis of malignant mesothelioma. The combined use of microscopy and immunohistochemistry is usually needed.

Although there may be some modest hope with the new therapeutic combinations of cytotoxic agents and cytokines,[18] survival remains very limited, and death from progression of the disease usually occurs within 2 years from cardiorespiratory failure.

The various modalities of therapy for malignant mesothelioma, surgery, radiotherapy, chemotherapy, and lately immunotherapy or cytokine therapy or a combination of the above, have been equally unsuccessful in curing the disease. At best, extension of a few months of survival after initial diagnosis can be objectively demonstrated in selected studies.[18]

Medical interventions remain of a supportive nature in providing relief of symptoms.

PREVENTION

Current practices of public health regarding the protection of workers against the risk associated with their job are legislated in each country.[60] The law establishes the standards of permissible exposure levels and health surveillance of the workers by periodic medical examinations. Principles of the regulatory approach are discussed in Chapter 55. At present, there is concern about the potential effects of relatively low level exposure in occupational and nonoccupational (home community) settings. This is discussed further in Chapter 56.

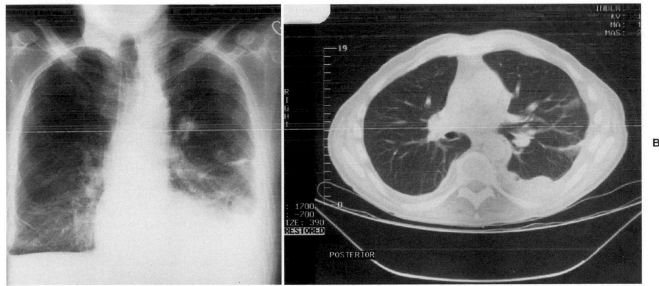

Fig. 20-1-15. Chest radiograph (**A**) and middle field CT scan in a long term asbestos-exposed plumber. On the chest radiograph, the right lung field shows pleural thickening and obliteration of the costodiaphragmatic angle suggestive of pachypleuritis. The reticulation of the right lower lung field on the radiograph is suggestive of asbestosis. On the left lung field of the radiograph, there is a clear obliteration of costodiaphragmatic angle, some opacities of the parenchyma, and some images of nodularities, which on the CT scan (**B**) are seen to be pleural based, thus highly suggestive of mesothelioma, which was proven by biopsy in this case.

REFERENCES

1. Antman K and Aisner J: *Asbestos related malignancy,* New York, 1987, Grune & Stratton.
2. Becklake MR: Asbestos-related diseases of the lung and other organs: their epidemiology and implications for clinical practice. *Am Rev Resp Dis* 144:187-227, 1976.
3. Boutin C, Viallat JR, and Rey F: Asbestose et atteintes pleurales de l'amiante. Encycl Med Chir, Paris, Poumon, U¹⁰, 4-1984, Masson.
4. Craighead JE, Abraham JL, Churg A, Green FHY, Kleinerman J, Pratt PC, Seemayer TA, Vallyathan V, and Weill H: The pathology of asbestos-associated diseases of the lung and pleural cavities: diagnostic criteria and proposed grading scheme, *Arch Pathol Lab Invest* 106:544-595, 1982.
5. Parkes WR: Asbestos related disorders, *Br J Dis Chest* 67:261-300, 1973.
6. Preger L (ed): *Asbestos related disease,* New York, 1978, Grune & Stratton.
7. Selikoff IJ and Lee DHK: *Asbestos and disease,* New York, 1978, Academic Press.
7a. Auribault M: Note sur l'hygiène et la sécurité des ouvriers dans les filatures et tissages d'amiante, *Bull Insp Trav Paris* 14:120, 1906.
8. Murray H: *Report, department, Commission on compensation of industrial disease,* Cd 3496, pp127-128, London, HMSO.
9. Marchand F: Uber eigentümliche pigment kristalle in den lungen, *Ver Deutsch Gesell* 17:223, 1906.
10. Jacob G, and Bohlig H: Lungenkrebserwartung der deutschen asbestarbeiter, *Krebsforrrsch Krebsbekampf* 3:130, 1959.
11. Wagner JC, Sleggs CA, and Marchand P: Diffuse pleural mesothelioma and asbestos exposure in North Wertern Cape Province, *Br J Ind Med* 17:160-171, 1960.
12. Landrigan PJ and Kazemi H, editors: The third wave of asbestosis disease: exposure to asbestos in the workplace. Public Health Control, *Ann NY Acad Sci* 643:1-628, 1991.
13. Selikoff IJ, and Churg J, (editors): Biological effects of asbestos, *Ann NY Acad Sci* 132:1-76, 1965.
14. Selikoff IJ and Hammond EC(editors): Health hazards of asbestos exposure, *Ann NY Acad Sci* 330:1-814, 1979.
15. Wagner JC, editor: *Biological effects of mineral fibres,* Lyons, France, 1980, WHO IARC scientific Pub No 30.
16. Anonymous. *Proceedings of the world symposium on asbestos,* Montréal, Canada, 1982, Canadian Asbestos Information Centre.
17. Wagner JC, editor: The biological effects of chrysotile, In *Accomplishment in oncology,* vol 1, #2, pp1-162, Philadelphia, 1986, J.B. Lippincott.
18. Jaurand MC, Bignon J, and Brochard P ed: International conference on: "Mesothelial cell and mesothelioma. Past, present and future," *Eur Respir Rev* 3:1-237, 1993.
19. Bégin R, Cantin A, and Massé S: Recent advances in the clinical assessment and pathogenesis of the mineral dust pneumoconiosis, *Eur Respir J* 2:988-1001, 1989.
20. Bégin R, Ostiguy R, Fillion R, and Groleau S: Recent advances in the early diagnosis of asbestosis, *Sem Roentgenol* 27:121-139, 1992.
21. Rom WN, Travis WD, and Brody AR: Cellular and molecular basis of the asbestos-related diseases, *Am Rev Respir Dis* 143:408-42, 1991.
22. Anonymous. Health Effects Institute-Asbestos Research: *Asbestos in public and commercial buildings: a literature review and synthesis of current knowledge,* HEI-AR, 141 Portland Street, suite 7100, Cambridge MA.
23. Zussman J: The mineralogy of asbestos, Michaels L and Chissick SS, editors: In *Asbestos: properties, applications, and hazards,* vol 1, chap 2, p 45, Chichester, UK, 1979, John Wiley.
24. Bignon J, Sébastien P, and Gaudichet A: Measurement of asbestos retention in human respiratory system related to health effects. In *Proceedings of the workshop on asbestos,* Gaithersburg, Maryland, Special Pub No506, pp 95-119, Washington DC, 1977, National Bureau of Standards.
25. Churg A and Green FHY: *Pathology of occupational lung disease,* ed 1, New York, 1989, Igaku-Shoin.
26. Sébastien P: La biométrologie des fibres inhalées, PhD thesis, Paris, 1982, Paris XII University.
27. Jaurand MC: Observations on the carcinogenicity of asbestos fibers, *Ann NY Acad Sci* 643:258-270, 1991.
28. Sébastien P and Bégin R: Mass, number and size of fibres in the pathogenesis of asbestosis in sheep, *Br J Exp Pathol* 71:1-10, 1990.
29. International Labor Office/University of Cincinnati: *International classification of radiographs of pneumoconiosis 1980,* No22, revised, Occupational safety and health series, Geneva, 1980, International Labor Office.
29a. Bégin R, Cantin A, Berthiaume Y, Boileau R, Bisson G, Lamoureux G, Rola-Pleszczynski M, Drapeau G, Massé S, Boctor M, Breault J, Péloquin S, and Dalle D: Clinical features to stage alveolitis in asbestos workers, *Am J Ind Med* 8:521-536, 1985.
30. Kamp DW, Graceppa P, Pryor WA, and Weitzman SA: The role of free radicals in asbestos-induced diseases, *Free Rad Biol Med* 12:293-315, 1992.
31. Mossman BT, Marsh JP, Sesko A, et al. Inhibition of lung injury, inflammation, and interstitial pulmonary fibrosis by polyethylene-conjugated catalase in a rapid inhalation model of asbestosis, *Am Rev Respir Dis* 141:1266-1271, 1990.
32. Cantin A, Allard C, and Bégin R: Increased alveolar plasminogen activator in early asbestosis, *Am Rev Respir Dis* 139:604-609, 1989.
33. Bégin R, Cantin A, and Massé S: Influence of continued asbestos exposure on the outcome of asbestosis in sheep, *Exp Lung Res* 17:971-984, 1991.
34. Bégin R, Cantin A, Drapeau G, Lamoureux G, Boctor M, Massé S, and Rola-Pleszczynski M: Pulmonary uptake of gallium-67 in asbestos exposed humans and sheep, *Am Rev Respir Dis* 127:623-630, 1983.
35. Bégin R, Ostiguy G, Filion R, Colman N, and Bertrand P: CT scan in early asbestosis, *Br J Ind Med* 50:689-698, 1993.
36. Viallat JR, Boutin C, Pietri JF, and Fondarai J: Late progression of radiographic changes in Canari chrysotile mine and mill exworkers, *Arch Environ Health* 38:54-58, 1983.
37. Bégin R, Boileau R, and Péloquin S: Asbestos exposure, cigarette smoking, and airflow limitation in long-term Canadian chrysotile miners and millers, *Am J Ind Med* 11:55-66, 1987.
38. Becklake MR, B Toyota, M Stewart, R Hanson, and J Hanley: Lung structure as a risk factor in adverse pulmonary response to asbestos, *Am Rev Respir Dis* 128:385-388, 1983.
39. Bégin R, Ménard H, Décarie F, and St-Sauveur A: Immunogenetic factors as determinants of asbestosis, *Lung* 165:159-163, 1987.
40. Bégin R, and Sébastien P: Alveolar dust clearance capacity as determinant of individual susceptibility to asbestosis: experimental observations, *Ann Occup Hyg* 33:279-282, 1989.
41. Bégin R, Cantin A, and Sébastien P: Chrysotile asbestos exposure can produce an alveolitis with limited fibrosing activity in a subset of susceptible sheep, *Eur Respir J* 3:81-90, 1990.
42. American Thoracic Society: The diagnosis of nonmalignant diseases related to asbestos, *Am Rev Respir Dis* 134:363-368, 1986.
43. Staples CA, Gamsu G, Ray CS, and Webb WR: High resolution computed tomography and lung function in asbestos-exposed workers with normal chest radiograph, *Am Rev Respir Dis* 139:1502-1508, 1989.
44. Task force on occupational respiratory disease [G. Ostiguy, chairman]. Health and welfare Canada. Ottawa: 1979, Canadian Government Publication, 35-48.
45. Harber P and Smitherman J: Asbestosis: diagnostic dilution, *J Occup Med* 33:786-793.
46. Hillerdal G: The pathogenesis of pleural plaques and pulmonary asbestosis: possibilities and impossibilities, *Eur J Respir Dis* 61:129-138, 1980.
47. Schwartz DA: New developments in asbestos induced pleural disease, *Chest* 99:191-198, 1991.
48. Rey F: La migration pleurale des fibres d'amiante. A propos d'une étude expérimentale chez le rat. Mémoire du diplôme d'études et de recherche en biologie humaine sous la direction de C Boutin. Marseille, France, 1990, Faculté de médecine de Marseille.

49. Epler GR, McLoud TC, and Gaensler EA: Prevalence and incidence of benign asbestos pleural effusion in a working population, *JAMA* 247:617-622, 1982.

50. Rosenstock L, Barnhart S, Heyer NJ, Pierson DJ, and Hudson LD: The relation among pulmonary function, chest roentgenographic abnormalities, and smoking status in an asbestos-exposed cohort. *Am Rev Respir Dis* 138(2):272-277, 1988.

51. Schwartz DA, Fuortes LJ, Galvin JR, Burmeister LF, Schmidt LE, Leistikow BN, Lamarte FP, and Merchant JA: Asbestos-induced pleural fibrosis and impaired lung function. *Am Rev Respir Dis* 141(2):321-326, 1990.

52. Bourbeau J, Ernst P, Chrome J, Armstrong B, and Becklake MR: The relationship between respiratory impairment and asbestos-related pleural abnormality in an active work force. *Am Rev Respir Dis* 142(4):649-656, 1988.

53. Oliver LC, Eisen EA, Greene R, and Sprince NL: Asbestos-related pleural plaques and lung function. NIOSH-00184515, *Am J Ind Med* 14(6):649-656, 1988.

54. Hughes JM and Weill H: Asbestosis as a precursor of asbestos related lung cancer: results of a prospective mortality study. *Br J Ind Med* 48(4):229-233, 1991.

55. Kipen HM, Lilis R, Suzuki Y, Valciukas JA, and Selikoff IJ: Pulmonary fibrosis in asbestos insulation workers with lung cancer: a radiological and histopathological evaluation. *Br J Ind Med* 44(2):96-100, 1987.

56. Sluis-Cremer GK and Bezuidenhout BN: Relation between asbestosis and bronchial cancer in amphibole asbestos miners. *Br J Ind Med* 46(8)537-540, 1989.

57. Rom WN, Travis WD, and Brody AR: Cellular and molecular basis of the asbestos-related diseases. *Am Rev Respir Dis* 143(2):408-422, 1991.

58. Bégin R, Gauthier JJ, Desmeules M, and Ostiguy G: Work related mesothelioma in Québec 1967-1990, *Am J Ind Med* 22:531-542, 1992.

59. Davis JM: Histogenesis and fine structure of peritoneal tumors produced in animals by injection of asbestos, *J Natl Cancer Inst* 52:1823-1833, 1974.

60. International Labor Bureau: *Asbestos. health risk and prevention.* Pub No 30, Geneva, 1974, International Labor Bureau.

PART **II**

Asbestos in buildings

Jonathan M. Samet
Rashid A. Shaikh

Sources and concentrations
Risks to custodial, maintenance, and other workers
Risks to general building occupants
Approaches to management
Summary

Asbestos, an established cause of malignant and nonmalignant diseases, has been used in a variety of construction materials since early in the century (Table 20-2-1). It is now present in many schools, public and commercial buildings, and residences.[1] The use of asbestos in the United States has decreased since 1973, coincident with the banning of certain applications by the U.S. Environmental Protection Agency. Nevertheless, the asbestos already in place will remain a potential source of exposure throughout the lifetimes of millions of buildings worldwide.

Because of its fibrous nature, heat resistance, and tensile strength, asbestos has been used for insulation, surface treatment, and as a component of cement products, floor tiles, and other materials (Table 20-2-1). This chapter briefly considers the problem of indoor asbestos, covering sources and concentrations, risks to workers and to general building occupants, and approaches to management. The topic of indoor asbestos has been covered more comprehensively in proceedings of several symposia, including a meeting held at Harvard in 1988,[2] a symposium on the possibility of a "third wave" of asbestos-related disease held by the Ramazzini Institute in 1990,[3] and a workshop on in-place management of asbestos held in 1993 by the Health Effects Institute—Asbestos Research in 1993 and anticipated to be published in *Applied Occupational and Environmental Hygiene* during 1994, and in a comprehensive report prepared by the Health Effects Institute—Asbestos Research, which was published in 1991.[1]

The potential for asbestos-containing materials in buildings that lead to worker and occupant exposures was first recognized about 20 years ago.[4] Experience with one building at Yale University showed that friable material containing asbestos could produce exposures comparable with those causing disease in asbestos workers. In the early 1970s, a significant and visibly recognizable problem of indoor contamination from friable sprayed-on asbestos coating was recognized in the Yale Art and Architecture Building.[5] An attempt was made to manage the asbestos in place, but removal eventually proved necessary.[4]

In the 1980s, concern about indoor asbestos largely focused on schools after apparently elevated concentrations were found in several school surveys. Adding to the concern about schools was the possibility of heightened risk for exposure during childhood, either because of inherent susceptibility or the lengthening of the interval over which disease could develop. In response to these concerns, the U.S. Congress enacted the Asbestos Hazard Emergency Response Act (AHERA) in 1986. AHERA mandated the U.S. Environmental Protection Agency to develop and implement a comprehensive regulatory framework of inspection, management, planning, and operations and maintenance activities, as well as appropriate abatement action, to control asbestos-containing materials in the nation's schools. In view of confusion about the AHERA regulations and public policy, many school systems removed asbestos-containing materials, generally at a great cost, and, at least in some instances, without adequate precautions to avoid contamination of buildings. As the costs of asbestos man-

Table 20-2-1. Asbestos-containing materials found in buildings

Subdivision	Generic name	Asbestos (%)	Dates of use	Binder/sizing
Surfacing material	Sprayed- or troweled-on	1-95	1935-1970	Sodium silicate, Portland cement, organic binders
Preformed thermal insulating products	Batts, blocks, and pipe covering			
	85% magnesia	16	1926-1949	Magnesium carbonate
	Calcium silicate	6-8	1949-1971	Calcium silicate
Textiles	Curtains* (theatre, welding)	60-65	1945-present	Cotton
Cementitious concrete-like products	Extrusion panels	8	1965-1977	Portland cement
	Corrugated	20-45	1930-present	Portland cement
	Flat	40-50	1930-present	Portland cement
	Flexible	30-50	1930-present	Portland cement
	Flexible perforated	30-50	1930-present	Portland cement
	Laminated (outer surface)	35-50	1930-present	Portland cement
	Pipe	20-15	1935-present	Portland cement
Paper products	Corrugated			
	High temperature	90	1935-present	Sodium silicate
	Moderate temperature	35-70	1910-present	Starch
	Indented	98	1935-present	Cotton and organic binder
	Millboard	80-85	1925-present	Starch, lime, clay
Asbestos-containing compounds	Caulking putties	30	1930-present	Linseed oil
	Adhesive (cold applied)	5-25	1945-present	Asphalt
	Joint compound		1945-1975	Asphalt
	Spackles	3-5	1930-1975	Starch, casein, synthetic resins
	Cement, insulation	20-100	1900-1973	Clay
	Cement, finishing	55	1920-1973	Clay
	Cement, magnesia	15	1926-1950	Magnesium carbonate
Flooring tile and sheet goods	Vinyl/asbestos tile	21	1960-present	Poly(vinyl)-chloride
	Asphalt/asbestos tile	26-33	1920-present	Asphalt
	Sheet goods/resilient	30	1950-present	Dry oils
Wall covering	Vinyl wallpaper	6-8	Unknown to present	—
Paints and coatings	Roof coating	4-7	1900-present	Asphalt
	airtight	15	1940-present	Asphalt

From Table 4-2 in the Health Effects Institute—Asbestos Research Report.[1]
*Laboratory aprons, gloves, cord, rope, fire blankets, and curtains may be common in schools.

agement mounted, so did attempts at recovery of such costs by lengthy and highly contentious litigation.

The Asbestos Hazard Emergency Response Act also required that the Administrator of the Environmental Protection Agency conduct a study to determine extent and condition of asbestos in public and commercial buildings, the extent of danger to human health, and appropriate means to respond to any such danger. In the Agency's 1988 report to Congress[6] in response to this mandate, the Administrator did not call for a regulatory approach but offered an agenda for research and education for more effective management of the problem. Based on a 1984 survey of U.S. buildings, the report estimated that 733,000 public and commercial buildings, 20% of the nation's total, had asbestos-containing material. About two-thirds of these buildings were projected to have some damage to this material. The Agency estimated that the cost of extending an AHERA-like program to all buildings would be about $50 billion.

In 1988, consistent with the emphasis on research in the Agency's report, the U.S. Congress also mandated that the Health Effects Institute, a nonprofit, nongovernmental agency in Cambridge, MA, address a charge that included the following tasks: (1) "to determine actual airborne (asbestos) levels prevalent in buildings," (2) "to characterize peak exposure episodes and their significance," and (3) "to evaluate the effectiveness of asbestos management and abatement strategies in a scientifically meaningful manner." In response, the Health Effects Institute—Asbestos Research was formed. Initially, the Institute convened its Literature Review Panel, which published a comprehensive report in 1991.[1] A research agenda directed at exposures of workers and general building occupants was developed and implementation was in progress when the Institute ceased operations in 1994 because of a lack of funding from private sector groups to match federal appropriations. Without targeted research funding directed at indoor asbestos, it now seems unlikely that any substantive gains will soon be made in understanding the health risks posed by indoor asbestos and in establishing the most effective and safest approaches for management.

Table 20-2-2. Asbestos-containing products found in buildings by physical state

Unbound asbestos in inorganic mixtures	Bound asbestos composites*	Asbestos textiles
Surface treatments†	Thermal systems insulation	Packings (valves and flanges)
Fireproofing (steel structures)	Insulating products: boiler covers, cements, pipe lagging	Plumbing cords and ropes
Acoustical applications	Vinyl tiles and floor coverings	Electrical wire insulation
Decorative surfaces	Ceiling tiles	
Equipment lagging	Ceiling and wall boards	
Moisture barrier	Cement products	
Dry applications	Papers (including pipe covering)	
Feathered (generally friable)	Acoustic plasters	
Wet applications	Spackling, patching, taping compounds	
Tamped (generally nonfriable		
Untamped		

Classification modified from a scheme used in the International Program on Chemical Safety, Environment Health Criteria *53:* Asbestos and Other Natural Mineral Fibres. United Nations Environment Program, International Labor Office, World Health Organization, Geneva (1986). Reprinted with permission from Table 4-3 in the Health-Effects Institute—Asbestos Research Report.[1]

*All generally nonfriable.

†Note that "surface treatments" in the United States also includes asbestos bound in cements and plasters. The use of the word "unbound" for these applications is European in origin.

SOURCES AND CONCENTRATIONS

Asbestos has been extensively used in building materials since the beginning of this century[1] (Table 20-2-1 and 20-2-2). The broad use categories are thermal and acoustic insulation, fire protection, and the reinforcement of building products. In addition to its use in acoustic ceiling tiles and vinyl floor tiles, asbestos has been used in paints and wall and ceiling plaster and to coat pipes, boilers, and steel structural beams.

Fibers may be released from asbestos-containing materials by the primary release mechanism: impact, abrasion, fallout, vibration, air erosion, and fire damage.[1]

Water damage and normal aging of binders leading to friability of the material increase the likelihood of release. Resuspension of asbestos-contaminated surface dust, secondary release, may contribute to airborne concentrations in buildings as well. Occupant activities are considered central in secondary release. The episodic nature of fiber release and gravitational settling reduce the likelihood that elevated concentrations will be detected with area-integrated monitoring.

An enlarging data base on airborne asbestos concentrations in buildings demonstrates extremely low average values under normal building use conditions.[1,7] Occupant risk is determined by exposures to airborne fibers rather than the presence of asbestos-containing materials in the building, which should be considered as the source of occupant exposure. Results of monitoring buildings for asbestos cannot be readily compared across studies because different sampling, analysis, and counting criteria have been used.[1] Phase-contrast microscopy (PCM), the most widely used method, has low resolving power so that fibers less than 0.25 μm in width cannot be visualized. Phase-contrast microscopy cannot distinguish between asbestos and other fibers, which are ubiquitous in the indoor environment. The transmission electron microscope (TEM), when used in conjunction with selective area diffraction and energy dispersive x-ray analysis, can be used to discriminate between fibers of different types of asbestos and also to distinguish between asbestos and other fibers. The higher resolving power of TEM in comparison with PCM allows visualization of the very thin fibers. Some investigators have prepared samples destined for TEM analysis by the so-called "indirect" method in which the filter is ashed and the residue dispersed and redeposited on a second filter before analysis by TEM is performed; this method appears to produce a higher fiber count than the alternative, the "direct" method in which the ashing step is omitted. Irrespective of the sample preparation method used, accurate TEM determinations require rigorous attention to quality, and interlab comparison studies indicate that not only do results vary among laboratories but even the technicians handling, preparing, and counting TEM-analyzed fibers may introduce important variation.[1]

Surveys conducted of asbestos concentrations in commercial buildings demonstrate very low fiber concentrations under normal conditions.[1,8,9] The Literature Review Panel Report published by the Health Effects Institute—Asbestos Research[1] compiled all published data as well as previously unpublished information on buildings sampled for litigation and for other purposes. The Report acknowledged that these data cannot be considered representative of U.S. buildings and that buildings with deteriorated asbestos-containing materials may have been subjected to remediation rather than sampling. The total data set included 1377 measurements made by TEM in 198 buildings. For fibers greater than 5 μm in length, which are considered most relevant to disease risk even though they constitute a minority of fibers in indoor air,[10] the mean and median concentrations were

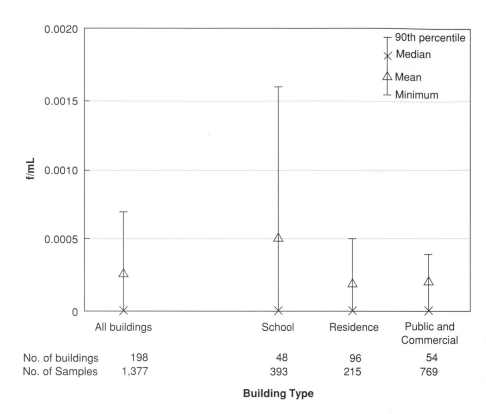

Building Type	No. of buildings	No. of Samples
All buildings	198	1,377
School	48	393
Residence	96	215
Public and Commercial	54	769

Fig. 20-2-1. Distribution of building average airborne concentrations of asbestos fibers greater than 5 μm for nonlitigation data by building type. (Reprinted with permission from the report of the Health Effects Institute.[1])

low, as were the 90th percentile values (Fig. 20-2-1). Most measurements were below the limit of detection but some buildings had fiber concentrations above levels in ambient air. Levels tended to be higher in schools, presumably reflecting the higher level of activity in schools in comparison with public and commercial buildings. The results from buildings that were sampled for litigation purposes were similar to those sampled for other reasons.

Rare individual buildings with levels much higher than the typical values in the data assembled by the Health Effects Institute—Asbestos Research have been reported. For example, as discussed previously, one of the first reports to draw attention to the problem of indoor asbestos described the Art and Architecture building at Yale University.[4] Levels measured by PCM were 0.02 fibers per cubic centimeter (f/cm^3) under quiet conditions and normal use and as high as 4 f/cm^3 after direct impact or during sweeping. With the much greater awareness of asbestos, such situations have not been described in the literature more recently and given the current social and legal climate, it is unlikely that such buildings would be reported in the scientific literature.

RISKS TO CUSTODIAL, MAINTENANCE, AND OTHER WORKERS

The widespread presence of asbestos-containing materials in buildings has appropriately raised concern that custodial and maintenance workers and workers in other trades may be exposed to asbestos as they perform their jobs. Lack of knowledge as to the presence of asbestos would increase the potential for exposure, but many of the routine duties

of workers in buildings could result in exposure, even if asbestos is known to be present. The use of contract services to provide custodial and maintenance services would appear to further increase the potential for exposure; contract workers may have less complete knowledge of the buildings where they work than would permanently based workers. Abatement workers and emergency personnel (e.g., firefighters) may be particularly likely to be exposed at high concentrations, although measurements have not been made.[1]

In addition to a few attempts to directly measure exposures of building service workers in the past, several groups of custodial and maintenance workers have been evaluated for evidence of asbestos exposure and related adverse respiratory effects. Findings in school custodial and maintenance workers in Boston, New York City, Wisconsin, and California have been described. Oliver and colleagues[11] conducted a cross-sectional survey of 120 custodians in Boston public schools. The survey population of 120 white men had a mean age of 57 years and a mean duration of work as a custodian of 27 years and included 52% of those eligible. Pleural plaques were found in 33% of the total group and in 21% of those denying other asbestos exposure. Multivariate analyses suggested an adverse effect of asbestos exposure on lung function.

From 1985 through 1987, Levin and Selikoff[12] surveyed 660 male school custodians in New York City, two-thirds of whom had started custodial work before 1965. Most (89%) reported working directly with asbestos-containing materials and the majority reported mixing asbestos, fixing asbestos, and removing asbestos. The chest x-rays were interpreted according to the ILO 1980 scheme with the finding that 28% had abnormal x-rays (11% parenchymal only, 12% pleural only, and 5% both parenchymal and pleural). The findings were similar in the group with asbestos exposure limited to New York City schools.

The findings from these two northeastern cities were confirmed in reports from Wisconsin and California. A state-wide survey of school workers in Wisconsin showed that about 11% had an abnormal chest radiograph as interpreted by a "B" reader certified by the National Institute for Occupational Safety and Health.[13] The mean years of school employment was 13 years. Balmes and colleagues[14] reported on findings from a surveillance program conducted from 1983 through 1985 in a large California school district. About 11% of the workers, who had worked for an average of 16 years, were classified as having radiographic abnormality considered as asbestos-related.

These studies have several potential limitations including use of a cross-sectional design without control subjects, lack of exposure data, and variable standardization of interpretation of chest radiographs. Additionally, pleural plaques are indicative of past exposures and not of the exposures associated with current work practices. Nevertheless, the studies provide evidence that the work practices of school custodial and maintenance workers through the 1970s resulted in sufficient exposure to have detectable health consequences. The scope of work activities involving asbestos-containing materials reported for these workers suggests that exposures may have been substantial for many.

Little information is available on past or current exposures of custodial and maintenance workers. The Literature Review Panel Report of the Health Effects Institute-Asbestos Research[1] summarized the available data through 1991. No comprehensive, recent data on custodial workers were identified. For maintenance workers, exposure estimates had been made by the CONSAD Research Corporation[15] (Table 20-2-3). The ranges of these estimates indicate a potential for significant exposure. There has also been concern that activities of custodial and maintenance workers may generate brief, relative high exposure episodes that might lead to significant exposures that would not be detected by routine monitoring, although the Health Effects Institute Literature Review Panel could not find evidence for such peaks.

The limited exposure data available for custodial and maintenance workers indicate that there is little potential for current exposures to asbestos-containing materials in buildings to cause asbestosis. However, the assumption of a non-threshold relationship between exposure and the occurrence of malignancy implies some risk for lung cancer and mesothelioma. Risks have not been specifically estimated for

Table 20-2-3. Representative exposure levels, absent respiratory protection, by construction activity

Construction activity	Representative TWA exposure levels, absent respiratory protection (f/ml)
New construction	
A/C pipe installation	0.02-0.06
A/C sheet installation	≤0.15
Roofing felt installation	ND-0.6
Asbestos abatement and demolition	
Removal	<0.01-<8 (pipe insulation) <0.01-<25 (spray-applied)
Encapsulation	0.03-0.28
Demolition	<0.01-11
Renovation/remodeling	
Drywall demolition	0.15-11
Remove built-up roofing	ND-0.2
Remove flooring products	0.02-0.04
Routine maintenance: commercial/residential	
Remove/repair/replace ceiling tiles	0.02-1.4
Repair HVAC or lighting	0.01-2.8
Other work above drop ceiling	0.01-2.8
Repair boilers	0.04-0.53
Repair plumbing	0.04-<0.1
Repair roofing	ND-0.3
Repair drywall	0.02-1.4
Repair flooring	0.02-0.04
Routine maintenance: general industry	
Gasket removal and installation	<0.1
Removal/repair of boiler insulation	<0.01-8
Removal/repair of pipe insulation	<0.01-<0.1
Miscellaneous maintenance activities	<0.01-2.8

From CONSAD[15], Table 4-20 in the Health Effects Institute—Asbestos Research Report.[1] With permission.
HVAC, Heating, ventilation, and air conditioning; *ND,* not detected; *TWA,* time-weighted average.

probable scenarios of exposure (Table 20-2-3). Using a cancer risk estimate based on the asbestos workers exposed at approximately 10 fiber/ml in the past, the Literature Review Panel Report[1] estimated that the permissible exposure limit of 0.1 fiber/ml of the U.S. Occupational Safety and Health Administration resulted in 2000 premature cancer deaths per million persons exposed for 20 years from age 25 to 45 years. A similar quantitative estimate was derived by Hughes and Weill.[16]

RISKS TO GENERAL BUILDING OCCUPANTS

During the 1980s, concern mounted about the potential for asbestos exposure of general building occupants, other than workers whose jobs might directly involve contact with asbestos-containing or contaminated materials. Potential routes of exposure for general building occupants included the "peaks" generated by activities of various trade workers, contamination of heating, ventilating, and air-conditioning systems, fiber release from impact and abrasion of accessible asbestos-containing materials, and resuspension of asbestos-contaminated surface dust. The concern about asbestos exposure to the general population of building occupants was sufficient to lead to the mandate from the U.S. Congress that created the Health Effects Institute—Asbestos Research. With over 700,000 public and commercial buildings nationwide estimated to contain asbestos, enormous costs were projected for management, particularly if removal was the principal strategy.

As concern about asbestos in public and commercial buildings mounted, risk assessments were carried out to gauge the magnitude of the hazard posed by asbestos-containing materials. The risks of exposure to general building occupants could not be directly assessed using epidemiologic approaches because of the anticipated low level of risk, the difficulty of quantifying exposure, the lengthy interval between exposure and the manifestation of increased cancer risk, and the impossibility of separating any contribution of indoor exposure to asbestos from other, much stronger causes of lung cancer. Trends of mesothelioma mortality and incidence rates, particularly in women, were evaluated as an indirect indicator of asbestos exposure through nonoccupational routes. The Literature Review Panel Report of the Health Effects Institute—Asbestos Research,[1] which evaluated trends in North America and Europe, did not find trends in women consistent with an effect of asbestos exposure in buildings. The report acknowledged the many limitations of this indirect approach to risk assessment.

Risk assessments have been accomplished more directly using the findings of the epidemiologic studies of workers historically exposed at levels that dramatically increased lung cancer risk and caused mesothelioma and asbestosis. A number of groups developed risk models using these data and applied the models to various exposure scenarios. For lung cancer, the general approach was to develop linear models for the excess relative risk associated with asbestos exposure in the workers; for mesothelioma, approaches based on the multistage model were used. Models were published by the Consumer Product Safety Commission,[17] the National Research Council's Committee on Nonoccupational Health Risks of Asbestiform fibers,[18,19] and by Doll and Peto[20] for the Health & Safety Commission in the United Kingdom.

These risk assessments were subject to substantial uncertainty because of the extremely limited information on levels of asbestos exposure to general building occupants. Assumptions were made as to the likely exposures or the upper limits of exposures sustained by building occupants. The Consumer Product Safety Commission Report considered risks of exposure at 0.01 fibers/ml, the National Research Council Committee on Nonoccupational Health Risks of Asbestiform Fibers considered exposures at 0.0004 and 0.002 fibers/ml, and Doll and Peto considered the consequences of 0.0005 fibers/ml. Because nonthreshold risk models were used, each of these risk assessments projected some elevation of lifetime cancer risk from exposure to asbestos at the assumed concentrations. Table 20-2-4 provides the risk estimates of the National Research Council committee as an example. Doll and Peto[20] estimated that exposure to a concentration of 0.0005 fibers/ml for 40 hours/week for 20 years would produce an additional lifetime risk of death of 1 per 100,000.

The Health Effects Institute—Asbestos Research report[1] provides the most recent risk assessment. In comparison with the earlier risk assessments, the Health Effects Institute—Asbestos Research estimates were based on a more substantial data base on exposures to building occupants; the estimates were similarly based on the epidemiologic studies of workers although an indirect approach was used for dose–response assessment. For the asbestos workers assumed at a level of about 10 fibers/ml, the lifetime cancer risk was estimated as about two in 10. This relationship was extended to scenarios of exposure based on the exposure data gathered by the Literature Review Panel. For the various scenarios of average exposure, only small increments in risk were projected (Table 20-2-5). These risk estimates

Table 20-2-4. Estimated individual lifetime risks from a continuous exposure to asbestos at 0.0004 fiber/cm^3 (a median dose) or 0.002 fiber/cm^3 (a high dose)

		Estimated individual lifetime risk ($\times 10^6$)	
Disease	Exposure group	Median exposure (0.0004 fiber/cm^3)	High exposure (0.002 fiber/cm^3)
Lung cancer	Male smoker	292	1459
Lung cancer	Female smoker	105	524
Lung cancer	Male nonsmoker	27	132
Lung cancer	Female nonsmoker	14	68
Mesothelioma	All groups	156	780

Based on corrected Table 7.2 from the National Research Council Report,[18] as corrected.

should be regarded as highly uncertain because of the assumption that an exposure–response relationship observed in highly exposed workers can be extrapolated to exposures at orders of magnitude lower; additionally, the exposure data base available remains extremely limited. Nevertheless, the Health Effects Institute—Asbestos Research report provides an indication of the scope of the risk for building occupants, suggesting that hundreds of cancer deaths at most may be attributed to asbestos exposure in U.S. buildings.

Table 20-2-5. Estimated lifetime cancer risks for different scenarios of exposure to airborne asbestos fibers*

Conditions	Premature cancer deaths (lifetime risks) per million exposed persons
Lifetime, continuous outdoor exposure	
0.00001 fiber/ml from birth (rural)	4
0.0001 fiber/ml (high urban)	40
Exposure in a school containing ACM, from age 5 to 18 years (180 days/yr, 5 hr/day)	
0.0005 fiber/ml (average)†	6
0.005 fiber/ml (high)†	60
Exposure in a public building containing ACM age 25 to 45 years (240 days/yr, 8 hr/day)	
0.0002 fiber/ml (average)†	4
0.002 fiber/ml (high)†	40
Occupational exposure from age 25 to 45	
0.1 fiber/ml (current occupational levels)‡	2000
10 fiber/ml (historical industrial exposures)	200,000

*This table represents the combined risk (average for males and females) estimated for lung cancer and mesothelioma for building occupants exposed to airborne asbestos fibers under the circumstances specified. These estimates should be interpreted with caution because of the reservations concerning the reliability of the estimates of average levels and of the risk assessment models. Reprinted with permission from Table 1-1 in the report of the Health Effects Institute—Asbestos Research.[1]
†The "average" levels for the sampled schools and buildings represent the means of building averages for the buildings reviewed herein (Fig. 20-2-1). The "high" levels for schools and public buildings, shown as 10 times the average, are approximately equal to the average airborne levels of asbestos recorded in approximately 5% of schools and buildings with asbestos-containing materials (ACM). If the single highest sample value were excluded from calculation of the average indoor asbestos concentration in public and commercial buildings, the average value is reduced from 0.00021 to 0.00008 fiber/ml, and the lifetime risk is approximately halved.
‡The concentration shown (0.1 fiber/ml) represents the permissible exposure limit (PEL) proposed by the U.S. Occupational Safety and Health Administration. Actual worker exposure, expected to be lower, will depend on a variety of factors including work practices, and use and efficiency of respiratory protective equipment.

APPROACHES TO MANAGEMENT

Asbestos remediation consists of methods that either leave asbestos in place, such as in-place management, enclosure, or encapsulation, or those that remove asbestos. During the 1980s, asbestos removal was often considered as the preferred remediation method. However, it is now recognized that a comprehensive operations and maintenance program to manage asbestos in place is the preferred course of action.

Asbestos removal involves strict isolation of the work area, protection of the workers, clean-up after removal, and disposal of the removed material. Isolation is generally achieved by physical separation with construction of barriers as well as by maintaining an air pressure differential. Removal is a difficult and expensive option, and, if improperly done, it can increase airborne fiber levels for varying periods of time. During the 1980s, the AHERA regulations were seemingly often interpreted as requiring asbestos removal from schools, and on the same basis, asbestos was removed from some public and commercial buildings.

It is now generally accepted that asbestos-containing material in buildings in good repair and undisturbed is unlikely to give rise to elevated airborne fiber concentrations, and, therefore, management of asbestos in place, rather than removal, is viewed as the best option.[21] Operations and maintenance (O&M) programs are being widely implemented today for the in-place management of asbestos-containing material and for control of asbestos exposures. An operations and maintenance program may be viewed as an administrative framework that prescribes the application of specific work procedures for activities that may disturb or damage asbestos-containing material, dust, or debris.[22] The work procedures include engineering controls, worker protection, and clean-up and disposal procedures.

A small, but increasing body of literature suggests that when executed according to well-designed plans, and by well-trained workers, operations and maintenance procedures are effective at reducing exposures to low levels in buildings. The Health Effects Institute—Asbestos Research[23] reported on airborne asbestos concentrations for 394 samples (191 area and 203 personal) collected during 106 jobs that were part of an operations and maintenance program at a hospital complex that contained a variety of asbestos-containing materials. The average concentrations, as determined by phase contrast microscopy, for personal and area samples were 0.11 and 0.02 fiber/ml. When the data were used to calculate 8-hour time weight average concentrations for personal samples, 95% were below 0.1 filter/ml and 99% were below 0.2 fiber/ml; 0.1 and 0.2 fiber/ml are the proposed and current permissible exposure limits, respectively, established by the Occupational Safety and Health Administration.

Perkins et al.[24] analyzed data on asbestos levels in the vicinity of glove bags during asbestos removal; the average of 430 samples taken at the glove bag was 0.037 fiber/ml whereas the average of 386 samples collected 15 to 20 feet from the glove bag was 0.028 fiber/ml. Corn et al.[25] analyzed approximately 500 area and personal air samples obtained in five buildings. Although arithmetic averages were not given, the information provided (the 8-hour time-weighted average and average work time) can be used to calculate the average fiber levels during electrical and plumbing activities, cable pulling, and heating, ventilating, and air conditioning system work; these averages were 0.0075, 0.0059, and 0.0074 fiber/ml, respectively. Nine hundred and sixteen area samples obtained in a large office building in Washington during a variety of operations and maintenance activities had an average value of 0.0059 fiber/ml.[26] Kaselaan and D'Angelo[27] summarized air monitoring data for 178 samples obtained in five commercial buildings; the averages in the buildings ranged from 0.011 to 0.073 fiber/ml. Price et al.[28] complied and analyzed data submitted to the Occupational Safety and Health Administration by a number of organizations; the mean of 1227 samples, weighted by volume, was 0.045 fiber/ml.

Little information is available regarding long-term ambient levels in buildings that have an operations and maintenance program. In one building that contained sprayed-on asbestos-containing material as well as thermal system insulation, air was sampled on nine occasions (328 samples) from 1985 to 1988; an operations and maintenance program was operational during this entire period.[23] The average for all fibers longer than 5 μm determined using the transmission electron microscope was 0.00004 fiber/ml.

As noted previously, asbestos operations and maintenance programs and work practices, which have evolved over the last 10 to 12 years, are now central in maintaining acceptable worker exposures at acceptable levels. Indeed, in earlier studies in buildings where stringent measures, in comparison with contemporary practices, were not taken,[5,29] or in recent simulation studies,[30] considerably higher levels of asbestos fiber exposure in the building environment have been demonstrated.

It thus appears that operations and maintenance programs are effective at keeping asbestos levels low; however, it has been noted by some observers that only a small proportion of all buildings—perhaps as few as 10%—presently have such programs in place. There may be substantial numbers of buildings where uncontrolled exposure is taking place and where workers and general building occupants are being exposed to unnecessary and preventable risk from asbestos.

SUMMARY

Health care providers and other health professionals may become involved with the problem of indoor asbestos in its clinical and public health dimensions. Clinicians may be asked about the need for surveillance of custodial and maintenance workers along with other trades who may come in contact with asbestos in schools, in public and commercial buildings, and in residences. These workers remain at risk for exposure, particularly if an effective operations and maintenance program has not been implemented. Past exposures of custodial and maintenance workers in schools resulted in pleural plaques and possibly reduced lung function; the limited measurement data indicate a potential for exposure at levels that are associated with unacceptable risks for lung cancer and mesothelioma. In obtaining an occupational history relevant to asbestos exposure, the clinician should fully cover custodial and maintenance work.

Policy on indoor asbestos has evolved substantially since the 1970s; the present thrust of the U.S. Environmental Protection Agency is toward in-place management with an operations and maintenance program. Health professionals may be drawn into the policy and legal aspects of the problem as experts on the medical consequences. These contentious dimensions of the problem have been addressed elsewhere.[7,31]

REFERENCES

1. Health Effects Institute Asbestos Research Literature Review Panel: *Asbestos in public and commercial buildings,* Cambridge, MA, 1991, Health Effects Institute—Asbestos Research.
2. Harvard University Energy and Environmental Policy Center: *Symposium on health aspects of exposure to asbestos in buildings,* Cambridge, MA, 1988, Harvard University.
3. Landrigan PJ and Kazemi H, editors: *The third wave of asbestos disease: exposure to asbestos in place. public health control,* p. 628, New York, 1991, The New York Academy of Sciences.
4. Sawyer RN: Yale art and architecture building: asbestos management revisited, *Appl Occup Environ Hyg,* 9:781-784, 1994.
5. Sawyer R: Asbestos exposure in a Yale building: analysis and resolution, *Environ Res* 13(1):146-168, 1977.
6. U.S. Environmental Protection Agency: *A citizen's guide to radon. The guide to protecting yourself and your family from radon.* Washington, DC, 1992, U.S. Government Printing Office.
7. Mossman BT et al: Asbestos: scientific developments and implications for public policy, *Science* 247:293-301, 1990.
8. Corn M et al: Airborne concentrations of asbestos in 71 school buildings, *Reg Toxicol Pharmacol* 13:99-114, 1991.
9. Chesson J et al: Airborne asbestos in public buildings, *Environ Res* 51:100-107, 1990.
10. Lippmann M: Asbestos and other mineral fibers, In Lippmann M, editor:*Environmental toxicants: human exposures and their health effects,* pp30-75, New York, 1992, Van Nostrand Reinhold.
11. Oliver LC, Sprince NL, and Greene R: Asbestos-related disease in public school custodians, *Am J Ind Med* 19:303-316, 1991.
12. Levin SM and Selikoff IJ: Radiological abnormalities and asbestos exposure among custodians of the New York City Board of Education, In Landrigan PJ and Kazemi H, editors: *The third wave of asbestos disease: exposure to asbestos in place. Public health control,* pp530-539, New York, 1991, The New York Academy of Sciences.
13. Anderson HA et al: A radiographic survey of public school building maintenance and custodial employees, *Environ Res* 59:159-166, 1992.
14. Balmes JR, Daponte A, and Cone JE: Asbestos-related disease in custodial and building maintenance workers from a large municipal school district, In Landrigan PJ and Kazemi H, editors: *The third wave of asbestos disease: exposure to asbestos in place. Public health control,* pp 540-549, New York, 1991, The New York Academy of Sciences.
15. CONSAD Research Corporation: *Economic analysis of the proposed revisions to the OSHA asbestos standards for construction and gen-*

eral industry, OSHA J-9-F-8-0033. Washington DC, 1990, U.S. Department of Labor.

16. Hughes JM and Weill H: Asbestos exposure—quantitative assessment of risk, *Am Rev Respir Dis* 133:5-13, 1986.

17. Consumer Product Safety Commission: *Report of the chronic hazard advisory panel on asbestos,* Washington, DC, 1983, United States Consumer Product Safety Commission Directorate for Health Sciences.

18. Committee on Nonoccupational Health Risks of Asbestiform Fibers: *Asbestiform fibers: nonoccupational health risks,* 1984, Board on Toxicology and Environmental Health Hazards, Commission on Life Sciences, National Research Council.

19. Breslow L, Brown S, and Van Ryzin J: Response (letter: risk from exposure to asbestos), *Science* 234:923, 1986.

20. Doll R and Peto J: *Asbestos: effects on health of exposure to asbestos,* Health and Safety Commission. London, 1985, Her Majesty's Stationery Office.

21. U.S. Environmental Protection Agency: *Managing asbestos in place: a building owner's guide to operations and maintenance programs for asbestos-containing materials,* Washington, DC, 1990, U.S. EPA, Office of Pesticides and Toxic Substances.

22. National Institute of Building Sciences: *The NIBS guidance manual: asbestos operations and maintenance,* Washington DC, 1992, NIBS.

23. Health Effects Institute-Asbestos Research (HEI-AR): *Asbestos in public and commercial buildings: supplementary analyses of selected data previously considered by the literature review panel,* Cambridge, MA, 1992, Health Effects Institute-Asbestos Research.

24. Perkins JL, Rose VE, and Cleveland MS: Analyses of PCM asbestos air monitoring results for a major abatement project, *Appl Occup Environ Hyg* 7(1)27-32, 1992.

25. Corn M, McArthur B, and Dellarco M: Asbestos exposures of building maintenance personnel, *Appl Occup Environ Hyg* 9:845-852, 1994.

26. Kinney P, Satterfield MH, and Shaikh RA: Airborne fiber levels during asbestos operations and maintenance work in a large office building, *Appl Occup Environ Hyg* 9:825-835, 1994.

27. Kaselaan & D'Angelo Associates Inc: *Worker exposure to asbestos resulting from small-scale short duration operations: an historical sample. prepared for real estate's environmental action league.* Haddon Heights, NJ, 1991, Kaselaan & D'Angelo Associates, Inc.

28. Price B, Crump KS, and Baird EC III: Airborne asbestos levels in buildings: maintenance worker and occupant exposures, *J Exp Anal Environ Epidemiol* 2(3):357-374, 1992.

29. Paik NW, Walcott RJ, and Brogan PA: Worker exposure to asbestos during removal of sprayed material and renovation activity in buildings containing sprayed material, *Am Ind Hyg Assoc J* 44(6):428-432, 1983.

30. Keyes DL, Chesson J, and Ewing WM: Exposure to airborne asbestos associated with simulated cable installation above a suspended ceiling, *Am Ind Hyg Assoc J* 52(11):479-484, 1990.

31. D'Agostino R, Jr. and Wilson R: Asbestos: the hazard, the risk, and public policy, In Foster KR, Bernstein DE, and Huber PW, editors: *Phantom risk,* pp183-210, Cambridge, MA, 1993, The MIT Press.

Chapter 21

MAN-MADE FIBERS AND NONASBESTOS FIBROUS SILICATES

James E. Lockey

The industrial use of naturally occurring, nonasbestos fibrous silicates, as well as man-made fibers, has been increasing, particularly since the banning of most asbestos products in the United States. The experience with the fibrous zeolite, erionite, in Turkey indicates that environmental exposure to other naturally occurring fibrous minerals can cause health abnormalities currently associated with occupational and environmental exposure to asbestos. The Mine Safety and Health Administration (MSHA) has listed over 150 minerals that can be expected to contain fibrous minerals or occur in a fibrous form.[1] Even though only a small percentage of these are under commercial exploitation, there are some indications of potential health risks. The production of various types of man-made fibers has increased markedly and, with the exception of man-made vitreous fibers (MMVFs) such as glass fiber and mineral wool, inadequate human health data are available. This chapter reviews the general determinants of fiber toxicity, and then discusses the health implications from exposure to the man-made fibers and nonasbestos fibrous silicates as listed in Box 21-1.

DETERMINANTS OF FIBER TOXICITY

The main determinants of fiber toxicity are the dose delivered to the target organ, the fiber dimension, and fiber durability.[2,3] The deposition of fiber within the lower respiratory system is dependent on fiber diameter and length. In general, fibers less than 3.5 μm in diameter and less than 200 μm in length are considered to be respirable in size. As such, they can be deposited within the lower respiratory system. Here, they are cleared through the mucociliary clearance mechanism or through macrophage translocation or fiber disintegration. The latter refers to dissolution of the surface and the chemical matrix of the fiber and/or the fracturing of the fiber perpendicular to the longitudinal plane into shorter segments. Short enough fibers can be engulfed by alveolar macrophages and subsequently translocated to the interstitium or the ciliated epithelium of the terminal bronchioles. An important difference between noncrystalline or amorphous man-made fibers and natural crystalline fibers such as erionite is that erionite cleaves along a longitudinal crystalline plane into thinner and thinner fibers, whereas amorphous man-made fibers cleave transversely.

Fiber dimensions are the second determinant of fiber toxicity. The Stanton hypothesis states that fiber dimension and durability are determinants of carcinogenic potential. When investigators used a pleura implantation technique in rats, variable degrees of carcinogenicity were seen with a variety of man-made and naturally occurring fibers, including potassium octatitanate, silicon carbide, halloysite, dawsonite, attapulgite, wollastonite, aluminum oxide, and glass fiber. The probability of induction of pleural sarcoma was best correlated with fibers 0.25 μm or less in diameter and greater than 8 μm in length. A high correlation was also seen for fibers up to 1.5 μm in diameter and greater than 4 μm in length.[4] Additional analysis indicated that the probability of inducing a tumor was related to the number of long, thin fibers as well as the type of particle.[5]

The pleural implantation and intraperitoneal injection animal models are sensitive methods for detecting the carcinogenic potential of different types of fibrous minerals.[6] These models, however, bypass the normal pulmonary defense mechanisms and, although sensitive, may not reflect the physiologic response of cells of the respiratory tract to inhalational exposures.

Fiber durability is the third determinant of fiber toxicity.[2,3,7] By modifying the quantity of stabilizers and modifiers in the production of MMVFs, for example, the physical characteristics can be changed according to their end-use requirements. Increases in stabilizers such as aluminum impart a greater degree of chemical durability.[8] Fibers that demonstrate stable surface characteristics and integrity within a cellular or extracellular milieu have the potential for prolonged "residence time" in lung tissue.

In vitro bioassays have demonstrated that, in general, fibrous minerals in comparison with nonfibrous mineral particulates with similar chemical analogs have an enhanced cytotoxic response in cells of the respiratory tract.[9] Short-term animal inhalational studies have correlated fiber toxicity to the persistence of cytotoxicity, inflammation, altered macrophage function, and persistence of the fiber particle within the lung.[10] A potential mechanism for fiber-induced carcinogenesis revolves around damage of cellular deoxyribonucleic acid (DNA) through production of oxygen free radicals, by formation of clastogenic factors, or missegregation of chromosomes in cells in mitosis.[11,12]

Fiber exposure indices have been proposed for lung cancer, mesothelioma, and interstitial fibrosis (Table 21-1). There appear to be critical length–diameter values for du-

---

Box 21-1. Man-made fibers and nonasbestos fibrous silicates

Man-made fibers

Carbon/graphite
Kevlar para-aramid
Silicon carbide fibers and whiskers
Aluminum oxide

Man-made vitreous fibers

Glass fiber
  Glass wool
  Continuous glass filament
  Special-purpose glass fiber
Mineral wool
  Rock wool
  Slag wool
Refractory ceramic fiber

Fibrous silicates

Palygorskite
  Attapulgite
  Sepiolite
Wollastonite
Zeolite
  Erionite

Minerals with potential fiber contamination

Vermiculite
Talc
Metal ore deposits

Table 21-1. Fiber exposure indices

Exposure index	Diameter boundary (μm)		Length boundary (μm)	
	Lower	Upper	Lower	Upper
Stanton fibers	—	1.5	4	—*
Pott fibers†	—	1	3	—
Lippmann fibers				
Asbestosis‡	0.15	2	2	—
Cancer§	0.15	—	10	—
Mesothelioma§	—	0.1	5	—

Adapted from Schneider T and Skotte J: Fiber exposure reassessed with the new indices, *Environ Res* 51:108-116, 1990. With permission.
*No boundary.
†Carcinogenic potential applies to fibers durable in vivo for longer than 3 years.
‡Total surface area of fibers within these dimensions.
§Number of fibers within these dimensions.

rable fibers and carcinogenic potential. For interstitial disease such as pulmonary asbestosis, the critical index may be the surface area of the fibers. In general fibers that are of respirable size have high aspect ratios (long and thin), and fibers that are durable in biologic fluids have a high potential for an adverse pulmonary health outcome.[4,13-15]

MAN-MADE FIBERS
Carbon/graphite fiber composites

Carbon fibers impregnated or mixed with resin binders are in increasing use as strong, heat-resistant, chemically inert, lightweight construction material. Carbon fiber composites have replaced traditional aircraft construction material and are being used more often in the automobile and sporting goods manufacturing industries. Combination with binders allows the material to be molded and machined. Carbon fibers are formed by heating carbonaceous pitch, rayon, or polyacrylonitrile fibers to 1200°C and consist of amorphous carbon (Fig. 21-1). When carbon fibers are heated above 2200°C, crystalline graphite fibers are formed.[16,17] Carbon/graphite fiber diameters range from 7 to 10 μm, but smaller diameter fibers can be produced, depending on the end-use application. The mechanical manipulation of carbon/graphite fiber composites, such as with sawing, sanding, and machining, can generate airborne particulates of respirable size. The fibers fracture crosswise while maintaining their original diameter. The result is the generation of airborne particulate aerosols with large variability in the percentage respirable fraction.[16] When exposed to temperatures from 900°C to 1100°C in composite burn tests small amounts of respirable-size fibers can be released. This is attributed to oxidation of the original fibers and a fibrillation effect.[18]

Intratracheal injection studies in rats of dust from several different graphite fiber composites used in the aerospace industry demonstrated a heterogenic response. Using

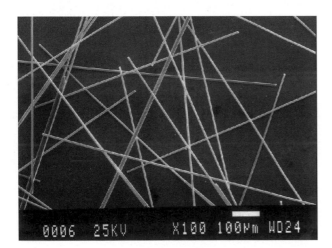

0006   25KV   X100 100μm WD24

Fig. 21-1. SEM photomicrograph of carbon fibers (Courtesy of T. Hesterberg, Ph.D.).

aluminum oxide particles as an inert control and α-quartz as a toxic control, three graphite fiber composite dusts demonstrated minimal toxicity and two demonstrated consistent toxicity as manifested by cytotoxicity for alveolar macrophages and total number of cells recovered from the lungs.[19] The histopathologic responses ranged between the aluminum oxide inert control and the toxic quartz control.[20] Mutagenicity studies of extracts of pitch-based carbon fibers have demonstrated positive clastogenic effects that were not seen in extracts of polyacrylonitrile-based carbon fibers.[21] An inhalation study in rats exposed to carbon fibers demonstrated only an increased number of particle-containing macrophages. The average fiber diameter to which the animals were exposed, however, was 7 μm, a size with limited lung penetration capability.[22]

As carbon fiber is a new manufacturing material, inadequate medical information is available in regard to potential latent or chronic health abnormalities. The results of a survey of workers involved in 8- to 10-μm-diameter carbon fiber production for 10 years demonstrated no abnormalities.[23]

The available data indicate a heterogenicity in potential health risk from exposure to carbon/graphite fibers and composites. The potential toxicity is dependent on the material used to synthesize the carbon/graphite fibers, fiber size (respirable versus nonrespirable), binder composition, percentage respirable fraction in particulate aerosol resulting from mechanical manipulation, and potential for the carbon/graphite fibers to absorb chemical contaminants.[19,21] Exposure levels for respirable-size carbon/graphite fibers should be maintained at or below 1 fiber per cubic centimeter (f/cc) and respirable composite particulates should be maintained below the current U.S. Occupational Safety and Health Administration (OSHA) respirable dust standard for nuisance dust until the various health aspects are adequately defined.

Kevlar para-aramid fibers

Kevlar para-aramid fibers have unique physical properties in terms of wear, heat resistance, and tensile strength that make them suitable for a variety of applications. Kevlar is Du Pont's registered trademark for its para-aramid fibers.[10] These are used as reinforcement agents in plastics, rubber, and fabric products and as friction material for automobile brake shoes. Intact Kevlar fibers are approximately 12 μm in diameter. The surface is covered with curled and tangled fibrils that are ribbonlike and mostly under 1 μm in width (Fig. 21-2). The fibrils have a tendency to peel from fibers and curl, twist, entangle, and interlock with other fibrils, forming mostly non–respirable-size clumps. Kevlar fibrils are composed of crystallites that form a tight bond to other fibrils along the longitudinal fiber axis. During manufacturing and end use, fibril levels range from 0.01 to 0.4 f/cc for an 8-hour time-weighted average (TWA).[24,25] Use of Kevlar para-aramid fibers in friction materials such as brake shoes produces extremely low levels of fibers in the dust generated.[26]

Intraperitoneal injection in rats exposed to Kevlar fibers produced an inflammatory granulomatous response.[27] Inhalation studies in rats exposed to ultrafine Kevlar fibrils over a 1- to 2-year period demonstrated a dose-related alveolar bronchiolarization at exposures of 25, 100, and 400 f/cc. At the 100- and 400-f/cc exposures slight fibrosis was noted along with persistent minimal fibrotic changes in the region of the alveolar ducts in the 400-f/cc 1-year recovery group of rats.[24] The fibrotic changes seen in this study may have been the result of overloading the pulmonary clearance mechanism, therefore facilitating a long-term inflammatory response.[10] A few of the animals also developed a cystic keratinizing squamous cell tumor that was believed to be a type of experimental tumor unique to rats.[24] Overall, the residence time of long Kevlar fibrils was believed to be decreased because of fiber-shortening mechanisms such as enzymatic attack at fibril defects.[28] A short-term inhalation bioassay in rats exposed to ultrafine Kevlar para-aramid fibrils indicated a reduced biopersistence in lung tissue because of low durability and rapid clearance. The initial acute inflammatory response was reversible within 1 month and there were no reported significant postexposure histopathologic effects.[10] No human health data are available on Kevlar fibril exposure.

The curved, ribbonlike configuration and reduced biopersistence of Kevlar fibrils in lung tissue reduce the potential fibrogenic and carcinogenic risks. As long as fibril concentrations are maintained near the level found in current commercial operations (0.5 f/cc or less), the potential health risk to humans should be minimal.

Silicon carbide fibers and whiskers

Silicon carbide (SiC), also called carborundum, is an artificially produced and widely used abrasive and refractory material. Commercially, silicon carbide is produced by combining silica and carbon in an electric furnace at 2400°C. Applications for silicon carbide include sandpaper, abrasive wheels, and refractory materials in boilers and foundry furnaces. During the production of silicon carbide crystals, silicon carbide fibers can be generated as a by-product. The fibers can also be preferentially produced as polycrystalline silicon carbide fibers and as monocrystalline silicon carbide whiskers (Figs. 21-3 through 21-5). Incorporation of silicon carbide fibers and whiskers in ceramics, ceramic composites, and metal matrix composites adds strength and toughness to the product. Exposure to silicon carbide fibers and whiskers can occur during the production process, during manufacturing of composite material, and during machining or finishing of composite parts.[29-32]

In vitro studies using mouse cell cultures of silicon carbide whiskers demonstrated equal or greater cytotoxic response compared with crocidolite asbestos.[30,33] A subacute inhalation study in rats exposed to silicon carbide whiskers at 630 f/cc and above demonstrated alveolar, bronchiolar,

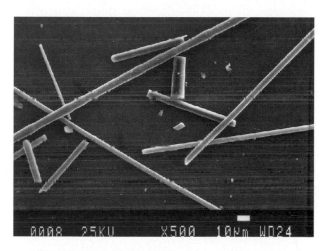

Fig. 21-3. SEM photomicrograph of silicon carbide fibers (Courtesy of T. Hesterberg, Ph.D.).

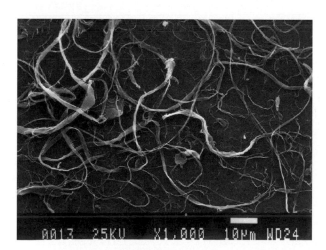

Fig. 21-2. SEM photomicrograph of Kevlar para-aramid fibers (Courtesy of T. Hesterberg, Ph.D.).

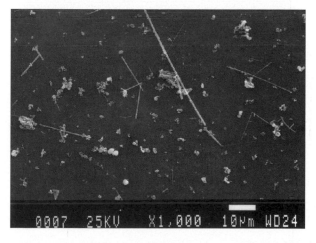

Fig. 21-4. SEM photomicrograph of silicon carbide whiskers) Courtesy of T. Hesterberg, Ph.D.).

and pleural thickening as well as adenomatous hyperplasia of the lung that was persistent over a 26-week recovery period.[29]

Inhalation studies in sheep exposed to silicon carbide dust have demonstrated that the particles are inert. The same material in a fibrous form produced a sustained moderate fibrosing alveolitis with increased fibronectin production and fibroblast growth activity.[34] The pneumoconiosis associated with the manufacturing of silicon carbide crystals is most likely associated with exposure to silicon carbide fibers and whiskers generated as a by-product, and quartz or the biologically more active tridymite and cristobalite formed in the thermal production process.[31,34]

Histologic review of lung specimens of workers involved with silicon carbide manufacturing has demonstrated silicotic nodules, ferruginous bodies, and nodular and irregular interstitial changes on chest radiographs, as well as pleural plaques.[35-37] In one worker with pneumoconiosis, fiber counts done by transmission electron microscopy for fibers longer than 5 μm demonstrated 39,300 fibers per milligram of dry lung; the mean diameter and length were 0.49 and 11 μm, respectively. Results indicate that silicon carbide fibers are durable and capable of persisting in human lung parenchyma at high concentrations.[32]

Respirable-size fibers have been found in airborne samples from silicon carbide production facilities. The fiber tends to be straight and needlelike and range from less than 1 to 2 μm in diameter and from 3 to 4 μm up to 30 μm in length.[31] Machining of metal matrix composites containing silicon carbide whiskers produced 8-hour TWA exposure concentrations of 0.031 f/cc. Machining of ceramic matrix composites produced 8-hour TWA exposures of up to 0.76 f/cc. The silicon carbide whiskers averaged 0.5 μm in diameter and 10 μm in length. Short-term exposure activities such as handling recycled materials have been associated with fiber counts up to 5 f/cc.[38] Because of these results, one producer of silicon carbide whisker composites set an internal exposure standard at 0.2 f/cc for an 8-hour TWA.[39]

The currently available data indicate that there is a potential for exposure to silicon carbide fibers and silicon carbide whiskers both during silicon carbide and silicon carbide composite production and when silicon carbide composites are machined and finished. Animal and human data indicate a fibrogenic and possible carcinogenic potential. Environmental exposure assessments in work environments should include measurements of airborne respirable fibers using both phase contrast light microscopy and electron microscopy.

Aluminum oxide fibers

Exposure to aluminum oxide (Al_2O_3) particles has been identified as a potential cause of pulmonary fibrosis in workers involved with the manufacturing of aluminum oxide abrasives.[40] An interesting case report raised the possibility that aluminum oxide fibers may play a role in aluminum oxide fibrosis (Fig. 21-6). A worker with 19 years of employment in the aluminum smelting industry and chest radiographic findings of interstitial fibrosis had 1.3×10^9 crystalline fibers per gram of dry lung tissue. The geometric mean length of the fibers was 1.0 μm and the width was 0.06 μm, with an aspect ratio of 16. The quantity of fibers was 10 times greater than the number of asbestos fibers found in chrysotile miners and millers with pulmonary asbestosis. A large aluminum oxide particulate burden was also found in the lung tissue. Although long, thin fibers are felt to be more fibrogenic than short ones, a large lung burden of short fibers can also represent a significant pulmonary hazard.[14,41] Additional studies are needed to determine

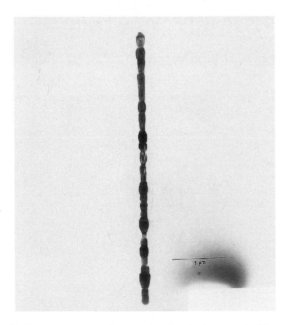

Fig. 21-5. TEM photomicrograph of a single crystal silicon carbide whisker (Courtesy of Owens-Corning Fiberglas).

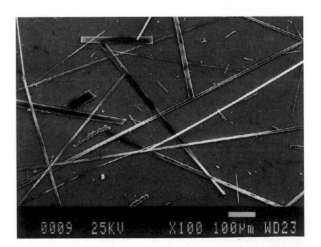

Fig. 21-6. SEM photomicrograph of aluminum oxide fibers (Courtesy of T. Hesterberg, Ph.D.).

the role crystalline aluminum oxide fibers play in regard to the potential for causing pulmonary fibrosis. As with MMVFs and silicon carbide, the potential for fiberization exists in production processes that involve molten material and air flow. Identification of potential fibers both in air samples and within lung tissue necessitates the use of sensitive analytic techniques such as electron microscopy with energy dispersive x-ray analysis.

MAN-MADE VITREOUS FIBERS

Man-made vitreous fiber production and use has been increasing over the last century. These fibers, also known as synthetic vitreous fibers or man-made mineral fibers, can be divided into three main groups: glass fiber (glass wool, continuous glass filament, and special-purpose glass fiber), mineral wool (rock wool and slag wool), and refractory ceramic fiber (Fig. 21-7). Glass wool, commonly known as fiberglass or fibrous glass, is used in home insulation. Depending on fiber diameter and chemical composition, MMVFs have unique physical properties that make them useful for over 35,000 applications. Typical end uses of glass wool and, to a lesser extent, slag and rock wools include insulation blankets, batts, and blowing wool as well as acoustic ceiling board and wall panels. Air-handling systems commonly use glass wool. Continuous glass filament is used in fabric and as a reinforcement agent in plastics. Refractory ceramic fibers are predominantly used in special industrial settings requiring high heat insulations, such as in petroleum refineries, chemical plants, and electrical utility plants.[3,42,43]

The term *man-made mineral fibers* is commonly used in the industrial, governmental, and trade literature. This term is inappropriate, however, for two reasons. (1) By definition a *mineral* is a chemical compound or element that results from inorganic processes of nature. (2) A mineral exists in a naturally occurring crystalline structure. The manufacturing process for MMVFs involves the melting of raw materials in a cupola with subsequent fiberization and rapid cooling. The rapid cooling accounts for the noncrystalline or vitreous structure of glass fiber, mineral wool, and refractory ceramic fiber. An important distinction between MMVFs and naturally occurring fibers such as asbestos and zeolite is the respective noncrystalline versus crystalline state. When MMVFs fracture, they break perpendicular to the longitudinal noncrystalline structure and become shorter in length, whereas asbestos fibers fracture parallel to the longitudinal crystalline planes into thinner filaments that maintain their overall length. This and other physical and chemical differences accounts for what is generally believed to be a substantially lower-order health risk for MMVFs in comparison with naturally occurring crystalline fibers that have high aspect ratios and are respirable in size.

Manufacturing process

Glass fiber is manufactured from silicon dioxide with varying amounts of stabilizers such as aluminum, titanium, and zinc and modifiers or fluxes such as sodium, potassium, calcium, barium, lithium, and manganese.[43] The physical properties of MMVFs such as thermal nontransference, resistance to corrosion and moisture, tensile strength, and elasticity can vary according to the amount and types of stabilizers and modifiers in the raw materials. The stabilizers impart a higher degree of chemical durability in relation to end-use applications. The vast majority of glass wool is fiberized through a rotary process producing discontinuous fibers with average diameters ranging from 3 to 15 μm. The production process, however, allows for wide variations in fiber size, resulting in fibers of less than 1 μm in diameter. The discontinuous glass wool is bound together by binding agents, predominantly phenol formaldehyde resins. A heat curing process converts binders to insoluble polymers. Other agents can be added in the production process as lubricants or antistatic and wetting agents. Glass wool is predominantly used for residential and commercial thermal and acoustic insulation (Box 21-2).

Continuous glass filament is produced by a more exacting continuous filament process that allows for little variation in the average fiber diameter, which ranges from 3 to 25 μm.[43] Continuous glass filament is used in textile fab-

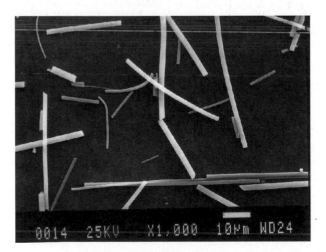

Fig. 21-7. SEM photomicrograph of slag wool. Rock wool, glass fibers, and refractory ceramic fibers are identical in appearance (Courtesy of Owens-Corning Fiberglas).

> ### Box 21-2. Industrial and commercial applications for glass wool
>
> Industrial and commercial insulation
> Residential insulation batts, blankets, and blowing wool
> Air-handling ducts
> Ceiling panels
> Acoustic panels
> Horticultural growing medium

Adapted from reference 43 with permission of TIMA, Inc.

Box 21-3. Industrial and commercial applications for special-purpose glass fiber

Aerospace and aircraft insulation
Battery separator media
Air and liquid filtration media
Special temperature, electrical, and acoustic applications

Adapted from reference 43 with permission of TIMA, Inc.

Box 21-4. Industrial and commercial applications for rock and slag wools

Acoustic ceiling tiles and wall panels
Fire protection
Residential insulation batts, blankets, and blowing wool
Industrial and commercial low- and high-temperature insulation
Horticultural growing medium

Adapted from reference 43 with permission of TIMA, Inc.

Box 21-5. Industrial and commercial applications for refractory ceramic fiber

Kiln and furnace insulation, blankets, and modular insulation
Refractory papers and felts
Refractory textiles
Castable insulation
High-temperature gaskets and joints
High-temperature filtration
Reinforcements

Adapted from reference 43 with permission of TIMA, Inc.

---

rics as well as plastic reinforcement agents, including the production of boat hulls and automobile parts. Special-purpose glass fibers are produced through a flame attenuation fiberization process and average less than 3 μm in diameter. These fibers are used in special applications requiring high thermal and acoustic insulation, such as in the aircraft industry (Box 21-3).

Slag and rock wools are produced by melting and fiberizing slag from metallic ore refining processes or rock.[43] The majority of mineral wool production in the United States is produced from slag. In Europe the majority is produced from igneous rock. The production occurs via a variation of the Downey process and the wheel centrifuge process that produces discontinuous fiber averaging 3.5 to 7 μm in diameter. Again, the nature of the production process allows for wide variations in the diameters of fibers, including those well within the respirable range. Mineral wool without binder is used as blown insulation and in the manufacture of ceiling tiles. Mineral wool with binder is principally used for insulation batts, boards, and blankets and for pipe coverings (Box 21-4).

Refractory ceramic fibers constitute 1% to 2% of worldwide MMVF production.[43] They are produced from melted kaolin clay, alumina/silica, or alumina/silica/zirconium through a steam-jet fiberization or wheel centrifuge process. The average diameters range from 1 to 5 μm. Products include bulk fiber, blankets, board, paper, and textile products (Box 21-5). Refractory ceramic fiber is used as insulation in high-temperature applications (2600°F). When exposed to temperatures exceeding 1800°F, refractory ceramic fiber partially converts to a type of crystalline silica, cristobalite.

Animal inhalation studies

Inhalation studies provide a good model for determining fiber toxicity, as they do not bypass the normal respiratory defense mechanisms. Two-year multidose (30, 150, and 240 f/cc) inhalation studies in rats exposed to two types of glass wool commercial insulation with an average diameter and length of 1 and 20 μm, respectively, demonstrated a mild pulmonary cellular response that appeared to be at least partially reversible upon removal from exposure. Initial results from one type of slag wool have yielded similar findings. The initial results of a rock wool inhalation study indicated the presence of minimal fibrosis at 145 and 247 f/cc.[44] An inhalation study of refractory ceramic fiber at a maximum tolerated dose of 250 f/cc has demonstrated mesothelioma, lung cancer, and pulmonary and pleural fibrosis in rats, and mesothelioma and pulmonary and pleural fibrosis in hamsters. A multidose inhalation study of refractory ceramic fiber in rats at 25, 75, and 120 f/cc demonstrated one mesothelioma and minimal fibrosis in the animals exposed to 75 and 120 f/cc. There was a pulmonary cellular response at 25 f/cc.[44] The pulmonary response of one type of MMVF with a specific chemical composition may not be applicable to another type because of a qualitative and/or quantitative difference in the stabilizers and modifiers. Comparison of one type of MMVF with another should take into consideration differences in size, chemical composition, and durability.

Health effects

Skin irritation is the most frequent health complaint from exposure to MMVFs.[45] The irritation is from mechanical injury from fibers greater than 4 to 5 μm in diameter. Fibers are capable of penetrating the stratum corneum and, at times, deeper into the epidermis. The usual symptom is intense itching of the skin without objective findings other than excoriation from scratching. This frequently occurs where bare skin comes in contact with surfaces contaminated with MMVFs, such as the forearm, where clothing is in tight contact with the skin, such as the neck area, and within skin folds. The intense pruritus is worse in hot, humid weather and is the result of the release of histamine or kinins. Other findings may include transient, small erythematous papules or vesicles and, less frequently, urticaria, petechiae, erosions, and rare nummular eczema. Approximately 5% of new workers involved with MMVF manufacturing reportedly leave employment within a few weeks because of this phenomenon. Studies of end users of MMVFs such as construction workers have demonstrated increased symptoms of skin irritation with increasing hours of fiber exposure per month. Individuals with dermatographism or atopic dermatitis may have difficulty tolerating MMVF exposure. A practical procedure to determine whether glass fiber is the etiologic agent is to sample for fiber from the affected skin area by using cellophane tape to lift adherent debris from the stratum corneum. Microscopic examination of the sample will demonstrate rodlike fibers. The use of loose-fitting, long-sleeved shirts and pants that are changed at work and washed daily but separately from other clothes will help prevent skin irritation. Proper work practices and environmental control measures are important preventive measures.

Man-made vitreous fibers can cause irritation of the eyes as well as the upper and lower airways. The occurrence of irritative symptoms varies according to exposure levels and job duties. In residential settings irritation from fiberglass is very unusual unless the material is improperly handled, installed, or repaired. For example, a family experienced a massive home contamination from improperly installed air-conditioning ducts lined with fiberglass.[46] Symptoms included nasal congestion and sneezing, cough and shortness of breath, and exacerbation of an asthmatic condition. The home was reoccupied after disposal of carpets, draperies, and upholstered furniture and vacuuming with filters capable of removing particles as small as 0.3 μm.

In MMVF manufacturing facilities studies have generally not identified an increase in upper and lower respiratory tract symptoms in comparison with findings in similar non-MMVF workers.[47] Fiber exposure levels in manufacturing plants are generally below 0.5 f/cc for an 8-hour TWA, and manufacturers routinely have in place environmental controls and work practice guidelines. Unusual dusty situations, however, have been associated with upper respiratory tract irritation. For secondary production facilities utilizing MMVF in product fabrication and for end users such as insulators and sheet metal workers, there is a potential for higher exposure. This can occur by manipulation of MMVFs such as with sawing, cutting, or sanding; installing or tearing out of insulation; and working with MMVFs in an enclosed space. Man-made vitreous fiber exposure levels of workers involved with installation of residential insulation products have been studied.[48] Mean 8-hour TWA airborne fiber concentrations were below 0.3 f/cc except for installers and feeders of loose fiberglass without binder (1.96 and 0.85 f/cc, respectively) and install-

ers of loose mineral wool (0.97 f/cc). Actual task length average exposures were higher. Exposure levels were substantially lower for installers of fiberglass and mineral wool batts and loose fiberglass blowing wool with binder. Construction workers using mineral wool demonstrated a correlation between upper respiratory tract symptoms and duration of exposure.[49] Previously measured mineral wool exposure levels varied from less than 0.05 to over 3 f/cc. The potential for increased exposure to respirable-size MMVFs exists when working with MMVFs with smaller average diameters, such as special-purpose glass fiber or refractory ceramic fiber.

Respiratory morbidity studies have generally failed to identify any adverse health trends in glass wool, slag wool, or rock wool manufacturing facilities.

The most recent follow-up of U.S. workers from seven MMVF production plants found no overall increase in small opacities on chest radiographs in comparison with a regional non–MMVF-exposed comparison group [23/1435 (1.6%) versus 2/305 (0.7%), respectively].[47] Of the radiographic changes identified, 21 of 23 were in workers from an ordinary- and fine-diameter glass wool manufacturing plant (average fiber diameter, over 3 μm and 1 to 3 μm, respectively) and a very fine-diameter glass wool manufacturing plant (average fiber diameter, less than 1 μm). The primary type of opacity was irregular and all were at 1/0 and 1/1 profusion levels as rated by the International Labor Organization system. At the ordinary- and fine-diameter manufacturing plant, there was an association with several exposure indicators at profusion category 1/0 but not at profusion category 1/1. The overall prevalence of radiographic change at the ordinary- and fine-diameter manufacturing plant was 5.9% versus 3.0% for the regional non–MMVF-exposed comparison group. This difference was not statistically significant.

The spirometric measurements indicated a healthy population with no relationship with exposure indicators or radiographic changes. Within this study there was significant intrareader and interreader variability in interpreting the chest radiographs, and the authors recommended that continued health surveillance was prudent, particularly in plants manufacturing fine-diameter fibers.

An ongoing morbidity study of current and former workers of refractory ceramic fiber manufacturing facilities has demonstrated a statistically significant increased prevalence of pleural changes.[50] Of the 23 workers with pleural changes, 21 had pleural plaques. In workers with more than 20 years since first employment, 11.4% (8/70) had pleural changes evident on chest radiographs. No interstitial changes were identified.

Limited morbidity data are available on the potential health effects of MMVFs on workers using these fibers in secondary production processes or on end users such as insulators. Previous asbestos exposure is a confounding factor in many of these secondary and end-user applications, especially in populations with 20 to 30 years from the time of initial employment, the population at risk for potential radiographic changes. Production workers with exposures of 15 years or more who were using rotary spun fiberglass for insulating appliances have been studied.[51] Fiber diameters ranged from 15 μm to less than 1 μm. The prevalence of irregular opacities, profusion $\geq 1/0$ to 2/1, in workers who reported no known exposure to asbestos and volunteered to participate in the study was 3.5% (10/284). When profusion category 0/1 was included, the prevalence was 7.7% (22/284). There was insufficient historical exposure information to calculate cumulative exposure indices. Some airborne asbestos fiber (0.25 f/cc or less) had been previously measured in the manufacturing facility.[52] These data indicate a need for additional health studies on product fabricators and end users of MMVFs with no previous confounding exposure to asbestos.

Mortality studies

There are large ongoing mortality studies on workers involved with glass fiber and mineral wool manufacturing. The results of these studies are updated approximately every 5 to 10 years. The U.S. study is conducted through the University of Pittsburgh and the European study is run through the International Agency for Research on Cancer (IARC).

The latest results of the U.S. study demonstrated an overall small but statistically significant increased risk of respiratory cancer (standardized mortality ratio, 112.1).[53] There was, however, no association with indicators of exposure such as fiber exposure estimates, time since first employment, or duration of employment. A subsequent case–control study of nine U.S. slag wool plants reported a definite association with increased lung cancer mortality and smoking but not with MMVF exposure.[54] A case–control study of a Newark, Ohio, glass fiber manufacturing facility reported that the excessive lung cancer reported for the facility may be partially due to differences in the prevalence of cigarette smoking in the local community versus the United States as a whole.[55]

The European study of glass fiber and mineral wool manufacturing facilities demonstrated an overall increase in lung cancer mortality using national but not local mortality rates.[56] A significant increase in lung cancer mortality using local mortality rates was found in workers involved in the earliest technologic phase of mineral wool production. The mortality ratios were substantially reduced in later production phases. Further analysis demonstrated an increasing trend between lung cancer and time since first employment but not with duration of employment in the mineral wool and glass wool cohorts.[57]

There has been no demonstrated increased risk of death from lung cancer or other causes associated with continuous glass filament manufacturing.[58] A mortality study of re-fractory ceramic fiber manufacturing workers is currently in progress through the University of Cincinnati.

A mortality study of workers involved with the use of glass wool and rock wool in the prefabricated house industry did not demonstrate any increase in lung cancer mortality.[59] The exposure for workers involved with direct handling of MMVFs ranged from 0.05 to 0.25 f/cc. The short time from initial exposure and the small number of workers in the cohort necessitate caution in interpreting the results. An extended follow-up study of the cohort is necessary before a definitive conclusion is warranted.

Overall, there does not appear to be persuasive evidence of any substantial increase in respiratory cancer risk in workers involved with glass fiber or mineral wool manufacturing based on the ongoing mortality studies. Exposure levels in these plants, however, generally average below 0.5 f/cc. Mortality results from these manufacturing facilities may not be applicable to product fabrication and end-user job tasks when potential exposure to MMVFs can be higher and when there are inadequate human health data.

The ongoing animal and human studies will continue to refine the database and the health risks associated with MMVF exposure. Based on previous available data, the IARC classified glass wool, rock wool, slag wool, and ceramic fiber as group 2B (possibly carcinogenic to humans).[12] The currently available data indicate the potential health risks of MMVFs are substantially lower than what has historically been associated with asbestos exposure. As a general class, glass fiber has the lowest order of health risk, followed by rock and slag wools, and then special-purpose glass fiber that has increased durability and refractory ceramic fiber. The vast majority of the human data, however, are from manufacturing facilities in which exposure levels have generally been below 0.5 f/cc. More emphasis should be placed on surveying product fabricators using MMVFs and end users who have not had previous opportunities for exposure to asbestos and where exposure levels to MMVFs can be potentially higher. In the interim it is important to maintain exposure levels at or below 1 f/cc and to have in place proper environmental controls, worker training, and work practice guidelines.

FIBROUS SILICATES
Attapulgite and sepiolite

Palygorskites are crystalline magnesium silicate clays with varying proportions of aluminum, magnesium, and iron. The two commercial mineral clays of the palygorskite group are attapulgite (Fig. 21-8) (palygorskite is referred to as *attapulgite* commercially) and sepiolite (Fig. 21-9). Attapulgite is produced throughout the world but predominantly from the Georgia–Florida region of the United States. Sepiolite is produced mostly in Spain.[60,61] Attapulgite and sepiolite are used in a variety of commercial products, in-

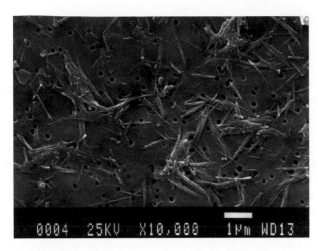

Fig. 21-8. SEM photomicrograph of attapulgite (Courtesy of T. Hesterberg, Ph.D.).

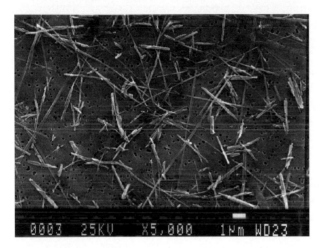

Fig. 21-9. SEM photomicrograph of sepiolite (Courtesy of T. Hesterberg, Ph.D.)

cluding absorption granulates, paint thickeners, and drilling muds, and as asbestos substitutes.[61] Attapulgite, sepiolite, and the aluminum silicate montmorillonite are also members of a group of absorbent clays known as fuller's earth.[62] The name *fuller's earth* is derived from its use for finishing and thickening ("fulling") wool cloth.[63] Attapulgite derived from different geological locations can have different physical and chemical properties, including fiber size distribution, surface properties, and mineral purity. Fibers measured in air samples from the Georgia attapulgite mine range from 0.1 to 2.5 μm in length and from 0.02 to 0.1 μm in diameter.[62] Other geologic sites can produce fibers with lengths exceeding 10 μm.[60]

Carcinogenesis studies of attapulgite from different geologic origins have produced variable results. Some ore specimens have been demonstrated to have carcinogenic and fibrogenetic potentials in animal intrapleural injection and inhalation studies.[60] Membranolytic activity, as deter-

mined by using human erythrocytes, varies among attapulgite specimens.[64]

Intratracheal instillation in rats of short attapulgite fibers obtained from a Florida deposit induced an alveolar inflammatory reaction with some indication of biopersistance within the alveolar structure.[65] Inhalational studies have been performed in sheep with attapulgite fibers obtained from ore sources in Florida with a mean length of 0.8 μm (range, 0.25 to 4 μm) and diameter of 0.02 μm. The animals demonstrated a macrophage and neutrophil alveolitis with peribronchiolar involvement.[66]

A case report suggested that attapulgite may cause pulmonary fibrosis.[67] A morbidity study of sepiolite workers in Spain, where the clay is used predominantly as pet litter, demonstrated an effect of clay dust on both forced expiratory volume in 1 second (FEV1) and forced vital capacity (FVC). No pleural plaques were noted on chest radiographs, but 20% of 218 workers had small opacities profusion category >1/0, as interpreted by at least one of two readers.[68] A study of workers in Turkey using meerschaum, a solid form of sepiolite, as a material for handicraft such as carved pipes was inconclusive because of confounding environmental exposures to tremolite asbestos and zeolite.[69] A mortality study of workers involved with mining and milling attapulgite clay in the Georgia–Florida area demonstrated no increase in mortality from nonmalignant respiratory disease. There was an increase in lung cancer deaths that were not associated with latency, duration of employment, or attapulgite exposure level. Lack of smoking data was a limitation in this study.[62]

Because of variation in the geologic deposits of palygorskite, the physical characteristics and biologic activities for each ore source should be characterized before commercial exploitation. Based on the limited animal and human data, it would be prudent to maintain exposure levels below the current OSHA respirable dust standard for nuisance dust, particularly for ore sources in which there is a potential for the generation of respirable fibers exceeding 8 to 10 μm in length.

Wollastonite

Wollastonite is a naturally occurring monocalcium silicate mineral found in various deposits throughout the world. The mineralogic structure of wollastonite can vary and certain deposits can be contaminated with other minerals. Wollastonite has potential uses in a variety of industrial applications, including ceramics and as an asbestos substitute in selected products (Fig. 21-10). The largest deposits are found in the United States, Mexico, and Finland.[70]

A long-term inhalational study in rats exposed to wollastonite produced an alveolar macrophage response that resolved with cessation of exposure. No neoplasms were found in the animals. The wollastonite came from a New York mineral source in which the acicular or needlelike fibers had length–diameter ratios ranging from 3 : 1 to 20 : 1.

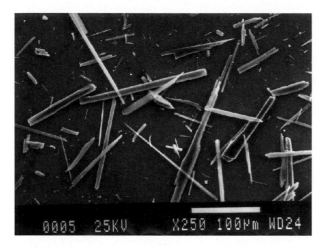

Fig. 21-10. SEM photomicrograph of wollastonite (Courtesy of T. Hesterberg, Ph.D.)

The animals were exposed to 360 f/cc, with the vast majority of fibers under 5 μm in length due to the aerosol generation technique. The lack of a fibrogenic or carcinogenic response to wollastonite was felt to be secondary to its biodegradability and lack of persistence in the lungs.[7,71] There were similar findings in an animal intraperitoneal injection model using wollastonite from India.[6]

A morbidity study of 46 workers exposed to wollastonite at a quarry for at least 10 years demonstrated irregular interstitial changes in 30% (profusion category, ≥1/0) as well as bilateral pleural thickening in 28% consistent with plaques. Airborne fiber concentrations at various quarry operations were high and ranged from 1 to 63 f/cc using scanning electron microscopy. There was also a potential exposure to limestone and silica.[70] From the same wollastonite quarry, one worker developed a "malignant retroperitoneal mesenchymal tumor" 30 years after initial wollastonite exposure.[72]

Results of a morbidity study of workers from a northern New York wollastonite deposit demonstrated no significant relationship between exposure and pulmonary function or radiographic changes. Approximately 36% of employees had over 15 years of exposure, and airborne fiber counts by phase contrast microscopy were 0.3 f/cc in the mine and 23 f/cc in the mill.[73] A follow-up study of the same cohort demonstrated a greater decline in peak flow over time in the high dust-exposed group of workers.[74]

Animal data indicate low carcinogenic and fibrogenic potentials for wollastonite, most likely because of its low durability. The results of the human morbidity studies are in conflict. This may be reflective of higher exposure levels in the study of Finnish wollastonite quarry workers. Of the various type of naturally occurring nonasbestos fibrous minerals, wollastonite has a low level of toxicity but very well may cause pleural and interstitial changes at exposure levels that are unusually high.

Zeolites

Zeolites are a group of hydrated aluminum silicate minerals that occur in fibrous and nonfibrous forms. Natural zeolite deposits are found throughout the Intermountain West, particularly in the Great Basin. The naturally occurring fibrous zeolite, erionite, splinters along a longitudinal plane into thinner fibers with extremely high aspect ratios. The majority of zeolites used in industrial applications are from commercial production of nonfibrous synthetic zeolites. These synthetic zeolites have no known identified health risks and are used for their selective absorptive and ion-exchange capabilities in the petrochemical and water purification and treatment industries.[75,76]

Animal studies have demonstrated that fibrous erionite is both a potent fibrogenic and carcinogenic agent.[77] Fibrous erionite from Oregon injected intraperitoneally in rats was more carcinogenic than chrysotile, amosite, and crocidolite asbestos.[78] Fibrous erionite from the village of Karain, Turkey, produced similar results.[79] Synthetic zeolite has not demonstrated carcinogenicity in mouse peritoneal injection studies.[80]

In the villages of Tuzköy and Karain, Turkey, exposure to fibrous erionite in the environment has been linked to both malignant and nonmalignant respiratory diseases. The zeolite erionite is found in the volcanic tuffs located in the Cappadocia region of central Anatolia, Turkey. In the past villagers had carved homes into these volcanic tuffs. The local villages have became tourist attractions because of these volcanic tuff rock dwellings, called "fairy chimneys."[81] An epidemic of malignant pleural and peritoneal mesotheliomas occurred in these villages with an incidence 1000 times higher than that within the general world population. There has also been an excess of lung neoplasms. Nonmalignant changes have included various pleural changes, such as pleural plaques and calcification, diffuse pleural thickening, benign pleural effusion, and diffuse interstitial fibrosis.[81-84]

Environmental samples have demonstrated erionite fibers in the building stones of homes and in soil as well as in lung tissue from affected villagers from central Anatolia, Turkey.[84,85] Airborne erionite levels have been low but most likely do not reflect historical indoor exposures that have potentially occurred since birth for some of the local residents.[83,84] A potential confounder has been chrysotile and tremolite asbestos fibers found in the area as well as in lung tissue from local residents.[84,86] Fibrous erionite has also been identified in the lung tissue of a heavy equipment operator from Nevada.[87]

The animal and human data indicate that the naturally occurring fibrous zeolite, erionite, is a potent fibrogenic and carcinogenic agent and is associated with pulmonary abnormalities currently related to commercial asbestos exposure. Exposure levels should be maintained at the current exposure standard for asbestos, 0.1 f/cc for an 8-hour TWA. Air sampling and analysis should be done in any area where there are geologic deposits of zeolite that are under consideration for disruption, such as earth moving during road construction projects.

MINERALS WITH POTENTIAL FIBER CONTAMINATION
Vermiculite

Vermiculite is a nonfibrous hydrated aluminum–iron–magnesium silicate mineral that expands many times its original size with the application of heat. The ore is shipped in its unexpanded form and expanded at regional expanding plants. The expanded vermiculite is used as insulation; as aggregate and fillers in cement and gypsum; as carriers for fertilizer, pesticides, and herbicides; and as soil conditioners and animal bulking agents. The main mining source in the United States was the vermiculite mine at Libby, Montana, which closed in 1990. Other commercial mining sources are South Carolina, Virginia, and South Africa.[88-90]

Ore from Libby is contaminated with a highly fibrous or asbestiform variety of actinolite and tremolite asbestos. Ore from Virginia contains a lower concentration of actinolite, mostly as short cleavage fragments with low aspect ratios. South African ore can contain low concentrations of nonfibrous anthophyllite and possibly small amounts of tremolite.[89,91] Morbidity and mortality studies of the miners and millers from Libby have demonstrated pulmonary abnormalities associated with the fibrous tremolite and actinolite found in this particular geologic location. These abnormalities include excess respiratory cancer, including mesotheliomas, as well as pleural and interstitial fibrotic changes visible on chest radiographs. The excess in cancer was related to cumulative fiber exposure.[92-96] A cluster of benign bloody pleural effusions was found in workers expanding the Libby ore. There was also a relationship between pleural changes on chest radiographs and cumulative tremolite fiber exposure.[97] A morbidity study of workers exposed mostly to a shorter nonasbestiform variety of tremolite and actinolite from South Carolina demonstrated parenchymal (profusion, $\geq 1/0$) and pleural changes in 4.7% and 8.1%, respectively, similar to what was found in a nonexposed comparison group.[98] Similar but fewer findings were noted in South African workers involved with vermiculite mining and processing.[91]

Pure vermiculite is an example of a silicate mineral that, from an exposure perspective, can be treated as a nuisance dust. However, the potential for vermiculite to be contaminated with amphibole asbestos warrants vigilance in characterizing raw ore sources and scrutinizing airborne particles for fiber contamination.

Talc

Pure talc is a hydrated magnesium silicate used for a variety of industrial and consumer applications. The potential health risk from industrial and consumer exposures to talc is covered in Chapter 22. Depending on the geologic location of the ore source, talc ore can exist as pure platy talc or with intergrowths of tremolite, actinolite, and anthophyllite primarily of the nonasbestiform variety as well as occasional chrysotile asbestos.[99] Homogeneous talc fibers as well as heterogenous talc anthophyllite fibers have also been identified.[98,100] As with vermiculite, routine monitoring of the ore source for fiber contamination will help control potential fiber-related pulmonary health abnormalities.

Metal ore deposits

Chrysotile as well as asbestiform and nonasbestiform tremolite and actinolite can be found near mineral deposits mined for copper, gold, silver, tungsten, lead, and zinc. Careful characterization of the ore source, particularly during the drilling of access tunnels or with stripping of overburden, will help control potential exposure to fibrous contaminant minerals.[101]

CONCLUSION

Under current OSHA standards man-made fibers and nonasbestos fibrous silicates are treated as dust not otherwise classified. They fall under the nuisance dust standard of 5.0 mg/m^3 for respirable dust and 15 mg/m^3 for total dust as an permissible exposure limit. Manufacturers of man-made fibers as well as some fabricators and end users have established their own, self-imposed internal guidelines. A new standard for MMVFs at 1 f/cc has been proposed by OSHA for the construction, maritime, and agricultural industries. As reviewed previously, the majority of exposures in the man-made fiber manufacturing industry are below 0.5 to 1 f/cc. These levels of exposure are technically feasible through environmental control measures.

Exposure levels can vary markedly in secondary and end-user applications. During the fabrication of both man-made and natural fiber-containing products, vigorous attention has to be given to controlling airborne fiber levels, proper worker training and work practice, and, as indicated, respiratory protection programs. Changing from work clothes into street clothes while at work will help prevent contamination of the home environment. Special attention should be given to work practices that require manipulation of fiber-containing products, such as sanding, power saw cutting, and recycling procedures, especially within enclosed spaces. This is especially applicable to natural and man-made fibers that are respirable in size and durable in biologic media, and, therefore, have the propensity for deposition and retention within the pulmonary parenchyma.

ACKNOWLEDGMENTS

The author would like to acknowledge the contribution of fiber photomicrographs by Frank D'Ovidio, Bill Miller, and Tom Hesterberg, Ph.D., Microstructural Analysis Laboratory, Mountain Technical Center, Littleton, Colorado, and Iris Ailin-Pyzik, Ph.D., and James Davis, Ph.D., Owens-Corning Science and Technology, Granville, Ohio.

REFERENCES

1. Bank W: *Asbestiform and/or fibrous minerals in mines, mills, and quarries,* Pub No 1980-603-120/34, Washington, DC, 1980, US Department of Labor, Mine Safety and Health Administration.
2. Lippmann M: Man-made mineral fibers (MMMF): human exposures and health risk assessment, *Toxicol Ind Health* 6:225-246, 1990.
3. Lockey JE and Wiese NK: Health effects of synthetic vitreous fibers, *Clin Chest Med* 13:329-339, 1992.
4. Stanton MF, Layard M, Tegeris A, et al: Relation of particle dimension to carcinogenicity in amphibole asbestoses and other fibrous minerals, *JNCI* 67:965-975, 1981.
5. Oehlert GW: A reanalysis of the Stanton et al. pleural sarcoma data, *Environ Res* 54:194-205, 1991.
6. Pott F, Ziem U, Reiffer FJ, et al: Carcinogenicity studies on fibres, metal compounds, and some other dusts in rats, *Exp Pathol* 32:129-152, 1987.
7. Bellmann B, Muhle H, Pott F, et al: Persistence of man-made mineral fibres (MMMF) and asbestos in rat lungs, *Ann Occup Hyg* 31:693-709, 1987.
8. Law BD, Bunn WB, and Hesterberg TW: Solubility of polymeric organic fibers and manmade vitreous fibers in Gambles solution, *Inhalation Toxicol* 2:321-339, 1990.
9. Mossman BBT and Sesko AM: In vitro assays to predict the pathogenicity of mineral fibers, *Toxicology* 60:53-61, 1990.
10. Warheit DB, Kellar KA, and Hartsky MA: Pulmonary cellular effects in rats following aerosol exposures to ultrafine Kevlar aramid fibrils: evidence for biodegradability of inhaled fibrils, *Toxicol Appl Pharmacol* 116:225-239, 1992.
11. Jaurand MC: Particulate-state carcinogenesis: a survey of recent studies on the mechanisms of action of fibres, *IARC Sci Publ* 90:54-73, 1989.
12. International Agency for Research on Cancer (IARC): *Man-made mineral fibres and radon,* IARC monographs on the evaluation of carcinogenic risk to humans, No 43, Lyon, France, 1988, IARC.
13. Pott F: Die Faser als krebserzeugendes Agens. *Zentralbl Bakteriol Hyg B* 184:1-23, 1987.
14. Lippmann M: Asbestos exposure indices, *Environ Res* 46:86-106, 1988.
15. Schneider T and Skotte J: Fiber exposure reassessed with the new indices, *Environ Res* 51:108-116, 1990.
16. Boatman ES, Covert D, Kalman D, et al: Physical, morphological, and chemical studies of dusts derived from the machining of composite-epoxy materials, *Environ Res* 45:242-255, 1988.
17. Donnet J-B and Bansal RC: *Carbon fibers,* international fiber science and technology series, vol 3, New York, 1984, Marcel Dekker.
18. Zumwalde RD and Harmison LT: *Carbon-graphite fibers: environmental exposures and potential health implications,* National Institute for Occupational Safety and Health (NIOSH) No 1WS-52.3, National Technical Information Service (NTIS) (No) PB 81-229692, Springfield, Va, 1980.
19. Martin TR, Meyer SW, and Luchtel DR: An evaluation of the toxicity of carbon fiber composites for lung cells *in vitro* and *in vivo, Environ Res* 49:246-261, 1989.
20. Luchtel DL, Martin TR, and Boatman ES: Response of the rat lung to respirable fractions of composite fiber-epoxy dusts, *Environ Res* 48:57-69, 1989.
21. Thomson SA: Toxicology of carbon fibers, *Appl Ind Hyg* (spec issue):29-33, 1989.
22. Owen PE, Glaister JR, Ballantyne B, et al: Subchronic inhalation toxicology of carbon fibers, *JOM, J Occup Med* 28:373-376, 1986.
23. Jones HD, Jones TR, and Lyle WH: Carbon fibre: results of a survey of process workers and their environment in a factory producing continuous filament, *Ann Occup Hyg* 26:861-868, 1982.
24. Lee KP, Kelly DP, O'Neal FO, et al: Lung response to ultrafine Kevlar aramid synthetic fibrils following 2-year inhalation exposure in rats, *Fundam Appl Toxicol* 11:1-20, 1988.

25. Merriman EA: Safe use of Kevlar aramid fiber in composites, *Appl Ind Hyg* (spec issue):34-36, 1989.
26. Jaffrey SAMT, Rood AP, and Scott RM: Fibrous dust release from asbestos substitutes in friction products, *Ann Occup Hyg* 36:173-181, 1992.
27. Brinkmann OA and Müller K-M: What's new in intraperitoneal test on Kevlar (asbestos substitute)?, *Pathol Res Pract* 185:412-417, 1989.
28. Kelly DP, Merriman EA, Kennedy GL, et al: Deposition, clearance, and shortening of Kevlar para-aramid fibrils in acute, subchronic, and chronic inhalation studies in rats, *Fundam Appl Toxicol* 21:345-354, 1993.
29. Lapin CA, Craig DK, Valerio MG, et al: A subchronic inhalation toxicity study in rats exposed to silicon carbide whiskers, *Fundam Appl Toxicol* 16:128-146, 1991.
30. Johnson NF, Hoover MD, Thomassen DG, et al: In vitro activity of silicon carbide whiskers in comparison to other industrial fibers using four cell culture systems, *Am J Ind Med* 21:807-823, 1992.
31. Scansetti G, Piolatto G, and Botta GC: Airborne fibrous and nonfibrous particles in a silicon carbide manufacturing plant, *Ann Occup Hyg* 36:145-153, 1992.
32. Dufresne A, Perrault G, Sébastien P, et al: Morphology and surface characteristics of particulates from silicon carbide industries, *Am Ind Hyg Assoc J* 48:718-729, 1987.
33. Vaughan GL, Jordan J, and Karr S: The toxicity, *in vitro,* of silicon carbide whiskers, *Environ Res* 56:57-67, 1991.
34. Bégin R, Dufresne A, Cantin A, et al: Carborundum pneumoconiosis, *Chest* 95:842-849, 1989.
35. Durand P, Bégin R, Samson L, et al: Silicon carbide pneumoconiosis: a radiographic assessment, *Am J Ind Med* 20:37-47, 1991.
36. Funahashi A, Schlueter DP, Pintar K, et al: Pneumoconiosis in workers exposed to silicon carbide, *Am Rev Respir Dis* 129:635-640, 1984.
37. Massé S, Bégin R, and Cantin A: Pathology of silicon carbide pneumoconiosis, *Mod Pathol* 1:104-108, 1988.
38. Bye E: Occurrence of airborne silicon carbide fibers during industrial production of silicon carbide, *Scand J Work Environ Health* 11:111-115, 1985.
39. Beaumont GP: Reduction in airborne silicon carbide whiskers by process improvements, *Appl Occup Environ Hyg* 6:598-603, 1991.
40. Jederlinic PJ, Abraham JL, Churg A, et al: Pulmonary fibrosis in aluminum oxide workers, *Am Rev Respir Dis* 142:1179-1184, 1990.
41. Gilks B and Churg A: Aluminum-induced pulmonary fibrosis: do fibers play a role?, *Am Rev Respir Dis* 136:176-179, 1987.
42. Pundsack FI: Fibrous glass manufacture, use, and physical properties. In LeVee WN, editor: *Occupational exposure to fibrous glass,* National Institute for Occupational Safety and Health Pub No 76-151, pp 11-18, Washington, DC, US Public Health Service, Department of Health, Education, and Welfare.
43. Nomenclature Committee of TIMA, Inc (Eastes W, editor): *Man-made vitreous fibers: nomenclature, chemical and physical properties,* rev ed 2, Stamford, Conn, 1993, TIMA, Inc.
44. Bunn WB, Bender JR, Hesterberg TW, et al: Recent studies of man-made vitreous fibers: chronic animal inhalation studies, *JOM, J Occup Med* 35:101-113, 1993.
45. Björnberg A: Glass fiber dermatitis, *Am J Ind Med* 8:395-400, 1985.
46. Newhall HH and Brahim SA: Respiratory response to domestic fibrous glass exposure, *Environ Res* 12:201-207, 1976.
47. Hughes JM, Jones RN, Glindmeyer HW, et al: Follow up study of workers exposed to man made mineral fibres, *Br J Ind Med* 50:658-667, 1993.
48. Lees PSJ, Breysse PN, McArthur BR, et al: End user exposures to man-made vitreous fibers: I. Installation of residential insulation products, *Appl Occup Environ Hyg* 8:1022-1030, 1993.
49. Petersen R and Sabroe S: Irritative symptoms and exposure to mineral wool, *Am J Ind Med* 20:113-122, 1991.

50. Lemasters G, Lockey J, Rice C, et al: Radiographic changes among workers manufacturing refractory ceramic fiber and products. *Ann Occup Hyg* (suppl 1) 38:745-751, 1994.

51. Kilburn KH, Powers D, and Warshaw RH: Pulmonary effects of exposure to fine fibreglass: irregular opacities and small airways obstruction, *Br J Ind Med* 49:714-720, 1992.

52. Bender JR: Pulmonary effects of exposure to fine fibreglass: irregular opacities and small airways obstruction, *Br J Ind Med* 50:381-382, 1993. Letter.

53. Marsh GM, Enterline PE, Stone RA, et al: Mortality among a cohort of U.S. man-made mineral fiber workers: 1985 follow-up, *JOM, J Occup Med* 32:594-604, 1990.

54. Wong O, Foliart D, and Trent LS: A case–control study of lung cancer in a cohort of workers potentially exposed to slag wool fibres, *Br J Ind Med* 48:818-824, 1991.

55. Chiazze L, Watkins DK, and Fryar C: A case–control study of malignant and non-malignant respiratory disease among employees of a fibreglass manufacturing facility, *Br J Ind Med* 49:326-331, 1992.

56. Simonato L, Fletcher AC, Cherrie JW, et al: The International Agency for Research on Cancer historical cohort study of MMMF production workers in seven European countries: extension of the follow-up, *Ann Occup Hyg* 31:603-623, 1987.

57. Boffetta P, Saracci R, Anderson A, et al: Lung cancer mortality among workers in the European production of man-made mineral fibers—a Poisson regression analysis, *Scand J Work Environ Health* 18:279-286, 1992.

58. Shannon HS, Jamieson E, Julian JA, et al: Mortality of glass filament (textile) workers, *Br J Ind Med* 47:533-536, 1990.

59. Gustavsson P, Plato N, Axelson O, et al: Lung cancer risk among workers exposed to man-made mineral fibers (MMMF) in the Swedish prefabricated house industry, *Am J Ind Med* 21:825-834, 1992.

60. Wagner JC, Griffiths DM, and Munday DE: Experimental studies with palygorskite dusts, *Br J Ind Med* 44:749-763, 1987.

61. Rödelsperger K, Brückel B, Manke J, et al: Potential health risks from the use of fibrous mineral absorption granulates, *Br J Ind Med* 44:337-343, 1987.

62. Waxweiler RJ, Zumwalde RD, Ness GO, et al: A retrospective cohort mortality study of males mining and milling attapulgite clay, *Am J Ind Med* 13:305-315, 1988.

63. Sakula A: Pneumoconiosis due to fuller's earth, *Thorax* 16:176, 1961.

64. Nolan RP, Langer AM, and Herson GB: Characterisation of palygorskite specimens from different geological locales for health hazard evaluation, *Br J Ind Med* 48:463-475, 1991.

65. Lemaire I, Dionne PG, Nadeau D, et al: Rat lung reactivity to natural and man-made fibrous silicates following short-term exposure, *Environ Res* 48:193-210, 1989.

66. Bégin R, Massé S, Rola-Pleszczynski M, et al: The lung biological activity of American attapulgite, *Environ Res* 42:328-339, 1987.

67. Sors H, Gaudichet A, Sébastien P, et al: Lung fibrosis after inhalation of fibrous attapulgite, *Thorax* 34:695-696, 1979.

68. McConnochie K, Bevan C, Newcombe RG, et al: A study of Spanish sepiolite workers, *Thorax* 48:370-374, 1993.

69. Baris YI, Sahin AA, and Erkan ML: Clinical and radiological study in sepiolite workers, *Arch Environ Health* 35:343-346, 1980.

70. Huuskonen MS, Tossavainen A, Koskinen H, et al: Wollastonite exposure and lung fibrosis, *Environ Res* 30:291-304, 1983.

71. McConnell EE, Hall L, and Adkins B: Studies on the chronic toxicity (inhalation) of wollastonite in Fischer 344 rats, *Inhalation Toxicol* 3:323-337, 1991.

72. Huuskonen MS, Järvisalo J, Koskinen H, et al: Preliminary results from a cohort of workers exposed to wollastonite in a Finnish limestone quarry, *Scand J Work Environ Health* 9:169-175, 1983.

73. Shasby DM, Petersen M, Hodous T, et al: Respiratory morbidity of workers exposed to wollastonite through mining and milling. In Lemen R and Dement JM, editors: *Dusts and disease*, pp 251-256, Park Forest South, Ill, 1979, Pathotox Publishers.

74. Hanke W, Sepulveda M-J, Watson A, et al: Respiratory morbidity in wollastonite workers, *Br J Ind Med* 41:474-479, 1984.

75. Sand B and Mumpton FA, editors: *Natural zeolites: occurrence, properties, use*, Oxford, England, 1978, Pergamon Press.

76. Rom WN, Casey KR, Parry WT, et al: Health implications of natural fibrous zeolites for the Intermountain West, *Environ Res* 30:1-8, 1983.

77. Suzuki Y: Carcinogenic and fibrogenic effects of zeolites: preliminary observations, *Environ Res* 27:433-445, 1982.

78. Davis JMG, Bolton RE, Miller BG, et al: Mesothelioma dose response following intraperitoneal injection of mineral fibres, *Int J Exp Pathol* 72:263-274, 1991.

79. Özesmi M, Patiroglu TE, Hillerdal G, et al: Peritoneal mesothelioma and malignant lymphoma in mice casued by fibrous zeolite, *Br J Ind Med* 42:746-749, 1985.

80. Suzuki Y and Kohyama N: Malignant mesothelioma induced by asbestos and zeolite in the mouse peritoneal cavity, *Environ Res* 35:277-292, 1984.

81. Baris YI, Sahin AA, Özesmi M, et al: An outbreak of pleural mesothelioma and chronic fibrosing pleurisy in the village of Karain/Ürgüp in Anatolia, *Thorax* 33:181-192, 1978.

82. Artvinli M and Baris YI: Malignant mesotheliomas in a small village in the Anatolian region of Turkey: an epidemiologic study, *JNCI* 63:17-22, 1979.

83. Baris YI, Saracci R, Simonato L, et al: Malignant mesothelioma and radiological chest abnormalities in two villages in central Turkey, *Lancet* 2:984-987, 1981.

84. Baris YI, Simonato L, Artvinli M, et al: Epidemiological and environmental evidence of the health effects of exposure to erionite fibres: a four-year study in the Cappadocian region of Turkey, *Int J Cancer* 39:10-17, 1987.

85. Sébastien P, Gaudichet A, Bignon J, et al: Zeolite bodies in human lungs from Turkey, *Lab Invest* 44:420-425, 1981.

86. Rohl AN, Langer AM, Moncure G, et al: Endemic pleural disease associated with exposure to mixed fibrous dust in Turkey, *Science* 216:518-520, 1982.

87. Casey KR, Shigeoka JW, Rom WN, et al: Zeolite exposure and associated pneumoconiosis, *Chest* 87:837-840, 1985.

88. Lockey JE: Nonasbestos fibrous minerals, *Clin Chest Med* 2:203-218, 1981

89. Moatamed F, Lockey JE, and Parry WT: Fiber contamination of vermiculites: a potential occupational and environmental health hazard, *Environ Res* 41:207-218, 1986.

90. Gamble JF: Silicate pneumoconiosis. In Merchant JA, editor: *Occupational respiratory diseases*, pp 243-285, Washington, DC, 1986, US Department of Health and Human Services, National Institute for Occupational Safety and Health publication no. 86-102.

91. Hessel PA and Sluis-Cremer GK: X-ray findings, lung function, and respiratory symptoms in black South African vermiculite workers, *Am J Ind Med* 15:21-29, 1989.

92. McDonald JC, McDonald AD, Armstrong B, et al: Cohort study of mortality of vermiculite miners exposed to tremolite, *Br J Ind Med* 43:436-444, 1986.

93. McDonald JC, Sébastien P, and Armstrong B: Radiological survey of past and present vermiculite miners exposed to tremolite, *Br J Ind Med* 43:445-449, 1986.

94. Amandus HE, Wheeler R, Jankovic J, et al: The morbidity and mortality of vermiculite miners and millers exposed to tremolite–actinolite: Part I. Exposure estimates, *Am J Ind Med* 11:1-14, 1987.

95. Amandus HE and Wheeler R: The morbidity and mortality of vermiculite miners and millers exposed to tremolite–actinolite: Part II. Mortality, *Am J Ind Med* 11:15-26, 1987.

96. Amandus HE, Althouse R, Morgan WKC, et al: The morbidity and mortality of vermiculite miners and millers exposed to tremolite–actinolite: Part III. Radiographic findings, *Am J Ind Med* 11:27-37, 1987.

97. Lockey JE, Brooks SM, Jarabek AM, et al: Pulmonary changes after exposure to vermiculite contaminated with fibrous tremolite, *Am Rev Respir Dis* 129:952-958, 1984.

98. McDonald JC, McDonald AD, Sébastien P, et al: Health of vermiculite miners exposed to trace amounts of fibrous tremolite, *Br J Ind Med* 45:630-634, 1988.

99. Dement JM and Zumwalde RD: Occupational exposures to talcs containing asbestiform minerals. In Lemen RA and Dement JM, editors: *Dusts and disease,* pp 287-306, Park Forest South, Ill, 1979, Pathotox Publishers.

100. Abraham JL: Non-commercial amphibole asbestos fibers and cleavage fragments in lung tissues of New York State talc miners with asbestosis and talcosis, *Am Rev Respir Dis* 141:A244, 1990.

101. Lockey JE and Parry WT: Health implications of naturally occurring mineral fibers. *Health Hazards Occup Environ* 7:1-7, 1984.

Chapter 22

NONFIBROUS INORGANIC DUSTS

Steven Short
Edward L. Petsonk

Silicates
  Montmorillonite clays
  Bentonite
  Fuller's earth
  Mica
  Sericite
  Illites
  Feldspar
  Feldspathoids
  Leucite
  Nepheline
  Diatomaceous earth
  Alunite
  Agate
  Talc
  Perlite
  Kaolin
  Volcanic ash
Metals
  Iron
  Barium
  Antimony
  Tin
  Chromite
Sedimentary compounds
  Calcium carbonate
  Oil shale
  Carbon
  Portland cement
  Gilsonite
  Slate
  Potash
  Gypsum
  Trona
  Phosphate
  Fluorspar
  Salt

This chapter will discuss the reported health effects from inhalational exposures to nonfibrous inorganic particulates, a heterogeneous group of materials. To focus the discussion of this chapter, it is necessary to briefly review human responses to inhaled agents. In general, the fate of particles after they are inhaled is determined by the physical composition of the dust, the particle sizes and shapes, and the concentration of the material inhaled. Water-soluble materials may dissolve and be absorbed on the mucosal surface or in the parenchyma. Virtually all insoluble particulates are cleared through a combination of mucociliary clearance and phagocytic cell migration into the lung airways or interstitium.

Organic and *inorganic* substances comprise the two broad classes of occupational exposures. Materials recently derived from plant, animal, or microbial sources (usually composed of complex molecules such as proteins, lipids, polysaccharides, or combinations of these) may initiate an immunologic response, which is manifest on subsequent exposures. Symptoms and lung dysfunction from organic dust can also be triggered by stimulation of lung or airway inflammation through activation of inflammatory cascades (e.g., grain fever, byssinosis, organic dust toxic syndrome). These are discussed in more detail in Chapters 17 and 25.

In contrast to organic dusts, there are various responses in human lungs and airways to inorganic dusts. Certain minerals, such as crystalline silica, and several metals and metal compounds (zinc, cobalt, beryllium, platinum, etc.), may also trigger inflammatory and immunologic responses analogous to those from organic dusts, resulting in symptoms and lung dysfunction. Inorganic fibrous materials also may initiate inflammation. The inflammation often persists and may result in symptoms and lung functional consequences. Conversely, other inorganic dusts, when inhaled in moderate concentrations, may be cleared from the respiratory tract without provoking marked acute or persistent inflammation or apparent structural change. The discussion in this chapter encompasses current knowledge of the respiratory health effects from inhalation and lung deposition of this latter group of relatively inert inorganic materials. Some of these substances have been categorized as "inert" dusts, although, as discussed below, high concentrations or prolonged inhalation frequently can provoke symptoms and an inflammatory response and may result in functional, structural, and/or radiographic abnormalities.

The group encompasses such diverse substances as graphite (coal is discussed separately in Chapter 23), sedimentary materials, and nonfibrous silicates. The discussion will be facilitated by classifying these materials into various categories based upon their mineralogy. This will also help in the recognition of associations between exposures to physicochemically related materials and the recognized health effects of the related compounds.

SILICATES

The two most abundant elements are oxygen and silicon, hence we have prolific supplies of silicate minerals and silica polymorphs, especially quartz. The affinity of oxygen for silicon, entailing a variety of bonding possibilities, results in many silicate forms. Silicate minerals have as their basic building block the silicate tetrahedron. This has a net negative charge of 4, which is satisfied by positively charged cations. This charge imbalance may be met by several monovalent and divalent cations, especially Li^+, Na^+, K^+, Ca^{2+}, Mg^{2+}, Fe^{2+}, and Mn^{2+}. Substitution with Al^{3+} results in a charge imbalance.[1]

The variety of silicate forms and structures are a result of the various structural possibilities that are created by the cationic charges of silicon and oxygen. In general, the silicates have low solubilities and slow dissolution rates, inherent properties that enable them to serve as fire retardants, fillers, cation exchangers, catalysts, and construction materials for use as building stone, road aggregate, and lightweight aggregate for concrete.

Silicates that occur in a sheet structure $(Si_2O_5)^2$, are utilized for their pliable consistency and adsorptive properties. Minerals in this group are products of erosion and weathering of rock structures and are major soil constituents. These clays exhibit a platy or flaky property and are soft and flexible with a relatively low specific gravity.[2]

Montmorillonite clays

Montmorillonite clays (montmorillonite, bentonite, attapulgite, and palygorskite), derive their name from Montmorillon, France, the origin of the clay mineral montmorillonite, but the term is now restricted to hydrated aluminum silicates.

Bentonite

Bentonite is a commercial term for clays containing montmorillonite minerals formed by the alteration of volcanic ash and has high absorptive properties.[2] In the United States, bentonite is produced in 12 states and derives its name from the clays at Fort Benton in Wyoming. The clay is ground, then dried in kilns, then bagged for shipping. The airborne concentration of free silica in the mill dust has been found to consist of appreciable amounts of cristobalite. Bentonite finds use as a foundry sand bond, a drilling mud, a filtering agent for wine and water, in water impedance, in animal feed, in pharmaceuticals, as a filler in paints and cosmetics, an additive to ceramic clays, as a fire retardant, as a catalyst in petroleum refining, and in carbonless copy paper.[1]

Pneumoconiosis has been documented in bentonite workers and is felt to be related to the free silica content (cristobalite) of the clay. The prevalence is not known. Symptoms of dyspnea and reductions of forced vital capacity (FVC), forced expiratory volume in 1 second (FEV1), and mid-maximum expiratory flow (MMEF) on spirometry have been observed in relation to bentonite exposure.[3]

Fuller's earth

Fuller's earth is a generic term for aluminum silicate clays. These adsorbent clays derive their name from their use in the process of "Fulling," which is the removal of grease from wool. Most uses of Fuller's earths derive from their adsorbent properties, although other uses are found in oil refining, as a binder in foundry molds, as a filter, and as a filler in cosmetics.

Several silicates are considered in the category of Fuller's earth, which vary in contaminants depending on their sedimentary origin. The amount of quartz in Fuller's earth varies from 0% to 20%. Fuller's earth (montmorillonite) from a plant in Illinois contained quartz, muscovite (1% to 2%), glauconite (1% to 2%), and amorphous silica (<1%).[4]

Mica

Mica refers to the family of minerals that are complex aluminum silicates associated with the alkaline metals of either iron and magnesium. They are characterized by the precision with which they split into thin sheets. They differ from the montmorillonites in that layers of mica cannot be expanded by water and thus have no adsorptive properties. Important groups of micas include the muscovites, phlogopite, lepidolites, and biotites. The only micas used commercially are muscovite and phlogopite. The predominant chemical composition is potassium aluminum silicate with variable amounts of magnesium, iron, and lithium.

Sheet mica has economic value due to its electrical and thermal properties. Its historical use was in the windows of stoves or as shades for oil lamps, but it continues to be utilized as liner for steam boilers, in optical instruments, in oil well drilling mud, as artificial snow and flocking for Christmas ornaments, in roofing material, as a filler for asphalt and plaster, in ceiling tile and wallboard joint cements, and electrical insulation. Fine particles of mica are used for lubrication and mold release in the manufacture of rubber products. Some talcum powders also contain mica.[5]

Mica pneumoconiosis is characterized radiographically by nodular and reticular interstitial infiltration both favoring the lower lung fields. Intense exposures to pure finely ground mica have been demonstrated on necroscopy to result in a fine interstitial fibrosis related to deposits of mica.[6]

Sericite

Sericite is a muscovite mica that occurs as minute scales and as fibrous aggregates. It is used as a fine facing sand in foundry molds. Questions regarding the toxicity of sericite have been raised[7] and have been supported with animal studies showing fibrosis when sericite was injected into lymph nodes of experimental animals.[8]

Illites

Illites are micas of secondary origin. They contain silicates of potassium, aluminum, iron, and magnesium, complexed with water. The minerals are the predominant alkali-bearing constituents in sedimentary clays, shales, and fireclays.

Feldspar

Feldspars are the largest group of minerals that make up the igneous rocks. They are composed of aluminum silicate in combination with potassium and sodium. There are two major groups of feldspars, the orthoclase or potassium based (microcline) and the plagioclase or sodium based (albite and anorthite). Feldspars are solid solutions of these components. Granite is a granular igneous rock with quartz, mostly feldspar, and small amounts of mica, hornblende, and pyroxene. Feldspars are used extensively in the ceramics industry and, when associated with quartz, they induce collagenous fibrosis of the lung. In the absence of quartz, feldspars are not felt to be pathogenic.[9]

Feldspathoids

Feldspathoids are chemically similar to feldspars in that they are also potassium, sodium, and calcium aluminum silicates. However, they contain two thirds less silica than the corresponding feldspar. The most common feldspathoids are leucite and nepheline.

Leucite

Leucite is a natural potassium aluminum silicate found in lava but not in rocks with quartz. It is not mined, but is a potential source of potash.

Nepheline

Nepheline is a silicate of sodium, potassium, and aluminum ($KNa_3Al_4Si_4O_{16}$), which occurs in crystalline form in the feldspars albite and microcline. It contains no free silica.

The major uses of nepheline are in the ceramics industry, as a filler for paints, and in Russia, where it is mined as a source of alumina for aluminum.

Although the silica (SiO_2) component of nepheline is not free, the milling process may result in exposures with fibrogenic potential, and result in a pneumoconiosis with a pattern of increased interstitial markings in the lower lung zones.[10] The toxicity of the material has not been adequately studied. Lungs from affected workers contained intraalveolar exudates of fibrin and branching plugs of connective tissue extending as far as the respiratory bronchioles.[11]

Diatomaceous earth

Diatomaceous earth resulted from deposits of diatoms (unicellular algae) that lived millions of years ago. The diatom has a skeleton of silica (SiO_2), which can be calcinized to crystalline silica by heating to 450°C. The crystalline forms consist of cristobalite, quartz, tridymite, and coesite, all of which have caused pulmonary fibrosis in experimental animal studies.[12,13]

Diatomaceous earth is used for its insulating and adsorbent properties and finds application in the lining of molds in the foundry industry, in filters, abrasives, lubricants, and explosives.

The crystalline forms are markedly fibrogenic and contain 65% to 90% free silica and result in clinical and radiographic changes of simple silicosis, including a risk of progressive massive fibrosis with greater exposures.[14]

Alunite

Alunite clay is a hydrated sulfate of aluminum and potassium, which is calcined and leached to yield potash (K_2SO_4). The residue is a crystalline aluminum silicate (mullite), which is highly adsorbent and has been packaged for retail use as cat litter.

There have been very few studies investigating the effects of alunite on workers. There is a suggestion that with heavy exposure, workers develop small irregular chest radiographic opacities throughout both lung fields.[15]

Agate

Agate is a fine grained, fibrous variety of chalcedony. Chalcedony is translucent to transparent, milky or grayish quartz with microscopic crystals arranged in slender fibers. It is mined in India, and the stones are processed to make decorative items like rings, beads, lockets, necklaces, paper weights, ink pots, cups, etc. After mining, the stones are dried in the sun for 3 to 4 days and then placed in a fire of burning cowdung cakes. The stones then are chipped into desired sizes and shapes and then ground on emery wheels to make the surface smooth. The smooth stones are polished with wet emery and agate dust in a rolling drum.[16]

A survey of 363 agate workers, tested with questionnaires and chest radiographs, showed that the length of time exposed to agate dust and the worker's age were related to the presence of radiographic changes of pneumoconiosis, thought to be silicosis.[16]

Talc

Talc in a pure form is a layered hydrous magnesium silicate with an ideal chemical composition of 63.5% SiO_2, 31.7% MgO, and 4.8% H_2O. It consists of a brucite sheet containing magnesium ions sandwiched between two silica sheets that are held together by relatively weak forces. Talc can be tabular, granular, fibrous, or platy, but it is usually crystalline, flexible, and soft.[17] Substitutions of ions may occur in the mineral lattice or the talc may be contaminated by other minerals.[18] Thus "talc" is not a uniform material.[19]

Commercial talc in the United States comes from over 10 states with the major portions obtained from New York, California, Texas, and Vermont. A problem encountered in studying many commercial talc deposits is that the ore bodies show nonuniformity in their mineralogy. Commercial talc is frequently contaminated with other minerals such as magnesite, dolomite, calcite, tremolite (fibrous and nonfibrous), pyrophillite, antigorite, lizardite, mica, anthophyllite, chlorite, and quartz.[20] In assessing the respiratory health effects of talc, it is important to distinguish effects of talc itself from those of contaminants (such as tremolite fibers).

Talc has a wide variety of uses in paint, paper, ceramics, cosmetics, roofing products, textile material, rubber, lubricants, corrosion proofing compositions, fire extinguishing powders, water filtration, insecticides, dusting powders, and asphalt products.[21,22] More than 500 different products are sold under the name "talc," with worldwide production of approximately 5 to 6 million tons per year. The major worldwide producers are Australia, Austria, China, France, and the United States.[23]

Lung microscopic pathology in workers who were exposed to nonasbestiform talc has revealed various forms of pulmonary fibrosis. Evaluation with polarized light has shown dense accumulations of birefringent dust particles in perivascular and peribronchiolar scars, with higher degrees of fibrosis found in lungs from workers who had prolonged exposure histories[24] (Fig. 22-1). Commonly, the micropathologic appearance of talc-induced lung damage is a stellate interstitial collection of dust-laden macrophages that extends, with varying degrees of fibrosis, from around respiratory bronchioles. The bronchiolitis reported with talc exposure has been associated with symptoms of cough, dyspnea, and phlegm production.[25]

Although initial investigators reported an increased risk of bronchogenic carcinoma in talc miners and millers,[26–28] newer studies, conducted on miners and millers who are exposed to more pure forms of talc, show differing results. There is a trend for higher mortality from nonmalignant respiratory disease (silicosis, silicotuberculosis, emphysema, and pneumonia), but in two independent studies bronchogenic cancer was not found to be elevated.[29,30]

In cross-sectional pulmonary function studies of talc miners and millers, the mean ratio of observed to predicted

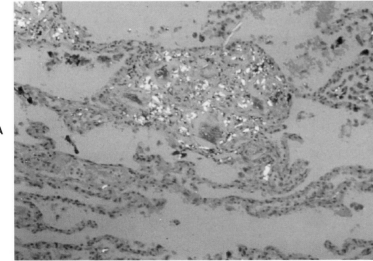
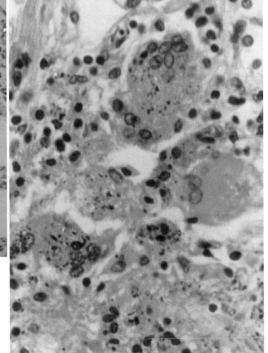

Fig. 22-1. Light microscopic pathology from lungs of talc-exposed worker, showing **A,** collections of birefringent talc crystals and associated interstitial inflammatory changes, and **B,** talc granulomas.

FEV1 and midexpiratory flow rates were significantly reduced, although the FVC as a percentage of predicted forced vital capacity was not different from 100%.[30]

Chest radiographs in the talc workers have revealed diffuse parenchymal opacities and pleural abnormalities, with the duration of talc exposure being associated with both small rounded and irregular opacities.[31,32] Rounded and irregular shadows seen radiographically have been related to the pathologic findings of numerous dust-laden macrophages intermingled with bundles of collagen.[32] It is unclear how much of the findings in talc-exposed workers are due to the talc itself or to contaminants in the talc, some of which have established fibrogenic and oncogenic properties. In many cases, the lung pathologic appearance suggests a mixed dust fibrosis. Mineralogic examination of lung tissue in some talc-exposed workers has revealed the presence of mica or mixed silicate pneumoconiosis, and it is felt that talcosis frequently represents disease associated with a variety of minerals that have talc as a common denominator.[33]

Perlite

Perlite is a noncrystalline silicate, occurring naturally as beads of volcanic glass. It occurs in volcanic ash deposits and can be contaminated by other volcanic ash components. When perlite beads are heated in an expansion facility, the beads soften and swell, creating a spongelike particle of low-density, high-surface area, and low-thermal conductivity. The expanded form can fracture and produce respirable dust. These spongelike particles are used as a soil conditioner, an inert carrier or filler, in filters and lightweight plaster, and to provide insulating properties.

Production of perlite became commercialized in 1946, with worldwide production reaching 1.5 million tons in 1983. In 1986 there were 42 producers operating 68 expansion plants in 33 states.[34]

Although perlite miners and expansion operators are exposed to respirable dusts, it is said that the particles are unlikely to persist in the lungs long enough to cause fibrosis.[35] Radiographic or spirometric abnormalities have not been documented to result from perlite exposure.[34,36,37]

Kaolin

Kaolin is a nonfibrous hydrated aluminum silicate with the chemical structure $Al_2O_3 \cdot 2SiO_2 \cdot 2H_2O$. It derives its name from the Chinese "Kau-Ling," which is a high ridge near Jauchau Fu, China, where the clay was first mined.[38] China stone and china clay are altered forms of granite, resulting from weathering and past geological activity. China stone is a hard rock retaining the quartz content of the original granite. Kaolin (China clay) is a soft white material derived from the feldspar component of the granite. The main component, kaolinite, is an aluminum silicate that is also present in several other clay varieties. Kaolinite particles take the form of pseudohexagonal platelets varying in width between 10 to less than 0.1 μm. Mining of the sedimentary deposits is usually done by forcing a high-powered water jet at the surface of an open pit mine face. This technique does not generate airborne dust until the slurry is dried.[39] Ancillary minerals present with kaolin include quartz, micas, oxides of titanium and iron, feldspars, and amorphous silicon dioxide.

Some kaolin is calcinized through removal of water by heating to 1000°C for 20 minutes. This calcinized clay contains a mixture of alumina and silica in an amorphous noncrystalline configuration that helps maintain the plate-like structure of the hydrated kaolin.[40]

Industrial uses for kaolin include the manufacture of paper products (80%), refractory materials, ceramics, and as a filler in plastics, rubber, and paints.

The jobs with the heaviest kaolin exposure are those involved in the processing of kaolin clay, such as milling, bagging, and loading. Traditionally the clay was dried in kilns to a moisture content of about 10%, then the dried clay was bagged and loaded for storage. More recently the kilns have been replaced with automated presses that dewater the clay under high pressure to a moisture content of 18%. Approximately 10% of the total production is shipped in slurry form.

Lung radiographic changes in kaolin workers have taken the form of both rounded and irregular small opacities.[41] On evaluation of the lung tissue, irregular radiologic changes are seen predominantly in the presence of kaolinite, whereas the rounded opacities are associated with a higher lung quartz content. All levels of profusion of simple pneumoconiosis, as well as progressive massive fibrosis (PMF) have been documented with kaolin exposure. This finding has been consistent in studies of large numbers of workers exposed in the mining and processing of kaolin. The main variables predictive of pneumoconiotic changes are age and cumulative years of work exposure in production.[42]

When compared with unexposed workers, kaolin workers show reductions in FVC, FEV1, and peak flow rate. Further, the group of workers with radiographic kaolin pneumoconiosis and PMF, but not those without PMF, had reduced spirometry results when compared with exposed workers who had no radiographic evidence of kaolin-induced lung disease.[38]

The potential for kaolin dusts to induce lung damage, in the absence of crystalline silica contamination, is not universally accepted.[43] As a result kaolin continues to be regarded as a "particulate not otherwise classified," a designation implying little fibrogenic potential.

Volcanic ash

Volcanic ash is released as a result of a volcano's explosive eruption, in contrast to effusive fluid flow of lava, as occurs in the Hawaiian chain of volcanoes. Limited information regarding the respiratory health effects of volcanic ash exposure existed prior to the Mount St. Helens volcanic eruption. That eruption, which occurred on May 18,

1980, sent a vertical cloud of ash and gas more than 20 km in the air in less than 10 minutes. This resulted in deposition of ash up to 70 mm or more in depth over a sparsely populated region surrounding the mountain and up to 10 mm in more populated centers to the west and southwest of the volcano's core.[44] The ash was characterized as belonging to the plagioclase (glass) mineral class of aluminum silicates and other oxides[45] (Fig. 22-2). More than 90% of the particles had an aerodynamic diameter of less than 10 μm and were thus within the respirable range. Peak levels of total suspended particles (TSP) were recorded in excess of 30,000 μg/m³, with the current Environmental Protection Agency emergency level for TSP being 1000 μg/m³.[46] The ash was found to have levels of crystalline-free silica in the range of 3% to 7%, including both quartz and cristobalite.

The toxicology of the ash was assessed in short term in vivo animal experiments, which were consistent with the pulmonary histologic findings in autopsy studies of two loggers who died following the eruption.[47] These findings suggest that volcanic ash is moderately fibrogenic and should be considered a pneumoconiosis risk in heavily exposed individuals. Other volcanic eruptions have occurred since the Mt. St. Helens eruption, although none with the degree of exposure to human populations. Ash samples from these eruptions have been evaluated and have similar quartz and elemental composition but different cytotoxicities. Differences in the cytotoxicities of volcanic ash appear more correlated with differences in the particle size distributions in each ash sample than differences in the mineralogic composition. Those samples with a greater proportion of small particles (i.e., more surface area per weight of ash sample) exhibited more cytotoxic activity.[48]

Health effects recorded in relation to the massive particulate exposure from Mt. St. Helens, which resulted in total darkness of Yakima, Washington, a city of 50,000 people 135 km northeast of the volcano, included irritation to the eyes and respiratory tract. Adverse respiratory effects were seen in persons with existing lung disease. Individuals with preexisting airway hyperresponsiveness experienced more severe respiratory distress and pulmonary impairment, and those with chronic mucus hypersecretion suffered exacerbations. In individuals with no previous respiratory history, potential responses included delayed-onset ash-induced mucus hypersecretion, obstructive airways disease, or "pneumo(vol)coniosis."[45]

Spirometric lung function of loggers exposed in the Mt. St. Helens area was followed for 4 years following the erup-

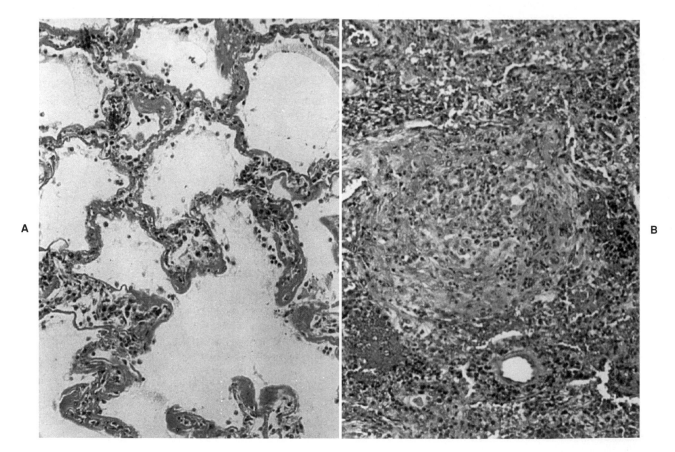

Fig. 22-2. Light microscopic pathology from lungs of logger heavily exposed to volcanic ash from Mt. St. Helens showing **A,** hyaline membrane formation, and **B,** intense interstitial inflammation with granulomas.

tion. These loggers were matched with nonexposed loggers over a similar time frame and prospectively followed. A transient decrease in FEV1 was noted, relative to the control group, over the first year of exposure, followed by gradual recovery as exposure levels decreased. The rate of decline in FEV1 was greatest in the highest exposure group, intermediate in the low exposure group, and lowest in the control group.[49]

METALS

A metal may be defined as "an element which under biologically significant conditions reacts by losing one or more electrons to form cations." Occupational exposures to the pure metallic forms (zero oxidation state) are rare, whereas exposures to the oxides or to multielement compounds, mainly salts, are more common.[50] The bioavailability and absorption of the metal depend on its solubility in biological fluids. The more insoluble the metal, the more likely it will be cleared by the mucociliary system. Soluble metal ions have the ability to be absorbed and interact with organic ligands, which can result in a number of toxic actions and health effects.[50] The group of metals discussed below have the common characteristic of being relatively inactive in the lung tissues. Additional discussion of the health effects of metal exposure is in Chapter 29.

Iron

Iron is a ubiquitous element, found in nature in a variety of ores, including oxides (hematite, limonite, magnetite) and sulfides (pyrites). Taconite and ocher are low-grade oxide ores in which iron is combined with silicates and quartz. Siderite is a carbonate iron ore mined in Britain. Emery consists primarily of aluminum oxide but also contains about 30% iron oxide and is used as an abrasive.

The use of metallic iron in items for domestic, agricultural, and military purposes dates from over 5000 years ago. By about 1000 BC, iron metallurgy was widely practiced. Worker exposure to iron-containing dusts and fumes increased dramatically in the latter half of the nineteenth and early twentieth centuries and is still common. However, industrial mechanization and diminished use of steel in many products have reduced the opportunity for worker exposure to ferrous metals. Additionally, the increased commercial use of structural materials made from hydrocarbons and synthetic fibers, as well as increasingly complex metal alloys, has directed attention to the effects of these exposures on industrial workers.

Inhalational iron exposures to workers may potentially occur during mining and beneficiation of ores, in smelting and throughout the steelmaking process, in foundries (see also Chapter 39) and fabrication shops, as well as during maintenance and repair operations such as cutting and welding. Iron oxide dust exposures may occur consequent to its use in pigments and as an abrasive for polishing silver and other articles.

Numerous studies of workers exposed to dusts and fumes containing iron in various forms have been performed. Zenker (1866) is said to have coined the term "siderosis" for the lung condition resulting from prolonged inhalation of iron or iron oxides. Unfortunately, the certainty of conclusions relative to the effects of metallic iron and iron oxides is tempered by the nearly invariable concurrence of other potentially toxic exposures.

Early studies of silver finishers concluded that although radiographic shadows can be seen after lung deposition of the radioopaque iron oxide, little clinically important fibrosis occurred.[51] Pathologic examination of the lungs of one finisher did show extensive emphysema. In another early study, radiographic changes of a fine reticulation, primarily in the lower lung zones, was observed in 15 of 171 iron and steel grinders and lathe operators, but no clear relationship of these changes to symptoms was noted.[52] Chest x-ray densities suggesting pneumoconiosis have been associated with exposures in steel foundry work. Gregory reported the findings from a series of radiographic surveys performed between 1950 and 1960 in 3059 workers at the Sheffield, England steel works. Overall, a condition that at that time was labeled "silicosis" was noted to develop in 64/1000 men per year. Radiographic changes characterized as "siderosis" developed after an average latency of 22 years and were more common among welders and burners, averaging 176 cases each year per 1000 men.[53]

Worth and Smidt compared pulmonary physiologic findings in a group of 720 iron workers with the results in 240 workers of similar age and smoking habits but without occupational exposures. Overall, the iron workers showed a significantly greater increase in residual volume (RV) and reduction in FVC with age than the controls. FEV1 was less clearly affected. Abnormality of the difference in oxygen tension between alveolar and arterial blood, but not airway resistance as determined by body plethysmography, was also associated with iron work. When compared with iron workers in other areas, those involved in smelting additionally showed evidence of airflow obstruction, with a reduced FEV1 and increased airway resistance (R_{aw}) and ratio of residual volume to total lung capacity (RV/TLC).[54]

Mining and milling of the various iron ores have also been shown to lead to risk to the respiratory system. Mining, however, leads to numerous exposures in addition to iron and its oxides (see Mining, Chapter 38). In Great Britain, the health effects in hematite miners in West Cumbria have been documented over many years and include massive lung fibrosis, advanced emphysema, tuberculosis, and lung carcinomas.[55] However, dust and fume controls have reportedly resulted in the virtual elimination of the occurrence of radiographic pneumoconiosis in these workers.[56] In Labrador, Canada, radiographic categories of pneumoconiosis are still significantly ($p < 0.05$) associated with cumulative and peak exposures to respirable dust and quartz in 1950 miners working an ore that is primarily hematite and magnetite with significant quartz contamination.[57] The proportion of Labrador miners found to have pneumoconiotic changes increased with age and tenure. Additionally, both FVC and FEV1 were reduced with increasing radiographic category. Estimates of cumulative iron oxide exposure, in contrast, did not predict the radiographic changes as closely ($p = 0.054$), suggesting that the iron may have contributed less than quartz to the chest x-ray findings.[58] Pham and colleagues recently reported findings in a group of 871 French iron ore mine workers followed for 5 years. After accounting for smoking, airflow obstruction increased in relation to underground mine work, although the functional loss was said to be less on average than seen in coal miners.[59] Lung cancer deaths in the French iron miners were also excessive, as were stomach cancers.[60] In China, where the introduction of ventilation and other dust controls has occurred more recently, death from nonmalignant respiratory diseases in hematite miners is still clearly increased in relation to age and dust indices.[61] Tuberculosis and silicosis are both commonly reported causes of death in these workers, as is lung cancer.[62]

The increased cancer risk noted in several studies of iron miners may be related to a number of potential factors, such as radon gas, diesel emissions, explosives, and silica. The relative roles of these, as well as the iron oxides in the cancer risk, are debated. A low-grade iron ore mined in Minnesota is associated with a fibrous silicate contaminant, the amphibole cummingtonite-grunerite. However, radiographic changes analogous to those seen with asbestos were not noted in one study of taconite miners.[63] Pyrite, a crystalline iron sulfide, is mined in Italy.[64] High dust exposure levels and pneumoconiosis have been present historically. Recent studies have documented that dust levels are lower and quartz contamination of dust is less than 2%, although diesel exhaust is present. Radiographic changes [International Labor Organization (ILO) Category 1 or 2] are still seen in 4.3% of the miners, but only minor reductions in vital capacity with exposure were noted, without airflow obstruction.[64]

Iron exposures also occur generally among welders and burners and have been associated with radiographic changes (see Chapter 42). Because of the complex welding environments with multiple concurrent exposures (NOx, ozone, asbestos, chromium and other metals, etc.), the specific contribution of iron and iron oxide to the symptoms and lung findings seen with welding exposures remains unclear. Recent studies in welders have failed to demonstrate significant increases in mortality from nonmalignant respiratory diseases, although lung cancer mortality was somewhat elevated.

In summary, inhalational exposure to iron and iron oxides can result in radiographic opacities, particularly at high exposure levels, related in part to the fact that the deposited iron is relatively radioopaque. Probably because it provokes less inflammation per milligram of deposited dust than many other agents, the degree of tissue reaction and functional effects related to iron and iron oxide exposures are generally modest. Concurrent exposures (silica, asbestos, NOx, other metals) can result in important lung disease.

Barium

Barium is derived from the greek "barys," which means heavy. The largest natural source of barium is barite ore, which is composed largely of barium sulfate. Barite crystals are embedded in the rock ore, which is found in beds or masses in limestone, shales, and other sedimentary formations. These white tabular crystals are obtained from the ore through a pulverizing process utilizing a mill that crushes the ore into a fine powder.[65]

Deposits of barite in the United States are found in South Carolina, Kentucky, Montana, Washington, Idaho, New Mexico, Utah, Nevada, Texas, Arizona, Wisconsin, California, and Missouri.[66] The largest use (85% to 95%) of barite is in the support of oil and gas well drilling. Barite is used to make a mud that has a heavy weight. This mud settles into the drilling hole and due to its weight helps to prevent a "blowing out" when the oil or gas is struck. Other uses for barium compounds include the brick, ceramic, and photographic industries. Barium is also used as a stabilizer in the manufacture of plastics, paints, rubber, ink, glass, linoleum, oil cloth, lubricating oils, jet fuels, and certain types of pesticides.

In 1980, approximately 10,000 people were potentially exposed to elemental barium in the workplace and about 474,000 to various barium compounds. Principal occupations with exposure include lithopone plant workers, barite millers, barite miners, ceramic workers, fluorescent lamp makers, glass makers, and metallurgists.[66]

The soluble forms of barium tend to be more injurious than the sulfate form. The ion is a potassium antagonist and symptoms of poisoning appear to result from the effects of barium-induced hypokalemia with potassium shifting across cell membranes. The hydroxide and oxide forms have strong alkaline properties that can cause severe burning to the eyes, mucous membranes, and skin. Barium chloride exerts a marked toxic effect, whereas the nitrate, oxide, and peroxide forms are somewhat less toxic. Barium carbonate and acetate are the least toxic forms.[67] There currently exist no regulatory exposure limits in the United States for barium sulfate, other than as a "particulate not otherwise classified." Very few studies have evaluated the respiratory effects following acute, intermediate, and chronic inhalation exposure to barium. A pneumoconiosis (baritosis) has been observed in workers exposed in the mining and milling of barium. Baritosis is not associated with pronounced respiratory symptoms or obvious impairment in many cases. Its incidence is unknown, with very few cases being reported, in spite of the large numbers of workers exposed to the dust each year. As with many other minerals, the question has been raised regarding the contribution of barium to the pneumoconiosis, in light of the potential exposures to silica and quartz in the mining and milling process. Laboratory rats exposed to mineral barytes containing up to 2% of SiO_2 and pure barium sulfate at moderate inhalation levels (3.6 mg barium/m^3) develop pulmonary lesions (perivascular and peribronchial sclerosis and focal thickening of interalveolar septa),[65] which, in association with the lung mineral content, result in radiographic changes and tend to corroborate the human findings.

Antimony

Stibnite is the principal ore of antimony and is found most abundantly in China, Mexico, Bolivia, Algeria, Portugal, France, and South Africa.[68] Antimony sulfide in the ore is typically smelted with limestone, sandstone, iron slag, coke, and powdered coal. A process termed roasting involves heating the stibnite in a rotary kiln, which volatilizes the metal and creates antimony oxide, a fine white dust with a mean particle diameter less than 1 μm. The oxide form is subsequently reduced to the metal in furnaces.

Antimony has been used since ancient times as a cosmetic and a constituent of bronzes and other alloys. Antimony has many other industrial and medical applications. Common industrial exposures occur during the mining, smelting, and refining of the ore in the production of alloys (with tin, lead, and copper), in the manufacture of abrasives, in the printing industry, in the compounding of rubber, in flameproofing compounds, in plating of vases and domestic vessels, and in the manufacture of paints, lacquers, enamels, glass, and pottery. Antimony compounds have been used medicinally since the time of the Roman empire. "Calcis vomitorum" was a preparation that induced vomiting, formed when wine was allowed to stand in goblets made from antimony alloys. "Powder of Algaroth" was a preparation of antimony oxychloride used during the Middle Ages to induce vomiting. In this century, antimony containing compounds have been successfully used to treat schistosomiasis and leishmaniasis.[69]

Chronic cough is the most common symptom noted by antimony exposed workers with mucous membrane irritation being a common complaint. Orange coloration of the teeth is a sign of antimony oxide exposure, and a particular dermatosis, with vesicular and at times pustular lesions, occurs in workers exposed to fumes near the furnaces.[70,71]

No specific pattern of pulmonary function abnormality was observed in workers with antimony exposure.[71]

Distinctive radiographic findings have been noted in workers who have had antimony exposure for 9 or more years. The pneumoconiotic lesions are characterized by diffuse punctate opacities, typically occurring in the mid-lung zones, having an opacity size of less than 1.0 mm and both rounded and irregular shapes. Higher degrees of radiographic profusion do occur, and conglomerate lesions have been observed in antimony-exposed workers with associated silica exposure, as in stibnite miners.[70]

Tin

The history of tin use as a metal is as ancient as that of copper and gold with tin smelting occurring in the neolithic age 5000 years ago. Tin is found in metal bearings, bronzes, specula, lead tin (Babbitt metal), and also is used in soldering, tinning (electroplating of sheet steel), and in the making of float glass (in which plate glass is floated and formed on a bath of molten tin).[72]

Ores are found in Malaysia, the United Kingdom, Thailand, Indonesia, Bolivia, Nigeria, Zaire, and Australia. Tin, like barium, iron, and antimony, has a high atomic weight, and this is felt to be one of the reasons it produces radiographic shadows.[73] Tin oxide occurs in two forms, stannous (SnO) and stannic (SnO_2). The stannic form is also known as the mineral cassiterite and is considered the form that results in the pneumoconiotic changes.[72,73]

Various processes are involved in tin metallurgy, including grinding, iron leaching, briquet making, smelting, and casting. In the mill, the raw ore is ground, then poured into a hydrochloride bath. The parent compound contains small quantities of other metals including iron, zinc, and sulfur. In the hydrochloride bath the iron is chemically attached to chloride to form iron chloride, which is eliminated by washing. The tin concentrate is then dried and mixed with a vegetable coal, borax, sodium borate, and calcium carbonate and again ground. This material is mixed with sodium sulfide, caustic soda, and molasses, then pressed into briquets that are smelted in an electric furnace, and the resulting metal is cast into bars. Pneumoconiosis has been identified in the grinding, briquet making, smelting, and casting processes, and in the bagging of tin oxide prior to transport to the smelter.[73]

Radiographic changes that occur with tin are termed stannosis. The findings characteristically mimic other "benign" pneumoconioses such as those due to barium and iron. Densities on the chest radiograph range in size from the typical 1 to 2 mm smaller nodules, to larger, softer lesions, with the hila at times also being unusually opaque[74] (Fig. 22-3). The opacities are not reported to be associated with symptoms or disability and demonstrate neither progression nor clearing after cessation of exposure. Abnormal spirometric lung function has not been identified in tin workers.[75]

Pathologic lung specimens of workers with stannosis reveal dust foci consisting of dense aggregates of dust-laden macrophages surrounding the respiratory bronchioles. Little of this dust is burned away with microincineration, but when lung sections are subsequently treated with concentrated hydrochloric acid, the dust disappears. There is little reticulin response or collagen formation in association with the dust-laden macrophages. As a result of these findings,

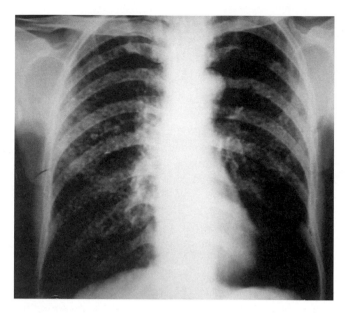

Fig. 22-3. Radiographic appearance of pneumoconiosis in a tin miner, revealing diffuse small rounded opacities typical of radiodense dusts.

tin has been historically classified as a "particulate not otherwise classified" leading to a "benign" pneumoconiosis.[76]

Chromite

Chromite is the only mineral ore of chromium and consists of the oxides of chromium and of iron (Cr_2O_3FeO). The ore exists in packed sheets of granules, 0.5 mm in diameter, intermixed in a silicate lattice of magnesium and aluminum feldspar, which gives the raw ore a mottled appearance.

Chromite exposure has been associated with chronic bronchitis,[77] asthma (due to a hypersensitivity to the chrome compounds)[78,79] interstitial fibrosis, nasal septal perforation,[80] ulceration of the skin, and intestinal and respiratory tract (nose, pharynx, and lung) cancers.[81–83]

Human epidemiologic studies have provided convincing evidence that zinc chromate is a potent carcinogen and there is some evidence that calcium chromate and chromium trioxide also constitute a cancer hazard in humans. Human studies have not selectively confirmed the carcinogenic potency for the other chromium compounds. Animal studies confirm the carcinogenic potency of calcium chromate and zinc potassium chromate and present strong evidence that chromates of lead and strontium are carcinogenic in animals. The significance of the water solubility for the carcinogenic potency of the chromates has not been clarified by animal studies.[84]

Current threshold limit values (TLV) are set at 0.05 mg/m^3 for chromium VI and chromite ore and 0.5 mg/m^3 for chromium II and III compounds. The TLVs are designed to prevent cancer as well as irritation and other respiratory symptoms. The relative risk of dying from a respiratory cancer has ranged from 20 to 40 times the rate for a control population. The risk seems highest shortly after the cohort was identified as being actively employed in the chromate industry, suggesting a short latent period and a potent carcinogenic effect.[85]

Pneumoconiosis that results from chromite mining exposure typically manifests as a very fine nodulation, less than 1 mm in diameter. Sparse, short, linear opacities of similar density to the nodules may be seen. The nodulation is finer in quality, though somewhat more radioopaque, than in simple coal worker's pneumoconiosis. Occasionally there is a mixture of rather large nodules 2 to 3 mm in diameter. This larger form of nodulation occurs both in men who give a history of pure chrome mining and in those with mixed mining service.[86]

SEDIMENTARY COMPOUNDS

Sedimentary carbonates, sulfates, and halides provide relatively pure minerals that have crystallized from concentrated solutions. A striking difference between these minerals and the silicate minerals is their more rapid dissolution. Silicate phases generally have low solubilities and slow dissolution rates, whereas sulfides are readily attacked in oxidizing conditions and many halides, carbonates, phosphates, hydroxides, and sulfates have high solubilities in weak acids and bases.[1] Based on the high solubility of many of these sedimentary compounds, there is dissolution and clearance from the pulmonary system, generally minimizing resulting pulmonary pathology.

Calcium carbonate

Calcium carbonate is an odorless, tasteless powder. It exists in nature as the mineral aragonite and calcite (limestone, chalk, and marble). Aragonite is changed to calcite when heated in dry air to about 400°C.

Calcium carbonate is used to manufacture quicklime, Portland cement, and paints. It is a component in dentifrices, cosmetics, foods, and pharmaceuticals. Portland cement is discussed later in this chapter. Exposure to calcium carbonate has not been associated with lung effects.[87,88]

Oil shale

Oil shale was first used as an energy source in the 1850s in Scotland.[89] In the United States, the industry devoted to recovering shale oil is relatively recent, and is located mainly in the Green River formation connecting the corners of Wyoming, Utah, and Colorado, where there are deposits containing an estimated 1.8 trillion barrels of oil. Other major deposits exist in Scotland and Estonia. The mineral is found in sedimentary rock, and is a gray-brown layered consistency known as marlstone. The oil (kerogen), which is contained in the rock is a mixture of organic material composed mainly of carbon, hydrogen, oxygen, sulfur, and nitrogen that accumulated millennia ago in freshwater lakes.[90]

Extraction of the oil from the shale deposits may involve open pit mining, underground room and pillar mines, or retorting. Underground retorting involves the heating of the oil underground to a temperature of 350° to 500°C, where it vaporizes and then is condensed into liquid oil in the collection process. Aboveground retorting involves a direct and indirect method. In the direct method, the oil shale is crushed and then ignited in a retort that creates an oil mist that is collected and condensed. The indirect method similarly involves creating an oil mist and a collection process. Porcelain balls are heated and introduced into the retort, or the outside of the retort is heated through burning of a recycled gas. The kerogen molecule that is collected is too large to be conventionally refined and thus is hydrogenated before refining to various petroleum products.[90]

Shale mining involves shattering of the deposits by drilling holes into the shale and placing explosives. Broken rock is loaded and transported to the processing area, where retorting is performed. The dust generated by shale mining and sorting has a free silica content of about 3% to 4%. The concentration of dust in the atmosphere of underground oil shale mines is also relatively low, but it is of relatively fine dispersion with up to 80% of the dust particles under 2 μm in size.[91] The low dustiness may be related to the soft claylike consistency of shale, which makes it less likely to break up into respirable particles.[92]

Reports of skin cancer in paraffin workers in the Scottish shale oil industry have been related to the carcinogens in the Scottish shale oil, which was produced for lighting, lubricating oils, and paraffin (kerosene). The majority of these skin cancers are believed to be caused by the by-products of thermal treatment of the mineral fuel.[93] The carcinogenic constituents of the shale oil are thought to be related to pyrolytic effects, which result in the generation of polycyclic aromatic hydrocarbons during retorting. In the early 1900s, "mulespinners" were noted to often die of scrotal cancer. From 1911 to 1938, 1631 men in England and Wales died of cancer of the scrotum. Of these men, 575 were textile workers, 121 chimney sweeps, and 45 workers who were engaged in the manufacture of coal gas, coke, and patent fuel. The tumors in textile workers were related to exposure to spindles that were lubricated with Scottish shale oil and then soaked the mulespinner's pants. Seaton identified two cases of peripheral squamous cell carcinoma of the lung in shale oil miners with pneumoconiosis and addressed the possibility that these tumors were related to lung deposition of the kerogens contained in shale dust.[92]

Pneumoconiosis related to the deposition of shale oil dusts in the lung is termed shalosis. The dust creates a granulomatous and fibrotic reaction in the lungs. This pneumoconiosis is similar clinically to coal workers' pneumoconiosis and silicosis and may progress to massive fibrosis even after the worker has left the industry.[92]

Pathologic changes identified in lungs with shalosis are characterized by vascular and bronchial deformation with irregular thickening of interalveolar and interlobular septa. In addition to interstitial fibrosis, most lung specimens with Kukersite (Estonian) shale pneumoconiosis show enlarged hilar shadows, related to the transport of oil shale dust to the hilar lymph nodes and subsequent development of well-defined sclerotic changes.[94]

Estonian shale workers have been found to have a prevalence of chronic bronchitis 2.5 times that of age-matched controls.[94] The effect of shale exposure on lung function has not been studied systematically, although a group of retired miners with shalosis had reductions in FEV1, FVC, and diffusion capacity of the lung for carbon monoxide (DLCO), when compared with retired miners without radiographic changes.

Carbon

Elemental carbon has found numerous uses in commerce and industry based upon its various properties. Aside from coal, which is discussed in Chapter 23, the two common forms are graphite (crystalline carbon) and carbon black, which is a partially decomposed form. Graphite is used in the manufacture of lead pencils, foundry linings, paints, electrodes, dry batteries, and in making crucibles for metallurgic purposes. Finely ground graphite has lubricant properties. Carbon black is used in automotive tires, pigments, plastics, inks, and other products. Other relatively pure carbon products include carbon fibers, which are used in a variety of goods, and carbon microspheres and elipses, which, among other uses, are inhaled by humans during radionuclide lung scanning.[95]

Natural graphite (also known as plumbago, as it was originally mistaken for lead) is mined throughout the world and is often contaminated with crystalline silica and silicates.[96] Even the purest form of natural graphite contains about 2% quartz. Deposits of graphite occur in veins and fissures in underground crystalline rocks. The mining of the ore consists of driving shafts and blasting the rock until a graphite vein is localized. The dislodged graphite is collected and loaded into buckets and hauled to the surface.

Artificial graphite is manufactured by the heating of coal or petroleum coke and generally contains no free silica. Inhalation of carbon dusts may occur during the mining and milling of graphite, as well as during the manufacture of artificial graphite. Carbon black is manufactured from fossil fuels through a variety of processes involving partial combustion or thermal decomposition. End use of numerous carbon products may also offer potential for exposure.

Radiographic shadows consistent with pneumoconiosis are still being reported among workers exposed to both natural and artificial graphite.[97,98] Clinically, workers with carbon black or graphite pneumoconiosis show similar findings to coal workers with radiographic changes of small rounded opacities predominantly in upper and mid-lung zones. Severe symptomatic cases with massive pulmonary fibrosis were reported in the past, particularly related to the manufacture of carbon electrodes for metallurgy, although recent reports emphasize that the implicated exposures are likely to be mixed dusts.[99]

Epidemiologic study of graphite miners also have suggested that the radiographic changes result from mixed dust exposures, including carbon, silica, and the host rock that envelopes the graphite.[100]

Portland cement

Portland cement, commonly called cement, is a manufactured mixture of raw components consisting of hydrated calcium silicates, aluminum oxide, magnesium oxide, iron oxide, calcium sulfate, clay, shale, sand, and other impurities.

Raw materials are crushed to a suitable size by being rolled and ground in a grinder. This powdered mixture is then calcinized in high temperature kilns to remove impurities and to facilitate the chemical reactions of certain substrates. After cooling, gypsum is added to moderate the chemical reaction of the finished product.

Cement is dependent on various physical changes and chemical reactions of the mineral constituents: (1) evaporation of free water, (2) release of combined water, (3) decomposition of carbonates (calcination), and (4) combination of the lime, silica, alumina, and other oxides. This process produces a combination of solid and liquid phases in the $CaO + SiO_2 + Al_2O_3$ system, which crystallizes to form a mixture of solid calcium silicates and calcium aluminate.[101]

Dusts inhaled during the manufacture of cement result from exposures in the quarrying and preparing of the raw materials, calcining and grinding clinker, blending with additives (mainly gypsum), packing, and shipping of the finished product.[102] Respirable quartz exposure risk is greatest in raw materials preparation, followed by the mixer, clinker, and finishing areas.

Radiographically, findings of both rounded and irregular opacities as well as pleural abnormalities have been identified in workers. Although in the past, asbestos was used in numerous cement products, the presence of the pleural plaques and irregular opacities seen in these workers was not considered to be related to known asbestos exposure.[103] Pathologic specimens of lungs with cement pneumoconiosis have shown pulmonary granulomas containing inclusions of cement.[103]

Pulmonary alveolar proteinosis (PAP) has also been reported to occur in cement dust-exposed workers. It is felt to be a result of dust overload, which provokes excessive secretion of surfactant and associated lipids from type II pneumocytes. Evaluation of lung tissue obtained from workers who developed PAP after the inhalation of cement dust has revealed increased numbers of inorganic particles (silicates found in cement dust). The mechanism for this reaction may be simply mechanical and not related to the presence of fibrogenic material, yet laboratory animals have developed PAP within 3 weeks of a single intratracheal instillation of silica dust.

Several studies have found significant deficits in the FEV1/FVC ratio in cement-exposed workers, although this has not been observed in all groups of workers.[104–106] The differences in the studies may be related to the intensity of exposure.

As with most other inorganic dusts discussed in this chapter, cement is classified as a "particulate not otherwise classified" by the American Conference of Government Industrial Hygienists with a time weighted average threshold limit value of 10 mg/m^3 for total dust.

Gilsonite

Gilsonite is a solidified hydrocarbon, also known as uintaite, which is a bitumen of the asphaltite class. It occurs as a solid black substance that runs in veins in the rock strata of the eastern Utah and Western Colorado Uinta Basin. The veins of gilsonite are believed to have been deposited through the distillation of viscous crude oil from nearby oil shale deposits.

Gilsonite was discovered during the 1860s by settlers who first thought it was coal, but noted that when they heated the substance, it melted. In attempts to market the substance, Samuel Gilson spent many years experimenting with the ore and subsequently named the substance gilsonite.

Gilsonite is mined using air-driven chipping hammers that chip ore from the vein. The ore falls by gravity to the bottom of the slope where a vacuum air lift system transports it to holding bins on the surface. The ore is processed through physical and mechanical processes that include drying, crushing, sizing, and packaging[107] (Fig. 22-4).

Current uses of gilsonite are in the manufacture of automotive body seam sealers, inks, paints, and enamels, in oil-well drilling fluids and cements, as an additive in sand molds in the foundry industry, as a component of asphalt, building boards, explosives, and in the production of nuclear grade graphite.[108]

Little is known of the health effects of gilsonite exposure. The workforce that is involved in the mining is relatively small. Exposure assessments have been completed, which evaluated components of gilsonite that might be harmful due to their chemical relationship to aliphatic hydrocarbons (branched alkanes, cycloalkanes, and/or olefins). Trace amounts of toluene, xylene, and alkyl-substituted naphthalenes have been detected, but no polynuclear aromatic hydrocarbons (PNAs) that could represent a carcinogenic risk. Low molecular-weight hydrocarbons (4 to 10 carbon paraffins and olefins), have been detected that range from nonquantifiable to 104 mg/m^3.[109]

Cross-sectional studies have indicated that gilsonite dust is a respiratory irritant, producing symptoms of cough and phlegm in workers with high exposures. Radiographic evi-

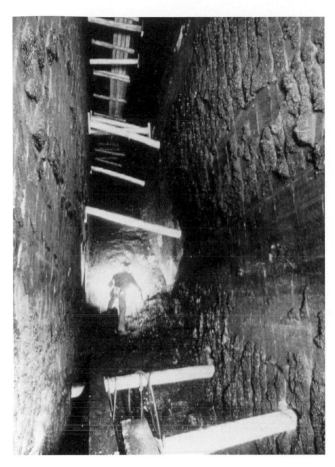

Fig. 22-4. Underground mining of gilsonite, western Colorado.

dence of pneumoconiosis was found in a population of gilsonite workers. Each of the workers identified with pneumoconiosis had worked more than 18 years in the gilsonite industry and had no prior exposure to respiratory hazards, which raises the possibility that inhalation of gilsonite dust may be associated with the development of pneumoconiosis. However, 25% (2/8) of the miners' respirable dust exposure measurements in this study exceeded the TLV for respirable quartz, increasing the likelihood of silicosis among gilsonite miners. Pulmonary function deficits were not identified in a cross-sectional study of gilsonite workers.[110]

Slate

Slate is a metamorphic rock, made up of various minerals, clays, and carbonaceous matter. The most common minerals found in slate are muscovite and quartz, which make up to 25% of Cornish slate and 30% of North Wales slate. Other silicates are also found, such as feldspar and kaolin. The color and texture of slate are variable, depending on the mixture of the sedimentary salts and carbonaceous matter. Mica slates are created when muscovite combines with aluminum silicates such as kaolin and feldspar. During the process of metamorphosis, these form a dense crystalline rock that possesses strength and the ability to be cleaved. The rock has natural cleavage planes that are orientated in relation to their crystalline structure. This ability to fracture and be mined in tabular form accounts for its economic importance. Various colors of slate result from the mixture of minerals: iron salts, red; chlorite, green; ferruginous and chlorite, purple; and carbonaceous material, black. Clay slates are comprised of silicate particles compressed by weight and pressure and cemented together by various salts. These slates are difficult to fracture along cleavage planes and are thus less economically important.[111]

Slate is used in roofing, dimension stone, floor tile, structural shapes such as panels and window sills, blackboards, pencils, billiard tables, and laboratory bench tops. Crushed slate is used in highway construction, tennis court surfaces, and lightweight roofing granules.

The lungs of miners exposed to slate dust have revealed localized areas of perivascular and peribronchial fibrosis, extending to macule formation and considerable interstitial fibrosis. Typical lesions are fibrotic macules of variable configuration intimately associated with small pulmonary blood vessels.

A variety of lung radiographic changes are identified in slateworkers. Because of the high quartz content of some slates and the adjacent rock strata, slateworkers' pneumoconiosis often has features of silicosis. Radiographically, Welsh slate workers show lesions typical of silicosis with small rounded opacities and progressive massive fibrosis, whereas Vermont slateworkers generally have a diffuse linear interstitial pulmonary abnormality identified.[112] Pneumoconiosis has been found in a third of workers studied in the slate industry in North Wales[113] and 54% of slate pencil makers in India.[114] Elemental composition analyzed by x-ray diffraction revealed a combination of minerals (Si, Al, K, Fe), providing evidence that slateworkers develop a mixed dust pneumoconiosis.

The prevalence of respiratory symptoms in slateworkers is high, and the proportion of workers with symptoms increases with the pneumoconiosis category, irrespective of smoking status. Diminished FEV1 and FVC are associated with increasing pneumoconiosis category, reductions in these values being evident even with simple pneumoconiosis. This implies that the effect of slate dust on the lung differs from that of coal-related pneumoconiosis.[115]

Potash

Potash (sodium and potassium chloride, sylvite) is a name given to mined potassium ores. It was the name originally given to the crude potassium carbonate obtained from wood ashes, which was mixed with water and the resulting solution evaporated to dryness in iron pots, hence potash.[116,117]

Potash exposure has been associated with nasal perforation,[117] but has not been related to pulmonary function changes.[118] Potash workers report more respiratory symptoms than control subjects, suggesting an irritant effect of the dust and/or mine environment.[118]

Gypsum

Gypsum is a hydrated calcium sulfate ($CaSO_4 \cdot 2H_2O$). It is used mainly in the manufacture of plasterboard, plaster of paris, and as a retarder in Portland cement. It occurs in a variety of forms: gypsite, an impure earthy form; alabaster, a fine-grained translucent form; and satin spar, a silky variety of selenite that is a transparent crystalline form. It is found in various states of purity, usually with other mineral deposits such as quartz, pyrites, carbonates, clays, and bituminous materials.

Several older studies suggested that gypsum dust was not a respiratory hazard, had no effects in producing pneumoconiosis,[119,120] and might even be protective in situations when quartz was inhaled.[121,122] Recent studies have not agreed with the previous findings, and have identified parenchymal changes in gypsum miners over the age of 35 and having at least 20 years of mining. Pneumoconiosis, quantified radiographically according to the ILO scale (see Chapter 7), was noted at a level of $\geq 1/0$ in 41 (31%) miners and category 2/1 in 3 (13%) of the miners evaluated.[123] The mines that recorded a high rate of pneumoconiosis were mining gypsum in layers of limestone and shale with the shale containing 30% quartz, and thus the greatest dust hazard appeared to be the quartz.

In contrast to the findings on chest films, questionnaire and lung function surveys in gypsum-exposed workers have not identified increased rates of respiratory abnormalities.[122,123]

Trona

Trona (sodium sesquicarbonate, $Na_2CO_3 \cdot NaHCO_3 \cdot 2H_2O$) is mined in underground deposits near Green River, Wyoming. The ore is processed to produce soda ash (sodium carbonate), which is used in the manufacture of glass, paper, detergents, and in other chemical applications.[124]

Trona dust is alkaline (pH 10.5), quite soluble, and induces irritation to the skin and mucous membranes, including the respiratory tract.

Pulmonary function surveys performed among miners exposed to trona dust found lung function to be within normal limits. There was a decline in FEV1 across the work shift in some workers, but when these workers were followed longitudinally for 5 years, they were not found to have an accelerated decrement in FEV1.

Symptoms questionnaires did detect eye and upper respiratory tract irritation to be quite common, but 23% of workers also reported lower respiratory symptoms of cough and phlegm.[124]

There are no known pneumoconiotic effects of trona dust.

Phosphate

Phosphate ore, the pure chemical compound defined as calcium phosphate $Ca_5(F,Cl)(PO_4)_3$, is mined and used to extract elemental phosphorus and phosphoric acid. Phosphoric acid is used in the manufacture of triple superphosphate fertilizer, ammonium phosphates, and inorganic phosphates, which are used in the production of soaps, dietary supplements, toothpaste, and evaporated milk. Elemental phosphorus is used in detergents, preservatives for food-grade chemicals, pesticides, rodent poisons, and ammunition.[125]

The processing of phosphate ore begins with the removal of the earth overburden. The ore is excavated by large draglines and broken up by high-pressure water jets, which carry the slurry to the beneficiation plant. There it is washed, sized, and subjected to flotation to remove sand and clays. The beneficiated form is processed further by being acidulated by reaction with sulfuric acid, which produces normal superphosphate fertilizer and phosphoric acid. Phosphoric acid may also be reacted with ammonia to produce monoammonium and diammonium phosphate fertilizers. Some phosphate rock is combined with coke and silica and processed in electric furnaces to extract elemental phosphorus.[126]

The process of refining phosphorus rock exposes the worker to several respiratory irritants, including phosphoric acid, phosphorus oxides, fluorides, and coal tar pitch volatiles.

Radiographic changes of pneumoconiosis are described in phosphate rock workers. These have been observed typically as small rounded opacities, but irregular opacities have also been reported. No pleural disease or mediastinum alterations have been described. Lung biopsies reveal extensive deposits of brownish crystalline material within the pneumoconiotic nodules, containing varying amounts of Ca, P, Fe, Mn, Si, Ti, Ba, Nb, and S. The data appear consistent with the development of a nonfibrogenic pneumoconioses in relation to phosphate rock exposure.[126,127]

Epidemiologic studies in worker populations have revealed increased prevalence of cough and chronic bronchitis, although lung function was not found to be affected by worker exposure to the process of mining or extracting the phosphorus.[128]

Fluorspar

Fluorspar (CaF_2) is a fluoride-containing mineral, which is used worldwide for high-temperature smelting and refining processes to make metals and alloys such as aluminum and steel.[129] It is used as a source of fluorine in the manufacture of chemicals such as hydrogen fluoride and various fluorinated hydrocarbons.

The mining of fluorspar occurs by removing epithermal veins of the material that exist in granite fissures that are from 1 inch to more than 50 feet wide. Higher-grade veins are usually narrow and have an average width of 4 to 5 feet, with an average fluorite content of 90%, and silica content of 5% to 6%. Wider low-grade veins have an average silica content of 15% to 20% with an average fluorite content of 60% to 70%. Nickel, chromium, beryllium, yttrium, samarium-147, and uranium are found in minor constituents of the rock and ore.[129]

Fluoride is absorbed by workers who are exposed to the mining and extraction of the mineral, and common complaints of exposure include burning epigastric discomfort and pain and stiffness of the spine and joints.[130]

Heavily exposed fluorspar miners accumulate a significant amount of fluorspar in the lungs, which has been confirmed with urine fluoride levels. No radiographic or pulmonary function changes have been confirmed in studies that have evaluated fluoride exposures on worker populations. However, the possibility of pulmonary effects of fluorspar dust needs further study.[131]

Salt

Sodium chloride is generally not considered a hazardous substance to the respiratory system. Salt miners were evaluated with spirometry, respiratory questionnaire, and chest x-ray in a cross-sectional survey of 259 white male workers in five salt mines using diesel mining equipment and five nondiesel salt mines. No increase in the prevalence of cough, phlegm, dyspnea, or obstruction was identified. The prevalence of pneumoconiosis was too low (one case of small rounded and one case of small irregular opacities) to analyze for dose-response relations.[132] Communities adjacent to alkaline lakes have been studied to determine if the exposure to the airborne alkaline dust had any effect on the respiratory health. Exposed residents were found to have significant increases in the prevalence of cough, wheeze, nasal irritation, and eye irritation when compared with the nonexposed group.[133] No changes in pulmonary function were detected in residents in relation to the exposure.[134]

REFERENCES

1. Cerling TE: Mineralogy of nonfibrous minerals with regard to health studies, Chapter 2. In Wagner WL, Rom WN, Merchant JA, editors, *Health issues related to metal and nonmetal mining,* pp 35-47, Boston, 1983, Butterworth.
2. Gamble J: *Silicate pneumoconiosis. Occupational respiratory diseases,* 1987. Pub No DHHS (NIOSH) 86-102, 243-285, 1987.
3. Phibbs BP, Sundin RE, and Mitchell RS: Silicosis in Wyoming bentonite workers. *Am Rev Respir Dis* 103:1-17, 1971.
4. McNally WD and Trostler IS: Severe pneumoconiosis caused by the inhalation of fuller's earth, *J Ind Hyg* 23:118-126, 1941.
5. Bowes DR, Langer AM, and Rohl AN: Nature and range of mineral dusts in the environment, *Phil Trans R Soc London* 86:593-610, 1977.
6. Davies D and Cotton R: Mica pneumoconiosis, *Br J Ind Med* 40:22-27, 1983.
7. Jones WR: Silicotic lungs, the minerals they contain, *J Hyg* 33:307-329, 1933.
8. Drinker CK, Field ME, and Drinker P: The cellular response of lymph nodes to suspensions of crystalline silica and to two varieties of sericite introduced through lymphatics, *J Ind Hyg* 16:160-164, 1934.
9. Mohanty GP, Roberts DC, King EJ, et al: The effect of feldspar, slate and quartz on the lungs of rats, *J Pathol Bacteriol* 65:501-512, 1953.
10. Olscamp G, Herman SJ, and Weisbrod GL: Nepheline rock dust pneumoconiosis, *Radiology* 142:29-32, 1982.
11. Barie HJ and Gosselin L: Massive pneumoconiosis from a rock dust containing no free silica, *Arch Environ Health* 1:31-39, 1960.
12. Bye E, Davies R, Griffiths DM, Gylseth B, and Moncrieff CB: In vitro cytotoxicity and quantitative silica analysis of diatomaceous earth products, *Br J Ind Med* 41:228-234, 1984.
13. Beskow R: Silicosis in diatomaceous earth factory workers in Sweden, *Scand J Respir Dis* 59:216-221, 1978.
14. Cooper WC and Jacobson G: A 21 year radiographic follow-up of workers in the diatomite industry, *J Occup Med* 19:563-566, 1977.
15. Musk AW, Greville HW, and Tribe AE: Pulmonary disease from occupational exposure to an artificial aluminum silicate used for cat litter, *Br J Ind Med* 37:367-372, 1980.
16. Mathur N, Gupta BN, Chandr H, et al: Pneumoconiosis risk assessment in agate workers, *Indiana J Chest Dis All Sci* 31:91-97, 1989.
17. Hildick-Smith GY: The biology of talc, *Br J Ind Med* 33:217-229, 1976.
18. Gibbs AE, Pooley FD, Griffiths DM, et al: Talc pneumoconiosis. A pathologic and mineralogic study, *Human Pathol* 23(12):1344-1354, 1992.
19. Gibbs AE, Pooley FD, and Griffiths DM: Talc pneumoconiosis. A pathologic and mineralogic study, *Human Pathol* 23:1344-1354, 1992.
20. Rohl AN, Langer AM, Selikoff IJ, et al: Consumer talcums and powders. Mineral and chemical characterization, *J Toxicol Envir Health* 2:255-284, 1976.
21. Weigeland E, Andersen A, and Baerheim A: Morbidity and mortality in talc-exposed workers, *Am J Ind Med* 17:505-513, 1990.
22. Weiss B and Boettner EA: Commercial talc and talcosis, *Arch Environ Health* 14, 1967.
23. Ferret J and Moreau P: Mineralogy and talc deposits, In Bignon J, editor: *Health related effects of phyllosilicates,* G21:147-158, NATO ASI Series, Berlin, 1990, Springer-Verlag.
24. Vallyathan NV and Craighead JE: Pulmonary pathology in workers exposed to nonasbestiform talc, *Human Pathol* 12:28-35, 1981.
25. Reijula K, Paakko P, Kerttula T, et al: Bronchiolitis in a patient with talcosis, *Br J Ind Med* 48:140-142, 1991.
26. Brown DP and Wagoner JK: Occupational exposure to talc containing asbestos. III. Retrospective cohort study of mortality, U.S. Dept. of HEW. (NIOSH) Pub No 80-15 31-30, 1980.
27. Kleinfeld M, Messite J, Kooyman O, et al: Mortality among talc miners and millers in New York State, *Arch Environ Health* 14:663-667, 1967.
28. Kleinfeld M, Messite J, and Zaki MH: Mortality experiences among talc workers. A follow-up study, *J Occup Med* 16:345-349, 1974.
29. Stille WT and Tabershaw IR: The mortality experience of upstate New York talc workers, *J Occup Med* 24:480-484, 1982.
30. Rubino GF, Scansetti G, Piolatto G, and Romano CA: Mortality study of talc miners and millers, *J Occup Med* 18:186-193, 1976.
31. Wegman DH, Peters JM, Boundy MG, and Smith TJ: Evaluation of respiratory effects in miners and millers exposed to talc free of asbestos and silica, *Br J Ind Med* 39:233-238, 1982.
32. Gamble JF, Fellner W, and Dimeo MJ: An epidemiologic study of a group of talc workers, *Am Rev Respir Dis* 119:741-753, 1979.
33. Gibbs AE, Pooley FD, Griffith DM, et al: Talc pneumoconiosis: a pathologic and mineralogic study, *Human Pathol* 23(12):1344-1354, 1992.
34. Cooper WC and Sargent EN: Study of chest radiographs and pulmonary ventilatory function in perlite workers, *J Occup Med* 28:199-206, 1986.
35. Elmes PC: Perlite and other 'nuisance' dusts, *J Royal Soc Med* 80:403-404, 1987.

36. Cooper WC: Radiographic survey of perlite workers, *J Occup Med* 17:304-307, 1975.

37. Cooper WC: Pulmonary function in perlite workers, *J Occup Med* 18:723-279, 1976.

38. Sepulveda MJ, Vallyathan V, Attfield MD, et al: Pneumoconiosis and lung function in a group of kaolin workers, *Am Rev Respir Dis* 127:231-235, 1983.

39. Sheers G: The China Clay Industry-Lessons for the future of occupational health, *Respir Med* 83:173-175, 1989.

40. Morgan WKC, Donner A, Higgins ITT, Pearson MG, et al: The effects of kaolin on the lung, *Am Rev Respir Dis* 138:813-820, 1988.

41. Wagner JC, Pooley FD, Gibbs A, et al: Inhalation of china stone and china clay dusts: relationship between the mineralogy of dust retained in the lungs and pathological changes, *Thorax* 41:190-196, 1986.

42. Kennedy T, Raylings W, Baser M, and Tockman M. Pneumoconiosis in Georgia kaolin workers, *Am Rev Respir Dis* 127:215-220, 1983.

43. American Conference of Governmental Industrial Hygienists: *Documentation of the threshold limit values,* ed 6, Cincinnati, 1991, ACGIH.

44. Bernstein RS, Baxter PJ, Falk H, et al: Immediate public health concerns and actions in volcanic eruptions: Lessons from the Mount St. Helens' eruption, *Am J Public Health* 6(suppl):25-37, 1986.

45. Green FHY, Bowman I, Castranova V, et al: Health implication of the Mount St. Helens eruptions: laboratory investigations, *Ann Occup Hyg* 26:921-933, 1982.

46. Baxter PJ and Ing R: Mount St. Helens eruptions, May 18 to June 12, 1980: an overview of the acute health impact, *JAMA* 246:2585-2589, 1981.

47. Green FHY, Vallyathan V, et al: Is volcanic ash a pneumoconiosis risk? *Nature* 293:216-217, 1981.

48. Cytotoxicity of volcanic ash: assessing the risk for pneumoconiosis. Leads from the MMWR, *JAMA* 255:2727-2728, 1986.

49. Bruist AS, Vollmer WM, Johnson LR, Bernstein RS, and McCamant LE: A four year prospective study of the respiratory effects of volcanic ash from Mt. St. Helens, *Am Rev Respir Dis* 133:526-534, 1986.

50. Nemery B: Metal toxicity and the respiratory tract, *Eur Respir J* 3:202-219, 1990.

51. McLaughlin ALG, Grout JLA, Barrie HJ, and Harding HE: Iron oxide dust and the lungs of silver finishers, *Lancet* 337-341, 1945.

52. Buckell M, Garrad J, Jupe MH, McLaughlin AIG, and Perry KMA: The incidence of siderosis in iron turners and grinders, *Br J Ind Med* 3:78-82, 1946.

53. Gregory J, Sheffield, and England DIH: A survey of pneumoconiosis at a Sheffield steel foundry, *Arch Environ Health* 20:385-399, 1970.

54. Worth G and Smidt U: Lung function in iron-workers, *Respiration* 26S:225-230, 1969.

55. Faulds J: Haematite pneumoconiosis in Cumberland miners, *J Clin Pathol* 10:187-199, 1957.

56. Craw J: Pneumoconiosis in the haematite iron ore mines of west cubria. A study of 45 years of control, *J Soc Occup Med* 32:53-65, 1982.

57. Moore E, Martin JR, Edwards AC, and Muir DCF: A case control study to investigate the association between indices of dust exposure and the development of radiologic pneumoconiosis, *Arch Environ Health* 42:351-355, 1987.

58. Martin JR, Muir DCF, Moore E, et al: Pneumoconiosis in iron ore surface mining in Labrador, *J Occ Med* 30:780-784, 1988.

59. Pham QT, Mur JM, Teculesu D, Chau N, Gabiano M, Gaertner N, et al: A longitudinal study of symptoms and respiratory function tests in iron miners, *Eur J Respir Dis* 69:346-354, 1986.

60. Chen SY, Hayes RB, Liang SR, Li QG, Stewart PA, and Blair A: Mortality experience of haematite mine workers in China, *Br J Med* 45:175-181, 1990.

61. Chen S-Y, Hayes RB, Wang J-M, Liang SR, and Blair Aaron: Non malignant respiratory disease among hematite mine workers in China, *Scand J Work Environ Health* 5:319-322, 1989.

62. Pham QT, Chau N, Patris A, Trombert B, Henquel JC, Geny M, and Teculescu D: Prospective mortality study among iron miners, *Cancer Detect Prevent* 449-453, 1991.

63. Clark TC, Harrington VA, Asta JM, Morgan WKC, and Sargent NE: Respiratory effects of exposure to dust in taconite mining and processing, *Am Rev Respir Dis* 121:959-966, 1980.

64. Franzinelli A, Gori B, Levante G, Belli S, Comba P, and Sartorelli E: Respiratory disorders and lung function impairment in pyrite miners, *Med Lav* 80:479-488, 1989.

65. U.S. Department of Health and Human Services, Agency for Toxic Substances and Disease Registry (ATSDR): *Toxicological profile for barium and compounds,* Atlanta, 1992, DHHS, ATSDR.

66. Timmreck TC and Shook G: Environmental health and occupational health implications of baritosis, a pneumoconiosis, *J Environ Health* 55:22-26, 1992.

67. Rumyantsev GI and Barium Compounds: In Israelson ZI, editor: *Toxicology of rare metals,* pp 118-124, Washington, 1963, National Science Foundation.

68. Browning E: *Toxicity of industrial metals,* London, 1961, Butterworth.

69. Cooper DA, Pendergrass EP, Vorwald AJ, Mayock RL, and Brieger H: Pneumoconiosis among workers in an antimony industry, *AJR* 103:495-508, 1968.

70. Oliver T: Health of antimony oxide workers, *Br Med J* 1:1094-1095, 1933.

71. Potkonjak V and Pavlovich M: Antimoniosis: a particular form of pneumoconiosis, *Int Arch Occup Environ Health* 51:199-207, 1983.

72. Sluis-Cremer GK, Thomas RG, Goldstein B, and Solomon A: Stannosis. A report of two cases, *S Afr Med J* 75:124-126, 1989.

73. Oyanguren H, Haddad R, and Maass H: Stannosis: benign pneumoconiosis owing to inhalation of tin dust and fume, *Ind Med Surg* 27:427-431, 1958.

74. Cole CWD, Davies JVSA, Kipling MD, and Ritchie GL: Stannosis in hearth tinners, *Br J Ind Med* 21:235-241, 1964.

75. Robertson AJ: Pneumoconiosis due to tin oxide, In King EJ and Fletcher CM, editors: *Industrial pulmonary diseases,* 7:168-184, London, 1960, Churchill.

76. Robertson AL, River D, Nagelschmidt G, and Duncumb P: Stannosis. Benign pneumoconiosis due to tin dioxide, *Lancet* 1089-1093, 1961.

77. Ballal SG: Respiratory symptoms and occupational bronchitis in chromite ore miners, Sudan, *J Trop Med Hyg* 89:223-228, 1986.

78. Broch C: Bronchial asthma caused by chromium trioxide, *Nord Med* 41:996-997, 1949.

79. Naidu VR and Rao RN: Occupational diseases in relation to the manufacture of dichromates, their prevention and treatment, *Indian Med Gaz* 83:431-433, 1948.

80. Kleinfeld M and Rosso A: Ulcerations of the nasal septum due to inhalation of chromic and acid mist, *Ind Med Surg* 34:242-243, 1965.

81. Mancuso TF: Occupational cancer and other health hazards in a chromate plant: a medical appraisal. II. Clinical and toxicologic aspects, *Ind Med Surg* 20:393-407, 1951.

82. Mancuso TF: Occupational cancer and other health hazards in chromate plant: a medical appraisal. I. Lung cancers in chromate workers, *Ind Med Surg* 20:358-363, 1951.

83. Bidstrup PL and Case RAM: Carcinoma of the lung in workmen in the bichromates producing industry, *Br J Ind Med* 13:260-264, 1956.

84. Langard S: Chromium carcinogenicity. A review of experimental data, *Sci Total Environ* 71:341-350, 1988.

85. Enterline PE: Respiratory cancer among chromate workers, *J Occup Med* 16:523-526, 1974.

86. Sluis-Cremer GK and Du Toit RSJ: Pneumoconiosis in chromite miners in South Africa, *Br J Ind Med* 25:63-67, 1968.

87. Beal AJ, Griffin OF, and Nagelschmidt G: *Safety in mines research establishment (SMRE).* Research report No. 72, 1956.

88. Hunter D: *The disease of occupations,* ed 5, p 916, London, 1975, The English Universities Press.

89. Seaton J, Lamb D, Rhind BW, Sclare G, and Middleton WG: Pneumoconiosis of shale miners, *Thorax* 36:412-418, 1981.

90. Rom WN, Lee JS, and Craft BF: Occupational and environmental health problems of the developing oil shale industry: a review, *Am J Ind Med* 2:247-260, 1981.

91. Kung VA: Morphological investigations of fibrogenic action of estonian oil shale dust, *Environ Health Perspect* 30:153-156, 1979.

92. Seaton A, Lamb D, Rhind Brown W, Sclare G, and Middleton WG: Pneumoconiosis of shale miners, *Thorax* 36:412-418, 1981.

93. Costello J: Morbidity and mortality study of shale oil workers in the United States, *Environ Health Perspect* 30:205-208, 1979.

94. Maripuu I: The prevalence of chronic bronchitis in workers of mechanized miners of the oil shale plant, *Ind Hyg Occup Pathol,* Valgus, Tallinn, Estonia SSR, 25, 1972.

95. Burch WM, Sullivan PJ, and McLaren CJ: Technegas—a new ventilation agent for lung scanning, *Nucl Med Commun* 7:865-871, 1986.

96. Merchant JA, Taylor G, and Hodous TK: Coal workers' pneumoconiosis and exposure to other carbonaceous dusts. In Merchant JA, editor: *Occupational respiratory diseases,* pp 329-384, Cincinnati, 1986, US Department of Health and Human Services (NIOSH) Pub No 86-102.

97. Jennison E. Personal communication, 1993.

98. Petsonk EL, Storey E, Becker PE, et al: Pneumoconiosis in carbon electrode workers, *J Occ Med* 30:887-891, 1988.

99. Hanoa R: Graphite pneumoconiosis. A review of etiologic and epidemiologic aspects, *Scand J Work Environ Health* 9:303-314, 1983.

100. Ranasinha DW and Uragoda CG: Graphite pneumoconiosis, *Br J Ind Med* 29:178-183, 1972.

101. McCunney RJ and Godefroi R: Pulmonary alveolar proteinosis and cement dust. A case report, *J Occup Med* 31:233-237, 1989.

102. Abrons HL, Sanderson WT, and Peterson MR: Respiratory effects of Portland cement dust, Morgantown, WV, 1988, U.S. Department of Health and Human Services (NIOSH), Pub No 86-226958.

103. Pimentel JC and Menezes AP: Pulmonary and hepatic granulomatous disorders due to the inhalation of cement and mica dusts, *Thorax* 33:219-227, 1978.

104. Yan CY, Huang CC, Chang IC, Lee CH, Tsai JT, and Ko YC: Pulmonary function and respiratory symptoms of Portland cement workers in southern Taiwan, *Kaohsiung J Med Sci* 9:186-192, 1993.

105. Abrons HL, Peterson MR, Sanderson WT, et al: Symptoms, ventilatory function, and environmental exposures in Portland cement workers, *Br J Ind Med* 45:368-375, 1988.

106. Kalacic I: Ventilatory lung function in cement workers, *Arch Environ Health* 26:84-85, 1973.

107. Jackson D: American gilsonite: mining solid hydrocarbon, *Engl Min J* 182:88-91, 1981.

108. Shushan L: Bonanza. The only place on earth where everybody knows what gilsonite is, *Stand Oiler* 1-5, 1983.

109. Kullman GJ, Doak CB, Keimig DG, Cornwell RJ, and Ferguson RP: Assessment of respiratory exposures during gilsonite mining and milling operations, *Am Ind Hyg Assoc J* 50(8):413-418, 1989.

110. Keimig DG, Castellan RM, Kullman GJ, and Kinsley KB: Respiratory health status of gilsonite workers, *Am J Ind Med* 11:287-296, 1987.

111. Craighead JE, Emerson RJ, and Stanley DE: Slateworkers' pneumoconiosis, *Human Pathol* 23:1098-1105, 1992.

112. Gibbs AR, Craighead JE, Pooley FD, et al: The pathology of slate workers' pneumoconiosis in North Wales and Vermont, In Dodgson J, McCallum RI, Bailey MR, et al, editors: *Inhaled particles VI,* pp 273-278, Oxford, 1988, Pergamon.

113. McDermott M, Bevan C, Cotes JE, Bevan MM, and Oldham PD: Respiratory function in slateworkers, *Bull Env Physiopathol Respir* 14:54, 1978.

114. Saiyed HN, Parikh KJ, Ghodasara NB, Sharma YK, Patel GC, et al: Silicosis in slate pencil workers: I. An environmental and medical study, *Am J Ind Med* 8:127-133, 1985.

115. Cochrane AL: An epidemiologist's view of the relationship between simple pneumoconiosis and morbidity and mortality, *Proc R Soc Med* 69:12-24, 1976.

116. Williams N: Potash ore and perforation of the nasal septum, *J Occup Med* 16:383-387, 1974.

117. Markham JW and Tan LK: Concentrations and health effects of potash dust, *Am Ind Hyg Assoc J* 42:671-674, 1981.

118. Graham BL, Dosman JA, Cotton DJ, et al: Pulmonary function and respiratory symptoms in potash workers, *J Occup Med* 26:209-214, 1984.

119. Riddell AR: Clinical investigations into the effects of gypsum dust, *Can Public Health J* 25:147-150, 1934.

120. Forbes JJ, Davenport SJ, and Morgis GG: Review of literature on dusts, *United States Department of the Interior, Bureau of Mines, Bulletin* 478;488, 1950.

121. Schepers GWH, Durkan TM, and Delahunt AB: Biological effects of calcinated gypsum dust, *Arch Ind Health* 12:329-347, 1955.

122. Schepers GWH and Durkan TM: Pathological study of the effects of inhaled gypsum dust on human lungs, *Arch Ind Health* 12:209-217, 1955.

123. Oakes D, Douglas R, Knight K, Wuseman M, and McDonald JC: Respiratory effects of prolonged exposure to gypsum dust, *Ann Occup Hyg* 26:833-840, 1982.

124. Rom WN, Greaves W, Bang KM, Hallthouser M, Campbell D, and Bernstein R: An epidemiologic study of the respiratory effects of trona dust, *Arch Environ Health* 86-92, 1983.

125. Checkoway H, Mathew RM, Hickey JLS, Shy CM, Harris RL, Hunt EW, and Waldman GT: Mortality among workers in the Florida phosphate industry, *J Occup Med* 27:885-892, 1985.

126. Dutton CB, Pigeon MG, Renzi PM, Feustel PJ, Dutton RE, and Renzi GD: Lung function in workers refining phosphorus rock to obtain elementary phosphorus, *J Occup Med* 35:1028-1033, 1993.

127. De Capitani EM: Prevalence of pneumoconioses among phosphate rock workers in Brazil. DHHS (NIOSH), 1990, Pub No 90-108, Part II: 1310-1311.

128. Samara N and Khraisha S: Lung functions in phosphate miners in Jordan: a pilot study, *Am J Ind Med* 16:297-304, 1989.

129. de Villiers AL and Windish JP: Lung cancer in a fluorspar mining community I. Radiation, dust and mortality experience, *Br J Ind Med* 21:94-109, 1964.

130. Desai VK, Bhavsar BS, Mehta NR, Saxena DK, and Kantharia SL: Symptomatology of workers in the fluoride industry and fluorspar processing plants. Fluoride research 1985, *Studies Environ Sci* 27:193-199, 1985.

131. Rees D, Rama DBK, and Yousefi V: Fluoride in workplace air and in urine of workers concentratin fluorspar, *Am J Ind Med* 17:311-320, 1990.

132. Gamble J, Jones W, and Hudak J: An epidemiological study of saltminers in diesel and non-diesel mines, *Am J Ind Med* 4:435-458, 1983.

133. McLaughlin ALG, Grout JLA, Barrie HJ, and Harding HE: Iron oxide dust and the lungs of silver finishers, *Lancet* 337-341, 1945.

134. Gomez SR, Parker RA, Dosman JA, and McDuffie HH: Respiratory health effect of alkali dust in residents near desiccated Old Wives Lake, *Arch Environ Health* 47:364-369, 1992.

Chapter 23

COAL

Michael Attfield
Gregory R. Wagner

Definition of agent
Utilization
History
Overview of effects
    Coal worker's pneumoconiosis
    Progressive massive fibrosis
    Silicosis
    Chronic airways obstruction
    Emphysema
    Other diseases
Risk factors and exposure response
    Effects on ventilatory function
Regulations
Placement considerations
Control methods
Controversies and future concerns

DEFINITION OF AGENT

Coal is comprised primarily of carbonaceous material, chiefly carbon, hydrogen, and oxygen, with some sulfur and many trace elements. However, most occupational exposures in coal mining include various mineral dusts, arising from the cutting of rock and dirt during coal extraction, as well as coal dust. Normally in underground mines, this "coal mine dust" contains between 30% and 40% noncoal minerals, of which 5% is silica, on average. In some situations, particularly for specific occupations such as surface drilling or underground roof bolting, the silica percentage can be much higher.

Mining generates dust particles in a wide range of sizes, lying generally between 1 and 50 μm. The fine dust (respirable dust) deposits in the peripheral regions of the lung and gives rise to coal worker's pneumoconiosis (CWP), silico-

sis, and emphysema. The complicated form of pneumoconiosis, progressive massive fibrosis (PMF), is often associated with disability and premature death. Larger particles (thoracic dust) deposit in the larger airways and can lead to airways obstruction and bronchitis, both of which may be important physiologically and clinically, given sufficient dust exposure.

The current U.S. coal mine dust exposure standards were established in 1969 to prevent advanced CWP. The standards were not designed to prevent other respiratory conditions resulting from dust exposure and, as discussed below, may not be effective for this purpose.

UTILIZATION

World production of coal in 1990 was 5697 million short tons.[1] The major producers in that year were China (22% of the total), the United States (19%), the former U.S.S.R. (15%), and East Germany (6%); India, Poland, Australia, and West Germany were each responsible for about 4%. In 1990, close to 1 billion short tons of coal were produced in the United States, most of which (87%) were used for power generation. Secondary uses for coal were for coke and as a raw material for the production of various chemicals. Currently, coal is little used for residential and commercial heating, although in 1950 the heating category accounted for about 25% of all consumption. Coal is not now used in transportation, though this use figured heavily in the past and may do so in the future (chemical conversion of coal to oil and gasoline).

Coal is obtained through both surface (strip) and underground mining. Since around 1950, U.S. surface production has risen rapidly from 140 to 600 million short tons of coal. This amount has surpassed that of underground mining, which has remained fairly level at 300 to 400 short tons.[1] Much of this rise in production has taken place in surface mines west of the Mississippi, with production in the east remaining relatively stationary. Bituminous coal has always comprised most of the coal extracted in the United States, but it is now in competition with western and southern subbituminous and lignite coals, production of which has risen from virtually zero in 1970 to about 330 million short tons in 1990. In contrast, anthracite mining, ever a small part of the industry, had declined to 4 million short tons by 1990.

Figure 23-1, which shows coal mine employment and production from 1950 to 1990, reveals the dramatic drop in employment that occurred after 1950 in the wake of mine mechanization. Production remained level despite many fewer workers.[1] Production and productivity has increased further in recent years, and the work force continues to decline.

Coal is produced in surface mines by removal of overburden, often using drilling, blasting, and bulldozer operations, followed by coal extraction and transportation. The risk to workers arises mostly from rock drilling, as dust exposures for other workers are generally low (1 mg/m^3 or below) because of the natural ventilation.[2] Although only a small minority of surface miners are drillers, their risk of disease can be high due to the intense exposures often experienced, mainly because of inadequate dust control methods and the practical difficulty in enforcing the dust standard.

In underground coal mining, the coal is reached by shafts and tunnels (headings), and the coal extracted using various types of coal cutting machines. There are two most commonly used techniques. One is the use of continuous miner machines, which are employed to extract the coal in "rooms," leaving pillars of coal to support the roof. A more modern method being used increasingly is the longwall face, which employs a cutter that takes out a long slice of the coal seam, leaving the roof to collapse behind it. Since the latter method is very productive, dust exposures can be difficult to control. In either method, each face (or section) employs about six miners per shift.

Among underground coal miners, it is the coal face workers who generally receive the most dust exposure,

with longwall miners being at the greatest risk due to the higher dust levels intrinsic to the method. Roof bolters, who drill into the rock, may be at risk from the silica dust. General principles of mining work are discussed further in Chapter 38.

HISTORY

Coal mining has been reported as far back as A.D. 852 in Europe. In America, coal was first discovered in 1673; the first reported production occurred in Virginia in 1748. There was an early appreciation that exposure to coal mine dust was hazardous to health. As noted by Meiklejohn,[3] George Steele commented in 1834, "It would afford me much gratification if any means could be devised as regards either prevention or remedy, whereby might be lessened the evils of a disease, the ravages of which, upon the most robust constitutions, I have every day cause to deplore."

Unfortunately, Steele's point of view was not shared by many of his later colleagues. In fact, it was not until one hundred years later, in 1940, that CWP was officially differentiated from silicosis for certification purposes in the United Kingdom. As late as 1960 it was being said, "The attitude of the medical profession in the United States has been, and still is, characterized by obscurantism and a persistent refusal to face the facts."[4]

Revelations following the 1968 Farmington mine disaster in West Virginia, however, brought home to the public the hidden human costs that were being paid by the coal miners, and federal legislation followed swiftly in an attempt to rectify the problems. The 1969 Coal Mine Health and Safety Act mandated four activities: first, a reduction in dust levels in underground mines to 3 mg/m^3, to be followed by a reduction to 2 mg/m^3 in 1972; second, the introduction of a radiologic surveillance program, whereby

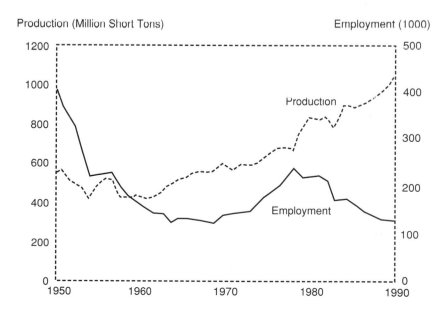

Fig. 23-1. Coal mining production and employment from 1950 to 1990.

miners with pneumoconiosis could work in lower dust environments and have their exposures monitored more frequently; third, research was to begin on preventing disease and accidents in the mines; fourth, a program for awarding medical and financial benefits to underground coal miners demonstrating certain signs of lung disease, caused or exacerbated by their coal mine employment, was instituted.

Epidemiologic research into the diseases of coal miners began in Britain around 1950, when the British Medical Research Council began a series of population studies in coal mining areas. These useful studies were complemented by a comprehensive epidemiologic investigation, the Pneumoconiosis Field Research, which began in 1952.[5] This massive study, which employed industrial hygienists stationed permanently at each mine to collect exposure measurements continuously, has provided an enormous amount of information about the extent of lung disease in coal miners in relation to dust exposure. In the United States, a parallel study was begun in 1970, following the mandate of the Coal Mine Health and Safety Act.[6] This study is continuing and has provided many findings of particular relevance to U.S. miners.

In addition to epidemiologic research, over the years a considerable amount of pathologic, clinical, and laboratory research has been undertaken on the lung diseases associated with coal mining. Much has concentrated on CWP and its causes.

OVERVIEW OF EFFECTS

Coal worker's pneumoconiosis is the disease unambiguously associated with exposure to coal mine dust. It is conventionally divided into two different entities, *simple* and *complicated pneumoconiosis,* with the distinction between the two generally reflecting the differing size of the lesions and their medical implications. *Progressive massive fibrosis,* a term often used synonymously for complicated pneumoconiosis, is the advanced stage of CWP; the risk of the development of PMF rises with the severity of simple pneumoconiosis.

Silicosis may also occur in coal miners, usually in response to exposure to high levels of crystalline silica. This is most often seen in drillers and roof bolters, who drill through rock strata adjacent to the coal seams, and in motormen, who apply sand to the tracks to gain traction when the wheels of the electric locomotives slip. Many underground miners may develop lesions of both silicosis and CWP from mixed dust exposure.

In mining, as in other dusty trades, dust exposure leads to a reduction in ventilatory function and to increased symptoms of cough, phlegm, and breathlessness. Given sufficiently high or sustained exposure, these effects may be clinically important.

Emphysema occurs in response to coal mine dust inhalation. Pathologically, the unique form is that which appears immediately surrounding the pigmented coal dust macule.

Autopsy studies in coal miners have shown that increasing severity of emphysema is observed in the lungs with increasing dust exposure.

It is important to understand that the terminology and definitions used in relation to lung disease arise from various sources, including medical, legal, epidemiologic, and pathologic, as well as lay terms. In the latter category, the term *Black Lung* generally refers to any lung disease or disorder associated with work in coal mining. The legal term, used in the 1969 Coal Mine Health and Safety Act, follows the lay definition. On the other hand, the medical, epidemiologic, and pathologic terminology usually refer to specific elements of disease defined in the context of each discipline.[7] Translation of these terms from one discipline to another is neither exact nor appropriate.

Other terms used, now only of historical interest, are *miners' phthisis, miners' asthma, anthracosis,* and *anthracosilicosis.* The latter term reflects the preoccupation with silica that characterized the early study of the etiology of CWP.

Coal worker's pneumoconiosis

Coal worker's pneumoconiosis has been defined as the deposition of dust in the lungs and the body's reaction to it. This includes the formation of macules, nodules, and lesions of PMF. It is detected in living miners by radiograph almost exclusively, the International Labor Organization (ILO) classification of the pneumoconioses being employed to define its severity (see Chapter 7).[8] Coal worker's pneumoconiosis is conventionally divided into two disease processes: *simple* and *complicated.*

Pathologically, the characteristic lesion of simple CWP is the dust *macule,* an inflammatory lesion near the respiratory bronchioles that is 1 to 5 mm in size, consisting of collections of dust-laden macrophages.[9] Reticulin is present in the macules, though there is minimal collagen. The distension or destruction of nearby alveolar walls leads to emphysema. With advancing disease, the macules tend to coalesce, and nodules are formed. In contrast to the macules, the nodules are firm and palpable, range in size from 2 to 10 mm, and show collagenous fibers. They are distinguishable from silica nodules by their pigmentation and by the pattern of collagen fibers, which is disorganized, as compared with the distinct whorled picture in silicotic nodules.

Chest radiographs of miners with simple CWP often reveal small opacities, which are the result of the attenuation of the x-ray beam by the inflammatory changes in the lung (macules and nodules) in association with the dust deposits. For the most part, there is a good correlation between the profusion of small opacities, as seen on the radiograph, and the number and size of the pathologic abnormalities.[10] It is clear, however, that a substantial degree of dust deposition has to take place before the effects are evident on the radiograph. Hence, the chest radiograph is not a sensitive indicator of early simple CWP.

Radiologically, simple CWP is classified according to the standardized system promulgated by the ILO.[8] Under this system, films are placed into major categories labeled 1, 2, and 3, determined by the increasing profusion of small opacities, with category 0 being used to indicate the absence of opacities. A secondary score (e.g., 2/1) is used to provide more detailed information on the opacity profusion within the major category. The opacities of simple CWP tend to be seen predominantly in the upper lung zones. The principal type of opacity seen lies in the 1.5 to 3 mm range (ILO type *q*), followed by the *p* type (<1.5 mm), with type *r* (3 to 10 mm) being the least frequent (and perhaps more associated with silicosis). Although rounded opacities have traditionally been associated with CWP, there has been an increased interest in, and reporting of, irregular opacity types *(s, t, u)*.[11]

Miners with simple CWP, particularly in its initial stages, may have little measurable physiologic abnormality and few clinical signs or symptoms. However, the condition is not to be ignored, for its presence is associated with greatly increased risk of developing the clinically important PMF. This risk rises with each increasing radiographic category of simple CWP. For instance, in one detailed study, the risk of developing PMF from ILO category 2 was about six times that for category 0.[12]

In general, studies have not shown particularly elevated mortality rates among individuals with radiographic simple CWP. This observation is mainly a reflection of the benign nature of simple CWP in its early stages, combined with a lack of statistical power to detect effects in the much smaller number of miners with category 2 and 3 CWP. It is important to note, however, that survival clearly decreases with increasing dust exposure, regardless of CWP status.[13]

Coal worker's pneumoconiosis frequently accompanied work in coal mining in the past. However, the dust control measures introduced in the United States since 1970 appear to have resulted in the reduction, but not the elimination,

of disease. Figure 23-2 shows the prevalence of ILO category 1 (or greater) by years in coal mining from 1971 to 1988 for U.S. underground miners.[14] For miners with 25 or more years in mining, whose radiographs were taken around 1971 (i.e., for miners who had worked predominantly before the 1969 Act), there was a 30% prevalence of CWP. Subsequently, the prevalences for that tenure group have dropped considerably, to below 20% between 1985 and 1988. Moreover, miners employed for 15 to 19 years have shown a threefold drop in prevalence, these being the group that in 1988 would have worked only under the lower dust conditions mandated by the 1969 Act. One disturbing trend, however, is the indication that disease rates may have risen between 1985 and 1988. This rise may reflect the effect of increased productivity, and hence elevated dust levels, that occurred in mines after 1985. Trends similar to those noted above have been seen for the prevalence of category 2 or greater.

Progressive massive fibrosis

Progressive massive fibrosis consists of large lesions (arbitrarily defined pathologically to be 2 cm or greater in diameter) comprised of dust particles, collagen, reticulin, and dust-engorged macrophages.[9] The lesions tend to occur in the upper regions of the lung and may be unilateral or bilateral and may be rounded or irregular in shape. They may contain cavities of black liquid. The presence of PMF is often associated with other disorders, including emphysema and bronchitis, and cardiovascular changes, such as cor pulmonale.

Radiographically, large opacities (i.e., 1 cm or greater according to the ILO definition) are indicative of PMF in individuals with a history of coal mining. However, there is some evidence that these opacities may be reflecting different entities, in some cases being homogeneous and in others being conglomerations of nodules. Silica exposure has been implicated in the latter type.[15] Since the large

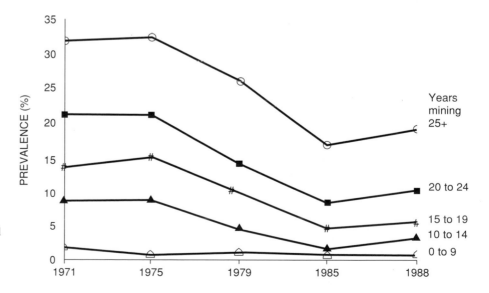

Fig. 23-2. Prevalence of CWP category 1 (or greater) in U.S. underground miners from 1970 to 1990. Year represents midpoint of time period.

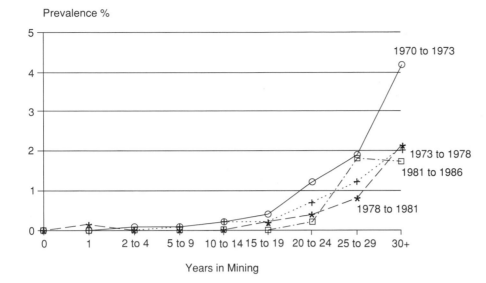

Fig. 23-3. Prevalence of PMF for U.S. underground coal miners for four timeperiods, 1970 to 1986.

opacities are not specific for PMF, other diseases, such as lung carcinoma and tuberculosis, should also be carefully considered, particularly in miners with risk factors for these other conditions. Unilateral lesions, those in atypical locations (e.g., lower lung zone), associated with few or absent small opacities or showing rapid progression, are less likely to represent PMF. Conversely, lesions that are bilateral and relatively symmetric, have been essentially stable for over one year, and occur in miners with prolonged dust exposures and preexisting simple CWP, are suggestive of PMF. Each miner's clinical presentation must be evaluated on an individual basis.

Individuals with PMF typically suffer from chest symptoms, including cough, phlegm, and dyspnea. Impairment and disability can range from minor to severe, with some affected individuals suffering premature mortality. PMF can develop after dust exposure ceases. Furthermore, although the risk of PMF development rises dramatically with each increasing category of simple CWP, it has been shown that some development will occur over 5 years even among miners with a normal initial chest radiography[16] and that the risk is proportional to dust exposure.

In industrialized countries, PMF is now seen much more rarely than in the past. An example of the reduction is seen in Fig. 23-3, which shows the U.S. prevalence rates for four time intervals covering the period from 1970 to 1986.[17] The data for the initial interval shown is applicable to miners who worked prior to the 1969 Act. It should be pointed out that this information may underestimate the true prevalence, as only working miners are included and affected individuals probably left the work force.

Despite the reductions in prevalence of simple CWP and PMF, brought about by the 1969 Coal Mine Health and Safety Act, a legacy of ill health remains. Figure 23-4 shows the number of death certificates with mention of CWP and silicosis for the years 1968 to 1987.[14]

There is no known effective treatment for reversing CWP. Affected individuals should minimize additional dust exposure to the extent possible. Care should be directed at stabilizing or improving overall pulmonary health. In China, therapeutic pulmonary lavage has been used for pneumoconiosis treatment, although its long-term efficacy in preventing disability has yet to be demonstrated.

If CWP is detected early, if dust exposure is reduced thereafter, and if no other lung disease is present, it is likely that many individuals with simple CWP will not suffer any noticeable ill health from the disease itself. This does not mean, however, that dust exposure is of no consequence. Development of simple CWP puts a miner at increased risk of PMF development with the concomitant likelihood of becoming disabled, perhaps even after retirement from mining. Moreover, as described below, dust exposure may lead to other lung diseases, often in conjunction with radiographically apparent CWP, but also frequently in its absence.

Silicosis

Silicosis occurs among coal miners, particularly among those occupations involving drilling into rock. In these cases the disease takes the forms experienced by workers in other industries who suffer excessive silica exposures (see Chapter 24).

Although pure silicosis cases are not common among coal miners, those that do occur have often been severe. For example, eleven cases of silicosis were discovered between 1978 and 1988, seven from a single hospital in West Virginia.[18] The ages of the men ranged from 25 to 51; they had been involved in drilling from 3 to 19 years. Two were suffering from acute silicosis, seven from accelerated silicosis, and two from chronic silicosis. Two had PMF. Two are known to have died shortly after diagnosis.

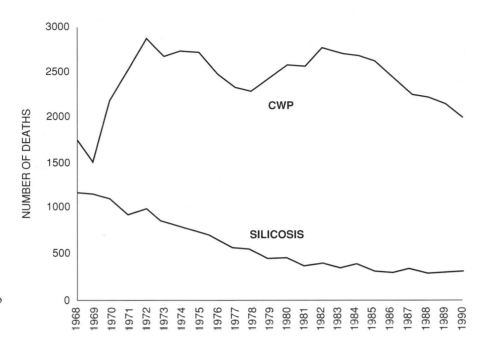

Fig. 23-4. Number of death certificates with mention of CWP or silicosis, 1968 to 1987. (Tabulated from NCHS multiple-cause of death tapes.)

Far more common than outright silicosis is the presence of silica nodules in the lung.[19] These nodules occur together with the lesions commonly associated with CWP (i.e., macules and nodules). The implication of their presence is not clear, though they have been linked with the development of PMF.

Chronic airways obstruction

Work in coal mining is associated with chronic airways obstruction (CAO) as defined by reduced ventilatory function and chest symptoms and also as revealed by pathologic findings of chronic bronchitis and emphysema. Chronic airways obstruction in miners is associated with increased rates of cough, sputum production, breathlessness, and wheezing. In general, the disease is clinically indistinguishable from CAO brought about by other exposures (e.g., smoking). The severity of CAO is dependent on the extent of dust exposure. There is evidence that coal face work can have an effect on ventilatory function that is similar to smoking ½ pack of cigarettes per day.[20]

Chronic airways obstruction in coal miners can occur together with radiographic CWP, or, importantly, in its absence. Hence, a radiograph that is negative for CWP should not be taken to imply the absence of lung disease resulting from coal mine dust exposure.

In general, the treatment and prognosis for CAO in coal miners in the absence of CWP is the same as for nonminers with CAO. The presence of CWP naturally worsens the prognosis.

Emphysema

It is well known that coal miners suffer from emphysema, although there has been debate about its nature and significance. *Focal emphysema* is the form most commonly associated with coal mining, which constitutes a 1 to 2 mm zone of tissue destruction around most of the dust macules. Focal emphysema differs from *centriacinar emphysema* only through its association with the macule and in its often more limited extent.

Emphysema, in general, tends to be more prevalent in coal miners as compared with nonminers and is associated directly with the degree of pneumoconiosis, with the amount of retained dust, with the cumulative prior dust exposure, and inversely with the forced expiratory volume in 1 second (FEV1) percent predicted.[21,22] These relationships imply that the emphysema caused by dust exposure can be important clinically.

Other diseases

Caplan-type opacities are one of a number of different forms of the uncommon "rheumatoid" pneumoconioses. Often appearing with rheumatoid arthritis, these diseases may progress rapidly.

Tuberculosis (TB) has long been associated with mining, mainly because of the miners' poor working and living conditions that occurred in the past. In addition, the presence of silicosis, and perhaps silica exposure alone, increases the risk of mycobacterial infection. With the rise of multiple drug-resistant TB, this issue is of growing importance, although little is currently known about the risk to workers.

No consistent evidence has been found that miners suffer excess mortality from lung cancer. In part, this may be due to the prohibition of smoking underground. However, studies on British and U.S. miners have revealed an elevated level of mortality from stomach cancer. No obvious explanation for this excess has been established, although it could be related to inhaled coal mine dust, which is then cleared and swallowed.

RISK FACTORS AND EXPOSURE RESPONSE

Detailed epidemiologic study relating the incidence of simple CWP to a number of indices of dust exposure in British miners has shown that the predominant factor of importance is simply the degree of mixed mine dust exposure.[23,24] Silica exposure, though long thought to be the critical exposure variable, was found to exert only a secondary influence (at levels around 5% of the mixed mine dust). The latter finding, although surprising initially since silica had long been known to be more toxic in vitro as compared with coal dust, was actually consistent with other epidemiologic findings in that workers exposed to dusts with minimal silica (washed coal and graphite dust) still developed CWP.

Coal rank, a categorization of coal related to hardness and increasing percentage carbon in the coal (going from low rank soft coals [subbituminous] to high rank [anthracite] coals), and which varies inversely with the percent silica, was found to be clearly related to incidence, with disease levels rising with increasing coal rank.[25-27]

To some extent, the rank effect may be a manifestation of the smaller and denser particles that arise from cutting the hard high rank coals, although that explanation does not appear to supply the full answer. One interesting line of research pursued on this topic involves detailed study of individual dust particles. It revolves around the hypothesis that silica particles in coal from lower rank regions are often occluded (thinly coated) by clay minerals and are thereby prevented from exerting their toxic effect on the cells, whereas occlusion occurs seldom in high rank coals because the rocks have been altered by the heating and folding that occurred in those regions.[28] Another theory under investigation involves the toxic effect of the free radicals

generated when rock is cleaved. Free radicals appear in greater concentrations in dusts from high rank coal.

Despite the strong associations between dust exposure and CWP incidence, observed in Britain, the United States, and other countries, there nevertheless remains a high degree of unexplained variability between mines. An intensive epidemiologic study has been made to discover the underlying causes of this variation, but the study has been unsuccessful as of 1994.[29]

The first exposure–response curve for simple CWP was developed on data for British mines and miners.[24] Apart from being the pioneering study, it is of importance in the United States because the results of the study featured heavily in the decision-making process for the current U.S. federal limit on dust in underground mines. The curve, which related 35-year predictions of risk of developing category 2 or greater simple CWP to dust concentration, suggested that zero incidence would be expected around 2 mg/m³. Later British studies of exposure–response for simple CWP confirmed the initial findings,[23] showed that the relationship for former miners was similar to that for current miners,[30] and revealed that smoking did not modify the relationship with dust exposure.[31] The implications of British epidemiologic data for U.S. coal miners and mining has been reviewed.[32]

In the United States, exposure–response relationships for simple CWP were developed for a cross-sectional cohort of working miners studied in 1970 to 1971,[25] the dust exposures being derived from special sampling exercises undertaken in certain U.S. mines in 1968 to 1969, and on data collected by mine operators after 1970.[33] Figure 23-5 shows the observed prevalences from this study by cumulative exposure and coal rank. The results indicated higher predictions of disease than did the British findings at equivalent dust levels. In particular, the prevalence estimate for a 40-year exposure to 2 mg/m³ in medium rank bituminous

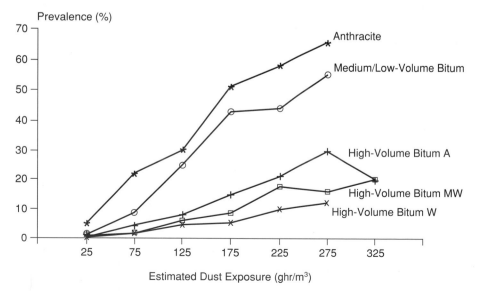

Fig. 23-5. Observed relationship between prevalence of CWP category 1 (or greater) and dust exposure and coal rank.

mines was about 12%. Another more recent U.S. study found a predicted prevalence of about 14% for the same exposure duration and level.[34] Although choice of statistical model is responsible for much of the difference between the later U.S. findings and the initial British predictions (the British model permitting a threshold, whereas the U.S. studies, like later British investigations, did not), it does not explain the entire increase. Factors such as mining methods, work practices, type of coal, dust sampling methods, x-ray readers, and x-ray classification may well have contributed to this discrepancy.

Although much of the older epidemiologic research concentrated exclusively on the profusion of rounded opacities, there has been increasing attention given to the irregular types. It is evident, however, that there is much interreader disagreement on classification of type, which makes study difficult. Some British findings have indicated that there is little prognostic difference between the two types, and thus the principal factor should remain the aggregate profusion score rather than type of opacity.[35]

In summary, the primary variables determining the risk of CWP are the level of mixed coal mine dust and coal rank. Silica is a secondary factor, unless present in large amounts, in which case silicosis will be the outcome.

An in-depth epidemiologic investigation of risk factors for PMF development in British miners revealed that mixed mine dust exposure and coal rank were the primary environmental factors, silica again being a secondary factor.[12,25,36] Other factors of import were category of simple CWP and age of miner. There were also indications that body mass and breathlessness had a bearing on PMF development.

These investigations did not include certain other variables that have long been an issue in PMF development. Of these, tuberculosis has received much attention, at one time being thought necessary for development of PMF. More recent evidence, however, has shown that many cases of PMF develop in the absence of infection.

Until 1989, no exposure–response curve was available for PMF. All previous analyses concentrated on categories of simple CWP as end points. Since that date several relationships have been derived for British miners. One of these relationships examined 5-year incidence of PMF in 52,280 man intervals of risk.[37] Logistic models relating risk of CWP development and progression to dust level, coal rank, age, and simple CWP category, were used to obtain predicted probabilities. These 5-year predicted probabilities were then compounded into 40-year working life risks of PMF development. For medium rank coal mines (such as those mined on the western side of the Appalachian divide), it is predicted that 0.71% of miners would develop PMF after 40 years at 2 mg/m³.

Exposure–response findings for PMF in U.S. coal miners have found cumulative dust exposure, coal rank, and age to be important predictors. Estimated prevalences for me-

dium rank bituminous miners who worked for 40 years in a 2 mg/m³ environment were 2.2% and 1.4% in two different studies.[25,34] Again, it is not clear exactly why the U.S. predictions are higher than those from the British studies, although, as mentioned earlier, it is likely that methodologic variations contribute to real effects of differences in environmental factors.

Effects on ventilatory function

Clear and consistent relationships have been found between dust exposure and ventilatory function in a number of studies by both British and U.S. researchers. These relationships have been detected through examination of absolute measures of function[38-40] and of longitudinal changes.[20,41] Effects were seen in all three smoking groups (never, former, and current), but no synergistic influence of smoking has been detected. This dust effect on ventilatory function is independent of the presence or absence of radiologic CWP.

Both $FEV1$ and forced vital capacity (FVC) appear to decline roughly in parallel with increasing dust exposure, though the $FEV1/FVC$ ratio also declined. This suggests that dust exposure leads to both an obstructive and a restrictive effect on the lung. Some findings suggest that miners, when starting work, experience an initially severe loss in lung function. This appears to be followed by a slower, more chronic decline.[42]

Findings from both sides of the Atlantic suggest that work at the coal face in underground mining may cause changes in $FEV1$ equivalent to the average effect of smoking one pack of cigarettes a day. In particular, severe effects have been demonstrated in one subgroup of coal miners who suffered moderately high exposures.[43] Moreover, a study of measures of indices of respiratory dysfunction (e.g., $FEV1 < 65\%$ of predicted) has shown that moderate to high levels of dust exposure may be as significant as smoking in smoking miners and of major health importance in nonsmokers.[44]

Symptoms of cough and phlegm also increase with dust exposure, both with and without cigarette smoking.[45] Chest symptoms were associated with lower $FEV1$ values, after accounting for age, smoking, dust exposure, and other factors.[39] Importantly, bronchitis and emphysema mortality has been shown to be related to increasing dust exposure, as manifested by 22-year survival, allowing for age.[13]

Airway responsiveness to dust exposure may be a risk factor for development of chronic obstructive pulmonary disease (COPD). Some initial analyses suggest that miners who are methacholine responsive tend to seek jobs having lower dust exposures.[46] This implies that those who work for long periods in the high-dust jobs may be better able to tolerate the dust. This self-selection would be expected to lead to bias toward underestimation of dust effect in exposure–response studies of lung function and dust exposure.

In summary, dust exposure, as well as smoking, is a risk factor for the development of respiratory symptoms and for ventilatory function decline. Smoking does not appear to modify the relationship of function with dust exposure. The exact pattern of temporal decline in function among those exposed to coal mine dust remains to be elucidated.

REGULATIONS

In the United States, dust levels in the coal mines are regulated by the Mine Safety and Health Administration of the Department of Labor (MSHA). A limit on mixed mine dust is used that varies with the proportion of silica in the dust. When silica comprises less than 5% of the coal mine dust, the standard is 2 mg/m^3 for an 8-hour time weighted average (TWA). When there is more than 5% silica, however, the dust limit is lowered, using the formula 10/% silica. Compliance samples are taken on designated "high risk" workers, who are usually those closest to the coal cutting machines. The rationale for this enforcement strategy is that if the high risk worker is in compliance, all other workers should be protected. Typically, five consecutive samples are taken every 2 months by the mine operator. Ever since the passage of the 1969 Act there have been complaints of irregularities in the sampling collection process. These culminated in the disclosure of widespread tampering in 1989. Since then, MSHA has acted to combat these problems.

The U.S. Occupational Safety and Health Administration (OSHA) regulates exposure in nonmining settings; the limit for coal dust is 2.4 mg/m^3 for dusts with 5% or less silica, and 10/(% quartz + 2) mg/m^3 for dusts with more than 5%, both being 8-hour TWA samples.

The World Health Organization recommends a mine-specific limit that can range from 0.5 to 4 mg/m^3, depending on risk factors for the mine, including coal rank and silica level. Internationally, a number of countries have limits in the 3.5 to 5 mg/m^3 range, applicable when silica is less than 5%, but many reduce the limit proportionately as the silica percentage rises above 5%. A few countries regulate solely on the basis of the silica percentage.

PLACEMENT CONSIDERATIONS

Although the physical demands of coal mining, with some notable exceptions, are not as strenuous as they were when coal was dug manually, miners have to be fit enough to vacate the mine speedily wearing a respirator in the case of fire or explosion. Consideration needs to be given to the placement of workers with existing lung disease to avoid as much as possible further dust exposure.

CONTROL METHODS

Engineering controls in underground mines center around ventilation and water sprays, with scrubbers playing a subsidiary role. Before full-time production can begin on a face, a dust suppression plan has to be drawn up,

tested, and approved by MSHA. This plan is reviewed periodically. Dust exposure is often reduced by miners through use of respirators and special helmets that supply filtered air, whereas remote operation of machines upwind has proved to be an effective way to reduce exposure. Surface operations tend to rely on natural ventilation, although it is essential that drilling machines be fitted with dust retaining skirts and that they use wet drilling. Closed cabs, with conditioned and filtered air, provide an excellent haven from the copious dust clouds of pure silica that can be liberated when drilling.

Underground miners in the United States are provided with a secondary disease prevention measure.[17] This is the Coal Workers' X-ray Surveillance Program (CWXSP), which is a federally run program that enables miners to receive periodic free chest x-rays. If pneumoconiosis is evident on the x-ray, the miner has the right to work in a low-dust job in the mine, at no immediate loss of pay. In addition, personal dust exposure is monitored frequently to confirm that exposures remain low. Unfortunately, this program has not been as successful as intended, due to low participation in the CWXSP and low rates of transfer. However, a campaign of education and streamlining of procedures has recently led to a substantial increase in participation.

CONTROVERSIES AND FUTURE CONCERNS

Despite the facts that coal mining is an ancient occupation and that its ill effects were noted early on, general agreement to reduce dust levels and to provide compensation for affected workers was extremely slow in coming. Today, however, there are few who would challenge the view that CWP is a real occupational disease of significance in coal mining. Unfortunately, the same cannot be said of other lung diseases and dust exposure. There still remains a vocal minority that doubts the severity of nonpneumoconiotic dust effects. Nevertheless, the continually gathering body of information is consistent in indicating that miners suffer from significant lung diseases other than pneumoconiosis as a result of their work in coal mining.

Prevention and control of coal mine dust-related lung disease depends primarily on effective control of exposure to coal mine dust. Nevertheless, secondary prevention strategies can be of value. The right to work in a low-dust job, based on free periodic examinations, is a desirable administrative mechanism for helping to prevent further progression of pneumoconiosis. However, the potential of this strategy to limit all occupational lung disease is hampered by its total focus on the chest radiograph. Consideration needs to be given to alternate secondary prevention strategies, possibly triggered by changes in pulmonary function over time.

Good progress has been made in reducing the prevalence and incidence of CWP over the years since the 1969 Coal Mine Health and Safety Act was passed. It is probable that the reduced dust levels have also led to concomitant reductions in other lung disease. Pressure to improve productivity in recent years, however, has led to higher dust levels, particularly because of the introduction of longwall mining methods. It would be unfortunate if the gains made after 1969 were reversed by this new phase in mining. All parties, including operators, miners, inspectors, and control engineers, will have to work together to maintain the past progress, to ensure that lung disease and its sad social effects can be eliminated once and for all.

REFERENCES

1. Energy Information Administration: *Coal data: a reference,* Washington DC, 1991, U.S. Department of Energy.
2. Amandus HE and Piacitelli G: Dust exposures at U.S. surface coal mines in 1982-1983. *Arch Environ Health* 42:374-381, 1987.
3. Meiklejohn A: History of lung diseases of coal miners in Great Britain: part I, 1800-1875, *Br J Ind Med* 8:127-137, 1951.
4. Morgan WKC: Coalworkers' pneumoconiosis: the clinical features. *Virginia Medical Monthly* 96:712-716, 1969.
5. Fay JWJ and Rae S: The pneumoconiosis field research of the national coal board, *Ann Occup Hyg* 1:149-161, 1959.
6. Attfield MD and Castellan RM: Epidemiological data on U.S. coal miners' pneumoconiosis, 1960 to 1988. *Am J Public Health* 82:964-970, 1992.
7. Weeks JL and Wagner GR: Compensation for occupational disease with multiple causes: the case of coal miners' respiratory disease. *Am J Public Health* 76:58-61, 1986.
8. International Labour Office: *International classification of radiographs of pneumoconiosis,* (revised edition), Occupational safety and health series no. 22, pp 1-48, Geneva, 1980, International Labour Office.
9. Kleinerman J, Green FHY, Laqueur W, et al: Pathology standards for coal workers' pneumoconiosis. *Arch Pathol Lab Med* 103:375-432, 1979.
10. Attfield MD, Vallyathan V, and Green FHY: Radiographic appearances of small opacities and their correlation with pathology grading of macules, nodules, and dust burden in the lungs. In Dodgson J, editor: *Inhaled Particles VII, Ann Occup Hyg* 38(suppl.1): 783-789, 1994.
11. Collins HPR, Dick JA, Bennett JG, et al: Irregularly shaped small shadows on chest radiographs, dust exposure, and lung function in coalworkers' pneumoconiosis, *Br J Ind Med* 45:43-55, 1988.
12. Maclaren WM, Hurley JF, Collins HPR, and Cowie AJ: Factors associated with the development of progressive massive fibrosis in British coalminers: a case-control study. *Br J Ind Med* 46:597-607, 1989.
13. Miller BG and Jacobsen M. Dust exposure, pneumoconiosis, and mortality of coal miners. *Br J Ind Med* 42:723-733, 1985.
14. Althouse RB, Castellan RM, and Wagner GR: Pneumoconioses in the United States: highlights of surveillance data from NIOSH and other federal sources, *Occ Med* 7:197-208, 1992.
15. Soutar CA and Collins HPR: Classification of progressive massive fibrosis of coalminers by type of radiographic appearance. *Br J Ind Med* 41:334-339, 1984.
16. Hurley JF, Alexander WP, Hazledine DJ, Jacobsen M, and Maclaren WM: Exposure to respirable coalmine dust and incidence of progressive massive fibrosis. *Br J Ind Med* 44:661-672, 1987.
17. Attfield MD and Althouse RB. Surveillance data on U.S. coal miners' pneumoconiosis, 1970 to 1986, *Am J Public Health* 82:971-977, 1992.
18. National Institute for Occupational Safety and Health: Request for assistance in preventing silicosis and deaths in rock drillers, *NIOSH Alert DHHS (NIOSH)* Publication no. 92-107, pp 1-13, Cincinnati, 1992, NIOSH.
19. Green FHY, Althouse R, and Weber KC: Prevalence of silicosis at death in underground coal miners. *Am J Ind Med* 16:605-615, 1989.
20. Attfield MD: Longitudinal decline in FEV1 in United States coalminers, *Thorax* 40:132-137, 1985.
21. Leigh J, Outhred KG, McKenzie HI, Glick M, Wiles AN: Quantified pathology of emphysema, pneumoconiosis, and chronic bronchitis in coal workers. *Br J Ind Med* 40:258-263, 1983.
22. Ruckley VA, Gauld SJ, Chapman JS, et al: Emphysema and dust exposure in a group of coal workers. *Am Rev Respir Dis* 129:528-532, 1984.
23. Hurley JF, Burns J, Copland L, Dodgson J, and Jacobsen M: Coal-workers' simple pneumoconiosis and exposure to dust at 10 British coalmines. *Br J Ind Med* 39:120-127, 1982.
24. Jacobsen M, Rae S, Walton WH, and Rogan JM: The relation between pneumoconiosis and dust exposure in British coal mines. In Walton WH, editor: *Inhaled Particles III,* pp 903-919, Old Woking, England, 1971, Unwin Brothers.
25. Attfield MD and Morring K: An investigation into the relationship between coalworkers' pneumoconiosis and dust exposure in U.S. coal miners. *Am Ind Hyg Assoc J* 53:486-492, 1992.
26. Robock K and Bauer HD: Investigations into the specific fibrogenicity of mine dusts in hardcoal mines of countries in the European Community. In Anonymous, editor: *Proceedings of the VIIth international pneumoconiosis conference, Part 1,* Pittsburgh, 1988, DHHS (NIOSH) publication no. 90-108, pp 280-283, Cincinnati, 1990, DHHS (NIOSH).
27. Walton WH, Dodgson J, Hadden GG, and Jacobsen M. The effect of quartz and other non-coal dusts in coalworkers' pneumoconiosis. In Walton WH, editor: *Inhaled Particles IV, Volume 2,* pp 669-689, Old Woking, England, 1977, Unwin Brothers.
28. Wallace WE, Harrison JC, Grayson RL, et al: Aluminosilicate surface contamination of respirable quartz particles from coal mine dusts and from clay works dusts, *Ann Occup Hyg* 38(suppl.1): 439-446, 1994.
29. Crawford NP, Bodsworth FL, and Dodgson J: A study of the apparent anomalies between dust levels and pneumoconiosis at several British collieries. In Walton WH, editor: *Inhaled Particles V,* pp 725-744, Oxford, United Kingdom, 1982, Pergamon.
30. Soutar CA, Maclaren WM, Annis R, and Melville AWT: Quantitative relations between exposure to respirable coalmine dust and coalworkers' simple pneumoconiosis in men who have worked as miners but have left the industry, *Br J Ind Med* 43:29-36, 1986.
31. Jacobsen M, Burns J, and Attfield MD: Smoking and coalworkers' simple pneumoconiosis. In Walton WH, editor: *Inhaled Particles IV,* pp 759-772, Oxford, 1977, Pergamon.
32. Attfield MD: British data on coal miners' pneumoconiosis and relevance to U.S. conditions, *Am J Public Health* 82:978-983, 1992.
33. Attfield MD and Morring K: The derivation of estimated dust exposures for U.S. coal miners working before 1970, *Am Ind Hyg Assoc J* 53:248-255, 1992.
34. Attfield MD: Prevalence of pneumoconiosis and its relationship to dust exposure in a cohort of U.S. bituminous coal miners and ex-miners. *Am J Ind Med* 1994, 27:137-151, 1994.
35. Miller BG, Campbell SJ, Cowie HA, et al: The natural history and implications of irregularly-shaped small shadows on coalminers' chest radiographs, report no. TM/90/01. pp 1-111, Edinburgh, Scotland, 1990, Institute of Occupational Medicine.
36. Becklake MR: Chronic airflow limitation: its relationship to work in dusty occupations, *Chest* 88:608-617, 1985.
37. Hurley JF and Maclaren WM: Dust-related risks of radiological changes in coalminers over a 40-year working life: report on work commissioned by NIOSH, report no. TM/87/09. pp 1-66, Edinburgh, Scotland, 1987, Institute of Occupational Medicine.
38. Attfield MD and Hodous TK: Pulmonary function of U.S. coal miners related to dust exposure estimates, *Am Rev Respir Dis* 14:605-609, 1992.
39. Rogan JM, Attfield MD, Jacobsen M, Rae S, Walker DD, and Walton WH: Role of dust in the working environment in development of

chronic bronchitis in British coal miners, *Br J Ind Med* 30:217-216, 1973.

40. Soutar CA and Hurley JF: Relation between dust exposure and lung function in miners and ex-miners, *Br J Ind Med* 43:307-320, 1986.

41. Love RG and Miller BG: Longitudinal study of lung function in coal miners. *Thorax* 37:193-197, 1982.

42. Seixas NS, Robins TG, Attfield MD, and Moulton LH: Exposure–response relationships for coal mine dust and obstructive lung disease following enactment of the Federal Coal Mine Health and Safety Act of 1969, *Am J Ind Med* 21:715-734, 1992.

43. Hurley JF and Soutar CA: Can exposure to coalmine dust cause a severe impairment of lung function? *Br J Ind Med* 43:150-157, 1986.

44. Marine WM, Gurr D, and Jacobsen M: Clinically important respiratory effects of dust exposure and smoking in British coal miners, *Am Rev Respir Dis* 137:106-112, 1988.

45. Rae S, Walker DD, and Attfield MD: Chronic bronchitis and dust exposure in British coalminers. In Walton WH, editor: *Inhaled Particles III*. pp 883-896, Old Woking, 1971, Unwin Brothers.

46. Mannino DM, Daniloff E, Peck A, and Petsonk EL: Do miners select jobs based on airway responsiveness? *Am Rev Respir Dis* 143:a264 (Abstract), 1991.

Chapter 24

SILICA

Gerald S. Davis

DEFINITIONS

Silicosis is a chronic diffuse interstitial fibronodular lung disease caused by long-term inhalation of dust containing free crystalline silica. Crystalline silica can cause several forms of silicosis and can also produce chronic industrial bronchitis among exposed workers. Silicosis may be associated with chronic indolent tuberculosis. Data suggest that silica exposure is linked to an increased risk for the development of lung cancer.

Silicosis is still a significant health problem in industrialized nations, although it is far less prevalent than it was from 1920 through 1945. Although national statistics may underestimate the problem, death certificate statistics compiled by the National Institute for Occupational Safety and Health (NIOSH) recorded 2152 deaths due to silicosis in the United States between 1975 and 1986.[1,2] Silicosis remains a common and disabling lung disease in developing nations where dust controls and other industrial hygiene measures have not yet been adopted to achieve a safe workplace.

Exposure to silica occurs by inhalation of dry mineral particles of respirable size (0.2 to 10 μm aerodynamic diameter). The element silicon (Si) is abundant and widely distributed in nature, comprising approximately 25% of the earth's crust. It is usually complexed with oxygen to form silica (SiO_2) or with other anions and oxygen to form various silicates. Silica (SiO_2) occurs in crystalline forms and in amorphous forms. Among the crystalline polymorphs, *quartz* is the most abundant and is the form usually associated with human disease. *Cristobalite* and *trydamite* are less common but are more biologically active on an equal weight basis and can cause disease with appropriate exposure. *Stishovite* and *coesite* appear to be less toxic. All of these crystalline forms have the same chemical formula, and all assume the shape of a tetrahedron (4 oxygen atoms shared by 2 silicon atoms), except stishovite, which is configured as an octahedron. The exact dimensions and shape of the crystal lattice differ among the polymorphs and may be related to fibrogenicity. The surface properties of the particles appear to be critical in conferring the biological properties of crystalline silica.

Natural stone may be almost pure crystalline silica, such as beach sand or sandstone, or it may be a mixture of silica particles with other minerals and silicates, as in granite, shale, or basalt. Working with these rocks may liberate respirable particles of crystalline silica, thus causing silicosis. Pneumoconioses, produced by silicates and other mixed dusts, are discussed elsewhere in this book.

The amorphous, noncrystalline forms of silica occur in nature as diatomaceous earth, the skeletons of marine organisms (see below) and as vitreous silica or volcanic glass. The amorphous forms of silica do not cause silicosis as readily as the crystalline forms and are classified as nuisance dusts. As discussed in relation to the diatomaceous earth industry, opinions differ as to the degree to which amorphous silica alone is hazardous. High-temperature processes may convert noncrystalline materials into crystalline forms, including cristobalite. This sequence occurs in the mining and processing of diatomaceous earth and in certain applications of ceramic fibers.[3] Hence, any occupational exposure to silica may potentially be hazardous if the intensity and duration of exposure are extensive.

EXPOSURE TO SILICA

The industries and avocations where there is a risk of silicosis are numerous; some of the more common ones are listed here (see box). These can be grouped broadly into trades where rock is drilled or removed from the earth (mining, quarrying), trades where silica-bearing stone is worked to produce other products (sculpting, cutting), jobs utilizing abrasives containing silica (tool grinding, sand blasting) or where abrasives are directed at a stone surface (building cleaning), and occupations where powdered silica is used as a raw material or an additive in manufacturing (glass, paint, plastics). The critical elements in all of these trades

---

Occupations with exposure to silica

Hard rock mining
Tunnel drilling
Stone quarrying
Stone crushing
Granite monument carving
Stone sculpting
Stone masonry
Foundry casting
Abrasive blasting
Tool grinding
Knife sharpening
Silica flour production
Diatomaceous earth production
Glass manufacture
Plastics manufacture
Paint manufacture
Pottery
Ceramic manufacture

---

are the crystalline free silica content of whatever dust aerosol may be generated, the concentration of particles in the air, and the duration of exposure (see Dose–effect–risk relationships in silicosis), as modified by the health and susceptibility of each worker. The nature of the industry and the work habits of the individual will affect greatly the interplay of these factors. Some of the more widespread exposures will be discussed in detail.

Hard rock mining

Underground mines for the extraction of ores and minerals, such as gold, tin, iron or coal, usually require drilling and removal of large quantities of bedrock to follow the valuable vein. Although coal causes a distinct pneumoconiosis (see Chapter 14), coal miners may also receive substantial exposure to silica as they remove hard bedrock surrounding the coal veins. The bedrock surrounding ores is usually shale, granite, basalt, or a similar stone that is rich in quartz and silicates. As tunnels and drifts are created along the ore veins, respirable particles of crystalline silica are generated by the destruction of the bedrock by mechanized drills and explosive blasting. Mining processes are described in Chapter 38.

Lung disease in miners, caused by dust, has been recognized since antiquity and was described by Hippocrates. Detailed discussions of the exposure conditions and disease in Cornish tin miners appeared in the 19th century. Extensive modern reports of silicosis in miners have included gold miners in South Africa,[4] iron-ore miners in Sweden,[5] and precious-metal miners in Canada.[6,7] A detailed discussion of the work conditions, exposure levels, and dust control methods in the coal mining industry has been published.[8]

Modern underground mining techniques, coupled with government safety regulations, have reduced, but not eliminated, the risk of silicosis. Automated machinery has improved work conditions for those remaining in mining industries in highly developed countries. Machines have replaced many workers, decreasing the number exposed, and have enabled some of those remaining workers to move back from the cutting face. Machinery permits larger tunnels to be dug and the removal of larger pieces of rock with less disintegration of stone. Better techniques for handling water and air permit greater application of wet-cutting methods and improved ventilation. These measures are expensive and require high technology. Developing countries still utilize human labor rather than machines to mine ores at relatively low cost in world-trade pricing. Silicosis in miners remains a tremendous public health problem in China, Eastern Europe, and parts of Africa and South America.

Tunnel drilling

Cutting tunnels for roads and rail lines through mountains or under rivers can expose tunnel drillers and caisson workers to extremely high levels of airborne silica. The work conditions are similar to mining, but the stone is often harder and with a higher silica content, and adequate ventilation may be more difficult. Silicosis received wide public attention in the United States in 1936 when almost 500 men died and 1500 were disabled near the town of Gauley Bridge, West Virginia, as a result of silica dust exposure that occurred while tunneling through a mountain.[9,10] Dust levels were so high that the men could see only a few feet before them. Adequate safety precautions were not taken, although the risk of silicosis was well recognized. This incident, along with recognition of major health problems in the granite industry, foundries, and other trades, led to public outcry and government regulations to protect workers from silicosis.

Granite quarrying and carving

Granite for building stone, cemetery monuments, and sculpture has been quarried from hills of Barre, Vermont since the late eighteenth century. The Barre, Vermont granite industry serves as an example of similar industries throughout the world. Granite is a hard igneous rock, whose strength, durability against weathering, and pleasing gray color and texture make it well suited for construction and decorative purposes. The respirable particles of Barre granite contain 9% to 14% free crystalline silica as quartz, 16% mica, 65% to 70% feldspar, and 6% other mixed silicates.[11] The first stage in processing is the removal of large blocks of granite from the mountainside. Using modern techniques, the stone in the mountain is drilled with water-immersed bits and is cut using high temperature oil-fueled torches; explosive blasting would weaken the material. There is low dust exposure in quarry work, since little fracturing of stone occurs. In former times, dry drilling, cutting, and blasting generated substantial dust and silicosis was prevalent among quarrymen. Quarry workers comprise about 10% of an industry that now employs approximately 1500 people.

The large blocks of quarried granite are transported to sheds for further processing by several large employers and many smaller businesses and family sheds. In the granite sheds, the rough stone is cut into smaller cubes for building stone and grave monuments, using large diamond saws. The blocks are then further shaped and polished with various abrasives to achieve a smooth surface. Memorial inscriptions are carved into the stone with hand or pneumatic chisels or "sandblasted" using iron-based, nonsilica abrasive. Carving of decorations or three-dimensional sculpture on blocks is accomplished using a combination of hand tools, hammers, and chisels, as well as air- and motor-driven power tools. Final smoothing and polishing is achieved with abrasives.

High levels of silica were common in the granite sheds in earlier times. During the nineteenth century most of the quarrying, cutting, and carving operations were performed by hand. Hand tools generate relatively little dust, particularly finely divided respirable particles, and thus silicosis

was probably not a major health problem. Mechanization changed the atmosphere dramatically. In the 1890s pneumatic drills and chisels, power saws, and grinders were developed. Edging saws, honing saws, and sandblasting were introduced in 1910 to 1915. The power tools permitted much more efficient production, and the industry prospered. The peak of employment in 1915 involved more than 15,000 workers in the industry. The new power tools generated large amounts of finely divided dust, made more dangerous by the close proximity of the craftsman to the cutting surface. The workers were aware of this hazard. The first labor strike occurred in 1909 over the use of the "bumper," described by a contemporary source as "a machine to which the union objected because it jeopardized the health of the worker on account of the large volume of dust it created."[12]

The health risks of dusty trades in general, and the granite industry in particular, became apparent during the 1920s, culminating in a report by Russell in 1929 from the U.S. Public Health Service.[13] The granite industry management group, workers unions, and the Vermont State Health Department worked together throughout the 1930s and 1940s to improve dusty conditions and create a safe working environment. Water that was sprayed on cutting and grinding surfaces kept dust down. Vacuum hose air extractors, positioned just above cutting surfaces, removed air-borne particles. Improved ventilation in closed sheds reduced ambient dust levels. Today, individual positive forced air respirator hoods are used for dusty tasks, such as abrasive blasting, in addition to these more general controls. Measured dust levels now fall within government standards and silicosis has been virtually eliminated from the granite industry.[14]

Foundry work

Casting of ferrous and nonferrous metals is often performed with molds of sand and clay. Hollow structures are produced by the insertion of a space-occupying core into the mold. In addition to the sand or ceramic used for the mold, the casting may be coated with silica flour powder to facilitate removal. Residue from the mold or core remains adherent to the casting, and its removal often requires mechanical means, which can aerosolize quantities of silica. The high temperatures endured by the molds may convert other forms of silica to the more toxic polymorph cristobalite, and quartz dust from the sand is liberated as well. Surveys indicate that silicosis is still a problem in the foundry industry.[15-17]

Ceramic materials, composed of various mixtures of aluminum silicates and other minerals and clays, are replacing pure silica or sand for forming foundry-mold facings. They are also being used for insulation and support structures in furnaces. The ceramic products may be less expensive and they provide better durability and finer resolution in the casting process. These materials may be powders or fibers and are generally composed of amorphous silica or silicates. Unfortunately, they are converted to cristobalite in the high temperature industrial furnaces used for casting, and substantial exposure to crystalline silica may occur. A survey of foundries utilizing ceramic fibers for furnace linings demonstrated that these fibers devitrify with high heat and undergo conversion to cristobalite during cooling; substantial airborne levels may be generated during removal of this insulation.[3] Ambient levels of crystalline silica exceeded permissible exposure levels in two foundries using aluminum silicate synthetic mullite to line molds.[18] At plant locations where molds were shaken out and residual casting material was ground off of the metal cast, dust levels measured 7- to 25-fold above permissible levels and were composed of 3% to 41% cristobalite.

Abrasive cleaning

Sandblasting is an important cause of silicosis.[19,20] Exposure occurs when a high pressure, air-driven stream of sand is directed against a steel or stone surface to clean or smooth the surface. Abrasive cleaning is widely used in shipyards to clean steel plates before painting, in boiler maintenance to scale and clean boilers, and similarly in other applications.[21] Without adequate dust controls, sandblasting can result in nodular silicosis in a relatively short period of exposure (5 to 7 years)[22] and can produce accelerated or acute silicosis. The use of sand in abrasive cleaning is declining in the United States, and its use in Great Britain and Europe has been outlawed. Abrasive sand has been replaced by iron carbide slag, steel shot, and other nonsiliceous particulates. However, if the target of abrasive cleaning is siliceous, even steel shot or other blasting media may be associated with a risk of silicosis. Thus, carving letters or other artwork into grave markers or monuments with an air driven stream of abrasive, and cleaning architectural stone, can expose the worker to hazardous dusts.

Silica flour production

Silica flour, sometimes called *tripoli*, is finely divided powdered silica, usually almost pure quartz, manufactured by crushing and milling quartzite ore, sand, or sandstone.[2] Silica flour is used as an additive or thickener in paints, plastics, and cosmetics, as an abrasive, and for other industrial applications. The fine powder is readily thrown up into a respirable aerosol, particularly since it is usually manufactured and utilized in dry form. Workers may be exposed to silica flour aerosols both during primary manufacture and during the secondary application of the raw material in other industries.

A survey of two silica flour mills in Illinois in 1979 revealed a significant problem in this industry.[23] In both mills, the mean respirable silica dust concentration for all inspections was more than 5 times the permitted limit. The samples proved to be 95% to 98% crystalline silica, with particle mass median aerodynamic diameters of 2.3 to 5.2 μm; more than 90% of the particles were in the respirable range. Twenty-three of 61 workers (37%) with more than 1 year of exposure had radiographic evidence of silicosis. Conglomerate lesions of progressive massive fibrosis (PMF) were found in seven cases, of whom six had less than 10 years of work exposure. Most workers with PMF, and a few with simple silicosis, had abnormal lung function attributable to their occupation. Other individual cases describe silicosis with less than 5 years of exposure to silica flour manufacture.[24] These surveys document that clinically significant silicosis can develop rapidly in response to silica flour and that high exposure levels to this material can occur in modern processing plants.

The respiratory hazards of silica flour should be considered in secondary industries that employ this material as an abrasive, a lubricant, or an additive. Specific occupations that may involve exposure to silica flour include fine polishing using tripoli as an abrasive, rubber goods manufacture, where the powder serves as a dry lubricant in molds and on the final product, plastics and paints, where silica flour is used as a thickening agent, and cosmetics manufacture, where the powder is used as a carrier for other materials. In many of these applications, the exposure may be limited to workers who empty bags of dry silica flour into machines where it will be combined with other ingredients. The exposures may episodic and brief, but intense.

Diatomaceous earth mining and milling

Diatomaceous earth (diatomite, kieselguhr) is a fine-grained material composed of the remains of microscopic marine and fresh-water plants known as diatoms. Their skeletons are composed of biologically synthesized amorphous silica. Deposits of diatomaceous earth throughout the world are mined to produce the commercial product, at an annual yield of approximately 1,800,000 tons.[25] In the United States, large deposits near Santa Barbara, California are the main source of this powder. Diatomaceous earth is widely used for liquid filtration and chromatography, as a filler in the manufacture of paints and other products, and as an insulating material. The diatomaceous earth may be used directly, as mined, after crushing and drying to a powder, or it may be calcined by heating to between 800° C and 1000° C. The calcining may done directly to the raw powder, or a flux of sodium bicarbonate or sodium chloride may be added. The raw diatomaceous earth contains approximately 4% quartz, presumably from natural rock sources. When the mined diatomaceous earth is heated and then cooled, some of the amorphous silica is converted to cristobalite. The plain-calcined and flux-calcined diatomaceous earth products contain 10% to 20% and 20% to 25% cristobalite, respectively.[26]

Major health problems in Californian diatomaceous earth miners and millers became apparent in the early 1930s and were described in the landmark report by Legge and Rosencrantz.[26a] They noted that:

The menace is due to vast clouds of dust which escape and endanger the immediate workers and are also disseminated by the prevailing winds over the district where the employees reside. At the mill the bag house is very dusty, as well as the packing quarters where the product is sacked; also where bricks are made by being sawed.

Pneumoconiosis by x-ray was present in 68.5% of the 108 workers surveyed with a clear dose–time–effect relationship. Disease developed in fewer than 5 years in many cases. Tuberculosis as well as silicosis was prevalent.

Remarkably, this occupational health problem was largely ignored or denied for 20 years. In 1952, the workers of the International Chemical Workers Union (AFL–CIO) went on strike at the Johns Manville diatomaceous earth plant in Lompoc, California and made health protection their key issue.[25] A public exposé, several federal and state surveys, and substantial worker pressure together resulted in recognition of the silicosis caused by this work environment. Extensive workplace dust control measures were undertaken and ambient dust levels were greatly reduced. Worker health surveys in the 1950s revealed a high prevalence of pneumoconiosis, including workers who had been exposed only to the raw, uncalcined diatomaceous earth. Abrams concluded that the amorphous form of this silica could cause symptomatic lung disease, although higher exposures were required for the crystalline materials.[27] Whether silicosis in diatomaceous earth workers is due to amorphous silica alone, the quartz fraction only, or a combined effect, remains controversial.

Modern studies show relatively little pneumoconiosis among Californian diatomaceous earth workers who began work after the imposition of dust controls. Chest radiographic evidence of compatible abnormalities (International Labor Organization [ILO] score 1/0 or greater) were found in 5% of 490 workers, with an association between the presence and degree of abnormality and the extent of exposure to total dust and to cristobalite.[28] A retrospective cohort mortality study shows an excessive rate of lung cancer and of nonmalignant respiratory disease (NMRD), excluding infectious disease and pneumonia, in this industry with a direct relationship to exposure intensity.[26] The excess respiratory disease was attributable to pneumoconiosis.

Other occupational exposures

Glass making may expose workers to several polymorphs of silica as a result of the high temperatures involved in the manufacturing process. Quartz abrasives are occasionally used in polishing glass articles. Refractory brick workers produce silica-rich products for use in high temperature furnaces employed in the steel and iron industries. These refractories often use crushed sandstone as a raw material and, therefore, an increased risk of silicosis may result.

The clay used for ceramics may have a high silica content and can expose commercial, artisan, or hobby pottery workers to silicosis. The china and ceramics industry, once notable for the incidence of silicosis, has been moving away from siliceous components in their products and has been using alumina rather than silica as a bed for firing articles, thus reducing the occupational hazard. The Dutch ceramic industry has observed a sizable reduction in the prevalence of silicosis among large industries with rigorous dust controls, whereas the disease remains common among workers in smaller family potteries.[30] A similar pattern of silicosis as a common disease in small workshops and a rare one in larger industries was found in Japan.[31]

Domestic and environmental exposures

Mild forms of chronic simple silicosis can occur from environmental or domestic exposures to silica dust. The Bedouin Arabs of the Sahara inhale dust from sandstorms throughout their lives. Some develop micronodular densities that are visible by chest radiograph and perivascular fibrosis in lung tissue without classic silicosis.[32,33] This simple pneumoconiosis does not appear to be associated with symptoms or clinical impairment. Dust storms in the Himalayas can produce radiographic silicosis among older villagers, some of whom demonstrate progressive massive fibrosis.[34]

HISTORY

Silicosis is an ancient disease, probably experienced, if not recognized, by neolithic miners and stone workers. Hippocrates (460 BC) and Pliny (70 AD) noted the association between mining, dust, and progressive lung disease in Greek and Roman times.[10] Silicosis was clearly defined by the sixteenth century, when Agricola[35] noted the "ailments of miners" and recognized the important role of water, or wet cutting, in reducing dust exposure.

Vivid evidence of silicosis as an ancient disease is provided by the sixteenth century Andean miners who dug for precious metals under the press of the conquering Spaniards.[36] Pneumoconiosis took a devastating toll on the lives of the Indians of South America who were forced to mine copper and gold at high altitude in the Andes mountains following the Spanish conquest. As many as 80,000 Indians were forced into the mines of Peru in the early seventeenth century, but 50 years later only 1674 were available for this labor. The miners climbed ladders down narrow shafts as deep as 1000 feet and returned carrying sacks of ore on their backs. No ventilation was available, and mines had to be closed when the air would no longer support life. The working lifespan of a miner has been estimated to be only 6 to 18 months under these conditions. Autopsy examination of lung tissue from 22 mummies, embalmed and buried about 1575 in a mountain mining community in

Chile, documented extensive pneumoconiosis.[36] Prominent fibrosis, emphysema, and an alveolar process resembling silico-proteinosis were found.

The effects of dust on the lungs of stonecutters were clearly known when Bernardo Ramazzini[37] published *De Morbis Artificum* (Diseases of Workers) in 1700:

We must not underestimate the maladies that attack stone-cutters, sculptors, quarrymen and other such workers. When they hew and cut marble underground or chisel it to make statues and other objects, they often breathe in the rough, sharp, jagged splinters that glance off; hence, they are usually troubled with cough and some contract asthmatic affections and become consumptive. . . . When the bodies of such workers are dissected, the lungs have been found to be stuffed with small stones.

Lung diseases associated with occupations that exposed the workers to stone dust often carried the names of the trades with which they were associated, such as "miners' asthma," "potters' rot," "grinders' consumption," or "stonemasons' disease." No clear distinction was made between tuberculosis (TB), common in the general population, and pneumoconiosis in dusty trades. It is likely that TB complicated silicosis, as was proven in the twentieth century when the diseases could be distinguished definitively.

Not only were the effects of stone dust on respiratory health apparent by the early nineteenth century, but the major concepts of mineral composition and of exposure intensity on the extent of disease were known as well. The poor health of the steel grinders of Sheffield, England, illustrated these concepts to Thackrah[38] in 1832 and to Clark[39] in 1835. A large iron- and steel-forging industry in the midlands employed thousands of workers at various tasks. Many of the pieces that were cast required grinding to remove burrs and to provide a final polish. The sandstone abrasive wheels used by the grinders generated large quantities of respirable silica.[38] Respiratory disease with early death was recognized among workers who ground forks "dry" with abrasive wheels, whereas less severe disease and longer life was apparent among knife sharpeners who used wet stones. The importance for better health of improved ventilation and spraying water onto the rock face in underground ore mines was also well known. Thus little is new in the industrial hygiene of dusty trades. It is remarkable that 100 years later the same observations, concerns, and solutions were being considered in the Vermont granite industry and in the mines of the American South and West.

The mineral causing pneumoconiosis that is associated with many dusty trades was identified by the late nineteenth century, and in 1870 Visconte coined the term *silicosis* to apply to this condition.[10] The clinical features and cause of silicosis had been clearly delineated by the early years of the twentieth century. The importance of the silica content of inhaled dust had been recognized, as Sir William Osler's[40] textbook of 1927 emphasized:

The inhalation of pure silica dust leads very rapidly to serious changes in the respiratory tract. This dust is most often encountered in mining operations and in potteries. In the pottery industry, however, only a few of the workmen are exposed to pure silica. The majority are exposed to the prepared clay, containing a small amount of silica, used in the manufacture of china, and as a result the irritating effects are of much slower evolution. Pure silica produces crippling effects in from six to eight years, while clay dust mixed with silica rarely incapacitates the worker in less than twenty to twenty-five years.[40]

Important historical events in the recognition and control of silicosis have continued throughout the twentieth century. The story is not over, as evidenced by the many current issues discussed throughout this chapter.

HEALTH EFFECTS RELATED TO SILICA EXPOSURE

Silica exposure can adversely affect human health by causing *silicosis* in several forms, by promoting chronic cough and mild airflow obstruction in the form of *industrial bronchitis,* by supporting chronic *tuberculosis* that may be difficult to cure, and by increasing the risk for *lung cancer.* All of these health effects are related to the intensity and the duration of exposure to silica (as detailed below), but the effects are also influenced by concomitant exposures, such as smoking, and by individual susceptibility. The relative and interactive roles of the multiple causative factors in each of these diseases is an area of active research.

Silicosis

Pulmonary silicosis is the classic disease caused by inhalation of crystalline silica particles. The diagnosis of silicosis is established by an appropriate exposure history coupled with characteristic chest radiographic abnormalities. In most instances, the diagnosis can be established for epidemiologic or legal purposes without the need for lung biopsy, but confirmation may be required for cases upon occasion. The severity of clinical impairment must be assessed by physiologic function testing and cannot be estimated by radiograph alone. Four clinical and pathologic varieties can be identified: *chronic simple silicosis, PMF, accelerated silicosis,* and *acute silicosis.* Simple silicosis is the most common variety and is largely identified as a radiographic abnormality that develops slowly after 5 to 10 or more years of exposure. The pathologic lesions may progress and coalesce to form the conglomerate lesions of PMF, with substantial associated clinical impairment. Accelerated silicosis, which is associated with high levels of dust exposure, appears to be a more rapidly progressive form of simple silicosis. Acute silicosis is a form of diffuse alveolar injury caused by intense silica exposure and is characterized by an outpouring of surfactant materials that fill the air spaces of the lung to produce a disease resembling pulmonary alveolar proteinosis.

Chronic nodular silicosis. Chronic silicosis is usually first recognized as a radiographic abnormality, rather than by symptoms or physiologic impairment. Specific categories and descriptions of radiographs that relate to silicosis are included in the classification scheme developed by the ILO and related groups[41,42] (see Chapter 7). Simple silicosis is manifest as diffuse rounded opacities (ILO classification type *p*, profusion 1/1–2/1), with an upper lobe predominance. This mild abnormality is illustrated in Fig. 24-1. The more extensive disease involves enlargement in nodule size and increased numbers of nodules (ILO type *p–q*, profusion 1/2–2/2), as shown in Fig. 24-2. Eggshell calcification of the hilar nodes is characteristic of silicosis, although only a small proportion of chest radiographs in silicosis will demonstrate such calcifications (Fig. 24-3) . Infrequently, simple nodular silicosis may calcify as well. With advanced disease, the discrete rounded opacities may coalesce and fuse to form large, irregularly shaped masses, as shown in

Fig. 24-4, thus qualifying for the label PMF. Subpleural nodules that may sometimes calcify are characteristic of silicosis and may be prominent on computed tomography (CT), even when they are not apparent on plain chest radiographs (Fig. 24-5). The degree of pulmonary function impairment is generally related to the severity of the radiographic abnormalities and possibly to the CT findings.[43] Many workers, with definite but mild radiographic abnormalities, will be asymptomatic and will demonstrate normal lung function.

Dyspnea with exertion is the most common symptom of silicosis and is usually of gradual onset and slow progression. Most workers with clinically evident silicosis are 40 years of age or older, because of the long exposure required to cause illness and the slow progression of the disease. Cough and sputum production are frequent, and many workers have associated bronchitis. Since many workers exposed to silica also smoke tobacco, it may be difficult to

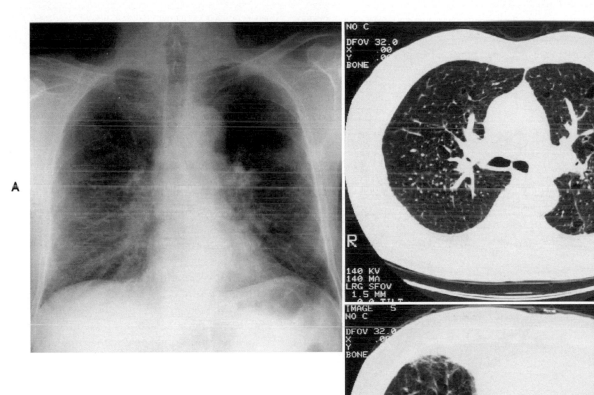

Fig. 24-1. A, Posteroanterior chest radiograph of a 72-year-old underground iron miner reveals simple silicosis. There is a pattern of small rounded opacities in moderate profusion seen throughout all lung zones. Calcium is apparent in the left hilar nodes. There is a 2 × 3 cm retrocardiac mass, which proved to be an adenocarcinoma. Lung tissue from this patient is shown in Fig. 24-6. **B,** High resolution CT scan at the level of the carina reveals a pattern of small rounded opacities with diffuse distribution. Calcium is apparent in the left hilar node region. **C,** A scan at the level of the heart reveals the 3 cm lung mass in the left lower lobe.

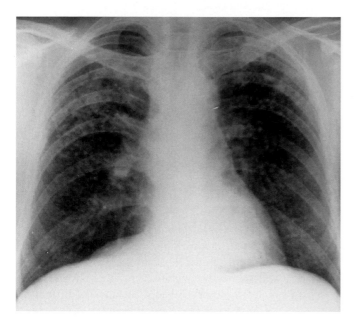

Fig. 24-2. Posteroanterior chest radiograph demonstrates simple nodular silicosis, but with larger opacities and greater profusion than are seen in Fig. 24-1. This man had exposure from 1926 to 1936 as a stonecutter in upstate New York, with no known dust exposure thereafter. The upper lung zone predominance of nodules is apparent. The hilar lymph nodes are enlarged.

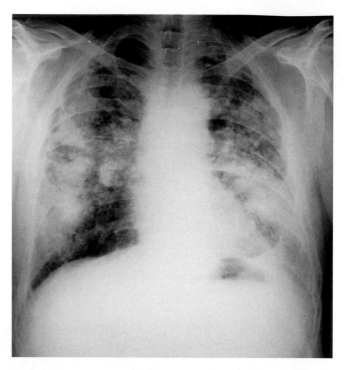

Fig. 24-4. Chest radiograph reveals complicated silicosis with progress massive fibrosis in a Barre, Vermont, granite cutter. Conglomerate masses with adjacent areas of hyperlucency are apparent. "Eggshell" calcification of hilar nodes can be seen. There is also calcification within the parenchymal masses and possible pleural calcification at the right apex.

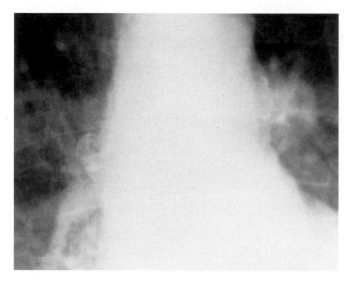

Fig. 24-3. Posteroanterior chest radiograph of an 86-year-old man with silicosis. The hilar lymph nodes reveal "eggshell" calcifications.

distinguish the symptoms of silicosis from those of chronic obstructive pulmonary disease (COPD). Rales and scattered wheezes may be found on physical examination of the chest, but often auscultation is normal despite relatively advanced silicosis. Digital clubbing is rare. Pulmonary function abnormalities in simple nodular silicosis are uncommon, but a mixed pattern of obstruction and reduction in lung vol-

umes has been noted in workers with more advanced disease.

Progressive massive fibrosis produces severe restriction, loss of pulmonary compliance, and hypoxemia. The course of the disease is often insidious, and progression can occur in the absence of continued exposure to silica. Shortness of breath may become disabling if PMF develops. Cor pulmonale is not common but may occasionally be found as an end-stage feature. Marked emphysema, then extensive silicosis, then pulmonary thromboembolism were the order of relative risk factors for cor pulmonale among South African gold miners.[44]

The pathognomonic lesion of silicosis is the silicotic nodule, found in lung tissue and in the involved lymphoid tissues, with surrounding fibrosis and other changes.[45] The typical silicotic nodule is composed of whorled collagen and reticulin centrally, with surrounding macrophages, fibroblasts, and lymphocytes, as shown in Fig. 24-6. Nodules are typically located near the respiratory bronchiole. This localization may be the result of the site of dust deposition in the lung, since initial deposition is nonuniform and is concentrated at alveolar duct bifurcations.[46,47] These sites are anatomically close to the respiratory bronchioles. The minimal lesion is a collection of macrophages with refractile dust particles concentrated within it. The developing silicotic nodule shows a distinct architecture centered

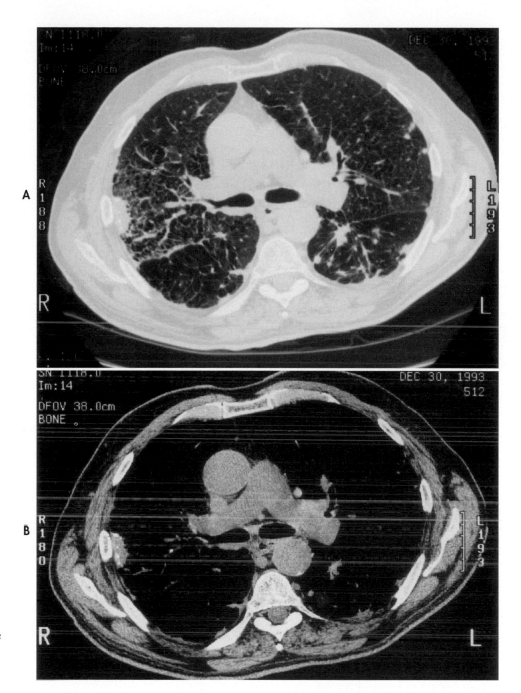

Fig. 24-5. A 73-year-old man with a history of employment in the granite industry in Vermont was evaluated for increased exercise dyspnea. Plain chest radiograph was nonspecific. **A,** High-resolution computed tomography, adjusted to optimize lung tissue density, demonstrates rounded opacities in low profusion. Multiple bilateral subpleural nodules are typical of silicosis. **B,** Calcification within the subpleural nodules, particularly at the right lateral chest, can be seen with the scan optimized for soft tissue density.

around cells and dust. Large macrophages are abundant at the center of the nodule and contain some dust. As nodules enlarge, whorled, concentric layers of collagen appear at the center of the lesion (see Fig. 24-6A). Smaller macrophages and many lymphocytes surround the central cells, and dust may move to the periphery as the lesion enlarges (see Fig. 24-6B). Epithelioid giant cells are a variable feature. Immunoglobulins have been discovered in silicotic nodules as well.[48] Typical granulomata rarely occur. Perinodular emphysematous regions may coalesce to form macroscopic blebs and can rupture to cause pneumothorax.

Silicosis can involve tissues outside the lung parenchyma if inhaled particles are carried to remote sites by lymphatic or hematogenous routes. The hilar lymph nodes, which drain lung tissue, are virtually always involved with typical silicotic nodules and abundant dust. Mediastinal lymph nodes are frequently involved, and supraclavicular nodes are sometimes involved, as secondary lymphatic drainage sites. Dust may occasionally be carried outside the thorax as well. A retroperitoneal mass caused by silicotic nodules was reported in a miner with pulmonary silicosis.[49] Small hepatic nodules can be found in the livers of individuals

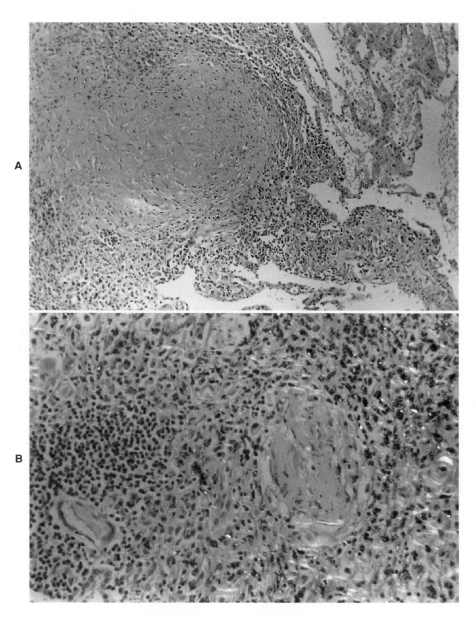

Fig. 24-6. A silicotic nodule appears adjacent to more normal lung tissue. This tissue was resected as part of a lobectomy performed for adenocarcinoma, as described in Fig. 24-1. **A,** There is a concentric, whorled collection of connective tissue at the center of the nodule, surrounded by an inflammatory infiltrate of macrophages and lymphocytes. The inflammatory cell influx and fibrosis can be seen streaming out into the interstitial space. **B,** A smaller nodule, viewed under polarized light microscopy, reveals bright refractile crystalline particles of silica and granite surrounding the connective tissue and an aggregate of lymphocytes adjacent to a small blood vessel.

exposed to silica by inhalation.[50] The extrathoracic localization of silica may be of interest in terms of systemic immune–inflammatory responses in silicosis, but these lesions do not appear to cause clinical disease within the target organs.

Laboratory abnormalities, reflecting polyclonal activation of humoral immunity, are common in silicosis but are nonspecific. Elevation of serum immunoglobulin levels, circulating immune complexes, rheumatoid factor, and antinuclear antibodies are sometimes observed.[51] It is unclear whether these diverse antibodies are related directly to the pathogenesis of tissue inflammation or are secondary phenomena that are the result of the disease. Other laboratory abnormalities are not usually found.

Accelerated silicosis. Accelerated silicosis is relatively rare but can develop in 2 to 5 years if exposure to free silica is intense.[23,52] Dyspnea is apparent early and soon becomes

disabling. The radiographic picture is of diffuse, small, irregular opacities, or reticulonodular opacities, rather than the upper-lobe nodular opacities that are typical of simple silicosis. Accelerated silicosis appears to be uniformly fatal within several years after the appearance of clinical signs.

Acute silicosis. Acute silicosis is a rare consequence of exposure to free silica at high concentrations, usually in tunneling through hard rock or sandblasting, or exposure to finely divided silica powder.[53-56] Acute silicosis presents with rapidly progressive dyspnea and respiratory insufficiency. Radiographically, acute silicosis appears as a diffuse, perihilar alveolar-filling process with ground-glass opacities. Upon pathologic examination, the alveolar spaces are filled with a lipid and proteinaceous exudate and cellular debris; damage to the epithelium is extensive. Thus acute silicosis more closely mimics pulmonary alveolar proteinosis than it does interstitial fibrosis, and acute silicosis is sometimes referred to as silicoproteinosis. Acute silicosis appears to be a uniformly fatal disease.

Bronchoalveolar lavage in silicosis. Bronchoalveolar lavage (BAL) provides a sample of cells and secretions from the alveolar air spaces of the lung, retrieved by the instillation and immediate withdrawal of a small volume of sterile saline solution through a flexible fiberoptic bronchoscope. This technique has been applied widely to research in human diffuse lung diseases and provides interesting insight into the events of silicosis at an alveolar level. Extensive studies of healthy human volunteers[57] reveal that normal BAL fluid contains mostly alveolar macrophages (AM) (10×10^4/ml, 85% of the cells), a minor fraction of lymphocytes (12%), few neutrophils, and rare eosinophils. The profiles of major protein and lipid constituents have been reported as well.[57a-57c]

Silica particles can be recovered in BAL fluids from exposed workers, and virtually all of the particles are found within AM that have phagocytosed them. The particles of quartz can be detected as bright crystals under polarized light microscopy or by electron probe analysis using scanning electron microscopy (SEM) with radiograph energy dispersive spectrometry.

A variety of abnormalities of BAL have been described in workers exposed to silica or in workers with silicosis. Workers with simple pneumoconiosis may have increased numbers of alveolar macrophages recovered by BAL,[58,59] and the production of IL-1, fibronectin, and high-energy oxygen products by these cells appears to be increased. Patients with silicosis,[60] asymptomatic granite workers,[61] and patients with mixed-dust pneumoconiosis,[62] do not evidence any increase in the proportions of neutrophils recovered by BAL. Notably, neutrophils are not a prominent feature of the tissue pathology of silicosis, and these cells may be less important in the pathogenesis of silicosis than other mononuclear inflammatory cell types. Some patients with advanced silicosis (progressive massive fibrosis) demonstrate increased neutrophils in BAL fluid. Patients with silicosis and asymptomatic granite workers show evidence of a slight increase in the proportion of lymphocytes recovered by BAL but show normal proportions of CD-4+ and CD-8+ cells.[57,61] Bronchoalveolar lavage fluid from silica-exposed granite workers contains increased concentrations of IgG, IgA, and IgM.[63] Workers with silicosis demonstrated significant increases in the number of Type-II cells recovered by BAL.[64]

The abnormalities found in human BAL fluid, in response to silica exposure, help to highlight important events in the pathogenesis of the disease and to place observations in animal models in perspective. The recovery of silica particles in BAL macrophages may confirm exposure if exposure is in doubt. More research is required to permit interpretation of BAL findings in the clinical management of individual patients.

Industrial bronchitis

Cough, sputum production, and mild airflow obstruction associated with occupational exposure to dusts or fumes has been termed *industrial bronchitis*.[65] This clinical syndrome is common among worker groups with exposure to silica. It may be difficult to define the limits of industrial bronchitis precisely, since it will overlap with the more common COPD caused by tobacco smoking and with symptoms produced by mild silicosis. Industrial bronchitis can be detected epidemiologically by respiratory symptoms in excess of those expected from smoking alone in a cohort of workers exposed to dust but who have no radiographic evidence of silicosis. Industrial bronchitis has been identified among German coal workers,[66,67] South African and Australian gold miners,[4,6,68] Indonesian granite workers,[68a] Indian agate workers,[69] and other groups. A recent metaanalysis of 13 studies among coal and gold miners confirmed an excess of bronchitic symptoms and obstructive physiology, even among nonsmokers.[70] There may be a synergistic effect between tobacco smoke and industrial pollutants to produce chronic bronchitis and air flow obstruction. Rats, into which intratracheal silica was administered, developed airflow obstruction on physiologic testing and pathologically showed small airways lesions.[71] Thus exposure to silica and other dusts at levels that appear not to cause overt silicosis can cause a form of chronic bronchitis.

Chronic pulmonary tuberculosis

The association between TB and silicosis has been well known since the nineteenth century. Although these two diseases were sometimes confused with one another, the advent of microbiologic techniques to identify tubercle bacilli permitted their clear distinction.[72] It soon became apparent that they often coexisted and that each disease influenced the course of the other. The combined disease is sometimes referred to as silicotuberculosis. The association between silicosis and increased susceptibility to TB has been demonstrated in hard rock miners, coal miners, granite workers, and other industrial groups.[73-75] Workers with established silicosis appear to be more susceptible than the general population to developing active TB when exposed and to a more chronic persistent form of TB after infection. It is not clear whether low levels of exposure to silica, without the development of overt silicosis, also predispose workers to TB. The rising rates of pneumoconiosis in developing countries as mining industries grow, coupled with the high prevalence of TB in those countries, focus attention for public health on the issue of silicotuberculosis.[76]

Silica potentiates the growth of *M. tuberculosis* in macrophage cultures in vitro,[77] but the organism also grows in such cell cultures without the addition of dust. Macrophages recovered from human workers exposed to silica and from animal models of silicosis demonstrate normal phagocytosis and killing of pyogenic bacteria.[61,78] It is possible that the immune–inflammatory responses that characterize silicosis create locations in which cells aggregate, and that these cells are particularly susceptible to infection by *Mycobacteria.*

The early radiographic changes are similar in both silicosis and TB, with progression of densities and infiltrates in upper lung zones; thus definitive diagnosis may be difficult. Tuberculosis in silicosis may be indolent and may progress slowly, with few organisms shed, and it may produce barely positive sputum smears or cultures. Silicosis predisposes to infection with both typical *M. tuberculosis* and atypical *Mycobacteria;* thus the species and drug sensitivity must be confirmed. Silicotuberculosis patients usually respond well to conventional antituberculous therapy in terms of clinical improvement and radiographic stabilization, but complete eradication of organisms may be impossible. Reactivation following an apparent cure is common in silicotuberculosis. For this reason many experts recommend multidrug treatment of silicotuberculosis patients, with isoniazide treatment for the rest of their lives.[74]

Lung cancer

Epidemiologic studies from around the world reveal an increased risk for lung cancer among workers exposed to silica.[79] Although the issue is complex, and reservations exist regarding the methodologies and populations of most studies, the balance of evidence favors this association. The statistical problems of confounding variables, such as smoking, radon, or hydrocarbon exposure, and of selection bias

in detection of pneumoconiosis cases, has been emphasized.[80] Selected reports are summarized in Table 24-1. The studies have used several approaches.

Retrospective cohort mortality (RCM) or retrospective cohort incidence (RCI) studies identified a group of workers exposed to silica in a particular industry (e.g., tin mining) and then sought the frequency of lung cancer as revealed by mortality reports or cancer registry statistics. The relative risk, or standardized mortality ratio (SMR), for workers was estimated by comparison within the industry (e.g., surface versus underground workers) or with contemporary general population statistics. In many studies, the cohort was defined by subjects listed with silicosis in a national or local registry. Other studies have used a case-referent or a case-control (CC) strategy, in which index cases of lung cancer were compared with matched noncancer control cases for the frequency of silica exposure or silicosis. Several studies used a large registry of all trades and determined the frequency of lung cancer among them by cross-indexing with a cancer registry.

The well-documented causal association between tobacco smoking and lung cancer complicates the analysis of each of these studies, although in most instances the investigators attempted to separate the effects of smoking from silica exposure. The degree of silica exposure (free silica content, intensity, duration) for each worker is rarely known and may vary widely across an industry, obscuring effects in workers with high exposures. Some authors have dealt

Table 24-1. Silicosis and lung cancer

	Nation	Number	Associated	SMR	Design	Smoke	Author, year	Reference
Miners, metal ores	United States	9912	Yes	1.73	RCM	Yes	Amandus, 1991	84
Miners, iron ore	China	6444	Yes		RCM	Yes	Chen, 1990	85
Miners, pottery	China	68000	Yes		RCM	No	Chen, 1992	81
Miners, tin ore	United Kingdom		Yes	4.4	RCM	Yes	Hodgson, 1990	83
Miners, gold	South Africa	2209	Yes		RCM	Yes	Hnizdo, 1991	82
Mixed silicosis	Italy (Sardinia)	724	Yes	1.29	RCM	No	Carta, 1991	86
Mixed silicosis	Italy (Genoa)	520	Yes	6.85	RCM	Yes	Merlo, 1990	89
Mixed silicosis	Italy (Veneto)	1313	Yes	2.39	RCM	Yes	Zambon, 1987	75
Mixed silicosis	Canada (Quebec)		Yes	3	RCM	No	Infante-Rivard, 1989	88
Mixed silicosis	Canada (Ontario)	1479	Yes	2.3	RCM	Yes	Finkelstein, 1987	87
Mixed silicosis	Japan	3335	Yes	6.03	RCM	Yes	Chiyotani, 1990	91
Mixed silicosis	Indonesia	1419	Yes	2.03	RCM	Yes	Ng, 1990	90
Granite workers	United States (VT)	5414	Yes	1.27	RCM	Yes	Costello, 1988	93
Granite workers	Indonesia	159	Yes	2.01	RCI	Yes	Chia, 1991	94
Diatomaceous earth	United States (CA)	2570	Yes	1.43	RCM	No	Checkoway, 1993	26
Foundry workers	Denmark	6144	Yes	1.3	RCI	Yes	Sherson, 1991	95
Slate workers	Germany		Yes		RCM	No	Mehnert, 1990	96
Ceramic workers	Sweden	280	Yes	2	RCI	No	Tornling, 1990	97
Dusty trades	United States (NC)	306	Yes	2.5	RCM	Yes	Amandus, 1992	98
Ceramic workers	Italy	72	Yes	2	CC	Yes	Lagorio, 1990	99
Mixed (necropsy)	South Africa	231	No			CC	Yes	Hessel, 1990	101
Mixed (silicosis)	Italy (Padova)	309	Yes	1.85	CC	Yes	Mastrangelo, 1988	102
Mixed exposures	Nordic countries	84,676	Yes		RCI	No	Lynge, 1986	103

Associated, Silicosis and lung cancer associated; *SMR*, standardized mortality ratio; *RCM*, retrospective cohort mortality study; *RCI*, retrospective cohort incidence study; *CC*, case-control or case-referent study; *Smoke*, adjusted for smoking.

with exposure intensity by distinguishing workers with silicosis (and presumed high exposure) from those with no radiographic or clinical disease. In several studies a higher incidence of lung cancer was documented among workers exposed during previous periods of high ambient dust as compared with a lower frequency among current workers employed since the institution of dust controls.

Cohort mortality studies of miners with silica exposure in the United States, the United Kingdom, Scandinavia, China, and South Africa have revealed a significant increase in mortality due to lung cancer,[81-83] with two- to fivefold increases in risk. Several of these studies were adjusted for the effects of smoking. A study of U.S. metal miners revealed a significantly increased age- and smoking-adjusted rate-ratio (SMR 1.96) for lung cancer among 369 silicotics as compared with 9543 nonsilicotics.[84] Underground tin miners in the United Kingdom experienced greater risk than their surface work colleagues.[85] Radon exposure may be an important variable for cancer risk in underground miners, as noted by several authors. The independent effects of silica, smoking, and radon radiation, and how they might interact, have not been clearly defined.

Reports from Italy, Canada, Japan, and Indonesia have identified an increased frequency of lung cancer among workers registered with silicosis.[86-90] The relative risk for lung cancer, as compared with the general population, ranged from 1.27 to 6.85, as shown in Table 24-1. These studies attempted to adjust for the effects of smoking and still documented a slight excess in cancer mortality. In all series, the dominant effect that produced cancer appeared to be smoking. Excess lung cancers were, however, found in never-smokers in two series.[91,92]

Granite workers have demonstrated a slightly increased lung cancer risk. In Vermont,[93] lung cancer mortality was increased in shed workers hired before 1940 but neither in those hired later nor in quarry workers. All workers who died of lung cancer were smokers. In Indonesia,[94] increased risk was observed after adjustment for smoking. California diatomaceous earth workers, exposed to amorphous silica and cristobalite rather than quartz, had a slightly increased lung cancer mortality rate (SMR 1.43), but full adjustment for smoking could not be made.[29] Danish foundry workers,[95] East German slate workers,[96] and Swedish ceramic workers[97] also evidenced an increased lung cancer risk in cohort studies. A retrospective analysis of lung cancer among North Carolina workers in the dusty trades revealed an increased risk associated with silica exposure (SMR 1.85), with adjustment made for smoking effects; the analysis included cases in nonsmokers.[98]

Case-referent studies have shown more confusing results, particularly in autopsy series. Lung cancer and silicosis were associated with one another among ceramic workers in Italy[99] but not in Holland.[100] Exposure to silica or silicosis was more frequent among lung cancer cases identified at autopsy than among matched controls in Italy[101] but not in South Africa.[102] The differences among these studies are not clear. The relative importance of small case series, low frequency of silicosis, incomplete adjustment for smoking, and the impact of genuine local effects in producing lung cancer have not been delineated.

The Nordic countries maintain registries of occupation and of cancer incidence. An extensive record linkage study tracked lung cancer among nearly 85,000 workers who were exposed to silica dust in Sweden, Finland, Norway, and Denmark.[103] Slight overall increases in relative risk were detected for workers in foundries, ore mining, and stone cutting, with substantial variation among countries. For example, mining carried increased risks in Sweden (SMR 3.28) and Finland (SMR 5.02), but no significantly increased risks in Norway or Denmark. The effects of radon exposure for miners, and smoking habits for all workers, were considered important cofactors, but could not be analyzed statistically.

All of these epidemiologic studies appear to generate comparable and mutually supportive conclusions, despite the differences of their methods and nations of origin. Exposure to high levels of silica dust (the level and duration of which was enough to cause overt silicosis in some workers) produces a two- to fourfold increased risk for lung cancer in tobacco smokers. This risk pertains to surface industry workers in granite sheds, foundries, and mills, as well as to underground miners, thus implicating a true effect of the mineral dust rather than an effect produced by radon daughters, trace elements, or other confounding carcinogens in the mine environment. Low levels of silica-dust exposure, obtainable in modern industry, probably do not increase cancer risk. Whether silica exposure produces an increased cancer risk for workers who do not smoke tobacco requires the study of more cases for greater statistical certainty. The effect of silica on enhancing lung cancer risk among smokers appears to be less than the risk for comparably exposed asbestos workers. Larger, ideally prospective, studies will be needed to determine whether silica exposure within levels that are regulated as safe for silicosis still cause a significantly increased lung cancer risk.

The mechanisms by which silica promotes lung cancer, or potentiates tobacco smoke as a cause of cancer, are not clear. Animal studies are being used to model cancer associated with silica exposure.[104] The mineral could act as a cocarcinogen that induces cancer, a cancer promoter that stimulates growth of transformed cells, a passive means of carrying tobacco carcinogens into the lung or impairing their clearance, or the mineral could alter immune surveillance mechanisms resulting in a failure to eliminate malignant cells when they arise. More research will be needed to determine which of these possibilities are important and the extent to which silica represents an important cancer risk for exposed workers.

DOSE–EFFECT–RISK RELATIONSHIPS IN SILICOSIS

The development of silicosis demonstrates a dose–effect relationship with exposure to silica dust. The factors that interact to influence the severity of silicosis are listed in the box. Most important among these factors are the intensity and duration of exposure to fibrogenic crystalline silica. The proportion of the dust represented by silica (free quartz), the percentage of particles of a size suitable for inhalation (respirable fraction), the concentration of dust in the air (number of particles or weight per unit volume), and the duration of exposure (work years) all interact to determine the prevalence and rapidity of progression of silicosis. Although individual variation and coincident exposures may influence silicosis, these factors are less important. Most workers will develop silicosis under similar exposure conditions.

The granite industry of Barre, Vermont, described in the Exposures to Silica section, provides an excellent opportunity to examine dose–effect–risk relationships in silicosis. A detailed survey of the Vermont granite sheds was conducted in 1924 to 1928 by the United States Public Health Service, just prior to the institution of extensive dust control measures.[13] There was a tremendous range of observed dust concentrations. Silicosis was defined by symptoms, physical examination findings, and chest radiograph abnormalities. A total of 166 workers with no evidence of TB were studied. The effects of exposure time and dust con-

centration were dramatic. The prevalence of silicosis was higher in those with greater dust concentration measured in their workplace, and the prevalence of silicosis increased with the length of employment. The dose–response relationships were clear. Fig. 24-7 shows a summary of the results observed by Russell and colleagues. None of the granite workers had definite silicosis with less than 5 years of employment. After 14 years in the industry, virtually every worker with high exposure had disease. Mortality among granite cutters was high; the average cumulative death rate for pneumatic tool operators was 50 per 1000 persons by age 50 years, as compared with about two deaths per 1000 for men in the general population.

Public awareness, and the results of this survey in 1929, sparked the development of effective dust controls and the prevalence of silicosis fell abruptly. This industry has been monitored and surveyed repeatedly over the past 60 years.[11,104a,105-110] The examinations by Graham and colleagues[111] of pulmonary function, chest radiographic changes, and mortality among Barre granite workers document that this industry now has dust exposure levels generally below federal limits and does not produce clinically apparent silicosis. The frequency of death due to silicosis in a cohort mortality study of 5414 workers, employed between 1950 and 1982 in the Barre, Vermont, granite industry, clearly demonstrates the effects of exposure intensity.[93] Workers employed before 1940 were exposed to high dust levels, exceeding 40 mppcf. Workers employed after the institution of dust controls in 1940 were exposed to levels below the current permissible exposure limit (PEL), less than 10 mppcf. Deaths due to silicosis and TB were common among workers hired before 1940, with SMRs that were 5 to 10 times those expected for the general U.S. population. Virtually no deaths due to silicosis were observed among workers who had exposure in the granite industry after dust control measures were instituted. Pulmonary function was preserved in current granite workers, with no loss over time beyond the expected effects of aging and smoking.[111] Chest radiographs from 972 workers revealed only 7 films with small rounded opacities that were suggestive of silicosis, and all of these were of mild degree.[14]

Studies of BAL materials from Vermont granite workers demonstrate dose–effect relationships within the current low-dust exposure levels. The recovery of alveolar macrophages with granite mineral particles was directly linked to the intensity of current exposure among 44 granite workers.[112] The intensity of exposure was estimated from personal sampling measurements of workers with similar jobs.[113] Workers with low levels of exposure (quarry workers, draftsmen) had relatively few macrophages with particulates, whereas workers with higher levels of exposure (cutters, polishers) had many cells with silica. Retired workers still exhibited evidence of BAL particulates, although fewer than current workers in comparable jobs. These relationships are illustrated in Fig. 24-8. The duration of em-

---

Factors contributing to the severity of silicosis

Variety of free-crystalline silica

Quartz
Cristobalite
Tridymite

Intensity of exposure

Concentration of dust in ambient air (mg/m^3, mmpcf)
Fraction of airborne dust that is respirable (<10 μm)
Fraction of respirable dust that is silica

Duration of exposure

Years of work in dusty trade
Portion of workday exposed to dust

Confounding influences

Coincident dust exposure (talc, silicates)
Coincident fume exposure (welding, foundry)
Tobacco smoking

Individual variation

Genetic susceptibility
Personal work habits
Use of respiratory protection
Coincident lung disease

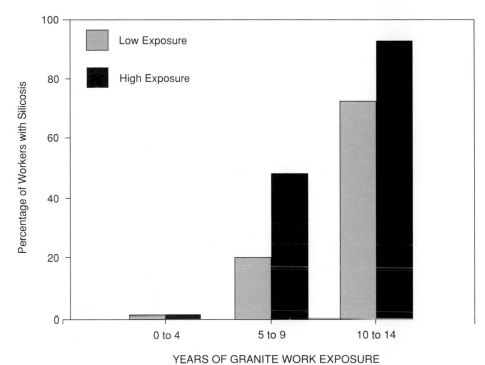

Fig. 24-7. The prevalence of silicosis in the granite industry in Barre, Vermont was reported by Russell and associates in 1929.[13] Their data demonstrated a clear dose–effect relationship. The percentage of individuals with silicosis is shown for workers with high-exposure jobs, as compared to low-exposure jobs, and with brief (0–4 years), moderate (5–9 years), or prolonged (10–14 years) of employment.

ployment was related significantly to the fraction of BAL cells with particles, but there was substantial individual variation. In addition to granite particle deposition, other studies in this worker population have shown a slightly increased proportion of lymphocytes[61] and raised immunoglobulin concentrations in BAL fluid,[63] indicating a subclinical response of the lung to this dust exposure. Other industries demonstrate dose–effect–risk relationships similar to that seen in the granite sheds.

PATHOGENETIC MECHANISMS OF SILICOSIS

The pathogenesis of silicosis is focused on interactions between lung cells and inhaled particles and the secondary responses triggered by this interaction. At exposure levels encountered in most occupational settings, the resident alveolar macrophage appears to be the most important lung cell that interacts with silica. At higher workplace exposure levels for humans, or in many of the exposures used to create silicosis by experiment in animals, a variety of lung cells appear to be affected directly by silica particles. Each of these events can be considered individually before attempting to fit them together into an integrated scheme.

Evidence must be drawn from human subjects, animal models, and in vitro studies to understand these processes. The sequence of events appears to proceed from injury to inflammation and then to fibrosis, often occurring simultaneously at different locations within the lung. Although many of these mechanisms appear to be common biologic responses to injury, silica produces a distinctive clinical and pathologic entity. Perhaps this is due to the particular way in which silica is localized within tissues in combination

with a more general injury–inflammation–fibrosis response at these specific sites.

Studies of the effects of silica exposure on a variety of specific cells and processes are summarized below. A proposed integrative pathogenic scheme is then presented.

Inhalation, deposition, and translocation of silica particles

Workers in dusty trades may inhale large amounts of mineral particles, much of it in the form of larger particles that do not reach the distal lung. Black sputum expectorated by coal miners, and gray phlegm from granite workers, are hallmarks of these trades. Even smaller particles, less than 5 to 10 μm in size, deposited in the alveoli may be cleared with reasonable efficiency, but a substantial fraction remains within the lung.

A standardized exposure of Fischer 344 rats to a respirable aerosol of quartz (40 mg/m^3) or cristobalite (10 mg/m^3) for 6 hr/day over 8 days has been used to study silica deposition, translocation, and mechanisms of disease.[78,115-117] When rats are exposed to silica by inhalation, most of the dust is deposited at alveolar duct bifurcations, but the alveolar macrophages recovered by BAL contain particles within several hours of dusting.[47] Both free particles and macrophages containing particles appear within the bronchiolar and alveolar interstitium within hours. Mucociliary clearance, interstitial lymphatics, and other transport mechanisms redistribute the dust over time. Although up to 80% of the initially-deposited dust is cleared within several months after this brief exposure, 20% or more remains within the lung indefinitely. Translocation to peri-

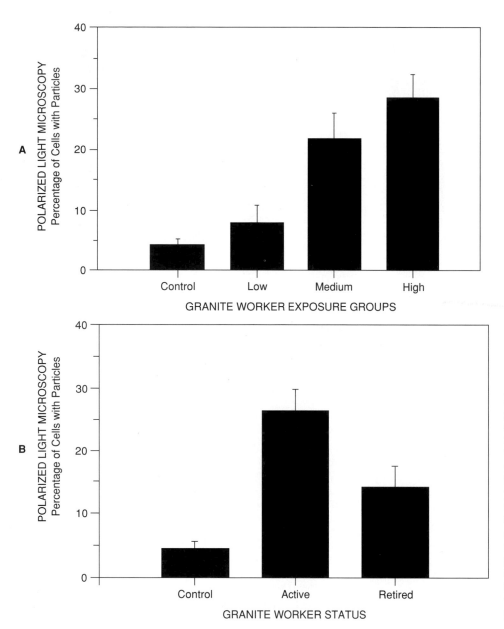

Fig. 24-8. A group of 44 Vermont granite industry workers and 42 unexposed healthy subjects volunteered for bronchoalveolar lavage.[112] The workers were classified by job type as experiencing low, medium, or relatively high exposure to dust. **A,** The percentage of cells containing refractile particles under polarized light microscopy showed a dose–effect relationship in regard to the intensity of granite dust exposure. **B,** All worker groups had higher fractions of lung cells with particles than were found in the control group, but active workers with current exposure had a higher percentage than retired workers.

bronchial, subpleural, and interstitial pulmonary sites, as well as to intrathoracic lymphoid tissues, continues.[118,119] Most of the clearance that will occur by direct mucociliary removal takes place immediately after inhalation, whereas translocation between the air space and the interstitium continues indefinitely.[120] The exchange appears to be bidirectional, with dust recirculating between both compartments. Accumulation in mediastinal and intrapulmonary lymphoid tissue continues for up to 1 year after dusting.

Silica particle toxicity

The biological response to silica appears to rest upon its crystalline nature and the highly reactive surface radical groups associated with the crystalline, rather than the amorphous, polymorphs. The reactivity of surface groups with biological materials, particularly internal or external cell membranes, may be the key element in toxicity. Three main types of sites for adsorption are found on a silica surface: silanols, siloxane bridges, and surface radicals related to mechanical cleavage of Si—O bonds. The surfaces formed by grinding or fracture appear to be highly reactive, whereas chemically generated surfaces are less so. Thus newly fractured stone may produce more toxic particles than old "weathered" silica, such as desert sand. Quartz demonstrates abundant, strongly-reactive surface sites, attributed to cleavage of the covalent Si—O bond, whereas amorphous silica contains few surface sites.[121] Cristobalite, the most biologically active isoform, contains the greatest number of these reactive groups.[122] More work is required to determine the exact ways in which the reactive surface groups modify biological materials to cause disease and to explain the differences in bioactivity among the silica isomorphs.

Silica particles react with cells in vitro to damage and lyse them by interaction with the external cell membrane. Although lysis of erythrocytes may be a useful means of studying particle surface radicals and particle–membrane interactions, the cell destruction probably bears little relation to in vivo events. Initial studies showed that silica, in contrast to latex or diamond particles, caused lysis of macrophages when added to them in vitro.[123] This toxicity can be greatly reduced if the particles are coated with surfactant lipids, as they would be after deposition in the lung.[124] Alveolar macrophages exposed to silica aerosols, recovered from animals and human workers, contain many particles but demonstrate normal viability, normal phagocytic function, and enhanced bacterial killing.[61,78] Although some macrophages may be injured or killed by silica, most appear to be stimulated. This discrepancy between in vitro and in vivo events may be explained by differences in dosage on a per-cell basis, by coating of particles, and possibly by other factors as well.

An important aspect of silica toxicity is its persistence in tissue. Little or no silica is dissolved in tissue, in contrast to many other minerals, and it appears to remain biologically active for a long time. Thus dust that remains in or is translocated through vulnerable tissues may continue to produce a local reaction throughout the lifetime of the host. Some of the silica becomes sequestered in hyalinized nodules or lymph nodes, and calcification may ultimately isolate this material.

Macrophages

Resident and recruited macrophages are key participants in the mechanisms of silicosis. These cells play a triple role in sequestering the mineral, transporting silica through the lung, and releasing pathogenetic mediators that alter the behavior of other cells. As noted, most of the silica particles can be found within macrophages soon after inhalation. Studies utilizing colored beads[125] and other materials have demonstrated the critical role macrophages play in transporting particles through the lung to regional lymph nodes.

Monocyte–macrophage recruitment (and possibly proliferation) into the lung is an important aspect of silicosis. Large numbers of these cells are apparent in the nodules found in lung tissue (see Fig. 24-6) and lymph nodes. The number of macrophages recovered by BAL or from the interstitium increases two- to fourfold over several months after silica exposure of rats.[78,115,117]

The macrophage responds to the ingestion of crystalline silica particles in vivo with activation and with the release of a wide variety of cytokines and other reactants. Macrophages, recovered from animals exposed to silica, exhibit increased cell surface ruffling and spreading, increased oxygen consumption, enhanced phagocytosis of inert particles and bacteria,[78] increased release of superoxide anion after stimulation,[126] increased expression of class II major histocompatibility antigens,[127] and enhanced secretion of cytokines. These are the features of stimulated or activated macrophages. Although airspace cells may be more easily recovered for research, the macrophages within the lung interstitium may be more important pathogenetically, and may show greater elaboration of selected cytokines.[117,128]

Macrophages from human subjects and animals with silica exposure or overt silicosis release a wide variety of materials that can influence the growth and function of other cells. Increased production by silica-exposed macrophages or monocytes has been reported for chemoattractants and activating substances for neutrophils, monocytes, and lymphocytes (interleukin-1 [IL-1],[127,129-134] tumor necrosis factor-α [TNF-α],[135-138] chemotactants[139]), and other miscellaneous substances. Arachidonic acid metabolites may also be up- or down-regulated.[140-142]

These potent materials can interact with many target cells.[143] Two of these, IL-1 and TNF-α, appear to be of critical importance in granuloma formation[144] and in the evolution of silicosis. Removal of TNF-α by antibody treatment early after animal exposure reduces fibrosis in silicosis,[145] whereas the addition of extra TNF-α augments the expression of disease. Mice, relatively deficient in TNF-α production, develop less silicosis than TNF-sufficient strains.[146]

Cytokines that are produced by macrophages that affect fibroblasts are also critical to the pathogenesis of silicosis. Macrophages from a variety of animal species and from man release factors that promote fibroblast proliferation and/or collagen production when exposed to silica in vitro or when recovered following in vivo exposure.[117,133,147-152] Platelet-derived growth factor (PDGF), insulinlike growth factor (IGF-1), IL-1, TNF-α, fibronectin, and probably other substances, appear to be important in this activity. The macrophage can be seen as the central element in the granulomatous inflammation and fibrosis that create silicosis.

Lymphocytes

Lymphocytes appear to be an essential part of silicosis as well. Large numbers of lymphocytes appear in the mixed mononuclear cell aggregates that surround the central hyaline in silicotic nodules. Discrete lymphoid nodules and hypertrophy of bronchial-associated lymphoid tissue appear in lung parenchyma of human cases and animal models of silicosis, and thoracic lymph nodes are strikingly enlarged. Increased numbers of lymphocytes are recovered by BAL and from the interstitium of animals with silicosis.[133,153] Human workers who have been exposed to silica or who have overt silicosis produce slightly increased numbers of lymphocytes in BAL fluid.[57,60] Thus there is tremendous hypertrophy of the lymphocyte population as part of this disease.

Most of the lymphocytes detected in lung tissue or recovered by BAL are T cells, although absolute numbers of B cells may be somewhat increased as well.[154,155] In animal models there is an increased predominance of CD4[+] T cells (helper/inducer T cells) as compared with normal, but CD8[+] (cytolytic/suppressor) cells are common as well. The

T cells appear to activate, as is evident by increased expression of IL-2 receptors.[153] Human BAL specimens have shown a normal ratio of CD4[+]:CD8[+] lymphocytes.[57]

The CD4[+] activated T cells may be responding to IL-1 and other cytokines released by macrophages. In a complimentary fashion, these same cells may be elaborating interferon-γ and other substances that recruit and activate macrophages. The importance of T cells for macrophage activation was demonstrated by silicosis in nude (thymic-deficient) mice, where the usual influx of macrophages was not observed.[156]

Immune response and lymphocyte function has been examined to a limited degree in human silicosis. Few observations have been made regarding lung lymphocytes or those within silicotic lymph nodes. Workers with silicosis demonstrate normal cutaneous reactivity to recall antigens and have normal proportions of lymphocyte populations in their blood.[157] Workers' peripheral blood lymphocytes have normal responses to recall antigens but show a slightly decreased proliferative response to a mitogen,[158] although the functional importance of this change is not clear. Silicosis patients demonstrate an increased prevalence of autoantibodies and a polyclonal increase in serum immunoglobulins[51,159]; healthy granite workers have slightly increased immunoglobulin concentrations in BAL fluid, but normal serum levels.[114] These observations suggest nonspecific systemic stimulation of humoral immune responses. It is not known whether this stimulation represents a part of the mechanism of disease or a secondary effect of it.

Neutrophils

Neutrophils are not prominent in the tissue lesions of silicosis. Human patients with silicosis or exposed workers do not demonstrate increased neutrophils in BAL fluid. Neutrophils are apparent in the BAL fluid of animals exposed to silica, particularly after high dosage or early in the course of the disease. Neutrophils could participate in tissue injury through the release of proteolytic enzymes and reactive oxygen species. Mechanisms for recruitment of neutrophils in animal models could include activation of complement, since complement-deficient mice evidence less neutrophil influx,[160] or generation of chemotactins such as leukotriene B4 (LTB4). Initial results of a study on the production of LTB4 show decreased production by macrophages in animals with silicosis.[141]

Mast Cells

Mast cells have received little attention in silicosis. These tissue leukocytes contain potent proinflammatory mediators and chemoattractants. Mice that are genetically deficient in mast cells developed less intense pulmonary abnormalities and less BAL neutrophil influx than mast-cell sufficient strains following intratracheal silica instillation.[161] The response was restored to normal after bone-marrow transplantation and engraftment of mast cells in the deficient mice.

Fibroblasts

Fibroblasts are mesenchymal cells responsible for collagen and elastin synthesis and, in part, for degradation during the course of normal connective tissue matrix turnover. The excessive amounts and abnormal locations of collagen within the silicotic nodule and the interstitium suggest excessive production and/or inadequate degradation by fibroblasts. Production of excess collagen begins almost immediately after silica exposure and proceeds excessively for at least 1 year.[162] The proportions of type I and type III collagen appear to be normal, although both are produced in excess.[163] Lung tissue from silicotic animals continues to exhibit excessive collagen production when cultured in vitro.[164] Elevated levels of enzymes, responsible for collagen crosslinking and for degradation, have been found in such animals.[165-167] As noted above, a variety of mediators produced by activated macrophages may stimulate fibroblast proliferation and collagen synthesis. It is not yet clear whether the fibroblasts in silicosis are phenotypically normal but increased in number or have undergone transformation into a more proliferative and synthetic type.

Alveolar epithelium

Acute injury to alveolar epithelial cells accompanies silicosis, particularly when the dose of silica is high. This injury is reflected as acute silicosis or silicoproteinosis in humans and in experimental animals. Histopathology of silicoproteinosis reveals alveolar spaces filled with a homogeneous eosinophilic proteinaceous material, cellular debris, and neutrophils. There is extensive damage to the type I epithelial cells, and hypertrophy and hyperplasia of type II cells.[56] Following the relatively high-dose, intratracheal instillation of silica in the rat, there was a tenfold increase in the amounts of phospholipid and surfactant protein A (SP-A) recovered by BAL, and a fraction of type II cells isolated from these animals showed hypertrophy.[168] After cristobalite inhalation, recovery of BAL lipids (nonpolar lipids, phospholipids, saturated phosphatidylcholine) was greatly increased, and the phosphatidylcholinephosphatidylglycerol ratio was decreased.[169] These findings indicate that the alveolar epithelium responds to silica injury with a tremendous hyperplasia of type II cells and with increased production of surfactant proteins and lipids.

There may be several pathways by which alveolar injury occurs in silicosis. The reactive radicals on the surface of silica particles could react directly with vulnerable type I epithelial cells. This may not occur if the alveolar dust burden is low and macrophages are able to phagocytose particles promptly after deposition. If the phagocytic capability of the resident macrophages were overwhelmed, silica particles could interact directly with parenchymal cells. Reactive oxygen species, elaborated by neutrophils and macrophages in response to particle ingestion or as result of indirect activation, as discussed, could also cause epithelial injury.[170] Quartz particles induced the elaboration of reactive oxygen metabolites (superoxide, hydrogen peroxide) from phagocytes in vitro, whereas nonfibrogenic particles did not.[171,172]

Apparent confirmation of the importance of reactive oxygen species is provided by the response of the lung. Antioxidant enzymes assist the degradation of reactive oxygen species and can be induced in the lung in response to oxidant stress. Rats exposed to cristobalite silica evidenced increased whole-lung steady-state expression of messenger ribonucleic acid (mRNA) for manganese superoxide dismutase (Mn—SOD) and glutathione peroxidase within 10 days.[173] Western blot analysis showed twofold increases Mn—SOD protein, and immunoelectronmicroscopy localized this protein to hypertrophied type II epithelial cells lining alveolar spaces.[174] Epithelial injury by reactive oxygen species may be an important mechanism in acute silicosis and possibly in the more chronic disease as well.

Integrated mechanisms of disease

The large amount of information accumulated about silicosis in human studies and animal models permits a scheme that may draw several mechanisms together. It is important not to oversimplify this scheme: multiple mechanisms may overlap; inflammatory pathways and mediators are often redundant; down-regulatory and proinflammatory influences often coexist or compete simultaneously. Little is known about down-regulating mechanisms in silicosis to add to this scheme. Although some of the ideas that follow are speculative, direct evidence for most of them is cited above. This hypothetical "story line" will undoubtedly need refinement as new information and ideas become available.

The silicotic nodule appears to be a paradigm for the mechanisms of chronic silicosis. The disease in toto could be viewed as the sum of many microscopic foci of injury, inflammation, and fibrosis, evolving in parallel. These nodules may be of different sizes and stages of development at different locations. Finally, the nodules merge or aggregate to form the large lesions of progressive massive fibrosis. The rate at which this process advances may be defined by a complex interaction among the type of silica, intensity of exposure, duration of exposure, genetic responsiveness of the host, and other factors.

Within the lung and the silicotic lesion, the cell types listed interact to produce disease. Resident and recruited macrophages ingest silica immediately after inhalation, unless exposure is massive. These phagocytes sequester the particles and contain them most or all of the time that the dust remains in the lung. Direct interactions between silica particles and other lung cells may also occur, leading to injury or stimulation, if there is a high level of exposure. The macrophages that contain the dust are stimulated to produce cytokines (e.g., IL-1β), which recruit and activate T cells.

These lymphocytes in turn recruit and activate a secondary population of monocyte-macrophages, which may be important proinflammatory participants, but which do not contain silica. The activated macrophages also produce cytokines that stimulate fibroblasts to proliferate and to produce increased amounts of collagen (e.g., TNF-α, PDGF, IGF-1). Both macrophage-derived products (e.g., LTB-4) and serum proteins (e.g., complement) may recruit neutrophils to these lesions. The neutrophils appear to be somewhat less important in human chronic silicosis than in more acute animal models.

It is possible that regional or systemic immunostimulation could augment these reactions. Silica reaches regional lymphoid tissues in large amounts and produces a hyperplastic reaction and granulomas. The polyclonal antibody responses and autoantibodies found in human silicosis, and the systemic "priming" of macrophages for cytokine secretion found in animal models,[138] could be reflections of systemic immunostimulation.

Substantial injury to lung structure may result from direct interaction with silica and from the secondary inflammatory process. The type I epithelial cell appears to be particularly vulnerable. The injury could be based on reactive oxygen species generated on silica particle surfaces or secreted by phagocytes. The type II cell appears to be less susceptible to injury and is able to generate effective antioxidant defenses, to proliferate, and to secrete increased amounts of its unique surfactant products. Higher doses of silica and more toxic isoforms increase the intensity of this injury response.

Future directions for research into the mechanisms of silicosis will involve additional animal studies in which the site and timing of cytokine production and response are defined more precisely in vivo. Manipulations with deficient strains or transgenic varieties of experimental animals should help clarify the importance of these mechanisms. Interventions that block mediators with antibodies, soluble receptors, or receptor antagonists, or block the mediators' transcription with antisense probes, will also provide insights into the ways the many active substances interact. It is hoped that a more precise understanding of these processes will permit opportunities for treatment in humans. Silicosis should continue to provide a useful model system for studies of chronic diffuse interstitial lung disease in which the etiologic agent is known, the dose can be controlled, the material can be tracked throughout the course of the pathogenic process, and the interactions of various cell types can be observed.

GOVERNMENT REGULATIONS RELATED TO CRYSTALLINE SILICA

Government agencies throughout the world have been concerned with establishing safe working conditions for those exposed to dusts containing crystalline silica almost since the dust's first recognition as a health hazard. Measurements of airborne dust became common during the early years of the twentieth century, and recommendations for apparently safe levels of exposure to dust were made as early as the 1920's.[13] Initial standards recommended exposure to no more than 10 mppcf of granite dust. These standards have been refined as the technology to measure airborne particulates and the understanding of health effects have improved.

Current standards are based on measurements of particles small enough to enter the lower respiratory tract. This limit for humans ranges from approximately 5 to 10 μm particles down to 0.1 to 0.3 μm mass median aerodynamic diameter. There has been substantial debate and controversy over exactly how to sample workplace air for respirable particles for regulatory purposes.[175] In general, these particles are defined on the basis of the collection profile of the sampling instruments used to capture them and may be considered to be particles less than 10 μm. Large particles may contribute inordinately to the weight of a total air or bulk sample and may have a somewhat different mineral composition than the smaller respirable particles. Current standards recommend that samples be collected with personal samplers from the breathing zone of workers. The important point is that regulatory standards are based on the mass of particles that may actually enter the lung.

Standards assume that it is primarily crystalline-free silica that confers health risk, and standards are based on the fraction of silica in a particular dust. As noted, finely divided quartz (silica flour, tripoli) is nearly pure crystalline silica, whereas granite dust contains approximately 10% quartz. The proportion of silica contained in a dust can be determined by physical and chemical analysis of a bulk or airborne dust sample, and the fraction is then applied to the personal air sample data. The isomorph of crystalline silica (quartz, cristobalite, tridymite) must also be determined. The American Conference of Governmental Industrial Hygienists recommended in 1962 a threshold limit value (TLV) for quartz, based on a percentage of the measured particle number, and in 1968 the Conference recommended a value based on size-selective gravidimetric measurements. The recommendations of 1986 specify a direct measurement of respirable quartz no greater than 0.1 mg/m^3 (100 μm^3) over a time-weighted average exposure of 8 hr/day.[175a] For example, a personal dust sample of respirable particles measuring 0.2 mg/m^3 and determined to contain 15% quartz would be recorded as an exposure to 0.03 mg/m^3 crystalline-free silica. United States federal regulatory agencies have continued to adopt this standard for quartz and half that level for cristobalite or tridymite, as shown in Table 24-2.[176] The 1975 U.S. National Institute for Occupational Safety and Health (NIOSH) recommendation for a lower level for respirable quartz (0.05 mg/m^3)[177] generated controversy[178] and has not been adopted.

Government standards provide benchmarks for industry and a mechanism for the regulation of workplace safety. The

Table 24-2. U.S. regulatory standards for silica

Crystalline silica isomorph	Maximum permissible exposure level
Quartz	0.10 mg/m^3
Tripoli (quartz, silica flour)	0.10 mg/m^3
Cristobalite	0.05 mg/m^3
Tridymite	0.05 mg/m^3

The permissible exposure limit (PEL) is defined as an 8-hour time weighted average (TWA) for the respirable silica fraction.[176]

absolute levels established, and the means for measuring them, carry tremendous economic impact. Lower permissible exposure levels are expensive in terms of equipment and modification of industrial practices; higher levels may be expensive in terms of human health and suffering. Reports suggest that the U.S. Maximum Permissible Exposure Level for quartz, 0.1 mg/m^3, appears to provide protection from silicosis in nonmining exposure when it is rigorously applied[14] and that modern industrial practices can achieve this level.[179] Many mining and surface industries, particularly in developing countries, exceed this exposure. Many believe that regulatory efforts should be directed toward applying and enforcing current standards rather than debating them.

PREVENTION OF SILICOSIS

Silicosis can be prevented by limiting the exposure of workers to levels of ambient dust that do not produce lung disease. This level can be achieved in modern industries, as documented by the examples presented previously. In granite sheds, iron foundries, silica-flour manufacture, abrasive cleaning, diatomaceous earth production, and other workplaces, silicosis has become rare as effective dust-control measures were instituted and enforced. The specific measures used in some of these industries are discussed. Some strategies for reducing the exposure of workers to respirable silica particles are listed in Table 24-3.

The respirable dust levels permitted by U.S. standards appear adequate to prevent the occurrence of classical silicosis, at least in above-ground work settings. It is not yet certain that all other long-term adverse health effects will be prevented by these same levels. Thus there may still exist an excess risk for bronchitis, lung cancer, or susceptibility to tuberculosis, even if true silicosis does not develop. Too little is known, and low-dust levels have been in place for too short a time in most industries to judge these other more subtle risks.

THERAPY OF SILICOSIS

No truly effective therapy is available for silicosis. Many approaches have been tried, and some may offer help for severally diseased patients. Because no simple remedies can be offered, the discussion that follows is largely theoreti-

Table 24-3. Strategies for reducing exposure to respirable silica

Strategy	Example from industry
Improve ventilation in the work space	Air exchanges in tunnel mines; filtration of factory air
Extract air directly from the cutting or grinding surface	Granite cutting and polishing; foundry cast grinding
Spray the cutting surface with water	Granite cutting and grinding; coal mine face boring
Provide personal respiratory protective devices	Respirators for clean-up workers
Provide independent personal air sources	Air hoods for sandblasters
Substitute machinery for human labor	Mine face boring; the "continuous miner"
Place machine operators at a distance	Remote control operators
Substitute nonsiliceous materials for silica	Iron carbide in abrasive cleaning; ceramic casting mold liners

---

> ### Theoretical strategies for the treatment of excessive silica exposure
>
> Physically remove dust from the lung by external means
> Enhance pulmonary transport to promote dust removal
> Render dust remaining in the lung less toxic
> Sequester dust in the lung at harmless locations
> Decrease the inflammatory response to mineral particles
> Reduce tissue fibrosis accompanying inflammation
> Repair or replace damaged tissue

cal. Logical analysis of therapeutic options may provide avenues for future investigation.

Treatment of workers who have received excessive exposure to silica could, in theory, be based on a variety of logical strategies as listed (see box). Most of these approaches have been tried with variable success. Several features of silicosis bear scrutiny when considering therapy. (1) Silicosis develops in direct relation to the intensity and duration of exposure to crystalline-free silica, thus workers who have received the highest exposures, and those who carry the greatest dust burden, should benefit most from therapy. (2) Tissue injury and response occur in close proximity to the injurious agent, silica particles. (3) The major anatomic site of disorganization appears to be the interstitium, thus particles in the interstitium could be considered to be the prime target for intervention. Nonetheless, airspace macrophages carry large quantities of dust years after exposure has ceased, and there may be an ongoing exchange of particles between air space and interstitial compartments. Massive short-term exposure provides a special case, since acute silicosis or silicoproteinosis appears to be a disease of primary alveolar epithelial injury rather than interstitial fibrosis. Thus more dust may be present in the air spaces than in cases of chronic silica exposure that has extended over decades. (4) Simple nodular silicosis usually involves mild functional impairment, whereas progressive massive fibrosis causes severe dysfunction and respiratory insufficiency. These observations suggest that therapy need not result in complete removal of all dust in order to be

helpful. Treatments would still be beneficial if they could reduce dust burdens and/or reduce the body's response to particles to the extent that potential massive fibrosis was converted into simple nodular silicosis.

Therapeutic whole lung pulmonary lavage has been employed as a technique for physically removing silica from the air spaces of the lung. This treatment has been directed primarily at workers who have received massive exposures or who have already developed acute silicosis. One case of mixed dust pneumoconiosis was treated in the United States with whole lung lavage without change in pulmonary function.[180] Studies of coal miners in China have reported that several grams of dust can be removed from the lung in this fashion, but no objective improvement in lung function has been observed.[181,182]

No treatments are available to enhance endogenous pulmonary transport mechanisms in order to promote the removal of silica from the lung. The critical target for this intervention would appear to be the transport of particles from the interstitium to the alveolus and from the alveolus to the bronchial mucociliary escalator. Expectoration of bronchial secretions does not appear to be a problem in silicosis. Augmentation of transport from the interstitium via lymphatics to sequestered lymphoid aggregates might also be useful.

Several strategies have been developed in an attempt to render inhaled silica less toxic. Aluminum powder, inhaled simultaneously with silica dust, was tested in animal studies in the 1930s and 1940s, with less fibrosis apparent in animals that received the aluminum treatment.[181] It was believed that aluminum salts and/or oxide interacted with the reactive surface groups on silica particles and rendered them less toxic. The effectiveness of aluminum lactate inhalation administered after the development of silicosis has been tested in a carefully documented model of silicosis in sheep.[183] The sheep that received aluminum therapy showed less silicosis and accelerated clearance of silica from their lungs. After World War II, the animal findings promoted enthusiasm for the inhalation of finely divided aluminum powder as a "preventive" in workers exposed to silica. A 4-year randomized controlled trial of aluminum powder inhalation in human pottery workers and miners was reported in 1956, but no objective beneficial results were detected.[184] Inhalation of MacIntyre Powder (finely divided aluminum and aluminum oxide) was used at some locations in Canadian mines from 1944 through 1979. Although animal results with aluminum treatment appear promising, aluminum toxicity may limit its application in humans.

No treatments are available to promote sequestration of dust at harmless locations within the body. The lung may employ this strategy, however, as silica is transported via lymphatics to regional and mediastinal lymph nodes, where it accumulates in large amounts. Although these nodes enlarge and calcify, they do not usually cause discomfort or clinical disease.

Corticosteroid treatment may be directed at reducing the inflammatory response to silica through its actions on lymphocytes, macrophages, and other cells. Although fibrosis dominates the tissues of advanced or complicated silicosis, substantial accumulations of lymphocytes and monocyte-macrophages are found to be part of the silicotic nodule. As discussed, these mononuclear cells are believed to be the directing force behind fibroblast proliferation and excessive collagen deposition. A beneficial result with steroid therapy, as made evident by radiographic and physiologic improvement, was reported for one patient with acute silicosis.[185] A trial of daily prednisolone for 6 months was carried out among 34 stone-crushing workers with silicosis in India.[186] Pulmonary function and gas exchange improved, and BAL inflammatory cell numbers decreased, from the beginning to the end of the trial. These and other anecdotal experiences, and this one trial, suggest that steroids may sometimes be helpful in patients with rapidly progressive silicosis. It is not clear whether any improvement is maintained, disease progression is delayed, or how long treatment must be continued in order for the worker to benefit. Experience with other inflammatory or cytotoxic agents has not been reported. Chinese researchers are engaged in the evaluation of several agents derived from traditional Chinese medicine that appear to be active in animal models and possibly in humans.[181] Compounds directed at blocking the effects of cytokines from macrophages or lymphocytes could be useful in silicosis. Although promising in the short-term animal studies, these approaches may be limited in humans by the slow progression of the disease and its course over decades.

No interventions yet known promote orderly internal repair and renewal of lung structure that has been destroyed. Lung transplantation is the ultimate extension of this strategy, which is the replacement of damaged tissue. Transplantation has become the final resort of therapy for many chronic diffuse diseases that are localized to the lung, and silicosis may be no exception. Lung transplantation for silicosis has been reported among case series of patients from many countries.[187-191] Lung transplantation is expensive, and access is severely limited by the availability of suitable organs. Most transplant programs limit therapy to younger patients, and severe silicosis is often not apparent until patients are in their 60s or 70s. This treatment should be considered for younger patients with severe impairment who give evidence of progressive disease.

General supportive care is the best that can be offered for many patients with chronic respiratory impairment due to silicosis. Pulmonary function and symptoms, rather than the appearance of the chest x-ray, should guide the assessment of severity. Useful treatment measures may include supplemental oxygen to maintain normal oxygen saturation, respiratory and limb muscle exercises to promote strength and endurance, bronchodilator medications if reversible airflow obstruction is present, and early antibiotic therapy for acute exacerbations. Smoking cessation is critical for patients who have not already quit. A high level of vigilance for TB should be maintained, since new signs may be subtle and this treatable complication will lead to accelerated loss of lung function. Whole lung lavage, corticosteroid therapy, and lung transplantation might be considered for patients with massive exposure and acute silicosis or relatively young patients with severe progressive disease (see box).

CONTROVERSIES AND FUTURE DIRECTIONS

Health problems related to silica remain with us in the modern world. Much work must still be done in order to prevent new disease, to develop effective therapy for those already suffering with silicosis, and to translate industrial hygiene measures from industrialized countries to meet the needs of developing nations. Several issues remain controversial and require further research.

Pathogenesis

A better understanding is needed of the critical steps leading from cell–particle contact to clinical silicosis. Improved understanding of the timing and the relative importance of different steps in the pathogenesis of the disease may permit focused interdiction. Many cytokines have been implicated in silicosis; it is not yet clear whether all of them

---

Treatment options for silicosis patients

General measures

Supplemental oxygen (if desaturation present)
Respiratory and limb muscle exercises
Bronchodilator medications (if reversible airflow obstruction present)
Early antibiotic therapy for acute exacerbations
Smoking cessation (if applicable)
Vigilance for tuberculosis

Special measures (for acute silicosis, severe progressive disease)

Whole lung lavage
Corticosteroid therapy
Lung transplantation

are essential or if some are less important secondary phenomena. Clarification of which cytokines are of greatest importance could provide strategies for treatment. The genetics of responsiveness to silicosis have received little attention. A great deal may be learned from a better understanding of why specific animal strains or human families are more sensitive to silicosis than others.

Clinical management

Prevention, rather than treatment, remains the clear choice for reducing silicosis, TB, industrial bronchitis, and lung cancer. Nonetheless, better therapies would be of great benefit to those already suffering with disease. More extensive evaluation of corticosteroid therapy for silicosis is warranted; small case series suggest short-term effectiveness in patients with relatively acute silicosis. The duration of the beneficial effect needs to be determined. A controlled trial to assess efficacy and safety of corticosteroid therapy in patients with more chronic disease may be necessary.

The usefulness of whole lung lavage in removing dust, and the physiologic benefits gained by this dust removal, should be assessed. Standardized treatment criteria, untreated comparison groups, and careful follow-up studies are needed. Inhalation of aluminum lactate shows promise for reducing silicosis in animals but may be too toxic for humans. Further studies are needed to determine whether aluminum compounds or other similar salts are effective in reducing silicosis and also are safe for human use. Selective drugs that interfere with essential mediators and with specific steps in the pathogenesis of silicosis could permit improved treatment for this disease.

Regulation and industrial hygiene

We must maintain continuing vigilance for excess exposure to silica in settings with well-known risks. Surveys of foundries, mines, and other industries continue to identify hazardous exposures despite effective regulations. This vigilance must include surveillance and regulation of industries but should also include education of employees about safe work practices. Workers must believe that dust exposure will be harmful, that prevention is effective, and that they share personal responsibility for a safe workplace.

We must maintain an alert posture for new industries that create unexpected risks. Increasing use of ceramic fibers, amorphous silica, and silica flour may create new risks of contracting an ancient disease in a modern high-technology setting. We must be particularly alert for the generation of cristobalite as a result of the high-temperature transformation of amorphous, apparently safe, silica materials.

Current ambient dust standards appear to be safe in providing protection from classical silicosis. The limits of respirable silica that provide safety from an excess risk of bronchogenic carcinoma, particularly in smokers, are not known. Current levels may be adequate, or more stringent

regulations may be required. In any event, smoking cessation will be more effective in lung-cancer risk reduction than lowering of the silica-TLV. Smoking cessation and prevention should receive high priority in workplaces with silica exposure.

Standards that are now accepted as safe in the industrialized world must be applied to developing nations. We must encourage the production of improved and inexpensive equipment for ventilation, for air extraction, and for the application of water to stone-cutting surfaces. Technical advances in equipment for better industrial hygiene should provide a tremendous boost for worker safety. This equipment must become cost-effective for all countries.

Silicosis has been with us for thousands of years and remains a major public-health problem in developing nations as we enter the twenty-first century. New ideas and new technologies, as well as continuing application of the many lessons learned over past centuries, are required to combat this disease.

REFERENCES

1. *U.S. Dept. of Labor Supplementary Data Systems. Publication PB86-129830*, Washington, D.C., 1983, National Technical Information Service.
2. Current trends: exposure trends in silica flour plants—United States, 1975-1986, *MMWR* 39:380-383, 1989.
3. Gantner BA: Respiratory hazard from removal of ceramic fiber insulation from high temperature industrial furnaces, *Am Ind Hyg Assoc J* 47:530-534, 1986.
4. Hnizdo E, Baskind E, Sluis Cremer GK: Combined effect of silica dust exposure and tobacco smoking on the prevalence of respiratory impairments among gold miners, *Scand J Work Environ Health* 16.411-422, 1990.
5. Jörgensen HS: Silicosis in the iron-ore mine in Kiruna, Sweden, and the future need for silicosis control, *Int Arch Occup Environ Health* 58:251-257, 1986.
6. Muir DC, et al: Silica exposure and silicosis among Ontario hardrock miners: III analysis and risk estimates, *Am J Ind Med* 16:29-43, 1989.
7. Verma DK, et al: Silica exposure and silicosis among Ontario hardrock miners: II exposure estimates, *Am J Ind Med* 16:13-18, 1989.
8. Short SR and Petsonk EL: Respiratory health risks among nonmetal miners, *Occup Med: State of the Art Reviews* 8(1):57-70, 1993.
9. Hearings Before a Subcommittee of the Committee on Labor. House of Representatives, 74th Congress. Anonymous, editor: *H.J. Res. 449. Jan 16, 17, 20, 21, 27-29, Feb 4, 1936*, Washington, D.C., 1936, U.S. Government Printing Office.
10. Corn JK: Historical aspects of industrial hygiene, II. silicosis, *Am Ind Hyg Assoc J* 41:125-133, 1980.
11. Theriault GP, et al: Dust exposure in the Vermont granite sheds, *Arch Environ Health* 28:12-17, 1974.
12. Piguet PF, Collart MA, Grau GE, Sappino AP, and Vassalli P: Requirement of tumour necrosis factor for development of silica-induced pulmonary fibrosis, *Nature* 344:245-247, 1990.
13. Russell AE, et al: *The health of workers in dusty trades. II. exposure to siliceous dust (granite industry)*, Washington, D.C., 1929, USGPO: Public Health Bulletin No. 269.
14. Graham WG, et al: Radiographic abnormalities in Vermont granite workers exposed to low levels of granite dust, *Chest* 100:1507-1514, 1991.
15. Ehrlich RI, Rees D, and Zwi AB: Silicosis in non-mining industry on the Witwatersrand, *S Afr Med J* 73:704-708, 1988.

16. Landrigan PJ, et al: Silicosis in a gray iron foundry: the persistence of an ancient disease, *Scand J Work Environ Health* 12:32-39, 1986.

17. Valiante DJ and Rosenman KD: Does silicosis still occur? *JAMA* 262:3003-3007, 1989.

18. Janko M, et al: Occupational exposure and analysis of microcrystalline cristobalite in mullite operations, *Am Ind Hyg Assoc J* 50:460-465, 1989.

19. Glindmeyer HW and Hammad YY: Contributing factors to sandblasters' silicosis: inadequate respiratory protection equipment and standards, *J Occup Med* 30:917-921, 1988.

20. Westerholm P, Ahlmark A, Maasing R, and Segelberg I: Silicosis and risk of lung cancer or lung tuberculosis: a cohort study, *Environ Res* 41:339-350, 1986.

21. Samimi B, Weill H, and Ziskind M: Respirable silica dust exposure of sandblasters and associated workers in steel fabrication yards, *Arch Environ Health* 29:61-66, 1974.

22. Silicosis: cluster in sandblasters—Texas, and occupational surveillance for silicosis, *MMWR* 39:433-437, 1990.

23. Banks DE, et al: Silicosis in silica flour workers, *Am Rev Respir Dis* 124:445-450, 1981.

24. Johnson WM and Busnardo MS: Silicosis following employment in the manufacture of silica flour and industrial sand, *J Occup Med* 35:716-719, 1993.

25. Abrams HK: Diatomaceous earth silicosis, *Am J Ind Med* 18:591-597, 1990.

26. Checkoway H, et al: Mortality among workers in the diatomaceous earth industry, *Br J Ind Med* 50:586-597, 1993.

26a. Legge RT and Rosencrantz E: Observations and studies on silicosis by diatomaceous silica, *Am J Public Health* 22:1055-1060, 1932.

27. Abrams HK: Diatomaceous earth pneumoconiosis, *Am J Pub Health* 44:592-599, 1954.

28. Harber P, et al: Radiographic findings in diatomaceous earth industry workers, *Am Rev Respir Dis* 147:901a 1993.

29. Reference deleted in proofs.

30. Swaen GM, Passier PE, and van Attekum AM: Prevalence of silicosis in the Dutch fine-ceramic industry, *Int Arch Occup Environ Health* 60:71-74, 1988.

31. Huang J, et al: Comprehensive health evaluation of workers in the ceramics industry, *Br J Ind Med* 50:112-116, 1993.

32. Bar Ziv J and Goldberg GM: Simple siliceous pneumoconiosis in Negev Bedouins, *Arch Environ Health* 29:121-126, 1974.

33. Nouh MS: Is the desert lung syndrome (nonoccupational dust pneumoconiosis) a variant of pulmonary alveolar microlithiasis? report of 4 cases with review of the literature, *Respiration* 55:122-126, 1989.

34. Norboo T, et al: Silicosis in a Himalayan village population: role of environmental dust, *Thorax* 46:341-343, 1991.

35. Agricola G: *De re metallica, book 1, 1556,* edition 12, San Francisco, 1912, Mining and Science.

36. Munizaga J, et al: Pneumoconiosis in Chilean miners of the 16th century, *Bull NY Acad Med* 51:1281-1293, 1975.

37. Ramazzini B: *De morbis artificum (diseases of workers),* New York, 1964, Hefner.

38. Thackrah CT: *The effects of arts, trades, and professions, and of civic states and habits of living on health and longevity: with suggestions for the removal of many of the agents which produce disease, and shorten the duration of life,* edition 2, London, 1832, Longman, Rees, Orme, et al.

39. Clark J: *A treatise on pulmonary consumption; comprehending an inquiry into the causes, nature, prevention, and treatment of tuberculosis and scrofulous diseases in general,* Philadelphia, 1835, Carey, Lea, and Blanchard.

40. Landis HRM: Pneumoconiosis. Osler W, McCrae T, and Funk EH, editors: *Modern medicine: Its theory and practice,* Philadelphia, 1927, Lea and Febiger.

41. *Radiographs of the pneumoconioses—1980,* Washington, D.C., 1980, International Labor Office.

42. Classification of radiographs of the pneumoconioses, *Med Radiogr Photogr* 57:1-17, 1981.

43. Begin R, et al: Lung function in silica-exposed workers. a relationship to disease severity assessed by CT scan, *Chest* 94:539-545, 1988.

44. Murray J, et al: Cor pulmonale and silicosis: a necropsy based case-control study, *Br J Ind Med* 50:544-548, 1993.

45. Craighead JE, et al: Diseases associated with exposure to silica and nonfibrous silicate minerals. silicosis and silicate disease committee, *Arch Pathol Lab Med* 112:673-720, 1988.

46. Brody AR, et al: Use of backscattered electron imaging to quantify the distribution of inhaled crystalline silica, *Scan Electron Microsc* 301-306, 1980.

47. Brody AR, et al: Deposition and translocation of inhaled silica in rats: quantification of particle distribution, macrophage participation, and function, *Lab Invest* 47:533-542, 1982.

48. Vigliani EC and Pernis B: Immunological aspects of silicosis, *Adv Tuberc Res* 12:230-279, 1963.

49. Tschopp JM, et al: Retroperitoneal silicosis mimicking pancreatic carcinoma in an Alpine miner with chronic lung silicosis, *Thorax* 47:480-481, 1992.

50. Liu YC, et al: Mineral-associated hepatic injury: a report of seven cases with X-ray microanalysis, *Hum Pathol* 22:1120-1127, 1991.

51. Doll NJ, et al: Immune complexes and autoantibodies in silicosis, *J Allergy Clin Immunol* 68:281-285, 1981.

52. Seaton A, et al: Accelerated silicosis in Scottish stonemasons, *Lancet* 337:341-344, 1991.

53. Buechner HA and Ansari A: Acute silicoproteinosis, *Dis Chest* 55:174-177, 1969.

54. Chapman EM: Acute silicosis, *JAMA* 98:1439-1441, 1932.

55. Dumontet C, et al: Acute silicosis due to inhalation of a domestic product, *Am Rev Respir Dis* 143:880-882, 1991.

56. Suratt PM, et al: Acute silicosis in tombstone sandblasters, *Am Rev Respir Dis* 115:521-529, 1977.

57. Cherniack RM, et al: Bronchoalveolar lavage constituents in healthy individuals, idiopathic pulmonary fibrosis, and selected comparison groups, *Am Rev Respir Dis* 141:s169-s202, 1990.

57a. Reynolds HY and Newball HH: Analysis of proteins and respiratory cells obtained from human lungs by bronchial lavage, *J Lab Clin Med* 84:559-573, 1974.

57b. Low RB, Davis GS, and Giancola MS: Biochemical analyses of bronchoalveolar lavage fluids of healthy human volunteer smokers and nonsmokers, *Am Rev Respir Dis* 118:863-875, 1978.

57c. Merrill WW, Goodenberger D, Strober W, Matthay RA, Naegel GP, and Reynolds HY: Free secretory component and other proteins in human lung lavage, *Am Rev Respir Dis* 122:156-161, 1980.

57d. Bell DY, Haseman JA, Spock A, McLennan G, and Hook GER: Plasma proteins of the bronchoalveolar surface of the lungs of smokers and nonsmokers, *Am Rev Respir Dis* 124:72-79, 1981.

57e. Gotoh T, Ueda S, Nakayama T, Takishita Y, Yasuoka S, and Tsubura E: Protein components of bronchoalveolar lavage fluids from nonsmokers and smokers, *Eur J Respir Dis* 64:369-377, 1983.

58. Begin RO, et al: Spectrum of alveolitis in quartz-exposed human subjects, *Chest* 92:1061-1067, 1987.

59. Cordeiro R: Pathogenic perspectives in the alveolitis of silicosis, *Sarcoidosis* 6:28-29, 1989.

60. Rom WN, et al: Characterization of the lower respiratory tract inflammation of nonsmoking individuals with interstitial lung disease associated with chronic inhalation of inorganic dusts, *Am Rev Respir Dis* 136:1429-1434, 1987.

61. Christman JW, et al: Mineral dust and cell recovery from the bronchoalveolar lavage of healthy Vermont granite workers, *Am Rev Respir Dis* 132:393-399, 1985.

62. Costabel U, et al: Lung and blood lymphocyte subsets in asbestosis and in mixed dust pneumoconiosis, *Chest* 91:110-112, 1987.

63. Calhoun WJ, et al: Raised immunoglobulin concentrations in bronchoalveolar lavage fluid of healthy granite workers, *Thorax* 41:266-273, 1986.

64. Schuyler MR, et al: Bronchoalveolar lavage in silicosis, *Lung* 157:95-102, 1980.

65. Morgan WKC: Industrial bronchitis, *Br J Ind Med* 35:285-291, 1978.

66. Ulmer WT: Chronic obstructive airway disease in pneumoconiosis in comparison to chronic obstructive airway disease in non-dust exposed workers, *Bull Physiopathol Respir (Nancy)* 11:415-427, 1975.

67. Ulmer WT and Reichel G: Epidemiological problems of coal workers' bronchitis in comparison with the general population, *Ann N Y Acad Sci* 200:211-219, 1972.

68. Holman CD, et al: Determinants of chronic bronchitis and lung dysfunction in Western Australian gold miners, *Br J Ind Med* 44:810-818, 1987.

68a. Ng TP, et al: An epidemiological survey of respiratory morbidity among granite quarry workers in Singapore: chronic bronchitis and lung function impairment, *Ann Acad Med Singapore* 21:312-317, 1992.

69. Rastogi SK, et al: A study of the prevalence of respiratory morbidity among agate workers, *Int Arch Occup Environ Health* 63:21-26, 1991.

70. Oxman AD, et al: Occupational dust exposure and chronic obstructive pulmonary disease. A systematic overview of the evidence, *Am Rev Respir Dis* 148:38-48, 1993.

71. Wright JL, Harrison N, Wiggs B, and Churg A: Quartz but not iron oxide causes air-flow obstruction, emphysema, and small airways lesions in the rat, *Am Rev Respir Dis* 138:129-135, 1988.

72. Rosner D and Markowitz G: Consumption, silicosis, and the social construction of industrial disease, *Yale J Biol Med* 64:481-498, 1991.

73. Prowse K and Cavanagh P: Tuberculosis in the Potteries 1971-1974, *Lancet* 2:357-359, 1976.

74. Snider DE: The relationship between tuberculosis and silicosis, *Am Rev Respir Dis* 118:455-460, 1978.

75. Zambon P, Simonato L, Mastrangelo G, et al: Mortality of workers compensated for silicosis during the period 1959-1963 in the Veneto region of Italy, *Scand J Work Environ Health* 13:118-123, 1987.

76. van Sprundel MP: Pneumoconioses: the situation in developing countries, *Exp Lung Res* 16:5-13, 1990.

77. Allison AC and D'Arcy Hart P: Potentiation by silica of the growth of Mycobacterium tuberculosis in macrophage cultures, *Br J Exp Pathol* 49:465-476, 1968.

78. Davis GS, et al: Alveolar macrophage stimulation and population changes in silica-exposed rats, *Chest* 80:8-10, 1981.

79. Pairon JC, et al: Silica and lung cancer: a controversial issue, *Eur Respir J* 4:730-744, 1991.

80. Spivack SD: Silica and lung cancer, *Lancet* 335:854-855, 1990.

81. Chen J, et al: Mortality among dust-exposed Chinese mine and pottery workers, *J Occup Med* 34:311-316, 1992.

82. Hnizdo E and Sluis Cremer GK: Silica exposure, silicosis, and lung cancer: a mortality study of South African gold miners, *Br J Ind Med* 48:53-60, 1991.

83. Hodgson JT and Jones RD: Mortality of a cohort of tin miners 1941-1986, *Br J Ind Med* 47:665-676, 1990.

84. Amandus H and Costello J: Silicosis and lung cancer in U.S. metal miners, *Arch Environ Health* 46:82-89, 1991.

85. Chen SY, et al: Mortality experience of haematite mine workers in China, *Br J Ind Med* 47:175-181, 1990.

86. Carta P, Cocco PL, and Casula D: Mortality from lung cancer among Sardinian patients with silicosis, *Br J Ind Med* 48:122-129, 1991.

87. Finkelstein M, et al: Mortality among workers receiving compensation awards for silicosis in Ontario 1940-1985, *Br J Ind Med* 44:588-594, 1987.

88. Infante-Rivard C, et al: Lung cancer mortality and silicosis in Quebec, 1938-1985, *Lancet* 2:1504-1507, 1989.

89. Merlo F, et al: Mortality from specific causes among silicotic subjects: a historical prospective study, *IARC Sci Publ* 105-111, 1990.

90. Ng TP, Chan SL, and Lee J: Mortality of a cohort of men in a silicosis register: further evidence of an association with lung cancer, *Am J Ind Med* 17:163-171, 1990.

91. Chiyotani K, et al: Lung cancer risk among pneumoconiosis patients in Japan, with special reference to silicotics, *IARC Sci Publ* 95-104, 1990.

92. Ziskind M, Weill H, Anderson AE, et al: Silicosis in shipyard sandblasters, *Environ Res* 11:237-243, 1976.

93. Costello J and Graham WG: Vermont granite workers' mortality study, *Am J Ind Med* 13:483-497, 1988.

94. Chia SE, et al: Silicosis and lung cancer among Chinese granite workers, *Scand J Work Environ Health* 17:170-174, 1991.

95. Sherson D, Svane O, and Lynge E: Cancer incidence among foundry workers in Denmark, *Arch Environ Health* 46:75-81, 1991.

96. Mehnert WH, et al: A mortality study of a cohort of slate quarry workers in the German Democratic Republic, *IARC Sci Publ* 55-64, 1990.

97. Tornling G, Hogstedt C, and Westerholm P: Lung cancer incidence among Swedish ceramic workers with silicosis, *IARC Sci Publ* 113-119, 1990.

98. Amandus HE, et al: Reevaluation of silicosis and lung cancer in North Carolina dusty trades workers, *Am J Ind Med* 22:147-153, 1992.

99. Lagorio S, et al: A case-referent study on lung cancer mortality among ceramic workers, *IARC Sci Publ* 21-28, 1990.

100. Meijers JM, et al: Epidemiologic studies of inorganic dust-related lung diseases in The Netherlands, *Exp Lung Res* 16:15-23, 1990.

101. Hessel PA, Sluis Cremer GK, and Hnizdo E: Silica exposure, silicosis, and lung cancer: a necropsy study, *Br J Ind Med* 47:4-9, 1990.

102. Mastrangelo G, et al: A case-referent study investigating the relationship between exposure to silica dust and lung cancer, *Int Arch Occup Environ Health* 60:299-302, 1988.

103. Lynge E, et al: Silica dust and lung cancer: results from the Nordic occupational mortality and cancer incidence registers, *J Natl Cancer Inst* 77:883-889, 1986.

104. Saffiotti U: Lung cancer induction by crystalline silica, *Prog Clin Biol Res* 374P51-69:51-69, 1992.

104a. Ashe HB and Bergstrom DE: Twenty-six years' experience with dust control in the Vermont granite industry, *Indust Med Surg* 33:73-78, 1964.

105. Ayer HE, et al: A monumental study—reconstruction of a 1920 granite shed, *Amer Ind Hyg Assoc J* 34:206-211, 1973.

106. Davis LK, et al: Mortality experience of Vermont granite workers, *Am J Ind Med* 4:705-723, 1983.

107. Eisen EA, Wegman DH, and Louis TA: Effects of selection in a prospective study of forced expiratory volume in Vermont granite workers, *Am Rev Respir Dis* 128:587-591, 1983.

108. Musk AW, et al: Pulmonary function in granite dust exposure: a four-year follow-up, *Am Rev Respir Dis* 115:769-776, 1977.

109. Theriault GP, Peters JM, and Fine LJ: Pulmonary function in granite shed workers of Vermont, *Arch Environ Health* 28:18-22, 1974.

110. Theriault GP, Peters JM, and Fine LJ: Pulmonary function and roentgenographic changes in granite dust exposure, *Arch Environ Health* 28:23-27, 1974.

111. Graham WGB, O'Grady RV, and Dubuc B: Pulmonary function loss in Vermont granite workers: A long-term follow-up and critical reappraisal, *Am Rev Respir Dis* 123:26-28, 1981.

112. Christman JW, et al: Effects of work exposure, retirement, and smoking on bronchoalveolar lavage measurements of lung dust in Vermont granite workers, *Am Rev Respir Dis* 144:1307-1313, 1991.

113. Eisen EA, et al: Estimation of long term dust exposures in the Vermont granite sheds, *Am Ind Hyg Assoc J* 45:89-94, 1984.

114. Reference deleted in proofs.

115. Absher MP, et al: Biphasic cellular and tissue response of rat lungs after eight-day aerosol exposure to the silicon dioxide cristobalite, *Am J Pathol* 134:1243-1251, 1989.

116. Hemenway DR, et al: Effectiveness of animal rotation in achieving uniform dust exposure and lung dust deposition in horizontal flow chambers, *Am Ind Hyg Assoc J* 44:655-658, 1983.

117. Sjostrand M, et al: Comparison of lung alveolar and tissue cells in silica-induced inflammation, *Am Rev Respir Dis* 143:47-52, 1991.

118. Absher MP, et al: Intrathoracic distribution and transport of aerosolized silica in the rat, *Exp Lung Res* 18:743-757, 1992.

119. Hemenway DR, et al: Comparative clearance of quartz and cristobalite from the lung, *Am Ind Hyg Assoc J* 51:363-369, 1990.

120. Vacek PM, et al: The translocation of inhaled silicon dioxide: an empirically derived compartmental model, *Fundam Appl Toxicol* 17:614-626, 1991.

121. Fubini B, et al: Chemical functionalities at the silica surface determining its reactivity when inhaled. Formation and reactivity of surface radicals, *Toxicol Ind Health* 6:571-598, 1990.

122. Fubini B, et al: Structural and induced heterogeneity at the surface of some SiO_2 polymorphs from the enthalpy of adsorption of various molecules, *Langmuir* 9:2712-2720, 1993.

123. Allison AC, Harington JS, and Birbeck M: An examination of the cytotoxic effects of silica on macrophages, *J Exp Med* 124:141-154, 1966.

124. Emerson RJ and Davis GS: Effect of alveolar lining material-coated silica on rat alveolar macrophages, *Environ Health Perspect* 51:81-84, 1983.

125. Harmsen AG, et al: The role of macrophages in particle translocation from lungs to lymph nodes, *Science* 230:1277-1280, 1985.

126. Cantin A, Dubois F, and Begin R: Lung exposure to mineral dusts enhances the capacity of lung inflammatory cells to release superoxide, *J Leukoc Biol* 43:299-303, 1988.

127. Struhar DJ, et al: Increased expression of class II antigens of the major histocompatibility complex on alveolar macrophages and alveolar type II cells and interleukin-1 (IL-1) secretion from alveolar macrophages in an animal model of silicosis, *Clin Exp Immunol* 77:281-284, 1989.

128. Bowden DH, Hedgecock C, and Adamson IYR: Silica-induced pulmonary fibrosis involves the reaction of particles with interstitial rather than alveolar macrophages, *J Pathol* 158:73-80, 1989.

129. Hurme M, Seppala IJ: Differential induction of membrane-associated interleukin-1 (IL-1) expression and IL-1 alpha and IL-1 beta secretion by lipopolysaccharide and silica in human monocytes, *Scand J Immunol* 27:725-730, 1988.

130. Kampschmidt RF, Worthington ML, and Mesecher MI: Release of interleukin-1 (IL-1) and IL-1-like factors from rabbit macrophages with silica, *J Leukoc Biol* 39:123-132, 1986.

131. Oghiso Y: Heterogeneity in immunologic functions of rat alveolar macrophages—their accessory cell function and IL-1 production, *Microbiol Immunol* 31:247-260, 1987.

132. Oghiso Y and Kubota Y: Enhanced interleukin-1 production by alveolar macrophages and increase in Ia-positive lung cells in silica-exposed rats, *Microbiol Immunol* 30:1189-1198, 1986.

133. Schmidt JA, et al: Silica-stimulated monocytes release fibroblast proliferation factors identical to interleukin-1. A potential role for interleukin-1 in the pathogenesis of silicosis, *J Clin Invest* 73:1462-1472, 1984.

134. Struhar D and Harbeck RJ: Anti-Ia antibodies inhibit the spontaneous secretion of IL-1 from silicotic rat alveolar macrophages, *Immunol Lett* 23:31-34, 1989.

135. Bissonnette E and Rola-Pleszczynski M: Pulmonary inflammation and fibrosis in a murine model of asbestosis and silicosis. Possible role of tumor necrosis factor, *Inflammation* 13:329-339, 1989.

136. Driscoll KE, et al: Pulmonary response to silica or titanium dioxide: inflammatory cells, alveolar macrophage-derived cytokines, and histopathology, *Am J Respir Cell Mol Biol* 2:381-390, 1990.

137. Dubois CM, Bissonnette E, and Rola-Pleszczynski M: Asbestos fibers and silica particles stimulate rat alveolar macrophages to release tumor necrosis factor. Autoregulatory role of leukotriene B4, *Am Rev Respir Dis* 139:1257-1264, 1989.

138. Mohr C, et al: Systemic macrophage stimulation in rats with silicosis: enhanced release of tumor necrosis factor-alpha from alveolar and peritoneal macrophages, *Am J Respir Cell Mol Biol* 5:395-402, 1991.

139. Lugano EM, Dauber JH, and Daniele RP: Acute experimental silicosis. Lung morphology, histology, and macrophage chemotaxin secretion, *Am J Pathol* 109:27-36, 1982.

140. Englen MD, et al: Stimulation of arachidonic acid metabolism in silica-exposed alveolar macrophages, *Exp Lung Res* 15:511-526, 1989.

141. Mohr C, et al: Reduced release of leukotrienes B4 and C4 from alveolar macrophages of rats with silicosis, *Am J Respir Cell Mol Biol* 7:542-547, 1992.

142. Mohr C, et al: Enhanced release of prostaglandin E2 from macrophages of rats with silicosis, *Am J Respir Cell Mol Biol* 6:390-396, 1992.

143. Kelley J: Cytokines of the lung: state of the art, *Am Rev Respir Dis* 141:765-788, 1990.

144. Kasahara K, et al: The role of monokines in granuloma formation in mice: The ability of interleukin-1 and tumor necrosis factor-α to induce lung granulomas, *Clin Immunol Immunopathol* 51:419-425, 1989.

145. Piguet PF, et al: Requirement of tumor necrosis factor for development of silica-induced pulmonary fibrosis, *Nature* 344:245-247, 1990.

146. Davis GS, et al: Altered patterns of lung lymphocyte accumulation in silicosis in cytokine-sufficient (C3H/HeN) and cytokine-deficient (C3H/HeJ-LPSd) mice, *Chest* 103:120S-121S, 1993.

147. Aalto M, Kulonen E, and Pikkarainen J: Isolation of silica-dependent protein from rat lung with special reference to development of fibrosis, *Br J Exp Pathol* 70:167-182, 1989.

148. Benson SC, Belton JC, and Scheve LG: Regulation of lung fibroblast proliferation and protein synthesis by bronchiolar lavage in experimental silicosis, *Environ Res* 41:61-78, 1986.

149. Brown GP, Monick M, and Hunninghake GW: Fibroblast proliferation induced by silica-exposed human alveolar macrophages, *Am Rev Respir Dis* 138:85-89, 1988.

150. Harrington JS, et al: The in-vitro effects of silica-treated hamster macrophages on collagen production by hamster fibroblasts, *J Pathol* 109:21-37, 1973.

151. Heppleston AG and Stiles JA: Activity of a macrophage factor in collagen formation by silica, *Nature* (London) 214:521-522, 1967.

152. Sjostrand M and Rylander R: Lysosomal enzyme activity and fibroblast stimulation of lavage from guinea pigs exposed to silica dust, *Br J Exp Pathol* 68:309-318, 1987.

153. Kumar RK, Li W, and O'Grady R: Activation of lymphocytes in the pulmonary inflammatory response to silica, *Immunol Invest* 19:363-372, 1990.

154. Kumar RK: Quantitative immunohistologic assessment of lymphocyte populations in the pulmonary inflammatory response to intratracheal silica, *Am J Pathol* 135:605-614, 1989.

155. Struhar D, Harbeck RJ, and Mason RJ: Lymphocyte populations in lung tissue, bronchoalveolar lavage fluid, and peripheral blood in rats at various times during the development of silicosis, *Am Rev Respir Dis* 139:28-32, 1989.

156. Hubbard AH: Role for T lymphocytes in silica-induced pulmonary inflammation, *Lab Invest* 61:46-52, 1989.

157. Schuyler M, Ziskind M, and Salvaggio J: Cell-mediated immunity in silicosis, *Am Rev Respir Dis* 116:147-151, 1977.
158. Schuyler MR, Ziskind MM, and Salvaggio J: Function of lymphocytes and monocytes in silicosis, *Chest* 75:340-344, 1979.
159. Jones RN, et al: High prevalence of antinuclear antibodies in sandblasters' silicosis, *Am Rev Respir Dis* 113:393-394, 1976.
160. Callis AH, et al: The role of complement in experimental silicosis, *Environ Res* 40:301-312, 1986.
161. Suzuki N, et al: Mast cells are essential for the full development of silica-induced pulmonary inflammation: a study with mast cell-deficient mice, *Am J Respir Cell Mol Biol* 9:475-483, 1993.
162. Reiser KM, et al: Experimental silicosis. I. Acute effects of intratracheally instilled quartz on collagen metabolism and morphologic characteristics of rat lungs, *Am J Pathol* 107:176-185, 1982.
163. Reiser KM, et al: Experimental silicosis. II. Long-term effects of intratracheally instilled quartz on collagen metabolism and morphologic characteristics of rat lungs, *Am J Pathol* 110:30-40, 1983.
164. Dauber JH, et al: Experimental silicosis: morphologic and biochemical abnormalities produced by intratracheal instillation of quartz into guinea pig lungs, *Am J Pathol* 101:595-612, 1980.
165. Poole A: Measurements of enzymes of collagen synthesis in rats with experimental silicosis, *Br J Exp Pathol* 66:89-94, 1985.
166. Poole A, et al: Collagen biosynthesis enzymes in lung tissue and serum of rats with experimental silicosis, *Br J Exp Pathol* 66:567-575, 1985.
167. Ramos C, et al: Collagen metabolism in experimental lung silicosis. A trimodal behavior of collagenolysis, *Lung* 166:347-353, 1988.
168. Kawada H, et al: Alveolar type II cells, surfactant protein A (SP-A), and the phospholipid components of surfactant in acute silicosis in the rat, *Am Rev Respir Dis* 140:460-470, 1989.
169. Low RB, et al: Alveolar type II cell response in rats exposed to aerosols of alpha-cristobalite, *Am J Pathol* 136:923-931, 1990.
170. Ghio AJ, et al: Hypothesis: is lung disease after silicate inhalation caused by oxidant generation, *Lancet* 336:967-969, 1990.
171. Gusev VA, et al: Effect of quartz and alumina dust on generation of superoxide radicals and hydrogen peroxide by alveolar macrophages, granulocytes, and monocytes, *Br J Ind Med* 50:732-735, 1993.
172. Nyborg P and Klockars M: Quartz-induced production of reactive oxygen metabolites by activated human monocyte-derived macrophages, *APMIS* 98:823-827, 1990.
173. Janssen YM, et al: Expression of antioxidant enzymes in rat lungs after inhalation of asbestos or silica, *J Biol Chem* 267:10625-10630, 1992.
174. Holley JA, et al: Increased manganese superoxide dismutase protein in type II epithelial cells of rat lungs after inhalation of crocidolite asbestos or cristobalite silica, *Am J Pathol* 141:475-485, 1992.
175. Hearl FJ and Hewett P: Problems in monitoring dust levels within mines, *Occup Med* 8:93-108, 1993.
175a. Documentation of the threshold limit values and biological exposure indices, 5th ed, Cincinnati, 1986, American Conference of Governmental Industrial Hygeinists.
176. Regulations for maximum permissible exposure levels of silica (quartz, cristobalite, tridymite, and tripoli), *Federal Register* 54:2521-2523, 1989.
177. Utidjian HMD: Recommendations for a crystalline silica standard, *J Occup Med* 17:775-781, 1975.
178. Morgan WKC: The walrus and the carpenter or the silica criteria standard, *J Occup Med* 17:782-783, 1975.
179. Cooper TC, et al: Successful reduction of silica exposures at a sanitary ware pottery, *Am Ind Hyg Assoc J* 54:600-606, 1993.
180. Mason GR, Abraham JL, and Hoffman L: Treatment of mixed dust pneumoconiosis with whole lung lavage, *Am Rev Respir Dis* 126:1102-1106, 1982.
181. Banks DE, et al: Strategies for the treatment of pneumoconiosis, *Occup Med* 8:205-232, 1993.
182. Tan KX. Observation of the therapeutic effect of whole lung lavage on silicosis and other pneumoconiosis, *Chin J Ind Hyg Occup Med* 8:220-222, 1990.
183. Begin R, et al: Aluminium inhalation in sheep silicosis, *Int J Exp Pathol* 74:299-307, 1993.
184. Kennedy MCS: Aluminum powder in the treatment of silicosis of pottery workers and pneumoconiosis of coal-miners, *Br J Ind Med* 13:85-101, 1956.
185. Goodman GB, et al: Acute silicosis responding to corticosteroid therapy, *Chest* 101:366-370, 1992.
186. Sharma SK, Pande JN, and Verma K: Effect of prednisolone treatment in chronic silicosis, *Am Rev Respir Dis* 143:814-821, 1991.
187. da Silva JP, et al: Transplante cardiopulmonar. experiencia clinica inicial (The heart-lung transplant. initial clinical experience), *Rev Port Cardiol* 12:951-955, 1993.
188. Dromer C, et al: Long-term functional results after bilateral lung transplantation. Bordeaux lung and heart-lung transplant group, *Ann Thorac Surg* 56:68-72, 1993.
189. Lung transplant group: single lung transplantation for end-stage silicosis: report of a case, *J Formos Med Assoc* 91:926-932, 1992.
190. Metras D, et al: Heart and heart-lung transplantation. 3 years' experience in Timone CHU (Marseilles 1985-1988), *Arch Mal Coeur Vaiss* 83:209-215, 1990.
191. Roman A, et al: Unilateral lung transplantation: the first 2 cases. group of lung transplantation of the university general hospital of the Vall d'Hebron, *Med Clin* 100:380-383, 1993.

Agents Causing Airway Disease

JOHN R. BALMES

Airway injury and inflammation as a result of inhaled toxins have not received much attention in traditional occupational lung disease texts that have focused on dust-induced lung parenchymal fibrosis. In this section acute and chronic effects on the airways of both sensitizers and irritants are discussed. Although exposure levels have been greatly reduced in the United States, cotton and other vegetable dusts remain a major cause of acute and chronic respiratory symptoms worldwide. Chapter 25 discusses byssinosis from an epidemiologic as well as a clinical perspective. Chapter 26, on occupational asthma, is by the same experienced authors who wrote Chapter 5 on bronchoprovocation techniques; together these two chapters provide a virtual blueprint of the ideal work-up of a case of suspected occupational asthma. Please note that Appendix B contains a list of key references documenting specific causes of occupational asthma. There has been considerable controversy over the years about whether so-called "industrial bronchitis" (i.e., chronic cough and sputum production in dust-exposed workers) is merely an adaptive phenomenon or can lead to chronic airflow limitation and respiratory impairment. Chapter 27 provides an insightful discussion of this issue and thoroughly documents that prolonged or repeated exposure to irritating dusts, vapors, mists, and fumes can lead to chronic airflow limitation.

Chapter 25

COTTON DUST

Robert M. Castellan

Cotton is grown primarily as a raw material for use in the production of textiles. Cotton fiber, referred to as *lint* in the industry, is the hairlike material that grows from the coat of the cotton seed during its development in the fruit, or boll, of the cotton plant. The lint itself is essentially pure cellulose, but it grows in a complex biological milieu within the boll and is exposed to additional sources of external contamination after the boll opens to the environment upon maturing in the field.

COTTON DUST

Cotton dust is a complex mixture and includes a variety of substances, many of which are biologically active. This is reflected in the U.S. Occupational Safety and Health Administration (OSHA) regulatory definition of cotton dust as "dust present in the air during the handling or processing of cotton, which may contain a mixture of many substances including ground up plant matter, fiber, bacteria, fungi, soil, pesticides, noncotton plant matter and other contaminants which may have accumulated during the growing, harvesting and subsequent processing or storage periods," exclusive of lubricating oil mist in weaving operations.[1] Detailed information on the complex botanical, chemical, and physical nature of cotton dust is available elsewhere.[2]

Factors that may affect variability of cotton dust composition include cotton variety, growing conditions, insect damage, field weathering, harvest methods, ginning practices, storage conditions, and differences in textile mill processes within and between mills. For example, in contrast to yarn preparation areas, airborne dust in weaverooms is characterized by substantial quantities of starchlike material derived from the sizing material applied to warp yarns. This marked difference in composition may underlie the differing slopes of exposure–effect relationships defined for gravimetrically measured airborne cotton dust in yarn preparation areas and in weaving areas of cotton textile mills.

SUMMARY OF EFFECTS

The inhalation of cotton (and flax and hemp) dust is associated with byssinosis, a respiratory disorder characterized by a temporal pattern of chest tightness and shortness of breath most prominent during the first shift worked after a weekend away from the job. These "Monday" symptoms have a gradual onset over several hours and are often accompanied by a reversible impairment of ventilatory function. After years of exposure, a fixed obstructive impairment may disable affected workers. Other health effects associated with occupational exposure to relatively high levels of cotton dust include mill fever and irritation of the ocular and nasal mucous membranes.

UTILIZATION
Cotton production

Over the past 2 centuries, aided in part by advances in the mechanization of cotton harvesting, ginning, and textile processing, cotton fiber production has increased tremendously. (Flax, from which linen is produced, now accounts for a relatively minor proportion of textile production, especially in the United States.) The current level of worldwide cotton consumption is on the order of 90 million bales, or approximately 45 billion pounds.[3] With a crop of approximately 18 million bales, the United States is second only to China in cotton production; other major cotton producers are Russia, India, Pakistan, and Brazil.[4]

American upland cotton *(Gossypium hirsutum)* accounts for the vast majority of the cotton grown in the United States. American Pima cotton *(G. barbadense),* which produces generally longer fibers, accounts for the remainder. Other major types of cotton *(G. arboreum* and *G. herbaceum)* have generally shorter fibers and are commercially grown elsewhere.

In the United States substantial amounts of cotton are still grown in the Southeast, where it was once exclusively concentrated. However, the "cotton belt" now extends across the southern portion of the continental United States. Although cotton continues to be produced in the southeastern coastal plain, major growing areas are currently located in the San Joaquin Valley of California, central Arizona, the Texas Panhandle, the south-central Mississippi River Valley, and the Rio Grande River Valley.

In addition to its status as a major producer of cotton, the United States is also a major consumer of cotton fiber. Although the market share of cotton (relative to synthetic fibers) declined in the 1970s, it has steadily increased over the past decade. Currently, U.S. mills consume about 9 million bales of cotton each year, still somewhat less than the 11 to 12 million bales consumed during a peak in the early years of World War II.[4]

Cotton processing

In the United States essentially all commercially grown cotton is harvested by machine, a process that has replaced hand-picking but that entrains much extraneous plant and other matter along with harvested seed cotton. The two major types of machine harvesting are (1) spindle picking, a process in which revolving metal spindles remove seed cotton from bolls, and (2) stripper harvesting, a process in which the entire boll and its seed cotton content is pulled from the plant. Compared with spindle picking, stripper harvesting tends to leave less fiber in the field, but it also generally results in higher levels of contamination of seed cotton by plant trash.

Ginning, which occurs in close proximity to the farms on which cotton is grown, is the process by which the lint is separated from the seed. At the gin, lint is also dried and cleaned of most large plant trash. Prior to leaving the gin, cotton lint is baled for entry into the market. In the United States, each bale is tagged with a unique warehousing identifier and a lint sample is obtained for classification.

Cotton classing has been largely automated over the past decade. In addition to a subjective grade determined by comparison with standards, objective instrument-determined classification parameters include color, trash content, length, strength, and micronaire (a measure of fiber fineness and maturity). Together with general economic factors of supply and demand, these criteria form the basis of the cotton trade (e.g., eligibility for government farm loans, cotton pricing, and purchase orders from cotton merchants and textile mills).

Cottonseed, with short fibers (linters) still attached, is shipped from cotton gins to cottonseed mills, where (1) linters are removed for use as cellulose fiber in applications (e.g., paper manufacture) that do not require longer fibers, (2) oil is separated from the seed for use in a myriad of food products, and (3) residual protein-containing seed material is processed into feed supplement for animals and organic fertilizers for horticultural use.

Upon arrival in cotton textile mills, bales of cotton are opened and blended to ensure appropriate consistency of the final product. Blended cotton lint undergoes mechanical action that enables much of the remaining large trash and foreign material to drop out of the fiber mass. During carding, rapid action by wire teeth mounted on large, rotating cylinders serves to separate, align, and gather the fibers into a loose, ropelike intermediate called sliver. Substantial quantities of smaller foreign material are released, much in the form of airborne dust. After carding, multiple slivers are blended and further cleaned in a process called drawing, which further increases the alignment of fibers. Finish sliver from drawing may be taken directly to spinning if open-end rotor spinning, a relatively recent development, is used. Otherwise, it is first processed through roving, which imparts a slight twist in the fiber, before going on to traditional ring spinning, which produces threadlike yarn. Bobbins of yarn are consolidated into continuous lengths in winding processes, and often individual yarns are plied in twisting processes prior to weaving into fabric. In the process of slashing, just prior to weaving, warp yarns are treated with a starchlike "size" to protect them from abrasion during high-speed weaving.

Although many textile mills are fully integrated and transform bale cotton into finished cloth, some restrict operations to yarn production. Mills also differ in the type of yarn and/or fabric they produce, and this may influence the respiratory health hazard faced by employees. Beyond variability in dust levels by mill or work area, respiratory hazard may relate to characteristics of the raw cotton processed (e.g., the grade or region of growth), whether a mill is processing 100% cotton or cotton–synthetic blend, and various wet treatments of lint or yarns (e.g., washing, dyeing, or mercerization). There is essentially no risk of byssinosis from processing final fabric after it has undergone hot and wet treatments.

Sweepings and other lint-containing wastes, including material collected in textile mill air filtration systems, are commercially valuable. Partially cleaned of debris and blended in specialized waste utilization mills, these materials are sold to other manufacturers for use in the production of mattress and upholstery padding, coarse mop yarn, and various other end products.

Population at risk

Recent estimates of the number of workers potentially exposed to cotton dust in the United States are not readily available. Based on data available from the mid- to late 1970s, it has been suggested that over a half million workers were potentially exposed, approximately 80% in textile industries (i.e., yarn manufacturing and fabric manufacturing) and 20% in the nontextile industries (e.g., ginning, classing, warehousing, cottonseed processing, and manufacturing of mattress and upholstery padding).[5]

These figures probably overestimate the true U.S. population currently at risk of respiratory disease from cotton dust, for two main reasons. First, a substantial portion of those exposed are probably not significantly exposed; and second, there has been a tremendous increase in automation over the past 15 years, so that far fewer workers are required to operate the increasingly modernized textile mills in the United States.

The global population of workers exposed to cotton dust dwarfs that in the United States. Domestic mills only process about 20% of the cotton consumed worldwide, and textile processing technology in many other major cotton-consuming countries is much less advanced, requiring many more workers. In the Far East alone there are estimated to be in excess of 6 million cotton textile workers.[6] Workers outside the United States are also generally exposed to substantially higher levels of cotton dust, particularly in developing countries, where dust levels are generally much less controlled and byssinosis is still quite prevalent.[7]

HISTORY

Documentation of respiratory disorders associated with the inhalation of dust from cotton and other vegetable fibers dates back to the early 1700s. Ramazzini is credited with the earliest written observations. In his treatise on occupational diseases, he wrote, "Those who card flax and hemp so that it can be spun and given to the weavers to make the fabric find it very irksome. For a foul and poisonous dust flies out from these materials, enters the mouth, then the throat and lungs, makes the workmen cough incessantly, and by degrees brings on asthmatic troubles".[8]

During the nineteenth century, coincident with the transformation of textile manufacturing from a cottage industry into a factory system, the occurrence of occupational respiratory disease among cotton textile workers became more frequently recognized and documented. The increasingly regular work schedule associated with the Industrial Revolution led to the recognition of a peculiar "Monday phenomenon" among cotton textile workers. This was characterized by symptoms of chest tightness and other breathing difficulties occurring predominantly on the first day back to work after a Sunday break.

Although some textile mill operators in the early 1800s suggested that workers' Monday symptoms resulted from weekend revelry,[9] the concept that inhalation of dust generated during the processing of cotton (and flax) was responsible for these symptoms became increasingly accepted. By 1877 the term byssinosis—after the Latin byssus, meaning "a fine cotton or linen"—first appeared in the published literature to emphasize the apparent causative role played by inhaled dust in the resulting respiratory disorder suffered by many cotton and linen textile mill workers.[10]

Midway through the present century modern epidemiologic methods began to be applied to the problem. Schilling and others presented scientifically defensible evidence indicating that byssinosis was induced by an unknown contaminant of the airborne cotton dust inhaled by cotton mill workers.[11] This evidence contributed to an enhanced recognition of the importance of controlling occupational exposure to cotton dust and stimulated continuing research to better define the nature and specific causes of byssinosis and related disorders.

CLINICAL EFFECTS
Byssinosis

The distinguishing feature of byssinosis is a relatively specific temporal pattern of chest tightness and shortness of breath occurring at work and most prominent during the first shift worked after a weekend or vacation away from the job. These "Monday" symptoms have a gradual onset over several hours and are typically accompanied by a reversible impairment of ventilatory function most often measured as a reduction in forced expiratory volume in 1 second (FEV1). After years of exposure, a fixed obstructive lung function impairment may disable affected workers.

Variable usage of the term byssinosis has at times led to misunderstanding and controversy. Whereas its use has sometimes been restricted to either acute[12,13] or chronic[14] respiratory effects, in more common usage it embraces both acute and chronic pulmonary effects caused by inhalation of cotton, flax, or hemp dust.[5]

Table 25-1. Schilling classification of byssinosis*

Grade	Criteria
0	No particular respiratory symptoms on the first day of the work week
½†	Chest tightness and/or other breathing difficulties on some first days of the work week
1	Chest tightness and/or other breathing difficulties on all first days of the work week
2	Chest tightness and/or other breathing difficulties on the first and subsequent days of the work week
3†	Grade 2 symptoms as well as symptoms of permanent incapacity (from standard questions regarding dyspnea)

*Grade is based on subjective responses to a modification of a questionnaire developed by the Medical Research Council Committee on Research into Chronic Bronchitis.[19]

†These two grades were later additions[18] to an earlier scheme[17] based on grades 0, 1, and 2.

An early clinical description, published prior to systematic epidemiologic study of the disease but based on a review of over 100 affected workers, emphasized the progressive nature of the disorder in outlining three stages of byssinosis, between which there was "no sharp distinction"[15]:

1. "The stage of irritation—. . . cough and a tight feeling in the chest . . . usually of temporary duration, passing off in one or two days, but the susceptibility returns during a short absence away from work. . . ."
2. "The stage of temporary disablement or incapacity—After . . . some ten or more years, the effects . . . become more persistent, and the operative suffers from early bronchitis or asthma, or both combined, associated with cough and mucous expectoration."
3. "The stage of total disablement or incapacity.—In this advanced stage there is chronic bronchitis, ... Cough is present with mucous or muco-purulent expectoration and shortness of breath on exertion. This condition is incurable and at this stage work in the dusty atmosphere becomes impossible . . . ."

For epidemiologic studies conducted in the 1950s, a standardized scheme for grading symptoms of byssinosis was developed and validated (Table 25-1). Initially, this scheme focused on the characteristic acute "Monday" symptoms.[16] Later, it was modified to include chronic dyspnea symptoms as well as acute respiratory symptoms,[17] and it remains in wide use.

Initial efforts to validate the symptoms grading scheme revealed that ventilatory capacity among cotton textile workers was progressively lower with higher grades of byssinosis, controlling for age and anthropomorphic measures, and that maximum voluntary ventilation measured during work on Monday compared with Thursday tended to be lower with higher grades of symptomatic byssinosis.[17]

In subsequent physiologic evaluation of the peculiar "Monday" symptoms of byssinosis, cotton textile workers became the first occupational group to be studied with pulmonary function measurements over the work shift. McKerrow and colleagues observed increased airways resistance, decreased peak expiratory flow, and decreased maximal breathing capacity over the work shift among cotton workers with byssinosis, with similar but much less marked changes observed in cotton workers without symptoms of byssinosis.[18] Similar later observations by Merchant and colleagues[20] are shown in Fig. 25-1, which clearly illustrates the lower baseline FEV1 associated with increasing grade of byssinosis, as well as the greater acute reductions in FEV1 over the work shift, particularly on Mondays, among individuals with byssinosis.

Although chest tightness and acute decline in lung function are generally associated, these clinical responses to cotton dust are sometimes discordant within individuals. Individuals who report chest tightness sometimes do not experience associated measurable declines in function, and individuals with functional declines sometimes do not report associated chest symptoms. Concern about the subjective basis of the Schilling scheme for grading byssinosis led to the development of a functional grading system[21-23] (Table 25-2), which has been adapted for use in employee monitoring and management programs.

Building on the Schilling and functional classification schemes, an expert committee of the World Health Organization (WHO) proposed an alternative classification scheme for the effects of cotton and other vegetable dusts.[24] The WHO scheme (Table 25-3) attempts comprehensiveness by separately classifying (1) byssinosis, in terms of the work-related "Monday" pattern of acute chest tightness or shortness of breath; (2) respiratory tract irritation, in terms of dust-related symptoms of cough and phlegm, including chronic bronchitis; and (3) lung function, in terms of both acute and chronic changes. Perhaps because of its relative complexity, the WHO classification scheme has not been widely used.

Mill fever

Some other clinical effects clearly associated with the inhalation of cotton dust are not generally considered to be manifestations of byssinosis. The most significant is mill fever, a systemic febrile illness with influenzalike symptoms that typically follows initial, intense exposures to cotton dust.[25] Symptoms are most intense 6 to 12 hours after exposure and frequently resolve within 1 day, or 2 to 3 days in the most severe cases. Workers develop tolerance with repeated exposure but may have a recurrence of mill fever after a particularly high-level exposure or upon return to work following a prolonged absence.

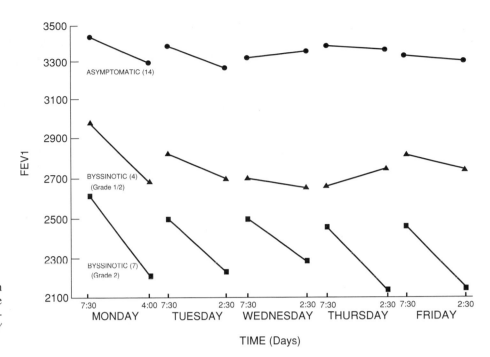

Fig. 25-1. Mean FEV1 values before and after the work shift and on each day of the workweek for 25 cotton textile mill workers with various grades of byssinosis. (Adapted from Merchant JA, Halprin GM, Hudson AR, et al: Evaluation before and after exposure—the pattern of physiologic response to cotton dust, *Ann NY Acad Sci* 221:38-43, 1974.)

Table 25-2. Functional classification of workers exposed to cotton dust

Functional grade	Baseline FEV1 (% of predicted value)	FEV1 decline (% of preshift)	Interpretation
$F_{0(a)}$	>80	<−5	No chronic impairment, minimal or no acute effect
$F_{0(b)}$	>80	−9 to −5	No chronic impairment, moderate acute effect
$F_{0(c)}$	>80	>−10	No chronic impairment, definite and marked acute effect
$F_{1(a)}$	60 to 79	<−5	Slight to moderate chronic impairment, minimal or no acute effect
$F_{1(b)}$	60 to 79	>−5	Slight to moderate chronic impairment, moderate to severe acute effect
F_2	<60	—	Moderate to severe chronic impairment

Adapted from references 21 through 23.

The generally controlled cotton dust levels in U.S. mills have apparently made mill fever a rare occurrence in this country, although occupational physicians in developing countries are still likely to deal with it on a regular basis, especially among new employees of cotton mills. Mill fever is generally considered a form of what has more recently been referred to as organic dust toxic syndrome or, more generically, as inhalation fever, discussed in more detail in Chapter 17.

The term *mattress-makers' fever* was given to a widespread outbreak of self-limited disease that appears to have been clinically identical to mill fever. This outbreak was notable in that, rather than affecting employees of textile mills, it affected poor rural families engaged in making mattresses for personal use from low-grade, stained cotton provided by a federally sponsored program intended to reduce a cotton surplus. Evidence suggesting that gram-negative bacteria (GNB) are a likely cause of mill fever, and possibly also a contributing factor in the etiology of acute and chronic pulmonary effects associated with byssinosis, resulted from an investigation of this outbreak.[26]

Asthma and weaver's cough

Although byssinosis with its characteristic "Monday" pattern of symptoms is the more common acute respiratory response, nonbyssinotic, immediate-onset, severe bronchoconstriction can occur upon exposure to cotton dust. This contrasts with the more gradual and generally mild to moderate reduction in ventilatory function typical of the acute byssinotic response to cotton dust.[27]

Individuals with a history of asthma may be at particular risk of asthmatic response when exposed to cotton dust, as illustrated by a case report of an individual with a history of childhood asthma who visited a cotton textile mill to investigate byssinosis.[28] It is widely accepted that most individuals with typical asthma would find it difficult to tolerate regular work in cotton dust, particularly at higher levels, although definitive studies have not been done to address this hypothesis.

Nonbyssinotic occupational asthma has not been systematically studied among workers exposed to cotton dust, except in response to obvious outbreaks. Such outbreaks have occurred primarily among weavers, and implicated etiologic agents include various materials used in the size used to coat the warp yarn (e.g., tamarind seed powder[29,30] and locust bean gum[31]), as well as airborne fungi from mildewed warp threads.[32,33]

Airway Hyperresponsiveness

Several studies have demonstrated an increase in airway responsiveness following exposure to cotton dust. Acute increases in nonspecific responsiveness occurring across a

Table 25-3. WHO classification of respiratory disorders from exposure to vegetable dusts causing byssinosis and respiratory tract irritation

Grade 0	No symptoms
Byssinosis	
Grade B1	Chest tightness and/or shortness of breath on most first days back at work
Grade B2	Chest tightness and/or shortness of breath on the first and other days of the work week
Respiratory tract irritation	
Grade RTI1	Cough associated with dust exposure
Grade RTI2	Persistent phlegm (on most days during 3 months of the year) initiated or exacerbated by dust exposure
Grade RTI3	Persistent phlegm initiated or made worse by dust exposure either with exacerbations of chest illness or persisting for 2 years or more
Lung function	
Acute changes	
No effect	Consistent FEV1 decline over work shift of 5% or less, or increase
Mild effect	Consistent FEV1 decline over work shift of 5% to 10%
Moderate effect	Consistent FEV1 decline over work shift of 10% to 20%
Severe effect	FEV1 decline over work shift of 20% or more
Chronic Changes	
No effect	Baseline ("Monday" preshift) FEV1 >80% of predicted value
Mild to moderate effect	Baseline ("Monday" preshift) FEV1 60% to 79% of predicted value
Severe effect	Baseline ("Monday" preshift) FEV1 <60% of predicted value

Adapted from World Health Organization (WHO) Study Group: *Recommended health-based occupational exposure limits for selected vegetable dusts*, WHO Technical Report Series No 684, Geneva, 1983, WHO.

Monday work shift have been shown in both byssinotic and nonbyssinotic cotton workers.[34] Carefully controlled experimental exposure studies have shown that this acute effect also occurs in previously nonexposed volunteers, regardless of atopic status (although the effect is more marked in atopic individuals), and that there is a direct association between the preexposure level of responsiveness and the magnitude of exposure-induced acute decline in lung function.[35] A recent study of cotton mill workers has shown that workers with byssinosis have increased nonspecific airway responsiveness compared with nonbyssinotic workers from the same mill, and that the mean cumulative dust exposure was greater among workers with airway hyperresponsiveness.[36]

The significance of increased airway responsiveness induced by cotton dust is uncertain. However, based on current general concepts of the pathogenesis of accelerated lung function decline, it may play an important role in the eventual development of chronic lung function impairment resulting from occupational exposure to cotton dust.

Byssinosis syndrome

Over the years a number of authorities have expressed a willingness to entertain the possibility that different clinical effects caused by exposure to cotton dust (e.g., mill fever and "Monday" symptoms) result from differences in dose, duration, and schedule of exposures, as well as from variability in host susceptibility,[25,37,38] rather than primarily from different etiologic agents within cotton dust. *Byssinosis syndrome,* a recently suggested term, is intended to emphasize the relatedness of various clinical effects induced by inhalation of cotton dust, including mill fever.[39] Morgan[13] pointed out that "the possibility still exists that mill fever and byssinosis are just variants of the same condition," and Kilburn similarly noted that "the differentiation of this [byssinotic] response from [mill fever] is not distinct and may be one of degree, not kind."[40]

This line of reasoning, together with the wide-ranging settings in which organic dust toxic syndrome is observed, suggests that byssinosis-like clinical effects might be anticipated in settings that do not involve exposure to cotton or other vegetable fibers. This possibility is illustrated by the reported "Monday" pattern of chest tightness associated with across-shift FEV1 declines observed in wool carpet workers exposed to endotoxin-contaminated dust.[41]

Summary

The unifying concept of byssinosis as a syndrome is countered by confusing terms such as *classic byssinosis, acute byssinosis, chronic byssinosis, and atypical byssinosis,* each of which is intended to individually relate to a different clinical response to cotton dust inhalation. In an attempt to bring some clarification, an expert committee met in 1986 and produced a consensus report of key effects caused by inhalational exposure to cotton dust.[42] A list of effects adapted from the summary report of the committee is shown in the box.

DIAGNOSTIC AND THERAPEUTIC CONSIDERATIONS

The diagnosis of byssinosis remains primarily based on symptoms and occupational exposure history, usually supplemented with results of pulmonary function testing. Occupational exposure to dust generated during the processing of cotton (or other vegetable fiber) is a prerequisite, although the necessary duration of the exposure is somewhat controversial. Although some observational epidemiologic studies suggest that years of exposure are necessary before the earliest acute symptoms of byssinosis (e.g., grade ½ "Monday" chest symptoms) occur in an individual worker, experimental exposure studies and a study of a captive population of workers in a prison cotton mill[43] suggest that, in some individuals, it should be possible to base a diagnosis on both acute symptoms and acute physiologic response within the first several weeks of employment in cotton processing mills. Indeed, since 1941 eligibility for compensation for byssinosis in Great Britain has been reduced from

---

> ### Clinical responses caused by cotton dust inhalation: the Manchester criteria
>
> *Mill fever (i.e., organic dust toxic syndrome)*
>
> *Chest tightness*
>
> "Monday" pattern with diminishing severity over workweek (i.e., classic symptom of byssinosis)
>
> Worsening and stable pattern over the week (uncommon; probably a form of occupational asthma)
>
> *Chronic bronchitis (chronic cough and phlegm after years of exposure)*
>
> *Pulmonary function effects*
>
> Gradual across-shift decline in ventilatory function (e.g., typical FEV1 decline associated with "Monday" symptoms)
>
> Accelerated annual decline in ventilatory function (chronic pulmonary impairment after years of exposure)
>
> Immediate and severe decline in ventilatory function (uncommon; probably a form of occupational asthma)
>
> *Airway hyperresponsiveness*
>
> Acute and reversible after a single exposure
>
> Chronic and possibly irreversible, after repeated exposures (may be pathogenically related to accelerated FEV1 decline)

The reference to Manchester derives from the location of the consensus committee meeting.

(Adapted from Rylander R, Schilling RSF, Pickering CAC, et al: Effects after acute and chronic exposure to cotton dust: the Manchester criteria, *Br J Ind Med* 44:577-579, 1987.)

---

10 years to no minimum period of work in specified areas of cotton mills.[44]

Acute physiologic response to cotton dust is most commonly assessed with standard spirometry performed before and after a work shift on the first day back following at least 2 days' absence from work. The preshift test provides a measure of chronic pulmonary impairment, although an assessment of reversibility requires retesting after administration of bronchodilators or other appropriate treatment.

Although a substantial dust-related decline in FEV1 may be obvious from testing done over a single work shift, smaller one-time decrements (those less than 20% and especially those less than 10%) may not be dust related, given expected variabilities in across-shift testing.[45] This has led to a recommendation that acceptance of an across-shift decline of small magnitude as being dust related should depend on consistency in the response over three consecutive test sessions.[24] This recommendation assumes relative consistency of dust exposures, and those responsible for interpreting the results of repeat testing should realize that variability in exposure between test days may contribute to inconsistency in across-shift FEV1 declines.

Spirometric assessment of acute obstructive effects has the advantages of being performed with relatively sturdy equipment that is widely available and often portable. However, standard spirometry is not entirely sensitive to acute airway responses induced by cotton dust, which have been alternatively assessed in research-based studies with partial flow–volume curves,[46] helium–oxygen spirometry,[47] measures of airways resistance,[18] and measures of thoracic impedance.[48]

A current or former cotton worker presenting with chronic respiratory symptoms (e.g., chronic productive cough, dyspnea, or persistent chest tightness) and chronic obstructive impairment can represent a diagnostic challenge. In such cases a diagnosis can sometimes be based on a convincing clinical history and/or past records indicating an initial pattern of "Monday" chest symptoms or documenting acute physiologic decrements measured across a work shift on the first day back to work after a weekend break. Some affected cotton workers, including those who may have worked 7 days a week without weekend breaks,[49] may not have experienced "Monday" symptoms. Without such history or physiologic evidence, byssinosis presents as typical chronic obstructive airways disease. As such, it is essentially impossible to clinically differentiate from chronic airways disease induced by the common habit of cigarette smoking, although it is important to be aware that smoking is generally associated with an increased susceptibility to and severity of effects induced by occupational exposure to cotton dust.[50] Chronic impairment in smoking cotton workers may be principally attributable to either dust exposure or tobacco smoke, depending on the relative duration and intensity of the exposures to the two agents.

Physical examination reveals no differentiating characteristics. Wheezing may be present especially in advanced cases but is often absent. Chest radiographs are not helpful, except to rule out the presence of other lung conditions, because byssinosis and other conditions caused by cotton dust inhalation do not have specific radiographic correlates. Likewise, there are no serologic or other clinical markers specific for byssinosis. Acute reactions to cotton dust are typically accompanied by a mild peripheral leukocytosis and, more prominently, by an influx of neutrophils to the airways, including the nasal mucosal surface.[27] Results of one study indicate that the increase in peripheral neutrophils roughly parallels the magnitude of acute FEV1 decline.[51]

The medical treatment of chronic respiratory symptoms and obstructive impairment associated with exposure to cotton dust is no different than that of chronic bronchitis and emphysema. A few limited research studies involving pharmacologic prevention and/or treatment of acute obstructive ventilatory effects have been published.[46,52-55] However, these studies offer no evidence to suggest that pharmacologic therapy should displace control of exposures and medical monitoring of workers in preventing chronic and irreversible obstructive pulmonary disease caused by cotton dust.

Readers should refer to other relevant chapters in this volume for information regarding the diagnosis and treatment of mill fever and immediate-onset occupational asthma in workers exposed to cotton dust.

PATHOLOGY

Tissue is rarely available for premortem diagnostic purposes. However, limited postmortem studies of compensated byssinotics and long-term cotton mill workers have clearly demonstrated that the airways are most prominently affected.[56-59] Findings attributable to the effects of cotton dust inhalation are essentially those of chronic bronchitis and include mucous gland hypertrophy and goblet cell hyperplasia, as well as smooth muscle hypertrophy. The issue of whether emphysema is associated with cotton dust inhalation remains controversial, although one recent article presented compelling evidence from an animal model and from a reanalysis of previously published human data.[60] In addition, so-called "byssinosis bodies" have been observed incidentally in the lungs of a minority of individuals with byssinosis, but there is no evidence that these have diagnostic or pathogenetic significance.[56]

PROGNOSIS AND COURSE OF ILLNESS

The most substantial health threat presented by occupational exposure to cotton dust is the potential for irreversible chronic impairment of pulmonary function and associated disability. Early clinical descriptions of byssinosis clearly indicate that chronic impairment and disability were considered a late stage of byssinosis.[15] Results of more recent studies have also generally documented a relationship

between chronic occupational exposure to cotton dust and reduced pulmonary function in cotton workers.[61] The effect of cigarette smoking on chronic (preshift) levels of FEV1 in cotton workers has generally been shown to be additive to that of cotton dust exposure.[50,62,63]

Although cotton workers experience accelerated lung function decline regardless of whether they have byssinosis, it has been shown that cotton workers with symptoms of byssinosis experience an accelerated loss of lung function compared with cotton workers without these symptoms.[64] In addition, recently produced evidence confirms the long-held notion that cotton workers with larger-magnitude acute (across-shift) reductions in FEV1 generally experience a more rapid chronic decline in FEV1.[65]

Substantially reduced dust concentrations in modern U.S. mills reduce the likelihood that intolerable acute reactions will be experienced or reported by workers. Lower dust concentrations also reduce the likelihood that obvious acute physiologic responses will be observed with a cross-shift spirometry monitoring. The possibility that lower dust levels may enable more susceptible workers to tolerate cotton mill work for longer periods has raised the concern that chronic effects of long-term exposure to cotton dust among textile workers may remain a problem even when acute effects are apparently under control.[42]

DOSE–EFFECT RISK RELATIONSHIPS
Cotton dust measured gravimetrically

A number of epidemiologic studies conducted primarily in textile mills have documented a gradient of increasing prevalence of byssinosis symptoms with increasing exposure to airborne cotton dust. The first report to do so was that by Roach and Schilling, who found that work area prevalences ranging up to 89% correlated well with exposures ranging from approximately 0.5 to 6 mg/m^3 total dust.[66] Furthermore, these same investigators observed that byssinosis prevalence correlated much more strongly with the medium-sized fraction and the protein content of cotton dust than with other size fractions (i.e., coarse or fine) or other compositional (i.e., cellulose or inorganic ash) fractions of dust.

Duration of exposure, a surrogate for cumulative exposure, was shown by Molyneux and Tombleson to be an important determinant of byssinosis, with prevalences, after adjustment for age, mill type, and sex, ranging from about 9% in those with less than 5 years' tenure to nearly 40% in those with over 40 years' tenure.[67] Shortly thereafter, Fox and colleagues reported that whereas the total dust (less fly) concentration correlated with byssinosis prevalence by work area, the estimated cumulative dust exposure provided a much stronger correlation.[68] An inverse relationship between increasing cumulative dust exposure and FEV1, controlling for age, sex, height, and smoking status, was also observed.

After finding that total dust concentrations in mills with

dust controls (i.e., local card exhaust and general air conditioning) were not associated with byssinosis risk,[62] Merchant and colleagues[69] reported a strong association between byssinosis prevalence and the airborne concentration of dust samples by vertical elutriator (Fig. 25-2), an area sampler designed to collect lint-free dust samples of aerodynamic size fraction similar to that deposited predominantly at and below the level of the trachea.[70] This major respiratory health study of cotton textile workers in the United States provided a basis for the comprehensive cot-

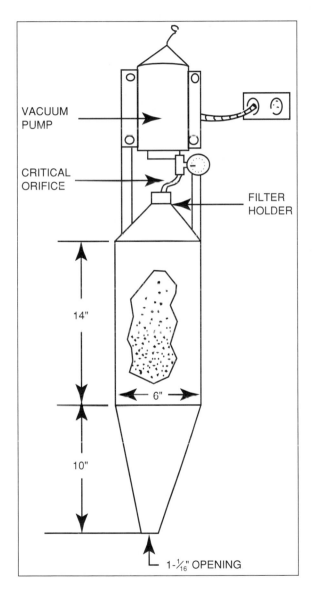

Fig. 25-2. Schematic representation of the vertical elutriator cotton dust sampler. Airflow is controlled by a critical orifice. An aerodynamically selected fraction of dust entering the bottom opening is collected on a filter after passing through a settling chamber. (Adapted from National Institute for Occupational Safety and Health (NIOSH): *Criteria for a recommended standard: occupational exposure to cotton dust,* Department of Health and Human Services Pub No (NIOSH) 75-118, Washington, DC, 1974, US Government Printing Office.)

ton dust standard first promulgated by OSHA in 1978, and OSHA-mandated routine environmental monitoring and enforcement of occupational exposure to cotton dust in textile mill work areas remain based on gravimetric measurement of airborne dust sampled by vertical elutriator. Fig. 25-3 illustrates the steeper dose–response slope for yarn preparation workers compared with that for slashing and weaving workers, which underlies the different permissible exposure limits (PELs) established by OSHA for these two different operations in cotton textile mills.

A recently completed longitudinal study has yielded evidence of a dust-related accelerated annual decline in FEV1 among yarn production workers during a period following promulgation of the comprehensive OSHA cotton dust standard in 1978.[65,71] Results from this study indicate that smokers in particular are at apparent risk for accelerated pulmonary function decline, even at dust levels equivalent to the current OSHA PEL for cotton dust in yarn preparation areas.

Despite the epidemiologically defined relationship between respiratory effects and exposure to cotton dust measured gravimetrically, it is universally acknowledged that the effects are caused by some biologically active material(s) carried in the dust. Substantial research has been conducted to identify the agent(s) in cotton dust responsible for byssinosis and related conditions.

Bacteria

The first published observation relevant to a possible etiologic role of microbial products in byssinosis was Ramazzini's description of the use of animal dung as an agent to facilitate the retting of flax and hemp: ". . . hemp and flax are macerated in stagnant, putrid waters and are first smeared with filth to hasten the necessary maceration when they are submerged under water, and so the particles that the carders breathe in must be poisonous and highly injurious to human beings."[8] The presence of large numbers of airborne GNB in cotton textile mills was initially described decades ago.[15] However, since cotton workers suffering from byssinosis were not apparently clinically infected, this observation received little attention at the time.

More recently, it has been observed that dust from chemically retted flax is much better tolerated by workers than that from biologically retted flax in terms of both "Monday" chest symptoms and acute decline in FEV1; experimental human exposure studies have confirmed this.[72] A plausible explanation for these observations is that microbes active in the biologic retting process are involved in the etiology of byssinosis.

Proteolytic enzymes. Proteolytic enzymes, predominantly of microbial origin, are known to be present in cotton dust. In a study of U.S. cotton textile mills, the airborne concentration of these enzymes correlated better with symptoms and acute physiologic signs of byssinosis than did coarse, fine, or total gravimetric dust concentrations.[73] A

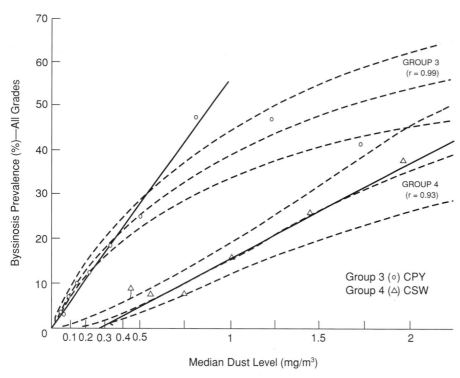

Fig. 25-3. Dose–response relationships between median gravimetric dust levels measured by vertical elutriator in various work areas and byssinosis prevalence of workers in those areas. Shown are linear regressions and probit curves (and 95% confidence limits) for cotton preparation and yarn (CPY) (group 3) and cotton slashing and weaving (CSW) (group 4) operations. (Adapted from Merchant JA, Lumsden JC, Kilburn KH, et al: Dose response studies in cotton textile workers, *JOM, J Occup Med* 15:222-230, 1973.)

similar study in British mills also found a correlation between byssinosis prevalence and airborne protease activity, but the correlation was not so strong and was no better than that for gravimetric dust.[74] Moreover, the relative paucity of byssinosis in waste cotton mill workers, despite the presence of substantial quantities of protease in the air of these mills, suggested that these enzymes were not involved in the etiology of byssinosis.[75] Although proteolytic enzymes present in cotton dust may not be involved in the etiology of "Monday" symptoms and physiologic changes, it has recently been suggested that they may play a role in the etiology of chronic bronchitis and possibly emphysema among cotton workers, perhaps acting synergistically with endotoxin.[76]

Endotoxin. The first scientific evidence suggesting that bacterial endotoxin may cause respiratory disease associated with the inhalation of cotton dust came from investigations of an outbreak of respiratory illness among mattress makers, discussed previously in the section on mill fever.[26] Pernis and colleagues[77] were the first to document the presence of endotoxin in cotton dust. Noting similarities to byssinosis, they reported that workers at a typhoid vaccine factory experienced transient low-grade fever and acute respiratory difficulties when intermittently exposed to substantial concentrations of airborne GNB. Based on results of animal and human experimental exposures, they concluded that endotoxin accounted for much of the acute response to cotton dust. Furthermore, they suggested that the phenomenon of endotoxin tolerance (and its ready loss) might account for the classic "Monday" temporal pattern of byssinosis symptoms. Later, the same group of investigators presented data

indicating that the prevalence of byssinosis in cotton workers was strongly correlated with endotoxin concentration but not with dust concentration in workplace air.[78]

Several experimental human exposure studies intended to closely mimic dust conditions experienced by textile mill workers have included measurements of airborne endotoxin. As a result of natural variation in the endotoxin contamination of cotton dust, series of exposures were created in which airborne endotoxin concentrations did not correlate with dust concentrations. In the absence of a dust effect, these studies have documented a clear relationship between endotoxin concentration and acute FEV1 decrement (Fig. 25-4), as well as an association of acute respiratory symptoms and fever with higher endotoxin concentration.[38,79,80]

Several observational epidemiologic studies based on commercial cotton and/or flax mills have investigated the possible association between occupational exposure to airborne endotoxin (or GNB, the natural source of endotoxin) and byssinosis. Cinkotai and colleagues presented the results of cross-sectional surveys that clearly correlated the prevalence of "Monday" chest symptoms with airborne viable GNB concentration and with airborne endotoxin concentration, but not with the concentration of airborne dust.[81,82] Ten years later a resurvey found a much lower prevalence of "Monday" chest symptoms and markedly reduced airborne concentrations of GNB that were not accompanied by a similar decline in airborne dust levels.[83] These findings were explained as possibly resulting from a change in dust quality related to the closure of mills that processed "dirty, coarse fibre."[84]

A survey of the Swedish cotton textile industry produced evidence that the prevalence of "Monday" chest symptoms by work area correlated more strongly with airborne GNB than with airborne dust.[85] Likewise, results of a study of cotton mill workers in Shanghai suggested an endotoxin effect (in the absence of a dust effect) on both baseline and across-shift decrements in FEV1, as well as on both acute and chronic chest symptoms.[86] Additionally, endotoxin exposure was associated with both symptomatic byssinosis and baseline FEV1 among Danish textile mill workers.[87] Finally, a preliminary report of a large survey of British textile workers also indicated that byssinosis symptom prevalence was more strongly correlated with endotoxin exposure than with dust exposure.[88]

One experimental study purporting to provide evidence against an etiologic role of endotoxin involved exposing human subjects to nebulized solutions of "endotoxin" prepared from *Enterobacter agglomerans,* a GNB frequently observed to predominate in cotton.[89] However, the "endotoxin" preparation used in the experiment was purified lipopolysaccharide, not complete endotoxin. With higher doses of purified lipopolysaccharide (LPS) or with "cell-bound" (complete) endotoxin from the same organism inhaled in amounts commensurate with endotoxin exposures in cardrooms, approximately half of exposed human subjects experienced FEV1 decrements and chest tightness.[90]

Plant products

Reasonably early in the modern era of byssinosis investigation, it had been suggested that a component of the cotton plant was an unlikely candidate for etiologic agent because taxonomically differing plants (e.g., cotton, flax, and hemp) had been implicated in byssinosis.[77] Nevertheless, a variety of biologically active compounds produced by the cotton plant have been investigated with respect to a possible etiologic role in causing byssinosis.

It is possible that the endotoxin exposure–response relationships for cotton dust might result from some other cotton dust component with a concentration that closely parallels that of endotoxin. Although concentrations of many cotton plant products do not appear to parallel that of endotoxin,[91,92] it has been suggested that concentrations of certain phytoalexins (e.g., cadelenes and lacinilenes), which are toxic plant compounds produced by the cotton plant in response to microbial infections, might roughly correlate with the endotoxin concentration.[93] However, unlike the situation with endotoxin, there is no existing human clinical or epidemiologic evidence to indicate that these phytoalexins play a causative role.

Research on many botanical compounds from cotton has been limited, but results of experimental human exposure studies involving the acute ventilatory response to card-generated dust from selected cottons provide evidence against a primary causal role for cotton bract, the brittle leaflike plant structures that subtend the boll and commonly contaminate harvested cotton,[94] for specifically measured plant components (e.g., gossypol, tannins, and terpenoid aldehydes),[95] and also for viable fungi that contaminate cotton lint.[38]

Additionally, although Buck and colleagues[96] reported the existence of an unidentified agent in cotton bract extract capable of inducing human bronchoconstriction in the relative absence of endotoxin, they did not seriously challenge the endotoxin causation hypothesis, stating that "possibly, however, where the bract constrictor agent and . . . endotoxin are present together, as they may be in mill dust, a synergistic action exists."

REGULATIONS
History of federal cotton dust regulations in the United States

The first federal regulation concerning cotton dust, established under the Walsh–Healy Act, regulated government contractors. It required that airborne exposures to cotton dust not exceed 1000 $\mu g/m^3$, measured as total dust. The initial OSHA cotton dust standard, established in 1971, merely adopted this 1000 $\mu g/m^3$ total dust limit as a PEL for cotton dust in general industry. In 1978, several years after the National Institute for Occupational Safety and Health (NIOSH) published a recommended occupational health standard for cotton dust,[23] OSHA promulgated a comprehensive occupational health standard for cotton dust in general industry.[97] Numerous administrative and judicial actions have been taken with respect to the 1978 OSHA cotton dust standard, culminating in a major OSHA revision of the standard in 1985.[1]

Of historical significance, the OSHA cotton dust standard provided the basis for an important decision by the U.S. Supreme Court concerning the cost of compliance with occupational safety and health regulations in the United States. In 1981 the Court upheld the OSHA standard by rejecting the concept that OSHA be required to apply cost–benefit considerations in the establishment of occupational health standards. Based on a provision of the Occupational Safety and Health Act, which states that each standard shall be set "which most adequately assures, *to the extent feasible,* on the basis of the best available evidence, that no employee will suffer material impairment of health or functional capacity . . ."[98] (emphasis added), the majority opinion indicated that *feasible* means "capable of being done, executed, or effected," and that costs of compliance with occupational safety and health standards should be considered part of the cost of doing business.[99]

Current Occupational Safety and Health Administration cotton dust regulations

The main OSHA regulatory requirements regarding cotton dust-exposed workers are listed by regulated industries

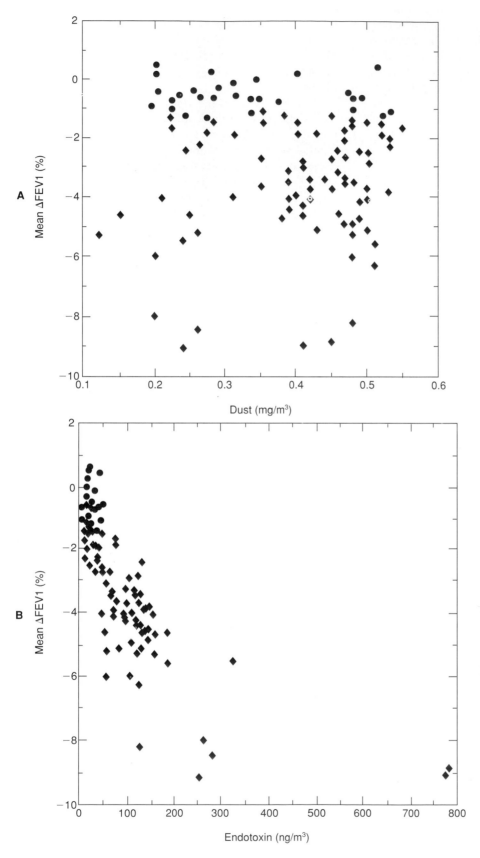

Fig. 25-4. Mean FEV1 change versus dust concentration **(A)**, endotoxin concentration **(B)**, and log endotoxin concentration. **(C)** determined from air samples collected by vertical elutriators, and proportion of exposed subjects with an FEV1 decrease of at least 5% versus log endotoxin concentration **(D)**. Each point represents the mean change in FEV1 for a group of 24 to 35 individuals over a 6-hour experimental exposure to card-generated cotton dust. (Adapted from Castellan RM, Olenchock SA, Kinsley KB, et al: Inhaled endotoxin and decreased spirometric values—an exposure–response relation for cotton dust. Reprinted, by permission of *The New England Journal of Medicine*, 317:605-610, 1987.) Continued on page 413.

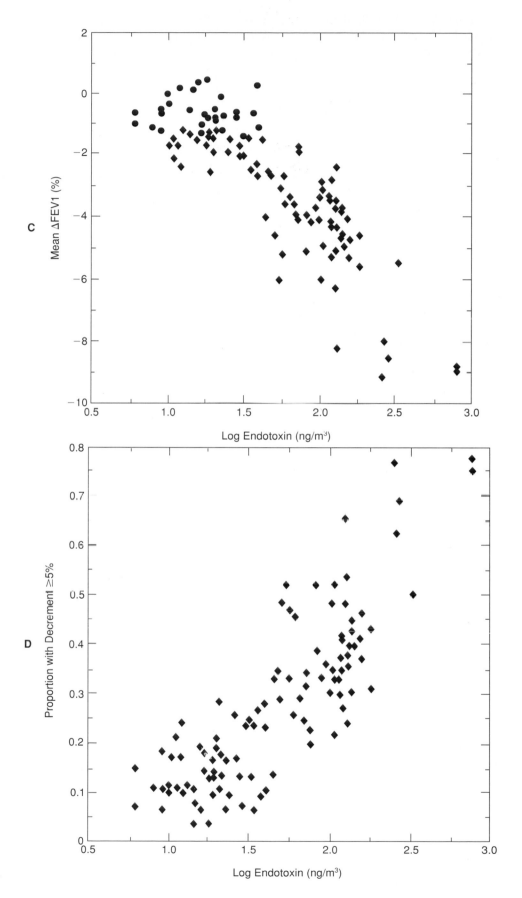

Fig. 25-4. Continued from page 412.

and processes in Table 25-4. Growing, harvesting, ginning, classing, warehousing, and knitting of cotton are not currently regulated. Handling and processing of woven or knitted cotton fabrics are likewise not regulated. Nontextile operations that are regulated are cottonseed processing and waste recycling and garnetting. Although cottonseed processing is not subject to a special PEL for cotton dust, employers in this sector of the industry are required to biannually monitor worker health status with symptoms questionnaires and across-shift spirometry testing. Employers must provide for biannual medical monitoring of workers in waste-recycling operations, and there is a 1000 μg/m^3 PEL for cotton dust in waste-recycling and garnetting industries.[100]

In cotton textile mill operations several different PELs apply, ranging from 200 μg/m^3 in yarn manufacturing to 750 μg/m^3 in slashing and weaving. Moreover, OSHA has specified that employers must monitor dust levels in these textile mill operations, annually for work areas at or below the PEL and semiannually for work areas above the PEL, and must post the results of the environmental monitoring. In addition, for employees exposed to cotton dust, cotton textile mill operators must establish a medical monitoring program under the supervision of a physician. Routine medical monitoring is to be done biannually for employees in work areas with dust levels at or below the action level and annually for those in work areas above the action level. Semiannual medical monitoring is mandated for workers with (1) an across-shift decline in FEV1 of 5% or more (or 200 ml or more), (2) an FEV1 less than 80% of that predicted, or (3) any significant change in symptoms, pulmonary function, or other diagnostic tests, based on comparisons with findings from previous examinations. Finally, the OSHA standard mandates referral to a physician for detailed pulmonary examination for workers who have an FEV1 less than 60% of that predicted.

The OSHA cotton dust standard specifies the standardized questionnaire to be used for routine medical monitoring and requires that each worker be graded for byssinosis according to the Schilling classification scheme (see Table 25-1). Spirometry testing is to be done before work, after returning from at least 35 hours away from dust, and then again after at least 4 and no more than 10 hours at the employee's usual workplace and typical exposure. Technicians must have completed a NIOSH-approved training course in spirometry. In addition, for evaluating pulmonary function test results, the published standard provides a table of predicted values for FEV1 and forced vital capacity (FVC) and specifies that a predicted value correction factor of 0.85 be used for black workers.

After the examination the employer is required to provide each worker with a copy of the physician's written opinion, containing (1) the medical examination and test results, (2) the physician's assessment regarding medical conditions that put the worker at increased risk of impairment from cotton dust exposure, (3) the physician's recommendations for the employee's limits to cotton dust exposure and for respirator use, and (4) a statement that the physician has informed the employee of any medical conditions that require further examination or treatment. The OSHA standard specifies that "specific findings or diagnoses unrelated to occupational exposure" not be revealed in this written opinion.[1]

EMPLOYEE PLACEMENT AND TRAINING

The OSHA cotton dust standard requires that regulated employers provide initial medical examinations to all new employees prior to placement and periodic examinations to all employees exposed to cotton dust (discussed previously). Although the OSHA standard does not specify employee placement or job transfer actions to be recommended to the employer by the supervising or examining physician,

Table 25-4. Key requirements of current OSHA regulations specific to cotton dust

Process	Permissible exposure limit*	Action level	Medical monitoring by employer	Other requirements
Nontextile operations				
Waste recycling and garnetting	1000 μg/m^3	None	Yes	No
Cottonseed processing	None	—	Yes	No
Textile mills				
Yarn manufacturing	200 μg/m^3	100 μg/m^3	Yes	Yes
Waste house operations	500 μg/m^3	250 μg/m^3	Yes	Yes
Slashing and weaving operations	750 μg/m^3	375 μg/m^3	Yes	Yes

*All permissible exposure limits are 8-hour time-weighted averages measured by vertical elutriator or equivalent sampler. Action levels determine the frequency of routine medical monitoring of exposed workers. Other requirements include environmental monitoring by employer, work practices, training, and posting. See text for exemptions of washed cotton from requirements of the Occupational Safety and Health Administration (OSHA) cotton dust standard.

general guidance based on the functional classification scheme (see Table 25-2) has been published[21-23] and is shown in Table 25-5.

The results of some studies suggest that atopic individuals are at somewhat greater risk for adverse acute respiratory reactions to cotton dust and that these acute reactions may be more severe.[87,101,102] Despite this, there is a significant overlap of distributions of acute FEV1 responses to cotton dust among atopic and nonatopic persons (Fig. 25-5). Thus, compared with early detection by direct assess-

Table 25-5. Recommended employee placement and medical monitoring based on functional classification of workers exposed to cotton dust*

Functional grade	Recommended actions
$F_{0(a)}$	No change; repeat medical monitoring in 12 months
$F_{0(b)}$	No change; repeat medical monitoring in 6 months
$F_{0(c)}$	Move to lower risk area; repeat medical monitoring in 6 months
$F_{1(a)}$	No change; repeat medical monitoring in 6 months
$F_{1(b)}$	Move to lower risk area; repeat medical monitoring in 6 months
F_2	Remove from cotton dust exposure; detailed pulmonary evaluation

*See Table 25-2. Adapted from references 21 through 23.

ment of symptoms and measurement of across-shift changes in FEV1 through the periodic medical monitoring required by OSHA, atopic status may not be very useful a priori to identify specific workers at risk for these acute responses to cotton dust. It has been suggested that, by selecting themselves out of exposure as a result of more severe acute symptoms early in the course of employment, atopic individuals may tend not to develop chronic impairment from cotton dust.[36] Definitive longitudinal studies have not been conducted to document the possible long-term risks of those with atopy or preexisting asthma.

Based on an early 1970s study of mills with relatively high dust levels, Merchant and colleagues[62] recommended that smokers be excluded from textile mill work areas with high concentrations of cotton dust. Recommendations contained in a recently published report of a longitudinal study of cotton textile workers similarly suggest that, at least until dust concentrations can be further lowered, smokers should be restricted from working in yarn-manufacturing areas of mills in order to prevent dust-induced chronic respiratory effects.[65,71] Physicians responsible for the respiratory health of cotton textile mill workers should actively promote smoking cessation and champion control of cotton dust, not just to the lowest level required to achieve compliance with the OSHA standard but to the lowest feasible level as recommended by NIOSH.[23] In addition to providing other training required by the OSHA standard,[1] employers should ensure that smokers are informed of the combined adverse effects of smoking and cotton dust exposure.

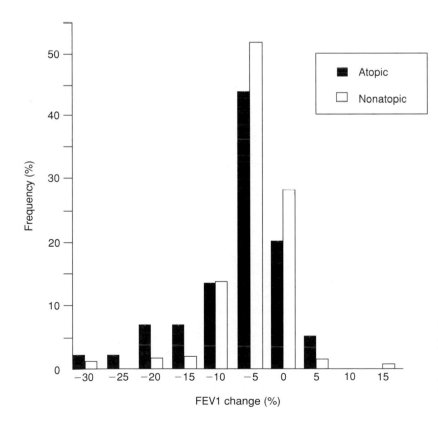

Fig. 25-5. Distribution of magnitudes of acute FEV1 responses to experimental cotton dust exposure for 59 atopic and 167 nonatopic volunteers. Atopy was defined as positive prick tests to at least 2 of 10 common environmental inhalant allergens. (Adapted from Sepulveda M-J, Castellan RM, Hankinson JL, et al: Acute lung function response to cotton dust in atopic and nonatopic individuals, *Br J Ind Med* 41:487-491, 1984.)

OTHER CONTROL METHODS
Dust control

Primary prevention through control of airborne dust in textile mills is the mainstay of current preventive action. Engineering controls for textile mills have advanced markedly in recent years, and a great deal of modern textile machinery is now typically designed and manufactured with enclosures and local exhaust systems. Moreover, some dust-generating processes of the past are being designed out of modern mill machinery. For example, the very dusty process of "picking," in which rolls of matted cotton lint were prepared for carding, is not required for modern chute-fed carding machines. Modern cotton textile manufacturers increasingly realize that state-of-the-art production of high-quality yarns depends on dust control, which provides an incentive for some degree of dust control beyond that of worker health protection alone.

As one might expect, standard industrial hygiene guidelines on general workplace ventilation and work practices (e.g., restrictions on sweeping and compressed air "blowdown" cleaning of machinery) apply to the control of worker exposures to cotton dust, as do standard guidelines on the use of respirators. Specific legal requirements applicable in the United States are outlined in the comprehensive OSHA cotton dust standard.[1]

Substitution, including pretreatment of cotton

One means of reducing cotton dust levels associated with the manufacture of cotton yarns and fabric is to substitute other materials for the cotton used in yarn manufacture. Since synthetic fibers are less dusty than cotton, the dust generation of yarn manufacturing processes is related largely to the proportion of cotton in the blend.[103] However, characteristics of the resulting fabric also relate to the proportion of cotton in the blend, and control of cotton dust is not generally a major factor in textile manufacturers' decisions regarding the use of cotton–synthetic blends.

Another form of substitution is to use prewashed cotton as a raw material for producing manufactured products. On the basis of epidemiologic and experimental evidence demonstrating an absence of toxicity, cotton that has been thoroughly washed for use in medical products is completely exempted from the OSHA cotton dust standard.[1,97] However, such severe washing removes natural waxes from the lint surface and adversely affects fiber characteristics required for the manufacture of quality yarns.

More recently, research has shown that mild washing of cotton physically removes dust and also markedly reduces the toxicity of dust remaining in the cotton.[104] On this basis mildly washed cotton has been partially exempted from the OSHA cotton dust standard.[1] However, even mild washing adversely affects processing qualities, though much less so than severe washing. Moreover, washing cotton involves substantial additional cost. As a result, the potential for widespread application of mildly washed cotton (e.g., beyond nonwoven materials and coarse yarns) currently appears to be limited.

Proposed limits for occupational exposure to endotoxin

Although current practice focuses on the control of exposure to gravimetric dust, Jacobs has suggested that consideration be given to establishing a general threshold limit value for airborne endotoxin,[105] and several published reports have suggested specific levels for limiting occupational exposure to airborne endotoxin exposure for the cotton textile industry,[106] for other specific industries,[107] or in general.[108,109]

Regulation of exposure to endotoxin represents a possible future approach to controlling byssinosis and related disorders among workers exposed to cotton dust. As a first step interlaboratory variability in endotoxin measurements on environmental dust samples must be better understood, and standardized methods for sample extraction and assay need to be defined and used. However, since current gravimetric dust monitoring, along with medical monitoring of exposed workers, has succeeded in providing substantial respiratory health protection for cotton textile mill workers,[110] it seems likely that regulation of exposure to cotton dust on a gravimetric basis will continue to be warranted for the foreseeable future.

REFERENCES

1. Occupational Safety and Health Administration: Occupational exposure to cotton dust, *Fed Regist* 50:51120-51179, 1985.
2. Committee on Byssinosis: Characterization of cotton dust. In: *Byssinosis: clinical and research issues,* pp 48-101, Washington, DC, 1982, National Research Council.
3. Barlowe RG: U.S. and world cotton outlook. In Whitton CL and Herndon CW Jr, editors: *Proceedings of the Cotton Economics and Marketing Conference,* pp 343-348, Memphis, 1992, National Cotton Council.
4. Dunavant WB Jr: Cotton supply and demand. In Funk T and Jones F, editors: *Proceedings of the Beltwide Cotton Production Conference,* pp 121-122, Memphis, 1992, National Cotton Council.
5. Merchant JA: Byssinosis. In Merchant JA, Boehlecke BA, and Pickett-Harner M, editors: *Occupational respiratory diseases,* Department of Health and Human Services (National Institute for Occupational Safety and Health) Pub No 86-102, pp 533-568, Washington, DC, 1986, US Government Printing Office.
6. Wegman DH: Describing the magnitude of the problem. Workgroup 1, *Am J Ind Med* 12:789-790, 1987.
7. Parikh JR: Byssinosis in developing countries, *Br J Ind Med* 49:217-219, 1992.
8. Ramazzini B: *Diseases of workers* (Translated from the Latin text *De morbis artificum* of 1713 by WC Wright), pp 257-259, New York, 1964, Hafner Publishing.
9. Mareska J and Heyman J: Enquête sur le travail et la condition physique et morale des ouvriers employés dans les manufactures de coton, à Gand, *Ann Soc Med Gand* 16(part 2):5-245, 1845 (Cited by Bouhuys A: *Breathing: physiology, environment and lung disease,* p 417, New York, 1974, Grune & Stratton).
10. Massoud A: The origin of the term "byssinosis," *Br J Ind Med* 21:162, 1964.
11. Schilling RSF: Byssinosis in cotton and other textile workers, *Lancet* 2:261-265 and 319-325, 1956.

12. Weill H: Problem solving in occupational airways disorders, *Chest* 79(suppl):1S-2S, 1981.
13. Morgan WKC: Byssinosis and related conditions. In Morgan WK and Seaton A, editors: *Occupational lung diseases,* pp 484-502, Philadelphia, 1995, WB Saunders.
14. Heyden S and Pratt P: Exposure to cotton dust and respiratory disease, *JAMA* 247:176, 1982. Letter.
15. Home Office: *Report of the departmental committee on dust in cardrooms in the cotton industry,* London, 1932, His Majesty's Stationery Office.
16. Schilling RSF, Hughes JPW, Dingwall-Fordyce J, et al: An epidemiological study of byssinosis among Lancashire cotton workers, *Br J Ind Med* 12:217-227, 1955.
17. Schilling RSF, Vigliani EC, Lammers B, et al: *A report on a conference on byssinosis,* International Congress Series No 62, pp 137-145, New York, 1963, Excerpta Medical Foundation.
18. McKerrow CB, McDermott M, Gilson JC, et al: Respiratory function during the day in cotton workers: a study in byssinosis, *Br J Ind Med* 15:75-83, 1958.
19. Shilling RSF: Worldwide problems of byssinosis, *Chest* 79(suppl):3S-5S, 1981.
20. Merchant JA, Halprin GM, Hudson AR, et al: Evaluation before and after exposure—the pattern of physiological response to cotton dust, *Ann NY Acad Sci* 221:38-43, 1974.
21. Ayer HE, Battigelli M, Fraser DA, et al: The status of byssinosis in the United States, *Arch Environ Health* 23:230-234, 1971.
22. Ayer HE: Byssinosis, *CRC Crit Rev Environ Control* 2:207-241, 1971.
23. National Institute for Occupational Safety and Health (NIOSH): *Criteria for a recommended standard: occupational exposure to cotton dust,* Department of Health and Human Services Pub No (NIOSH) 75-118, Washington, DC, 1974, US Government Printing Office.
24. World Health Organization (WHO) Study Group: *Recommended health-based occupational exposure limits for selected vegetable dusts,* WHO Technical Report Series No 684, Geneva, 1983, WHO.
25. Holness DL, Taraschuk IG, and Goldstein RS: Acute exposure to cotton dust—a case of mill fever, *JAMA* 247:1602-1603, 1982.
26. Neal PA, Schneiter R, and Caminita BH: Report on acute illness among rural mattress makers using low grade, stained cotton, *JAMA* 119:1074-1082, 1942.
27. Merchant JA, Halprin GM, Hudson AR, et al: Responses to cotton dust, *Arch Environ Health* 30:222-229, 1975.
28. Hamilton JD, Germino VH, Merchant JA, et al: Byssinosis in a nontextile worker, *Am Rev Respir Dis* 107:464-466, 1973.
29. Murray R, Dingwall-Fordyce J, and Lane RE: An outbreak of weaver's cough associated with tamarind seed powder, *Br J Ind Med* 14:105-110, 1957.
30. Tufnell PG and Dingwall-Fordyce J: An investigation into the acute respiratory reaction to the inhalation of tamarind seed preparations, *Br J Ind Med* 14:250-252, 1957.
31. Vigliani EC, Parmeggiani L, and Sassi C: Studio de un epidemia di bronchite asmatica fra gli operi di una tessiture di cotone, *Med Lav* 45:349-378, 1954.
32. Collis EL: The occurrence of an unusual cough among weavers of cotton cloth, *Proc R Soc Med* 8:108-112, 1915.
33. Middleton EL: Weaver's cough, *J Ind Hyg* 8:428-435, 1936.
34. Haglind P, Bake B, and Belin L: Is mild byssinosis associated with small airways disease?, *Eur J Respir Dis* 64:449-459, 1983.
35. Jacobs RR, Boehlecke BA, Van Hage-Hamstein M, et al: Bronchial reactivity, atopy, and airway response to cotton dust, *Am Rev Respir Dis* 148:19-24, 1993.
36. Fishwick D, Fletcher AM, Pickering CAC, et al: Lung function, bronchial reactivity, atopic status, and dust exposure in Lancashire cotton mill operatives, *Am Rev Respir Dis* 145:1103-1108, 1992.
37. Rylander R: Bacteria as etiologic agents in byssinosis and other lung disease, *Eur J Respir Dis* 63(suppl 123):34-46, 1982.
38. Castellan RM, Olenchock SA, Hankinson JL, et al: Acute bronchoconstriction induced by cotton dust: dose-related responses to endotoxin and other dust factors, *Ann Intern Med* 101:157-163, 1984.
39. Rylander R: Organic dusts and lung reactions—exposure characteristics and mechanisms for disease, *Scand J Work Environ Health* 11:199-206, 1985.
40. Kilburn KH: Byssinosis and other diseases of textile workers. In Rom WN, editor: *Environmental and occupational medicine,* pp 359-365, Boston, 1992, Little, Brown.
41. Ozesmi M, Aslan H, Hillerdal G, et al: Byssinosis in carpet weavers exposed to wool contaminated with endotoxin, *Br J Ind Med* 44:479-483, 1987.
42. Rylander R, Schilling RSF, Pickering CAC, et al: Effects after acute and chronic exposure to cotton dust: the Manchester criteria, *Br J Ind Med* 44:577-579, 1987.
43. Bouhuys A, Wolfson RL, Horner DW, et al: Byssinosis in cotton textile workers. Respiratory survey of a mill with rapid labor turnover, *Ann Intern Med* 71:257-269, 1969.
44. Rooke GB: Compensation for byssinosis in Great Britain, *Chest* 79(suppl):124S-127S, 1981.
45. Ghio AJ, Castellan RM, Kinsley KB, et al: Changes in forced expiratory volume in one second and peak expiratory flow rate across a work shift among unexposed blue collar workers, *Am Rev Respir Dis* 143:1231-1234, 1991.
46. Bouhuys A, Mitchell CA, Schilling RSF, et al: A physiological study of byssinosis in colonial America, *Trans NY Acad Sci* 35:537-546, 1973.
47. Sepulveda MJ, Hankinson J, Castellan RM, et al: Helium—oxygen spirometry in experimental cotton dust exposure, *Lung* 162:347-356, 1984.
48. Sepulveda MJ, Hankinson J, Castellan RM, et al: Cotton-induced bronchoconstriction detected by a forced random noise oscillator, *Br J Ind Med* 41:480-486, 1984
49. Morgan PGM and Ong SG: First report of byssinosis in Hong Kong, *Br J Ind Med* 38:290-292, 1981.
50. Office on Smoking and Health: Cotton dust exposure and cigarette smoking. In: *The health consequences of smoking. cancer and chronic lung disease in the workplace—a report of the Surgeon General,* pp 399-439, Washington, DC, 1985, US Government Printing Office.
51. Rylander R, Haglind P, and Butcher BT: Reactions during the work shift among cotton mill workers, *Chest* 84:403-407, 1983.
52. Bouhuys A: Prevention of Monday dyspnea in byssinosis: a controlled trial with an antihistamine drug, *Clin Pharmacol Ther* 4:311-314, 1963.
53. Zuskin E, Valic F, and Bouhuys A: Byssinosis and airway responses to exposure to textile dust, *Lung* 154:17-24, 1976.
54. Zuskin E and Bouhuys A: Protective effect of disodium cromoglycate against airway constriction induced by hemp dust extract, *J Allergy Clin Immunol* 57:473-479, 1976.
55. Fawcett IW, Merchant JA, Simmonds SP, et al: The effect of sodium cromoglycate, beclomethasone diproprionate and salbutamol on the ventilatory response to cotton dust in mill workers, *Br J Dis Chest* 29:29-38, 1978.
56. Edwards C, MacArtney J, Rooke G, et al: The pathology of the lung in byssinosis, *Thorax* 30:612-623, 1975.
57. Rooke GB: The pathology of byssinosis, *Chest* 79(suppl):67S-71S, 1981.
58. Pratt PC, Vollmer RT, and Miller JA: Epidemiology of pulmonary lesions in nontextile and cotton textile workers: a retrospective autopsy analysis, *Arch Environ Health* 35:133-138, 1980.
59. Moran TM: Emphysema and other chronic lung disease in textile workers: an 18-year autopsy study, *Arch Environ Health* 38:267-276, 1983.

60. Milton DK, Godleski JJ, Feldman HA, et al: Toxicity of intratracheally instilled cotton dust, cellulose, and endotoxin, *Am Rev Respir Dis* 142:184-192, 1990.

61. Beck GJ and Schachter EN: The evidence for chronic lung disease in cotton workers, *Am Stat* 37:404-412, 1983.

62. Merchant JA, Kilburn KH, O'Fallon WM, et al: Byssinosis and chronic bronchitis among cotton textile workers, *Ann Intern Med* 76:423-433, 1972.

63. Merchant JA, Lumsden JC, Kilburn KH, et al: An industrial study of the biological effects of cotton dust and cigarette smoke exposure, *J Occup Med* 15:212-221, 1973.

64. Beck GJ, Schachter EN, and Maunder LR: The relationship of respiratory symptoms and lung function loss in cotton textile workers, *Am Rev Respir Dis* 130:6-11, 1984.

65. Glindmeyer HW, Lefant JJ, Jones RN, et al: Cotton dust and across-shift change in FEV1 as predictors of annual change in FEV1, *Am J Respir Crit Care Med* 149:584-590, 1994.

66. Roach SA and Schilling RSF: A clinical and environmental study of byssinosis in the Lancashire cotton industry, *Br J Ind Med* 17:1-9, 1960.

67. Molyneux MKB and Tombleson JBL: An epidemiological study of respiratory symptoms in Lancashire mills, 1963-66, *Br J Ind Med* 27:225-234, 1970.

68. Fox AJ, Tombleson JBL, Watt A, et al: A survey of respiratory disease in cotton operatives. Part II. Symptoms, dust estimations, and the effect of smoking habit, *Br J Ind Med* 30:48-53, 1973.

69. Merchant JA, Lumsden JC, Kilburn KH, et al: Dose response studies in cotton textile workers, *J Occup Med* 15:222-230, 1973.

70. Corn M: Methods to assess airborne concentration of cotton dust, *Am J Ind Med* 12:677-686, 1987.

71. Glindmeyer HW, Lefante JJ, Jones RN, et al: Exposure-related declines in the lung function of cotton textile workers: relationship to current workplace standards, *Am Rev Respir Dis* 144:675-683, 1991.

72. British Occupational Hygiene Society: A basis for hygiene standards for flax dust, *Ann Occup Hyg* 23:1-26, 1980.

73. Tuma J, Parker L, and Braun DC: The proteolytic enzymes and the prevalence of signs and symptoms in US cotton textile mills, *J Occup Med* 15:409-413, 1973.

74. Cinkotai FF: The size-distribution and protease content of airborne particles in textile mills cardrooms, *Am Ind Hyg Assoc J* 37:234-238, 1976.

75. Chinn DJ, Cinkotai FF, Lockwood MG, et al: Airborne dust, its protease content and byssinosis in "willowing" mills, *Ann Occup Hyg* 19:101-108, 1976.

76. Milton DK and Chawla RK: Cotton dust contains proteolytic and elastolytic enzymes not inhibited by alpha-1-protease inhibitor, *Am J Ind Med* 9:247-260, 1986.

77. Pernis B, Vigliani EC, Cavagna G, et al: The role of bacterial endotoxins in occupational diseases caused by inhaling vegetable dusts, *Br J Ind Med* 18:120-129, 1961.

78. Cavagna G, Foa V, and Vigliani EC: Effects in man and rabbits of inhalation of cotton dust or extracts and purified endotoxins, *Br J Ind Med* 26:314-321, 1969.

79. Castellan RM, Olenchock SA, Kinsley KB, et al: Inhaled endotoxin and decreased spirometric values—an exposure–response relation for cotton dust, *N Engl J Med* 317:605-610, 1987.

80. Rylander R, Haglind P, and Lundholm M: Endotoxin in cotton dust and respiratory function decrement among cotton workers in an experimental cardroom, *Am Rev Respir Dis* 131:209-213, 1985.

81. Cinkotai FF, Lockwood MG, and Rylander R: Airborne microorganisms and prevalence of byssinotic symptoms in cotton mills, *Am Ind Hyg Assoc J* 38:554-559, 1977.

82. Cinkotai FF and Wittaker CJ: Airborne bacteria and the prevalence of byssinotic symptoms in 21 cotton spinning mills in Lancashire, *Ann Occup Hyg* 21:239-250, 1978.

83. Cinkotai FF, Seaborn D, Pickering CAC, et al: Airborne dust in the personal breathing zone and the prevalence of byssinotic symptoms in the Lancashire textile industry, *Ann Occup Hyg* 32:103-113, 1988.

84. Cinkotai FF, Rigby A, Pickering CAC, et al: Recent trends in the prevalence of byssinotic symptoms in the Lancashire textile industry, *Br J Ind Med* 45:782-789, 1988.

85. Haglind P, Lundholm M, and Rylander R: Prevalence of byssinosis in Swedish cotton mills, *Br J Ind Med* 38:138-143, 1981.

86. Kennedy SM, Christiani DC, Eisen EA, et al: Cotton dust and endotoxin exposure–response relationships in cotton textile workers, *Am Rev Respir Dis* 135:194-200, 1987.

87. Sigsgaard T, Pedersen OF, Juul S, et al: Respiratory disorders and atopy in cotton, wool, and other textile mill workers in Denmark, *Am J Ind Med* 22:163-184, 1992.

88. Niven RM, Horan MA, Pickering CAC, et al: Endotoxin exposure and respiratory symptoms in cotton and man-made fibre textile workers, *Am Rev Respir Dis* 143:A103, 1991.

89. Jamison JP and Lowry RC: Bronchial challenge of normal subjects with the endotoxin of *Enterobacter agglomerans* isolated from cotton dust, *Br J Ind Med* 43:327-331, 1986.

90. Rylander R, Bake B, Fischer J, et al: Pulmonary function and symptoms after inhalation of endotoxin, *Am Rev Respir Dis* 140:981-986, 1989.

91. Bell AA: Natural products content of cotton bracts and mill dust: tannins. In Jacobs RR and Wakelyn PJ, editors: *Cotton dust: proceedings of the Tenth Cotton Dust Research Conference,* pp 37-41, Memphis, 1986, National Cotton Council.

92. Bell AA, Stipanovich RD, Elzen GW, et al: Natural products content of cotton bracts and mill dust: volatile terpenes and terpenoid aldehydes. In Jacobs RR and Wakelyn PJ, editors: *Cotton dust: proceedings of the Tenth Cotton Dust Research Conference,* pp 30-36, Memphis, 1986, National Cotton Council.

93. Greenblatt GA and Bell AA: Natural products of cotton bracts and mill dust: lacinilenes and cadalenes. In Jacobs RR and Wakelyn PJ, editors: *Cotton dust: proceedings of the Tenth Cotton Dust Research Conference,* pp 23-29, Memphis, 1986, National Cotton Council.

94. Castellan RM, Brashears AD, Cocke JB, et al: Removal of bract prior to harvest: effects on cardroom dust levels and acute human ventilatory responses. In Wakelyn PJ and Jacobs RR, editors: *Cotton dust: proceedings of the Tenth Cotton Dust Research Conference,* pp 101-104, Memphis, 1986, National Cotton Council.

95. Rylander R: Plant constituents of cotton dust and lung effects after inhalation, *Eur Respir J* 1:812-817, 1988.

96. Buck MG, Wall JH, and Schachter EN: Airway response to cotton bract extracts in the absence of endotoxin, *Br J Ind Med* 43:220-226, 1986.

97. Occupational Safety and Health Administration: Occupational exposure to cotton dust. Final mandatory occupational safety and health standards, *Fed Regist* 43:27351-27417, 1978.

98. 91st Congress: Public Law 91-596, Section (6)(b)(5), 1970.

99. Excerpts from court decision on health standards, *NY Times* June 18:B8, 1981.

100. Occupational Safety and Health Administration, U.S. Department of Labor: *Code of federal regulations,* 29 CFR 1910.1000, Table Z-1, revised July 1, 1994.

101. Jones RN, Butcher BT, Hammad YY, et al: Interaction of atopy and exposure to cotton dust in the bronchoconstrictor response, *Br J Ind Med* 37:141-146, 1980.

102. Sepulveda MJ, Castellan RM, Hankinson JL, et al: Acute lung function response to cotton dust in atopic and nonatopic individuals, *Br J Ind Med* 41:487-491, 1984.

103. Jacobs RR: Strategies for prevention of byssinosis, *Am J Ind Med* 12:717-728, 1987.

104. Castellan RM: Evaluation of acute human airway toxicity of standard and washed cotton dusts. In Wakelyn PJ, Jacobs RR, and Kirk IW, editors: *Washed cotton: washing techniques, processing charac-*

teristics, and health effects, pp 41-52, New Orleans, 1986, US Department of Agriculture.

105. Jacobs RR: Airborne endotoxins: an association with occupational lung disease, *Appl Ind Hyg* 4:50-56, 1989.

106. Rylander R: The role of endotoxins for reactions after exposure to cotton dust, *Am J Ind Med* 12:687-697, 1987.

107. Palchak RB, Cohen R, Ainsle M, et al: Airborne endotoxin associated with industrial-scale production of protein products in gram-negative bacteria, *Am Ind Hyg Assoc J* 49:420-421, 1988.

108. Popendorf W: Report on agents, *Am J Ind Med* 10:251-259, 1986.

109. Committee on Organic Dusts: The Committee on Organic Dusts—a presentation, Sweden, 1991, International Commission of Occupational Health.

110. Merchant JA: Byssinosis: progress in prevention, *Am J Public Health* 73:137-138, 1983.

Chapter 26

OCCUPATIONAL ASTHMA

Jean-Luc Malo
André Cartier

HISTORICAL BACKGROUND

Although it is generally thought that Ramazzini was the first to describe the occurrence of occupational asthma (OA) in "sifters and measurers of grain" in 1713, his description corresponds more to farmer's lung than to OA and was preceded by a much earlier (1555) and comparable description of respiratory disease due to threshing grain by Olaus Magnus.[1] Several causes of OA due to high-molecular-weight (e.g., castor bean and vegetable gums) and low-molecular-weight (e.g., wood dust) agents were described between 1920 and 1960. Isocyanates, the most common cause of OA, were incriminated in 1951 by Fuchs and Valade.[2] The 1970s and 1980s saw an improvement in the means of investigation. Specific inhalation challenges were introduced by Pepys and Hutchcroft,[3] and peak expiratory

flow rate (PEFR) monitoring was introduced by Burge and colleagues a few years later.[4,5]

DEFINITION

Occupational asthma can be defined as a "disease characterized by variable airflow limitation and/or airway hyperresponsiveness due to causes and conditions attributable to a particular occupational environment and not to stimuli encountered outside the workplace."[6] Two types of OA are recognized, depending on whether or not it develops after a latency period. Occupational asthma with a latency period is characterized by a variable time during which "sensitization" takes place (although the immunologic basis for this remains unknown in most instances of OA caused by low-molecular-weight agents). Occupational asthma without a latency period may be termed *irritant-induced asthma,* an example of which is the "reactive airways dysfunction syndrome" (RADS) described by Brooks and collaborators in 1985.[7] Besides the types of OA, there are also "asthma-like" syndromes not covered in this chapter, such as byssinosis, effects of exposure to grain dust, and the airway disease seen in workers in aluminum refineries.

PATHOPHYSIOLOGY

There are several pathophysiologic features common to both nonoccupational asthma and OA. Occupational asthma can be used as a model of asthma, extrinsic asthma being similar to OA caused by high-molecular-weight agents and intrinsic asthma being closer to OA caused by low-molecular-weight agents. The common pathophysiologic characteristic is airway inflammation. The subject of airway inflammation in asthma is reviewed in Chapter 13.

The pathophysiology of OA has been studied in humans, and animal models have also been developed. In humans the initial focus was on the distinction between immediate and late asthmatic reactions. Late or atypical reactions are common after exposure to low-molecular-weight agents, whereas isolated immediate or dual reactions are the rule after challenges with high-molecular-weight agents.[3,8] Bronchoalveolar lavage studies revealed the influx of eosinophils and neutrophils after late reactions to toluene di-

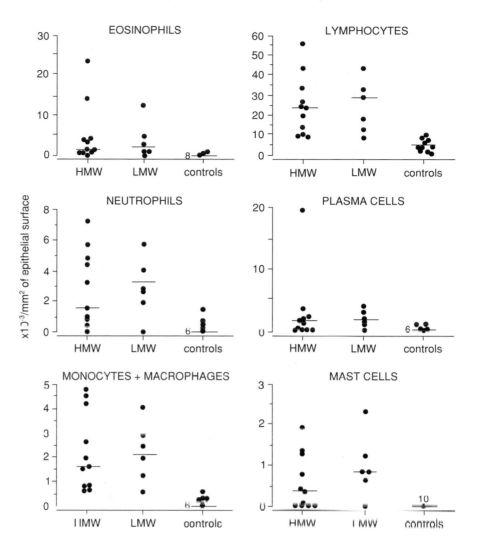

Fig. 26-1. Comparative cell differentials of bronchial biopsies from patients with asthma induced by high-molecular-weight or low-molecular-weight agents and controls. There was a significant increase in all inflammatory cell counts except plasma cells in patients with occupational asthma, compared with controls. Median values are shown by the horizontal lines. Figures indicate the number of points at the specific place. (Adapted from Boulet LP, Boutet M, Laviolette M, et al: Airway inflammation after removal from the causal agent in occupational asthma due to high and low molecular weight agents, *Eur Respir J* 7:1567-1575, 1994.

isocyanate (TDI).[9] Sloughing of epithelial cells has also been detected after late asthmatic reactions due to plicatic acid, the active product in western red cedar.[10] More recently, it has become possible to examine bronchial biopsies of subjects with OA during and after exposure.[11,12] There is an increase in all cell types as compared with normal controls (Fig. 26-1). Eosinophils and lymphocytes show evidence of activation.[13] Bronchial biopsies of subjects with OA seen 3 to 24 weeks after the end of exposure also show evidence of persistent inflammation, such as extensive epithelial desquamation, ciliary abnormalities of the epithelial cells, smooth muscle hyperplasia, and increased subepithelial fibrosis (Fig. 26-2). There is, however, no difference in the degree of bronchial biopsy findings depending on whether the agent is of high or low molecular weight.

The mechanism of OA caused by high-molecular-weight agents is immunoglobulin E (IgE) dependent. It is therefore logical to assume that the hypothesized inflammatory process that, in some cases, has been confirmed for common aeroallergens would also apply to this category of occupational agent. The mechanism of OA resulting from exposure to low-molecular-weight agents is still a controver-

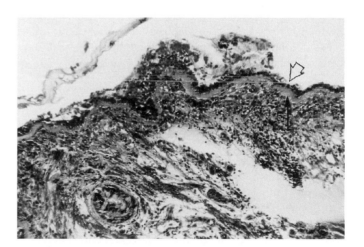

Fig. 26-2. Light micrograph of a bronchial biopsy of a patient with occupational asthma showing epithelial desquamation *(open arrow)* with remaining basal cells still attached to a thickened basement membrane *(solid arrow)*. Numerous inflammatory cells are seen in edematous subepithelial connective tissue. Original magnification, ×400. (Courtesy of Dr. Michel Boutet, Hôpital Laval and Université Laval, Quebec City.)

sial subject. Antibody-dependent immunity does not seem to be a key feature. Several studies have been conducted in recent years by Fabbri's group on OA caused by isocyanates.[14] Lymphocytes are thought to play a major role in the pathophysiology of asthma. An increased number of activated T lymphocyte subclasses have been detected in subjects with OA caused by TDI.[13] These findings, coupled with the fact that the percentage of the CD8 T cell class is altered after inhalation challenges with TDI,[15] seem to suggest that lymphocytes are involved in the pathophysiology of isocyanate-induced asthma. Di Stefano and coworkers[99] recently examined the presence of mast cells in the epithelium and the lamina propria of patients with OA due to TDI. There were significantly more mast cells in those who had developed symptoms less than 5 years after exposure began as compared with those who had been exposed for longer intervals. This may suggest an individual susceptibility to the development of OA due to isocyanates. An imbalance between the cholinergic and β-adrenergic functions has been proposed as the genesis of asthma and OA. Exposure of rat trachea to TDI resulted in a diminished response to isoproterenol and an increased response to methacholine, which suggests that this hypothesis could apply to this type of OA.[16] Recently, there has been a growing interest in the possibility that inflammation can be mediated through neurogenic stimulation. Exposure of guinea pigs to TDI enhances airway responsiveness to substance P and decreases neutral endopeptidase, a modulator of substance P.[17]

Several animal models of OA caused by diisocyanates, acid anhydrides, plicatic acid, and platinum salts have been developed.[18] The production of antibodies has been demonstrated, although sensitization via inhalation has been difficult to achieve. Exposure to isocyanates via inhalation has resulted in functional and histopathologic airway alterations. Changes were observed a few hours after the end of exposure, which makes these findings difficult to interpret because humans take much longer to develop OA due to TDI.

EPIDEMIOLOGIC STUDIES

The incidence of OA is on the rise, as reflected by the number of cases referred and/or accepted for medicolegal compensation[19] and the number of cases reported by sentinel physicians.[20] The causes of this increase are unknown, although it may reflect increased recognition of the problem. In the 1978 Social Security Disability Survey of 6000 U.S. respondents, 15% of those who mentioned that asthma was a personal medical condition also said that asthma was negatively affected by their workplace.[21] In a survey of 94 asthmatic patients discharged from three Michigan hospitals in 1990, 3% met the criteria for having definite OA and 12% to 25%, probable and possible OA, which suggests that the prevalence of OA in adult asthmatic subjects is in the range of 3% to 20%.[22]

Most epidemiologic surveys of OA have so far been of the cross-sectional type and have assessed the prevalence of the condition.[23] The main pitfall of this approach is that it is likely to be influenced by the healthy-worker effect. It is to be expected that this bias is more pronounced in the case of OA than for slowly progressing conditions such as pneumoconiosis. Asthma symptoms can be very troublesome and even life threatening,[24] and it is likely that many subjects leave the workplace before a survey can be conducted. Another difficulty lies in the diagnostic tools for assessing prevalence. Surveys rely on questionnaires, immunologic testing, assessment of airway caliber, measurement of airway responsiveness and PEFR monitoring. These tests are used alone or in combination in a stepwise fashion that leads to identifying cases that can then be confirmed by specific inhalation challenges (Fig. 26-3). As a rule of thumb, the prevalence of OA due to high-molecular-weight agents varies from 2% to 5%,[25-27] whereas it is more on the order of 5% to 10% in the case of low-molecular-weight agents.[28,29] These figures result from studies in which a combination of tools was used and the final diagnosis was

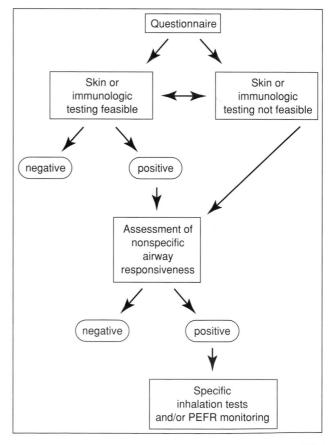

Fig. 26-3. Stepwise assessment of occupational asthma in epidemiologic surveys, with distinction of surveys conducted in workers exposed to high-molecular-weight agents, for whom skin or immunologic testing is feasible because these tests can be performed, and in those exposed to low-molecular-weight agents, for whom these tests are not feasible. (PEFR, Peak expiratory flow rate.)

confirmed by specific inhalation challenges (Fig. 26-3). Medical surveys should include environmental and individual risk factors, which can play a role in the natural history of the development of OA (Fig. 26-4) (see the section on the natural history).

DIAGNOSIS
Clinical assessment

Every patient with asthma should be questioned about his or her current and past workplaces. Persistent asthma can certainly be attributable to past exposure. The answers to two important questions point to the possibility of OA. What is the patient's job? What products does he or she come into contact with at work? If the medical history reveals that the patient is a nurse, possible exposure to a sensitizing product such as psyllium should be considered. Being an asthmatic and being exposed to polyurethane at work should also suggest the possibility of OA. Databases of high-risk jobs and products can be obtained from national agencies (the National Institute for Occupational Safety and Health [NIOSH] in the United States).[30] An interesting database was developed in France; physicians there have access to a databank based on jobs and causal agents by using an electronic information service, called MINITEL.[31] A list of all known causes of OA was recently published[32] and updated (see Appendix B). Agents are usually classified according to molecular weight. Several features summarized in Table 26-1 differentiate between the two types (high and low molecular weight) of agents. Overall, the most common causes of OA are isocyanates among low molecular-weight agents and flour for high-molecular-weight agents. The nature of all products present in the

workplace, not only those handled by the patient, should be obtained by requesting Material Safety Data Sheets. There could be products that have not been listed as known causes of OA, which does not preclude the possibility of OA. Besides agents causing chest symptoms, those causing ocular and nasal symptoms should be investigated. It is the authors' experience that these symptoms are more common in cases of OA due to high-molecular-weight rather than low-molecular-weight agents. Chest symptoms can be atypical, as is the case for asthma. Patients frequently experience cough and are treated for bronchitis of unknown etiology before the diagnosis of asthma is made. At the onset of symptoms, improvement on weekends and vacations is generally the rule. However, after a while, symptoms persist even through these short periods away from work. Improvement over weekends and during vacations is therefore not a satisfactory way to determine the presence of OA.[33] Finally, it is to be remembered that, as is the case with other medical conditions, questionnaires are sensitive, but they are not specific tools, as is apparent when results are compared with the final diagnosis. In a prospective study of 162 individuals, the positive predictive value of a clinical questionnaire was 63%, but the negative predictive value was 83%.[34]

Environmental assessment

Although air sampling can be done at the workplace, the most important information is whether or not a product is actually present. In many instances a causal agent can be released into the air in minute amounts, which makes its detection difficult even with sophisticated instruments. Product information is often difficult to obtain, so good

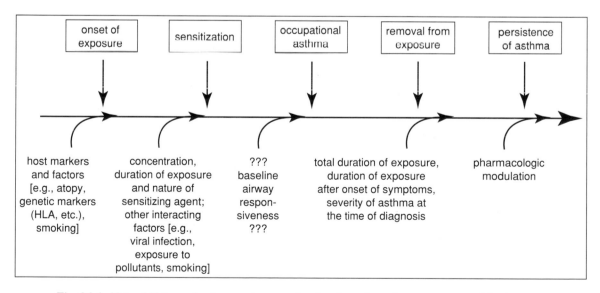

Fig. 26-4. Natural history of asthma and occupational asthma. At each step represented in the open boxes, several factors listed below the horizontal line can play a role. (Adapted from Malo J-L, Ghezzo H, D'Aquino C, et al: Natural history of occupational asthma: relevance of type of agent and other factors in the rate of development of symptoms in affected subjects, *J Allergy Clin Immunol* 90:937-943, 1992. With permission.)

Table 26-1. Characteristics of high- and low-molecular-weight agents

Characteristic	High molecular weight	Low molecular weight
Physical		
Size	<1000-5000 daltons	>1000-5000 daltons
Examples of agents	Proteins, enzymes, gums, and flour	Isocyanates and Western red cedar (plicatic acid)
Physiopathologic		
Humoral mechanism	Immunoglobulin E	Absent
Clinical and functional		
Temporal patterns of reaction on specific inhalation challenges	Isolated immediate or dual	Late or atypical
Epidemiologic		
Interval between onset of exposure and symptoms	Long	Short
Prevalence in high-risk populations	<5%	>5%
Model	"Extrinsic asthma"	"Intrinsic asthma"

communication should be established with the employer, the manufacturers of the suspected products, and local, regional, and national health and safety agencies. A recent study showed that the total dose of the product (in this instance, TDI) is more significant than either the concentration or the duration of exposure in causing an asthmatic reaction.[35] Time-weighted average exposure may be more important once symptoms appear, whereas peak levels are probably more important in causing a "sensitization" to the product. The level that provokes symptoms in already sensitized workers is lower than what would cause sensitization. Many instruments cannot detect low levels, particularly the minute amounts that can cause asthmatic symptoms in some workers. Air sampling at workplaces, however, can serve several purposes, as suggested by Reed and coworkers.[36] It can confirm exposure as the cause of the disease; it can be used to investigate a plant where OA has been found; it can be part of a longitudinal monitoring of the worksite or can investigate the spread of an allergen from the plant to the community; and it can establish risk levels. One other purpose can be added to this list: ensuring that workers are not exposed to "irritant" concentrations (above threshold limit values) of a product. This kind of exposure can result in RADS, a form of OA (discussed in a later section), if very high concentrations of a gas or aerosol are present, or nonspecific exacerbation of preexisting asthma if levels are high, but not to the extent of causing RADS. General air sampling in a workplace does not usually provide an accurate reflection of what workers are actually exposed to, particularly if they are at any distance from the sampling apparatus. However, personal samplers have been developed to overcome this problem. With such an apparatus aerosols, mists, and dusts are sampled on filters or membranes that are then examined through various radioimmunoassay methods in the case of protein-derived materials[36] or through analytical chemical methods (e.g., gas chromatography or high-performance liquid chromatography) in the case of low-molecular-weight agents such as diisocyanates, acid anhydrides, formaldehyde, colophony, and metals.[37]

Immunologic assessment

Occupational asthma with a latency period is believed to be mediated through immunologic sensitization, although the exact mechanism remains unknown for low-molecular-weight agents. The mechanism of OA due to high-molecular-weight agents is IgE dependent, as for extrinsic asthma due to common aeroallergens. Skin tests and/or assessment of the specific IgE can be performed for high-molecular-weight agents.[38] As with common asthma, a positive test reflects sensitization but not necessarily the presence of disease. The combination, however, of a positive skin test and airway hyperresponsiveness (see the section on the natural history of OA) is highly suggestive of OA (with an approximately 80% probability).[26,39] An IgE- or IgG-dependent mechanism has not been consistently seen with low-molecular-weight agents (isocyanates, for example).[40] These agents can cause sensitization through a hapten-mediated effect. The role of lymphocytes or other immunologic mechanisms remains unclear. Although the presence of specific antibodies does not confirm a diagnosis of OA, the information can be a useful adjunct for several reasons: (1) the absence of skin reactivity to well-characterized antigens virtually excludes the possibility of OA in workers exposed to high-molecular-weight agents, and (2) the presence of specific antibodies in a worker not affected by asthma should suggest a close follow-up to ensure that he or she does not develop OA later.

Physiologic assessment

The presence of airway obstruction with demonstrable reversibility after inhaling a bronchodilator is a confirmatory step for asthma. If there is no significant airway obstruction, the demonstration of increased airway responsiveness is suggestive of OA (see Chapter 5). Pre- and postshift assessments of forced expiratory volume in 1 second (FEV1) are not sensitive or specific enough to be useful in the investigation of OA.[41] Serial PEFR monitoring has been proposed for the investigation and assessment of both asthma[42,43] and OA.[4,5] Several patterns of worsening in PEFR have been described: hourly, diurnal, and day by day.[41] The sensitivity and specificity of PEFR monitoring as compared with the "gold standard," specific inhalation challenges, vary from 72% to 89%, depending on the study.[44,45] The PEFR graphs can be generated by plotting individual values or maximum, mean, and minimum values (Fig. 26-5). Recording PEFR twice a day is clearly not sufficient compared with doing so four or six times per day.[46] There are several pitfalls to PEFR monitoring: it requires good collaboration and honesty on the part of the patient, the interpretation requires specific expertise and is based on "eyeballing,"[47] and it is difficult at times to distinguish between a nonspecific irritant exacerbation of asthma at work and OA. The recent availability of instruments that can store data such as the time of recordings on computer chips or that can record both PEFR and FEV1, which is more sensitive and specific than PEFR alone in detecting airway obstruction, may improve the methodology. Combining PEFR and assessment of airway responsiveness for periods at work and away from work may, at times, improve the diagnostic yield,[48] although, in a more general way, it does not seem to add anything to the monitoring by PEFR alone.[45,49]

The use of nonspecific and specific challenges is discussed in Chapter 5.

PREVENTION AND SURVEILLANCE
Natural history of occupational asthma[50]

The natural history of OA can be illustrated as in Fig. 26-4. Atopy is a well-known predisposing factor to asthma and OA caused by high-molecular-weight agents such as detergent enzymes,[51] laboratory animal-derived antigens,[52] psyllium,[25] guar gum,[26] and snow crab.[53] The predictive value is not very strong, however, as only one third of atopic subjects exposed to laboratory animals developed symp-

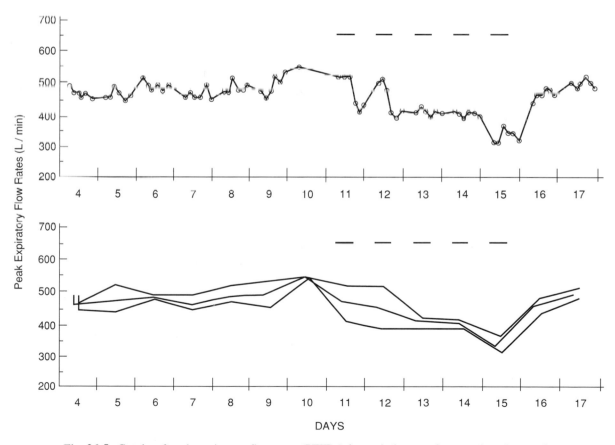

Fig. 26-5. Graphs of peak expiratory flow rates (PEFRs) for periods away from work and at work (horizontal bars). Individual results plotted in the upper section and maximum, mean, and minimum daily values in the lower graph are according to the method proposed by Burge et al.[4,5] The progressive weekly pattern of falls in PEFR is shown during a week spent at work.

toms of asthma on exposure to the agent.[52] Smoking is not a predisposing factor in OA caused by plicatic acid, the active agent in western red cedar,[54] but it is a risk factor (mean relative risk, 5) in workers exposed to platinum salts.[55] The effect of smoking is controversial in the case of high-molecular-weight agents.[56]

Anecdotal reports have suggested an association between spills of isocyanates and the likelihood of developing asthma symptoms.[57] However, these episodes could be identified as OA or reactive airways dysfunction syndrome (RADS) (see the following). Some association has been found between the concentration of exposure to colophony,[58] western red cedar,[59] and flour,[60] on the one hand, and the presence of symptoms on exposure to the causal agent on the other. However, this information is derived from cross-sectional studies that could have been affected by a healthy-worker survival bias. The nature of the occupational agent can also play a role in the rate of development of symptoms, as shown in Fig. 26-6; more workers exposed to western red cedar and isocyanates develop work-related symptoms in the first 2 years of exposure than do those exposed to high-molecular-weight agents. However, after 5 years of exposure, the rate for developing symptoms is similar for high-molecular-weight agents and isocyanates.[61]

Once sensitization has occurred, airway hyperresponsiveness is required in order to develop OA. It is unlikely that asthma is a predisposing factor in the development of OA resulting from low-molecular-weight agents. Although this information was gathered retrospectively in all studies, most workers who develop OA did not have a history of asthma before exposure began. We observed workers exposed seasonally to snow crab. Several of them had normal airway responsiveness before the seasonal exposure began. After starting work, they progressively developed airway hyperresponsiveness that persisted for several months.[53] In a prospective study Chan-Yeung and Desjardins found that four workers who developed OA due to western red cedar did not have airway hyperresponsiveness before exposure.[62]

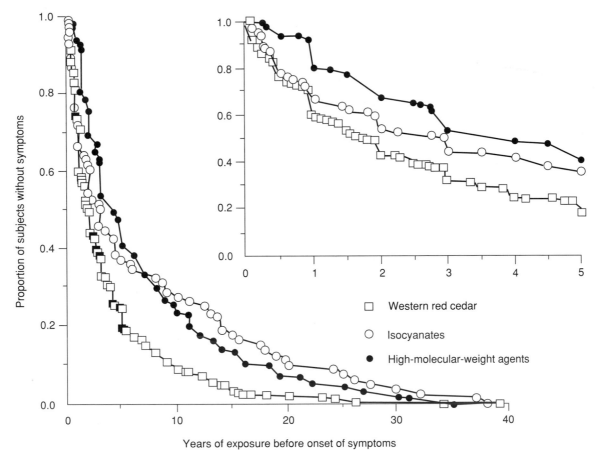

Fig. 26-6. Survival curves showing the proportion of patients in whom a diagnosis of occupational asthma was confirmed who are still without symptoms according to the number of years of exposure before the onset of symptoms. The magnified portion of the curve covering the first 5 years is shown in the upper right. Patients with occupational asthma due to isocyanates or western red cedar develop symptoms more rapidly than those with occupational asthma due to high-molecular-weight agents. After 1 to 2 years this phenomenon slows in the group with asthma caused by isocyanates.

Several retrospective studies, summarized in Table 26-2, have demonstrated a persistence of asthmatic symptoms, airway obstruction, and hyperresponsiveness in subjects with OA after they were removed from exposure. This was originally suggested by Chan-Yeung[63] and has since been confirmed by multiple investigators studying subjects exposed to various occupational agents.[64-70] Most studies have also shown that the total duration of exposure, the duration of exposure after the onset of symptoms, and the severity of the asthma at the time of diagnosis were all determinants of prognosis. A plateau of improvement has been shown to occur approximately 2 years after cessation of exposure in workers with OA due to snow crab.[71] If exposure continues, there is a deterioration in the asthmatic condition; in patients with western red cedar asthma, wearing a conventional face mask while still continuing to work does not diminish the risk.[72] It is unknown, however, whether wearing more protective respirators would prevent deterioration of asthma.

Strategies: primary, secondary, and tertiary prevention[73]

In terms of primary prevention, it is tempting to exclude atopic workers from exposure to high-molecular-weight agents. Although this can be done ethically through direct counseling (e.g., trying to dissuade young atopic persons from taking specific jobs that will expose them to laboratory animals), the practice cannot be applied to whole populations. In laboratory animal workers the risk of developing symptoms is not sufficiently high (approximately one third of workers) to justify excluding atopic persons.[52,74] Persuading employees to stop smoking in industries in which smoking has been identified as a significant risk factor appears reasonable. Keeping the concentration of the possible occupational agents low and avoiding spills also seem reasonable. It is, however, unrealistic to count on replacement products changing the picture of OA in the next few years. For example, no effective replacement product has been found for isocyanates. For secondary prevention,

routine skin testing with high-molecular-weight occupational agents is feasible and can identify subjects who have become immunologically sensitized and who should be followed up more closely in terms of the development of airway hyperresponsiveness and asthma symptoms. In workers exposed to low-molecular-weight agents, routine questionnaires coupled (preferably) with assessment of airway responsiveness could prove useful in detecting individuals at an early stage of the disease. In the authors' experience questionnaires can be sensitive, but they are not specific enough for this purpose. Preliminary results show that combining the tools might be the best strategy. In one study the workers who developed OA due to spiramycin were those who had had both a positive questionnaire and increased airway responsiveness.[75]

Tertiary prevention focuses on early diagnosis. Once the diagnosis of OA is made, it is important to remove the affected worker from exposure as quickly as possible. If this is done, it is less likely that the worker will be left with permanent sequelae of asthma and airway responsiveness requiring medication. If this is not possible, efforts should be made to diminish exposure. It is not known whether taking antiinflammatory preparations is any help once removal from exposure has occurred. However, retrospective evidence shows that patients taking antiinflammatory preparations are left with the same level of airway hyperresponsiveness as those on the usual bronchodilators only.

MEDICOLEGAL ASPECTS

There are several reasons that it is important to confirm the diagnosis of OA.[76] Missing the diagnosis may well mean that a worker will continue to be exposed to the agent causing the asthma, with all the medical consequences that this implies.[72] A diagnosis of OA can also have significant social and financial consequences.[77-79] Unlike pneumoconiosis, OA frequently affects young people, and advising them to quit their job has a major impact, as it implies retraining for a new occupation. It has been shown that the quality of life of patients with OA is slightly but signifi-

Table 26-2. Retrospective evidence for the persistence of symptoms and airway hyperresponsiveness after removal from the offending agent

Agent	No. of patients	Duration of follow-up (yr)	Persistence of symptoms (%)	Persistence of hyperresponsiveness (%)	Reference
Red cedar	38	0.5-4	29	38/38 (100%)	63
Red cedar	75	1-9	49	25/33 (76%)	64
Colophony	20	1.3-3.8	90	7/20 (35%)	65
Isocyanates	12	1-3	66	7/12 (58%)	66
Snow crab	31	0.5-2	61	28/31 (90%)	67
Snow crab	31	4.8-6	100	26/31 (84%)	71
Various	32	0.5-4	93	31/32 (97%)	67
Isocyanates	50	>4	82	12/19 (63%)	68
Isocyanates	20	0.5-4	50	9/12 (75%)	69
Isocyanates	22	1	77	17/22 (77%)	70

Table 26-3. American Thoracic Society guidelines for assessing impairment and disability in patients with asthma and occupational asthma

	Score				
	0	1	2	3	4
FEV1 (% of predicted value)	≥80	70-79	60-69	50-59	<50
Reversibility of airway obstruction or degree of airway responsiveness					
Reversibility (% change in FEV1)	≤10	10-19	20-29	≥30	—
PC20 (mg/ml)	≥16	2-16	0.25-2	≤0.25	—
Medication need					
Bronchodilators	None	Occasional (not daily)	Daily	Daily	—
Cromolyn	None	Occasional course (1-3/yr)	Daily	—	—
Inhaled steroid	None	Occasional course (1-3/yr)	Low dose daily	High dose daily	High dose daily
Systemic steroid	None	None	None	Occasional course (1-3/yr)	Daily
Summary impairment/disability rating class					
Class	0	I	II	III	IV	V
Total score	0	1-3	4-6	7-9	10-11	Asthma not controlled

From American Thoracic Society: Guidelines for the evaluation of impairment/disability in patients with asthma, *Am Rev Respir Dis* 147:1056-1061, 1993. *FEV1*, Forced expiratory volume in 1 second; *PC20*, Provocative concentration of methacholine causing a fall of 20% in FEV1 (PC 20).

cantly less satisfactory than that of control asthmatic patients.[80] Although it is of the utmost importance to offer retraining programs (for either the same employer or another one) or early retirement with financial compensation, the efficacy and cost of these programs must also be considered. In Quebec it has been estimated that it takes, on average, 8 months from the time a claim is made to the Workers' Compensation Board until compensation is awarded, which is too long for most patients. A single case of OA costs roughly $50,000 Canadian, approximately half of which is spent on temporary rehabilitation programs and the other half on permanent disability. For all of these reasons, it is important to ensure that the diagnosis is accurate.

As already discussed, OA can lead to permanent asthma even after removal from exposure, so it is reasonable that affected workers be offered compensation. Compensation scales designed for pneumoconiosis and fixed airway obstruction are inadequate for OA.[81] A scaling system specific to OA was designed and has been used in Quebec since 1985.[82] An official statement of the American Thoracic Society recently presented guidelines for assessing impairment and disability in persons with asthma.[83] The guidelines involve the level of airway obstruction on baseline spirometry, the level of airway responsiveness, and the severity of asthma as assessed by the patient's minimum medication needs. A summary of these guidelines is presented in Table 26-3.

A VARIANT OF OCCUPATIONAL ASTHMA: REACTIVE AIRWAYS DYSFUNCTION SYNDROME

Reactive airways dysfunction syndrome, also referred to as *irritant-induced asthma*,[84] is characterized by the presence of nonspecific airway hyperresponsiveness in persons who had no previous history of asthma. Although this syndrome was included in a recently published definition of OA,[85] it is different from typical OA in that there is no latency period for the development of symptoms. Other publications had previously described a similar type of syndrome after toxic inhalation of various products besides chlorine, such as ammonia, acid, fumes, and sulfur dioxide.[86-90] Cases of RADS had also been described after population exposures.[91] This condition consists of the development of respiratory symptoms (e.g., cough, wheezing, and dyspnea) in the minutes or hours after a single accidental inhalation of high concentrations of an irritating gas, aerosol, or particulate. A small percentage of exposed persons are left with "asthmalike" symptoms.[92] It was recently proposed that the definition of *RADS* be extended to include a similar condition that can occur after more than one ac-

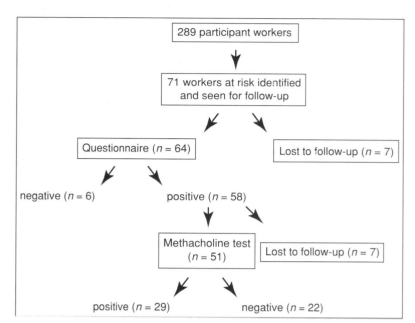

Fig. 26-7. Survey of 289 workers exposed to chlorine in a paper mill. Seventy-one workers were identified as being at risk; 64 underwent a questionnaire, and 51 underwent methacholine testing approximately 1 year after being symptomatic due to exposure to high concentrations of chlorine; 29 developed airway hyperresponsiveness. (Adapted from Chan-Yeung M, Lam S, Kennedy SM, et al: Persistent asthma after repeated exposure to high concentrations of gases in pulpmills, *Am J Respir Crit Care Med* 149:1676-1680, 1994. With permission.)

cidental exposure.[93,94] This often occurs in workplaces such as paper and pulp mills.[94] Kern found that there is a dose-dependent relationship between the intensity of exposure and the likelihood of developing permanent symptoms, reduction in airway caliber, and hyperresponsiveness.[95] Besides respiratory symptoms, systemic symptoms that can persist for several days after exposure have been described.[96] Up to 50% of persons at moderate to high risk of exposure can develop long-lasting airway hyperresponsiveness, as was documented 1 year after an exposure event (Fig. 26-7).[97] The pathologic features of RADS have seldom been described, but they seem to differ from those of asthma. In a series of five cases, greater subepithelial fibrosis was demonstrated[98] (Fig. 26-8), than is typically seen in asthma. Reversibility of airway obstruction after inhaling a bronchodilator is less likely than in OA with a latency period.[98]

CONCLUSION

Occupational asthma is the most common occupational respiratory illness. Because of the significant medical and social consequences, the diagnosis should be carefully confirmed. Prevention programs should be set up in high-risk workplaces. Permanent impairment and disability are common. Occupational asthma is a model of asthma in general, from the epidemiologic point of view, the natural history of sensitization and asthma can be described prospectively; from a pathophysiologic point of view, OA caused by high-molecular-weight agents is a model of "extrinsic asthma," whereas OA due to low-molecular-weight agents may be a type of "intrinsic asthma."

ACKNOWLEDGMENT

J-L Malo is a research scholar with the Fonds de la Recherche en Santé du Québec and the Université de Montréal School of Medicine.

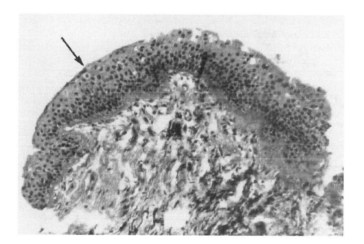

Fig. 26-8. Light micrograph of a bronchial biopsy of a patient with reactive airways dysfunction syndrome, 1 year after the inhalational accident, showing significant squamous cell metaplasia of the epithelium with dysplasia *(arrow)*. Large and dark nuclei at the luminal surface of the epithelium can be seen. Subepithelial fibrosis can also be seen. Original magnification, ×400. (Courtesy of Dr. Michel Boutet, Hôpital Laval and Université Laval, Quebec City.)

REFERENCES

1. Pepys J: Historical aspects of occupational asthma. In Bernstein IL, Chan-Yeung M, Malo J-L, et al, editors: *Asthma in the workplace,* pp 5-27, New York, 1993, Marcel Dekker.
2. Fuchs S and Valade P: Étude clinique et expérimentale sur quelques cas d'intoxication par le Desmodur T (diisocyanate de toluylene 1-2-4 et 1-2-6), *Arch Mal Prof* 12:191-196, 1951.
3. Pepys J and Hutchcroft BJ: Bronchial provocation tests in etiologic diagnosis and analysis of asthma, *Am Rev Respir Dis* 112:829-859, 1975.
4. Burge PS, O'Brien IM, and Harries MG: Peak flow rate records in the diagnosis of occupational asthma due to isocyanates, *Thorax* 34:317-323, 1979.

5. Burge PS, O'Brien IM, and Harries MG: Peak flow rate records in the diagnosis of occupational asthma due to colophony, *Thorax* 34:308-316, 1979.

6. Bernstein DI, Bernstein IL, Malo J-L, et al: Definition and classification. In Bernstein IL, Chan-Yeung M, Malo J-L, et al, editors: *Asthma in the workplace,* pp 1-4, New York, 1993, Marcel Dekker.

7. Brooks SM, Weiss MA, and Bernstein IL: Reactive airways dysfunction syndrome (RADS); persistent asthma syndrome after high level irritant exposures, *Chest* 88:376-384, 1985.

8. Perrin B, Cartier A, Ghezzo H, et al: Reassessment of the temporal patterns of bronchial obstruction after exposure to occupational sensitizing agents, *J Allergy Clin Immunol* 87:630-639, 1991.

9. Fabbri LM, Boschetto P, Zocca E, et al: Bronchoalveolar neutrophilia during late asthmatic reactions induced by toluene diisocyanate, *Am Rev Respir Dis* 136:36-42, 1987.

10. Lam S, LeRiche J, Phillips D, et al: Cellular and protein changes in bronchial lavage fluid after late asthmatic reaction in patients with red cedar asthma, *J Allergy Clin Immunol* 80:44-50, 1987.

11. Saetta M, Di Stefano A, Maestrelli P, et al: Airway mucosal inflammation in occupational asthma induced by toluene diisocyanate, *Am Rev Respir Dis* 145:160-168, 1992.

12. Saetta M, Maestrelli P, Di Stefano A, et al: Effect of cessation of exposure to toluene diisocyanate (TDI) on bronchial mucosa of subjects with TDI-induced asthma, *Am Rev Respir Dis* 145:169-174, 1992.

13. Bentley AM, Maestrelli P, Saetta M, et al: Activated T-lymphocytes and eosinophils in the bronchial mucosa in isocyanate-induced asthma, *J Allergy Clin Immunol* 89:821-828, 1992.

14. Fabbri LM, Ciaccia A, Maestrelli P, et al: Pathophysiology of occupational asthma. In Bernstein IL, Chan-Yeung M, Malo J-L, et al, editors: *Asthma in the workplace,* pp 61-92, New York, 1993, Marcel Dekker.

15. Finotto S, Fabbri LM, Rado V, et al: Increase in numbers of CD8 positive lymphocytes and eosinophils in peripheral blood of subjects with late asthmatic reactions induced by toluene diisocyanate, *Br J Ind Med* 48:116-121, 1991.

16. Borm PJA, Bast A, and Zuiderveld OP: In vitro effect of toluene diisocyanate on beta adrenergic and muscarinic receptor function in lung tissue of the rat, *Br J Ind Med* 46:56-59, 1989.

17. Sheppard D, Thompson JE, Scypinski L, et al: Toluene diisocyanate increases airway responsiveness to substance P and decreases airway neutral endopeptidase, *J Clin Invest* 81:1111-1115, 1988.

18. Bernstein DI: Animal models of occupational asthma. In Bernstein IL, Chan-Yeung M, Malo J-L, et al, editors: *Asthma in the workplace,* pp 93-101, New York, 1993, Marcel Dekker.

19. Lagier F, Cartier A, and Malo J-L: Statistiques médico-légales sur l'asthme professionnel au Québec de 1986 à 1988 (Medico-legal statistics on occupational asthma in Quebec between 1986 and 1988), *Rev Mal Respir* 7:337-341, 1990.

20. Meredith SK, Taylor VM, and McDonald JC: Occupational respiratory disease in the United Kingdom 1989: a report to the British Thoracic Society and the Society of Occupational Medicine by the SWORD project group, *Br J Ind Med* 48:292-298, 1991.

21. Blanc P: Occupational asthma in a national disability survey, *Chest* 92:613-617, 1987.

22. Timmer S and Rosenman K: Occurrence of occupational asthma, *Chest* 104:816-820, 1993.

23. Malo J-L and Chan-Yeung M: Population surveys of occupational asthma. In Bernstein IL, Chan-Yeung M, Malo J-L, et al, editors: *Asthma in the workplace,* pp 145-170, New York, 1993, Marcel Dekker.

24. Fabbri LM, Danieli D, Crescioli S, et al: Fatal asthma in a subject sensitized to toluene diisocyanate, *Am Rev Respir Dis* 137:1494-1498, 1988.

25. Bardy JD, Malo J-L, Séguin P, et al: Occupational asthma and IgE sensitization in a pharmaceutical company processing psyllium, *Am Rev Respir Dis* 135:1033-1038, 1987.

26. Malo J-L, Cartier A, L'Archevêque J, et al: Prevalence of occupational asthma and immunologic sensitization to psyllium among health personnel in chronic care hospitals, *Am Rev Respir Dis* 142:1359-1366, 1990.

27. Malo J-L, Cartier A, L'Archevêque J, et al: Prevalence of occupational asthma and immunological sensitization to guar gum among employees at a carpet-manufacturing plant, *J Allergy Clin Immunol* 86:562-569, 1990.

28. Séguin P, Allard A, Cartier A, et al: Prevalence of occupational asthma in spray painters exposed to several types of isocyanates, including polymethylene polyphenylisocyanates, *JOM, J Occup Med* 29:340-344, 1987.

29. Malo J-L and Cartier A: Occupational asthma in workers of a pharmaceutical company processing spiramycin, *Thorax* 43:371-377, 1988.

30. Seta JA, Young RO, Bernstein IL, et al: Compendium III. The United States national exposure survey (NOES) data base. In Bernstein IL, Chan-Yeung M, Malo J-L, et al, editors: *Asthma in the workplace,* pp 627-634, New York, 1993, Marcel Dekker.

31. Perrin B, Dhivert H, Godard P, et al: The telematic information service (MINITEL) on occupational asthma in France. In Bernstein IL, Chan-Yeung M, Malo J-L, et al, editors: *Asthma in the workplace,* pp 635-638, New York, 1993, Marcel Dekker.

32. Chan-Yeung M and Malo J-L: Compendium I. Table of the major inducers of occupational asthma. In Bernstein IL, Chan-Yeung M, Malo J-L, et al, editors: *Asthma in the workplace,* pp 595-623, New York, 1993, Marcel Dekker.

33. Malo J-L, Ghezzo H, L'Archevêque J, et al: Is an open questionnaire a satisfactory means for diagnosing occupational asthma?, *J Allergy Clin Immunol* 85:251, 1990.

34. Malo J-L, Ghezzo H, L'Archevêque J, et al: Is the clinical history a satisfactory means of diagnosing occupational asthma?, *Am Rev Respir Dis* 143:528-532, 1991.

35. Vandenplas O, Cartier A, Ghezzo H, et al: Response to isocyanates: effect of concentration, duration of exposure, and dose, *Am Rev Respir Dis* 147:1287-1290, 1993.

36. Reed CE, Swanson MC, and Li JTC: Environmental monitoring of protein aeroallergens. In Bernstein IL, Chan-Yeung M, Malo J-L, et al, editors: *Asthma in the workplace,* pp 249-275, New York, 1993, Marcel Dekker.

37. Lesage J and Perrault G: Environmental monitoring of chemical agents. In Bernstein IL, Chan-Yeung M, Malo J-L, et al, editors: *Asthma in the workplace,* pp 277-298, New York, 1993, Marcel Dekker.

38. Grammer LC and Patterson R: Immunologic evaluation of occupational asthma. In Bernstein IL, Chan-Yeung M, Malo J-L, et al, editors: *Asthma in the workplace,* pp 125-143, New York, 1993, Marcel Dekker.

39. Cockcroft DW, Murdock KY, Kirby J, et al: Prediction of airway responsiveness to allergen from skin sensitivity to allergen and airway responsiveness to histamine, *Am Rev Respir Dis* 135:264-267, 1987.

40. Cartier A, Grammer L, Malo J-L, et al: Specific serum antibodies against isocyanates: association with occupational asthma, *J Allergy Clin Immunol* 84:507-514, 1989.

41. Burge PS: Physiologic assessment of occupational asthma. In Bernstein IL, Chan-Yeung M, Malo J-L, et al, editors: *Asthma in the workplace,* pp 171-188, New York, 1993, Marcel Dekker.

42. Epstein SW, Fletcher CM, and Oppenheimer EA: Daily peak flow measurements in the assessment of steroid therapy for airway obstruction, *Br Med J* 1:223-225, 1969.

43. Turner-Warwick M: On observing patterns of airflow obstruction in chronic asthma, *Br J Dis Chest* 71:73-86, 1977.

44. Perrin B, Lagier F, L'Archevêque J, et al: Occupational asthma: vallidity of monitoring of peak expiratory flow rates and non-allergic bronchial responsiveness as compared to specific inhalation challenge, *Eur Respir J* 5:40-48, 1992.

45. Côté J, Kennedy S, and Chan-Yeung M: Sensitivity and specificity of PC 20 and peak expiratory flow rate in cedar asthma, *J Allergy Clin Immunol* 85:592-598, 1990.

46. Malo J-L, Côté J, Cartier A, et al: How many times per day should peak expiratory flow rates (PEFR) be assessed when investigating occupational asthma?, *Thorax* 48:1211-1217, 1993.

47. Côté J, Kennedy S, and Chan-Yeung M: Quantitative versus qualitative analysis of peak expiratory flows in occupational asthma, *Thorax* 48:48-51, 1993.

48. Cartier A, Pineau L, and Malo J-L: Monitoring of maximum expiratory peak flow rates and histamine inhalation tests in the investigation of occupational asthma, *Clin Allergy* 14:193-196, 1984.

49. Perrin B, Lagier F, L'Archevêque J, et al: Occupational asthma: validity of monitoring of peak expiratory flow rates and non-allergic bronchial responsiveness as compared to specific inhalation challenge, *Eur Respir J* 5:40-48, 1992.

50. Chan-Yeung M and Malo J-L: Natural history of occupational asthma. In Bernstein IL, Chan-Yeung M, Malo J-L, et al, editors: *Asthma in the workplace,* pp 299-322, New York, 1993, Marcel Dekker.

51. Mitchell CA and Gandevia B: Respiratory symptoms and skin reactivity in workers exposed to proteolytic enzymes in the detergent industry, *Am Rev Respir Dis* 104:1-12, 1971.

52. Slovak AJM and Hill RN: Does atopy have any predictive value for laboratory animal allergy? A comparison of different concepts of atopy, *Br J Ind Med* 44:129-132, 1987.

53. Cartier A, Malo J-L, Forest F, et al: Occupational asthma in snow crab-processing workers, *J Allergy Clin Immunol* 74:261-269, 1984.

54. Chan-Yeung M, Vedal S, Kus J, et al: Symptoms, pulmonary function, and bronchial hyperreactivity in western red cedar workers compared with those in office workers, *Am Rev Respir Dis* 130:1038-1041, 1984.

55. Venables KM, Dally MB, Nunn AJ, et al: Smoking and occupational allergy in workers in a platinum refinery, *Br Med J* 299:939-942, 1989.

56. Venables KM: Epidemiology and the prevention of occupational asthma, *Br J Ind Med* 44:73-75, 1987. Editorial.

57. Butcher BT, Jones RN, O'Neil CE, et al: Longitudinal study of workers employed in the manufacture of toluene diisocyanate, *Am Rev Respir Dis* 116:411-421, 1977.

58. Burge PS, Edge G, Hawkins R, et al: Occupational asthma in a factory making flux cored solder containing colophony, *Thorax* 36:878-834, 1981.

59. Vedal S, Chan-Yeung M, Enarson D, et al: Symptoms and pulmonary function in western red cedar workers related to duration of employment and dust exposure, *Arch Environ Health* 41:179-183, 1986.

60. Musk AW, Venables KM, Crook B, et al: Respiratory symptoms, lung function, and sensitisation to flour in a British bakery, *Br J Ind Med* 46:636-642, 1989.

61. Malo J-L, Ghezzo H, D'Aquino C, et al: Natural history of occupational asthma: relevance of type of agent and other factors in the rate of development of symptoms in affected subjects, *J Allergy Clin Immunol* 90:937-943, 1992.

62. Chan-Yeung M and Desjardins A: Bronchial hyperresponsiveness and level of exposure in occupational asthma due to western red cedar *(Thuja plicata):* serial observations before and after development of symptoms, *Am Rev Respir Dis* 146:1606-1609, 1992.

63. Chan-Yeung M: Fate of occupational asthma. A follow-up study of patients with occupational asthma due to western red cedar *(Thuja plicata), Am Rev Respir Dis* 116:1023-1029, 1977.

64. Chan-Yeung M, Lam S, and Koener S: Clinical features and natural history of occupational asthma due to western red cedar *(Thuja plicata), Am J Med* 72:411-415, 1982.

65. Burge PS: Occupational asthma in electronics workers caused by colophony fumes: follow-up of affected workers, *Thorax* 37:348-353, 1982.

66. Paggiaro PL, Loi AM, Rossi O, et al: Follow-up study of patients with respiratory disease due to toluene diisocyanate (TDI), *Clin Allergy* 14:463-469, 1984.

67. Hudson P, Cartier A, Pineau L, et al: Follow-up of occupational asthma caused by crab and various agents, *J Allergy Clin Immunol* 76:682-687, 1985.

68. Rosenberg N, Garnier R, Rousselin X, et al: Clinical and socioprofessional fate of isocyanate-induced asthma, *Clin Allergy* 17:55-61, 1987.

69. Mapp CE, Corona PC, de Marzo N, et al: Persistent asthma due to isocyanates. A follow-up study of subjects with occupational asthma due to toluene diisocyanate, *Am Rev Respir Dis* 137:1326-1329, 1988.

70. Lozewicz S, Assoufi BK, Hawkins R, et al: Outcome of asthma induced by isocyanates. *Br J Dis Chest* 81:14-27, 1987.

71. Malo J-L, Cartier A, Ghezzo H, et al: Patterns of improvement on spirometry, bronchial hyperresponsiveness, and specific IgE antibody levels after cessation of exposure in occupational asthma caused by snow-crab processing. *Am Rev Respir Dis* 138:807-812, 1988.

72. Côté J, Kennedy S, and Chan-Yeung M: Outcome of patients with cedar asthma with continuous exposure, *Am Rev Respir Dis* 141:373-376, 1990.

73. Bernstein DI: Surveillance and prevention. In Bernstein IL, Chan-Yeung M, Malo J-L, et al, editors: *Asthma in the workplace,* pp 359-372, New York, 1993, Marcel Dekker.

74. Newill CA, Evans R, and Khoury MJ: Preemployment screening for allergy to laboratory animals: epidemiologic evaluation of its potential usefulness, *JOM, J Occup Med* 28:1158-1164, 1986.

75. Malo J-L and Cartier A: Occupational asthma in workers of a pharmaceutical company processing spiramycin, *Thorax* 43:371-377, 1988.

76. Malo J-L: The case for confirming occupational asthma: why, how much, how far?, *J Allergy Clin Immunol* 91:967-970, 1993.

77. Marabini A, Ward H, Kwan S, et al: Clinical and socioeconomical features of subjects with red cedar asthma—a follow up study, *Chest* 104:821-824, 1993.

78. Gannon PFG, Weir DC, Robertson AS, et al: Health, employment, and financial outcomes in workers with occupational asthma, *Br J Ind Med* 50:491-496, 1993.

79. Malo J-L, Dewitte JD, Cartier A, et al: The Quebec system of compensation for occupational asthma: description, effectiveness and cost, *Rev Mal Respir* 10:313-323, 1993.

80. Malo J-L, Dewitte JD, Cartier A, et al: Quality of life of subjects with occupational asthma, *J Allergy Clin Immunol* 91:1121-1127, 1993.

81. Chan-Yeung M: Evaluation of impairment/disability in patients with occupational asthma, *Am Rev Respir Dis* 135:950-951, 1987.

82. Chan-Yeung M and Malo J-L: Occupational asthma, *Chest* 91:130S-136S, 1987.

83. American Thoracic Society: Guidelines for the evaluation of impairment/disability in patients with asthma, *Am Rev Respir Dis* 147:1056-1061, 1993.

84. Brooks SM and Bernstein IL: Reactive airways dysfunction syndrome or irritant-induced asthma. In Bernstein IL, Chan-Yeung M, Malo J-L, et al, editors: *Asthma in the workplace,* pp 533-549, New York, 1993, Marcel Dekker.

85. Bernstein IL, Chan-Yeung M, Malo J-L, et al: Definition and classification of asthma. In Bernstein IL, Chan-Yeung M, Malo J-L, et al, editors: *Asthma in the workplace,* pp 1-4, New York, 1993, Marcel Dekker.

86. Härkönen H, Nordman H, Korhonen O, et al: Long-term effects of exposure to sulfur dioxide, *Am Rev Respir Dis* 128:890-893, 1983.

87. Flury KE, Ames DE, Rodarte JR, et al: Airway obstruction due to inhalation of ammonia, *Mayo Clin Proc* 58:389-393, 1983.

88. Rajan KG and Davies BH: Reversible airways obstruction and interstitial pneumonitis due to acetic acid, *Br J Ind Med* 46:67-68, 1989.

89. Boulet LP: Increases in airway responsiveness following acute exposure to respiratory irritants. Reactive airway dysfunction syndrome or occupational asthma?, *Chest* 94:476-481, 1988.

90. Luo JC, Nelsen KG, and Fischbein A: Persistent reactive airway dysfunction syndrome after exposure to toluene diisocyanate, *Br J Ind Med* 47:239-241, 1990.

91. Weill H, George R, Schwartz M, et al: Late evaluation of pulmonary function after acute exposure to chlorine gas, *Am Rev Respir Dis* 99:374-379, 1969.

92. Brooks SM, Weiss MA, and Bernstein IL: Reactive airways dysfunction syndrome. Case reports of persistent airways hyperreactivity following high-level irritant exposures, *J Occup Med* 27:473-476, 1985.

93. Kennedy SM, Enarson DA, Janssen RG, et al: Lung health consequences of reported accidental chlorine gas exposures among pulpmill workers, *Am Rev Respir Dis* 143:74-79, 1991.

94. Salisbury DA, Enarson DA, Chan-Yeung M, et al: First-aid reports of acute chlorine gassing among pulpmill workers as predictors of lung health consequences, *Am J Ind Med* 20:71-81, 1991.

95. Kern DG: Outbreak of the reactive airways dysfunction syndrome after a spill of glacial acetic acid, *Am Rev Respir Dis* 144:1058-1064, 1991.

96. Courteau JP, Cushman R, Bouchard F, et al: A survey of construction workers repeatedly exposed to chlorine in a pulpmill over a 3-6 month-period. I. Exposure and symptomatology, *Occup Environ Med* 51:219-224, 1994.

97. Bhérer L, Cushman R, Courteau JP, et al: A survey of construction workers repeatedly exposed to chlorine over a 3-6 month-period in a pulpmill. II. Follow-up of affected workers with questionnaire, spirometry and assessment of bronchial responsiveness 18 to 24 months after exposure ended, *Occup Environ Med* 51:225-228, 1994.

98. Gautrin D, Boulet LP, Boutet M, et al: Is reactive airways dysfunction syndrome (RADS) a variant of occupational asthma?, *J Allergy Clin Immunol* 93:12-22, 1994.

99. Di Stefano A, Saetta M, Maestrelli P, et al: Mast cells in the airway mucosa and rapid development of occupational asthma induced by toluene diisocyanate, *Am Rev Respir Dis* 147:1005-1009, 1993.

Chapter 27

AGENTS CAUSING CHRONIC AIRFLOW OBSTRUCTION

Susan M. Kennedy

Examples of mixed-exposure situations
    Nonoccupational mixed exposures
    Occupational mixed exposures
Work-related chronic obstructive pulmonary disease:
  evidence
    Workplace-based studies
      Is chronic obstructive pulmonary disease an independent outcome of exposure to fibrogenic dusts (e.g., coal, silica, or asbestos)?
      Exposures to complex dusts or mixed dust, gas, and fume combinations
      Exposure to compounds believed to be "nuisance dusts"
    Population-based studies
Exposure patterns associated with nonspecific chronic obstructive pulmonary disease
Controversial questions
Summary and conclusions

Many texts on occupational pulmonary disease use the general heading *other pneumoconioses* to refer to the interstitial response to mixed dust exposures or to exposures to uncommon specific dusts and the heading *industrial bronchitis* to refer to nonspecific combined airway responses to "dust." However, for the most part, current knowledge does not permit a clear differentiation among the response patterns of the lung when it encounters mixed dust, fume, and gas exposures. Exceptions to this generalization form the majority of standard textbook chapters include specific interstitial fibrosis patterns associated with coal, silica, and asbestos exposures (the "classic" pneumoconioses); granulomatous interstitial reactions associated with some metals

(e.g., beryllium or cobalt); asthma due to specific agents (e.g., occupational asthma); other immunologically mediated lung diseases (e.g., hypersensitivity pneumonitis); and specific respiratory cancers. In addition, due to the presence of large, concentrated industrial groupings, a few substances that cause a mixed pulmonary response (e.g., coal dust exposure in coal mining or cotton dust exposure in cotton textile production) have been studied in sufficient detail to provide a reasonably complete picture of the spectrum of pulmonary disease attributable to these substances (although, even for these substances, there remains considerable controversy about the nature of exposure–response relationships).

Despite the attention given to these specific pulmonary response patterns or to responses to a few single substances, the majority of workers who may be exposed to dusts in the course of their work are exposed to mixtures of various types of dusts (inorganic and organic), as well as to gases, fumes, and, possibly, temperature extremes. Therefore, given the embryonic state of knowledge about specific pulmonary responses under these circumstances, it is still necessary to consider a category of either *nonspecific etiologic agents* or *nonspecific pulmonary responses* in any textbook on occupational pulmonary disease. This chapter addresses this mixed exposure–mixed response enigma by examining work-related chronic obstructive pulmonary disease (COPD), the quintessential nonspecific pulmonary response to inhaled substances.

EXAMPLES OF MIXED-EXPOSURE SITUATIONS

Mixed exposures are the norm rather than the exception in the occupational and environmental exposure setting. Some examples are listed in Table 27-1. Cigarette smoke is perhaps the most well-studied mixed exposure, and, although it provides a useful example of a complex exposure, it lacks an important characteristic of mixed exposures in the occupational setting, namely, that exposures in workplaces tend to be variable over time as well as having complex characteristics at any one time. Even in occupations

Table 27-1. Environmental sources of mixed exposures: examples

Nonoccupational
Cigarette smoke

Specific industries
Construction and demolition
Mining and smelting
Manufacturing of complex products (e.g., furniture or ceramics)
Food processing
Animal confinement

Specific jobs
Maintenance workers
Firefighters and emergency response workers
Casual or transient workers

that are thought of as having a single dust exposure (e.g., coal mining), potential exists for exposure to other substances (often gases or fumes) that may modify the pulmonary response to the primary mineral dust.

Nonoccupational mixed exposures

Cigarette smoking is perhaps the best example of a mixed inhaled exposure. It contains complex particulate and gaseous phases, and the pathophysiologic responses to whole smoke and to fractions of cigarette smoke have been studied extensively. However, even though much is known about the cellular and tissue responses from experimental and clinical studies, it is still not possible to explain exposure–response relationships in the smoking population with any degree of precision, nor is it possible to explain why one smoker will develop chronic bronchitis with airflow limitation or emphysema and others will not. As such, it provides a reasonable model from which to compare information relevant to the anticipated pulmonary response to occupational mixtures of dust and gases.

Despite similarities between cigarette smoke and mixed occupational exposures, there are some important differences. Cigarette smoke contains a powerful stimulant, nicotine, which acts acutely as a bronchodilator. On the other hand, many industrial mixed-exposure situations include exposure to silica or asbestos, both of which cause fibrosis at the level of the small airways and the interstitium.[1]

Occupational mixed exposures

It would be impossible to list all of the industries and occupations in which mixed exposures are found. Examples of industries include construction (which, at various stages, may lead to exposure to asbestos, other fibrous materials, solvents, pigments, ceramics, cements, wood dust, welding fumes, metal and polymer fumes, vehicle exhaust, asphalt and other petroleum products, and temperature extremes); mining, smelting, and mineral processing (for which exposures similar to those found in construction are present, as well as exposure to the ore-containing materials); manufacturing of composite or complex materials (e.g., rubber, furniture, clay, or ceramic products); and food processing and animal confinement (which may include exposure to extremely complex mixtures of both organic and inorganic substances).

Some job categories (regardless of industry) are also more likely than others to be associated with mixed exposures, maintenance work being perhaps the most common. Maintenance employees in most industries (even so-called "clean" industries such as service, sales, health care, and education) may be exposed intermittently (or sequentially) to solvents, metal fumes and dusts, mineral oil products, organic mixtures, and temperature extremes. In part because of their mixed exposures, maintenance workers have tended to be excluded from occupational cohort studies.[2,3] Other examples of specific jobs with diverse and complex exposures include firefighters, emergency response workers, demolition workers, and general laborers.

Finally, mixed exposures can occur not only as a result of working in a job or industry in which varied or variable exposures may occur, but also as a result of being an underemployed or transient worker. Workers who change jobs frequently may not be exposed or may have only a single exposure in any one job, but may, over the course of several decades, be exposed to many differing substances, with an overall effect similar to that if the worker were employed in a single industry with mixed exposures. Such workers are generally systematically excluded from most occupational health studies; thus few systematic data are available on this group.

WORK-RELATED CHRONIC OBSTRUCTIVE PULMONARY DISEASE: EVIDENCE

Chronic obstructive pulmonary disease is the generic term given to the final common pathway resulting from numerous initiating events. The pathogenesis and clinical course of this disease are discussed in Chapter 16. The essential clinical component of the disease is airflow limitation, due to airway obstruction and loss of elastic recoil in the parenchyma.[4] The principal early pathologic component of the disease is an inflammatory response in the peripheral airways.[5] This inflammatory response can lead to fibrotic lesions in the parenchyma, narrowing of the air passages, or emphysema. The latter two responses are generally called COPD; the former is generally called pneumoconiosis. In a single-exposure situation (e.g., if a miner is exposed to high concentrations of only one type of asbestos dust and not to fumes or irritating gases), chances are that one response pattern will predominate (in this example, the miner may develop fibrotic parenchymal disease). However, in the presence of mixed exposures, all three response patterns may occur, to a greater or lesser extent.

This section examines the evidence that COPD, manifested by a reduction in measures of airflow in the lung [e.g., reduced ratio of forced expiratory volume in 1 second to forced vital capacity (FEV1/FVC ratio), FEV1, or flow rates at low lung volumes], occurs in association with two types of exposure conditions: first, with exposures that are traditionally believed to cause pneumoconiosis, and second, with mixed exposures from which pneumoconiosis is not generally believed to result. In addition, large community-based or aggregate industrial population-based studies are discussed, as they provide evidence of the overall impact of this disease.

Workplace-based studies

Is chronic obstructive pulmonary disease an independent outcome of exposure to fibrogenic dusts (e.g., coal, silica, or asbestos)? As other chapters of this book examine the pneumoconioses in detail, this section discusses only the evidence for or against the hypothesis that exposures that can cause pneumoconiosis can also cause COPD.

Although many studies have shown that coal dust exposure is associated with increased symptom rates for cough and phlegm production,[6-9] there have been conflicting reports about whether dust exposure alone (i.e., in the absence of cigarette smoking) is responsible for airflow limitation. Several studies have shown no correlation between the presence of symptoms and either fibrotic lesions on chest radiographs or physiologic measures of airway obstruction.[6-8,10] These studies, conducted in the 1960s, clarified that increased sputum production (the clinical correlate of increased bronchial mucous gland number and size) is not inevitably associated with either radiographic fibrosis or airflow obstruction. They did not clarify the relationship, if any, between dust exposure and chronic airflow limitation. This was principally due to an inability to study a sufficient number of nonsmoking miners, a lack of data with which to classify workers into differing actual dust exposure levels, and the necessity to rely on an outcome measure (i.e., radiographic fibrosis) as a surrogate for exposure.

Studies in which nonsmoking and smoking miners have been investigated separately provide clearer information about the possible effects of dust on airways (Table 27-2). Among surface coal miners with very little radiographic fibrosis, Fairman and colleagues[11] found significant airway obstruction (defined as having an FEV1/FVC ratio less than two standard deviations below expected) in 6.6% of nonsmoking miners and 18.9% of smoking miners. In a study of 8555 U.S. soft-coal miners using an identical criterion for significant airway obstruction, Kibelstis and coworkers[9] found this outcome in 6.3% of nonsmoking miners and 17.8% of smoking miners. Marine et al.[12] analyzed the results in 3380 British coal miners who were either current smokers or lifetime nonsmokers. They found a significant relationship between cumulative dust exposure and FEV1 below 80% of that predicted and for FEV1 below 65% of that predicted in both smokers and nonsmokers. The prevalence rates for FEV1 under 80% were 10.5% for nonsmok-

ers and 17.4% for smokers in the lowest exposure group and 20.6% for nonsmokers and 31.8% for smokers in the medium- to high-exposure group. A significant negative interaction was reported between the effects of age and dust exposure, suggesting that the effect of dust was more pronounced in younger workers. In a 1993 publication Oxman and associates[13] reported the results of an overview analysis of the evidence from all available quantitative studies of the relationship between inorganic dust exposure and COPD (published between 1966 and 1991), in which the effects of both dust exposure (measured quantitatively) and smoking were taken into account. Thirteen suitable reports were retrieved; these covered the results from three coal-mining cohorts and one gold-mining cohort. From their aggregate analysis of the coal-mining cohorts, these authors concluded that after roughly 35 years of work at a mean coal dust exposure level of 2 mg/m^3, approximately 8% of nonsmoking coal miners (and 6.6% of smoking miners) could be expected to experience a loss of FEV1 below 80% of the predicted level, and 1.2% of nonsmoking coal miners (and 2.3% of smoking miners) would suffer an FEV1 level below 65% of that predicted. Even more recently, Seixas and collaborators[14,15] reported on the relationship between dust exposure and obstructive lung disease in a population of 1185 U.S. underground coal miners who started mining after 1970, when dust exposure regulations required a reduction in coal dust levels. They found no consistent relationship between cumulative dust exposure level and FVC, but a significant decrease in both FEV1 and FEV1/FVC ratio in relation to exposure level (with estimated decline in FEV1 of −5.7 ml for each mg/m^3-year of exposure). The exposure–response relationship was modeled best with a nonlinear exposure term, suggesting that the added effect of many additional years of dust exposure is not as strong as the effect of dust in the initial years of exposure. As found in the study of British miners,[12] examination of those who had never smoked revealed a negative interaction between dust exposure and age, such that the association between increasing cumulative dust exposure and decreased FEV1 was seen only in the under-50 age groups. Among the nonsmoking miners the frequency of having an FEV1 less than 80% of the predicted value ranged from 7.4% in the low-exposure category to 14.3% in the high-exposure category (compared to 28.1% among smokers in the high-exposure group.[14] Longitudinal analysis of lung function decline in a subset of the same population confirmed a rapid initial loss in FEV1 associated with cumulative dust exposure (−35-ml FEV1 decline per mg/m^3-year of cumulative exposure in miners over age 25, in the initial 2 to 4 years of employment) but no subsequent dust-associated decline over the next 10 to 14 years.[15]

Studies of gold miners suggest an even stronger relationship between dust exposure level and airflow obstruction in hard-rock mining compared to coal mining (Table 27-2). In Oxman and colleagues' reanalysis of results from a South

Table 27-2. Exposure to fibrogenic dusts: studies of airflow obstruction

Reference	Population	Airflow obstruction measure	Exposure measure	Relationship between exposure and outcome	Interaction between exposure and smoking	Prevalence of obstruction	
						Nonsmokers	Smokers
12	British coal miners (n = 3380)	1. FEV1 <80% 2. FEV1 <65%	Cumulative dust over previous 10 years	Significant dose-related effect of exposure on all levels of airflow obstruction in smokers and non-smokers	No statistical interaction between smoking and dust; Effect of medium or high dust exposure similar to effect of current smoking for FEV1 <80%; Effect of smoking greater than effect of dust for FEV1 <65%; Effect of dust exposure more severe in younger smokers	Low dust: 0.5% High dust: 24.6%	17.4% 45.8%
11	U.S. surface coal miners (n = 1171)	FEV1/FVC <2 SD below that expected	Years of employment	No relationship between years as a surface miner and FEV1	No statistical interaction	No bronchitis: 6.2% With bronchitis: 8.5%	16.1% 25.6%
9	U.S. coal miners, face and surface (n = 8555)	FEV1/FVC <2 SD below that expected	Surface workers compared to face workers	Little difference in airflow obstruction between surface and face miners	N/A	6.3%	17.8%
14 and 15	U.S. coal miners first employed after 1970 (n = 1185)	FEV1 <80%	Cumulative dust exposure	Significant dose-response relationship between cumulative-exposure airflow obstruction; Effect of cumulative exposure on FEV1 greatest in miners under age 30; Longitudinal decline in FEV1 greatest in the first 5 years of employment	N/A	10.8%	11.7%

Continued.

16	South African gold miners (n = 2209)	FEV1 between 95% and 99% lower CL with normal VC	Cumulative dust exposure	Significant dose-response relationship between increased dust and FEV1, similar in all smoking categories	No interaction between dust and smoking with respect to FEV1 in total group. Interaction between dust and smoking only in miners with marked airflow obstruction
17	Australian gold miners (n = 1093); nickel smelter workers (n = 324, controls)	FEV1/FVC <70 plus chronic bronchitis symptoms	Duration of work in underground gold mining	Significant dose-response relationship between both measures of obstruction and increased exposure duration	N/A
22	34 lifetime nonsmoking Canadian chrysotile miners versus 21 nonexposed manual workers	Upstream conductance and resistance at low lung volumes	Asbestos miners versus non-asbestos-exposed workers	Decreased Gus at low lung volume in miners with increasing severity as extent of alveolitis and asbestosis increases	N/A
23	U.S. asbestos insulators (n = 416)	Airflow rates	Insulators versus reference values (Michigan)	Significantly decreased FEV1 and FEF75-85 in all smoking categories	N/A
24	U.S. construction and shipyard workers with diaphragmatic plaques (n = 64)	Airflow rates	Asbestos workers versus reference values (Michigan)	Significantly decreased FEV1 in nonsmokers. Significantly decreased FEV1/FVC in smokers and nonsmokers	N/A
25	U.S. boilermakers (n = 534)	FEV1/FVC%	Years in trade	Significantly decreased FEV1/FVC% associated with >20 yr in the trade. Effects not associated with job status as a welder versus other jobs in the trade	N/A

Table 27-2. Exposure to fibrogenic dusts: studies of airflow obstruction—cont'd

Reference	Population	Airflow obstruction measure	Exposure measure	Relationship between exposure and outcome	Interaction between exposure and smoking	Prevalence of obstruction	
						Nonsmokers	Smokers
27	Canadian asbestos insulators over age 50 (employed, $n = 59$; retired, $n = 29$)	Both FEV1 and FEV1/FVC% <95% lower CL	Insulators compared to reference population	35% had airflow obstruction Obstruction associated with diffuse pleural abnormality and with history of work in pulp mills	N/A		
28	U.S. asbestos union members with normal radiographs ($n = 113$)	Airflow rates	Years in trade	Significantly decreased FEV1/FVC% and FEF25-75% in workers with >20 yr in the trade Relationship between duration of employment and FEV1 greater in workers with <20 yr employment	Effect of smoking additive with asbestos Effect of >20 yr employment approximately equal to that of smoking		
29	Canadian asbestos miners ($n = 983$)	FEV1 % predicted	Many exposure–time variables	Airflow limitation associated with exposure, weighted for residence time in the lung, suggesting increased effect of earlier exposure	No statistical interaction seen		
30	U.S. wollastonite miners ($n = 108$); electrical plant workers ($n = 86$, controls)	Airflow rates	Cumulative exposure; miners versus controls	Significant association between FEV1/FVC% and cumulative exposure Longitudinal decline in peak flow related to cumulative exposure	Dose–response relationship more pronounced in nonsmokers		

FEV1, Forced expiratory volume in 1 second; *FVC*, forced vital capacity; *CL*, confidence limit; *VC*, vital capacity; *Gus*, upstream conductance; *FEF75-85*, forced expiratory flow rate from 75-85% of expired volume.

African gold-mining cohort[13,16] (to allow direct comparison with the coal-mining cohorts also reanalyzed by these authors), the estimated effect of cumulative dust exposure from this mining environment on airflow obstruction was approximately one order of magnitude greater than that seen in the coal-mining cohorts. This differential was more pronounced among nonsmokers than smokers. In an original analysis of results from the same South African cohort, Hnizdo and colleagues[16] reported additive effects of smoking and dust exposure on FEV1 level and categorical measures of obstructive lung disease, with departures from additivity (toward a synergistic effect) in the groups with marked airflow obstruction. Synergy between the effects of smoking and mining dust was also suggested in a population of workers from a Western Australian gold-mining district, reported by Holman et al.,[17] although stable estimates for an interaction effect were not possible when examining airflow obstruction as a categorical outcome. The overall prevalence of obstructive lung disorder (FEV1/FVC ratio, <0.7) in the white male segment of this population ($n =$ 1363) was 11.3%. Chronic bronchitis together with this obstructive disorder was approximately five times more prevalent for gold miners with over 20 years underground compared to nonminers, after adjustment for age and smoking habits.

The case–control study design was applied by Becklake and collaborators[18] to evaluate predictors of emphysema in South African gold miners. From 419 autopsy examinations of miners with at least 1 year in gold mining and no history of exposure to coal or asbestos who died in 1980 or 1981, 44 subjects with definite emphysema (grade 2 or higher) were compared to 42 subjects with no emphysema (grade 0 to 0.5). Detailed smoking and work histories were available for these miners from the time they entered mining. The results indicated that smoking early in life (20 cigarettes per day prior to 1960) was associated with a 30-fold increase in emphysema risk, and 20 years of working in a high-dust exposure job was associated with a 13-fold increase in emphysema risk. These relationships were not altered by taking into consideration other clinical factors such as the presence of symptoms, silicosis grade, or bronchial wall mucous gland hyperplasia, nor were any of these features significant independent predictors of emphysema.

In contrast to these studies of coal and gold miners, in a study of a selected group of iron miners,[19] generally negative associations between underground mining exposures and lung function were reported. A one-fifth random sample of a population of French iron miners with normal chest radiographs and no cardiovascular disease ($n = 1167$) was studied prospectively for 10 years (only 522 were still available at the time of follow-up). As no comparison population was studied, the effect of exposure could only be evaluated by comparing underground to surface miners. The results suggested little difference in lung function decline between these groups. A relationship was seen, however, between DLCO and duration of employment underground of about the same magnitude as that seen for cigarette smoking.

Airflow obstruction in association with asbestos exposure has also been the subject of several recent reports. It has been demonstrated that the early pathologic lesion associated with asbestos exposure is small airway wall inflammation and fibrosis,[20] and animal studies have shown a strong correlation between asbestos-induced increased airway wall thickness and reduced airflow rates.[21] It is not surprising, therefore, that in addition to pneumoconiosis, airflow obstruction has been found in studies of asbestos-exposed workers.[22-26] In a study of Canadian chrysotile miners,[22] specific airway conductance at low lung volumes was found to be reduced in nonsmoking miners compared to nonsmoking manual workers without asbestos exposure. Similar, but more pronounced, effects were seen among smokers. However, no differences were seen in simple spirometry between exposed and nonexposed groups in this study. Significant reductions in both FEV1 and forced expiratory flow rate from 75% to 85% of expired volume (FEF75-85) were reported by Kilburn and colleagues[23] among nonsmoking asbestos insulators compared to nonsmoking population controls; in a subsequent study of 79 men with diaphragmatic plaques as the only radiographic abnormality,[24] these authors reported airflow obstruction but no evidence of restriction among both nonsmokers and smokers, at a level significantly greater than that seen in population controls. In a prevalence study of boilermakers, Demers et al.[25] found airflow obstruction that was associated with increasing years in the trade and with both pleural and parenchymal radiographic abnormalities, and was not accounted for by other exposures. This is consistent with the results of our study of construction insulators over age 50,[27] in which the authors found significant airflow obstruction in one third of the population that was associated with diffuse pleural abnormalities. In our study, however, airflow obstruction also appeared to be associated with other, nonasbestos exposures, particularly with a history of construction work at pulp mill sites. This emphasizes the point made earlier that few working populations are truly exposed to a single substance and that multiple exposures may be the norm rather than the exception, even when the scientific report is focused on a single exposure.

Two studies have documented a stronger relationship between asbestos exposure early in working life and subsequent airflow obstruction. In a cross-sectional study of 113 asbestos workers with normal chest radiographs, Hall and Cissik[28] found that the regression coefficients associated with years of asbestos work, for models of FVC, FEV1, FEF25-75, and peak expiratory flow rate (PEFR), were all significantly greater in the subset of workers with less than 20 years of exposure than in workers with longer exposure, suggesting a stronger dose–response relationship in the earlier years of exposure than in the later years. Similarly,

Copes and colleagues[29] found that exposures received early in a worker's career were more important than recent exposure in relation to airflow limitation among a population of 983 Canadian miners.

Finally, wollastonite, a fibrous monocalcium silicate mineral, has also been shown to impair airway function. A study of 108 wollastonite miners and millers, reported by Hanke and coworkers,[30] compared these workers to a control population of electronic components factory workers. The results showed no exposure-related increase in respiratory symptoms, but significant dose–response relationships for FEV1, FEV1/FVC ratio, and PEFR in relation to cumulative dust exposure. No exposure effect was seen for FVC. The dose–response relationship between FEV1/FVC ratio and dust exposure continued to be significant when nonsmokers alone were analyzed. Longitudinal rates of decline in FEV1 over a 6-year period in the exposed population were −49 ml/yr for nonsmokers and −75 ml/yr for smokers.

In summary, numerous studies of workers employed in industries generally believed to be associated with single exposures to potentially fibrogenic dusts have demonstrated that airflow obstruction is also a significant outcome of prolonged employment in these industries. The effect on airflow was generally seen in both smokers and nonsmokers employed in these industries, and the combined effect of dust exposure and smoking was most often reported to be additive (or less than additive) rather than multiplicative (although some studies suggested a synergistic effect between silica exposure and smoking). In most of these studies, exposure duration (or cumulative exposure) has been used as the primary exposure dose measure. As dust exposure duration in mining and mineral processing is correlated with exposure duration to other irritant gases or fumes in these worksites, it is not yet possible to differentiate the potential role played by mixed exposures in the development of the airflow obstruction reported to be associated with fibrogenic dust exposure in these industries.

Exposures to complex dusts or mixed dust, gas, and fume combinations. Steelworks, foundries, blast furnaces, smelters, and coke ovens are examples of environments with more obvious mixed mineral dust and fume exposures. Temperature extremes are also generally found in these work environments. Several studies have implicated a connection between these mixed mineral dust and fume exposures and chronic airflow obstruction (Table 27-3). Manfreda and colleagues[31] studied 241 hard-rock (zinc, copper, and nickel) miners and smelter workers from northern Manitoba and compared these to a general-population sample of 382 men. They found increased prevalence rates for cough and sputum in nonsmoking underground miners and in smoking miners and smelter workers, and slightly reduced levels of pulmonary function, especially in exposed smokers compared to the general-population smokers. Increased prevalence rates for airflow in the abnormal range

were seen only in the smelter workers (both nonsmokers and smokers, although statistically significant only among smoking smelter workers).

Studies of welders generally do not demonstrate restrictive impairment due to pneumoconiosis unless there is a concomitant history of asbestos or silica exposure; however, evidence suggestive of airway abnormalities has been reported in this group. A Swedish study of nonsmoking metal arc shipyard welders compared to men with no welding history, conducted by Hjortsberg and associates,[32] demonstrated evidence of small airway obstruction among nonsmoking welders. In both cross-sectional and longitudinal surveys of 609 British shipyard welders and caulkers/ burners,[33,34] FEV1 and other measures of airflow limitation were found to be reduced in association with the duration of time spent welding in confined spaces. In the initial cross-sectional study this effect was seen only among smokers. In a subsequent longitudinal follow-up investigation the average rate of decline in FEV1 was −44 ml/yr in welders compared to −21 ml/yr in other tradesmen. In regression models, taking both age and smoking into account, the additional effect on FEV1 decline of work as a welder or caulker/burner was approximately equal to the effect of being a smoker or recent exsmoker; however, there was also significant interaction between these effects. Among the exposed subset atopy was also significantly related to an annual decline in FEV1; this relationship was not seen among the nonexposed tradesmen. In an earlier study of British arc welders from the automotive and related industries, who generally work in open booths or spaces, abnormalities indicative of small airway obstruction were also found, but in this case only among the smoking subset when compared to nonwelding subjects from the same factories.[35]

In a clinical–pathologic correlation study among patients about to undergo lung resection surgery, we compared lung function and airway pathology among 19 subjects with a work history of 10 or more years in mining ($n = 10$) or in a job with exposure to mixed mineral dust or fume in a nonmining environment ($n = 9$), to 19 nonexposed subjects individually matched for age and smoking history.[36] All but one of the miners were hard-rock miners; most of the nonmining exposed workers were welders, smelter workers, or foundry workers. Significant reductions in lung function and small airway wall fibrosis and increased mucous cells were seen in the exposed group. The pathologic changes were seen almost exclusively in the mixed exposed group, although the functional changes were seen in both groups.

Mixed exposures to mineral dusts and fumes are often found together with exposures to combustion products, gases, and organic vapors. For example, in rubber products manufacturing industries the principal dust exposures are carbon black and talc, but additional exposures are found to gaseous, liquid, and particulate aerosols from curing processes. In a series of studies in this industry, reported in 1976 by Fine and Peters,[37-40] both curing and production

Table 27-3. Mixed mineral dust and fume exposure: relationship between exposure and outcome in studies controlling for the effects of smoking

Reference	Population	Airflow obstruction measure	Exposure measure	Relationship between outcome and exposure	Interaction between exposure and smoking
31	Canadian miners and smelter workers ($n = 241$); general-population controls ($n = 382$)	Airflow rates below lower 95th percentile in controls	Miner, smelter worker, or control	Significant reduction in airflow rates in exposed smokers, most prominent among smelter workers. Decreased airflow rates in association with increased duration of employment (miners only)	Positive interaction between smelter work and smoking in relation to airflow obstruction
35	British engineering factory welders ($n = 258$); matched controls ($n = 258$)	Airflow rates	Welder or control	No difference between welders and controls for the total group	Small reductions in flow rates at low lung volumes in a subset of smoking welders
33	British shipyard welders and caulker/burners ($n = 607$)	Airflow rates	Average total welding fume exposure	Significantly reduced airflow rates associated with average exposure in smokers and ex-smokers. Positive interaction between welding exposure and age effects on airflow	Effects of welding exposure on airflow seen in smokers only
34	British shipyard welders and caulker/burners, follow-up of study 33 ($n = 488$)	FEV1 slope (over 7 yr of follow-up)	Welder, caulker/burner, or other trade	Annual decline in FEV1 2 times greater in welders or caulker/burners than in other trades	Significant positive interaction between smoking and exposure
38 and 39	U.S. rubber manufacturing workers (curing, $n = 121$; production, $n = 65$; controls, $n = 189$)	Airflow rates; FEV1 slope (over 1 yr of follow-up)	Job type or duration of exposure	Significantly decreased FEV1/FVC associated with production work. Significantly decreased FEV1 associated with increasing years of exposure to dust. Steeper FEV1 slope associated with increased years of employment in curing department	N/A

FEV1, Forced expiratory volume in 1 second; *FVC,* forced vital capacity.

workers were found to have exposure duration-related decreases in FEV1 and increases in the prevalence of chronic bronchitis symptoms.

An equally complex mixed inorganic and organic exposure situation, in which temperature extremes also play a role, is seen in firefighting. The range of reported exposures in this profession include carbon monoxide, hydrogen chloride, hydrogen cyanide, formaldehyde, nitrogen oxides, sulfur dioxide, and particulates.[41] Mineral dust is a less likely component of this exposure mixture. A number of studies, although not all, have reported both acute and chronic airflow obstruction among firefighters.[42-45] Among firefighters studied as a part of the U.S. Normative Aging Study,[45] employment as a firefighter was associated with an effect

on the 5-year rate of decline in FEV1 approximately one half that of being a cigarette smoker (i.e., -12 ml/yr for firefighting versus -21 ml/yr for smoking).

Complex exposure mixtures of predominantly organic components are more typically found in occupations associated with agriculture and food processing. Some of the more well-studied agricultural industries include grain handling, animal confinement, and animal feed production.[3,46-49] These are covered in detail in Chapter 36. However, it is worth reiterating here that, in addition to the immunologically mediated responses to organic components of these exposure mixtures, nonspecific COPD, essentially indistinguishable from that seen in mixed mineral dust and fume exposures, is seen in studies of workers exposed to mixed organic dusts and fumes. Linear regression coefficients similar to those associated with cumulative grain dust exposure level in relation to age- and smoking-adjusted annual declines in FEV1 were reported in longitudinal studies of workers in the grain elevator industry[48] and the animal feed production industry.[3] One study of retired grain handlers[49] has found evidence of moderate to severe airflow obstruction (FEV1 below 65% of that predicted) in 40% of nonsmokers and 50% of smokers in this population. These rates were significantly elevated over those found in a comparison population, with the between-group difference being more pronounced among the nonsmokers. Despite the reduced level of FEV1 (which was associated with cumulative dust exposure)[48] and increased prevalence of obstructive disease in this group after retirement, the average rate of decline in FEV1 over the previous 15 years was no more rapid than that seen in the comparison group, indicating that the differential in FEV1 level between these groups must have occurred earlier in the working life of this cohort. Large rates of FEV1 decline in the initial few years of employment were also seen among grain handlers studied by Zejda and colleagues.[50]

No clear general conclusions emerge from these varied studies of mixed exposures, except to reiterate that a number of studies do show a significant relationship between these exposures and COPD. Some features of the relationship between COPD and mixed organic dust exposures are similar to those seen for mineral dust exposures; that is, an additive or less than additive effect in combination with smoking and a more rapid decline in lung function in the earlier exposure years. The mixed mineral dust and fume exposures appear to behave somewhat differently, in that a significant interaction between the effects of smoking and exposure is more likely to be seen. These general conclusions are based on evidence from very few studies, however, and whether they will be supported or refuted as additional evidence becomes available remains to be seen.

Exposure to compounds believed to be "nuisance dusts". At varying time periods numerous dusts have been referred to as "nuisance dusts," including carbon black, iron, and grain. As discussed briefly already and in greater detail elsewhere,[46] the notion that grain dust may be simply a nuisance dust has been clearly shown to be false, although its previous designation as such serves to emphasize the changing nature of our understanding about the effects of occupational exposures.

The concept of a dust exposure representing only a nuisance refers to the possibility that exposure to the substance alone (i.e., in the absence of other biologically or chemically active substances) leads to no harmful pathologic reaction in the body. Unfortunately for scientists who wish to study this possibility, few workers are ever exposed to these dusts alone. For example, considerable carbon black exposure occurs in the rubber industry, but, as discussed, it is usually not encountered without exposure to other sub-

stances. Iron dust may be present in iron mining and welding exposures but, again, seldom in the absence of other exposures. The question remains, however, what are the effects of "pure" exposures to these types of substances?

Some investigators have looked at the pulmonary effects of iron dust or iron oxide exposure by comparing lung function among workers with and without siderosis. *Siderosis* is the term applied to the radiographic appearance of iron particles in the lungs of electric arc welders. Prevalence rates for this radiographic feature vary across studies but tend to be related to age and years of employment.[51] Most studies that have examined both radiographic appearance and pulmonary function in welders have found no relationship between these two measures.[51-53] This has been interpreted as evidence against an adverse effect of welding exposures and as support for using the term *nuisance dust* in relation to iron dust exposure. This interpretation is erroneous, because the finding of an absence of a relationship between two possible outcomes of exposure simply suggests that the pathway leading to these two outcomes is unlikely to be the same. In fact, in a pathologic, physiologic, and radiologic correlation study of 52 cases of atypical pneumoconiosis, Gaensler and colleagues[54] found that the most important histologic determinant of lung function in these cases was the integrity of the lung tissue between the nodules, not the number or extent of fibrotic foci themselves. Thus studies comparing workers with and without radiographic pneumoconiosis are not sufficient to provide evidence that the exposure either is or is not benign. This can only be done by a study design that compares outcomes in groups with differing exposure levels. Such studies are complicated by the fact that iron dust is not the only exposure present in welding fume, and it is almost completely impossible to isolate the effects of iron dust from the effects of welding gases and fumes.

Tin represents a similarly radiopaque dust that leads to radiographically and pathologically evident nodules in tin miners (i.e., stannosis). As with siderosis, the presence of radiographic stannosis does not appear to be associated with pulmonary function abnormalities. Although several small, mostly negative, studies (comprising cases of stannosis or selected groups of tin-exposed workers) were reported in the 1950s and 1960s,[55-57] there do not appear to be any large cross-sectional or longitudinal studies that have examined populations of tin-exposed workers with comparison to non-exposed groups, from which conclusions could be drawn about whether or not this exposure is benign.

One large-population study of workers exposed to carbon black[58] reported radiographically evident nodules in only 6 of 396 workers with 10 or more years of exposure. Reductions in airflow rates were found in association with dust exposure, but this effect was considerably lesser in magnitude than that seen with cigarette smoking. A recently published study of workers from 18 carbon black manufacturing plants in seven European countries[59,60] reported carbon black exposure levels in excess of the allowable limits for inhalable dust in several job categories, as well as exposure to carbon monoxide and trace levels of sulfur dioxide in this industry. The results indicated that exposed workers had significantly reduced flow rates in association with increasing respirable dust levels, most prominent among nonsmokers.

The majority of studies of pure carbon black exposure have been conducted using animal models.[61-64] In general, the results of studies in which carbon black (and/or other apparently nonreactive particles such as titanium dioxide or aluminum oxide) is instilled or aerosolized into animal lungs indicate reduced pulmonary clearance of particulate and enhanced susceptibility to infection by pathogens as a result of exposure to these substances at levels close to the regulated nuisance dust standards set by most jurisdictions. Therefore, although the dusts themselves may be relatively nonreactive in lung tissue, airway pathology in workers exposed to these dusts may occur as a result of both combined exposures to dusts and other irritant exposures and the inflammation associated with respiratory infections.

To summarize, the clinical and epidemiologic studies of workers exposed to iron, tin, or carbon black dust alone suggest little or no relationship between isolated exposure to these dusts and spirometry outcomes. On the other hand, the evidence from animal models would predict that airway abnormalities may ensue in situations in which exposures to these dusts occur in combination with other dusts or other irritant gases or fumes. Epidemiologic studies of welders, rubber manufacturing workers, and carbon black manufacturing workers in which airflow obstruction is seen confirm the predictions of the animal models with respect to toxicity of these nuisance dusts in mixed-exposure situations.

Population-based studies

The objective of this chapter is to examine evidence for COPD in relation to mixed exposures in the workplace, and the argument has been put forward that the majority of workplace exposures occur in combinations, not singly. However, despite this stated objective, the emphasis here so far has been on studies that have attempted to examine single exposures or single industry types. The common work history, which may include exposure to a wide variety of dusts, gases, or fumes, with varying time–exposure profiles (from periods of time with little or no exposure to other brief or extended periods with exposure peaks or more extensive cumulative exposure), does not lend itself to study in specific cohorts. However, further evidence regarding the effects of this type of exposure can be inferred from broad-based population studies, of which there have been a number in recent years (Table 27-4).

Exposure to dust and to gases or fumes was evaluated in a U.S. cross-sectional population-based study reported by Korn and colleagues[65] in 1987. The population consisted of a random sample of white adults ($n = 8515$) from six U.S. cities, selected to represent cities with differing levels of ambient air pollution. Significantly increased relative odds were seen for symptoms of cough, phlegm, wheezing, and breathlessness in relation to dust exposure, with no evidence of interaction with cigarette smoking. Similar increased relative odds were seen for these symptoms in association with gas or fume exposure, but only for former and current smokers. Chronic obstructive pulmonary disease, defined as having an FEV1/FVC ratio of 0.6 or less, was increased in association with dust exposure, but not with fume exposure alone.

Bakke and associates[66] reported the results of a cross-sectional population cohort study, drawn from the Norwegian county of Hordaland. Occupational exposure was evaluated using job title, with jobs evaluated as having no, moderate, or high airborne exposure (considering dusts, fumes, mists, and gases together). In addition, reported exposure to seven specific agents was evaluated. Significantly increased prevalence odds ratios were seen for airflow obstruction based on spirometry alone and for a clinical diagnosis of obstructive lung disease, in relation to airborne exposure in the present job or in the job held the longest. A dose–response trend was also seen in relation to exposure rated in three categories of increasing exposure potential. Odds ratios relating clinically diagnosed obstructive lung disease and each of the seven specific exposures were all greater than 1, but were statistically significant only for quartz, metal gases (platinum, chromium, and nickel), aluminum production and processing, and welding.

The French pollution atmosphérique et affections respiratoires (chroniques) (PAARC) study,[67] a community-based cross-sectional study of over 16,000 residents from seven French towns, was specifically designed to measure the effects of air pollution on lung health; therefore, households headed by a "manual worker" were excluded in order to rule out persons with potential for heavy workplace exposures. Thus it provides a population in which to evaluate the possible respiratory effects of light to moderate workplace dust, fume, or gas exposure in jobs that would not be classified as manual work. Participants were classified as *exposed* if they responded positively to the question "Were you exposed to dust, gases, or chemical fumes?" in the current or past jobs. In all, 34% of men and 23% of women were so classified. All analyses were adjusted for the effects of age, smoking, social class, air pollution, and education level. Exposed men and women had significantly more symptoms (approximate increases in the range of 50%) of chronic cough, chronic bronchitis, dyspnea, and wheezing. For exposed men significant reductions in FEV1/FVC and FEF25-75/FVC ratios were seen, which were similar in magnitude to the differences observed between nonsmokers and former smokers and approximately one third of the magnitude of differences observed between current light smokers and nonsmokers. This same pattern was

Table 27-4. Population-based studies: relationship between exposure and airflow obstruction in studies controlling for the effects of smoking

Reference	Population	Airflow obstruction measure	Exposure measure	Relationship between outcome and exposure	Interaction between exposure and smoking
65	Sample of residents from six U.S. cities (n = 8515)	FEV1/FVC <0.6	Questionnaire: job with potential exposure to dust and gas or fume	Increased relative odds for airflow obstruction associated with dust alone (OR = 1.7) and with dust and fumes combined (OR = 1.6)	No statistical interactions seen
66	Stratified sample of residents of Hordaland county, Norway (n = 714)	Positive clinical history plus FEV1/FVC <0.7	Questionnaire: job with potential "airborne exposure" (three levels)	Increased relative odds for obstruction associated with high-level exposure jobs (OR = 3.6) Effect of exposure more pronounced in older workers	No statistical interactions seen
67	Residents from 24 areas of seven French cities (excluding households headed by a "manual worker") (n = 12,182)	Airflow rates	Questionnaire: exposed to dust, gases, or chemical fumes in any job	FEV1/FVC significantly reduced in exposed group Effect of exposure most pronounced in older subjects	Magnitude of exposure effect approximately half the magnitude of the effect of smoking No interaction seen
68	Sample of residents of Beijing, China, not using coal for heat (n = 1094)	Airflow rates	Questionnaire: cumulative exposure (three levels) to dust and to gas or fume	Significant reduction in FEV1 and FEF25-75 associated with exposure to dust (compared to no exposure) Significant dose—response trend for FEV1 related to increasing gas or fume exposure among exposed subjects	Effects of exposure to dust most pronounced among exsmokers Significant interaction between smoking and dust exposure on FEV1/FVC
69	Workers from 11 Paris factories (n = 556)	FEV1 slope (over 12 yr of follow-up)	Technical survey: exposure to dust (five levels), gases (two levels), or heat (three levels)	More rapid decline in FEV1 associated with dust alone, heat alone, and gas in combination with dust and/or heat Steeper slopes among unskilled workers Workers in the 30-39 age group had higher initial FEV1 but equally steep slopes as for older workers	N/A
70	Random sample of residents of Cracow, Poland (n = 1679)	FEV1 slope (over 13 yr of follow-up)	Questionnaire: history of exposure to dusts, variable temperature, or chemicals	More rapid decline in FEV1 associated with prolonged exposure to variable temperature and acute exposure to irritating gases Effects of exposure most pronounced in those exposed for relatively short periods	No statistical interactions seen Size of exposure coefficients in regression models greater than the size of smoking coefficients

FEV1, Forced expiratory volume in 1 second; *FVC,* forced vital capacity; *OR,* odds ratio; *FEF25-75,* forced expiratory flow rate from 25% to 75% of expired volume.

observed when analysis was restricted to men without a history of wheezing or asthma. Among men with such a history, the opposite effect was seen (i.e., the exposed group had somewhat better lung function than the unexposed group). Among women no significant relationships were seen between any of the spirometric measures and occupational exposure. Neither were any significant relationships seen between FEV1 or FEF25-75 and smoking in these women. In contrast to the results for men, stratifying the analysis of women according to history of wheezing or asthma showed a greater effect of exposure on the FEV1/FVC ratio among those with an asthmatic history. No interactions between occupational exposure and smoking or air pollution were seen for symptoms or lung function in either men or women among these nonmanual workers.

A recent study by Xu and colleagues[68] examined a random sample of 3606 Beijing, China, adults between the ages of 40 and 69 years. Increased relative odds (in the range of a 30% increase) were seen for symptoms of cough, phlegm, and breathlessness in association with both exposure to dust and exposure to gases or fumes. Wheezing was not associated with dust exposure but was significantly associated with gas or fume exposure, with an odds ratio of 1.6 (95% confidence interval, 1.2 to 2.2). Dose–response trends were seen for all symptoms (i.e., chronic bronchitis, breathlessness, and wheezing) in relation to both dust and gas or fume exposure. No interactions were seen between the effects of smoking and exposure. The effects of exposure on lung function was evaluated only in the 1094 subjects who reported no coal stove home heating, as earlier analysis of this population had shown this to be a significant predictor of lung function deficits. In this subgroup without coal stove heating, a small reduction in FEV1 was seen in those with dust exposure (most prominent among former smokers); the same effect was not seen in association with any gas or fume exposure. However, a dose–response trend for decreasing FEV1 in association with increasing cumulative exposure (defined by three categories, taking into consideration both intensity and duration of exposure) was seen in association with gas or fume exposure, but not with dust exposure. This dose–response trend was most evident among those with some exposure potential (i.e., comparing high-, medium-, and low-exposure groups, excluding those with no exposure); the low-exposure group had lung function values that were higher than those seen in the group with no exposure.

Two large longitudinal studies have also been conducted that offer the opportunity to examine the role of occupational exposure on lung function changes over time. Kauffmann and associates[69] reported results from a cohort of Paris area workers tested in 1960 and followed up in 1972 to 1973. Of the 1002 men tested originally, 556 were available and provided acceptable spirometry at the follow-up period. Detailed occupational exposure information, obtained on the first survey, was used to assign the workers to groups exposed to dust (three intensity categories) or gas

or heat (two intensity categories each). When these exposures were evaluated independently, a significant relationship was seen between change in FEV1 over the study period and dust exposure level (with a significant dose–response trend), exposure to gas only at the highest exposure level and exposure to heat. Combinations of these exposure groupings showed that the longitudinal decline in FEV1 increased with exposure combinations as follows (in men with no change in smoking habit): no exposure or exposed only to slight dust or only to gases, −44 ml/yr; exposed to noticeable dust, −50 ml/yr; exposed to heat, −59 ml/yr; exposed to noticeable dust and heat, −56 ml/yr; and exposed to noticeable dust and high levels of gases and heat, −67 ml/yr.

The longitudinal change in ventilatory function over a 13-year period in relation to occupational exposures was also assessed by Krzyzanowski and colleagues among a sample of Cracow, Poland, residents.[70,71] Of 1193 men and 1485 women tested in 1965, 58% of the men and 66% of the women were available for follow-up testing in 1981. History of exposure to dusts, chemicals, and variable temperature was assessed from interviews in 1968, 1973, and 1981. The most striking findings of this study were significant associations between FEV1 decline and exposure to variable temperature and exposure to chemicals (both prior to 1968 and in 1973) among the men studied. Dust exposure alone was not associated with a significantly elevated rate of decline in FEV1. A similar association with variable temperature was also seen among the women studied. The magnitude of these effects was greater than that seen for cigarette smoking in both sexes, and no interaction was observed between exposure indicators and smoking. The authors suggested that reporting of exposure to variable temperature is likely to be more accurate (i.e., less misclassified) than reporting of exposure to dust or chemicals. As random misclassification of exposure invariably leads to a reduction in the magnitude of any relationship seen between exposure and disease, this relative lack of exposure misclassification for temperature variability could account, in part, for the stronger association seen between lung function decline and this exposure parameter. Increases in respiratory symptoms over the same 13-year period (studied in a slightly larger proportion of participants than for the lung function analysis) showed a stronger relationship between increased symptoms and dust exposure among both men and women, and chemical exposure among women.[71]

Although the case-control study design lends itself to evaluating mixed or multiple exposures, this design has rarely been used to examine the relationship between industrial exposures and COPD. In a notable exception Kjuus and colleagues[72] compared lifetime work histories among 36 emphysema patients and 72 referents (matched for age and smoking history) in a community hospital in an industrial area of Norway. They found a significantly elevated risk ratio (RR = 3; 95% confidence interval, 1.2 to 7.5) for exposed subjects developing emphysema, with exposure defined as 10 or more years of employment in a polluted job. From the job history examples given by the investigators, "polluted" jobs included a wide variety of jobs (and industries) in which potential for dust or fume exposure was present. As over 80% of both cases and referents were heavy cigarette smokers, this study does not shed light on the potential for emphysema development for industrial exposures in the absence of cigarette smoking, but does suggest that the combination of smoking and industrial workplace pollution increases the risk for emphysema. An attempt to examine the dose–response relationship in this study by comparing the RR in three duration categories (less than 10 years, 10 to 24 years, and at least 25 years in a polluted job) did not show a significant dose–response trend. The authors suggested that this may have been due either to insufficient statistical power of the study or to the possibility that workers who develop shortness of breath may remove themselves to cleaner jobs.

The results of these population-based studies support the general impressions derived from the workplace-based studies with respect to the combined effects of exposures to cigarette smoking, dusts, and gases or fumes. Although the evidence is not completely uniform, combinations of exposure types appear to add to the risk for COPD, but in a less than completely additive fashion. Interaction (or multiplication) of effects was seldom seen. Exposures to dusts alone tended to be the most likely single-exposure type to be associated with increased airflow obstruction,[69] whereas when workplace exposure was reported to be to gases or fumes alone, an interaction with smoking was more likely to be seen.[65]

EXPOSURE PATTERNS ASSOCIATED WITH NONSPECIFIC CHRONIC OBSTRUCTIVE PULMONARY DISEASE

Most of the workplace- and population-based studies discussed here indicate, at least in a general way, that COPD occurring in association with occupational exposures will be more pronounced as the cumulative exposure burden increases. Although, in the past decade, epidemiologists have defined *cumulative exposure* for a specific substance more precisely as the product of exposure duration and exposure intensity for that substance, these studies suggest that a broader view of cumulative exposure burden that incorporates at least additive effects for dusts and fumes, gases, and temperature extremes, should be considered for mixed exposure. This relationship with cumulative exposure is also clearly true for cigarette smoking, as heavy smokers are more likely to develop COPD than light smokers. However, as with cigarette smoking, this relationship between cumulative exposure burden and COPD risk is by no means sufficient to characterize risk. Recent studies have suggested the necessity to examine other exposure patterns and characteristics (e.g., peak exposures, combination exposures,

early responses, and particle size distributions), as they influence pulmonary responses. This is especially true in mixed-exposure situations, in which a simple relationship with cumulative dust burden is unlikely to be sufficient to explain the response.

Several studies have suggested that, in addition to overall career cumulative exposure burden, exposures early in the working life appear to play a particularly important role in inducing persistent airflow obstruction. This has been reported in coal mining,[12,14] asbestos exposure,[28,29] and grain handling,[49,50] and in association with cigarette smoking.[18,73] It is possible that this finding in epidemiologic studies is simply a reflection of the normal industrial practice of starting a new employee in the job with higher potential exposure and to the inevitable later self-selection of exposure-susceptible persons into jobs with lesser exposures. However, Seixas' report[14] of this phenomenon among young coal miners who started employment in mining after the introduction of new dust control measures suggests that this may not be simply an effect of excessively high exposure levels early in the worker's life. The general-population profile for lung function change in adults shows an increase in FEV1 up to approximately age 17 to 22, a plateau for approximately 8 to 10 years, and a linear decline thereafter.[74,75] One can speculate that irritant exposure during the end of the growth phase and during the plateau phase (whether it be to cigarette smoke or to a similar mixed industrial exposure) may ultimately be more harmful than later exposure, if it has the effect of initiating the decline phase at an earlier point in time. This effect has been seen in relation to cigarette smoking in a large Dutch population-based study[76]; further clarification of the role of early occupational exposure remains for future studies.

The importance of particle size fractions with respect to pulmonary deposition has been studied extensively; however, with the exception of fiber exposures, it has seldom been possible to take this factor into consideration in epidemiologic studies of occupational airflow obstruction unless exposure measurements have been historically divided into respirable and nonrespirable fractions. Other subdivisions of the respirable fraction may also be important. For example, submicron particles (or particulate fumes) have been implicated in the development of the pulmonary toxicity associated with dust overload.[61] It is possible that particle size may also play a role in the enhanced effect of dust–fume mixtures seen in some of the population-based studies. The increasing number of studies in which exposure assessment science and epidemiology are used concurrently will perhaps shed further light on this issue.

Differences in the profile of exposure intensity over time is also recognized as a potential source of variability in the evaluation of occupational exposure–response relationships. In several industries airflow rates have been shown to be related to the frequency of peak exposures over a threshold as well as to cumulative exposure.[2,77,78] This raises the possibility that chronic clinically relevant airway abnormalities may derive from the combination of repeated acute inflammatory episodes over a background of chronic low-grade airway inflammation, even though the consequences of one or the other event alone may be less clinically detectable. Some of the discrepancies between studies that have looked for possible synergy between dust and gases or fumes or between workplace exposures and cigarette smoking in both population- and industry-based studies may be due in part to differences in exposure intensity–time profiles. Again, this remains to be investigated in future studies.

CONTROVERSIAL QUESTIONS

It would not be appropriate to leave this discussion of COPD as the nonspecific response of the lung to a dirty environment without posing some of the still unanswered or controversial questions about this topic. As COPD is a disease that develops slowly and generally causes impairment only among the elderly, the definitive answers to some of these questions and controversies will necessarily require the passing of additional time. Occupational COPD that exists among the current elderly population is the result of exposures many years ago, and epidemiologic study of even these workers is hampered by the fact that the elderly are more difficult to study once they leave the workforce.

Most of the studies summarized throughout this chapter have reported statistically significant reductions in airflow rates among groups of exposed workers compared to nonexposed workers. Symptoms of cough, phlegm, and wheezing are variably reported to be increased or not increased. The relevance of these findings with respect to disability and clinical outcome is strongly debated.[79-81] Studies of coal miners have addressed this issue[12,82] and have shown "clinically relevant" airflow obstruction even among nonsmoking miners; however, this question is not resolved by studies of active workers. Rather, stronger evidence as to whether or not exposure-related reductions in airflow rates among currently working populations lead to disability is found from three additional sources. First, mortality studies have now demonstrated a clear association between reduced FEV1 level and subsequent early death from respiratory and nonrespiratory diseases. This was suggested by Higgins' study of a mining community[83] and further supported by two comprehensive prospective population-based studies among British[84] and French[85] men. In considering the previously described association between occupational exposure early in the working career and greater subsequent airflow obstruction, it is of interest that both these British and French population studies of COPD found that a more rapid decline in FEV1 early in adulthood was associated with an even greater relative risk for early mortality.

A second source of evidence is found from the few studies that have followed exposed cohorts into the postretirement years[36,49] and have shown increased prevalence rates of moderate to severe airflow obstruction and associated activity limitation[49] compared to nonexposed groups with similar smoking histories. Finally, evidence is obtained from the examination of work histories from autopsy-proven cases of emphysema compared to cases with no emphysema. Among gold miners[18] emphysema was shown to be related independently to age, smoking, and duration of exposure to high-dust jobs; among a general population sample[72] in which emphysema cases were matched to noncases on age and smoking history, emphysema was found to be related to work in a "polluted" job, with an exposures odds ratio of 3. The weight of evidence from these three sources that clinically relevant chronic airflow obstruction can and does result from workplace exposures to mixed dust and fume or gas exposures is now very strong.

A second unresolved and debated question deals with the relative impact of cigarette smoking and occupational exposures in the development of COPD. Given the evidence in some studies of interactions between smoking and work exposures, the question remains, what will be the impact on exposure-related respiratory morbidity and mortality of the current trend toward reduction in cigarette smoking prevalence? No definite answer is available from the current literature, although it would appear that for some exposures with a strong synergistic effect (e.g., predominantly gas or fume exposures) a marked reduction in exposure-related morbidity should occur, whereas for other exposures with little evidence of interaction (e.g., grain or coal dust) the reduction in exposure-related morbidity is unlikely to be as dramatic.

SUMMARY AND CONCLUSIONS

This chapter has addressed the issue of mixed occupational exposures leading to the nonspecific pulmonary response characterized by chronic airflow limitation or COPD. Although most of the scientific work in the field of occupational lung diseases has focused on specific responses to single agents, it is argued that much of the occupational and environmental exposures that occur are not well described by these specific responses. Evidence from epidemiologic studies (and some pathologic studies) is presented that suggests that clinically relevant COPD occurs not only in response to exposures typically thought to be fibrogenic only (e.g., gold, coal, or asbestos) but also in many other complex and mixed exposure situations, including mineral dust and fume and mixtures of organic and inorganic exposures. Evidence from community-based studies suggests that the combination of dust and gas or fume exposure may be more potent than dust alone in leading to this outcome. Other recent evidence suggests that although the total dust burden accumulated over time is important in predicting the risk for COPD, other aspects of the exposure should be considered in evaluating COPD risk. These include exposures early in the work career (for which an increasing body of evidence is emerging suggesting that this is especially significant), peak exposures, and the combination of dust plus irritant gas and fume exposures.

The natural inclination to classify the universe as a way of explaining or understanding leads to a proliferation of disease designations to describe rare individual cases or small groups of cases in which pulmonary impairment appears to be related to work in a dusty job. Thus, long lists of specific pneumoconioses, bronchitides, and pneumonitides are tempting as a way to describe specific reactions to isolated substances. This divisive approach may also be necessary to the pursuit of molecular or cellular responses to specific agents. However, as humans are rarely exposed to isolated substances, this chapter has attempted to provide a counterbalance to this understandable need to classify by examining the nonspecific common features of the pulmonary response to many complex work environments.

REFERENCES

1. Churg A and Wright JL: Small airway lesions in patients exposed to nonasbestos mineral dusts, *Hum Pathol* 14:688-693, 1983.
2. Diem JE, Jones RN, Hendrick DJ, et al: Five-year longitudinal study of workers employed in a new toluene diisocyanate manufacturing plant, *Am Rev Respir Dis* 126:420-428, 1982.
3. Smid T, Heederik D, Houba R, et al: Dust and endotoxin related respiratory effects in the animal feed industry, *Am Rev Respir Dis* 146:1474-1479, 1992.
4. Hogg JC, Macklem PT, and Thurlbeck WM: Site and nature of airway obstruction in chronic obstructive lung disease, *N Engl J Med* 278:1355-1360, 1968.
5. Cosio M, Ghezzo H, Hogg JC, et al: The relations between structural changes in small airways and pulmonary function tests, *N Engl J Med* 298:1277-1281, 1978.
6. Ulmer WT: The relationship between dust exposure and chronic bronchitis and emphysema. In Shapiro HA, editor: *Pneumoconiosis, proceedings of the international conference, Johannesburg 1969*, pp 328-336, Cape Town, South Africa, 1969, Oxford University Press.
7. Rasmussen DL: Patterns of physiological impairment in coal workers pneumoconiosis, *Ann NY Acad Sci* 200:455-464, 1972.
8. Ryder RC, Lyons JP, Campbell H, et al: Bronchial mucous gland status in coal workers' pneumoconiosis, *Ann NY Acad Sci* 200:370-380, 1972.
9. Kibelstis JA, Morgan EJ, Reger R, et al: Prevalence of bronchitis and airway obstruction in American bituminous coal miners, *Am Rev Respir Dis* 108:886-893, 1973.
10. Higgins ITT, Oldham PD, Cochrane AL, et al: Respiratory symptoms and pulmonary disability in an industrial town, *Br Med J* 20:904-910, 1956.
11. Fairman RP, O'Brien RJ, Swecker S, et al: Respiratory status of surface coal miners in the United States, *Arch Environ Health* 32:211-215, 1977.
12. Marine WM, Gurr D, and Jacobsen M: Clinically important respiratory effects of dust exposure and smoking in British coal miners, *Am Rev Respir Dis* 137:106-112, 1988.
13. Oxman AD, Muir DCF, Shannon HS, et al: Occupational dust exposure and chronic obstructive pulmonary disease, *Am Rev Respir Dis* 148:38-48, 1993.
14. Seixas NS, Robins TG, Attfield MD, et al: Exposure–response relationships for coal mine dust and obstructive lung disease following enactment of the federal Coal Mine Health and Safety Act of 1969, *Am J Ind Med* 21:715-734, 1992.
15. Seixas NS, Robins TG, Attfield MD, et al: Longitudinal and cross-sectional analyses of coal mine dust and pulmonary function in new miners, *Br J Ind Med* 50:929-937, 1993.
16. Hnizdo E, Baskind E, and Sluis-Cremer GK: Combined effect of silica dust exposure and tobacco smoking on the prevalence of respiratory impairments among gold miners, *Scand J Work Environ Health* 16:411-422, 1990.
17. Holman CDJ, Psaila-Savona P, Roberts M, et al: Determinants of chronic bronchitis and lung dysfunction in Western Australian gold miners, *Br J Ind Med* 44:810-818, 1987.
18. Becklake MR, Irwig L, Kielkowski D, et al: The predictors of emphysema in South African gold miners, *Am Rev Respir Dis* 135:1234-1241, 1987.
19. Pham QT, Teculescu D, Bruant A, et al: Iron miners—a ten year follow-up, *Eur J Epidemiol* 8:594-600, 1992.
20. Craighead J, Abraham J, Churg A, et al: The pathology of asbestos-associated diseases of the lungs and pleural cavities: diagnostic criteria and proposed grading schema, *Arch Pathol Lab Med* 106:541-595, 1982.
21. Wright JL, Tron V, Wiggs B, et al: Cigarette smoke potentiates asbestos-induced airflow abnormalities, *Exp Lung Res* 14:537-548, 1988.
22. Begin R, Boileau R, and Peloquin S: Asbestos exposure, cigarette smoking, and airflow limitation in long-term Canadian chrysotile miners and millers, *Am J Ind Med* 11:55-66, 1987.
23. Kilburn KH, Warshaw RH, Einstein K, et al: Airway disease in nonsmoking asbestos workers, *Arch Environ Health* 40:293-295, 1985.
24. Kilburn KH and Warshaw RH: Abnormal pulmonary function associated with diaphragmatic pleural plaques due to exposure to asbestos, *Br J Ind Med* 47:611-614, 1990.
25. Demers RY, Neale AV, Robins T, et al: Asbestos-related disease in boilermakers, *Am J Ind Med* 17-327-339, 1990.
26. Rodriquez-Roisin R, Merchant JA, Cochrane GE, et al: Maximal expiratory flow volume curves in workers exposed to asbestos, *Respiration* 39:158-165, 1980.
27. Kennedy SM, Vedal S, Muller N, et al: Lung function and chest radiograph abnormalities among construction insulators, *Am J Ind Med* 20:673-684, 1991.
28. Hall SK and Cissik JH: Effects of cigarette smoking on pulmonary function in asymptomatic asbestos workers with normal chest radiographs, *Am Ind Hyg Assoc J* 43:381-386, 1982.
29. Copes R, Thomas D, and Becklake MR: Temporal patterns of exposure and non-malignant pulmonary abnormality in Quebec chrysotile workers, *Arch Environ Health* 40:80-87, 1985.
30. Hanke W, Sepulveda M-J, Watson A, et al: Respiratory morbidity in wollastonite workers, *Br J Ind Med* 41:474-479, 1984.
31. Manfreda J, Sidwall G, Maini K, et al: Respiratory abnormalities in employees of the hard rock mining industry, *Am Rev Respir Dis* 126:629-634, 1982.
32. Hjortsberg U, Orbaek P, and Arborelius M. Small airways dysfunction among nonsmoking shipyard arc welders, *Br J Ind Med* 49:441-444, 1992.
33. Cotes JE, Feinmann EL, Male VJ, et al: Respiratory symptoms and impairment in shipyard welders and caulker/burners, *Br J Ind Med* 46:292-301, 1989.
34. Chinn DJ, Stevenson IC, and Cotes JE: Longitudinal respiratory survey of shipyard workers: effects of trade and atopic status, *Br J Ind Med* 47:83-90, 1990.
35. Hayden SP, Pincock AC, Hayden J, et al: Respiratory symptoms and pulmonary function of welders in the engineering industry, *Thorax* 39:442-447, 1984.
36. Kennedy SM, Wright JL, Pitman RG, et al: Pulmonary function and peripheral airway pathology in patients with mineral dust or fume exposure, *Am Rev Respir Dis* 132:1294-1299, 1985.
37. Fine LJ and Peters JM: Respiratory morbidity in rubber workers. I.

Prevalence of respiratory symptoms and disease in curing workers, *Arch Environ Health* 31:1-5, 1976.

38. Fine LJ and Peters JM: Respiratory morbidity in rubber workers. II. Pulmonary function in curing workers, *Arch Environ Health* 31:6-10, 1976.

39. Fine LJ and Peters JM: Respiratory morbidity in rubber workers. III. Respiratory morbidity in processing workers, *Arch Environ Health* 31:136-140, 1976.

40. Fine LJ and Peters JM: Respiratory morbidity in rubber workers. IV. Respiratory morbidity in talc workers, *Arch Environ Health* 31:195-200, 1976.

41. Trietman RD, Burgess WA, and Gold A: Air contaminants encountered by firefighters, *Am Ind Hyg Assoc J* 41:796-802, 1980.

42. Musk AW, Peters JM, Bernstein L, et al: Pulmonary function in firefighters: a six-year follow-up in the Boston Fire Department, *Am J Ind Med* 3:3-9, 1982.

43. Horsfield K, Guyatt AR, Cooper FM, et al: Lung function in West Sussex firemen: a four year study, *Br J Ind Med* 45:116-121, 1988.

44. Minty BD, Royston D, Jones JG, et al: Changes in permeability of the alveolar–capillary barrier in firefighters, *Br J Ind Med* 42:631-634, 1985.

45. Sparrow D, Bosse R, Rosner B, et al: The effect of occupational exposure on pulmonary function, *Am Rev Respir Dis* 125:319-322, 1982.

46. Chan-Yeung M, Enarson D, and Kennedy SM: State of the art. grain dust induced lung disease, *Am Rev Respir Dis* 145:476-487, 1992.

47. Zejda JE, Hurst TS, Rhodes CS, et al: Respiratory health of swine producers. Focus on young workers, *Chest* 103:702-709, 1993.

48. Huy T, de Schiffer K, Chan-Yeung M, et al: Grain dust and lung function: dose–response relationships, *Am Rev Respir Dis* 144:1314-1321, 1991.

49. Kennedy SM, Dimich-Ward H, Desjardins A, et al: Respiratory health among retired grain elevator workers, *Am J Respir Crit Care Med* 150:59-65, 1994.

50. Zejda JE, Pahwa P, and Dosman J: Decline in spirometric variables in grain workers from start of employment: differential effect of duration of follow-up, *Br J Ind Med* 49:576-580, 1992.

51. Attfield MD and Ross DS: Radiological abnormalities in electric arc welders, *Br J Ind Med* 35:117-122, 1978.

52. Stanescu DC, Pilat L, Gavrilescu N, et al: Aspects of pulmonary mechanics in arc welders siderosis, *Br J Ind Med* 24:143-147, 1967.

53. Fawer RF, Ward Gardner A, and Oakes D: Absences attributed to respiratory diseases in welders, *Br J Ind Med* 39:149-152, 1982.

54. Gaensler EA, Carrington CB, Coutu RE, et al: Pathological, physiological, and radiological correlations in the pneumoconioses, *Ann NY Acad Sci* 200:574-607, 1972.

55. Schuler P, Cruz E, Guijon C, et al: Stannosis. Benign pneumoconiosis owing to inhalation of tin dust and fume, *Ind Med Surg* 27:432-435, 1958.

56. Dicken DY and Scott MJ: An investigation into health conditions in a tin smelter, *Med J Malaya* 16:1-13, 1961.

57. Cole CWD, Davies JVSA, Kipling MD, et al: Stannosis in hearth tinners, *Br J Ind Med* 21:235-241, 1964.

58. Crosbie WA. The respiratory health of carbon black workers, *Arch Environ Health* 41:346-353, 1986.

59. Gardiner K, Trethowan NW, Harrington JM, et al: Respiratory health effects of carbon black: a survey of European carbon black workers, *Br J Ind Med* 50:1082-1096, 1993.

60. Gardiner K, Trethowan NW, Harrington JM, et al: Occupational exposure to carbon monoxide and sulphur dioxide during the manufacture of carbon black, *Ann Occup Hyg* 36:363-372, 1992.

61. Oberdorster G, Ferin J, Finkelstein G, et al: Increased pulmonary toxicity of ultrafine particles? II. Lung lavage studies, *J Aerosol Sci* 21:384-387, 1990.

62. Jakab GJ: The toxicologic interactions resulting from inhalation of carbon black and acrolein on pulmonary antibacterial and antiviral defenses, *Toxicol Appl Pharmacol* 121:167-175, 1993.

63. Lee PS, Gorski RI, Hering WE, et al: Lung clearance of inhaled particles after exposure to carbon black generated from a resuspension system, *Environ Res* 43:364-373, 1987.

64. Strom KA, Johnson JT, and Chan TL: Retention and clearance of inhaled submicron carbon black particles, *J Toxicol Environ Health* 26:183-202, 1989.

65. Korn RJ, Dockery DW, Speizer FE, et al: Occupational exposures and chronic respiratory symptoms. A population-based study, *Am Rev Respir Dis* 136:298-304, 1987.

66. Bakke PS, Baste V, Hanoa R, et al: Prevalence of obstructive lung disease in a general population: relation to occupational title and exposure to some airborne agents, *Thorax* 46:863-870, 1991.

67. Krzyzanowski M and Kauffmann F: The relation of respiratory symptoms and ventilatory function to moderate occupational exposure in a general population, *Int J Epidemiol* 17:397-406, 1988.

68. Xu X, Christiani D, Dockery C, et al: Exposure–response relationships between occupational exposures and chronic respiratory illness: a community-based study, *Am Rev Respir Dis* 146:413-418, 1992.

69. Kauffmann F, Drouet D, Lellouch J, et al: Occupational exposure and 12-year spirometric changes among Paris area workers, *Br J Ind Med* 39:221-232, 1982.

70. Krzyzanowski M, Jedrychowski W, and Wysocki M: Occupational exposures and changes in pulmonary function over 13 years among residents of Cracow, *Br J Ind Med* 45.747-754, 1988.

71. Krzyzanowski M and Jedrychowski W: Occupational exposure and incidence of chronic respiratory symptoms among residents of Cracow followed for 13 years, *Int Arch Occup Environ Health* 62:311-317, 1990.

72. Kjuus H, Istad H, and Langard S: Emphysema and occupational exposure to industrial pollutants, *Scand J Work Environ Health* 7:290-297, 1981.

73. Jaakkola MS, Ernst P, Jaakkola JKJ, et al: Effect of cigarette smoking on evolution of ventilatory lung function in young adults: an eight year longitudinal study, *Thorax* 46:907-913, 1991.

74. Burrows B, Cline MG, Knudson RJ, et al: A descriptive analysis of the growth and decline of the FVC and FEV1, *Chest* 83:717-724, 1983.

75. Sherrill DL, Lebowitz MD, Knudson RJ, et al: Continuous longitudinal regression equations for pulmonary function measures, *Eur Respir J* 5:452-462, 1992.

76. van der Lende R, Kok T, Peset R, et al: Longterm exposure to air pollution and decline in VC and FEV1, *Chest* 80(suppl):23-26, 1981.

77. do Pico GA, Reddan W, Anderson S, et al: Acute effects of grain dust exposure during a work shift, *Am Rev Respir Dis* 128:399-404, 1983.

78. Kennedy SM, Enarson DA, Janssen RG, et al: Lung health consequences of reported accidental chlorine gas exposures among pulp-mill workers, *Am Rev Respir Dis* 143:74 79, 1991.

79. Morgan WKC: Editorial: on dust, disability, and death, *Am Rev Respir Dis* 134:639-641, 1986.

80. Becklake MR. Occupational pollution, *Chest* 96(suppl):372-378, 1989.

81. Morgan WKC and Seaton A: Forum. Coal mining, emphysema, and compensation revisited, *Br J Ind Med* 50:1051-1053, 1993.

82. Soutar C, Campbell S, Gurr D, et al: Important deficits of lung function in three modern colliery populations. Relations with dust exposure, *Am Rev Respir Dis* 147:797-803, 1993.

83. Higgins ITT: Chronic respiratory disease in mining communities, *Ann NY Acad Sci* 200:197-210, 1972.

84. Peto R, Speizer FE, Cochrane AL, et al: The relevance in adults of air-flow obstruction, but not of mucus hypersecretion, to mortality from chronic lung disease. Results from 20 years of prospective observation, *Am Rev Respir Dis* 128:491-500, 1983.

85. Annesi I and Kauffman F: Is respiratory mucus hypersecretion really an innocent disorder? A 22-year mortality survey of 1,061 working men, *Am Rev Respir Dis* 134:688-693, 1986.

Agents Causing Other Respiratory Disease

MARC B. SCHENKER

Agents not predominantly causing airway or interstitial disease are included in this section. In general, these agents may be classified as those causing cancer, infectious disease, or other respiratory disease. Chapters 34 and 35 cover agents that cause lung cancer and upper airway cancers, respectively. Because of the extensive data on cancers due to ionizing radiation and diesel exhaust and the other respiratory diseases associated with these exposures, these topics are briefly addressed in Chapter 34 and covered in detail in separate chapters. A general discussion of occupational infectious organisms is in Chapter 32, whereas additional information can be found in the chapters in Section VIII that address industries for which this is a particular hazard (agriculture, hospitals and laboratories). Other respiratory diseases are included in the chapter on acute gaseous exposures (Chapter 30), which may result in mucous membrane irritation to pulmonary edema, depending on the gas characteristics and exposure specifics. Finally, organic solvents (Chapter 28), and metals (Chapter 29) may cause a spectrum of responses in the lungs and systemically. The reader is referred to other sources for a more complete discussion of nonrespiratory effects.

Chapter 28

ORGANIC SOLVENTS

Marc B. Schenker
Jeffrey A. Jacobs

Solvents are substances widely used in many industrial processes and also found in many commercial household products. The potential for exposure thus includes occupational and nonoccupational settings. Early industries relied on a few organic solvents, but modern industries use hundreds of different agents. Organic solvents are used for extraction of fats and oils, degreasing, dry cleaning, and the manufacturing of a wide range of products, including paints, adhesives, plastics, textiles, electronics, and semiconductors.

Solvents have many properties that make them useful and ubiquitous in human activities, however, they have many potentially adverse health effects. These adverse effects primarily include central nervous system toxicity, dermatitis, and hematologic, liver, and renal damage. Adverse health effects have been documented in standard references and medical literature in the form of case reports, animal

toxicology studies, and epidemiologic research.[1-6] Patients exposed to solvents frequently complain of respiratory tract symptoms, which typically include chest tightness, shortness of breath, or cough after acute exposure. These symptoms are often ascribed to the chemical in question if the history of exposure is convincing, but there is surprisingly little research on acute respiratory illness following solvent exposure despite the general acknowledgement by physicians that this condition exists.[4,7] This chapter presents the physical properties and categories of solvents and the major uses and occupations of greatest exposure. The chapter critically reviews the existing data on solvent-induced respiratory effects. Studies reviewed are based on a Medline search from 1966 to the present for articles on solvents and pulmonary effects, a Toxline search for similar references, and searches for references on specific chemicals.

What is a solvent?

A solvent is defined as any substance capable of dissolving another substance to form a uniformly dispersed mixture or solution. Solvents may be classified as either polar or nonpolar. Water, a polar solvent, readily dissolves polar substances, and nonpolar solvents more readily dissolve nonpolar compounds, including most hydrocarbons. In industrial processes, water is often incapable of dissolving a large number of substances and therefore organic liquids are used. The expressions "industrial solvents" or organic solvents are conventionally applied to these organic liquids.[6,8]

In this chapter the authors have defined a solvent as a "simple organic substance that is a liquid at room temperature, and under standard atmospheric conditions is able to dissolve a wide range of organic compounds."[4] The authors have used this definition because it adequately reflects the nature of solvents typically used in industry. Whereas there are exceptions to this definition, for the majority of chemicals the definition is appropriate.

Categories of solvents

The organic solvents used in industry are generally arranged in groups according to their chemical classifications. The members of each group of solvents typically exhibit similarities in chemical and solvent characteristics. Solvents used in industry, however, typically include impurities that may affect their properties, and solvent mixtures are commonly used. For this study we have organized the chemicals into eight major groups based on their chemical structure. This classification follows the organization scheme generally used for organic solvents.[4,6,8]

The first category consists of open carbon structures termed *aliphatic hydrocarbons*. These compounds may be either saturated hydrocarbons (alkanes) or unsaturated hydrocarbons, which contain one or more double bonds (alkenes) or one or more triple bonds (alkynes). Those compounds containing four or fewer carbon atoms are gases at room temperature, whereas those with five or more carbon atoms are liquids. Compounds with more than 15 carbon atoms are solids.

Cyclic hydrocarbons are saturated or unsaturated ring compounds with three or more carbon atoms. These compounds behave in a manner similar to the aliphatics, but the compounds are less inert. Many of the cyclic hydrocarbons are metabolized to compounds with low toxicity. Petroleum solvents containing relatively high concentrations of these compounds include gasoline, diesel fuel, mineral spirits, and kerosene.

The *aromatic hydrocarbons* are compounds characterized by the presence of one or more benzene (6 carbon) rings. Aromatics include coal tar-derived hydrocarbon solvents. Benzene has been studied in particular, with exposure typically causing central nervous system depression and hepatic, renal, and bone marrow disorders.[9]

Halogenated hydrocarbons are both saturated and unsaturated hydrocarbon chains that have one or more substituted halogens (fluorine, chlorine, bromine, iodine, astatine). The halogens generally impart stability and nonflammability to the compounds. Examples of chlorinated hydrocarbons include carbon tetrachloride, trichloroethylene, and methyl chloroform. Compounds containing fluorine tend to be the least toxic of the group. The most frequently experienced toxic effects of the halogenated hydrocarbons are central nervous system toxicity and dermatitis. Respiratory toxicity has been most commonly studied with these agents.

Alcohols are hydrocarbon compounds that contain a substituted hydroxyl (-OH) group and glycols are dihydrated alcohols. Alcohols are widely used as industrial solvents. The most common adverse effect of this group, which includes ethanol, is central nervous system (CNS) depression. Central nervous system depression increases with increasing molecular weight, but volatility decreases as the molecular weight increases. Thus inhalation hazards decrease with the heavier compounds.

Ketones are compounds represented by the general formula R—CO—R, where the oxygen atom forms a double bond with a carbon atom. Because of their excellent solvent properties and low cost, ketones are used in large quantities in industry. Examples of ketones include acetone and methyl ethyl ketone, which are liquids at room temperature. Formaldehyde is a gas at room temperature, and becomes formalin when mixed with water. It is a respiratory irritant that has been shown to produce asthma in high concentrations.[10,11]

Esters are formed by the reaction of an acid and an alcohol, and the properties in part reflect the parent alcohol. The esters have irritating effects on the skin and respiratory tract and they also exhibit anesthetic properties. Examples include methyl- and ethyl-acetate.

Ethers are composed of two hydrocarbons joined by an oxygen atom. Ethers have a high solvent capability for fats, greases, and oils, and they are commonly used in industry for extractions.

Properties of solvents

Two important characteristics of organic solvents, and determinants of their toxicity, are volatility and lipophilicity. Most organic solvents are highly volatile, readily evaporating into the atmosphere, which enables them to enter the body through respiration. The solvents are also able to enter through the skin when the dermis is in direct contact with the liquid; this amount is negligible, however, when the skin is exposed only to air containing solvent vapors.[12]

Organic solvents are generally stable and do not react when in contact with solid materials such as metals and plastics. However, variations in temperature or pressure may cause chemical instability in some solvents; other solvents will react with foreign materials under certain conditions. For example, ultraviolet energy from welding may cause chlorinated hydrocarbons to break down into a variety of corrosive chemicals, including potent respiratory toxins such as phosgene (Fig. 28-1).[13]

Solvents with substantial vapor pressures at room temperature generally have detectable odors. These odors may be pleasant, as in the case of coal tar hydrocarbon solvents,

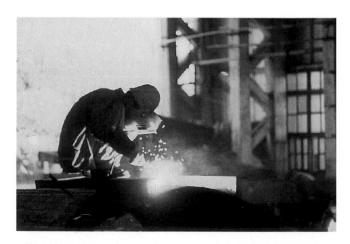

Fig. 28-1. Ultraviolet energy from welding may cause chlorinated hydrocarbons to break down into a variety of corrosive chemicals including potent respiratory toxins such as phosgene.

or objectionable. Absorption of solvents onto dust particles, or dissolution in mist droplets, may impart the solvent odor to the aerosol.

When inhaled, the solvent vapors must traverse the highly polar, watery mucous barrier lining, which is the respiratory tract epithelium. Because most solvents are nonpolar, the majority of inspired solvent reaches the alveoli where they can be absorbed into the bloodstream. These vapors are then absorbed through passive diffusion along their concentration gradient and are distributed among the various body tissues according to the substance's lipophilicity. A portion of the vapor is enzymatically transformed into metabolites with polar functions and is finally excreted into the urine after being conjugated with water-soluble molecules such as glucuronic acid and sulfate ions.[12]

Solvent-related toxicity of the central nervous system (CNS) and of the liver and kidney is believed to occur through the generation of highly reactive intermediates, which bind to cellular proteins, membranes, or DNA. For example, carbon tetrachloride has been shown to cause hepatic and renal damage through the formation of the trichloromethyl (CCl3•) radical, which binds directly to microsomal lipids and other cellular macromolecules, which in turn contribute to the breakdown of membrane structure and disrupt cell energy processes and protein synthesis.[14]

Solvents used in industry commonly contain chemical impurities that affect their properties. These impurities also may result in a wide spectrum of clinical responses and make the interpretation of health effects studies difficult.

SOURCES OF EXPOSURE

Solvents have a wide variety of applications in the home, the office, and in industry. They may be used for the selective dissolution of one substance from a mixture (i.e., chemical extraction), for reduction of the viscosity of a substance, or as a feed stock for the production of synthetics.[4] Solvents are used in paints, adhesives, glues, coatings, degreasing and cleaning agents, and in the production of dyes, polymers, plastics, textiles, printing inks, agricultural products, dry cleaning agents, and pharmaceuticals (Figs. 28-2 and 28-3).[3,5] Solvents also are commonly used in the manufacturing of numerous products such as electronics components and semiconductors (Fig. 28-4). The chemical industry estimates that over 18 billion kilograms of organic solvents were produced in the United States in 1992.[15]

The U.S. National Institute for Occupational Safety and Health's (NIOSH) National Occupational Hazard Survey estimated that approximately 10 million workers in the United States are potentially exposed to organic solvents.[3] Many workers are at risk for exposure because organic solvents are ubiquitous in modern society. For example, because of its many uses, benzene is widespread in the environment. A prominent source of atmospheric benzene in the United States was gasoline filling station pumps before the installation of vapor recapture devices on the delivery hoses.

In 1980, an estimated 37 million people in the United States were exposed to benzene vapors at self-service gasoline stations.[9]

Other solvents to which many workers are exposed include the halogenated hydrocarbons tetrachloroethylene (PCE), trichloroethylene (TCE), and carbon tetrachloride (CCl4). NIOSH estimated that 500,000 workers in the United States may be at risk of exposure to tetrachloroethylene; many of these workers are employed in the 20,000 U.S. drycleaning establishments.[16] About 40% to 45% of the estimated 227 million kilograms of PCE produced annually is used by drycleaners.[17]

In addition, NIOSH has estimated that 3.5 million workers in the United States are exposed to TCE, with the majority of high exposures ascribed to metal degreasing operations. Other potential exposures occur in the manufacturing process of disinfectants, pharmaceuticals, dyes, per-

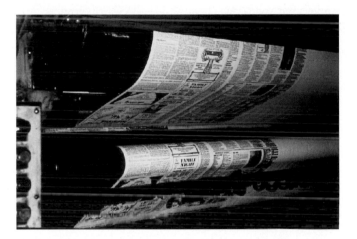

Fig. 28-2. Solvents are heavily used in the printing industry. In a cross-sectional study of printing-industry workers, printers had significantly more eye, airway, and neurological symptoms than controls.

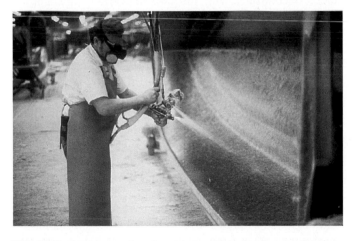

Fig. 28-3. A large study of styrene polymerization workers revealed acute mucous membrane irritation of the upper respiratory tract to be a common occurrence.

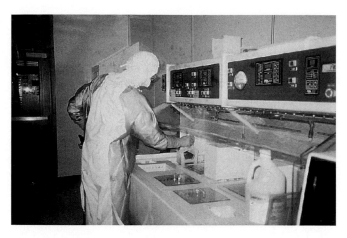

Fig. 28-4. Solvents are commonly used in the manufacturing of numerous products such as electronic components and semiconductors.

fumes, and soaps. Mechanics, oil processors, printers, resin makers, rubber cementers, shoe makers, textile and fabric cleaners, and varnish workers have an increased likelihood of TCE exposure.[18]

According to a survey from 1981 to 1983, approximately 60,000 workers in the United States were exposed to CCl_4, with workers employed in industries that manufacture CCl_4 at the greatest risk of exposure. This includes air transportation workers, automobile mechanics, hazardous waste workers, pesticide applicators, and steel mill and blast furnace operators. Phaseout of CCl_4 will decrease the number of exposures.[14]

The versatility of solvents results in their widespread use in the industrialized and industrializing countries of the world. Uses in industrializing countries range from simple processes, such as degreasing and cleaning, printing, and gluing, to more technical production processes, such as electronics and semiconductor manufacturing (see Chapter 43) (Fig. 28-4).[19] Exposures may be particularly high in small, uncontrolled work places in industrializing countries, such as shoe and paint manufacturing. Reliable estimates of populations exposed to solvents in the developing countries do not exist.

Respiratory and other health effects of solvent exposure depend on the actual dose received. Physiologically-based pharmacokinetic models have suggested that absorption occurs in the conducting airways and in the alveoli, with the majority of absorption taking place in the alveoli.[20] Determination of solvent dose is generally based on the toxicity of the agent, the vapor concentration in the workplace, and the duration of exposure, although more complex models have been developed that include factors such as workload (pulmonary ventilation), solubility coefficients, and the type and degree of biotransformation.[21] Whereas substantial exposure may occur from cutaneous contact, this is generally less hazardous than respiratory toxicity. Vapor concentrations may be measured by air sampling when this expertise

is available. Biologic markers exist for some solvents, although the markers (usually metabolites) may have a short biologic half-life and may have low specificity in epidemiologic studies with less controlled conditions.[22] Biologic markers may also fail to identify local toxicity of solvent exposure, such as may occur at the alveoli. The small fraction of some solvents eliminated via the urine is another limiting factor in their use as biomarkers.[23]

MECHANISM OF INJURY AND EFFECT
Animal studies

Studies of solvent exposure in animals have demonstrated effects in both the conducting and respiratory airways. When exposed to high levels of acetone over 48 hours, the lungs of guinea pigs showed congestion of interalveolar capillaries with extravasation of red blood cells into the alveolar spaces. As the concentration of the acetone vapor increased, pulmonary congestion became more marked.[24] Similarly, a small proportion of rats and all guinea pigs died of pulmonary edema after 40 hours of continuous exposure to styrene vapors.[25]

Whereas respiratory effects are most dramatic with high-level exposures, other studies have shown that pulmonary damage is not confined to high doses, but may occur at concentrations close to the Threshold Limit Values (TLVs). The upper respiratory tract mucosa of rats exposed to low concentrations of white spirit vapor (a mixture of paraffins, napthenes, and alkyl aromatic hydrocarbons) displayed an inflammatory cell infiltrate in the nasal cavity, trachea, and larynx.[26] In addition, the epithelial lining of the nasal cavity and trachea showed loss of cilia, basal cell hyperplasia, and squamous metaplasia. Low level exposures of rats to p-xylene have induced alterations in pulmonary microsomal membrane structures without histologic changes noted.[27] Following one day of exposure, conjugated diene levels were elevated, while total phospholipid levels were decreased, indicating lipid peroxidation of cell membranes. These changes returned to baseline levels several days after exposure had ceased. Decreased levels of pulmonary surfactant were also observed, an outcome noted in other inhalation studies using TCE, CCl_4, and gasoline vapors. The decrease in extracellular surfactant levels caused by CCl_4 is assumed to be caused by an inhibition of surfactant synthesis.

CLINICAL MANIFESTATIONS
Nonrespiratory health effects

The most commonly reported symptoms attributed to acute solvent exposure are CNS depression and narcosis. The nerve cells, because of their lipid content, are sensitive to organic solvents that have crossed the blood-brain barrier.[3] People exposed to acute high-level concentrations of solvents typically show signs of disorientation, euphoria, and confusion, which may progress to unconsciousness, convulsions, and death from respiratory or cardiovascular collapse if exposure is not terminated. In the majority of subjects, recovery from CNS effects is rapid and complete following removal from exposure.[2]

The liver is another common site of organic solvent toxicity, with exposure leading to fatty degeneration, cirrhosis (alcohol), and hepatic necrosis (halogenated hydrocarbons). Because the liver's cytochrome p-450 enzymes are a prominent site of biotransformation for these substances, bioactivated compounds, such as free radicals, can easily react with cellular macromolecules and membrane proteins to cause extensive cell damage and death.[25]

The kidney is also affected by certain solvents, with lower levels of exposure leading to glycosuria, aminoaciduria, and polyuria, and increasing levels causing cell necrosis.[25] The proximal convoluted tubules are sensitive to solvents, particularly the halogenated hydrocarbons, which exert their effects by a combination of direct cellular toxicity and ischemia secondary to vasoconstriction.[25]

The bone marrow is affected by exposure to certain solvents, most notably benzene. Chronic exposure to benzene, resulting in aplastic anemia, has been recognized since the beginning of the twentieth century. This pancytopenia is thought to occur in a dose-dependent fashion by action on a precursor stem cell in the bone marrow. Benzene's hematopoietic effects also include aplastic anemia and leukemia, with a latency period for leukemia of 5 to 15 years after first exposure.[9]

In addition to systemic effects, localized skin injury may be caused by the defatting action of organic solvents. The lipid-soluble skin layers become cracked, chapped, and vulnerable to other harmful irritants, sensitizers, and infections.[5]

Human chamber studies

While there have been several human chamber studies performed to ascertain the health effects of solvents, the majority of these studies have focused only upon CNS toxicity. Other studies have used chambers to measure both the dermal and respiratory absorption of certain solvents.[28,29]

One experimental study, measuring lung function after a 6-hour exposure to toluene, documented increased complaints of both nasal and ocular irritation at 100 ppm.[30] However, nasal mucus flow was unchanged and no pulmonary function decrements were noted by the investigators. At this level of exposure there were reported complaints of neurotoxicity (dizziness, headache, and feelings of intoxication) by the volunteers, consistent with CNS effects occurring at levels lower than respiratory effects.[30] Another study exposed subjects to n-butyl acetate with results indicating only minimal irritation of eyes, as measured by eye redness, and slight decrements in pulmonary function.[31]

A study of asthmatics exposed to volatile organic solvent vapors for 90 minutes at levels up to 25 mg/m^3 revealed a significant decrease in forced expiratory volume in 1 second (FEV1) among subjects during exposure to the highest concentration of solvent vapors[32]; however, this value was not significantly different from the value found after sham exposure and no change in airway hyperresponsiveness to histamine challenge was observed.

Volunteers exposed to several commercial aerosol sprays showed significant immediate falls in airflow that were consistent with small airway obstruction.[33] The sprays contained mixtures of solvents including freons, alcohols, and chlorinated hydrocarbons. Pulmonary function changes were generally reproduced by exposure to the pure solvents in the aerosols. The authors also observed workshift changes in pulmonary function in beauticians and suggested that the decline in function was caused by solvents in the hair sprays. Other investigators have not observed pulmonary function changes in beauticians[34,35]; the presence of respiratory effects from hair sprays remains controversial.

Controlled exposures to formaldehyde have generally failed to demonstrate airway obstruction or hyperresponsiveness. A double-blind, random exposure study of 15 asthmatics to 2 ppm formaldehyde for 40 minutes revealed no significant increase in airway obstruction or methacholine responsiveness as compared with air exposure.[36] Another study of nonsmoking asthmatics who were exposed to 3 ppm formaldehyde for 3 hours also failed to demonstrate any change in pulmonary function or nonspecific airway responsiveness.[37] When respirable carbon particles were included in the chamber exposure protocol, minimal changes in forced vital capacity (FVC) and FEV1 were noted (<5%), along with 10% decreases in forced expiratory flow FEF25-75%, which were thought to be indicative of increased airway tone. It was hypothesized that formaldehyde adsorbed on respirable particles was the cause of greater pulmonary effect than formaldehyde alone.[38] Similarly, exposure of 15 asthmatics to 0.85 mg/m^3 (0.69 ppm) formaldehyde for 90 minutes resulted in no change in pulmonary function or in bronchial reactivity as measured by histamine responsiveness.[39]

Case reports

Generally, solvents are not thought to cause asthma or to act as pulmonary sensitizers although solvents have been shown to cause mucous membrane irritation (Table 28-1). However, a variety of respiratory disease cases caused by solvent exposures have been described in the literature. Reported respiratory outcomes have included both restrictive and obstructive processes (including asthma).

Several cases and case series of asthma attributed to occupational formalin exposure have been reported in the literature.[10,40] Formaldehyde is recognized as a sensory irritant, and exposure causes a dose-related burning sensation of the eyes, nose, and throat.[41,42] Two of these cases demonstrated a positive response (drop in FEV1) after formalin provocation challenge. The duration of asthmatic response

Table 28-1. Case reports of occupational respiratory disease caused by solvent exposure

Reference	Industry	Number of subjects	Chemicals	Effects	Comments
Hendrick and Lane 1975 [40]	Hospital staff	2	Formalin	Asthma	1/2 cases with > 20% drop in FEV upon inhalation of 25% formalin
Porter 1975[43]	Hospital worker (neurology resident)	1	Formalin	Pulmonary edema	15 hours of exposure to formalin
Hendrick and Lane 1977[10]	Dialysis unit workers	28	Formalin	8/28 Workers with symptoms of wheeze/cough	FEV1% > 70% in all cases
Hellquist et al. 1983[48]	Spray painters	10	Toluene Isobutylacetate	10/10 Abnormal nasal histology	Effect not related to exposure
Schikler et al. 1984[46]	Solvent abusers	62	Toluene	Elevated residual volume	No difference between cases/controls in VC and FEV1
Bakinson and Jones 1985[49]	Industrial gassing cases	129	Methylene chloride Xylene Toluene Styrene	25% Respiratory symptoms	Heavy exposures
Bottomley et al. 1993[47]	Organic chemical manufacturing	1	Toluene Xylene	⇓ FVC 61% of predicted	Atypical scleroderma syndrome

FEV1, Forced expiratory volume in 1 second; *FVC,* forced vital capacity; *VC,* vital capacity.

appeared to be dependent on the extent of the exposure and the authors suggested that formalin acts as an agent that induces increased airway hyperresponsiveness. Another case involved an episode of pneumonitis occurring after 17 hours of exposure to formalin in a pathology lab.[43] Pulmonary function tests were decreased in this patient 2 days after exposure, but began to return to predicted levels 1 month after exposure.

Another case of pulmonary edema, attributed in this instance to PCE exposure, occurred when a laundry worker was overcome by vapors and lost consciousness.[44] The authors hypothesized that the mechanism of pulmonary edema in this case was the result of the direct toxic effects of the breakdown products of PCE, such as phosgene, CCl_4, and hydrochloric acid. The findings of diffuse alveolar damage with interstitial pulmonary fibrosis have also been produced in rats receiving intraperitoneal injections of CCl_4.[45]

Habitual solvent inhalers (glue sniffers) have been reported to develop pathologic microscopic abnormalities similar to those seen in experimental panlobular emphysema. The obstructive nature of this process was demonstrated with pulmonary function testing, which showed residual volumes of inhalers to be significantly higher than controls.[46] More recently, an unusual case of a sclerodermatous syndrome with restrictive lung disease has been re-

ported in a worker with a 32-year history of exposure to organic solvents.[47]

A Swedish analysis revealed symptoms and nasal biopsies in 10 male spray painters.[48] The source of the case series was unclear from the publication and some selection bias may have occurred. The subjects were exposed to solvents, primarily toluene and isobutylacetate, at concentrations well below the threshold limit values (TLVs). They also were exposed to low concentrations of dusts including chromium and zinc oxides. Three cases had nasal symptoms and four had cough, but the analysis did not control for smoking and symptoms were unrelated to exposure. Histologic examination of nasal mucosa revealed abnormalities in all 10 cases, with the average graded score of nasal pathology significantly higher than in a control population of 25 men.

A British study analyzed 118 industrial gassings caused by toluene, xylene, styrene, and methylene chloride between 1961 and 1980.[49] The cases had severe exposures with four deaths and 40% becoming unconscious. Coughing, dyspnea, and chest tightness were associated with exposure in about one-third of the solvent-exposed cases. The highest number of respiratory symptoms occurred following xylene exposure and the lowest number occurred after methylene chloride gassings.

Table 28-2. Population-based studies of worker complaints of respiratory symptoms secondary to solvent exposure

Reference	Study type	Industry	Number of subjects	Chemicals	Effects	Comments
Lebowitz 1977[54]	Cross-sectional	Multiple occupations	1195	Solvents	⇑ respiratory symptoms, abnormal lung function	Multiple comparisons, exposure based on JEM, not validated
Heederik et al. 1989[51]	Cross-sectional	Multiple occupations	828	Organic solvents	⇑ Respiratory symptoms, ⇑ CNSLD	Multiple comparisons, exposure based on JEM, not validated
Heederik et al. 1990[52]	Cohort	Residents	804	Organic solvents	No ⇑ CNSLD	Exposure based on JEM; low prevalence solvent exposure
Le Moual et al. 1994[55]	Cross-sectional	Residents	20,000	Organic solvents	⇓ FEV1	Exposure based on JEM; effect in men and women; dose response present
Post et al. 1994[53]	Cohort	Residents	804	Organic solvents	⇑ CNSLD incidence	Exposure based on JEM and full work history

CNSLD, Chronic nonspecific lung disease; *FEV1,* forced expiratory volume in 1 second; *JEM,* job exposure matrix.

EPIDEMIOLOGY

Despite frequent worker complaints of respiratory symptoms secondary to solvent exposure, few epidemiologic studies have been performed to investigate this phenomenon (Tables 28-2 to 28-4). The majority of studies concerning the health effects of solvents have concentrated on the central and peripheral nervous systems, and on liver and kidney toxicity.[50] In addition, the epidemiologic studies of respiratory effects commonly have been limited by inadequate exposure data.

Population-based studies. Population-based epidemiologic studies have suggested that occupational solvent exposure may be associated with respiratory symptoms, impaired pulmonary function, or respiratory disease (Table 28-2). In the longitudinal Zutphen study of middle-aged Dutch men, occupational exposures to solvents were classified by a job-exposure matrix.[51] Solvent exposure was independently associated with an increased prevalence of wheeze, dyspnea, cough, sputum, and physician diagnosis of chronic nonspecific lung disease (CNSLD) after controlling for age and cigarette smoking. The association was also present after excluding asthmatics from the population. A stronger association was observed for respiratory symptoms and CNSLD with paint exposure than with exposure to organic solvents, suggesting that the other respiratory toxins in paints (e.g., epoxy resins, isocyanates, and fillers) may be more potent causes of adverse respiratory effects among painters than the solvents. In a prospective followup of this cohort, solvent exposure was not associated with an increased incidence of CNSLD, although the analysis was limited by low statistical power.[52] An update of this population showed that the increased risk of CNSLD among solvent-exposed workers persisted after adjustment for dust exposure.[53]

Another population-based community study in Tucson, Arizona, showed an increased prevalence of respiratory symptoms and pulmonary function impairment associated with solvent exposure among men in age- and smoking-adjusted groups.[54] An analysis of the French Cooperative PAARC survey has also shown a significant association in men and women of occupational solvent exposure, derived from a job-exposure matrix, and age- and smoking-adjusted reduction in FEV1.[55]

These community-based studies are limited by their reliance on self-reported occupational history and the possibility of mixed or confounded exposures. There is also the possibility of chance associations caused by multiple comparisons (Type I errors). However, the studies provide important and consistent evidence that solvent exposures may cause respiratory symptoms or impaired pulmonary function in the general population, independent of the effects of cigarette smoking.

Occupational morbidity studies. Several occupational epidemiologic studies have reported mucous membrane irritation effects, but they are less conclusive in demonstrating respiratory symptoms or change in pulmonary function associated with solvent exposure (Table 28-3). In a cross-sectional study of workers in the printing industry, printers had significantly more eye, airway, and neurological symptoms than controls. These complaints consisted of eye, nose, and throat irritation and were reported to be more prevalent at work than after work. However, no differences in

Table 28-3. Occupational morbidity studies of solvent exposure

Reference	Study type	Industry	Number of subjects	Chemicals	Effects	Comments
Larson 1964[34]	Cross-sectional	College student	142 (analyzed) 219 (volunteered)	Hair spray	No significant effect on midexpiratory flow rate	Study only followed young women; may not have observed an effect of prolonged exposure to hair spray. Mixed exposure
Selikoff 1975[59]	Cross-sectional	Painters	485	Mixed	⇑ Respiratory symptoms, ⇓ pulmonary function	No control, mixed exposure
Lorimer et al. 1976[7]	Cohort	Styrene polymerization	494	Styrene	⇑ Lower respiratory symptoms, ⇑ prevalence of FEV1/FVC <75% for high exposure group	
Sabroe and Olsen 1979[62]	Cross-sectional	Cabinetry, carpentry	418	Lacquer	⇑ Respiratory symptoms current lacquers	Possible selection bias
Alexandersson et al. 1982[66]	Cross-sectional	Carpenters	47	Formaldehyde	⇓ FEV1, ⇑ closing volume % compared to control	
Baelum et al. 1982[56]	Cross-sectional	Printers	104	Solvents	⇑ Eye, CNS and airway symptoms; no difference in PFTs	
Jedrychowski 1982[63]	Cross-sectional	Styrene and methylmethacrylate plant	1137 683 Controls 454 Cases	Styrene methylmethacrylate	2× Risk of lung obstruction (<80% predicted FEV1)	Mixed exposures
Levine et al. 1984[69]	Cross-sectional	Morticians	90	Formaldehyde	No differences in PFT parameters	Oregon/Michigan male reference population
Burge et al. 1985[11]	Case series	Printers Plastics industry	15	Formaldehyde	3 Workers with occupational asthma; 6 workers developed immediate asthmatic reactions	Levels used in specific challenge test were higher than typical environmental levels
Johnson et al. 1985[79]	Cross-sectional	Iron/steel foundry	450	Phenolformaldehyde MDI Silica	⇑ Respiratory symptoms in foundry workers; ⇓ mean FEV1 and FEF25-75%	Exposure to other known respiratory toxins (MDI)

Reference	Study type	No.	Population	Exposure	Results	Comments
Alexandersson et al. 1987[57]	Cross-sectional	159	Car painters	Isocyanates (HDI)	⇑ Closing volume %; no difference in FEV1 or FVC	Mixed exposure
Alexandersson et al. 1988[70]	Cross-sectional	56	Woodworkers	Formaldehyde Butanol Ethanol Toluene Xylene	No ⇑ respiratory symptoms, small ⇓ FVC, ⇓ FEV1	Mixed exposure; low solvent exposure
Horvath et al. 1988[77]	Cross-sectional	363	Particle board	Formaldehyde Respirable dust	⇑ Eye, respiratory symptoms; ⇑ FEF25-75 in exposed	Confounding with respirable dust particles
Imbus and Tochilin 1988[80]	Cross-sectional	176	Strandboard production	Formaldehyde Wood dust	No change in PFT over workshift	Mean levels of formaldehyde <0.1 ppm; no control group
White and Baker 1988[60]	Cross-sectional	225	Construction	Mixed	⇑ Nasal irritation, cough; ⇓ FEV1 in smokers	Mixed exposure; possible selection bias
Alexandersson and Hedenstierna 1989[67]	Longitudinal cohort	67	Woodworkers	Formaldehyde Wood dust	⇑ FEF25-75% over workshift in exposed; ⇑ CV% in nonsmokers	PFT decrements were reversed after 4 weeks of nonexposure
Holness and Nethercott 1989[68]	Cross-sectional	122	Funeral service workers	Formaldehyde	⇑ Eye/nose irritation, chronic bronchitis and SOB in exposed; no difference in PFT between exposed and unexposed	Mean levels of formaldehyde = 0.36 ppm
Kilburn et al. 1989[71]	Cross-sectional	230	Histology technicians	Formaldehyde Xylene Toluene Chloroform	⇓ FVC, ⇓ FEV1	Mixed exposure; volunteers, possible selection bias; external control
Harving et al. 1990[39]	Human exposure chamber study	15	Asthmatics	Formaldehyde	No change in FEV1, specific airway resistance (SRAW)	Maximum chamber levels of formaldehyde of 0.85 mg/m³ may be too low to produce changes in lung parameters
Malaka and Kodama 1990[65]	Cross-sectional	186	Plywood	Formaldehyde Respirable dust	⇑ symptoms of cough, phlegm, asthma; ⇓ FEV1	Possible recall bias; asthma defined by questionnaire; possible effect of dust exposure

Continued.

Table 28-3. Occupational morbidity studies of solvent exposure—cont'd

Reference	Study type	Industry	Number of subjects	Chemicals	Effects	Comments
Nunn et al. 1990[78]	Cohort	Urea formaldehyde Resin	293	Formaldehyde Phenol	No difference in respiratory symptoms or PFT decrements between cohorts	
Angerer et al. 1991[64]	Cross-sectional	Floor laying workers	62	Toluene Petroleum Hydrocarbons Ethyl acetate Methanol Acetone	⇓ FEV1, PEF, FEC, cross-shift in floor-laying workers	Mixed exposure; limited size; smoking interaction
Khamgoankar and Fulare 1991[74]	Cross-sectional	Anatomy and pathology	148	Formaldehyde	⇑ Productive cough, breathlessness and chest tightness in exposed, ⇓ FVC, FEV1% in exposed	Only 1 measurement taken after 2 days of nonexposure; no cross-shift measurements
Chia et al. 1992[73]	Cross-sectional	Medical students	339	Formaldehyde	⇑ Eye, nose, throat irritation in exposed group; no differences between groups in FVC or FEV1	Mean level of formaldehyde = 0.74 ppm (personal sampling)
Ulfvarson et al. 1992[57]	Cross-sectional	House painters	9	Glycols Esthers Ethers	⇓ FVC, ⇓ FEV1, ⇓ PEF	Small sample size; possible confounding exposure (isothiazolinine)
Wieslander et al. 1993[61]	Cross-sectional	House painters	475	VOC	⇓ FEV1, FVC, abnormal methacholine in sample	No control for confounders; low VOC, high dust
	Nested case-control	Residents	563	Newly painted dwellings	⇑ Respiratory symptoms	No exposure assessment; no difference in clinical findings
Akbar-Khanzadeh et al. 1994[75]	Cross-sectional	Medical students	34	Formaldehyde	⇑ eye, nose, throat symptoms in exposed; ⇓ FVC in exposed	Small decrement in FVC (1.4%)

CNS, Central nervous system; *FEC,* forced expiratory capacity; *FEF,* forced expiratory flow; *FEV1,* forced expiratory volume in 1 second; *FVC,* forced vital capacity; *MDI,* metered-dose inhalers; *PEF,* peak expiratory flow; *PFT,* pulmonary function test; *SRAW,* specific airway resistance.

pulmonary function were found between the two groups (FVC, FEV1, and FEV1/FVC).[56]

A study of car spray painters exposed to solvents, dusts, and isocyanates documented frequent complaints of eye, nose, and throat irritation in the exposed group, but no differences in FVC or FEV1. Closing volume % was significantly higher in the exposed population than in the nonexposed group, suggestive of "small airways disease."[57] However, potential exposure to isocyanates, a known cause of pulmonary toxicity including airway obstruction, prevents any conclusion regarding the independent effects of solvent exposure in this population.

An investigation of respiratory function among house painters also revealed a significant amount of mucous membrane irritation.[58] In addition, FVC, FEV1, and peak expiratory flow (PEF) in painters reporting a nuisance from the paints were reduced as compared with painters not reporting a nuisance. This reduction, however, was not thought to be associated with solvent exposures, but to be caused by derivatives of isothiazolinone.

A cross-sectional study of 485 current and former members of a painters' union in the United States found a high prevalence of respiratory tract irritation symptoms among the painters, particularly those who worked with epoxy materials.[59] Conclusions from this study with respect to the effects of solvent exposure are limited by the selection of volunteers for the study, the absence of a dose-response or external control, and the potential exposure to other respiratory toxins such as epoxy.

Another study of 225 male painters' union members in the United States revealed increased nose irritation and frequent cough associated with increasing number of weeks worked with solvent paints in the previous year.[60] Years of painting were also associated with reduced FEV1, and there was evidence of an interaction with cigarette smoking in this analysis. The low response rate of volunteers in this study (37%), potential exposure to respiratory toxins other than organic solvents, and possible failure to control adequately for confounding exposures preclude conclusions regarding the effect of solvents on the outcomes studied.

A study of questionnaire responses, pulmonary function, and methacholine challenge tests in 236 house painters and 239 unexposed control workers showed a nonsignificant tendency toward more respiratory symptoms in the exposed painters.[61] In a subset analysis of the painters there was increased cross-shift decline in spirometry and increased bronchial hyperresponsiveness. However, exposure measurements for the painters revealed low concentrations of total volatile organic compound (VOC), formaldehyde, and ammonia and high total dust exposures. It is therefore difficult to relate the respiratory findings to solvent exposures, although the interaction of solvents with the dust exposure cannot be excluded.

A Danish study of respiratory symptoms among cabinet makers and carpenters showed an increased prevalence of cough, phlegm, and dyspnea on exertion among the lacquerers as compared with the nonlacquerers.[62] As with the other studies of painters, potential exposure to other respiratory toxins limits the interpretation with regard to organic solvents.

In a large study of styrene polymerization workers, the authors found acute mucous membrane irritation of the upper respiratory tract to be a common occurrence (18%).[7] Eleven percent of workers also complained of wheezing or chest tightness and 19% had complaints of chronic bronchitis. When stratified according to smoking status, six percent of the nonsmokers had symptoms consistent with chronic bronchitis. Pulmonary function testing of these workers disclosed that 35% had FEV1/FVC % less than 75%, with nonsmokers comprising about one third of the total. Because of these findings, the possibility was raised that styrene, in addition to its mucous membrane effects, may also cause clinically significant lower respiratory tract irritation; however, the absence of controls limits the interpretation of this study.

A Polish study of 454 workers from a styrene and methylmethacrylate plant compared respiratory symptoms and function to 683 control workers exposed to low concentrations of methanol, phenol, and carbon monoxide.[63] Exposures were high to both styrene (range 0.06 to 31.81 mg/m^3) and methyl methacrylate (range 0.20 to 382.2 mg/m^3). No difference in the prevalence of respiratory symptoms was observed, but lung obstruction (<80% predicted FEV1) was significantly more common in the exposed workers than in the controls (45% versus 18%). The effect of the styrene/methyl methacrylate exposure was greater than the effect of smoking on lung obstruction, and there was no observed interaction of smoking and the chemical exposure.

Floor laying workers subjected to inhalation exposure to adhesives containing toluene, petroleum hydrocarbons, ethyl acetate, methanol, and acetone also had increased respiratory complaints during work. Symptoms were reported by 23% of the subjects who complained of dyspnea and 50% who noted rhinitis. There was no difference in lung function between this group and the controls; however, when the groups were stratified by smoking status, all lung function values for smoking floor laying workers were observed to decrease over the workshift, whereas almost all values for the control group increased. This deterioration in lung function (particularly FEV1 during a work shift) of the smoking floor layer group was thought to be caused by the combination of cigarette smoke and solvent vapors.[64]

Several studies have also concentrated on inhalation exposure to formaldehyde and respiratory effects. In a cross-sectional study of 186 plywood workers, formaldehyde exposure (average 1.13 ppm) was associated with increased complaints of cough, phlegm production, asthma, chronic bronchitis, and colds. Across-shift decrements in pulmonary function were not observed for either the exposed or nonexposed population; however, baseline mean FEV1 (-0.04

L) and FEV1% (−2.2%) values for the exposed population were significantly lower than for the referent population after adjusting for respirable dust.[65]

A study of carpentry shop workers revealed an increased prevalence of upper airway irritation in the exposed workers as opposed to the nonexposed controls, with typical symptoms including eye and throat burning with chest tightness.[11] Pulmonary function testing was performed on each subject both before and after work, with significant decreases of both FEV1 ($\bar{x}$ = 0.17 L) and FEV1/FVC% ($\bar{x}$ = 2.4%) in the exposed population. These findings were consistent with a slight obstructive airway pattern.[66] These woodworkers were examined 5 years later and a reduction of 0.15 L in FEF25-75 and a 3% increase in closing volume percent (CV%) in the exposed population was noted to occur over a work shift. Significant decreases in FEV1% also were observed in the exposed population over the 5-year interval; however, these decreases returned to normal after 4 weeks of nonexposure and it was postulated that formaldehyde caused the transient pulmonary function impairment over the work shift, but that the impairment was reversible following cessation of exposure.[67]

Symptoms of chronic bronchitis, dyspnea, and eye, nose, and throat irritation were reported more frequently by 84 funeral service workers when compared in a cross-sectional study to 38 nonexposed controls. The mean formaldehyde level measured was 0.36 ppm (area sample) and the level ranged from 0.08 to 0.81 ppm. There were no significant differences in baseline pulmonary function testing between exposed and nonexposed participants.[68] A cross-sectional study of West Virginia morticians also led to the same conclusions, as the pulmonary function of the exposed population compared favorably with the reference population of unexposed Oregon and Michigan men.[69]

A study of spray painters exposed to acid-hardening lacquers containing formaldehyde demonstrated increased symptoms of eye, nose, and throat irritation following an 8-hour work shift at exposure levels slightly lower than the TLV (Fig. 28-5).[70] FEV1 was decreased by 0.21 L and FVC was decreased by 0.24 L in the exposed group as compared with the nonexposed control group; however, no change in lung function was observed postshift in the exposed workers.

A study of female histology technicians, who were chronically exposed to formaldehyde and xylene, revealed reductions in pulmonary function.[71] The major functional change in these workers was a steeper decrement in vital capacity and lung flows among subjects aged 20 to 60 years as compared with the control population. The contribution of a "healthy worker effect" in this cross-sectional investigation is unknown. Whereas the results of this study suggest that there may be a low-magnitude reduction of pulmonary function following chronic exposure to formaldehyde combined with other organic solvents, a prospective investigation of medical students exposed to formaldehyde

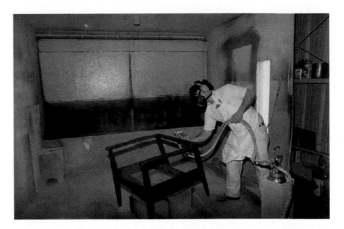

Fig. 28-5. Spray painters may be exposed to several solvents plus other respiratory toxins such as isocyanates.

at <1 ppm (peak exposures < 5 ppm) revealed eye and nose irritation associated with exposure but no evidence of increased airway obstruction, even among asthmatics.[72] A cross-sectional study of medical students in Singapore reported similar findings of increased mucous membrane irritant complaints after dissection without decrements in FVC or FEV1. Personal sampling for formaldehyde showed the mean concentration to be 0.74 ppm formaldehyde, with a peak value of 1.2 ppm.[73] However, another cross-sectional study of 148 anatomic and histopathologic workers showed pulmonary function decrements with increased complaints of productive cough, breathlessness, and chest tightness in the exposed group. The mean concentration of formaldehyde presented to the exposed group was 1.00 ppm. Forced vital capacity was reduced by 17% and the FEV1% was reduced by 23% as compared with the nonexposed population. These figures were not adjusted for smoking-status.[74] Small decrements in FVC (−1.4%), with an increase in FEV1% (1.6%) were observed in 34 nonsmoking medical students and instructors as compared with 14 participants who were not exposed to formaldehyde. The mean concentration of formaldehyde in the anatomy laboratory was 1.24 ppm (time-weighted average[TWA], breathing zone) found in 32 samples ranging from 0.07 to 2.94 ppm. Mean FEV1 decrement in the exposed subjects (−0.03%) was less than the loss seen in the nonexposed population. There were also increased complaints of eye, nose, and throat irritation in the exposed group.[75] A population-based study of children and adults exposed to 60-120 ppb formaldehyde indoors revealed higher prevalence rates of asthma and chronic bronchitis than among residents in homes with lower exposures.[76] The effects were greater in children than in adults and were greater with simultaneous environmental tobacco smoke exposure. Formaldehyde concentrations were measured with passive samplers in the homes.

Several studies have focused on respiratory exposure to formaldehyde in industry, but many are confounded by exposures to other respiratory toxins. A cross-sectional study compared 109 particleboard workers to 254 food-processing workers at nearby facilities. The mean level of formaldehyde (personal sampling) found in the particleboard facility was 0.62 ppm as compared with 0.05 ppm in the food-processing plants. The study showed increased complaints of cough, phlegm production, and burning of eyes, nose, and throat in the exposed population. Baseline pulmonary function testing failed to disclose any differences between the two groups, but statistically significant decrements in FEV1% and FEF25-75 across a work shift were observed in the exposed group that were not evident in the reference population. These effects may be confounded by the presence of respirable particles of wood dust, which may combine with formaldehyde and assist in transporting the highly polar compound (formaldehyde) lower into the respiratory tree, where it can exert influence.[77]

A 6-year cohort study of 164 workers exposed to formaldehyde failed to disclose any differences in respiratory symptoms or pulmonary function decrements when compared to other plant manufacturing workers not exposed to formaldehyde. Exposure to formaldehyde was assessed using area and personal monitoring samples and was assigned in a matrix from low (0.1 to 0.5 ppm) to high (above 2.0 ppm) according to job description.[78]

Another industrial study assessing formaldehyde effects compared 78 workers from an iron and steel foundry with 372 railway yard workers, who were not significantly exposed to contaminants at work. There was a statistically significant increase in complaints of sputum production, breathlessness, and chest tightness among the smoking foundry workers as compared with smokers among the unexposed participants. Mean FEV1, FVC, and FEF25-75 were also lower for foundry workers than for controls, after adjusting for age, height, and smoking status. It is difficult, however, to attribute this decrease to formaldehyde because of other respiratory exposures in the foundry cohort, including diphenyl methane diisocyanate (MDI).[79]

A cross-sectional study of 176 workers in the phenol-formaldehyde-resin coated wood industry revealed no association of cross-shift pulmonary function and formaldehyde exposure, but formaldehyde concentrations were low ($\leq$ 0.05 ppm) and the effects of confounding exposures (wood dust) or selection bias could not be excluded.[80]

In summary, the epidemiologic studies of formaldehyde-exposed subjects yield evidence of eye and nose irritation consistent with controlled chamber exposures. Asthma has been observed following high-level occupational exposures to formaldehyde (>5 ppm), but has not been seen with occupational or controlled chamber exposures to lower concentrations. This suggests that high concentrations of the water soluble formaldehyde are necessary to penetrate deeply into the lungs, which is consistent with the absence of increased airway hyperresponsiveness following chamber exposures to <5 ppm. Chronic effects on pulmonary function that are observed following long-term, low-level

exposure to formaldehyde may be caused by mixed exposures, and require further investigation.

Occupational mortality studies. A Swedish mortality study of over 50,000 members of the Painters' Union showed increased mortality from chronic obstructive pulmonary disease (COPD) (Table 28-4).[81] Standard mortality ratios (SMRs) for the painters ranged from 141 to 162 with an increase associated with increasing years since entry into the Union. Some of this increase may have been caused by cigarette smoking, although the lung cancer mortality did not show the same elevation (SMRs 124 to 132). An analysis of occupational mortality in California revealed increased mortality from lung cancer among painters and plasterers (adjusted SMR = 136, 95% confidence interval [CI] 115 to 160), but no increase in COPD mortality in this group (adjusted SMR = 94, 95% CI 62 to 136).[82] A Swedish asthma mortality study also failed to show increased smoking-adjusted asthma mortality among painters (SMR = 104, 95% CI 58 to 150).[83] Inferences regarding solvent effects in studies of painters must be made with caution because of exposure to other known respiratory toxins such as isocyanates and particles.

A retrospective cohort mortality study of over 15,000 workers in the plastics industry, who were exposed to styrene, documented a slightly elevated SMR for emphysema of 118 for the cohort as compared with the U.S. reference population, but there was no dose-response effect on emphysema mortality because low TWA exposures had a larger SMR than higher exposures (166 versus 57). Other exposures or lifestyle factors may also have been responsible for the increased number of deaths caused by emphysema.[84]

Several studies have outlined mortality rates in workers exposed to formaldehyde. Mortality studies in formaldehyde-using and formaldehyde-producing industries have generally not shown elevated SMRs for noncancerous respiratory causes, despite higher exposures to formaldehyde in the workplace.

Among 1132 white, male, New York state embalmers, the proportional mortality rate (PMR) was lower (PMR = 77) for deaths caused by respiratory system ailments (excluding cancer) than in the U.S. male reference population.[85] A British mortality study of 7680 workers in the plastics industry revealed an SMR of 102 (95% CI, 90 to 117) for diseases of the respiratory system. Exposure was not measured, but was estimated on the basis of job classification. Approximately one-third of the cohort was estimated to have "high" formaldehyde exposure (>2 ppm) on a regular basis.[86]

A retrospective cohort mortality study of more than 26,000 American formaldehyde-industry workers failed to demonstrate an elevated SMR for emphysema in the cohort (SMR = 94) when compared to the U.S. reference population. The highest SMR was observed in the individuals exposed to less than 0.5 ppm formaldehyde per year

Table 28-4. Occupational mortality studies of respiratory disease caused by solvent exposure

Reference	Study type	Industry	Number of subjects	Chemicals	Effects	Comments
Engholm and Englund 1982[81]	Retrospective cohort	Painters	30,580	Various paint chemicals	⇑ COPD mortality; SMR = 141-162	Swedish reference population
Walrath and Fraumeni 1983[85]	Mortality cohort	White male embalmers	1132	Formaldehyde	PMR respiratory system deaths = 77	U.S. reference population
Acheson et al. 1984[86]	Mortality cohort	Chemical and plastics	7680	Formaldehyde	SMR = 102 (95% CI = 90-117) for disease of respiratory system	British reference population
Singleton and Beaumont 1989[82]	Mortality study	Painters Plasterers	147	Unknown	No ⇑ mortality from COPD; ⇑ mortality from lung cancer; adjusted SMR = 136	Unknown exposures
Stewart et al. 1990[88]	Cohort	Producers and users of formaldehyde	26,561	Formaldehyde	Workers <1 year, SMR emphysema = 174; SMR asthma = 214. Workers > 1 year, SMR emphysema = 90; SMR asthma = 23	No dose effect
Wong 1990[84]	Retrospective cohort	Reinforced plastic	15,908	Styrene	SMR emphysema = 118	U.S. reference population; multiple exposures
Torén et al. 1991[83]	Mortality study	Painters	20 (deaths)	Unknown	No ⇑ in smoking-adjusted asthma mortality	Unknown exposures
Blair et al. 1986[87]	Retrospective cohort	Producers and users of formaldehyde	26,561	Formaldehyde	Workers <1 year, SMR emphysema = 94; SMR unexposed = 98. Workers > 1 year, SMR emphysema = 133 in group exposed to <0.5 ppm formaldehyde/year	U.S. reference population; no dose effect
Dosemeci et al. 1991[89]	Retrospective cohort	Producers and users of formaldehyde	14,861	Phenol formaldehyde	Emphysema rates for white men; exposed = 0.9, unexposed = 1.5	U.S. reference population

CI, Confidence interval; *COPD*, chronic obstructive pulmonary disease; *PMR*, proportional mortality ratio; *SMR*, standardized mortality ratio.

(SMR =133), with higher exposures demonstrating less than expected mortality (SMR = 92).[87] The same cohort was also analyzed in terms of duration of employment, with workers exposed less than one year having higher mortality rates for emphysema (SMR = 174) and asthma (SMR = 214) than those individuals who worked more than one year (SMRs = 90 and 23, respectively). It was postulated that the elevated rates for the short-term workers were likely caused by lifestyle risk factors rather than by exposure to formaldehyde.[88] Finally, a segment of this cohort who were engaged in the production of phenol was also examined. The SMR for emphysema was not found to be elevated, with (phenol- and formaldehyde-) exposed individuals having a rate of 0.9 for developing emphysema (95% CI, 0.6 to 1.3), as compared with the nonexposed population (odds ratio [OR] = 1.5, 95% CI, 0.9 to 2.4).[89]

Several limitations must be recognized when considering the mortality studies discussed previously. These include possible survivor bias or healthy worker effect, inaccuracy of death certificates for respiratory disease mortality, and possible confounding exposures. Nevertheless, the data are consistent in not showing excess respiratory disease mortality associated with occupational exposure to formaldehyde.

Indoor environments. Some studies of indoor environments have indicated an association of solvent exposure and respiratory symptoms, but potentially confounding exposures cloud the interpretation of these investigations. A comprehensive review of this subject is beyond the scope of this chapter. In general, organic solvents in the home environment occur at low concentrations and occur substantially below concentrations in the industrial environment.[90] A Swedish case-control study of 44 asthmatics and 45 random controls revealed significantly higher concentrations of total volatile organic compounds (VOCs), low boiling point VOCs, toluene, and xylene in the homes of the asthmatics.[91] No differences were present for respirable dust, relative air humidity, or room temperature. The concentration of low boiling point VOCs was correlated with the presence of bacteria in the bedroom air, and was related to 1-octen-3-ol, a microbial volatile emitted from molds and bacteria. The authors hypothesized that microbial growth was the etiologic factor that was possibly mediated via VOCs.

In another preliminary report, symptoms were analyzed in a nested case-control study of 3600 subjects living in Uppsala, Sweden.[61] There were 563 individuals selected out of the study population of 3600. Occupants living in newly painted dwellings reported significantly higher prevalences of airway irritation and awakening because of chest tightness than did occupants of buildings not recently painted. Subjects working in newly painted buildings also reported more wheezing and attacks of dyspnea at rest than did controls. A U.S. study of residential formaldehyde exposure in homes insulated with urea formaldehyde foam insulation compared 29 exposed children and 58 matched control children. No differences in respiratory symptoms or function were observed.[92]

These studies raise the possibility that VOCs emitted from water-based paints induce nasal irritation and airway symptoms, but additional studies measuring exposure and excluding potential confounding factors are needed. Caution is necessary in interpreting the results of these studies because of possible selection factors in the study populations.

CONCLUSIONS

The data on acute respiratory effects secondary to solvent exposure are limited. There is reasonable evidence of a dose-dependent relationship between exposure and mucous membrane irritation and this outcome is consistent with animal toxicologic studies. Population-based epidemiological studies using job-exposure matrices have shown an independent association of solvent exposure and both respiratory symptoms and reduced pulmonary function, confirmation of these findings is necessary in hypothesis-testing studies. There have been only a few studies of pulmonary function and solvent exposure and these also have been limited by mixed exposures, potential response biases, and absent exposure data. Mortality studies have generally not shown an association of respiratory disease mortality and solvent-exposed occupations (e.g., painting), but there are serious limitations in mortality studies to investigating nonmalignant disease outcomes and the absence of an observed association in these data does not exclude solvent-associated morbidity or mortality. Similar considerations exist for the studies of mortality among formaldehyde-exposed workers.

The most consistent clinical and toxicologic data for solvent-mediated respiratory effects are collected following acute massive exposures and from acute and chronic exposure to a few selected agents, such as formaldehyde. A possible interaction of solvent exposure and cigarette smoking has been suggested by some investigators, but has not been observed in all studies. In general, studies of pulmonary function impairment following solvent exposure are limited and inconsistent. Animal and human chamber studies suggest that solvent-mediated toxicity of the CNS occurs at lower concentrations than respiratory effects, but respiratory outcomes have rarely been studied along with CNS outcomes and quantitative comparisons of both outcomes are necessary. Studies of the potential mechanisms of solvent-mediated respiratory effects have been limited and the effects may be related to a wide range of mechanisms. Solvent-mediated respiratory toxicity is biologically plausible and further research is needed to characterize the specific chemical and individual factors associated with an increased risk, the mechanisms of effect, and possible interactions with other respiratory toxins.

ACKNOWLEDGMENTS

This work was supported by NIOSH Cooperative Agreement #U07/CCU906162-05 and NIEHS Center #ES05707-04.

REFERENCES

1. Lundberg I, Hogstedt C, Lidén, and Nise G: Organic solvents and related compounds. In Rosenstock L and Cullen MR, editors: *Textbook of clinical occupational and environmental medicine,* pp 766-784, Philadelphia, 1994, WB Saunders.
2. Andrews LS and Snyder R: Toxic effects of solvents and vapors. In Amdur MO, editor, *Casarett and Doull's toxicology: the basic science of poison,* New York, 1991, Pergamon Press.
3. National Institute of Occupational Safety and Health: *NIOSH current intelligence bulletin 48: organic solvent neurotoxicity,* Cincinnati, 1987 U.S. Department of Health and Human Services, Public Health Service, Centers for Disease Control, National Institute of Occupational Safety and Health, DHHS (NIOSH) Pub No 87-104.
4. Gerr F and Letz R: Solvents. In Rom WN, editor: *Environmental and occupational medicine,* Boston, 1992, Little, Brown.
5. U.S. Congress Office of Technology Assessment: *Neurotoxicity: identifying and controlling poisons of the nervous system: new developments in neuroscience,* pp 296-311, Washington, D.C., 1990, Congress of the U.S., Office of Technology Assessment.
6. International Labor Office: Industrial solvents. In Parmeggiani L, editor: *Encyclopedia of occupational health and safety,* pp 2085-2088, Geneva, Switzerland, 1994; International Labor Office.
7. Lorimer WV, Lilis R, Nicholson WJ, et al: Clinical findings of styrene workers: initial findings, *Environ Health Perspect* 17:171-181, 1976.
8. Alliance of American Insurers: Handbook of Organic Industrial Solvents, 6th ed. Schaumburg, IL, 1987, Alliance of American Insurers.
9. Snyder R, Witz G, and Goldstein BD: The toxicology of benzene, *Environ Health Perspect* 100:293-306, 1993.
10. Hendrick DJ and Lane DJ: Occupational formalin asthma, *Br J Ind Med* 34:11-18, 1977.
11. Burge PS, Harries MG, Lam WK, O'Brien IM, and Patchett PA: Occupational asthma due to formaldehyde, *Thorax* 40:255-260, 1985.
12. Sato A and Nakajima T: Pharmacokinetics of organic solvent vapors in relation to their toxicity, *Scand J Environ Health* 13:81-93, 1987.
13. Andersson HF, Dahlberg JA, Wetterström R: Phosgene formation during welding in air contaminated with perchloroethylene, *Ann Occup Hyg* 18:129-132, 1975.
14. Agency for Toxic Substances and Disease Registry: *Case studies in environmental medicine: carbon tetrachloride toxicity.* Atlanta, 1992, U.S. Department of Health and Human Services, Public Health Service.
15. Chemical production resumed growth in 1992 (production by the U.S. Chemical Industry), *Chem Eng News* 71(26):40-47, 1993.
16. Agency for Toxic Substances and Disease Registry: *Case studies in environmental medicine: tetrachloroethylene toxicity,* Atlanta, 1990, U.S. Department of Health and Human Services, Public Health Service.
17. Cleaner dry cleaners (search to replace dangerous solvents used by dry cleaners), *Time* 140:26, 1992.
18. Agency for Toxic Substances and Disease Registry: *Case studies in environmental medicine: trichloroethylene toxicity.* Atlanta, 1990, U.S. Department of Health and Human Services, Public Health Service.
19. Schenker M: Occupational lung diseases in the industrializing and industrialized world due to modern industries and modern pollutants, *Tubercle and Lung Disease* 73:27-32, 1992.
20. Johanson G: Modelling of respiratory exchange of polar solvents, *Ann Occup Hyg* 35:323-339, 1991.
21. Pezzagno G, Ghittori S and Imbriani M: Respiratory measurements of occupational exposure to industrial solvents, *Giornale Italiano di Medicina del Lavoro* 7:17-34, 1985.
22. Pezzagno G, Imbriani M, Ghittori S, and Capodaglio E: Urinary concentration, environmental concentration, and respiratory uptake of some solvents: effect of the work load, *Am Ind Hyg Assoc J* 49:546-552, 1988.
23. Wigaeus E, Holm S, and Astrand I: Exposure to acetone: uptake and elimination in man, *Scand J Work Environ Health* 7:84-94, 1981.
24. Specht H, Miller JW, and Valner PJ: *Acute response of guinea pigs to the inhalation of dimethyl ketone (acetone) vapor in air.* Division of Industrial Hygiene, 1939, National Institutes of Health.
25. Lu FC, editor: *Basic toxicology: fundamentals, target organs, and risk assessment,* Washington, D.C., 1991, Hemisphere Publishing.
26. Riley AJ, Collings AJ, Browne NA, and Grasso P: Response of the upper respiratory tract of the rat to white spirit vapour, *Toxicol Lett* 22:125-131, 1984.
27. Silverman DM and Schatz RA: Pulmonary microsomal alterations following short-term low level inhalation of *p*-xylene in rats, *Toxicology* 65:271-281, 1991.
28. Johanson G and Boman A: Percutaneous absorption of 2-butoxy-ethanol vapour in human subjects, *Br J Ind Med* 48:788-792, 1991.
29. Stewart RD, Dodd HC, Baretta ED, and Schaffer AW: Human exposure to styrene, *Arch Environ Health* 16:656-662, 1968.
30. Andersen E, Lundqvist GR, Molhave L, et al: Human response to controlled levels of toluene in six-hour exposures, *Scand J Work Environ Health* 9:405-418, 1983.
31. Iregren A, Lof A, Toomingas A, and Wang Z: Irritation effects from experimental exposure to n-butyl acetate, *Am J Ind Med* 24:727-742, 1993.
32. Harving H, Dahl R, and Molhave L: Lung function and bronchial reactivity in asthmatics during exposure to volatile organic compounds, *Am Rev Respir Dis* 143:751-754, 1991.
33. Skuric Z, Zuskin E, and Valic F: Effects of aerosols in common use on the ventilatory capacity of the lung, *Int Arch Arbeitsmed* 34:137-149, 1975.
34. Larson RK: A study of mid-expiratory flow rate in users of hair spray, *Am Rev Resp Dis* 90:786-788, 1964.
35. Sharma OP and Williams MH: Thesaurosis—pulmonary function studies in beauticians, *Arch Environ Health* 13:616-618, 1966.
36. Witek Jr T, Schachter EN, Tosun T, Beck GJ, and Leaderer BP: An evaluation of respiratory effects following exposure to 2.0 ppm formaldehyde in asthmatics: lung function, symptoms, and airway reactivity, *Arch Environ Health* 42:230-237, 1987.
37. Sauder LR, Green DJ, Chatham MD, and Kulle TJ: Acute pulmonary response of asthmatics to 3.0 ppm formaldehyde, *Toxicol Ind Health* 3:569-578, 1987.
38. Green DJ, Bascom R, Healey EM, et al: *Acute pulmonary response in healthy, nonsmoking adults to inhalation of formaldehyde, and carbon, J Toxicol Environ Health* 28:261-275, 1989.
39. Harving H, Korsgaard J, Pedersen OF, Molhave L, and Dahl R: Pulmonary function and bronchial reactivity in asthmatics during low-level formaldehyde exposure, *Lung* 168:15-21, 1990.
40. Hendrick DJ and Lane DJ: Formalin asthma in hospital staff, *Br Med J* 1:607-608, 1975.
41. Kane LE and Alarie Y: Evaluation of sensory irritation from acrolein-formaldehyde mixtures, *Am Ind Hyg Assoc J* 39:270-274, 1978.
42. Committee on Aldehydes, Board on Toxicology and Environmental Health Hazards, Assembly of Life Sciences, National Research Council: *Formaldehyde and other aldehydes,* Washington, D.C., 1981, National Academy Press.
43. Porter JAH: Acute respiratory distress following formalin inhalation, *Lancet* 603-604, 1975.
44. Patel R, Janakiraman N, and Towne WD: Pulmonary edema due to tetrachloroetylene, *Environ Health Perspect* 21:247-249, 1977.
45. Anttinen H, Oikarinen A, Puistola U, Paakko P, and Ryhanen L: Prevention by zinc of rat lung collagen accumulation in carbon tetrachloride injury, *Am Rev Respir Dis* 132:536-540, 1985.

46. Schikler KN, Lane EE, Seitz K, and Collins WM: Solvent abuse associated pulmonary abnormalities, *Adv Alcohol Substance Abuse* 3:75-81, 1984.

47. Bottomley WW, Sheehan-Dare RA, Hughes P, and Cunliffe WJ: A sclerodermatous syndrome with unusual features following prolonged occupational exposure to organic solvents, *Br J Dermatol* 128:203-206, 1993.

48. Hellquist H, Irander K, Edling C, and Ödkvist LM: Nasal symptoms and histopathology in a group of spray-painters, *Acta Otolaryngol* 96:495-500, 1983.

49. Bakinson MA and Jones RD: Gassings due to methylene chloride, xylene, toluene, and styrene reported to Her Majesty's Factory Inspectorate 1961-1980, *Br J Ind Med* 42:184-190, 1985.

50. Englund A, Ringen K, and Mehlman MA, editors: *Advances in modern environmental toxicology, vol II: occupational health hazards of solvents,* Princeton, NJ, 1982, Princeton Scientific Publishing.

51. Heederik D, Pouwels H, Kromhout H, and Kromhout D: Chronic nonspecific lung disease and occupational exposures estimated by means of a job exposure matrix: the Zutphen study, *Int J Epidemiol* 18:382-389, 1989.

52. Heederik D, Kromhout H, Burema J, Biersteker K, and Kromhout D: Occupational exposure and 25-year incidence rate of non-specific lung disease: the Zutphen study, *Int J Epidemiol* 19:945-952, 1990.

53. Post WK, Heederik D, Kromhout H, and Kromhout D: Occupational exposures estimated by population specific job exposure matrix and 25 year incidence rate of chornic nonspecific lung disease (CNSLD): the Zutphen study, *Eur Resp J* 7:1048-1055, 1994.

54. Lebowitz MD: Occupational exposures in relation to symptomatology and lung function in a community population, *Environ Res* 14:59-67, 1977.

55. Le Moual N, Orlowski E, Schenker MB, et al: Occupational exposures estimated by means of job exposure matrices in relation to lung function in the PAARC survey. Abstract presented at Tenth International Symposium Epidemiology in Occupational Health, September 1994, Como, Italy.

56. Baelum J, Andersen I, and Molhave L: Acute and subacute symptoms among workers in the printing industry, *Br J Ind Med* 39:70-74, 1982.

57. Alexandersson R, Hedenstierna G, and Kolmodin-Hedman B: Exposure, lung function, and symptoms in car painters exposed to hexamethyldiisocyanate and biuret modified hexamethyldiisocyanate, *Arch Environ Health* 42:367-373, 1987.

58. Ulfvarson U, Alexandersson R, Dahlzvist M, et al: Temporary health effects from exposure to water-borne paints, *Scand J Work Environ Health* 18:376-387, 1992.

59. Selikoff IJ: *Investigations of health hazards in the painting trades,* Report to the National Institute for Occupational Safety and Health, contract CDC 99-74-91, New York, 1975 Environmental Sciences Laboratory, Mount Sinai School of Medicine.

60. White MC and Baker EL: Measurements of respiratory illness among construction painters, *Br J Ind Med* 45:523-531, 1988.

61. Wieslander G, Norbäck D, Edling C, et al: Emission of volatile organic compunds (VOC) from water based paints—a contributing cause of respiratory symptoms and bronchial hyperresponsiveness? In *Proceedings of the international conference on volatile organic compounds in the environment,* pp 447-453, London, 1993, Lonsdale Press.

62. Sabroe S and Olsen J: Health complaints and work conditions among lacquerers in the Danish furniture industry, *Scan J Soc Med* 7:97-104, 1979.

63. Jedrychowski W: Styrene and methyl methacrylate in the industrial environment as a risk factor of chronic obstructive lung disease, *Int Arch Occup Environ Health* 51:151-157, 1982.

64. Angerer P, Marstaller H, Bahemann-Hoffmeister A, et al: Alterations in lung function due to mixtures of organic solvents used in floor laying, *Int Arch Occup Environ Health* 63:43-50, 1991.

65. Malaka T and Kodama AM: Respiratory health of plywood workers occupationally exposed to formaldehyde, *Arch Environ Health* 45:288-294, 1990.

66. Alexandersson R, Hendenstierna G, and Kolmodin-Hedman B: Exposure to formaldehyde: effects on pulmonary function, *Arch Environ Health* 37:279-284, 1982.

67. Alexanderson R and Hedenstierna G: Pulmonary function in wood workers exposed to formaldehyde: a prospective study, *Arch Environ Health* 44:5-11, 1989.

68. Holness DL and Nethercott JR: Health status of funeral service workers exposed to formaldehyde, *Arch Environ Health* 44:22-28, 1989.

69. Levine RJ, DalCorso RD, Blunden PB, and Battigelli MC: The effect of occupational exposure on the respiratory health of West Virginia morticians, *J Occup Med* 26:91-98, 1984.

70. Alexandersson R, Hedenstierna G, and Kolmodin-Hedman B: Respiratory hazards associated with exposure to formaldehyde and solvents in acid-curing paints, *Arch Environ Health* 43:222-227, 1988.

71. Kilburn KH, Warshaw R, and Thornton JC: Pulmonary function in histology technicians compared with women from Michigan: effects of chronic low dose formaldehyde in a national sample of women, *Br J Ind Med* 46:468-472, 1989.

72. Uba G, Pachorek D, Bernstein J, et al: Prospective study of respiratory effects of formaldehyde among healthy and asthmatic medical students, *Am J Ind Med* 15:91-101, 1989.

73. Chia SE, Ong CN, Foo SC, and Lee HP: Medical students' exposure to formaldehyde in a gross anatomy dissection laboratory, *J Am Coll Health* 41:115-119, 1992.

74. Khamgaonkar MB and Fulare MB: Pulmonary effects of formaldehyde exposure, *Indian J Chest Dis Allied Sci* 33:9-13, 1991.

75. Akbar-Khanzadeh F, Vaquerano MU, Akbar-Khanzadeh M, and Bisesi MS: Formaldehyde exposure, acute pulmonary response, and exposure control options in a gross anatomy laboratory, *Am J Ind Med* 26:61-75, 1994.

76. Krzyzanowski M, Quackenboss JJ, and Lebowitz MD: Chronic respiratory effects of indoor formaldehyde exposure, *Environ Res* 52:117-125, 1990.

77. Horvath EP, Anderson H, Pierce WE, Hanrahan L, and Wendlick JD: Effects of formaldehyde on the mucous membranes and lungs, *JAMA* 259:701-707, 1988.

78. Nunn AJ, Craigen AA, Venables KM, and Newman-Taylor AJ: Six year follow up of lung function in men occupationally exposed to formaldehyde, *Br J Ind Med* 47:747-752, 1990.

79. Johnson AJ, Chan-Yeung M, MacLean L, et al: Respiratory abnormalities among workers in an iron and steel foundry, *Br J Ind Med* 42:94-100, 1985.

80. Imbus HR and Tochilin SJ: Acute effect upon pulmonary function of low level exposure to phenol-formaldehyde-resin-coated wood, *American Ind Hyg Assoc J* 49:434-437, 1988.

81. Engholm G and Englund A: Cancer incidence and mortality among Swedish painters. In Englund A, Ringen K, and Mehlman MA, editors: *Advances in modern environmental toxicology, vol II: occupational health hazards of solvents,* pp 173-185, Princeton, NJ, 1982, Princeton Scientific Publishing.

82. Singleton JA and Beaumont JJ: *COMS II California occupational mortality, 1979-1981 adjusted for smoking, alcohol, and socioeconomic status,* Special report from the University of California at Davis to the California Department of Health Services, December 1989.

83. Torén K, Hörte L, and Järvholm B: Occupation and smoking adjusted mortality due to asthma among Swedish men, *Br J Ind Med* 48:323-326, 1991.

84. Wong O: A cohort mortality study and a case-control study of workers potentially exposed to styrene in the reinforced plastics and composites industry, *Br J Ind Med* 47:753-762, 1990.

85. Walrath J and Fraumeni JF: Mortality patterns among embalmers, *Int J Cancer* 31:407-411, 1983.

86. Acheson ED, Gardner MJ, Pannett B, et al: Formaldehyde in the British chemical industry, *Lancet* 1(8377):611-661, 1984.

87. Blair A, Stewart P, O'Berg M, Gaffey W, and Walrath J: Mortality among industrial workers exposed to formaldehyde, *J Natl Cancer Inst* 76:1071-1084, 1986.

88. Stewart PA, Schairer C, and Blair A: Comparison of jobs, exposures, and mortality risks for short-term and long-term workers, *J Occup Med* 32:703-708, 1990.

89. Dosemeci M, Blair A, Stewart PA, Chandler J, and Trush MA: Mortality among industrial workers exposed to phenol, *Epidemiology* 2:188-193, 1991.

90. Wallace LA: Volatile organic compounds. In Samet JM and Spengler JD, editors: *Indoor air pollution: a health perspective,* pp 253-272, Baltimore, 1991, The Johns Hopkins University Press.

91. Norbäck D, Björnsson E, Widström J, et al: Asthma symptoms in relation to volatile organic compounds (VOC) and bacteria in dwellings. In *Proceedings of the International Conference on Volatile Organic Compounds in the Environment,* pp 377-386, London, 1993, Lonsdale Press.

92. Norman GR, Pengelly LD, Kerigan AT, and Goldsmith TH: Respiratory function of children in homes insulated with urea formaldehyde foam insulation, *Can Med Assoc J* 134:1135-1138, 1986.

Chapter 29

METALS

Lee S. Newman

This chapter amalgamates the existing body of information concerning the effects of metals and metalloids on the respiratory tract of humans. Elements on the periodic table are defined as metals based on their physical and/or chemical traits. Some elements, like arsenic and antimony, are referred to as "metalloids" because they share properties of both metals and nonmetals. From the pulmonary perspective, many metals and metalloids can produce adverse effects on the respiratory tract following their inhalation as either metal fumes (oxides) or dust. Gaseous metal compounds and organometallic compounds, such as the carbonyls, are particularly toxic. Dissecting the effects of various metals is made difficult by their variety, their capacity to exist at different valences, and their ability to form complex or alloyed particles and to combine with nonmetallic elements, such as carbon or silica. The emphasis in this chapter will be on those elements that have metallic properties, omitting mineral dusts that produce the classic pneumoconioses such as coalworkers' pneumoconiosis, silicosis, and asbestosis. These topics are discussed elsewhere in the text. The chapter will summarize key features of metal exposures and effects in comprehensive tables, emphasizing key aspects in the text. Table 29-1 summarizes the common sources of exposure.

METAL TOXICITY

Table 29-2 lists principal routes of metal absorption, distribution, excretion, and mechanisms of toxicity. In general, we have only a primitive understanding of the mechanisms by which a metal's physicochemical properties produce biological consequences for the human respiratory tract. Humans who are occupationally or environmentally exposed to metals rarely inhale the pure metal but are exposed to compounds composed of multiple metals, multiple elements (such as metal salts), or binary metal compounds, such as oxides, halides, or carbides. The chemical species assumed by the metal often dictate its toxicologic properties and in some cases may help predict the biological consequences. For example, metal compounds of higher solubility tend to dissociate and are transported as metal ions deeply into the lung parenchyma, whereas more insoluble metals tend to

Text continued on page 480.

Table 29-1. Sources of exposure to metals and metalloids associated with respiratory tract effects

Metal	Group	Common ores, alloys, and compounds	Occupational exposures
Aluminum (Al)	IIIA	Ores: bauxite, corundum (α-Al_2O_3) Alloys: zinc, copper, magnesium, manganese, silicon, beryllium Compounds: metal, hydroxide, oxides, salts, organoaluminums, alkyaluminum halides	Bauxite ore converted to alumina ($Al_2O_3 \cdot H_2O$) through autoclaving, calcining reduction in electrolytic cell or "pot" Building materials Cables Utensils Laboratory equipment Abrasives Glass manufacture Textiles Printing inks Paper manufacture Welding Incendiary agents (organoaluminums) Catalysts (alkylaluminum halides)
Antimony (Sb)	VA	Ores: stibnite (Sb_3S_3), cervantite, jamesonite, kermesite, valentinite, livingstonite Alloys: lead, copper Compounds: antimony trioxide (Sb_2O_3), trisulfide (Sb_2S_3), trichloride, antimony potassium tartrate, antimony pentoxide, sodium antimony dimercaptosuccinate, Stibine (SbH_3, odorless gas)	Ceramics Glass ware Pigments Medication Lead solders Lead storage batteries Munitions Tobacco
Arsenic (As)	VA	Ores: copper, lead, and gold ore by-product (sulfide ores) Alloys: lead Compounds: inorganic arsenic, e.g., trioxide, trichloride, pentoxide, sodium arsenite, arsenic acid, arsenates; organic arsenic (e.g., arsanilic acid, methylarsonic acid, arsenobetaine; arsine [A_sH_3, garlic odor gas])	Fungicides Insecticides Paints Wood preservatives Weed killers Lead–arsenic alloys Human and veterinary medicine Computers Communications equipment Semiconductors
Barium (Ba)	IIA	Ores: witherite ($BaCO_3$), barite ($BaSO_4$) Alloys: steel additive Compounds: barium sulfide, hydroxide, chloride, nitrate, sulfate; halide salts (volatile)	Brick and tile refractories Paints Paper coating Rubber, vinyl Ceramics Glass Sugar refineries Insecticides, rodenticides Medical diagnosis
Beryllium (Be)	IIA	Ores: beryl, euclase, phenakite, chrysoberyl, bertrandite Alloys: copper, aluminum, nickel Compounds: metal, salts, oxide	Nuclear weapons parts Nonsparking tools and dies Dental alloys in crowns and bridges Missile components Nuclear reactor components Automobile ignition systems Electronics Computers Extraction from bertrandite and beryl ores Metal reclamation smelting operations Laser tubes, x-ray windows Aircraft brakes, parts
Boron (B)		Alloys: steel additive Compounds: hydrides of boron: diborane (B_2H_6), pentaborane (B_5H_9), decaborane ($B_{10}H_{14}$)	High energy aerospace fuel Nuclear reactor neutron moderate Steel alloy hardener Abrasive fire proofing Textiles Glass production Plastic polymerization catalyst Fungicides Bactericides

Continued.

Table 29-1. Sources of exposure to metals and metalloids associated with respiratory tract effects—cont'd

Metal	Group	Common ores, alloys, and compounds	Occupational exposures
Cadmium (Cd)	IIB	Ores: zinc, lead, copper (sulfide ores) Alloys: electroplated on steel Compounds: cadmium sulfide, cadmium selenide, cadmium stearate, cadmium oxide, cadmium carbonate, cadmium sulfate, cadmium chloride; organometallic compounds (e.g., cadmium thiocarbamate)	Smelting and refining process Scrap metal recovery Corrosion-resistant metal, production for engines Welding Electroplating on iron and on steel Nickel–cadmium battery production Soldering and brazing (cadmium alloys) Electrical parts manufacture Paint pigments Ceramics Plastics Insecticides Pesticides Veterinarian pharmaceuticals Dental amalgams Nonsparking tools Tobacco smoke
Chromium	VIB	Ores: chromite (trivalent) Alloys: iron, nickel, manganese, molybdenum Compounds: ferrous chromite, trivalent chromic oxide, chromic sulfate, hexavalent chromic acid, monochromates, dichromates, lead chromate, barium chromate, sodium and potassium chromate or dichromate, chromium acetate, chromic citrate, zinc chromate, calcium chromate, strontium chromate	Plating industry Tanning leather Dyeing industry Cement Cartography Engraving, lithography Coal and oil combustion Blueprint development Refractory and furnace emissions Water contamination due to fly ash or industrial effluent
Cobalt (Co)	VIII	Ores: smaltite, cobaltite, erythrite (silver, lead, nickel, copper, iron ores) Alloys: steels, "super-alloys" Compounds: metal, cobalt oxide, cobalt tetraoxide, cobalt chloride, cobalt sulfide and sulfate, carbides, carbonyls	Silver and copper mining Roasting process followed by leaching and electrolysis High temperature alloys, magnets, cemented carbide tools Manufacturing of "hard metal" tools Wearing off of grinders, drills, and cutting tools Catalysts Glass and ceramic pigments Paints, lacquers, varnishes Electroplating of nickel Filaments for lamps Automotive exhaust systems Radiation therapy Catalysts in oxidation reactions Electronics Plastics manufacture Printing ink manufacture Textile industry Chemical and petroleum industries Animal feed manufacture Aircraft manufacture High technology industries Burning of fuel oil and coal Production and use of metal alloys and tungsten carbides
Copper (Cu)	IB	Ores: cuprite (Cu_2O), chalcocite (Cu_2S), chalcopyrite ($CuFeS_2$), malachite [$Cu_2CO_3 \cdot Cu(OH)_2$], azurite [$2CuCO_3 \cdot Cu(OH)_2$] Alloys: zinc, tin, beryllium, cobalt, nickel, silver, cadmium Compounds: elemental copper, native copper, copper oxides, carbonates, sulfides, sulfate	Crushing, roasting, smelting Metal reclamation Preparation of alloys including brass and bronze Paint pigments Fungicides, insecticides Plumbing industry Electrical industry Roofing Electroplating

Continued.

Table 29-1. Sources of exposure to metals and metalloids associated with respiratory tract effects—cont'd

Metal	Group	Common ores, alloys, and compounds	Occupational exposures
Iron (Fe)	VIII	Ores: hematite (Fe_2O_3), magnetite (Fe_3O_4), siderite ($FeCO_3$), limonite ($Fe_2O_3 \cdot H_2O$) Alloys: steel (iron alloy) containing carbon, chromium, nickel, molybdenum, manganese, other metals Compounds: inorganic: iron oxides, carbonates, disulfides, sulfate, chlorides; organic: carbonyls (e.g., iron pentacarbonyl [Fe(CO)5])	Catalyst Fuel additive Pigment Magnetic tape, abrasive, and polish production Steel mills and foundries Steel grinding Oxyacetylene and electric arc welding Steel, silver, glass, and stone polish Boiler cleaning Ore mining and crushing Emery abrasive preparation Earth pigment preparation
Lead (Pb)	IVA	Ores: galena (lead sulfide), anglesite (lead sulfate), cerrusite (lead carbonate) Alloys: antimony, copper, tin Compounds: inorganic leads (e.g., lead sulfide, lead acetate, lead chloride); organoleads (e.g., tetramethyllead)	Pipe and ammunition manufacture Lead refining Mining and smelting operations North American air pollution Storage battery manufacture Pigments
Lithium (Li)	IA	Ores: spodumene Compounds: lithium salts (e.g., lithium stearate, lithium hydride)	Aerospace and pharmaceutical alloys Experimental rocket fuel propellant Organic chemical production Alkaline storage batteries Automotive lubricating greases
Magnesium (Mg)	IIA	Ores: brucite, dolomite, carnalite, kieserite, magnesite, olivine, periclase, seawater extraction Alloys: various steels, zirconium, titanium, uranium Compounds: magnesium carbonate, chloride, oxide, elemental Mg	Automotive industry Aerospace industry Boating industry Pharmaceuticals Hand tools Batteries
Manganese (Mn)	VIIB	Ores: pyrolusite (MnO_2), iron ores, silicates, coal, crude oil Alloys: major use in steels, ferrous, non-ferrous alloys Compounds: magnesium dioxide (tetravalent); permanganates (+7), organometallic forms (e.g., methylcyclopentadienyl manganese tricarbonyl [MTT], cyclopentadienyl manganese tricarbonyl [CMT])	Dry-cell batteries Steel manufacture Incendiary devices, matches Ceramics and glass pigments Chemical industry Dyes, inks, paints Mining and ore smelting Plant manufacturing of manganese and steels alloys Foundry workers Electric arc welders Antiknock gasoline additive
Mercury (Hg)	IIB	Ores: cinnabar (red sulfide), fossil fuels Compounds: inorganic mercury (e.g., elemental mercury, divalent salts [halides, nitrates, sulfates]); organic mercury (e.g., alkylmercury compounds, phenylmercury, methoxyalkylmercury, methylmercury dicyandiamide, methylmercury chloride)	Electronic components Scientific equipment Catalyst in polyurethane manufacturing Explosive production Metallurgic laboratories Solder for dry batteries High-frequency induction furnaces Electrolysis process Pharmaceuticals Dental amalgam production Photoengraving Paints Metal smelting Fungicides, algaecides Paper pulp preservative

Continued.

Table 29-1. Sources of exposure to metals and metalloids associated with respiratory tract effects—cont'd

Metal	Group	Common ores, alloys, and compounds	Occupational exposures
Nickel (Ni)	VIII	Ores: sulfide ores, oxide ores Alloys: cadmium, aluminum, chromium, iron Compounds: nickel oxide, hydroxide, subsulfide, chloride, sulfate, carbonate; nickel carbonyl [Ni(CO)4]	Steel manufacture Nickel–cadmium batteries Automotive and aircraft parts Jet engines and turbines Electrical equipment, magnets Refining process Automotive parts Machinery parts Electroplating Catalysts Power plants Tobacco smoke
Osmium (Os)		Ores: by-product of platinum extraction Alloys: iridium Compounds: metallic osmium, osmium tetroxide (osmic acid), osmium salts	Fountain pens Watches Engraving tools Annealing Electron microscopy Histologic staining Finger printing
Phosphorus (Pb)		Ores: yellow phosphorus, white phosphorus, red phosphorus Compounds: elemental phosphorus, phosphoric acid, phosphorus trichloride, pentachloride, pentasulfate, metal phosphides, phosphorus oxychloride, phosphine (PH_3), organophosphate (insecticides)	Fireworks Munitions Incendiary devices Chemical production Detergent Fertilizers Animal feed Pharmaceuticals Insecticides Rodenticides Pesticides Acetylene production Phosphorus production Photography Engraving Semiconductor industry Acetylene gas welding Match production
Platinum (Pt)	VIII	Ores: nickel, copper-containing ores Alloys: cobalt, rhodium, iridium Compounds: elemental platinum, platinum salts (e.g., chloroplatinates, tetrachloroplatinates, hexachloroplatinates)	Magnets Catalysts Corrosion resistance Automotive industry Chemical industry Petroleum industry Electrical industry Jewelry industry Pharmaceutical industry Ceramics industry Dental industry Plastic industry
Rare earths (lanthanides)	III	Ores: monazite, or produced in nuclear fission of uranium, thorium, plutonium Alloys: iron, magnesium, aluminum, in combination with each other (e.g., didymium = Pr + Nd) Compounds: in addition to alloys and as elements, salts (e.g., chlorides, citrates)	Arc lamps (cerium) Lighter flints Munitions Lenses Welders' protective goggles Nuclear reactors Color ceramics Vacuum tube gas absorber

Continued.

Table 29-1. Sources of exposure to metals and metalloids associated with respiratory tract effects—cont'd

Metal	Group	Common ores, alloys, and compounds	Occupational exposures
Selenium (Se)	VIA	Ores: sulfide ore by-product (copper-refining) Alloys: multiple metal alloys Compounds: selenium dioxide, selenium trioxide, selenous acid, selenic acid, selenium oxychloride, selenite and selenate salts, elemental selenium hydrogen selenide, dimethylselenide	Electronics industry Photoelectric cells Rectifiers Ceramics industry Pigments Rubber manufacture
Silver (Ag)	IB	Ores: argentite Alloys: copper, aluminum, antimony, cadmium, chrome, nickel, lead Compounds: silver nitrate, silver lactate, silver acetate, silver picrate, silver halides	Jewelry Coins Utensils Inks Steel coating in telephone equipment Photography Solder
Thallium (T l)	IIIA	Ores: crookesite, lorandite, zinc and lead ores, fossil fuels, by-product of cadmium production Alloys: silver, lead, mercury Compounds: thallous sulfate, thallous nitrate, thallous acetate, thallium oxides, thallous carbonate, thallous sulfide	Optic lenses Low temperature thermometers Pigments Semiconductors Catalyst for organic reactions Insecticide Rodenticide Fungicide Depilatory Mining, refining, burning coal Ambient air
Tin (Sn)	IVA	Ores: cassiterite, tinstone (SnO_2), tin sulfides Alloys: phosphor brass, light brass, high tensile brass (copper, zinc, tin), gun metal, die casting alloys, pipe metals, pewter, bronze (tin, copper), antimony Compounds: in addition to alloys, inorganic tins (e.g., dioctyltin, dibutyltin, dimethyltin, triorganotins)	Alloy preparation Metal coating and plating Insecticides, fungicides Antihelminthics Ceramics Glass Inks Metal shops Scrap metal recovery Mining Foundry Pigments Textiles Solders Furnaces Reducing agent Rubber, plastics industries Chemical industry
Titanium (Ti)	IVB	Ores: ilmenite, rutile Alloys: aluminum, tin, iron, vanadium Compounds: inorganic forms (e.g., titanium dioxide, chloride, tetrachloride, phosphate, nitrate, sulfate, calcium titanate, iron titanate, sodium titanate); organometallic forms (e.g., alkyltitanate, aryltitanate) especially titanocene	Aerospace industry Defense industry Cobalt-cemented carbide cutting tools Drill tips Welding rods Electrodes Lamp filaments Magnets Paints Smoke screens Cosmetics Topical ointments Surgical appliances

Continued.

Table 29-1. Sources of exposure to metals and metalloids associated with respiratory tract effects—cont'd

Metal	Group	Common ores, alloys, and compounds	Occupational exposures
Tungsten (W) (wolfram)	VIB	Ores: wolframite, scheelite Alloys: "hard metals," steel, with chromium, cobalt Compounds: tungsten trioxide, tungstic acid, sodium tungstate, ammonium paratungstate, tungsten carbide	Crushing and milling of ore Metallurgic operations Light bulb filaments Textile pigments Production of tungsten carbide
Uranium (U)		Ores: $^{238}U \gg ^{235}U \gg ^{234}U$, natural isotopes in carnatite, and other ores Compounds: elemental uranium, uranium oxides, halides, uranium hydrides, sulfates, carbonates, nitrates, uranium hexafluoride (UF_6, gas), mostly in tetravalent and hexavalent forms	Nuclear power reactor fuel Nuclear powered submarines Photography Ceramics colorant Armaments Mining
Vanadium (V)	VB	Ores: phosphate rock, clays, carnatite, magnetite, fossil fuels Alloys: titanium, special steels and alloys Compounds: halides (e.g., pentafluoride, tetrachloride, dichloride, trichloride, oxovanadium chloride); vanadium pentoxide, vanadates, metavanadates; vanadium carbonyls	Mining Production Steel alloys Jet engines Aircraft Hardened steels Catalyst Synthetic rubber production Photographic chemicals Coal combustion Crude oil Heavy sulfur fuel Gas, oil, coal furnaces
Zinc (Zn)	IIB	Ores: sphalerite, wurzite (sulfide ores) Alloys: copper, nickel, aluminum, galvanized iron, bronze, brass; contaminated by lead and cadmium Compounds: in addition to alloys, zinc oxide, salts (e.g., zinc sulfate, zinc ammonium sulfate, zinc chloride); organic zinc compounds (e.g., carbamates)	Paint Rubber products Pigments Ceramic glazes Glass Paper production Cosmetics Pharmaceuticals Dentistry Smelting Brass founding Galvanized iron production Welding Electroplating Flux Wood preservative Smoke bombs Dental cement Textiles Deodorant
Zirconium (Zr)	IVB	Ores: ilmenite, rutile, magnetite, monazite, quartz, beach sands, widely distributed as zircon ($ZrO_2 \cdot SiO_2$) or baddeleyite (ZrO_2) Alloys: copper, nickel, cobalt, manganese, silicon, niobium–tantalum; hafnium frequently present as well Compounds: elemental zirconium, zirconium dioxide (zirconia), zirconium silicate, zirconium salts, (e.g., sodium zirconium lactate, zirconium tetrachloride [$ZrCl_4$, gas])	Ceramics Glass manufacture Furnace bricks Nuclear reactor shields High temperature and water repellent textiles Abrasives in optics industry Dyes and pigments Catalyst in organic chemical reactions Arc lamps Munitions Ointments—poison ivy Antiperspirants (ceased)

Table 29-2. Routes of occupational exposure, absorption, distribution, and toxicity of metals

Metal	Principal routes of exposure and absorption	Distribution and excretion	Mechanisms of toxicity
Aluminum (Al)	Lungs, slight gastrointestinal absorption	Prolonged lung retention; distributes to bone, muscle, spleen, liver; urinary excretion	Al^{3+} interacts with enzyme systems, including adenylate cyclase, phosphodiesterases and hexokinases High affinity for DNA, RNA, and nucleotides Injury to microtubules and filaments resulting in neurofibrillary degeneration
Antimony (Sb)	Lungs	Prolonged lung retention; distributes to thyroid, adrenal, liver, kidney; urinary (pentavalent) or fecal (trivalent) excretion	Stibine binds to hemoglobin, leading to hemolysis Myocardial injury Fatty degeneration of liver
Arsenic (As)	Dependent upon the chemical and physical form of compound; routes include gastrointestinal, lung, or skin	Prolonged lung retention; retention in skin, hair, nails, thyroid, bone, teeth; widely distributed; urinary, fecal excretion	Biotransformed to pentavalent arsenites that bind to proteins and sulfhydryl groups and inhibit cellular enzyme systems Arsenic and arsine bind to hemoglobin leading to hemolysis Induction of chromosomal aberrations
Barium (Ba)	Lungs, gastrointestinal (soluble forms), respiratory tract (free barium ion)	Retention in bone, eye; fecal, urinary excretion	Dependent upon solubility; soluble salts do not result in occupational toxicity Potassium antagonist, blocks K^+ channels of Na–K pump in cell membranes
Beryllium (Be)	Lungs, much less via skin	High lung, liver, spleen, and bone distribution and retention; mucociliary clearance and urinary excretion	Direct irritant and chemical effects Serving as an antigen, induces specific cellular immune response Inhibits enzyme activities, including phosphatases, kinases, dehydrogenases, in some cases through competitive inhibition of Mg^{2+} or K^+ Induces infidelity of DNA replication
Boron (B)	Lungs	High lung retention	Irritative due to exothermic properties of diborane Neurogenic effects Hypersensitivity response
Cadmium (Cd)	Lungs and gastrointestinal tract, amount depends upon size of particles and solubility; more gastrointestinal absorption if iron deficient	High lung retention, distributes to liver, kidney, muscle; excretion via feces, urinary tract, saliva, bile, hair, nails; crosses placenta	Related to the absence of homeostatic control and tendency of cadmium to bind thiol groups, especially metallothionein in plasma Inactivates multiple enzyme systems Binds DNA and RNA Disturbance of calcium metabolism

Metal	Absorption	Distribution and Excretion	Effects
Chromium (Cr)	Lungs, poor gastrointestinal and dermal absorption; hexavalent>>trivalent forms	Distribution depends on valence; retained in lymph nodes, lungs, kidney, liver, spleen; urinary excretion	Effects on enzyme systems (hexavalent chromium) Interacts with nucleic acids and binds to DNA, affecting DNA synthesis (hexavalent chromium converted to trivalent chromium) Effects on cell cycle (hexavalent chromium) Mutagenic (hexavalent chromium) Strong oxidizers that are corrosive and irritating (hexavalent chromium)
Cobalt (Co)	Gastrointestinal, lungs	Distributes to liver, kidney, cardiovascular system; urinary excretion; rapid lung clearance following inhalation	Effects on cellular systems through oxidation or serving as an adjuvant, bound to endogenous proteins Interferes with some oxidation steps of citric acid cycle Inhibits tyrosine iodinase in thyroid (a cause of goiter) Increases erythropoietin release Induction of delayed-type hypersensitivity responses in the skin Induction of infidelity of DNA replication in vitro, mutagenic
Copper (Cu)	Gastrointestinal (mostly stomach), lungs	Retention in liver; later in brain, heart, kidney, muscle, and liver; biliary excretion, little urinary excretion; crosses placenta	Catalyst for a number of enzymatic reactions within the body involved with iron absorption and synthesis of hemoglobin Can cause hemolysis Copper salts induce infidelity of DNA replication in vitro
Iron (Fe)	Gastrointestinal	Bound to hemoglobin, myoglobin, iron-requiring enzymes, iron-storage proteins ferritin, hemosiderin, transferrin; accumulates in liver, spleen, kidney, heart, muscle; low excretion, usually via feces, skin, hair, nails, blood, low urinary excretion	Excessive intake can result in hemochromatosis and hemosiderosis Iron loading results in organ-specific pathologic alterations Possible cocarcinogenic effects
Lead (Pb)	Varies with particle size, chemical form, lung clearance mechanism; exposure through lungs and gastrointestinal tract	Largest body burden is in bone, lesser amounts in blood, soft tissue; fecal, urinary excretion, also milk, sweat, hair, nails; crosses placenta	Inhibition of delta-aminolevulinic acid dehydrogenase Free erythrocyte protoporphyrin elevation in red cells Alterations in neurotransmitter systems Degenerative changes in proximal renal tubules, mitochondrial swelling
Magnesium (Mg)	Lungs, gastrointestinal, with rapid lung absorption	Widely distributed; urinary excretion	Divalent cation for the function of biological systems, bound to proteins and phosphates Cofactor in many enzyme systems, including metalloenzymes Interaction with calcium

Continued.

Table 29-2. Routes of occupational exposure, absorption, distribution, and toxicity of metals—cont'd

Metal	Principal routes of exposure and absorption	Distribution and excretion	Mechanisms of toxicity
Manganese (Mn)	Gastrointestinal, lungs	Accumulates in liver, kidney, brain, bone; fecal excretion, mucociliary clearance, milk; crosses placenta	Reduced in the respiratory tract to form soluble manganese salts absorbed in blood stream, resulting in potential toxicity to other organs Alterations in neurotransmitter levels
Mercury (Hg)	Efficient lung absorption, some skin absorption, poor gastrointestinal absorption, but varies greatly with form of mercury (e.g., organic, inorganic)	Widely distributed, prefers epithelial cells and glandular tissue, throid, salivary glands, liver, pancreas, sweat glands, brain; fecal and urinary, sweat excretion	Binds covalently with high affinity for sulfur and sulfhydryl groups in proteins, as well as with $-CONH_2$, $-NH_2$, $-COOH$, and $-PO_4$ groups Inhibits many enzyme systems in the body, altering cellular function Induces allergic sensitivity Immunologic mechanism for some forms of mercury toxicity
Nickel (Ni)	Lungs, depending on solubility; inorganic nickel through gastrointestinal tract; through skin for nickel sulfate	Accumulates in kidneys, liver, lungs, pituitary; urinary, fecal excretion; crosses placenta	Transport via albumin, nickeloplasmin (α-macroglobulin), serum Genotoxic effects, inducing infidelity in DNA synthesis and mutagenesis in some organisms and cell types Induces a delayed type hypersensitivity response Apparent irritant effects (especially nickel carbonyl) Ingested elemental metal is relatively nontoxic
Osmium (Os)	Lungs	Lung retention	Lipophilic Fatty degeneration of renal tubules
Phosphorus (P)	Gastrointestinal, lungs (vapor), skin absorption	Bone accumulation; urinary excretion	Chlorinated forms may liberate chlorine gas upon inhalation
Platinum (Pt)	Lungs	High lung retention; long-term in kidney, liver, muscle, spleen; urinary excretion	Acts as antigen, inducing specific antibody response
Rare earths (lanthanides)	Lungs, gastrointestinal	Accumulates in liver, bone; fecal, urinary excretion	Interferes with mitochondrial ATP Inhibits activity of key intracellular enzyme systems Anticoagulant properties
Selenium (Se)	Lungs, gastrointestinal, skin	Widely distributed; biotransformed in liver	Toxicity related to inhalation of hydrogen selenide gas Essential trace element part of enzyme systems (e.g., glutathione peroxidase) Biotransformation in the liver to excretable metabolites Both irritant and allergic properties (urticarial response) Interacts with metals (e.g., arsenic, cobalt, mercury, lead, copper, platinum, silver, tellurium, thallium)

Metal	Absorption	Distribution and excretion	Effects
Silver (Ag)	Gastrointestinal, lungs	Accumulates in liver, less in spleen, lung, muscles, skin, brain; fecal excretion	Silver salts are caustic Hepatic, renal, bone marrow necrosis after intravenous injection Argyria, due to deposits of silver granules in tissue, toxic effect none to minimal, depending upon organ of deposition
Thallium (Tl)	Gastrointestinal, skin, lungs, rapid absorption	Widely distributed, highest in kidney; retention in hair; fecal, urinary, hair excretion	Interfere with enzymatic systems, especially with reactive sulfhydryl groups Disrupt mitochondria in animal muscle and peripheral nervous tissue Thallium ion similarities to potassium ion results in toxicity Uncouples oxidative phosphorylation, inhibits multiple enzyme systems
Tin (Sn)	Common inorganic tin compounds poorly absorbed through gastrointestinal tract, lungs; organotins absorbed through skin readily	Increase accumulation in lungs with age; also stored in bone, kidney; urinary excretion	Major toxicity associated with organotins, causing irritation, burns Inorganic tin inhibits 5-aminolevulinic deydratase Dialkyltin reacts with thiols, affecting mitochondrial enzymes Interference with calcium metabolism, and calcium-related enzymes
Titanium (Ti)	Poorly absorbed through lungs, gastrointestinal tract	High lung and lymph node retention; urinary excretion	Titanium tetrachloride, oxychloride cause irritation and burns Generally considered to be of low toxicity
Tungsten (W)	Gastrointestinal and lung absorption rapid	Distributed to spleen, kidney, bone; small fraction retained in bone; urinary excretion	Low toxicity
Uranium (Ur)	Lungs, gastrointestinal tract, but high density of particles greatly limits ability to reach lung parenchyma; transport depends upon solubility; water-soluble uranium compounds penetrate skin	Most retained in bone; urinary excretion as uranyl-bicarbonate and uranyl-citrate complexes	Binds to plasma proteins or forms bicarbonate complexes filtered by kidney, resulting in uranyl ion release toxic to tubular epithelium Toxicity may be due to chemical properties and ionizing radiation
Vanadium (V)	Lung absorption high for soluble compounds, poor gastrointestinal absorption	Widely distributed, urinary excretion	Interferes with metabolism of amino acids containing sulfur Inhibition of enzymes including acid and alkaline phosphatase and kinases Enzyme stimulation including adenylate cyclase
Zinc (Zn)	Gastrointestinal absorption is variable, lung data limited	Widely distributed, excreted in feces, urine, sweat	Involved in enzyme systems including metalloenzymes, alkaline phosphatase, alcohol dehydrogenase, carbonic anhydrase Cofactor for enzymes involved in DNA, RNA, protein synthesis Irritant properties of zinc chloride may be result of formation of HCl Metal fume fever may result from induction of inflammatory cytokines in the lungs Chromosomal anomalies in leukocytes following zinc workplace exposures
Zirconium (Zr)	Lungs, skin	Widely distributed, lung retention; urinary excretion	Generally considered to be of low toxicity Induction of a delayed-type hypersensitivity (cell-mediated immune) response

DNA, Deoxyribonucleic acid; *RNA*, ribonucleic acid.

be deposited in the airways. Metal ions have a strong tendency to associate with organic molecules found within tissues at physiologic pH. The capacity to bind covalently, both extra- and intracellularly, can have grim implications for the organism.

Metal toxicity can be both direct and indirect. For example, certain metals interact directly with functional molecules, such as sulfhydryl groups, or directly bind and alter deoxyribonucleic acid (DNA) as a potential mechanism for metal carcinogenesis. Some metals serve as co-enzymes, thereby disrupting normal enzymatic activity within the lung. Some metals become antigenic, by binding to low–molecular-weight endogenous peptide. Yet another mechanism of pulmonary toxicity, especially among the so-called "transition metals," such as iron and copper, hinges upon the ability of metals to change oxidation stage (losing electrons), thus catalyzing oxidation reactions, enhancing potential toxicity through oxygen free radical species generation.[1-6]

The mechanisms of toxicity associated with specific metals are summarized in Table 29-1. Unfortunately, in many circumstances the mechanisms by which metals cause pathologic changes remain enigmatic. Many published reports perpetuate the mystery by referring to "irritant mechanism." This is an uninformative term that underscores our limited understanding. Ultimately, we must learn more about the biochemical, chemical, immunologic, and molecular events to better identify, prevent, and treat metal-induced diseases.

MEASURING EXPOSURE

Information about inhalational exposure is extremely important to recognition of metal-induced lung disorders. Many of the inhalable metals can be measured and identified with high specificity using industrial hygiene monitoring (see Chapter 11). Whereas detailed assessment of exposure and of dose may be helpful, some metal-induced lung diseases are immunologically mediated and may be provoked by low levels of exposure. In such cases, reliance on air samples may be misleading.

Biological monitoring can help make the link between exposure and diagnosis. Examples include the detection of metals in biological specimens like lung, urine, and blood, or specimens of immunologic assessment, by in vivo and in vitro methods.

Analysis of the mineral content of tissue specimens can provide specific data confirming exposure. The traditional approach to such an analyses combines light microscopy and bulk tissue analysis, but sufficient amounts of lung tissue are often obtainable only through open lung biopsy or at the time of autopsy. More modern microprobe mineral analyses can be performed on smaller specimens, including bronchoalveolar lavage cells, to determine the metal content of particles retained within the lungs.[7-11]

Light microscopy is a logical starting point when one has histopathology available as is often the case with the parenchymal forms of metal-induced lung disease. But metal particles are not characteristic enough for pathologists to discriminate types of metals by light microscopy alone. Some pathogenic particles are too small to be seen with the light microscope. More recent developments using transmission electron microscopy (EM) and scanning electron microscopy (SEM) on paraffin sections allow the enumeration of size, number, and distribution of particles. Such EM techniques can be combined to advantage with analytic tools such as energy-dispersive x-ray spectroscopy using a microprobe (EDXM).[10,11] Studies with SEM/EDXM, laser probes, ion probes, or proton-induced x-ray emission show that such techniques can identify metals with high sensitivity and specificity within small specimens of lung tissue. Such data support the conclusion that an individual has been exposed and has retained metal within the lung. It is sometimes more difficult to determine which metal particles may be causing disease, as some may be present in normal lungs or may be "innocent bystanders." Because metals vary in their pulmonary retention, some disease-inducing metals may disappear after the damage has been done. For example, highly soluble cobalt causes disease but is usually absent from the lung by the time that mineral analysis is performed. Thus, one must proceed with caution in interpreting the results of mineral analyses. The information must be placed in the clinical context with the constellation of other data from the workplace and clinical evaluation that lead to the conclusion of workplace-related exposure and disease.

Other biological markers of exposure to metals include the urine and blood assays. In most circumstances such tests do not reflect the inhaled dose and generally will not prove metal-induced respiratory tract disease, although they may confirm that exposure has occurred. A variety of metals can be detected with a high degree of reliability in blood or urine, including aluminum, arsenic, cadmium, chromium, cobalt, lead, manganese, mercury, nickel, and vanadium.[12] A note of caution: both false-positive and false-negative results occur. Before obtaining urinary or blood levels for a specific metal, the clinician should consider the analytic and kinetic factors pertinent to detection of specific metals of interest. Detection limits vary by analytic technique, laboratory, and metal. The level of metal that will be detected will vary with the dose, the absorption, the rate of excretion, and the time since last exposure.[13,14] Conditions under which the specimens are collected can also influence the results. One must be scrupulous in avoiding contamination from work clothes. Specimen containers must be properly voided of all trace elements.

Measuring the immunologic response to metals represents another form of biological monitoring that may help confirm pathogenically relevant exposure or, in some cases, help make the specific diagnosis. Measurement of metal-specific antibodies by methods such as the enzyme-linked immunosorbent assay (ELISA) can, if positive, confirm exposures to metals including cobalt, nickel, and chromium.[15-18] In the proper clinical context, they help confirm the cause of disorders such as asthma and dermatitis. Demonstration of serum antibodies to a metal does not always prove causation, and a negative in vitro antibody response does not exclude the diagnosis of metal-induced respiratory tract disease. Analogously, skin tests for immediate type hypersensitivity to metals, such as prick and scratch tests, are poorly standardized, but can, in experienced hands, help confirm the exposure and diagnosis when positive.

Cellular immune responses to certain metal antigens can be measured in bronchoalveolar lavage (BAL) or blood as a means of confirming the diagnosis of metal-induced lung diseases. The best example of this is chronic beryllium disease in which immunologic evaluation has become pivotal in making the specific diagnosis.[19-22] Analogously, skin patching test can be helpful in demonstrating delayed type hypersensitivity responses to metal salts.[23,24] Most metal salts are poorly standardized, are not part of the standard patch test "tray," but are in common use among occupational dermatologists. In some cases of suspected metal-induced asthma, specific bronchoprovocation testing has been used in research to prove causation. Clinical application of such specific challenges must be performed with great caution, preferably in centers experienced in their use.

As summarized in Table 29-3, the identification of respiratory tract exposure to metal may be helped by considering other organs that may be involved, especially the skin.

CLINICAL APPROACH TO METAL-INDUCED RESPIRATORY TRACT DISEASE

Recognition of metal-induced respiratory tract disease generally begins with clinical suspicion fueled by clues from one of several directions: (1) the patient presents with lung disease and offers a history of occupational or environmental exposure to one or more of the metals outlined in Table 29-3; (2) chest radiographic abnormalities suggest a possible underlying lung disease due to metals, such as evidence of pneumoconiotic type densities; (3) pathologic changes seen on transbronchial or open lung biopsy specimens, sometimes associated with abundant particulate material, raise suspicion of an inhalational source. Respiratory tract diseases associated with metal or metalloid exposure are diverse and include adult respiratory distress syndrome (ARDS), chronic obstructive pulmonary disease (COPD), asthma, tracheobronchitis, alveolar proteinosis, interstitial fibrosis, lung and nasal cancer, and acute inhalational fever syndromes (Table 29-3).

A careful occupational and environmental history is the first step toward diagnosis. It is important to ask if the workplace or inhalational exposures are associated with the patient's chief complaint. Because of the long latency for many metal-induced diseases, a chronological list of all jobs is important. In addition to collecting the names of metals and metal compounds, one should inquire about the spe-

cific job tasks and types of metal work performed, such as welding, grinding, sanding, smelting, polishing; the nature of the exposures, such as dust or fumes; conditions of exposure, such as the perceived adequacy of ventilation, use of respiratory protection, and clean-up or dust-disturbing practices. The history should include hobbies and habits that can result in metal exposure outside of work, including whether an individual smokes tobacco and whether a spouse is in a metal-related trade.

If the clinical history suggests metal exposure in the workplace, additional information can help to confirm it. Obtain Material Safety Data Sheets (MSDS), and review them for the possible presence of metals that induce adverse health effects. Discussions with the plant safety or industrial hygiene personnel can be extremely helpful in certain circumstances. Worksite investigations frequently provide information unobtainable at the time of an office visit. In light of the often complex array of exposures in the workplace, it may be necessary to then perform an industrial hygiene investigation with air monitoring or review previous sampling data. Epidemiologic assessment of the workforce for evidence of excess respiratory symptomatology is time consuming but often critical for helping industry recognize the need to improve primary and secondary preventive measures.

Although traditional clinical tools, such as the physical examination, chest imaging, and pulmonary physiology, help us form a diagnosis and assess disease severity, these tools are generally too nonspecific to link exposure to disease. Environmental and biologic measures of exposure can lend greater specificity to the more general clinical diagnosis (see "Measuring Exposure").

SPECIFIC RESPIRATORY TRACT EFFECTS CAUSED BY METALS

The remainder of this chapter will consider those metals for which there is sufficient medical evidence linking them to respiratory tract disease, or for which the respiratory tract serves as a major route of absorption resulting in systemic toxicity.

It is important to bear in mind a number of general principles that pertain to the effects of metals on the respiratory tract.

- First, not every metal causes respiratory tract injury. For example, radiodense metals may induce chest radiographic opacities that are not necessarily associated with underlying pulmonary injury. Similarly, although a number of metals, including beryllium, platinum, gold, and nickel can induce cellular or humoral immune system hypersensitivity, not every form of a particular metal will have the same antigenic properties.
- Second, metal and metalloid exposure that is sufficient to cause disease is not limited to workers in the traditional industries like mining and metallurgy (see Table 29-1).

Text continued on p. 488.

Table 29-3. Summary of nonmalignant respiratory and extrathoracic disorders associated with metal or metalloid exposure

Respiratory tract disease	Aluminum (Al) (13)	Antimony (Sb) (51)	Arsenic (As) (33)	Barium (Ba) (56)	Beryllium (Be) (4)	Boron (B) (5)
Airways						
Rhinitis/nasal injury/sinusitis		X	X		X	X
Tracheitis	X	X			X	
Acute bronchitis	X	X			X	X
Bronchiolitis	X					
Bronchiectasis					X	
Chronic bronchitis	X	X	X	X		
Asthma/reactive airways	X					X
Parenchyma						
Acute pneumonitis or pulmonary edema	X	X	X		X	X
Interstitial fibrosis	X			X	X	
Granulomatous pneumonitis	X			X	X	
Benign pneumoconiosis		X		X		
Emphysema						
Metal fume fever/inhalational fever			X			X
Other respiratory effects	Pulmonary alveolar Proteinosis; potroom asthma					
Other organ effects						
Skin	X	X	X		X	
Eyes		X	X			X
Oropharyngeal		X	X			
Cardiovascular		X	X		X	
Hepatic		X	X		X	X
Gastrointestinal		X	X			
Renal	X	X	X		X	X
Lymphatic/hematologic		X [hemolysis (SbH$_3$)]	X [hemolysis (AsH$_3$)]		X	X
Musculoskeletal/rheumatologic					X	X
Peripheral nervous system			X			
Central nervous system	X	X	X			X
Comments		Reproductive toxicity				Effects from boranes; metallic boron non-toxic

Continued.

Table 29-3. Summary of nonmalignant respiratory and extrathoracic disorders associated with metal or metalloid exposure—cont'd

Respiratory tract disease	Cadmium (Cd) (48)	Chromium (Cr) (24)	Cobalt (Co) (27)	Copper (Cu) (29)	Gold (Au) (79)
Airways					
Rhinitis/nasal injury/sinusitis	X (anosmia)	X	X	X	X
Tracheitis	X	X			
Acute bronchitis	X	X	X		
Bronchiolitis			X		
Bronchiectasis					
Chronic bronchitis		X	X		
Asthma/reactive airways		X	X		
Parenchyma					
Acute pneumonitis or pulmonary edema	X	X	X	X	
Interstitial fibrosis	X (after acute injury)		X	X	X
Granulomatous pneumonitis			X	X	X
Benign pneumoconiosis					
Emphysema	X	X (Oxide)			
Metal fume fever/inhalational fever	X			X	
Other respiratory effects			Giant cell interstitial pneumonitis	Lung cancer among "vineyard sprayer's lung" cases	Hypersensitivity pneumonitis (nonoccupational)
Other organ effects					
Skin		X	X	X	X
Eyes		X	X	X	
Oropharyngeal	X (dental discoloration)	X		X	X
Cardiovascular			X		
Hepatic	X	X			
Gastrointestinal	X			X	
Renal	X	X		X	
Lymphatic/hematologic	X			X	
Musculoskeletal/rheumatologic	X				
Peripheral nervous system					
Central nervous system	X				
Comments	"Itai-Itai disease"			Green hair, skin, teeth	

Continued.

Table 29-3. Summary of nonmalignant respiratory and extrathoracic disorders associated with metal or metalloid exposure—cont'd

Respiratory tract disease	Iron (Fe) (26)	Lead (Pb) (82)	Lithium (Li) (3)	Magnesium (Mg) (12)	Manganese (Mn) (25)
Airways					
Rhinitis/nasal injury/sinusitis			X	X	
Tracheitis					
Acute bronchitis					X
Bronchiolitis					
Bronchiectasis					
Chronic bronchitis					X
Asthma/reactive airways					
Parenchyma					
Acute pneumonitis or pulmonary edema	X (iron carbonyl)		X		X
Interstitial fibrosis					
Benign pneumoconiosis	X				
Emphysema					
Metal fume fever/inhalational fever				X	X
Other respiratory effects	Lung cancer risk possibly due to iron oxide or other coexposures	Inhalation results in systemic absorption and extrathoracic toxicity			Inhalation results in systemic absorption and extrathoracic toxicity; increased risk of pneumonia
Other Organ Effects					
Skin					X
Eyes				X	X
Oropharyngeal					
Cardiovascular					
Hepatic	X (iron carbonyl)	X			
Gastrointestinal		X			
Renal		X			
Lymphatic/hematologic		X			X
Musculoskeletal/rheumatologic		X			X
Peripheral nervous system		X			
Central nervous system	X (iron carbonyl)	X			X
Comments	Shared exposures to SiO$_2$; secondary hemosiderosis				

Continued.

Table 29-3. Summary of nonmalignant respiratory and extrathoracic disorders associated with metal or metalloid exposure—cont'd

Respiratory tract disease	Mercury (Hg) (80)	Nickel (Ni) (28)	Osmium (Os) (76)	Phosphorus (P) (15)	Platinum (Pt) (78)
Airways					
Rhinitis/nasal injury/sinusitis	X	X (cancer)	X		X
Tracheitis	X		X	X	
Acute bronchitis	X		X	X	
Bronchiolitis	X				
Bronchiectasis					
Chronic bronchitis				X	
Asthma/reactive airways		X	X	X	X
Parenchyma					
Acute pneumonitis or pulmonary edema	X	X	X	X	
Interstitial fibrosis	X	X			
Benign pneumoconiosis					
Emphysema					
Metal fume fever/inhalational fever		X			
Other respiratory effects	Mercury embolism	Lung cancer; eosinophilic pneumonia			
Other Organ Effects					
Skin	X	X	X	X	X
Eyes	X		X		X
Oropharyngeal	X		X	X	X
Cardiovascular					
Hepatic		X			
Gastrointestinal	X			X (PH$_3$)	
Renal	X	X	X		
Lymphatic/hematologic					
Musculoskeletal/rheumatologic	X	X		X	
Peripheral nervous system					
Central nervous system	X	X	X	X (PH$_3$)	
Comments				"Phossy Jaw"	

Continued.

Table 29-3. Summary of nonmalignant respiratory and extrathoracic disorders associated with metal or metalloid exposure—cont'd

Respiratory tract disease	Rare earths (lanthanides) (Cerium, Ce, 58) (Yttrium, Yb, 39) (Terbium, Tb, 65)	Selenium (Se) (34)	Silver (Ag) (47)	Thallium (Tl) (81)	Tin (Sn) (50)
Airways					
Rhinitis/nasal injury/sinusitis		X	X		X
Tracheitis		X	X		X
Acute bronchitis		X			X
Bronchiolitis					
Bronchiectasis					
Chronic bronchitis			X		
Asthma/reactive airways		X			
Parenchyma					
Acute pneumonitis or pulmonary edema		X		X	X
Interstitial fibrosis	X			X	
Granulomatous pneumonitis	X				
Benign pneumoconiosis	X				X
Emphysema					
Metal fume fever/inhalational fever					
Other respiratory effects				Respiratory muscle failure due to neuromuscular toxicity	
Other Organ Effects					
Skin	X	X	X	X (alopecia)	X
Eyes	X		X		X
Oropharyngeal		X	X		X
Cardiovascular				X	
Hepatic				X	
Gastrointestinal		X		X	
Renal				X	
Lymphatic/hematologic	X				
Musculoskeletal/rheumatologic				X	
Peripheral nervous system				X	X
Central nervous system		X		X	
Comments		Red teeth, hair, nails; garlic odor	Argyria		Toxicity due to organic tin

Continued.

Table 29-3. Summary of nonmalignant respiratory and extrathoracic disorders associated with metal or metalloid exposure—cont'd

Respiratory tract disease	Titanium (Ti) (22)	Uranium (Ur)(92)	Vanadium (V) (23)	Zinc (Zn) (30)	Zirconium (Zr) (40)
Airways					
Rhinitis/nasal injury/sinusitis			X	X	
Tracheitis					
Acute bronchitis	X (TiCl$_4$)		X	X	
Bronchiolitis			X	X	
Bronchiectasis					
Chronic bronchitis			X	X	
Asthma/reactive airways		X	X	X	
Parenchyma					
Acute pneumonitis or pulmonary edema	X (TiCl$_4$)	X		X	X (ZrCl$_4$)
Interstitial fibrosis	X			X	X
Granulomatous pneumonitis	X				X
Benign pneumoconiosis	X				
Emphysema			X		
Metal fume fever/inhalational fever	X			X	
Other respiratory effects	Pleural thickening; bronchial polyposis		Pneumonia		
Other organ effects					
Skin		X	X	X	X
Eyes		X	X	X	
Oropharyngeal			X	X	
Cardiovascular					
Hepatic					
Gastrointestinal				X	
Renal		X	X		
Lymphatic/hematologic				X	
Musculoskeletal/rheumatologic			X	X	
Peripheral nervous system					
Central nervous system			X		
Comments			Green tongue	Most toxicities due to ZnCl$_2$; shared exposure with Cd	

This chapter emphasizes the many and varied sources of exposure, both in and outside of the workplace.

- Third, although some metals induce respiratory tract disease in a dose–response fashion, others produce idiosyncratic effects that do not obey conventional exposure–response principles.
- Fourth, much of the medical literature on metals and the respiratory tract is composed of case reports, only occasionally supported by population-based epidemiologic investigations. It is a literature plagued by multiple workplace exposures producing potential interactions among inhaled toxic materials.
- Fifth, many case descriptions lack histopathologic information and rely on insensitive and nonspecific clinical tools, such as spirometry and chest radiography.

The modern clinician and researcher would be well-advised to consider the published metals literature as only a guide and not as dogma. There is more respiratory tract disease due to metals than is presently realized. Some of the isolated case reports in the literature warrant further, more in-depth investigation of exposed worker populations.

TOXICITY OF SPECIFIC METALS
Aluminum

A spectrum of respiratory tract effects has been attributed to aluminum dust and fume exposure, including asthma, chronic bronchitis, pulmonary fibrosis, granulomatous lung disease, pulmonary alveolar proteinosis, lung cancer, and, in the case of organoaluminum compounds, acute tracheobronchitis, pneumonitis, and pulmonary edema.[25] Some of these effects can be directly attributed to aluminum compounds, while others may be due to the other toxic agents encountered in smelting, welding, or "potroom" electrolysis processes.

In 1936, Frostadt recognized that potroom exposures in aluminum refineries induced asthma.[26] Since that time, many investigators have described the development of cough, wheezing, chest tightness, and leukocytosis with and without eosinophilia among potroom workers, symptoms recently reviewed by Abramson and colleagues.[27,28] Unfortunately, bronchial hyperreactivity may persist even after removal from exposure, although in many cases the use of powered air-purifying respirators or reduction of exposure helps symptoms. Thus, the best approach is to effect primary preventive strategies. The annual incidence of potroom asthma is estimated to be approximately 2%; however the high turnover of workers may result in underestimates. Risk factors for potroom asthma may include prior bronchitis, atopy, cigarette smoking, prior pleurisy, and prior pertussis. High levels of fluoride in the workplace and in urine specimens appear to be associated with cross-shift decrements in airflow. Despite numerous studies, the exact relationship between specific workplace exposures and development of potroom asthma remains obscure.[27]

An excess frequency of COPD has been found among workers with a variety of potential aluminum exposures in different industries. Because of the cross-sectional design of most of the studies, this has not been a consistent finding.[27] When chronic disease has been described, authors report increased frequency of worker symptoms of chronic bronchitis, mucus production, and functional evidence of airflow limitation and emphysema. Taken in composite, it appears that aluminum workers have more respiratory symptoms than control subjects, with productive cough, shortness of breath, chest tightness, and wheezing. Cigarette smoking may have confounded some studies of aluminum smelter workers. The dose–response relationship has been difficult to study, in part because of limitations of the industrial hygiene data.[29-33]

A single case report of pulmonary alveolar proteinosis following aluminum dust exposure in an aluminum rail grinder adds aluminum to the list of potential environmental causes for that disorder.[34]

In the 1940s, investigators first reported radiographic evidence of interstitial fibrosis among aluminum powder workers in Europe.[35,36] Subsequently, numerous case series and case reports have supported the assertion that aluminum, aluminum powder, fume from aluminum arc welding, potroom fumes, and dust from aluminum polishing and abrasive manufacturing induce interstitial fibrosis.[37-43] The interstitial disease is typically described as having an upper lung zone predominance with a reticular pattern. In many of the reported cases, the fibrosis has been progressive over the course of several years, often leading to death. Although the experimental animal data vary, they show that diffuse interstitial fibrosis can occur in animals exposed to pure forms of aluminum oxides and other aluminum compounds.

Although in general aluminum does not induce hypersensitivity responses, the dermatology literature and immunologic studies suggest that aluminum compounds can induce a delayed type hypersensitivity response in a small number of individuals.[44] Individual case reports indicate that sarcoidosis-like granulomatous lung disease can be caused by aluminum[45] or can produce foreign-body type granulomas in the lungs.[46] Interestingly, in a case of sarcoid-like granulomatosis in a chemist who worked with aluminum powders, DeVuyst and colleagues not only demonstrated the presence of aluminum particles within the granulomas but showed the lavage cells to be predominantly CD4$^+$ T-helper lymphocytes. Aluminum sulfate and aluminum chloride stimulated blood lymphocytes to proliferate in vitro, supporting a pathogenic role for cell-mediated immune response to aluminum.[45]

A number of cancer mortality studies reveal an increased relative risk of lung cancer for aluminum workers, whereas others find no such risk among the aluminum smelter workers. It is difficult to discern from these studies whether aluminum or aluminum oxides themselves are carcinogenic, given the presence of other known carcinogens in the aluminum workplace.[47-51]

Flameless atomic absorption, spectrometry, and neutron activation analysis can be used to detect aluminum in serum, whole blood, and urine with the latter generally providing a better indication of exposure. Energy-dispersive x-ray microanalysis and ion beam analyses can detect aluminum within tissue specimens.

Antimony

This metal of antiquity shares many of the toxic properties of arsenic. In the sentinel work on antimony poisoning and the respiratory tract, Renes[52] reported on illness among workers engaged in the mining and smelting of antimony sulfide ore. Illness began shortly after the smelter commenced operation. In the first 5 months, 69 of 78 employees visited the plant's physician due to occupationally associated rhinitis, nasal septal perforation, laryngitis, tracheitis, and/or acute pneumonitis. In six individuals, chest radiographs were taken after particularly heavy smelter fume exposures lasting 2 to 12 hours. All six showed perihilar infiltrates that reportedly improved away from exposure.

In 1966, Taylor reported acute respiratory tract effects from inhalation of antimony trichloride. Workers exposed to fumes developed either acute upper respiratory tract irritative symptoms, delayed onset of gastrointestinal symptoms, or delayed onset of respiratory tract symptomatology 8 hours after exposure.[53] Although hydrochloric acid vapor may have produced some initial irritant and burn symptoms, the fume contained up to 73 mg/m^3 of antimony. Urinary levels for the metal were high. High inhalational exposure to SbCl$_5$ can result in pulmonary edema and death.[54]

In addition to acute respiratory symptoms, antimony is considered a cause of "benign" pneumoconiosis.[55,56] Cooper and colleagues observed that the physiologic impact of antimony pneumoconiosis seemed minimal.[55] In one of the few pathology studies, lung tissue showed macrophages with many intracellular particles but without evidence of fibrosis.[57] In 1963 and 1964 McCallum and colleagues found chest radiographic evidence of pneumoconiosis in 8.5% of workers but with no associated pulmonary function deficits. Small rounded opacities involved all areas of the lung, without forming conglomerate masses.[55,56]

Chronic antimony exposure has been implicated as a cause of COPD. In 1983 Potkonjak and Pavlovich reported airflow obstruction or a mixed obstructive and restrictive pattern in one quarter of antimony-exposed workers.[58] Chronic cough was the most common symptom.

A slight excess risk of lung cancer has been observed among smelter workers who have been exposed to antimony trioxide.[59] Experimental animals develop lung cancer following antimony trioxide exposure, as well.

Treatment of antimony toxicity includes the use of dimercaprol.

Arsenic

This infamous metal has found medicinal, industrial, and sinister application for over 2,000 years.

In addition to being a major avenue for absorption leading to systemic toxicity, the respiratory tract is itself a target organ for inorganic arsenic and arsine. With both acute and chronic exposures, arsenic-exposed workers experience irritant symptoms of the skin, mucus membranes, and conjuctiva. In particular, arsenic workers may develop hoarseness, nasal congestion, oropharyngeal inflammation, increased lacrimation, tongue pain, and perforation of the nasal septum. Cessation of exposure generally leads to resolution of these symptoms.

High dose inhalation of inorganic arsenic compounds or arsine can cause acute onset of cough, dyspnea, and chest pain. This may evolve into acute noncardiogenic pulmonary edema and respiratory failure.[60,61] Pulmonary edema can also result from arsenic-induced myocardial injury with associated cardiac dilitation.[62] Lundgren and colleagues described chronic upper respiratory tract symptoms in Swedish smelter workers exposed to arsenic trixode as well as to sulfur dioxide.[63] Dyspnea develops in some workers as a consequence of the anemia caused by chronic arsine exposure.

The International Agency for Research on Cancer (IARC) classifies arsenic and arsenic compounds as Group 1 human carcinogens (see Table 29-4). An excess rate of respiratory tract cancers is found in major epidemiologic studies. Arsenic exposure plus cigarette smoking has been shown in one study to have a multiplicative effect.[64-74]

Diagnosis of occupational arsenic poisoning starts with knowledge of the work history and of the amount and type of arsenic compound to which the individual has been exposed. Illness among co-workers is an important piece of the occupational history. Blood levels for arsenic are generally poorly reflective of body burden. Biologic assays of hair, nails, and urine have been used in studies of industrial arsenic toxicity[75]; however, the levels may be difficult to relate to occupational exposure because of the presence of arsenic in food, water, and ambient air. Results from laboratories that offer hair and nail testing should be scrutinized carefully because of inconsistent results.[76]

Treatment of arsenic inhalation is supportive. Some authors have suggested the use of dimercaprol (British antilewisite, BAL) in the presence of severe respiratory symptomatology.[77] The advantages and disadvantages of chelation therapy have been recently reviewed.[78]

For medical screening purposes in the workplace, blood arsenic levels generally correlate poorly with exposure. Urinary arsenic excretion is superior and has been shown by some authors to correlate with airborne arsenic.[79] Quantitative 24-hour urine arsenic determinations are the most reliable method and may be helpful in medical screening and in diagnosis. Measurement of monomethylarsonic acid (MMA) and dimethylarsinic acid (DMA), methylated deri-

Table 29-4. International Agency for Research on Cancer (IARC) classification of carcinogenicity of metals*[64,111,134]

Metal	Comment	IARC class†	Species	Types of malignancy
Aluminum (Al)	Production (associated risk; may not be caused by aluminum)	1	Human	Lung, bladder, lymphosarcoma, reticulosarcoma, pancreatic, leukemia, esophageal, stomach, urinary bladder
Arsenic (As)	Arsenic and arsenic compounds	1	Human	Skin, liver, angiosarcoma, intestinal, bladder, meningioma, kidney, lung, colon, gastrointestinal, renal, hematolymphatic, stomach
			Animal	Lung, stomach, renal
Beryllium (Be)	Beryllium and beryllium compounds	1	Human	Lung
			Animal	Lung, osteosarcoma
Cadmium (Cd)	Cadmium and cadmium compounds	1	Human	Prostatic, nasopharyngeal, colorectal, lung, genitourinary, renal
			Animal	Testicular, pancreatic, lung, prostatic
Chromium (Cr)	Chromium metal	3	Human	Lung, gastrointestinal, stomach, pancreatic
	Trivalent chromium compounds	3		
	Hexavalent chromium compounds	1	Animal	Bronchial
Iron (Fe)	Iron and steel founding	1	Human	Lung, digestive, stomach, genitourinary, prostatic, renal, leukemia, urogenital
Lead (Pb)	Lead and inorganic lead compounds	2B	Human	Digestive, stomach, lung, renal, bladder, brain
	Organolead compounds	3		
			Animal	Renal, lung, liver, kidney
Mercury (Hg)	Methylmercury compounds	2B	Human	Lung, brain, liver, esophagus
	Metallic mercury and inorganic mercury compounds	3	Animal	Kidney, renal, stomach
Nickel (Ni)	Nickel and nickel compounds	1	Human	Nasal cavity, lung, laryngeal, respiratory tract
			Animal	Muscular, renal, testicular, ocular, trachea, lung

*Data shown are for those metals where information on IARC classification of carcinogenicity was available. At the time of writing, the following metals were not classified: Sb, Ba, B, Ca, Co, Cu, Au, Li, Mg, Mn, Os, P, Pt, Yb, Ce, Se, Th, Sn, Ti, Ur, V, Z, and Zr.

†Group 1 = the agent is carcinogenic to humans. Group 2A = the agent is probably carcinogenic to humans (limited evidence in humans, sufficient evidence with animals). Group 2B = the agent is possibly carcinogenic to humans (limited evidence in humans in the absence of sufficient evidence in animals; inadequate or absent evidence in humans but sufficient in animals; sometimes based on limited evidence in animals). Group 3 = the agent is not classifiable as to its carcinogenicity to humans. Group 4 = the agent is probably not carcinogenic to humans (evidence suggesting a lack of carcinogenicity in humans and in experimental animals).

vates of inorganic arsenic, can help distinguish those body levels of arsenic that may come from ingestion of water or seafood.

The key to prevention of respiratory toxicity due to arsenic centers around appropriate workplace ventilation, industrial hygiene monitoring, medical screening, and recognition that mishandling of chemicals can liberate highly toxic trivalent arsinates and particularly hazardous arsine gas.

Barium

By virtue of its high atomic number, barium is radioopaque and associated with the development of what is generally considered to be a benign pneumoconiosis, "baritosis."[80,81] This conditions develops following the inhalation of fine ground barium sulfate. In general there are no respiratory symptoms, and no pulmonary function abnormalities based on spirometry. Chest x-rays show sharply circumscribed small nodules without conglomerate mass formation. The nodular opacities have been described as either rounded or reticular, and are evenly distributed in the lungs. With removal from exposure to barium, there is gradual improvement in the number of nodular opacities. Interestingly, although there is little published on the histologic appearance of occupational baritosis, biopsies from patients who have aspirated barium sulfate during radiographic procedures open speculation as to whether barium is truly inert. Záková and Svoboda described a patient who aspirated barium 2 months prior to his death in whom foreign body granulomas and localized areas of fibrosis developed in the areas of retained barium within the pulmonary interstitium. Similar lesions were observed in rabbits exposed to the same contrast medium.[82] Barium granulomas have been described in other case reports.[83] It is reasonable to conclude that whereas inhaled barium sulfate is of low toxicity it has the potential to induce a mild fibrotic and foreign body granulomatous response in humans.

Beryllium

In addition to the occupational exposures listed in Table 29-1, nonoccupational, environmentally induced beryllium disease occurred in communities surrounding beryllium extraction plants in the 1940s and 1950s. Second-hand exposure cases in family members continue to occur.[84-86] Historically, beryllium was used in the manufacture of fluorescent and neon lights, leading Hardy and colleagues to recognize "Salem sarcoid" as a consequence of beryllium exposure.[87]

The exposure–response relationship involved in the development of beryllium lung disease has been the subject of controversy for over 40 years. Early studies of residents in the communities surround the beryllium extraction plant suggested that low levels of exposure could produce chronic beryllium disease (CBD), in seeming defiance of principles of dose–response.[88] Sterner and Eisenbud thus postulated a "hypersensitivity" mechanism for beryllium disease. When the United States industry adopted the 1949 Atomic Energy Commission inhalational exposure standard (see Table 29-5), the acute form of beryllium pneumonitis largely disappeared.[89] That standard did not eliminate the chronic form of beryllium disease. Studies conducted in the 1980s and 1990s show that CBD continues to occur in industry and develops in some individuals even at extremely low levels of exposure.[19,20,90] It has been commonly held for 40 years that beryllium hypersensitivity and disease occur without regard to magnitude of exposure. Our understanding of this concept has changed as a result of recent epidemiologic investigations showing that the risk of disease is related to work task and magnitude of past exposure[20,91-101] Beryllium sensitization and lung disease continue to occur even in industries attempting to comply with existing exposure standards. All principal forms of beryllium have been implicated, including the beryllium copper alloy that contains only 1 to 4% beryllium. The ore itself is thought to be nontoxic but epidemiologic studies of miners have not been performed.

The inhalational effects of beryllium include acute pneumonitis, tracheobronchitis, chronic beryllium disease, and an increased risk of lung cancer.

The acute pneumonitis common in the 1940s and 1950s has largely disappeared with improved workplace controls of exposure. It is unclear from review of the early reports whether the acute disease was a chemical pneumonitis or an early, aggressive form of beryllium-specific cellular immune response, or both. Interestingly, acute disease progresses to chronic granulomatous lung disease in up to one third of cases.[101]

Patients with CBD, formerly known as "berylliosis" or "chronic berylliosis," develop insidious onset of dyspnea on exertion, cough, fatigue, and in some cases weight loss and anorexia. Some patients present with a more precipitous course. Other symptoms may include fever, arthralgias, night sweats, chest pain. Usually the disease is limited to the lungs, with interstitial and endobronchial involvement, and the thoracic lymph nodes, but it may affect skin, liver, spleen, myocardium, skeletal muscle, salivary glands, kidney, and bone. Latency from time of first beryllium exposure to the development of clinically obvious disease ranges from a few months to 40 years.[19,20,101,102]

Chest radiographs range from being completely normal to demonstrating small nodular opacities throughout the lung fields sometimes with more upper lobe predominance, and formation of conglomerate masses as the disease progresses. Mediastinal adenopathy is observed on approximately one third of chest radiographs. Pleural reaction occurs in more advanced stages of disease, often adjacent to areas of greatest parenchymal involvement.[103-105] A recent study of thin-section computed tomography (CT) demonstrated four predominant findings on CT scans: small ill-defined nodules, septal lines, areas of ground-glass attenuation, and adenopathy.[103]

Physiologic alterations in CBD include airflow obstruction, or a mixed pattern of obstruction and restriction. Later in the course of disease, restrictive physiology predominates. The most sensitive indicator of physiologic embarrassment due to beryllium disease is the demonstration of worsening gas exchange during maximum exercise testing.[106]

Histopathologic examination in this disease demonstrates noncaseating granulomas with mononuclear cell infiltrates and varying degrees of interstitial pulmonary fibrosis.[84,107] The pulmonary histologic appearance is indistinguishable from sarcoidosis. The demonstration of beryllium in tissue from beryllium workers does not necessarily prove that beryllium has caused the disease, and the absence of beryllium from tissue analyses does not exclude the diagnosis, especially in light of the hypersensitivity mechanism underlying this disorder.[108] Hence, the current diagnostic approach relies more on biologic markers of immunopathogenesis and the demonstration of typical histopathology.

The major differential diagnostic dilemma is to separate workers with suspected CBD from sarcoidosis, a multisystem granulomatous disorder of unknown cause.[108] Historically, it was difficult to distinguish sarcoidosis from CBD because of the lack of specific and reliable discriminating tools. The beryllium lymphocyte transformation test, also called the beryllium lymphocyte proliferation test (BeLPT), is now a standard part of the clinical armamentarium for beryllium disease diagnosis in the United States.[22] The test quantitates the beryllium-specific cellular immune response based on cell uptake of radiolabeled DNA precursors. The BeLPT identifies over 90% of individuals who have CBD.

Table 29-5. Regulatory standards for metals associated with respiratory tract disorders

Metal	ACGIH TLVs			OSHA PELs		
	TWA* (mg/m³)	STELs† (mg/m³)	Comment	TWA* (mg/m³)	STELs† (mg/m³)	Comment
Aluminum (Al)	10		Metal dust	15		Total dust
	5		Pyro powders	5		Respirable fraction
	5		Welding fumes	5		Pyro powders
	2		Soluble salts	5		Welding fumes
	2		Alkyls	2		Soluble salts
	10		Oxides	2		Alkyls
Antimony (Sb)	0.5		Compounds	0.5		Compounds
	0.5		Trioxide			
Arsenic (As)	0.01		Elemental and inorganic compounds	0.5		Organic compounds
Barium (Ba)	0.5		Soluble compounds	0.5		Soluble compounds
	10		Sulfate	10		Sulfate—total dust
				5		Sulfate—respirable fraction
Beryllium (Be)	0.002			0.002 ppm	0.005 ppm (30 mins)	
Boron (B)	10		Oxide	10		Oxide—total dust
	10		Tribromide-ceiling limit	5		Oxide—total dust
	2.8		Trifluoride-ceiling limit			
Cadmium (Cd)	0.01		Elemental and compounds; total dust/particulate			
	0.002		Respirable fraction of dust			
Chromium (Cr)	0.5		Metal	1		Metal
	0.5		Chromium II compounds	0.5		Chromium II compounds
	0.5		Chromium III compounds	0.5		Chromium III compounds
	0.05		Chromium VI compounds, water soluble			
	0.05		Chromium VI compounds, certain water insoluble			
Cobalt (Co)	0.05		Metal dust and fume	0.05		Metal, dust, and fume
	0.1		Carbonyl	0.1		Carbonyl
	0.1		Hydrocarbonyl	0.1		Hydrocarbonyl
Copper (Cu)	0.2		Fume	0.1		Fume
	1		Dust and mists	1		Dust and mists
Iron (Fe)	5		Oxide fume	10		Oxide dust and fume (total particulate)
	0.23	0.45	Pentacarbonyl	0.8	1.6	Pentacarbonyl
	1		Soluble salts	1		Soluble salts
Lead (Pb)	0.15		Inorganic dust and fume			
	0.15		Arsenate			
Lithium (Li)	0.025		Hydride	0.025		Hydride
Magnesium (Mg)	10		Oxide fume	10		Oxide fume—total dust
				5		Oxide fume—respirable fraction
Manganese (Mn)	5		Dust and compound			Compounds
	1	3	Fume	1	3	Fume
	0.1		Cyclopentadienyl tricarbonyl	0.1		Cyclopentadienyl tricarbonyl

Continued.

Table 29-5. Regulatory standards for metals associated with respiratory tract disorders—cont'd

Metal	ACGIH TLVs			OSHA PELs		
	TWA* (mg/m³)	STELs† (mg/m³)	Comment	TWA* (mg/m³)	STELs† (mg/m³)	Comment
Mercury (Hg)	0.01	0.03	Alkyl compounds	0.01	0.03	Alkyl compounds
	0.05		All forms except alkyl-vapor	0.05		Vapor
	0.1		Aryl and inorganic compounds			Aryl and inorganic compounds
Nickel (Ni)	1		Metal	0.007		Carbonyl
	1		Insoluble compounds	1		Metal and insoluble compounds
	0.1		Soluble compounds	0.1		Soluble compounds
	0.12		Carbonyl			
	1		Sulfide roasting, fume, and dust			
Osmium (Os)	0.0016	0.0047	Tetroxide	0.002	0.006	Tetroxide
Phosphorus (P)	0.1		Yellow	0.1		Yellow
	0.63		Oxychloride	0.6		Oxychloride
	0.85		Pentachloride	1		Pentachloride
	1	3	Pentasulfide	1	3	Pentasulfide
	1.1	2.8	Trichloride	1.5	3	Trichloride
Platinum (Pt)	1		Metal	1		Metal
	0.002		Soluble salts	0.002		Soluble salts
Rare earths						
Yttrium (Yb)		1	Metal and compounds		1	
Cerium (Ce)	1					
Selenium (Sc)	0.2		Compounds	0.2		Compounds
	0.16		Hexafluoride	0.4		Hexafluoride
Thallium (Th)	0.1		Elemental and soluble compounds	0.1		Soluble compounds
Tin (Sn)	2		Metal	2		Inorganic compounds except oxides
	2		Oxide and inorganic compounds except SnH_4	0.1		Organic compounds
	0.1	0.2	Organic compounds	2		Oxides
Titanium (Ti)	10		Dioxide	10		Dioxide—total dust
				5		Dioxide—respirable fraction
Uranium (Ur)	0.2	0.6	Soluble and insoluble compounds	0.05		Soluble compounds
				0.2	0.6	Insoluble compounds
Vanadium (V)	0.05		Pentoxide as V_2O_5; respirable dust or fume	0.05		Respirable dust V_2O_5
				0.05		Fume V_2O_5
Zinc (Z)	5	10	Oxide fume	5	10	Oxide fume
	10		Oxide dust	10		Oxide—total dust
				5		Oxide—respirable fraction
Zirconium (Zr)	5	10	Compounds	5	10	Compounds

*Concentration for a normal 8-hour work day and a 40-hour work week.
†Fifteen-minute exposure, which should not be exceeded at any time during a work day even if 8 hours TWA is within the TLV.
ACGIH, American Conference of Governmental Industrial Hygienists (1993–1994 #1138); *OSHA,* U.S. Occupational Safety and Health Administration (1989 #1139); *PELs,* permissible exposure limits; *STELs,* short-term exposure limit; *TLV,* threshold limit value; *TWA,* time-weighted average.

A small subset of individuals has normal blood beryllium lymphocyte transformation tests to beryllium but abnormal BAL beryllium lymphocyte transformation tests, revealing the intrapulmonary beryllium-specific cell-mediated immune response. Some individuals with repeatedly abnormal blood beryllium lymphocyte transformation tests do not have CBD, but are beryllium sensitized. Longitudinal data suggest that over half of these individuals progress to develop CBD. Thus, the BeLPT can identify people in preclinical stages of this disorder and can also be used to screen for beryllium disease among individuals with so-called "sarcoidosis." Under some circumstances, individuals with CBD have falsely negative BAL beryllium lymphocyte transformation tests due to inhibitory effects of alveolar macrophages or due to the effect of corticosteroids.

The current diagnostic criteria for CBD required an individual to have (1) a history of beryllium exposure, (2) demonstration of a beryllium-specific cell-mediated immune response, and (3) granulomas and/or mononuclear cell infiltrates, in the absence of evidence for infection. In addition to its use in clinical diagnosis, the blood BeLPT is helpful in the medical screening of populations of beryllium-exposed workers.[20,92] Compared with other tests used conventionally in medical screening programs, the blood BeLPT is more sensitive than symptoms reporting, physical examination, lung mechanics, diffusing capacity, or chest radiograph. This test also has high negative and positive predictive values.[20,91,109]

A recent study suggests that individuals with beryllium disease share a common allelic substitution in the HLA-DP gene that serves as a marker of beryllium disease risk.[100,110] These data present the strongest evidence to date that beryllium disease results from both exposure to beryllium and a genetic difference that may confer susceptibility. In the future, there may be a role for use of genetic markers of beryllium sensitivity.[100,110] At this time there is no place for such testing, until further research is conducted. The details of the immunology and immunopathogenesis of beryllium disease have been reviewed elsewhere.[84,101]

Beryllium disease is treated with oral corticosteroids. Although the earlier literature suggests that low-dose steroids are usually effective, more current experience suggests that a sizable subset of individuals requires high doses of prednisone (30 to 60 mg/day) to control the progression of disease. Second line immunosuppressive medications and lung transplantation should be considered in such circumstances if there is no response to prednisone. If diagnosed early, mild disease may not require steroid therapy until clinical symptoms and gas exchange abnormalities occur. Clinical monitoring for disease progression is best performed using measures of gas exchange such as arterial blood gases at rest and at maximum exercise.

In early cohort studies of workers from two extraction and production facilities, a slight excess of lung cancer deaths was observed. Subsequent studies of workers from seven beryllium plants confirmed a small statistically significant excess mortality for lung cancer. Using cases of beryllium disease from the U.S. Beryllium Case Registry, investigators have shown an excess in lung-related cancer mortality. This was especially observed among those who had previous acute beryllium disease. A recent IARC working group reclassified beryllium as a Group 1 human carcinogen (see Chapter 34). Experimental animal data also support the tumorigenicity of beryllium (see Table 29-4).[113]

In light of the carcinogenesis data and studies of Kreiss and colleagues showing work task-related risk for CBD, there is good reason to push for tight regulatory controls over beryllium emissions in the workplace, for diligence on the part of industry in reducing exposure to the lowest possible levels, and for screening exposed workers with the blood BeLPT.

Boron

Although metallic boron is considered nontoxic, the boranes (boron hydrides) are highly toxic, particularly to the respiratory and neurologic systems.

Diborane (B_2H_6) produces the most significant respiratory toxicity although pentaborane and to a lesser extent decaborane can affect the respiratory tract as well. Our understanding of the respiratory tract effects stems from studies in the 1950s on boron use by laboratory workers[112] and boron hydride workers[113] and in the production of high energy fuels.[114] The respiratory tract effects of the boranes include acute pneumonitis that may be due to a chemical toxicity or be the results of secondary infection, an asthma-like condition with severe variable air flow obstruction, pulmonary edema, and transient respiratory insufficiency associated with neuromuscular collapse due to effects of borane hydride.

Cordasco and colleagues studied workers exposed to experimental space fuels, confirming earlier observations that diborane produces the majority of respiratory toxicity, with respiratory symptomatology noted in fewer individuals exposed to decaborane or pentaborane.[114] In their study, diborane caused chest tightness, dyspnea, nonproductive cough, and wheezing that lasted 3 to 5 days in most patients. In a second group of patients with subacute exposures, cough and chest tightness were the predominant symptoms.[113] On physical examination the acute and subacute exposure cases developed inspiratory and expiratory rhonchi. These authors also report on three "chronic diborane patients" who had persistent wheezing, dyspnea, chest tightness, and dry nonproductive cough. The dyspnea was worse with exertion and the wheezing was aggravated by exertion in two and constant in one individual. In these chronic cases the authors observed inspiratory and expiratory rales without rhonchi. Some developed hypoxemia at rest and with exercise. Chest radiographs, when abnormal, generally showed increased bronchovascular markings.

Although the original report of boron hydride toxicity by Rozendaal[112] suggested that "metal fume fever" may develop, careful review of this literature favors a chemical pneumonitis, with development of radiographic evidence of consolidation during the acute phases, resolving within several days.

In addition to removal from exposure, treatment includes management of the neuromuscular symptoms, protection of the airway, and supplemental oxygen. In the cases of air flow obstruction, corticosteroids and bronchodilators may be helpful. Prevention of this condition requires special handling and storage of boron and the boranes with appropriate avoidance of contact with water.

Cadmium

Inhalation of cadmium fumes, principally cadmium oxide in welding, smelting, and soldering, produces respiratory symptoms within 24 hours of the exposure. Patients develop shortness of breath, fever, fatigue, and can progress to profound respiratory insufficiency with pulmonary edema, and death.[115-117] The acute lung disorder has been described as both a chemical pneumonitis and as noncardiogenic pulmonary edema. In individuals who have survived such episodes, late sequelae, such as intersitital fibrosis in a peribronchial and perivascular distribution and the development of emphysema may occur.[118-123] The lethal exposure is estimated to be approximately 50 mg Cd/m^3 for 1 hour (cadmium oxide dust) or one-half hour (for fume).[116]

Common upper respiratory tract complaints in chronically exposed workers include chronic rhinitis and anosmia. With chronic low dose inhalational exposure, cadmium can cause emphysema, with dose-related decrements in lung function and diffusing capacity compared to control subjects.[124,125] Cadmium workers experience increased mortality due to nonmalignant respiratory disorders.[126-130]

There is limited evidence of cadmium and cadmium compound carcinogenicity in humans (see Chapter 34). Exposure to the oxide has been associated with increased risk of respiratory as well as prostatic cancer.[131] In a study of cadmium-nickel battery workers in Sweden, excesses of nasopharyngeal, lung prostatic, and colorectal cancer were reported.[132] In a study of 6,995 workers exposed to cadmium in Britain, excesses of lung cancer and prostatic cancer were reported.[133] IARC has found the evidence for carcinogenicity in animals to be sufficient.[134] The significance of cadmium as a human carcinogen remains controversial.[135]

Treatment of chronic cadmium intoxication has been advocated with use of intravenous calcium gluconate and subcutaneous vitamin D. Chelators will have difficulty reaching and binding cadmium that is mostly already bound to metallothionein. The exception may be very early in acute cadmium poisoning.[136] At this time neither the use of British antilewisite or ethylenediaminetetraacetic acid is recommended for treatment of cadmium toxicity. Monitoring of urine cadmium levels may reflect excessive body burdens in some individuals but does not correlate well with either the magnitude of exposure or disease severity.[137] Other investigators have shown that urinary cadmium levels do provide a good measure of excessive cadmium exposure.[116] Periodical medical examinations of cadmium-exposed workers should include inquiry into gastrointestinal complaints, rhinitis, and anosmia. Teeth should be inspected for yellow discoloration, and in some cases cadmium-related proteinuria may be detected by urinalysis. Periodic pulmonary function tests may be helpful in detecting serial decline in airflow. Prevention is best effected by adherence to recommended industrial hygiene standards. Because of prolonged retention of cadmium in the body, current permissible exposure limits may not be protective for workers with long tenure.

Chromium

Hexavalent chromium compounds in general have higher toxicity than trivalent chromium compounds. The most common acute chromium toxicity in the workplace is the induction of nasal mucosal irritation, ulceration, and septal perforation. In 1827, "chrome holes" were first described on the hands and arms of workers exposed to dichromates. These penetrating ulcers can involve the nasal septum, crusting over in some cases but forming chronic ulcers with intermittent purulent discharge in others. Lindberg and Hedenstierna reported the development of nasal septal ulceration and perforation at relatively low levels of exposure to chromic acid, within current threshold limit values (TLVs).[138,139] In addition to nasal mucosal symptoms, low level exposures to hexavalent chromium compounds can induce gingivitis, conjunctivitis, and keratitis. Workers frequently complain of chronic bronchitis, rhinitis, and sinusitis with formation of nasal polyps as well, in some instances.[140-143] Chronic pharyngitis and tracheitis occur with acute or chronic exposures.

Other respiratory tract effects related to higher levels of acute exposure include acute chromium-induced pneumonitis,[140] pleuritis with pleural effusion,[144] and a metal fume fever pattern of illness in ferrochrome workers exposed to fresh chromium oxide.[145]

Pulmonary sensitization from hexavalent and to a lesser extent from trivalent chromium compounds can result in asthma. Asthma from chromium compounds has been described among those exposed to chromium bicarbonate, chromite ore, chromic acid, and chrome spray paints. It is seen both with and without coexisting allergic contact dermatitis.[140,146-149] In some cases, chromium-specific skin prick tests, patch tests, and radioallergosorbent tests (RASTs) have been reported.

Epidemiologic studies of occupational cohorts exposed to chromium indict it as a carcinogen (see Chapter 34). Hexavalent chromium in particular has been associated with increased lung cancer mortality and is considered a Group 1 human carcinogen by IARC (see Table 29-4).[150-153]

Key to the prevention of toxicity due to chromic acid and other chromates is to avoid skin and inhalational contact in the workplace. It is important to recognize that the permissible exposure limits (PELs) listed in Table 29-5 are not protective for all workers, especially those who develop hypersensitivity responses (dermatitis, asthma) or nasal mucosal and upper respiratory irritative symptoms.

Cobalt

With acute high exposures to cobalt fumes, a form of chemical pneumonitis and pulmonary edema can develop.

Problems encountered in relation to chronic cobalt exposure, especially among tungsten carbide workers, include occupational asthma, hypersensitivity pneumonitis, giant cell interstitial pneumonitis (GIP), bronchiolitis obliterans, and interstitial fibrosis. There is substantial overlap with some of these outcomes occurring concomitantly. The term "hard metal disease" is an unfortunate label that blurs the distinctions among these hard metal-related conditions. As such, it is probably more appropriate to discuss each clinicopathologic condition in relation to cobalt exposure rather than emphasize the term "hard metal disease."

Respiratory tract irritant symptoms and reticulonodular infiltrates due to hard metal exposure were reported first in Germany in the 1940s and 1950s.[154,155] Later, Fairhall and colleagues noted symptoms of bronchitis, rhinitis, and conjuctivitis among tungsten carbide workers in the United States.[156] Many of these workers also developed pruritis as seen earlier by Jobs and Ballhausen.[154]

Hard metal-associated asthma produces the typical symptoms of cough, wheezing, and shortness of breath.[154,157] In some instances, patients with cobalt-related asthma also develop manifestations of hypersensitivity pneumonitis.[158] The asthmatic response typically has a delayed onset of approximately 4 to 6 hours.[158] At first, workers may report improvement in asthma and pruritis symptoms with time off work. The latency between first exposure and the development of symptoms varies from 6 to 48 months.[157] Asthma may result from exposure to cobalt metal dust, as occurs when milling cobalt metal, as well as in relation to tungsten carbide.

Development of a clinical pattern likened to chronic hypersensitivity pneumonitis occurs subacutely with the insidious onset of nonproductive cough, exertional dyspnea, and weight loss, or with acute respiratory and systemic symptoms associated with workplace exposures. Clinical findings may include dry rales and irregular or rounded opacities on the chest radiograph. Although the clinical pattern is that of hypersensitivity pneumonitis, pathologic findings generally have not shown granulomas but appear more as either desquamative interstitial pneumonitis or GIP, with or without bronchiolitis obliterans, and varying degrees of interstitial fibrosis.[158,159] The histology may vary and even overlap. In some cases, the clinical course may be misdiagnosed as a viral infection. Removal from work leads to

improvement in symptoms, with recrudescence upon return to work. Over time, return to work produces less acute symptoms but gradually increasing dyspnea as the condition becomes more chronic. Lung volumes become restrictive and diffusing capacity falls. In some instances, the administration of corticosteroids may produce clinical and radiographic improvement, but some individuals are left with end-stage interstitial fibrosis as a result of repeated episodes of pneumonitis.[157,160]

GIP described by Liebow[161] was not initially associated with cobalt exposure. Abraham and Spragg made the link among occupational exposure, pulmonary pathology, and BAL in a patient with GIP[9,157,162,163] and other investigators have confirmed this association.[157,162,163] A history of cobalt and hard metal exposure should be carefully explored whenever GIP is found on lung biopsy. At the end stage of GIP, patients can develop pulmonary hypertension and cor pulmonale and increasingly severe interstitial fibrosis and honeycomb lung. A subset of patients experiences a rapidly progressive and sometime fatal interstitial fibrosis akin to that seen with idiopathic pulmonary fibrosis.

In the event that tissue mineral analyses are performed on lung biopsies of hard metal workers, tungsten will be found and cobalt may be absent because of cobalt's high solubility and rapid transit from the lung. Experimental animal studies and human case series' workers exposed purely to cobalt confirm that cobalt, not the tungsten, causes GIP, desquamative interstitial pneumonitis, and interstitial fibrosis pattern of disease in these workers.[157,159,164-166]

Despite inconsistencies and methodologic limitations of in vitro immunologic studies, the dermatology literature clearly documents allergic contact dermatitis in tungsten carbide alloy workers.[167] and shows that cobalt salts can induce delayed-type hypersensitivity responses by patch testing.[168] Individuals who are sensitized to cobalt often react to nickel as well. In vivo studies using cobalt salts have shown positive lymphocyte proliferative responses in individuals who have positive patch test reactions.[23,169,170] These data suggest a cell-mediated immune mechanism, although some asthma patients develop cobalt specific-IgE based on modified RAST.[171] Alternatively, nonimmunologic mechanisms may contribute to the development of cobalt-related respiratory conditions.[172]

Copper

Copper fumes and dust can cause nasal passage and upper airway irritation and copper sulfate has been implicated in "vineyard sprayer's lung." Copper fumes may be a cause of metal fume fever, but in general there have been few reports of respiratory tract illness related to copper, especially given its common use in industry.

Nasal and pharyngeal irritant symptoms are common among workers exposed to high levels of copper fume and dust, and can cause nasal ulceration and nasal septal perforation.[173] Workers polishing copper plates have reported coryzal symptoms with malaise, fever, and nasal congestion.[174] A more dramatic form of febrile illness has been reported among workers exposed to copper welding fumes in a copper factory and with copper acetate exposure.

Vineyard sprayer's lung. A form of interstitial lung disease known as "vineyard sprayer's lung" has been well-described among Portuguese vineyard workers who spray an antimildew agent referred to as "Bordeaux mixture." This aerosolized solution includes 1:2.5% copper sulfate neutralized.[175]

With prolonged, intermittent exposure, usually over the course of several years, sprayers develop dyspnea, weight loss, productive cough, fatigue, and gradually progressive chronic respiratory insufficiency. Several forms of this respiratory condition have been described. (1) "Subclinical forms" in which asymptomatic individuals have abnormal chest radiographs show small nodular densities in the lung bases corresponding to hyalinized granulomas similar to those seen in silicosis but in the absence of any silica exposure. (2) "Active forms" or "acute exacerbations of subclinical forms" develop either acutely or insidiously. Individuals with insidious onset present with fatigue, anorexia, weight loss, and dyspnea. Chest radiographs show a diffuse miliary or nodular pattern. Granulomas are seen on biopsy. In the acute cases, individuals report recurrent respiratory infections, fever, and purulent sputum, sometimes with hemoptysis. Chest radiographs show nodular and reticular infiltrates and consolidation that can lead to cavitation. (3) "Chronic forms," which include (a) small nodules that form conglomerate masses and pulmonary massive fibrosis in the upper lung fields, and (b) "diffuse progressive fibrosis," characterize histologically progressive interstitial fibrosis as well as foreign body type granulomas.[175-177] Hyalinized granulomas may also form in the nasal and bronchial mucosa. Interestingly, in all of these patterns, the lung tissue is densely infiltrated with copper.

Other organs may be involved in this condition, with hyalinized granulomas in the kidney and thoracic lymph nodes, and hepatic involvement with fibrosis, cirrhosis, angiosarcoma, and portal hypertension. In some cases, non-caseating type granulomas have been observed, raising the possibility of a cellular immune mechanism underlying this condition.

In one clinical series of 33 cases of vineyard sprayer's lung, 21% developed lung cancer.[176] In a review of over 20,000 autopsies of rural workers who died in a wine-producing region of Portugal, 832 cases of the vineyard sprayer's lung were detected among 4,100 individuals who had lung pathology. Of the autopsied patients who had evidence of vineyard sprayer's lung, 108 also had lung cancer.[175,178]

Pathologic lesions consistent with vineyard sprayer's lung have been reproduced experimentally in guinea pigs using the Bordeaux mixture itself as well as with organocupric and organosulfuric fungicides. Interestingly, in a 1966 study in which albino rats received endotracheal or inhalational exposures to metallic copper dust or copper oxide dust they developed diffuse nodular and interstitial fibrotic lung disease.[179]

The mechanism underlying vineyard sprayer's lung has not been carefully studied. Whether it represents a form of delayed-type hypersensitivity to a copper-containing antigen or results from other inflammatory mechanisms remains to be elucidated.

Removal from exposure improves the prognosis for some vinesprayers, especially those who have had the acute episodes or who have subclinical disease. Without removal from exposure, the majority of patients progress to the more chronic forms, although a subset of individuals with subclinical disease may remain asymptomatic despite radiographic abnormalities.

Reviews on copper toxicity report a clinical pattern consistent with metal fume fever in workers exposed in a paint factory where copper oxide was crushed, in welders exposed to copper fumes, and in a copper factory.[180] Inhalational fever due to copper warrants further study.

Gold

Although occupational inhalational exposures have not resulted in illness, the condition referred to as "gold lung" warrants mention given the similarity it shares with a number of respiratory disorders due to inhaled metals, such as beryllium. Use of gold in pharmaceuticals can cause interstitial pulmonary fibrosis and hypersensitivity pneumonitis. Recent research implicates a cell-mediated immune response to gold salts in the pathogenesis of this condition.[98,181-184] Allergic contact dermatitis, stomatitis, and glomerulonephritis have been reported. Patch testing with gold salt solutions can confirm a delayed-type hypersensitivity response in individuals with gold-related skin conditions.

Iron

In considering the respiratory tract effects of iron and iron oxides, it is critical to recognize that many workers exposed to iron are simultaneously exposed to other dusts such as asbestos and silica. Differentiating pure siderosis from mixed dust pneumoconiosis can be difficult.

Siderosis resulting from the inhalation of iron oxides occurs in a variety of settings, including the manufacture of iron oxide, the preparation of emery rock for grinders and adhesives, the use of emery wheels, the preparation of pigments, and the polishing of jewelry or silver with "rouge." Welders frequently encounter iron oxide fumes, especially if working in confined spaces on boilers, tanks, or below ship deck. In most major case series of workers with siderosis, little or no respiratory tract morbidity or mortality is found.[185-188] However, case reports and small case series raise the possibility that under some circumstances iron oxide can cause respiratory symptoms such as cough and sputm production, with associated physiologic abnormalities.[189-192] Earlier studies often failed to note smoking status or could not exclude concomitant exposures to fibrogenic dusts. Nonetheless, the more recent literature suggests that siderosis is not a benign condition in all patients, although it generally causes little fibrosis or physiologic impairment.

In pure siderosis, chest radiographs demonstrate fine dense linear opacities without conglomerate masses. Kerley's B-lines are observed if iron accumulates in interlobular septa. As the lymph nodes accumulate iron as well, they may appear more radiodense but not enlarged. The opacities generally develop after many years of metallic iron dust or iron oxide fume exposure, although in some cases high intensity exposures over as little as 3 years can cause radiograph abnormalities.[185] The differential diagnosis for this radiographic abnormality includes exposure to other radiodense dusts such as tin, antimony, or barium. The fine linear opacities of siderosis can be mistaken for asbestosis but appear different from the typical nodular patterns seen with silicosis or coal workers' pneumoconiosis. In some circumstances, the radiographic abnormalities seen in siderosis gradually improve or clear following removal from exposure.[193,194]

Unfortunately the medical literature has only limited information concerning the histopathology in individuals with siderosis. In those welders, miners and others with suspected siderosis versus mixed dust pneumoconiosis, the use of microanalytic techniques such as SEM/EDXM help determine which metals or other particles are present in the regions of pulmonary pathology.[192] In workers exposed to iron oxides, careful attention should be given to the occupational history and lung histology to determine whether other potentially injurious dusts have been inhaled.

Many epidemiologic mortality studies of iron ore miners observed increased risks of lung cancer. Similarly, excess lung cancer mortality has been seen among ferrous foundry workers and in the steel industry.[194-200] Among the studies of miners, some implicate iron oxides as lung carcinogens, although it is also possible that the iron oxides are cocarcinogens or that some of the risk may be due to other exposures, including radon.[200]

Iron carbonyl (pentacarbonyliron, C_5FeO_5) is a colorless, pyrophoric liquid that forms F_2O_3, $Fe_2(CO)^9$ + CO in air. Generated during the manufacturing process for powdered iron cores for radios and televisions and used as a catalyst and automotive fuel additive, iron carbonyl is a potential respiratory tract hazard. Inhalation causes acute toxicity similar to nickel carbonyl, producing pulmonary irritant symptoms and some cases of pulmonary edema.

Lead

Lead has been included in this chapter because of the importance of the respiratory tract as a major route of exposure. With the possible exception of an association with increased lung cancer risk, there have been no published reports of lead toxicity for the respiratory tract.

IARC has categorized lead compounds as possible human carcinogens and organolead compounds as not classifiable (Table 29-2). The basis for these determinations has been summarized in a recent monograph.[64] There have been multiple epidemiologic studies of workers exposed to lead and lead compounds including workers in smelters and in battery production. The majority of these studies showed excess rates of respiratory cancers, not reaching statistical significance. Most studies have not shown an association between either the magnitude or duration of exposure to lead and rate of respiratory cancer. Potential confounding factors include tobacco smoke and arsenic.[201,202]

Prevention of lead poisoning requires recognition of the potential sources of exposure and of the signs and symptoms of this condition. From a pulmonary perspective, it should be remembered that disease continues to occur because of inadequate ventilation and inappropriate respiratory protection from inhalable lead.

Lithium

Lithium hydride is an irritating gas that can produce coughing and sneezing.[203] It has also been associated with the development of acute pulmonary edema in a worker exposed in a confined space.[204]

Magnesium

Fresh, insoluble magnesium oxide (MgO) can produce a pattern of inhalational fever analogous to the metal fume fever seen with zinc oxide. In a group of seven foundry workers, recurring bouts of inhalational fever followed the introduction of a new technique that exposed workers to magnesium oxide fumes. The symptoms were felt to be due to alkaline effects of the oxide on the small airways. In that case series, the one individual with highest exposure developed a more prolonged pneumonitis.[205] High levels of exposure to both soluble and insoluble magnesium salts can irritate mucus membranes, producing rhinitis and conjunctivitis.

Manganese

An inhalational fever like metal fume fever has been described in relation to inhaled manganese dioxide fumes and aerosols.[14] Others report acute chemical pneumonitis.[206]

Even in the absence of manganese-induced pneumonitis, occupational and inhalational exposure to manganese appears to be a risk factor for development of pulmonary infections. Increased mortality rates for pneumonia were observed in the general population following the opening of a manganese smelter in Norway in the 1920s In 1946, researchers showed an increased annual incidence of pneumonia among potassium permanganate workers who inhaled magnesium oxide dusts. Manganese dioxide dust induces an inflammatory response in the lungs, altering dust clearance and alveolar macrophage function. Such effects may result in increased susceptibility to bacterial pathogens.

With chronic inhalation of respirable size manganese oxide particles, workers also develop a subacute or chronic pneumonitis, sometimes with acute or subacute occurrence of lobar pneumonia, pulmonary hemorrhage, fever, and dyspnea with or without bacterial pneumonia. Some cases have developed pulmonary fibrosis, as well.[14]

Mercury

Mercury is a group IIB metal long recognized for its high potential toxicity through observation of mercury-exposed miners and hatters who treated the fur used in felt hats with mercury nitrate. Although there have been fewer reports of "hatter's shakes" and workers becoming "mad as a hatter" since the 1950s, there are many other uses for mercury that result in work-related illness (Table 29-1).

The respiratory tract is both a major route of absorption and a target organ for mercury's acute and chronic effects.

Exposure to mercury vapor, especially in confined spaces, causes severe airway irritation with development of tracheobronchitis, bronchiolitis, pneumonitis, and in some cases pulmonary edema and death. Typically there is a several hour delay in the onset of cough, dyspnea, fever, and nausea. Additional symptoms include chest tightness followed by intense shivering, diaphoresis, and agitation often with crampy abdominal pain. At the time of presentation, patients often have bilateral inspiratory rales at the lung bases. Chest x-rays may show an alveolar filling pattern predominantly in the lower lung fields. In some studies, the pulmonary function test abnormalities seen in association with acute mercury exposure have an obstructive pattern. In one case series, restriction and marked abnormalities of diffusing capacity and gas exchange were observed.[207] Pathologic evidence of pulmonary edema with proteinaceous exudates in alveolar spaces, cellular infiltration, and formation of hyaline membranes is seen. Central nervous system symptoms also develop in severe cases.[207-209]

Severe cases die within 2 to 3 days, although many recover if provided with supportive care. Corticosteroids are administered but the benefit is based on anecdotal evidence.

For those surviving the acute tracheobronchitis and pneumonitis, chronic interstitial fibrosis may develop over the following weeks, with a desquamative interstitial pneumonitis pattern of cellular infiltration, alveolar Type II cell hyperplasia, fibrosis, and honeycombing.[161,210] Radiographic evidence of chronic interstitial lung disease may occur without acute episodes. The pathology underlying these x-ray findings have not been confirmed.[211,212] Under most circumstances, exposure to mercury vapor does not cause permanent lung disease. Intravenous administration of metallic mercury, as seen among drug abusers who combine elemental mercury with narcotics, causes an acute febrile illness with associated wheezing, chills, dyspnea, and pleuritic chest pain. Chest radiographs demonstrate the radiodense elemental mercury in a branching pattern of small spherules, often with accumulation of mercury in the right ventricle. Occupational occurrence of mercury embolization is rare, but could occur with accidental inoculation through lacerations.

Diagnosis of acute or chronic mercury poisoning relies on careful occupational and environmental history taking. Whereas whole blood estimates of mercury may be helpful, urinary mercury levels have tended to show great variability and correlate poorly with level of environmental exposure and level of toxicity. In the acute scenario, bacterial and viral pneumonia and causes of cardiogenic and noncardiogenic pulmonary edema must be considered.

The use of British antilewisite (2-3-dimercaptopropanol) or other chelating agents are advocated for the treatment of acute mercurial poisoning. D-Penicillamine may be helpful for treatment of chronic mercury poisoning although there is controversy in the literature regarding its use. A 1-day course of oral D-penicillamine may help diagnostically, if it shows a rise in the amount of mobilizable mercury. Renal dialysis may be helpful in the face of renal toxicity.[213]

Nickel

Nickel compounds cause a range of respiratory tract effects that includes acute pulmonary edema, chemical pneumonitis, pulmonary hemorrhage, asthma, eosinophilic pneumonia (Löeffler's syndrome), and nasosinal and lung cancer.

Acute respiratory effects of nickel carbonyl take two forms, initial and delayed.[214-217] Usually the initial symptoms are mild and improve with removal from exposure. They may include headache, dizziness, and sometimes nausea with emesis. In the delayed reaction, individuals develop retrosternal chest pain, chest tightness, cough, dyspnea, fatigability, and gastrointestinal symptoms. Target organs are the lung, liver, and brain with death resulting from the development of pulmonary edema, atelectasis, and hemorrhage, due to massive necrosis. There is rapid infiltration of the lung interstitium with fibrosis.[218] As the condition progresses, individuals report increasing shortness of breath with nonproductive cough sometimes with abrupt deterioration. Laboratory findings include leukocytosis, elevated urinary nickel concentrations, and occasionally slight elevation of hepatic enzymes. Chest radiographs may show irregular linear opacities or diffuse irregular nodules, pulmonary edema, and on rare occasion pleural effusions. Treatment is supportive. Corticosteroids and bronchodilators are used although there have been no controlled trials of these medications. Dithiocarb (sodium diethyldithiocarbamate) has been shown to be helpful in chelating nickel. Antabuse (tetraethylthiuram) may also be effective. D-Penicillamine and dimercaprol have lower efficacy.[219] Although it has been reported that patients who survive nickel carbonyl poisoning have a slow but successful recovery, published reports with long-term follow-up of such individuals cannot be found. Similarly, the possibility of chronic central nervous system injury from nickel carbonyl has not been studied. In some, a toxic myocarditis develops.[216]

Case reports over the past 25 years demonstrate that nickel salts cause asthma. McConnell first described asthma due to nickel sulfate exposure in a metal-plate worker, in whom specific bronchoprovocation tests using nickel sulfate reproduced the patient's symptoms.[220] In addition, that individual was shown to have circulating nickel-specific antibodies. Subsequently, Block and Yeung described a metal polisher who had a history of contact dermatitis and new onset of asthma at age 60 having worked for 49 years grinding and polishing irregularities on nickel surfaces of car bumpers. Bronchoprovocation with nickel sulfate and using work environment dust produced immediate falls in the patient's forced expiratory volume in 1 second (FEV1). Prick testing with nickel sulfate solution produced a wh●l. Patch testing with dust collected from the work environment was negative.[221] Whereas the patient described by McConnell had evidence of IgG or IgM antibodies based on hemagglutinin reaction to nickel-coated erythrocytes, hemagglutination studies and gel diffusion studies were negative in the Block and Yeung case.[221] Malo and colleagues subsequently described a metal-plating factory worker in whom peak flow rates suggested a work-related pattern of airflow obstruction. Prick tests with nickel sulfate elicited an immediate reaction. Bronchoprovocation with nickel sulfate showed an immediate asthmatic response. Using nickel sulfate bound to human serum albumin in a RAST, the authors demonstrated specific IgE antibody.[16] In another electroplater, Novey and colleagues described the new onset of asthma and confirmed nickel sulfate-specific response on bronchoprovocation, but interestingly observed both an acute and a 3-hour delayed drop in FEV1. This individual had a positive modified-RAST for nickel sulfate. Interestingly, this individual reacted immediately to chromium sulfate fumes and had a positive modified RAST to chromium sulfate.[18] The evidence suggests that nickel causes asthma, usually involving a humoral immune response. It is not known how commonly nickel asthma occurs in industry.

Two groups have described cases of pulmonary eosinophilia (Löffler's syndrome) associated with nickel sensitivity.[222,223] The workers were exposed to nickel carbonyl. In addition to developing pulmonary infiltrates and eosinophilia one patient developed an eczematous dermatitis. Patch testing showed extreme sensitivity to nickel. Removal from exposure to nickel led to symptomatic relief and resolution of the skin lesions.[222] Tschumy described a fireman who developed eosinophilic pneumonia following smoke inhalation, noting that nickel and chromium were among the metal-plated materials in the fire.[224]

The carcinogenic properties of nickel carbonyl were first described in the 1920s. Since then, multiple clinical and epidemiologic investigations of the carcinogenicity of nickel have shown excess occupational risks of lung, nasal, and laryngeal cancer.[153,225-229]

Osmium

Heating osium (e.g., osmium tetraoxide) liberates a fine fume that irritates mucous membranes and generates a bromine-like odor. Immediate symptoms include eye pain, excessive lacrimation, halos seen around lights, cough, symptoms sometimes evolving into pneumonia, and symptoms of asthma.[230] Even with brief exposures, workers have experienced nasal, laryngeal, tracheal, as well as bronchial symptoms with chest tightness and airflow limitation. Perhaps because the irritant symptoms are so immediate, workers are quick to avoid concentrated osmium tetraoxide. With improved ventilation, symptoms resolve.[230]

Phosphorus

Many phosphorus compounds are potent respiratory tract and mucous membrane irritants, even producing frank burns. Red phosphorus dust has been associated with acute chemical pneumonitis. Phosphorus oxychloride ($POCl_3$), phosphorus trichloride (PCl_3), and phosphorus pentachloride (PCl_5) act in a manner analogous to chloride gas, producing direct chemical irritant effects on the airways with associated cough and chest tightness, wheezing, and asthma-like symptoms.[231] In addition to these chlorophosphorus compounds, phosphoric acid and phorphorus pentasulfide cause respiratory tract irritation and, with high exposures, pulmonary edema. Although a rare occurrence, the accidental liberation of phosphine gas can cause rapidly fatal noncardiogenic pulmonary edema.[232]

Platinum

The respiratory tract toxicity of platinum can be divided into upper and lower respiratory effects. In 1911 Karasek and Karasek first described the development of rhinorrhea, sneezing, dyspnea with cyanosis, and skin irritation among photographic studio workers. Three decades later, such symptoms were demonstrated in over half of the workers in platinum refineries who were exposed to complex platinum salts as dust or as fine spray.[233] Other upper respiratory tract symptoms include itching of the throat, pallet, and nasal congestion. The lower respiratory tract symptoms progress to wheezing, cough, and dyspnea. Now recognized as having platinum-induced asthma, workers noted improvement and even resolution of symptoms within an hour of leaving the factory, although some workers awakened during the night with symptoms. Skin lesions are common among platinum asthma cases, with contact dermatitis, pruritis, eczema, and in some cases urticaria and even angioedema. Workers with platinum asthma may show evidence of mild peripheral blood eosinophilia. Roberts renamed this condition "platinosis," reporting 60% of platinum refinery and laboratory workers developing skin problems with or without respiratory symptoms, and the remainder demonstrating conjunctival and mucous membrane inflammatory symptoms and signs.[234] He hypothesized that the salts were acting as allergens, showing that scratch test reactivity to sodium chloroplatinate correlated with symptomatic platinosis. Subsequently, this condition has been described among solderers, jewelers, electroplaters, refinery workers, principally in response to ammonia tetrachloroplatinite (II) and ammonia hexachloroplatinate (IV). Elemental platinum does not elicit this response.[235,236] The upper respiratory, asthmatic, and dermatologic symptoms occur in 20 to 100% of platinum salt-exposed workers.

The underlying mechanism appears to be principally a Type I immediate onset IgE response but possibly with an IgG component. Interestingly, the relationship between duration of exposure, onset of symptoms, and skin test positivity is highly variable. As is commonly the case with metals that cause asthma, RASTs can be positive in patients with and without disease,[237,238] thus marking exposure or sensitization but not necessarily disease. In an epidemiologic study of IgE antibody responses to platinum in a refinery, Murdoch and colleagues used skin prick testing and RAST to measure sensitivity to platinum, palladium, and rhodium salts in 306 platinum refinery workers.[239] Of the 306 workers 38 had positive skin prick test to the platinum salts. Total IgE levels were elevated in 63% of these prick test-positive workers. Of those with positive skin tests, 62% also had a positive RAST. Only 2.5% of those workers with negative skin tests had positive RAST tests. In general, platinum sensitization develops within the first year of exposure, sometimes within the first few weeks. Once sensitized, individuals become hypersensitive to extremely small amounts of salts, although the exact threshold of this reactivity is unknown.

Some authors indicate that chronic platinum salt exposure may result in pulmonary fibrosis. Roberts[234] observed increased bronchovascular markings on radiographs from 16 of 21 platinosis cases. One of these individuals clearly had pulmonary fibrosis. Whether this was a result of a hypersensitivity pneumonitis type response is not known. Chronic exposure leads to exacerbation of platinum hypersensitivity once an individual has been sensitized. As such, it is generally recommended that individuals with this condition avoid further exposure.

Additional management of platinum-induced asthma attacks involves the usual forms of asthma management in addition to restriction of further exposure. Prevention should revolve around limiting inhalation and dermal exposure in the workplace. Atopic individuals may develop sensitization to platinum and related compounds more quickly than nonatopic individuals.[240] In either circumstance, workers deserve equal protection from exposure, and medical monitoring that centers around the early recognition of upper respiratory, asthmatic, and dermatologic conditions.

Although general laboratory tests and pulmonary function tests do not distinguish platinum-induced asthma from other forms of asthma, a number of specific tests can be employed in identifying sensitized workers. It should be recognized, however, that skin prick test, RAST, and other tests designed to identify IgE antibody have variable sensitivity and variable specificity. Thus although a positive test confirms sensitization, the data must be placed in context with the skin and respiratory tract manifestations of the patient. Negative tests do not exclude the possibility of platinum allergy. Workers exposed to platinum salts who present with the signs and symptoms discussed above should be considered to have platinum allergy until proven otherwise, and a trial of removal from exposure may be warranted.

Biologic monitoring of plasma platinum concentrations may help prevent toxicity in patients receiving *cis*-platinum as a cancer chemotherapeutic agent when administered parenterally, but such tests are less helpful in the occupational setting.

While metallic platinum dusts have a threshold limit value of 1.0 mg/m^3, the TLV for soluble platinum salts is 0.002 mg/m^3 to help prevent sensitization and respiratory effects from developing. Such levels are not protective for already-sensitized workers.

Rare earths (lanthanides)

The lanthanide series of metals, also termed "rare earth," is a complex group of metals mainly in the atomic number range of 57 to 71, part of the group III transition metals. They share similar molecular features and are extremely difficult to isolate from one another. The rare earths include yttrium (Y) atomic number 39; lanthanum (La) atomic number 57; cerium (Ce) atomic number 58; praseodymium (Pr) atomic number 59; neodymium (Nd) atomic number 60; promethium (Pm) atomic number 61; samarium (Sm) atomic number 62; europium (Eu) atomic number 63; gadolinium (Gd) atomic number 64; terbium (Tb) atomic number 65; dysprosium (Dy) atomic number 66; holmium (Ho) atomic number 67; erbium (Er) atomic number 68; thulium (Tm) atomic number 69; ytterbium (Yb) atomic number 70; and lutetium (Lu) atomic number 71.

In the 1950s, Gardener suggested that small reticular nodular opacities seen on x-rays of workers were the result of exposure to rare earth oxides and fluorides.[241] Subsequently, there have been multiple case reports and small case series relating lung disease to exposures to cerium oxide or to various mixtures of rare earths in the glass manufacturing, lens polishing, and photoengraving industries.[242-246] In most of these cases, the workers developed restrictive, obstructive, or mixed physiologic abnormalities, with or without respiratory tract symptoms. Unfortunately, in the majority of these cases no lung histology was available. In one case of a lens polisher, granulomatous pneumonitis was found. In one photoengraver, interstitial fibrosis was noted in a peribronchiolar and peribronchial distribution.[243,245] In symptomatic cases, the patients range from having dyspnea to extreme dyspnea on exertion, productive cough with clinical evidence of cyanosis, dry rales, and associated hypoxemia in addition to restriction. In an interesting report from Sulotto and colleagues[246] a photoengraver with restrictive physiology and abnormal gas exchange showed a marked increase in gallium scan lung uptake, increased bronchoalveolar lavage cellularity, and extremely high levels of Ce, La, Nd, Sm, Tb, Yb, and Lu in lavage by neutron activation analysis. Unfortunately no histopathology was available in this case; however the evidence strongly favored an ongoing inflammatory process due to rare earth, even 17 years after last exposure.

Little is known about the natural history of this condition or its response to therapy. There is variability in the clinical, radiographic, and pathologic appearance that may be due to different mixtures of rare earths inhaled by these individuals. In some cases the radiograph opacities may be indicative of a truly "benign pneumoconiosis" (Table 29-6), but in the 16 published cases, significant physiologic alterations occurred in rare earth pneumoconiosis.

Selenium

Although elemental selenium is considered harmless, it burns when it comes in contact with air and generates red selenium dioxide fumes that have a characteristic garlic odor. Inhalation of such fumes produces symptoms of cough, substernal chest pain, and, with sufficient exposure, pulmonary edema. Whereas selenium dioxide represents the more common exposure risk in industry, there is potential contact with hydrogen selenide gas (selenium anhydride) as a result of industrial accidents, with leakage from gas cylinders and among laboratory workers. Acute involvement of mucus membranes produces excessive tearing, rhinitis, sneezing, cough, and chest tightness.[247,248] Of particular note is the potential for delayed development of pulmonary edema 6 to 8 hours following the exposure.[249-252] In one

notable case report, Schecter and colleagues described an individual who developed severe dyspnea with cough and asthma symptoms, pneumomediastinum, and subcutaneous emphysema associated with both obstructive and restrictive physiologic decrements, gradual improvement but persistent respiratory embarrassment 3 years after exposure.[247]

Biologic monitoring for selenium is performed by testing urine levels.

Prevention is achieved by controlling the processes that involve exposure of heated selenium to air, with appropriate control of ventilation, provision of eye protection and respirators, and storage of selenium away from potential contact with acids or with water.

Silver

Although there have been reports of toxicity from the "company" silver keeps (i.e., cadmium, fluoride, iron oxides used in the polishing of silver), silver itself is not recognized as a significant human respiratory tract toxin.[253-255] Argyria is a nontoxic discoloration of skin that can involve the airways.

Two studies have reported respiratory tract complaints among workers exposed to silver nitrate, silver oxide, silver chloride, and silver cadmium oxide powders. In one study, one third of workers developed cough, wheezing, chest tightness, and irritation symptoms affecting the eyes, nose, and throat.[256] In a second study, 56% of workers reported mucosal irritation symptoms. One third reported chest tightness, wheezing, and cough especially after exposure to silver crystal, powder, and melting. Epistaxis was common in individuals exposed to silver crystal.[257]

Thallium

In a number of cases, individuals with thallium intoxication have developed interstitial fibrosis. Unfortunately in these instances it is difficult to distinguish whether cardiogenic edema was present.[258,259] One reported case devel-

Table 29-6. High radiodensity metals*

Metal	Pneumoconiosis	Atom number	Atomic weight
Titanium		22	47.88
Vanadium		23	50.94
Iron	Siderosis	26	55.85
Zirconium		40	91.22
Tin	Stannosis	50	118.71
Antimony		51	121.75
Barium	Baritosis	56	137.33
Hafnium		72	178.49
Rare Earth Metals (Lanthanides)		39–71†	88.91
			174.97

*The metals listed can potentially produce pneumoconiotic opacities due to their radiodensity. In addition to producing a so-called "benign" pneumoconiosis, metals listed also may cause pathologic responses in the lungs (see text).

†Includes 14 elements ranging in atomic number from 58 to 71. Sometimes included as well are lanthanum (La) atomic number 57, atomic weight 138.91, and yttrium (Y) atomic number 39, atomic weight 88.91.

oped both central and peripheral neurological complications of thallium intoxication associated with the development of adult respiratory distress syndrome. Animal studies have shown the development of pulmonary edema and alveolar hemorrhage in a dog model of thallium intoxication. Because thallium interferes with the peripheral nervous system and with muscle contractility, it can cause respiratory arrest due to respiratory muscle paralysis.[260]

Treatment involves competitively inhibiting thallium with potassium chloride and potassium ferrichexacyanoferrate (Prussian blue), and with supportive measures for those demonstrating respiratory, renal, or other organ system failure.

Tin

Individuals exposed to metallic tin, tin oxide dust, or fumes can develop dense bilateral nodular infiltrates due to the high radiopacity of tin, called stannosis[261-268] (Table 29-6). Such radiographic abnormalities can be extremely common. In Robertson and Whitaker's study of 215 smelter workers, 121 developed radiographic evidence of stannosis at a tin refinery.[263] These individuals had no clinical abnormalities apart from abnormal chest radiographs. X-ray diffraction analyses confirm that tin oxide was the predominant metal or mineral present in the few cases of stannosis that have been autopsied. This literature is hindered by the relatively few pathologic specimens examined. Grossly the lungs show numerous 1 to 3 mm gray rounded densities along intralobular septae and subpleurally. Microscopically, macrophages are found to contain large numbers of dust particles within the pulmonary interstitium. Dust particles accumulate in hilar nodes. Macules can form in the perivascular and peribronchiolar tissue, analogous to those seen in silicosis and coal workers' pneumoconiosis. Conglomerate masses and massive fibrosis have not been described. Tin oxide crystals show strong birefringence. In describing pathologic changes due to stannic oxide, Dundon and Hughes[264] observed increased connective tissue (fibrosis) surrounding "pigment-choked lymphatics" lightly infiltrated with both large and small mononuclear cells without nodulation or hyalinization. These nodules are generally irregular in shape. Their shape, density, and profusion are associated with the dose of exposure. Thus, although there may be some subtle pathologic alterations in the perilymphatic regions, most authors contend that stannosis is nonetheless a benign process.

Although it is commonly stated that there are no pulmonary symptoms or other clinical abnormalities in patients with this condition, most methods used to study such workers have been relatively insensitive. In addition, careful review of early cases fuels speculation that this disease may produce both symptoms and physiologic alterations in some instances. For example, one of the early cases described by Spencer and Wycoff[267] had shortness of breath of 1 to 2 years duration, rales at the lung bases, normal airflow, but low vital capacity. This individual also had what was felt to be hypertensive heart disease with mild congestive failure, but this report cannot exclude the possibility of the restrictive physiology being due to the underlying stannosis. In another sentinel case, a worker with 24 years of exposure had expiratory rales in the left lung, with normal lung capacity.[265] Interestingly, the first published case of "benign pneumoconiosis due to tin oxide" in the English literature included no clinical history and no histopathology despite the authors' coinage of the term "benign pneumoconiosis."[266,269] In this paper they noted that whereas "some of these dusts may cause a non-progressive low grade chronic inflammation, in general, they have little effect on connective tissue causing little fibrosis and never progressing to true nodulation. However, if there are old fibrosis scars in the lungs many of these 'non-specific' dusts may collect in increased amounts around the scars, such collections being secondary to the fibrosis."[269,270]

The bulk of the evidence supports the conclusion that tin has low toxicity for the lungs. When significant physiologic impairment is observed among tin workers other fibrogenic dusts should be considered in a differential diagnosis. Nonetheless, clinicians and researchers should keep an open mind to the possibility of tin being nonbenign in some cases. Further study is warranted.

Organotin compounds produce conjuctival, mucous membrane, upper respiratory and skin irritation, and burns, with trialkyltins being the most toxic. The major target organ is the central nervous system.

No specific treatment is required for stannosis. Treatment of organic tin poisoning includes management of cerebral edema if it develops and removal from exposure as well as appropriate treatment for burns if they have occurred. Ventilatory control as well as appropriate protection of skin, eyes, and the respiratory tract are warranted to avoid toxicity from the organotins.

Titanium

Titanium and titanium dioxide are generally considered inert and nontoxic, based on early reports of humans exposed to titanium oxides. Medical reviews have been dismissive of the studies that purport to show titanium-related radiographic changes, on the basis that worker exposed to titanium may have been exposed to silica, asbestos, or other fibrogenic or granuloma-causing minerals. Nonetheless, more recent publications suggest that even though respiratory tract toxicity is rare related to titanium, it probably does occur in some individuals. Moschinski and colleages identified chest radiographic abnormalities consistent with pulmonary fibrosis in 3 of 15 titanium oxide-exposed workers.[155] Elo and co-workers found titanium dioxide in mildly fibrotic lung tissue in three workers from a factory processing titanium dioxide. In a later study of the lung biopsies from these two cases plus a third individual, these authors identified evidence of mild fibrosis in alveolar septi and elevated numbers of electron-dense titanium dioxide particles in alveolar macrophage lysosomes.[271] Greenish pigmentation to the lungs was found in a perivascular and a peribronchial distribution as well as in the subpleural, pleural, and interstitial regions with some evidence of bronchiolar hyperplasia along with the mild fibrotic change observed.[271,272] Four other workers had radiographic abnormalities suggestive of pneumoconiosis.[272] These workers had a history of 9 to 10 years of exposure. Symptoms included cough, fever, and increasing dyspnea, which initially waxed and waned in a work-related pattern.

In a related set of observations, Garabrandt and co-workers observed a high frequency of pleural plaques (10% to 22%) among titanium metal production workers. In the population of 209 workers studied, there were no differences found in the frequency of respiratory tract symptoms among high and low exposure groups, but there was a greater annual decrement in FEV1 among workers in the reduction area. Although asbestos exposure was common for many of these workers and might potentially explain some of the pleural plaques seen on radiographs, pleural disease correlated with the duration of titanium manufacturing employment. When the authors controlled for asbestos exposure, titanium exposure alone conferred a 3.8-fold increased risk of pleural disease on workers with 10 or more years of employment when compared with titanium workers with less than 5 years' employment.[273] A subsequent cross-sectional study of 398 workers exposed to titanium dioxide showed no radiographic evidence of pulmonary fibrosis and no pleural plaques at two titanium dioxide-producing plants.[274] In a study of a titanium oxide paint factory in Nigeria, restrictive physiology occurred commonly among exposed workers. Half of the workforce experienced airways symptoms.[275] Recently, Moran and colleagues identified six individuals in whom skin, lung, synovial, and muscle tissue showed high levels of accumulated titanium. In three of the cases, patients presented with shortness of breath and one with cough. The chest radiograph showed diffuse "fibrosis" in one and restrictive physiology in another. One of these individuals was a painter with hypothesized exposure to titanium oxide, one worked in a paper mill, and another in a titanium dioxide plant. SEM/EDXM confirmed that the extensive deposits of birefringent material was titanium. These pathologists report that the lesions seen were unlike those of either talc or silicosis. Bronchopneumonia developed in adjacent areas of lung in these workers.

One of the consistent criticisms of such manuscripts in the past has been the difficulty in controlling for the potential confounding effect of other fibrogenic minerals.[14] In addition, studies of titanium dust from ilmenite (iron titanium oxide) in Ceylon showed no chest radiographic abnormalities,[276] with a similar negative finding in a study of chest radiographs of 207 titanium dioxide processing plant workers with ilmenite exposure.[277] Although they did not ob-

serve an excess of radiographic abnormalities in that cohort, airflow obstruction was more common in the workforce than expected, even when controlling for smoking status. Potential exposures included titanium dioxide, titanium tetrachloride, and other liberated by-products.[277] Examination of lung biopsies by Schmitz-Moorman and colleagues demonstrated aggregates of particulate material around respiratory bronchioles and in the alveolar walls with no evidence of fibrosis.[278] The majority of published studies with experimental animals exposed to titanium dioxide favor the conclusion that it has little or no fibrogenic potential.[279] However slight degrees of fibrosis have been described in some of these studies.[280,281]

Besides the controversy over fibrosis, other investigators have suggested that pulmonary deposition of titanium may, in some circumstances, result in granulomatous lung disease. Redline and colleagues described a patient who spent 13 years as a furnace feeder in a titanium production plant who developed exertional dyspnea with a work-related pattern of symptoms, reticulonodular infiltrates, restrictive physiology, and evidence of noncaseating granulomas on lung biopsy.[282] The authors report that on two of four occasions the patient's blood lymphocytes showed a positive in vitro stimulation to titanium chloride with stimulation indexes of 2.0 and 2.1, with negative lymphocyte transformation test to other metals. Although the data presented in support of a cellular immune response to titanium chloride are marginal, the evidence associating titanium particles with granulomas merits attention. Another case of diffuse granulomatous disease in a worker exposed to titanium dioxide abrasive had been previously reported by Angebalut and co-workers, with evidence of the mineral in the lungs and in the sarcoidal lesions.[283]

In contrast to titanium and titanium dioxide, titanium tetrachloride inhalation can have profound effects on the bronchial tree, producing severe irritation, bronchitis, chemical pneumonitis, and endobronchial polyposis.[284,285] Liquid titanium tetrachloride can burn the skin and mucous membranes of the laryngx, trachea, and bronchi.[286]

In a single epidemiologic study of cancer outcomes for titanium dioxide workers, Chen and Fayerweather observed no statistically significant associations between titanium dioxide exposure and lung cancer incidence among 1,576 workers exposed during the interval of 1956 through 1985 and from 1935 through 1983 for cancer mortality.[274]

Tungsten

Tungsten has been the victim of guilt by association. Hard metal disease develops in individuals exposed to tungsten carbide as a result of cobalt exposure, not tungsten. There is no known respiratory tract disease directly attributed to tungsten. However, intratracheal administration of tungsten dust in guinea pigs can induce an acute interstitial infiltrate with perivascular cellular accumulation. With chronic exposure, obliterative bronchiolitis and peribronchial and perivascular fibrosis are seen in experimental animals, although some studies of tungsten dust in inhalational models have observed no biologic reaction in the absence of cobalt.[287,288]

Uranium

The principal long-term toxicity to the respiratory tract of exposure to uranium and its by-products is lung cancer. Howland reported on the acute toxic effects of uranium hexafluoride (UF_6) from a 1944 accident in which one of 21 workers died within 15 minutes due to burns from the degradation products uranium oxyfluoride and hydrogen fluoride. Another died in 70 minutes with acute respiratory distress. Most of the other exposed individuals developed chemical burns to the respiratory tract, skin, and eyes. Some developed pulmonary edema as well as renal tubular damage.[289]

Whereas animals exposed to alpha radiation in the lungs develop emphysema and interstitial fibrosis, the complicated exposures of miners and other uranium-exposed workers make it difficult to distinguish among possible causes of emphysema and pulmonary fibrosis. Archer and co-workers have reported pulmonary function abnormalities among uranium miners as well as increased lung cancer risk.[290,291] A more recent study of New Mexico uranium miners that controlled for cigarette smoking showed an association between reduced airflow and duration of underground uranium mining. Of the miners studied, 9% had abnormal chest radiographs credited to silicosis.[292]

Vanadium

Acute respiratory tract effects of vanadium have been recognized since the early 1900s when Dutton described vanadium ore grinders who developed hematologic derangements associated with anorexia, cachexia, and severe cough often with hemoptysis.[293] In 1919, Alice Hamilton observed a high prevalence of cough among ore grinders in a ferrovanadium production plant.[294] Multiple subsequent studies have verified that vanadium oxide dusts can induce acute upper and lower airway irritation with bronchitis as the predominant symptom.[295-299] In general, the cough symptom resolves several weeks after removal from exposure. Chronic bronchitis occurs less commonly, often developing after recurrent episodes of acute bronchitis.

Other upper respiratory tract effects include irritation of the mucous membranes of the nose and throat. Nasal irritation can become severe enough to result in epistaxis. Chronic rhinitis is an extremely common symptom among vanadium workers, as is stinging of the throat. A green-black discoloration of the tongue occurs with chronic exposures.[298]

Vanadium dust, vanadium pentoxide, and vanadate cause asthma.[298,300-303] Pulmonary function tests document decrements in airflow that reverse after removal from exposure. Chest pain and chest tightness are common symptoms

among the patients with either the bronchitis or asthmatic responses to vanadium. Zens and Burg exposed normal subjects to 0.25 mg/m^3 of vanadium pentoxide for 8 hours. These volunteers developed cough within the next 24 hours that resolved within 10 days. Spirometry was not adversely effected. However, when workers were exposed to the ash of oil-fired boilers that contained over 15% vanadium, marked drops in FEV1 and forced vital capacity (FVC) were seen within 24 hours, recovering within a month.[298]

In 1946, Wyers presented 10 illustrative cases of workers with exposure to vanadium pentoxide dust from a crushing operation. In addition to all 10 having chronic bronchitis, dyspnea, and in some cases hemoptysis, with clinical findings of rales and rhonci, he described abnormal chest radiographics in some of these individuals with reticular opacities later evolving into emphysema; 3 of the 10 cases developed pneumonia. There was no comment on their smoking histories. Although vanadium's atomic number is close to that of iron, most other studies have not observed any evidence of radiographic opacities due to the radiodensity of vanadium, possibly due to its rapid translocation from the lungs into the blood and urine. Unfortunately there is a paucity of lung histologic data on vanadium-exposed workers. Levy and colleagues, in studying boiler makers' bronchitis, noted that of 65 chest x-rays examined, 18 were abnormal, 9 showing increased parenchymal markings. The interstitial radiographic abnormality did not correlate with a history of previous asbestos exposure.[295] Other investigators have not observed increased interstitium markings.[302,304]

Urinary monitoring is helpful, especially if performed within 2 weeks of last exposure.[305]

Zinc

Probably the most common toxic effect of zinc is metal fume fever due to inhalation of zinc oxide fume (see Chapter 17). Long-term pulmonary sequela from the inhalation of zinc oxide have not been reported. Although still unknown, the proposed mechanisms underlying metal fume fever bear mentioning here because of the potential insights they offer related to other forms of zinc respiratory tract toxicity. It has been suggested, for example, that metal fume fever is a result of an acute inflammatory response involving release of inflammatory cytokines. In some circumstances, it may induce an antibody-specific immune response.[306] Either mechanism may ultimately be relevant to the reports of other zinc compounds producing interstitial pneumonitis, fibrosis, and asthma.[307,308]

Most zinc salts are relatively innocuous with the important exception being zinc chloride ($ZnCl_2$) which is caustic and burns eyes and skin.[309,310] Airway irritant effects of zinc chloride were recognized in World War II when smoke bombs were produced by heating zinc chloride. When it is volatilized into fine particles, severe upper airway irritation is experienced. In some cases, fatal pulmonary edema or secondary bronchopneumonia occurs. Associated with such injuries is profound sluffing of mucous membranes of the nasopharynx, larynx, trachea, and bronchi, due to the strong necrotizing effect of the fume.[311-314] Individuals surviving the acute pulmonary edema and chemical pneumonitis may succumb subacutely to a desquamative form of interstitial pulmonary fibrosis.[313,315]

The risk of zinc chloride inhalational lung injury from smoke bombs remains an active problem in industry, especially in the military.[314,316,317] Interestingly, in two soldiers participating in military exercises, inhalation of $ZnCl_2$ resulted in an unusually slow, progressive onset of adult respiratory distress syndrome, ending in respiratory failure and death, and associated interstitial fibrosis. Three survivors tended to have low FEV1 1 year following the accident.

Radiographic densities can persist even after symptomatic recovery from zinc chloride inhalation.[318,319] Some authors suggest the early administration of intravenous and nebulized acetyl-cysteine in the treatment of acute inhalational injury due to zinc chloride. The infusion of acetyl-cysteine increases urinary zinc excretion and decreases plasma concentration.[313]

Malo and Cartier[320] suggest that zinc oxide fumes may produce an asthmatic response, although the contribution of other metals in galvanized metal cannot be fully excluded from the reported cases. Interestingly, bronchoprovocation testing with welding fumes from galvanized metal not only mimics the symptoms of metal fume fever in some individuals, but has reproduced a systemic allergic response with angioedema and urticaria in one welder.[321] The delayed pattern of response reported in both papers suggests that an antigen may be responsible in these welding fume-exposed individuals.[320,321]

Excess risk of lung cancer mortality has been observed among workers exposed to zinc chromate in the chromate pigment industry. Although these workers are exposed to zinc oxide powder as well chromate, the zinc itself is generally not considered the causative agent in development of malignancy.[150,153,322]

Zirconium

Reed studied 22 workers exposed to zirconium fumes for 1 to 5 years in the process of purifying and reducing zirconium metal. Fifteen were asymptomatic. Five had chronic bronchitis, and four had slight increase in peripheral lung markings but no granulomatous disease was observed. No pneumoconiosis was found. An earlier case of pulmonary granulomatous disease in the chemical engineer from the plant was later determined to have chronic beryllium disease based on autopsy results.[323,324] Hadjimichael and Brubaker studied 32 workers with 1 to 17 years of exposure to zirconium metal reactor parts and observed no spirometric or radiographic differences compared to control subjects.[325] A study of chest radiographs in 136 workers with an average of 4.4 years of exposure to ilmenite, routile, and zircon revealed only one worker with radiographic evidence of small opacities.[276]

McCallum hypothesized that the radiographic opacities seen in eight men at a zirconium processing plant adjacent to an antimony smelter may have been the result of zirconium exposure.[56] Analogously, Cooper and colleagues found abnormal chest radiographs in eight workers who inhaled mixed dusts of zirconium, antimony, and coal or furnace brick. The radiographic abnormalities were described as simple pneumoconiotic nodules.[55]

More recent case series and case reports support the notion that although zirconium-related lung toxicity may be rare, it does occur. Bartter and colleagues reported on the development of pulmonary fibrosis in a lens grinder who mixed zirconium oxide powder with water used in the polishing of optical lenses. After a latency of 15 years, this individual developed slowly progressive chest radiographic changes consistent with pneumoconiosis and on open lung biopsy was found to have interstitial fibrosis, honeycomb lung, and birefringent particles. Energy dispersive x-ray microanalysis with scanning electron microscopy demonstrated high concentrations of zirconium compounds. Other potential causes of fibrosis were excluded. The patient had rales, clubbing, irregular small opacities in the lower lobes, and restrictive physiology with a gas exchange abnormality.[326] Interestingly, there were no granulomas and attempts at zirconium lymphocyte transformation testing using blood and bronchoalveolar lavage lymphocytes were negative, although details of those assays were not provided.

A recent report by Romeo and colleagues suggests that both pulmonary fibrosis and granulomatous lung disease may occur in some zirconium-exposed workers.[327] One patient worked for 28 years in a refractory brick factory with exposures to zirconium dioxide, zirconium silicate, baddeleyite, as well as to alumina, kaolin, and corundum. Spirometry and arterial blood gases were normal, but diffusing capacity was slightly reduced. Chest radiographs showed bilateral rounded opacities. Transbronchial lung biopsy showed interstitial fibrosis, alveolar cell hyperplasia, and PAS-positive weakly birefringent particles in alveolar and interstitial macrophages. Neutron activation analysis revealed elevated levels of zirconium. A second individual worked for 8 years in a foundry with exposure to zirconium silicate ($ZrSiO_4$). Chest radiographs showed diffused irregular opacities. Transbronchial biopsies demonstrated multiple noncaseating granulomas that contained PAS-positive, birefringent particles in the interstitial macrophages. They found relatively low levels of zirconium in the lung biopsy as measured by neutron activation analysis. This individual was asymptomatic and had normal lung function tests and arterial blood gases. The authors acknowledge that these individuals did not have pure exposures to zirconium, but were also exposed to low levels of silica and cristobalite.

REFERENCES

1. Leonard A and Lauwerys R: Mutagenicity, carcinogenicity, and teratogenicity of cobalt metal and cobalt compounds, *Mut Res* 239:17-27, 1990.
2. Moorhouse CP, Halliwell B, Grootveld M, et al: Cobalt (II) ion as a promoter of hydroxyl radical formation under physiologic conditions: differential effects of hydroxyl radical scavengers, *Biochim Biophys Acta* 843:261-268, 1985.
3. Newman LS: Pulmonary toxicology. In Sullivan JB Jr and Kreiger GR, editors: *Hazardous materials toxicology: clinical principles of environmental health,* pp 124-144. Baltimore, 1991, Williams & Wilkins.
4. Halliwell B and Gutteridge JMC: Oxygen toxicity, oxygen radicals, transition metals, and disease, *Biochem J* 219:1-14, 1984.
5. Martell AE: Chemistry and metabolism of metals relevant to their carcinogenecity, *Environ Health Perspect* 40:27-34, 1981.
6. Aust SD, Moorehouse LA, and Thomas CE: Role of metals in oxygen radical reactions, *J Free Rad Biol Med* 1:3-25, 1985.
7. Baker D, Kupke KG, Ingram P, et al: Microprobe analysis in human pathology, *Scan Electron Microsc* 3:659-680, 1985.
8. Johnson NF, Haslam PL, Dewar A, et al: Identification of inorganic dust particles in bronchoalveolar lavage macrophages by energy dispersive X-ray microanalysis, *Arch Environ Health* 41:133-144, 1986.
9. Abraham JL and Spragg RG: Documentation of environmental exposure using open biopsy, transbronchial biopsy, and bronchoalveolar lavage in giant cell interstitial pneumonia (GIP), *Am Rev Respir Dis* 119(Part 2 Suppl)(2):197 (Abstract), 1979.
10. Roggli VL, Ingram P, Linton RW, et al: New techniques for imaging and analyzing lung tissue, *Environ Health Perspect* 56:163-183, 1984.
11. Jones Williams W and Wallach ER. Laser microprobe mass spectrometry (LAMMS) analysis of beryllium, sarcoidosis, and other granulomatous diseases, *Sarcoidosis* 6:111-117, 1989.
12. Aitio A, Järvisalo J, Riihimäki V, et al: Biologic monitoring. In Zenz C, editor: *Occupational medicine: principles and practical applications,* ed. 2, pp 178-197, Chicago, 1988, Yearbook Medical.
13. Alexandersson R: Tungsten, cobalt, and their compounds. In Zenz C, editor: *Occupational medicine: principles and practical applications,* ed. 2, pp. 624-630, Chicago, 1988, Yearbook Medical.
14. Stokinger HE: The metals. In Clayton GD and Clayton FE, editors: *Patty's industrial hygiene and toxicology, Volume IIA, toxicology,* 3rd ed., pp 1493-2060, New York, 1981, Wiley Interscience.
15. Newman L, Storey E, and Kreiss K: Immunologic evaluation of occupational lung disease. In Rosenstock L, editor: *Occupational medicine: state of the art reviews,* pp 345-372. Philadelphia, 1987, Hanley and Belfus.
16. Malo J, Cartier A, Doepner M, et al: Occupational asthma caused by nickel sulfate, *J Allergy Clin Immunol* 69:55-59, 1982.
17. Shirakawa T, Kusaka Y, Fujimura N, et al: The existence of specific antibodies to cobalt in hard metal asthma, *Clin Allergy* 18:451-460, 1988.
18. Novey HS, Habib M, and Wells ID: Asthma and IgE antibodies induced by chromium and nickel salts, *J Allergy Clin Immunol* 72:407-412, 1983.
19. Newman LS, Kreiss K, King TE Jr., et al: Pathologic and immunologic alterations in early stages of beryllium disease: Re-examination of disease definition and natural history, *Am Rev Respir Dis* 139:1479-1486, 1989.
20. Kreiss K, Newman LS, Mroz MM, et al: Screening blood test identifies subclinical beryllium disease, *J Occup Med* 31:603-608, 1989.
21. Rossman MD, Kern JA, Elias JA, et al: Proliferative response of bronchoalveolar lymphocytes to beryllium: A test for chronic beryllium disease, *Ann Intern Med* 108:687-693, 1988.
22. Mroz MM, Kreiss K, Lezotte DC, et al: Re-examination of the blood lymphocyte transformation test in the diagnosis of chronic beryllium disease, *J Allergy Clin Immunol* 88:54-60, 1991.
23. Veien NK and Svejgaard E: Lymphocyte transformation in patients with cobalt dermatitis, *Br J Dermatol* 99:191-196, 1978.
24. Räsänen, Sainio H, Lehto M, et al: Lymphocyte proliferation test as a diagnostic aid in chromium contact sensitivity, *Contact Dermatitis* 25:25-29, 1991.
25. Kilburn KH: Chapter 32. Pulmonary and neurologic effects of aluminum. In Rom WN, editor: *Environmental and occupational medicine,* ed. 2, pp 465-473, Boston, 1992, Little Brown.
26. Frostadt EW: Fluoride intoxication in Norwegian aluminum plant workers, *Tidsskr Nor Laegeforn* 56:179-182, 1936.
27. Abrahamson MJ, Wlodarczyk JH, Saunders NA, et al: Does aluminum smelting cause lung disease?, *Am Rev Respir Dis* 139:1042-1056, 1989.
28. Wergeland E, Lund E, and Waage JE: Respiratory dysfunction after potroom asthma, *Am J Industr Med* 11:627-636, 1987.
29. Chan-Yeung M and Lam S: Occupational asthma: State of the art, *Am Rev Respir Dis* 133:686-703, 1986.
30. Kaltreider NL, Elder MJ, Cralley LV, et al: Health survey of aluminum workers with special reference to fluoride exposure, *J Occup Med* 14:531-541, 1972.
31. Chan-Yeung M, Wong R, Maclean L, et al: Epidemiologic health study of workers in an aluminum smelter in British Columbia: Effects on the respiratory system, *Am Rev Respir Dis* 127:465-469, 1983.
32. Kilburn KH and Warshaw RH: Occupational asthma and airways dysfunction in aluminum workers, *Am Rev Respir Dis* 141:A79, 1990.
33. Discher DP and Breitenstein BD: Prevalence of chronic pulmonary disease in aluminum potroom workers, *J Occup Med* 18:379-386, 1976.
34. Miller RR, Churg AM, Hutcheon M, et al. Pulmonary alveolar proteinosis and aluminum dust exposure, *Am Rev Respir Dis* 130:312-315, 1984.
35. Goralweski G: Die aluminum lunge: Eine neue gewerbeerkrankung, *Z Gessmte Inn Med* 2:665-673, 1947.
36. Mitchell J, Manning GB, and Molyneaux M: Pulmonary fibrosis in workers exposed to finely powdered aluminum, *Br J Industr Med* 18:10-21, 1960.
37. McLaughlin AIG, Kazantzis G, King E, et al: Pulmonary fibrosis and encephalopathy associated with the inhalation of aluminum dust, *Br J Industr Med* 19:253-263, 1962.
38. DeVuyst P, Dumortier P, Rickert F, et al: Occupational lung fibrosis in an aluminum polisher, *Eur J Respir Dis* 68:131-140, 1986.
39. Gilks B and Churg A: Aluminum-induced pulmonary fibrosis: Do fibers play a role?, *Am Rev Respir Dis* 136:176-179, 1987.
40. Vallyathan V, Bergeron WN, Robichaux PA, et al: Pulmonary fibrosis in an aluminum arc welder, *Chest* 81:372-374, 1982.
41. Shaver CG and Riddell AR: Lung changes associated with the manufacture of alumina abrasives, *J Industr Hyg Tox* 29:145-157, 1947.
42. Shaver C: Pulmonary changes encountered in employees engaged in the manufacture of alumina abrasives, *Occup Med* 5:718-728, 1948.
43. Jederlinic PJ, Abraham JL, Churg A, et al: Pulmonary fibrosis in aluminum oxide workers: Investigation of 9 workers with pathologic examination and microanalysis in 3 of them, *Am Rev Respir Dis* 142:1179-1184, 1990.
44. Burrows D and Adams RM: Metals. In Adams RM, editor: *Occupational skin diseases,* ed. 2, pp. 349-350, Philadelphia, 1990, W.B. Saunders.
45. DeVuyst P, Dumortier P, Schandené L, et al: Sarcoid-like lung granulomatosis induced by aluminum dusts, *Am Rev Respir Dis* 135:493-497, 1987.
46. Chen WJ, Monnat R, Chen M, et al: Aluminum induced pulmonary granulomatosis, *Hum Pathol* 9:705-711, 1978.
47. Gibbs GW and Horowitz I: Lung cancer mortality in aluminum reduction plant workers, *J Occup Med* 21:347-353, 1979.

48. Andersen A, Dahlberg BE, Magnus K, et al: Risk of cancer in the Norwegian aluminum industry, *Int J Cancer* 29:295-298, 1982.

49. Rockette HE and Arena VC: Mortality studies of aluminum reduction plant workers: potroom and carbon department, *J Occup Med* 25:549-557, 1983.

50. Mur JM, Moulin JJ, Meyer-Bisch C, et al: Mortality of aluminum reduction plant workers in France, *Int J Epidemiol* 16:257-264, 1987.

51. Simonato L: Carcinogenic risk in the aluminum production industry: An epidemiological overview, *Med Lev* 72:266-276, 1981.

52. Renes LE: Antimony poisoning in industry, *Industr Hyg Occup Med* 7:99-108, 1953.

53. Taylor PJ: Acute intoxication from antimony trichloride, *Br J Industr Med* 23:318-321, 1966.

54. Cordasco EM: Newer concepts in the management of environmental pulmonary edema, *Angiology* 25:590-601, 1974.

55. Cooper DA, Pendergrass EP, Vorwald AJ, et al: Pneumoconiosis among workers in an antimony industry, *Am J Roentg* 103:495-508, 1968.

56. McCallum RI: Detection of antimony in process workers' lungs by x-radiation, *Trans Soc Occup Med* 17:134-138, 1967.

57. Gross P, Brown JHU, Westrick ML, et al: Toxicologic study of calcium halophosphate phosphors and antimony trioxide. I. acute and chronic toxicity and some pharmacologic aspects, *Arch Industr Health* 11:473-478, 1955.

58. Potkonjak V and Pavlovich M: Antimoniosis: a particular form of pneumoconiosis. I. Etiology, clinical, and x-ray findings, *Int Arch Occup Environ Health* 51:199-207, 1983.

59. NIOSH: *Criteria for a recommended standard: occupational exposure to antimony,* Washington, D.C., 1977, U.S. Government Printing Office [DHEW (National Institute for Occupational Safety and Health) Pub No 77-222.

60. Pinto S and McGill CM: Arsenic trioxide exposure in industry, *Ind Med Surg* 22:281-287, 1953.

61. Pinto S, Petronella SJ, Johns DR, et al: Arsine poisoning: a study of 13 cases, *Arch Ind Hyg Occup Med* 1:437-451, 1950.

62. Gorby MS: Arsenic poisoning, *West J Med* 149:308-315, 1988.

63. Lundgren AKD, Richtnér NG, and Sjöstrand T: Changes of respiratory tract in workers of Rönskär smelting works probably due to arsenic trioxide intoxification, *Nord Med* 46:1556-1560, 1951.

64. International Agency for Research on Cancer, In *Evaluation of the carcinogenic risk of chemicals to humans. Silica and some silicates,* pp 39-144, Lyon, 1987, IARC.

65. Welch K, Higgins I, Oh M, et al: Arsenic exposure, smoking, and respiratory cancer in copper smelter workers, *Arch Environ Health* 37:325-335, 1982.

66. Lee-Feldstein A: Cumulative exposure to arsenic and its relationship to respiratory cancer among copper smelter employees, *J Occup Med* 28:296-302, 1986.

67. Lee-Feldstein A: Arsenic and respiratory cancer in humans: follow-up of copper smelter employees in Montana, *JNCI* 170:601-609, 1983.

68. Enterline PE and Marsh GM: Cancer among workers exposed to arsenic and other substances in a copper smelter, *Am J Epidemol* 116:895-911, 1982.

69. Wall S: Survival and mortality pattern among Swedish smelter workers, *Int J Epidemiol* 9:73-87, 1980.

70. Hill AB and Faning EL: Studies in the incidence of cancer in a factory handling inorganic compounds of arsenic: I. Mortality experience in the factory, *Br J Industr Med* 5:1-6, 1948.

71. Lee AM and Fraumeni JF Jr: Arsenic and respiratory cancer in man: an occupational study, *JNCI* 42:1045-1052, 1969.

72. Ott MG, Holder BB, and Gordon HL: Respiratory cancer and occupational exposure to arsenicals, *Arch Environ Health* 29:250-255, 1974.

73. Sobel W, Bond GG, Baldwin CL, et al: An update of respiratory cancer in occupational exposures to arsenicals, *Am J Ind Med* 13:263-270, 1988.

74. Persajgen G, Bergman F, Klominek J, et al: Histological types of lung cancer among smelter workers exposed to arsenic, *Br J Ind Med* 44:454-458, 1987.

75. Schroeder HA and Balassa JJ: Abnormal trace metals in man: arsenic, *J Chronic Dis* 19:85-106, 1966.

76. Barrett S: Commercial hair analysis. Science or scam?, *JAMA* 254:1041-1045, 1985.

77. Inishi N, Tsuchiya K, Vahter M, et al: Arsenic. In Friberg L, Nordberg GF, and Voulk VB, editors: *Handbook on the toxicology of metals, Volume II: Specific metals,* ed. 2, pp. 43-83, Amsterdam, 1986, Elsevier Science Publishers B.V.

78. Dart RC: Arsenic, In Sullivan JB Jr. and Krieger GR, editors: *Hazardous materials toxicology: clinical principles of environmental health,* pp. 818-823, Baltimore, 1992, Williams & Wilkins.

79. Nelson MK: Arsenic trioxide production. In Carnow BW, editor: *Health effects of occupational lead and arsenic exposure,* Washington, D.C., 1976, U.S. Government Printing Office.

80. Arrigoni A: Pneumoconiosis, *Pneumoconiosi Da Bario Med Lavoro* 24:461-468, 1933.

81. Doig AT: Baritosis: A benign pneumoconiosis, *Thorax* 31:30-39, 1976.

82. Záková N and Svoboda M: Morphological changes in the lungs following bronchography with barium sulphate, *Acta Universitatis Carolinae Medica* 11:125-135, 1965.

83. Mital OP, Narang RK, Misra US, et al: Barium granuloma following bronchography: a case report, *Indian J Chest Dis* 17(1); 55-57, 1975.

84. Rose CS and Newman LS: Hypersensitivity pneumonitis and chronic beryllium disease, In Schwarz MI and King TE Jr., editors: *Interstitial Lung Disease,* ed. 2, pp. 231-253, St. Louis, 1993, Mosby Yearbook.

85. Lieben J and Metzner F: Epidemiological findings associated with beryllium extraction, *Am Ind Hyg Assoc J* 20:494-499, 1959.

86. Newman LS and Kreiss K: Non-occupational chronic beryllium disease masquerading as sarcoidosis: identification by blood lymphocyte proliferative response to beryllium, *Am Rev Respir Dis* 145:1212-1214, 1992.

87. Hardy HL and Tabershaw IR: Delayed chemical pneumonitis in workers exposed to beryllium compounds, *J Ind Hyg Toxicol* 28:197-211, 1946.

88. Sterner JH and Eisenbud M: Epidemiology of beryllium intoxication, *Arch Ind Hyg Occup Med* 4:123-151, 1951.

89. Eisenbud M and Lisson J: Epidemiological aspects of beryllium-induced nonmalignant lung disease: a 30-year update, *J Occup Med* 25:196-202, 1983.

90. Cullen MR, Kominsky JR, Rossman MD, et al: Chronic beryllium disease in a precious metal refinery: clinical epidemiologic and immunologic evidence for continuing risk from exposure to low level beryllium fume, *Am Rev Respir Dis* 135:201-208, 1987.

91. Kreiss K, Wasserman S, Mroz MM, et al: Beryllium disease screening in the ceramics industry: blood lymphocyte test performance and exposure-disease relations, *J Occup Med* 35:267-274, 1993.

92. Kreiss K, Mroz MM, Zhen B, et al: Epidemiology of beryllium sensitization and disease in nuclear workers, *Am Rev Respir Dis* 148:985-991, 1993.

93. Curtis GH: Cutaneous hypersensitivity due to beryllium, *Archs Dermatol Syph* 64:470-482, 1951.

94. Hanifin JM, Epstein WL, and Cline MJ: In vitro studies of granulomatous hypersensitivity to beryllium, *J Invest Dermatol* 55:284-288, 1970.

95. Saltini C, Winestock K, Kirby M, et al: Maintenance of alveolitis in patients with chronic beryllium disease by beryllium-specific helper T cells, *N Engl J Med* 320:1103-1109, 1989.

96. Epstein PE, Dauber JH, Rossman MD, et al: Bronchoalveolar lavage in a patient with chronic berylliosis: evidence for hypersensitivity pneumonitis, *Ann Intern Med* 97:213-216, 1982.

97. Bargon J, Kronenberger H, Bergmann L, et al: Lymphocyte transformation test in a group of foundry workers exposed to beryllium and non-exposed controls, *Eur J Respir Dis* 69 (Suppl 136):211-215, 1986.

98. Romagnoli P, Spinas GA, and Sinigaglia F: Gold-specific T cells in rheumatoid arthritis patients treated with gold, *J Clin Invest* 89:254-258, 1992.

99. Sinigaglia F, Scheidegger D, Garotta G, et al: Isolation and characterization of Ni-specific T cell clones from patients with Ni-contact dermatitis, *J Immunol* 135:3929-3932, 1985.

100. Newman LS: To Be^{2+} or not to Be^{2+}: Relating immunogenetics to occupational exposure, *Science* 262:197-198, 1993.

101. Finkel AJ, Hamilton A, and Hardy HL: Beryllium. In Finkel AJ, editor: *Hamilton & Hardy's industrial toxicology,* pp 26, Boston, 1983, John Wright.

102. Kreibel D, Brain JD, Sprince NL, et al: The pulmonary toxicity of beryllium, *Am Rev Respir Dis* 137:464-473, 1988.

103. Newman LS, Buschman DL, Newell JD Jr., et al: Beryllium disease: assessment with CT, *Radiology* 190:835-840, 1994.

104. Weber AL, Stoeckle JD, and Hardy HL: Roentgenologic patterns in long-standing beryllium disease: report of eight cases, *AJR* 93:879-890, 1965.

105. Aronchick JM, Rossman MD, and Miller WT: Chronic beryllium disease: diagnosis, radiographic findings, and correlation with pulmonary function tests, *Radiology* 163:677-682, 1987.

106. Pappas GP and Newman LS: Early pulmonary physiologic abnormalities in beryllium disease, *Am Rev Respir Dis* 148:661-666, 1993.

107. Freiman DG and Hardy HL: Beryllium disease: the relation of pulmonary pathology to clinical course and prognosis based on a study of 130 cases from the U.S. Beryllium Case Registry, *Hum Pathol* 1:25-44, 1970.

108. Newman LS: Beryllium disease and sarcoidosis: clinical and laboratory links, *Sarcoidosis,* in press.

109. Kreiss K, Wasserman S, Mroz MM, et al: Beryllium disease screening in the ceramics industry: blood test performance and exposure-disease relations, *J Occup Med* 35:267-274, 1993.

110. Richeldi L, Sorrentino R, and Saltini C: HLA-DPβ1 Glutamate 69: a genetic marker of beryllium disease, *Science* 262:242-244, 1993.

111. Meeting of the IARC working group on beryllium, cadmium, mercury, and exposures in the glass manufacturing industry, *Scan J Work Environ Health* 19(5):360-363, 1993.

112. Rozendaal HM: Clinical observations on the toxicology of boron hydrides, *Arch Industr Hyg Occup Med* 42:57-260, 1951.

113. Lowe HJ and Freeman G: Boron hydride (borane) intoxication in man, *Arch Industr Hyg Occup Med* 16:523-533, 1957.

114. Cordasco EM, Cooper RW, Murphy JV, et al: Pulmonary aspects of some toxic experimental space fuels, *Dis Ches* 41:68-74, 1962.

115. Lucas PA, Jarivalla AG, Jones JH, et al: Fatal cadmium fume inhalation, *Lancet* 2:205, 1980.

116. Friberg L, Piscator M, Nordberg GF, et al: *Cadmium in the environment,* Cleveland, 1974, CRC Press.

117. Bulmer FMR, Rothwell HE, and Frankish ER: Industrial cadmium poisoning, *J Can Public Health* 29:19-26, 1938.

118. Blejer HP and Caplan PE: *Occupational health: aspects of cadmium fume poisoning,* ed. 2, California, 1971, Bureau of Occupational Health and Environmental Epidemiology.

119. Buxton R: Respiratory function in men casting cadmium alloys. II. The estimation of the total lung volume, its subdivisions, and mixing coefficient, *Br J Ind Med* 13:36-40, 1956.

120. Bonnell JA, Cazantzis G, and King E: A follow-up study of men exposed to cadmium oxide fumes, *Br J Ind Med* 16:135-147, 1959.

121. Lane RE and Campbell HCB: Fatal emphysema in two men making a copper-cadmium alloy, *Br J Ind Med* 11:118-122, 1954.

122. Hirst RN Jr., Perry HM Jr., Cruz MG, et al: Elevated cadmium concentration in emphysematous lungs, *Am Rev Respir Dis* 108:30-39, 1973.

123. Townshend RH: Acute cadmium pneumonitis: A 17-year follow-up, *Br J Ind Med* 39:411-412, 1982.

124. Davison AG, Newman-Taylor AJ, Darbyshire J, et al: Cadmium fume inhalation and emphysema, *Lancet* 2:663-667, 1988.

125. Edling C, Elinder CG, and Randma E: Lung function in workers using cadmium containing solders, *Br J Ind Med* 43:657-662, 1986.

126. Armstrong BG and Kazantzis G: Prostatic cancer and chronic respiratory and renal disease in British cadmium workers: a case-controlled study, *Br J Ind Med* 42:540-545, 1985.

127. Kazantzis G, Lam TH, and Sullivan KR: Mortality of cadmium-exposed workers, *Scand J Work Environ Health* 14:220-223, 1988.

128. Wäälkes MP, Coogan TP, and Barter RA: Toxicologic principles of metal carcinogenesis with special emphasis on cadmium, *Crit Rev Toxicol* 22:175-201, 1992.

129. Martin FM and Witschi HP: Cadmium-induced lung injury: cell kinetics in long-term effects, *Toxicol Appl Pharmacol* 80:215-227, 1985.

130. Snider GL, Lucey EC, Faris B, et al: Cadmium chloride-induced air space enlargement with interstitial pulmonary fibrosis is not associated with the destruction of lung elastin: implication for the pathogenesis of human emphysema, *Am Rev Respir Dis* 137:918-923, 1988.

131. Piscator M: Role of cadmium in carcinogenesis with special reference to cancer of the prostate, *Environ Health Perspect* 40:107-120, 1981.

132. Kjellström T, Friberg L, and Rhanster B: Mortality and cancer morbidity among cadmium-exposed workers, *Environ Health Perspect* 28:199-204, 1979.

133. Kazantzis G and Armstrong BG: A mortality study of cadmium workers in 17 plants in England, In Wilson D and Volpe RA, editors: *Proceedings of the fourth international cadmium conference, Munich,* pp 139-142, London, 1982, Cadmium Association.

134. International Agency for Research on Cancer (IARC): Monographs on the evaluation of the carcinogenic risk of chemicals to humans, vol. 23, In *Some metals and metallic compounds,* vol 23, pp 139-142, Lyon, 1980, IARC.

135. Doll R: Occupational cancer: problems in interpreting human evidence, *Ann Occup Hyg* 28:291-305, 1984.

136. Wäälkes MP, Wahba ZZ, and Rodriguez RE: Cadmium. In Sullivan JB Jr. and Krieger GR, editors: *Hazardous materials toxicology clinical principals of environmental health,* pp 845-852, Baltimore, 1992, Williams & Wilkins.

137. Lauwerys RB, Roels HA, Regniers M, et al: Significance of cadmium concentration in blood and urine of workers exposed to cadmium, *Environ Res* 20:375-391, 1979.

138. Lindberg E and Hedenstierna G: Chrome plating: symptoms, findings in the upper airways, and effects on lung function, *Arch Environ Health* 38:367-374, 1983.

139. Kleinfeld M and Rosso A: Ulcerations of the nasal septum due to inhalation of chromic acid mist, *Ind Med Surg* 34:242-243, 1965.

140. Mancuso TF and Hueper WC: Occupational cancer and other health hazards in a chromate plant: a medical appraisal. I. Lung cancers in chromate workers, *Ind Med Surg* 20:358-363, 1951.

141. Mancuso TF: Occupational cancer and other health hazards in a chromate plant: a medical appraisal. II. Clinical and toxicologic aspects, *Ind Med Surg* 20:393-407, 1951.

142. Burrows D, ed: *Chromium: metabolism and toxicity,* Boca Raton, 1983, CRC Press.

143. Agency for Toxic Substances and Disease Registry (ATSDR): Toxicological profile for chromium, In *Department of Health and Human Services,* Atlanta, 1989, Public Health Service, NTIS Report No PB/89/236665/AS.

144. Meyers JB: Acute pulmonary complications following inhalation of chromic acid mist, *Ind Hyg Occup Med*:742-747.

145. Stoke J: Metal fume fever in ferro-chrome workers, *Central Afr J Med* 23(2):25-28, 1977.

146. Smith AR: Chrome poisoning with manifestations of sensitization: Report of a case, *JAMA* 97:95-98, 1931.

147. Joules H: Asthma from sensitization to chromium, *Lancet* 2:182-183, 1932.

148. Card WI: A case of asthma sensitivity to chromates, *Lancet* 2:1348-1349, 1935.

149. Kaplan I and Zeligman I: Urticaria and asthma from acetylene welding, *Arch Dermatol* 88:188-194, 1963.

150. Davies JM: Lung cancer mortality among workers making lead chromate and zinc chromate pigments at 3 English factories, *Br J Ind Med* 41:158-169, 1984.

151. Hayes RB: Review of occupational epidemiology of chromium chemicals and respiratory cancer, *Sci Total Environ* 71:331-339, 1988.

152. Norseth T: The carcinogenicity of chromium and its salts, *Br J Ind Med* 43:649-651, 1986.

153. International Agency for Research on Cancer (IARC): Monographs on the evaluation of the carcinogenic risk of chemicals to humans, vol. 23, In *Some metals and metallic compounds,* vol 23, pp 205-323, Lyon, 1980, IARC.

154. Jobs H and Ballhausen C: Powder metallurgy as a source of dust from the medical and technical standpoint, *Bertrauensartz Krankenkasse* 8:142-148, 1940.

155. Moschinski G, Jurisch A, and Reinl W: Die lungenveranderunegn bei sinterhartmetall arbeitern, *Arch Gewerbepathol Gewerbehyg:* 697-721, 1959.

156. Fairhall LT, Castberg HT, Carrosso NJ, et al: Industrial hygiene aspects of the cemented tungsten carbide industry, *Occup Med* 4:371-379, 1947.

157. Cugell DW, Morgan WKC, Perkins DG, et al: The respiratory effects of cobalt, *Arch Int Med* 150:177-183, 1990.

158. Coates EO Jr., Sawyer HJ, Rebuck JW, et al: Hypersensitivity bronchitis in tungsten carbide workers, *Chest* 64:390, 1973.

159. Coates EO and Watson JHL: Diffused interstitial lung disease in tungsten carbide workers, *Ann Int Med* 75:709-716, 1971.

160. Figueroa S, Gerstenhaber B, Welch L, et al: Hard metal interstitial pulmonary disease associated with a form of welding in a metal parts coating plant, *Am J Industr Med* 21:363-373, 1992.

161. Liebow VA: Definition and classification of interstitial pneumonias in human pathology, *Prog Respir Res* 8:1-33, 1975.

162. Demedts M, Gheysens B, Nagels J, et al: Cobalt lung in diamond polishers, *Am Rev Respir Dis* 130:130-135, 1984.

163. Auchincloss JH, Abraham JL, Gilbert R, et al: Health hazards of poorly regulated exposure during manufacture of cemented tungsten carbides and cobalt, *Br J Ind Med* 49:832-836, 1992.

164. Fischbein A, Abraham JL, and Horowitz SF: Hard metal disease: A multi-disciplinary evaluation of two cases, *NY State J Med* 11:600-603, 1986.

165. Balmes JR: Respiratory effects of hard metal dust exposure, *J Occup Med* 2:327-344, 1986.

166. Kusaka Y, Yokoyama K, Sera Y, et al: Respiratory diseases in hard metal workers: An occupational hygiene study in a factor, *Br J Ind Med* 43:474-485, 1986.

167. Burrows D and Adams RM: Metals. In Adams RM, editor: *Occupational skin diseases,* ed 2, pp 364-366, Philadelphia, 1990, W.B. Saunders Company.

168. Rystedt I and Fisher T: Relationship between nickel and cobalt sensitization in hard metal workers, *Contact Dermatitis* 9:195-210, 1983.

169. Al-Tawil NG, Marcusson JA, and Moller E: In vitro testing for cobalt sensitivity: an aid to diagnosis, *Acta Derm Venereol* 64:203-208, 1984.

170. Kusaka Y, Nakano Y, Cherakowa T, et al: Lymphocyte transformation with cobalt in hard metal asthma, *Ind Health* 27:155-163, 1989.

171. Cherakowa T, Kusaka Y, Fujimura N, et al: Occupational asthma from cobalt sensitivity in workers exposed to hard metal dust, *Chest* 95:29-37, 1989.

172. Demedts M and Ceuppens JL: Respiratory diseases from hard metal or cobalt exposure: solving the enigma, *Chest* 95:2-3, 1989.

173. Brodskii I: In Patty FA, editor: *industrial hygiene and toxicology,* vol 2, ed 2, p 1037, New York, 1963, Intrascience Publisher.

174. Gleason RP: Exposure to copper dust, *Am Ind Hyg Assoc J* 29:461-462, 1968.

175. Cortez PJ and Marques F: Vineyard sprayer's lung: a new occupational disease, *Thorax* 24:678-688, 1969.

176. Avila R: Epidemiologic aspects of suberosis and vineyard sprayer's lung, *Broncho-Pneumologie* 30:50-60, 1980.

177. Villar TG: Vineyard sprayer's lung: clinical aspect, *Am Rev Respir Dis* 110:545-555, 1974.

178. Cortez PJ and Villar TG: Pulmonary granulomatoses due to inhaled particles. In *Proceedings of the international pneumoconiosis conference,* p 465, Bucharest, 1971, Apimondia Publishing House.

179. Kuznetsov GB: Fibrogeneous effect of copper dust and copper oxide on the lungs in experimental conditions, *Gig Truda Profess Zabolev* 10:22-27, 1966.

180. Cohen SR: A review of the health hazards from copper exposure, *J Occup Med* 16:621-624, 1974.

181. Evans RB, Ettensohn DB, Fawaz-Estrup F, et al: Gold lung: Recent developments in pathogenesis, diagnosis, and therapy, *Sem Arth Rheum* 16:196-205, 1987.

182. McCormick J, Cole S, Lehirir B, et al: Pneumonitis caused by gold salts therapy: evidence for the role of cell-mediated immunity in its pathogenesis, *Am Rev Respir Dis* 122:145-152, 1980.

183. Winterbauer RH, Wilske KR, and Whellis RF: Diffuse pulmonary injury associated with gold treatment, *N Engl J Med* 294:919-921, 1976.

184. Geddes DM and Brostoff J: Pulmonary fibrosis associated with hypersensitivity to gold salts, *Br Med J* 2:1444, 1976.

185. Kleinfeld M, Messite J, Keoyman O, et al: Welders' siderosis: a clinical, roentgenographic, and physiological study, *Arch Environ Health* 19:70-73, 1969.

186. Stanescu DC, Pilat L, Gavrilescu N, et al: Aspects of pulmonary mechanics in arc welders' siderosis, *Br J Ind Med* 24:143-147, 1967.

187. Doig MB and McLaughlin ALG: X-ray appearance of the lungs of electric arc welders, *Lancet* i:771-775, 1936.

188. Albu P and Popescu HI: Lung scanning in occupational siderosis, *Am Rev Respir Dis* 107:291-294, 1973.

189. Charr R: Pulmonary changes in welders: a report of three cases, *Ann Intern Med* 44:806-812, 1956.

190. Friede E and Rachow DO: Symptomatic pulmonary disease in arc welders, *Ann Intern Med* 54:121-127, 1961.

191. Meyer E, Kratzinger SF, and Miller WH: Pulmonary fibrosis in arc welders, *Arch Environ Health* 15:462-468, 1967.

192. Funahashi A, Schlueter DP, Pintar K, et al: Welder's pneumoconiosis: Tissue elemental microanalysis by energy dispersive x-ray analysis, *Br J Ind Med* 45:14-18, 1988.

193. Doig AT and McLaughlin ALG: Clearing of x-ray shadows in welders' siderosis, *Lancet* i:789-791, 1948.

194. Morgan WKC and Kerr HD: Pathologic and physiologic studies of welder's siderosis, *Ann Intern Med* 55:293-305, 1963.

195. Faulds JS and Stewart MJ: Carcinoma of the lung in haematite miners, *J Pathol Bacteriol* 72:353-365, 1956.

196. Wagoner JK, Miller RW, Lundin FE, et al: Unusual cancer mortality among a group of underground metal miners, *N Engl J Med* 269:284-289, 1963.

197. Jörgensen HS: A study of mortality from lung cancer among miners in Kiruna, 1959-1970, *Work Environ Health* 10:126-133, 1973.

198. Lawler AB, Mandel JS, Schuman LM, et al: A retrospective cohort mortality study of iron ore (hematite) in minerals in Minnesota, *J Occup Med* 27:507-517, 1985.

199. Mur J-M, Meyer-Bisch C, Pham QT, et al: Risk of lung cancer among iron ore miners: a proportional mortality study of 1,075 deceased miners in Lorraine, France, *J Occup Med* 29:762-768, 1987.

200. Boyd JT, Doll R, Faulds JS, et al: Cancer of the lung in iron ore (hematite) miners, *Br J Ind Med* 27:97-104, 1970.

201. Gerhardsson L, Lundström N-G, Nordberg G, et al: Mortality and lead exposures: a retrospective cohort study of Swedish smelter workers, *Br J Ind Med* 43:707-712, 1986.

202. Sweeney MH, Beaumont JJ, Waxweiler RJ, et al: An investigation of mortality from cancer and other causes of death among workers employed at an East Texas chemical plant, *Arch Environ Health* 41:23-28, 1986.

203. Spiegl CJ, Scott JK, Steinhardt H, et al: Acute inhalation toxicity of lithium and anhydride, *AMA Arch Ind Health* 14:468-470, 1956.

204. Cordasco EM, Kosti H, Vance JW, et al: Pulmonary edema of noncardiac origin, *Arch Environ Health* 11:588-596, 1965.

205. Hartmann AL, Hartmann W, and Bühlmann AA: Magnesium oxide as a cause of metal fume fever, *Schweiz Med Woch* 113:766-770, 1983.

206. Morichau-Beauchant G: Pneumonies manganiques, *J Fr Medé Chir Thorac* 18:300-312, 1964.

207. Levin M, Jacobs J, and Polos PG: Acute mercury poisoning and mercurial pneumonitis from gold ore purification, *Chest* 94:554 556, 1988.

208. Milne J, Christophers A, and DeSilva P: Acute mercurial pneumonitis, *Br J Ind Med* 27(4):334-338, 1970.

209. Haddad JK and Stenberg E Jr: Bronchitis due to acute mercury inhalation, *Am Rev Respir Dis* 88:543, 1953.

210. Hallee TJ: Diffuse lung disease caused by inhalation of mercury vapor, *Am Rev Respir Dis* 99:430-436, 1969.

211. Liles R, Miller A, and Lerman Y: Acute mercury poisoning with severe chronic pulmonary manifestation, *Chest* 88:306-309, 1985.

212. Snodgrass W, Sullivan JB Jr., Rumack BH, et al: Mercury poisoning from home gold ore processing: use of penicillamine and dimercaprol, *JAMA* 246:1929-1931, 1981.

213. Sunderman FW: Clinical response to therapeutic agents in poisoning from mercury vapors, *Ann Clin Lab Sci* 8:259-269, 1978.

214. Sunderman FW and Kincaid JF: Nickel poisoning II. Studies on patients suffering from acute exposure to vapors of nickel carbonyl, *JAMA* 155:889-894, 1954.

215. Amor AJ: Toxicology of carbonyls, *J Ind Hyg* 14:216-221, 1932.

216. Zhicheng S: Acute nickel carbonyl poisoning: A report of 179 cases, *Br J Ind Med* 43:422-424, 1986.

217. Hackett RL and Sunderman FW: Acute pathological reactions to administration of Ni(CO)₄, *Arch Environ Health* 14:604-613, 1967.

218. Bayer O: Beitrag zur toxikologic, klinik und pathologischen anatomie der nickelkarbonylbergiftung, *Arch Gewerbepath Gewerbehyg* 9:592-606, 1938.

219. Sunderman FW: Kelation therapy in nickel poisoning, *Ann Clin Lab Sci* 11:1-8, 1981.

220. McConnell LH, Fink JN, Schlueter DP, et al: Asthma caused by nickel sensitivity, *Ann Intern Med* 78.888-890, 1973.

221. Block G and Chan-Yeung M: Asthma induced by nickel, *JAMA* 247:1600-1602, 1982.

222. Sunderman FW and Sunderman FW Jr.: Löffler's syndrome associated with nickel sensitivity, *Arch Intern Med* 107:149-152, 1961.

223. Arvidsson H and Bogg A: Transitory pulmonary infiltrations: Löffler's syndrome; acute generalized dermatitis, *Acta Dermat-venereol* 39:30-34, 1959.

224. Tschumy W Jr.: Pulmonary infiltration with eosinophilia (Löffler's syndrome) due to smoke inhalation: report of a case in comment on pathogenesis, *Ann Intern Med* 49:665-672, 1958.

225. Grandjean P, Andersen O, and Nielsen GD: Carcinogenecity of occupational nickel exposures: an evaluation of the epidemiologic evidence, *Am J Ind Med* 13:193-209, 1988.

226. Becker N, Claud J, and Frentzel-Beyme R: Cancer risk of arc welders exposed to fumes containing chromium and nickel, *Scand J Work Environ Health* 11:75-82, 1985.

227. Doll R, Morgan G, and Speizer FE: Cancers of the lung and nasal sinus in nickel workers, *Br J Cancer* 24:623-632, 1970.

228. Sorahan T: Mortality from lung cancer among a cohort nickel cadmium battery workers: 1946-1984, *Br J Ind Med* 44:803-809, 1987.

229. Sunderman FW Jr: A review of the carcinogenicities of nickel, chromium, and arsenic compounds in man and animals, *Prev Med* 5:279-294, 1976.

230. McLaughlin AIG, Milton R, and Perry KMA: Toxic manifestations of osmium tetraoxide, *Br J Ind Med* 3:183-186, 1946.

231. Wason S, Gomolin I, Mariam S, et al: Phosphorus trichloride toxicity: preliminary report, *Am J Med* 77:1039-1042, 1984.

232. Rubitsky HJ and Myerson RM: Acute phosphorus poisoning, *Arch Intern Med* 83:164-178, 1949.

233. Hunter D, Milton R, and Perry KMA: Asthma caused by the complex salts of platinum, *Br J Ind Med* 2:92-98, 1945.

234. Roberts AE: Platinosis: a five-year study of the effects of soluble platinum salts on employees in a platinum laboratory and refinery, *Arch Ind Hyg Occup Med* 4:549-559, 1951.

235. Pepys J, Pickering CAC, and Hughes EG: Asthma due to inhaled chemical agents: complex salts of platinum, *Clin Allergy* 2:391-396, 1972.

236. Hughes EG: Medical surveillance of platinum refinery workers, *J Soc Occup Med* 30:27-30, 1980.

237. Cromwell O, Pepys J, Parish WE, et al: Specific IgE antibodies to platinum salts in sensitized workers, *Clin Allergy* 9:109-117, 1979.

238. Biagini RE, Bernstein IL, Gallagher JH, et al: The diversity of reaginic immune responses to platinum and palladium metallic salts, *Allergy Clin Immunol* 76:794-802, 1985.

239. Murdock RD, Pepys J, and Hughes EG: IgE antibody responses to platinum group metals: a large scale refinery survey, *Br J Ind Med* 43:37-43, 1986.

240. Seiler HG and Siegel H: *Handbook on toxicity of inorganic compounds,* pp 341-344, New York, 1988, Marcel Dekker.

241. Schepers GWH, Delahant AB, and Redlan AJ: An experimental study of the effects of rare earths on animal lungs, *AMA Arch Ind Health* 12:297-300, 1955.

242. Heuck F and Hoschek R: Cer-pneumoconiosis, *AJR* 104:777-783, 1968.

243. Sinico M, Le Bouffant L, Paillas J, et al: Pneumoconiose due au cérium: documents anatomopathologiques, *Arch Mal Profess* 43:249-252, 1982.

244. Husain MH, Dick JA, and Kaplaen YS: Rare-earth pneumoconiosis, *J Soc Occup Med* 30:15-19, 1980.

245. Vocaturo G, Colombo F, Zanoni M, et al: Human exposure to heavy metals: rare earth pneumoconiosis in occupational workers, *Chest* 83:780-783, 1983.

246. Sulotto F, Romano C, Berra A, et al: Rare-earth pneumoconiosis: a new case, *Am J Ind Med* 9:567-575, 1986.

247. Schecter A, Shanske W, Stenzler A, et al: Acute hydrogen selenide inhalation, *Chest* 77:554-555, 1980.

248. Motley HL, Ellis MM, and Ellis MD: Acute sore throats following exposure to selenium, *JAMA* 109(21):1718-1719, 1937.

249. Buchan RF: Industrial selenosis: a review of the literature, report of five cases, and a general bibliography, *Occup Med* 3:439-456, 1947.

250. Dudley HC and Miller JW: Toxicology of Selenium: VI. Effects of subacute exposure to hydrogen selenide, *J Ind Hyg Toxicol* 23(10):470-477, 1941.

251. Adelson L and Sunshine I: Fatal hydrogen sulfide intoxication: report of three cases occurring in a sewer, *Arch Pathol* 81:375-380, 1966.

252. Diskin CJ, Tomasso CL, Alper JC, et al: Long-term selenium exposure, *Arch Int Med* 139:824-826, 1979.

253. Harding HE: Fibrosis in the lungs of a silver finisher, *Br J Ind Med* 5:70-73, 1948.

254. McLaughlin AIG, Grout JLA, Barrie HJ, et al: Iron dust in the lung of silver finishers, *Lancet* 1:337-341, 1945.

255. Chien PT: Metallic copper and silver dust hazards, *Ind Hyg Assoc J* 40:747, 1979.

256. Rosenman KD, Moss A, and Kon S: Argyria: clinical implications of exposure to silver nitrate and silver oxide, *J Occup Med* 21:430-435, 1979.

257. Rosenman KD, Seixas N, and Jacobs I: Potential nephrotoxic effects of exposure to silver, *Br J Ind Med* 44:267-272, 1987.

258. Davis LE, Standefer JC, Kornfeld M, et al: Acute thallium poisoning: toxicological and morphological studies of the nervous system, *Ann Neurol* 10:38-44, 1981.

259. Hologgitas J, Ullucci P, and Driscoll J: Thallium elimination kinetics in acute thallotoxicosis, *J Anal Toxicol* 44:68-73, 1980.

260. Roby DS, Fein AM, Bennet RH, et al: Cardiopulmonary effects of acute thallium poisoning, *Chest* 85:236-240, 1984.

261. Oyanguren H, Haddad R, and Maass H: Stannosis: benign pneumoconiosis owing to inhalation of tin dust and fume. I. Environmental and experimental studies, *Ind Med Surg* 27:427-429, 1958.

262. Robertson AJ, Rivers D, Nagelschmidt G, et al: Stannosis: benign pneumoconiosis due to tin dioxide, *Lancet* I:1089-1095, 1961.

263. Robertson AJ and Whitaker PH: Radiological changes in pneumoconiosis due to tin oxide, *J Fac Radiol* 6:224-233, 1955.

264. Dundon CC and Hughes JP: Stannic oxide pneumoconiosis, *Am J Roent* 63:797-812, 1950.

265. Cutter HC, Faller WW, Stocklen JB, et al: Benign pneumoconiosis in a tin oxide recovery plant, *J Ind Hyg Toxicol* 31:139-141, 1949.

266. Pendergrass EP and Pryde AW: Benign pneumoconiosis due to tin oxide: case report with experimental investigation of radiographic density of tin oxide dust, *J Ind Hyg Toxicol* 30:119-123, 1948.

267. Spencer GE and Wycoff WC: Benign tin oxide pneumoconiosis, *Ind Hyg Occup Med* 10:295-296, 1954.

268. Cole CWD, Davies JVSA, Kipling MD, et al: Stannosis in hearth tinners, *Br J Ind Med* 21:235-241, 1964.

269. Pendergrass EP and Leopold SS: Benign pneumoconiosis, *JAMA* 127:701-705, 1945.

270. Belt TH: The pathology of pneumoconiosis: a review, *Am J Med Sci* 188:418-435, 1934.

271. Elo R, Määtä K, Uksila E, et al: Pulmonary deposits of titanium dioxide in man, *Arch Pathol* 94:417-424, 1972.

272. Määtä K and Arstila AV: Pulmonary deposits of titanium dioxide in cytologic and lung biopsy specimens: light and electron microscopic x-ray analysis, *Lab Invest* 33:342-346, 1975.

273. Garabrandt DH, Fine LJ, Oliver C, et al: Abnormalities of pulmonary function in pleural disease among titanium metal production workers, *Scand J Work Environ Health* 13:47-51, 1987.

274. Chen JL and Fayerweather WE: Epidemiologic study of workers exposed to titanium dioxide, *J Occup Med* 30:937-942, 1988.

275. Oleru UG: Respiratory and non-respiratory morbidity in a titanium oxide paint factor in Nigeria, *Am J Ind Med* 12:173-180, 1987.

276. Uragoda CG and Pinto MRN: An investigation into the health of workers in an ilmenite extraction plant, *Med J Aust* 1:167-169, 1972.

277. Daum S, Anderson HA, Lilis R, et al: Pulmonary changes among titanium workers, *Proc R Soc Med* 70:31-32, 1977.

278. Schmitz-Moorman P, Hörlein H, and Hanefeld F: Lungenveranderungen bei titandioxyd staub exposition, *Beitr Silikose ForschungQ* 80:1-17, 1964.

279. Dale K: Early effects of quartz and titanium dioxide dust on pulmonary function and tissue: an experimental study on rabbits, *Scand J Respir Dis* 54:168-184, 1973.

280. Lee KP, Trochimowicz HJ, and Reinhardt CF: Pulmonary response of rats exposed to titanium dioxide (TiO_2) by inhalation for two years, *Toxicol Appl Pharmacol* 79:179-192, 1985.

281. Grandjean E, Turrian H, and Nicod JL: The fibrogenic action of quartz dusts, *Arch Ind Health* 14:421-441, 1956.

282. Redline S, Barna BP, Tomashefski JF, et al: Granulomatous disease associated with pulmonary deposition of titanium, *Br J Ind Med* 43:652-656, 1986.

283. Angebault M, Berland M, Parent G, et al: Toxicité pulmonaire du bioxyde de titane, risque lié au ponchee des mastics, *Arch Mal Prof Med Tray* 40:501-508, 1979.

284. Lawson JJ: The toxicity of titanium tetrachloride, *J Occup Med* 3:7-12, 1961.

285. Park T, DiBenedetto R, Morgan K, et al: Diffuse endobronchial polyposis following a titanium tetrachloride inhalation injury, *Am Rev Respir Dis* 130:315-317, 1984.

286. Finkel AJ, Hamilton A, and Hardy HL: Titanium, In Finkel AJ, editor: *Hamilton and Hardy's industrial toxicology*, pp 136-137, Boston, 1983, John Wright/PSGE.

287. Lundgren K-D and Swensson A: Experimental investigations using method of Miller and Sayers on the effect upon animals of cemented tungsten carbides and powders used as raw material, *Acta Med Scand* 145:20-27, 1953.

288. Delahant AB: An experimental study of the effects of rare metals on animal lungs, *Arch Ind Health* 12:116-120, 1955.

289. Moore RH and Kathren RL: A World War II uranium hexafluoride inhalation event with pulmonary implications for today, *J Occup Med* 27:753-756, 1985.

290. Archer VE, Brinton HP, and Wagoner JK: Pulmonary function of uranium miners, *Health Phys* 10:1183-1194, 1964.

291. Archer VE, Wagoner JK, and Lundin FE Jr: Lung cancer among uranium miners in the United States, *Health Phys* 25:351-371, 1973.

292. Samet JM, Young RA, Morgan MV, et al: Prevalence survey of respiratory abnormalities in New Mexico uranium miners, *Health Phys* 46:361-370, 1984.

293. Dutton LF: Vanadiumism, *JAMA* 56:1648, 1911.

294. Finkel AJ, Hamilton A, and Hardy HL: Vanadium, In Finkel AJ, editor: *Hamilton and Hardy's industrial toxicology*, pp 139-141, Boston, 1983, John Wright/PSGE.

295. Levy BS, Hoffman L, and Gottsegen S: Boilermakers' bronchitis: Respiratory tract irritation associated with vanadium pentoxide exposure during oil-to-coal conversion of a power plant, *J Occup Med* 26:567-570, 1984.

296. Sjöberg SG: Vanadium bronchitis from cleaning oil-fired boilers, *Arch Ind Health* 12:505-512, 1955.

297. Sjöberg SG: Follow-up investigation of workers at a vanadium factory, *Acta Med Scand* 154:381-386, 1956.

298. Lees REM: Changes in lung function after exposure to vanadium compounds in fuel oil ash, *Br J Ind Med* 37:253-256, 1980.

299. NIOSH: Criteria for a Recommended Standard: Occupational exposure to vanadium, Publ No 77-222, Washington, DC, 1977, U.S. Government Printing Office [DHEW (National Institute for Occupational Safety and Health)].

300. Musk AW and Tees JG: Asthma caused by occupational exposure to vanadium compounds, *Med J Aust* 1:183-184, 1982.

301. Kiviluoto M: Observations of the lungs of vanadium workers, *Br J Ind Med* 37:363-366, 1980.

302. Williams N: Vanadium poisoning from cleaning oil-fired boilers, *Br J Ind Med* 9:50-55, 1952.

303. Browne RC: Vanadium poisoning from gas turbine, *Br J Ind Med* 12:57-59, 1955.

304. Debrock HE and Mackle W: Exposure to europium-activated yttrium orthovanadate, *J Occup Med* 10:692-696, 1968.

305. Kawai T, Seiji K, Watanabe T, et al: Urinary vanadium as a biological indicator of exposure to vanadium, *Int Arch Occup Environ Health* 61:283-287, 1989.

306. Farrell AJ: Metal oxides. In Sullivan JB Jr. and Kreiger GR, editors: *Hazardous materials toxicology*, pp 921-927, Baltimore, 1992, Williams & Wilkins.

307. Blanc P, Wong H, Bernstein MS, et al: An experimental human model of metal fume fever, *Ann Intern Med* 114:930-936, 1991.

308. Gordon T, Chen LC, Fine JM, et al: Pulmonary effects of inhaled zinc oxide in human subjects, guinea pigs, rats, and rabbits, *Am Ind Hyg Assoc J* 53:503-509, 1992.

309. McCord CP and Kilker CH: Zinc chloride poisoning, *JAMA* 76:442-443, 1921.

310. du Bray ES: Chronic zinc intoxication, *JAMA* 108:383-385, 1937.

311. Evans EH: Casualities following exposure to zinc chloride smoke, *Lancet* 2:368-370, 1945.

312. Macauley MB and Mant AK: Smoke-bomb poisoning: a fatal case following the inhalation of zinc chloride smoke, *J RAMC* 110:27-32, 1964.

313. Milliken JA, Waugh D, and Cadish ME: Case report: acute interstitial pulmonary fibrosis caused by a smoke bomb, *Can Med Assoc J* 88:36-39, 1963.

314. Hjortsberg U, Nise G, Orbae KP, et al: Bronchial asthma due to exposure to potassium aluminum tetrafluoride, *Scand J Work Environ Health* 12:223, 1986.

315. Hjortsø E, Qvist J, Budm I, et al: ARDS after accidental inhalation of zinc chloride smoke, *Intensive Care Med* 14:17-24, 1988.

316. Matarese SL and Matthews JI: Zinc chloride (smoke bomb) inhalational lung injury, *Chest* 89:308-309, 1986.

317. Pedersen C, Hansen CP, and Grønfeldt W: Zinc chloride smoke poisoning following employment of smoke amunition, *J Dan Med Assoc (Copenhagen)* 146:2397, 1984.

318. Johnson FA and Stonehill RB: Chemical pneumonitis from inhalation of zinc chloride, *Dis Chest* 40:619-624, 1961.

319. Pare CMB and Sandler M: Smoke-bomb pneumonitis: description of a case, *J RAMC* 100:320-322, 1954.

320. Malo J-L and Cartier A: Occupational asthma due to fumes of galvanized metal, *Chest* 92:375-377, 1987.

321. Farrell FJ: Angioedema and urticaria as acute- and late-phase reactions to zinc fume exposure, with associated metal fume fever-like symptoms, *Am J Ind Med* 12:331-337, 1987.

322. Sheffet A, Thind I, Miller AM, et al: Cancer mortality in a pigment plant utilizing lead and zinc chromates, *Arch Environ Health* 37:44-52, 1982.

323. Reed CE: Effects of the lungs of industrial exposure to zirconium dust, *Arch Ind Health* 13:578-581, 1956.

324. Finkel AJ, Hamilton A, and Hardy HL: Zirconium. In Finkel AJ, editor: *Hamilton and Hardy's industrial toxicology,* p 145, Boston, 1983, John Wright/PSGE.

325. Hadjimichael OC and Brubaker RE: Evaluation of an occupational exposure to a zirconium-containing dust, *J Occup Med* 23:543-547, 1981.

326. Bartter T, Irwin RS, Abraham JL, et al: Zirconium compound-induced pulmonary fibrosis, *Arch Intern Med* 151:1197-1201, 1991.

327. Romeo L, Cazzadori A, Botempini L, et al: Zirconium interstitial lung disease: case reports, In Hurych J, Lesage M, and David A, editors: *8th international conference on occupational lung diseases,* vol 3, pp 1016-1020, Prague, Czech Republic, 1993, Czech Medical Society and Geneva: International Labour Office.

Chapter 30

ACUTE GASEOUS EXPOSURE

George L. Delclos
Arch I. Carson

"Those who deal with burning or liquefied sulphur contract coughs, dyspnoea, hoarseness, and sore eyes. . . . When sulphur has been liquefied over a fire or still more when it is burning, this volatile acid rises in fumes. When these fumes are taken in by the mouth they occasion the afore-said ailments, and especially they excite coughing and sore eyes. For the tender and delicate texture of the lungs and eyes is peculiarly liable to injury from a pungent acid. . . .

There is a well-known anecdote of an unfaithful wife who, when her husband came home, hid her lover under the bed; to cover up her crime she threw over him a garment that had been cleaned with sulphur, but by this she betrayed herself, for the lover was choked by the smell of fresh sulphur and could not help coughing and sneezing violently."

BERNARDINO RAMAZZINI
DE MORBIS ARTIFICUM DIATRIBA, 1713[1]

This chapter addresses the health effects of acute exposures to toxic gases and vapors, which can present in the emergency center setting, often following an inadvertent spill or emission or under conditions of inadequate ventilation. Although most of the focus is on exposure to individual gases, some concepts regarding the effects of exposure to gas mixtures, specifically smoke inhalation, are also included. Although "fume" is a term often used as a synonym for a specific gas or vapor, in the strictest sense its use should be limited to metal particles formed by the condensation of vapors from heated metals. Since they behave as particles, their mass median aerodynamic diameter will be the principal determinant of the site of deposition and location of injury. Dusts, mists, and fumes behave as aerosols, and are addressed in Sections V through VII. Discussion of health effects of more chronic, lower level exposures to gases and vapors, although certainly of public health interest, is also beyond the scope of this chapter.

Although acute gas exposure incidents most commonly involve a single individual or small groups of workers, examples of exposure of entire communities, with tragic outcomes, are well documented in the medical literature and through the media. Thus, the release of methyl isocyanate gas, a potent and deadly irritant, from a pesticide plant in Bhopal, India in 1984,[2] or of naturally occurring carbon dioxide gas, a simple asphyxiant, from a volcanic lake in Lake Nyos, Cameroon in 1986[3,4] serve as recent reminders that, despite technological advances in the control of hazardous gas and vapor emissions, there are still instances where sudden exposure to toxic inhalants may be unleashed and result in the loss of lives.

DEFINITION OF AGENT

Inhalation is one of the major routes through which materials can enter our body. It has been estimated that, when measured as volume, we take in approximately 5,000 times more air than either water or food over a lifetime.[5] In addition, however, numerous other substances, some of them potentially toxic, are present in the atmosphere along with air. Airborne materials can be classified into aerosols or gases and vapors. *Aerosols* are defined as any collection of solid particles or liquid droplets of small enough particle size to remain suspended in air for a period of time. *Gases* are fluids that tend to expand indefinitely and therefore have no independent volume or shape. A gas can be transformed into the liquid or solid state only by increasing its pressure and/or decreasing its temperature. *Vapors* are substances that, under room temperature and pressure, exist normally as a solid or liquid. However, there are molecules at the surface of this liquid or solid that, because of high individual kinetic energies, tend to continuously leave the surface and enter the gaseous phase. For any given temperature and pressure, the number of vapor molecules remains constant, as does the pressure exerted by these molecules (vapor pressure). Both gases and vapors can be referred to using the more general term *gaseous*.

The spectrum of health effects of an acute exposure to a gas or vapor is broad and dependent on the exposure characteristics and physicochemical properties of the toxic agent, as well as on specific host factors. The medical literature provides a large body of knowledge regarding the immediate effects of an acute exposure; less well established, and recently an area of scientific interest, are the long-term consequences of single or multiple exposures to high levels of a single gas or mixture of gases.

In general, a gas or vapor may predominantly impact the respiratory system or simply use the lungs as a route of entry to other target organs. Acute respiratory effects can vary from mild mucosal irritation to fatal respiratory failure, usually by asphyxiation or massive pulmonary edema. Long-term effects reported to date include persistent airways dysfunction with[6] or without subsequent sensitization[7]; rarely, chronic respiratory failure as a consequence of bronchiolitis obliterans[8] or bronchiectasis[9,10] occurs. Pulmonary fibrosis, as a sequela to noncardiogenic pulmonary edema, is probably very rare in these circumstances.[11] The systemic toxicities of a gas exposure will depend on the target organ system affected. Most often these will consist of acute neurologic effects, hepatic or renal dysfunction, or acute hematologic emergencies.

Exposure to hazardous gases and vapors is regulated primarily by the Occupational Safety and Health Administration (OSHA), in the occupational setting, and by the Environmental Protection Agency (EPA), which regulates exposure of the general public through various statutes.

EXPOSURE
Magnitude of the problem

In a recent analysis of 32,933 reports to the American Association of Poison Control Centers Toxic Exposure Surveillance System, inhalation was the most common route of exposure in both occupational (43.6% of reports) and environmental (61.4% of reports) settings.[12] Exposure to fumes, gases, and/or vapors was responsible for most of the fatalities in both settings, primarily from exposure to hydrogen sulfide (occupational) and carbon monoxide (environmental). Similarly, of 4,756 workplace deaths investigated by OSHA from 1984 to 1986, 233 (4.9%) were due to asphyxiation and poisoning (excluding trench cave-ins); the majority of these were caused by toxic gases and simple asphyxiants.[13]

Most of the literature dealing with smoke exposure centers around the effects of accidental exposure in fires, explosions, industrial accidents, or transportation mishaps. Over 8,000 fire fatalities occur annually in the United States. Of these, 80% can be attributed to the acute inhalation of toxic products of combustion.[14] This proportion seems to hold true for different regions of the country and hospitals serving different segments of the population. The proportion of fire fatalities due primarily to toxic respiratory tract injury ranges between 70% and 89%.[15–20]

Population at risk

The sources of potential exposure to toxic respiratory gases and vapors are numerous and by no means limited to the workplace. Several thousand new chemical products are introduced into the world marketplace every year, targeted for use in occupational, community, and/or residential settings. Many of these materials are capable of becoming airborne and entering the body through the lungs. Because of the almost ubiquitous presence of chemicals in our daily lives, the population at risk for accidental exposure to dangerous levels of certain toxic gases and vapors could theoretically include any member of a modern society, as end product users. It is, therefore, difficult to accurately estimate numbers of persons at risk for acute exposure to single gases and vapors. In the occupational setting, some idea of the number of U.S. workers at risk can be obtained by combining estimates of exposure to the most commonly cited agents (Table 30-1), based on two separate surveys conducted by the National Institute for Occupational Safety and Health (NIOSH), the 1972–1974 National Occupational Hazard Survey (NOHS), and the 1981–1983 National Occupational Exposure Survey (NOES).[21,22] This is likely to underestimate the true figures given the limited number of chemicals considered, the lack of consideration of exposure to mixtures, the exclusion from the survey of very small businesses (where safety practices may be lacking), and the age of the data. Table 30-2 presents a partial list of occupations commonly associated with a potential for exposure to respiratory asphyxiants and irritants.

Table 30-1. Estimates of U.S. workers exposed to common gases and vapors with respiratory toxicity

	NOHS*	NOES†
Asphyxiants		
Carbon dioxide	447,416	192,401
Carbon monoxide	—	68,434
Hydrogen sulfide	15,422	94,923
Cyanides	41,740	134,716
Acrylonitrile	55,698	81,691
Irritants		
Ammonia	1,168,429	805,962
Sulfur dioxide	51,398	55,033
Hydrogen fluoride	68,886	189,051
Chlorine	220,544	4,768
Phosgene	5,729	2,358
Oxides of nitrogen	11,419	18,737

*National Occupational Hazards Survey, 1971-1974.[21]
†National Occupational Exposure Survey, 1981-1983.[22]

Measurement of exposure

Concentrations of gas may be expressed as a volume-to-volume measurement (e.g., parts per million [ppm]):

$$ppm = gas\ volume/air\ volume$$

Alternatively, concentration may be presented on a mass per unit volume basis in which gas weight, usually in milligrams, for a given volume of air, usually expressed as cubic meters, is reported (mg/m^3). These two units of measurement can be interconverted by the equations:

$$ppm = mg/m^3 \times 24.5/MW\ (at\ 25°\ C\ and\ 760\ mm\ Hg)$$

or

$$mg/m^3 = ppm/24.5 \times MW$$

where MW is the molecular weight of the substance of concern.

Permissible exposure levels, such as those recommended by the American Conference of Governmental Industrial Hygienists (ACGIH) or mandated by OSHA and EPA, will usually be expressed in these units (see Regulatory Aspects, below).

Warning properties

One key consideration regarding dangerous gases and vapors relates to the degree with which they make their presence known to potential victims. This phenomenon is referred to as the "warning properties" of a substance, and comprises its potential to stimulate the senses of persons who encounter it. In general, gases or vapors that have a very strong or otherwise noticeable odor even at very low concentrations or are very irritating to mucous membranes or the eyes, or have vivid colors, are said to have good warning properties. Warning properties themselves may be

Table 30-2. A partial listing of occupations with potential for toxic gas and/or vapor exposures

Occupation	Gas or vapor
Aircraft workers	Solvents
	Thinners
	Paints
	Hydrogen fluoride
Animal handlers, zookeepers	Disinfectants
	Cleaners
	Deodorants
	Insecticides
	Germicides
Artists	Paints
	Thinners
	Solvents
	Polishes
Automobile workers, mechanics	Gasoline
	Solvents
	Cleansers
	Alkalis
	Formaldehyde
	Paints
Bakers	Carbon dioxide
Battery makers	Alkali
	Solvents
	Sulfuric acid
Bookbinders	Formaldehyde
	Solvents
	Thinners
Bronzers	Ammonia
	Solvents
	Cyanides
	Hydrochloric acid
	Sulfur dioxide
Carpenters, furniture makers	Acid bleaches
	Solvents
	Polishes
	Formaldehyde
	Acrylonitrile
Carpet makers, upholsterers	Solvents
	Cleaners
	Formaldehyde
Chemical workers	Acids
	Alkalis
	Cleaners
	Disinfectants
	Formaldehyde
	Ammonia
	Phosgene
	Cyanides
	Nitriles
	Hydrogen sulfide
	Hydrogen fluoride
Clerks	Solvents
	Formaldehyde
Degreasers	Alkalis
	Solvents
Dentists	Disinfectants
	Formaldehyde
Dry cleaners	Acetic acid
	Ammonia

Continued.

Table 30-2. A partial listing of occupations with potential for toxic gas and/or vapor exposures—cont'd

Occupation	Gas or vapor
Dry cleaners	Solvents
Dye makers	Solvents
	Acids
	Alkalis
Electricians	Solvents
	Varnishes
Electronics, semiconductor workers	Acids
	Alkalis
	Ammonia
	Arsine
	Phosphine
	Solvents
Entomologists	Pesticides
	Fungicides
	Disinfectants
Farmers, florists	Disinfectants
	Fungicides
	Pesticides
	Solvents
	Herbicides
	Ammonia
	Oxides of nitrogen
Firefighters, policemen	Smoke
	Cyanides
	Carbon monoxide
	Carbon dioxide
	Nitriles
	Acrolein
	Oxides of nitrogen
	Solvents
	Hydrochloric acid
Food processors	Bleaches
	Acetic acid
	Disinfectants
Hairdressers	Formaldehyde
	Antiseptics
	Cosmetics
	Dyes
Healthcare workers	Solvents
	Disinfectants, sterilizing agents
	Formaldehyde
Histology technicians	Formaldehyde
	Solvents
Jewelers	Acids
	Cyanides
	Formaldehyde
Laundry workers	Bleaches
	Alkalis
	Fungicides
	Germicides
	Hydrogen fluoride
	Chlorine
Loggers	Formaldehyde glue
	Pesticides
	Fungicides
Longshoremen	Insecticides
	Fumigants
	Petroleum, tar

Continued.

Table 30-2. A partial listing of occupations with potential for toxic gas and/or vapor exposures—cont'd

Occupation	Gas or vapor
Painters	Acids
	Alkalis
	Solvents
	Thinners, strippers
	Paints
Pharmaceutical industry	Disinfectants
Platers	Acids
	Organic vapors
Printers	Solvents
	Alkalis
	Thinners
	Acids
Railroad workers	Acids
	Solvents
	Formaldehyde
Sewer workers	Chlorine
	Disinfectants
	Hydrogen sulfide
	Methane
	Ammonia
	Carbon dioxide
Shoemakers	Formaldehyde
	Ammonia
	Solvents
	Polish
Swimming pool workers	Chlorine
Textile workers	Solvents
	Bleaches
	Formaldehyde
Welders	Solvents
	Smoke
	Phosgene
	Ozone
	Hydrogen fluoride
	Oxides of nitrogen

important preventors of injury in that they alert bystanders to a danger, or repel them from the area of potential exposure. If these effects occur at concentrations lower than those producing adverse health effects, then the warning properties are said to be protective. Environmental or host factors that alter perception may mask a substance's warning properties and thereby increase the potential for harm. For example, darkness may render nitrogen dioxide, usually an orange brown gas, entirely invisible. Likewise, the presence of carbon disulfide (CS_2) vapors in the air may mask the characteristic rotten egg odor of hydrogen sulfide.

Monitors, detectors, and dosimeters

Because many harmful gaseous substances have poor warning properties or are subject to masking, devices have been developed to supplement the senses in the early detection of low concentrations. When available, which unfortunately is often not the case, the information provided by these devices can be invaluable in defining the nature and extent of exposure, allowing the clinician to anticipate the likely clinical evolution of an injured worker. *Detectors* are devices that undergo a sudden transformation when exposed to the substance of interest. This change then serves as a signal to the presence of a dangerous gas. Detectors often employ a paper strip that has been impregnated with a chemical matrix that changes color when the gas in the air reacts with it. This principle is sometimes employed in badges that are worn near a worker's breathing zone. A color change signals that some exposure has occurred. Detector badges are available for a variety of gaseous substances, including arsine, hydrogen cyanide, hydrogen sulfide, and phosgene. Once reacted, detectors cannot be reused. *Monitors* are devices that continuously sample the air for the presence of a contaminant. They are usually set for a particular threshold concentration that, when surpassed, causes an alarm to sound or lights to flash. They may also be used as a continuous recorder of environmental levels, and are usually installed in fixed locations providing area measurements. *Dosimeters* are devices that are worn by potentially exposed workers. They absorb gaseous materials that may be recovered and analyzed, or in some way undergo progressive changes over a period of time, so that later the total exposure can be assessed.

Detectors, monitors, and dosimeters are designed to be sensitive, but often lack the specificity or precision desirable for the assessment and reconstruction of a given exposure. For this reason, more accurate sampling methods have been developed that utilize calibrated airflow pumps and standardized analyses for determination of airborne contaminant concentration. Industrial hygienists are particularly trained to employ or recommend the appropriate techniques for the particular workplace or environmental setting of concern. Special training and skills allow the industrial hygiene professional to apply critical analytical practices to the assessment and remediation of airborne hazards in the workplace.

EFFECTS OVERVIEW AND GENERAL MECHANISMS
General classification

Based on the site and mechanism of injury, a classification of acute gaseous exposure can be constructed that is useful in clinical practice (see box, top of next column). Depending on the type of gas, the respiratory system may either be the primary target organ of injury (respiratory toxicant) or merely serve as a route of exposure for gases that exert their main effects on other target organs (systemic toxicant), such as the central nervous and hematologic systems. Exposure may be to a known single agent (e.g., following a release from an ammonia or chlorine tank car). In this case the immediate toxicity of the agent is reasonably easy to identify, based on information from the medical literature, material safety data sheets, or consultation with poison control centers. The consequences of exposure to mix-

---

General classification of acute inhalational toxicants

I. Respiratory toxicants

  A. Single agents
    1. Asphyxiants
      a. Simple
      b. Chemical
        i. Agents that decrease O_2-carrying capacity
          —Carbon monoxide
          —Hydrogen sulfide
          —Oxides of nitrogen
        ii. Agents that inhibit tissue oxygen utilization
          —Hydrogen cyanide
          —Hydrogen sulfide
          —Acrylonitrile
    2. Irritants
      a. High solubility gases
        —Ammonia
        —Sulfur dioxide
        —Formaldehyde
        —Chlorine (intermediate solubility)
      b. Low solubility gases
        —Oxides of nitrogen
        —Phosgene
        —Ozone
  B. Mixtures
    1. Smoke inhalation
    2. Other

II. Systemic toxicants

  A. Nervous system: solvent vapors
  B. Other systems: arsine

---

tures of gases or vapors, (e.g., household cleaning products, smoke inhalation or following a release from a chemical waste line) may be less well defined, and therefore difficult for the clinician to predict. In these cases, the effects may represent the summation of the individual toxicities of one or more gases in the mixture, or there may be interaction (potentiation or antagonistic action) among the various agents.[23]

Determinants of injury

For injury to the respiratory tract to occur as a consequence of acute exposure to a respiratory toxicant, several determinants come into play. These determinants can be divided into factors relating to the gaseous agent and host factors (see box on page 519). The net effect of the interaction among these various determinants will define the likelihood, severity, and type of injury.

Physical and chemical properties of the toxicant. The physical state and chemical properties of the toxicant are important determinants of the pathogenesis of the injury.

Asphyxiant gases exert their effect either by reducing the partial pressure of oxygen in ambient air (simple asphyxi-

---

Determinants of injury

Toxicant factors

Physical and chemical properties
Intensity (concentration/duration) of exposure

Host factors

Defense mechanisms
Ventilatory parameters
Preexisting health status

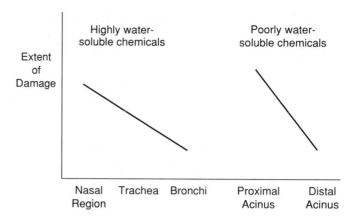

Fig. 30-1. Gradients of injury to the respiratory tract caused by inhaled respiratory irritants, which depend on the water solubility of the gas, especially at lower concentrations. At very high gas concentrations, however, damage tends to involve the entire respiratory tract, with loss of the gradient. (Adapted from Dungworth DL: Noncarcinogenic responses of the respiratory tract to inhaled toxicants, In McClellan RO, Henderson RF, editors: *Concepts in inhalation toxicology.* New York, 1989, Hemisphere. With permission.)

ants) or by influencing oxygen utilization at the cellular or subcellular level (chemical asphyxiants).

Virtually any gas can behave as a simple asphyxiant if its ambient concentration is great enough to decrease the fraction of inspired oxygen (FIO_2) to levels that cause a decrease in arterial oxygen saturation. Generally, humans are able to tolerate drops in FIO_2 from 0.21 to around 0.16 without significant symptoms. Greater decreases lead to tachypnea, tachycardia, lack of coordination, fatigue, altered mental status, and ultimately, at levels below 0.06, seizures and cardiopulmonary arrest.[24]

Chemical asphyxiants may interfere with the oxygen-carrying capacity of hemoglobin (e.g., carbon monoxide, hydrogen sulfide, oxides of nitrogen or hydrogen cyanide), or decrease tissue oxygenation by blocking the cytochrome oxygen transport chain (hydrogen cyanide, hydrogen sulfide, acrylonitrile) in the mitochondria.

Irritant gases are characterized by their ability to injure the tissue with which they come in direct contact, causing inflammation. Irritant injury may be produced by extreme alterations in pH at the cell membrane surface (acid gases), by nonspecific chemical reaction with membrane and intracellular components (lipid peroxidation, alkylation, hydrolysis), or by specific toxic effects on cellular or tissue systems (enzyme inhibition, pharmacologic effect). The spectrum of pathology produced may range from mild, transient hyperemia with increased interstitial and intraluminal secretions, to massive edema and extensive tissue destruction and denudation.[25,26] The repair process routinely involves cell proliferation in the damaged tissues as a common response to toxic injury, and may ultimately resolve with permanent alterations of the anatomy and physiology of the respiratory system.[23,27–29] Animal studies have confirmed the relationship between a single exposure to one or a combination of substances and the development of chronic progressive lesions.[23]

When dealing with irritant gases, the intrinsic *water solubility* of the gas is an important element in defining the anatomic site of cytotoxic injury within the respiratory system. Highly water-soluble gases, such as ammonia, sulfur dioxide, and acidic gases, possess a high affinity for cells and epithelia rich in water content. These cells are predominantly found lining the conjunctiva and upper respiratory

tract, including the nasal passages, nasal and oropharynx, and laryngotracheobronchial region. It will be primarily these structures, following a proximal to distal gradient, that will sustain and manifest the irritation produced by highly soluble gases, especially at lower exposure ranges (Fig. 30-1).[30] Patients may present acutely with findings of conjunctivitis, lacrimation, rhinitis, epistaxis, pharyngitis, laryngotracheitis, bronchitis, and/or bronchospasm. Pathological lesions produced by irritant injury of the airways include ciliated epithelial cell destruction with replacement by nonciliated Clara cells, increased epithelial permeability, goblet cell emigration and hyperplasia, and hyperresponsiveness to both secretory and contractile stimuli.[30–32] These lesions appear to occur in a focal distribution after acute inhalation injury, the reasons for which are not well understood.[25,30] Recent data support that, in some cases, these may be followed by the development of temporary or chronic airway hyperreactivity or other persistent pulmonary function changes.[6,29,33–35] The increase in epithelial permeability seen in irritant inhalation injury has been postulated as a principal determinant in allowing access of toxicants to the underlying sensory neural network, with the resulting development of airway hyperreactivity.[6,36]

Poorly water-soluble gases (also termed deep lung irritants), on the other hand, will tend to bypass water-rich epithelia and produce irritation of cells relatively low in water content, such as those found in the bronchioloalveolar region. Here too, the site of injury will follow a cranial to caudal gradient, with proximal acinar structures more likely to sustain damage than the distal acini.[37,38] The respiratory bronchiole may be a particularly significant site of irritant injury due to its influence on pulmonary performance, which may become more significant as the aging process progresses, despite the tendency to overlook compromise at this level when utilizing usual tests of pulmonary function.[39] Common examples of deep lung irritants include oxides of nitrogen, phosgene, and ozone. The most serious acute injury, typically associated with deep lung irritants, is noncardiogenic pulmonary edema, also variably described in the literature as chemical pneumonitis or pneumonia, hemorrhagic edema, diffuse alveolar damage, or adult respiratory distress syndrome. Although damage to the alveolar epithelium, and specifically to the Type I pneumocyte, ultimately leads to alveolar edema, recent data concerning oxidant injury suggest that the earliest damage occurs at the level of the alveolar capillary endothelium, possibly due to polymorphonuclear leukocyte-controlled release of free oxygen radicals.[40] This leads to a "leaky capillary" state and production of interstitial edema. Leukocyte activity is probably not strongly correlated with the degree of alveolar epithelial damage,[31,41,42] although considerable species differences exist in the intensity of all these responses.[23]

As long as integrity of the alveolar epithelial wall is maintained, the interstitial fluid accumulation is handled predominantly by the lymphatics. However, as injury progresses, the integrity of the alveolar epithelium is lost, pulmonary surfactant layer composition is altered, and flooding of the alveoli with protein-rich fluid occurs.[43,44] The time course for this series of events is usually from 3 to 12 hours following the exposure, so that clinical manifestation of pulmonary edema is characteristically delayed. In some instances, the delay can be as long as up to 72 hours. In keeping with these observations, it is believed that alveolar injury occurring only to the Type I cells will usually resolve with only mild to moderate lung lesions; on the other hand, combined injury to both Type I and Type II cells is much more harmful and can lead to fatal lung damage.[23]

Intensity of exposure. Notwithstanding the physical and chemical properties of a gas, the intensity of exposure is a major factor, if not the crucial factor, in determining injury, both for asphyxiant as well as irritant gases. Intensity, in turn, is dependent on *concentration* and *duration* of the acute exposure. In general, at lower levels of exposure intensity, irritant gases will produce cytotoxicity following the previously described solubility-dependent general principles. However, as exposure intensity increases, the gradient of injury becomes less obvious and the sites of involvement spread in both caudal and cranial directions. Thus, given enough intensity of exposure, any irritant gas has the capability of producing inflammatory damage to the entire respiratory tract.[32]

Host factors. The aforementioned physicochemical properties and exposure characteristics of the inhaled gas interact with various host factors to establish the probability, nature, location and severity of injury. Among these is the presence of local defense mechanisms that, when intact,

attempt to contain damage. Reflex maneuvers such as cough, sneeze, or bronchoconstriction may serve to limit the penetration of an agent. The nasal passages and upper airways act as potent scrubbers of highly soluble gases, such as sulfur dioxide.[30] The lining of the airways, largely composed of epithelium covered by a blanket of water-rich mucin, can act to neutralize the effects of inhaled toxins. This fluid also contains a variety of immunochemical mediators, such as lysozyme, complement, and other secretory proteins, which may also have a role in the detoxification of gases.[30]

Changes in certain ventilatory parameters, such as oronasal or oral breathing, or increased minute ventilation like that seen during exercise or sudden bursts of activity (as in an emergency evacuation) may increase the depth of penetration of an inhaled gas or vapor.[45,46]

The presence of underlying disease can also modulate the impact of acute inhalation injury. Patients with underlying coronary artery disease are more susceptible to the effects of carbon monoxide intoxication, with earlier precipitation of angina or cardiac rhythm disturbances at lower levels of carboxyhemoglobin than the general population. Asthmatics and persons with preexisting chronic obstructive pulmonary disease may be more prone to exacerbations following a nonspecific irritant exposure, or the severity of the injury may be worse, and resistance to infectious disease may be temporarily impaired.[47–49] The role of atopy as a predisposing condition to long-term irritant-induced airways disease is less well established.[29,50]

Gaseous mixtures: the case of smoke inhalation

The earliest written accounts of the detrimental effects resulting from exposure to toxic smokes date to the Middle Ages. In 1273, the first recorded smoke abatement law was passed in England, due to fears that smoke was detrimental to health, and in 1306 a royal proclamation was signed, prohibiting the burning of coal in London.[51] More recently, other disasters have intensified research interest in the injurious effects of inhaling concentrated products of combustion, including the 1967 deaths of three Apollo astronauts trapped in a sealed space capsule when an otherwise minor electrical fire occurred.

The first widely recognized indications that toxic gases, rather than heat and flame, were the major agents of death in fires came following the Cleveland Clinic fire in 1929, and the Coconut Grove fire in Boston in 1943.[52] In both of these incidents large numbers of people perished, and yet few were actually burned. In a study of over 200 fires in Boston, personal sample measurements of smoke components were obtained in firefighters.[53] The substances assayed included carbon monoxide, carbon dioxide, hydrochloric acid, nitrogen dioxide, hydrogen cyanide, benzene, acrolein, and particulates. Both carbon monoxide and acrolein were found to be present at hazardous levels in a high percentage of the fires. Specifically, acrolein was present at above the ACGIH short-term exposure limit (STEL)[54] in over half of the fires, and above the immediately dangerous to life and health (IDLH) level, adopted by NIOSH and OSHA,[55] in 10% of the incidents. Acrolein has been demonstrated to rapidly produce pulmonary edema at concentrations as low as 10 ppm.[56]

Pulmonary lesions seen in smoke inhalation victims have included bacterial pneumonias,[16-18,20,57] denuding of airway epithelium,[17] bronchial plugging with debris,[17] bronchospasm,[16,58] chronic bronchitis,[59] permanent bronchial stenosis,[59] tracheobronchitis and bronchiolitis,[17,18,20] intraalveolar hemorrhage,[17] focal atelectasis,[17,18] emphysema,[18] reduced residual volume and functional residual capacity,[15,20,60] and pulmonary edema.[15,20]

Although fire victims represent a group exposed to extremely high concentrations of complex combustion gases and particulates over a relatively short period of time, they make up only one end of the spectrum of persons exposed to thermal decomposition products of polymers. Others are exposed to more specific thermally induced airborne contaminants wherever chemically defined polymeric materials are subjected to hot manufacturing processes, as in the injection molding, reaction curing, match metal die pressing, or other open thermal plastics forming industries.[61-63] Plastics pyrolysis products contain many of the same toxic and reactive species found in any "fresh smokes," including the presence of particulates that may act as carriers of otherwise harmless toxic gases into the deep lung regions. In the case of equipment overheating or accidental exposures or releases, significant inhalation doses may be delivered. These include aldehydes, organic and mineral acids, free radicals, and carbonaceous particulates.[62 67] Several reports have described the appearance of respiratory symptoms and eye irritation in workers exposed to hot plastic forming processes.[68] Reported respiratory symptoms range from acute asthmalike symptoms[61,69] to long-term shortness of breath, chest tightness,[70] productive cough, and decreased resistance to respiratory infections.[71]

Numerous accidental or routine exposures common in the occupational setting may also involve inhalation of hazardous levels of toxic gas mixtures. These include but are not limited to engine exhausts, welding and torch cutting fumes, oxidant atmospheres generated by intense electromagnetic fields, static electricity, electrical arcs, or ultraviolet light, and refuse combustion or incineration effluent.

CLINICAL EVALUATION AND MANAGEMENT

A number of factors related to both exposure and clinical presentation can complicate the evaluation and management of an acute gaseous exposure. Accidental exposures are difficult to anticipate, and may require the evaluation of multiple casualties in a short period of time. The identity and toxicity of the agent may not be known, especially if exposure was to a mixture of chemicals. Quantitative measures of exposure are rarely available, and estimates are

therefore largely based on individual accounts of what transpired. This information, although crucial, can be difficult to weigh, particularly when the initial medical evaluation is performed months or years after the exposure incident. Time of onset varies for the different clinical manifestations, and the accurate diagnosis of long-term sequelae may be elusive.[28] Clinical management of the acute presentation and at a time remote from the exposure must be considered separately. For patients presenting at the time of the exposure or shortly thereafter, the emphasis of the evaluation is on assessment and treatment of acute manifestations. For patients who present with respiratory symptoms some time after the exposure, issues generally revolve around accurately diagnosing the sequelae of the exposure, addressing causation, determining impairment, and implementing an appropriate treatment plan.

Acute presentation: general management principles

The assessment and treatment of a patient presenting in the acute phase of an inhalation injury will be guided by the immediate goals of maintaining life support, decontamination, and stabilizing the injury.[72-74]

Accidental inhalation exposures are commonly associated with additional factors such as contaminant-drenched skin and clothing, fractures or other physical injuries, altered consciousness or mental state, thermal or chemical surface burns, or hypothermia. These may act to delay or confuse appropriate assessment and treatment of the inhalation injury itself. It is important to maintain a high index of suspicion for respiratory injury in any accident where gases, vapors, mists, liquid sprays, submersion, smoke, fire, or explosions are involved. Any chemical exposure occurring within a confined or poorly ventilated space (such as a tank, vessel, vault, hold, silo or otherwise unventilated room) should be particularly suspect for inhalation injury because of the potential for development of high air concentrations of contaminants.

The rescue of a chemically injured or asphyxiated victim is a potentially dangerous endeavor that requires specific training, equipment, and advance planning, in addition to common sense. This activity is usually best left to those who have had approved hazardous materials ("hazmat") training and drills, and who are familiar with the location and substances present at an accident site (e.g., industrial fire brigades, or emergency response teams).[72]

Whether responding to a victim at the site of an accident or receiving that person in an emergency facility, immediate attention must be paid to assuring an adequate airway, and maintenance of respiratory and circulatory function. It is important to remember that chemical contamination of the victim may continue to worsen the exposure and may secondarily expose rescuers or health care providers. Precautions should therefore be taken to avoid secondary exposures to health care personnel by the use of appropriate personal protective equipment. Decontamination of the victim should begin as soon as life support is assured, or intercurrently if possible.[72]

Prompt determination of the identity, physicochemical properties, and associated health effects of the exposure is necessary to guide appropriate diagnosis, prognosis, and treatment. In the case of industrial or transportation accidents, Material Safety and Data Sheets (MSDS) may be available at the scene or nearby and should be consulted as early as possible after notification of the accident. Container labels may provide chemical names, trade names, code numbers, or useful information or telephone numbers. The Chemical Transportation Emergency Center (CHEMTREC), a service of the Chemical Manufacturers Association (1-800-424-9300), and/or the local poison control center may be able to rapidly provide useful information by telephone or facsimile. These services are often accessible through the 911 emergency network.

Once emergency medical assistance has been instituted attention turns to the extent and severity of the injury, which will be determined by toxicant and host factors (see box, Determinants of injury). A detailed eyewitness account of the events leading up to and surrounding the exposure is essential to estimate its toxic potential. A chronology of symptoms and exposure events should be elicited from exposed individuals (even mildly exposed or asymptomatic persons), including all aspects of the sensorium (sight, smell, taste, sound, sensation). Special attention should be paid to symptoms of eye, nose, or throat irritation, chest pain, chest tightness, shortness of breath, coughing, wheezing, or hemoptysis. This information may often be as valuable to the assessment as the identification of the chemicals themselves. Past medical history should focus on proximal acute and chronic illnesses and medications that might affect cardiopulmonary reserve, healing response, or diagnostic tests.

The physical examination should be targeted at identifying evidence of asphyxia and/or tissue irritation. Signs of asphyxia include shortness of breath, tachypnea, rapid pulse, cyanosis, and altered mental status. Irritant inhalation can present as conjunctival erythema, nasal and pharyngeal hyperemia or bleeding, hoarseness, stridor, wheeze, rhonchi, rales, shallow breathing, or traces of exposure substances or burns on the face around the nose or mouth. Any suspicion of an exposure to a deep lung irritant (respiratory symptoms, air monitoring data, identified gas release, or change in personal detector badge color), or intense exposure to a soluble irritant, should be sufficient to trigger careful monitoring for the development of delayed, life-threatening pulmonary compromise, including noncardiogenic pulmonary edema, laryngeal edema, or other severe obstructive defect.[75]

Diagnostic testing, in symptomatic cases, should include arterial blood gas analysis to assess oxygenation, ventilation, and acid–base status. A complete blood cell count and serum chemistries may detect the presence of hemolysis,

acute renal, or hepatic dysfunction. Venous blood can yield information regarding presence of methemoglobin, carboxyhemoglobin, sulfhemoglobin, or cyanohemoglobin. Arterial samples are not necessary for these determinations. Serum analyses may reveal traces of the exposure substances or their metabolites, thus verifying internal exposure, and can help quantify the degree of tissue destruction or electrolyte abnormalities. Chest radiographs can show evidence of pulmonary edema, air trapping, atelectasis, or secondary infection. An unremarkable chest radiograph in the initial hours after presentation, however, does not rule out the possibility of pulmonary edema, which may be delayed up to 72 hours in onset.[75,76] Decreases in serial spirometry or peak expiratory flow determinations may alert the clinician to the appearance of pulmonary edema or airway obstruction.

Treatment of severe respiratory injuries requiring hospitalization should be based on principles of critical care and treatment of specific toxicities, the detailed discussion of which is beyond the scope of this chapter. Ambulatory victims of acute gas inhalation injury should also be carefully assessed, recognizing that there may be delay in the onset of specific symptomatology. The appearance of progressive shortness of breath and/or deterioration of spirometric indices over the course of a few minutes or hours suggest the need for treatment in a facility possessing the full medical armament required for intravenous therapy, tracheal intubation, mechanical ventilation, and specialty consultation. Symptomatic persons with negative findings should at least be observed for several hours following exposure.[28] Symptoms of respiratory irritation may be treated by the use of analgesics and bronchodilators, as needed. Scheduled topical inhaled steroids, systemic steroid taper, or nonsteroidal antiinflammatory agents are reported to be useful during the initial inflammatory phase of repair,[40,76] although no clinical trials have been conducted. Prompt diagnosis and treatment of secondary infection are essential; the use of prophylactic antibiotics, however, is not clearly justified. Despite a few case reports,[77,78] the benefits of corticosteroids in limiting the extent of pulmonary damage due to inhalation injury has not been convincingly demonstrated in humans, with the possible exception of nitrogen dioxide-induced bronchiolitis obliterans.[79,80] However, internationally there are significant differences of opinion regarding their routine use in these settings.[76]

Follow-up should be early and frequent (usually daily until progression toward recovery is evident and then weekly). Clinicians should note that many inhalation injuries will resolve completely within days of the exposure, signaling a superficial epithelial injury. However, more severe injuries may require prolonged treatment (6 to 8 weeks or longer) to allow for reepithelialization and stabilization of subepithelial structural compartments.[25,30,32,75] Chest radiography may be helpful in identifying certain residual effects of the acute injury, including bronchiectasis

(Fig. 30-2), bullae, atelectasis, or nonspecific interstitial patterns associated with bronchiolitis obliterans.[81] The emergence of bronchiolitis obliterans as a complication of an irritant exposure, best described following nitrogen dioxide exposure[80,82] and sulfur dioxide,[77] usually occurs within 2 to 6 weeks of the incident. It is characterized by the appearance of fever, cough, and dyspnea, an obstructive ventilatory pattern, a reduced diffusing capacity, and nonspecific nodular and infiltrative changes on the chest radiograph. Examination of open lung biopsy specimens will reveal obliterative changes of small bronchioles, coupled with cellular infiltrates and a variable degree of peribronchial fibrosis. Most cases reported in the literature describe eventual recovery, which may be aided by a course of corticosteroid treatment.[80,83,84]

The patient can usually be returned to work as soon as physically able, but precautions should be taken to avoid irritant inhalant exposures, both occupational and environmental, until a point of maximum medical improvement is reached.

Considerations for specific agents

Simple asphyxiants. These are agents that displace the oxygen normally present in the air to levels that may disturb physiologic or metabolic functioning. They include such common industrial gases as nitrogen (N_2), carbon dioxide (CO_2), methane (CH_4), helium (He), hydrogen (H), freons, or normal air when oxygen is removed by combustion or biologic decay processes. These oxygen deficient environments may occur wherever compressed gases are released, or in confined spaces or unventilated areas which have been closed for a period of time. Symptoms of simple asphyxia are those of hypoxemia, i.e., tachypnea, tachycardia, cyanosis, or altered mental status. The appropriate emergency response is (1) safe rescue of the victim(s) with removal from further exposure and (2) cardiopulmonary resuscitation with supplemental oxygen. Ideally these two steps can take place simultaneously. Any patient who has experienced loss of consciousness from an anoxic event is at risk for permanent damage, primarily to the central nervous system, and should be evaluated despite uneventful resuscitation.

Chemical asphyxiants. These agents are longer acting and may require special treatments. Nonetheless, the principles of first response described above for simple asphyxiants apply in this case as well.

Carbon monoxide (CO) is an incomplete product of combustion present in high concentration in engine exhaust, and in furnace, foundry, kiln, wood or coal stove, or other combustion process stack emissions. It is produced in smaller quantities by the process of arc welding or explosives detonation. CO is used as a reducing agent in metallurgy and as an organic synthesis raw material.[85] It is routinely present in the atmosphere of structural fires, and a common cause of incapacitation and death in fire victims.[75,76] CO is a chemical asphyxiant in that it binds to hemoglobin (carboxyhemoglobin) with a high affinity and alters the hemoglobin–oxygen dissociation curve making it more difficult for oxygen to be released at the level of the tissues. In addition, it is a metabolic poison that binds to and inhibits the action of the cytochrome oxygen transport chain within cellular mitochondria and therefore blocks tissue respiration.[86] These mechanisms are particularly consequential for tissues sensitive to the effects of anoxia (e.g., heart, kidney, brain); persons with underlying coronary artery disease may be particularly susceptible. This is a reversible process when carbon monoxide exposure has ceased. The half-life of carbon monoxide in the tissues is 5 to 6 hours when breathing room air, about 90 minutes when breathing 100% oxygen at sea level, and can be reduced to less than 30 minutes by the use of hyperbaric oxygen therapy, thus decreasing the potential for permanent toxic effects.

Hydrogen cyanide (HCN), acrylonitrile, and other nitriles are widely used in industry in chemical, plastics, and rubber manufacturing processes. They may be present in the metal treating and electroplating industries, and are sometimes used as solvents, extractants, fumigants, or pesticides.[85] The cyanides are metabolic poisons, HCN being the most rapidly acting and potent. They form nonfunctional he-

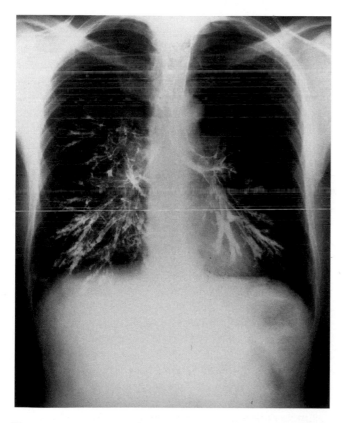

Fig. 30-2. Bilateral bronchogram showing cylindrical bronchiectasis in a young man 16 months following a high-level ammonia release that resulted when a tank truck crashed on a busy Houston freeway in 1976.

moglobin complexes (cyanohemoglobin), but their primary toxicity is inhibition of cytochrome oxidase at the level of the tissue mitochondria, both locally in the respiratory system and systemically. Respiration is essentially shut down and, depending on the degree, can result in temporary loss of tissue function, cell death, or major system failure. Treatment must be initiated very rapidly (at the time of exposure if possible) and consists of specific antidotal therapy designed to competitively trap the cyanate ion in a nontoxic excretable form thus protecting cytochrome oxidase.[86] The standard cyanide antidote kit uses blood hemoglobin as a cyanide trap. A newer treatment involves the use of hydroxocobalamin, a vitamin B_{12} relative, to trap the cyanate ion as harmless cyanocobalamin.[87] Oxygen therapy, including hyperbaric treatment, can be of use primarily to minimize the detrimental effects of the artificially induced anemia.

Hydrogen sulfide (H_2S) is widely distributed in the industrial and natural environment. It is found in greatest abundance in the petroleum and natural gas industries where it is a natural contaminant removed during the refining process. H_2S is a raw material used in the production of sulfuric acid and in sulfation processes. It is generated by the decay of sulfur-containing organic matter and may be a hazard in sewers, septic tanks, animal confinement sheds, and manure bins.[85] H_2S, like cyanide, is a metabolic poison that binds to hemoglobin (sulfhemoglobin), but, more importantly, it blocks the cytochrome chain in the tissue mitochondria and can lead to similar effects. Hydrogen sulfide is much more soluble in lipid-rich tissues and therefore has a predilection for producing its toxicities in the central nervous system.[88] It is easily recognized by its characteristic rotten egg odor, but even at low concentrations it produces rapid paralysis of the sense of smell and thus its own detection.

Because of its rapid action on the central nervous system, hydrogen sulfide is known to cause "knockdowns," where an individual or group of workers may be suddenly rendered unconscious by a release or a plume of gas and will collapse "as if a switch were thrown on a mechanical doll."[89] They characteristically awaken again just as suddenly with no apparent acute effects, although recent studies have described possible long-term neurologic deficits.[90]

The treatment for hydrogen sulfide exposure is similar to that for cyanide in that it is trapped to inhibit its action on the cytochrome chain. The traditional cyanide antidote kit can be effectively used to produce methemoglobin, forming a stable complex with the toxicant that is then eliminated gradually by endogenous biochemical processes. However, thiosulfate is of no use in the case of hydrogen sulfide poisoning. Oxygen therapy, including hyperbaric treatment, is employed for reasons similar to those discussed for cyanide.

Hydrogen fluoride (HF). Hydrogen fluoride, also referred to as hydrofluoric acid, is the starting material for the chemical synthesis of most fluorine compounds and fluorinated plastics. It is used as a catalyst in the paraffin alkylation process, as a fumigant, and is a byproduct of the aluminum and uranium processing industries. HF is also used in research laboratories, in semiconductor manufacturing, and by artisans in etching glass or removing silica deposits from metal castings.[85]

HF is a severe irritant that can cause very painful burns of the skin and eyes as well as inhalation injury. Symptoms are characteristically delayed. It has the propensity to penetrate deep into tissues at the site of contact where it complexes with cellular and humoral calcium ion leading to possibly severe electrolyte disturbances, precipitating cardiac arrhythmias, subsurface bone dissolution, and barrier compromise.

The treatment for hydrogen fluoride inhalation injury is immediate administration of aerosolized calcium gluconate (as a 2.5% solution), and monitoring of serum ionized calcium levels. Electrocardiograms should be performed to evaluate early signs of the cardiac effects of hypocalcemia, such as a prolonged Q-T interval. Attention should also be given to the skin and eyes, which are almost certainly involved in the case of an inhalation exposure. Any location where HF is routinely used or where exposures may occur should have appropriate antidote preparations on hand and persons trained in their use.

Arsine (AsH_3). Arsine gas is a contaminant sometimes found in the chemical, smelting, and refining industries. It can be present in metal pickling, drossing, or plating operations, and can be produced whenever inorganic arsenic compounds have occasion to contact sources of nascent hydrogen.[85]

Arsine is a commonly used gas in semiconductor manufacturing (see Chapter 43). When inhaled, arsine is absorbed by the lungs into the bloodstream and sets up a chain reaction of events leading ultimately to massive intravascular hemolysis, producing the triad of hemoglobinuria within hours, jaundice within hours to days, and oliguric renal failure. Arsine is also toxic to the pulmonary vasculature and can produce pulmonary edema. Treatment is supportive with attention to respiratory function, oxygen carrying capacity, and renal function.[85]

Phosgene ($COCl_2$). Phosgene is a deep lung irritant that produces insidious development of pulmonary edema. It is a raw material in the production of dyes, plastics, and isocyanate precursors. It may also be produced in small amounts in any situation where chlorinated hydrocarbon residues (solvents, refrigerants, cleaning fluids, etc.) and oxygen are subjected to intense heat, as in welding, brazing, soldering, or torch cutting operations (see Chapter 42).[85,91]

Smoke inhalation. Observations on fire victims, primarily gleaned from autopsy studies, show common factors in the pathogenesis of smoke inhalation, typical of irritant lung injury, to include paralysis of cilia of the airway epithelium, with mucostasis; upper airway obstruction, from epithelial edema, laryngeal edema, and bronchospasm; and small airway closure with air trapping and/or atelectasis.[59,60,92] In patients, within the first few hours following exposure, radiographic changes, including signs of pulmonary edema, perivascular fuzziness, and peribronchial cuffing, may be present.[81] Immediate inactivation of pulmonary surfactant has been observed in some cases,[15,92] and has been shown to persist, or worsen, over a period of up to three weeks due to injury to alveolar Type II cells.[93] Early lung volume and ventilatory studies may indicate reduction in functional residual capacity and residual volume with no noticeable abnormalities in the major spirometric indices. After 72 hours, airflow obstruction abnormalities are the primary features, limited to late volume-dependent flows in mild cases, but extending to defects in the forced expiratory volume in 1 second (FEV1), in more severe cases.[94,95] These changes may not correlate with symptoms or other signs of respiratory deterioration.[94] This array of alterations produced in the airways and the alveolar septa may disrupt the normal defense mechanisms of the host, making these areas prime sites for bacterial invasion, leading to purulent bronchitis or bronchopneumonia, a common complication in the burn or smoke inhalation patient, especially if surface burns are present.[47,48,57,92]

Assessment of a remote gaseous exposure

Frequently, occupational and pulmonary physicians are asked to evaluate workers with persistent respiratory symptoms and a remote history of gaseous exposure. Not uncommonly, these referrals occur in the context of impairment evaluations, where disability income, expense compensation, or recovery of monetary damages is at stake. Circumstances may dictate the need to establish causation of the perceived respiratory impairment in light of a single past exposure nestled within a lifetime of other minor toxic inhalation exposures, or even to apportion its contribution to the impairment. The evaluation may be further complicated by the presence of personal factors that can also be causal or aggravating in nature, such as preexisting respiratory disease or a significant smoking history.[49] In addition, recall bias on the part of the patient regarding the events at the time of the exposure, the opportunity for secondary gain, the time elapsed from the occurrence of injury, and psychologic factors associated with the injury or its impact on the life of the patient and family, may all act to obscure the careful fact finding necessary to accomplish the major goals to the best advantage of the patient's health.

The primary goals of remote inhalation injury assessment, therefore, may include (1) establishing a diagnosis, (2) addressing causation, (3) determining degree of respiratory impairment and its long-term stability, and (4) specifying the most appropriate therapy for maximizing function while minimizing symptoms.

In the majority of cases, following an acute inhalation injury, most patients are likely to have reached a point of maximum medical improvement by approximately 8 weeks following the injury.[30,32] In a recent review of irritant inhalational exposures reported to a poison control center, persistent symptoms beyond 2 weeks was reported by only 6% of subjects; both preexisting lung disease and cigarette smoking were significant risk factors for the prolonged symptomatology.[96] Exceptions to this generalization can occur, however, when the initial injury is subsequently complicated by reactive airways dysfunction syndrome, airway strictures, fibrosing bronchiolitis obliterans, bronchiectasis, slowly resolving adult respiratory distress syndrome (ARDS), chronic rhinitis and sinusitis, or neurological deficits, among others.

An *accurate diagnosis* is the most important element in these types of evaluations. Once a diagnosis has been reached, the establishment of causation must rely on sound scientific and epidemiologic studies, or in their absence, sound medical, scientific, and epidemiologic principles. Central to the identification of causal or aggravating factors is a careful review of all available information, to accurately assess the significance of the exposure and the temporal relationships between that exposure and the subsequent development of disease.

Reconstruction of the original exposure usually requires obtaining a detailed description of the exposure incident and pertinent events relating to nature, intensity, and duration of the exposure, use of personal protective equipment, and symptoms or recollections about the injury itself. Objective documentation of the exposure or accident, when available, is always helpful in establishing its significance. A continuous chronologic history of subsequent symptoms and medical interventions (including emergency medical care at the time of injury), symptom triggers, remedies, and a description of how symptoms have impinged on normal functioning, is necessary. Medical records, biopsy material, injury reports, incident investigation reports, and MSDSs covering this period should be conscientiously reviewed.

Accurate details regarding a patient's *preexposure status* are crucial, focusing on health status (especially previous respiratory conditions), baseline activity level, workplace functionality at the time of the injury, professional experience level, work history stability, smoking history, prior episodes of exposure or inhalation injury, and family history of atopy, asthma, or other respiratory disease. In this regard, medical records covering the preinjury period should also be sought and examined as objective documentation. A sense should be gained of the patient's avocational interests, including hobbies, physical exercise, and sports activities and the degree to which they have been affected by the development of symptomatology. A directed physical examination, with emphasis on inspection of the mucous membranes of the eyes, nose, and mouth, auscultation of the lungs and heart, and neurologic function (including mental status) should be performed.

Determination of respiratory impairment should be based on published guidelines,[97,98,99] whenever possible. Of note are recently published guidelines by the American Thoracic Society for the assessment of respiratory impairment for asthma,[99] which are also applicable to patients with reactive airways dysfunction syndrome. These clinically practical guidelines consist of two steps: (1) establishing an accurate diagnosis, based on compatible respiratory symptomatology and objective evidence of reversible airflow obstruction; and (2) impairment assessment, based on a triad of postbronchodilator FEV1 level, degree of bronchial hyperresponsiveness, and amount of medication. Furthermore, they recognize that impairment level may vary over time, and that it is influenced by the adequacy of treatment. For a more in-depth discussion of impairment assessment in occupational and environmental respiratory disease, refer to Chapter 53.

All pulmonary function tests should be performed with meticulous attention to quality control (Chapter 4). Spirometry, with confirmation by measurement of full lung volumes, may reveal the presence of obstructive or restrictive ventilatory defects, and is particularly useful when obtained serially to monitor clinical course. Postbronchodilator spirometry and/or nonspecific bronchial challenge testing with methacholine or histamine can provide objective evidence of the degree of reversibility of airflow obstruction and bronchial hyperresponsiveness that is central to the diagnosis of reactive airways dysfunction (RADS). In cases where there is a disparity between the degree of respiratory symptoms and objective findings by physical examination and laboratory testing, cardiopulmonary exercise testing may be useful in establishing the level of achievable exertion and its limiting factors (Chapter 4). Finally, in any case that involved loss of consciousness or prolonged anoxia, neuropsychiatric studies can be of value in distinguishing organic central nervous system damage from psychological phenomena.

EPIDEMIOLOGY

Since acute gaseous exposure usually occurs suddenly and without warning, such as in the case of an accidental spill or inadvertent release of a gas or vapor cloud, the literature is sparse with regard to well-designed studies of exposure and response. In humans, this literature consists mostly of individual case reports and case series of persons exposed to one or more irritant inhalational agents. These uncontrolled studies have been useful in describing the clinical presentation and evolution of patients, especially in the acute setting. They have also been of value in generating hypotheses of the chronic sequelae of acute exposure to gaseous agents. There have been very few cross-sectional and longitudinal studies of exposed populations, however. Important questions remain, especially with respect to the long-term consequences and management of these patients. In recent years, one of the areas of greatest uncertainty has been in regards to whether survivors of acute exposures to high levels of irritant agents ultimately are at risk for, or in fact develop, persistent respiratory symptoms and/or airways disease. If this does occur, the actual rates of occurrence (i.e., prevalence and incidence) of these complications are largely unknown.

Surveillance systems and exposure surveys, such as the NOHS and NOES, in general have been more helpful in identifying populations at risk for chronic, low level exposures to gases and vapors than groups at risk for acute, short-term exposures. In a large population-based random sample of 8,515 adults from six U.S. cities, Korn and colleagues found a higher prevalence of chronic respiratory symptoms among those with a history of occupational exposure to gases or fumes, after accounting for smoking.[96] No significant exposure–response relationships, however, could be demonstrated. Recently, promising use of poison control center data as a surveillance measure for acute respiratory illness, including that resulting from irritant exposure, and as a source for follow-up of these cases, has been reported.[12,49,100]

Despite the methodologic limitations, a growing body of literature nonetheless suggests that, at least in some survivors of an acute gaseous exposure, the natural history may not necessarily be one of eventual resolution of symptoms over the short-term, but rather may be characterized by the persistence of symptoms, demonstrable bronchial hyperresponsiveness, respiratory impairment, and, ultimately, a variable degree of disability.

Experimental studies in both animals and humans support the concept that acute irritant exposures can lead, at least initially, to acute bronchial hyperresponsiveness; this has been studied most extensively with sulfur dioxide,[101–103] ozone,[104,105] and nitrogen dioxide.[106]

In 1970, Gandevia described acute inflammatory bronchoconstriction following exposure to a variety of respiratory irritants. Although recovery over weeks to months was the rule, he noted that permanent pulmonary injury could also occur, although not much detail was provided.[107]

Harkonen and colleagues followed a group of seven men, acutely exposed to sulfur dioxide following a pyrite dust explosion, for 4 years.[108] Maximal decrease in spirometric indices—forced vital capacity (FVC), FEV1, and forced expiratory flow at 25% to 75% (FEF25–75)—was observed 1 week following the accident. After 4 years, all study subjects complained of exertional dyspnea, and histamine challenge testing was positive in four subjects. Reversible airflow obstruction 5 years after an exposure to liquid ammonia has also been reported,[109] as has the development of bronchiectasis following ammonia burns[9,110] and smoke inhalation.[10]

In 1985, Brooks and colleagues reported a series of 10 patients, all of whom had a history of single, high-level inhalation exposures to different irritant agents and demonstrable bronchial hyperreactivity by methacholine challenge.[6] This clinical entity was termed RADS, and initial criteria established for its diagnosis included (1) absence of preexisting asthmalike disease; (2) exposure to high concentrations of a known irritant gas, vapor, fume, aerosol or dust; (3) abrupt onset of symptoms within at most a 24-hour period, with persistence of asthmalike symptoms for at least 3 months; (4) exclusion of other respiratory disorders; and (5) a positive response to nonspecific bronchial challenge testing. Since then, RADS has also been referred to as irritant-induced occupational asthma[29] and nonallergic occupational asthma.[50]

Subsequent to the initial study by Brooks, several additional reports of similar events have surfaced, and the list of inciting agents has grown. Irritant gases or vapors implicated to date include uranium hexafluoride,[6] floor sealant,[6,111] ammonia-containing spray paint,[6] hydrazine,[6] acids,[6,29] metal coat remover,[6] bleaching agent,[35] sulfuric acid,[35] hydrochloric acid,[35] perchloroethylene,[35] toluene diisocyanate,[35] sulfur dioxide,[112] calcium oxide,[29] chlorine,[113] phosgene,[29] diphenyl methane diisocyanate,[29] glacial acetic acid,[114] and diesel exhaust.[115] In 1989, Tarlo described a series of 154 workers evaluated for potential occupational asthma.[29] Of the 105 workers felt to have either definite or possible occupational asthma, 25 (24%) were considered to have either definite or possible irritant-induced asthma. Unlike the series described by Brooks et al.,[6] however, irritant exposures were not limited necessarily to a single high-level exposure; a few of the workers reported more than one significant exposure over time. The original criteria of Brooks et al. were, therefore, modified to reflect this.

In most case series of RADS where this was addressed, atopy has not been felt to represent a predisposing factor.[6,29,114] However, there have been reports of sensitization developing after exposure to irritant levels of known sensitizers,[7] particularly isocyanates. The larger clinical series of RADS have also reported a higher prevalence of ever-smoking in those persons meeting the diagnostic criteria for RADS.[6,29] Whether this is because smokers have a higher preexposure prevalence of positive responses to methacholine at baseline (possibly because of lower baseline airway caliber),[116,117] or because smokers, despite normal preexposure bronchial responsiveness are more likely to develop subsequent, symptomatic bronchial hyperreactivity is not known.

Follow-up studies of persons after acute chlorine exposure incidents have produced conflicting findings. In the first half of this century, studies of U.S. survivors of World War I chlorine gassings were conducted by both the Army and Veterans Administration.[118,119] A subset of veterans was found to have a variety of chronic respiratory disorders that were felt to be possibly or probably related to the wartime chlorine exposure. However, further useful information was limited by the coexistence of high rates of other respiratory disorders, notably tuberculosis and complications of the influenza pandemic, poor quality chest radiography and the lack of periodic, valid pulmonary function tests.

Jones and colleagues[120] performed serial clinical evaluations over a 6-year period in a group of 60 adults following a chlorine gas exposure from a train derailment. Although preexposure pulmonary function data were not available and bronchial challenge testing was not performed, no cases of new onset asthma, persistent respiratory symptomatology, or longitudinal decline in lung function attributable to the chlorine exposure were detected in this fairly large group. These findings contrast with a more recent study by Schwartz and colleagues,[33] who obtained full pulmonary function studies on a group of 13 construction workers over a 12-year period following a liquid chlorine spill in a pulp mill. Pulmonary function profiles performed within 24 hours of the exposure were remarkable for a high prevalence of obstructive ventilatory defects and evidence of air trapping. During the follow-up period, airflow obstruction persisted, but the evidence of air trapping tended to resolve. In fact, a residual volume below the lower limit of normal was described in 67% of subjects by the end of the study period. No other significant longitudinal changes in spirometric indices or lung volumes were encountered. Although increased reactivity to methacholine was present in 5 of the 13 (38%) subjects, this was felt to be consistent with expected rates given the high prevalence of ever-smokers (over 90%) in the group. An additional case report described persistent reactive airway disease in an atopic man following an acute chlorine gas leak in an enclosed environment.[110]

Aside from some experimental studies, few reports have addressed the issue of exposure–response relationships between an acute irritant exposure and the subsequent development of chronic airways disease. This is not surprising given the rare availability of measured exposure levels at the time of an accident or spill, and the difficulties inherent in reconstruction of those levels. Possibly the best supporting evidence derives from a study by Kern[114] in an investigation of 51 of 56 hospital employees exposed to a spill of 100% glacial acetic acid. The evaluation consisted of a respiratory symptom questionnaire and methacholine challenge; preexposure respiratory status was verified by review of preemployment health histories. Exposures were estimated by an industrial hygienist blinded to the clinical data, and categorized as low, medium, and high exposure levels. The Brooks et al.[6] clinical criteria for RADS were satisfied by no persons in the low exposure group, and by 3.3% and 21.4% of those persons in the medium and high exposure groups, respectively. The odds ratio for RADS in the highest exposure category was 9.8, although the 95% confidence interval included the null.

One of the worst industrial accidents leading to a large-scale community toxic exposure took place in 1984, in Bhopal, India.[121] Approximately 30 tons of methyl isocyanate, a potent ocular and respiratory irritant used in the manufacture of carbamate pesticides, were released via an exothermic reaction that resulted from operational and equipment malfunction. Wind direction and a temperature inversion favored the spread of a low-lying vapor cloud in the direction of nearby heavily populated parts of the city. Although the exact number is unknown, it is estimated that approximately 2,500 or more persons perished in the first several hours and days after the release, predominantly from pulmonary edema. In the days that followed, an estimated 100,000 persons sought medical attention for symptoms related to the exposure. Irritative ocular complaints, including photophobia, lacrimation, and corneal erosions were common; fortunately, progression to permanent eye injury was unusual.[2] Of several hundred patients hospitalized with respiratory complaints, over 80% had clinical and/or radiographic evidence of pulmonary edema.[122] In the first few months following the release, persistent respiratory symptomatology and restrictive (78%), obstructive (29%), and/or resting oxygen uptake abnormalities (55%) were reported in a group of 82 patients who survived the exposure.[123] Evidence of more chronic respiratory injury has centered on the findings of fibrosing bronchiolitis obliterans[2] in some of the Bhopal victims. Although studies of the long-term consequences of this terrible exposure continue, epidemiologic investigations have been largely hampered by the lack of adequate exposure information and definition of the follow-up population.[2]

Several factors limit the inferences that can be made from the literature to date regarding the possibility that acute irritant gas or vapor exposures can lead to long-term airways dysfunction or asthma. First, none of the studies to date has been able to provide objective data on preexposure pulmonary function; more specifically, no information exists on the preexposure level of bronchial reactivity. This is not surprising given the usual inability to predict when or how an accident will occur. No prospective occupational studies have been conducted of worker groups in whom preemployment bronchial reactivity was measured before following the population over time to see whether irritant exposures would lead to the de novo appearance of chronic respiratory symptoms or changes in airway reactivity. As both Brooks[50] and Kennedy[34] note, research along these lines would add important information to our understanding of nonimmunogenic mechanisms involved in the development of asthma. Other factors that have limited research on this topic include the lack of a consistent definition of occupational asthma,[124] uncertainty regarding the distribution of bronchial responsiveness to methacholine or histamine in the general nonasthmatic population,[34] quality control issues in pulmonary function testing in general and with methacholine challenge testing in particular,[50] bias in the selection of study populations, recall bias of exposed symptomatic subjects, and the frequent lack of quantitative exposure data at the time of an acute irritant exposure.[124]

In summary, experimental data support the conclusion that irritant exposure can lead to demonstrable increases in airway response. An increasing number of case reports and case series document instances of single or recurrent exposures to various high-level irritant gases, vapors, smokes, or fumes that are subsequently followed, in an uncertain proportion of those exposed, by the development of asthma-like symptoms and compatible functional changes that may last for months to years. Atopy does not appear to predispose to irritant-induced asthma; smoking, on the other hand, may be an important risk factor. The few epidemiologic studies to date, however, yield somewhat conflicting data regarding the long-term respiratory function outcomes following a significant irritant exposure.

REGULATORY ASPECTS

In the United States, regulatory control of exposure to hazardous levels of gaseous materials depends largely on the population at risk. In the occupational setting, standards are promulgated and enforced by OSHA, under the Department of Labor (see Chapter 55); for potential exposure of the general public, this is largely the responsibility of the EPA, currently a free-standing agency (see Chapter 56). Other federal agencies, such as the Department of Transportation, have established additional regulations that are pertinent. In addition to federal law, individual states may have separate regulations, usually either equal to or more stringent than federal standards, that address exposure to various gaseous materials. At the international level, several countries have established their own occupational exposure levels, based on a variety of sources.

An excellent resource to consult for these levels is the Registry of Toxic Effects of Chemical Substances (RTECS), developed and routinely updated by NIOSH; this is now available in CD-ROM format.[125] However, it should be remembered that permissible exposure levels are mainly useful in the control of predictable exposures; they are of relatively little value in the context of an unanticipated exposure to high levels of a toxic inhalant. Employer responsibility and worker knowledge of specific chemical hazards, coupled with the implementation of safe work practices (e.g., work in confined spaces) and the establishment of emergency preparedness procedures are much more important in the prevention and mitigation of the impact of these kinds of industrial accidents. These same principles apply in the home and community, where access to asphyxiants and chemical mixtures (e.g., natural gas, household cleaning agents) is a part of daily life.

OSHA has the regulatory authority to protect workers from exposure to noxious gases and vapors, a function that the agency seeks to accomplish through the development and enforcement of occupational health standards. These standards define permissible exposure limits (PELs) for individual gases and vapors, as well as for other chemicals and physical agents. The majority of PELs for individual agents are described either under the Z-tables of the air contaminants standard (29CFR 1910.1000), or in substance-specific standards, such as those for acrylonitrile (29CFR1910.1045), ethylene oxide (29CFR 1910.1047), and formaldehyde (29CFR 1910.1048).

In addition to defining exposure limits, substance-specific standards address broader aspects of hazardous exposure control, including exposure monitoring programs, medical surveillance, use of personal protective equipment, worker education and training, and recordkeeping. Other OSHA standards are applicable to toxic gas and/or vapor exposure as well. The hazard communication standard (29CFR 1910.1200), also referred to as a "right-to-know" regulation, defines procedures for worker notification, in part through access to MSDS, and training in the use of workplace chemicals. Standard 29CFR1910.1450 regulates occupational exposure to hazardous chemicals in laboratories, requiring that employers develop and implement a chemical hygiene plan describing procedures, instruments, personal protective equipment, and work practices targeted at protecting workers from potential health hazards while working in the laboratory setting. In 1993, OSHA also promulgated a new standard regulating work in confined spaces (29CFR 1910.146), an environment particularly conducive to poor ventilation and responsible for numerous fatalities or near fatalities in the past.[13]

Community exposure to air, soil, and water contaminants in the United States is regulated mainly by EPA. A number of statutes define EPA's responsibilities; several of these are applicable to exposures either to gases or to materials capable of generating potentially hazardous vapors. Through the Toxic Substances Control Act of 1976 (TSCA), chemical manufacturers and processors are required to compile data on the health effects and safety of new chemicals, and to notify the Environmental Protection Agency prior to the introduction of any new product. The Resource Conservation and Recovery Act of 1976 (RCRA) created a new hazardous waste control program, and established standards for the storage, transport, and disposal of hazardous waste; these regulations also mandate worker training, emergency response plans, and safe handling procedures.

Finally, the Department of Transportation, through the Hazardous Materials Transportation Act, is responsible for regulating the packaging, handling, and shipment of substances potentially hazardous to workers and the general public. Issues such as warning labels, preventive practices, and response to accidental spills or leaks are covered under this Act.

CONTROL METHODS

Anticipation and preparedness are key concepts in the control and prevention of acute exposures to gaseous materials and their consequences. Primary prevention measures are largely based on a hierarchical approach to safety in the workplace, and include engineering controls, administrative controls, and personal protection.

1. Engineering controls may include substitution of less hazardous materials, provision of adequate general and local exhaust ventilation, or redesign of potentially hazardous processes and work practices.
2. Administrative controls chiefly consist of development, implementation, and periodic review of safe standard operating procedures (SOPs), particularly in situations involving work in confined spaces and instances where hazardous materials are handled.
3. Personal protection, although not a substitute for engineering and administrative controls, includes availability of emergency respiratory protection and regular use of respirators during potentially dangerous routines.
4. Workers and the general community have the right to know which substances are present in their environment and their associated hazards, and should have access to practical information on these materials.

Advance emergency response planning is the cornerstone in the mitigation of the effects of an industrial or community disaster. Table 30-3 provides a list of national telephone information and technical support resources useful during hazardous materials emergencies. Key elements of planning consist of anticipating an accident, formulating a plan, performing drills, and accident investigation. The Agency for Toxic Substances and Disease Registry (ATSDR) has published a set of practical guidelines that describe a step-by-step approach to the management of hazardous materials incidents.[72–74]

RESEARCH NEEDS

In general, we have a good understanding of the immediate consequences of acute exposures to single gases or toxic vapors. Greater insight into the mechanisms of injury and effects of exposure to mixtures of gases is needed, especially in view of the increasing number of new chemical mixtures introduced to the marketplace. The main questions that persist, however, refer to the long-term consequences of acute gaseous exposures.

In 1985, the National Heart, Lung and Blood Institute convened a workshop to identify strategies for investigating the relationship between occupational exposures and airflow obstruction.[124] Several areas of needed research were identified and many of these were relevant to the topic of respiratory irritant exposure. Most of these needs remain relevant. From a nomenclature standpoint, it is still unclear whether reactive airways dysfunction syndrome is a part of the spectrum of asthma, although there appears to be a growing consensus to consider it so, hence, the increasing use of terms such as "nonallergic" or "irritant-induced" asthma. Asthma prevalence and severity are increasing na-

Table 30-3. Telephone information and technical support references

Resource	Contact		Services provided
CHEMTREC (Chemical Transportation Emergency Center)	1-800-424-9300		24-hour emergency number. Connection with manufacturers and/or shippers who will provide advice on handling, rescue gear needed, decontamination considerations, etc. Also provides access to Chlorine Emergency Response Plan (CHLOREP)
ATSDR (Agency for Toxic Substances and Disease Registry)	1-404-639-0615		24-hour emergency number for health-related support in hazardous materials emergencies, including on-site assistance, if necessary
Bureau of Explosives	1-202-639-2222		24-hour emergency number for hazardous materials incidents involving railroads
Emergency Planning and Community Right-to-Know Information Hotline	1-800-535-0202		8:30 A.M.-7:30 P.M. (EST) Provides information on SARA Title III. Provides list of extremely hazardous substances and planning guidelines
EPA (Environmental Protection Agency) Regional Offices	Region I CT, ME, MA, NH, RI, VT	(617) 565-3698	Environmental response team available for technical assistance
	Region II NJ, NY, PR, VI	(212) 264-0504	
	Region III DE, DC, MD, PA, VA, WV	(215) 597-0980	
	Region IV AL, FL, GA, KY, MS, NC, SC, TN	(404) 347-3454	
	Region V IL, IN, MI, MN, OH, WI	(312) 886-7579	
	Region VI AR, LA, NM, OK, TX	(214) 655-6760	
	Region VII IA, KS, MO, NE	(913) 236-2850	
	Region VIII CO, MT, ND, SD, UT, WY	(303) 293-1720	
	Region IX AM SAMOA, AZ, CA, GU, HI, NV, Trust Territory of the Pacific Isl., Marshall Isl., Palau, Ponape	(415) 974-7460	
	Region X AK, ID, OR, WA	(206) 442-2782	
National Animal Poison Control Center	1-217-333-3611		24-hour consultation concerning animal poisonings or chemical contamination. Provides an emergency response team to investigate incidents and perform laboratory analysis
National Response Center	1-800-424-8802		For reporting transportation incidents where hazardous materials are responsible for death, serious injury, property damage in excess of $50,000, or continuing danger to life and property

tionally; the contribution of occupational and environmental exposures to this change in pattern remains unclear.[126] However, the contribution of occupational airways diseases to the burden of all occupational respiratory disease seems to be increasing. This may be in part due to declining rates of more classic occupational lung diseases, such as the pneumoconioses, or possibly to increased recognition of occupational asthmagens by physicians. Better surveillance and reporting systems, including use of poison control centers and their national networking capabilities, are needed to allow the identification, not only of new cases of irritant-induced airways disease, but also of the populations at risk, so that accurate estimates of prevalence and incidence can be established.

To accurately characterize persons at risk for long-term airways sequelae, a greater understanding of the role of host factors such as preexisting asthma and atopic status, preexposure level of bronchial responsiveness and smoking, as well as better characterization of exposure intensity during these acute episodes, is needed. Ideally, this could be achieved by carefully designed prospective studies in which these variables were measured at baseline, and then the population followed over time with meticulous investigation of irritant exposure events. In reality, the sample size needed to generate a sufficient number of events would probably be extremely large and, therefore, difficult to achieve.

For the past several years, a considerable amount of research has been published regarding mechanisms of asthma induction, especially with regards to the role of inflammation mediators and epithelial injury, through bronchoalveolar and bronchial lavage studies and examination of bronchial biopsy specimens. It is likely that several of the findings will be applicable to irritant-induced airways disease as well. More recently, there has been interest in evaluating the response of the nasal and upper airway passages to various irritants, such as capsaicin and environmental tobacco smoke, through the use of nasal lavage analysis following both nonspecific and specific challenges.[127–129] Information derived from these types of studies may be applicable to the study of airway response to similar agents. Furthermore, the extrapolation of results and concepts derived from the study of high level irritant exposure to the evaluation of effects of more chronic, lower level exposure to irritants in the workplace and community could be extremely valuable.

Finally, the recently published, clinically practical guidelines for the evaluation of impairment/disability for asthma should be welcomed by physicians who often have to evaluate patients some time after an accidental spill or release has occurred.[99] They allow useful information to be generated regarding level of impairment, while recognizing that asthma, including irritant-induced asthma, can change over time, and, therefore, so can the level of impairment. There is a need, however, to periodically reassess these guidelines, so that their validity can be established.

REFERENCES

1. Ramazzini B and Wright WC trans. Diseases of workers. In *De morbis artificum diatriba*, 1713, Chicago, 1940, University of Chicago.
2. Weill H: Disaster at Bhopal: the accident, early findings and respiratory health outlook in those injured, *Bull Eur Physiopathol Respir* 23:587-590, 1987.
3. Wagner GN, Clark MA, Koenigsberg EJ, and Decata SJ: Medical evaluation of the victims of the 1986 Lake Nyos disaster, *J Forensic Sci* 33:899-909, 1988.
4. Baxter PJ, Kapila M, and Mfonfu D: Lake Nyos disaster, Cameroon, 1986: the medical effects of large scale emission of carbon dioxide? *Br Med J* 298:1437-1441, 1989.
5. Phalen RF and Prasad SB: Morphology of the respiratory tract. In McClellan RO and Henderson RF, editors: *Concepts in inhalation toxicology,* New York, 1989, Hemisphere.
6. Brooks SM, Weiss MA, and Bernstein IL: Reactive airways dysfunction syndrome (RADS). Persistent asthma syndrome after high level irritant exposures, *Chest* 88:376-384, 1985.
7. Moller D, McKay RT, Bernstein IL, and Brooks SM: Persistent airways disease caused by toluene diisocyanate, *Am Rev Respir Dis* 134:175-176, 1986.
8. King TE: Bronchiolitis obliterans, *Lung* 167:69-93, 1989.
9. Hoeffler HB, Schweppe HI, and Greenberg SD: Bronchiectasis following pulmonary ammonia burn, *Arch Pathol Lab Med* 106:686-687, 1982.
10. Slutzker AD, Kinn R, and Said SI: Bronchiectasis and progressive respiratory failure following smoke inhalation, *Chest* 95:1349-1350, 1989.
11. Wright JL and Churg A: Diseases caused by metals and related compounds, fumes and gases. In Churg A and Green FHY, editors: *Pathology of occupational lung disease*. New York; 1988, Igaku-Shoin.
12. Litovitz T, Oderda G, White JD, and Sheridan MJ: Occupational and environmental exposures reported to poison centers, *Am J Public Health* 83:739-743, 1993.
13. Suruda A and Agnew J: Deaths from asphyxiation and poisoning at work in the United States, *Br J Ind Med* 46:541-546, 1989.
14. Birky MM, Paabo M, Levin BC, Womble SE, and Maler D: *Development of recommended test method for toxicological assessment of inhaled combustion products.* Final report to products research committee. Washington, DC, 1980, National Bureau of Standards.
15. Achauer BM, Allyn PA, Furnas DW, and Bartlett RH: Pulmonary complications of burns: the major threat to the burn patient, *Ann Surg* 177:311-319, 1973.
16. DiVincenti FC, Basil MC, Pruitt A, and Reckler JM: Inhalation injuries, *J Trauma* 11:109–117, 1971.
17. Phillips AW, Tanner JW, and Cope O: Burn therapy: IV. Respiratory tract damage (an account of the clinical, x-ray and postmortem findings) and the meaning of restlessness, *Ann Surg* 158:799–811, 1963.
18. Sochor FM and Mallory GK. Lung lesions in patients dying of burns, *Arch Pathol* 75:303-308, 1963.
19. Stone HH, Rhame DW, Corbitt JD, Given KS, and Martin JD: Respiratory burns: a correlation of clinical and laboratory results, *Ann Surg* 165:157-168, 1967.
20. Zikria BA, Weston GC, Chodoff M, and Ferrer JM: Smoke and carbon monoxide poisoning in fire victims, *J Trauma* 12:641-655, 1972.
21. National Institute for Occupational Safety and Health: *National occupational hazard survey, 1972-1974,* Cincinnati, OH, 1976, National Institute for Occupational Safety and Health, Department of Health and Human Services.
22. National Institute for Occupational Safety and Health: *National occupational exposure survey, 1981-1983,* Cincinnati, OH, 1984, National Institute for Occupational Safety and Health, Department of Health and Human Services.
23. Witschi H: Responses of the lung to toxic injury, *Environ Health Perspec* 85:5-13, 1990.
24. Wilkenfeld M: Simple asphyxiants. In Rom WN, editor: *Environmental and occupational medicine,* Boston, 1992, Little, Brown.
25. Hulbert WC, Man SFP, Rosychuk MK, Braybrook G, and Mehta JG: The response phase—the first six hours after acute airway injury by SO_2 inhalation: an in vivo and in vitro study, *Scanning Microsc* 3:369-378, 1989.
26. Summer W and Haponik E: Inhalation of irritant gases, *Clin Chest Med* 2:273-287, 1981.
27. Rajini P, Gelzleichter TR, Last JA, and Witschi H: Alveolar and airway cell kinetics in the lungs of rats exposed to nitrogen dioxide, ozone, and a combination of the two gases, *Toxicol Appl Pharmacol* 121:186-192, 1993.
28. Schwartz DA: Acute inhalational injury, *Occup Med: State Art Rev* 2:297-318, 1987.
29. Tarlo SM and Broder I: Irritant-induced occupational asthma, *Chest* 96:297-300, 1989.
30. Man SFP and WC Hulbert: Airway repair and adaptation to inhalation injury. In Loke J, editor: *Pathophysiology and treatment of inhalation injuries,* New York, 1988, Marcel Dekker.

31. Kleeberger SR and Hudak BB: Acute ozone-induced change in airway permeability: role of infiltrating leukocytes, *J Appl Physiol* 72:670-676, 1992.

32. Prien T and Traber DL: Toxic smoke compounds and inhalation injury—a review, *Burns* 14:451-460, 1988.

33. Schwartz DA, Smith DD, and Lakshminarayan S: The pulmonary sequelae associated with accidental inhalation of chlorine gas, *Chest* 97:820-825, 1990.

34. Kennedy SM: Acquired airway hyperresponsiveness from nonimmunogenic irritant exposure, *Occup Med: State Art Rev* 7:287-300, 1992.

35. Boulet LP: Increases in airway responsiveness following acute exposure to respiratory irritants. Reactive airway dysfunction syndrome or occupational asthma? *Chest* 94:476-481, 1988.

36. Sheppard D: Mechanisms of airway responses to inhaled sulfur dioxide, In Loke J, editor: *Pathophysiology and treatment of inhalation injuries,* New York, 1988, Marcel Dekker.

37. Pinkerton KE, Mercer RH, Plopper CG, and Crapo JD: Distribution of injury and microdosimetry of ozone in the ventilatory unit of the rat, *J Appl Physiol* 73:817-824, 1992.

38. Dungworth DL: Noncarcinogenic responses of the respiratory tract to inhaled toxicants, In McClellan RO and Henderson RF, editors: *Concepts in inhalation toxicology,* New York, 1989, Hemisphere Publishing Corporation.

39. Bates DV: The respiratory bronchiole as a target organ for the effects of dusts and gases, *J Occup Med* 15:177-180, 1973.

40. Loick HM, Traber LD, Tokyay R, et al: Thromboxane receptor blockade with BM-13,177 following toxic airway damage by smoke inhalation in sheep, *Eur J Pharmacol* 248:75-83, 1993.

41. Pino MV, Stovall MY, Levin JR, et al: Acute ozone-induced lung injury in neutrophil-depleted rats, *Toxicol Appl Pharmacol* 114:268-276, 1992.

42. Bhalla DK, Rasmussen RE, and Daniels DS: Adhesion and motility of polymorphonuclear leukocytes isolated from the blood of rats exposed to ozone: potential biomarkers of toxicity, *Toxicol Appl Pharmacol* 123:177-186, 1993.

43. Mengel RG, Bernard W, Barth P, Von Wichert P, and Muller B: Impaired regulation of surfactant phospholipid metabolism in the isolated rat lung after nitrogen dioxide inhalation, *Toxicol Appl Pharmacol* 120:216-223, 1993.

44. Paterson JF, Hammond MD, Montgomery MR, et al: Acute ozone-induced lung injury in rats: structural-functional relationships of developing alveolar edema, *Toxicol Appl Pharmacol* 117:37-45, 1992.

45. Alarie Y, Lin CK, and Geary DL: Sensory irritation evoked by plastic decomposition products, *Am Ind Hyg Assoc J* 35:654, 1974.

46. Barrow CS, Alarie Y, and Stock MF: Sensory irritation and incapacitation evoked by thermal decomposition products of polymers and comparisons with known sensory irritants, *Arch Environ Health* 33:79-89, 1978.

47. Gilmour MI and Selgrade MJK: A comparison of the pulmonary defenses against streptococcal infection in rats and mice following O_3 exposure: differences in disease susceptibility and neutrophil recruitment, *Toxicol Appl Pharmacol* 123:211-218, 1993.

48. Jakab GJ: The toxicologic interactions resulting from inhalation of carbon black and acrolein on pulmonary antibacterial and antiviral defenses, *Toxicol Appl Pharmacol* 121:167-175, 1993.

49. Blanc PD, Galbo M, Hiatt P, and Olson KR: Morbidity following acute irritant inhalation in a population-based study, *J Am Med Assoc* 266:664-669, 1991.

50. Brooks SM: Occupational and environmental asthma, In Rom WN, editor: *Environmental and occupational medicine,* Boston, 1992, Little, Brown.

51. Clayton GD: Air pollution. In Patty FA, editor: *Industrial hygiene and toxicology,* ed 2, vol. I, New York, 1958, Interscience.

52. Hartzell GE, Packham SC, and Switzer WC: Toxic products from fires, *Am Ind Hyg Assoc J* 44:248-255, 1983.

53. Treitman RD, Burgess WA, and Gold A: Air contaminants encountered by firefighters, *Am Ind Hyg Assoc J* 41:796-802, 1980.

54. American Conference of Governmental Industrial Hygienists: *1993-1994 threshold limit values for chemical substances and physical agents and biological exposure indices,* Cincinnati, OH, 1993, American Conference of Governmental Industrial Hygienists.

55. Department of Labor: *NIOSH/OSHA pocket guide to chemical hazards.* Washington, DC, 1978, US Government Printing Office.

56. Deichmann WB and Gerarde HW, editors: *Symptomatology and therapy of toxicological emergencies,* New York, 1964, Academic Press.

57. Foley FD, Moncrief JA, and Mason AD: Pathology of the lung in fatally burned patients, *Ann Surg* 167:251-264, 1968.

58. Lloyd EL and MacRae WR: Respiratory tract damage in burns, *Br J Anaesth* 43:365-379, 1971.

59. Beal DD, Lambeth JT, and Conner GH: Follow-up studies on patients treated with steroids following pulmonary thermal and acrid smoke injury, *Laryngoscope* 78:396-403, 1968.

60. Horovitz JH: Abnormalities caused by smoke inhalation, *J Trauma* 19:915-916, 1979.

61. Frostling H: Degradation products of plastics-analytical, occupational and toxicologic aspects, *Scand J Work Environ Health* 8:9-12, 1982.

62. Pfaffli P: Degradation products of plastics: polyethylene and styrene-containing thermoplastics-analytical, occupational and toxicologic aspects, *Scand J Work Environ Health* 8:27-43, 1982.

63. Sangha GK, Matijak M, and Alarie Y: Toxicologic evaluation of thermoplastic resins at and above processing temperatures, *Am Ind Hyg Assoc J* 42:481-485, 1981.

64. Boettner EA and Ball GL: Thermal degradation products from PVC film in food-wrapping operations, *Am Ind Hyg Assoc J* 41:513-522, 1980.

65. Bouley G, Dubreuil A, Jouany JM, and Boudene C: Effet du pyrolysat de matiere plastique polypropylenique sur les mechanismes de defense de l'appareil respiratoire, *Bull Eur Physiopathol Respir* 17:903-910, 1981.

66. Eckardt RE and Hindin R: The health hazards of plastics, *J Occup Med* 15:808-819, 1973.

67. Hoff A and Jacobson S: Degradation products of plastics-analytical, occupational and toxicologic aspects. II. Analysis of volatile products, *Scand J Work Environ Health* 2:12-27, 1982.

68. Maintz G and Werner L: Zur wirkung von kunststoffen auf den atemtrakt: literaturubersicht. Z, *Gesamte Hyg* 29:2-10, 1983.

69. Polakoff PL, Lapp NL, and Reger R: Polyvinyl chloride pyrolysis products: a potential cause for respiratory impairment, *Arch Environ Health* 30:269-271, 1975.

70. National Institute for Occupational Safety and Health: Health Hazard Evaluation: Overheating at switches in Goshen, Indiana, 1979, HHE-79-133:CDC-PHS-DHEW.

71. Marsh GM: Mortality among workers from a plastics producing plant: a matched case-control study nested in a retrospective cohort study, *J Occup Med* 25:219-230, 1983.

72. Agency for Toxic Substances and Disease Registry: *Managing hazardous materials incidents: vol. I—emergency medical systems: a planning guide for the management of contaminated patients,* US-GPO/ATSDR, 1993.

73. Agency for Toxic Substances and Disease Registry: *Managing hazardous materials incidents: vol. II—hospital emergency departments: a planning guide for the management of contaminated patients,* US-GPO/ATSDR, 1993.

74. Agency for Toxic Substances and Disease Registry: *Managing hazardous materials incidents: vol. III—medical management guidelines for acute chemical exposures,* USGPO/ATSDR, 1993.

75. Clark WR: Smoke inhalation: diagnosis and treatment, *World J Surg* 16:24-29, 1992.

76. Kulling P: Hospital treatment of victims exposed to combustion products, *Toxicol Lett* 64/65:283-289, 1992.

77. Galea M: Fatal sulfur dioxide inhalation, *Can Med Assoc J* 91:345-347, 1964.

78. Chester EH, Kaimal PJ, Payne CB, and Kohn PM: Pulmonary injury following exposure to chlorine gas. Possible beneficial effects of steroid treatment, *Chest* 72:247-250, 1977.

79. Douglas WW, Hepper NGG, and Colby TV: Silo-filler's disease, *Mayo Clin Proc* 64:291-304, 1989.

80. Horvath EP, doPico GA, Barbee RA, and Dickie HA: Nitrogen dioxide-induced pulmonary disease, *J Occup Med* 20:103-110, 1978.

81. Teixidor HS, Rubin E, Novick GS, and Alonso DR: Smoke inhalation: radiologic manifestations, *Radiology* 149:383-387, 1983.

82. Ramirez JR and Dowell AR: Silo-filler's disease:nitrogen dioxide-induced lung injury, *Ann Intern Med* 74:569-576, 1971.

83. Epler GR: Silo-filler's disease: a new perspective [editorial], *Mayo Clin Proc* 64:368-370, 1989.

84. Seggev JS, Mason UG, Worthen S, Stanford RE, and Fernandez E: Bronchiolitis obliterans. Report of three cases with detailed physiologic studies, *Chest* 83:169-174, 1983.

85. Key MM, Henschel AF, Butler J, Ligo RN, and Tabershaw IR, editors: *Occupational diseases: a guide to their recognition,* USGPO/NIOSH/77-181, 1977.

86. Amdur MO, Doull J, and Klaassen CD, editors: *Casarett and Doull's toxicology: the basic science of poisons,* ed 4, New York, 1991, Pergamon Press.

87. Forsyth JC, Mueller PD, Becker CE, et al: Hydroxocobalamin as a cyanide antidote: safety, efficacy and pharmacokinetics in heavily smoking normal volunteers, *J Toxicol Clin Toxicol* 31:227-294, 1993.

88. Reiffenstein RJ, Hulbert WC, and Roth SH: Toxicology of hydrogen sulfide, *Annu Rev Pharmacol Toxicol* 109-134, 1992.

89. Glass DC: A review of the health effects of hydrogen sulphide exposure, *Ann Occup Hyg* 34:323-327, 1990.

90. Guidotti TL: Central nervous system toxicity from hydrogen sulfide, *Occup Environ Med Rpt* 6:3-4, 1992.

91. Bradley BL and Unger KM: Phosgene inhalation: a case report, *Texas Med* 78:51-53, 1982.

92. Cohen MA and Guzzardi LJ: Inhalation of products of combustion, *Ann Emerg Med* 12:628-632, 1983.

93. Head JM: Inhalation injury in burns, *Am J Surg* 139:508-512, 1980.

94. Cooke NT, Cobley AJ, and Armstrong RF: Airflow obstruction after smoke inhalation, *Anaesthesia* 37:830-832, 1982.

95. Petroff PA, Hander EW, Clayton WH, and Pruitt BA: Pulmonary function studies after smoke inhalation, *Am J Surg* 132:346-351, 1976.

96. Korn RJ, Dockery DW, Speizer FE, Ware JH, and Ferris BG: Occupational exposures and chronic respiratory symptoms. A population-based study, *Am Rev Respir Dis* 136:298-304, 1987.

97. American Medical Association: *Guidelines to the evaluation of permanent impairment,* ed 4, Chicago, 1993, American Medical Association.

98. American Thoracic Society Ad Hoc Committee on Impairment/Disability Criteria: Evaluation of impairment/disability secondary to respiratory disorders, *Am Rev Respir Dis* 134:1205-1209, 1986.

99. American Thoracic Society: Guidelines for the evaluation of impairment/disability in patients with asthma, *Am Rev Respir Dis* 147:1056-1061, 1993.

100. Blanc PD, Rempel D, Maizlish N, Hiatt P, and Olson KR: Occupational illness: case detection by poison control surveillance, *Ann Intern Med* 111:238-244, 1989.

101. Dixon M, Jackson DM, and Richards IM: Changes in the bronchial reactivity of dogs caused by exposure to sulfur dioxide, *J Physiol* 337:89-99, 1983.

102. Riedel F, Kramer M, Scheibenbogen C, et al: Effects of SO_2 exposure on allergic sensitization in the guinea pig, *J Allergy Clin Immunol* 82:527-534, 1988.

103. Wolff RK, Osminski G, and Newhouse MT: Acute exposure of symptomatic steelworkers to sulfur dioxide and carbon dioxide: effects on mucociliary transport, pulmonary function, and bronchial reactivity, *Br J Ind Med* 41:499-505, 1984.

104. Golden JA, Nadel JA, and Boushey HA: Bronchial hyperirritability in healthy subjects after exposure to ozone, *Am Rev Respir Dis* 118:287-294, 1978.

105. Holtzman MJ, Cunningham JH, Sheller JH, et al: Effect of ozone on bronchial reactivity in atopic and non-atopic subjects, *Am Rev Respir Dis* 120:1059-1067, 1979.

106. Mohsenin V: Effect of vitamin C on NO_2-induced airway hyperresponsiveness in normal subjects. A randomized double-blind experiment, *Am Rev Respir Dis* 136:1408-1411, 1987.

107. Gandevia B: Occupational asthma, Parts I-II, *Med J Aust* 2:332-335,372-376, 1970.

108. Harkonen H, Nordman H, Korhonen O, and Winblad I: Long-term effects of exposure to sulfur dioxide. Lung function four years after a pyrite dust explosion, *Am Rev Respir Dis* 128:890-893, 1983.

109. Flury KE, Dines DE, Rodarte JR, and Rodgers R: Airway obstruction due to inhalation of ammonia, *Mayo Clin Proc* 58:389-393, 1983.

110. Kass I, Zamel N, Dobry CA, and Holzer M: Bronchiectasis following ammonia burns of the respiratory tract. A review of two cases, *Chest* 62:282-285, 1972.

111. Lerman S and Kipen H: Reactive airways dysfunction syndrome, *Am Fam Phy* 38:135-138, 1988.

112. Rabinovitch S, Greyson ND, Weiser W, and Hoffstein V: Clinical and laboratory features of acute sulfur dioxide inhalation poisoning: two-year follow-up, *Am Rev Respir Dis* 139:556-558, 1989.

113. Moore BB and Sherman M: Chronic reactive airway disease following acute chlorine gas exposure in an asymptomatic atopic patient, *Chest* 100:855-856, 1991.

114. Kern DG: Outbreak of the reactive airways dysfunction syndrome after a spill of glacial acetic acid, *Am Rev Respir Dis* 144:1058-1064, 1991.

115. Wade JF and Newman LS: Diesel asthma. Reactive airways disease following overexposure to locomotive exhaust, *J Occup Med* 35:149-154, 1993.

116. Du Toit JI, Woolcock AJ, Salome CM, Sundrum R, and Black JL: Characteristics of bronchial hyperresponsiveness in smokers with chronic air-flow limitation, *Am Rev Respir Dis* 134:498-501, 1986.

117. Kennedy SM, Burrows B, Vedal S, Enarson DA, and Chan-Yeung M: Methacholine responsiveness among working populations. Relationship to smoking and airway caliber, *Am Rev Respir Dis* 142:1377-1383, 1990.

118. U.S. Army: *Medical aspects of gas warfare,* vol 14, Medical Department of the United States Army in the World War. Washington, 1926, Government Printing Office.

119. Gilchrist HL and Matz PB: The residual effects of warfare gases: the use of chlorine gas, with report of cases, *Med Bull VA* 9:229-270, 1933.

120. Jones RN, Hughes JM, glindmeyer H, and Weill H: Lung function after acute chlorine exposure, *Am Rev Respir Dis* 134:1190–1195, 1986.

121. Melius JM: The Bhopal disaster, In Rom WN, editor: *Environmental and occupational medicine,* Boston, 1992, Little, Brown.

122. Sharma S, Narayanan PS, Sriramachari S, Vijayan VK, Kamat SR, and Chandra H: Objective thoracic CT scan findings in a Bhopal gas disaster victim, *Respir Med* 85:539-541, 1991.

123. Kamat SR, Patel MH, Pradhan PV, et al: Sequential respiratory, psychologic, and immunologic studies in relation to methyl isocyanate exposure over two years with model development, *Environ Health Perspect* 97:241-253, 1992.

124. Brooks SM and Kalica AR: Strategies for elucidating the relationship between occupational exposures and chronic air-flow obstruction, *Am Rev Respir Dis* 135:268-273, 1987.

125. CCINFOdisc, Series C2 (RTECS) [CD-ROM].MS-DOS version. Ontario (Canada), 1993, Canadian Centre for Occupational Health and Safety.

126. Schenker MB, Gold EB, Lopez RL, and Beavmont JJ: Asthma mortality in California, 1960-1989: demographic patterns and occupational associations, *Am Rev Respir Dis* 147:1454-1460, 1993.

127. Bascom R: The upper respiratory tract: mucous membrane irritation, *Environ Health Perspect* 95:39-44, 1991.

128. Bascom R, Kagey-Sobotka A, and Proud D: Effect of intranasal capsaicin on symptoms and mediator release, *J Pharmacol Exp Ther* 259:1323-1327, 1991.

129. Willes SR, Fitzgerald TK, and Bascom R: Nasal inhalation challenge studies with sidestream tobacco smoke, *Arch Environ Health* 47:223-230, 1992.

Chapter 31

IONIZING RADIATION AND THE LUNGS

Otto G. Raabe
Jerrold T. Bushberg

The interaction of ionizing radiation on lung tissue can cause acute or chronic injury and may lead to various types of radiation-induced lung cancer. At high doses typically associated with radiation therapy or severe external exposure accidents, acute inflammatory changes may manifest over the first week. This may be followed by chronic fibrosis in those regions where the regenerative capacity of the tissue has been destroyed. Individuals who survive these high level exposures, as well as those who are exposed to lower doses, may have an increased risk of cancer. The probability of occurrence is dose and dose-rate dependent. This chapter reviews the characteristics of ionizing radiation, sources of exposure, dosimetry, occupational exposure standards, and both neoplastic and nonneoplastic biologic responses. These principles are employed in selected review of occupational exposure cases to illustrate their application.

PHYSICAL PRINCIPLES
Ionizing radiation

Ionizing radiation includes both subatomic particles and electromagnetic waves (or photons) with enough energy to effect the removal of an orbital electron from neutral atoms changing them to charged atoms called ions. Ionization is the initiating phenomenon in a complex sequence of events within living tissue that may lead to biologic alterations or cellular damage. This review does not consider other forms of radiation that are not ionizing, such as infrared radiation, ultraviolet radiation, microwaves, electrical fields, and magnetic fields. These forms of nonionizing radiation may also cause biologic effects.

Electromagnetic radiation

Electromagnetic radiation (EMR) is a term applied to waves of oscillating electric and magnetic fields that are mutually dependent and perpendicular to each other and their direction of propagation (Fig. 31-1). EMR radiates outward from its point of origin at the speed of light ($\sim 3 \times$

10^8 m/sec) and is characterized by its *wavelength* (λ), defined as the distance between any two corresponding points on adjacent waves or alternatively by its *frequency* (ν) defined as the number of waves that pass a given point per unit time. Frequency and wavelength are inversely proportional and expressed in units of cycles/sec (or Hertz, abbreviated Hz) and meters, respectively. EMR extends from the very low frequencies associated with electric power transmission (60 Hz) to cosmic radiation ($\sim 10^{24}$ Hz) in a continuous *electromagnetic spectrum* (Fig. 31-2) that (in order of increasing energy, frequency, and decreasing wavelength) includes radio and TV broadcasts, microwaves, visible light, x-rays and γ-rays. The characteristics of radiation interaction with matter change dramatically as a function of energy (frequency). High energy EMR often exhibits a corpuscular behavior in its interaction with matter so that it can be treated as consisting of small bundles of energy called photons ($E_{emr} = h\nu$ where h is Planck's constant). Energy of ionizing EMR is typically expressed in very small energy units known as electron volts (eV). One electron volt is defined as the kinetic energy acquired by an electron as it traverses a potential difference of 1 V in a vacuum. EMR beyond the far ultraviolet region of the spectrum (~ 10 eV) has sufficient energy to ionize atoms and thus is referred to as ionizing radiation. EMR below this level (such as microwaves and radio waves) is referred to as *nonionizing radiation* and deposits its energy in matter via atomic and molecular excitation.

Electromagnetic radiation interactions. Ionizing EMR interacts with matter several ways, with the most important being (arranged in order in increasing probability as a function of photon energy) *Rayleigh scattering, photoelectric absorption, Compton absorption or scattering,* and *pair production.*[1]

In Rayleigh scattering (also called elastic or classic scattering) photons are scattered through small deflection angles with virtually no loss of energy. This type of interaction is of little radiobiologic consequence. It is associated with very low photon energies and occurs infrequently ($<5\%$) for photons with energies above 100 keV.

Compton scattering is the predominate interaction of medium energy photons (~ 100 to 1000 keV) with tissue. The

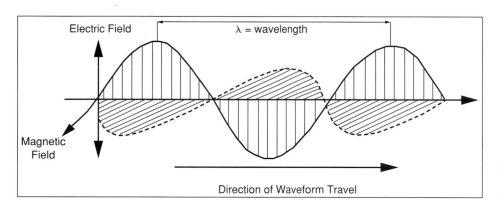

Fig. 31-1. Illustration of the electric and magnetic field components of electromagnetic radiation.

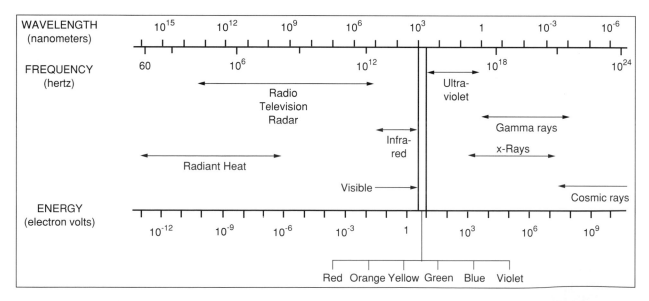

Fig. 31-2. Illustration of the spectrum of electromagnetic radiation. Only radiation with energies above ultraviolet are forms of ionizing radiation.

incident photon (E_0) interacts with an outer (valence) electron that is ejected from the atom. The kinetic energy of the ejected *Compton electron* (E_e) will be dependent upon the energy of the incident photon and the angle of the scattering event. As the angle of the deflection is increased, the energy transferred to the electron increases. The incident photon is scattered with lower energy (E_{sc}). In general, the fraction of energy given to the scattered photon is large for low energy incident photons and small scattering angles. The ejected electron deposits its energy via excitation and ionization as its electrostatic charge field interacts with neighboring atoms. The scattered photon (depending on its energy and the atomic number of the material) may undergo subsequent Compton interactions and/or deposit the balance of its energy by photoelectric absorption.

In photoelectric absorption the photon is completely absorbed as its energy is transferred to an orbital electron (typically an inner K or L shell). The electron is subsequently ejected with a kinetic energy equal to the incident photon energy minus the binding energy of the ejected electron. The vacancy left by the ejection of this electron is filled by an electron transition from an outer shell. The vacancy left from this transition is filled by an electron with even lower binding energy. This process is continuous until the atom reestablishes electronic neutrality.

When an electron transitions to an orbit closer to the nucleus, its binding energy is increased, which is offset with an equal decrease in energy emitted by the atom as either a photon (called a *characteristic x ray*) or the ejection of an electron (called an *Auger electron*). The x ray has a "characteristic" energy equal to the difference in binding energies of the transitioning electron's initial and final shell. Auger electron emission is an alternative to characteristic x-ray emission in which the energy, otherwise emitted as a characteristic x-ray, is transferred to an orbital electron. The orbital electron is subsequently ejected with a kinetic energy equal to the characteristic x-ray energy minus the ejected electron's binding energy. The radiobiologic significance of photoelectric absorption is the production of energetic photoelectrons and low energy characteristic x-rays (and/or Auger electrons) that deposit their energy locally, thus increasing the dose to surrounding cells. This local dose distribution pattern (referred to as *microdosimetry*) may have relevance with respect to some biologic effects that occur with cells.

When very high energy photons (>1.022 MeV) interact with high Z material, pair production may occur. Pair production refers to the instantaneous creation of an electron-positron pair as an energetic photon is converted from energy to matter under the influence of the atomic nucleus. The mass–energy conversion follows Einstein's famous equation of mass–energy equivalence: $E = mc^2 = 931$ MeV/u. The 1.02 MeV threshold for this interaction is equivalent to the rest mass energy of the electron–positron pair. The probability of pair production (as compared with Compton scattering) does not become important until photon energies exceed 2 MeV. Energy in excess of the 1.02 MeV threshold needed to create the mass of two electrons appears as the kinetic energy of motion of the electron–positron pair. The positron deposits its energy in the same manner as the electron (excitation and ionization), but its fate is very different. Once an ordinary electron has deposited its kinetic energy it becomes part of the "free electron pool." In contrast, once the positron comes to rest it interacts violently with an electron converting their mass to pure energy resulting in the emission of two oppositely directed 0.511 MeV photons. These photons, referred to as *annihilation radiation,* will undergo subsequent Compton and photoelectric interactions as previously described.

The probability of photoelectric absorption is proportional to Z^3/E^3 where Z is the atomic number of the attenuating material and E is the energy of the incident photon. The probability of Compton interaction is relatively independent of Z and inversely related to incident photon energy ($1/E$). Thus, relative to photoelectric absorption, the probability of Compton scattering increases with incident photon energy. The arithmetic sum of linear attenuation coefficients for all interaction mechanisms provides the total. At low photon energies (<30 keV) photoelectric interactions dominate the attenuation process. However, at energies typically associated with exposures from radiation producing machines or γ-rays, Compton scattering predominates.[1]

Attenuation of electromagnetic radiation. The interaction of EMR with matter is a random process of absorption and/or scattering called *attenuation*. The *linear attenuation coefficient* (μ) is the probability that a photon will be attenuated as it traverses a given distance, typically expressed in units of inverse centimeters (cm^{-1}). A μ of 0.2 cm^{-1} for 80 keV photons in tissue, for example, signifies that, for a large number of 80 keV photons (say 10,000), approximately 20% (or 2,000) will be attenuated as the photons traverse a thickness of 1 cm. The actual relationship is *not* linear, however, but rather follows an exponential relationship as a function of the depth of penetration. This is expressed mathematically as

$$I = I_0 e^{-\mu x} \tag{1}$$

where the incident photon intensity (I_0) is reduced to I after traversing a distance x. For example, if the linear attenuation coefficient for 100 keV photons in tissue was 0.16 cm^{-1}, the number of photons transmitted through 10 cm of tissue would be

$$I = I_0 e^{-(10 \text{ cm})(0.16 \text{ cm}^{-1})} = 0.2 I_0 \tag{2}$$

so that (on average) 20% of the photons would be transmitted though a 10 cm thickness of tissue.

Particulate radiation

Particulate radiations are various forms of high-speed subatomic particles of matter that by virtue of their kinetic energy of motion can directly or indirectly cause the ionization of atoms (Table 31-1). Important forms of particulate radiations include alpha radiation (α^{2+}), beta radiation (β^-), and positron radiation (β^+) that originate from the nuclei of atoms during radioactive decay, neutrons (n^0) that are produced in nuclear fission and fusion, and electron radiation (e^-) that originates from extranuclear orbital electrons. α particles are equivalent to helium-4 (^{4}He) nuclei that are typically emitted from the nuclei of larger unstable atoms having a high number of protons (high atomic number or Z) and higher total number of nucleons (A). The mass of nuclear particles is measured in atomic mass units (u) where the mass of an electrically neutral atom of carbon-12 (^{12}C) equals exactly 12 u.

α particles are emitted with high kinetic energies (4 to 8 MeV). However, their range is limited to a few centimeters in air and <100 μm in tissue and thus cannot even penetrate the cornified (or "dead") layer of the skin. Considering their limited range in tissue, exposure to an α radiation source is clinically significant only when there is the possibility of internal contamination.

β particles and positrons are simply electrons (negatively and positively charged, respectively) that are emitted from the nucleus during radioactive decay. These electrons can travel several meters in air and, depending on their energy, can penetrate several centimeters in tissue.

Neutrons (n^0) are much less frequently encountered in the workplace environment but can be produced by the spontaneous fission of some heavy unstable (radioactive) elements such as californium-252 (^{252}Cf) that can fission spontaneously or as the result of high-energy photon interactions with matter (photonuclear reactions). Major sources of neutrons include both nuclear fission (as occurs in nuclear reactors) and fusion (as occurs in thermonuclear weapons). Neutrons are approximately 2000 times the mass of an electron and have no net charge. A 1-MeV neutron has an average depth of penetration of 2.5 cm in tissue. Although the electrical neutrality of the neutron precludes it from interacting electrostatically like charged particles, its mass and kinetic energy allow it to interact with protons and small nuclei in a classic "billiard ball"-like interaction resulting in recoil protons or nuclei recoil with transferred kinetic energy. These recoil protons or nuclei have a positive charge and deposit their energy via excitation and ionization in a manner similar to α particles.

Excitation, ionization, and radiative losses. Charged particles interact with matter and lose their kinetic energy via *excitation, ionization,* and/or *radiative losses.* Excitation occurs when the columbic field of a charged particle approaches close enough to an atom's orbital electrons to allow the transfer of some of the particle's kinetic energy either by electrostatic attraction (as for α particles) or by electrostatic repulsion (as for β particles). This energy increase may cause one or more orbital electrons to be temporarily promoted to high-energy states.

If the transferred energy exceeds the binding energy of the orbital electron, ionization can occur in which the orbital electron is ejected from its parent atom and an ion pair is created. In some cases the removed electrons receive enough kinetic energy to ionize other atoms in a process called *secondary ionization.* These secondary electrons are then called *delta (δ) rays.*

A β particle or energetic electron can undergo a radiative type of energy loss when it traverses an atom close enough to have its path deflected by the electrostatic charge field from a positively charged nucleus. The deflection causes a decrease its kinetic energy, which is instantaneously emitted as an electromagnetic radiation photon (x-ray) called *bremsstrahlung,* a German word meaning "braking radiation."

Specific ionization and linear energy transfer. *Specific ionization* refers to the number of ion pairs (IP) produced per unit path length of the incident radiation expressed in IP/mm. The specific ionization of β particles in air is about 100 IP/mm. The higher the electrostatic charge and the slower the radiative particle, the greater the specific ionization. For example, the specific ionization of a 7.69-MeV α particle reaches a maximum of approximately 7000 IP/mm of air as the particles slow, allowing the electrostatic field generated by the 2+ charge to interact at a given location for a longer period of time. The specific ionization maximum characteristic of heavy charged particle interaction with matter is referred to as the *Bragg peak.* The rapid decrease in specific ionization on either side of the Bragg peak is exploited in radiation oncology, allowing large radiation doses to be delivered to a tumor volume at a particular depth in tissue while keeping the dose to surrounding healthy tissue as low as possible.

Another important distinction between light (e.g., electrons) and heavy (e.g., α) charged particles is their *path length* and *range* in matter. The path length is defined as the actual distance traveled by a charged particle before it comes to rest with respect to its surroundings. The range of a particle is defined as its depth of penetration into matter.

Table 31-1. Fundamental properties of particulate radiation

Particle	Symbol	Relative charge	Mass (u)
Alpha	α^4 (^{4}He^{2+})	+2	4.00277
Proton	p^1 (H$^+$)	+1	1.00759
Electron (beta minus)	e^-, β^-	−1	0.00055
Positron (beta plus)	e^+, β^+	+1	0.00055
Neutron	n^0	0	1.00898

A light charged particle like an electron or a β undergoes multiple scattering events resulting in a sparse ionization pattern over a tortuous path. In this case the devious path length far exceeds the net range. A heavier charged particle, such as an α, is not as easily deflected and produces a dense and nearly linear ionization track. The path and range of a heavy charged particle are approximately equal.

When the specific ionization (IP/mm) is multiplied by the ionization potential (about 34 eV/IP) of the material the result is the energy deposition per unit path length, referred to as the *linear energy transfer* or LET (eV/mm). The LET of a particular type of radiation specifies the intensity of the energy deposition pattern, which in turn is a critical element in determining the radiobiologic consequence of a particular exposure. In general, "high LET" radiation refers to heavy charged particles (e.g., αs and protons) that produce dense ionization tracks and "low LET" radiation refers to photons (x-rays and γ-rays) and electrons (β⁺, β⁻, and e⁻) in which the energy deposition pattern and the radiobiologic damage per unit dose are less severe. The intensity of biologic alterations or damage associated with different types of ionizing radiation can be indicated by a radiation weighting factor, w_R, or quality factor, Q, which is a function of LET. Table 31-2 summarizes the LET and w_R values for the common forms of ionizing radiation.[2]

Radioactivity

Terms and definitions. The nucleon total of an atom is the sum of the nuclear protons and neutrons *(A)*. Only certain combinations of neutrons and protons in the nucleus form stable atomic nuclei. At low atomic numbers *(Z)*,

Table 31-2. Linear energy transfer (LET) and radiation weighting factors (w_R) for various types of radiation*

Type of radiation	LET (keV/μm)	Radiation weighting factor (w_R)
x-rays		
γ-rays	<2	1
β particles and electrons†		
Protons (<2 MeV)	~20	5
Neutrons (energy dependent)	20-80	5-20
α particles and other multiple charged particles	~100	20
HZE space particles§	>200	20

*The radiation weighting factor is also called the quality factor, Q. For radiations principally used in medical imaging (x-rays, γ-rays, β particles) w_R = 1, thus the absorbed dose and equivalent dose are equal (i.e., 1 Gy = 1 Sv). Adapted from 1990 Recommendations of the International Commission on Radiological Protection.[2]
†w_R = 1 for electrons of all energies except for Auger electrons emitted from nuclei bound to deoxyribonucleic acid (DNA) for which a higher quality factor may be used.
§High atomic number (Z) and high energy particles.

stable nuclides have a ratio of neutrons-to-protons (n/p) of ~1:1. As the atomic number increases, the neutron to proton ratio of stable nuclides increases to ~1.5:1. The additional neutrons (relative to the number of protons) provide the required nuclear strong force necessary to compensate for the increased electrostatic repulsion between the protons in the nucleus. Stable nuclei with the proper balance of nucleons fall on the so called "line of stability" when the atomic number (proton number) is plotted against the number of neutrons *(A–Z)* in the nucleus (Fig. 31-3). On either side of this line lie unstable or radioactive nuclides that have either too many or too few neutrons (relative to the number of protons), called "neutron rich" or "neutron poor," respectively.

Radioactive nuclei will spontaneously undergo nuclear transformation with the emission of energy (particulate emissions and/or EMR) to achieve a lower (more stable) nuclear energy state. This process of spontaneous nuclear transformation is referred to *radionuclide decay, nuclear disintegration or transformation,* and/or *radioactivity.* The radionuclide undergoing transformation is referred to as the *parent* nuclide and the transformed (more stable) nuclide is called the *daughter.* Although the daughter is more stable than its parent it may still be relatively unstable with respect to its ground state and also be radioactive. Successive transformations will occur in a so-called *decay chain,* possibly yielding several radioactive *progeny,* until a stable nuclide is reached. There are many naturally occurring radioactive nuclides, such as radon-222 (^{222}Ra), that are continually being produced from decay chains in which the parent, such as uranium-238 (^{238}U), at the beginning of the series has a physical half-life comparable to the age of the earth (4.5 billion years). The ^{238}U decay series is shown in Fig. 31-4.

The quantity of radioactive material expressed as the number of radioactive atoms undergoing nuclear transformation per unit time is called *activity.* The traditional unit of activity is the *curie* (Ci), which is defined as 3.7×10^{10} disintegrations per second (dps), the decay rate of 1 g of pure radium-226 (^{226}Ra). Although the curie is still the most commonly used unit of activity in the United States, the majority of the world's scientific literature has converted to the newer Systeme International (SI). The SI unit for activity is the *becquerel* (Bq), named for Henri Becquerel, who discovered radioactivity in 1896. The becquerel is defined as one dps. Since a curie is a large quantity of activity, metric prefixes are typically used to refer to smaller quantities that are commonly encountered in laboratory and environmental settings. The most commonly encountered prefixes and their symbol and equivalence in Bq are given in Table 31-3.

Nuclear transformation is a random process, thus it is not possible to predict from moment to moment which radioactive atoms will decay. However, observation of a large number of radioactive atoms over a period of time allows the average rate of nuclear transformation to be established.

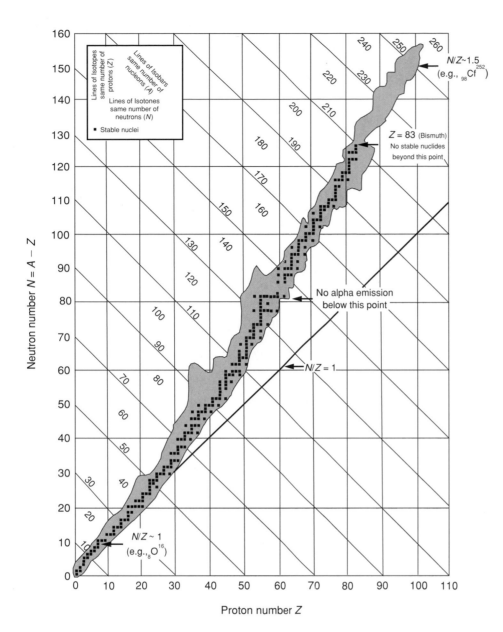

Fig. 31-3. Nuclide line of stability. The shaded area represents the range of known nuclides. The stable nuclides are indicated by small black squares, whereas all other locations in the shaded area represent radioactive (i.e., unstable) nuclides. Note that all nuclides with $Z > 83$ are radioactive.

This average rate is expressed mathematically as the *decay constant* (λ), which is the fraction of the number of radioactive atoms remaining in a sample that decay per unit time. The number of radioactive atoms *(N)* remaining in a sample after a period of time *(t)* can be easily calculated from the relationship

$$N_t = N_0 e^{-\lambda t} \qquad (3)$$

where N_0 is the initial number of radioactive atom in the sample. Another useful relationship related to the decay constant is the physical *half-life* ($T_{p_{1/2}}$). The half-life is defined as the time required for one half of the radioactive atoms in a sample to decay. After one half-life the number of radioactive atoms in a given sample has been reduced by one half. After two half-lives the number of radioactive atoms has been reduced to one fourth ($\frac{1}{2} \times \frac{1}{2} = \frac{1}{4}$), and

so on. The decay constant and physical half-life are unique to each radionuclide and are related as follows

$$\lambda = (\ln_e 2)/T_{p_{1/2}} = 0.693/T_{p_{1/2}} \qquad (4)$$

Physical half-lives are immutable constants that, depending on the radionuclide, range from a fraction of a second to billions of years. A useful rule is that after 10 half-lives the quantity of radioactivity has been reduced to $\sim 1/1000$ of its original amount; after 20 half-lives the amount is reduced by $\sim 1/1,000,000$.

A related and directly analogous term is the *biologic half-life* ($T_{b_{1/2}}$), defined as the time required for one-half of a given quantity of radioactivity to be eliminated from the body or from a specified organ of the body via physiologic processes. Although independent of the physical half-life, the biologic half-life is dependent upon the chemical form

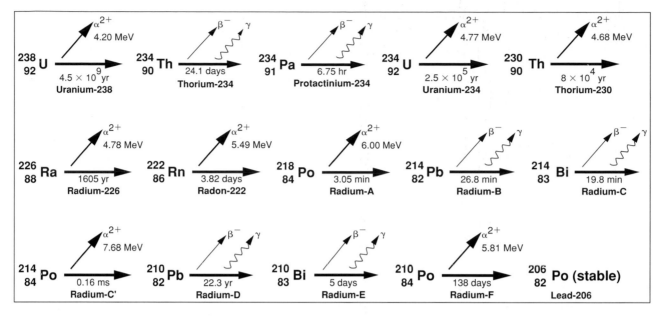

Fig. 31-4. Schematic representation of the uranium-238 natural decay series.

Table 31-3. Units and prefixes associated with various quantities of radioactivity

System	Quantity	Symbol	dps (Bq)	dpm
Traditional	Curie	Ci	3.7×10^{10}	2.22×10^{12}
	Millicurie	mCi (10^{-3} Ci)	3.7×10^{7}	2.22×10^{9}
	Microcurie	μCi (10^{-6} Ci)	3.7×10^{4}	2.22×10^{6}
	Nanocurie	nCi (10^{-9} Ci)	3.7×10^{1}	2.22×10^{3}
	Picocurie	pCi (10^{-12} Ci)	3.7×10^{-2}	2.22
SI	Becquerel	Bq	1	60
	Millibecquerel	mBq (10^{-3} Bq)	10^{-3}	6×10^{-2}
	Kilobecquerel	kBq (10^{3} Bq)	10^{3}	6×10^{4}
	Megabecquerel	MBq (10^{6} Bq)	10^{6}	6×10^{7}
	Gigabecquerel	GBq (10^{9} Bq)	10^{9}	6×10^{10}

dpm, Disintegration per minute; *dps,* disintegration per second; *SI,* Systeme International.

of the radionuclide, route of entry into the body, and various metabolic processes. This concept will be discussed in greater depth as it relates to the metabolic pathways of radionuclides deposited in the lung. The combination of the physical and biologic half-lives results in an *effective half-life* ($T_{e_{1/2}}$), which is related to $T_{p_{1/2}}$ and $T_{b_{1/2}}$ as follows:

$$\frac{1}{T_{e_{1/2}}} = \frac{1}{T_{p_{1/2}}} + \frac{1}{T_{b_{1/2}}} \tag{5}$$

If either $T_{p_{1/2}}$ or $T_{b_{1/2}}$ is substantially different from one another the smaller one will effectively predominate in the elimination of the radioactivity.

Modes of radioactive decay. Most radionuclides of interest to occupational medicine decay in one or more of the following ways: α emission, β (β^{-}) emission, positron (β^{+}) emission, electron capture, or isomeric transition.[1]

α *decay.* α decay typically occurs with heavy radionu-

clides ($A > 150$) and is often followed by the emission γ-rays and characteristic x-rays. αs are emitted at fixed, discrete energies (in the range of 4 to 8 MeV) that are a specific characteristic of a given decay scheme. For example, the α particles from ^{222}Rn are all emitted with a kinetic energy of 5.49 MeV. This kinetic energy, together with the mass–energy equivalence of the α particle itself, represents a significant decrease in the daughter's energy relative to the parent. α decay can be generalized in the following way:

$$_{Z}^{A}X \rightarrow _{Z-2}^{A-4}Y + _{2}^{4}He^{2+}(\text{alpha particle}) + \text{energy} \tag{6}$$

Example:

$$_{86}^{222}Rn \rightarrow _{82}^{214}Pb + _{2}^{4}He^{2+} + 5.59 \text{ MeV} \tag{7}$$

^{222}Rn is a radioactive noble gas in the uranium-238 (^{238}U) decay chain (Fig. 31-4) that decays with a half-life of 3.8

days to polonium-218 (^{218}Po), followed by several other α and β decays, eventually leading to stable lead-206 (^{206}Pb). ^{222}Ra and its decay products are the most significant sources of exposure to naturally occurring radionuclides. The risks of radon exposure are discussed in detail later in this chapter.

β decay. β^- decay typically occurs with radionuclides that occupy the "neutron-rich" side of the line of stability, such as radionuclides produced as the result of nuclear fission (i.e., fission products). In β decay an energetic electron and an *anti-neutrino* ($\acute{\upsilon}$) are emitted from the nucleus producing a daughter nuclide with one less neutron and one more proton. One way to think of this transformation is as the conversion of a neutron to a proton with the emission of the β particle. The anti-neutrino is an ultralight, uncharged subnuclear particle that carries away a portion of the kinetic energy associated with the β decay. On average, the distribution of kinetic energy between the β^- and the anti-neutrino is 1/3 and 2/3, respectively. However, unlike α decay in which the kinetic energy of the emitted particle was fixed, the kinetic energy of β particles spans from zero to a maximum, which is characteristic of a particular radionuclide's decay scheme. The result is a nuclide with the same mass number, A (referred to as an isobaric transition), and a lower n/p ratio closer to the line of stability. β decay can be generalized in the following way:

$$^A_Z X \rightarrow ^A_{Z+1} Y + \beta^- + \acute{\upsilon} + \text{energy} \qquad (8)$$

Example:

$$^{32}_{15} P \rightarrow ^{32}_{16} S + \beta^- + \acute{\upsilon} + 1.7 \text{ MeV} \qquad (9)$$

The β^- particles will be emitted with a spectrum of energies ranging from zero to a maximum of 1.71 MeV (E_{max}) and an average energy (E_{avg}) of $\sim 1/3$ E_{max}.

Positron decay. Positron (β^+) decay is opposite of, but in some ways similar to β decay. β decay typically occurs with radionuclides that are "neutron deficient" (i.e., have low n/p ratios). The decay sequence results in the emission of a positron and a *neutrino* (υ) with kinetic energy that is shared between the positron and the neutrino in a fashion analogous to β decay. The net result is a daughter nuclide with one additional neutron, one less proton, thus keeping the same atomic mass number, A (isobaric), and a higher n/p ratio closer to the line of stability. Positron decay can be generalized in the following way:

$$^A_Z X \rightarrow ^A_{Z-1} Y + \beta^+ + \upsilon + \text{energy} \qquad (10)$$

Example:

$$^{18}_9 F \rightarrow ^{18}_8 O + \beta^+ + \upsilon + 0.635 \text{ MeV (kinetic energy}$$
$$\text{followed by 1.022 MeV annihilation radiation)}$$
$$\qquad (11)$$

The β^+ particles will be emitted with a spectrum of energies from zero to E_{max} and an average energy equal to $\sim 1/3$ E_{max} in a manner that is directly analogous to β decay. However, the fate of the positron is substantially different from that of the β, resulting in annihilation radiation, as described above.

Electron capture decay. The classic Bohr model of the atom describes electrons in fixed discrete orbits about a dense positively charged nucleus. However, in the quantum-mechanical model of the atom the position of orbital electrons is best described by a probability density function in which there is a finite probability that, at any moment in time, an orbital electron may be found at a specified location in the atom, even near the nucleus. Electron capture decay, as the name implies, occurs when the nucleus captures an orbital electron. The net result of this process is similar to, and in fact competes with, positron decay by producing a daughter nuclide with one additional neutron, one less proton, and an increase in the n/p ratio bringing it closer to the line of stability. The excess energy is emitted as a γ-ray or transferred by a process called internal conversion to another orbital electron (e^-) that is energetically ejected from the atom. Electron capture decay can be generalized in the following way:

$$^A_Z X + e^- \rightarrow ^A_{Z-1} Y + \gamma \text{ and/or } e^- + \text{energy} \qquad (12)$$

Example:

$$^{111}_{49} In \rightarrow ^{111}_{48} Cd + \gamma \text{ and/or } e^- + 1.1 \text{ MeV} \qquad (13)$$

Isomeric transition. During other types of radioactive decay a daughter is often formed in an excited (i.e., excess energy) state. γ-rays are emitted as the daughter nucleus undergoes an internal rearrangement and transitions from the excited state to a lower energy state. This process is referred to as *isomeric transition* as there is no change in atomic number, mass number, or neutron number and occurs between two energy states. Often, in place of γ-rays, energy may be internally converted and transferred to an orbital electron within the same atom. The electron (e^-) is subsequently ejected with a kinetic energy equal to the available energy minus the electron's binding energy. These *internal conversion electrons* have radiobiologic significance because they are typically of higher energy than Auger electrons and result in a higher local radiation dose than would have resulted from simple γ-ray emission.

Once created, most excited states transition nearly instantaneously to a lower energy state with the simultaneous emission of a γ-ray. In some cases the excited state persists for longer periods of time with half-lives that range from $\sim 10^{-12}$ seconds to more than 100 years. These excited states are called *metastable* or isomeric states and are denoted by the letter m after the atomic mass number (e.g.,

Technetium-99m [^{99m}Tc]). Decay by isomeric transition can be generalized in the following way:

$$^{Am}_Z X \rightarrow {}^A_Z X + \gamma \text{ and/or } e^- + \text{energy} \qquad (14)$$

Example:

$$^{99m}_{43} Tc \rightarrow {}^{99}_{43} Tc + \gamma \text{ and/or } e^- + 142 \text{ keV} \qquad (15)$$

^{99m}Tc is the primary radionuclide used in diagnostic nuclear medicine because of its relatively short half-life (6.02 hours), ideal photon energies for external imaging, and the relatively few particulate emissions associated with its decay.

Radiation exposure and dose

Radiation exposure. The term *radiation exposure,* although often used in a very general way, has a very precise meaning when used in reference to radiation fields. Exposure, measured in traditional units of *roentgens* (R), is defined as the quantity of x- or γ-radiation required to liberate 2.58×10^{-4} coulombs of charge per kilogram (C/kg) of air at standard temperature and pressure. The roentgen is named in honor of Wilhelm Conrad Röentgen, the german physicist who discovered x-rays in 1895. The SI unit for exposure is expressed directly in its base units of C/kg. The application of the term exposure is somewhat limited in that it is defined only for ionization of air associated with electromagnetic radiation. Nonetheless, exposure is a useful quantity to describe the intensity of a ionizing EMR field and many radiation survey instruments are designed and calibrated to measure radiation fields in units of exposure. Radiation fields are often expressed as an exposure rate (R/hr or mR/min).

Absorbed dose. Although it is useful to be able to measure a radiation field in terms of its ability to ionize air, the potential biologic damage will result from the energy that is actually absorbed in tissue. This quantity is expressed as the *absorbed dose (D),* defined as the energy deposited by ionizing radiation (photons and particulate) per unit mass (of any substance). The traditional unit for absorbed dose is the rad, an acronym for "*rad*iation *a*bsorbed *d*ose." One rad is equal to the 0.01 Joule *(J)* deposited per kilogram of any material. The SI unit for absorbed dose is the *gray (Gy),* which is equal to 1 J/kg, thus, 100 rads equals 1 Gy.[2,3]

Equivalent dose. Some types of radiations have a greater potential to produce biologic damage per unit dose than others. As discussed previously, high LET radiation produces a more intense ionization track than low LET radiation. The *equivalent dose* weights the absorbed dose using a *radiation weighting factor* (w_R) to account for this difference. The absorbed dose *(D)* in Gy is multiplied by the appropriate radiation weighting factors to obtain the

equivalent dose *(H).* The SI unit for equivalent dose is the *sievert (Sv).* Thus

$$H(Sv) = D(Gy) \times w_R \qquad (16)$$

Values for w_R recommended by the International Commission on Radiological Protection[2] (ICRP) for commonly encountered types of radiation together with their associated LET are listed in Table 31-2. The traditional unit for equivalent dose (often referred to as dose equivalent) is the *rem,* an acronym for "*r*oentgen *e*quivalent in *m*an" (or mammals). In this case the radiation weighting factor is replaced by the traditional term, the *quality factor (Q),* which is also specific for different types of radiations and multiplied by the rad to yield rems (rem = rad × Q). There are 100 rem in 1 Sv. The quality factor *(Q)* and the radiation weighting factor (w_R) are essentially equivalent.[2]

Effective dose. Just as the intensity of the ionization track depends upon the LET of the radiation, the risk of a given exposure is also dependent upon the relative radiosensitivity of the tissue being irradiated. In addition, there is a need to be able to assign a risk from an exposure that involves partial body or selective organ exposure rather than total body irradiation. In 1990 the ICRP established tissue-specific *organ weighting factors* (w_T), which, when multiplied by the equivalent dose, incorporate an estimate of the relative radiosensitivity (for radiogenic cancer induction and genetic effects) of the tissue being irradiated. These weighting factors are an attempt to assign specific risk factors for organs in which there is sufficient radiobiologic data to support such an assessment. When the equivalent dose for each organ irradiated is multiplied by its appropriate weighting factors and summed over all organs exposed the result is called the *effective dose* (H_E) expressed as

$$H_E = \Sigma w_T \times H_T(Sv) \qquad (17)$$

The effective dose is expressed in units of sieverts (Sv) or, in traditional units, rem. The organ dose weighting factors adopted by the ICRP-60[2] are shown in Table 31-4. Before 1990, the ICRP had established different w_T values that, when applied as shown above, were referred to as the *effective dose equivalent.* Many regulatory agencies, including the U.S. Nuclear Regulatory Commission (NRC), have not as yet adopted the ICRP report 60 w_T values and are currently using earlier estimates[3] of w_T in their regulations. The organ weighting factor for the whole lung is 0.12, of which a factor of 0.08 is assigned to the bronchial epithelium and 0.04 is assigned to the rest of the lung tissue. This means that if radiation-induced cancer occurs following whole-body exposure to ionizing radiation, there is expected to be a 12% chance that radiation-induced neoplasm will occur in the lung and an 8% chance that it will occur in cells of the bronchial epithelium.

The traditional units of the roentgen, rad, rem, and curie are still in common use in the United States. However, virtually all published scientific literature and the majority of the world's scientific community have switched over to the SI system of units. These traditional units and their SI equivalents are summarized in Table 31-5.

Sources of exposure to ionizing radiation

Exposure to ionizing radiation is an inevitable consequence of life on earth. There are naturally occurring

Table 31-4. Organ dose weighting factors (w_T) assigned by the International Commission on Radiological Protection (ICRP-60)

Tissue organ	w_T
Gonads	0.20
Stomach	0.12
Colon	0.12
Lung (bronchial epithelium)	0.12(0.08)
Red bone marrow	0.12
Breast	0.05
Esophagus	0.05
Bladder	0.05
Liver	0.05
Thyroid	0.05
Bone surfaces	0.01
Skin	0.01*
Remainder	0.05

Adapted from 1990 Recommendations of the International Commission on Radiological Protection.[2]

*Applied to the mean equivalent dose over the entire skin.

sources of radiation and radioactivity that have existed on the planet since its formation. In addition, there are technology enhanced sources that also add to the total dose received. The average per capita effective dose in the United States (from all sources exclusive of smoking) is ~3.6 millisieverts (mSv) (360 mrem) per year.[4] Approximately 80% of this exposure, ~3 mSv (300 mrem), is from naturally occurring (or "background") sources, whereas 20%, 0.6 mSv (60 mrem), is from technologic enhancements of naturally occurring sources and radiation-producing machines, the vast majority of which are diagnostic x-ray procedures (Fig. 31-5). It is important to remember that these "averages" apply to the population as a whole, and thus the dose to a particular individual will depend on a variety of specific exposure factors that are discussed in greater detail below.

Naturally occurring radiation sources. Naturally occurring radiation sources include *cosmic rays, cosmogenic radionuclides,* and *primordial radionuclides* and their decay products. Details about these radiation sources can be found in National Committee on Radiation Protection and Measurement (NCRP) Report No. 94.[5]

Cosmic rays consist primarily of extremely high energy (mean energy ~10 billion eV) particulate radiation (primarily protons) and high energy γ-rays. When the particulate radiations collide with the earth's atmosphere a shower of "secondary" radiations is produced, which includes high-energy electrons and photons. The average per capita dose from cosmic radiation is 0.27 mSv (27 mrem) per year or ~7% of natural background. Exposure to cosmic radiation increases with altitude as there is less atmosphere to absorb

Table 31-5. Radiologic quantities: the Systems International units and equivalents in traditional units

Radiation quantity (customary term)	Description of quantity	Traditional unit (abbreviation)	SI unit (abbreviation)	Symbol	Equivalent relationships among quantities
Exposure	Amount of ionization per unit mass of air due to x-rays and γ-rays	Roentgen (R)	coulombs/kg (C/kg air)	X	$1\ R = 2.58 \times 10^{-4}$ C/kg air
Absorbed dose	Amount of energy imported by radiation to a unit mass	Radiation absorbed dose (rad)	gray (Gy)	D	1 rad = 10 mGy 100 rad = 1 Gy 1 J/kg = 1 Gy
Equivalent dose (dose equivalent)	A measure of radiation-specific biologic damage in man	Radiation equivalent in man (rem)	sievert (Sv)	H	H (Sv) = $w_R \times D$ (Gy) H (rem) = $Q \times D$ (rad) 1 rem = 10 mSv 100 rem = 1 Sv
Effective dose (effective dose equivalent)	A measure of radiation and organ system-specific damage in man	Radiation equivalent in man (rem)	sievert (Sv)	H_E	H_E (Sv) = $\sum_T w_T H_T$ (Sv) H_E (rem) = $\sum_T w_T H_T$ (rem)
Activity	Amount of radioactive material expressed as the nuclear transformation rate	curie (Ci)	becquerel (Bq)	A	$1\ Ci = 3.7 \times 10^{10}$ Bq 1 Bq = 1 sec^{-1} (dps) 37 mBq = 1 pCi 37 kBq = 1 μCi 37 MBq = 1 mCi 37 GBq = 1 Ci

SI, Systeme International.

the radiation, so populations at high elevations receive higher cosmic doses. For example, people living in Leadville, Colorado, at 3,200 m above sea level receive ~1.25 mSv/yr (125 mrem/yr) or five times the average exposure at sea level.

A fraction of the secondary particulate cosmic radiation collides with stable atmospheric nuclei making them radioactive. These cosmogenic radionuclides contribute very little [~0.004 mSv/yr (0.4 mrem/yr) or less than 1%] to natural background radiation. The majority of this component of natural background is from the formation of carbon-14 (^{14}C) and tritium (^{3}H).

Terrestrial radioactive material that has been present on earth since its formation is called primordial radionuclides. Population exposure from primordial radionuclides comes from external exposure, inhalation, and incorporation of radionuclides into the body. The decay chains of uranium-238 (^{238}U), $T_{p_{1/2}} = 4.5 \times 10^9$ years (uranium series) and thorium-232 (^{232}Th), $T_{p_{1/2}} = 1.4 \times 10^{10}$ years (thorium series), produce several dozen radionuclides that together with potassium-40 (^{40}K), $T_{p_{1/2}} = 1.3 \times 10^9$ years are responsible for the majority of the external terrestrial average equivalent dose rate of 0.28 mSv/yr (28 mrem/yr) or ~9% of natural background. Some regions of the country with high concentration of primordial radionuclides produce equivalent dose rates as high as 25 mSv/yr (2,500 mrem/yr).

Radon-222 (^{222}Rn) and its decay products, which are constituents of the ^{238}U decay series (Fig. 31-4), are the most significant source of natural background radiation exposure. Once inhaled, the majority of the dose is deposited in the tracheobronchial region by its short lived daughters rather than by ^{222}Rn itself. Radon concentrations in the environment vary widely due to differences in ^{238}U concen-

tration in the soil and differences in ventilation and construction of buildings. All other factors being equal, buildings with less ventilation will tend to have higher radon concentrations and, thus, higher level of background radiation exposure.

Exposure to ^{222}Rn in the United States results in an average equivalent dose to the bronchial epithelium of 24 mSv/yr (2.4 rem/yr).[6] A tissue w_T of 0.08 for the bronchial epithelium (Table 31-4) yields an effective dose rate of ~2 mSv/yr (200 mrem/yr) or ~68% of natural background. The average indoor air concentration of ^{222}Rn in the United States is ~55 Bq/m^3 (1.5 pCi/L). However, levels can exceed 2.75 kBq/m^3 (75 pCi/L) in poorly ventilated buildings with high concentrations of ^{238}U in the soil. The point at which remediation is recommended to reduce ^{222}Rn levels remains controversial. For example, the U.S. Environmental Protection Agency (EPA)[7] and NCRP[8] have set different action levels beyond which they recommend reducing ^{222}Rn concentrations; they are 147 and 294 Bq/m^3 (4 and 8 pCi/L), respectively.

The second largest source of natural background radiation exposure comes from the ingestion of food and water that contain primordial radionuclides (and their decay products) of which potassium-40 (^{40}K) is the most significant. Altogether this pathway is responsible for an average effective dose rate of 0.4 mSv/yr (40 mrem/yr), or ~13% of natural background.

Technology-based radiation exposure. The most significant source of exposure to technology based (or "manmade") radiation sources in the United States is from medical diagnosis and therapy.[9] Diagnostic x-ray and nuclear medicine examinations account for ~0.39 mSv/yr (39 mrem/yr) and 0.14 mSv/yr (14 mrem/yr), respectively. Ra-

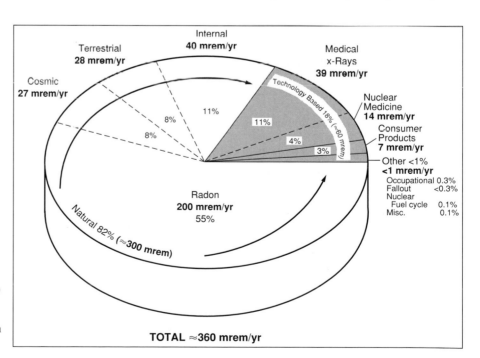

Fig. 31-5. The percentage contribution of various radiation sources to the total average effective dose equivalent (360 mrem/yr) in the U.S. population. Divide mrem/yr by 100 to obtain mSv/yr. (Adapted from the National Committee on Radiation Protection and Measurement.[4])

diation therapy, while delivering a significantly larger dose per patient, exposes many fewer patients. Thus, it does not significantly contribute to the average dose, which is calculated based on the total U.S. population.

Population exposure also occurs from enhanced natural sources such as radon dissolved in domestic water supplies, building materials like granite, brick, and concrete that contain higher concentrations of primordial radionuclides, and their decay products (e.g., uranium, thorium, and potassium) than would be found in other materials like wood. These and others sources typically referred to as "consumer products" may account for as much as 0.07 mSv/yr (7 mrem/yr).[10]

Other sources, such as fallout from nuclear weapons testing, operation of nuclear power facilities, and occupational exposures, although in some cases have received a lot of attention by the media, in fact contribute very little (<1%) to population background exposure.[11]

Inhalation toxicology and radionuclide dosimetry

Inhalation and particle deposition.   The risk associated with the deposition in the respiratory tract of inhaled radioactive airborne particles depends upon the pattern of deposition and subsequent cellular irradiation. Initial deposition depends on anatomic and physiologic factors as well as on particle size distribution (considering both aerodynamic and diffusive behavior of airborne particles within the respiratory airways). Cellular irradiation depends upon the pattern of deposition, type of radiation emitted by the particles and their radioactivity (mass and specific activity), rate of decay of the radionuclides involved (half-lives), and retention and redistribution of radioactive material within the lung with time after deposition. These are affected by the elemental and radiologic characteristics of a radionuclide, the chemical form, and the numbers, sizes, and distribution of particles in the lung.[12,13]

The behavior of inhaled airborne particles in the respiratory airways and their alternative fates of either deposition in the various airway regions (nasopharyngeal airways, mouth, oral pharynx, larynx, tracheobronchial airways, respiratory bronchioles, and pulmonary parenchyma) or exhalation depend upon the aerodynamic and diffusive behavior of the airborne particles and upon physiologic and anatomic factors. Particle aerodynamic behavior depends on particle physical density, shape, size distribution, electrostatic charge, and hygroscopicity or deliquescence. The diffusive behavior favors smaller particles that readily undergo Brownian motion. Physiologic factors include breathing patterns, breathing rate, tidal volume (TV), functional residual capacity (FRC), air flow dynamics in the airways, and variations in relative humidity and temperature within the respiratory tract. The exact anatomy of the airways from nose or mouth to the lung parenchyma including the diameters, lengths, and branching angles of airway segments also influences airborne particles particle deposition.[13,14]

The collection in the respiratory tract of inhaled airborne particles and the initial regional pattern of these collected particles is called deposition. Inhaled particles that pass the head airways region (HAR) of the respiratory tract during inhalation may deposit in the tracheobronchial region (TBR) or the gas exchange region (GER) of the lung. The magnitude of this deposition will depend upon aerodynamic and diffusive particle sizes, respiratory mechanics, and anatomic relationships. Of particular importance is the deposition of particles associated with inhalation via the mouth rather than the nose, since the deposition of particles in the deep lung is enhanced for particles in the aerodynamic diameter range from 1 to 10 μm. The deposition of inhaled airborne particles in the nasopharyngeal region during nasal breathing is much higher for all sizes than the deposition that occurs in the oropharyngeal head airways during mouth breathing. Specifically, larger particles that normally are collected in the nasopharyngeal portion of the head airways during breathing via the nose may pass the epiglottis and larynx and deposit in the lung during breathing via the mouth.[14,15]

The five principal physical mechanisms that may lead to the deposition of inhaled particles in the respiratory tract include electrostatic attraction, physical interception, inertial impaction, gravitational settling, and Brownian motion (diffusion). All particles that come in contact with the moist wall of the airways are deposited. Most airborne particles are electrostatically charged by the airborne particles generation processes, and these charged particles may be attracted to the wall of the airway by the image-charge effect. However, the overall influence of charge on the deposition of most airborne particles is probably small. Likewise, the noninertial incidental contact of a particle with the wall of the airways leads to deposition by interception, but this process is most important for elongated particle shapes such as fibrous airborne particles. The most important physical processes associated with inhalation deposition of radioactive airborne particles are impaction, gravitational settling, and Brownian diffusion. In each of these deposition processes, the simple physical contact of small airborne particles with the surface of the respiratory airways leads to irreversible sticking and removal from the airstream (deposition).[13]

Deposition by gravitational settling occurs throughout the respiratory tract due to the influence of the earth's gravity on small particles suspended in air. The settling rate of small particles increases proportionally to the square of the aerodynamic diameter. Gravitational deposition is especially important in the distal regions of the bronchial airways and in portions of the gas exchange region.

Inertial impaction is the dominant mechanism of deposition of particles larger than 3 μm in aerodynamic diameter, which occurs primarily in the head airways or tracheobronchial airway regions. In this process the airborne particles, because of their inertia, do not follow changes in direction or speed of air streamlines and they may collide with the wall of the airway. For example, if air is directed toward an airway surface (such as a branch carina) but the forward velocity is suddenly reduced because of the change in flow direction caused by the obstruction of the surface, inertial momentum may carry larger particles across the air streamlines and collide with the moist surface of the tract where they are deposited. Aerodynamic separation of this type may be characterized in terms of the average inspiratory flow rate and the square of the aerodynamic diameter.

Unlike impaction and settling that increase with increasing particle size, deposition by Brownian diffusion increases with decreasing size and depends on the diffusive diameter (related to the physical diameter of a sphere) rather than the aerodynamic diameter. The diffusive diameter is sometimes called the thermodynamic diameter since it depends upon the thermal molecular energy of the air molecules. Diffusional deposition in the gas exchange region of the lung is the predominant collection mechanism for particles smaller than 0.5 μm physical diameter. Deposition by diffusion can also occur in the nose, mouth, and pharyngeal airways for very small particles (primarily those smaller than 0.01 μm).[16]

Utilizing the specific details of these controlling factors, theoretical models of regional deposition have been developed to predict the fate of inhaled particles of various types. Carefully collected data from experiments with human volunteers provide the basis for verifying these predictions.[17,18] Overall, inhalable airborne particles consist primarily of particles or droplets smaller than about 10 μm in aerodynamic equivalent diameter since larger particles deposit primarily in the head airways if breathed.

Even with carefully developed theoretical models and with the support of reliable deposition data, it is not possible to predict exactly the quantitative regional deposition of particles of a given inhaled airborne particles in a particular person. Considerable variability in respiratory parameters may occur among individuals in the population,

particularly when healthy adults are contrasted with children, or women are contrasted with men. Biologic variability between individuals, differences in health, confounding factors such as cigarette smoking, differences that relate to age or breathing styles, as well as inherent differences in airway sizes can cause differences in the fraction of inhaled airborne particles that may deposit in the airways and in the quantity of particulate mass that is actually breathed. However, for the purposes of radiation and occupational safety, reasonable predictions must be made using the available models and data employing certain simplifying assumptions concerning biologic factors.

The most widely used models of regional deposition and lung dosimetry versus particle size for radioactive particles have been developed by the International Commission on Radiological Protection.[19-21] These models use representative values for normal respiratory parameters described as "reference man."[22] Assumed values for a typical adult include a body weight of 70 kg, height of 175 cm, and body surface area of 1.8 m². For typical deposition calculations particles are assumed to be insoluble, stable, and spherical with physical densities of 1 g/cm³. The inhalation deposition of particles of different size during nasal inhalation at 15 breaths per minute (BPM) with a TV of 1450 ml is represented in Fig. 31-6 based upon the results of Morrow et al.[19] with the addition of the diffusive deposition of small particles as predicted by Cheng et al.[16]

The inhalation of deliquescent or hygroscopic radioactive airborne particles will alter the deposition characteristics since these particles will tend to grow rapidly in size in the humid environment of the respiratory tract.

Dosimetry. If the irradiation of the lung occurs from external penetrating radiation as from x-rays or γ-rays, the dosimetry depends upon quantitative evaluation of the exposure conditions and estimation of the absorbed dose. The lung irradiation ends when the external exposure ends. On the other hand, if radioactive airborne particles are inhaled that deposit in the lung, the irradiation of the lung begins

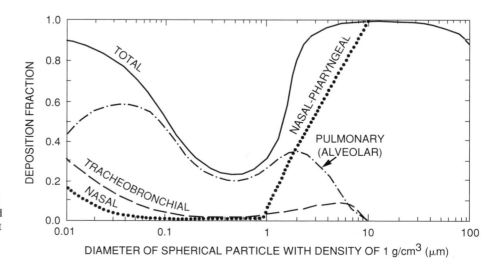

Fig. 31-6. Plot of estimated deposition fraction versus particle size for airborne particles of physical density 1 g/cm³ (the aerodynamic equivalent diameter) inhaled via the nose by a representative person at rest breathing at a rate of 15 breaths per minute with a tidal volume of 750 ml.

with that exposure and continues for as long as the radioactive materials remain in the lung tissue. After initial deposition of particles associated with inhaled airborne particles, these particles are subjected to various biologic, physical, and chemical processes including dissolution into body fluids with absorption by the blood, uptake by cells by phagocytosis or pinocytosis, and movement with mucus and body fluids. The term clearance is used to describe the translocation, transformation, and removal of deposited particles from the various regions of the respiratory tract. The temporal distribution of uncleared deposited particles or their resultant transformation products is called retention.[13,14] The irradiation of the lung and other tissues occurs during the retention of deposited particles as the radioactive nuclei decay and emit ionizing radiation. This irradiation may be protracted if the physical half-life ($T_{p_{1/2}}$) of the radionuclides is long and if the biologic retention half-time ($T_{b_{1/2}}$) is also long.[12]

Airborne radioactive particles may consist of droplets and/or water-soluble components that will readily dissolve in body fluids soon after deposition. Ultimate clearance of dissolved materials will be via the systemic circulation with transfer to and irradiation of other organs of the body. Relatively insoluble particles deposited in the ciliated region of the tracheobronchial airways are moved with mucus flow toward the epiglottis where they are swallowed or expectorated. This process is relatively efficient in that most particles deposited in the TBR are probably cleared within a few hours to 1 day postexposure. A few percent of the insoluble particles that deposit in the bronchial airways may lodge on tissue surfaces rather than joining the mucus clearance flow. More protracted irradiation would be associated with particles exhibiting delayed clearance from the bronchial airways.[12]

Insoluble particles deposited in the nonciliated bronchioles or the alveoli of the GER are not rapidly cleared from the lung. Most are engulfed by and phagocytized by scavenger pulmonary alveolar macrophage cells recruited in the GER, and some of these cells may ultimately enter the TBR mucous flow, but this does not seem to be a rapid process in human lungs and requires up to 3 years to effectively clear half of GER deposited insoluble particles. Some of the macrophages may enter the pulmonary lymph circulation and be transported to tracheobronchial lymph nodes, but this also is a slow process requiring up to 1 year for clearance of half of the deposited particles from the GER. In addition, many particles become trapped within the interstitial tissue of the lung. Consequently, very insoluble particles (e.g., particles of plutonium dioxide) are tenaciously retained in the GER. Consequently, clearance by dissolution becomes an important process even for sparingly soluble particles (e.g., fused aluminosilicate particles).[13]

In radiation dosimetry, the word dose refers specifically to the radiation absorbed dose to tissue measured in units of energy deposited per unit mass of tissue (Gy). Dosage refers to the amount of radioactive material (Bq) that enters the lung or is deposited. Content refers to the amount (Bq) retained in the lung after intake. Since the irradiation of the lung proceeds after inhalation deposition, a single brief exposure may initiate an extended period of chronic irradiation of the lung that depends in duration on radioactive half-life and lung retention of the deposited radioactive particles. Insoluble radioactive particles with long residence times in the lung chronically irradiate the lung for extended periods after inhalation exposure, and may also irradiate surrounding tissues. The controlling variable in the dose–response relationship is the tissue concentration of the radioactive material and the corresponding radiation dose per unit time to the cells. Dose rate, d, is proportional to tissue concentration.[12]

Cumulative absorbed dose, D, is derived from the time integral of concentration (or dose rate), and for protracted irradiation is correlated to elapsed time post intake; it can be calculated as the mathematical product $t\bar{d}$, where t is the elapsed time after intake and $\bar{d}$ is the time-weighted average dose rate. The effectiveness of radiation exposure per unit of dose may vary widely at different dose rates.

The dose to the whole lung from deposited radioactive particles can be computed from the reported lung content and retention information. The initial absorbed dose rate (Gy/day) averaged over the whole total lung for a single brief inhalation exposure is given by:

$$d_0 = 13.8 \; a_0 \bar{E}_r / m \tag{18}$$

where a_0 is the initial lung content (MBq), E_r is the average ionizing radiation energy (MeV) deposited in lung tissue per radioactive disintegration, m is the mass (g) of the lung including associated circulating blood, and 13.8 is a constant correcting the dimensional units. For reference man, the adult lung mass with the normal complement of circulating blood is estimated as 1,000 g or 1.4% of the body weight. The time-weighted average dose rate from exposure to any given post-exposure time is calculated by

$$\bar{d} = d_0 \left(\int_0^{t_r} R(\theta)\delta\theta \right)/t_r = d_0(1 - e^{-\lambda t_r})/\lambda t_r \tag{19}$$

where $R(\theta)$ is the lung retention function, t_r is the elapsed retention time, and θ the surrogate time variable; the right side of Eq. (19) is the expression used for a single component exponential retention function with effective clearance constant, λ, given by ln 2 divided by the effective half-time of retention in the lung.[23]

Occupational exposure standards

The standards for exposure of the lung to ionizing radiation have been developed primarily from analysis of lung cancer incidence in the Japanese atomic bomb survivors.[6] In those cases exposure of the lung and the rest of the body to penetrating γ-radiation and neutrons occurred almost instantaneously following the atomic bomb detonation. Those individuals that received doses significantly greater than 5 Sv probably did not survive the blast, heat, or acute radiation effects. Among the survivors, lung cancer incidence was slightly elevated later in the lives of the exposed individuals. Linear risk models with a lifetime risk for lung cancer of about 4.8×10^{-3}/Sv (4.8×10^{-5}/rem) represent these observations after a correction for lower dose rates.[2] For external exposure to γ-radiation, lung cancer represents about 12% of whole-body lifetime cancer risk. For this reason it has been assigned a tissue weighting factor of $w_T = 0.12$ in calculation of the cancer effective dose for cancer induction (Table 31-4). Two thirds of this risk has been assigned to the cells of the bronchial epithelium, which are the site of many lung cancers that occur in people.

Federal and State occupational exposure standards for radiation exposure of the lung in the nuclear industry are based upon the recommendations of the NCRP and of the ICRP. Earlier standards allowed an annual dose of 15 rem/yr for each year of a 50-year work career based upon a calculated limit of 1.5 rad/yr for α irradiation with $Q = 10$.[24] A Q (or w_R) of 20 is now recommended for α radiation, so that the old standard becomes 30 rem/yr. The newer recommendations based upon risk calculations allow an effective committed dose of 0.05 Sv/yr, which for the whole lung with $w_T = 0.12$ yields 0.05 Sv/yr ÷ 0.12 = 0.42 Sv/yr = 42 rem/yr. From these basic standards the annual limit of intake (ALI) and the derived air concentration (DAC) limit for the workplace can be calculated for soluble and insoluble forms of each radionuclide. Standards for exposure of the general public are normally set at 10% of those for nuclear workers.[3]

For the α radiation exposure of the bronchial epithelium from inhaled radon decay products, the current standard is based upon an exposure that is limited to 4 working level months (WLMs) (explained on page 550) per year.[25] An exposure of 4 WLM/yr yields an equivalent dose of 0.52 Sv/yr (52 rem/yr) to the lining cells of the bronchial epithelium. With $w_R = 0.08$ for the bronchial epithelium, the effective dose is 0.52 Sv/yr × 0.08 = 0.04 Sv/yr.

These exposure standards are intended to minimize the risk of development of lung cancer during a normal lifetime for radiation-induced lung cancer.[26] Nonneoplastic injury of the lung is not considered in these standards because much higher doses are required for nonneoplastic lung injury. The risks that are assigned above to radiation exposure are based upon a hypothetical linear dose–response model that applies at lower doses and dose rates than have been observed in occupational exposures. Analysis of protracted irradiation from internally deposited radionuclides clearly shows nonlinearity with lower than expected risks at lower doses. There are currently no documented cases of radiation-induced lung cancer in anyone whose radiation

exposure was *below the recommended standards,* even though hundreds of workers have been exposed to a variety of irradiations including α irradiation from inhaled plutonium dioxide. Almost all lung cancer in our society can be traced to cigarette smoke.[27]

Radon and progeny

All of the earth's atmosphere contains low concentrations of radioactive airborne particles and gases associated with various naturally occurring radionuclides. Of particular interest are radioactive isotopes of the inert gas, radon, formed in the earth's mantle by α decay of radium. Radium-226, a radioactive decay product of long-lived ^{238}U, occurs naturally in all the soils and rock on the surface of the earth at concentrations of about 40 Bq/kg (Fig. 31-4). Consequently, it is also naturally found in groundwater and the human body, usually in trace amounts (about 1 Bq per person). When ^{226}Ra undergoes radioactive decay (half-life 1600 years) it forms gaseous ^{222}Rn, which can percolate through and diffuse out of the soil or rock and into the air. This process has definite temporal limits since the half-life of ^{222}Rn is only about 3.8 days. However, enough radon reaches the earth's atmosphere to provide an average concentration of about 10 Bq/m^3 in outdoor air in the most populated parts of the world. Much lower concentrations occur over the oceans and in cold polar locations. The ^{222}Rn decays in air to radioactive, metallic (nongaseous) decay products that form radioactive aerosols having very small particle sizes. In addition to ^{226}Ra, small amounts of ^{224}Ra, a decay product of ^{232}Th, and ^{223}Ra, a decay product of ^{235}U, are also found on the earth leading to the atmospheric release of the radon gas isotopes, thoron, ^{220}Rn, and actinon, ^{219}Rn, respectively. However, the concentrations of airborne thoron and actinon, as well as their decay products, are usually negligible in comparison of the ^{222}Rn and its decay products.

As each ^{222}Rn gas atom in air decays by emitting α radiation it forms an atom of radioactive polonium, ^{218}Po (called radium-A, half-life about 3 minutes). This metallic atom quickly oxidizes and forms the center of a particulate molecular cluster of about 8 Å in diameter. When it decays emitting α radiation, a series of short-lived decay products is formed in air. These also form particulate clusters. This radon decay process is shown schematically in Fig. 31-4. The long-lived lead isotope ^{210}Pb (half-life 22.3 years) provides negligible radioactivity to the atmospheric aerosols and is, in effect, virtually nonradioactive compared to its short-lived progenitors. The radon progeny clusters represent the smallest airborne particles normally found in ambient air. In addition, these clusters attach upon contact to other, larger airborne particles to an extent that depends upon the concentration and sizes of these larger particles. Typically, more than 90% of airborne radon decay progeny are associated with particles smaller than 0.5 μm in aerodynamic diameter.[27a]

Upon inhalation, the airborne particles containing radon decay products will deposit upon contact onto the surfaces of the respiratory airways. Because of their diffusivity, the very small molecular clusters will tend to deposit in the head airways or in the trachea and bronchial airways of the lung.[28] Other somewhat larger particles may reach the alveolar region of the lung, as well. Because of their short radioactive half-lives, the deposited short-lived radon progeny quickly decay to ^{210}Pb before being cleared from the respiratory tract and irradiate the respiratory epithelium. Of primary concern in this regard is the irradiation of the bronchial epithelium by the highly ionizing alpha radiation emitted by radium-A (^{218}Po) and radium-C' (^{214}Po). Since radon itself is an inert gas, it is not appreciable absorbed into the respiratory airways during inhalation and is mostly exhaled. Occasionally an atom of radon gas may decay and emit α radiation in air present in the lung irradiating the epithelium, but the fraction of the dose contributed by the radon itself is small compared to that associated with the deposited decay product particles. Because naturally occurring radon decay products are found in ambient air both outdoors and within buildings, the lung is continually irradiated by α radiation. In fact, the lung is the most highly irradiated organ of the human body of a typical person from natural background radiation sources at about 24 mSv/yr.[6] Persons chronically exposed over extended periods of employment to high levels of airborne radon decay products such as are found in uranium mines have developed bronchiogenic carcinoma at incidence rates that significantly exceeded the expected rates in either smokers or nonsmokers. It has been suggested that some lung cancer cases among the general public are caused by lung irradiation from naturally occurring radon progeny.[29] Others have suggested that the typical exposures of the general population are too small to result in radiation-induced lung cancer during a normal human lifetime.

Given sufficient time and other favorable conditions, the decay products of ^{222}Rn will come into radioactivity equilibrium with the radon with each of the short-lived decay products having the same activity concentration in the air as the ^{222}Rn. However, this ideal equilibrium is rarely attained in air containing elevated levels of radon so that measurement of the radon gas concentration does not precisely indicate the concentration of decay products unless that state of disequilibrium is known. Since essentially all of the biologically important radiation dose to the respiratory epithelium is derived from the α-emitting radon decay products, it has been customary to describe their air concentration in special units called the *working level* (WL). The WL unit is defined as any combination of the short-lived radon progeny in 1 L of air that will ultimately yield in the emission of 130,000 MeV of total α radiation energy. Air having a ^{222}Rn concentration of 3.7 kBq/m^3 with the progeny in secular equilibrium would represent 1 WL. The exposure associated with a typical work month in a uranium mine 170 hours at 1 WL is called an exposure of 1 WLM. Dosimetric models indicate that the nominal dose to the bronchial epithelium associated with inhalation of radon decay product aerosols by a uranium miner is about 6 mGy/WLM.[30,31,32,32a] Assuming an α radiation quality factor of 20, this yields about 120 mSv/WLM. With a cancer weighting factor of 0.08 for the bronchial epithelium, the effective dose for cancer induction is about 10 mSv/WLM.[33]

BIOLOGIC EFFECTS
Introduction

There have been few reports of biologic effects in the respiratory system associated with occupational radiation exposures. Wing et al.[34] reported an apparent association between radiation worker exposure and increased incidence of lung cancer, but cigarette smoking by workers probably explains those findings. In contrast, Gilbert et al.[35] showed an inverse relationship among nuclear workers with fewer lung cancers associated with higher exposure doses. Cases of radiation-induced lung cancer in people are limited to special groups of individuals that received very high exposures, far exceeding the current radiation exposure limits for nuclear workers. Medical patients who received high doses of medical x-rays or γ irradiation for cancer treatment or alkylosing spondylitis sustained high radiation exposures to lung tissue that led to nonneoplastic injury and elevated incidence of lung cancer, as also did the survivors of the atomic-bomb explosions that occurred in 1945 in Nagasaki and Hiroshima, Japan, who were exposed almost instantaneously to subfatal doses of high dose-rate γ-rays and some neutron fluxes.[6] Although cigarette smoking is responsible for most of the lung cancer cases that have been observed in the Japanese survivors, there is a small but significant increase in observed cases at the higher radiation doses.

The primary occupational data relating biologic effects to occupational exposure to ionizing radiation are those associated with exposure to radon and progeny in underground mines, especially uranium mines. Uranium miners and other underground miners inhaled large quantities of radon decay product aerosols that deposited in the bronchial airways and irradiated the epithelium with α radiation.[35a] Both smoking and nonsmoking uranium miners have been found to have significantly elevated incidences of bronchogenic carcinoma associated with increased inhalation exposure to airborne radon decay products. These data indicate a compounding, not a simple addition, of lung cancer risks from inhaled tobacco smoke and α irradiation for inducing bronchogenic carcinoma.

Potential human risks and the form of the dose–response relationships can be predicted from the results of inhalation toxicology studies conducted with laboratory animals. Life-time studies of the toxicity in purebred beagles of inhaled radioactive particles of both α-emitting and β-emitting radionuclides have been conducted at the Pacific Northwest Laboratory (PNL) in Richland, Washington,[36,37] and at the Inhalation Toxicology Research Institute (ITRI) in Albuquerque, New Mexico.[38] These studies provide quantitative dose–effect and response data that can be used to predict human risks from inhaled radionuclides. In these studies inhalation exposures of young adult beagles were usually nose only, single, individual, and brief (usually less than 1 hour). Particle size distributions usually involved particles in the range of 1.0 to 3.0 μm in aerodynamic diameter, so that the inhaled particles deposited readily in the lung parenchyma as well as in the conductive airways with modest nasal deposition. The lung was the main target organ of the resultant effects, although other organs were sometimes involved. After intake the beagles were given lifetime care. The endpoint was death, either spontaneous or by euthanasia when death was imminent. The beagle studies of particular interest are those involving plutonium dioxide (PuO_2) airborne particles at PNL and airborne particles of fission-product radionuclides entrapped in fused aluminosilicate particles (FAP) at ITRI. The form of the dose–response relationships can be evaluated using data from these studies. In addition, by use of the method of lifespan normalization,[39] human risks and dose–response relationships can be predicted.

Respiratory tract risk from inhaled radionuclides depends upon both the pattern and timing of exposure dose and the dose–response relationships governing the possible adverse responses to irradiation of the lung tissues from particles lodged in the lung. The response depends strongly on the dose rate, d, of absorbed ionizing radiation.[40] Other tissues may also be at risk from indirect irradiation from the particles or because of translocation of the inhaled radioactive material from the lung to other organs of the body. Age at intake has an important influence on the lifetime occurrence of an effect since it influences the time available for induction and maturation of an effect.

Although the exact response may vary with the microdistribution of dose (especially for α irradiation), the dose rate can be expressed in terms of the mean energy deposited in the tissue of interest. This may be the whole lung including its normal content of circulating blood or it may be the bronchial epithelium. Since the dose rate to lung may change with time after intake due to clearance and radioactive decay, the time-weighted average dose rate, $\bar{d}$ was used. This $\bar{d}$ is an independent variable that can be determined retrospectively in an analysis of dose–response data or it can be predicted prospectively for risk assessment purposes based upon initial tissue concentration and known clearance rates. It has been shown to be practicable whether dose rate is increasing, decreasing, or relatively constant with respect to elapsed time.[40a]

Dose–response relationships have the general form that the independent risk distribution attributable to irradiation for a given effect has a probability density, $f(t,\bar{d})$, and cumulative risk function, $F(t,\bar{d})$, which are distributed with respect to elapsed time, t, but depend on average dose rate,

$\bar{d}$, forming three-dimensional mathematical response surfaces. The cumulative risk for a single effect is the independent probability (values between zero and one) of an individual succumbing to the specified response (e.g., dying of radiation-induced lung cancer) assuming that there are no other possible effects. At a given average dose rate

$$\Pr[T \leq t\backslash\bar{d}] = F(t,\bar{d}) = \int_0^t f(u,\bar{d})\delta u \quad (20)$$

where $t = A - E$ with A the age of the individuals at risk, E is their age at the beginning or time of the exposure, and T is the specific survival time from initial exposure until each individual succumbs.[40-42]

A simple regression model utilizes a response relationship given by

$$t_m = K_m \bar{d}^{-s} \quad (21)$$

or in logarithmic coordinates with ln the natural logarithm by

$$\ln t_m = \ln K_m - s \ln \bar{d} \quad (22)$$

where $\bar{d}$ is the average dose rate to the lung, t is the elapsed time to death after initial exposure, K is a characteristic parameter associated with level of risk, radionuclide, and exposure conditions, and s is the negative slope of the logarithmic form of the function. Maximum likelihood methods can be used to fit the log-linear function, Eq. (22), to experimental data.[43] With the median value of $K = K_m$ obtained from regression analysis, the resulting time, $t = t_m$, is the median time to death for exposed individuals. The geometric scale factor, σ_g, obtained from the fit using various probability density functions, provides a measure of the spread of the probability distribution function (the clustering of the cases) about the fitted median lines.

Separate regression risk distributions can be used for nonneoplastic radiation injury and for radiation-induced lung cancer, respectively. In this absolute risk model, all eventually succumb to the specified response (e.g., dying of radiation-induced cancer) given enough time in the absence of competing risks or natural deaths.

A risk distribution can be normalized with respect to the life spans of mammalian species by defining a dimensionless time, $t^* = t/L$ where L is the nominal life span of each species. This yields a normalized median K_m^* given as a function of the normalized dose rate, $\bar{d}^*$, where $\bar{d}^* = \bar{d}L$, and $K_m^* = K_m L^{(s-1)}$. When the parameters of Eq. (22) and σ_g have been established, it can be scaled among mammalian species by normalization of the species life spans to yield the form of Eq. (22) utilizing the appropriate nominal life span: 75 years for people and 14 years for beagles.[39]

The distribution of deaths associated with natural life span is a mixture of the various causes including various forms of both communicable and noncommunicable diseases (including some cases of lung cancer or lung impairment) and is commonly represented utilizing a Gompertz function.[39a] The form of this function is given by

$$F_1(t) = 1 - \exp[h_0(1 - e^{\psi t})/\lambda\psi] \qquad (25)$$

where the parameters h_0 and ψ can be evaluated from unexposed population records.

When several fatality risk distributions are superimposed in the time and dose-rate space, the occurrence (overall or dependent risk) of one effect at a specific average dose rate is a fraction, Ω, of individuals who succumb to that effect based upon the temporal convolution of all risks. It is calculated by integrating the product of the respective survivorship fractions $[1.0 - F(t,\overline{d})]$ and the instantaneous hazard rate of that effect. The hazard rate is the fraction of survivors at risk per unit time, $f(t,\overline{d})/[1.0 - F(t,\overline{d})]$. For example, the occurrence of effect 1 is given by

$$\Pr[T_i \leq t, T_{\neq i} > T_i] = \Omega_i(t,\overline{d}) =$$
$$\int_0^t (1 - F_1)(1 - F_2)(1 - F_3)\, h_i(u,\overline{d})\, \delta u \qquad (24)$$

where the 1, 2, and 3 subscripts refer to three separate independent risk distributions and death is the common endpoint. In this analysis effect 1 is spontaneous death from those causes associated with natural life span, effect 2 is death associated with radiation-induced lung cancer, and effect 3 is death from radiation-induced nonneoplastic lung injury.[39,40]

Nonneoplastic biologic response

Humans whose lungs were irradiated by high doses of x-rays and γ-rays (hundreds to thousands of rem) during the treatment of breast cancer or alkylosing spondylitis demonstrate serious damage to lung biochemical balance and tissue integrity.[44-49] Pulmonary surfactant levels are abnormal.[50] Pneumonitis and pulmonary edema ensue.[51] Functional capacities are impaired.[52] Fibrotic changes proceed as a later developing effect.[53,54]

Coggle et al.[55] reviewed the data on humans and animals and found that acute radiation pneumonitis develops within 6 months in persons or animals exposed to >8 Gy (800 rem) of low LET radiation (γ, x-rays, β particles). This is a progressive process beginning with an exudative phase (3 to 8 weeks) and continuing to an inflammatory response that includes intraalveolar and septal edema with desquamation of the epithelial and endothelial cells and type II cell hyperplasia. Pulmonary surfactant levels are elevated with a fall in compliance and abnormal gas exchange values. Complete respiratory failure is common at the higher doses. The resolution of the early inflammatory response is followed by progressive fibrosis depending in its severity on the dose delivered to the lung.

In the beagle studies of inhaled radioactive airborne particles, early deaths at high doses were associated with pulmonary insufficiency from acute radiation pneumonitis, pulmonary edema, and later development of pulmonary fibrosis.[56] The dose-rate/time/response models for these radiation pneumonitis deaths up to 1,000 days postinhalation exposure for beagles exposed to airborne particles of $^{239}PuO_2$ and of $^{238}PuO_2$ at PNL and of $^{90}Sr + ^{90}Y$ FAP and of $^{144}Ce + ^{144}Pr$ FAP at ITRI have been evaluated by Raabe and Goldman.[57] Their results are shown in Fig. 31-7. Doses of several thousand cGy (rad) are required to cause death from nonneoplastic radiation injury of the lung. Similarly large doses would apply to human lungs when the irradiation is protracted following lung deposition of relatively insoluble forms of radionuclides.

Neoplastic biologic response

Human exposures, primarily to penetrating low LET γ radiation (a small neutron dose was also involved) associated with the atomic bombing of Hiroshima and Nagasaki in 1945, have led to the development of significantly increased occurrence of lung cancer among the survivors.[6,58] These exposures were single acute exposures that occurred instantaneously at the time of the detonation of the bombs. BEIR-V[6] has reviewed the age dependence of the radiation risks and has indicated a somewhat increased sensitivity in individuals exposed in childhood. The relative risk rose for both smokers and nonsmokers and was higher for females than for males, but most of the cases were among the male smokers. The risk appeared elevated even at 0.1 Sv (10 rad). From these data the International Commission of Radiological Protection estimated a linear overall lifetime fatal lung cancer risk of 0.01/Sv for exposed adults.[2]

The exposure of uranium miners and other workers to elevated levels of airborne radon decay products has led to significantly increased incidence of lung cancer from this protracted exposure of the bronchial epithelium to high LET α radiation.[35a,59,60] Although both nonsmokers and smokers had elevated relative risk, most of the cases were among the smokers, and an important compounding of the risks from smoking and radon exposures is clearly shown in the data.[61] The data indicate that the combined exposure to carcinogenic levels of airborne radon decay products and cigarette smoke increases the lung cancer risk well above that for nonsmokers exposed to high levels of radon and above that for smokers who have not been exposed to high levels of radon.[35a] In addition the latent period is shortened by the combined exposures.[35a] A linear risk model estimates 350 cases per million person-WLM or 3.5×10^{-4}/WLM.[35a] At 0.12 Sv (12 rem) to the bronchial epithelium per WLM, the equivalent lifetime risk is 0.003/Sv. This is about one third of the risk per sievert for exposure of the whole lung by γ-rays in the atomic bomb survivors.

Land et al.[58] contrasted the histologic types of lung cancer found in Japanese A-bomb survivors and American ura-

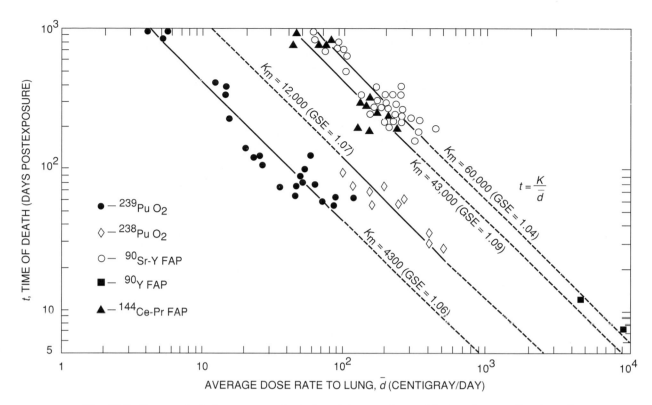

Fig. 31-7. Time to death from nonneoplastic lung injury as observed in beagles as a function of average dose rate to lung after inhalation deposition of radioactive airborne particles of selected types. The plutonium particles irradiate the lung with α radiation, whereas the others deliver β radiation. Human lung injury risks are predicted to be approximately the same as for beagles.

nium miners. The proportion of squamous cell carcinoma was found to be related to cigarette smoking in both groups. Small-cell carcinoma appeared to be more likely to be radiation-induced than adenocarcinomas in both populations, but the risk of both types was increased by the radiation exposures.

Inhalation carcinogenesis studies with beagles. Inhalation carcinogenesis studies with beagles tend to emphasize protracted irradiation of the lung following inhalation deposition of relatively insoluble forms of radionuclides. This type of protracted irradiation should not be expected to yield a dose–response relation similar to those obtained with acute, brief, or instantaneous irradiation exposures of the lung. In the beagle studies, lung cancers in beagles caused by α particles from ^{239}Pu were usually described as bronchioalveolar carcinomas. Lung cancers caused by β particle irradiation in beagles exposed to the insoluble ^{90}Sr + ^{90}Y FAP were primarily described as hemangiosarcoma, but hemangiosarcomas in tissues adjacent to lung were also found to be a major cause of death. Hahn[62] has reviewed the types of lung cancer found in laboratory animals from inhalation exposures to carcinogenic materials including airborne radioactive particles.

^{239}PuO$_2$ in beagles. The first lifetime study of inhaled α radiation emitting ^{239}PuO$_2$ in beagles at PNL, described by Park et al.,[63] Bair and Willard,[64] Park et al.,[36] West and

Bair,[56] Bair et al.,[65] and Dagle et al.,[65a] utilized single 10 to 30 minute nose-only exposures of 58 beagles that varied in age from about 6 to 43 months. Count median diameters (CMD) ranged from 0.1 to 0.65 μm with geometric standard deviations from 2.1 to 2.3, equivalent to activity median aerodynamic diameters (AMAD) from about 2 to 12 μm. Initial long-term lung (gas-exchange region) burdens were from about 10 to 2,000 kBq in three dosage groups. The second lifetime study of inhaled ^{239}PuO$_2$, described by Park and Staff[37] involved single 5 to 30 minute nose-only exposures of 116 beagles that varied in age from about 14 to 21 months. Inhaled particles had an average AMAD of 2.3 μm and geometric standard deviation of 1.9. Initial long-term lung burdens were from about 0.1 to about 200 kBq. There were 20 sham-exposed controls in this lifetime study. The doses for the two ^{239}Pu-dioxide studies were separately computed from the reported lung burdens and retention information. The life-span occurrences of lung cancer and lung injury for these two studies were combined as summarized in Fig. 31-8 with each beagle coded by cause of death along with fitted three-dimensional regression models. In Fig. 31-8 the third dimension, the probability density of cases, is indicated by the grouping of the data points. Utilizing life-span normalization of the beagle data, the predicted risk distributions for people consequent to inhalation exposure to ^{239}PuO$_2$ are shown in

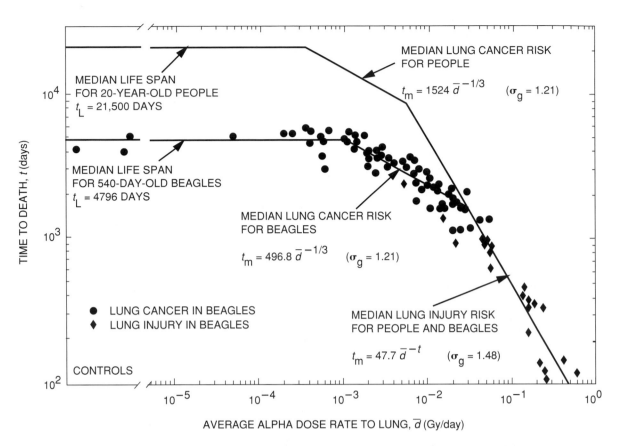

Fig. 31-8. Plot of the distribution of beagle deaths with lung cancer or lung injury after inhalation deposition of airborne particles of $^{239}PuO_2$ as a function of time-weighted average alpha radiation dose rate to whole lung showing the median risk functions observed and the predicted human median risk of lung cancer and injury obtained by life-span normalization.[40]

two dimensions in Fig. 31-8 along with the risk distributions for beagles.

The three separate risks of death associated with the $^{239}PuO_2$ studies can be mathematically separated to yield separate occurrence (overall risk) of death with lung injury limited to the highest dose rates and normal life-span deaths at the very lowest dose rates. The three causes of death intersect and interrelate in such a way as to separately predominate over different ranges of average dose rate. At high dose rate lung injury predominates. At low dose rates deaths are associated with causes associated with natural aging. The lung cancer risk predominates over the intermediate dose rates. The predicted lung cancer risk for people after inhalation of $^{239}PuO_2$ is shown in three dimensions in Figure 31-9.[23]

Life-span effective threshold. Although the independent risk of death with radiation-induced lung cancer approaches unity with time (all ultimately succumb at every nonzero dose rate) when there are no other causes of death, at lower dose rates it takes longer to reach any specified level of risk. This varying latent period may exceed the natural life span, resulting in a life-span effective threshold for cancer induction as shown in Fig. 31-9. This effective threshold occurs

at a lifetime cumulative dose to the lung of about 1 Gy for ^{239}Pu α radiation or about 20 Sv (2000 rem).

Gilbert et al.[66] and Dagle et al.[67] used proportional hazards models to describe the hazard rate for lung cancer for beagles in Study 2. Their hazard rate was based on induction of lung cancer rather than death. They fit their models as a function of time (beagle age) and calculated cumulative dose to lung as a function of retention time. They found a lung cancer hazard rate that was proportional to a baseline hazard rate associated with unexposed beagles and a factor $(1 + kD^2)$, where k is a fitted constant and D is the cumulative dose. This hazard rate that rapidly rises as cumulative dose increases is qualitatively similar to the rapidly rising hazard rate of the regression model, although the approach is quite different. The results of the studies of these investigators support the concept of the effective threshold since their dose–response function is nonlinear and close to background at low doses.

^{144}Ce FAP in beagles. The β radiation $^{144}Ce + {}^{144}Pr$ FAP study, described by Cuddihy and Boecker[68] and Hahn et al.,[69] involved single 4 to 76 minute nose-only exposures of beagles from 12 to 14 months of age. The exposures occurred between 1967 and 1971. Airborne particles of fused

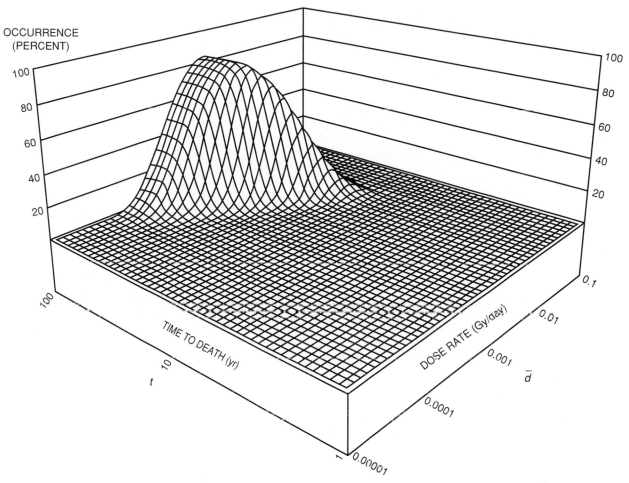

OCCURRENCE (PERCENT)

TIME TO DEATH (yr)

DOSE RATE (Gy/day)

TIME AFTER INTAKE & AVERAGE ALPHA DOSE RATE TO LUNG (LOG SCALES)

Fig. 31-9. Predicted lifetime occurrence of human deaths with radiation-induced lung cancer from $^{239}PuO_2$ deposited in the lungs at age 20 years based upon dose–responses observed in beagles using life-span normalization for interspecies scaling.

aluminosilicate particles (FAP) were formed by heating air-borne particles of ^{144}Ce-labeled montmorillonite clay to temperatures exceeding 1,100°C to entrap the radionuclide into relatively insoluble spherical particles.[57] The resulting airborne particles had AMAD that ranged from 1.4 to 2.8 μm with geometric standard deviations about equal to 2. The experimental design involved 110 beagles with equal numbers of both sexes divided among eight dosage levels with average initial pulmonary content from 4.4 to 3550 kBq. In addition there were 15 control dogs exposed to non-radioactive cerium in fused aluminosilicate particles.

The distribution of lung cancer and radiation lung injury deaths in the ^{144}Ce + ^{144}Pr FAP study are shown in Fig. 31-10 with each beagle coded by cause of death. The most striking result for the β-irradiated lung is that the negative slope $s = 2/3$ for radiation-induced lung cancer, so that β irradiation effectiveness drops at lower dose rates more rapidly than does α effectiveness in inducing lung cancer. In this two-dimensional plot the third dimension, the risk distribution, is reflected by the clustering of the individual

cases. Also shown in Fig. 31-10 is the scaled prediction of the median risks to people from radiation-induced lung cancer and injury following inhalation at age 20 years of insoluble particles containing ^{144}Ce + ^{144}Pr. A three-dimensional plot of the predicted lung cancer risk for people after inhalation of ^{144}Ce + ^{144}Pr in insoluble particles is shown in Fig. 31-11.

The three causes of death, natural life span causes, radiation-induced lung injury, and radiation-induced lung cancer, are seen to intersect and interrelate in such a way as to separately predominate over different ranges of dose rate. The independent risk distribution of fatal radiation-induced lung cancer (Fig. 31-11) is circumscribed by the other risks. Radiation pneumonitis deaths are limited to the highest dose rates because at intermediate dose rates radiation-induced lung cancer deaths occur before pneumonitis can fully develop. Lung cancer predominates at intermediate dose rates and in Fig. 31-11 is seen to be low both at low dose rates (because of deaths associated with natural life span) and at high dose rates (because of deaths from

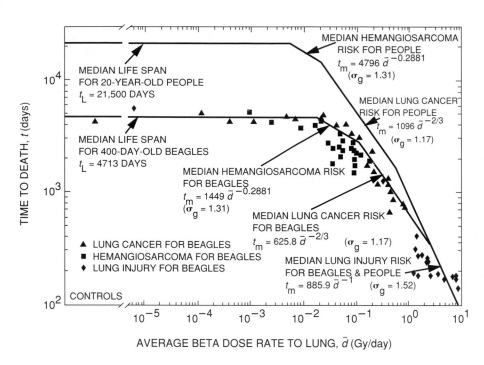

Fig. 31-10. Distribution of beagle deaths with lung cancer or injury after inhalation deposition of particles of ^{144}Ce + ^{144}Pr in fused aluminosilicate particles (FAP) as a function of time-weighted average β radiation dose rate to whole lung with the median risk functions and the predicted human median lung cancer and lung injury risks.

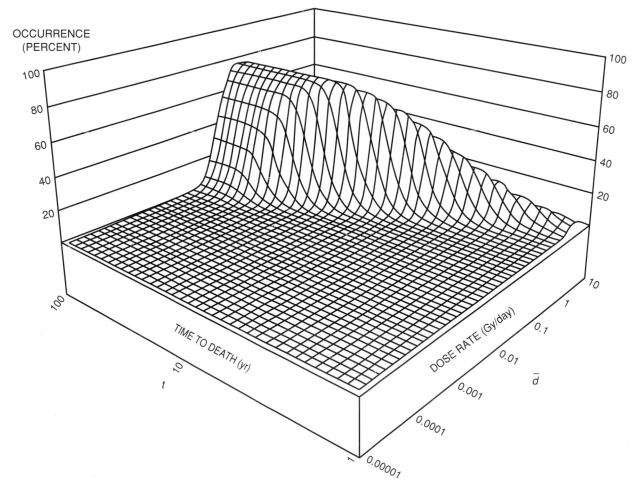

Fig. 31-11. Predicted lifetime occurrence of human deaths with radiation-induced lung cancer from ^{144}Ce + ^{144}Pr in particles deposited in the lungs at age 20 years based upon beagle studies after life-span normalization for interspecies scaling.

radiation pneumonitis). The existence of a minimum latent period for cancer is the result of competing noncancer risks.

Although the independent risk of fatal radiation-induced cancer approaches unity with time (all ultimately succumb at every nonzero dose rate) when there are no other causes of death, at lower dose rates it takes longer to reach any specified level of risk. This varying latent period may exceed the natural life span, resulting in a type of life span effective threshold for cancer induction. This effective threshold occurs at about 20 Gy (for β radiation) or 20 Sv (2,000 rem).

CASE STUDIES OF THE HEALTH RISKS OF RADON

Numerous studies have documented the significant lung cancer risks associated with extended occupational exposure to high levels of airborne radon decay products in uranium mining and other types of mining, and in uranium mills. Excess lung-cancer occurrence has been found in uranium miners in the United States, Canada, France, and Czechoslovakia. Excess lung cancer from exposures to radon progeny has also been reported among Swedish metal miners, British iron and tin miners, Newfoundland fluorspar miners, Chinese tin miners, and American metal miners. Epidemiologic studies of many thousand of miners have been conducted. These results have been summarized by the National Academy of Sciences.[35a] An example of one study of 3,363 male uranium miners in the Colorado plateau, there were 185 lung cancer deaths (5.5%) compared with 38 (1.1%) expected.[70] The dose–response relationship for α radiation-induced lung cancer as a function of cumulative exposure (WLM) is shown for the Colorado Plateau uranium mines in Fig. 31-12.[35a] Although the exposure to radon decay products can be highly carcinogenic for exposures well above 100 WLM (about 12 Sv or 1200 rem to the bronchial epithelium), according to these data exposures

smaller than about 50 to 100 WLM may not result in elevated incidence of lung cancer. This apparent effective threshold for radiation-induced lung cancer is consistent with, although somewhat smaller than, the predicted effective threshold at about 1 Gy (20 Sv) for exposure to airborne particles of $^{239}PuO_2$ discussed in the preceding section. Biological Effects of Ionizing Radiation (BEIR-IV)[32] suggested a linear dose–response risk of 350 per 10^6 WLM (3.5×10^{-4}/WLM) of exposure based upon the dose–response for fatal lung cancer such as shown in Fig. 31-12.

A consistent and important aspect of the cases of lung cancer in miners is the elevated combined effect associated with exposures to carcinogenic levels of radon progeny and cigarette smoking. Cigarette smoke and inhaled radon progeny both preferentially target the basal cells of the bronchial epithelium. Squamous cell carcinoma is the most common cancer type of induced cancer. Together carcinogenic levels of radon progeny and cigarette smoke lead to the acceleration of the development of bronchiogenic carcinoma and a marked elevation in cancer occurrence above that expected for either agent acting alone. The resulting carcinogenic action exceeds the additive combination of risks if they acted independently. Even with the combined insult, the high doses of α radiation involved in all of the cases suggest that the promoting action of cigarette smoke accelerates the induction of lung cancer at carcinogenic levels of inhaled radon progeny, while lower levels of α irradiation have little impact on the combined carcinogenic and promoting actions of cigarette smoke.

The acceleration and mutual reinforcement of carcinogenic action between inhaled cigarette smoke and radon decay products led to an early assessment that indicated that virtually all the cases of lung cancer in U.S. uranium miners were in smokers.[61] However, Roscoe et al.[71] showed significant elevations in lung cancer incidence among 516 white male miners who never smoked cigarettes, pipes, or

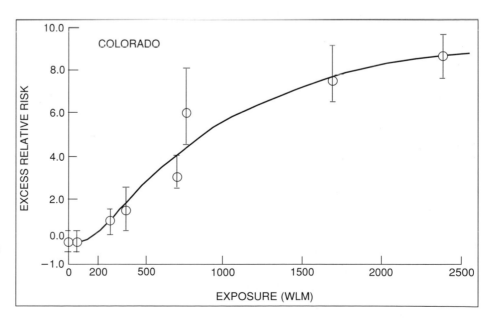

Fig. 31-12. Observed excess relative fatal lung cancer risk among male uranium miners in the Colorado Plateau study group as a function of exposure to airborne radon decay products in working level months (WLM). (Adapted from Biological Effects of Ionizing Radiation–IV.[32])

cigars. They provided case histories for 14 white, nonsmoking uranium miners who died of lung cancer in this cohort (2.7%). Only 1.1 deaths were expected (0.2%), yielding a standardized mortality ratio of 12.7 with 95% confidence limits of 8.0 and 20.1. The exposures among the 14 deaths ranged from 465 to 16,467 WLM. It is noteworthy that the smallest exposure among these 14 cases was 465 WLM, equivalent to an α radiation dose 3 Gy (60 Sv). These data suggest that higher radiation doses were required to induce lung cancer among the nonsmokers, but the cohort was too small to positively confirm this possibility.

SUMMARY

The lung is the organ of the body that receives the largest annual exposure from natural sources of ionizing radiation, namely from inhaled airborne radon decay products that preferentially irradiate the bronchial epithelium at about 24 mSv/year. But the lung is relatively insensitive to these and additional exposure to ionizing radiation. Large doses are required to yield appreciable risk of nonneoplastic injury or lung cancer, and there appear to be effective thresholds for both of these types of responses, at least in the case of protracted exposures from radionuclides deposited in the lung subsequent to inhalation of airborne radioactive particles. Both acute exposures to penetrating radiation and protracted exposures to radionuclides deposited in the lung can cause neoplastic and nonneoplastic adverse effects, but the doses required are much higher in the case of protracted exposures. An acute dose of 5 to 8 Sv (500 to 800 rem) can biochemically disrupt the lung and cause appreciable injury to tissues manifesting acute pulmonary pneumonitis and delayed pulmonary fibrosis. Protracted exposures extending over months or years for irradiation of lung tissue by radionuclides deposited in the lung must exceed 20 Sv to result in similar systemic injury. Likewise, the dose required to yield a significant and observable risk of lung cancer appears to be lower for acute exposure than for protracted exposures. The studies of the Japanese survivors of the atomic bombs exploded in Japan in 1945 show a nearly linear lifetime risk of lung cancer at about 0.01/Sv, although it is difficult to demonstrate that there is any risk below an acute exposure to 0.1 Sv (10 rem). In contrast, protracted exposures to radionuclides deposited in the lung that extend over months and years demonstrate an effective threshold at about 20 Sv, such that virtually no cancer risk occurs at lifetime doses smaller than 20 Sv (2000 rem) to lung tissue. The exposure of miners to high concentrations of airborne radon decay products yields a risk that has been described by a linear relationship, i.e., 350 per 10^6 person-WLM. But the data indicate that there may be an effective threshold at a lifetime exposure of about 50 to 100 WLM.

REFERENCES

1. Evans RD: *The atomic nucleus,* New York, 1955, McGraw-Hill.
2. ICRP: *1990 recommendations of the International Commission on Radiological Protection,* ICRP Publication 60 Oxford, 1991, Pergamon Press.
3. ICRP: *Recommendations of the international commission on radiological protection,* ICRP Publication 26. Oxford, 1977, Pergamon Press.
4. NCRP: National Council on Radiation Protection and Measurement. *Ionizing radiation exposure of the population of the United States,* NCRP Report No. 93, Bethesda, Md., 1987, National Council on Radiation Protection and Measurement.
5. NCRP: National Council on Radiation Protection and Measurement. *Exposure of the population of the United States and Canada from natural background radiation,* NCRP Report No. 94, Bethesda, Md., 1987, National Council on Radiation Protection and Measurement.
6. BEIR V: Committee on the Biological Effects of Ionizing Radiations. *Health effects of exposure to low levels of ionizing radiation,* Washington, DC, 1990, National Academy Press.
7. EPA: *A citizens' guide to radon, what it is and what to do about it,* OPA-86-004, Washington, DC, 1986, Environmental Protection Agency and Department of Health and Human Services.
8. NCRP: National Council on Radiation Protection and Measurement. *Control of radon in houses,* NCRP Report No. 103, Bethesda, Md., 1989, National Council on Radiation Protection and Measurement.
9. NCRP: National Council on Radiation Protection and Measurement. *Exposure of the U.S. population from diagnostic medical radiation,* NCRP Report No. 100, Bethesda, Md., 1989, National Council on Radiation Protection and Measurement.
10. NCRP: National Council on Radiation Protection and Measurement. *Exposure of the U.S. population from consumer products and miscellaneous sources,* NCRP Report No. 95, Bethesda, Md., 1987, National Council on Radiation Protection and Measurement.
11. NCRP: National Council on Radiation Protection and Measurement. *Public radiation exposure from nuclear power generation in the United States,* NCRP Report No. 92, Bethesda, Md., 1987, National Council on Radiation Protection and Measurement.
12. Raabe OG: Physical properties of aerosols affecting inhalation toxicology. In Sanders CL, Cross FT, Dagle GE, and Mahaffey JA, editors: *Pulmonary toxicology of respirable particles,* pp 1-28, CONF-791002, Springfield, Va., 1880, U.S. Department of Energy, National Technical Information Service.
13. Raabe OG: Deposition and clearance of inhaled aerosols. In Witschi HR, and Nettesheim P, editors: *Mechanisms in respiratory toxicology,* pp 27-76, West Palm Beach, FLa., 1982, CRC Press.
14. Raabe OG: Deposition and clearance of inhaled particles, In Gee JBL, Morgan WKC, and Brooks SM, editors: *Occupational lung diseases,* pp 1-37, New York, 1984, Raven Press.
15. Hatch TE and Gross P: *Pulmonary deposition and retention of inhaled aerosols.* New York, 1964, Academic Press.
16. Cheng YS, Yanada Y, Yeh HC, and Swift DL: Diffusional deposition of ultrafine aerosols in a human nose cast, *J Aerosol Sci* 19:741-752, 1989.
17. Heyder J, Arbruster L, Gebhart J, Grein E, and Stahlhofen W: Total deposition of aerosol particles in the human respiratory tract for nose and mouth breathing, *J Aerosol Sci* 6:311-328, 1975.
18. Stahlhofen W, Gebhart J, and Heyder J: Experimental determination of the regional deposition of aerosol particles in the human respiratory tract, *Am Ind Hyg Assoc J* 41:385-398, 1980.
19. Morrow PE, Bates DV, Fish BR, Hatch TF, and Mercer TT: Deposition and retention models for internal dosimetry of the human respiratory tract (Report of the International Commission on Radiological Protection: ICRP: Task Group on Lung Dynamics), *Health Phys* 12:173-207, 1964.
20. James AC, Birchall A, Cross FT, Cuddihy RG, and Johnson JR: The current approach of the ICRP task group for modeling doses to respiratory tract tissues, *Health Phys* 57, Suppl.1:271-282, 1989.

21. ICRP: *Human respiratory tract model for radiological protection,* International Commission on Radiological Protection, ICRP Publication 66, Oxford, 1994, Pergamon Press.

22. Snyder WS: (Chairman, Task Group of ICRP Committee 2). *Report of the task group on reference man,* International Commission on Radiological Protection Publication 23, Oxford, 1975, Pergamon Press.

23. Raabe OG and Park JF: Lung injury and cancer risk from inhaled ^{239}PuO$_2$, *Radiat Res* 1995 (submitted for publication).

24. NCRP: National Council on Radiation Protection and Measurement. *Basic radiation protection criteria,* NCRP Report No. 39 Bethesda, Md., 1971, National Council on Radiation Protection and Measurement.

25. ICRP: *Limits for inhalation of radon daughters by workers,* International Commission on Radiological Protection, ICRP Publication 32, Oxford, 1981, Pergamon Press.

26. ICRP: *Lung cancer risk from indoor exposures to radon daughters,* International Commission on Radiological Protection, ICRP Publication 50, Oxford, 1987, Pergamon Press.

27. Surgeon General of the United States: *Reducing the health consequences of smoking: 25 years of progress,* Rockville, Md., 1989, U.S. Department of Health and Human Services, Public Health Service.

27a. Raabe OG: Concerning the interactions that occur between radon decay products and aerosols, *Health Phys* 17:177–185, 1969.

28. George AC and Breslin AJ: Deposition of natural radon daughters in human subjects, *Health Phys* 13:375-378, 1967.

29. Al-Affan IA and Haque AK: Transformation of lung cells from inhalation of radon daughters in dwellings: a preliminary study, *Int J Radiat Bio* 56(4):413-422, 1989.

30. James AC, Jacobi W, and Steinhausler F: Respiratory tract dosimetry of radon and thoron daughters: the state-of-the-art and implications for epidemiology and radiobiology. In *Radiation hazards in mining: control, measurement and medical aspects,* Golden, Co., 1981, Colorado School of Mines.

31. James AC: Lung dosimetry, In Nazaroff WW and Nero AV Jr, editors: *Radon and its decay products in indoor air,* pp 259-308, New York, 1988, John Wiley.

32. BEIR IV: Committee on the Biological Effects of Ionizing Radiations. *Health risks of radon and other internally deposited alpha-emitters,* Washington, DC, 1988, National Academy Press.

32a. Birchall A and James AC: Uncertainty analysis of the effective dose per unit exposure from radon progeny and implications for ICRP risk-weighting factors, *Radiat Prot Dosim* 53(1–4):133–140.

33. ICRP: *Protection against radon-22 at home and at work,* International Commission on Radiological Protection, ICRP Publication 65, Oxford, 1994, Pergamon Press.

34. Wing S, Shy CM, Wood JL, Wolf S, Cragle DL, and Frome EL: Mortality among workers at Oak Ridge National Laboratory: evidence of radiation effects in follow-up through 1984, *JAMA* 265(11):1397-1402, 1991.

35. Gilbert ES, Petersen GR, and Buchanan JA: Mortality of workers at the Hanford site: 1945-1981, *Health Phys* 56:11-25, 1989.

35a. Beir IV: Committee on the Biological Effects of Ionizing Radiations. *Health risks of radon and other internally deposited alpha-emitters,* Washington, DC, 1988, National Academy Press.

36. Park JF, Bair WJ, and Busch RH: Progress in beagle dog studies with transuranium elements at Battelle-Northwest, *Health Phys* 22:803-810, 1972.

37. Park JF and Staff: *Pacific Northwest Laboratory annual report for 1984 to the DOE Office of Energy Research: Part 1: biomedical sciences,* PNL-8500 Pt. 1. Springfield, Va., 1993, National Technical Information Service.

38. Boecker BB, Muggenburg BA, Miller SC, and Coors TA, editors: *Annual report on long-term dose-response studies of inhaled or injected radionuclides 1988-89,* LMF-128, Albuquerque, 1990, Inhalation Toxicology Research Institute.

39. Raabe OG, Rosenblatt LS, and Schlenker RA: Interspecies scaling of risk for radiation-induced bone cancer, *Int J Radiat Biol* 57:1047-1061, 1990.

39a. Gross AJ and Clark VA: *Survival distributions: reliability applications in the biological sciences.* New York, 1975, John Wiley.

40. Raabe OG: Scaling of fatal cancer risks from laboratory animals to man, *Health Phys* 57(Suppl 1):419-432, 1989.

40a. Raabe OG: Comparison of the carcinogenicity of the radium and bone-seeking actinides, *Health Phys* 46:1241–1258, 1984.

41. Lee ET: *Statistical methods for survival data analysis,* Belmont, Ca., 1980, Lifetime Learning Publications.

42. Raabe OG: Three-dimensional dose-response models of competing risks and natural life span, *Fund Appl Toxicol* 8:465-473, 1987.

43. Kalbfleisch JD and Prentice RL: *The statistical analysis of failure time data,* New York, 1980, John Wiley.

44. Boushy SF, Helgason AH, and North LB: The effect of radiation on the lung and bronchial tree, *Am J Roentgenol Radium Ther Nucl Med* 108(2):284-292, 1970.

45. Davis SD, Yankelevitz DF, and Henschke CI: Radiation effects on the lung: clinical features, pathology, and imaging findings, *Am J Roentgenol* 159(6):1157-1164, 1992.

46. Frija J, Ferme C, Baud L, Gisselbrecht C, Miot C, Fermand JP, and Laval-Jeantet M: Radiaton-induced lung injuries: a survey by computed tomography and pulmonary function tests in 18 cases of Hodgkin's disease, *Eur J Radiol* 8(1):18-23, 1988.

47. Fennessy JJ: Irradiation damage to the lung, *J Thoracic Imaging* 2(3):68-79, 1987.

48. Gibson PG, Bryant DH, Morgan GW, Yeates M, Fernandez V, Penny R, and Breit SN: Radiation-induced lung injury: a hypersensitivity pneumonitis? *Ann Intern Med* 109:288-291, 1988.

49. Gross NJ: The pathogenesis of radiation-induced lung damage, *Lung* 159:115-125, 1981.

50. Hallman M, Maasilta P, Kivisaari L, and Mattson K: Changes in surfactant in bronchoalveolar lavage fluid after hemithorax irradiation in patients with mesothelioma, *Am Rev Respir Dis* 141:998-1005, 1994.

51. Rothwell RI, Kelly SA, and Joslin CA: Radiation pneumonitis in patients treated for breast cancer, *Radiother Oncol* 4(1):9-14, 1985.

52. Slavin JD Jr, Friedman NC, and Spencer RP: Radiation effects on pulmonary ventilation and perfusion, *Clin Nucl Med* 18(1):81-82, 1993.

53. Kaufman J, Gunn W, Hartz AJ, Fischer M, Hoffman RG, Schlueter DP, and Komanduri A: The pathophysiologic and roentgenologic effects of chest irradiation in breast carcinoma, *Int J Radiat Oncol Biol Phys* 12(6):887-893, 1986.

54. Molls M, Herrmann TH, Steinberg F, and Feldmann HJ: Radiopathology of the lung: experimental and clinical observations, *Recent Results Cancer Res* 130:109-121, 1993.

55. Coggle JE, Lambert BE, and Moores SR: Radiation effects in the lung, *Environ Health Perspect* 70:261-291, 1986.

56. West JE and Bair WJ: Plutonium inhalation studies, V: radiation syndrome in beagles after inhalation of plutonium dioxide, *Radiat Res* 22:489-506, 1964.

57. Raabe OG and Goldman M: A predictive model of early mortality following acute inhalation of PuO$_2$ aerosols, *Radiat Res* 78:264-277, 1979.

58. Land CE, Shimosato Y, Saccomanno G, Tokuoka S, Auerbach O, Tateishi R, Greenberg SD, Nambu S, Carter D, Akiba S, Keehn R, Madigan P, Mason TJ, and Tokunaga, M: Radiation-associated lung cancer: a comparison of the histology of lung cancers in uranium miners and survivors of the atomic bombings of Hiroshima and Nagasaki, *Radiat Res* 134:234-243, 1993.

59. Burkart W: Radiation biology of the lung: recent progress in understanding cancer induction and non-stochastic effects of inhaled radon daughters, hot particles and other radionuclides, *Sci Total Environ* 89(1-2):v-ix, 1-230, 1989.

60. Polednak AP, Keane AT, and Beck WL: Estimation of radiation doses to the lungs of early uranium processing plant workers, *Environ Res* 28:313-328, 1982.

61. Saccomanno G, Archer VE, Saunders RP, James, LA, and Beckler PA: Lung cancer of uranium miners on the Colorado Plateau, *Health Phys* 10:1195-1201, 1964.

62. Hahn FF: Carcinogenic responses of the lung to inhaled materials, In McClellan RO and Henderson RF, editors: *Concepts in inhalation toxicology,* pp 313-346, New York, 1989, Hemisphere Publishing.

63. Park JF, Willard DH, Marks S, West JE, Vogt GS, and Bair WJ: Acute and chronic toxicity of inhaled plutonium in dogs, *Health Phys* 8:651-657, 1962.

64. Bair WJ and Willard DH: Plutonium inhalation studies IV: mortality in dogs after inhalation of ^{239}PuO$_2$, *Radiat Res* 16:811-821, 1962.

65. Bair WJ, Metivier H, and Park JF: Comparison of early mortality in baboons and dogs after inhalation of ^{239}PuO$_2$, *Radiat Res* 82:588-610, 1980.

65a. Dagle GE, Sanders CL, Park JF, and Mahaffey JA: Pulmonary carcinogenesis with inhaled plutonium in rats and dogs, In Sanders CL, Cross FT, Dagle GE, and Mahaffey JA, editors: *Pulmonary toxicology of respirable particles,* CONF-791002, pp 601-615, Springfield, Va., 1980, National Technical Information Service.

66. Gilbert ES, Park JF, and Buschbom RL: Time-related factors in the study of risks in animals and humans, *Health Phys* 57(Suppl 1):379-385, 1989.

67. Dagle GE, Park JF, Gilbert ES, and Weller RE: Risk estimates for lung tumours from inhaled ^{239}PuO$_2$, ^{238}PuO$_2$, and ^{239}Pu(NO$_3$)$_4$ in beagle dogs, *Radiat Protect Dosimetry* 26:173-176, 1989.

68. Cuddihy RB and Boecker BB: Controlled administration of respiratory tract burdens of inhaled radioactive aerosols in beagle dogs, *Toxicol Appl Pharmacol* 25:597-605, 1973.

69. Hahn FF, Benjamin SA, Boecker BB, Chiffelle TL, Hobbs CH, Jones RK, McClellan RO, Pickrell JA, and Redman HC: Primary pulmonary neoplasms in beagle dogs exposed to aerosols of ^{144}Ce in fused-clay particles, *J Natl Cancer Inst* 50:675-679, 1973.

70. Waxweiler RJ, Roscoe RJ, Archer VE, Thun MJ, Wagoner JK, and Lundin FE: Mortality follow-up through 1977 of the white underground uranium miners cohort examined by the United States Public Health Service. In Gomez M, editor: *International conference, radiation hazards in mining: control, measurement, and medical aspects,* pp 823-830, New York, 1981, Society of Mining Engineers of the American Institute of Mining, N\Metallurgical, and Petroleum Engineers, Inc.

71. Roscoe RJ, Steenland K, Halperin WE, Beaumont JJ, and Waxweiler RJ: Lung cancer mortality among nonsmoking uranium miners exposed to radon daughters, *JAMA* 262(5):629-633, 1989.

Chapter 32

INFECTIOUS ORGANISMS

Julie Louise Gerberding

Occupational exposures constitute an important cause of respiratory infections among otherwise healthy adults. Many common infections are readily transmitted from one person to another in the worksite, especially under conditions of crowding and poor ventilation. Inhalation of more unusual pathogens from environmental or animal reservoirs is another significant mode of acquiring occupational respiratory infections. Although virtually all communicable respiratory diseases can be present in the workplace, those that are highly prevalent and have a large impact on productivity, those with a high potential for serious outbreaks, and those that require special prevention or control interventions are emphasized in this chapter.

UPPER RESPIRATORY INFECTIONS
The common cold

Epidemiology. The common cold is a self-limited viral illness and is the most frequent cause of absenteeism from work in the United States. A number of viral pathogens, including rhinoviruses (30%), coronaviruses (10%), influenza virus, parainfluenza virus, respiratory syncytial virus, and adenoviruses (15% to 20%) are etiologic, but in approximately 40% of cases, the causative agent cannot be isolated,[1] The large numbers of implicated viruses and immunologically distinct subtypes account for the high incidence of these infections (two to four colds per year among healthy adults).

Household contact with young children is a major source of exposure to the common cold. Secondary transmission among adults in the workplace or other sites of crowding then ensues. Respiratory syncytial virus is an important source of nosocomial outbreaks, affecting up to 50% of adult care providers in some reports.[2] Studies of human volunteers have clearly demonstrated the importance of direct mucosal inoculation of infectious secretions carried on the hands from one person to another in rhinovirus transmission.[3] Inhalation of aerosols generated through coughing or sneezing may also be important modes of cold virus transmission. Fomites (such as drinking glasses, telephone receivers, and shared office equipment) are not known to be important vectors of transmission, but viruses can be recovered from environmental surfaces for several hours after deposition.

Clinical manifestations. Symptoms of the common cold are independent of the causative agent and include rhinorrhea, congestion, dry cough, sneezing, pharyngeal irritation, and laryngitis. The constellation of typical symptoms and signs is sufficient for diagnosis, and specific laboratory tests are not indicated. Although low-grade fever is not unusual, high fever, lymphadenopathy, or the presence of a productive cough should prompt a search for alternative diagnoses. Bacterial infections may complicate viral upper respiratory infection. Sinusitis, otitis media, and streptococcal pharyngitis are the most common infections in this category. Not surprisingly, seasonal variations in the incidence of each of these parallel that of the common cold.

Treatment, prevention, and control. Specific antiviral therapy is not yet available for the common cold. A myriad of prescription and over-the-counter products are helpful for treating cold symptoms. A major challenge for the clinician is to avoid the use of antibiotic agents for these viral infections, even when the patient requests treatment. Decongestants and antihistamines, alone or in combination, as well as lozenges, expectorants, and antipyretics are useful alternatives for most. Antibiotic treatment of sinusitis is directed against the most likely etiologic organisms (Table 32-1). Among adults, *Streptococcus pneumoniae, Hemophilus influenzae, Branhamella catarrhalis,* and oral anaerobes (especially in odontogenic sinusitis) are the most common organisms.[4] Oral treatment with trimethoprim-sulfamethoxazole, amoxicillin-clavulanic acid, or cephalosporins active against β-lactamase-producing organisms (e.g., cefixime) for 7 to 10 days is appropriate.[5] The spectrum of organisms responsible for otitis media in adults is similar to that found in sinusitis, and treatment recommendations are identical (Table 32-1).[5]

Colds are difficult to prevent, especially since the period of virus shedding is highly variable and precedes the onset of symptoms. Restriction of those with cold symptoms from the workplace could reduce spread but is unlikely to completely eliminate occupational transmission. Moreover, the cost of such an approach in terms of days lost from work would be enormous. Avoidance of hand contact with oral and nasal mucosal surfaces or secretions could reduce the potential for person-to-person spread, but is very difficult (if not impossible) to accomplish. Handwashing after contact with nasal secretions may be a more practical solution. The use of tissues for containing coughs and sneezes is also a sensible but unproven intervention. Nosocomial transmission of respiratory syncitial virus can be contained by clustering infected children and employing barrier protection to minimize hand and conjunctival contamination of health care providers.[6]

Bacterial pharyngitis

Epidemiology. Group A streptococcal pharyngitis is the most common bacterial cause of acute pharyngitis among adults. Streptococcal pharyngitis is a highly contagious upper respiratory infection spread directly from person to person through contaminated droplet secretions. Crowding dramatically facilitates transmission, as evidenced in several reports of massive outbreaks among military recruits and in institutional settings.[7] Nosocomial transmission between patients and their health care providers has also been documented.

Group A *Streptococcus pyogenes* is the most common etiology of streptococcal respiratory infections, but other streptococcal serogroups, including groups C and G, have been associated with both endemic and epidemic cases.[8] A pharyngeal carrier state may persist for weeks to months

Table 32-1. Empiric treatment of bacterial respiratory infections in adults

Diagnosis	Etiology	Suggested regimens
Sinusitis	*S. pneumoniae*	Amoxicillin*‡
Otitis media	*H. influenzae*	Amoxicillin clavulanate
	Oral anearobes	Trimethoprim-sulfamethoxazole
	(*S. aureus*)	Penicillinase-resistant penicillin
Exudative pharyngitis	Group A,C,G streptococci	Benzathine penicillin G, penicillin V, erythromycin†
	C. diphtheriae	Erythromycin†
	N. gonnorheae	Ceftriaxone im
	Viral infections	None
	Infectious mononucleosis	None
Typical pneumonia	*S. pneumoniae*	Penicillin,‡ amoxicillin
	H. influenzae	Amoxicillin,* amoxicillin clavulanate, trimethoprim-sulfamethoxazole
	(*L. pneumophilia*)‡	Erythromycin†
	Oral anaerobes	Clindamycin, penicillin
Atypical pneumonia	*Mycoplasma pneumoniae*	Erythromycin,† doxycycline
	Legionella pneumophilia	Erythromycin† ± rifampin
	Chlamydia pneumoniae	Doxycycline
	Chlamydia psittaci	Erythromycin†
	Coxiella burnetii	

*Use alternate agent when β-lactamase-producing strains of *H. influenzae* are suspected.

†Newer macrolides (azithromycin, clarithromycin) are also effective, but clinical experience is limited.

‡Use alternate agent (vancomycin, erythromycin, cepahlosporin, dependent on local resistance patterns) in geographic locales where high level resistance to penicillin is anticipated.

following untreated infections. However, the quantitative titer of organisms in the nasopharynx declines over time, and characteristic virulence markers, including M-protein, are usually lost. For these reasons, persons with chronic infection are much less likely to transmit streptococci to susceptibles than are acutely infected individuals.

Clinical syndromes. Typically, streptococcal pharyngitis presents with a relatively abrupt onset of sore throat, fever, tachycardia, and myalgias with or without chills. Mild symptoms indistinguishable from viral pharyngitis can also be seen. Tonsillar and posterior pharyngeal exudates, temperature greater than 101° F, and tender cervical lymphadenopathy are highly suggestive but by no means pathognomonic. Precise diagnosis is dependent on culturing the organism from the throat. The yield of this procedure is increased by swabbing the oropharynx, nasopharynx posterior to the uvula, and tonsils or tonsillar fossae. The appearance of β-hemolytic colonies sensitive to bacitracin on sheep blood agar plates is sufficient for a presumptive diagnosis. Tests that detect streptococcal antigens present on throat swabs are also available. The sensitivity of these tests varies from 60% to 95%, but their specificity is usually quite good and they can provide an inexpensive method for rapid diagnosis.[9] One cost-effective approach is to obtain two throat swabs initially. If the rapid test of the first swab is negative, the second swab should be sent for culture. If the rapid test is positive, a presumptive diagnosis can be made without obtaining the more expensive throat culture. Neither antigen tests nor cultures reliably distinguish carriers from those with acute infection.

The incidence of local suppurative complications (peritonsillar abscess, acute otitis media, acute sinusitis) as well as invasive disease (cellulitis, pneumonia, bacteremia) and toxic shock syndrome associated with streptococcal infection has increased in the last decade.[10-14] This increase in clinical severity is highly correlated with a change in the prevalence of strains producing pyrogenic exotoxins and other virulence factors. The incidence of poststreptococcal rheumatic fever also increased in the 1980s, especially among white suburban children, but appears to have subsequently declined.[15]

In addition to the common cold viruses, infectious mononucleosis, acute human immunodeficiency virus (HIV), infection, adenovirus, herpangina, and herpes simplex virus infections should be included in the differential diagnosis of pharyngitis among adults.[7] Gonorrhea and syphilis should not be overlooked among sexually active persons. In the United States, nasopharyngeal diphtheria is extremely uncommon, especially among healthy adults, but recent outbreaks among Native Americans and urban alcoholic patients have occurred.[16]

Treatment, prevention, and control. Streptococcal pharyngitis should be treated with antibiotics (Table 32-1). The goal of treatment is to prevent local supportive complications and the development of acute rheumatic fever. *S. pyogenes* remains exquisitely sensitive to penicillin, and parenteral penicillin (1.2 MU benzathine penicillin im) is the treatment of choice.[5] Oral treatment (penicillin V 250 tid) is an acceptable and potentially safer alternative, but achieving compliance for the full 10 days necessary to adequately prevent rheumatic fever is problematic for many patients. Erythromycin (250 mg po qid) is an acceptable alternative for penicillin-allergic patients. Azithromycin has been approved for treatment of streptococcal infection, but its efficacy in preventing rheumatic fever has not been established. Higher doses of oral antimicrobials are necessary to treat suppurative complications.

Asymptomatic contacts of employees with streptococcal pharyngitis do not require evaluation or treatment unless they have a history of rheumatic fever and are not receiving long-term prophylaxis. In homes where an individual with a history of rheumatic fever resides, household contacts of persons with group A streptococcal infection should receive prophylaxis with penicillin or erythromycin.[17,18]

Pertussis

Epidemiology. The number of reported cases of pertussis (whooping cough) in the United States steadily declined until the early 1980s but has gradually increased since.[19,20] The most common causative agent, *Bordatella pertussis,* remains endemic and is highly contagious, with attack rates in excess of 70% among susceptible contacts. At least three factors contribute to the persistence of this infection. First, large numbers of children are not vaccinated, either due to poor access to health care services or (in an increasing number of cases), a reluctance of parents to have children immunized because of concerns about adverse effects associated with the vaccine. Second, vaccine-mediated immunity wanes over time, so that many individuals become susceptible in early adulthood. Finally, infection is often undiagnosed and therefore untreated, so that sources of contagion persist in the community for relatively long time intervals and serve as reservoirs for transmission to other susceptibles.

Clinical syndromes. The classic three-phase (catarrhal, paroxysmal, and convalescent) pertussis illness seen in infants and children is rare among infected adults. Older children and adults more typically develop a severe bronchitic illness that may last for weeks to months. The diagnosis is all too often delayed and a significant proportion of cases goes unrecognized. Nasopharyngeal swabs (preferably calcium alginate or dacron) should be directly plated on selective media to enhance the diagnostic yield of bacterial cultures. A positive culture for *B. pertussis* (or more rarely *B. paraperpertussis* or *B. bronchiseptica*) is conclusive in a patient with a compatible illness. Unfortunately, cultures are relatively insensitive, especially late in the course, after antimicrobial therapy, and/or among those previously vaccinated.

Treatment, prevention, and control. Early treatment can attenuate the severity of infection and may be life-saving among infants. Erythromycin (500 mg qid) for 2 weeks is recommended for adults (Table 32-1).[5] The organism is eradicated after the fourth day of treatment but relapse is common if less than 14 days of therapy are completed. Trimethoprim-sulfamethoxazole is an acceptable alternative. Employees can return to work after 5 days of treatment, if they are otherwise doing well and agree to complete the full 14 day antibiotic course.[21] Close contacts should be treated prophylactically with erythromycin (500 mg qid for adults) for 14 days, even if prior immunization is documented.

Pertussis vaccine is efficacious in preventing infection among infants and children.[22] The incidence of serious adverse reactions to pertussis vaccine is actually quite low and may be further reduced with use of acellular vaccine products. Routine vaccination of adults is not yet recommended because the disease is rare. During outbreaks of infection in health care facilities when widespread vaccination was used as a control measure, more than 50% of adult recipients noted prominent local reactions.[21]

Influenza

Epidemiology. Influenza is an extremely common self-limited respiratory illness caused by types A, B, and rarely C influenza virus.[23,24] Adults are susceptible to recurrent episodes because the antigenic structure of these viruses changes frequently, leading to new epidemics. Influenza is a highly contagious airborne infection spread by the respiratory route. Virus can be detected in the respiratory tract 1 to 2 days before until 5 to 6 days after the onset of symptoms. Epidemics occur annually in the winter months, peak in 2 to 3 weeks, and subside over 2 to 3 months. Outbreaks within a community are heralded by increased absenteeism from work, increased hospitalizations for respiratory illness, and, subsequently, by excess mortality due to secondary pneumonias. Attack rates within the community range from 10% to 30% but may be much higher in closed populations.

Clinical syndromes. Influenza is an acute febrile illness that usually presents with the abrupt onset of systemic symptoms (fatigue, myalgia, chills, and headache) followed by upper respiratory tract symptoms.[25] Clinically apparent primary influenza pneumonia is rare in healthy adults but more common in elderly or debilitated patients. In these patients, secondary community-acquired bacterial pneumonias may complicate the clinical course and account for a significant proportion of the high morbidity and mortality of influenza epidemics.

Treatment, prevention, and control. Annual influenza vaccination is recommended for all persons at risk for complications, including persons aged 65 and older and those with chronic underlying diseases (congenital or acquired heart disease, chronic pulmonary diseases, chronic renal disease, diabetes, chronic anemias, or immunosuppression).[26] Persons providing essential community services, including health care personnel, at increased risk of exposure to or transmission of influenza are also candidates for immunization.

Amantadine and ramantidine are effective in the prophylaxis of influenza A but not influenza B.[27,28] To be effective, prophylaxis must be implemented at the onset of an outbreak and continued daily for its duration. The effect of amantadine and vaccination is additive. Amantadine can therefore be instituted at the time of immunization and continued for 2 weeks to provide protection until antibody is produced. Amantadine (200 mg/day) is also a useful therapy when taken for 3 to 5 days at the onset of symptoms and continued for 48 hours after resolution, but is not routinely recommended for otherwise healthy adults. The dose should be reduced to 100 mg/day in those over 65 years old and should be adjusted commensurate with creatinine clearance in those with impaired renal function.[29] Ramantidine is also effective and may have fewer central nervous system side effects.

LOWER RESPIRATORY TRACT INFECTIONS
Bacterial pneumonias

Epidemiology. Viruses are probably the most common cause of pneumonia in all age groups, although, in most cases, the etiologic agent is not established with certainty.[30,31] Primary influenza virus pneumonia should be suspected during community outbreaks, especially when compatible systemic and upper respiratory symptoms and signs are present. Adenoviruses (types 4, 7, 3, and 14) are associated with outbreaks of pneumonia and acute respiratory disease (cough, pharyngitis, regional lymphadenopathy) among military recruits and other closed populations.[32] Epidemics of the more common community-acquired bacterial pneumonias are unusual, even among closed populations. Nevertheless, sporadic cases of occupational transmission and occasional outbreaks in work settings make important contributions to the incidence of these infections.

Overall, *Streptococcus pneumoniae* is the most common bacterial cause of pneumonia among adults of all ages, accounting for about 70% of cases.[30,31,33] Person-to-person transmission of pneumococci occurs via droplets. Young children in the home are the primary source of strains colonizing adults, although transmission among adults in occupational settings is documented. Once the oropharynx is colonized, a type-specific antibody response develops and is associated with clearance of the carrier state.[34] Disease is actually unusual in the presence of normal pulmonary defense mechanisms. Tobacco use, viral or other intercurrent respiratory infections (including influenza and measles), age, and underlying diseases predispose to the development of pneumonia.

Hemophilus influenzae accounts for 2% to 18% of cases of community-acquired pneumonia in adults but is rare in the absence of compromised host defenses.[35] The organism is often isolated in the sputum of persons with chronic bronchitis and obstructive pulmonary disease, and, not surprisingly, *H. influenzae* is associated with pneumonia in these patients. Alcoholism is also a predisposing factor in many series. *Staphylococcus aureus,* pyogenic streptococci, and gram-negative enteric pathogens are rare causes of pneumonia among healthy employees.

Mycoplasma pneumoniae is not limited to young adults but is more common between the ages of 5 and 40 and accounts for approximately 50% of pneumonias among college students and military recruits.[36,37] This infection is more common in the fall and increases in incidence every 3 to 5 years, especially in northern communities. *Chlamydia pneumoniae* also produces pneumonia in young adults, at least in some geographic areas.[38-42]

Legionella spp. are important causes of both sporadic cases and outbreaks of pneumonia in the community and in health care settings.[43,44] The attack rate for *L. pneumophilia,* the agent responsible for Legionnaire's diseases, ranges from 1% to 7% in the community, but the rate may be higher among cigarette smokers, those with impaired pulmonary host defenses, and the elderly.

Legionellae are ubiquitous in both natural and man-made aquatic environments. They multiply in free-living ameoba, and recent epidemiologic evidence suggests that the presence of both legionellae and an ameobic host is necessary to perpetuate a water-borne outbreak.[45] Aerosols generated by cooling towers, humidifiers, aquafiers, nebulizers, hot-water storage tanks, showers, water faucets, and air conditioners are major sources of human infections. Excavation at construction sites and landfills can also produce infectious aerosols. Nosocomial transmission of legionellae occurs, usually via infected potable water, and accounts for up to 30% of cases of nosocomial pneumonia during outbreaks.[44,46] Otherwise healthy health care providers may experience asymptomatic seroconversion or a mild febrile illness (Pontiac fever) but rarely acquire pneumonia. Person-to-person transmission of legionellae has not been observed.

Clinical syndromes. The history of the presenting illness often provides helpful clues to the etiology of pneumonia. The onset of typical community-acquired bacterial pneumonia is abrupt, sometimes with an upper respiratory prodrome, and is often heralded by rigors. Fever, productive cough, tachypnea, and pleuritic chest pain are common associated features. Chest auscultation will demonstrate signs of airway consolidation and often pleural effusion. A chest radiograph is useful in most cases but not essential in those with mild illness. The responsible organism, usually *S. pneumoniae* or, less commonly, *H. influenzae* or other gram-negative organisms, can often be presumptively diagnosed by microscopic examination of expectorated sputum stained with Gram's stain. Blood cultures should be obtained when invasive disease is suspected, and lumbar puncture to evaluate meningeal fluid is imperative when meningeal signs are apparent. Small pleural effusions are not unusual and not all require diagnostic thoracentesis. If fever persists more than 72 hours, if the effusion is large, accumulates rapidly, or causes respiratory compromise, or if the patient deteriorates, then diagnostic thoracentesis is indicated. Empyemas require drainage.

The onset of atypical pneumonia is more often subacute and preceded by a viral-like prodrome.[36] Fever, headache, malaise, and dry cough are also characteristic. Pleuritic chest pain is unusual. Chest examination may be normal or demonstrate a variety of abnormalities. The chest x-ray is also nonspecific although lobar consolidation and large effusions are unusual. Platelike atelectasis, small nodular densities, and hilar adenopathy suggest mycoplasmic infection but are also described in patients with *C. pneumoniae*. The presence of bullous myringitis is also a clue to the diagnosis of mycoplasma.

The presentation of Legionella pneumonia is variable, and may have features of both typical and atypical pneumonia.[47] Among hospitalized cases, abrupt onset of a systemic prodrome (myalgia, headache, and fatigue) followed by high fever and rigors is usual. Tachypnea and a relative bradycardia are also common signs. Cough may be dry or productive of scant amounts of sputum. Pleurisy is present in up to one third of cases. A myriad of extrapulmonary manifestations are associated with the full-blown clinical syndrome. Altered mental status, delirium, and neuropathies are sometimes so conspicuous that acute encephalopathy is the initial diagnostic impression. Gastrointestinal symptoms (diarrhea, nausea, vomiting) are also prominent. Disseminated intravascular coagulation, rhabdomyolysis, respiratory distress, shock, and acute renal failure are rare complications that contribute to mortality in sicker patients.

Treatment, prevention, and control. Empiric therapy of typical acute bacterial pneumonia should include coverage for *S. pneumoniae* (Table 32-1).[5] Until recently, penicillin, ampicillin, or similar β-lactam drugs were the preferred therapies. However, the prevalence of penicillin-resistant pneumococci is increasing in the United States, and penicillin therapy is no longer reliable for treatment for all cases of pneumococcal infection.[5,48] Uncomplicated cases of pneumonia caused by strains relatively resistant to penicillin (MIC 0.1 to 0.9 μg/ml) can be treated with parenteral penicillin unless central nervous system infection or localized abscesses are present. Infection caused by strains highly resistant to penicillin (MIC ≥1 μg/ml) must be treated with an alternative agent. Simultaneous resistance to cepahlosporins, erythromycin, and/or trimethoprim-sulfamethoxazole is increasing in some regions, and treatment should be based on knowledge of the local pneumococcal antimicrobial resistance profile. When in doubt, vancomycin is usually a good choice for empiric therapy, but a second agent must be added if gram-negative or anaerobic infections are included in the differential diagnosis. Erythromycin is the drug of choice for treating legionellosis (Table 32-1). It is also effective treatment for other common bacterial causes of atypical pneumonia and for most but not all strains of pneumococcus in the United States.

Preventing bacterial pneumonia is a difficult challenge. Workers at risk for pneumococcal and hemophilus infections should be immunized, although the efficacy of this approach among patients at highest risk is debated. Influenza immunization could eliminate a major risk factor for both primary and secondary bacterial pneumonias. Occupational exposures to potential pathogens should be reduced with proper ventilation and respiratory protection.

Unusual causes of occupational pneumonia

A careful occupational history should be obtained from all adults with pneumonia, especially in cases where the presentation is atypical, because occupational exposure causes many otherwise rare pneumonias. Public health authorities should be notified if an occupational source is suspected so that an epidemiologic investigation to identify transmission routes and other susceptibles may commence.

Bird handlers are at increased risk for infection with *Chlamydia psittaci*.[49] Most birds can harbor this organism, and human infections have been linked to parrots, parakeets, budgerigars, pigeons, ducks, chickens, turkeys, and more exotic birds. Infected birds may be asymptomatic or evidence signs of illness (lassitude, ruffled feathers, anorexia). Transmission is more frequent following exposure to symptomatic birds. The organism is present in the secretions, excreta, feathers, and tissues of birds and is usually transmitted through the respiratory route, although bite wounds have been implicated. Even relatively brief exposures can result in transmission of this pathogen.

Occupational contact with animals is also a clue to the etiology of several unusual pneumonias.[50] *Francisella tularensis* is the bacteria responsible for tularemia (rabbit fever).[51] This organism is ubiquitous in nature and has been isolated from mammals (rabbits, squirrels, deer, muskrats, cattle, sheep), birds, reptiles, and fish. Transmission occurs via direct inoculation, through aerosolization, or via various tick species that excrete the organism in their feces.[52] Rabbits are the most common source of infection and, not surprisingly, hunters, trappers, and veterinarians are at greatest risk. Inhalation pneumonia is a special risk for laboratory personnel who process specimens containing the organism without appropriate ventilation and containment procedures.

Sylvatic plague *(Yersinia pestis)* is present in a large number of animal species, particularly rodents. Humans acquire the infection through contact with rodents or their fleas, or from exposure to domestic pets infected through contact with wild animals.[53] Most cases of plague pneumonia in the United States are a consequence of septicemic or bubonic infection; person-to-person spread through infectious aerosols (pneumonic plague) is rare. However, the potential for respiratory transmission to susceptibles is high, especially in hospital settings, if the diagnosis is delayed and case isolation is not implemented during the period of contagion.

Anthrax is an extremely unusual cause of pulmonary infection in the United States but is an important problem in developing countries.[54] Agricultural cases arise from direct contact with animals, via insect vectors, and rarely, from ingestion of contaminated meat. Industrial anthrax (woolsorter's disease) is usually caused by inhalation of airborne anthrax spores contained in the hides, skins, or bones of infected animals being processed for commercial use.[55]

Several fungal pulmonary infections may have an occupational source.[56,57] Although they are often opportunistic pathogens in immunocompromised persons, pulmonary disease in otherwise healthy adults can occur. In nature, *Histoplasma capsulatum* grows well in moist soil fertilized with bird and bat feces. Infection is endemic in the Ohio River valley, midatlantic, and southeastern states. Inhalation follows excavation, cleaning, spelunking, or other activities that disturb infected soil. The initial pulmonary infection may be asymptomatic or suggest a viral infection. In most cases the illness is self-limited, but progressive disease, dissemination, and reactivation are serious sequels in some patients.

The soil is also the source of infections caused by *Coccidioides immitis*. This organism is prevalent in arid climates in regions of California and the southwest. Inhalation of airborne arthrospores produces a mild, self-limited respiratory illness (valley fever) that usually escapes detection unless clustering occurs. The majority of infections are asymptomatic. Progressive pulmonary, extrapulmonary, and disseminated diseases are serious complications of coccidiomycosis infection. Archaeologists, construction workers, and other outdoor employees are at increased risk. Laboratory personnel who handle cultures of the organism must exercise extreme caution to avoid inhaling the highly infectious mold form.

Blastomyces dermatiditis is a fungal organism present in the soil and decomposing organic material. Inhalation sometimes produces an acute, usually self-limited, pneumonia.[58,59] More typically, the disease is chronic and indolent, with progressive pulmonary or extrapulmonary manifestations. Although there is no clear-cut occupational predisposition, infections usually occur among hunters, woodsman, and persons enjoying recreational activities in wooded endemic areas.

The epidemiology of cryptococcal pneumonia is not well-defined. Although the organism *(Cryptococcus neoformans)* can be cultured from a variety of sources, including pigeon feces and the bark of eucalyptus trees, no evidence directly links environmental exposure to infection. Although cryptococcal infection is usually acquired through inhalation, most pulmonary infections are asymptomatic.

Cryptococcal infiltrates are nodular and well-defined densities sometimes confused with malignancies. Diffuse involvement is unusual in the absence of immunosuppression.

Tuberculosis

Epidemiology. Tuberculosis is caused by *Mycobacterium tuberculosis* and, rarely today, by *Mycobacterium bovis*. The incidence of tuberculosis began to increase in the mid-1980s, after years of steady decline.[60,61] Attrition of public health services, the concurrent HIV epidemic, and crowding of homeless individuals in shelters are important factors contributing to the resurgence in tuberculosis.

Tuberculosis is transmitted by inhalation of aerosolized droplet nuclei contained in the respiratory secretions of patients with active respiratory disease. Droplets are produced as a consequence of speech, coughing, sneezing, and even singing. Droplets suspended in the air desiccate and become infectious by virtue of their smaller particle diameter, which promotes escape from mucociliary clearance and deposition in the alveoli. Tuberculosis is not highly communicable, and prolonged exposure is usually required. Overall, less than 50% of household contacts of a sputum smear positive case will acquire infection, but close proximity increases the risk. Health care personnel, prison attendants, and other public service workers in settings where infected persons are housed are at risk for acquiring tuberculosis (see Chapter 44). Most other workers are not at risk unless close and sustained contact with an untreated person with active disease occurs in the workplace.

Clinical syndromes. The initial presentation of pulmonary tuberculosis is dependent on the interaction between the cellular immune and hypersensitivity responses to infection.[62] Initial infection in neonates often disseminates, and confers a high risk of meningitis and fatality. Infection in young children produces a localized infiltrate, often with hilar adenopathy, that may be entirely asymptomatic or confused with acute bacterial pneumonia. Teenagers and young adults are at higher risk for rapid progression to active disease, usually apical cavitary disease, than are older adults or young children. Primary infection is usually asymptomatic in mature adults. Primary infection in the elderly usually presents as lower lobe consolidation with hilar adenopathy and, again, can be confused with acute bacterial or aspiration pneumonia.

Asymptomatic dissemination to the gastrointestinal tract, bone, genitourinary tract, and other extrapulmonary sites may follow the initial infection. Infection is contained by the host's immune response at this stage, but reactivation may later ensue. The risk for reactivation is highest in the first year after exposure (5%) and declines thereafter (10% lifetime risk). However, aging, immunosuppression, intercurrent illness, alcoholism, and chronic malnutrition can increase the probability of reactivation or dissemination. In persons without severe immunosuppression, reactivation tuberculosis is usually manifest as upper lobe pulmonary cavitary disease, but virtually any organ system can be involved. In persons with acquired immunodeficiency syndrome (AIDS) or other forms of severe cellular immunodeficiency, diffuse or localized pulmonary infiltrates, with or without hilar adenopathy, are typical features of reactivation. Widespread dissemination and even bacteremia are not unusual sequels.

Prevention and control. Tuberculin skin testing allows diagnosis of prior exposure to tuberculosis in immunologically healthy adults by assessing delayed hypersensitivity to tuberculin antigens. The Mantoux test, performed by injecting 5 TU (0.0001 mg of polysorbate-stabilized purified protein derivative [PPD] in 0.1 ml solution) intracutaneously with a 26- or 27-gauge needle to raise a wheal on the volar forearm, is the best test for diagnosing tuberculosis exposure.[63] The reaction is read at 48 to 72 hours. The presence of more than 10 mm induration indicates a positive test, 5 to 10 mm indicates an indeterminate result, and less than 5 mm is negative. In HIV-infected persons, any reaction greater than 5 mm induration is read as positive. In persons with remote infection, the initial test may be falsely negative. A second test (two-step test) applied after 7 to 14 days may boost the hypersensitivity response. A positive "booster" test should not be interpreted as evidence of skin test conversion. In surveillance programs, two-step testing is sometimes employed for those not tested in the past 2 years to establish an accurate baseline assessment of tuberculosis risk.

A positive PPD test means an individual has been exposed to tuberculosis in the past and is at risk for disease. A baseline chest radiograph should be performed on all persons with newly diagnosed PPD positivity.[64] If the x-ray suggests active disease, sputum samples should be obtained, stained for acid-fast bacilli, and cultured for mycobacteria. Treatment should be implemented immediately if the index of suspicion is high. Public health officials should be notified to institute case management and evaluation of contacts in the home and work environment.

If the radiograph is negative, prophylactic treatment with isoniazid to suppress or eradicate latent organisms may be appropriate.[64] Persons with recent infection (skin test converters), reactors with negative sputum cultures but chest x-ray findings suggestive of past infection, immunosuppressed persons, household contacts of persons with active disease, and reactors under age 35 are candidates for prophylactic treatment. The risk of isoniazid-induced hepatotoxicity in older but otherwise healthy patients may exceed the expected benefit derived from preventing reactivation, but the treatment decision should be individualized.

M. tuberculosis is a relatively slow growing organism, and prolonged courses of therapy are necessary to cure infection (Table 32-2).[64-67] Combination treatment with isoniazid, rifampin, and pyrazinamide is the most common regimen for treating active pulmonary disease. If the epide-

Table 32-2. Initial treatment of tuberculosis*

Regimen	Drugs	Usual daily adult dose†	Duration‡ (months)
I§	Isoniazid	300 mg po or im	6-9
	Rifampin	600 mg po or iv	6-9
	Pyrazinamide	25 mg/kg po	2
II	Isoniazid	300 mg po or im	9-12
	Rifampin	600 mg po or iv	9-12
III	Rifampin	600 mg po or iv	12-18
	Ethambutol	15-25 mg/kg po	12-18
IV	Isoniazid	300 mp po or im	18-24
	Ethambutol	15-25 mg/kg po	18-24

*In areas where multiple drug resistance is not uncommon, initial therapy should be based on local resistance patterns after consultation with local public health officials.

†Intermittent rather than daily treatment regimens have also been proven efficacious and are more convenient for patients undergoing directly observed therapy.

‡Longer treatment may be required if clinical response is slow.

§Ethambutol (15-25 mg/kg) is added when the patient is at risk for isoniazid and/or rifampin resistance.

miology of infection suggests a potential for isoniazid resistance, then ethambutol is added to the initial regimen.

In some areas of the United States, a dramatic increase in the prevalence of multiple-drug resistant tuberculosis was noted in the late 1980s.[68] These strains of mycobacteria were efficiently disseminated in the community, in prisons, and in health care institutions. Failure to recognize drug resistance, implement proper treatment, and properly isolate infectious cases contributed to this problem. Treatment guidelines for drug-resistance mycobacterial infections must be individualized.[66,67] Empiric treatment should be designed to cover the most likely strains, but sensitivity testing is imperative to guide subsequent treatment decisions.

A major factor contributing to the resurgence of tuberculosis in most communities is the failure to achieve patient adherence to the treatment regimen. Increasing support for programs that provide directly observed therapies has already had a favorable impact on the incidence of tuberculosis in some communities. Studies of shorter treatment regimens and less frequent dosing are in progress and may improve patient compliance.

Case identification and treatment of cases and contacts are the main thrusts of tuberculosis control in the United States. Quarantine and isolation are not required. However, patients with untreated active infection should be housed in private rooms that meet ventilation standards for respiratory isolation. Protective masks are recommended for health care personnel in contact with active cases, but their value in preventing occupational transmission has not been proven. Concerns about spread of multiple-drug-resistant tuberculosis to health care personnel prompted efforts to heighten requirements for personal protection equipment in health care settings. Although the final federal recommendations have not yet been promulgated, high-energy particulate air filter (HEPA) respirators are likely to be required for some patient-care contacts (see Chapter 59).[69,70]

REFERENCES

1. Gwaltney JM Jr: Virology and immunology of the common cold. *Rhinology* 23:265-271, 1985.
2. Hornstrup MK, Trommer B, Siboni K, Nielsen B, and Kamper J: Nosocomial respiratory syncytial virus infections in a paediatric department. *J Hosp Infect* 26:173-179, 1994.
3. Hendley JO and Gwaltney JM Jr: Mechanisms of transmission of rhinovirus infections, *Epidemiol Rev* 10:243-258, 1988.
4. Gwaltney JM Jr, Scheld WM, Sande MA, and Sydnor A: The microbial etiology and antimicrobial therapy of adults with acute community-acquired sinusitis: a fifteen-year experience at the University of Virginia and review of other selected studies, *J Allergy Clin Immunol* 90:457-461, 1992.
5. Sanford JP, Gilbert D, Sande MA, and Gerberding JL: *Guide to antimicrobial therapy,* Dallas, TX, 1994, Antimicrobial Therapy.
6. Madge P, Paton JY, McColl JH, and Mackie PL: Prospective controlled study of four infection-control procedures to prevent nosocomial infection with respiratory syncytial virus, *Lancet* 340:1079-1083, 1992.
7. Ylikoski J and Karjalainen J: Acute tonsillitis in young men: etiological agents and their differentiation, *Scand J Infect Dis* 2:169-174, 1989.
8. Fox K, Turner J, and Fox A: Role of beta-hemolytic group C streptococci in pharyngitis: incidence and biochemical characteristics of Streptococcus equisimilis and Streptococcus anginosus in patients and healthy controls, *J Clin Microbiol* 31:804-807, 1993.
9. Wegner DL, Witte DL, and Schrantz RD: Insensitivity of rapid antigen detection methods and single blood agar plate culture for diagnosing streptococcal pharyngitis, *JAMA* 267:675-695, 1992.
10. Hoge CW, Schwartz B, Talkington DF, Breiman RF, MacNeill EM, and Englender SJ: The changing epidemiology of invasive group A streptococcal infections and the emergence of streptococcal toxic shock-like syndrome. A retrospective population-based study, *JAMA* 269:384-389, 1993.
11. Musser JM, Kapur V, Peters JE, et al: Real-time molecular epidemiologic analysis of an outbreak of Streptococcus pyogenes invasive disease in US Air Force trainees, *Arch Pathol Lab Med* 118:128-133, 1994.
12. Colman G, Tanna A, Efstratiou A, and Gaworzewska ET: The serotypes of Streptococcus pyogenes present in Britain during 1980-1990 and their association with disease, *J Med Microbiol* 39:165-178, 1993.
13. Ferrieri P and Kaplan EL: Invasive group A streptococcal infections, *Infect Dis Clin North Am* 6:149-161, 1992.

14. Stevens DL: Invasive group A streptococcus infections, *Clin Infect Dis* 14:2-11, 1992.
15. Sergent JS: Acute rheumatic fever, *Transact Am Clin Climatol Assoc* 104:15-23, 1992.
16. Harnisch JP, Tronca E, Nolan CM, Turck M, and Holmes KK: Diphtheria among alcoholic urban adults. A decade of experience in Seattle, *Ann Intern Med* 111:71-82, 1989.
17. Meira ZM, Mota C de C, Tonelli E, Nunan EA, Mitre AM, and Moreira NS: Evaluation of secondary prophylactic schemes, based on benzathine penicillin G, for rheumatic fever in children, *J Pediatr* 123:156-158, 1993.
18. Berrios X, del Campo E, Guzman B, and Bisno AL: Discontinuing rheumatic fever prophylaxis in selected adolescents and young adults. A prospective study, *Ann Intern Med* 118:401-406.
19. Hodder SL and Mortimer EA Jr: Epidemiology of pertussis and reactions to pertussis vaccine, *Epidemiol Rev* 14:243-267, 1992.
20. Herwaldt LA: Pertussis in adults. What physicians need to know, *Arch Intern Med* 151:1510-1512, 1991.
21. Weber DJ and Rutala WA: Management of healthcare workers exposed to pertussis, *Infect Control Hosp Epidemiol* 15:411-415, 1994.
22. Guide for Adult Immunization: *ACP task force on adult immunization and infectious diseases society of america,* ed 3, Philadelphia, 1994, American College of Physicians.
23. McIntosh K, Halonen P, and Ruuskanen Ö: Report of a workshop on respiratory viral infections: epidemiology, diagnosis, treatment, and prevention, *Clin Infect Dis* 16:151-164, 1993.
24. Ortiz CR and La Force FM: Prevention of community acquired pneumonia, *Med Clin North Am* 78:1173-1183, 1994.
25. Nicholson KG: Clinical features of influenza, *Semin Respir Infect* 7:26-37, 1992.
26. Prevention and control of influenza: Part 1. Vaccines. Recommendations of the Advisory Committee on Immunization Practices, *MMWR* 42:1-14, 1993.
27. Betts RF: Amantadine and rimantadine for the prevention of influenza A, *Semin Respir Infect* 4:304-310, 1989.
28. Monto AS and Arden NH: Implications of viral resistance to amantadine in control of influenza A, *Clin Infect Dis* 15:362-367, 1992.
29. Somani SK, Degelau J, Cooper SL, Guay DR, Ehresman D, and Zaske D: Comparison of pharmacokinetic and safety profiles of amantadine 50- and 100-mg daily doses in elderly nursing home residents, *Pharmacotherapy* 11:460-466, 1991.
30. Fang GD, Fine M, Orloff J, et al: New and emerging etiologies for community-acquired pneumonia with implications for therapy. A prospective multicenter study of 359 cases, *Medicine* 69:307-316, 1990.
31. Berman S: Acute respiratory infections, *Infect Dis Clin North Am* 5:319-336, 1991.
32. Lehtomaki K, Leinonen M, Takala A, Hovi T, Herva E, and Koskela M: Etiological diagnosis of pneumonia in military conscripts by combined use of bacterial culture and serological methods, *Eur J Clin Microbiol Infect Dis* 7:348-354, 1988.
33. Ostergaard L and Andersen PL: Etiology of community-acquired pneumonia. Evaluation by transtracheal aspiration, blood culture, or serology, *Chest* 104:1400-1407, 1993.
34. Gwaltney JM Jr, Sande MA, Austrian R, and Hendley JO: Spread of Streptococcus pneumoniae in families. II. Relation of transfer of S. pneumoniae to incidence of colds and serum antibody, *J Infect Dis* 132:62-68, 1975.
35. Wallace RJ Jr, Musher DM, and Martin RR: Hemophilus influenzae pneumonia in adults, *Am J Med* 64:87-93, 1978.
36. Martin RE and Bates JH: Atypical pneumonia, *Infect Dis Clin North Am* 5:585-601, 1991.
37. Foy HM: Infections caused by Mycoplasma pneumoniae and possible carrier state in different populations of patients, *Clin Infect Dis* 17:Suppl 1:S37-46, 1993.
38. Almirall J, Morato I, Riera F, et al: Incidence of community-acquired pneumonia and Chlamydia pneumoniae infection: a prospective multicentre study, *Eur Respir J* 6:14-18, 1993.
39. Pacheco A, Gonzalez-Sainz J, Arocena C, Rebollar M, Antela A, and Guerrero A: Community acquired pneumonia caused by Chlamydia pneumoniae strain TWAR in chronic cardiopulmonary disease in the elderly, *Respiration* 58:316-320, 1991.
40. Wreghitt TG: Pneumonia due to Chlamydia pneumoniae strain TWAR, *Clin Infect Dis* 17:926, 1993.
41. Grayston JT: Infections caused by Chlamydia pneumoniae strain TWAR, *Clin Infect Dis* 15:757-761, 1992.
42. Ekman MR, Grayston JT, Visakorpi R, Kleemola M, Kuo CC, and Saikku P: An epidemic of infections due to Chlamydia pneumoniae in military conscripts, *Clin Infect Dis* 17:420-425, 1993.
43. Davis GS and Winn WC Jr: Legionnaires' disease: respiratory infections caused by Legionella bacteria, *Clin Chest Med* 8:419-439, 1987.
44. Lowry PW and Tompkins LS: Nosocomial legionellosis: a review of pulmonary and extrapulmonary syndromes, *Am J Infect Control* 21:21-27, 1993.
45. Vandenesch F, Surgot M, Bornstein N, et al: Relationship between free amoeba and Legionella: studies in vitro and in vivo, *Int J Med Microbiol* 272:265-275, 1990.
46. Hart CA and Makin T: Legionella in hospitals: a review, *J Hosp Infect* 18 Suppl A:481-489, 1991.
47. Granados A, Podzamczer D, Gudiol F, and Manresa F: Pneumonia due to Legionella pneumophila and pneumococcal pneumonia: similarities and differences on presentation, *Eur Respir J* 2:130-134, 1989.
48. Breiman RF, Butler JC, Tenover FC, Elliott JA, and Facklam RR: Emergence of drug-resistant pneumococcal infections in the United States, *JAMA* 271:1831-1835, 1994.
49. Kirchner JT and Boyarsky SA: Chlamydia psittaci. An uncommon cause of community-acquired pneumonia, *Arch Family Med* 2:997-1001, 1993.
50. Weinberg AN: Respiratory infections transmitted from animals, *Infect Dis Clin North Am* 5:649-661, 1991.
51. Evans ME, Gregory DW, Schaffner W, and McGee ZA: Tularemia: a 30-year experience with 88 cases, *Medicine* 64:251-269, 1985.
52. Scofield RH, Lopez EJ, and McNabb SJ: Tularemia pneumonia in Oklahoma, 1982-1987, *J Oklahoma State Med Assoc* 85:165-170, 1992.
53. Pneumonic plague—Arizona, 1992: *MMWR* 41:737-739, 1992.
54. Abramova FA, Grinberg LM, Yampolskaya OV, and Walker DH: Pathology of inhalational anthrax in 42 cases from the Sverdlovsk outbreak of 1979, *Proc Natl Acad Sci U.S.A.* 90:2291-2294, 1993.
55. Enticknap JB, Galbraith NS, Tomlinson AJ, and Elias-Jones TF: Pulmonary anthrax caused by contaminated sacks, *Br J Ind Med* 25:72-74, 1968.
56. Davies SF: Fungal pneumonia, *Med Clin North Am* 78:1049-1065, 1994.
57. Sarosi GA: Community-acquired fungal diseases, *Clin Chest Med* 12:337-347, 1991.
58. Bradsher RW: Blastomycosis, *Clin Infect Dis* 14 Suppl 1:S82-90, 1992.
59. Vaaler AK, Bradsher RW, and Davies SF: Evidence of subclinical blastomycosis in forestry workers in northern Minnesota and northern Wisconsin, *Am J Med* 89:470-476, 1990.
60. Cantwell MF, Snider DE Jr, Cauthen GM, and Onorato IM: Epidemiology of tuberculosis in the United States, 1985 through 1992, *JAMA* 272:535-539, 1994.
61. Barnes PF and Barrows SA: Tuberculosis in the 1990s, *Ann Intern Med* 119:400-410, 1993.
62. Korzeniewska-Kosela M, Krysl J, Muller N, Black W, Allen E, and FitzGerald JM: Tuberculosis in young adults and the elderly. A prospective comparison study, *Chest* 106:28-32, 1994.
63. Diagnostic standards and classification of tuberculosis. *Am Rev Respir Dis* 142:725-735, 1990.

64. Bass JB Jr, Farer LS, Hopewell PC, et al: Treatment of tuberculosis and tuberculosis infection in adults and children. American Thoracic Society and The Centers for Disease Control and Prevention, *Am J Respir Crit Care Med* 149:1359-1374, 1994.

65. Brausch LM and Bass JB Jr: The treatment of tuberculosis, *Med Clin North Am* 77:1277-1288, 1993.

66. Iseman MD: Treatment of multidrug-resistant tuberculosis, *N Engl J Med* 329:784-791, 1993.

67. Initial therapy for tuberculosis in the era of multidrug resistance: recommendations of the Advisory Council for the Elimination of Tuberculosis, *JAMA* 270:694-698, 1993.

68. Bloch AB, Cauthen GM, Onorato IM, et al: Nationwide survey of drug-resistant tuberculosis in the United States, *JAMA* 271:665-671, 1994.

69. Adal KA, Anglim AM, Palumbo CL, Titus MG, Coyner BJ, and Farr BM: The use of high-efficiency particulate air-filter respirators to protect hospital workers from tuberculosis. A cost-effectiveness analysis, *N Engl J Med* 331:169-173, 1994.

70. Guidelines for preventing the transmission of Mycobacterium tuberculosis in health-care facilities, *MMWR* 43:1-132, 1994.

Chapter 33

DIESEL EXHAUST

Eric Garshick
Marc B. Schenker

DEFINITION
Classification

Physical state. Diesel exhaust is not a single compound but is made up of thousands of chemicals.[1-3] It can be broadly divided into a gaseous phase and a particulate phase, with each phase made up of organic and inorganic compounds. The vapor phase includes carbon monoxide, sulfur dioxide, various oxides of nitrogen (NO_x), various aldehydes (such as acrolein, formaldehyde, and acetaldehyde), and other hydrocarbons. The particulate phase consists of clusters of respirable inorganic particles made mostly of carbon. Adsorbed to these particles are numerous complex organic compounds, mainly polycyclic aromatic hydrocarbons (PAH) and related chemicals (Table 33-1). Primary particles formed during combustion aggregate to form spongelike clusters and chains, most with diameters of up to 0.1 to 0.2 μm (Fig. 33-1).[4] Respirable particles of this size (<5 to 10 μm) are readily inhaled into the alveolar part of the lung.

The distribution of various chemicals in diesel engine exhaust depends on numerous factors (Table 33-2). One factor, the composition of diesel fuel, can significantly influence emissions. Diesel fuel contains aliphatic hydrocarbons of 9 to 28 carbon atoms and boils at 160° C to 390° C.[3,5] Diesel fuel No. 1 is similar to kerosene and contains predominantly normal alkanes with very low levels of PAH.

Diesel fuel No. 2, used in engines in mobile service, is similar to European automotive diesel fuel and may contain less than 5% or as much as 10% PAH. Diesel fuel No. 4 (or marine diesel, which is more viscous than diesel fuel No. 2), may also contain variable amounts of PAH and has a higher sulfur content than other grades. Diesel fuel No. 4 is used for stationary engines in continuous high load service, barges, and railroad engines.[5] The greater the aromatic content of the fuel, the greater the emissions of particles and PAH.[3,6,7] A higher fuel sulfur content is also associated with increased particle emissions.[3] Lubricating oil may also be a source of particle and PAH emissions due to potential oil leakage into the combustion chamber, particularly in older engines.[2] PAHs accumulate in diesel engine oil during fuel combustion.[8] Additives that improve the ignition quality of the fuel, oxidation inhibitors, and corrosion inhibitors also influence particle emissions[9] and may either increase or decrease emissions.[2]

Table 33-1. Various chemicals in diesel exhaust[1-3]

Gas phase	Formaldehyde, acrolein, acetaldehyde, oxides of nitrogen, sulfur dioxide, carbon monoxide, C_1-C_{18} hydrocarbons, two to four ring PAHs, nitrated and oxygenated C_1-C_{10} hydrocarbons
Particulate phase	PAH compounds, PAH ketones, PAH carboxaldehydes, PAH acid anhydrides, hydroxy-PAHs, PAH quinones, nitro-PAH

PAH, Polycyclic aromatic hydrocarbon.

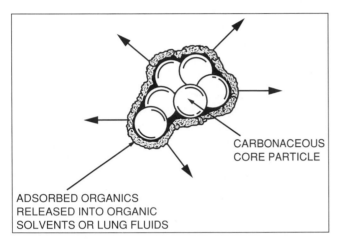

Fig. 33-1. Schematic representation of a diesel exhaust particle. (Adapted from Wolff et al.[4])

Diesel engine design (such as type of fuel injection) and operating conditions can also influence the chemical composition of diesel exhaust.[2] In general, at high engine loads, PAH and particle emissions increase, and increasing the ratio of fuel to air also leads to more emissions. However, when the amount of oxygen available for combustion is increased, more NO_x is formed. Cold starts, as compared with starting a warm engine, lead to more PAH and particle emissions.[6,8] Compared with emissions from gasoline engines with catalytic converters, diesel engine particle emissions are 30 to 100 times greater, and, consequently, there are more PAH compounds since these are associated with particles.[10-12] Levels of carbon monoxide and nitrogen oxides are similar for both light duty diesel and gasoline engines with catalytic converters.[3]

The International Agency for Research on Cancer regulatory classification. In the late 1970s, there was increased concern about the potential health effects of diesel exhaust. Diesel equipment use in underground mines was increasing.[13] As a result of rising fuel costs associated with gasoline-powered vehicles, it was projected that diesel-powered vehicles would constitute 18% of light-duty vehicle sales in the United States by 1985 and as much as 25% by the turn of the century.[14,15] The conclusions of a

Table 33-2. Factors influencing emissions from diesel engines

Factor	Result
Diesel fuel composition	
Increase in aromatic content	Increase in PAH, particles
Increase in sulfur content	Increase in particles
Various fuel additives	May increase or decrease particle emissions
Lubrication oil	May contribute to PAH emissions if leaks into combustion chamber
Engine operating conditions	
Increased load	Increase in PAH, particles
Increase in fuel-to-air ratio	Increase in PAH, particles
Decrease in fuel-to-air ratio	Increase in NO_x
Older engines	Increase in PAH, particles
Cold starts	Increase in PAH, particles

PAH, Polycyclic aromatic hydrocarbon.

1977 workshop on underground diesel use in mines[13] sponsored by the National Institute of Occupational Safety and Health (NIOSH) and a 1981 National Research Council report[14] commissioned by the U.S. Environmental Protection Agency (EPA), the Department of Energy, and the Department of Transportation were that no firm conclusions could be reached about the carcinogenic and noncarcinogenic health effects of diesel exhaust exposure in humans. Additional research was suggested. However, projections made in the 1970s regarding light-duty vehicle diesel use in the United States were not correct, with considerably fewer light-duty diesel-powered vehicles in use and now projected to be in service by the year 2000.

Following these reports epidemiologic studies in railroad workers were completed suggesting that diesel exhaust may be a human lung carcinogen.[16,17] Inhalation studies in rats[18-23] exposed to high levels of diesel exhaust have also resulted in lung tumors. On the basis of these reports, in 1988 NIOSH recommended that whole diesel exhaust be regarded as a potential occupational carcinogen.[24] Later studies in humans in motor exhaust-related occupations,[25,26] bus garage workers,[27] and dock workers[28] support this conclusion.

The International Agency for Research on Cancer (IARC)[3] has concluded that there is sufficient evidence for the carcinogenicity of whole diesel exhaust in experimental animals. There was inadequate evidence in animals for the vapor phase alone (with particles removed). Accordingly, there was sufficient evidence in animals for the carcinogenicity of extracts of diesel exhaust particles. In humans, there was limited evidence for the carcinogenicity of diesel exhaust. Based on these conclusions in human populations and on the results in animals, IARC classified diesel exhaust as a Group 2A human carcinogen, meaning that diesel exhaust is probably carcinogenic to humans. For gasoline exhaust, IARC felt that there was inadequate evidence for carcinogenicity.

Brief summary of human health effects

The health effects of diesel exhaust are due to exposure to both the vapor and particle phases. Exposure to diesel exhaust causes irritation of the eyes.[29,30] The odor of diesel exhaust is characteristic and is not tolerated by some.[31,32] Mucous membrane irritation, headache, and nausea have been reported after acute exposure.[33,34] Although there have been recent cases of asthma attributable to diesel exhaust,[35] other chronic effects on lung function and respiratory symptoms have not been documented in humans. Short-term reductions in pulmonary function across a work shift due to diesel exhaust exposure have been reported in stevedores[36] but not in bus garage workers[33] or coal miners.[37]

Since diesel particles are respirable, studies of the relationship between cancer and diesel exhaust exposure have focused on the occurrence of lung cancer. As noted, there is evidence based on epidemiologic studies in occupationally exposed workers that suggests that whole diesel exhaust is a human lung carcinogen.[16,17,25-28] However, only limited measurements of actual diesel exhaust exposure are available in these studies, and analysis was based mainly on job title. Consequently, it is not possible to conclude from human studies the level of diesel exhaust exposure experienced by these workers that resulted in the observed lung cancer risk. The occurrence of bladder cancer in humans due to exposure to diesel exhaust has also been studied, but a causal relationship is far less clear than for lung cancer.[3]

UTILIZATION AND SOURCES OF EXPOSURE
Occupational exposures

In 1983 NIOSH estimated that approximately 1.35 million workers were occupationally exposed to the combustion products of diesel fuel.[24] Occupations with potential exposure include mine workers, bridge and tunnel workers, railroad workers, loading dock workers, truck drivers, forklift drivers, farm workers, auto, truck, and bus maintenance garage workers, firefighters in fire stations, and operators of heavy construction equipment (see box).[3,24,38]

Diesel engines are used in underground coal, metal, and nonmetal mines throughout the world. They are used to power underground locomotives, mining utility vehicles, shuttle vehicles, and a variety of specialty vehicles used in coal mines such as load-haul-dump units.[39,40] In 1970 and 1971 there were 3,000 diesel-powered units in United States metal and nonmetal underground mines, and by 1976 there were 4,400 units in service.[13] In U.S. underground coal mines in 1977 there were only 162 pieces of diesel equipment in service,[13] with 2,224 units in service by 1993.[41] Diesel-powered heavy equipment is also used in surface mining operations. In U.S. surface coal mines in 1993 there were 25,910 diesel-powered units projected to be in service,

> **Occupations with potential exposure to diesel exhaust**
>
> Workers in mines with diesel-powered equipment
> Bus and diesel truck garage workers
> Other diesel vehicle repair workers
> Truck drivers
> Railroad workers who work around operating trains
> Railroad locomotive repair workers
> Forklift and other drivers of diesel vehicles
> Operators of heavy construction equipment
> Farm workers operating diesel equipment
> Ferry and dock workers
> Bridge and tunnel workers
> Firefighters

including drills, scrapers, backhoes, graders, trucks, bulldozers, and front-end loaders.[42] In 1993 there were 10,635 workers employed in U.S. underground metal and nonmetal mines and 50,262 workers in underground coal mines. In surface coal mining operations there were 36,398 workers, and in other surface mining operations there were 85,117 workers.[42] Other U.S. estimates of nonroad diesel use include 2.5 million tractors used in agriculture and 1.5 million units of heavy construction equipment.[43] In 1993 there were 18,004 diesel-powered locomotives in service in the United States in Class I Railroads.[44] In addition, in 1991 there were an estimated 318,000 diesel buses that were registered, roughly 50% of all bus registrations.[45,46] Individuals engaged in operating and maintaining these vehicles are among those potentially exposed to diesel exhaust. The degree of exposure experienced by an individual worker will vary depending on proximity to the source of the exhaust, the degree of local ventilation, the condition of the engine, and how the engine is operated.

Since the major concern of recent epidemiologic studies has been the occurrence of lung cancer in diesel exhaust-exposed workers, the focus of occupational exposure assessment has been on respirable particle measurement rather than on constituents from the gaseous phase of diesel exhaust. However, there has been difficulty in determining the precise contribution of diesel exhaust to respirable particles inhaled by a potentially exposed worker, even when personal sampling is done. Respirable particles inhaled by a worker include not only those derived from diesel engines, but also cigarette particulate and other particles generated as a result of the worker's job or workplace environment, such as sand, dirt, coal dust, and fibers. Thus, total respirable particulate values reported in workers with potential exposure to diesel exhaust can overestimate actual exposure. Two occupationally exposed groups most extensively investigated illustrating this point are railroad workers[47-50] working on and around operating trains and mechanics and truck drivers in the trucking industry.[51,52]

In railroad workers, cigarette smoke was found to account for a substantial proportion of total respirable particulate matter. As part of an epidemiologic study,[16,17] both diesel-exposed and unexposed railroad workers had respirable particles measured by personal sampling.[47] Clerks (diesel unexposed workers) had a mean respirable particulate level of 125 μg/m^3 unadjusted for cigarette smoke and a level of 42 μg/m^3 when cigarette particulate was subtracted, a reduction of 66% (Table 33-3). In locomotive repair shops, diesel machinists had a mean respirable particulate level of 147 μg/m^3 when cigarette particulate was considered, a reduction of 23%, and yard engineers and firemen exposed to diesel exhaust from operating trains had a mean level of 69 μg/m^3 when cigarette particulate was considered, a reduction of 36% compared with total respirable particulate (Table 33-3). Thus, cigarette smoke can account for a large fraction of the emissions of respirable particles, particularly if sources of other respirable particles are low.

In railroad workers, the extent that respirable particles adjusted for cigarette smoke represented diesel exhaust exposure depended on job location and duties (Table 33-3).[47,49,53]

It has been suggested that a more specific marker of diesel exhaust exposure is particle-associated organic matter, adjusted for cigarette particulate.[49] Organic matter associated with diesel particles can be extracted from the particles by using a solvent (dichloromethane) and expressed as weight per cubic meter of air. However, measurement of extractable matter is complex and costly, and because small amounts are measured (extractable percentage by weight varied from 16% to 49% of the collected respirable particles in one study),[49] there is more error possible. Contaminants from other combustion sources (such as kerosene heaters and stoves) may also contribute to extractable matter, such as in the clerks, who did not have exposure to diesel, but who had a similar concentration of extractable matter as the freight brakemen who are exposed to diesel exhaust from operating trains (Table 33-3).

In a study of trucking industry workers (road drivers, local drivers, dock workers, and mechanics) elemental carbon, which is derived from the core of the diesel exhaust particle, was chosen as the principal marker of diesel exhaust exposure.[51,52] The contribution of elemental carbon to tobacco smoke was only 1.5% to 2% in exposure chamber studies, making it unlikely that cigarette particulate would contribute significantly to measurements of elemental carbon. The contribution of particles from other combustion sources (gasoline, propane) to elemental carbon was also small relative to diesel exposure, as was the contribution of "background" particles to elemental carbon levels.[51]

Elemental carbon was found to be about 20% of respirable particles, allowing the estimation of exposure to diesel exhaust particles (Table 33-4).[51,52] Mechanics and dock workers had the highest exposure to diesel exhaust, whereas truck drivers had lower levels of exposure. The exposure of truck drivers (based on elemental carbon) is lower than exposure to diesel exhaust in the railroad industry (based on adjusted respirable particulate). Organic carbon was also measured in the trucking industry and correlated only moderately with elemental carbon for nonsmokers in various job

Table 33-3. Total respirable particulate, respirable particulate adjusted for cigarette particulate, and extractable matter adjusted for cigarette particulate (in μg/m^3)

Job category	*n*	Total respirable mean (SD)	Adjusted respirable mean (SD)	*n*	Adjusted extractable mean
Clerks	59	125 (75)	42 (36)	36	7.2
Signal maintainer	13	69 (39)	58 (33)	14	23
Engineers, fireman					
Freight	55	115 (67)	94 (55)	37	30
Yard	50	108 (109)	69 (70)	21	16
Passenger	23	75 (52)	51 (35)	20	24
Brakeman, conductor					
Freight conductor	62	126 (65)	69 (52)	48	30
Freight brakeman	21	145 (80)	102 (62)	16	7.9
Passenger	35	111 (62)	104 (58)	33	27
Yard	32	180 (117)	114 (76)	23	17
Hostler	8	231 (134)	224 (130)	8	33
Shop					
Electrician	42	256 (332)	192 (248)	15	44*
Machinist	110	191 (146)	147 (120)	35	79*
Supervisor, laborer, Other	24	244 (141)	155 (83)	22	43

Adapted from Woskie SR, Smith TJ, Hammond SK, Schenker MB, Garshick E, and Speizer FE: Estimation of the diesel exposures of railroad workers: I. current exposures, *Am J Ind Med* 13:381-394, copyright © 1988, Wiley-Liss, Inc., a subsidiary of John Wiley & Sons, Inc.[47] and Hammond et al.[49]

*Winter sample only for adjusted extractable matter. In summer, adjusted extractable matter for electricians = 30 μg/m^3 (*n* = 16) and for machinists = 32 μg/m^3.

groups (r = 0.62 to 0.71). The correlation between respirable dust and elemental carbon was also moderate (r = 0.84). As with railroad workers, there were potential sources of organic carbon in the workplace other than diesel exhaust, such as grease, oil, and degreasing solvents. The use of elemental carbon as a marker of diesel exhaust exposure presumably avoided confusing exposure to diesel exhaust with exposure to these other sources of organic carbon. It is clear that the degree a particular marker of diesel exhaust exposure actually represents true exposure depends on the nature of all sources of respirable particles in the workplace.

Only measurements of respirable dust exist for workers in other industries. It is not known the extent that diesel exhaust contributed to these measurements since other sources of respirable particles are also found in these work areas (such as coal dust in mines). Consequently, measurements of respirable particles in coal miners exposed to diesel exhaust have varied considerably, with a mean of 2,000 $\mu g/m^3$ obtained by personal sampling in one study,[37] and means of 930 to 2,730 $\mu g/m^3$ by personal sampling and area levels of 0 to 16,100 $\mu g/m^3$ over six mines in another study.[54] In salt miners, mean personal exposure levels were 560 to 590 $\mu g/m^3$.[55] In stevedores exposed to diesel trucks, mean respirable dust levels of 230 $\mu g/m^3$ were reported[56] and in a tunnel construction site with diesel construction equipment mean levels of 1,160 $\mu g/m^3$ were reported.[57] In four diesel bus garages, mean personal respirable dust levels of 120 to 610 $\mu g/m^3$ were measured.[33]

Within a given industry, the extent of diesel exhaust exposure may vary considerably depending on working conditions and job title. Truck mechanics[51] and locomotive repair shop workers[47] had mean exposures in cold weather roughly two or more times the warm weather levels, likely due to reduction in the degree of repair shop ventilation in cold weather. Railroad repair shop workers also had exposure levels roughly 1.5 to 2.5 times greater than engineers, conductors, brakemen, and firemen.[47] The extent of diesel exhaust exposure over a worker's lifetime can vary even if the worker held the same job title. In the railroad industry, the diesel engines first introduced in the 1950s were said to be "smokier" than locomotives introduced during the

Table 33-4. Exposure to respirable diesel exhaust particles ($\mu g/m^3$) in the trucking industry

	n	Elemental carbon mean (SE)	Estimated diesel particulate
Dock workers	54	31.3 (2.45)	156.5
Mechanics	80	26.6 (4.1)	133.0
Local drivers	56	5.4 (0.9)	27.0
Road drivers	72	5.1 (0.4)	25.5

Adapted from Zaebst et al.,[51] based on the assumption that elemental carbon is 20% of respirable dust.

1960s.[48] Smaller railroads tended to use these older diesel locomotives more than the larger U.S. railroads. Diesel repair shop design also changed throughout the years, and based on historical measurements of nitrogen dioxide, measurements of diesel exhaust constituents may have been tenfold higher in older shops that were busier and more poorly ventilated.[48] Constituents of the gaseous phase of diesel exhaust have also been measured in various workplaces (Table 33-5). These reported values demonstrate that occupational exposure to diesel exhaust may vary considerably.

Environmental exposure

Combustion products of fossil fuels contribute to air pollution, and motor vehicles are major sources of suspended

Table 33-5. Summary of exposure to gaseous constituents of diesel exhaust in various occupational environments

Work area	Exposure	Reference
Six coal mines	Short-term area samples Mean NO_x: 0-5.2 ppm Mean NO_2: 0-0.9 ppm Mean CO: 3.4-23.2 ppm	54
Salt mines	Calculated mean exposure Mean NO_2: 0.2-2.5 ppm	55
Six potash mines	Personal samples Mean NO_2: 0.7-3.2 ppm Area samples Mean CO: 5-9 ppm Aldehydes: 0.1-4 ppm	58
Ferry stevedores	Personal and area samples Mean CO: 2.23 ppm Mean formaldehyde: 0.03 ppm Mean NO_x: 1.12 ppm	56
Four bus garages	Personal samples Mean NO_2: 0.13-0.56 ppm	33
Railroad roundhouses	Area samples Formaldehyde: mean 0.16 ppm (0-0.8 ppm) Acrolein: mean 0.03 ppm (0-0.2 ppm) NO_x: mean 2.55 ppm (0-10 ppm)	59
Locomotive cabs	Formaldehyde: mean 0.01 ppm (0-0.1 ppm) Acrolein: mean 0.01 ppm (0-0.1 ppm) NO_x: mean 2.35 ppm (0-2.0 ppm)	

particulate matter, carbon monoxide, NO_x, and hydrocarbons that react with NO_2 to form ozone. These pollutants are not unique to diesel exhaust. However, changes in diesel vehicle use would have the potential to significantly contribute to ambient concentrations of respirable particles. In 1980, Bradow[60] estimated that 15% of the fine particles in U.S. cities were from mobile sources, mostly due to diesel-powered vehicles. Based on estimates that 20% of the light duty vehicles in the United States would become diesel powered, Cuddihy and co-workers[61] estimated at a roadside with 10,000 vehicles/hr passing, the total particle level would be 35 $\mu g/m^3$, and 100 m from the highway, the particle level would be 6 $\mu g/m^3$. In a Manhattan street canyon, with the assumption that 40% of the vehicles were diesel (based on conversion of all taxis to light-duty diesel vehicles), there would be an estimated particle level of 30 $\mu g/m^3$. These estimates were based on emission rates for diesel vehicles manufactured in the early 1980s, rather than on current standards. Total particles include respirable particles plus larger particles, but, as previously noted, most of the particles derived from diesel exhaust would be respirable. In comparison, in six eastern U.S. cities, depending on the degree of industrialization and urbanization, measured mean total particle levels between 1977 and 1985 were 34.1 to 89.9 $\mu g/m^3$, mean levels of respirable particles averaged 18.2 to 46.5 $\mu g/m^3$, and mean levels of fine particles (<2.5 μm) ranged from 11.0 to 29.6 $\mu g/m^3$ between 1979 and 1985.[62]

Thus, when compared with actual measured average levels of ambient particles, it was predicted that diesel-powered vehicles could significantly contribute to particulate air pollution in urban areas if there was an increase in diesel-powered light-duty vehicles.

In a study done in 1984 in Vienna, Austria a tracer element was put in diesel fuel to help measure ambient concentrations of particles attributable to diesel.[63] Seven percent of motor vehicles in Vienna were diesel powered, mostly trucks and buses. The mass concentrations of diesel particles varied between 10 and 26 $\mu g/m^3$. The usual background diesel particle level was estimated to be 11 $\mu g/m^3$ and increased by 5.5 $\mu g/m^3$ for each 500 diesel vehicles passing by per hour. These measurements also suggest that diesel-powered vehicles can significantly contribute to urban particulate air pollution.

The forecasted increase in U.S. light duty vehicles did not occur, both as a result of the increase in gasoline supply and drop in price, and reliability difficulties with diesel automobile engines. In 1991 only 8,154 diesel cars were sold in the United States, representing 0.16% of all new car sales.[64] In 1992, this number fell to 5,177 diesel-powered new cars, representing 0.06% of all new car sales. In contrast, in 1981, new car diesel sales peaked at 520,788 cars, 6.1% of sales. In other countries, diesel-powered cars make up a greater proportion of new vehicles (Table 33-6),[46] with up to 25% of the new cars sold in France in 1991 powered by a diesel engine. However, heavy duty trucks and buses in the United States are still commonly diesel powered (Table 33-7).[65] For buses, of the total 1991 diesel bus registration noted previously, 51,312 buses are in public transit systems, most of which are urban diesel buses.[66] The total number of diesel buses is projected to increase such that by 2000, 568,000 diesel buses will be registered. It is estimated that by 2019, all school buses registered will be diesel powered, with a total registration of 1,250,782 diesel-powered buses.[45] Thus, the regulation of diesel-powered light-duty vehicles is more of a concern in Europe, whereas in the United States, current regulations have targeted mainly heavy duty trucks and buses.

Table 33-6. Number of diesel vehicles and percent of new car sales in selected countries in 1991[46]

Country	Diesel vehicles	New car sales in 1991 (%)
France	811,333	25.5
Germany	711,347	15.3
Italy	121,044	7.4
Spain	258,328	14.6
U.K.	140,190	11.3
Japan	805,792	8.3

Table 33-7. Estimated number of diesel vehicles in the United States, and percent total registrations in each vehicle class in 1993, 1995, and 2000[65]

| | Cars | Light duty | Heavy duty trucks | | |
			Light	Medium	Heavy
1993	1,219,000	757,000	1,106,000	1,131,000	1,531,000
	(0.93%)	(1.5%)	(20.7%)	(49.1%)	(99.5%)
1995	1,106,000	864,000	1,288,000	1,231,000	1,600,000
	(0.81%)	(1.6%)	(22.9%)	(53.9%)	(99.6%)
2000	1,314,000	1,163,000	1,675,000	1,491,000	1,773,000
	(0.90%)	(1.8%)	(27.0%)	(62.55)	(99.9%)

EFFECTS OVERVIEW AND GENERAL MECHANISMS
Nonneoplastic effects

Effects in humans. Diesel exhaust is often visible as black smoke with a characteristic odor coming from the tailpipe of a diesel vehicle. Early research focused on the chemicals in diesel exhaust that were responsible for the odor, and attempts were made to characterize the public's response to odor by establishing rating scales for odor intensity.[31,32,67] The exact chemicals responsible for the odor of diesel exhaust have not been identified.[68] However, it was estimated that at least 200 chemicals can contribute to an "oily-kerosene odor" and over 2,000 chemicals can cause a "smoky-burnt" odor.[67] The study of the recognition of the odor of diesel exhaust in humans was halted by the EPA in the late 1970s when it was recognized that diesel particles had significant potential for adverse health effects.

Diesel exhaust can also cause eye, nose, and throat irritation. Acetaldehyde, formaldehyde, and acrolein are constituents of diesel exhaust whose irritant effects are well described.[69] The levels of formaldehyde reported in the previous section during occupational exposure to diesel exhaust are sufficient to result in irritation of the eyes, nose, and throat. In addition, other diesel exhaust constituents may be responsible for irritant effects, such as nitric acid (from NO_2) or sulfur dioxide. Various diesel exhaust constituents may also interact to contribute to mucous membrane irritation.[70,71] Acute decrements in lung function have also been described after exposure to diesel exhaust,[36] as have case reports of asthma.[35] Although formaldehyde is also a rare cause of occupational asthma,[72] and sulfur dioxide inhalation can cause bronchoconstriction, there is little information on the specific levels of exposure to diesel exhaust that have resulted in irritant effects or acute effects on lung function. In particular, the potential interaction of diesel particles and various constituents in the gaseous phase to cause acute irritant symptoms and acute changes in lung function is unknown.

Effects in animals.
Acute effects in animals. Pattle and co-workers[30] exposed mice, guinea pigs, and rabbits to undiluted diesel exhaust under varying load and fuel-air ratios that resulted in high concentrations of NO_2 (12 to 51 ppm), formaldehyde (6.0 to 154 ppm), carbon monoxide (0.056% to 0.17%), and particles (53 to 1,070 mg/m^3). Exposure was generally 5 hours per day for 7 days per week. Varying numbers of animals died, with autopsies showing pulmonary edema and variable amounts of tracheal and bronchial damage. At the higher levels of exposure to carbon monoxide, death was due to carbon monoxide poisoning. The levels of diesel exhaust constituents reported here are much higher than reported during usual occupational exposures, but it is possible that during exposure in an enclosed, poorly ventilated area there would be unusually high levels of concentrations of these diesel exhaust constituents.

Short-term exposure to diesel exhaust diluted with air has also been assessed in animals. Cats exposed to diluted diesel exhaust for 28 consecutive days, for 20 hours per day, at an average particle concentration of 6.4 mg/m^3, NO of 6.13 ppm, NO_2 of 2.13 ppm, and SO_2 of 2.10 ppm had no significant changes in total lung capacity (TLC), vital capacity (VC), dynamic compliance, and diffusion capacity compared with a control group of cats.[73] Compared with the controls, the exposed cats had a slightly greater residual volume (RV). The maximum expiratory flow rates at 50%, 25%, and 10% of the VC were diminished compared with the controls but were significant only for the maximum expiratory flow rate at 10% of the VC. No animal died as a result of exposure. When the animals were sacrificed, the lungs of the exposed cats were charcoal gray with some lungs containing 0.5- to 1.0-mm black foci on the pleural surface. There were black pigmented alveolar macrophages in the alveoli and adherent to the mucosa of the trachea, bronchi, and bronchioles. Macrophages were also found throughout the lung, but mostly in peribronchiolar locations with focal hypertrophy of the alveolar lining cells and interstitium. The tracheobronchial nodes contained aggregates of black pigment. In rats exposed by the same investigator to similar concentrations of diesel exhaust constituents for 28 days, black, particle-laden pulmonary macrophages, with occasional focal accumulations of polymorphonuclear leukocytes, and a possible thickening of the alveolar membrane were also noted.[74]

Similar findings, as well as goblet cell hypertrophy, were noted in guinea pigs exposed to diesel exhaust for up to 8 weeks using the same experimental set-up, with similar concentrations of diesel exhaust constituents.[75] Pulmonary function was also examined at 4 weeks in guinea pigs exposed to irradiated exhaust, to simulate atmospheric photochemical reactions.[75] Pulmonary flow resistance during tidal breathing was increased compared with controls. In rats after 9 weeks of exposure to diesel exhaust at a particle concentration of 6.0 mg/m^3, focal aggregations of particle-laden macrophages were seen near terminal bronchi with polymorphonuclear leukocytes. There was also type II alveolar cell proliferation and alveolar wall thickening.[76] These short-term experiments of animal exposure to diesel exhaust at levels well above those reported in occupationally exposed groups indicate that expiratory flows can be decreased, and that diesel particles in macrophages are found throughout the lung and in tracheobronchial lymph nodes.

Chronic effects in animals. In rats exposed to diesel exhaust for 12 months at a mean particle level of 2.01 mg/m^3, 9.7 ppm NO, 1.6 ppm NO_2, 0.83 ppm SO_2 for 7 hours per week, 5 hours per day, there were also collections of particle-laden macrophages throughout the lungs.[77] Some of these macrophages were found within the walls of respiratory bronchioles with increased numbers of fibroblasts, but there was no fibrosis and no abnormalities of pulmonary function noted. In another study, Takaki et al. exposed rats for nearly 29 months for 16 hours per day for 6 days per week to diesel exhaust from a light-duty diesel engine (at particle levels of 0.1, 0.4, 1.1, and 2.3 mg/m^3) and a heavy-duty diesel engine (at particle levels of 0.1, 0.4, 1.1, and 2.3 mg/m^3).[21] There was a dose-dependent deposition of anthracotic pigment, proliferation of type II alveolar cells and bronchiolar epithelial cells, and interstitial fibrosis.

In cats exposed to diesel exhaust 8 hours per day, 7 days per week for 27 months, peribronchiolar fibrosis with an increase in lymphocytes, fibroblasts, and interstitial macrophages containing diesel particles was noted, as well as bronchiolar metaplasia.[78] For the first 61 weeks the mean diesel particle level was 6.34 mg/m^3, mean NO_2 was 2.68 ppm, and mean SO_2 was 2.12. Thereafter, the mean diesel particle level was 11.70 mg/m^3, mean NO_2 was 4.37 ppm, and mean SO_2 was 5.03 ppm.

Pulmonary function was studied in these cats, and at the end of 2 years, there were reductions in TLC, forced vital capacity (FVC), functional residual capacity (FRC), RV, and diffusion capacity compared to a control group.[79] The forced expiratory volume in 0.5 second (FEV0.5%) was no different between exposed and control cats. Pulmonary function was also studied in rats exposed to diesel particulate at a level of 1.5 μg/m^3 for 20 hours per day, 5.5 days per week.[80] No differences in pulmonary function were noted after 267 days compared with control rats. In contrast, after 612 days, maximal expiratory flow at 40% and 20% of the FVC and the FRC were greater in the exposed animals.[81] In another study after 1 year of exposure to diesel exhaust at 4.24 mg/m^3 for 19 hours per day 5 days per week, both rats and hamsters exhibited a significant increase in airway resistance.[82] These results indicate that at very high levels of exposure over several years in animals, diesel exhaust inhalation results in interstitial inflammation and peribronchiolar fibrosis. Pulmonary function abnormalities noted are generally consistent with these pathologic findings, with variable findings regarding airway function.

Neoplastic effects

Effects in humans. The neoplastic effects postulated in humans as a result of diesel exhaust exposure are the occurrence of lung cancer and bladder cancer. Studies of lung cancer and diesel exhaust exposure in humans have been limited by difficulty in identifying a population with well-defined exposure to diesel exhaust and limited ability to consider the effects of cigarette smoking. However, an elevated risk of lung cancer was found in a case-control study in U.S. railroad workers whose exposure was characterized by an industrial hygiene survey.[16] After adjusting for cigarette smoking and asbestos, there was a relative odds of 1.41 (95% CI 1.06, 1.88) for lung cancer and work in a diesel exhaust-exposed job. A retrospective cohort study in U.S. railroad workers examining lung cancer mortality between 1959 and 1980 had similar results, with a relative risk of

1.45 (95% CI 1.11, 1.89) in workers with the longest duration of diesel exhaust exposure.[17] In another study, for workers with self-reported work in a motor exhaust-related occupation (not only diesel exhaust related), there was a smoking adjusted odds ratio of 1.5 (95% CI 1.2, 1.9) for 10 or more years of work.[25] An increased relative risk has also been reported in diesel bus garage workers based on a derived index of diesel exhaust exposure[27] and in stevedores.[28] Steenland and co-workers also reported an elevated lung cancer risk in road drivers who drove mostly diesel trucks.[26,52] Taken together, with other studies that will be discussed, human epidemiologic studies support the conclusion that diesel exhaust is a human carcinogen.

Exposure assessments in studies of bladder cancer have even further relied on the indirect assessment of diesel exhaust exposure by using next-of-kin or self-reported occupation as an index of exposure without validation by an industrial hygiene survey. It is presumed that exposure to respirable diesel particles with adsorbed polycyclic aromatic PAHs might lead to an increased risk of bladder cancer due to the excretion of urinary carcinogens.[83] An association between bladder cancer and work as a truck driver and other motor vehicle exhaust occupations has been found.[84-86] However, it is difficult to determine whether diesel exhaust exposure alone is responsible or some other unmeasured factor. A further discussion of the evidence linking diesel exhaust exposure to bladder cancer is beyond the scope of this chapter.

Effects in animals and bioassays. In 1955, Kotin et al.[87,88] painted extracts of diesel exhaust and automobile exhaust particles on the skin of mice, which resulted in skin papillomas and skin carcinomas. As part of a diesel emissions research program established by the U.S. EPA, extracts of diesel and gasoline exhausts were found to be mutagenic and carcinogenic in a variety of short-term tests.[89,90] For example, in the *Salmonella* bioassay (Ames Assay), both diesel and gasoline exhaust extracts were found to have both direct (without metabolic activation) and indirect mutagenic activity.[91] These observations have been confirmed by many others,[14] including in environmental samples of diesel exhaust collected from locomotive repair shops[50] and from heavy duty trucks.[92] Benzo[a]pyrene, the PAH that has been used as an epidemiologic marker for exposure to combustion products,[93] is responsible for some of the indirect mutagenic activity in diesel exhaust. However, many other classes of direct and indirect mutagens have been noted, such as alkyl-PAHs, nitro-PAHs, oxynitro-PAHs, and oxy-PAHs.[68,94] Nitro-PAHs are formed in diesel exhaust due to the reaction of nitrogen oxides with PAH compounds.[95]

Mutagens are capable of being released from diesel particles by serum, lung cytosol, and simulated pulmonary surfactant,[96,97] suggesting that organics are biologically available once inhaled and bound onto a particle. Deoxyribonucleic acid (DNA) adducts have also been noted in the lungs of rats exposed to diesel exhaust, indicating that alterations to genetic material can occur in vivo as a result of exposure.[98] Although Mauderly and co-workers[19] demonstrated a dose-dependent increase in the prevalence of lung tumors in rats exposed to diesel soot concentrations of 0.35, 3.5, or 7.0 mg/m^3 for 30 months for 7 hours per day, 5 days per week (control rate = 0.9%; 0.35 mg/m^3 = 1.3%; 3.5 mg/m^3 = 3.6%; 7.0 mg/m^3 = 12.8%), there was no dose-dependent increase in lung adducts noted in rats exposed for 12 weeks at the same exposure levels.[98]

Brightwell et al. also found a dose–response relationship between exposure to diesel exhaust and lung tumors in rats.[20] At 6.6 mg/m^3 for 16 hours per day, 5 days per week for 24 months the tumor prevalence was 38% in rats; at 2.2 mg/m^3 the tumor prevalence was 9.7%, and at 0.7 mg/m^3 there was a tumor prevalence of 0.7%. Takaki et al.[21] (see also Ishinishi et al.[23]) also found a dose–response relationship for lung cancer with exposure of rats to exhaust from a heavy duty diesel engine after 30 months of exposure. Heinrich et al.[18] studied one exposure level and found a tumor prevalence of 18% in 95 rats exposed to a particle level of 4.24 mg/m^3 for 19 hours per day, 5 days per week for 140 weeks.

The observation that lung tumor rates increase with increasing particle exposure in rats independent of DNA adduct formation suggests that at lower levels of diesel particle exposure the mechanism of lung tumor induction may be different than at higher levels. With higher, prolonged levels of inhaled particles, lung clearance mechanisms become impaired and particle-laden macrophages accumulate in the lung.[99,100] In one study,[100] in rats exposed at a mean level of diesel exhaust of 4.1 mg/m^3 for 7 hours per day, 5 days per week, for 18 weeks had a diesel particle mean clearance half-time of 165 days, compared with a clearance half time of 99 days at an exposure level of 940 µg/m^3. Exposure to carbon black can also result in an inhibition of particle clearance as observed with diesel exhaust exposure.[101] At high diesel particle lung burdens, clearance decreases[102] and chronic active inflammation is observed, with an increased number of lymphocytes.[18,19] It is possible that at the high levels of exposure to diesel exhaust that caused lung cancer in animals, a nonspecific effect due to the diesel particle is responsible. Supporting this conclusion is the observation that rats exposed to titanium dioxide (devoid of any adsorbed organics) at 250 mg/m^3 for 2 years developed lung cancer.[103] At lower exposure levels, other mechanisms perhaps related to the organic material may be more important. Exposure to filtered diesel exhaust has not resulted in lung cancer.[18]

DISEASE: CLINICAL MANIFESTATIONS
Noncancer effects

Acute exposure: Odor, eye irritation, and respiratory symptoms. In human exposure studies it was noted that the increase in reported diesel exhaust odor intensity was an exponential function of the increase in the concentration of diesel exhaust.[67] The response to the odor of diesel exhaust was variable, although in general, as the odor rating increased, greater percentages of individuals objected to or requested a reduction of the odor.[32] Linnell and Scott[31] had six individuals smell diluted diesel exhaust and noted that dilution factors varied greatly, from 140 to 475, to achieve the odor detection threshold. Accordingly, the concentrations of each of the exhaust constituents varied considerably at the odor threshold. The concentration of formaldehyde was 0.012 to 0.088 ppm, the concentration of acrolein ranged from 0.011 to 0.046 ppm, and the concentration of NO_2 was 0.11 to 2.28 ppm. In 1965 Battigelli exposed six subjects to three concentrations of diesel exhaust for 10 minutes.[29] The mean NO_2 concentration ranged from 1.3 to 4.2 ppm, the mean SO_2 concentration ranged from 0.2 to 1 ppm, and formaldehyde and acrolein were less than 0.1 ppm and 0.05 ppm at each exposure level, respectively. When exposed by inhalation only, the subjects complained only of a slightly abnormal taste. With eye exposure at the highest exposure level, 50% discontinued exposure before 10 minutes. At the lowest level, none discontinued exposure, but some experienced eye irritation with the onset of irritation after 6 minutes of exposure. At the higher levels of exhaust reported by Pattle et al.[30] (previously described), the time until intolerable eye irritation occurred in a human subject was very brief, ranging from 5.5 to 20 seconds. It is also possible that the odor and irritative effects of diesel exhaust can occur at lower levels than expected due to the constituents acting together.[70,71]

Most of what is known about acute exposure to diesel exhaust in humans comes from anecdotal reports. For example, it was observed that in a ferry, when the engines were not run at optimal speed, that "black smoke" was emitted and the crew reported headaches and light-headedness.[104] Particularly in cold mornings, it was noted in a London bus garage that when the buses were started, a lacrimatory mist was produced.[105] Kahn and co-workers reviewed 13 cases of acute overexposure to diesel exhaust[34] based on reports from five underground coal mines in Utah and Colorado between 1974 and 1985. Interviews in 1986 revealed 12 had experienced symptoms of mucous membrane irritation, headache, and light-headedness. Eight miners reported nausea, and four reported a sensation of unreality ("being high") and heartburn. These symptoms resolved within 24 to 48 hours.

To describe the acute effects of diesel exhaust on respiratory symptoms, Gamble et al.[33] studied 232 male workers in four diesel bus garages. Workers with the highest exposure to respirable particles (≥0.31 mg/m^3) reported significantly more work-related cough, itchy or burning eyes, headache, difficult or labored breathing, chest constriction, and wheeze when compared with workers with lower exposures, adjusting for age and cigarette smoking. However, there was no specific marker of diesel exhaust measured. It is not known the extent that nondiesel particles contributed to the measured respirable particles. For workers whose NO_2 values were above 0.3 ppm, there was also more work-related itchy or burning eyes, difficult or labored breathing, chest constriction, and wheeze. Compared with a group of lead acid battery workers, the prevalence of symptoms reported as "sometimes" or "often" related to work were significantly higher for burning eyes, headaches, difficult or labored breathing, nausea, and wheeze while at work.

In a smaller study of 17 ferry stevedores involved in transporting both diesel trucks and gasoline-powered vehicles compared with 11 office worker controls,[106] the stevedores had a higher prevalence of wheeze, chest tightness, nasal complaints, chest pain, and eye irritation. However, there were more smokers among the stevedores and some of these symptoms might have been attributable to smoking. The concentrations of NO_2 and SO_2 were both less than 0.25 ppm, and respirable particle levels were not measured. In an iron ore mine where diesel vehicles were used underground, more underground workers who were smokers noted chest pressure and difficulty "getting air" than the nonsmoking underground workers.[107] The underground smokers also had more episodes of productive cough lasting 3 weeks over several winters than the smokers who worked above ground.

These reports indicate that exposure to diesel exhaust in occupationally exposed workers may cause symptoms of eye, upper respiratory mucous membrane irritation, and respiratory symptoms usually attributable to lower respiratory tract involvement. The study by Gamble and co-workers[33] in bus garage workers suggests that there is an effect of occupational exposure to diesel exhaust on respiratory tract symptoms. However, the contribution of diesel exhaust to respirable particles in these studies is uncertain, since these workplace exposures are complex and involve exposure to other sources of respirable dust. It is also possible that the reporting of these symptoms may be modified by concomitant cigarette smoking, but little specific information is available to better evaluate this.

Acute exposure: pulmonary function. Changes in pulmonary function across a work shift in 60 coal miners who worked in diesel-equipped mines and in 90 underground coal miners who worked in nondiesel mines were compared by Ames and co-workers.[37] In both groups of miners, the FVC and FEV1 significantly declined over a work shift, but there was no significant difference in decline between miners at the diesel and nondiesel mines. In an analysis adjusting for age, respirable dust, and years of underground mining in both smokers and nonsmokers, there was no independent effect of work in a diesel-equipped mine on shift-related changes in pulmonary function. NO_2 levels averaged 0.2 ppm, formaldehyde averaged 0.3 ppm, and respirable dust averaged 2000 $\mu g/m^3$ in the miners in the diesel-equipped mines. In the unexposed group, mean respirable dust exposure was 1400 $\mu g/m^3$.

No significant changes in FVC and FEV1 were noted across a work shift in ferry workers involved in transporting diesel trucks and gasoline vehicles when compared with controls.[106] Gamble and co-workers[33] (discussed previously) were also not able to relate changes in spirometry to shift worked, respirable particle level, or NO_2 level. In contrast, Ulfvarson et al.[36] found significant declines in FVC and FEV1 across a shift in 23 cargo shipworkers exposed to diesel truck exhaust who had not had any exposure to diesel exhaust for the previous 10 days. When the experiment was repeated in workers without diesel exhaust exposure for 5 days, the FVC again significantly declined over a shift, but the FEV1 did not. The concentration of total particles (not only respirable particles) ranged from 0.13 to 1000 mg/m^3, formaldehyde levels ranged from less than 0.03 to 0.5 ppm, and NO_2 levels ranged from 0.06 to 1.0 ppm. In other studies[56,57] filters were put on diesel equipment and shift-related decrements in FVC were not observed.

Three railroad workers developed asthma following more acute exposure to diesel locomotive exhaust.[35] The workers were riding immediately behind the lead engine of a train (second locomotive) such that exhaust was blown continually into their locomotive cabs. Two of the men had never smoked, one was an exsmoker, and all had jobs with previous diesel exposure. None had any history of asthma or respiratory disease, except one who had seasonal rhinitis. One worker who had peak flow monitoring had a decrement in peak flow noted when he was riding behind the lead locomotive. All had reversible airflow obstruction and evidence of nonspecific bronchial hyperreactivity.

These studies indicate that reversible changes in pulmonary function can occur in relation to exposure to diesel exhaust, although it is not possible to relate this to specific levels of exposure. At exposure levels that were likely to be relatively high three railroad workers developed asthma. Taken together, these reports indicate that reversible airflow obstruction and persistent bronchial hyperreactivity are possible following diesel exhaust exposure.

Chronic exposure. Studies of the chronic effects of diesel exhaust exposure have been conducted in miners and bus garage workers (Table 33-8). There has been no consistent association between work in a job with diesel exhaust exposure and decreased pulmonary function attributable to chronic exposure. However, of the four cross-sectional studies described (Table 33-8), three reported an association between diesel-exposed jobs and respiratory symptoms (such as cough and phlegm). The levels of particle exposure reported in these studies are much greater than the levels of respirable particles attributable to diesel in trucking industry workers and railroad workers, and dust exposure was generally higher in the mines compared with the bus garage. However, interpretation of these dust levels is hindered by their lack of specificity for diesel exhaust and surely reflects considerable nondiesel dust.

Table 33-8. Effects of chronic exposure to diesel exhaust: noncarcinogenic effects

Population	Outcome	Reference
550 underground and 273 surface coal miners matched on age, smoking status, and years underground to miners from nondiesel mines	At underground diesel mines, significantly more persistent cough (23.6%) compared with controls (16.5%); more exacerbations of cough and phlegm (21.7% vs 16.2%); decreased FVC and FEV1 in both underground and surface diesel mine workers compared with controls; no relation to years of work; exposure: respirable dust 0.4-16.1 mg/m^3 area samples; 0.93-2.73 mg/m^3 personal; personal NO$_2$ 0.13-0.22 ppm	54
630 miners from 6 potash mines	No consistent relationship between respiratory symptoms or pulmonary function with exposure (years of exposure; cumulative dust; NO$_2$ levels; prevalence of mine diesel use); exposure: personal total dust 9-23 mg/m^3; total dust to respirable dust ratio of 2 to 11; personal NO$_2$ 0.1 to 3.3 ppm	58
259 salt miners in 5 salt mines	Cumulative NO$_2$ exposure, respirable particulate, years of exposure were predictors of chronic phlegm, adjusting for age and smoking; no effects noted on pulmonary function; exposure: average respirable particulate 0.2-0.7 mg/m^3; NO$_2$ 0.3-2.5 ppm	55 108
Longitudinal change in PFT and respiratory symptoms over 5 years in 280 underground coal miners in diesel-use mines and 838 miners in nondiesel underground mines	No difference in PFT change between groups; no increase in respiratory symptoms in miners in diesel-use mines; exposure: no data reported; reported as "low"	109
283 diesel bus garage workers in 4 garages in 2 cities	Years worked was a significant predictor of FVC and FEV1, adjusting for age and smoking; more cough, phlegm, wheeze compared with a reference blue-collar population; exposure: mean respirable particulate 0.16-0.61 mg/m^3 across garages; NO$_2$ 0.13 0.56 ppm	110

FEV1, Forced expiratory volume in 1 second; *FVC,* forced vital capacity; *PFT,* pulmonary function test.

Although these studies are reported as representing chronic exposure, work in diesel-exposed jobs was relatively short. Reger and co-workers[54] in 550 underground and 273 surface workers reported a short duration of exposure to diesel exhaust, a mean of 4.7 years spent in underground (mining) by the workers at the underground diesel-use mines. In potash miners,[58] the mean duration of work in a diesel-use mine varied between 5 and 14 years, depending on the mine. The salt miners had only a mean 10.6 years of mine work.[55,108] In the bus garage, there was a mean of only 8.7 years of work. It is possible that the effects on pulmonary function and respiratory symptoms observed were not attributable to the long-term effects of diesel exhaust but to some other factor since exposure was relatively short. Since shift-related effects of diesel exhaust exposure on respiratory symptoms and pulmonary function have been noted (as discussed in the previous sections), it is also possible that the results reported actually represent a more acute effect of exposure.

Thus, these studies of pulmonary function and respiratory symptoms in relation to chronic exposure to diesel exhaust have been limited by the study of populations with a relatively short duration of exposure. Furthermore, the study of only active workers will make it more difficult to detect an effect of diesel exhaust in cross-sectional studies because of the healthy worker effect.

Only one longitudinal study with a relatively short follow-up (5 years) has been done in diesel exhaust-exposed workers. There was no relationship between diesel-exposed job, lung function, and respiratory symptoms.[109] It is possible that this study was not adequately analyzed because decline in lung function was not adjusted for level of lung function in the analysis. Additional studies in populations with a longer duration of diesel exhaust exposure are needed.

Carcinogenic effects

Lung cancer. Until recently, the study of lung cancer and diesel exhaust exposure was limited by failure to consider the latency and duration of exposure sufficient for the development of lung cancer.[14] Studies of the occurrence of lung cancer and diesel exhaust exposure have been conducted among various occupational cohorts (railroad workers, truck drivers, other transport workers), and in the general population (with cases of lung cancer obtained from hospitals or from cancer registries). Studies of specific occupational cohorts have also been limited by lack of industrial hygiene exposure data, with such data limited to the U.S. railroad industry[47-50] and trucking industry.[51,52] In studies of other occupational groups, job title or a derived index have been used to indicate exposure. In studies based on hospital or registry-based cases, self-reported exposure to diesel exhaust or usual work in a job exposed to vehicle exhaust have been used. Such lack of precision in the ascertainment of exposure would make it more difficult to detect an effect of diesel exhaust exposure on lung cancer occurrence. As a consequence, in some studies with the least precise definition of exposure, elevated point estimates of lung cancer risk have been reported, but with wider confidence intervals than in the studies with the better exposure assessments.

In the U.S. railroad industry, diesel engine use became more prevalent after 1950 such that by 1959, 95% of the locomotives in service were diesel powered. Railroad workers in the United States also have their own retirement system (the U.S. Railroad Retirement Board) that maintains computerized work records, generally starting in 1959, and mortality records. As a result, these records could be utilized as a source of exposure to diesel exhaust (based on yearly job history from 1959 through death and retirement) and as a death registry. Jobs with exposure to diesel exhaust were workers on operating trains (engineers, firemen, brakemen, conductors) and workers engaged in the repair and maintenance of diesel locomotives. In a case-control study, 1,256 incident cases of lung cancer (based on death certificate) were collected over 12 months in 1981 to 1982 and matched by age to workers dying of causes other than cancer or accidents.[16] Smoking histories were obtained from next-of-kin by mail questionnaire and telephone contact. An important potential confounding exposure was asbestos, since the steam locomotives replaced by the diesel locomotives were insulated with asbestos.[111] The workers engaged in the repair of diesel locomotives in the repair sheds and roundhouses would have been exposed to asbestos previously while repairing the steam locomotives. However, adjusting for asbestos exposure and smoking, workers age ≤64 years at death with 20 years of work in a diesel-exposed job had an elevated odds ratio of 1.41 (95% CI = 1.06, 1.88) of dying of lung cancer.

In a related retrospective cohort study of 55,407 railroad workers aged 40 to 64 in 1959, mortality was ascertained from 1959 through 1980.[17] The workers with the longest potential duration of diesel exhaust exposure, workers aged 40 to 44 with a 1959 job title indicating work in a diesel exhaust-exposed job, had a relative risk of dying of lung cancer of 1.45 (95% CI = 1.11, 1.89). Workers with slightly less exposure, aged 45 to 49 in 1959, had a relative risk of 1.33 (95% CI = 1.03, 1.73). For both the case-control study[16] and retrospective cohort study[17] industrial hygiene data were used to characterize exposure (described previously and in Table 33-3).[47,48] It was not possible to consider smoking in this retrospective study, but the adjustment for smoking did not appreciably change the odds ratio for lung cancer in the case-control study. Respirable particles adjusted for cigarette smoke were used as the marker of diesel exposure. It is likely that exposure to diesel exhaust from locomotives was higher shortly after diesel engines were introduced into the railroad compared with the exposures reported when sampling was done for the epidemiologic studies. However, reported current exposure levels for respirable particles were considerably less than the exposure levels where lung cancer was observed to occur in animal exposure studies.

Gustavsson et al. studied men who had worked in five bus garages in Stockholm from 1945 through 1970 using a nested case-control design.[27] Diesel-powered buses were first introduced in Stockholm in the 1930s, and, after 1945, all buses with combustion engines were diesel. Exposure to diesel exhaust was estimated by industrial hygienists rather than measured, with calculations based on the number of buses in the garages, garage ventilation and air volume of the garages, and job types and work practices. No cigarette smoking information was available. Details of the estimation of diesel exposure were not presented, but exposure was graded on a scale of five levels with each increase in scale corresponding to a 50% increase in intensity. An index of cumulative exposure to diesel exhaust was calculated for each worker by multiplying the exposure level for each work period by the duration in years. Past exposure to asbestos was also estimated based on historical measurements of asbestos fibers obtained during brake repair operations. As the diesel exhaust exposure index increased, the relative risk of lung cancer increased. At the highest exposure index, the relative risk of lung cancer was 2.43 (95% CI = 1.32, 4.47), and no such increase was observed using a similar index for asbestos exposure.

The mortality of 6,071 stevedores in Sweden employed for at least 6 months between 1961 and 1974 was determined through 1980.[112] Diesel-powered trucks were first used in Swedish ports in the late 1950s, with a rapid increase in use in the 1960s. No formal assessment of exposure to diesel exhaust was made, and exposure to both gasoline and diesel exhausts was likely. An elevated standard mortality rate (SMR) for lung cancer was found (SMR = 132; 95% CI = 105, 166) with a greater increase in lung cancer risk over time compared with the Swedish male population. A later case-control study among Swedish dock workers was conducted in an attempt to refine the assessment of exposure and adjust for smoking.[28] Exposure to diesel exhaust was estimated based on diesel fuel consumption and number of workers in each Swedish port, and the cases and controls were selected from male dock workers employed for at least 6 months from 1950 to 1974, with case ascertainment starting in 1960 through 1982. Based on

50 cases and 154 referents with complete information available and adjusting for smoking (yes/no), there was an increase in the odds ratio for lung cancer with increasing exposure for three indices of exposure (years since diesel equipment was used in a port, estimates of cumulative fuel consumption, and years that fuel use was above a minimum level in a port), consistent with an exposure–response relationship. However, the confidence limits for all the point estimates of the odds ratios for lung cancer except one did not achieve statistical significance.

Lung cancer in motor vehicle occupations was studied in 1,444 male hospital-based cases of lung cancer and 1,893 controls using data pooled from three studies carried out by the National Cancer Institute between 1976 and 1983.[25] Overall, these individuals would have had exposure to exhaust from both diesel and nondiesel sources. It was not possible to measure exposure to various exhausts, and consequently exposure was assessed by job title, with exposure defined as work in any motor vehicle exhaust-associated occupation. Job and smoking history information was obtained by interview of the cases and controls. For any motor exhaust-related occupation, the odds ratio for lung cancer was 1.5 (95% CI = 1.2, 1.9) with 10 or more years of employment in a motor vehicle-related occupation, adjusting for age and smoking. In truck drivers with 10 or more years of employment, the odds ratio was 1.5 (95% CI = 1.1, 1.9). These truck drivers also would have had exposure to both diesel and nondiesel exhausts. Diesel trucks were introduced into trucking in the 1950s and 1960s, and, according to Steenland et al.,[27] trucking companies would have completed the transition to diesel trucks by 1960, while independent drivers and nontrucking companies would have completed the transition later.

In another study in workers exposed to motor vehicle exhausts, Steenland and co-workers[27,52] studied 994 male lung cancer deaths in 1982 and 1983 in Teamsters who had filed claims for pension benefits (requiring at least a 20 year Teamster membership). Work history and smoking history were obtained from next-of-kin, and job category was also available from Teamster records. For long-haul drivers (who likely would have driven mostly diesel trucks) with 18 or more years of employment after 1959, the odds ratio for lung cancer was 1.55 (95% CI = 0.97, 2.47), adjusting for age, smoking, and asbestos. Teamsters with 35 years or more employment whose main job was a diesel truck driver had a relative odds of lung cancer of 1.89 (95% CI = 1.04, 3.42), adjusting for age, smoking, and asbestos. For gasoline truck drivers, the relative odds for lung cancer was less, 1.34, and did not achieve conventional levels of significance (95% CI = 0.81, 2.22).

Boffetta et al. reported on the 2-year mortality of 378,622 men between 1982 and 1984 in the American Cancer Society prospective study of cancer.[113] The analysis of lung cancer mortality was based on the self-report of diesel exhaust exposure. Adjusting for age, smoking, and other oc-

cupational exposures (such as the self-report of exposure to asbestos, coal tar and pitch, and gasoline exhausts), the relative risk for lung cancer with ≥16 years of diesel exposure was 1.21 (95% CI = 0.94, 1.56). For truck drivers reporting diesel exhaust exposure, the relative risk was 1.22 (95% CI = 0.77, 1.95).

Boffetta and co-workers also reported the results of a case-control study with cases drawn from patients with lung cancer in 18 hospitals in six U.S. cities.[114] There were 2,584 cases of lung cancer between 1969 and the late 1980s matched to at least one control based on age, sex, hospital, and year of interview to obtain smoking and usual occupation. In 1985 and thereafter, information on the self-report of diesel exhaust exposure was obtained (477 cases). Exposure was graded as "probable" in individuals with usual work in railroads (although it is clear that all railroad workers are not exposed to diesel exhaust) and in a variety of motor vehicle-related occupations. For individuals with probable exposure to diesel exhaust the odds ratio for lung cancer was 1.31 (95% CI = 1.09, 1.57), and for those reporting a usual occupation as a truck driver the odds ratio was 1.31 (95% CI = 1.03, 1.67). However, after adjusting for cigarette use, age, race, and date of interview, the odds ratio for lung cancer was reduced to 0.95 (95% CI = 0.78, 1.16) and 0.88 (95% CI = 0.67, 1.15), for individuals with probable exposure and for truck drivers, respectively. For self-reported diesel exhaust exposure, the odds ratio for lung cancer was 1.21, adjusting for smoking, age, and other potential confounding variables (asbestos, education, race), but also did not achieve statistical significance (95% CI = 0.73, 2.02). This latter study by Boffetta et al.[114] illustrates the potential impact of the adjustment for the potential confounding effects of cigarette smoking. The odds ratio for the effect of diesel exposure was greatly reduced when the effects of smoking were considered. However, in both of the studies by Boffetta and co-workers,[113,114] there also was considerable misclassification of diesel exhaust exposure, making it more difficult to detect an effect of exposure on lung cancer.

In a study from France, 1,260 male cases of lung cancer and 2,084 controls matched on age and hospital were collected between 1976 and 1980.[115] This study was based on occupational history and was adjusted for smoking history obtained by interview, transport equipment operators (odds ratio = 1.35; 95% CI = 1.05, 1.75) and motor vehicle drivers (odds ratio = 1.42; 95% CI = 1.07, 1.89). Risk did not increase with duration of work. In Detroit, incident cases of lung cancer were collected in men between 1984 and 1987, and occupational history and smoking information were collected by interview with the subject or a surrogate.[116] Adjusting for smoking, for drivers of heavy trucks the odds ratio of lung cancer for white men with 20 or more years of work was 2.5 (95% CI = 1.4, 4.4). For drivers of light trucks with 20 or more years of work, the odds ratio was 2.1 (95% CI = 0.9, 4.6). For both drivers of heavy and light trucks, there was a significant increase in odds ratio for lung cancer with increasing years of work. It is unclear from both of these studies precisely which exposure in these motor vehicle-related jobs was responsible for the increased odds ratios.

The studies reviewed in this section support the conclusion that diesel exhaust exposure in humans results in lung cancer. In railroad workers and truck drivers, the relative risk was in the range of 1.4 to 1.5, or a 40% to 50% increased risk. However, the precise definition of exposure has varied among studies, and the effects of confounding by cigarette smoke or other, unmeasured factors can influence the magnitude of the risk observed. There is insufficient exposure information in human epidemiologic studies to adequately estimate the risk of lung cancer for a given level of diesel exhaust exposure or to explore relationships between dose and latency. However, as a whole, the human epidemiologic literature is in agreement with the findings of the animal studies that indicate whole diesel exhaust is a lung carcinogen.

REGULATIONS

Environmental emissions of diesel exhaust in the United States are regulated by the Clean Air Act Amendments of 1990. This act promulgates emission standards for passenger cars, including hydrocarbon, NO_x, and particle emissions. These standards require roughly an 80% reduction in particle emissions from diesel-fueled passenger cars, phased in beginning in 1994.[118] Emission standards are also set for light duty and heavy duty trucks. The sulfur content of diesel fuel available for trucks, buses, and cars will also be reduced to no more than 0.05% by weight, whereas diesel fuels in the 1980s had an average sulfur content of roughly 0.28% to 0.22%.[45,119] The reduction in fuel sulfur content will lead to reductions in particle, SO_2, and sulfate emissions and will reduce engine wear. For new urban buses, a particle standard below that of other heavy-duty vehicles was promulgated.[120] An urban bus engine is usually rebuilt two or three times since the engine wears out long before the bus is ready for retirement.[121] After 1994, when older urban buses (operating in metropolitan areas with 1980 populations of 750,000 or more) have their engines rebuilt, the Clean Air Act specifies various retrofit/rebuild requirements to control particle emissions. The EPA is also empowered to regulate nonroad diesel vehicles and within 5 years to regulate emissions from all new locomotives.

In underground coal mines the current standard for respirable particles, not specifically from diesel exhaust, is 2,000 $\mu g/m^3$.[40] Permitted exposure limits for various vapor phase constituents of diesel exhaust are based on the 1972 threshold limit values adopted by the American Conference of Governmental Industrial Hygienists.[122] These guidelines set ceiling values for formaldehyde of 2 ppm and ceiling values for NO_2 of 5 ppm. In 1992, the Mine Safety and Health Administration (MSHA) issued an advance notice of rule making[123] to ask the public to submit comments regarding establishing specific diesel particulate standards in mines. It was recognized that the current respirable particulate standard may not be adequate given the results of the animal inhalation studies and the human epidemiologic studies. MSHA was also involved in the rule-making process to revise mine air quality standards for vapor phase emissions.[40]

CONTROL METHODS

General approaches to the control of diesel emissions include changes in engine design, such as combustion chamber configuration and fuel injection timing, exhaust aftertreatment, and fuel modifications.[124] It is anticipated that to meet diesel particle emission standards, exhaust aftertreatment devices will be needed, such as traps without catalysts, traps with catalysts, and flowthrough oxidation catalysts.[45,124] Proper engine maintenance is important to control particle emissions, such as replacement of dirty air cleaners. A reduction in air available for combustion will increase soot emissions. Diesel engines in coal mines must operate with exhaust gas temperatures less than 77° C, which can be achieved by the use of water scrubbers.[125] Particle emissions are reduced by the scrubber and additional filters.

FUTURE NEEDS AND CONTROVERSIES
Noncancer effects

Although short-term effects on pulmonary function and respiratory symptoms have been noted following diesel exhaust exposure, there is a paucity of studies in occupationally exposed cohorts documenting an effect of chronic exposure. Longitudinal studies of occupationally exposed cohorts (such as miners) are needed with documentation of levels of exposure before a chronic effect of exposure on pulmonary function and respiratory symptoms can be determined.

Cancer effects

The available animal and human studies and the results of short-term bioassays support the conclusion that diesel exhaust is a lung carcinogen in humans. Since diesel engines were introduced in most industries after World War II and during the 1950s, only recently have cohorts of exposed workers suitable for epidemiologic study become available. Studies of lung cancer risk are needed in workers with most of their working lives exposed to diesel exhaust, with exposure and confounding effects (such as from tobacco smoke) well characterized. This is necessary to refine estimates of the human risk of lung cancer as a result of exposure.

Nevertheless, considerable effort has been spent using both animal and human epidemiologic data to determine "unit risk," the estimated lifetime risk of lung cancer from inhalation of 1 μg/m^3 of diesel exhaust particulate matter. Such estimates would be useful in setting standards to regulate diesel exhaust. It has been the opinion of some that the current human epidemiologic studies are not adequate to estimate unit risk.[126] Estimates of this risk vary widely, ranging from 0.6-2 $\times$ 10^{-3} to 8 $\times$ 10^{-5}, based on the assumptions made regarding human dose and by extrapolating results of animal bioassays to humans.[126] The higher estimates of unit risk are based on human epidemiologic studies and reflect the uncertainty of the available human exposure data.

REFERENCES

1. Schuetzle D: Sampling of vehicle emissions for chemical analysis and biological testing. *Environ Health Perspect* 47:65-80, 1983.
2. Scheepers PTJ and Bos RP: Combustion of diesel fuel from a toxicological perspective. I. Origin of incomplete combustion products, *Int Arch Occup Environ Health* 64:149-161, 1992.
3. IARC: *IARC monographs on the evaluation of carcinogenic risks to humans,* vol 46: *Diesel and gasoline engine exhausts and some nitroarenes,* Lyon, 1989, IARC.
4. Wolff RK, Henderson RF, Snipes MB, Sun JD, Bond JA, Mitchell CE, Mauderly JL, and McClellan RO: Lung retention of diesel soot and associated organic compounds, In Ishinishi N, Koizumi A, McClellan RO, and Stober W, editors: *Carcinogenic and mutagenic effects of diesel engines,* pp 199-211, Amsterdam, 1986, Elsevier.
5. IARC: *IARC Monographs on the evaluation of carcinogenic risks to humans,* vol 45: *Occupational exposures in petroleum refining; crude oil and major petroleum fuels,* Lyon, 1989, IARC.
6. Williams DJ, Milne JW, Quigley SM, and Roberts DB: Particulate emissions from 'in-use' motor vehicles-II. diesel vehicles, *Atmos Environ* 23:2647-2660, 1989.
7. Williams PT, Abbass MK, and Andrews GE: Diesel particulate emissions: the role of unburned fuel, *Combust Flame* 75:1-24, 1989.
8. Stenberg U, Alsberg T, and Westerholm W: Emission of carcinogenic components with automobile exhausts, *Environ Health Perspect* 47:53-56, 1983.
9. Docekal B, Krivan V, and Pelz N: Trace and minor characterization of diesel soot, *Fresenius J Anal Chem* 343:873-878, 1992.
10. Schuetzle D and Frazier JA: Factors influencing the emission of vapor and particulate phase components from diesel engines, In Ishinishi N, Koizumi A, McClellan RO, and Stober W, editors: *Carcinogenic and mutagenic effects of diesel engines,* pp 41-63, Amsterdam, 1986, Elsevier.
11. Holmberg B and Ahlborg U: Consensus report: mutagenicity and carcinogenicity of car exhausts and coal combustion emissions, *Environ Health Perspect* 47:1-30, 1983.
12. McClellan RO: Health effects of exposure to diesel particles, *Annu Rev Toxicol* 27:279-300, 1987.
13. Barrett RE: The federal viewpoint, In *National Institute of Occupational Safety and Health. Proceedings of a workshop on the use of diesel equipment in underground coal mines,* pp 6-12, DHHS (NIOSH) Pub No 82-122, 1982.
14. National Research Council: *Health effects of exposure to diesel exhaust,* Washington, DC, 1981, National Academy Press.
15. Cuddihy RG, Griffith WC, and McClellan RO: Health risks from light-duty diesel vehicles, *Environ Sci Technol* 18:14A-21A, 1984.
16. Garshick E, Schenker MB, Muñoz A, Segal M, Smith TJ, Woskie SR, Hammond SK, and Speizer FE: A case-control study of lung cancer and diesel exhaust exposure in railroad workers, *Am Rev Respir Dis* 135:1242-1248, 1987.
17. Garshick E, Schenker MB, Muñoz A, Segal M, Smith TJ, Woskie SR, Hammond SK, and Speizer FE: A retrospective cohort study of lung cancer and diesel exhaust exposure in railroad workers, *Am Rev Respir Dis* 137:820-825, 1987.
18. Heinrich U, Muhle H, Takenaka S, Ernst H, Fuhst R, Mohr U, Pott F, and Stober W: Chronic effects on the respiratory tract of hamsters, mice, and rats after long-term inhalation of high concentrations of filtered and unfiltered diesel engine emissions, *J Appl Toxicol* 6:383-395, 1986.
19. Mauderly JL, Jones RK, Griffith WC, Henderson FR, and McClellan RO: Diesel exhaust is a pulmonary carcinogen in rats chronically exposed by inhalation, *Fund Appl Toxicol* 9:208-221, 1987.
20. Brightwell J, Fouillet X, Cassano-Zoppi AL, Gatz R, and Duchosal F: Tumours of the respiratory tract in rats and hamsters following chronic inhalation of engine exhaust emissions, *J Appl Toxicol* 9:23-31, 1989.
21. Takaki Y, Kitamura S, Kuwabara N, and Fukuda Y: Long-term inhalation studies of exhaust from the diesel engine in F-34 rats: the quantitative relationship between pulmonary hyperplasia and anthracosis, *Exp Pathol* 37:56-61, 1989.
22. Iwai K, Udagawa T, Yamagishi M, and Yamada N: Long-term inhalation studies of diesel exhaust on F344 rats. Incidence of lung cancer and lymphoma, In Ishinishi N, Koizumi A, McClellan RO, Stober W, editors: *Carcinogenic and mutagenic effects of diesel engines,* pp 349-360, Amsterdam, 1986, Elsevier.
23. Ishinishi N, Kuwabara N, Nagase S, Suzuki T, Ishiwata S, and Kohno T: Long term inhalation studies on effects of diesel exhaust from heavy and light duty diesel engines on F344 rats, In Ishinishi N, Koizumi A, McClellan RO, and Stober W, editors: *Carcinogenic and mutagenic effects of diesel engines,* pp 329-348, Amsterdam, 1986, Elsevier.
24. National Institute of Occupational Safety and Health: *Current intelligence bulletin 50. Carcinogenic effects of exposure to diesel exhaust,* DHHS (NIOSH) Pub No 88-116, 1988.
25. Hayes RB, Thomas T, Silverman DT, Vineis P, Blot WJ, Mason TJ, Pickle LW, Correa P, Fontham ETH, and Schoenberg JB: Lung cancer in motor exhaust-related occupations, *Am J Ind Med* 16:685-695, 1989.
26. Steenland NK, Silverman DT, and Hornung W: Case-control study of lung cancer and truck driving in the teamsters union, *AJPH* 80:670-674, 1990.
27. Gustavsson P, Plato N, and Lidstrom EB: Lung cancer and exposure to diesel exhaust among bus garage workers, *Scand J Work Environ Health* 16:348-354, 1990.
28. Emmelin A, Nystrom L, and Wall S: Diesel exhaust exposure and smoking. A case-referent study of lung cancer among Swedish dock workers, *Epidemiology* 4:237-244, 1993.
29. Battigelli M: Effects of diesel exhaust, *Arch Environ Health* 10:165-167, 1965.
30. Pattle RE, Stretch H, Burgess F, Sinclair K, and Edginton JAG: The toxicity of fumes from a diesel engine under four different running conditions, *Br J Ind Med* 14:47-55, 1957.
31. Linnell RH and Scott WE: Diesel exhaust composition and odor studies, *J Air Pollut Cont Assoc* 12:510-515, 1962.
32. Hare CT and Springer KJ: *Public response to diesel engine exhaust odors.* Final Report to Environmental Protection Agency Contract No. EPA 70-44; PB 204 012. San Antonio, 1971, Southwest Research Institute.
33. Gamble J, Jones W, and Minshall S: Epidemiological-environmental study of diesel bus garage workers: acute effects of NO$_2$ and respirable particulate on the respiratory system, *Environ Res* 42:201-214, 1987.
34. Kahn G, Orris P, and Weeks J: Acute overexposure to diesel exhaust: report of 13 cases. *Am J Ind Med* 13:405-406, 1988.
35. Wade JF and Newman LS: Diesel asthma. Reactive airways disease following overexposure to locomotive exhaust, *JOM* 35:149-154, 1993.

36. Ulfvarson U, Alexandersson R, Aringer L, Svensson E, Hedenstierna G, Hogstedt C, Holmberg B, Rosen G, and Sorsa M: Effects of exposure to vehicle exhaust on health, *Scand J Work Environ Health* 13:505-512, 1987.

37. Ames RG, Attfield MD, Hankinson JL, Hearl FJ, and Reger RB: Acute respiratory effects of exposure to diesel emissions in coal miners, *Am Rev Respir Dis* 125:39-42, 1982.

38. Froines JR, Hinds WC, Duffy RM, LaFuente EJ, and Liu WV: Exposure of fire fighters to diesel emissions in fire stations, *Am Ind Hyg Assoc J* 48:202-207, 1987.

39. Emissions and control technology work group: In *National Institute of Occupational Safety and Health. Proceedings of a workshop on the use of diesel equipment in underground coal mines,* pp 149-175, DHHS (NIOSH) Pub No 82-122, 1982.

40. Mine Safety and Health Administration: *Report of the mine safety and health administration advisory committee on standards and regulations for diesel-powered equipment in underground coal mines,* Report to the Secretary of Labor, July 1988.

41. Diesel Inventory for Coal Mines, personal communication, U.S. Bureau of Mines, July 1993.

42. Personal communication, Mine Safety and Health Administration.

43. Office of Air and Radiation, Environmental Protection Agency: *Nonroad engine and vehicle emission study report,* EPA 460/3-91-02 PB 92-126960, 1991.

44. Association of American Railroads: *Railroad facts,* Washington, DC, 1993.

45. Office of Mobile Sources and Office of Air and Radiation, environmental Protection Agency: *Regulatory impact analysis. Control of sulfur and aromatics contents of on-highway diesel fuel,* Washington, DC, PB 93-207660, 1990.

46. American Automobile Manufacturers Association: *World motor vehicle data,* Detroit, 1993.

47. Woskie SR, Smith TJ, Hammond SK, Schenker MB, Garshick E, and Speizer FE: Estimation of the diesel exposures of railroad workers: I. current exposures, *Am J Ind Med* 13:381-394, 1988.

48. Woskie SR, Smith TJ, Hammond SK, Schenker MB, Garshick E, and Speizer FE: Estimation of the diesel exposures of railroad workers: II. national and historical exposures, *Am J Ind Med* 13:395-404, 1988.

49. Hammond SK, Smith TJ, Woskie SR, Leaderer BP, and Bettinger N: Markers of exposure to diesel exhaust and cigarette smoke in railroad workers, *Am Ind Hyg Assoc J* 49:516-522, 1988.

50. Hammond SK, Smith TJ, Woskie SR, Braun AG, Lafleur A, Liber H, Garshick E, Schenker MB, and Speizer FE: Railroad diesel exhaust: concentration and mutagenicity, *Appl Occup Environ Hyg* 8:955-963, 1993.

51. Zaebst DD, Clapp DE, Blade LM, Marlow DA, Steenland K, Hornung RW, Scheutzle D, and Butler J: Quantitative determination of trucking industry workers' exposures to diesel exhaust particles, *Am Ind Hyg Assoc J* 52:529-541, 1991.

52. Steenland K, Silverman D, and Zaebst D: Exposure to diesel exhaust in the trucking industry with possible relationships with lung cancer, *Am J Ind Med* 21:887-890, 1992.

53. Spengler JD, Dockery DW, Turner WA, Wolfson JM, and Ferris BG: Long-term measurements of respirable sulfates and particles inside and outside homes, *Atmos Environ* 15:23-30, 1981.

54. Reger R, Hancock J, Hankinson J, Hearl F, and Merchant J: Coal miners exposed to diesel exhaust emissions, *Ann Occup Hyg* 26:799-815, 1982.

55. Gamble J, Jones W, and Hudak J: An epidemiological study of salt miners in diesel and nondiesel mines, *Am J Ind Med* 4:435-458, 1983.

56. Ulfvarson U and Alexandersson R: Reduction in adverse effect on pulmonary function after exposure to filtered diesel exhaust, *Am J Ind Med* 17:341-347, 1990.

57. Ulfvarson U, Alexandersson R, Dahlquist M, Ekholm U, and Bergstrom B: Pulmonary function in workers exposed to diesel exhausts: the effect of control measures, *Am J Ind Med* 19:283-289, 1991.

58. Attfield MD, Trabant GD, and Wheeler RW: Exposure to diesel fumes and dust at six potash mines, *Ann Occup Hyg* 26:817-831, 1982.

59. Heino M, Ketola R, Makela P, Makinen R, Niemela R, Starck J, and Partanen T: Work conditions and health of locomotive engineers, *Scan J Work Environ Health* 4(suppl 3):3-14, 1978.

60. Bradow RL: Diesel particle emissions, *Bull NY Acad Med* 56:797-816, 1980.

61. Cuddihy RG, Griffith WC, Clark CR, and McClellan RO: *Potential health and environmental effects of light duty vehicles II.* Albuquerque, 1981, Inhalation Toxicology Research Institute, Lovelace Biomedical and Environmental Research Institute.

62. Dockery DW, Pope CA, Xu X, Spengler JD, Ware JH, Fay ME, Ferris BG, and Speizer FE: An association between air pollution and mortality in six U.S. cities, *N Engl J Med* 329:1753-1759, 1993.

63. Horvath H, Kreiner I, Norek C, Preining O, and Georgi B: Diesel emissions in Vienna, *Atmos Environ* 22:1255-1269, 1988.

64. *Ward's Automotive Yearbook,* Detroit, 1993, Wards Communications.

65. Department of Energy: *Motor Fuel Consumption Model Fourteenth Periodical Report,* DOE/OR/21400—H12, 1988.

66. American Public Transit Association: *Transit fact book,* p 26, Washington, DC, 1992.

67. Levins PL: *Review of diesel odor and toxic vapor emissions,* DOT-TSC-NHTSA-81-9. PB81-212961, U.S. Department of Transportation, 1981.

68. Scheepers PTJ and Bos RP: Combustion of diesel fuel from a toxicological perspective. II. Toxicity, *Int Arch Occup Environ Health* 64:163-177, 1992.

69. National Academy of Science: *Formaldehyde and other aldehydes,* Washington, DC, 1981, National Academy Press.

70. Kane LE and Alarie A: Evaluation of sensory irritation from acrolein-formaldehyde mixtures, *Am Ind Hyg Assoc J* 39:270-274, 1978.

71. Kane LE and Alarie Y: Interactions of sulfur dioxide and acrolein as sensory irritants, *Toxicol Appl Pharmacol* 48:305-315, 1979.

72. Burge PS, Harries MG, Lam WK, O'Brien IM, and Patchett PA: Occupational asthma due to formaldehyde, *Thorax* 40:255-260, 1985.

73. Pepelko WE, Mattox JK, Yang YY, and Moore W: Pulmonary function and pathology in cats exposed 28 days to diesel exhaust, *J Environ Pathol* 3:449-458, 1980.

74. Pepelko WE: Effects of 28 days exposure to diesel engine emissions in rats, *Environ Res* 27:16-23, 1982.

75. Wiester MJ, Ilitis R, and Moore W: Altered function and histology in guinea pigs after inhalation of diesel exhaust, *Environ Res* 22:285-297, 1980.

76. White HJ and Garg BD: Early pulmonary response of the rat lung to inhalation of high concentrations of diesel particles, *J Appl Toxicol* 1:104-110, 1981.

77. Green FHY, Boyd RL, Danner-Rabovsky J, Fisher MJ, Moorman WJ, Ong TM, Tucker J, Vallaythan V, Whong WZ, Zoldak J, and Lewis T: Inhalation studies of diesel exhaust and coal dust in rats, *Scan J Work Environ Health* 9:181-188, 1983.

78. Hyde DM, Plopper CG, Murnane RD, Warren DL, Last JA, and Pepelko WE: Peribronchiolar fibrosis in lungs of cats chronically exposed to diesel exhaust, *Lan Invest* 52:195-206, 1985.

79. Moorman WJ, Clark JC, Pepelko WE, and Mattox J: Pulmonary function in cats following long-term exposure to diesel exhaust, *J Appl Toxicol* 5:301-305, 1985.

80. Gross KB: Pulmonary function testing of animals chronically exposed to diluted diesel exhaust for 267 days, *Environ Int* 5:331-337, 1981.

81. Gross KB: Pulmonary function testing of animals chronically exposed to diluted diesel exhaust, *J Appl Toxicol* 1:116-123, 1981.

82. Heinrich U, Muhle H, Takenaka S, Ernst H, Fuhst R, Mohr U, Pott F, and Stoeber W: Chronic effects on the respiratory tract of hamsters, mice, and rats after long-term inhalation of high concentrations of filtered and unfiltered diesel engine emissions, *J Appl Toxicol* 6:383-395, 1986.

83. Schenker MB, Kado NY, Hammond SK, Samuels SJ, Woskie SR, and Smith TJ: Urinary mutagenic activity in workers exposed to diesel exhaust, *Environ Res* 57:133-148, 1992.

84. Hoar SK and Hoover R: Truck driving and bladder cancer mortality in rural New England, *J Natl Cancer Inst* 74:771-774, 1985.

85. Silverman DT, Hoover RN, Albert S, and Graff KM: Occupation and cancer of the lower urinary tract in Detroit, *J Natl Cancer Inst* 70:237-245, 1983.

86. Silverman DT, Hoover RN, Mason TJ, and Swanson GM: Motor exhaust-related occupations and bladder cancer, *Cancer Res* 46:2113-2116, 1986.

87. Kotin P, Falk HL, and Thomas M: Aromatic hydrocarbons. II. Presence in the particulate phase of gasoline-engine exhausts and the carcinogenicity of exhaust extracts, *Arch Ind Health* 11:164-177, 1955.

88. Kotin P, Falk HL, and Thomas M: Aromatic hydrocarbons. III. Presence in the particulate phase of diesel-engine exhausts and the carcinogenicity of exhaust extracts, *Arch Ind Health* 11:113-120, 1955.

89. Lewtas J, Bradow RL, Jungers RH, Harris BD, and Zweidinger RB: Mutagenic and carcinogenic potency of extracts of diesel and related environmental emissions: study design, sample generation, collection, and preparation, *Environ Int* 5:383-387, 1981.

90. Nesnow S and Lewtas J: Mutagenic and carcinogenic potency of extracts of diesel and related environmental emissions: summary and discussion of the results, *Environ Int* 5:425-429, 1981.

91. Claxton LD: Mutagenic and carcinogenic potency of diesel and related environmental emissions: Salmonella bioassay, *Environ Int* 5:389-391, 1981.

92. Salmeen IT, Gorse RA, and Peirson WR: Ames assay chromatograms of diesel exhaust particles from heavy duty trucks on the road and from passenger cars on a dynamometer, *Environ Sci Technol* 19:270-273, 1985.

93. Speizer FE: Assessment of the epidemiological data relating lung cancer to air pollution, *Environ Health Perspect* 47:33-42, 1983.

94. Wei ET and Shu HP: Nitroaromatic carcinogens in diesel soot. A review of laboratory findings, *Am J Pub Health* 73:1085-1088, 1983.

95. Henderson TR, Li AP, Royer RE, and Clark CR: Increased cytogenicity and mutagenicity of diesel fuel after reaction with NO_2, *Environ Mut* 3:211-220, 1981.

96. King LC, Kohan MJ, Austin AC, Claxton LD, and Huisingh JL: Evaluation of the release of mutagens from diesel particles in the presence of physiological fluids, *Environ Mut* 3:109-121, 1981.

97. Keane MJ, Xing SG, Harrison JC, Ong T, and Wallace WE: Genotoxicity of diesel-exhaust particles dispersed in simulated pulmonary surfactant, *Mut Res* 260:233-238, 1991.

98. Bond JA, Mauderly JL, and Wolff RK: Concentration- and time-dependent formation of DNA adducts in lungs of rats exposed to diesel exhaust, *Toxicology* 60:127-135, 1990.

99. Pritchard JN: Dust overloading causes impairment of pulmonary clearance: evidence from rats and humans, *Exp Pathol* 37:39-42, 1989.

100. Griffis LC, Wolff RK, Henderson RF, Griffith WC, Mokler BV, and McClellan RO: Clearance of diesel soot particles from rat lung after a subchronic diesel exhaust exposure, *Fund Appl Toxicol* 3:99-103, 1983.

101. Strom KA, Johnson JT, and Chan TL: Retention and clearance of inhaled submicron carbon black particles, *J Toxicol Environ Health* 26:183-202, 1989.

102. Creutenberg O, Bellmann B, Heinrich U, Fuhst R, Koch W, and Muhle H: Clearance and retention of inhaled diesel exhaust particles, carbon black, and titanium dioxide in rats, *J Aerosol Sci* 21:455-458, 1990.

103. Trochimowicz HJ, Lee KP, and Reinhardt CF: Chronic inhalation exposure of rats to titanium dioxide dust, *J Appl Toxicol* 8:383-385, 1988.

104. Culip WD: Sick boat, sick sailors. Casco Bay Weekly, Portland, Maine, September 20, 1990.

105. Commins BT, Waller RE, and Lawther PJ: Smoke in a London diesel bus garage. An interim report, *Br Med J* 29:753-754, 1956.

106. Purdham JT, Holness DL, and Pilger CW: Environmental and medical assessment of stevedores employed in ferry operations, *Appl Ind Hyg* 2:133-139, 1987.

107. Jorgensen H and Svensson A: Studies on pulmonary function and respiratory tract symptoms of workers in an iron ore mine where diesel trucks are used underground, *JOM* 12:348-354, 1970.

108. Gamble JF and Jones WG: Respiratory effects of diesel exhaust in salt miners, *Am Rev Respir Dis* 128:389-394, 1983.

109. Ames GR, Reger RB, and Hall DS: Chronic respiratory effects of exposure to diesel emissions in coal mines, *Arch Environ Health* 39:389-394, 1984.

110. Gamble J, Jones W, and Minshall S: Epidemiological-environmental study of diesel bus garage workers: chronic effects of diesel exhaust on the respiratory system, *Environ Res* 44:6-17, 1987.

111. Garshick E, Schenker MB, Woskie SR, and Speizer FE: Exposure to asbestos among active railroad workers, *Am J Ind Med* 12:399-406, 1987.

112. Gustafsson L, Wall S, Larsson LG, and Skog B: Mortality and cancer incidence among Swedish dock-workers—a retrospective cohort study, *Scand J Work Environ Health* 12:22-26, 1986.

113. Boffetta P, Stellman SD, and Garfinkel L: Diesel exhaust exposure and mortality among males in the American Cancer Society prospective study, *Am J Ind Med* 14:403-415, 1988.

114. Boffetta P, Harris R, and Wynder EL. Case-control study on occupational exposure to diesel exhaust and lung cancer risk, *Am J Ind Med* 17:577-591, 1990.

115. Benhamou S, Benhamou E, and Flamant R: Occupational risk factors of lung cancer in a French case-control study, *Br J Ind Med* 45:231-233, 1988.

116. Swanson GM, Lin CS, and Burns PB: Diversity in the association between occupation and lung cancer among black and white men, *Cancer Epidemiol Bio Prev* 2:313-320, 1993.

117. Netterstrom B: Cancer incidence among urban bus drivers in Denmark, *Int Arch Occup Environ Health* 61:217-221, 1988.

118. Waxman HA. Wetstone GS, and Barnett PS: Cars, fuels, and clean air: a review of title II of the clean air act amendments of 1990, *Environ Law* 2:1947-2019, 1991.

119. Federal Register: Part 80. Regulation of fuels and fuel additives, 40 CFR Ch. 1 (7-1-92 Edition), 370-391.

120. Federal Register: vol 58, No. 55. 40 CFR Part 86. Control of air pollution from new motor vehicles and new motor vehicle engines; particulate emission regulations for 1993 model year buses, particulate emission regulations for 1994 and later model year urban buses, test procedures for urban buses, and oxides of nitrogen emission regulations for 1998 and later model year heavy-duty engines, 1993, 15781-15802.

121. Federal Register: vol 58, No. 75. Retrofit/rebuild requirements for 1993 and earlier model year urban buses; fuel quality regulations for certification diesel test fuel. 40 CFR Parts 85 and 86, 1993, 21359-21401.

122. American Conference of Governmental Industrial Hygienists: *Threshold limit values for substance in workroom air adopted by ACGIH for 1972,* Cincinnati, 1972.

123. Federal Register: vol 57, No. 3. Permissible exposure limit for diesel particulate. 30 CFR Parts 58 and 72, 1992, 500-503.

124. Walsh MP: Review of motor vehicle emission control measures and their effectiveness, In Mage D and Zali O, editors: *Motor vehicle air pollution. Public health impact and control measures,* Geneva, Switzerland, 1992, Division of Environmental Health, World Health Organization and Ecotoxicology Service, Department of Public Health, Republic and Canton of Geneva. With permission.

125. Taylor LD and Thakur PC: Recent developments in coal mining technology and their impact of miners' health, In Banks DE, editor: *Occupational medicine: state of the art reviews. The mining industry* 8(1):109-126, 1993.

126. Chen C and Pepelko WE: Quantitative assessment of cancer risk from exposure to diesel engine emissions, *Reg Toxicol Pharm* 17:52-65, 1993.

Chapter 34

OCCUPATIONAL CAUSES OF LUNG CANCER

Kyle Steenland
Dana Loomis
Carl Shy
Neal Simonsen

Agents
  Silica
  Asbestos
  Products of the combustion of fossil hydrocarbons
    Soot
    Diesel engine exhausts
    Coke oven emissions
    Coal gas and coal tar volatiles
  Radon progeny
  Arsenic
  Acrylonitrile
  Bis-chloromethyl ether
  Chromium
  Beryllium
  Nickel
  Cadmium
Attributable risk

In this chapter the authors will focus on agents determined by the International Agency for Research on Cancer (IARC) to be definite (Group 1) or probable (Group 2A) lung carcinogens (Table 34-1). Exposure to these agents usually occurs in occupational settings, although two of these agents also occur commonly in the general environment, radon in homes and diesel fumes. The lung cancer risk due to environmental exposures to these agents will be covered elsewhere in this text (see Chapters 31 and 33).

Given the abundance of literature on the agents in Table 34-1, the authors will not provide a complete overview but rather highlight the major findings and major outstanding issues for each agent. Human epidemiology will be stressed, and animal data will be only briefly mentioned.

It should be noted that lung cancer is a disease that has many causes, and it is difficult to separate out the specific roles of the agents considered in this chapter from other more common exposures (primarily smoking) and also from possible genetic factors. Human epidemiology remains a rather crude tool, and we are only able to detect lung carcinogens that are strong enough to stand out above background.

The usual study design is a "cohort study" in which the lung cancer rates of an exposed group are compared with a nonexposed group. Often the exposure has occurred in the past and the follow-up for lung cancer mortality or incidence covers the time from first exposure to the present. A lung cancer rate ratio, sometimes called a relative risk, is then calculated. Rate ratios higher than the null value of 1.0 indicate that the exposed group has a higher lung cancer rate than the nonexposed. Frequently the nonexposed group is the general population, and in this situation the lung cancer mortality rate ratio is usually called a standard mortality ratio (SMR).

Generally we can assume some level of exposure to the agent in question among the exposed workers with the nonexposed referent group, often the general population, assumed to have little or no exposure. Issues of comparability of the two groups regarding other factors ("confounders") that might cause lung cancer, such as smoking, must also be addressed. Ideally, actual levels of exposure have been measured in the workplace, so that we can determine if more exposure results in more disease via a dose-response analysis.

Sometimes instead of a cohort design the reverse approach is used and we compare the past exposures of a group with lung cancer to the past exposures of a group without lung cancer in a "case-control study." Again con-

Table 34-1. Definite and probable lung carcinogens as classified by the International Agency for Research on Cancer (IARC)*

Agent	Animal evidence	Human evidence	IARC reference number
Probable			
Acrylonitrile	Sufficient	Limited	1979, 1987[191,16]
Diesel exhaust	Sufficient	Limited	1989[192]
Silica	Sufficient	Limited	1987[81]
Definite			
Arsenic	Inadequate	Sufficient	1980, 1987[173,16]
Asbestos	Sufficient	Sufficient	1977, 1987[193,16]
Bis-chloromethyl ether (BCME)	Sufficient	Sufficient	1974, 1987[194,16]
Beryllium	Sufficient	Sufficient	1993[177]
Cadmium	Sufficient	Sufficient	1993[177]
Chromium VI	Sufficient	Sufficient	1990[162]
Coke oven and coal gasification fumes	Sufficient	Sufficient	1984, 1987[79,16]
Nickel	Sufficient	Sufficient	1990[162]
Radon	Sufficient	Sufficient	1988[129]
Soot	Sufficient	Sufficient	1985, 1987[80,16]

*Agents classified as definite or probable carcinogens based primarily upon evidence at other sites, but with some evidence of lung carcinogenesis, have generally been omitted (e.g., formaldehyde, sulfuric acid mists). The U.S. National Institute for Occupational Safety and Health (NIOSH) considers all agents on this list to be carcinogenic, whereas the U.S. Occupational Safety and Health Administration (OSHA) considers all carcinogenic with the exception of silica, diesel exhaust, nickel, chromium, and beryllium (OSHA has no standard for soot; chromium VI is actively under consideration). Environmental tobacco smoke has been omitted but is covered elsewhere in the text.

founding and dose–response are important issues. Occupational case-control studies are often done within an exposed cohort and are then called "nested" case-control studies. The measure of association in a case-control study is the odds ratio, again sometimes called a relative risk. The odds ratio is the ratio of the odds of exposure in the diseased versus the nondiseased group, with a value greater than 1.0 indicating the exposed group is at greater risk of lung cancer.

In determining whether an agent does indeed cause lung cancer, common sense principles should be followed. Important criteria are the strength of the association (usually the magnitude of the relative risk), the consistency of effect across studies, a positive dose–response, biologic plausibility, and a correct temporal sequence (exposure precedes disease).[1]

It is important to consider the role of smoking because it is such a strong risk factor for lung cancer. Heavy smokers have a 20-fold risk compared with never smokers. The lifetime risk of smokers is on the order of 1 in 10, whereas the lifetime risk of never smokers is on the order of 1 in 200. Hence, differences in smoking between the exposed group and the nonexposed group can cause different lung cancer rates, and if unevaluated such confounding may cause the epidemiologist to falsely conclude that the occupationally exposed cohort has an excess lung cancer risk.

However, both theoretic and empiric data suggest that actual smoking differences between exposed and nonexposed rarely result in rate ratios greater than about 1.4 (40% excess risk for the exposed group).[2] For example, suppose 40% of the exposed are current or former smokers, suppose that these ever smokers have a relative risk of 10 compared with nonsmokers, and suppose that only 30% of the nonexposed are ever smokers. The resulting rate ratio or relative risk that will be observed due to smoking alone will be $[0.6(1) + 0.4(10)]/[0.7(1) + 0.3(10)]$ or 1.24. These theoretic calculations are supported by several studies in which investigators have looked at relative risks adjusted and unadjusted for smoking and found that they generally change very little and virtually never to the extent that an unadjusted 40% excess risk is reduced to no excess risk after adjustment.[3,4] A positive dose–response for the agent in question is another strong indicator that an overall excess risk for the exposed is not due to smoking alone, since it is unlikely that differences in smoking increase in parallel with differences in exposure level.

Smoking can interact with exposure to cause a higher lung cancer risk than would be expected by adding the risks of smoking and exposure together. For example, if the relative risk of smoking is 10 and the relative risk of exposure absent smoking is 5, then a relative risk of 15 for smoking and exposure together (versus neither) would indicate an additive model on a relative risk scale. On the other hand, a relative risk of 50 for exposed smokers would indicate a multiplicative model. A multiplicative model implies that the relative risk for the occupational exposure is the same for smokers and nonsmokers. This similarity of risks for smokers and nonsmokers indicates there is no "effect modification"; that is, the effect of the occupational carcinogen is not modified by the presence or absence of a third factor (smoking).

Two general points can be made about the interaction between smoking and the agents considered here. First, the observed interactions generally fall somewhere in between additive and multiplicative, regardless of the agent.[5,6] Second, there is frequently insufficient data to characterize the nature of the interaction, even when there are numerous studies with good smoking data for a given agent. This is true because lung cancer among nonsmokers is so rare. Therefore it is difficult to determine with any precision the lung cancer risk of nonsmokers, and hence it is difficult to distinguish it statistically from the risk for smokers.

Finally, it is also important to consider latency (time since first exposure) in evaluating the lung cancer risk of a given agent. Solid tumors usually do not develop until 10 to 20 years after exposure, and if the cohort in question has been exposed only recently, then no excess lung cancer risk would be expected. Investigators must take care to avoid false negative results from studing cohorts with insufficient potential latency.

AGENTS
Silica

Silica is among the most common minerals on earth, making up a substantial part of the earth's crust (see Chapter 24). Silica exists in two forms, crystalline and amorphous. It is the crystalline form (also called free silica) that is of concern. There is currently no evidence that amorphous silica causes either lung fibrosis or cancer.

Crystalline silica is made up of three minerals, quartz, tridymite, and cristobalite, with quartz being by far the most common. All have the same molecular formula, $(SiO_2)_n$. High exposures are common in foundry workers, miners, quarrymen, and sandblasters. Low exposures may occur whenever mixed dusts are breathed, but the general population is not considered to be exposed to levels sufficient to cause disease. The U.S. Occupational Safety and Health Administration (OSHA) limit for airborne quartz is 100 $\mu g/m^3$.

There are an estimated 1.7 million U.S. workers exposed to crystalline silica[7] outside of the mining industry. Some of the principal industries in which exposure occurs, other than mining, are masonry and stonework (130,000 workers), concrete and gypsum (65,000), and pottery (29,000 workers). Sandblasters are one occupation with very high exposure levels. Silica is a common exposure among miners but is highly variable depending on the silica content of the ore.

Silica has been long known to cause progressive granulomatous and fibrotic disease in the lung. It is known that silica is toxic to pulmonary macrophages that engulf the silica particles, and a variety of chemotactic and toxic substances released from lysed macrophages result in the collagen production which causes fibrosis.

The suspicion that silica may cause lung cancer first arose as the result of cancer found among silica-exposed rats used as controls in experiments testing the carcinogenicity of other substances.[8] Recent data indicate that inhaled silica can cause lung cancer in rats at relatively low doses (1 mg/m^3).[9] In rats inhaled silica causes both fibrosis and lung cancer, whereas in mice silica causes fibrosis but not lung cancer, and in hamsters it causes neither. The mechanism by which silica induces lung cancer in animals is not clear, whether directly through effects on the deoxyribonucleic acid (DNA) or indirectly by promoting growth of already initiated cells. Silica can cause chromosomal aberrations and transformation in vitro.[10] The strong immunologic response in the lung induced by silica particles and their toxicity to macrophages releases a number of substances (e.g., lysosomal enzymes), which may promote not only fibrosis but also cancer.[8]

The animal experiments sparked a large number of epidemiologic investigations in the last two decades. IARC has summarized the data in 1987,[11] whereas more recent reviews of the literature may be found in Pairon[12] and Goldsmith.[13] A general summary of the evidence is that the studies of silica-exposed workers suggest an increased lung cancer risk but are not consistent. The evidence for a lung cancer association is stronger for the many studies of workers with silicosis. Most of these (see below) have shown elevated lung cancer risk, often statistically significant and often beyond the range of excess risk that might be caused by confounding by smoking or other occupational exposures.

Cohort and case-control studies of silicotics are shown in Table 34-2 (studies in mines that might involve confounding exposures, autopsy, and proportionate mortality studies that may involve possible selection biases, as well as data from presentations or proceedings, are omitted from Table 34-2). A weighted average (inverse variance weighting) of the relative risks for these 15 studies gives a combined (inverse-variance weighted) relative risk of 3.74 (95% confidence interval [CI] 3.47 to 4.02). There is substantial heterogeneity between studies, as might be expected from different populations with different definitions of silicosis and therefore different entry criteria. These data suggest that either the relatively high doses of silica that are required to cause silicosis in turn result in lung cancer or that some aspect of the fibrotic disease itself accounts for the observed excess lung cancer risk. Generally the data are insufficient to determine which is the case. Although data for lung cancer among nonsmoking silicotics are sparse, there are indications that nonsmoking silicotics and smoking silicotics are at increased risk of lung cancer.[7,24,26]

Table 34-3 lists the larger studies of silica-exposed workers. All are studies where high exposure to silica occurred, as documented through actual measurements or an observed high prevalence of silicosis. Emphasis has been placed on studies without confounding exposures (for example, foundry studies are not included, and mining studies with appreciable levels of radon or arsenic are omitted). The studies in Table 34-3 suggest a moderate excess, with a combined (inverse-variance weighted) relative risk of 1.32

Table 34-2. Cohort and case-control studies of silicotics

Study	Lung cancer SMR or OR (95% CI)	Control for smoking; comment
Westerholm (1986)[14]	SMR = 4.4 (2.95-8.10)	Yes; 712 men compensated for silicosis from 1959-1977
Kurppa et al. (1986)[15]	SMR = 3.12 (2.30-4.14)	No; 961 men diagnosed 1935-1977 in Finland, consistent across industries
Forastiere et al. (1986)[16]	OR = 3.9 (1.8-8.3)	Yes; 72 cases, area of pottery industry, OR = 1.4 (0.7-2.8) for exposed nonsilicotics
Mastrangelo et al. (1988)[17]	OR = 1.9 (1.1-3.2)	Yes; 309 cases, area in Italy with quarries, OR = 0.9 for exposed nonsilicotics
Finkelstein et al. (1987)[18]	SMR = 3.02 (1.73-4.89)	No; 276 silicotics not employed in mines or foundries in Canada
Zambon et al. (1987)[19]	SMR = 2.28 (1.69-3.02)	Yes; smoking explains some of excess, 1234 men diagnosed 1959-1963, in Italy
Infante-Rivard et al. (1989)[20]	SMR = 3.47 (3.11-3.90)	Yes; 1165 silicotics compensated in Quebec 1938-985
Merlo et al. (1990)[21]	SMR = 6.85 (4.47-10.00)	Yes; 520 silicotics diagnosed in Italian hospital 1961-1980
Tornling et al. (1990)[22]	SMR = 1.88 (0.85-3.56)	No; 280 silicotic ceramic workers in Sweden
Ng et al. (1990)[23]	SMR = 2.03 (1.35-2.93)	Yes; 1419 men in a silicosis registry, estimated 50% of excess due to smoking
Chiyotani et al. (1990)[24]	SMR = 6.03 (5.39-6.77)	Yes; 3355 hospitalized pneumoconiosis patients, SMR = 2.22 for never smokers
Amandus et al. (1991)[25]	SMR = 2.6 (1.8-3.6)	Yes; 760 silicotics diagnosed 1930-1983 in North Carolina
Amandus and Costello (1991)[26]	SMR = 1.96 (1.19-3.23)	Yes; U.S. miners x-rayed 1951-1961, silicotics compared with 9543 nonsilicotics
Hnizdo and Sluis-Cremer (1991)[27]	OR = 0.9 (0.5-1.6)	Yes; nested case-control study among miners, OR = 3.9 (1.2-12.7) for silicosis of hilar gland
Chia et al. (1991)[28]	SMR = 2.01 (0.92-3.81)	Yes; 104 silicotic granite cutters registered between 1980 and 1984 in Singapore
Carta et al. (1991)[29]	SMR = 1.29 (0.8-2.0)	Yes; 724 silicotics diagnosed 1964-1970

CI, Confidence intervals; *OR*, odds ratio from case-control studies; *SMR*, standardized mortality ratio from cohort studies.

(95% CI 1.23 to 1.41), but with substantial heterogeneity between studies (again, as might be expected). Results of dose–response analyses were inconsistent in the seven studies that included dose–response analyses.

In summary the data to date support a view that either silica or silicosis entails an excess risk of lung cancer, with data for silicotics showing stronger evidence of an effect than the data for silica exposure alone. Although the data for silica exposure alone are inconsistent, the weight of the evidence is positive. It is possible that the mineralogic characteristics of crystalline silica vary sufficiently such that some varieties of silica induce lung cancer, but some do not.

Asbestos

Although use of asbestos (see Chapter 20) has been increasingly restricted as its dangers became known, the National Institute for Occupational Safety and Health (NIOSH) estimates that approximately 700,000 U.S. workers were exposed to asbestos, primarily maintenance and construction workers exposed to asbestos insulation and mechanics exposed to asbestos in brake linings.[7] Nicholson et al.[43] estimated that from 1940 to 1979, 27.5 million workers were potentially exposed, of whom 18.8 million had exposure in excess of the equivalent of 2 months in primary manufacturing of asbestos. Twenty-one million exposed workers were estimated to be alive in 1980. These authors estimated that excess lung cancer deaths caused by asbestos exposure would occur at the rate of about 5,400 annually in the mid-1990s and gradually decrease until the year 2030.

Asbestos refers to a variety of hydroxylated silicate minerals. These minerals are said to exist in an asbestiform or fibrous "habit" when the mineral has grown in one dimension to form long thin crystals. For the purpose of regulation OSHA has restricted its definition of asbestos to asbestiform fibers greater than 5 μm with aspect (length to width) ratios of at least 3 to 1.[44] In general it is believed that the long thin fibers are more pathogenic.[45] The current OSHA standard is 0.1 fibers/ml.[44]

Asbestos minerals are divided into two broad groups, serpentine and amphibole. Serpentine asbestos is called chrysotile, and the amphibole family includes crocidolite, anthophyllite, amosite, actinolite, and tremolite. All types of asbestos are known to cause lung cancer in humans. There is some debate about mesothelioma. There is considerable evidence that the risk of mesothelioma may be lower among workers exposed to chrysotile than among workers exposed to amphiboles. Some have suggested that the mesothelioma observed among chrysotile-exposed workers may have been caused by the small amounts of tremolite that invariably contaminate chrysotile.

Although asbestos has been shown to cause cancer in both animals and humans, the exact mechanism remains un-

Table 34-3. Selected studies of silica-exposed workers

Study	Lung cancer SMR, PMR, or OR (95% CI)	Control for smoking; comment
Davis et al. (1983)[30]	PMR 1.3 (1.0-1.6)	No; 969 dead granite workers, no trend with estimated dust exposure
Steenland and Beaumont (1986)[31]	PMR = 1.19 (0.97-1.46) PCMR = 1.09 (0.89-1.33)	No; 1905 dead granite cutters with high levels of silica exposure and silicosis before 1950
Neuberger et al. (1986)[32]	SMR = 1.48 (1.22-1.74)	No; 1630 Austrians exposed to nonfibrous dust, no change in SMR after excluding foundries
Costello and Graham (1988)[33]	SMR = 1.16 (0.96-1.39) SMR = 1.27, shed workers	No; 5,414 granite workers employed 1950-1982, high exposures, especially for shed workers
Guenel et al. (1989)[34]	SMR = 2.00 (1.49-2.69)	No; 2071 Danish stone workers with high historical rates of silicosis, 44 incident lung cancers
Koskela et al. (1990)[35]	SMR = 1.56 (1.05-2.21) SMR = 2.81, 25+ yr emp	No; but smoking habits probably similar to referents, 1,026 granite workers, 31 lung cancers
Siemiatycki et al. (1990)[36]	OR = 1.3 (1.0-1.8) OR = 1.7 for 20+ yr exp	Yes; cases ($n = 161$) restricted to nonadenocarcinoma (no risk for adenocarcinoma, $n = 37$)
Winter et al. (1990)[37]	SMR = 1.34 (1.03-1.73)	Yes; 3,669 pottery workers aged <60, surveyed for dust and smoking in 1970-1971, positive dose-response
Merlo et al. (1991)[38]	SMR = 1.51 (1.04-2.12) SMR = 1.77, hired < 1957	Yes; 1,022 brick workers, high historical silica exposure and silicosis excess, 28 lung cancers
Hnizdo and Sluis-Cremer (1991)[39]	OR = 1.97 (1.17-3.30)	Yes; case-control study among 2,209 gold miners, + dose–response, 77 cases, low radon exposure
McLaughlin et al. (1992)[40]*	OR = 2.1 (0.7-7.0) OR = 0.5 (0.3-1.0) OR = 0.7 (0.2-2.3)	Yes; case-control studies among Chinese pottery, tungsten, and iron workers, ORs for high silica versus none, dose–response for tungsten miners
Steenland and Brown (1995)[41]	SMR = 1.13 (0.93-1.36)	Yes; 3,328 gold miners, high historical exposures, no dose–response, low radon or arsenic
Checkoway et al. (1993)[42]	SMR = 1.43 (1.09-1.84)	No; 2,570 diatomaceous earth miners with high past exposures, 59 lung cancers, positive dose–response

CI, Confidence interval; *OR,* odds ratio from case-control studies; *PMR,* proportionate mortality ratio; *SMR,* standardized mortality ratio.
*95% CIs calculated from raw data and adjusted ORs. Tin miner data omitted because of arsenic confounding.

clear.[46] Asbestos is not a classic gene mutagen in bacterial systems, although it does have the capacity to induce gross chromosomal aberrations and transformation in mammalian cells. Asbestos may induce cancer directly in humans by these mechanisms, or by the production of free radicals consequent to immune response, and the subsequent action of these free radicals on DNA. Asbestos may also act as a promoter to increase the growth of already initiated cells. Although asbestos acts together with cigarette smoke in causing many lung cancers, it is clear that asbestos can cause lung cancer in nonsmokers as well. Inhalation studies among rats have shown that both serpentine and amphibole fibers cause both fibrosis, lung cancer, and mesothelioma.[47,48]

The dangers of asbestos first became known in the 1940s, largely from animal studies and case reports, but were not widely recognized except perhaps within the industries producing asbestos.[49] The first major human studies showing a lung cancer effect were published in England in 1955[50] and in the United States in 1964.[51]

Asbestos is much like silica in that cohort studies of subjects with asbestosis have shown a consistent and high rate ratio for lung cancer. Table 34-4 shows the results of cohort studies of asbestotics or men with radiographic abnor-

malities. Rate ratios ranged from 3.5 to 9.1, beyond the range of possible confounding by smoking. The combined relative risk (inverse-variance weighting) for these studies is 6.25 (95% CI 5.49 to 7.12) with substantial heterogeneity between studies.

Cohort studies of workers exposed to asbestos have shown a consistent excess of lung cancer. Table 34-5 lists the larger cohort studies, concentrating on those with some estimate of dose, and citing only the most recent update. The combined relative risk from Table 34-5 (inverse-variance weighting) is 1.88 (95% CI 1.81 to 1.96), again with substantial heterogeneity between studies. Those cohorts with lower exposures tend to exhibit lower risks, and dose–response analyses conducted within specific studies usually show a positive dose–response. Several of the studies shown in Table 34-5 include estimates of a linear dose–response in the form of a prediction equation in which the rate ratio (RR) or SMR for lung cancer between exposed and nonexposed is equal to 1.0 + (slope × fiber/ml-years). OSHA estimated an average slope across eight studies as 0.01 (95% CI 0.003 to 0.03).[44] It should be noted that estimation of historical dose is generally a problem because most studies have few historical measurements. Even in those studies that have the most historical data,[50,58,73,75]

Table 34-4. Cohort studies of asbestotic workers

Study	Lung cancer SMR (95% CI)	Control for smoking; comments
Liddell and McDonald (1980)[52]	SMR 3.50 (2.73-4.42)	Some; 4,559 chrysotile miners, SMR for men with less than normal x-rays versus general population, unchanged compared with men with normal x-rays, few smoking differences between normals or abnormals
Berry (1981)[53]	SMR = 9.1 (7.5-11.0)	Some; 665 certified asbestotics, 109 lung cancers, smoking data suggested asbestotics smoked only slightly more than referent group
Finkelstein et al. (1981)[54]	SMR = 7.9 (3.9-14.1)	No; 172 compensated cases, 11 lung cancers
Cookson et al. (1985)[55]	SMR = 5.1 (3.2-7.9)	No; 354 compensated asbestotics, 21 lung cancers, degree of profusion on x-ray predicted lung cancer but estimated cumulative exposure did not
Coutts et al. (1987)[56]	SMR = 7.40 (4.69-11.10)	No; 155 compensated asbestotics, 23 lung cancers
Hughes and Weil (1991)[57]	SMR = 4.33 (1.98-8.21)	Yes; 77 exposed men with abnormal x-rays ≥1/0 profusion, internal analyses confirmed risk

CI, Confidence interval; ***SMR,*** standardized mortality ratio.

counts by asbestos fiber occur only as of the 1960s, whereas earlier data are in units of millions of particles of dust per cubic foot (mppcf), and conversion of one to the other is difficult. Side-by-side measurements in the early 1960s have generally shown a poor correlation between the two.

For asbestos, like silica, the argument can be made that lung cancer cannot occur with preceding fibrosis. This hypothesis is difficult to assess epidemiologically because (1) those with fibrosis are those who also had higher doses, and higher doses would be expected to cause more lung cancer; and (2) few studies have good data on the three variables necessary to test this hypothesis (i.e., dose, radiographic changes, and smoking).[76] Recent studies with reasonably good data on these three variables suggest that only those with observable radiographic changes develop lung cancer.[52,57,71,77] However, each of these three studies has its own limitations, and very large populations are needed to truly confirm a negative hypothesis (that those without fibrosis do not get lung cancer). In summary, the human epidemiology is too sparse at this point to definitively decide this question.

OSHA's 1986 regulation did not differentiate between types of asbestos. Although chrysotile is cleared from the lung earlier than amphibole asbestos and although there is controversy regarding whether chrysotile can cause mesothelioma, there is neither consistent evidence that any one fiber type is more carcinogenic to the lung than any other, nor is there evidence that different fiber types exhibit different dose–response relationships.

In conclusion, asbestos is a known lung carcinogen for which the data are abundant. Most of the epidemiologic studies showing a lung cancer effect have been of workers exposed at very high historical levels, several orders of magnitude higher than most current levels. Little excess lung cancer is expected to result from the low levels of exposure of today, although there continues to be controversy regarding the potential of very low levels of exposure to cause mesothelioma.[78]

Products of the combustion of fossil hydrocarbons

Coal, petroleum, oil shale, and natural gas have been extensively used in industry since the early nineteenth century as energy sources and chemical feedstocks. These fossil hydrocarbons are complex compounds that vary widely in their chemical and physical properties. IARC has identified several products and processes related to heating or burning coal or petroleum as definite or probable lung carcinogens. The substances include soot, diesel engine exhaust products, coal tars, and emissions from coke ovens, coal gasification stills and iron, steel, and aluminum production operations.[79-81]

These hydrocarbon-derived products are highly variable, complex mixtures, rather than chemically specific substances. Epidemiologic studies show excess lung cancer risk among workers exposed to them. However, epidemiologic methods do not allow the specific constituents that cause cancer in humans to be identified. All of the substances considered here contain polynuclear aromatic compounds, some of which have been shown to be carcinogenic in animals, and these are generally suspected as the carcinogenic constituents.[79,80,82] Nevertheless, attribution of the carcinogenic effects of these mixtures to specific agents is speculative.

Soot. Soot is a particulate by-product of the incomplete combustion of carbon-containing materials, including wood, paper, and a variety of other products. The particulate phase of diesel engine exhaust may be considered a form of suspended soot (see below). During combustion, soot deposits on the walls of chimneys and fireboxes of combustion apparatus, and historically most occupational exposures have occurred during maintenance of these components. There is no specific OSHA standard for soot.

Table 34-5. Selected cohort studies of asbestos workers

Study	Lung cancer SMR (95% CI)	Control for smoking; comment
Selikoff et al. (1979)[51]	SMR = 4.06 (3.93-4.98)	Yes; 17,800 insulation workers, 429 lung cancers, OSHA (1986) estimated dose–response as SMR = 1 + 0.02 × f/ml-yr
Henderson and Enterline (1979)[58]	SMR = 2.70 (2.07-3.45)	No; 1075 men retired 1941-1967, 63 lung cancers, in an asbestos factory, OSHA estimated SMR = 1 + 0.005 × f/ml-yr
Finkelstein (1983)[18a]	SMR = 7.4 (4.4-11.6)	No; 241 men hired before 1960, 19 lung cancers, OSHA (1986) estimated SMR = 1 + 0.048 × f/ml-yr
McDonald et al. (1983)[59]	SMR = 1.05 (.77-1.42) (20+ yrs since hire)	No; 4,137 men in chrysotile/amphibole textile plant, 59 lung cancers, dose–response SMR = 1 + 0.051 × f/ml-yr
McDonald et al. (1984)[60]	SMR = 1.49 (1.18-1.87)	No; 3,641 in chrysotile friction products, 73 lung cancers, no dose–response, average level 2 mpcf
Newhouse et al. (1985)[61]	SMR = 2.96 (2.62-3.33)	No; 5,100 textile plant workers, 233 lung cancers, positive dose–response by low, medium, high jobs
Peto et al. (1985)[50]	SMR = 1.31 (1.10-1.55) (principal cohort)	No; 3,211 men in chrysotile textile plant, 132 lung cancers, OSHA (1986)[44] estimated SMR = 1 + 0.005 × fiber/ml-yr
Seidman et al. (1986)[62]	SMR = 4.97 (4.05-6.03)	No, 820 men in amosite factory, 102 lung cancers, no dose data but OSHA estimated SMR = 1 + 0.045 f/ml-yr
Hughes and Weill (1987)[63]	SMR = 1.34 (1.14-1.45) (>20 yr since hire)	Some; 5,492 chrysotile textile plant workers, OSHA (1986)[44] estimated SMR = 1 + 0.011 × f/ml-yr
Gardner et al. (1988)[64]	SMR = 2.05 (1.65-2.51)	No; 4,825 amosite factory workers, 93 lung cancers, positive dose–response by 4 exposure levels
Armstrong et al. (1988)[65]	SMR = 2.64 (2.15-3.64)	No; 6,915 crocidolite miners with brief exposures to 20-100 f/ml, 91 lung cancers, 30% lost to follow-up
Newhouse and Sullivan (1989)[66]	SMR = 1.04 (0.88-1.18)	No; 12,571 in chrysotile friction products, low doses, 242 lung deaths, OSHA estimate SMR = 1 + 0.001 × f/ml-yr
Piolatto et al. (1990)[67]	SMR = 1.1 (0.69-1.67)	No; 1,058 chrysotile miners, 22 lung cancers, no dose–response analysis, ⅓ of cohort with >400 f/ml-yr
Neuberger and Kundi (1990)[68]	SMR = 1.04 (0.79-1.41)	Yes; 2,816 workers at chrysotile cement plant after 1950, 49 lung cancers, low exposures, no dose analysis
Botta et al. (1991)[69]	SMR = 2.68 (2.18-3.26)	No; 2,608 men in chrysotile/crocidolite cement plant, 100 lung cancers, few exposure data
Cheng and Kong (1992)[70]	SMR = 3.15 (1.95-4.81)	Some; 1,072 workers in chrysotile plants, 21 lung cancers, positive dose–response by job categories
Sluis-Cremer et al. (1992)[71]	SMR = 1.72 (1.32-2.21)	No; 7,317 miners mining amosite and crocidolite, 63 lung cancers, no dose–response analyzed
Raffn et al. (1993)[72]	SMR = 1.82 (1.48-2.20)	No; 8,000 men in chrysotile/amosite cement plant, 104 lung cancers, exposures 10-800 f/ml in 50s
McDonald et al (1993)[73]	SMR = 1.33 (1.22-1.45)	Yes; 11,379 men exposed to chrysotile in mines/mills, 20+ yr latency, 545 lung cancers, follow-up 1951-1988
Dement et al. (1994)[74]	SMR = 1.76 (1.49-2.09)	Some; 3041 in chrysotile textile plant, update of Dement (1983),[75] dose–response SMR = 1 + 0.011 f/ml-yr

CI, Confidence interval; *OSHA,* U.S. Occupational Safety and Health Administration; *SMR,* standardized mortality ratio.

Extracts of coal and oil shale soots are carcinogenic in animals.[81] The evidence that soot is a human lung carcinogen comes principally from more recent epidemiologic studies of European chimney sweeps in which a twofold to threefold lung cancer risk was observed.[83,84]

Diesel engine exhausts. Diesel exhaust has recently been shown to be a lung carcinogen in animals (see Chapter 33).[85] The particulate phase of the exhaust rather than the gas phase appears to be implicated.

Human epidemiologic studies are difficult to conduct because it is difficult to substantiate the level of exposure to diesel fumes, particularly for populations exposed in the past. Very few historical sampling data exist. Diesel exhaust is a complex mixture of substances, characterized by polycyclic aromatic hydrocarbons surrounding an elemental car-

bon core. The gas phase includes carbon monoxide and nitrogen oxides. Past sampling techniques used carbon monoxide, nitrogen dioxide, or respirable particulate as surrogate measures of diesel exhaust. Recently, however, the measurement of elemental carbon has been used in conjunction with epidemiologic studies.[86] This measure is more specific to diesel exhaust and is of negligible significance in cigarette smoke, for example.

Outside of mining, there were approximately 1.34 million U.S. workers exposed to diesel exhaust in the early 1980s, principally in the trucking and construction industry.[87] The main occupations with substantial exposure are long-haul truck drivers, truck mechanics, miners in mines with diesel engines, railroad workers, and heavy equipment operators. There is currently no OSHA standard specifically for diesel exhaust, although there are standards for components of the exhaust such as carbon monoxide or nitrogen dioxide. The U.S. Environmental Protection Agency (EPA) regulations have been gradually tightened over the last decade to diminish the amount of diesel exhaust permitted from trucks.

Recent studies of diesel-exposed populations have improved on earlier ones because smoking data have been collected, and an attempt has been made to measure diesel exhaust currently and then extrapolate back to likely historical levels. Table 34-6 lists more recent studies that have had relatively good documentation of exposure or have been based on self-reported diesel exposure. Most have been able to adjust for smoking as well. These studies would indicate a combined relative risk of about 1.28 (95% CI 1.13 to 1.44) for diesel exposed populations versus nonexposed populations. These studies are reasonably consistent, so that the weight of the evidence to date tends to confirm IARC's 1992 judgment that occupational diesel exhaust is a probable lung carcinogen.

Coke oven emissions. Coke is produced by carbonizing bituminous coal through destructive distillation (see Chapter 39). Coke is used principally as a fuel for blast furnaces in the production of ferrous metals. Since the early part of this century, the by-products of the distillation process have also been recovered for use. Coal gas and coal tars, the principal by-products, are considered in subsequent sections.

Like other fossil hydrocarbons, the composition of coal is complex and variable. Its distillation produces a wide array of substances in solid and gaseous phases. These include carbon monoxide, hydrogen sulfide, aromatic amines, and polynuclear aromatic compounds. Within coke plants, exposures to particulate emissions and polynuclear aromatic compounds are highest on the top side of the coke oven where the coal is loaded.[79,94] The OSHA standard for coke oven emissions is 150 $\mu g/m^3$ in the benzene-soluble particulate fraction.

Compelling evidence of the carcinogenicity of coke oven fumes to the lung was presented by Lloyd from a study of 3530 male coke plant workers in the United States.[95] Compared with all steelworkers, men who had worked in the coke plant had an SMR of 1.70 for all respiratory cancers, which increased to 2.48 for men employed at the coke oven itself. Exposures to coke oven emissions were presumed to be highest at the top of the oven, and men who had worked exclusively in that location had an SMR for lung cancer of 7.31 compared with all steelworkers. Virtually all lung cancer mortality among workers in the coke plant was among nonwhite men, who were preferentially assigned to tasks requiring work on top of the ovens.

The large excess lung cancer risk among coke oven workers was seen in expanded studies of U.S. coke plants and was shown to be related to cumulative exposure to a measure of exposure to coal tar pitch volatiles.[96,97] The results of more recent studies of coke oven workers in Brit-

Table 34-6. Recent studies of lung cancer and diesel exhaust

Study	Lung cancer SMR (95% CI) or OR	Control for smoking; comment
Gustafsson et al. (1986)[88]	SMR = 1.32 (1.05-1.66) 6000 stevedores versus general population	Yes; via later case-control study (Emmelin[88a] et al, 1993) which found highest risk for highest exposed based on 50 cases and diesel fuel consumption survey, SRR for lung cancer incidence = 1.68 (1.36-2.07)
Garshick et al. (1987)[89]	OR = 1.41 (1.06-1.88) long-term railroad workers versus nonexposed	Yes; 1,256 cases, 20+ years exposed, parallel exposure survey of job categories, findings similar in subsequent cohort study
Boffetta et al. (1988)[90]	SMR = 1.18 (0.97-1.44) self-reported versus nonexposed	Yes; self-reported diesel exposure in Am. Cancer Soc. cohort of 1 million, 174 exposed lung cancers deaths, RR increased with duration of exposure, SMR = 1.24 for truck drivers, SMR = 1.59 for railroad workers
Gustavsson et al. (1990)[91]	SMR = 1.15 (0.67-1.84) garage workers versus nonexposed	No; but internal analysis showed highest risk for 695 bus garage workers highly exposed (OR = 2.4), parallel exposure survey, 17 lung cancer deaths
Steenland et al. (1990)[92]	OR = 1.89 (1.04-3.42) long-haul diesel truck drivers versus nonexposed	Yes; 996 cases in Teamsters union, risk highest for mechanics and drivers, parallel exposure survey, next-of-kin report of engine type, OR = 1.55 for long-haul drivers based on Teamster records
Boffetta et al. (1990)[93]	OR = 1.21 (0.78-2.02)	Yes; 477 cases, self-reported diesel exposure, + trend with increasing duration

CI, Confidence interval; *OR,* odds ratio; *RR,* rate ratio; *SMR,* standardized mortality ratio; *SRR,* standard rate ratio.

ain and the Netherlands are consistent with these findings from the United States, although with apparently smaller excesses of lung cancer.[98,99]

Coal gas and coal tar volatiles. Coal gas has been a major residential and industrial fuel since the late nineteenth century in countries where natural gas is scarce, notably in Europe. In the United States, there has been no widespread production of coal gas for fuel in the twentieth century, although some small-scale production occurred during the 1970s, following sharp increases in natural gas prices.

Because of the common origins of coke and coal gas and the related processes used to produce them, the epidemiologic literature describing the effects of these agents overlaps, but there have been relatively few studies of workers in plants operated exclusively for coal gasification without coke production. A study by Doll of men in the London gas works indicated that mortality from lung cancer was about twice that expected for men in the coal carbonization process where the potential for exposure to coal gas is greatest, but not elevated for those who worked in other areas.[100,101]

Coal tars are the heavy fraction of the by-products of coal distillation. Coal tars are used in crude form as a fuel, but the majority are refined for use in formulating other products, including pharmaceutical preparations, creosote wood preservatives, roofing and paving tars, coatings, insulation, oils, and carbon black products. Coal tar pitches are an important class of refined coal tar used widely in roofing and paving products, protective coatings, and as a binder in other products.

IARC's determination that there is sufficient evidence that coal tars and coal-tar pitches are carcinogenic to humans is based largely on excess skin cancer among exposed workers.[80] There is limited epidemiologic evidence of excess lung cancer among workers potentially exposed to coal-tar derivatives, including tar distillery workers,[102] roofers,[103] pavers,[104] aluminum reduction potroom workers,[105-107] and iron and steel foundry workers.[80] Exposures to coal-tar volatiles have not been well characterized in these studies, and it is likely that the workers in them were also exposed to other carcinogenic substances. One recent study of aluminum potroom workers exposed to coal tar pitch volatiles did include a detailed assessment of exposure and showed a significant positive dose–response between coal tar pitch volatiles and lung cancer.[65a] The potroom workers in this study had been exposed until the 1970s to levels of 1 to 3 mg/m^3 coal tar pitch volatiles (benzene-soluble fraction). The OSHA standard for coal-tar pitch volatiles is 0.2 mg/m^3.

Radon progeny

Radon (^{222}Rn) is a radioactive noble gas formed during the radioactive decay series through which uranium (^{238}U) decays to stable lead (see Chapter 31). The radioactive decay of radon gas itself produces short-lived radioactive isotopes of bismuth, polonium, and lead, known as radon progeny or "radon daughters." Unlike radon gas, which is chemically inert, the radon progeny are metal ions that adhere to particles suspended in the air. When inhaled these particles are deposited on the surface of the respiratory tract where they irradiate surrounding tissues with α particles. Like other ionizing radiations, the α particles emitted by radon progeny can break chromosomes. Chromosome breaks can lead to heritable cytogenetic change (translocations) capable of inducing or possibly promoting tumors through a multistage process. Thus, concern about the carcinogenic effects of radon exposure centers primarily on the radon progeny ^{218}Po, ^{214}Pb, ^{214}Bi, and ^{214}Po, rather than on radon itself. In most studies, ambient exposure to radon progeny is measured in working levels (WLs) and cumulative exposure is expressed in working level months (WLMs) (the product of exposure level in WLs and the number of 170-hour "working months" of exposure). One WL is any combination of radon progeny in air, which ultimately releases 1.3×10^5 MeV of energy during decay. Exposure to radon progeny is also sometimes expressed in picocuries/liter, a unit measuring decay; 0.005 WLM is approximately equal to the progeny in equilibrium with 1 pCi/L of radon. The current standard for radon exposure in mines is 4 WLM per year.

Occupational exposures to radon and its progeny occur in underground mining for uranium and other metals, in processing ores and radioactive materials, and in some caves and public spas. Most uranium mines in the United States closed by the 1980s and although other types of mines remain in operation and uranium mining continues elsewhere, the number of currently exposed miners in the United States is relatively small. There is potential exposure to large numbers of workers in poorly ventilated buildings. Although radon concentrations in buildings are far lower than in mines, the long periods of time that people spend at home and at work can result in significant cumulative exposures, although generally far less than a miner's exposure. A person spending 70 years in a residence and 45 years working-lifetime in buildings, both with the U.S. average radon concentration of 1.5 pCi/L[108] would accumulate approximately 20 WLM of exposure to radon progeny from the home and approximately another 5 WLM from buildings. By comparison, the median exposure to a uranium miner in the United States has been about 430 WLM.

Most of the direct epidemiologic evidence concerning the carcinogenicity of radon and its progeny comes from studies of underground miners. As early as 1879, European pathologists identified the characteristic lung lesions of the Erz Mountain miners as tumors.[109] Various causative agents for the tumors were suggested, including silica, metal ore dusts, fungi, genetic factors, and radioactivity—then recently discovered.[110]

Uranium extraction began to expand rapidly following World War II as a result of nuclear weapons production. In response to concern about the potential hazards of this new industry, the U.S. Public Health Service initiated a prospective study of a cohort of approximately 3,300 underground uranium miners in the Colorado Plateau region who were initially examined in 1950.[111] This cohort has been followed for nearly 40 years, using a variety of methods.[112] The initial results from the Colorado Plateau cohort study, reported in the middle 1960s, indicated a marked and statistically significant excess of lung cancer mortality among underground uranium miners, with mortality increasing with cumulative radon exposure.[113,114]

In subsequent decades results similar to those from the Colorado Plateau study were reported from many studies of cohorts of uranium miners and in other groups of metal miners worldwide.[115-125] In all of the major cohorts of miners that have been studied, mortality increases monotonically with cumulative exposure in WLM. The excess relative risk of lung cancer among miners is generally between 1% and 2% per WLM.[126] These data and data from animal experiments[127,128] provide convincing evidence that exposure to radon and its progeny is capable of inducing lung tumors in humans.[129]

The observation of excess lung cancer mortality at low cumulative exposures (less than 50 WLM) is an important finding in several studies of miners.[116-118,121,123,130] These risks and the linear fit of the dose–response function can be taken as supporting the view that radon carcinogenesis is a stochastic process with no risk threshold.[131] With this presumption, data from studies of miners with very large cumulative exposures have been used to estimate risks for individuals exposed at much lower levels in homes and workplaces.

Another important observation in studies of miners is that lung cancer risk appears to be a function of both radon and tobacco smoke acting "synergistically" among people with both exposures. In most studies the combined effects of joint exposure to radon and cigarette smoke are greater than the sum of both agents acting alone but less than their product. On the other hand, significantly elevated lung cancer risk has also been observed in nonsmoking uranium miners.[118,132]

The distribution of lung cancer histologic types has also been considered at some length in the literature concerning the carcinogenic effects of exposure to radon. Several studies of miners have suggested a predominance of small-cell undifferentiated carcinoma.[115,133,134] The most extensive data come from the Colorado Plateau cohort. Early reports[134] indicated that over 50% of the lung cancers identified among Colorado Plateau uranium miners were small-cell undifferentiated tumors, compared with some 20% among the general population of cases.[135] However, more recent studies of this group suggest that the proportion of small-cell tumors has declined with time and the numbers

of squamous and small-cell tumors are now roughly equal, at 36% and 32%, respectively.[136] All histologic types of lung cancer show an increase with increasing dose of radon progeny, however.[108,137]

Arsenic

Arsenic, an element commonly present in the earth's crust, occurs in organic and inorganic forms (See Chapter 29). Inhaled inorganic arsenic is a well-established human lung carcinogen, and inorganic arsenic also causes skin cancer after ingestion. Inorganic arsenic may occur as arsenate [As(V)] or arsenite [As(III)]. Metabolism of As(V) results in As(III), which is then detoxified by methylation.

Arsenic is unusual in that there is inadequate animal evidence of its carcinogenicity, whereas the human epidemiologic data are quite strong. Arsenic appears to interfere with DNA repair and has been shown to cause chromosomal aberrations, but it does not cause mutations in bacterial systems. Inhalation studies in rodents have been negative, but some studies with intratracheal injection have had positive results.[138]

The principal occupations exposed to substantial inorganic arsenic levels in the past are workers in copper smelters, workers manufacturing arsenical pesticides, and some miners. In the early 1980s there were an estimated 58,000 U.S. workers exposed to airborne arsenic, outside of the mining industry.[87] The current OSHA standard for airborne inorganic arsenic is 10 $\mu g/m^3$. There is some evidence that inorganic arsenic in drinking water is carcinogenic; excess lung cancer has been found in Taiwan in association with drinking water contamination, as well as excess cancers of the skin, liver, kidney, and bladder.[138]

The principal human epidemiologic studies are shown in Table 34-7. These studies show a consistent lung cancer risk at high levels, with a clear dose–response. The combined relative risk (inverse variance weighted) from these studies is 2.74 (2.54 to 2.97), with substantial heterogeneity. Hertz-Piccioto and Smith[139] have discussed the shape of the dose–response curve for arsenic. It would appear from the epidemiologic data that the excess lung cancer risks in worker population are primarily due to high exposures, which occurred largely in the past. No excess lung cancer occurred in the study by Enterline et al.[140] at smelters where exposures were estimated to be at the current OSHA level, 10 $\mu g/m^3$.

Acrylonitrile

Acrylonitrile is a colorless, volatile, flammable liquid with the chemical formula $CH_2CH—CN$. Acrylonitrile currently serves primarily as a key component in acrylic fibers used in textile manufacturing and is also used in pipes, fittings, and other products. NIOSH estimates that in the early 1980s, 335,000 U.S. workers were potentially exposed to acrylonitrile on the job, primarily via inhalation.[87] Absorbed acrylonitrile is primarily excreted through the urine

Table 34-7. Inorganic arsenic and lung cancer

Study	Lung cancer SMR (95% CI) or OR	Control for smoking; comment
Ott et al. (1974)[141]	SMR = 3.45 (2.11-5.32)	No; 603 men in pesticide plant, 20 lung cancers, 100-5000 $\mu g/m^3$ in 1940s-1950s, + dose–response
Lee-Feldstein (1986)[142]	SMR = 2.85 (2.57-3.16)	No; 8,000 workers at copper smelter, 302 lung cancers, + dose–response, range of exposure 400-62,000 mg/m^3
Enterline et al. (1987)[140]	SMR = 1.31 (1.07-2.65)	Yes; 6,000 workers at 8 copper smelters, 93 lung cancers, excess seen only at the one plant with the highest mean exposure (69 $\mu g/m^3$), other plants had 7-13 $\mu g/m^3$
Enterline et al. (1987)[140]	SMR = 1.98 (1.64-2.38)	No; 2,800 workers at copper smelter, 104 lung cancers, positive dose–response, 10-2,100 $\mu g/m^3$ exposures
Taylor et al. (1989)[143]	OR = 15.2 (4.9-52.7)	Yes; case-control study among tin miners, 107 cases, positive dose–response, mean exposures 420 $\mu g/m^3$ before 1951, 10-60 $\mu g/m^3$ thereafter
Jarup et al. (1989)[144]	SMR = 3.73 (3.04-4.50)	Yes; via later case-control study of 107 cases (Jarup and Pershagen, 1991[144a]), 3,900 in cohort at copper smelter, + dose–response, exposures 50-50,000 $\mu g/m^3$ before 1940, 50-5,000 $\mu g/m^3$ in 1940s, 50-200 $\mu g/m^3$ thereafter

CI, Confidence interval; *SMR,* standardized mortality ratio.

following metabolism by the liver. The OSHA standard is 2 ppm time-weighted average (TWA).

The similarity of acylonitrile's chemical structure with that of vinyl chloride monomer raises concerns regarding carcinogenicity. Most, but not all, bacterial studies involving acrylonitrile provide indications of mutagenicity, and rats exposed to acrylonitrile by inhalation or ingestion have shown elevated tumor rates, although rates were elevated for sites other than the lung.

A finding of 8 lung cancers versus 4.4 expected (rate ratio of 1.83, 95% CI 0.78 to 3.68) in a cohort of workers at an acrylic fiber plant prompted initial concern about lung carcinogenicity.[145] IARC reviewed acrylonitrile in 1987 at which time eight studies of exposed cohorts were available. In these studies, evidence of lung carcinogenicity was limited. Positive studies were generally based on small numbers and were not statistically significant.

Since 1987, there have been three relevant studies with reasonable sample size. A further follow-up through 1984 of the original cohort studied by O'Berg et al.[146,197] failed to observe a substantial lung cancer excess for either incidence or mortality (standardized incidence ratio [SIR] and SMR of 1.06). Collins et al.[148] reported on 1774 acrylonitrile-exposed workers employed between 1951 and 1973 at one acrylonitrile and one acrylic fiber production plant. The SMR for lung cancer was 1.00. Results using an internal reference population were similar. Swaen et al.[149] followed 2842 Dutch workers employed at 8 plants producing or using acrylonitrile. The SMR for lung cancer was 0.82 (95% CI, 0.47 to 1.33). Neither the studies of Collins et al. nor those of Swaen et al. showed a consistent dose–response.

In summary, animal studies indicate that acrylonitrile is a carcinogen but not a lung carcinogen. The evidence from cohort studies does not indicate that acrylonitrile exposure is strongly related to lung cancer but does not rule out a small increase in lung cancer risk.

Bis-chloromethyl ether

Bis-chloromethyl ether (BCME) is a colorless, very volatile liquid with the chemical formula $ClCH_2OCH_2$. BCME is not a naturally occurring substance. It occurs as a contaminant in chloromethyl methyl ether (CMME), used since the 1940s as an intermediary in the manufacture of a limited number of specialized products such as some pesticides and industrial solvents. Contamination can result in BCME concentrations ranging as high as 10% in CMME.[150] CMME contaminated with BCME will be referred to hereafter as chloromethyl ether (CME).

The occurrence of three cases of small cell lung cancer among 45 workers from the same facility in a Philadelphia chemical plant during 1962 eventually spawned a host of studies addressing the potential carcinogenicity of CME.

Although investigations of the Philadelphia plant were under way, animal studies implicated BCME as a lung carcinogen. BCME proved to be a potent carcinogen, causing lung cancer in rodent inhalation studies; purified CMME was markedly less carcinogenic.[151]

The studies on the Philadelphia plant workers revealed a threefold lung cancer excess for exposed workers.[152-154] Elevated lung cancer incidence was also noted at a California CME production plant.[155,156] Rates for five other U.S. CME plants showed little elevation.[156,157] Outside the United States, highly elevated lung cancer mortality was observed in German,[158] U.K.,[159] Chinese,[160] and French workers[161] exposed to CME.

Summarizing data to date, a total of 3,332 workers probably exposed to CME have been studied worldwide, among whom 24.1 lung cancers were expected during the period of follow-up. A total of 98 cases was actually observed, yielding an observed-to-expected ratio of 4.1. Studies have typically exhibited a marked dose–response and a histologic specificity for small-cell tumors. Fortunately, industrial hygiene control measures have drastically reduced the potential for CME exposure, probably accounting for the sharp decline in RRs beginning in the 1970s among U.S. and French CME plant workers under study.

Chromium

Chromium is a metal that can exist in any oxidation state between -2 and $+6$ (see Chapter 29). Most chromium compounds contain the metal in the $+3$ (trivalent) or $+6$ (hexavalent) state, and most natural chromium is found as oxides in chromite ore.

Chromium adds rust and acid resistance, as well as hardness to alloys. Foremost among these alloys is stainless steel, which accounted for 82% of all chromium consumed in the United States in 1987.[162] Numerous occupations entail opportunities for exposure to chromium. The most important include production of stainless steel, other chrome alloys, chromate, and chrome-containing pigments, chrome plating, and welding (of stainless steel). NIOSH estimates that in the early 1980s, 551,000 workers in the United States were exposed to hexavalent chromium, which is the principal cause of concern.[87] OSHA considers Cr(VI) to be carcinogenic, and the OSHA standard for chromic acid and chromates containing Cr(VI) is 0.1 mg/m^3. Historical exposures in chromate production and chromate plating were generally 10 times higher than the current standard.[162]

The oxidation state of chromium profoundly affects its physiologic properties. Cr(VI) readily infiltrates cells through normal ionic transport channels; Cr(III) apparently cannot and thus is poorly absorbed. Reduction of hexavalent to trivalent chromium at intracellular conditions releases oxidizing agents, which probably account for the consistent genotoxicity of hexavalent compounds in laboratory tests. Exposure to Cr(VI) has also been associated with chromosomal aberrations, mutations, and—in rats and mice—increased incidence of lung tumors following inhalation. Although other oxidation states have been more poorly studied, mammalian cell mutation and animal exposure studies of Cr(III) and metallic chromium are consistently negative.[162,163]

Over 50 epidemiologic investigations addressing lung cancer in occupational groups exposed to chromium compounds have appeared to date. Extensive tabulations of study results are available in the IARC review.[162] The largest and best-designed studies of chromium production workers, producers of chromate paints, and chromate plating workers are included in Table 34-8. Chromate production potentially exposes workers to many chromium species, including water-soluble and -insoluble forms of Cr(VI) and Cr(III), so lung cancer excesses in chromate workers cannot be clearly attributed to one species of the metal. Chrome pigments expose workers to hexavalent chromium, primarily in the form of lead or zinc chromate. Platers are potentially exposed to a variety of other carcinogens, including nickel. Takahashi and Okubo[164] found similarly elevated SMRs in platers using metals other than chromium (1.7) and in chromium-exposed platers (1.9), indicating that substances such as nickel may be involved in the lung cancer excesses seen in the chrome plating industry.

The epidemiologic evidence plainly establishes that workers involved in most major industrial uses of chromium are at increased risk of lung cancer. Those studies that addressed tobacco smoke, asbestos, and nickel exposure ruled out these factors as the major source of the observed association. The overall relative risk (inverse variance weighted) from Table 34-8 is 2.77 (2.52 to 2.90).

Beryllium

Occupational exposure to beryllium occurs in mining, extraction and refining of beryllium ore, in some metallurgic operations, in the manufacture of ceramics, electronic

Table 34-8. Selected cohort studies of chromium-exposed workers

Study	SMR (95% CI)	Control for smoking; comment
Enterline (1974)[165]	SMR = 9.43 (7.33-11.93)	No; respiratory cancer
Hayes et al. (1979)[165a]	SMR = 2.03 (1.55-2.63)	No; respiratory cancer, chromate plant, increase with duration
Alderson et al. (1981)[167]	SMR = 2.42 (2.00-2.90)	Some; U.K. chromate plant, heavy smokers rarer in cohort than in referents
Satoh et al. (1981)[168]	SMR = 9.23 (6.27-13.10)	No; chromate producers, increase with duration
Korallus et al. (1982)[169]	SMR = 2.10 (1.56-2.76)	No; respiratory cancer, chromate plant
Frentzel-Beyne (1983)[170]	SMR = 2.04 (1.23-3.19)	No; pigment plant, maximum risk at high exposure
Davies (1984)[171]	SMR = 1.82 (1.37-2.43)	No; 3 pigment plants, no increase at low exposures, smoking prohibited in workplace
Sorahan et al. (1987)[172]	SMR = 1.50 (1.17-1.89)	No; chrome and nickel platers, increase with duration
Hayes et al. (1989)[166]	SMR = 1.43 (0.93-2.13)	No; pigment workers, increase with duration
Takahashi and Obuko (1990)[164]	SMR = 1.87 (0.81-3.69)	Some; platers, 1.7 for platers using other metals, estimated 30% increase due to smoking

CI, Confidence interval; *SMR,* standardized mortality ratio. Results are for lung cancer mortality unless otherwise noted in comments.

equipment, nonferrous foundry products, aerospace equipment and tools and dies, in the machining, molding, grinding, cutting, and fabrication of beryllium alloys, and in the electroplating and atomic energy industries (see Chapter 29).[173] NIOSH estimates that 44,000 workers were potentially exposed to beryllium dust or fumes in the United States in the early 1980s.[87] Prior to the introduction of an 8-hour TWA limit of 2 $\mu g/m^3$ in 1949 and to avoid berylliosis, beryllium exposures were considerably higher than this limit (which is still the OSHA standard). A study of a U.S. beryllium-alloy plant conducted in 1947 to 1948 by NIOSH showed beryllium concentrations ranging from 411 $\mu g/m^3$ in the general air surrounding mixing operations to 43,000 $\mu g/m^3$ in the breathing zone of alloy operations.[174] Control measures were introduced throughout U.S. plants after 1949, and exposure levels were reduced markedly. Extraction plants and machine shops, for example, were able to maintain exposure levels below the 2 $\mu g/m^3$ limit.[174]

In its 1980 review of the experimental evidence for the carcinogenicity of beryllium, IARC concluded that there is sufficient evidence that beryllium metal and several beryllium compounds are lung carcinogens in rats and monkeys.[173] In particular, beryllium metal, beryllium–aluminum alloy, beryl ore, beryllium chloride, beryllium fluoride, beryllium hydroxide, and beryllium sulfate produced lung tumors in rats exposed by inhalation or intratracheally. Beryllium oxide and beryllium sulfate produced lung tumors in monkeys following intrabronchial implantation or inhalation. On reviewing epidemiologic studies conducted prior to 1980, IARC concluded that the evidence for increased lung cancer risk from occupational exposure to beryllium was limited, based on the three epidemiologic studies then available. Although each of these three studies showed excess lung cancer, IARC judged that it could not evaluate the contribution of beryllium to the observed lung cancer excess because the overall risk was small, the majority of cases occurred in a subgroup with very short employment in the beryllium industry, and data on the contribution of potential confounding factors were inadequate.[173]

Since the 1980 IARC review, two additional and larger cohort mortality studies have been reported, in each of which a significant excess of lung cancer was observed. Steenland and Ward[175] expanded the mortality follow-up of the Beryllium Case Registry cohort to include 689 women and men of all races. The lung cancer SMR was 2.00 (95% CI, 1.33 to 2.89). Lung cancer SMRs were greater among cohort members with acute beryllium disease (SMR = 2.32) than among those with chronic disease (SMR = 1.57). Based on limited smoking data (32% of the cohort) and the magnitude of the observed excess, the authors believed it would be unlikely that smoking was a major confounder of the observed excess lung cancer. The authors also argued that selection bias was minimized in this study because persons who died prior to entry into the registry were excluded, and only five persons were found to have cancer prior to

entry into the registry on review of registry records, and none of these had lung cancer.

Ward et al.[176] reported the results of a cohort mortality study of 9,225 male workers from seven beryllium plants in Ohio and Pennsylvania. The overall SMR for lung cancer was 1.24 (95% CI, 1.10 to 1.39). Cohorts having a high SMR for pneumoconiosis and therefore presumably higher beryllium exposure consistently also had an elevated SMR for lung cancer. Lung cancer SMRs increased with increasing latency. After a smoking-adjustment based on limited smoking data, the authors concluded that smoking was unlikely to fully account for the observed excess. The SMR at the plant with the highest exposures and longest latency remained elevated (smoking-adjusted SMR = 1.49). The authors note that the major difficulty in interpreting the smoking-adjusted SMRs is that smoking data were collected in the late 1960s, although most of the lung cancer cases (94%) occurred among workers hired in the 1940s and 1950s, when the smoking prevalence in the cohort may not have been very different from that in the national population.

In 1993, a working group of the IARC concluded that the evidence was now sufficient to conclude that beryllium is carcinogenic to humans.[177]

Nickel

The principal current uses of nickel are in the production of stainless and heat-resistant steels, nonferrous alloys, and superalloys (see Chapter 29). Other major uses of nickel and nickel salts are in electroplating, in catalysts, in the manufacture of nickel–cadmium batteries, in coins, in coated electrodes and filler wire used in welding, and in certain pigments and electronic products.[162] Data from NIOSH[87] indicate that about 147,000 workers in the United States were exposed to nickel and nickel compounds in the early 1980s (metallic nickel and nickel alloys excluded). Historically, highest occupational exposures, exceeding 0.2 mg/m^3, occurred in refining of nickel, grinding of high nickel alloys, production and processing of wrought nickel and nickel alloys, production of soluble nickel salts, production of nickel–cadmium batteries, and in polishing and grinding of stainless steel.[162] The OSHA standard is 0.1 mg/m^3 for soluble compounds and 1 mg/m^3 for nickel metal and insoluble nickel compounds.

IARC concluded that there is sufficient evidence in experimental animals for the carcinogenicity of metallic nickel, nickel monoxide and hydroxides, and crystalline nickel sulfides.[162] The experimental evidence for the carcinogenicity of nickel alloys, nickel carbonyl, nickel salts, nickel arsenicals, nickel antimonide, nickel selenides, and nickel telluride was judged to be limited.

From epidemiologic studies of nickel-exposed workers, IARC considered the evidence sufficient for the carcinogenicity of nickel sulfate and for "the combinations of nickel sulfides and oxides encountered in the nickel refining industry."[162] However, the evidence in humans for the carcinogenicity of metallic nickel and nickel alloys was deemed to be inadequate.[162]

The most current and comprehensive review of carcinogenic effects among nickel-exposed workers is presented in the 1990 report of the International Committee on Nickel Carcinogenesis in Man.[178] This report presents updated analyses of nine cohort studies and one case-control study of nickel workers and adds to or supersedes previous publications on most of these. Lung cancer and nasal cancer were consistently and significantly increased at nickel refineries among workers involved in sintering, calcining, leaching, milling, and grinding of nickel ores, and among workers in hydrometallurgy and electrolysis at these facilities. Using data from Table 83 of this report, which summarizes 13 relevant studies, the inverse-variance weighted average of the SMRs is 1.34 (95% CI, 1.28 to 1.40).

In contrast to these positive results, cohort mortality studies of workers engaged in the manufacture of high-nickel alloys showed no consistent significant overall excess of lung cancer,[178] and positive studies were often potentially confounded by other lung carcinogens. The role of nickel in lung cancer excesses observed among stainless steel welders is also unclear, as these welders are also exposed to chromium VI.

Cadmium

Cadmium is principally used in electroplating for the manufacture of automotive, aircraft, and electronic parts, marine equipment, and industrial machinery (see Chapter 29). The next largest use for cadmium is in the production of cadmium compounds that serve as stabilizers for plastics and as pigments. Cadmium is also widely used as the negative electrode in nickel–cadmium storage batteries and is combined with other metals in alloys for high-speed bearings, in welding rods and in reactor control rods.[179,180] Most exposure to cadmium and its compounds occurs in the working environment via inhalation. In the past, cadmium concentrations in workplaces were high; air levels of 1 to 10 mg/m^3 were found in alkaline battery factories in the 1950s, but with modern technology, it is possible to reduce air cadmium concentrations to less than 0.02 mg/m^3.[180] NIOSH estimates that 250,000 workers were exposed to cadmium in the early 1980s.[87] The current OSHA standard is 0.1 mg/m^3 for cadmium fumes (cadmium oxides), and 0.2 mg/m^3 for cadmium dust.

Experimentally, cadmium induces tumors of the prostate,[181] lymphocytic leukemia,[182] and lung tumors[183]; all tumors were induced in rats, and the incidence of tumors was dose dependent.

Until recently, the various epidemiologic studies of cadmium-exposed workers did not enable any definite conclusion to be reached due to concomitant exposures to other occupational carcinogens, mainly nickel and arsenic.[184]

Several cohort mortality studies have been conducted at a U.S. plant where cadmium oxide, sulfide, and metal were recovered from the waste of lead and zinc smelters since 1926; arsenic content of feedstock was reduced to 1.0% to 2.0% after 1940 and arsenic exposures were localized to one building.[185] Stayner et al.[186] extended the analysis of this cohort through 1984 and found a lung cancer relative risk of 1.49 (95% CI, 0.96 to 2.22); the relative risk increased with estimated cumulative exposure to cadmium and was statistically significant for workers in the highest exposure category (RR = 2.72, 95% CI, 1.24 to 5.18). To control for the potential confounding effect of arsenic, Stayner et al.[186] divided the 576 cadmium exposed workers in this cohort into two groups, those employed prior to 1940 and those employed in 1940 and later. The latter workers had little or no exposure to arsenic but, nevertheless, had a significant excess of lung cancer. In a subsequent nested case-control analysis of this cohort, Stayner et al.[187] reported a significant trend of increased lung cancer with increasing estimated cumulative cadmium exposure.

In 1993, a working group of the IARC concluded that there now was sufficient evidence in humans for the carcinogenicity of cadmium.[177]

ATTRIBUTABLE RISK

There are approximately 90,000 lung cancer deaths per year among U.S. men and approximately 100,000 newly diagnosed cases per year. The comparable figures for U.S. women are approximately 45,000 and 60,000. Nicholson et al.[43] have estimated that approximately 6,000 male lung cancer cases are now occurring annually in the United States because of occupational exposure to asbestos (and correspondingly, about 600 female cases). Other investigators have suggested that the total may be approximately half this number. Using our estimated proportions of U.S. workers exposed as well as our estimated relative risks, the authors estimate that an additional 3,000 male and 300 female cases occur annually because of past exposure to lung carcinogens other than asbestos (excluding occupational exposure to indoor radon, a potential hazard for which data are lacking). Overall, then, the authors estimate that approximately 9% of male lung cancers and 2% of female lung cancers in the United States are attributable to exposure to occupational lung carcinogens. These estimates are in fairly good agreement with earlier estimates.[190]

In general, estimates of the proportion of a disease resulting from a specific exposure are calculated using the population attributable risk percent (PAR%). This statistic is calculated as

$$\text{PAR\%} = \frac{P_e (R - 1)}{1 + P_e (R - 1)} \times 100$$

where P_e is the proportion of the population exposed, and R is the relative risk of the disease (lung cancer) from the exposure. Multiple exposures can be incorporated into their formula to obtain an overall PAR %. Limited data on the distribution of exposures in the general population (P_e) often prevent accurate assessment of the PAR%. Furthermore, uncertainties in estimated relative risk of lung cancer from specific exposures (e.g., asbestos) will affect the estimate. Finally, interactions of multiple causes of lung cancer (e.g., family history, cigarette smoking, diet) will change the proportion of cases attributable to a specific cause such as occupational exposure.

Estimates of the proportion of lung cancer caused by occupational exposures will therefore vary depending on which data and assumptions are used in the process. Any estimates should be considered as approximate.

REFERENCES

1. Hill A: The environment and disease: association or causation, *Proc R Soc Med* 58:295-300, 1965.
2. Axelson O and Steenland K: Indirect methods of assessing the effects of tobacco use in occupation studies, *Am J Ind Med* 13(1):105-118, 1988.
3. Siemiatycki J, Wacholder S, Dewar R, et al: Degree of confounding bias related to smoking, ethnic group, and socioeconomic status in estimates of the association between occupation and cancer, *J Occup Med* 30:617-625, 1988.
4. Blair A, Hoar S, and Walrath J: Comparison of crude and smoking-adjusted standardized mortality ratios, *J Occup Med* 27:881-884, 1985.
5. Steenland K and Thun M: The interaction of smoking and occupation in the causation of lung cancer, *J Occup Med,* 282:110-118, 1986.
6. Saracci R: The interactions of tobacco smoking and other agents in cancer etiology, *Epidemiol Rev* 8:175-194, 1987.
7. NIOSH: Work related diseases surveillance report, DHHS (NIOSH) publication 91-113, Cincinnati, OH, 1991, NIOSH.
8. Saffioti U: Lung cancer induction by crystalline silica, In D'Amato R, Slaga T, Farland W, et al, editors: *Relevance of animal studies to the evaluation of human cancer risk,* pp 51-69, New York, 1992, Wiley Liss.
9. Muhle H, Takenadka S, Mohr U, et al: Lung tumor induction upon long-term low-level inhalation of crystalline silica, *Am J Ind Med* 15:343-346, 1989.
10. Hesterberg T, Oshimura M, Brody A, et al: Asbestos and silica induce morphological transformation of mammalian cells in culture: a possible mechanism, In Goldsmith D, Winn D, and Shy C, editors: *Silica, silicosis, and cancer,* pp 415-422, New York, 1986, Praeger.
11. IARC: *Overall evaluations of carcinogenicity: an updating of IARCH Monographs 1-12, Supplement 7,* Lyon, France, 1987, IARC.
12. Pairon J, Brochard P, Jaurand M, et al: Silica and lung cancer: a controversial issue, *Eur Respir J* 4:730-744, 1991.
13. Goldsmith D: Silica exposure and pulmonary cancer, In Samet J, editor: *Epidemiology of lung cancer,* pp 245-298, New York, 1994, Marcel Dekker.
14. Westerholm P, Ahlmark A, Massing R, et al: Silicosis and the risk of lung cancer, *Environ Res* 41:339-350, 1986.
15. Kurppa K, Gudbergsson H, Hannunkari I, et al: Lung cancer among silicotics in Finland, In Goldsmith D, Winn D, Shy C, editors: *Silica, silicosis, and cancer,* New York, 1986, Praeger.
16. Forastiere F, Lagorio S, Michelozzi P, et al: Silica, silicosis, and lung cancer among ceramic workers: a case-referent study, *Am J Ind Med* 10:363-370, 1986.
17. Mastrangelo G, Zambon P, Simonato L, et al: A case-referent study investigating the relationship between exposure to silica dust and lung cancer, *Int Arch Occup Environ Health* 60:299-302, 1988.
18. Finkelstein M, Liss G, Krammer F, et al: Mortality among workers receiving compensation awards for silicosis in Ontario 1940-1985, *Br J Ind Med* 44:588-594, 1987.
18a. Finkelstein M, Mortality among long term employees of an Ontario asbestos-cement factory, *Orit J Ind Med* 40:138-144, 1983.
19. Zambon P, Simonato L, Mastrangelo G: Mortality of workers compensated for silicosis during the period 1959-1963 in the Veneto region of Italy, *Scand J Work Environ Health* 13:118-123, 1987.
20. Infante-Rivard C, Armstrong B, Petitclerc M, et al: Lung cancer mortality and silicosis in Quebec, 1938-85, *Lancet* 23-30:1504-1507, 1989.
21. Merlo F, Doria M, Fontana L, et al: Mortality from specific causes among silicotic subjects, *IARC Sci Publ* 97:105-11, 1990.
22. Tornling G, Hogstedt C, and Westerhom P: Lung cancer incidence among Swedish ceramic workers, *IARC Sci Publ* 97:75-81, 1990.
23. Ng T, Chan Shiu, and Lee J: Mortality of a cohort of men in a silicosis register: further evidence of an association with lung cancer, *Am J Ind Med* 17:163-171, 1990.
24. Chiyotani K, Saito K, Okubo T, et al: Lung cancer risk among pneumoconiosis patients in Japan, with special reference to silicotics, *IARC Sci Publ* 97:95-104, 1990.
25. Amandus H, Shy C, Wing S, et al: Silicosis and lung cancer in North Carolina dusty trades workers, *Am J Ind Med* 20:57-70, 1991.
26. Amandus H and Costello J: Silicosis and lung cancer in U.S. metal miners, *Arch Env Health* 46:82-89, 1991.
27. Hnizdo E and Sluis-Cremer G: Silica exposure, silicosis, and lung cancer: a mortality study of S. African gold miners, *Br J Ind Med* 48:53-60, 1991.
28. Chia S, Chia K, Phoon W, et al: Silicosis and lung cancer among Chinese granite workers, *Scan J Work Environ Health* 17:170-174, 1991.
29. Carta P, Cocco P, and Casula D: Mortality from lung cancer among Sardinian patients with silicosis, *Br J Ind Med* 48:122-129, 1991.
30. Davis L, Wegman D, Monson R, et al: Mortality experience of Vermont granite workers, *Am J Ind Med* 4:705-723, 1983.
31. Steenland K and Beaumont J: A proportionate mortality study of granite cutters, *Am J Ind Med* 9:189-201, 1986.
32. Neuberger M, Kundi M, Westphal G, et al: The Viennese dusty workers study, In Goldsmith D, Winn D, and Shy C, editors: *Silica, silicosis, and cancer,* pp 415-422, New York, 1986, Praeger.
33. Costello J and Graham W: Vermont granite workers' mortality study, *Am J Ind Med* 13:483-497, 1988.
34. Guenel P, Hojberg G, and Lynge E: Cancer incidence among Danish stone workers, *Scan J Work Environ Health* 15:265-270, 1989.
35. Koskela R, Klockars S, Jarvinen E, et al: Cancer mortality of granite workers 1940-1985, *IARC Sci Publ* 97:43-53, 1990.
36. Siemiatycki J, Gerin M, Dewar R, et al: Silica and cancer associations from a multicancer occupational exposure case-referent study, *IARC Sci Publ* 97:29-42, 1990.
37. Winter P, Gardner M, Fletcher A, et al: A mortality follow-up study of pottery workers: preliminary findings on lung cancer, *IARC Sci Publ* 97:83-84, 1990.
38. Merlo F, Costantini M, Reggiardo G, et al: Lung cancer risk among refractory brick workers exposed to crytalline silica: a retrospective cohort study, *Epidemiology* 2:299-305, 1991.
39. Hnizdo E and Sluis-Cremer G: Silica exposure, silicosis, and lung cancer: a mortality study of S. African gold miners, *Br J Ind Med* 48:53-60, 1991.
40. McLaughlin J, Chen J, Mustafa D, et al: A nested case-control study of lung cancer among silica exposed workers in China, *Br J Ind Med* 49:167-171, 1992.
41. Steenland K and Brown D: Mortality study of gold miners exposed to silica and nonasbestiform minerals, *Am J Ind Med* 27:217-229, 1995.
42. Checkoway H, Heyer N, Demers P, et al: Mortality among workers in the diatomaceous earth industry, *Br J Ind Med* 50:586-597, 1993.

43. Nicholson W, Perkel G, and Selikoff I: Occupational exposure to asbestos: population at risk and projected mortality—1980-2030, *Am J Ind Med* 3:259-311, 1982.

44. Code of Federal Regulations 29: *OSHA: Occupational Exposure to Asbestos, Proposed Rulemaking, Parts 1910 and 1926,* Washington, DC, 1986, Government Printing Office.

45. Stanton M, Layard M, and Tegeris A: Relation of particle dimension to carcinogenicity in amphibole asbestoses and other fibrous minerals, *J Natl Cancer Inst* 7:965-975, 1981.

46. Walker C, Everitt J, and Barrett C: Possible cellular and molecular mechanisms for asbestos carcinogenicity, *Am J Ind Med* 21:253-273, 1992.

47. Davis J, Beckett S, Bolton R, et al: Mass and number of fibers in the pathogenesis of asbestos-related lung disease in rats, *Br J Cancer* 37:673, 1978.

48. Wagner J, Berry G, Skidmore J, et al: The effects of the inhalation of asbestos in rats, *Br J Cancer* 29:252-269, 1974.

49. Enterline P: Changing attitudes and opinions regarding asbestos and cancer 1934-1965, *Am J Ind Med* 20:685-700, 1991.

50. Peto J, Doll R, Hermon C, et al: Relationship of mortality to measures of environmental asbestos pollution in an asbestos textile factory, *Ann Occup Hyg* 29:305-355, 1985.

51. Selikoff I, Hammond E, and Seidman H: Mortality experience of insulation workers in the US and Canada, 1943-1976, *Ann NY Acad Sci* 330:91-116, 1979.

52. Liddell F and McDonald J: Radiological findings as predictors of mortality in Quebec asbestos workers, *Br J Ind Med* 37(3):257-267, 1980.

53. Berry G: Mortality of workers certified by pneumoconiosis medical panels as having asbestosis, *Br J Ind Med* 38:130-137, 1981.

54. Finkelstein M, Kusiak R, and Suranyi G: Mortality among workers receiving compensation for asbestosis in Ontario, *J Can Med Assoc* 125(3):259-262, 1981.

55. Cookson W, Musk A, Glancy J, et al: Compensation, radiographic changes, and survival in applicants for asbestosis compensation, *Br J Ind Med* 42:461-468, 1985.

56. Coutts I, Gilson J, Kerr I, et al: Mortality in cases of asbestosis diagnosed by a pneumoconiosis medical panel, *Thorax* 42:111-116, 1987.

57. Hughes J and Weill H: Asbestosis as a precursor of asbestos-related cancer: results of a prospective study, *Br J Ind Med* 48:229-233, 1991.

58. Henderson V and Enterline P: Asbestos exposure: factors associated with excess cancer and respiratory disease mortality, *Ann NY Acad Sci* 330:117-126, 1979.

59. McDonald A, Fry J, Woolley A, et al: Dust exposure and mortality in an American factory using chrysotile, amosite, and crocidolite, *Br J Ind Med* 40:368-374, 1983.

60. McDonald A, Fry J, Woolley A, et al: Dust exposure and mortality in an American chrysotile friction plant, *Br J Ind Med* 41:151-157, 1984.

61. Newhouse M, Berry G, and Wagner J: Mortality of factory workers in east London 1933-1980, 1985.

62. Seidman H, Selikoff I, and Gelb S: Mortality experience of amosite asbestos factory workers: dose-response relationships 5-40 years after onset of short-term work exposure, *Am J Ind Med* 10:479-514, 1986.

63. Hughes J, Weill H, and Hammad Y: Mortality of workers employed in two asbestos cement manufacturing plants, *Br J Ind Med* 44:161-174, 1987.

64. Gardner M, Powell C, Gardner A, et al: Continuing high lung cancer mortality among ex-amosite factory workers and a pilot study of individual anti-smoking advice, *J Soc Occup Med* 38:69-72, 1988.

65. Armstrong B, Doklerk N, Musk A, et al: Mortality in miners and millers of crocidolite in western Australia, *Brit J Ind Med* 45:5-13, 1988.

65a. Armstrong B, Tremblay C, Baris D, et al: Lung cancer mortality and polynuclear aromatic hydrocarbons: a case-cohort study of aluminum production workers in Arvida, Quebec, Canada, *Am J Epidemiol* 139:250-262, 1994.

66. Newhouse M and Sullivan K: A mortality study of workers manufacturing friction materials: 1941-1986, *Br J Ind Med* 46:176-179, 1989.

67. Piollato G, Negri E, La Vecchia C, et al: An update of cancer mortality among chrysotile asbestos miners in Balangero, northern Italy, *Br J Ind Med* 47:810-814, 1990.

68. Neuberger M and Kundi M: Individual asbestos exposure: smoking and mortality—a cohort study in the asbestos cement industry, *Br J Ind Med* 47:615-620, 1990.

69. Botta M, Magnani C, Terracini T, et al: Mortality from respiratory and digestive cancers among asbestos cement workers in Italy, *Can Detect Prevent* 15:445-447, 1991.

70. Cheng W and Kong J: A retrospective mortality cohort study of chrysotile asbestos products workers in Tianjin 1972-1987, *Environ Res* 59:271–278, 1992.

71. Sluis-Cremer G, Liddell F, Logan W, et al: The mortality of amphibole miners in S. Africa, 1946–1980, *Br J Ind Med* 49:566-575, 1992.

72. Raffn E, Lynge E, and Korsgaard B: Incidence of lung cancer by histological type among asbestos cement workers in Denmark, *Br J Ind Med* 50:85-89, 1993.

73. McDonald J, Liddell F, Dufresne A, et al: The 1891-1929 birth cohort of Quebec chrysotile miners and millers: mortality to 1976-1988, *Br J Ind Med* 50:1073-1081, 1993.

74. Dement J, Brown D, and Okun A: Follow-up study of crysotile asbestos workers: whort mortality and case-control analysis, *Am J Ind Med* 26:431-443, 1994.

75. Dement J, Harris R, Symons M, et al: Exposures and mortality among chrysotile asbestos workers, *Am J Ind Med* 4:421-433, 1983.

76. Browne K: Is asbestos or asbestosis the cause of the increased risk of lung cancer in asbestos workers?, *Br J Ind Med* 43:145-149, 1986.

77. Slius-Cremer G and Bezuidenhout B: Relations between asbestosis and bronchial cancer in amphibole asbestos miners (letter), *Br J Ind Med* 47:215-216, 1990.

78. Health Effects Institute: *Asbestos in public and commercial buildings.* Boston, 1991, Health Effects Institute.

79. IARC: *Polynuclear aromatic compounds, part 2, carbon blacks, mineral oils, and some nitroarenes, Monograph 33,* Lyon, France, 1984, IARC.

80. IARC: *Polynuclear aromatic compounds, part 4, bitumens, coal-tars and derived products, shale-oils, and soots, Monograph 35,* Lyon, France, 1985, IARC.

81. IARC, *Silica and some silicates, Monograph 42,* Lyon, France, 1987, IARC.

82. IARC, *Polynuclear aromatic compounds, part 3, industrial exposures in aluminum production, coal gasification, coke production, and iron and steel founding, Monograph 34,* Lyon, France, 1984, IARC.

83. Hogstedt C, Andersson K, Frenning B, et al: A cohort study on mortality among long-time employed Swedish chimney sweeps, *Scand J Work Environ Health* 8(suppl. 1):72-78, 1982.

84. Hansen ES, Olsen JH, and Tilt B: Cancer and non-cancer mortality of chimney sweeps in Copenhagen, *Int J Epidemiol* 11:356-361, 1983.

85. Ishinishi N, Koizumni A, McClellan R, and Stober W (editors): *Carcinogenic and mutagenic effects of diesel engine exhaust,* New York, 1986, Elsevier.

86. Zaebst D, Clapp D, Blade L, et al: Quantitative determination of trucking-industry workers to diesel exhaust particles, *Am Ind Hyg Assoc J* 52:529-541, 1991.

87. NIOSH: *National Occupational Exposure Survey,* DHHS (NIOSH) 89-103, Cincinnati, OH, 1990, NIOSH.

88. Gustafsson L, Wall S, Larsson L, et al: Mortality and cancer incidence among Swedish dock workers: a retrospective cohort study, *Scan J Work Environ Health* 12:22-26, 1986.

88a. Emmelin A, Nystrom L, and Wall S: Diesel exhaust and smoking: a case-referral study, *Epidemiol* 4:237-244, 1993.

89. Garshick E, Schenker M, Munoz A, et al: A case-control study of lung cancer and diesel exposure in railroad workers, *Am Rev Respir Dis* 135:1242-1248, 1987.

90. Boffetta P, Stellman, S, and Garfinkel L: Diesel exhaust exposure and mortality among males in the American Cancer Society Prospective Study, *Am J Ind Med* 14:403-415, 1988.

91. Gustavsson P and Reuterwall C: Mortality and incidence of cancer among Swedish gas workers, *Br J Ind Med* 169-174, 1990.

92. Steenland K, Silverman D, and Hornung R: Case-control study of lung cancer and truck driving in the Teamsters Union, *Am J Pub Health* 80(6):670-674, 1990.

93. Boffetta P, Harris R, and Wynder E: Case-control study on occupational exposure to diesel exhaust and lung cancer risk, *Am J Ind Med* 17:577-591, 1990.

94. Fannick N, Gonshor L, and Shockley J: Exposure to coal tar pitch volatiles at coke ovens, *Am Ind Hyg Assoc J* 33:461-468, 1972.

95. Lloyd J: Long term mortality study of steelworkers. V. Respiratory cancer in coke plant workers, *J Occup Med* 13:53-68, 1971.

96. Redmond C: Cancer mortality among coke oven workers, *Environ Health Perspect* 52:67-73, 1983.

97. Mazumdar S, Redmond C, Sollecito W, et al: An epidemiological study of exposure to coal tar pitch volatiles among coke oven workers, *J Air Poll Control Assoc* 25:382-389, 1975.

98. Hurley J, Archibald R, Collings P, et al: the mortality of coke workers in Britain, *Am J Ind Med* 4:691-704, 1983.

99. Swaen G, Slangen J, Volovics A, et al: Mortality of coke plant workers in the Netherlands, *Br J Ind Med* 48:130-135, 1991.

100. Doll R: The causes of death among gas-workers with special reference to cancer of the lung, *Br J Ind Med* 9:180-185, 1952.

101. Doll R, Vessey M, Beasley R, et al: Mortality of gasworkers—final report of a prospective study, *Br J Ind Med* 29:394-406, 1972.

102. Maclaren W and Hurley J: Mortality of tar distillation workers, *Scand J Work Environ Health* 13:404-411, 1987.

103. Hammond EC, Selikoff IJ, Lawther PL, and Seidman H: Inhalation of benzopyrene and cancer in man, *Ann NY Acad Sci* 271:116-124, 1976.

104. Hansen E: Mortality of mastic asphalt workers, *Scand J Work Environ Health* 17:20-24, 1991.

105. Rockette H and Vena V: Mortality studies of aluminum reduction plant workers: potroom and carbon department, *J Occup Med* 25:549-557, 1983.

106. Gibbs G and Horowitz I: Lung cancer mortality in aluminum reduction plant workers, *J Occup Med* 21:347-353, 1979.

107. Spinelli J, Band P, Svirchev L, et al: Mortality and cancer incidence in aluminum reduction plant workers, *J Occup Med* 33:1150-1155, 1991.

108. Samet JM: Radon and lung cancer, *J Natl Cancer Inst* 81:745-757, 1989.

109. Greenberg M and Selikoff I: Lung cancer in the Schneeberg mines: a reappraisal of the data reported by Harting and Hesse in 1879, *Am Occup Hyg J* 37:5-14, 1993.

110. Hueper W: *Occupational tumors and allied diseases*, Vol 2, pp 435-468, Springfield, IL, 1942, Charles Thomas.

111. Archer V, Magnuson H, Holaday D et al: Hazards to health in uranium mining and milling, *J Occup Med* 4:55-60, 1962.

112. Hornung R and Meinhardt T: Quantitative risk assessment of lung cancer in U.S. uranium miners, *Health Phys* 52:417-430, 1987.

113. Wagoner J, Archer V, Carroll B, et al: Cancer mortality patterns among US uranium miners and millers, 1950 through 1962, *J Natl Cancer Inst* 32:787-801, 1964.

114. Wagoner J, Archer V, Lundin F, et al: Radiation as the cause of lung cancer among uranium miners, *N Engl J Med* 273:181-188, 1965.

115. Damber L and Larsson L: Combined effects of mining and smoking in the causation of lung carcinoma: a case-control study in northern Sweden, *Acta Rad Oncol* 21:305-313, 1982.

116. Howe G, Nair R, Newcombe H, et al: Lung cancer mortality (1950-1980) in relation to radon daughter exposure in a cohort of workers at the Eldorado Beaverlodge uranium mine, *J Natl Cancer Inst* 77:357-362, 1986.

117. Morrison H, Semenciw R, Mao Y, et al: Cancer mortality among a group of fluorospar miners exposed to radon progeny, *Am J Epidemiol* 128:1266-1275, 1988.

118. Radford E and St Clair Renard K: Lung cancer in Swedish iron miners exposed to low doses of radon daughters, *N Engl J Med* 310:1485-1494, 1984.

119. Sevc J, Tomasek L, Kunz E, et al: A survey of the Chechoslovak follow-up of lung cancer mortality in uranium miners, *Health Phys* 64:355-369, 1993.

120. Solli H, Andersen A, Stranden E, et al: Cancer incidence among workers exposed to radon and thoron daughters at a niobium mine, *Scand J Work Environ Health* 11:7-13, 1985.

121. Tinmarche M, Raphalen A, Allin F, et al: Mortality of a cohort of French uranium miners exposed to relatively low radon concentrations, *Br J Cancer* 67:1090-1097, 1993.

122. Hodgson J and Jones R: Mortality of a cohort of tin miners, 1941-86, *Br J Ind Med* 47:665-676, 1990.

123. Woodward A, Roder D, McMichael A, et al: Radon daughter exposures at the Radium Hill uranium mine and lung cancer rates among former workers, 1952-1987, *Cancer Causes Control* 2:213-220, 1991.

124. Samet J, Pathak D, Morgan M, et al: Lung cancer mortality and exposure to radon progeny in a cohort of New Mexico underground uranium miners, *Health Phys* 61:745-752, 1991.

125. Xuan X, Lubin J, Li J, et al: A cohort study in southern China of tin miners exposed to radon and radon decay products, *Health Phys* 64:120-131, 1993.

126. Samet JM and Hornung RW: Review of radon and lung cancer risk, *Risk Anal* 10:65-75, 1990.

127. Cross F, Palmer R, Filipy R, et al: Carcinogenic effects of radon daughters, uranium ore dust and cigarette smoke in beagle dogs, *Health Phys* 42:33-52, 1982.

128. Cross F, Palmer R, Busch R, et al: Development of lesions in Syrian golden hamsters following exposure to radon daughters and uranium ore dust, Health Phys lung carcinoma: a case-control study in northern Sweden, *Acta Rad Oncol* 21:305-313, 1982.

129. IARC: *Man-made mineral fibres and radon, Monograph 43,* Lyon, France, 1988, IARC.

130. Sevc J, Kunz E, and Placek V: Lung cancer in uranium miners and long-term exposure to radon daughter products, *Health Phys* 30:433-437, 1976.

131. National Council on Radiation Protection and Measurements (NCRP): *Evaluation of occupational and environmental exposure to radon and radon daughters in the U.S., Report 78,* Bethesda, Md, 1984, NCRP.

132. Roscoe R, Steenland K, Halperin W, et al: Lung cancer mortality among nonsmoking uranium miners exposed to radon daughters, *JAMA* 262:629-633, 1989.

133. Horacek J, Placek V, and Sevc J: Histologic types of bronchogenic cancer in relation to different conditions of radiation exposure, *Cancer* 40:832-835, 1977.

134. Saccomanno G, Archer V, Saunders R, et al: Lung cancer of uranium miners on the Colorado plateau, *Health Phys* 10:1195-1201, 1964.

135. Rosenow E and Carr D: Bronchogenic carcinoma, *CA* 29:233-244, 1979.

136. Saccomanno G, Huth GC, Auerbach O, et al: Relationship of radio-active radon daughters and cigarette smoking in the genesis of lung cancer in uranium miners, *Cancer* 62:1402-1408, 1988.

137. Archer V, Saccomanno G, and Jones J: Frequency of different histologic types of bronchogenic carcinoma as related to radiation exposure, *Cancer* 34:2056-2060, 1974.

138. Smith A, Hopenhayn-Rich C, Bates M, et al: Cancer risks from arsenic in drinking water, *Environ Health Perspect* 97:259-267, 1992.

139. Hertz-Piccioto I and Smith A: Observations on the dose-response curve for arsenic exposure and lung cancer, *Scan J Work Environ Health* 19:217-226, 1993.

140. Enterline P, Marsh G, Esmen N, et al: Some effects of cigarette smoking, arsenic, and SO$_2$ on mortality among US copper smelter workers, *J Occup Med* 29:831-838, 1987.

141. Ott M, Holder B, and Gordon H: Respiratory cancer and occupational exposure to arsenicals, *Arch Environ Health* 29:250-255, 1974.

142. Lee-Feldstein: Cumulative exposure to arsenic and its relationship to respiratory cancer among copper smelter employees, *J Occup Med* 28:296-302, 1986.

143. Taylor P, Qiao Y, Schatzkin A, et al: Relation of arsenic exposure to lung cancer among tin miners in Yunnan Province, China, *Br J Ind Med* 46:881-886, 1989.

144. Jarup L, Pershagen G, and Wall S: Cumulative arsenic exposure and lung cancer in smelter workers: a dose-response study, *Am J Ind Med* 15:31-41, 1989.

144a. Jarup L and Pershagen G: Arsenic exposure, smoking, and lung cancer in smelter workers—a case-control study, *Am J Epidemiol* 134:545-551, 1991.

145. O'Berg M: Epidemiologic study of workers exposed to acrylonitrile, *J Occup Med* 22:245-252, 1980.

146. Chen J, Fayerweather W, Pell S: Mortality study of workers exposed to dimethylformamide and/or acrylonitrile, *J Occup Med* 30:819-821, 1988.

147. Chen J, Fayerweather W, Pell S: Cancer incidence of workers exposed to dimethylformamide and/or acrylonitrile, *J Occup Med* 30:813-818, 1988.

148. Collins J, Page L, Caporossi J, et al: Mortality patterns among employees exposed to acrylonitrile, *J Occup Med* 31:368-371, 1989.

149. Swaen G, Bloemen L, Twisk J, et al: Mortality of workers exposed to acrylonitrile, *J Occup Med* 34:801-809, 1992.

150. Van Duuren B: Comparison of potency of human carcinogens: vinyl chloride, chloromethyl ether and bis(chloromethyl)ether, *Environ Res* 49:143-151, 1989.

151. Van Duuren B, Sivak A, Gosldschmidt B, et al: Carcinogenicity of haloethers, *J Natl Cancer Inst* 43:481-486, 1969.

152. Weiss W: Lung cancer due to chloromethyl ethers: bias in cohort definition, *J Occup Med* 31:102-105, 1989.

153. Defonso L and Kelton S: Lung cancer following exposure to CMME, *Arch Environ Health* 31:125-130, 1976.

154. Maher K and DeFonso L: Respiratory cancer among CMME workers, *J Natl Cancer Inst* 78:839-843, 1987.

155. Lemen R, Johnson W, Wagoner J, et al: Cytologic observations and cancer incidence following exposure to BCME, *Ann NY Acad Sci* 271:71-80, 1976.

156. Collingwood KW, Pasternack B, and Shore R: An industrywide study of respiratory cancer in chemical workers exposed to chloromethyl ethers, *J Natl Cancer Inst* 78:1127-1136, 1987.

157. Pasternak B, Shore R, and Albert R: Occupational exposure to CMME, *J Occup Med* 19:741-746, 1977.

158. Theiss A, Hey W, and Zeller H: Zur toxikologie von Dichlorodimethylather, *Zentralbl Arbeitsmed* 23:97-102, 1973.

159. McCallum R, Woolley V, and Petrie A: Lung cancer associated with CMME manufacture, *Br J Ind Med* 40:384-389, 1983.

160. Xue S and Liang Y: Occupational health in industrialization and modernization, WHO Collaborating Center for Occupational Health, Shanghai, China 2:75-80, 1988.

161. Gowers D, L DeFonso, P Schaffer, et al: Incidence of respiratory cancer among workers exposed to chloromethyl-ethers, *Am J Epidemiol* 137:31-42, 1993.

162. IARC: *Chromium, nickel, and welding, Monograph 49,* Lyon, France, 1990, IARC.

163. Cohen M, Kargacin B, Klein C, et al: Mechanisms of chromium carcinogenicity and toxicity, *Crit Rev Toxicol* 23:255-281, 1993.

164. Takahashi K and Okubo T: A prospective study of chromium plating workers in Japan, *Arch Environ Health* 45:107-111, 1990.

165. Enterline P: Respiratory cancer among chromate workers, *J Occup Med* 16:523-526, 1974.

165a. Hayes R, Lillienfeld A, and Snell L: Mortality in chromium chemical production workers: a prospective study, *Int J Epidemiol* 8:365-374, 1979.

166. Hayes R, Sheffet A, and Spirtas R: Cancer mortality among a cohort of chromium pigment workers, *Am J Ind Med* 16:127-133, 1989.

167. Alderson M, Rattan N, and Bidstrup L: Health of workmen in the chromate-producing industry in Britain, *Br J Ind Med* 38:117-124, 1981.

168. Satoh K, Fukuda Y, Torii K, et al: Epidemiological study of workers engaged in the manufacture of chromium compounds, *J Occup Med* 23:835-838, 1981.

169. Korallus U, Lange H, Neiss A, et al: Relationship between environmental hygiene control measures and mortality from bronchial cancer in the chromate producing industry (Ger), *Arbeitsmed Socialmed Praventivmed* 17:159-167, 1982.

170. Frentzel-Beyne: Lung cancer mortality of workers employed in chromate pigment factories, *J Can Res Clin Oncol* 105:183-188, 1983.

171. Davies J: Lung cancer mortality among workers making lead chromate and zinc chromate pigments in three English factories, *Br J Ind Med* 41:158-169, 1984.

172. Sorohan T, Burges D, and Waterhouse J: A mortality study of nickel/chromium platers, *Br J Ind Med* 44:250-258, 1987.

173. IARC: *Some metals and metallic compounds, Monograph 23,* Lyon, France, 1980, IARC.

174. NIOSH: *Criteria for a recommended standard-occupational exposure to beryllium.* NIOSH Document No. HSM 72-10268, Washington, DC, 1972, U.S. Department of Health, Education, and Welfare.

175. Steenland K and Ward E: Lung cancer incidence among patients with beryllium disease: a cohort mortality study, *J Natl Cancer Inst* 83:1380-1385, 1991.

176. Ward E, Okun A, Ruder A, et al: A mortality study of workers at seven beryllium plants, *Am J Ind Med* 22:885-904, 1993.

177. IARC: *Beryllium, cadmium, mercury and exposures in the glass manufacturing industry, Monograph 58,* Lyon, France, 1993, IARC.

178. ICNCM (International Committee on Nickel Carcinogenesis in Man): Report of the International Committee on Nickel Carcinogenesis in Man, *Scand J Work Environ Health* 16:1-84, 1990.

179. IARC: *Cadmium, nickel, some epoxides, miscellaneous industrial chemicals and general considerations on volatile anaesthetics, Monograph 11,* Lyon, France, 1976, IARC.

180. Schaller K and Angerer J: Biological monitoring in the occupational setting—relationship to cadmium exposure, In Nordberg G, Herber R, and Alessio L, editors: *Cadmium in the human environment: toxicity and carcinogenicity,* pp 53-63, Lyon, France, 1992, IARC.

181. Waalkes M, Rehm S, Perantoni A, et al: Cadmium exposure in rats and tumours of the prostate, In Nordberg G, Herber R, and Alessio L, editors: *Cadmium in the human environment: toxicity and carcinogenicity,* pp 391-400, Lyon, France, 1992, IARC.

182. Waalkes M, Rehm S, Sass B, et al: Induction of tumours of the haematopoietic system by cadmium in rats, In Nordberg G, Herber R, and Alessio L, editors: *Cadmium in the human environment: toxicity and carcinogenicity,* pp 401-404, Lyon, France, 1992, IARC.

183. Heinrich U: Pulmonary carcinogenicity of cadmium by inhalation in animals, In Nordberg G, Herber R, and Alessio L, editors: *Cadmium*

in the human environment: toxicity and carcinogenicity, pp 405-414, Lyon, France, 1992, IARC.

184. Boffetta P: Methodological aspects of the epidemiological association between cadmium and cancer in humans, In Nordberg G, Herber R, and Alessio L editors: *Cadmium in the human environment: toxicity and carcinogenicity,* pp 425-434, Lyon, France, 1992, IARC.

185. Thun M, Schnorr T, and Halperin W: Mortality from lung and prostatic cancer in U.S. cadmium workers, presented at the Workshop on Cadmium and Cancer, Oxford, England, September 29-October 1, 1986.

186. Stayner L, Smith R, Thun M, et al: A dose-response analysis and quantitative assessment of lung cancer risk and occupational cadmium exposure, *Ann Epidemiol* 2:177-194, 1992.

187. Stayner L, Smith R, Schnorr T, et al: Letter, *Ann Epidemiol* 3:114-116, 1993.

188. Doll R and Peto R: The causes of cancer: quantitative estimates of avoidable risks of cancer in the U.S. today, *J Natl Cancer Inst* 66:1191-1308, 1981.

189. Morabia A, Markowit S, Garibaldi K, et al: Lung cancer and occupation: results of a multicenter case-control study, *Br J Ind Med* 49:721-727, 1992.

190. Vineis P, Thomas T, Hayes R, et al: Proportion of lung cancers in males due to occupation in different areas of the U.S., *Int J Cancer* 42:851-856, 1988.

191. IARC, *Some aromatic amines, hydrazine and related compounds, N-nitroso compounds, and miscellaneous alkylating agents, Monograph 4,* Lyon, France, 1974, IARC.

192. IARC, *Asbestos, Monograph 14,* Lyon, France, 1977, IARC.

193. IARC, *Some monomers, plastics, and synthetic elastomers, and acrolein, Monograph 19,* Lyon, France, 1979, IARC.

194. IARC, *Diesel and gasoline engine exhausts and some nitroarenes, Monograph 46,* Lyon, France, 1989, IARC.

Chapter 35

AGENTS CAUSING OTHER RESPIRATORY CANCERS

Thomas L. Vaughan

Specific agents causing other upper airway cancers
  Tobacco
  Alcohol
  Nickel compounds
  Chromium compounds
  Other agents
    Mustard gas
    Thorotrast
Industries and occupations associated with other respiratory
  cancers
  Wood industry
  Leather boot and shoe manufacture and repair
  Isopropyl alcohol manufacture
Other agents or industries suspected of causing other
  respiratory cancers
  Agents
    Formaldehyde
    Asbestos
    Acid mists
  Industries
    Textile industry
    Painting
    Baking and pastry cooking

In 1994 it was projected that 218,600 persons in the United States would have been newly-diagnosed with cancer of the respiratory system or oral cavity, and over 166,000 would have died from one of these diseases (Table 35-1).[55] Tumors of the lung and bronchus accounted for most of the new cancers (78.7%) and an even larger proportion of deaths (92.1%). Thus it is not surprising that lung cancer has been the focus of many of the studies that have examined the association between environmental agents and can-

cer of the respiratory system. However, any inhaled environmental agent reaching the lung must first pass through, and potentially expose, the upper respiratory tract, where the mucosa of the oral cavity and extrinsic larynx comes in direct contact with ingested agents as well. Consequently cancers of the upper respiratory system and oral cavity also are important sites of cancer caused by environmental agents.

In some instances specific causal agents have been identified; in others an increased risk has been strongly linked to work in an industry or particular occupation, but the actual causal agent or agents have not been identified with certainty. There are also a number of agents or types of work for which there is reason to suspect an increased risk for other respiratory cancers, but where conclusive evidence is lacking. These three situations are discussed separately.

The carcinogenicity classification by the International Agency for Research on Cancer (IARC) is given when it is available. The IARC periodically convenes international working groups to review published information relating to the risk of cancer associated with exposure to an agent or work situation and to qualitatively assess the probability that such exposure is carcinogenic in humans. The classifications and definitions used are: group 1 (sufficient evidence of carcinogenicity), group 2A (probably carcinogenic), group 2B (possibly carcinogenic), group 3 (not classifiable), and group 4 (probably not carcinogenic).

In interpreting results from epidemiologic and animal studies, it is particularly important to assess the relationship between dose and cancer risk. Some of the strongest associations may reflect relatively high historic exposures or exposure levels and patterns found primarily in developing countries, whereas some negative results may be due to a low level of exposure in the study population.

It is also important to keep in mind potential synergism between agents. For example, simultaneous exposure to both carcinogenic chemicals and particles may be especially damaging to the respiratory tract. Chronic exposure to particles can cause stasis of the mucociliary clearance system,

Table 35-1. Cancers of the respiratory system and oral cavity: estimated new cases and deaths in the United States during 1994

Site	New cases (%)	Deaths (%)
Lung	172,000 (78.7)	153,000 (92.1)
Larynx	12,500 (5.7)	3,800 (2.3)
Pharynx	9,200 (4.2)	4,000 (2.4)
Other oral cavity	20,400 (9.3)	3,925 (2.4)
Nasopharynx, sinonasal cavities, other and unspecified	4,500 (2.1)	1,400 (0.8)
Total	218,600 (100.0)	166,125 (100.0)

From Boring CC, Squires TS, Tong T, et al: Cancer Statistics 1994, *CA Cancer J Clin* 44:18-19, 1994.

resulting in prolonged exposure to carcinogens that may be present on the particles or in the ambient air. Long-term particle exposure, with resulting chronic irritation and increased rates of cellular proliferation, may also promote neoplasms initiated by other agents.

The various exposures and cancers discussed in this chapter are summarized in Table 35-2, which describes specific agents that have been linked with an increased risk of other (nonbronchogenic) respiratory cancers, and Table 35-3, which describes industries and occupations that have been associated with these cancers.

SPECIFIC AGENTS CAUSING OTHER UPPER AIRWAY CANCERS
Tobacco

Products formed during the burning of tobacco are carcinogenic for every site within the respiratory system, and have been classified by IARC as group 1 carcinogens.[1] Over 3,800 individual compounds have been identified in tobacco smoke of which at least 43 are known to be animal carcinogens.[1]

The strength of the association between tobacco smoking and cancer risk at each site in the upper respiratory system in humans appears to depend largely on the extent to which the particular tissue is exposed. Thus current cigarette smokers have 10 or more times the risk of never-smokers for carcinomas of the oral cavity, pharynx, and larynx[2,3]; whereas for the sinonasal cavities and nasopharynx, where exposure is usually less direct, the relative risk among current cigarette smokers is much lower—on the order of two to three.[4-6]

As with lung cancer, the risk for upper respiratory cancers tends to drop rapidly after smoking cessation. For example, ten years after quitting, the risk for laryngeal cancer is only about 20% of what it would have been with continued smoking, although it is still higher than for lifetime nonsmokers.[3] It appears that the use of filter cigarettes decreases the risk associated with smoking as compared with nonfilter cigarette smokers but only to a mild degree.[3]

Table 35-2. Agents suspected of causing other respiratory and oral cavity cancers

Agent	Cancer site	IARC group, comment
Tobacco	Sinonasal cavities	1
	Nasopharynx	Highest risk for pharynx, oral cavity, and larynx
	Pharynx	
	Oral cavity	
	Larynx	
Alcohol	Sinonasal cavities (?)	1
	Nasopharynx (?)	Highest risk for pharynx, oral cavity, and larynx
	Pharynx	
	Oral cavity	
	Larynx	
Nickel compounds	Sinonasal cavities	1
		Highest risk associated with smelting and refining activities; exposure to metallic nickel possibly carcinogenic
Chromium[VI] compounds	Sinonasal cavities	1
Mustard gas	Pharynx	1
	Larynx	
Thorotrast	Sinonasal cavities	
Formaldehyde	Sinonasal cavities (?)	2a
	Nasopharynx (?)	Possibly carcinogenic only in presence of particulates
Asbestos	Larynx (?)	1
		IARC classification based on increased risk for lung cancer; risk for laryngeal cancer not established
Acid mists	Larynx (?)	

IARC, International Agency for Research on Cancer.

Table 35-3. Industries and occupations associated with other respiratory and oral cavity cancers

Industry or occupation	Cancer site	IARC group, comment
Wood: furniture making	Sinonasal cavities	1 Very high risk for adenocarcinomas
Wood: carpentry	Sinonasal cavities Nasopharynx	2b
Wood: logging, pulp, and paper, sawmill	Sinonasal cavities (?) Nasopharynx (?)	3 More recent studies support these associations
Leather boot and shoe manufacturing	Sinonasal cavities	1 Highest risk for adenocarcinomas; no increased risk found in U.S. studies
Isopropyl alcohol manufacturing	Sinonasal cavities Larynx (?)	1
Textile manufacturing	Sinonasal cavities Nasopharynx (?) Pharynx (?) Larynx (?)	2b
Painting	Sinonasal cavities (?) Pharynx (?) Larynx (?)	1 IARC classification based on increased risk for lung cancer; risk for other respiratory cancers not established
Baking and pastry cooking	Sinonasal cavities (?) Nasopharynx (?)	

IARC, International Agency for Research on Cancer.

There is little evidence that cigar and pipe smoking are important risk factors for upper respiratory cancer. However, long-term snuff users, who place the ground tobacco between the cheek and gums, have a greatly increased risk of oral cancer at the site of placement and may be at higher risk for laryngeal cancer as well.[7] This has been a particularly common practice in parts of the Southeastern United States, where a large fraction of oral cancers among women have been attributed to this practice.[8]

Alcohol

As is the case with tobacco, alcohol (or some component in alcoholic drinks) appears to be carcinogenic for every site in the mouth and upper respiratory system with which it comes in contact. The IARC has determined that there is sufficient evidence to classify alcohol drinking as carcinogenic in humans (group 1).[9]

The sites at highest risk appear to be the mouth, oropharynx, and hypopharynx, for which heavy drinkers have approximately nine times the risk of nondrinkers or occasional drinkers after the effects of tobacco are taken into account.[10] Consistent with the presumed amount of direct exposure, the relative risk associated with long-term frequent consumption of alcohol is about six for the extrinsic larynx, but only about two for the glottis and subglottis.[10] There is some indication that alcohol intake also increases the risk for nasopharyngeal and sinonasal carcinomas, although this has not been firmly established.[5,6]

The mechanism(s) through which the drinking of alcoholic beverages increases cancer risk are not known with certainty, and there is inadequate evidence for the carcinogenicity of alcohol or alcoholic beverages in animals.[9] Some of the postulated mechanisms include the presence of carcinogens in alcoholic beverages, the effects of carcinogenic metabolites of alcohol (primarily acetaldehyde), a reduction in the availability of nutrients which may inhibit cancer, and a reduction in the ability to detoxify carcinogens.[10] A number of studies have attempted to identify differences in risk associated with the different types of alcoholic beverages, but these have not been conclusive.

Nickel compounds

The primary use of nickel is in its metallic form as a component of stainless steel and other alloys. It is an important element in a number of electrical applications, such as nickel–cadmium batteries and is used as a catalyst as well.[11] The U.S. National Institute for Occupational Safety and Health (NIOSH) estimated that in the mid-1970s 1.5 million workers in the United States were exposed to nickel compounds while mining, refining, and producing nickel-containing products.[12] Community exposure to nickel compounds through food, air, and water also occurs but at levels much lower than in the workplace.[11]

Nickel compounds have been conclusively demonstrated to be carcinogenic to the sinonasal cavity and lung in humans (IARC group 1) (see Chapter 18).[11] The risk of sinonasal cancer is the highest, over one-hundredfold, among long-term workers involved in nickel smelting and refining, where the dominant exposures are to nickel sulfate, nickel sulfides, and nickel oxides.[11,13] This was particularly the case in the early 1900s when exposures were the highest. There is insufficient evidence from studies of nickel ore miners to determine whether they are at higher risk for sinonasal cancers.

The mechanisms by which nickel increases cancer risk probably depend on the particular compound. The soluble compounds appear able to affect directly deoxyribonucleic acid (DNA) during in vitro studies, yielding increased frequencies of chromosomal aberrations, sister chromatid exchanges, and, in some cases, gene mutations.[11]

Exposure to metallic nickel occurs in steel and alloy production and in the welding of nickel-containing metals (see Chapter 42). Although experimental animal studies involving intratracheal instillation have demonstrated that metallic nickel is carcinogenic, there is not yet convincing epidemiologic evidence of an increase in sinonasal cavity cancer caused by exposure to metallic nickel. The IARC has thus classified metallic nickel as possibly carcinogenic to humans (group 2B).[11]

The occupational exposure limits for airborne nickel that were developed by the U.S. Occupational Safety and Health Agency (OSHA) in 1987, based on a time-weighted average, are 1.0 mg/m^3 for metallic nickel, 0.1 mg/m^3 for soluble nickel compounds, and 0.007 mg/m^3 for nickel carbonyl.[11]

Chromium compounds

Chromium is produced from chromite ore and is used in the production of stainless steel and other alloys, in chrome plating as a pigment, in leather tanning, and in a wide range of chemicals.[11] Occupational exposure to chromium compounds occurs in the production of these materials and in welding of chromium-containing metals (see Chapter 42).

The carcinogenicity of chromium depends on its oxidative state. The IARC has classified chromium [VI] compounds as carcinogenic in humans (group 1).[11] However, chromium [III] and metallic compounds, which are not absorbed in the respiratory tract as readily as chromium [VI] compounds, were judged as not having sufficient evidence from human and animal studies to be able to classify them (group 3).

A number of in vitro tests in human and other mammalian cells indicate that chromium[VI] compounds have direct effects on DNA, which include inducing mutations, sister chromatid exchanges, and aberrations.[11] In contrast, there was little evidence of genomic effects for chromium [III] compounds.

Most of the epidemiologic studies demonstrating chromium [VI] carcinogenicity involve increased risk of lung cancer (see Chapter 34). However, there is substantial evidence, from studies of workers involved in primary chromate production, chromate pigment production, and chromium plating, that such compounds increase the risk of sinonasal cavity cancer as well.[11] The largest number of deaths were reported from a cohort study of 896 workers in a chromium manufacturing plant in Japan, in which six

of 31 respiratory cancer deaths were attributed to sinonasal cancer.[14]

The OSHA limits on the time-weighted average airborne concentrations are 0.5 mg/m^3 for soluble chromium, chromic and chromous salts, and 1.0 mg/m^3 for chromium metal and insoluble salts.[11]

Other agents

Mustard gas. There is strong evidence that workers involved in the manufacture of mustard gas (sulfur mustard) during the second world war are at higher risk of upper respiratory cancers, as well as lung cancer (see Chapter 34). In a cohort study of over 3,000 male and female workers in Britain, large and significant excess risk was observed for deaths from cancer of the larynx, pharynx, and other upper respiratory sites.[15] The IARC has classified this agent as a human carcinogen (group 1).[16]

Thorotrast. Thorotrast (thorium dioxide) is a radioactive contrast medium that was used in the 1930s and 1940s for cerebral angiography and other radiologic procedures. Follow-up studies of patients who received injections have demonstrated it to be carcinogenic for a number of sites, most notably the liver and hematopoetic system, where the majority of the chemical is deposited. It also appears to be carcinogenic for the sinonasal cavities, but not for other upper respiratory sites.[17]

INDUSTRIES AND OCCUPATIONS ASSOCIATED WITH OTHER RESPIRATORY CANCERS
Wood industry

Work in the wood industry includes a wide range of activities, including tree planting and harvesting, milling, the manufacture of wood products, such as particle board and plywood, the production of pulp and paper, construction carpentry, and finish carpentry. Consequently there is a wide range of potentially hazardous exposures to persons in this industry (see Chapter 37). It is also a common industry, with over three million people in the United States estimated to be employed in jobs entailing contact with raw or processed wood.

Wood dust is the most commonly encountered agent among woodworkers. Operations performed on wood can create dust in two ways— by shattering lignified wood cells, and by chipping out whole cells or groups of cells. The significance of this distinction is that the shattering of cells results in a finer particle size distribution and a higher fraction of respirable particles than does chipping. Sanding operations produce shattered cells almost exclusively, whereas sawing and milling of wood produces chipping as well as shattering. In addition, wood that has densely-packed cells (i.e., hardwood) and wood that is less elastic (i.e., dry wood) are more likely to be shattered during processing. These general principles appear to be confirmed by industry sampling. Lower mean total and respirable dust levels have been found more frequently in greenwood processing at sawmills than in furniture and cabinet-making shops where dried lumber and hardwoods are used. Facilities that have both wet and dry wood components (e.g., plywood and particleboard manufacturing) appear to have intermediate exposures.

Approximately 200 species of trees are used in the industry, and each contributes its own unique blend of chemicals that make up the wood. Different processes involved in wood processing contribute their own chemicals to the mix of agents to which wood workers may be exposed. Some of these chemicals include pesticides used in saw mills and carpentry, various bleaching and digesting agents used in the pulp and paper industry, and formaldehyde, which is used extensively in the production of particle board and plywood. Exposure to metal dust may occur during the sharpening of saw blades. The most common blade materials are tungsten carbide, high-speed steel, and stellite, some of which contain cobalt and chromium.

Workers may be exposed directly to these chemicals, or they may be exposed by the inhalation of wood dust particles containing them. In addition to the potential carcinogenic effects of chemicals in ambient air and those adhered to wood particles, exposure to wood dust itself may increase cancer risk by means of chronic irritation and resulting increased cell turnover.

A greatly increased risk (over one hundredfold) of adenocarcinomas of the sinonasal cavity among English furniture makers was discovered in the late 1960s.[18] Based on this and numerous additional studies in several countries, which have confirmed a large risk of adenocarcinoma of the sinonasal cavity, the IARC has classified work in furniture and cabinet-making as being carcinogenic in humans (group 1).[16]

Work in carpentry and joinery was classified by IARC in 1987 as being possibly carcinogenic in humans (group 2B).[16] This was based on the moderate risks of adenocarcinomas and/or squamous cell carcinomas of the sinonasal cavity reported in studies from western Europe and North America. A more recent case-control study in western Washington state found that carpenters in the construction industry had approximately five times the risk of nasopharyngeal cancer, and that this risk increased in long-term workers and in those who were first exposed in the more distant past.[19] A case-control study, using data from the New Zealand cancer registry, also shows evidence of increased nasopharyngeal cancer risk among carpenters.[20]

In their 1987 review, the IARC concluded that there was insufficient evidence to determine whether work in the pulp and paper, logging and sawmill industries was associated with increased risk of cancer (group 3).[16] However, recent studies from New Zealand and Thailand reported fourfold to sixfold increases in the risk of nasopharyngeal cancer among loggers.[20,21] A study of squamous cell carcinomas of the sinonasal cavity, occurring in western Washington state, found a twofold increase in risk among loggers and

an eightfold increase in risk among woodworking machine operators in the lumber and wood product manufacturing industry.[19] A national linkage study in Sweden reported that men employed in fiberboard plants had a fourfold increase in nasopharyngeal cancer risk.[22] Finally, a mortality study of pulp and papermill workers in New Hampshire reported a 75% excess risk of cancers of the buccal cavity and pharynx.[23]

In summary, since the initial report linking furniture making with excess incidence of sinonasal cavity adenocarcinomas, substantial evidence has accumulated indicating that woodworkers other than furniture makers are at increased cancer risk, that woodworkers have higher rates of squamous cell carcinomas of the sinonasal cavity as well as adenocarcinomas, and that the neighboring nasopharynx is probably also a site of carcinogenicity. However the great diversity of exposures within the various facets of the industry, across countries, and over time, makes it difficult to identify the specific agents associated with the increased risk. Thus this remains an active area of research.

Leather boot and shoe manufacture and repair

Significant changes have occurred in the boot and shoe industry since the 1950s, with synthetic components increasingly replacing leather and other natural products. Nevertheless, traditional materials and manufacturing processes are still used in some locations. The highest levels of exposure to leather dust tend to occur during hand finishing operations (scouring and roughing) and during edge trimming and cutting.[24] Exposure to a wide variety of chemical compounds, including solvents, formaldehyde, and dyes, may also occur during the application of cleaners, adhesives, and finishes.

Epidemiologic studies from the Denmark, Italy, England, Switzerland, and France have convincingly demonstrated that persons employed in the manufacture and repair of leather boots and shoes experience a much higher incidence of sinonasal cavity cancers, particularly adenocarcinomas, than the general population.[16,25,26] The IARC concluded that there was sufficient evidence to classify work in this industry as carcinogenic in humans (group 1).[16]

There is some evidence that the highest risk appears to occur in those exposed to the highest concentrations of leather dust.[27] Thus although the causal agent responsible for the increased risk of cancers of the sinonasal cavity is not known with certainty, and exposure to multiple chemical agents is likely to occur among workers in this industry, it appears that leather dust plays a lead role. This would be consistent with the associations that have been established between sinonasal cavity cancer and wood and textile dusts. It is of interest that elevated rates of sinonasal cavity cancer have not been documented in studies of this industry in the United States.[28] The reason for this discrepancy is not known.

Isopropyl alcohol manufacture

Workers involved in manufacturing isopropyl alcohol by the strong-acid process have been found to have increased risk of developing sinonasal cancers and perhaps laryngeal cancer as well.[29,30] The IARC has classified this evidence, together with strongly supporting evidence from nonhuman studies, as sufficient to conclude that the exposures in this process are carcinogenic in humans (group 1). The actual etiologic agent is probably diethyl sulfate, an alkylating agent which is an intermediate in the process, and for which there is strong animal evidence of carcinogenicity.[16] Isopropyl oils, which are by-products in the manufacturing process, may also be contributing factors, but these oils have not been adequately studied.[16]

OTHER AGENTS OR INDUSTRIES SUSPECTED OF CAUSING OTHER RESPIRATORY CANCERS
Agents

Formaldehyde. Formaldehyde is a common chemical found in both the occupational and residential environments. Much of the formaldehyde produced in the United States is used in resins which bind together wood products, such as plywood, fiberboard, and particle board. Other common uses include as an embalming fluid, an antiseptic, and a finishing treatment in the textile industry. Occupational exposures can occur in the actual production of formaldehyde, in the production of products in which formaldehyde is a component, and in the use of formaldehyde-containing products (e.g., in the construction industry). A major source of residential formaldehyde exposure is wood products that are used in home construction. Measured concentrations have tended to be higher in smaller residences with higher surface-to-volume ratios and in residences with less infiltration of outside air, such as in mobile and manufactured homes. An additional source of residential exposure is from tobacco smoke.

The carcinogenicity of formaldehyde in rats and mice has been firmly established from experimental studies. However, its role in human cancer is still controversial, even after the completion of over three dozen epidemiologic studies. The site at which formaldehyde is most likely to cause human cancer is the nasopharynx, where studies of persons exposed in both the work and residential environments have most consistently suggested a moderate (two- to threefold) increase in risk.[4,31,32] There is also substantial, although less consistent, evidence that formaldehyde increases the risk of sinonasal carcinomas as well.[31-33] The IARC reviewed the epidemiologic evidence in 1987 and classified formaldehyde as a probable human carcinogen (group 2A).[16]

Asbestos. Exposure to asbestos in the occupational or residential setting is well-documented as causally-related to cancers of the pleura and lung in humans (see Chapters 18 and 20). The role of asbestos in causing laryngeal cancer is more controversial. Authors attempting to review and sum-marize results from diverse studies have reached opposite conclusions,[34,35] and more recent reports have not clarified the issue.[36-38] It appears that if asbestos is indeed etiologically related to laryngeal cancer, the strength of the relationship is more moderate than with lung or pleural cancer.

Acid mists. Occupational exposure to sulfuric and other strong inorganic acids has been suggested to increase laryngeal cancer risk in a number of studies. A community-based case-control study found an almost sevenfold increase in risk associated with long-term exposure to high levels of sulfuric acid, after adjustment for the effects of smoking and alcohol.[39] Two industry-based studies also found significant elevations in risk, although of lower magnitude.[40,41] Barriers to more firmly establishing a causal relationship between laryngeal cancer and acids in general, or sulfuric acid in particular, include the multitude of simultaneous exposures that occur in industrial processes in which strong acids are used, and the relatively small number of exposed workers that can be studied. Nevertheless, the published studies, although few, have been remarkably consistent in their results. Together with the biologic plausibility that long-term irritation of laryngeal tissue by acid exposure may increase cell turnover and thus increase cancer risk, these results suggest that acid exposure is likely to be a causal factor in laryngeal cancer.

Industries

Textile industry. Over ten million people are employed worldwide in the manufacture of textile products.[42] The processes involved include fiber production and preparation, fabric production, and dyeing and finishing. Exposure to cotton and wool dust, especially during fiber preparation, is pervasive in the industry. Other exposures include bacteria and endotoxins, the many types of dyes (including benzidine-derived dyes), and formaldehyde.

There is consistent evidence that work in this industry may increase the risk of sinonasal cavity cancer. The IARC has classified exposures in this industry as possibly carcinogenic in humans (group 2B).[47] This classification was based on an assessment of results published before 1990, in which all five cohort studies of textile workers and three of four case-control studies demonstrated an approximate doubling of risk in men and/or women. Studies after 1990 have tended to confirm these findings and also to raise the possibility that risk may be increased in other upper respiratory sites, including the nasopharynx, oropharynx and larynx.[43-48] The etiologic agent(s) responsible for excess risk of upper respiratory cancers among textile workers are unknown but may relate to chronic irritation from long-term dust exposure.

Painting. Painters in the construction and metal industries are potentially exposed to literally thousands of chemicals that may be in paints and other finishing compounds. These include pigments, solvents, binders, and preservatives, many of which are potentially carcinogenic. Occupational exposures experienced by painters are considered by the IARC as carcinogenic in humans (group 1).[49] This conclusion is based mainly on the elevated risk of lung cancer demonstrated in several cohort and case-control studies (see Chapter 18). However, there is also accumulating evidence that painters may also be at higher risk for upper respiratory cancers. Sites for which multiple studies have indicated twofold or higher risks associated with painting or exposure to paints, include the larynx,[37,50,51] the pharynx and oral cavity,[52,53] and the sinonasal cavities.[45,54] Nevertheless, for each study suggesting higher risks, there have been one or more studies indicating no increase in risk. Thus the association between painting and respiratory cancers other than lung cancer must still be considered unproven.

Baking and pastry cooking. Persons working as bakers and pastry chefs are potentially exposed to polycyclic aromatic hydrocarbons from products formed during cooking, *N*-nitroso compounds from cooking byproducts and fungi-contaminated flour, and flour dusts. Studies in France and Denmark have both reported large excess risks (fourto eightfold) of sinonasal cavity cancers among bakers and pastry cooks, whereas a study in China has reported a more moderate excess risk for nasopharyngeal cancer.[25,36,45] Thus these preliminary studies indicate that persons in these occupations may be exposed to upper respiratory carcinogens; however, additional studies are needed to confirm these associations and identify, if possible, the causal agents.

REFERENCES

1. International Agency for Research on Cancer: *IARC Monographs* vol 38, Lyon, 1986.
2. La Vecchia C, Bidoli E, Barra S, et al: Type of cigarettes and cancers of the upper digestive and respiratory tract, *Can Causes and Control* 1:69-74, 1990.
3. Falk RT, Pickle LW, Borwn LM, et al: Effect of smoking and alcohol consumption on laryngeal cancer risk in coastal Texas, *Can Res* 49:4024-4029, 1989.
4. West S, Hildesheim A, and Dosemeci M: Non-viral risk factors for nasopharyngeal carcinoma in the Philippines: results from a case-control study, *Inter J Cancer* 55:722-727, 1993.
5. Nam JM, McLaughlin JK, and Blot WJ: Cigarette smoking, alcohol and nasopharyngeal carcinoma: a case-control study among U.S. whites, *JNCI* 84:619-622, 1992.
6. Strader CS, Vaughan TL, and Stergachis A: Use of nasal preparations and the incidence of sinonasal cancer, *J Epidem Commun Health* 42:243-248, 1988.
7. Mattson ME and Winn DM: Smokeless tobacco: association with increased cancer risk. *NIC Monographs* 8:13-16, 1989.
8. Winn DM, Blot WJ, Shy CM, et al: Snuff dipping and oral cancer among women in the southern United States, *NEJM* 304:745-749, 1981.
9. International Agency for Research on Cancer: *IARC Monographs* vol 44, Lyon, 1988.
10. Blot WJ: Alcohol and cancer, *Can Res* 52:2119s-2123s, 1992.
11. International Agency for Research on Cancer: *IARC Monographs* vol 49, Lyon, 1990.
12. NIOSH: Criteria for a recommended standard: occupational exposure to inorganic nickel, DHEW–NIOSH Doc. No. 77-164, Washington, D.C., 1977, U.S. Government Printing Office.
13. International Committee on Nickel Carcinogenesis in Man: Report of the international committee on nickel carcinogenesis in man, *Scand J Work Environ Health* 16:1-84, 1990.
14. Satoh K, Fukuda Y, Torii K, et al: Epidemiologica study of workers engaged in the manufacture of chromium compounds, *J Occup Med* 23:835-838, 1981.
15. Easton DF, Peto J, and Doll R: Cancers of the respiratory tract in mustard gas workers, *Brit J Indus Med* 45:652-659, 1988.
16. International Agency for Research on Cancer: *IARC Monographs* suppl 7, Lyon, 1987.
17. Andersson M and Storm HH: Cancer incidence among Danish thorotrast-exposed patients, *JNCI* 84:1318-1325, 1992.
18. Macbeth R: Malignant disease of the paranasal sinuses, *J Laryngol* 79:592-612, 1965.
19. Vaughan TL: Occupation and squamous cell cancers of the pharynx and sinonasal cavity, *Amer J Indus Med* 16:493-510, 1989.
20. Kawachi I, Pearce N, and Fraser J: A New Zealand cancer registry-based study of cancer in wood workers, *Cancer* 64:2609-2613, 1989.
21. Sriamporn S, Vatanasapt V, Pisani P, et al: Environmental risk factors for nasopharyngeal carcinoma: a case-control study in northeastern Thailand, *Can Epidem Biomarkers Preven* 1:345-348, 1992.
22. Malker HSR, McLaughlin JK, Weiner JA, et al: Occupational risk factors for nasopharyngeal cancer in Sweden, *Brit J Indus Med* 47:213-214, 1990.
23. Schwartz E: A proportionate mortality ratio analysis of pulp and paper mill workers in New Hampshire, *Brit J Indus Med* 45:234-238, 1988.
24. International Agency for Research on Cancer: *IARC Monographs* vol 25, pp 260-266, Lyon, 1981.
25. Olsen JH: Occupational risks of sinonasal cancer in Denmark, *Brit J Indus Med* 45:329-335, 1988.
26. Comba P, Battista G, Bille S, et al: A case-control study of cancer of the nose and paranasal sinuses and occupational exposures, *Amer J Indus Med* 22:511-520, 1992.
27. Merler E, Baldasseroni A, Laria R, et al: On the causal association between exposure to leather dust and nasal cancer: further evidence from a case-control study, *Brit J Indus Med* 43:91-95, 1986.
28. Decoufle P, Walrath J: Nasal cancer in the U.S. shoe industry: does it exist? *Amer J Indus Med* 605-613, 1987.
29. Lynch J, Hanis NM, Bird MG, et al: An association of upper respiratory cancer with exposure to diethyl sulphate, *J Occup Med* 21:333-341, 1979.
30. Alderson MR and Rattan NS: Mortality of workers on an isopropyl alcohol plant and two MEK dewaxing plants, *Brit J Indus Med* 37:85-89, 1980.
31. Blair A, Saracci R, Stewart PA, et al: Epidemiologic evidence on the relationship between formaldehyde exposure and cancer, *Scand J Work Environ Health* 16:381-393, 1990.
32. Partanen T: Formaldehyde exposure and respiratory cancer—a meta-analysis of the epidemiologic evidence, *Scand J Work Environ Health* 19:8-15, 1993.
33. Luce D, Gerin M, LeClerc A, et al: Sinonasal cancer and occupational exposure to formaldehyde and other substances, *Inter J Cancer* 53:224-231, 1993.
34. Smith AH, Handley MA, and Wood R: Epidemiological evidence indicates asbestos causes laryngeal cancer, *J Occup Med* 499-507, 1990.
35. Liddell FDK: Laryngeal cancer and asbestos, *Brit J Indus Med* 47:289-291, 1990.
36. Zheng W, Blot WJ, Shu XO, et al: Diet and other risk factors for laryngeal cancer in Shanghai, China, *Amer J Epidem* 136:178-191, 1992.
37. Wortley P, Vaughan TL, Davis S, et al: A case-control study of occupational risk factors for laryngeal cancer, *Brit J Indus Med* 49:837-844, 1992.
38. Muscat JE and Wynder EL: Tobacco, alcohol, asbestos and occupational risk factors for laryngeal cancer, *Cancer* 69:2244-2251, 1992.

39. Soskolne CL, Jhangri GS, Siemiatycki J, et al: Occupational exposure to sulfuric acid in southern Ontario, Canada, in association with laryngeal cancer, *Scan J Work Environ Health* 18:225-232, 1992.

40. Steenland K, Schnorr T, Beaumont J, et al: Incidence of laryngeal cancer and exposure to acid mists, *Brit J Indus Med* 45:766-776, 1988.

41. Soskolne CL, Zeighami EA, Hanis NM, et al: Laryngeal cancer and occupational exposure to sulfuric acid, *Amer J Epidem* 120:358-369, 1984.

42. International Agency for Research on Cancer: *IARC Monographs* vol 48, Lyon, 1990.

43. Comba P, Battista G, Belli S, et al: A case-control study of cancer of the nose and paranasal sinuses and occupational exposures, *Amer J Indus Med* 22:511-520, 1992.

44. Haguenoer JM, Cordier S, Morel C, et al: Occupational risk factors for upper respiratory tract and upper digestive tract cancers, *Brit J Indus Med* 47:380-383, 1990.

45. Luce D, Leclerc A, Morcet JF, et al: Occupational risk factors for sinonasal cancer: a case-control study in France, *Amer J Indus Med* 21:163-175, 1992.

46. Merletti F, Boffetta P, Ferro G, et al: Occupation and cancer of the oral cavity and oropharynx in Turin, Italy, *Scand J Work Environ Health* 17:248-254, 1991.

47. Ahrens W, Jockel KH, Patzak W, et al: Alcohol, smoking and occupational factors in cancer of the larynx: a case-control study, *Amer J Indus Med* 20:477-493, 1991; International Agency for Research on Cancer: *IARC Monographs* vol 47, Lyon, 1989.

48. Zheng W, McLaughlin JK, Gao YT, et al: Occupational risks for nasopharyngeal cancer in Shanghai, *J Occ Med* 34:1004-1007, 1992.

49. International Agency for Research on Cancer: *IARC Monographs* vol 47, Lyon, 1989.

50. Brown LM, Mason TJ, Pickle LW, et al: Occupational risk factors for laryngeal cancer on the Texas gulf coast, *Can Res* 48:1960-1964, 1988.

51. Dubrow R and Wegman DH: Cancer and occupation in Massachusetts: a death certificate study, *Amer J Indus Med* 6:207-230, 1984.

52. Huebner WW, Schoenber JB, Kelsey JL, et al: Oral and pharyngeal cancer and occupation: a case-control study, *Epidemiology* 3:300-309, 1992.

53. Lynge E and Thygesen L: Use of surveillance systems for occupational cancer: data from the Danish national system, 17:493-500, 1988.

54. Olsen JH, Jensen SP, Hink M, et al: Occupational formaldehyde exposure and increased nasal cancer risk in man, *Inter J Can* 639-644, 1984.

55. Boring CC, Squires TS, Tong T, et al: Cancer statistics 1994, *CA Cancer J Clin* 44:18-19, 1994.

Industries Associated with Respiratory Disease

MARC B. SCHENKER

Many industries are associated with a wide range of occupational respiratory hazards. The approach to diagnosing or treating a patient with respiratory disease, who works in one of these industries, may require consideration of several different exposures or respiratory diseases. For example, respiratory toxins in agriculture include inorganic and organic dusts (including endotoxins and fungal spores), various gases (e.g., NO_2, H_2S, NH_3, and CO), infectious agents (e.g., tuberculosis, Q fever, coccidiomycosis), pesticides, solvents, fuels, and other chemicals. Those who are responsible for health care or medical surveillance in one of these industries will benefit from reading these industry chapters. Additional detail on the diagnosis and treatment of specific disease entities can be found in Sections II and IV, and more detailed information on specific exposures can be found in Sections V through VII. For example, acute gaseous exposures are a specific hazard in agriculture and are covered in Chapter 30. Section VIII also includes chapters on the respiratory hazards associated with work in the environmental extremes of underwater diving and aerospace.

Chapter 36

AGRICULTURE

John J. May
Marc B. Schenker

Over the past 4 decades there have been considerable changes in agriculture in the United States. The number of farms has declined by 30% and many of the remaining farms are financially threatened (Fig. 36-1). Paradoxically, this has occurred in the face of remarkable increases in efficiency and productivity. With the use of agrichemicals, fertilizers, mechanization, and improved crops, agricultural production now requires only about a third of the total hours of labor that it required in the past. The average farmer's productivity has increased sixfold. Concomitantly, the agricultural workforce has declined from 6.8 million to 2.8 million workers.[1] This total does not include the seasonal and migrant population, which may be of equal or greater size. Those currently occupied in farming represent 2.5% of the total U.S. workforce. Of the surviving farms, two thirds are small, owner-operated businesses, which rely heavily on the labor of the owner and family members. It is this group of farms that is decreasing in number most rapidly. Large family and commercial operations comprise less than 5% of all American farms, yet these account for almost 50% of the total gross cash farm income and over 50% of the expenditures for farm labor. Agricultural production on many of these larger operations often involves commodities that require more intensive manual labor to produce.

In areas where intensive manual labor is needed, it is usually provided by seasonal workers. Virtually 80% of all hired farmworkers are seasonal with more than half working fewer than 75 days per year. Some of these seasonal workers are year-round residents who seek temporary employment or take on an added job when agricultural workers are needed by local producers. Often the number of workers required, or the salaries being offered, will dictate the need for migrant workers.

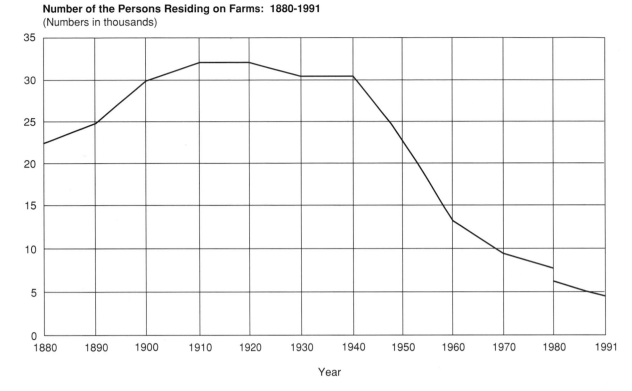

Number of the Persons Residing on Farms: 1880-1991
(Numbers in thousands)

Fig. 36-1. U.S. Census Bureau statistics document the marked decline in the number of Americans living on farms. (Adapted from Dacquel LT and Dahmann DC: Residents of farms and rural areas: 1991. In *Current Population Reports, P20-472*, p 3, Fig. 1, U.S. Bureau of the Census, 1993.)

Estimates of the size of the migrant and seasonal work force range from 750,000 to between 2.7 and 5 million workers.[2] The migrant and seasonal workers are predominantly young, Hispanic men from the United States and Mexico. There are small percentages of foreign-born farmworkers from other Latin American, Caribbean, and Asian countries. Most of these workers have low levels of education and are non-English speaking. Among U.S.-born farmworkers, the majority are white with about one third Hispanic and a small percentage of African-Americans. Twelve percent of all agricultural workers (20% of foreign-born workers) are unauthorized. Workers spend an average of about one half of the year performing agricultural work, and half of the family incomes are below the poverty level despite many families with two wage earners. Among agricultural workers who migrate, patterns of migration may be complex but generally fan out in three streams from Texas, Southern California, and Florida.

Despite the decline in the number of farms and farmers, American agriculture remains a massive industry that is of great economic importance to the United States. In recent years, total farm assets have been nearly $800 billion and annual gross income approximately $190 billion. Agricultural exports are of particular significance to the nation's international balance of trade. In an increasingly overpopulated world, the productivity of American farmers may un-

Table 36-1. Size of agricultural workforce relates inversely to level of development[3]

	Nigeria	India	Egypt	Jamaica	Mexico
Agricultural production (% GDP)	36	31	17	5	9
Labor force (%)	65.5	67.1	41.5	27.9	31.2
GDP per capita	$290	$350	$600	$1500	$2490

Adapted from the world bank: *World development report 1992: development and the environment*, Tables 1 and 3, New York, 1992, Oxford University Press.
GDP, Gross Domestic Product (1990).

fortunately begin to assume political as well as economic significance.

Globally, agriculture is no less significant than it is in the United States. In developing nations the relative inefficiency of agriculture makes farm production of vital concern. Large segments of the population are required for agricultural labor, sometimes up to 85% of the working population. Thus a considerable proportion of all people are involved in some aspect of farming (Table 36-1). In the countries where productivity is relatively low, agriculture is likely to account for a large proportion of the country's gross domestic product. It is in these nations where over 20% of all trade is, of necessity, in agricultural products.

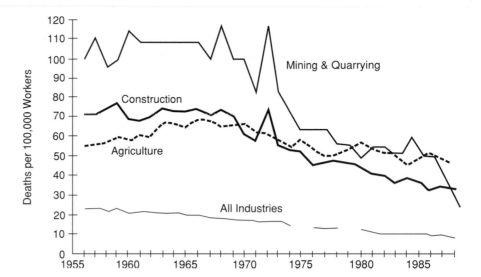

Fig. 36-2. National Safety Council data showing work accident death rates from 1955 to 1988 in the nation's three most hazardous industries. (Adapted from May JJ: Agriculture—work practices and health consequences, vol 14. In Petty TL and Cherniak RM, editors: *Seminars in respiratory medicine,* p 3, Fig. 1, 1993. New York, Thieme Medical Publishers.)

The inadequacy of local food production forces many developing countries to import basic foodstuffs and these nations account for more than half of the world's agricultural imports.

The inability of the developing world to feed itself is a cause for considerable concern. By the year 2035, the world's population will reach 9 billion, at the current rate of population growth. Consumption of food is likely to double over this period of time. Efforts of those working in agriculture to meet this demand are likely to focus on increasing the efficiency of agricultural production in the less developed areas of the world. Ninety-two percent of the increased production since 1970 is due to increased yields and 8% is due to increased land use.[3] With this intensification of farming come problems with water consumption and quality, runoff of agrichemicals, increased mechanization, and disposal of animal wastes. Some of these problems will become major issues for the entire community and many will remain particular hazards only for those working in agriculture.

This chapter focuses on the various respiratory hazards that may be encountered in the agricultural environment. The likelihood of exposure to such hazards varies with the type of farming and the jobs undertaken by the agricultural worker. As noted previously, this is a remarkably heterogeneous workforce, which includes the owners or managers of large farming operations, seasonal and migrant farmworkers, those involved in the handling, storage and initial processing of agricultural produce, the owners and operators of smaller family farms, and family members who contribute full- or part-time assistance.

These individuals as a group share a workplace that is often substantially less regulated than that of many other American workers. The problems and abuses experienced by the migrant workforce have been well publicized and range from child labor to inadequate sanitation and exposure to potentially harmful agrichemicals. The smaller family farm makes up the majority of farms in the country. Most

of these farms employ fewer than 11 workers and thus are exempted from inspection and regulation by the U.S. Occupational Safety and Health Administration (OSHA). This has likely contributed to the problems of antiquated, poorly-guarded equipment, suboptimal handling of chemicals, and routine exposure to noise, dust, and gas levels that are not acceptable elsewhere in industry. Thus throughout most agricultural production, there is a pattern of ineffectual or nonexistent safety regulation and inadequate worker education superimposed upon a diversified and inherently hazardous workplace.

OVERVIEW OF AGRICULTURAL HEALTH AND SAFETY

In addition to the respiratory problems described in this chapter, workers in agriculture may experience an increased rate of other occupational health problems. The most obvious are the problems of acute traumatic injury and death. Figures compiled by the National Safety Council[4] clearly underestimate the rates of injury,[5] yet these figures are sufficient to document rates of occupational fatality and injury that equal those of mining and construction. In contrast to the rates in mining and construction, rates in agriculture show little evidence of decline (Fig. 36-2). A large proportion of these injuries result from interactions with farm machinery. In a series of state-based surveys, the farm tractor is consistently the most dangerous machine, generally accounting for 50% to 55% of all farm fatalities, which is a situation that has not changed in several decades.[6] Despite clear evidence from other countries that rollover protective structures prevent most fatalities,[7] two thirds of American tractors are without these. In New York State the average age of the tractors on dairy farms is 20.3 years, ± 11.7 years, and 73% of the tractor fleet is over 10 years of age. Farmers also suffer injury and fatality from power takeoff devices, feedwagons, and a number of other mechanical devices.

Farm equipment also appears to inflict chronic injury

upon workers. Several studies document increased rates of noise-induced hearing loss in this population, appearing in some by their mid-twenties.[8] Chronic vibration related to long hours of tractor driving appears to correlate with symptomatic back disease in a dose-related fashion.[9]

Exposure of agricultural workers to agrichemicals may lead to direct toxicity in some cases. Exposure has also been increasingly associated with the occurrence of certain malignancies, particularly non-Hodgkin's lymphoma.[10] A number of other malignancies appear to occur at increased rates in agricultural workers. These include some leukemias, Hodgkin's lymphoma, multiple myeloma, and cancers of the brain, testicle, prostate, and stomach.[11] In most of these cases little is known about potential causative factors.

Those who work in agriculture are at risk for a variety of other health problems. Farmers and farmworkers have particular problems with dermatologic diseases, including cancers, which are often related to ultraviolet light exposure, zoonosis, and contact dermatitis.[2] These individuals also experience higher rates of osteoarthritis than nonfarmers.[12] Finally, these individuals, particularly farm owners and operators, have substantially increased rates of suicide when compared with nonfarm populations.[13]

Despite this litany of significant occupational health problems, respiratory disease remains one of the most common and important issues for those working in the agricultural field. The remainder of this chapter will review characteristics of this work environment that represent particular hazards and their impact on the respiratory health of the agricultural worker. It will become apparent to the reader that much remains to be learned about respiratory disease. This is particularly true in the case of farmworker populations where few studies of respiratory disease have been reported. The majority of the existing data is derived from clinic-based or convenience samples of farmworkers.[14]

SOURCES OF EXPOSURE
Spectrum of work environments

Field work. The vast majority of agricultural work is done outdoors. Most plants grow in outdoor environments, and large numbers of farmworkers perform fieldwork in growing and harvesting operations for labor-intensive crops such as fruits, vegetables, and horticultural products. Exposures in agricultural fields may be different from those in specialized environments, such as confinement houses, silos, and barns, but there have been few industrial hygiene surveys of exposures to field workers.[15] The major exposures of concern in fieldwork are dusts and agricultural chemicals. Although exposures to organic dusts may occur in outdoor agricultural environments, inorganic dusts represent a greater respiratory hazard in fieldwork than in most indoor agricultural environments.[15]

Thirty percent of the earth is silica, and crystalline silica

concentrations may be 10% to 20% or higher in dust samples collected from outdoor agricultural exposures. Further, clinically significant exposures to various silicates may occur from agricultural fieldwork. These exposures include nonfibrous silicate materials known to cause pulmonary fibrosis, including mica and clay silicates.[16,17] Respirable fibrous minerals have also been identified in samples collected in agricultural areas.[18] Finally, total dust concentrations in agricultural fields may be high, commonly exceeding general industry standards for nuisance dusts.[15,19]

Airborne mineral dust concentrations vary with many factors, including local geology, rainfall, winds, crops grown, and agricultural practices.[18] Exposures may be particularly high in dry, semiarid and desert climates, and in windy areas.[18,20] Agricultural practices may affect dust exposures. For example, in fruit crops tall foliage may collect dust during the dry growing season, which is subsequently aerosolized during harvesting with potential exposure to workers.[15] Many types of agricultural machinery disturb soils and crops with aerosolization of organic and mineral dusts.

Exposures to pesticides may also occur in fieldwork settings. Many minerals such as talc, zeolite, kaolin, and vermiculite are used as fillers and carriers for pesticides, with potential human exposure.[18] Exposures to pesticides may occur during harvesting, transport, and storage of agricultural products. Workers may be exposed directly from aerial application or from a variety of agricultural spray equipment ranging from large electrostatic sprayers to backpack spray equipment.

Confinement house. In recent decades the approach to animal husbandry has changed markedly. Efforts aimed at maximizing the efficient use of both barn space and labor have resulted in animals being gathered in progressively larger numbers into relatively smaller spaces. This approach first gained popularity on poultry farms but subsequently has been employed in the raising of sheep, young beef cattle (veal), and particularly in the raising of hogs.

Swine confinement farming has become a major industry in midwestern states such as Iowa and Nebraska, and it is estimated that 700,000 persons are employed in this industry nationwide. Animals receive all of their care (feeding, washing, and veterinary services) within one or a series of several buildings, where they literally spend their entire lives. Often the pigs are born in farrowing units, proceed through nursery-growing units, and end up in finishing buildings. The relative numbers of animals, feed consumption, and ventilation in these units vary and this may affect the results of published environmental studies.

The issues of ventilation, method of feeding, and manure disposal are major determinants of the worker's exposure in the confinement house. These buildings have traditionally been tightly constructed in an effort to reduce heating expense. Although there is an increasing awareness of the importance of adequate ventilation, most structures do not provide this. This in part reflects the conventional view that confinement house dust is simply a nuisance. It is now clear that ambient levels of both dusts and gases are potentially harmful to workers.[21]

Large numbers of densely packed animals generate substantial amounts of manure; across the country confinement operators must deal with nearly 500 million wet tons annually. This material contains proteins, carbohydrates, and fats that undergo anaerobic microbial degradation. The degradative process results in the generation of a series of malodorous and some potentially noxious gases.[22] Initial designs of confinement facilities used collection tanks under slotted floors in the animal pens to accumulate manure. Intermittently this material would be agitated to resuspend the solids prior to pumping out the tank. Unfortunately this practice would also drive heavier-than-air gases, such as hydrogen sulfide, up into the breathing zone of animals and workers—sometimes with disastrous results.[23]

In modern systems manure is pumped via an underground pipe to manure retention "ponds" and tanks that are usually located adjacent to the building. These manure storage areas still generate significant amounts of carbon dioxide, carbon monoxide, methane, ammonia, and hydrogen sulfide, and thus they represent a potential threat to workers in the adjoining area.[24,25] Between 1985 and 1995 more than 20 workers have died in the United States as a result of such exposures.[26]

Dairy barn. Most other work environments in agriculture have not been studied as thoroughly as the confinement building. The dairy barn is to some degree a confinement area, although the concentration of animals, degree of ventilation, method of feeding, and handling of manure are likely to differ substantially. These buildings are usually older and, of necessity, more ventilated. The cows may be confined to small stalls or may be allowed to roam freely in an enclosed space (free stall), but the density of animals does not approach that seen in poultry or swine confinement. Feed generally consists of a combination of hay and silage (preserved grasses or corn). The use of hay may be associated with considerable dust generation depending on the method of preparation and storage.[27] It appears that the mode of storage and of feeding hay to animals may help account for the variation in rates of allergic alveolitis in different parts of the world.[28] These rates are particularly high in Finnish farmwomen, for example, who feed the cows by shaking out the hay in small, tightly closed barns.[29] The dust arising from the hay may be heavily laced with microorganisms, particularly thermophilic actinomyces and *S. rectovirgula (M. faeni)*.[30]

In addition to bacteria and fungi, hay dust can be heavily contaminated with mites (storage mites), which are similar to, although antigenically discreet from, house dust mites. Depending on the season and the methods of storage of the feed, these arachnids may be found in extremely high concentrations both in the feed and suspended in the air of the barn.[31,32]

A major source of dust generation in the barn is the bedding chopper. Using a series of rotating blades, this gasoline-powered device reduces bales of hay into short lengths of straw and blows this material into the animals' stalls to serve as bedding. This twice-daily process is potentially an extremely dusty one. The dust problem is exacerbated by the usual practice of selecting hay bales that have become overgrown with microbes and are thus unsuitable for feed.

Silo. Along with the manure storage area, the silo provides some of the most potentially serious respiratory hazards in the agricultural environment. Farms with significant numbers of livestock usually rely upon some type of silo for storage of feed. A variety of relatively airtight structures can serve for such storage. These include upright tower silos, inground pits, and even huge plastic bags. Within the silo, recently harvested grasses or chopped corn are tightly compressed, squeezing out most of the air. Any remaining oxygen is rapidly consumed by the actively metabolizing plant cells. As the milieu becomes anaerobic, increasing amounts of lactate and other organic acids are generated. With the accumulation of these acids, the pH of the environment falls, microbial overgrowth is suppressed, and spoilage is prevented. Any portions of this material that remain exposed to air are rapidly overgrown with a progression of bacteria and fungi.[33]

This process may initially generate nitrogen dioxide and other oxides of nitrogen. When this occurs in a closed tower silo (Fig. 36-3), levels of NO_2 may rise abruptly over the ensuing 24 hours. Typically these levels may remain significantly elevated for 96 hours or longer after silo filling is completed. During this period the silo poses a grave threat to any worker who might attempt to enter and even to those who are working in buildings connected to the base of the silo.[34] Generally these gases escape through the small doors that extend up the side of the silo and fill the metal chute that encloses the doors as well as the ladder by which they are accessed. Farmers often enter the silo immediately upon completion of filling to level the silage and cover it with a plastic sheet. If this entry has been delayed by 12 or more hours, or if the filling process has taken several days, potentially toxic levels of NO_2 may be encountered in the chute on the way up the silo and particularly after crawling through the door onto the silage bed. Unfortunately the generation of these gases is unpredictable, and farmers who are simply following usual work practices may encounter high levels when in past years there had been little or no silo gas. This potential hazard exists with any type of ensiled feed, although the risk appears to be highest with corn silage.[35]

Although the recently-filled silo represents the gravest threat to workers, the about-to-be-emptied silo also represents a hazard. During the period of storage, any silage that has remained in a relatively anaerobic environment is not likely to spoil. Silage at the surface, however, is exposed to

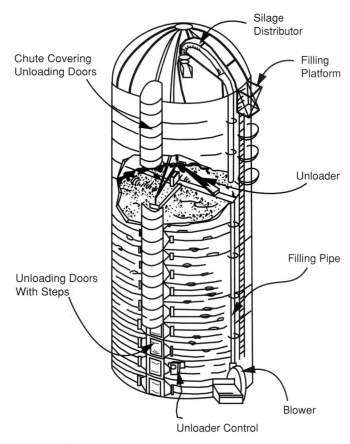

Fig. 36-3. The upright concrete stave silo is the most common type of silo. Chopped silage is blown through the filling pipe to the top of the silo where the distributor disperses it evenly. Access to the headspace is provided through the chute using the rungs placed on each of the vertically arranged unloading doors. Feeding from the silo is done by initially lowering the unloading mechanism onto the silage bed and thereafter activating it from the silo base. This device gathers the uppermost silage and sprays it through the open silo door and down the chute into a waiting feed wagon. Adapted from Zwemer FL, Pratt DS, and May JJ: Silo filler's disease in New York state, *Am Rev Resp Dis* 146:651, 1992, Fig. 1.

oxygen and thus will become contaminated as the levels of bacteria and fungi progressively increase.[33] Before the farmer can initiate the mechanical unloading of feed, the uppermost layer of spoiled silage must be removed by hand. This unenviable task generally takes an hour or more, during which time several tons of material are forked out of the top of the silo, down the chute, eventually to be dumped. If the cap material has dried, this task can be enormously dusty; sometimes a worker cannot see farther than 1 to 2 feet through the dust. Individuals who experience this type of exposure often will suffer an acute, febrile, flulike illness, organic dust toxic syndrome (ODTS), occurring 6 to 12 hours after completion of the silo opening job.[36]

Finally, brief mention should be made of "oxygen-limited" silo systems. Whereas in theory all silage is oxygen-limited, these upright silos are constructed of enameled metal plates with rubber seals around each plate in an effort to exclude all air strictly. By design these closed spaces have no oxygen and tend to trap the oxides of nitrogen and other toxic gases. These silos have barriers to prevent entry into the headspace above the silage. Ill-advised attempts to circumvent these barriers are likely to result in fatal asphyxia. Similarly, farmers have lost their lives attempting to repair the unloading mechanism at the base of these silos because to gain access to the device the farmer must crawl partly into a closed space.

Grain elevator. The processing of grains produced in the midwestern regions of North America usually involves storage in some type of grain elevator. This storage process entails weighing and grading the grain initially. Subsequently it is dried and stored until transfer to another elevator or to the customer. Grain is accumulated locally at country elevators, then shipped to larger terminal elevators for additional processing. Finally the grain may be stored at large transfer elevators prior to final shipping. A variety of grains, including oats, barley, wheat, rye, corn, and others, may be stored at elevators while awaiting transport.

Despite their silolike appearance, these large storage structures do not rely upon anaerobic conditions for the preservation of grain. Although grain stored in elevators may experience some microbial contamination, there is usually insufficient moisture for serious spoilage to take place. Additionally the use of fumigants such as aluminum phosphide suppresses bacterial and fungal growth.

Each manipulation of the grain results in further abrasion of the kernels and generation of dust. By one estimate, three to four pounds of dust are generated for each ton of grain handled. In addition to kernel components, grain dust contains small amounts of inorganic particles, pollens, insect and mammalian matter, and microbial contaminants, both fungal and bacterial.[37] The nature and size distribution of the particles varies with the type of grain, the season, and the abatement practices of the elevator operator.

Specific substance exposures

Toxic gases. As noted, there is some potential for harmful exposure to gases on many farms. These gases range in toxicity from irritants and potential asphyxiants to gases that are inherently highly toxic.

Ammonia. Ammonia, which has a threshold limit value (TLV) of 25 ppm, is particularly prevalent in association with animal waste from confinement operations. In these settings, levels may exceed 100 ppm.[38] Because of the marked water solubility of this gas, these quantities might be expected to cause symptoms of mucus membrane irritation in workers. Additionally, ammonia is adsorbed to dust particles that are sufficiently small to enter the respiratory system.[21]

Potential exposure to ammonia occurs when farmers work with anhydrous ammonia. This liquid has a boiling point of minus 28° F. It is transported, stored, and used in its liquid form. Anhydrous ammonia is more than 80% nitrogen and is used to boost the nitrogen content of soil. Typically an applicator tank is towed behind the tractor with a series of "knives" and associated tubing, which allows the ammonia to be injected into the soil in late fall or early spring. Occasionally farmers will add anhydrous ammonia to silage as it is being blown into the silo in an effort to increase the nitrogen content in the feed. When accidentally released into the environment, anhydrous ammonia usually dissipates rapidly. It can, however, exclude oxygen, particularly in a closed environment or in especially humid weather. Of greater concern is the fact that this material is strongly alkaline and an intense desiccant. Highly soluble in water, anhydrous ammonia forms ammonium hydroxide and then immediately dissociates into free hydroxyl ions. These can cause dermal burns, severe corneal burns, mucous membrane irritation and pulmonary injury with exposure.[39] Injuries to the lung include the adult respiratory distress syndrome, bronchiolitis obliterans, and possible late bronchiectasis. Exposures occur most commonly when transferring the liquid from one tank to another or when the lines or coupling devices on the application tank fail.

Carbon dioxide. Carbon dioxide may be generated in a number of agricultural processes. Usually these processes relate to the storage of some type of organic material. Ambient CO_2 levels may be elevated in some of the closed spaces used for storage such as the recently-filled silo, manure storage tanks, composting areas, or fruit chilling and storage buildings. Levels as high as 4000 ppm CO_2 have been documented in these settings.[22] In animal confinement settings, carbon dioxide presents a threat only if the ventilation system fails. In these instances, CO_2 may function as an asphyxiant by virtue of its specific gravity, displacing ambient oxygen from the worker's breathing zone.

Methane. Methane is another potential asphyxiant generated in manure storage areas.[40] Methane is related to the presence of methanogenic anaerobic bacteria in the environment, a phenomenon that has been used to advantage by some farmers who heat or even generate electricity with "biogas." Methane is lighter than air (specific gravity 0.55) and thus represents little hazard in open storage areas such as manure ponds. In a closed system, methane may exclude oxygen from the environment and, at levels above 5%, also represents some hazard because of possible explosion. Despite its potential as an agent of asphyxia, there is little solid evidence of serious injury or death in farmers caused by methane. Methane is usually found in combination with more toxic gases, which almost certainly account for the majority of worker injuries. In the one incident where deaths were attributed to methane, there are inadequate data to indicate that methane, rather than the more likely culprit hydrogen sulfide, was to blame.[24]

Hydrogen sulfide. The most toxic gas that is likely to be encountered in the agricultural workplace is hydrogen sulfide. This gas, which is generated in manure storage facilities, has several properties that combine to make it particularly dangerous. The specific gravity of H_2S is high so that the gas tends to accumulate along the surface of the manure slurry. In this setting it may significantly reduce the amount of oxygen available to a worker. Hydrogen sulfide has a strong "rotten egg" odor, which should serve as a warning to exposed individuals. At higher concentrations (>100 ppm), however, H_2S will rapidly inactivate the olfactory nerve, in effect rendering the gas odorless.[41] At low levels (50 to 200 ppm) the gas can cause irritation of the eyes and mucosal surfaces. At concentrations exceeding 300 ppm, the gas has been found predictably to cause pulmonary edema in animals and there is evidence of concurrent inhibition of surfactant activity.[42] Levels in excess of 600 ppm may be extremely toxic, exerting a cyanidelike uncoupling of oxidative metabolism, which can rapidly immobilize the victim, who dies of acute respiratory failure soon thereafter.[43] In manure facilities, this occurs either when a worker unwisely enters the storage area itself[25] or when a worker is near a slurry being mechanically agitated before pumping.[23]

Nitrogen dioxide. The heavier-than-air characteristic of this toxic gas also contributes to the hazard of nitrogen dioxide and related compounds. These compounds are generated with the conversion of nitrate to nitrite in recently ensiled plant material. Within 12 to 24 hours of filling a silo, various oxides of nitrogen may accumulate in sufficient concentrations to injure seriously an exposed worker.[44] In some test silos, levels of NO_2 have exceeded 1000 parts per million (ppm).[45] In the typical upright or "tower" silo this gas may persist in high concentrations for a week or longer. In these instances the gases may leak into the chute that encloses the silo's access ladder. Workers entering the chute or even working in the small shed at the base of the silo may encounter oxides of nitrogen at toxic levels. In addition to the inherent toxicity of these compounds, their accumulation in the chute and above the silage bed serves to displace oxygen from the breathing zone, thus superimposing the risk of extreme hypoxia.

The generation of high levels of NO_2 in recently-filled silos is an unusual and unpredictable occurrence that may develop without an apparent change in the farmer's usual practices. Silo gas production generally relates to the levels of nitrate in the ensiled feed. Nitrate levels are higher in certain crops such as corn, sudangrass, and sorghum. In addition, growing conditions such as heavy fertilization, wet, cloudy, cool growing seasons, immaturity at harvest, and cutting the plant close to the ground all increase the level of plant nitrates.

Carbon monoxide. This odorless, colorless gas is primarily encountered with internal combustion engines that are used with inadequate ventilation. Although this hazard might seem obvious, the use of such engines in closed buildings is common on many farms. Elevated levels of carbon monoxide have been recorded when gasoline-powered bedding choppers are used inside barns,[46] with some types of feed wagons in dairy barns, and notably in some animal confinement buildings.[47] In this setting CO generation from manure and gas-powered heating units can occasionally yield significant amounts of CO. High pressure spray devices that are routinely used to wash the inside of these buildings have been responsible for carbon monoxide intoxication of several workers.[48]

Organic dusts. The dusts generated in enclosed agricultural settings vary somewhat in composition depending upon the actual source. However there is a general pattern that applies to all of these dusts. Agricultural dust is actually a combination of suspended inorganic and organic matter, the former being primarily composed of various silicates. The organic dust contains fragments of microbial, plant, insect, and mammalian material. Each of these may contribute compounds of biologic significance.

Dust in confinement houses, silos, and barns may be heavily laced with both bacteria and fungi.[49,50] The bacteria are both gram-positive and gram-negative organisms. In stored feed, these organisms tend to grow in large numbers as long as there is sufficient moisture and oxygen. Eventually further growth is suppressed as the feed dries out, but this gives rise to conditions favoring aerosolization of these organisms. The presence of high levels of gram-negative organisms in agricultural dust adds the potential hazard of endotoxin exposure.

Endotoxin. The outer layer of gram negative organisms is a combination of polysaccharide side chains attached to a lipid component (lipid A) of the cell membrane. This lipopolysaccharide compound (LPS) is generically referred to as endotoxin and is recognized to have a multiplicity of biologic effects. These effects include activation of complement and alveolar macrophages, release of potent cytokines, and eventual capillary leak in the lung.[51,52] Studies in animal models demonstrate granulocyte accumulation in both the airspace and interstitium following endotoxin inhalation.[53] Clinically it is recognized that occupational inhalation of endotoxin can induce fever and constriction of airways.[54] Studies in cotton mills have provided evidence suggesting a prominent role for inhaled endotoxin in the symptoms of byssinosis. In these studies, levels ≥ 90 EU/m^3 appeared to cause significant biologic activity in exposed workers.[55] In many agricultural exposures, endotoxin levels far in excess of 90 EU/m^3 have been measured.[50,56] Thus workers in dairy barns using bedding choppers, workers in swine confinement buildings, and workers removing spoiled "cap" silage or cleaning out corn cribs are routinely at risk of potentially toxic inhaled doses of endotoxin. In confinement workers these levels of endotoxin correlate better with respiratory symptoms than with measures of total or respiratory dust.[57]

β-1,3 glucan. Less understood are the cell wall components of certain molds also found in agricultural dust. β-1,3 glucan is one of the most active of these glucan components. This compound is similar to endotoxin in its broad range of biologic activities. β-1,3 glucan is capable of complement activation, activation of macrophages, and stimulation of cytokine release.[58,59] Preliminary studies in exposed animals suggest that aerosolization of purified β-1,3 glucan elicits less neutrophil response than endotoxin. In fact the glucan may in some way act to moderate the endotoxin effect when both are aerosolized.[60] The issue is further complicated because glucans also have the capability of reacting in the limulus lysate test, which has been traditionally used for quantitation of endotoxin. This raises questions regarding relative contributions of endotoxin versus the β-glucans in some of the reactions to agricultural dust that have been reported.

Mycotoxins. These potent toxins are generated by several species of fungi found in the farm environment. Generally these are fairly stable compounds that may accumulate in feeds and remain long after the fungus itself has died. Affected crops include corn, cottonseed, and peanuts, among others. The best example of mycotoxins are the aflatoxins, a group of toxins produced by various *Aspergillus* species, particularly in hot, dry conditions of feed storage. These compounds may remain active even after exposure to high temperatures. They can affect both animals and humans following either inhalation or ingestion. Aflatoxin B$_1$ has been associated with hepatic inflammation and hepatocarcinoma.

Other mycotoxins that may be encountered include the trichothecenes, including deoxynivalenol and T-2 toxin, which can induce nausea, vomiting, and cardiac arrhythmias. Satratoxin is found in the spores of *Stachybotrys* and has been associated with hematopoetic and immune suppression. The ochratoxins, produced by *Penicillium* and *Aspergillus* are known to have renal toxicity. *Fusarium* species can also produce the zearalenone toxins, which have been associated with immunosuppression and reproductive complications in animals.

Studies of these agents are generally incomplete and their significance in relation to pulmonary toxicity is unclear. At least some of the mycotoxins are readily absorbed following inhalation. As a class the mycotoxins are remarkably potent, producing significant biologic effects at nanogram or microgram doses.[61]

Early reports of a febrile illness following exposure to high levels of agricultural dust was referred to as "pulmonary mycotoxicosis."[62] There is no compelling evidence to support mycotoxins as being a cause of organic dust toxic syndrome. This reaction is more likely caused by inhalation of either endotoxin or β-1,3 glucan.[63] In one study mycotoxins were systematically measured during this exposure and only trace amounts of deoxynivalenol were noted. These were unrelated to responses in dust-exposed workers.[50]

Biologic agents

Bacteria. As noted above both gram-negative and gram-positive bacteria are virtually ubiquitous in the agricultural workplace. In the manure slurry the presence of large numbers of gram negatives has yielded fulminant aspiration pneumonias in workers overcome by toxic fumes.[25] However, of greater significance to most persons working in this environment, is inhalational exposure to bacterial bioaerosols. Much of the recognized biologic activity of organic dusts relates to the presence of bacteria and their components.

Large numbers of bacteria become aerosolized when contaminated feed is disturbed. An example of this occurs when the silage cap from a silo is removed prior to the initiation of feeding. This cap material contains large numbers of both gram-positive bacilli and various gram negatives, thermoactinomyces, and fungi. The size and distribution of these populations vary with the depth into the silage bed. Gram-positive organisms, predominantly *Bacillus* species, account for greater than 99% of bacteria in the most superficial layers of silage. At a depth of 20 cm the percentage of gram-positive organisms falls to 11% and gram negatives, such as *Pseudomonas* and *Citrobacter* species, comprise 56% of all bacteria, with the remainder being *Corynebacterium* species. Still deeper (45 cm) the *Bacillus* again predominates.[33] When this cap material is removed, substantial quantities of bacteria may be aerosolized depending upon the moisture content of the silage. Levels of bacteria as high as $10^9/m^3$ have been documented in the dust generated by this process.[50] Similar findings have been documented in the dust produced by bedding choppers in some barns.[56]

Dust arising from the manipulation of feed such as hay in dairy barns has been associated with farmer's lung disease in a minority of farmers. The risk is determined in part by the levels of thermophilic actinomycetes generated in the dust.[27] When feed is moist and generates sufficient heat ($>40°$ C), the growth of various thermophiles is favored. Thus the cutting of hay in rainy weather, storage in moist conditions, or even high humidity facilitates the growth of organisms such as *Streptomyces rectovirgula* (*Micropolyspora faeni*), *Thermoactinomyces vulgaris,* and *Aspergillus* species.

Another setting in which bacterial aerosols are routinely encountered by workers is within the confinement house. Here the major component of the dust is usually feed particles; however, suspended fecal particles are also a substantial contributor. Gram-positive bacteria are seen in particularly high concentrations in some confinement house settings.[64] In nursery units, dried fecal matter comprises a higher portion of the particles suspended in the air and gram-negative content rises.[65] These particles tend to be considerably smaller (0.4 μm to 2.0 μm) than the feed particles and thus are eminently respirable. Bacteria make up as much as 50% of the fecal particles.[65] Quantitation of the bacterial content of swine feces shows a marked predominance of gram positives (*staphylococcus, streptococcus, lactobacillus*) with a smaller population of gram-negative coliform bacteria.[66] Despite these lesser numbers, suspended levels of bacteria are often sufficiently high (3.5 $\times$ $10^3/m^3$)[64] to permit deposition of substantial numbers of endotoxin-coated gram negatives at the small airway and alveolar level.

Fungi. A wide variety of fungi are found in feeds. Fungal growth begins when crops are still in the field; levels of fungal spores in the range of $10^8/m^3$ have been measured adjacent to combine harvesters.[67] Studies in Scotland have documented a progression of species of fungi in stored feed. Samples of hay showed a shift from "field species," *Aureobasidium, Cephalosporium, Cladosporium,* and *Fusarium,* to "storage species," such as *Penicillium* and *Aspergillus.*[68]

Agricultural workers are exposed to fungi in the same ways as noted above for bacteria. Levels of fungi in confinement-building suspended dust tend to be an order of magnitude lower than the levels of bacteria, and are in the range of 10^3 colony-forming units/m^3. Predominant species are *Alternaria, Fusarium, Cladosporium,* and *Aspergillus.*[65] The numbers of fungi encountered in work with spoiled feed tend to be substantially higher. Viable organisms in the range of $10^8/m^3$ have been measured during the opening of tower silos.[50] Quantitative cultures of the cap silage suggest that most of these aerosolized fungi are *Aspergillus fumigatus,* which are found within the top 20 cm of the silage bed.[33] Concentrations of spores up to $10^7/m^3$ have been discovered in nonventilated grain elevators, with species such as *Ustilago, Aspergillus, Mucor,* and *Cladosporium* predominating.[37] The progression from field fungi to storage fungi mentioned above has also been demonstrated in grain elevators.

Mites. Various species of insects are known to live in stored grain and hay. The presence of the grain weevil *Sitophilus granaris* may account for asthmatic reactions in some elevator workers.[69] These reactions have also been shown to occur in response to storage mites found in stored grain.[70]

Better defined is the role of storage mites in the barn setting. Studies from Scotland, Scandanavia, and Wisconsin have implicated storage mites as significant allergens in farmers who experience symptoms of rhinitis, conjunctivitis, and asthma following work in the barn.[68,71,72]

These mites are antigenically discrete from the better known house dust mite, *Dermatophagoides pteronyssinus.* The species most commonly implicated in this problem are *Glycyphagus (Lepidoglyphus) destructor, Tyrophagus longior* and *putrescentiae,* and *Acarus farris.* These mites may be found in a variety of stored feeds but seem most commonly associated with hay stored in barns. The mites eat various species of fungi found in the feed as well as the grain itself. The size of the mite population seems to par allel that of the thermophilic and mesophilic fungi, which multiply in the stored feed and reach peak numbers in October and November. Thereafter the numbers of viable mites decline and the ratio of dead to living mites increases.[68] Of interest are reports of storage mites inhabiting the dust of farmhouses.[73] In these situations an occupational allergy may become even more difficult to control as it becomes an environmental allergen in the home.

Inorganic dusts. Total dust exposures on farms are commonly above the nuisance level of 10 mg/m^3 and may be generated by an enormous variety of farm tasks and agricultural materials or products. High total dust exposures may occur from both indoor and outdoor farm tasks, although the actual exposure of the farmer will vary with time spent at a specific task, use of personal protective devices, and other factors.[19] Outdoor tasks such as ploughing, sowing, harrowing, and haymaking generate high dust concentrations. Dust generation will vary with many geologic and meteorologic factors such as rainfall, wind, soil composition, and cover. A tractor cabin with a filter system will decrease dust exposure, but the system must be maintained and must be properly functioning. Indoor dusts may be generated by animal movements, feeding, and transfer of grains and other products.

Whereas most studies have focused on the organic components of dust exposure on farms, a few investigations have measured inorganic dust levels. Tillage work is associated primarily with inorganic dust generation (70% to 95%), with total concentrations of 60 mg/m^3 observed and high quartz concentrations (11% to 66%) in the respirable fraction (<5 μm aerodynamic diameter).[19] Inorganic dust exposures have also been demonstrated in the prairie provinces of Western Canada from soil and crop interactions with farm machinery.[18] Measurements in California grape orchards showed average total airborne dust concentrations of 21 mg/m^3. Airborne quartz concentrations ranged from 70 to 105 μg/m^3, and were correlated with quartz concentrations in the soil and on foliar dusts.[15]

The major inorganic dust component of concern is crystalline silica or quartz, but exposures to many other fibrogenic inorganic dusts may occur as a result of agricultural activities. These include nonfibrous silicates known to cause pulmonary fibrosis, including mica and clay silicates.[16-18] Exposure may also occur to naturally occuring fibrous minerals such as fibrous zeolite.[18]

Although there are limited data on inorganic dust exposure of farmers, a few case reports and epidemiologic studies suggest that restrictive lung changes and pneumoconiosis may occur from occupational and environmental exposures. Silicate pneumoconiosis was found in six California farmworkers and one rural resident.[17] Analysis of particles in the lungs revealed primarily potassium and aluminum silicates (clays and micas) with less than one tenth of the particles being silicon dioxide. It was postulated that clay silicates that were used as pesticide vehicles, or agri-

cultural activities, were the source of the exposures. Soil analyses showed a composition similar to the particles in the lungs. Other case reports have demonstrated pneumoconiosis among farmers from diverse geographic regions and agricultural practices.[74,75] In one case, pulmonary fibrosis was associated with mica, talc, and silica in the lung tissue.[76] Analysis of soils from the farmer's storehouse revealed similar minerals.

Few epidemiologic studies have been performed on the effects of inorganic dust exposures among farmers. The incidence and prevalence of chronic bronchitis is increased among farmers, with etiologic studies implicating agricultural exposures.[77] Whereas the most commonly identified risk factor is grain dust, the contribution of other particulate and nonparticulate exposures is unknown. A study of rice mill workers in Malasia found an increased prevalence of respiratory symptoms and nodular opacities in 15% of the workers.[78] Total dust concentrations ranged from 2.3 to 5.4 mg/m^3 and, although rice husk is an organic dust, it is known to have a high silica content. An epidemiologic study of California farmworkers revealed increased restrictive pulmonary function among grape workers that was consistent with an effect of elevated silica concentrations in this work environment.[79]

More research is needed to characterize the determinants and levels of inorganic dust exposure among agricultural workers. Epidemiologic studies are also needed to assess the prevalence of restrictive lung disease caused by agricultural exposures.

Chemicals. The best known agrichemical with implications for the lung is the dipyridyl herbicide paraquat. Widely used in agriculture, this compound is available as a liquid concentrate and it is this form that causes most intoxications. Many intoxications follow deliberate ingestions, but there have been numerous cases of illness following incidents related to the mixing of the solution or the practice of blowing through a sprayhead to clear it. Severe irritation of the oropharynx may follow careless exposure to paraquat mists, but there is little evidence that this type of exposure can lead to serious pulmonary injury.[80] Subsequent to ingestion of one or more ounces of the concentrate, severe irritation of oropharynx and esophagus are followed by transient falls in both renal and hepatic function. Of more concern, however, is the fulminant pulmonary inflammation, which results in loss of capillary integrity and diffuse alveolar damage with the eventual influx of fibroblasts. This damage seems to be mediated in part by oxygen radicals generated by the paraquat. The administration of supplemental oxygen, which is needed to support most of these patients, seems to contribute synergistically to the paraquat injury.[81]

With the notable exception of paraquat, the pulmonary effects of exposure to most specific agrichemicals is uncertain. However, workers in agriculture are likely to have some contact with other chemicals that are known to have pulmonary toxicity. Many of these workers may be exposed to diesel exhaust fumes on a regular basis (see Chapter 33). In addition, most farmers do their own equipment repair and this often includes some welding (see Chapter 42), for which there is likely to be less protection than in most industrial settings. Exposure to certain organic solvents, potential aspiration of gasoline, and other compounds also represent real respiratory hazards on a farm (see Chapter 28).

Infectious organisms (see Chapter 32). There are a variety of zoonotic and other infections that have the potential to infect agricultural workers. However the problem of occupationally-acquired pulmonary infections is largely a theoretical one. An exception to this is tuberculosis, which represents a significant threat to some groups of workers in agriculture, particularly migrant workers. In a study of migrants in North Carolina, high rates of skin test positivity were found. A reactive purified protein derivative (PPD) test was present in 33% of Hispanic workers, 54% of African-American migrants, and 76% of Haitian workers. Active tuberculosis was found in black migrants at rates 300 times those expected.[82]

Fungal infections such as histoplasmosis and coccidiodomycosis may occur among exposed workers in endemic areas. Tularemia pneumonia has been described in workers exposed to high levels of grain dust. It seems likely to be related to contamination with rodent feces. There is some small risk of psittacosis among workers at fowl confinement facilities. Like brucella, this seems to be a significantly greater hazard for those working in packing houses than those involved in raising the animals.

Exposure dose issues

Gases adsorbed to particulate. As the number of environmental studies in the agricultural workplace increase, it becomes important to determine permissible levels of exposure for various agents. Threshold limits have been defined for many of the gases that can be encountered in farming. Although these limits are based upon work in other industrial settings, they should be applicable to agriculture in virtually every case. The possible exception to this applicability is the situation of gases adsorbed to dust particles. This seems to be most significant in the case of ammonia, although hydrogen sulfide adsorbed to dust might also represent a potential problem. The binding of ammonia to dust particles (3.9 mg nitrogen per gram of dust) in the confinement house setting has been well documented.[65] Concern has been raised that this phenomenon may permit penetration of this otherwise highly soluble gas beyond the upper airways, causing possible injury at the small airway and alveolar level. There are no human studies available to resolve this question with regard to ammonia bound to organic dust. Animal studies seem to suggest adverse effects from the combination of NH_3 with respirable confinement building dust. Pigs were exposed in chambers to moderate levels of ammonia and relatively high levels of organic dust

over a number of weeks. When compared to those exposed to dust or NH_3 alone, the dust plus NH_3 group showed no specific lesions on histologic examination. However this group was noted to have significantly reduced rates of weight gain.[83]

Inspirable versus respirable versus total dust. The problem of TLVs on organic dust is less clear than that of limits on gases. Because work exposures have been less studied, it is unknown whether limits proposed for some organic dusts, such as cotton or grain, apply equally to environments such as combining, confinement work, and barn exposures. Similarly it is unclear whether the biologically active organic dusts should be measured as total dust or respirable dust. Many of the components of these dusts are capable of producing local pathologic responses or systemic absorption of inflammatory mediators following deposition on virtually any mucosal surface. Thus penetration to levels in the vicinity of the terminal airways is not necessarily a determinant of the dust's toxic potential. In some cases "inspirability" may be of equal or greater significance than "respirability." Some authors argue that since the composition of most agricultural dusts is similar, measurements of total dust alone are sufficient to describe workers' exposures.[84]

Host phenomena. There is evidence that host factors play a significant role in moderating the effects of agricultural environmental exposures. Currently the specifics of most host factor interactions are incompletely described. For example, the determinants of the hypersensitivity pneumonitis response remain poorly understood (see Chapter 14). A majority of exposed workers experience no problems with farmer's lung disease (FLD). A small proportion of farmers may develop either positive precipitins or increased proportions of lymphocytes in their alveolar lavage without having actual pneumonitis.[85] An even smaller number will actually develop FLD. One determining factor is the level of organisms aerosolized in the barn,[27] although the risk seems to relate only indirectly to this. The actual initiation of the hypersensitivity response in farmers who may have had similar exposures for years is unexplained. Preliminary data from animal studies suggest that an intercurrent viral infection in the host may be required to trigger the evolution of active pulmonary inflammation.[86]

Cigarette smoking is another important host factor. It is recognized that the prevalence of hypersensitivity pneumonitis is higher in nonsmokers than in smokers.[87] This phenomenon is not well explained but could relate to alterations in the immune response of cigarette smokers. It is known, for example, that cytokine production by the alveolar macrophages of smokers is diminished.[88] Similarly, there is a reduction in smoker's lymphocyte response to various mitogens.[89] The interaction of one or several of these cigarette-mediated alterations seems to provide smokers with a degree of protection from both sensitization (that is, antibody production) and disease activation.

Although FLD provides the clearest example of the interaction of environmental and host factors, similar issues arise with many of the other respiratory problems seen in agriculture. Often documentation of such phenomena is complicated by the "healthy worker effect." In the grain industry, rates of long term ill-effects among workers may be reduced because of the early departure of sensitized workers. Factors such as smoking, storage mite allergy, and non-specific bronchial hyperreactivity appear to increase the worker's risk.[69] A number of ill-defined host factors seems to determine the risk of developing long-term reductions in pulmonary function in grain and confinement workers. Determinants of the risk of mite sensitization, ODTS reactions, and other responses to dust and fumes in the agricultural work environment need to be better defined.

Studies of exposure

Animal confinement. The confinement work environment has been better studied than most agricultural exposures. There are several toxic gases that can be present in the confinement house environment. To a large degree, these relate to the proximity of stored manure. Ammonia (average 33 ppm), carbon dioxide (1600 ppm), carbon monoxide (9.1 ppm), and hydrogen sulfide (1.4 ppm) are all generated by the digestion of manure.[21] Hydrogen sulfide and carbon dioxide both have specific gravities greater than that of air (1.19 and 1.53, respectively) and thus tend to remain in higher concentrations near the surface of the manure. However, there is some dispersal of these gases from up-drafting because of the body heat of the animals and distribution of the gases by area ventilation. Higher levels of these gases can be found in areas immediately adjacent to the building's exhaust fans.[90]

The most dangerous of these gases is H_2S. There are limited data suggesting that the usual concentrations of this gas are less than 2 ppm in the confinement setting. Additional data are available from measurements following incidents in which injury or death of animals or humans occurred. These measurements often relate to agitation and pumping of the manure slurry. In this setting, levels in the range of 400 ppm have been documented.[23]

Carbon dioxide is generated in manure storage facilities, but the majority of CO_2 in confinement buildings is from respiration of the animals. Levels of CO_2 encountered in the confinement house setting relate to the density of the animals and indirectly to the level of ventilation in the building. For this reason, levels in farrowing and nursery buildings tend to be roughly 30% higher (approximately 1800 ppm) than those in finishing buildings (1300 ppm).[21] Carbon dioxide levels may climb abruptly over a period of several hours if the confinement building's ventilation system fails. Levels may rise enough to affect both the workers and the animals.

Carbon monoxide has been found in the confinement setting, occasionally at significantly elevated levels. In nearly all cases this is a result of the incomplete combustion of hydrocarbons.[47] Initially this was attributed to the use of kerosene and propane heaters during the winter. More recently carboxyhemoglobin levels as high as 75.8% have been observed following routine washing in the building with gasoline-powered pressure washers.[48]

Workers in these facilities are routinely exposed to moderate levels of organic dust.[65,91] Levels of total dust average 3 to 5 mg/m³ in the farrowing and nursery buildings. One large study[49] showed similar levels for finishing buildings in Europe, whereas an American study described levels of 15 mg/m³ in these buildings.[65] Between 6% and 20% of this dust by weight is respirable, with the higher proportions being found in the nursery and farrowing buildings. These levels can rise appreciably during periods of activity.[91] This dust is a combination of feed particles, animal epithelium, particles of dried manure, pollen grains, and microbial organisms—particularly bacteria.[65,92] The latter components account for much of the endotoxin routinely found in this dust. Levels ranging from 3000 to 40,000 EU/m³ have been recorded in this environment.[57] An added feature of confinement house dust is the phenomenon of adsorption of potentially toxic gases, such as ammonia, to the dust particles.[65]

Several studies have demonstrated that the method of feeding can significantly affect the levels of dust in confinement buildings. In studies of swine buildings, scattering of feed on the floor, indoor grinding of feed, and the use of high moisture corn all contributed to higher levels of organic dust.[93] The use of covered feeders, filled from overhead via a closed spout, seems to generate less dust. Finally the practice of adding fat supplements to the animals' diet has been used to reduce dust. Studies reported by Chiba et al.[94] have demonstrated a 21% reduction of aerial dust in confinement buildings where 2.5% animal fat was added to the feed. Further increases of animal fat up to 5.0% and 7.5% resulted in decreases of 50% and 53% of total dust, respectively. There was an associated 60% reduction in ammonia levels and a 75% reduction in aerosolized bacterial colony-forming units with the highest level of fat supplement.[94]

Barns. Environmental measurements performed in barns have been reported to a limited degree. These studies relate to the dust generated with the use of a bedding chopper. This activity can generate levels of total area dust ranging from 9 to 40 mg/m³ with personal samplers detecting 10 to 70 mg/m³. This dust was found to have a high endotoxin content of 300 to 27,000 EU/mg. This resulted in levels of respirable endotoxin of 150 to 4000 EU/m³.[56] Added features of this exposure include histamine levels of up to 7.0 ng/mg dust and transient elevations of carbon monoxide in excess of 500 ppm.[46,95]

Aeroallergen studies have been reported in relatively quiet barns as well as following the use of a bedding chopper. Using radioallergosorbent test (RAST) inhibition techniques, high levels of *M. faeni, Thermoactinomyces vulgaris,* and *Aspergillus fumigatus* were noted; levels of dust and storage mites were among the highest noted. These levels are at least one hundred times the levels found in most other environments.[32] During the use of the bedding chopper, these levels increased roughly fiftyfold and then promptly returned to baseline after the job was completed.[96]

Silos. The level of toxic gases in the headspace of nonoxygen-limited silos is usually at or near zero. In a recently-filled silo, however, various oxides of nitrogen may accumulate at levels well above those designated by the U.S. National Institute for Occupational Safety and Health (NIOSH) as "immediately hazardous to life and health." Nitrogen dioxide levels of 200 ppm or above have been measured within the initial week of ensiling.[45]

There are some data on the dust levels generated when a silo is being prepared for unloading. Often the spoilage extends one or more feet down into the silage bed and this material must be manually thrown down from the top of the silo. Studies in a few such silos have shown great variability in dust levels depending upon the amount of moisture in the silage. When heavy dust is encountered, total dust may exceed 100 mg/m^3 and respirable levels may be in the range of 20 mg/m^3. Viable thermophilic bacteria in the dust can be in the range of 10^9 per cubic meter or more. Thermophilic fungi levels of 10^8/m^3 have been measured.[50] Levels of endotoxin are similarly elevated with dusty silos generating total dust endotoxin of up to 88,000 EU/m^3 and respirable endotoxin of 13,000 EU/m^3.[50]

Grain dust. Dust levels in grain elevators have been significantly reduced in recent years. Previously, levels of total dust above 100 mg/m^3 were documented. Total dust levels tended to be in the 10 to 25 mg/m^3 range, albeit with considerable variation. Certain jobs, particularly those involving housekeeping and maintenance, were associated with the highest dust exposures. Levels of respirable dust generally fell in the range of 0.5 to 5 mg/m^3.[97] Dust limits of 10 mg/m^3 were established in Canada in the late 1970s, and in the two decades since then there has been a notable decline in dust levels; many elevators are approaching or achieving the current target of 4 mg/m^3 (Fig. 36-4). Up to 40% of the particulate is sufficiently small to be classified as respirable dust. The fraction of respirable dust tends to be higher with certain grains, such as barley and wheat, and lower for corn.

Grain dust is a complex mixture of organic and inorganic matter. Approximately 20% of the dust is inorganic and the major component is quartz, which accounts for about 6% of the total dust. This proportion tends to be somewhat higher in country elevators where the grain has not been thoroughly cleaned. The organic component contains fractured grain particles, pollen and other plant material, insect parts, mites, mammalian debris, and large numbers of microorganisms and spores. These microorganisms are predominantly bacteria. The most prevalent fungi are yeasts, *Aspergillus, Penicillium,* and *Ustilago*.[98] Additionally chemical compounds, ranging from mycotoxins and plant enzymes to fumigants and pesticide residues, may be present. Not surprisingly, this material exhibits considerable biologic activity, which includes complement activation[99] and stimulation of alveolar macrophage chemotactic factors.[100] In vivo, this dust can cause an acute febrile reaction[101] and acute decrements in spirometric performance.[102]

EPIDEMIOLOGY OF OCCUPATIONAL RESPIRATORY DISEASE IN AGRICULTURE

The epidemiology of occupational lung disease in agriculture has been studied in a few areas, particularly in grain workers. Many other areas are less understood and, for some problems, little or no consistent data are available.

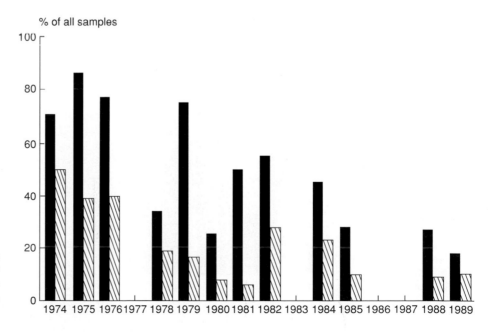

Fig. 36-4. Based upon personal total dust samples from Vancouver terminal grain elevator workers, 1974-1989, this figure shows the declining proportion of samples in excess of 10 mg/m^3 (solid bars) or 4 mg/m^3 (hatched bars). Total number of samples: 781. Adapted from Chan-Yeung M, Enarson DA, and Kennedy SM: The impact of grain dust on respiratory health, *Am Rev Resp Dis* 145:485, 1992, Fig. 1.

Silo filler's disease

The literature describing respiratory disease following NO_2 inhalation, silo filler's disease, consists primarily of case reports and small series. Douglas described a series of 17 farmers exposed to silo gas who were seen at the Mayo Clinic over a period of 32 years.[34] Eleven of these cases had evidence of lung injury and one ultimately died. The victims were all men, aged 34 ± 14 years. The majority of incidents occurred during the month of September and involved the storage of corn.

The only population-based study of this problem was done in New York where a statewide database on all hospital discharge diagnoses was used to identify all hospitalized cases of silo filler's disease over a 6-year period. Fifteen such cases were identified and confirmed by chart reviews. These victims resembled the Mayo Clinic cases in sex (100% men) and age (31 ± 11 years). The New York cases also occurred in the fall, 80% in September and October, and involved the storage of corn in 18 of 20 (90%) instances. Using data from the New York census of agriculture, the rate of serious cases of silo-filler's disease was calculated to be 5.0 per 100,000 exposed workers per year.[35] The New York cohort experienced 20% mortality.

Manure gas intoxication

There have been limited epidemiologic data on intoxication by manure gas. A surveillance system for traumatic occupational fatalities, devised by NIOSH, reports 22 deaths during 1980-1989.[26] This probably represents an underestimate since workers younger than 16 years were excluded. Donham has estimated the size of the worker population at risk during that period to be 500,000.[23] Thus a rough estimate of the incidence of fatal exposures is in the range of 0.5 per 100,000 exposed workers per year. The majority of reported incidents have occurred in the late spring through early fall (Fig. 36-5). Virtually all victims described in the reported cases are men. Most episodes involve either

deliberate or accidental entry into the facility, or work immediately adjacent to such a unit, while the manure is agitated. Several reports describe additional fatalities caused by entry during ill-conceived rescue efforts.

Farmer's lung disease (FLD)

The epidemiology of FLD is perhaps the most studied area in the field of agricultural lung disease. Unfortunately the studies performed since 1975 have yielded results that are so widely divergent that it is still difficult to define the prevalence of this disorder. As noted by Depierre, in ten such studies, the prevalence ranges from 4.2 to 170 cases per 1000 workers.[28] Most would agree that the rate of antibody positivity in the farm population is actually in the range of 5% to 20% and that considerably less than 1% of farmers actually develop hypersensitivity pneumonitis. However substantial confusion remains in the literature.

A major problem in the epidemiologic studies is the case definition. Many of the earlier studies sought only a history of fever or respiratory symptoms occurring several hours after work with dusty feed. A review of these cases shows that when findings of chest auscultation, radiographs, or spirometry are available, these are all negative in the majority of cases identified.[103] Such cases would better fit the criteria of ODTS than farmer's lung. It is now recognized that the former is a more common disorder.[104] Thus much of the FLD described in articles that relied heavily on the history of the illness was probably misdiagnosed.

There are other factors that may help to account for the marked variance in these studies. It is clear that FLD prevalence is influenced by climate. Regions where there are heavy rainfall and high humidity are at considerably greater risk for microbial overgrowth in stored hay and other feeds. Cold climates necessitate tight barns and decreased barn ventilation increases the likelihood of dust-related problems. Regional differences in farming methods and farm size also can account for significant differences. Farms that

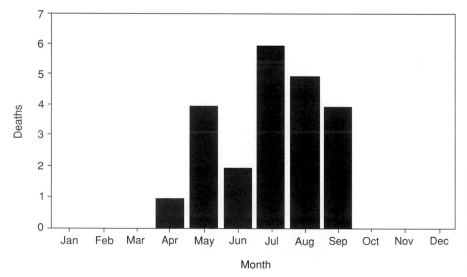

Fig. 36-5. Seasonal pattern of fatal manure gas intoxications, 1980-1989, as recorded by occupational fatality data from the National Institute for Occupational Safety and Health. Adapted from Anonymous: Fatalities attributed to entering manure waste pits—Minnesota, 1992, *MMWR*, 42:328, 1993, Fig. 1.

employ hay-drying systems have significantly less thermophilic actinomycete aerocontamination.[27] Some studies have revealed that farm size or herd size are determinants of risk for FLD and are likely to be related to exposure intensity.[105] Another major determinant of disease prevalence is cigarette smoking. Numerous studies have documented significantly lower rates of serum precipitins and of clinical disease in smokers.[106]

Finally it should be noted that alveolitis, in response to inhalation of dust from hay and other feeds, is not the only source of hypersensitivity pneumonitis seen in agricultural workers. This disorder can affect workers exposed to dust in the cultivation of mushrooms, tea, tobacco, certain types of grapes, and a variety of other plant products. Workers in the poultry industry may respond to a variety of avian antigens.

Asthma, airway hyperresponsiveness

The problem of allergic response, either immediate or delayed, to exposures in the barn work environment has been studied in many agricultural populations. The earliest studies were conducted in Scotland, where 30% of 290 farmers described allergic symptoms related to barn work.[107] Seventy-one percent of these symptomatic farmers had skin-prick tests that were positive to storage mite antigen. Subsequent studies in Britain described allergic symptoms in 21% of farmers after working in stored grain. Fifty-nine percent of these had IgE reactive to storage mites.[108] Swedish farmers on the island of Gotland were surveyed with questionnaires and a subsample underwent skin and RAST testing. This population had a rate of atopy of 16%, and 6.2% of farmers appeared to have symptoms related to specific storage mite allergy.[71] In a study using nasal challenge in dairy farmers, Finnish researchers noted an 18% prevalence rate.[109] These workers also described common reactions to cattle epithelium. Studies of storage mite reactivity in Denmark suggest positive skin tests in 5.8% and positive RAST in 4.6% of farmers. This population showed a strong correlation between positive testing for storage mites and positive testing for house dust mites.[73] Few studies have been performed on this problem outside of Europe. A study in Wisconsin used combined skin test and RAST testing on a cohort of 120 farmers. Fifty-six percent of the farmers had some allergen reactivity. Specific barn allergens (danders and storage mites) accounted for a third of these allergic responses.[72]

Considering the diversity of climates described and the variation in farming practices, barn construction, and ventilation, it is not surprising that some divergence in rates has been found. There have been differences in the case definitions, methods of testing, and antigens employed. Despite these differences, it seems that a significant number of people around the world suffer occupational allergy related to plant antigens, animal danders, and storage mites in particular.

Other sources of airway hyperresponsiveness are encountered in agriculture, including several studies in grain workers. A small proportion of these workers demonstrate an increased airway response to specific components of the grain dust (mites, molds) and others may demonstrate only nonspecific reactivity.[69] Additionally some grain workers experience a measurable cross-shift fall in forced expiratory volume in 1 second (FEV1) and forced vital capacity (FVC), which differ from nonspecific bronchial hyperresponsiveness, but seems to correlate with long-term reductions in pulmonary function. The rates of asthma in this population are not greater than controls, suggesting an early exodus from the job by affected workers.[69]

Many of these reactions seem to be caused by nonspecific irritant responses to agricultural dusts. Another potential factor that produces reactions is agrichemicals. A study of Canadian grain farmers suggested a relationship between pesticides and the occurrence of asthma in farmers.[110] Interestingly the pesticides involved were all insecticides that inhibit cholinesterase and thus might be expected to increase bronchoconstriction.

Bronchitis

The problem of bronchitis related to agricultural work was initially studied in the setting of grain elevators. Later studies addressed this issue in grain farmers, confinement house workers, and dairy farmers. Despite reduced rates of cigarette smoking, all of these populations experienced an abnormally high prevalence of chronic cough with excessive sputum production.

Grain workers may experience a dose-related, acute cross-shift fall in peak flow and a gradual reduction in FEV1 over the initial two weeks of exposure.[111] Many experience some related cough and dyspnea. Much of this is reversible initially but recurs with seasonal resumption of grain-dust exposure.[112] Chronically, approximately 20% of nonsmoking and up to 50% of smoking elevator workers develop cough and phlegm. Their risk increases, both with smoking and with intensity of grain-dust exposure, in an additive fashion.[69] Pulmonary function may be somewhat reduced, particularly with high levels of dust, smoking, and evidence of initial airway hyperreactivity.[113] Rates of atopy are reduced in these workers, suggesting a significant "healthy worker effect" with migration of atopics out of the industry, probably within the initial years of their employment.[69]

The situation is similar in confinement-house workers. Studies in both swine[57] and poultry[114] confinement document high rates of chronic cough and phlegm (up to 50%) that appear related to smoking as well as to length and intensity of exposure. Here also the overall effect on pulmonary function appears to be marginal. A comparative study done in Denmark indicates that these individuals experience higher rates of respiratory symptoms than those who work in combined swine and dairy operations. The latter, in turn, have more bronchitis than dairy farmers.[115] Several studies demonstrate that even workers in the dairy environment have measurably more bronchitis than nonfarm controls.[77] Thus the industry provides a series of differing work environments that vary primarily in terms of the intensity and constancy of exposure to agricultural dust. The rates of chronic bronchitis and other respiratory symptoms seem to reflect the extent of the dust exposure (Table 36-2).

PREVENTION

The major recognized respiratory threats to agricultural workers are toxic gases and organic dusts. The gases are only rarely present in life-threatening levels and usually are found (with the possible exception of ammonia in confinement facilities) in low concentrations. The dusts may be generated in high quantities with specific tasks but tend generally to be elevated in most agricultural settings. However for most workers these dusts do not represent an immediate threat to life.

The optimal approaches to protection from these diverse hazards are exactly the same as those used in other industries: prevention, ventilation, and avoidance (see Chapter 60). In the case of agricultural toxic gases prevention is less feasible than avoidance, whereas for dusts the converse is true. The final (and least desirable) method of prevention is personal protective equipment, which continues to play an important role in many agricultural settings. This topic is covered in greater depth elsewhere in this text (see Chapter 59) but will be mentioned when appropriate for specific agricultural hazards.

The major toxic gas hazards described earlier in this chapter are hydrogen sulfide, nitrogen dioxide, and carbon monoxide. The other gases likely to be encountered by an agricultural worker are primarily irritants or gases with potential asphyxiant capabilities. It is unrealistic to believe that personal protective equipment can play any significant role in dealing with these hazards. Protection from these gases requires a self-contained breathing apparatus, which is unlikely to be available on a farm and even less likely to be adequately maintained in this setting. Finally the access to some of the sites where gas may be encountered, such as the top of a silo, is too limited to permit use of these devices.

Similarly there are problems in devising realistic approaches to preventing the generation of most of these toxic gases. The biologic processes used in agriculture naturally give rise to H_2S, NO_2, and CO. It is unlikely that these can be altered in any way to ensure that the gases will not be produced. In the case of carbon monoxide this is only partly true since a large portion of the CO encountered may arise from the use of internal combustion engines and malfunctioning heater units. Prevention may be directed at these obvious sources of ambient carbon monoxide. Otherwise, safety measures must be based upon worker recognition of the potential hazard and appropriate avoidance. In the case of these gases, this is a realistic approach. After a silo has been filled, the blower can be left on for the brief time that may be required for capping. Thereafter the silo does not need to be reentered in the following several weeks when NO_2 may be present.[34] In the case of H_2S that is generated in manure storage facilities, workers can remove themselves from the area on the rare occasions when the agitator is being used. Should mechanical problems arise, workers must recognize that the area can only be entered under strict closed-space safety procedures.[26] Ventilation may be of some use with these toxic gases and should be the first measure used in the event of a worker's being overcome. The effectiveness of these efforts will vary with the particular situation. It is known, for example, that the ability of a silo blower to remove NO_2 effectively decreases substan-

Table 36-2. Relation of farming type to respiratory symptoms (%)*

	Type of farming				
	No animals (287)	Dairy (203)	Dairy and pig (316)	Pig (369)	p (χ^2 test)
Age over 50	53.8	43.1	65.8	54.5	<0.01
Smoking	35.1	41.9	37.1	35.7	NS
Full-time employment on farm	37.8	88.5	77.8	81.4	<0.01
Hay fever	8.1	7.6	9.6	13.3	NS
Asthma	7.5	5.5	6.4	10.9	NS
Treatment for asthma	2.2	1.5	3.6	5.3	NS
Cough and daily production of phlegm	18.6	17.5	28.4	32.0	<0.01
Shortness of breath	14.4	12.5	19.0	23.1	<0.01
Wheezing	16.0	13.5	27.1	26.2	<0.01
Dry cough	22.8	20.6	28.2	37.2	<0.01
Symptoms (shortness of breath, wheezing, or cough) during work in animal house	—	7.4	11.6	28.3	<0.01

*Rate of respiratory symptoms relates to type of farming exposure. NS, not statistically significant. From Iversen M, Dahl R, Korsgaard J, Hallas T, and Jensen EJ: Respiratory symptoms in Danish farmers: an epidemiologic study of risk factors, *Thorax* 43:874, 1988, Table 3 BMJ Publishing Group. With permission.

tially with increasing height of headspace above the silage bed.

The issue of rescue attempts when workers have been overcome by fumes always needs to be addressed with those working in the farm setting. Ill-advised efforts to rescue fellow workers from silos, manure pits, and other closed spaces often result in the loss of additional lives. There are numerous reports of multiple deaths, often in the same family, occurring in this situation.[23,24] Workers need to recognize the enormous danger associated with entry into a space that has already immobilized one or more persons. Measures aimed at optimizing ventilation and prompt summoning of rescue personel trained in closed-space rescue are the proper interventions.

Agricultural dusts do not present the same immediate threat as do the gases discussed above; dust presents a challenge because of its ubiquity. It is unrealistic to rely on a worker to avoid situations of potential dust exposure. However as avoidance becomes a less effective strategy, prevention assumes a more significant role. In many situations there are steps that can effectively prevent dust generation. Some of these steps relate to various work practices. Permitting adequate drying of cut grasses in the field before baling can markedly reduce the levels of actinomyces and other microorganisms generated when this material is later used for feed or bedding. Addition of fat to the diet of animals in confinement facilities has been found to reduce significantly the ambient dust levels.[94] Capping of silage material with a plastic sheet will reduce spoilage. Use of a chain or some other inorganic material to keep the sheet in place is preferrable to the more common practice of blowing up additional silage. Sometimes alterations to equipment or to the way it is used can prevent dust generation. Pouring a quart of water on the cut surface of a hay bale prior to use in a bedding chopper has been shown to reduce the associated dust levels by 85%. The use of covered feed troughs that are filled through enclosed spouts will reduce dust in confinement houses.

Ventilation may be a valuable adjunct to preventive efforts aimed at both gases and dust. The use of fans in barns and confinement houses can help to abate both the levels of toxic fumes and organic dusts. Older buildings often have generous, albeit ill-designed ventilation. Newer buildings, particularly in colder climates, may be more tightly insulated and thus have higher levels of humidity, carbon dioxide, and ambient dust. In such structures attention to the use of fans and other methods of ventilation will not only protect workers but will also often increase production.

The final protective measure that should be employed by agricultural workers is appropriate personal respiratory protection. Studies have shown that properly fitted, half-face air-purifying respirators can prevent exacerbations of farmer's lung in susceptible individuals who are exposed to high levels of agricultural dust.[116] Similar results have been achieved with helmet-type, powered air-purifying respirators.[117] The use of respirators in this population may be more challenging than in some other groups. Many of these workers have no access to appropriate fitting, instruction, and maintenance of respirators. For this reason it is common to recommend the use of NIOSH-approved, disposable dust respirators. Although not optimal, these disposable dust respirators are more practical for most agricultural settings where fitting and maintenance are not likely to be reliable. There are no systematic investigations currently available to support this recommendation.

REFERENCES

1. Dacquel LT and Dahmann DC: Residents of farms and rural areas: 1991. *U.S. Bureau of the Census, Current Population Reports, P20-472,* p. 24, Washington, D.C., 1993, U.S. Government Printing Office.
2. Schenker MB and McCurdy SA: Occupational health among migrant and seasonal farmworkers: the specific case of dermatitis, *Am J Ind Med* 18:345-351, 1990.
3. The world bank: *World development report 1992: development and the environment,* New York, 1992, Oxford University Press.
4. The National Safety Council: Accident facts. Chicago, 1991, National Safety Council.
5. Pratt DS, Marvel LH, Darrow D, et al: The dangers of dairy farming: the injury experience of 600 workers followed for two years, *Am J Ind Med* 21:637-650, 1992.
6. Etherton JR, Myers JR, Jensen RC, Russell JC, and Braddee RW: Agricultural machine-related deaths, *Am J Public Health* 81:766-768, 1991.
7. Thelin A: Epilogue: agricultural occupational and environmental health policy strategies for the future, *Am J Ind Med* 18:523-526, 1990.
8. Marvel ME, Pratt DS, Marvel LH, Regan M, and May JJ: Occupational hearing loss in New York dairy farmers, *Am J Ind Med* 20:517-531, 1991.
9. Crist W and Dupuis H: Untersuchung der Moglichkeit von gesundlichen Schaigungen im Bereich der Wirbelsaule bei Schlepperfahren, *Med Welt* 36.1919-1920, 1968.
10. Zahm SH, Weisenburger DD, Babbitt PA, et al: A case-control study of non-Hodgkin's lymphoma and the herbicide 2,4-dichlorophenoxy-acetic acid (2,4-D) in eastern Nebraska, *Epidemiology* 1:349-356, 1990.
11. Blair A and Zahm SH: Cancer among farmers, *Occup Med State Art Rev.* 6:335-354, 1991.
12. Croft P, Coggon D, Cruddas M, and Cooper C: Osteoarthritis of the hip: an occupational disease in farmers, *Brit Med J* 304:1269-1272, 1992.
13. The Minnesota Department of Health: An analysis of suicides among those who resided on farms in five north central states, 1980-1985, Daymond J and Gunderson P, editors: Washington, D.C., 1985 Office of Educational Research and Improvement, U.S. Department of Education.
14. Mobed K, Gold E, and Schenker MB: Occupational health problems among migrant and seasonal farmworkers, *West J Med* 157:367-373, 1992.
15. Popendorf WJ: Mineral dust in manual harvest operations. In Kelley WD, editor: *Agricultural respiratory hazards,* vol 2, pp 101-116, Cincinnati, 1982, American Conference of Governmental Industrial Hygienists.
16. Silicosis and Silicate Disease Committee: Diseases associated with exposure to silica and nonfibrous silicate minerals, *Arch Pathol Lab Med* 112:673-720, 1988.
17. Sherwin RP, Barman JL, and Abraham JL: Silicate pneumoconiosis of farm workers, *Lab Invest* 40:576-582, 1979.

18. Green FHY, Yoshida K, Fick G, et al: Characterization of airborne mineral dusts associated with farming activities in rural Alberta, Canada, *Int Arch Occup Environ Health* 62:423-430, 1990.

19. Louhelainen K, Kangas J, Husman K, and Terho EO: Total concentrations of dust in the air during farm work, *Eur J Respir Dis* 152(suppl):73-79, 1987.

20. Brambilla C, Abraham J, Brambilla E, Benirschke K, and Bloor C: Comparative pathology of silicate pneumoconiosis, *Am J Pathol* 96:149-170, 1979.

21. Donham KJ and Popendorf WJ: Ambient levels of selected gases inside swine confinement buildings, *Am Ind Hyg Assoc J* 46:658-661, 1985.

22. Muehling AJ: Gases and odors from stored swine wastes, *J Animal Sci* 30:526-531, 1970.

23. Donham KJ, Knapp LW, Monson R, and Gustafson K: Acute toxic exposure to gases from liquid manure, *J Occ Med* 24:142-145, 1982.

24. Fatalities attributable to methane asphyxia in manure waste pits—Ohio, Michigan, *MMWR* 38:583-586, 1989.

25. Osbern L and Crapo R: Dung lung: a report of a toxic exposure to liquid manure, *Ann Int Med* 95:312-314, 1981.

26. Fatalities attributed to entering manure waste pits—Minnesota, 1992, *MMWR* 42:325-329, 1993.

27. Dalphin JC, Pernet D, Reboux G, et al: Influence of mode of storage and drying of fodder on thermophilic actinomycete aerocontamination in dairy farms of the Doubs region of France, *Thorax* 46:619-623, 1991.

28. Depierre A, Dalphin JC, Pernet D, et al: Epidemiological study of farmer's lung in five districts of the French Doubs province, *Thorax* 43:429-435, 1988.

29. Terho EO, Heinonen OP, Lammi S, and Laukkanen V: Incidence of clinically confirmed farmer's lung in Finland and its relation to meteorological factors, *Eur J Resp Dis* 152(suppl):47-56, 1987.

30. Terho EO and Lacey J: Microbiological and serological studies of farmer's lung in Finland, *Clin Allergy* 9:43-52, 1979.

31. Cuthbert O, Brostoff J, Wraith D, and Brighton W: Barn allergy: asthma and rhinitis due to storage mites, *Clin Allergy* 9:229-236, 1979.

32. Campbell AR, Swanson MC, Fernandez-Caldas E, et al: Aeroallergens in dairy barns near Cooperstown, New York and Rochester, Minnesota, *Am Rev Resp Dis* 140:317-320, 1989.

33. Dutkiewicz J, Olenchock SA, Sorenson WG, et al: Levels of bacteria, fungi, and endotoxin in bulk and aerosolized corn silage, *App and Environ Microbiol* 55:1093-1099, 1989.

34. Douglas WW, Hepper NGG, and Colby TV: Silo filler's disease, *Mayo Clin Proc* 64:291-304, 1989.

35. Zwemer FL, Pratt DS, and May JJ: Silo filler's disease in New York state, *Am Rev Resp Dis* 146:650-653, 1992.

36. May J, Stallones L, Darrow D, and Pratt D: Organic dust toxicity (pulmonary mycotoxicosis) associated with silo unloading, *Thorax* 41:919-923, 1986.

37. Farant JP: Assessment of dust nature and levels in the grain industry. In Cockroft DW and Dosman JA, editors: *Principles of health and safety in agriculture,* pp 178-191, Boca Raton, Fla., 1990, CRC Press.

38. Day DL, Hansen EL, and Anderson S: Gases and odors in confinement swine buildings, *Trans Am Soc Agric Eng* 8:118-121, 1965.

39. Millea TP, Kucan JO, and Smoot EC: Anhydrous ammonia injuries, *J Burn Care Rehab* 10:448-453, 1989.

40. Lapp HM, Schulte DD, Sparling AB, and Buchanan LC: Methane production from animal wastes, *Can Agric Engin* 17:97-102, 1975.

41. Milby T: Hydrogen sulfide intoxication—review of the literature and a report of an unusual accident resulting in two cases of nonfatal poisoning, *J Occup Med* 4:431-437, 1962.

42. Green FHY, Schurch S, De Sanctis GT, et al: Effects of hydrogen sulfide exposure on surface properties of lung surfactant, *J Appl Physiol* 70:1943-1949, 1991.

43. Haggard H and Henderson Y: The influence of hydrogen sulfide on respiration, *Am J Physiol* 61:289-297, 1922.

44. Wang LC and Burris RH: Mass spectrometric study of nitrogenous gases produced by silage, *Agric Food Chem* 8:239-242, 1960.

45. Lowry T and Schuman LM: Silo-filler's disease—a syndrome caused by nitrogen dioxide, *JAMA* 162:153-160, 1956.

46. Jones W, Dennis J, May J, et al: Dust control during bedding chopping, *Appl Occup Environ Hyg* (in press).

47. Donham KJ, Carson TL, and Adrian BR: Carboxyhemoglobin values in swine relative to carbon monoxide exposure: guidelines for monitoring animal and human health hazards in swine confinement buildings, *Am J Vet Res* 43:813-816, 1982.

48. Kahler M, Kuhse W, Wintermeyer L: Unintentional carbon monoxide poisoning from indoor use of pressure washers–Iowa, January 1992-January 1993, *MMWR* 42:777-785, 1993.

49. Attwood P, Brouwer R, Ruigewaard P, et al: A study of the relationship between airborne contaminants and environmental factors in Dutch swine confinement buildings, *Am Ind Hyg Assoc J* 48:745-751, 1987.

50. May JJ, Pratt DS, Stallones L, et al: A study of dust generated during silo opening and its physiologic effects on workers. In Dosman JA and Cockcroft DW, editors: *Principles of health and safety in agriculture,* pp 76-79, Boca Raton, Fla., 1989, CRC Press.

51. Morrisson D and Rylan J: Endotoxin and disease mechanisms, *Annual Rev Med* 38:417-432, 1978.

52. Burrell R, Lantz R, and Hinton D: Mediators of pulmonary injury induced by inhalation of bacterial endotoxin, *Am Rev Resp Dis* 137:100-105, 1988.

53. Venaille T, Snella MC, Holt PG, and Rylander R: Cell recruitment into lung wall and airways of conventional and pathogen-free guinea pigs after inhalation of endotoxin, *Am Rev Resp Dis* 139:1356-1360, 1989.

54. Rylander R, Bake B, Rischer J, and Helander I: Pulmonary function and symptoms after inhalation of endotoxin, *Am Rev Resp Dis* 140:981-986, 1989.

55. Castellan RM, Olenchock SA, Hankinson JG, et al: Acute bronchoconstriction induced by cotton dust: dose-related responses to endotoxin and other dust factors, *Ann Int Med* 101:157-163, 1984.

56. Olenchock S, May J, Pratt D, Piacitelli L, and Parker J: Presence of endotoxins in different agricultural environments, *Am J Ind Med* 18:279-284, 1990.

57. Zejda J, Barber E, Dosman J, et al: Respiratory health status in swine producers relates to endotoxin exposures in the presence of low dust levels, *J Occup Med* 36:49-56, 1994.

58. Czop J, Valiante N, and Janusz M: Phagocytosis of particulate activators of the human alternative complement pathway through monocyte beta-glucan receptors, *Prog Clin Biol Res* 297:287-296, 1989.

59. Sherwood E, Williams D, McNamee R, et al: Enhancement of interleukin-1 and interleukin-2 production by soluble glucan, *Int J Immunopharmacol* 9:261-267, 1987.

60. Rylander R and Fogelmark B: Inflammatory responses by inhalation of endotoxin and (1-3)-β-D-glucan, *Am J Indust Med* 25:101-102, 1994.

61. Sorenson WG: Mycotoxins as potential occupational hazards, *J Indust Microbiol* 31(suppl):205-211, 1990.

62. Emanuel DA, Wentzel FJ, and Lawton BR: Pulmonary mycotoxicosis, *Chest* 67:293-297, 1975.

63. Malmberg P and Rask-Andersen A: Organic dust toxic syndrome, *Sem Resp Med* 14:38-48, 1993.

64. Clark SR, Rylander R, and Larsson L: Airborne bacteria, endotoxin, and fungi in dust in poultry and swine confinement buildings, *Am Indust Hyg Assoc J* 44:537-541, 1983.

65. Donham KJ, Scallon L, Popendorf WJ, et al: Characterization of dusts collected from swine confinement buildings, *Am Ind Hyg Assoc J* 47:404-410, 1986.

66. Salanitro JP, Blake IG, and Muirhead PA: Isolation and identification of fecal bacteria from adult swine, *Appl Envir Microbiol* 33:79-84, 1977.

67. Popendorf W, Donham K, Easton D, and Silk J: A synopsis of agricultural respiratory hazards, *Am Ind Hyg Assoc J* 46:154-161, 1985.

68. Cuthbert OD and Jeffrey IG: Barn allergy: an allergic respiratory disease of farmers, *Sem Resp Dis* 14:73-82, 1993.

69. Chan-Yeung M, Enarson D, and Kennedy S: The impact of grain dust on respiratory health, *Am Rev Resp Dis* 145:476-487, 1992.

70. Blainey AD, Topping MD, Ollier S, and Davies RJ: Allergic respiratory disease in grain workers: the role of storage mites, *J Allergy Clin Immunol* 84:296-303, 1989.

71. van Hage-Hamsten M, Johansson SGO, and Hogland S: Storage mite allergy is common in a farming population, *Clin Allergy* 15:555-564, 1985.

72. Marx JJ, Twiggs JT, Ault BJ, Merchant JA, and Fernandez-Caldas E: Inhaled aeroallergen and storage mite reactivity in a Wisconsin farmer nested case-control study, *Am Rev Resp Dis* 147:354-358, 1993.

73. Iversen M, Korsgaard J, Hala T, and Dahl R: Mite allergy and exposure to storage mites and house dust mites in farmers, *Clin Exp Allergy* 20:211-219, 1990.

74. Dynnik VI, Khizhniakova LN, Baranenko AA, Makotchenko VM, and Okseniuk IM: Silicosis in tractor drivers working on sandy soils on tree farms, *Gig Tr Prof Zabol* 12:26-28, 1981.

75. Fennerty A, Hunter AM, and Smith AP: Silicosis in a Pakistani farmer, *Br Med J* 287:698-699, 1983.

76. Gylseth B, Stettler L, Mowe G, Skaug V, and Lexow P: A striking deposition of mineral particles in the lungs of a farmer: a case report, *Am J Ind Med* 6:231-240, 1984.

77. Dalphin JC, Bildstein F, Pernet D, Dubiez A, and Depierre A: Prevalence of chronic bronchitis and respiratory function in a group of dairy farmers in the French Doubs province, *Chest* 95:1244-1247, 1989.

78. Lim HH, Domala Z, Joginder S, et al: Rice millers' syndrome: a preliminary report, *Br J Ind Med* 41:445-449, 1984.

79. Gamsky TE, McCurdy SA, Samuels SJ, and Schenker MB: Reduced FVC among California grape workers, *Am Rev Respir Dis* 145:257-262, 1992.

80. Fitzgerald GR, Barniville G, Black J, et al: Paraquat poisoning in agricultural workers, *J Irish Med Assoc* 71:336-342, 1978.

81. Fisher HK, Clements JA, and Wright RR: Enhancement of oxygen toxicity by the herbicide paraquat, *Am Rev Resp Dis* 107:246-252, 1973.

82. Ciesielski SD, Seed JR, Esposito DH, and Hunter N: The epidemiology of tuberculosis among North Carolina migrant farm workers, *JAMA* 265:1715-1719, 1991.

83. Curtis SE, Anderson CR, Simon J, et al: Effects of aerial ammonia, hydrogen sulfide and swine-house dust on rate of gain and respiratory tract structure in swine, *J Animal Sci* 41:735-739, 1975.

84. Rylander R: Organic dusts and cell reactions, *Semin Resp Med* 14:15-19, 1993.

85. Cormier Y, Belanger J, Beaudoin M, et al: Abnormal bronchoalveolar lavage in asymptomatic dairy farmers. study of lymphocytes, *Am Rev Resp Dis* 130:1046-1049, 1984.

86. Cormier Y, Assayag E, and Tremblay G: Viral infection enhances lung response to *Micropolyspora faeni*, *Am J Indust Med* 25:79-80, 1994.

87. Warren CPW: Extrinsic allergic alveolitis: a disease commoner in nonsmokers, *Thorax* 32:567-569, 1977.

88. Yamaguchi E, Okazaki N, Itoh A, et al: Interleukin-1 production by alveolar macrophages is decreased in smoker, *Am Rev Resp Dis* 140:397-402, 1989.

89. Daniele R, Dauber J, Altose M, Rowlands D, and Gorenberg D: Lymphocyte studies in asymptomatic cigarette smoker. a comparison between lung and peripheral blood, *Am Rev Resp Dis* 116:997-1005, 1977.

90. Brannigan PG and McQuitty JB: The influence of ventilation on distribution and dispersal of atmospheric gaseous contaminants, *Can Agric Engin* 13:69-75, 1971.

91. Thelin A, Tegler O, and Rylander R: Lung reactions during poultry handling related to dust and bacterial endotoxin levels, *Eur J Respir Dis* 65:266-271, 1984.

92. Cormier Y, Tremblay G, Meriaux A, Brochu G, and Lavoie J: Airborne microbial contents in two types of swine confinement buildings in Quebec, *Am Ind Hyg Assoc J* 51:304-309, 1990.

93. Holness D, O'Blenis E, Sass-Kortsak A, Pilger C, and Nethercott J: Respiratory effects and dust exposures in hog confinement farming, *Am J Indust Med* 11:571-580, 1987.

94. Chiba LI, Peo ER, and Lewis AJ: Use of dietary fat to reduce dust, aerial ammonia and bacterial colony forming particle concentrations in swine confinement buildings, *Trans Am Soc Ag Engin* 30:464-468, 1987.

95. Siegel PD, Olenchock SA, Sorenson WG, et al: Histamine and endotoxic contamination of hay and respirable hay dust, *Scan J Work Envir Health* 17:276-280, 1991.

96. Pratt DS, May JJ, Reed CE, et al: Massive exposure to aeroallergens in dairy farming: radioimmunoassay results of dust collection during bedding chopping with culture confirmation, *Am J Indust Med* 17:103-104, 1990.

97. Farant J and Moore C: Dust exposures in the Canadian grain industry, *Am Ind Hyg Assoc J* 39:177-194, 1978.

98. Smalley EB, Burkholder WE, Caldwell RW, et al: Microbial flora and fauna of respirable dust from grain elevators, Publication no: 86-104, 1986, Department of Health and Human Services (NIOSH).

99. Olenchock A, Mull J, and Major P: Extracts of airborne grain dust activate alternative and classical complement pathways, *Ann Allergy* 44:23-28, 1980.

100. Von Essen S, Robbins R, Thompson A, et al: Mechanisms of neutrophil recruitment to the lung by grain dust exposure, *Am Rev Resp Dis* 138:921-927, 1988.

101. doPico G, Flaherty D, Bhansall P, and Chavaje N: Grain fever syndrome induced by airborne grain dust, *J Allergy Clin Immunol* 69:435-443, 1982.

102. doPico G, Reddan W, Anderson S, et al: Acute effects of grain dust exposure during a work shift, *Am Rev Resp Dis* 128:399-404, 1983.

103. Grant IW, Blyth W, Wardrop V, et al: Prevalence of farmer's lung in Scotland: a pilot survey, *Brit Med J* 1:530-534, 1972.

104. Malmberg P, Rask-Andersen A, Hoglund S, Kolmodin-Hedman B, and Guernsey JR: Incidence of organic dust toxic syndrome and allergic alveolitis in Swedish farmers, *Int Arch Allergy Appl Immunol* 87:47-54, 1988.

105. Cormier Y, Belanger J, and Durand P: Factors influencing the development of serum precipitins to farmer's lung antigen in Quebec dairy farmers, *Thorax* 40:138-142, 1985.

106. Kusaka H, Homma Y, Ogasawara H, et al: Five year follow-up of micropolyspora faeni antibody in smoking and nonsmoking farmers, *Am Rev Resp Dis* 140:695-699, 1989.

107. Cuthbert OD, Jeffery IG, McNeil HB, Wood J, and Topping M: Barn allergy among Scottish farmers, *Clin Allergy* 14:197-206, 1984.

108. Blainey A, Topping M, Ollier S, and Davies R: Respiratory symptoms in arable farmworkers: role of storage mites, *Thorax* 43:697-702, 1988.

109. Terho EO, Husman K, Vohlonen I, Rautalahti M, and Tukiainen H: Allergy to storage mites or cow dander as a cause of rhinitis among Finnish dairy farmers, *Allergy* 40:23-26, 1985.

110. Senthilselvan A, McDuffie HH, and Dosman JA: Association of asthma with the use of pesticides, *Am Rev Resp Dis* 146:884-887, 1992.

111. James AL, Zimmerman MJ, Ee H, Ryan G, and Musk AW: Exposure to grain dust and changes in lung function, *Br J Ind Med* 47:466-472, 1990.

112. Broder I, Mintz S, Hutcheon MA, Corey PN, and Kuzyk J: Effect of layoff and rehire on respiratory variables in grain elevator workers, *Am Rev Resp Dis* 122:601-608, 1980.

113. Tabona M, Chan-Yeung M, Enarson DA, et al: Host factors affecting longitudinal decline in spirometry among grain elevator workers, *Chest* 85:782-786, 1984.

114. Morris PD, Lenhart SW, and Service WS: Respiratory symptoms and pulmonary functions in chicken catchers in poultry confinement units, *Am J Ind Med* 19:195-204, 1991.

115. Iversen M, Dahl R, Korsgaard J, Hallas T, and Jensen EJ: Respiratory symptoms in Danish farmers: an epidemiologic study of risk factors, *Thorax* 43:872-877, 1988.

116. Muller-Wenning D and Repp H: Investigation on the protective value of breathing masks in farmer's lung using an inhalation provocation test, *Chest* 95:100-105, 1989.

117. Nuutinen J, Terho EO, Husman K, et al: Protective value of powered dust respirator helmet for farmers with farmer's lung, *Eur J Respir Dis* 152:212-220, 1987.

Chapter 37

FORESTRY PRODUCTS

Moira Chan-Yeung
Jean-Luc Malo

Since the beginning of civilization, human beings have relied on forest products for food, shelter, clothing, and fuel. At present, 90% of persons in developing countries rely on firewood for cooking and heating. In industrialized countries, wood is chiefly used as a building material and as a source of pulp for making paper. The total world softwood harvest was 1.29 billion cubic meters in 1991, of which Canada's share is 12.6% and the United States' share is 24%.[1] It is estimated that by the year 2000, the demand will reach 4 to 5 billion cubic meters.[2] The manufacture of forest products is a major industry in the United States and Canada. In 1990 the Canadian forest industry was directly responsible for 275,000 jobs, and the corresponding figure for the United States was about 400,000.[3] The total number of workers employed in forest products industries in North America is difficult to estimate because of the diversity of these industries.

FOREST PRODUCTS INDUSTRIES

After timber is harvested by cutting, bucking, and sawing from the woods or timberlands, it is transported to wood products plants or chemical products plants.

There are thousands of forest products, but most can be classified into one of two main groups, wood products or chemical products. Wood products are made directly from wood, whereas chemical products are manufactured by breaking down wood cells through chemical processes.

Other forest products are derived from the bark, fruit, gum, leaves, and saps of trees. It has been estimated that each person in the United States uses enough forest products yearly to make a tree 100 feet tall and 16 inches in diameter.[4] Forest products are shown in Fig. 37-1.

Wood products

Woods are generally classified as hardwood or softwood, depending on the kind of tree. Softwood trees stay green throughout the year. Hardwood trees lose their leaves every autumn. This classification does not indicate the hardness of the wood. Most softwoods can be sawed, planed, or bored easily and are chiefly for structural use. Such woods include cedar, Douglas fir, hemlock, and pine. Hardwoods have beautiful grain patterns and are widely used for floors, furniture, and paneling. Such woods include birch, maple, oak, walnut, and mahogany.

Other types of wood products are plywood, veneers, particle boards, hardboards, and insulation boards. Plywood consists of thin layers of wood glued together in such a way that the grain pattern of each layer is at right angle to the next one. This arrangement gives plywood several advantages over lumber. It shrinks, swells, and warps less and can be nailed near the edges without splitting. Hardwood veneers can be glued to softwood lumber combining the advantages of both types of wood. Plywood and veneers are used widely in the construction and furniture industries. Particle board is made from small pieces of wood left over in sawmills and paper mills. These small pieces are mixed with an adhesive and pressed into a board. Most particle boards are covered with veneers for furniture and cabinet making. Hardboards are harder than solid wood and are used in making furniture and cabinets. Hardboards are made by exploding chips of wood into fibers which are then matted, dried, and compressed into a board.

Chemical products

Wood cells consist of cellulose, lignin, and hemicellulose. Cellulose gives wood its strength and structure, whereas lignin holds the fibers together. Paper, films, plastics, and fibers such as rayon and acetate, are made from cellulose. These products do not look or feel like wood.

To make paper, wood chips are "cooked" in various chemical solutions to form a pulp. The pulp is washed and passed through a series of screens to remove unwanted materials. It is then bleached, washed, and matted into a sheet. A machine squeezes the sheet between rollers and dries it to form paper or paperboard.

Fibers and films are made from wood by treating sheets of cellulose with chemical solutions that turn it into a thick liquid. The liquid is forced through tiny holes or slits and is treated with chemicals to make specific fibers and films. Plastics are made by combining cellulose with chemicals such as acetate and acetate butyrate. These compounds are molded into simple shapes that are then made into various plastic products, such as toys.

EXPOSURES IN DIFFERENT FOREST PRODUCTS INDUSTRIES

Wood dust. Workers are exposed to different types of wood dust in the "primary" industries such as sawmills, planer mills, and shake and shingle mills. However, many workers are employed in "secondary" industries such as cabinet and furniture factories, carpentry, construction trades, wood carving, jewelry and musical instrument making, and teaching of woodworking trades. Individuals can also be exposed to wood dust while pursuing hobbies.

Living plants growing on bark. Loggers, wood cutters, and sawmill workers who are involved in debarking may be exposed to lichens, liverworts, and mosses growing on the surface of the bark. These plants produce chemical compounds such as sesquiterpene lactones, which are known to create sensitization.[5]

Molds growing in wood chips, sawdust, or bark. Many different types of molds grow on wood chips, bark, and sawdust. Wood trimmers, workers in woodrooms of pulpmills, and cork workers are exposed to these molds on their jobs.

Other chemical compounds used in industries. In wood products industries, chemicals are often used. In sawmills, chemicals are used to preserve wood particularly for those species that do not produce chemicals with fungicidal properties. The timber is either sprayed or dipped into a tank of wood preservative. Workers can be exposed to high concentrations of these chemicals, for example, pentachlophenates, which have been used extensively in sawmills for several years. In plywood, veneer, and particle board plants, workers are often exposed to urea formaldehyde and phenol formaldehyde that are found in adhesives and glues. In some plants that produce composition boards, strips of wood are adhered to each other by a resin that contains diphenyl methane diisocyanate (see Chapter 26).

In chemical product industries, workers are exposed to numerous chemicals. For example, in pulpmills, workers are exposed to chemicals such as sodium sulfide, sulfite and carbonate for the digestion of fibers, and bleaching agents.

Gases and fumes. Pulpmill workers are at risk for exposure to gases such as sulfur dioxide, hydrogen sulfide, methyl mercaptan, chlorine, and chlorine dioxide (see Chapter 30).

Hard metals. In sawmills, sawfilers are at risk for exposure to fumes containing hard metals (see Chapter 29). Although the bodies of saw blades used in the lumber industry are usually made of saw steel, the saw tips are made of a hard metal alloy that is welded or soldered to the saw blades. Stellite has been introduced, which has a higher concentration of cobalt and chromium than the tungsten carbide tips that have been used previously.

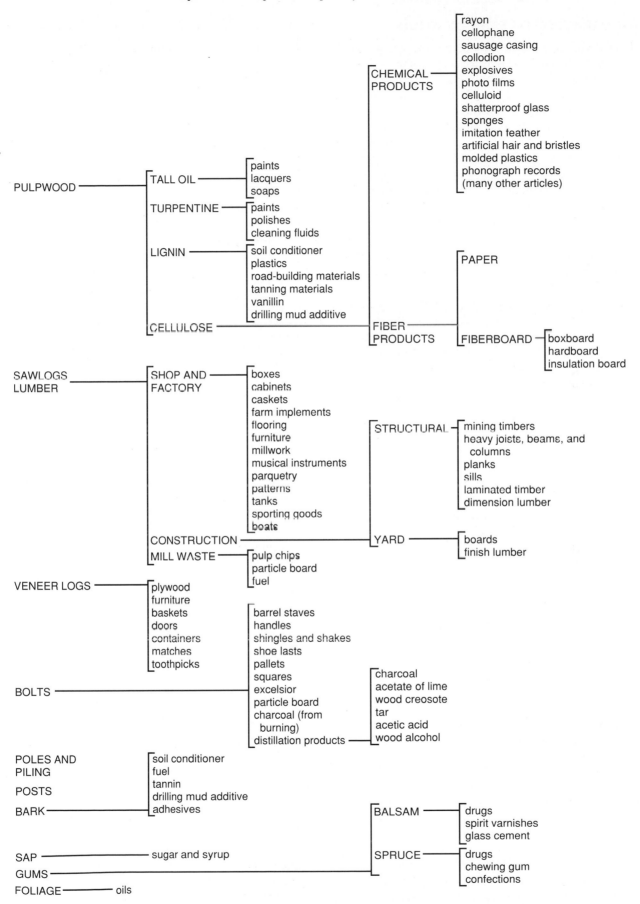

Fig. 37-1. Products that come from trees.

CHEMICAL CONSTITUENTS OF WOOD

About 20 wood species were found to be responsible for most of the health problems associated with wood-dust exposure.[6] Dust particles not only cause symptoms arising from mechanical irritation of skin and mucous membranes, but often induce sensitization, which yields to allergic contact dermatitis and asthma. Certain species of wood produce general symptoms such as headache, nausea, vomiting, and cardiac arrhythmia. The sensitization and toxic properties of wood dust are a result of the presence of many chemical compounds in the heartwood of trees. The compounds often protect the wood against fungi, bacteria, and insects. Some of the compounds are by-products of the biologic function of living trees, which are of no further use for the trees and are stored in the dead cells of the heartwood, giving the heartwood a different color. The quantity of chemicals may vary seasonally, with differing geographic location, and among different trees of the same species growing in the same area. The box on this page shows the chemical constituents of woods and their pharmacologic properties. The alkaloids, flavonoids, and glycosides are the properties that are responsible for the toxic symptoms and the systemic and cardiac effects. The benzoquinones and naphthoquinones and the phenolic compounds, including the catechols, are sensitizers in low concentrations and irritants in high concentrations. The majority of chemicals that act as sensitizers affect the skin more than the respiratory tract. For more information, refer to the excellent monograph by Hausen.[6]

RESPIRATORY DISEASES CAUSED BY EXPOSURES IN FOREST PRODUCTS INDUSTRIES

Many health hazards are associated with forest products industries. Skin diseases such as primary skin irritation, contact urticaria, and contact dermatitis are more common than respiratory diseases in these industries.[6] Vibration white finger syndrome is a common health problem among loggers and wood cutters. The actual prevalence and incidence of these diseases are not known. In this chapter, only respiratory diseases will be discussed.

Occupational asthma and rhinitis

Many types of wood dust have been implicated as causes of occupational asthma and rhinitis. The extent to which they are used in construction and in furniture industries is not known. A study of asthma mortality in Swedish men showed that it was significantly increased among wood-working machine operators with a smoking-adjusted standardized mortality ratio of 226 (95% confidence interval [CI] 108-344).[7]

Most of the cases of occupational asthma caused by wood dusts were published as case reports, with the exception of occupational asthma caused by the Western ce-

---

Wood constituents and their effects

Sensitizers

Benzoquinones and naphthoquinones
Phenols
Catechols
Sesquiterpene lactones
Stilbenes
Terpenes

Irritants

Anthraquinones
Minerals
Saponins

Toxic reaction, systemic effects, and cardiac symptoms

Alkaloids
Flavonoids
Glycosides

Adapted from Hausen B: Woods injurious to human health—a manual, Table 2, Berlin, 1981, Walter de Gruyter & Co., Publishers, Medical Department.

---

dar *(Thuja plicata),* which has been studied extensively in terms of the clinical picture, pathogenesis, outcome, prevalence, and risk factors. Western red cedar asthma will be discussed as an example.

Western red cedar *(Thuja plicata).* Western red cedar is an important wood species in the Pacific Northwest region of North America, particularly in the coastal areas. Cedar has been used extensively for poles, shakes, shingles, and lumber for exterior construction because of its known high durability. Red cedar asthma affects sawmill workers, shingle and shake mill workers, workers in remanufacturing plants, carpenters, construction workers, and cabinet makers.

Chemical composition of Western red cedar. Cedar wood extractive may be separated by steam distillation into volatile and nonvolatile fractions (see box on page 641).[8,9] The volatile fractions account for only 1% to 1.5% of the heartwood, whereas the nonvolatile fractions account for 5% to 15%. The volatile fractions contain at least nine compounds, some of which have interesting chemical properties. The tropolones, for example, are excellent natural fungicides and are likely to be responsible for the resistance of the wood against decay. The tropolones were found to have beta-adrenergic receptor-blocking properties.[10] Nezucone, an aromatic compound in red cedar, was found to produce an asthmatic reaction in an inhalation challenge test.[11] The significance of the tropolones and nezucone in the pathogenesis of red cedar asthma has yet to be determined in clinical studies. On the other hand, plicatic acid (PA), a nonvolatile compound, constitutes about 90% by weight of the nonvolatile components. It has a molecular weight of

Composition of Western red cedar extract

Volatile components

    Methyl thujate
    Thujic acid
    Tropolones
        β, Thujaplicinol
        γ, Thujaplicin
        β, Thujaplicin
        α, Thujaplicin
        β, Dolabrin
    Nazukone
    Carvacrol methyl ether

Nonvolatile components (water soluble)

    Phenolic fraction
        Plicatic acid
        Plicatin
        Thujaplicatin
        Thujaplicatin methyl ether
        Other lignans
    Nonphenolic fraction
        Pectic acid
        Starch
        Hemicellulose
        Arabinase
        Simple sugars

Adapted from Barton GM and MacDonald BF: The chemistry of utilization of Western red cedar. Publication No. 1023, Department of Fisheries and Forestry, 1971, Ottawa Department of Forestry.

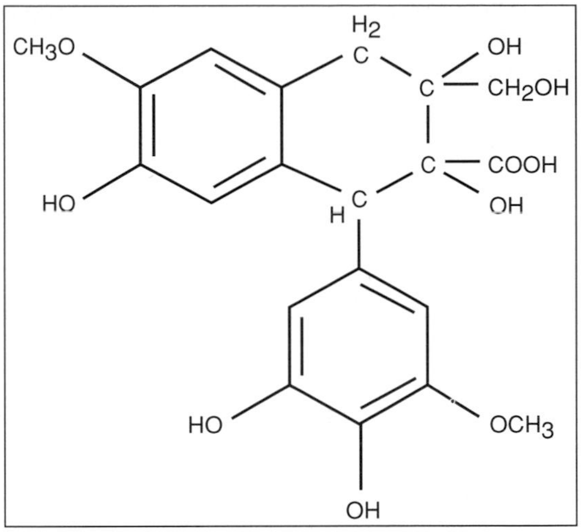

Fig. 37-2. Structural formula of plicatic acid.

440 daltons; the structural formula is shown in Fig. 37-2. PA is the primary chemical compound causing red cedar asthma.[12]

Clinical picture. The clinical picture of patients with red cedar asthma is characteristic. Many patients have worked with other wood dusts without respiratory symptoms. After a period of steady exposure to Western red cedar, usually between 6 weeks to 3 years, but sometimes as long as 10 years, patients develop cough, chest tightness, and wheeze. About half of the patients also have rhinitis. Some patients experience rhinorrhea several weeks before the onset of respiratory symptoms. In the majority of patients, respiratory symptoms occur initially after work and at night, waking them with cough and wheeze. Later, cough, wheeze, and dyspnea occur during the day, and the nocturnal symptoms become more distressing. The symptoms improve during weekends and holidays initially; with continued exposure the symptoms become persistent with no remission. At that stage, many patients complain of cough and wheeze immediately on exposure.

The characteristics of patients with red cedar asthma have been studied by Chan-Yeung et al.[12,13] The affected subjects are mostly nonatopic subjects and nonsmokers. These features are different than those in patients with asthma caused by high molecular weight (HMW) agents,

in whom atopy and smoking are probably important predisposing host factors.

Inhalation challenge tests with an extract of Western red cedar or PA induce three main types of asthmatic reaction: isolated immediate, isolated late, and biphasic or continuous asthmatic reaction. Systemic or alveolar reaction has not been observed. Unlike occupational asthma caused by HMW compounds, the proportion of patients with late asthmatic reaction is high (89.2%), manifested either as isolated late or part of the biphasic or continuous reaction. While the usual timing of the onset of late asthmatic reaction is 4 to 6 hours after inhalation challenge, it can be as early as 2 hours or as late as 12 hours. Some patients develop asthmatic reaction immediately after challenge and do not recover in the usual 1 to 2 hour period before the development of the late asthmatic reaction. These atypical reactions have been described by Perrin et al.[14] The lung function tests show airflow obstruction immediately after challenge, which persists for more than 24 hours. Recurrent nocturnal asthma lasting several nights after one single inhalation challenge test has been documented.[15]

Diagnosis. As with other types of occupational asthma, the diagnosis of red cedar asthma is based on a combination of history taking and objective evidence showing that exposure to red cedar dust causes acute respiratory symptoms and lung function changes. In general, any individual who is exposed to red cedar dust in the workplace or in the pursuit of a hobby and who develops asthma, should be suspected of suffering from red cedar asthma.

Skin tests and immunologic tests are not helpful in confirming the diagnosis of red cedar asthma. Both crude red cedar extract and PA or PA–human serum albumin (PA–HSA) conjugate failed to produce reactions on skin testing. Specific IgE antibodies to PA–HSA conjugate were detected in only 30% of the red cedar asthma patients who were diagnosed by inhalation challenge test[16] and they were also detected in 6% of exposed workers without respiratory symptoms.[16]

Prolonged recording of peak expiratory flow rate (PEFR) every 2 hours during waking hours for 2 weeks at work and 1 week away from work has been proven by Côté et al.[17] to be both sensitive and specific in the diagnosis of red cedar asthma when compared with the results of the specific challenge test with PA. Although serial measurements of nonspecific bronchial hyperresponsiveness (NSBH) have been used effectively together with prolonged recording of PEFR in the diagnosis of other types of occupational asthma, Côté et al.[17] did not find that the addition of serial measurements of NSBH improves the sensitivity and specificity of PEFR recording.

Specific challenge tests can be performed either by using fine red cedar dust or by using a crude extract of red cedar dust or plicatic acid. The exposure test with fine red cedar dust can be performed using the simple method described by Pepys and Hutchcroft[18] by pouring the dust from one container to another or by a more sophisticated method that allows for controlling the concentration and the size of particles, as described by Cloutier et al.[19] This type of exposure test has proven useful in confirming the diagnosis of red cedar asthma. The specific challenge test can also be performed by aerosolization of the crude red cedar extract or with PA.[12] At present plicatic acid is not available commercially.

Outcome of patients with red cedar asthma. The majority of patients with red cedar asthma failed to recover several years after they left exposure. A follow-up study was conducted on 232 patients at an average period of 4 years after the diagnosis was made.[13] Of the 136 patients who left the industry and were no longer exposed to red cedar dust, only 55 (40.4%) recovered completely, whereas the remaining 81 (59.6%) continued to experience attacks of asthma of varying severity. The mean lung function results at the time of diagnosis and the degree of NSBH as reflected by the mean PC_{20}, were significantly higher among the asymptomatic group as compared with the symptomatic group. These findings suggest that the patients in the asymptomatic group were diagnosed at an earlier stage of the disease. This observation was confirmed by the significantly shorter duration of symptoms before diagnosis among asymptomatic patients as compared with symptomatic patients. Race, smoking status, immediate skin reactivity, and the presence of specific IgE antibodies did not influence the outcome of the disease.

Of the 96 patients who continued to work with red cedar, 47 were exposed daily, whereas 41 were exposed intermittently. They all had respiratory symptoms and required medication. Both groups of patients demonstrated a reduction in forced expiratory volume in 1 second (FEV1) and forced vital capacity (FVC) and an increase in NSBH upon follow-up examination, although the differences failed to reach the level of statistical significance.[13]

The results of the follow-up study emphasize the importance of early diagnosis and early removal from exposure in the management of patients with red cedar asthma. Removal from exposure should be complete since partial removal did not prevent the deterioration of symptoms and lung function.

Pathogenesis. Red cedar asthma is a prototype of asthma caused by exposure to a low molecular weight (LMW) compound, PA. The pathogenetic mechanism is not entirely clear. The clinical feature of red cedar asthma is one of an allergic disease. Red cedar asthma affects only a small proportion of exposed workers[20]; a small amount of exposure can trigger a severe attack of asthma in sensitive subjects, and there is a latent period between the onset of exposure and the onset of symptoms. However, investigations have failed to distinguish specific immunologic mechanism(s) that is (are) responsible for the onset of symptoms.

Inhalation challenge tests result in PA-induced late asthmatic reaction, either alone or as a component of biphasic asthmatic reaction preceded by an immediate component. It is now generally recognized that specific IgE antibodies mediate both immediate and late asthmatic reaction in asthma caused by HMW allergens. However, skin tests with extract of Western red cedar, PA, and PA–HSA conjugate did not produce immediate wheal and flare reaction in patients and controls.[12] Specific IgE antibodies were found in only 30% of the patients with proven red cedar asthma.[17]

Lam et al.[21] examined the sequence of cellular and protein changes after late asthmatic reaction induced by PA acid in patients with red cedar asthma by bronchoalveolar lavage; the results were compared with healthy subjects. The late asthmatic reaction was associated with an increase in eosinophils and albumin in the lavage fluid and was associated with an increase in the sloughing of bronchial epithelial cells. Although there was a slight increase in neutrophils 48 hours after challenge, neutrophil infiltration was not a prominent feature earlier. Multiple bronchial biopsies were carried out in three of the patients 24 hours after inhalation challenge. The major findings were denudation of the bronchial epithelium, a thickened basement membrane, and infiltration of eosinophils in the bronchial epithelium and submucosa. The occurrence of these inflammatory changes was associated with the development of NSBH. Inflammatory mediators, predominantly histamine, and LTE_4 were found in the bronchoalveolar lavage fluid during the immediate asthmatic reaction induced by PA challenge.[22] The findings of airway inflammation and increase in NSBH during the late asthmatic reaction and the release of inflammatory mediators during immediate bronchoconstriction, are similar to patients with asthma induced by HMW allergens.

Immunologic mechanisms other than the Type I allergic reaction may be responsible for the onset of asthma. Frew et al.[23] reported the stimulation of lymphocytes in patients with red cedar asthma by PA or PA–HSA, as demonstrated by increased thymidine uptake. Moreover, staining of the bronchial mucosa in these patients showed an increase in activated T lymphocytes, suggesting that lymphocytes play a role in the pathogenesis of the disease.[24]

Prevalence. Table 37-1 shows the prevalence of occupational asthma in workers exposed to red cedar dust in different studies.[20,25-27] Ishizaki et al.[25] described asthma in 3.4% of the 1321 furniture factory workers exposed to red cedar dust in Japan. Brooks et al.[26] reported a higher prevalence (13.5%) of work-related asthma among shake mill workers. In 1978, Chan-Yeung et al.[20] reported the prevalence of red cedar asthma in workers in four cedar sawmills was 1.6% and the rate in former cedar mill workers was 4%. In a later cross-sectional study[27] on 652 workers in another cedar sawmill, Chan-Yeung et al. found a prevalence of 4.1% as compared with 1.6% in office workers. A close relationship exists between the prevalence of work-related asthma and the level of dust exposure; the higher the dust concentration, the higher the prevalence of work-related asthma.[26,28] The higher prevalence of work-related asthma, shown in the study by Brooks et al.,[26] is caused by the higher dust levels encountered in the shake mills.

Chan-Yeung et al.[29] examined the workers in their study annually for 3 years after the initial study and again after 6 years. The prevalence of red cedar asthma, defined as specific responsiveness to PA, was 1.68%. During the subsequent 6 years, six workers developed red cedar asthma at a rate of one worker per year, which is an incidence of 0.3% per year. The level of exposure in this sawmill was low, with few personal samples above 2 mg/m^3. In this study, the researchers were unable to demonstrate that NSBH is a predisposing host factor.

Occupational asthma caused by other wood dusts

Most cases in the literature of occupational asthma caused by other wood dusts were published as case reports (Table 37-2). The diagnoses were made by inhalation challenge test or by history and positive skin test reaction to the appropriate extracts of wood dust.

Aqueous extracts of some wood dust such as Abirucana,[31] African maple wood,[32] African zebrawood,[33] Kejaat wood,[34] mahogany,[35] and Quillaja bark[36] produced immediate wheal and flare reaction on skin testing in sensitive subjects. In some patients specific IgE antibodies were demonstrated in the sera using the radioallergosorbent test (RAST) method. In these patients, the type I allergic reaction is likely to be responsible for the asthma reaction. However aqueous extracts of other wood dusts such as California red wood,[37] Cedar of Lebanon,[38] Central American walnut,[39] Cocabolla,[40] Eastern white cedar,[41] and Iroko[42,43] failed to yield positive immediate skin reaction or specific IgE antibodies; precipitating antibodies were not detected in the sera of affected subjects. The pathogenetic mechanism of asthma induced by these wood dusts is likely to be similar to red cedar asthma. One or several of the chemical compounds present in these trees may be the causative agent(s).

Malo et al.[44] described 11 individuals with work-related asthma from 10 different sawmills of northwestern and southwestern Quebec and northern Maine where coniferous trees such as spruces, firs, and pines are cut into boards. Although the causative agent is not identified in each case, the study illustrates that many cases of occupational asthma caused by wood dust exposure are not recognized.

The prevalence of occupational asthma caused by wood dust exposure is not known. A study was conducted on furniture workers exposed to rimu, Dacrydium cupressinum, in Wellington, New Zealand.[45] About 10% of workers had a history compatible with work-related asthma confirmed by appropriate changes in the PEFR recording. Nouaigui et al.[46] reported 5.6% of 197 woodworkers in four plants in Tunisia had asthma. The type of wood the workers were exposed to was not documented in the report.

Occupational asthma caused by other agents present or used in the forest products industries

Woodworkers can also be sensitized to other living organisms growing on the wood, such as molds, and can develop asthma. Côté et al.[47] reported a case of occupational asthma in a plywood factory worker caused by a mold of Neurospora species growing on the wood in wet conditions. This worker had a positive skin reaction and bronchial reaction to challenge with an extract of the mold and the wood dust extract.

A number of chemicals encountered in the forest products industries can cause occupational asthma (see Chapter 26). Examples of these chemicals include phenol formaldehyde and urea formaldehyde[48] in the plywood plants, and chromium and cobalt exposure[49] among sawfilers in sawmills.

Irritant-induced asthma

Reactive airways dysfunction syndrome (RADS) or irritant-induced asthma was first described by Brooks et al.[50] in 10 subjects who developed cough, wheeze, and shortness of breath either immediately or within a few hours of a single exposure to high levels of irritant vapors, gas, fumes, or smoke. None of the subjects had any previous history of respiratory disease. Since this report was published there have been many reports of irritant-induced asthma caused by exposure to high concentrations of a variety of different chemicals, gases, and fumes.[51-60] In several instances, the subjects had multiple exposures rather than a single exposure.[51,54]

Workers in pulpmills, particularly maintenance workers and those working in bleach plants, and construction workers at pulpmill sites are at risk for repeated "gassings." Kennedy et al.[61] have shown that these workers who were at risk for repeated gassing had a higher prevalence of

Table 37-1. Epidemiologic studies of workers exposed to Western red cedar

Year	Site	Type of industries	Subjects	Age (mean or range)	Smoker (%)	Chronic cough (%)	Chronic phlegm (%)	Wheeze (%)	Work-related asthma (%)	Lung function FEV1	Lung function FVC	Dust concentration (mg/m³ or range)	Reference
1973	Japan	Furniture	1797	17-60	NA	NA	NA	NA	3.4%	NA	NA	NA	25
1978	Vancouver, British Columbia	Cedar sawmill	405	36.8	53.8	27.4	30.4	13.1	1.1	101%*	98.5%*	NA	20
		Former cedar mill	65	45.9	57.0	23.1	29.7	6.2	4.9			NA	
		Other wood dust	187	42.1	48.7	18.2	17.1	8.6	0	104%*	103.4%*		
1981	Washington State, United States	Cedar	74	NA	NA	20.2†			13.5	Cross-shift decrease in FEV1 greater in WRC workers		4.7 ± 7.45	26
		Other wood dust	58	NA	NA	26.4			5.2			1.3 ± 3.10	
		No wood dust	22	NA	NA	9.0			0			NA	
1984	Vancouver, British Columbia	Cedar sawmill	511‡	44 ± 14	38.2	16.9	16.4	14.7	4.1	−206 ml§	−163 ml§	0-6	27
		Office	394‡	43 ± 12	30.7	8.9‖	12.0‖	12.7	1.6‖				

*Nonsmokers only.
†Chronic bronchitis (%).
‡White males only.
§Effect of cedar dust exposure versus no exposure adjusted for age, height, and smoking differences.
‖Differences between cedar sawmill and office workers statistically significant $p < 0.05$.
FEV1, Forced expiratory volume in 1 second; *FVC*, forced vital capacity; *NA*, not available; *WRC*, Western red cedar.

Table 37-2. Wood dusts causing occupational asthma

| Species name | Common name | Number of subject | Diagnostic test | | | | Reference |
			Inhalation	Skin test	Serology	Other features	
Balfourodendron riedelianum	Pau marfim	1	Immediate	Negative	Positive RAST	—	30
Caesalpinia echinata	Fernam bouc	12	Immediate in one	Negative	NA	—	101
Cedra libani	Cedar of Lebanon	6	NA	Negative in five / Positive in one	Negative ppt	—	38
Chlorophora excelsa	Iroko	1	Late	Positive immediate	Negative ppt	—	42, 43
Cinnamomum zeylanicum	Cinnamon bark	9/40	NA	NA	NA	—	102
Dalbergia nigra	Palisander	1	Late	Positive immediate	NA	—	103
Dalbergia retusa	Cocobolla	3	NA	Positive immediate / Positive patch test	NA	Responded to hyposensitization	40
Diospyros crassiflora	Ebony	1	Late	Negative	NA	—	104
Fraxinus americana specific IgE	Ash wood	1	Immediate	Negative	Negative	—	105
Gonystyllus bacanus	Ramin	1	Late	Negative	Negative ppt	Decrease diffusing capacity on challenge	106
Juglans olanchana	Central American walnut	1	Biphasic	Negative	Negative ppt / Negative RAST	—	39
Microberlinia	African zebra	1	Biphasic	Positive immediate	Negative ppt	↑ Leukocytes, ↑ neutrophils on challenge	33
Myrocarpus fastigiatus	Cabreuva	1	Late and systemic	NA	NA		107
Nesorgordonia papaverifera	Kotibe	1	Late	NA	NA	—	108
Pouteria	Abirucana	2	NA	Positive immediate	Negative ppt	—	31
Pterocarpus angolensis	Kejaat	1	NA	Positive immediate	NA	Responded to hyposensitization	34
Sequoia sempervirens	California redwood	2	Biphasic	Negative	Negative ppt	—	37
Tanganyike aningre	—	3	Immediate	Positive immediate	Negative ppt	—	109
Thuja occidentalis	Eastern white cedar	1	Late	NA	Negative specific IgE	Plicatic acid present in extract of wood	41
Thuja plicata	Western red cedar	(see text)	Biphasic immediate	Negative	Positive RAST in 30%	—	110–113
Triplochiton scleroxylon	Obeche or African maple	2	Immediate	Positive immediate	Positive specific IgE	—	32
NA	Mahogony	1	Late	Negative	Positive ppt	—	35
NA	Oak	1	Immediate	Negative	Positive ppt	—	35
NA	Quillaja bark	1	Immediate	NA	Positive	—	36

NA, not available; *ppt*, precipitins; *RAST*, Radioallergosorbent test.

wheezing and lower lung function as compared to unexposed workers. A subsequent study of first-aid records from the company confirmed that those with gassing episodes, who required first aid treatment, had lower lung function and a more rapid lung function decline than those without such episodes.[62] This observation has been substantiated by other investigators.[63,64] Bherer et al.[65] studied a group of 71 construction workers in Quebec who were repeatedly exposed to chlorine over a 3 to 6 month period in pulpmills and found that 23% of those in the moderate and high-risk groups had evidence of bronchial obstruction and 41% in the same group had NSBH 18 to 24 months after exposure had ended.

Cases of asthma have been reported after recurrent "gassing" episodes by Chan-Yeung et al.[66] The histologic findings in the bronchial biopsies performed on these patients were similar to the findings for patients with allergic asthma and red cedar asthma, with the exception that there were few T lymphocytes. However, the study by Gautrin et al.[67] showed that patients with RADS had considerable subepithelial fibrosis on bronchial biopsies and less airway reversibility to an inhaled beta-2 adrenergic agent than those with occupational asthma with a latency period.

There is still a great deal to be learned about RADS or irritant-induced asthma with regard to the pathogenesis, predisposing host factors, and the natural history of the disease.

Hypersensitivity pneumonitis

Hypersensitivity pneumonitis often affects sawmill trimmers and pulp and papermill workers in the woodroom and sometimes affects farmers who handle wood chips (Table 37-3). The antigens responsible for these diseases are often not the wood dust themselves, but the molds growing in the wood dust or on the bark of the wood, such as *Cryptostroma corticale* in maple bark disease,[68,70] *Penicillium frequentans* in suberosis,[71] graphium and pullularia on redwood bark in sequoisis,[72] *Alternaria* in woodmills,[73] *Aspergillus* and *Thermoactinomyces vulgaris* in moldy wood chips,[74,75] and rhizopus or paecilomyces in wood trimmers disease in Sweden.[76-78] Of the different types of hypersensitivity pneumonitis, maple bark disease and wood trimmer's disease have been better investigated than the others. Maple bark disease was first described in 1932 by Towey et al.[68] and later by Emanuel et al.[69,70] in workers in the woodrooms of paper mills. The workers were involved in peeling bark from maple logs infected with fungal spores, which were identified as *Cryptostroma corticale*. The patients presented with fever, night sweats, cough, and shortness of breath. Chest radiographs showed diffuse parenchymal infiltrations. The histologic features of lung biopsy performed on these patients were compatible with those of hypersensitivity pneumonitis with granulomata, multinucleated giant cells, histocytes, and mononuclear cell infiltration affecting the alveolar wall and bronchiolar wall.

High levels of precipitating antibodies against the extracts of this fungus were found in the sera of these patients. A study of 37 men employed in a papermill was carried out over a period of 2½ years.[79] Five men were found to have active maple bark disease, nine had subclinical disease, and four had positive serologic test. Dust concentration in the woodroom was high, and a high percentage of the dust consisted of mold spores. The introduction of dust control measures led to a reduction in the spore count and a reduction in the incidence of maple bark disease.[79]

Wood trimmers' disease was described among sawmill workers in Sweden in the late 1960s when conventional outdoor wood drying during the summer was changed to artificial indoor wood drying in special kilns.[76] Spores of the molds Rhizopus and Paecilomyces, which grew on the wood when it was wet, were found in high concentrations in the sawmills.[77] A survey from 1976 to 1978 revealed that in 10 out of 17 Swedish sawmills employing 280 workers, about 50% of the wood trimmers had antibodies precipitating primarily to the Rhizopus antigens, whereas 10% to 20% had suffered symptoms compatible with hypersensitivity pneumonitis.[77] The level of exposure to Rhizopus was found to be high in affected workers ($>10^7$ cfu/m^3).[78] Hedenstierna et al.[80] measured lung function on 66 wood trimmers after a month of no exposure and then 3 months and 27 months later. In comparison with a nonexposed group, wood trimmers had lower FVC even after 1 month of no exposure. There was a further reduction in FVC after 3 months of work and it remained at that level 27 months later. The reduction in FVC was more obvious at the sawmills that had higher air concentrations of organic dust than at other sawmills. The authors concluded that wood trimmers may develop restrictive pulmonary dysfunction, which could be the result of heavy mold exposure. In British Columbia, six cases of hypersensitivity pneumonitis have been observed from the inland sawmills where spruce, pine, fir, and hemlock are being processed. In three cases, precipitating antibodies were found in the sera against *Aspergillus fumigatus* and *Thermoactinomyces vulgaris*.[75]

In other cases, antibodies to extracts of wood dust were found that indicate that certain wood dusts also contain antigens capable of inducing hypersensitivity pneumonitis.[81] However, it is difficult to exclude fungi as an etiologic agent in this study. Hypersensitivity pneumonitis-like reactions have also been reported among workers exposed to diphenylmethane diisocyanate in wood chip board workers.[82]

Chronic bronchitis with and without airflow obstruction

Exposure to wood dust causes not only bronchial asthma in a proportion of workers but an increased prevalence of chronic cough and phlegm production (Tables 37-1 and 37-4). There is controversy about whether chronic airflow limi

Table 37-3. Hypersensitivity pneumonitis in woodworkers

Species name	Common name	Exposure or job	Number of subjects	Causal agent	X-ray	Lung function	Biopsy	Serology	Inhalation	Others	Reference
								Diagnostic tests			
NA	Maple	Woodroom pulpmill	5	Cryptostroma corticale	Diffuse infiltrate	↓VC	Chronic interstitial pneumonitis *C. corticale*, spores +	ND	ND	—	68-70
NA	Cork	Cork factory	20/63	Penicillium frequentans	Fine mottling	↓VC	Granulomata in 7/7	Positive ppt to *P. frequentans* in 13/16	Positive in 4/5 (late asthmatic and alveolar)	—	71
Sequoia sempervirens	Redwood	Sawyer	1	Graphium pullularia	Diffuse haziness	↓VC, TLC O₂ desaturation with exercise	Granuloma multinucleated histocytes	Positive ppt to graphium and pullularia	ND	—	72
NA	NA	Woodroom papermill	2	Alternaria	Localized infiltrate	↓VC, TLC and DLCO	Chronic interstitial pneumonitis	Positive ppt to alternaria in 2	ND	—	73
Populus tiemuloides	Aspen	Woodroom pulpmill	40	Thermophilic actinomycetes	Diffuse infiltrate	↓DLCO in 2	ND	Positive ppt to *M. faeni* in 5 positive ppt to *T. vulgaris* in 1	ND	—	74
NA	Spruce, pine	Wood trimmers	60	Rhizopus microsporus Paecilomyces vaviotti	ND	ND	ND	IgG antibodies to *R. microsporus P. vaviotti*	ND	Correlation between airborne spore levels and IgE levels	76,77
Gonyctylus bancanus	Ramin	Woodworkers	1	Ramin dust	Normal	↓DLCO	ND	ND	Positive (alveolar)	—	80

NA, Not available; *ND*, not done; *ppt*, precipitin; *TLC*, total lung capacity; *VC*, vital capacity.

Table 37-4. Epidemiologic studies of workers exposed to other wood dusts

Year	Site	Type of facility	Wood dust	n	Age (years)	Smoker (%)	Chronic cough	Chronic phlegm	Wheeze	Asthma	Pulmonary function		Dust concentration (mg/m³)	Reference
											FEV1	FVC		
1980	Manchester, United Kingdom	Furniture factory	Different types	66	NA	NA	NA	NA	NA	NA	−80 ml*	−120 ml*	0.1-8.29	83
		Office		11	NA	NA	NA	NA	NA	NA	+10 ml	−20 ml		
1981	Vermont, United States	10 Woodworking comp.	Hardwoods	354	220 < 35, 126 > 35	49.7	NA	NA	NA	NA	106% 103%†	107% 102%†	L = 0-5 mg-yr/m‡	84
			Pine	220	145 < 35, 75 > 35	45.0	NA	NA	NA	NA	102% 96%	102% 100%	H = 10 + mg-yr/m‡	
1985	Toronto, Ontario	Cabinetmaker	Different types	50	45.3	70.9	29%	38%	NA	NA	92.8%‡	94.6%‡	1.8 ± 1.5 mg/m‡	85
			Not exposed	49	49.3	75.5	29%	20%	NA	NA	90.1%	96.3%		
1987	Turin, Italy	Furniture factories	Different types	15	47.9	12.2 pk/year	100%	100%	NA	NA	2.17 L§	3.71 L§	NA	86
			Different types	20	47.0	8.3 pk/year	NA	NA	NA	NA	2.90 L	3.99 L		
			Not exposed	53	47.8	12.4 pk/year	NA	NA	NA	100% BH	3.35 L	4.30 L		
1987	Wellington, New Zealand	Furniture	rimu (Dacrydium cupressinum)	44	33	36	30	30	25	10‖	NA	NA	1-25.4 mg/m‡	45
			Not exposed	38	33	32	5	16	9	0	NA	NA	3.6 mg/m	
1988	Tunisie	Sawmill	Different types	134	<20 years experience	54.5	NA	NA	NA	5.6%	94%¶	97%¶	10.7-11.7 mg/m‡	46
				63	>20 years experience	65.1					86%	90%		
1989	Lucknow, India	Sawmills	Sheesham (Dolbergia sissoo) Mango (Mangifera indica)	109	26.4	70.6	NA	NA	NA	NA	1.8%#	28.4%**		114
1992	Umtata, Transkei	Not exposed		88	28.7	42.0	NA	NA	NA	NA	2.2%#	0**		87
		Furniture factory	Pine	Men 77	34.9	0	5.5	15.2	10.3††	NA	90.4%††	93.2%††	NA	
				Women 68	32.3	0					94.5%††	97.9%		
			Fiberboard	Men 77	33.8	0	2.1	9.4	3.9		106.3%	103.4%		
		Bottling factory (not exposed)		Women 75	33.7	0					100.0%	100.9%		

*Preshift and postshift on Monday, furniture versus office workers statistically significant (p < 0.05).
†Nonsmokers only (low versus high exposure; L, low exposure; H, high exposure.
‡Exposed workers significantly lower than unexposed workers (p < 0.05).
§Adjusted for duration of exposure, age, and height; BH, bronchial hyperresponsiveness.
‖History and PEFR monitoring.
¶Adjusted for smoking, <20 years exposure significantly higher than >20 years exposure (p = 0.05).
#Obstruction versus defect.
**Restriction versus defect.
††Difference between exposed and unexposed statistically significant (p < 0.05).

FEV1, Forced expiratory volume in 1 second; *FVC*, forced vital capacity; *NA*, not available.

tation develops as a result of exposure to wood dust. Little information is available on this subject except for the case of Western red cedar workers.

Chan-Yeung et al.[20] reported that the prevalence of chronic cough and phlegm were significantly higher among cedar sawmill workers than among those breathing other types of wood dust such as hemlock and fir. Lung function tests were also lower among cedar workers as compared with workers exposed to other types of wood dust. In a later study, Chan-Yeung et al.[27] compared respiratory symptoms in cedar sawmill workers with office workers who had no exposure to wood dust. The odds ratios of cough and phlegm in cedar workers as compared with office workers were 2.18 and 1.44, respectively ($p > 0.001$ and 0.05, respectively, controlled for age and smoking). In addition, cedar workers had significantly lower lung function as compared with office workers after adjusting for differences in age, height, race, and smoking habits. The decrease in lung function was not caused by the increased prevalence of asthma in cedar mills since exclusion of these subjects from analysis failed to influence the results. The annual decline in lung function in cedar workers was also significantly greater than the control group,[81] suggesting that workers exposed to Western red cedar may have chronic airflow obstruction. Brooks et al.[26] also reported a higher prevalence of chronic cough and phlegm in shake mill (cedar) workers and in planer mill (noncedar) workers than in workers who were not exposed to wood dust. Lung function results were not presented.

There have been several epidemiologic studies of the respiratory health effects of exposure to wood dusts other than Western red cedar (Table 37-4). Furniture workers exposed to different types of wood dust had a significantly greater cross-shift fall in FEV1 than a group of unexposed workers.[83] Whitehead[84] conducted an epidemiologic study on 354 workers exposed to hardwood dust (mostly maple) and on 220 workers exposed to varying levels of softwood dust (pine). These workers did not have exposure to other industrial agents such as adhesives and finishing agents. Although an unexposed group was not studied as controls, workers in the category of high exposure to both hard wood and pine dust were associated with two to four times the prevalence of low PEFRs as compared with those who were exposed to lower levels of dust, irrespective of their smoking habits. These findings indicated that both hardwood and softwood exposure is associated with airflow obstruction. Holness et al.[85] studied 50 cabinet workers exposed to different types of wood dust and 50 controls. Woodworkers reported more cough, phlegm, and wheeze but their mean lung function did not differ significantly from the controls. Woodworkers, however, had a significant acute decline in lung function over a workshift. A positive correlation was found between baseline lung function and the degree of exposure. Paggiaro et al.[86] studied respiratory symptoms and lung function of 239 workers exposed to wood dust in a

furniture plant. Significantly higher prevalence rates of cough, phlegm, and wheeze in nonsmoking workers were found as compared to the control group derived from a population sample. Although mean lung function results were within normal limits, a lower FEV1% was found in subjects with more years of employment, which suggested a dose responsive relationship. Shamssain[87] demonstrated that exposure to pine and fiber board dust was associated with a higher prevalence of chest symptoms and lower lung function among furniture factory workers in Umtata, Republic of Transkei, as compared with a group of unexposed subjects.

The results of most of the previously mentioned studies have shown that exposure to different types of wood dust is associated with chronic respiratory symptoms and with some impairment of lung function as compared with those who are unexposed. A dose response relationship was observed between the level of exposure and the level of lung function in some studies, which indicates that this relationship was significant. Further studies on woodworkers with specific exposure to individual species of wood are necessary in order to delineate the respiratory effects of exposure.

Adenocarcinoma of nasopharynx

Prolonged exposure to wood dust has been associated with adenocarcinoma of the nasopharynx (see Chapter 35). This was first reported among furniture workers in the area around High Wycombe, England by Macbeth in 1965.[88] The proportion of these workers with adenocarcinoma of the nasopharynx was significantly higher than the rest of the population. This finding was confirmed among woodworkers in southern England by Hadfield.[89] Subsequent studies in Europe, the United States, and Australia have shown similar results.[6,90-94] In England and France, adenocarcinoma of the nasopharynx in woodworkers has become a prescribed disease.[6]

The latent periods between exposure and the development of adenocarcinoma of nasopharynx ranged from 28 to 45 years.[6] Affected workers' age was between 45 and 65 years. It has been postulated that particles of inhaled wood dust are trapped in the mucus and are not being carried away if there are no cilia to propel them. Any carcinogen in the wood dust has prolonged contact with the mucous membrane of the anterior turbinate of the ethmoid sinus. Possible carcinogens in wood dust include metabolites of molds and fungi, tar, tannins and tannic acids, and aldehydes.[6,95]

Lung cancer

Toren et al.[96] in a case-referent study of papermill workers in Sweden, reported an increase in mortality from lung cancer (odds ratio = 2.0) among the maintenance workers. Maintenance workers in Swedish paper and pulpmills were also found to have a higher mortality from malignant mesothelioma, which is probably because of exposure to asbestos.[97] There are other studies indicating an increased risk of lung cancer among paper and pulpmill workers.[98-100] The increase in lung cancer mortality in these maintenance workers is likely the result of exposure to asbestos.

PREVENTION OF RESPIRATORY DISEASES CAUSED BY WOOD DUST EXPOSURE

Primary prevention of respiratory diseases from wood dust lies in the reduction of exposure, as is the case for other types of inorganic or organic dust. The development of chronic obstructive lung disease or malignancy is dose-dependent. Even in respiratory diseases caused by sensitization, such as occupational asthma, a dose response relationship has been found between the prevalence of the disease and the level of dust exposure, as the case for red cedar dust.[26,27] Improved ventilation in the workplace is useful, particularly the institution of local exhaust ventilation, which may provide a more economic and effective means of reducing exposure. However, it may not be always effective, especially for workers who are sensitized to wood dust.

Another means of prevention exists in the evaluation of potential employees, at which time attempts are made to identify workers that are at high risk of developing occupational respiratory disease. In the case of occupational asthma caused by wood dust exposure, little is known about predisposing risk factors. When agents induce asthma through an IgE-dependent mechanism, atopy is a risk factor for sensitization. However, wood dust such as red cedar dust induces asthma through a non-IgE mechanism and atopy is not important.[12,13] There is also little evidence to suggest that NSBH predisposes to occupational asthma,[27] rather it is the result of the disease.[13] Even if a predisposing factor is known, protection of the worker from adverse health effects must be balanced with the worker's rights to employment.

After a worker has become sensitized to components of wood dust, he or she may develop asthmatic symptoms upon exposure to levels of dust below the permissible concentration. Removal from exposure is the treatment of choice. The use of personal protection may enable sensitized workers to return to work only in some circumstances. There are many types of respirators and it is beyond the scope of this chapter to review them (see chapter 58). The worker should be properly evaluated for the use of the most appropriate respirator and should be followed up regularly for assessment. The use of medications may be necessary in addition to the use of a protective device to prevent attacks of asthma. If there are deterioration in symptoms and lung function despite the above measures, the worker should be completely removed from exposure to prevent the occurrence of severe symptoms.

SUMMARY AND RESEARCH NEEDS

In this chapter, the respiratory effects of exposures encountered in the forest products industries were reviewed. Many wood dusts can lead to asthma and rhinitis by sensitization, by Type I allergic reaction, or by undetermined immunologic and nonimmunologic mechanisms. There are different chemicals in the forest products industries that can also lead to occupational asthma, particularly in the pulpmills. Exposure to gases such as chlorine in this setting has been shown to result in RADS or irritant-induced asthma. As with other types of occupational asthma in forestry industries, little is known about the pathogenesis, natural history, and prevalence of the disease. The dose response relationship between exposure and sensitization and asthma is unknown for the majority of agents. Hypersensitivity pneumonitis occurs often as a result of exposure to molds in the wood dust or bark of the trees. In North America, hypersensitivity pneumonitis in forest industries is uncommon as compared with Scandinavian countries. In many instances, the etiologic agent in hypersensitivity pneumonitis is unknown. Chronic bronchitis, with or without airflow obstruction unrelated to smoking, is common among exposed workers. However, epidemiologic studies relating to the chronic effect of wood dust exposure are scarce.

Although wood is extensively used worldwide in many different industries, respiratory health effects are generally poorly studied and poorly understood, as are the effects of exposure to other types of organic dusts. There is a considerable body of knowledge of various chemical constituents of different types of wood. Alternatively, the constituent responsible for asthmatic reactions is unknown for most cases of occupational asthma caused by wood dust exposure. Multidiscplinary research involving wood chemists, immunologists, and clinicians may be rewarding in our understanding of the pathogenesis of different respiratory diseases arising from wood dust exposure. Research into the health effects of exposure in forestry industries deserves more emphasis.

REFERENCES

1. FAO food and agriculture of the United Nations, 1981-1991, 1993, FAO Yearbook Forest Products.
2. Cibula EJ: Trends in timber supply and trade—an information review, London, 1980, HMSO.
3. Department of commerce IT administration, 1993, U.S. Industrial Outlook.
4. World Book Encyclopedia, vol 6, Toronto, 1988, World Book.
5. Mitchell JC, Fritig B, and Singh B: Allergic contact dermatitis from *Frullania* and compositae: the role of sesquiter pene lactones, *J Invest Dermatol* 54:233-237, 1970.
6. Hausen B: Woods injurious to human health—a manual, Berlin, 1981, Walter de Gruyter.
7. Torén K, Sèllsten G, and Jèrvholm B: Mortality from asthma, chronic obstructive pulmonary disease, respiratory system cancer, and stomach cancer among paper mill workers: a case-referent study, *Am J Ind Med* 19:729-737, 1991.

8. Gardner JA: Chemistry and utilization of Western red cedar. Department of Forestry Publication No. 1023, 1963, Ottawa Department of Forestry.

9. Barton GM and MacDonald BF: The chemistry of utilization of Western red cedar. Publication No. 1023, Department of Fisheries and Forestry, 1971, Ottawa Department of Forestry.

10. Belleau B and Burba J: Occupancy of adrenergic receptors and inhibition of catechol o-methyl transferase by toropolones, *J Med Chem* 6:755-759, 1963.

11. Shida T, Mimaki K, Sasaki N, Nakagawa Y, and Hattovi O: Western red cedar asthma: occurrance in Oume City, Tokyo and results of inhalation test using "nezucone" aromatic substance of Western red cedar, *Areugi Jap J Allergology* 20:915-921, 1971.

12. Chan-Yeung M, Barton G, MacLean L, and Grzybowski S: Occupational asthma and rhinitis due to Western red cedar (*Thuja plicata*), *Am Rev Respir Dis* 108:1094-1102, 1973.

13. Chan-Yeung M, MacLean L, and Paggiaro PL: Follow up study of 232 patients with occupational asthma caused by western red cedar (*Thuja plicata*), *J Allergy Clin Immunol* 79:792-796, 1987.

14. Perrin B, Cartier A, Ghezzo H, et al: Reassessment of the temporal patterns of bronchial obstruction after exposure to occupational sensitizing agents, *J Allergy Clin Immunol* 87:630-639, 1991.

15. Cockcroft DW, Cotton DJ, and Mink JT: Nonspecific bronchial hyperreactivity after exposure to Western red cedar, *Am Rev Respir Dis* 119:505-510, 1979.

16. Tse KS, Chan H, and Chan-Yeung M: Specific IgE antibodies in patients with occupational asthma due to western red cedar (*Thuja plicata*), *Clin Allergy* 12:249-258, 1982.

17. Côté J, Kennedy S, and Chan-Yeung M: Sensitivity and specificity of PC_{20} and peak expiratory flow rate in cedar asthma, *J Allergy Clin Immunol* 85:592-598, 1990.

18. Pepys J and Hutchcroft BJ: Bronchial provocation tests in etiologic diagnosis and analysis of asthma, *Am Rev Respir Dis* 112:829-859, 1975.

19. Cloutier Y, Lagier F, and Lemieux R: New methodolgy for specific inhalation challenges with occupational agents in powder form, *Eur Respir J* 2:769-777, 1989.

20. Chan-Yeung M, Ashley MJ, and Corey P: A respiratory survey of cedar mill workers. I. prevalence of symptoms and pulmonary function abnormalities, *J Occup Med* 20:323-327, 1978.

21. Lam S, LeRiche J, Phillips D, and Chan-Yeung M: Cellular and protein changes in bronchial lavage fluid after late asthmatic reaction in patients with red cedar asthma, *J Allergy Clin Immunol* 80:44-50, 1987.

22. Chan-Yeung M, Chan H, Salari H, and Lam S: Histamine and leukotrienes release in bronchial fluid during plicatic acid-induced bronchoconstriction, *J Allergy Clin Immunol* 84:762-768, 1989.

23. Frew AJ, Chan H, and Chan-Yeung M: Specificity of antigen-induced T cell proliferation in Western red cedar asthma, *J Allergy Clin Immunol* 91:A314, 1993.

24. Frew AJ, Chan H, Lam S, and Chan-Yeung M: Bronchial inflammation in occupational asthma due to Western red cedar, *Am J Resp Crit Care Med* (in press), 1995.

25. Ishizaka T, Shida T, Miyamoto T, et al: Occupational asthma from Western red cedar dust (*Thuja plicata*) in furniture factory workers, *J Occup Med* 15:580-585, 1973.

26. Brooks SM, Edwards JJ, Apol A, and Edwards FH: An epidemiologic study of workers exposed to Western red cedar and other wood dust, *Chest* 80(suppl):30-32, 1981.

27. Chan-Yeung M, Vedal S, Kus J, et al: Symptoms, pulmonary function, and bronchial hyperreactivity in Western red cedar workers compared with those in office workers, *Am Rev Respir Dis* 130:1038-1041, 1984.

28. Vedal S, Chan-Yeung M, Enarson D, et al: Symptoms and pulmonary function in Western red cedar workers related to duration of employment and dust exposure, *Arch Environ Health* 41:179-183, 1986.

29. Chan-Yeung M, Vedal S, and Kennedy SM: A longitudinal study of red cedar sawmill workers, *Am Rev Respir Dis* 141:A80, 1990.

30. Bascomba A, Burches E, Almodovar A, Rojas D, and Hemandez FD: Occupational rhinitis and asthma caused by inhalation of Balfourdendron riedelianum (Pau Marfim) wood dust, *Allergy* 46:316-318, 1991.

31. Booth BH, LeFoldt RH, and Moffitt EM: Wood dust hypersensitivity, *J Allergy Clin Immunol* 57:352-357, 1973.

32. Hinojosa M, Moneo I, Domingues J, et al: Asthma caused by African maple (*Triplochiton scleroxylon*) wood dust, *J Allergy Clin Immunol* 74:782-786, 1984.

33. Bush R, Yunginger JW, and Reed C: Asthma due to African zebrawood (*Microberlinia*) dust, *Am Rev Respir Dis* 227:601-604, 1978.

34. Ordman D: Wood dust as an inhalant allergen: bronchial asthma caused by Kejaat wood (*Pterocarpus angolensis*), *S Afr Med J* 23:973-975, 1949.

35. Sosman AJ, Schlueter DP, Fink JN, and Barboriak JJ: Hypersensitivity to wood dust, *N Engl J Med* 281:977-980, 1969.

36. Raghuprasad PD, Brooks SM, Litwin A, et al: Quillaja bark (soap bark) induced asthma, *J Allergy Clin Immunol* 65:285-287, 1980.

37. Chan-Yeung M and Abboud R: Occupational asthma due to California redwood (*Sequoia sempervirens*) dusts, *Am Rev Respir Dis* 114:1027-1031, 1976.

38. Greenberg M: Respiratory symptoms following brief exposure to Cedar of Lebanon (*Cedra Libani*) dust, *Clin Allergy* 2:219-224, 1972.

39. Bush RK and Clayton D: Asthma due to Central American walnut (*Juglans olanchana*) dust, *Clin Allergy* 13:389-394, 1983.

40. Eaton KK: Respiratory allergy to exotic wood dust, *Clin Allergy* 3:307-310, 1973.

41. Cartier A, Chan H, Malo J-L, et al: Occupational asthma caused by Eastern white cedar (*Thuja occidentalis*) with demonstration that plicatic acid is present in this wood and is the causative agent, *J Allergy Clin Immunol* 77:639-645, 1986.

42. Azofra J and Olaquibel JM. Occupational asthma caused by Iroko wood, *Allergy* 44:156-158, 1989.

43. Pickering CAC, Batten JL, and Pepys J: Asthma due to inhaled wood dusts. Western red cedar and Iroko, *Clinical Allergy* 2:213-218, 1972.

44. Malo JL, Cartier A, and Boulet LP: Occupational asthma in sawmills of Eastern Canada and United States, *J Allergy Clin Immunol* 78:392-398, 1986.

45. Norrish AE, Beasley R, Hodgkinson EJ, and Pearce N: A study of New Zealand wood workers: exposure to wood dust, respiratory symptoms, and suspected cases of occupational asthma, *N Z Med J* 105:185-187, 1992.

46. Nouaigui H, Gharbi R, M'Rizak N, et al: Etude transversale de la pathologie respiratoire hez les travailleurs du bois en Tunisie, *Arch Mal Prof* 49:69-75, 1988.

47. Côté J, Chan H, Brochu G, and Chan-Yeung M: Occupational asthma caused by exposure to neurospora in a plywood factory worker, *Br J Ind Med* 48:279-282, 1991.

48. Cockcroft DW, Hoeppner VH, and Dolovich J: Occupational asthma caused by cedar urea formaldehyde particle board, *Chest* 82:49-53, 1982.

49. Nemery B: Metal toxicity and the respiratory tract, *Eur Respir J* 3:202-219, 1990.

50. Brooks SM, Weiss MA, and Bernstein IL: Reactive airways dysfunction syndrome (RADS): persistent asthma syndrome after high level irritant exposures, *Chest* 88:376-384, 1985.

51. Boulet LP: Increases in airway responsiveness following acute exposure to respiratory irritants: reactive airway dysfunction syndrome or occupational asthma? *Chest* 94:476-481, 1988.

52. Flury KE, Dines DE, Rodarte JR, and Rodgers R: Airway obstruction due to inhalation of ammonia, *Mayo Clin Proc* 58:389-393, 1983.

53. Kern DG: Outbreak of the reactive airways dysfunction syndrome after a spill of glacial acetic acid, *Am Rev Respir Dis* 144:1058-1064, 1991.

54. Tarlo SM and Broder I: Irritant-induced occupational asthma, *Chest* 96:297-300, 1989.

55. Murphy D, Fairman R, Lapp NL, and Morgan WKC: Severe airways disease due to the inhalation of fumes from cleaning agents, *Chest* 69:372-376, 1976.

56. Porter JAH: Acute respiratory distress following formalin inhalation, *Lancet* 2:603-604, 1975.

57. Promisloff RA, Phan A, Lenchner GS, and Cichelli AV: Reactive airway dysfunction syndrome in three police officers following a roadside chemical spill, *Chest* 98:928-929, 1990.

58. Stenton SC, Kelly CA, Walters EH, and Hendricks DJ: Induction of bronchial hyperresponsiveness following smoke injury, *Br J Dis Chest* 82:436-438, 1988.

59. Wade JF and Newman LS: Diesel asthma: reactive airways disease following overexposure to locomotive exhaust, *J Occup Med* 35:149-154, 1993.

60. Brooks SM and Bernstein IL: Reactive airways dysfunction syndrome or irritant-induced asthma, In Bernstein IL, Chan-Yeung M, Malo JL, and Bernstein DI, editors: *Asthma in the workplace*, pp 533-550, New York, 1993, Marcel Dekker.

61. Kennedy SM, Enarson DA, Jannsen RG, and Chan-Yeung M: Lung health consequences of reported accidental chlorine gas exposures among pulpmill workers, *Am Rev Respir Dis* 143:74-79, 1991.

62. Salisbury DA, Enarson DA, Chan-Yeung M, and Kennedy SM: First-aid reports of acute chlorine gassing among pulpmill workers as predictors of lung health consequences, *Am J Ind Med* 20:71-81, 1991.

63. Henneberger PK, Ferris BG, and Sheehe PR: Accidental gassing incidents and the pulmonary function of pulpmill workers, *Am Rev Respir Dis* 148:63-67, 1993.

64. Courteau JP, Cushman R, Bouchard F, et al: A survey of construction workers repeatedly exposed to chlorine in a pulpmill over a 3-6 month period. I. Exposure and symptomatology, *Occup Environ Med* 51:219–225, 1994.

65. Bherer L, Cushman R, Courteau J-P, et al: A survey of construction workers repeatedly exposed to chlorine over a 3-6 month period in a pulpmill. II. follow-up of affected workers with questionnaire, spirometry, and assessment of bronchial responsiveness 18 to 24 months after exposure ended, *Occup Environ Med* 51:225–228, 1994.

66. Chan-Yeung M, Lam S, Kenndy SM, and Frew AJ: Persistent asthma after repeated exposure to high concentrations of gases in pulpmills, *Am J Respir Crit Care Med* 149:1676–1680, 1994.

67. Gautrin D, Boulet L-P, Boutet M, et al: Is reactive airways dysfunction syndrome (RADS) a variant of occupational asthma? *J Allergy Clin Immunol* 93:12–22, 1994.

68. Towey JW, Sweany HC, and Huraon WH: Severe bronchial asthma apparently due to fungus spores found in maple bark, *JAMA* 99:453-459, 1932.

69. Emanuel DA, Lawton BR, and Wenzel FJ: Pneumonitis due to Coniosporium corticale, *N Engl J Med* 266:333-337, 1962.

70. Emanuel DA, Wenzel FJ, and Lawton BR: Pneumonitis due to Cryptostroma corticale (maple-bark disease), *N Engl J Med* 274:1413-1418, 1977.

71. Pimentel JC and Avila R: Respiratory disease in cork workers (Suberosis), *Thorax* 28:409-423, 1973.

72. Cohen HI, Merigan TC, Kosek JC, and Eldridge F: Sequoiosis: a granulomatous pneumonitis associated with redwood sawdust inhalation, *Am J Med* 43:784-794, 1967.

73. Schlueter DP, Fink JN, and Hensley GT: Wood-pulp workers' disease: a hypersensitivity pneumonitis caused by Alternaria, *Ann Intern Med* 77:907-914, 1972.

74. Thiede WH, Banaszak EF, Fink JN, Unger GF, and Scanlon GT: Hypersensitivity studies in popple (aspen tree) peelers, *Chest* 67:405-407, 1975.

75. Enarson DA and Chan-Yeung M: Characterization of health effects of wood dust exposures, *Am J Ind Med* 17:33-38, 1990.

76. Belin L: Clinical and immunological data on "wood trimmer's disease" in Sweden, *Eur J Respir Dis* (suppl 107) 61:169-176, 1980.

77. Belin L: Health problems caused by actinomycetes and molds in the industrial environment, *Allergy* (suppl 40) 3:24-29, 1985.

78. Belin L: Sawmill alveolitis in Sweden, *Int Archs Allergy Appl Immunol* 82:440-443, 1987.

79. Wenzel FJ and Emanuel DA: The epidemiology of maple bark disease, *Arch Environ Health* 14:385-389, 1967.

80. Hedenstierna G, Alexandersson R, Belin L, Wimander K, and Rosen G: Lung function and Rhyzopus antibodies in wood trimmers: a cross-sectional and longitudinal study, *Int Arch Occup Environ Health* 58:167-177, 1986.

81. Howie AD, Boyd G, and Moran F: Pulmonary hypersensitivity to Ramin (Gonystylus bancanus), *Thorax* 31:585-587, 1976.

82. Vandenplas O, Malo J-L, Dugas M, et al: Hypersensitivity pneumonitis-like reaction among workers exposed to diphenylmethane diisocyanate (MDI), *Am Rev Respir Dis* 147:338-346, 1993.

83. Al Zuhair YS, Whitaker CJ, and Cinkotai FF: Ventilatory function in workers exposed to tea and wood dust, *Brit J Indust Med* 38:339-345, 1981.

84. Whitehead LW, Ashikaga T, and Vacek P: Pulmonary function status of workers exposed to hardwood or pine dust, *Am Ind Hyg Assoc J* 42:178-186, 1981.

85. Holness DL, Sass-Kortsak AM, Pilger CW, and Nethercott JR: Respiratory function and exposure effect relationships in wood dust-exposed and control workers, *J Occup Med* 27:501-506, 1985.

86. Paggiaro P, Vellutini M, Viegi G, et al: Indagine epidemiologica trasversale sui sintomi e la funzione respiratoria nei lavoratori di un mobilificio, *G Ital Med Lav* 8:145-148, 1986.

87. Shamssain MH: Pulmonary function and symptoms in workers exposed to wood dust, *Thorax* 47:84-87, 1992.

88. Macbeth P: Malignant disease of the paranasal sinuses, *J Laryng Otol* 79:592-612, 1965.

89. Hadfield EH: A study of adenocarcinoma of the paranasal sinuses in wood workers in the furniture industry, *Ann Royal Coll Surgeons* 46:301-319, 1970.

90. Acheson ED, Cowdell RH, and Rang E: Adenocarcinoma of the nasal cavity and sinuses in England and Wales, *Brit J Indust Med* 29:21-30, 1972.

91. Acheson ED, Cowdell RH, Hadfield E, and Macbeth RG: Nasal cancer in woodworkers in the furniture industry, *Brit J Med* i:587-596, 1968.

92. Andersen HC, Andersen I, and Solgaard J: Nasal cancers, symptoms and upper airway function in woodworkers, *Br J Indust Med* 34:201-207, 1977.

93. Ironside P and Matthews J: Adenocarcinoma of the nose and paranasal sinuses in woodworkers in the state of Victoria, Australia, *Cancer* 36:1115-1121, 1975.

94. Kauppinen TP, Partanen TJ, Nurminen MM, et al: Respiratory cancers and chemical exposures in the wood industry: a nested case-control study, *Br J Ind Med* 43:84-90, 1986.

95. Black A, Evans JC, Hadfield EH, et al: Impairment of nasal mucociliary clearance in woodworkers in the furniture industry, *Br J Ind Med* 31:10-17, 1974.

96. Toren K, Sallsten G, and Jarvholm B: Mortality from asthma, chronic obstructive pulmonary disease, respiratory system cancer, and stomach cancer among paper mill workers: a case-referent study, *Am J Ind Med* 19:729-737, 1991.

97. Jarvholm B, Malker H, Malker B, Ericksson J, and Sallsten G: Pleural mesotheliomas and asbestos exposure in the pulp and paper industries: a new risk group identified by linkage of official registers, *Am J Ind Med* 13:561-567, 1988.

98. Milham S and Demers R: Mortality among pulp and paper workers, *J Occup Med* 26:844-846, 1984.

99. Jappinen P, Hakulinen T, Pukkala E, Tola S, and Kurppa K: Cancer incidence of workers in the Finnish pulp and paper industry, *Scand J Work Environ Health* 13:197-202, 1987.

100. Solet D, Zoloth SR, Sullivan C, Jeweet J, and Michaels DM: Patterns of mortality in pulp and paper workers, *J Occup Med* 31:627-630, 1989.

101. Hausen B and Herrmann B: Bowmaker's disease: an occupational disease in the manufacture of bows for string instruments, *Deutsche Medizinische Wochenschrift* 115:169-173, 1990.

102. Uragoda CG: Asthma and other symptoms in cinnamon workers, *Brit J Ind Med* 41:224-227, 1984.

103. Godnic-Cvar J and Gomzi M: Case report of occupational asthma due to palisander wood dust and bronchoprovocation challenge by inhalation of pure wood dust from a capsile, *Am J Ind Med* 18:541-545, 1990.

104. Maestrelli P, Mercer G, and Dal Vecchio L: Occupational asthma due to ebony wood *(Diospyros crassiflora)* dust, *Ann Allergy* 59:347-349, 1987.

105. Malo J-L and Cartier A: Occupational asthma caused by exposure to ashwood dust *(Fraxinus americana)*, *Eur Resp Dis* 2:385-387, 1989.

106. Howie AD, Boyd G, and Moran F: Pulmonary hypersensitivity to Ramin *(Gonystylus bancanus)*, *Thorax* 31:585-587, 1976.

107. Innocenti A, Romeo R, and Mariano A: Asthma and systemic toxic reaction due to cabreuva (Myrocarpus fastigiatus Fr. All.) wood dust. *Med del Lavoro* 82:446-450, 1991.

108. Reques FG and Fernandez RP: Asthme professionel à un bois exotique. *Rev Mal Resp* 5:71-73, 1988.

109. Paggiaro PL, Cantalupi R, Filieri M, et al: Bronchial asthma due to inhaled wood dust: *Tanganyika aningre, Clin Allergy* 11:605-610, 1981.

110. Milne J and Gandevia B: Occupational asthma and rhinitis due to western (Canadian) red cedar *(Thuja plicata). Med J Aust* 2:741-744, 1969.

111. Gandevia B and Milne J: Occupational asthma and rhinitis due to western cedar *(Thuja plicata)* with special reference to bronchial reactivity, *Br J Ind Med* 27:235-244, 1970.

112. Blainey AD, Graham VA, Phillips MJ, and Davies RJ: Respiratory tract reactions to western red cedar, *Human Toxicology* 1:41-51, 1981.

113. Mue S. Ise T, Ono Y, and Akasaka K: A study of western red cedar induced asthma, *Ann Allergy* 34:296-304, 1975.

114. Rastogi SK, Gupta BN, Husain T, and Mathur N: Respiratory health effects from occupational exposure to wood dust in sawmills, *Am Ind Hyg Assoc J* 50:574-578, 1989.

Chapter 38

MINING

N. LeRoy Lapp

The purpose of this chapter is to familiarize the reader with the variety of underground and surface occupations in the mining industry. It will also provide an awareness of some of the substances, other than coal and silica dust, to which these miners may be exposed. This information will assist the physician in obtaining a more precise estimate of occupational exposures and understanding the relative energy expenditures required in various jobs. It is not intended to present a detailed discussion of the hazards of these exposures; this can be found in Chapters 23, 24, 30, 31, and 33. The descriptions of occupations in this chapter represent a compilation of several sources and the author's own knowledge gleaned from interviewing miners over the past nearly three decades.[1,2]

COAL MINING
Composition of coal

It is customary to classify coal into various ranks. The oldest, hardest, and highest rank coal is anthracite. This is followed by bituminous, subbituminous, and lignite, which is the softest and is only slightly harder than peat.[3,4] Anthracite coal was found almost exclusively in northeastern Pennsylvania. It is no longer economically feasible to mine anthracite coal in any appreciable quantities. Bituminous coal varies from the relatively soft coal that is mined in the Colorado and Utah plateau to the relatively hard subbituminous coal that is found in the central Pennsylvania region. Prevalence rates of pneumoconiosis in the United States appear to vary in proportion to the rank of coal mined.[4-6]

Coal mining operations

The conventional mining cycle involves five steps: (1) cutting, (2) drilling, (3) blasting, (4) loading and hauling, and (5) roof bolting and auxiliary services.[7] Before World War II the coal miner performed a majority of these tasks with little mechanical assistance. He was responsible for producing his allotted "16 tons" per day. This involved cutting a slot, generally at the bottom of the coal seam, with a giant saw to provide expansion during the shooting. A hand-held or mobile drill was used to drill a series of holes into the coal seam that permitted insertion of "black powder," or blasting charge, which fractured the seam. After an appropriate interval, during which the mine was cleared of the blast dust and fumes, the miner returned to load out the coal with a pick and shovel into a buggy or mine car. He was responsible to set his own posts to provide support for the roof under which he worked. This method of mining is used today in only a few small, nonunion mines.

The coal industry in the United States underwent extensive mechanization after World War II. The mining cycle was considerably shortened and production was markedly increased by the use of continuous mining. This type of mining combines the unit operations of cutting, drilling, blasting, and loading into one operation. The number of men employed in the industry fell from around 400,000 in 1948 to about 85,000 in 1964 as a result of mechanization.[3]

Room and pillar mining

Most coal mining in the United States, Great Britain, and the rest of Europe today is carried out by mechanical means. The traditional method of mining coal in the United States was, until the past 20 years, the room and pillar system (Fig. 38-1). This system involves driving a vertical shaft from the surface to the coal seam. Subsequently, a series of horizontal tunnels, or headings, are driven into the coal seam. These are then connected by lateral communicating tunnels. Extraction of the supporting coal pillars is undoubtedly the most hazardous occupation in the room and pillar method of coal mining. As the coal mining proceeds, some large pillars of coal are then left to support the rock strata above the mine and presumably avoid subsidence of the surface. This means of mining was economically feasible in relatively shallow mines with thick seams of coal such as those in western Pennsylvania and northern West Virginia.

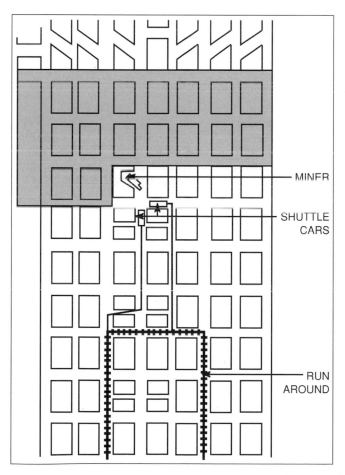

Fig. 38-1. Diagram of the layout of the room and pillar system of coal mining. (Adapted from Stefanko R: Room and pillar mining. In Bise CJ, editor: *Coal mining technology theory and practice,* pp 101-126, Littleton, Colo, 1983, Society of Mining Engineers of American Institute of Mining, Metallurgical, and Petroleum Engineers. With permission.)

Longwall mining

Recent competition in the world coal market has caused a shift in the United States to the longwall system, which had been the usual method of coal mining in Great Britain and the rest of Europe (Fig. 38-2). This system involves driving a vertical shaft to the coal seam, then creating parallel ingress and egress tunnels. A coal "plow" is pulled along the longwall face between the parallel tunnels, which may range from several hundred to upwards of 800 to 1000 feet apart. The longwall is supported by hydraulic roof supports, which are advanced as the coal is mined. When the coal has been removed, the hydraulic supports are moved forward and the roof behind is allowed to collapse. This method of mining eliminates the necessity of leaving large pillars of valuable coal to support the roof as the mining operation progresses. The advantages of longwall mining have been summarized by Stefanko[8] as (1) improved safety, (2) higher extraction rates, (3) greater flexibility in mining under a poorer roof, (4) better subsidence control, and (5) elimination of the need for roof bolting and many ventilation controls.

RELATIONSHIP OF JOBS TO DUST EXPOSURE

Dust formation is an inherent feature of most mining processes. Dust sampling has generally shown that the closer to the coal face the occupation is, the higher the airborne dust concentrations.[9] Thus, it is reasonable to classify underground coal mining occupations with regard to proximity to the dust-generating face. The dust levels in the mine atmosphere decrease as one moves farther away from the face.[10]

Face occupations

The "face occupations" in underground coal mines are those in which the dust levels are the highest. In the *premechanization* era they included those listed in the box on page 657 and discussed here.

The *cutting machine operator* operates a hand-held or mobile machine that saws a channel, usually along the bottom of the coal face. He starts an endless chain equipped with teeth that travel around the edge of a cutter bar. He moves levers to advance the cutter bar into and across the face. He may replace dull teeth and make minor repairs to the machine using a wrench and hand tools.

A *drilling machine operator* is one who operates a mounted or unmounted drill to bore blasting holes in the coal seam at a working face. He positions and stabilizes the machine, using jacks, and lowers the drill shaft into position. He moves levers to start and advance the drill into coal or rock formation. He stops the drill to install additional drill stems. He observes the operation to detect binding or stoppage of the drill. The worker removes the drill when a specified depth has been reached. He may replace worn or broken parts, using hand tools, and lubricates equipment (Fig. 38-3).

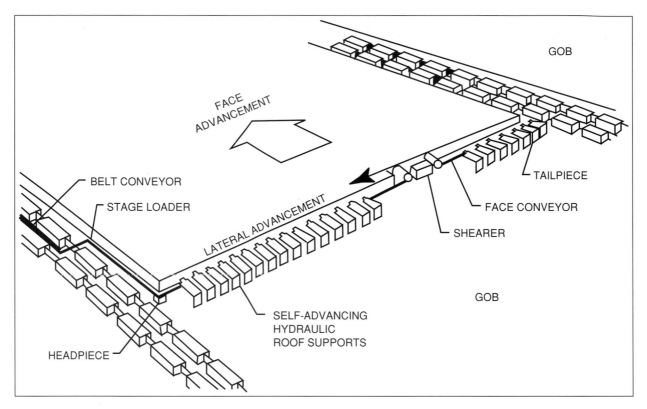

Fig. 38-2. Diagram of the layout of a longwall system of coal mining. Gob, loose waste left in the mine. (Adapted from Stefanko R: Longwall and shortwall mining. In Bise CJ, editor: *Coal mining technology theory and practice*, pp 127-170, Littleton, Colo, 1983, Society of Mining Engineers of American Institute of Mining, Metallurgical, and Petroleum Engineers. With permission.)

The *shot firer (dynamiter)* determines the strength and pattern of blast required and charges and detonates explosives in underground mines to fracture or separate stone or minerals from solid formations. He studies the formation to determine the amount, type, and location of explosive charge required. He then inserts dynamite, ammonium nitrate, black powder, or slurries into blast holes and compacts the charge using a tamping rod. He positions the assembled primer and blasting cap in the hole at a depth that will cause the most effective explosion, connects electric wire to the primer and covers the charge or fills blast holes with clay, drill chips, sand, or other material. He tamps material to secure the charge and prevent the force of blast from escaping through the blast hole. Prior to firing, he inspects the blasting area to ensure that safety laws are observed and signals workers to clear the area.

A *coal digger* or *hand loader* works in an underground mine performing any combination of the following tasks. He shovels coal or rock into cars or onto conveyors, pushes loaded mine cars from the working face to the haulage road, and couples them together for transportation to surface. He may position and adjust bits on drill shafts and place cables, jacks, roof bolts, and related equipment in specific locations.

In the *mechanized* room and pillar or longwall mines, the face operations with highest dust concentrations are less labor intensive.

The *continuous miner operator* operates a self-propelled, continuous mining machine to mine coal underground. This includes driving the machine into position at the working face, moving levers to advance a ripper bar or boring head into the face of the coal seam, and starting the machine to gather coal and convey it to the mine floor or directly into a shuttle car. He may move a lever to raise and lower the hydraulic safety bar that supports the roof above the machine until roof bolters complete their work. He may repair, oil, and adjust the machine and change the cutting teeth, using a wrench or other hand tools.

The *continuous miner helper* keeps track of the electrical cable supplying the continuous mining machine to avoid its being cut. He also observes the roof for signs of movement or imminent rock fall. He ensures that a buggy is available to receive the coal that is cut. He also assists the continuous miner operator in oiling, adjusting, and repairing the machine and changing the cutting teeth.

A *loading machine operator* operates a mounted machine with hydraulic arms that gather up coal produced by the continuous mining machine that has fallen loose onto

Mining occupations

Coal mining

FACE OCCUPATIONS
    Cutting machine operator
    Drilling machine operator
    Shot firer (dynamiter)
    Coal digger or hand loader
    Continuous miner operator
    Continuous miner helper
    Loading machine operator
    Loading machine helper
    Timberman
    Section foreman
    Roof bolter
    Longwall mining machine operator
    Longwall mining machine helper (tailer)

OCCUPATIONS WITH INTERMITTENT FACE EXPOSURE
    Brattice man
    Beltman
    Chute loader
    Motorman
    Rock duster
    Shuttle car operator

OCCUPATIONS AWAY FROM THE FACE
    Dispatcher
    Cager
    Mine inspector (fire boss)

SURFACE OCCUPATIONS AT UNDERGROUND MINES
    Coal washer
    Surface driller
    Driller helper

Metal and nonmetal mining

    Stope miner
    Grizzly man
    Slusher or slusher hoist operator
    Scraper
    Skip tender
    Diamond driller
    Sampler
    Mucker
    Breaker (crusher)
    Barring-down worker
    Trammer
    Concreter

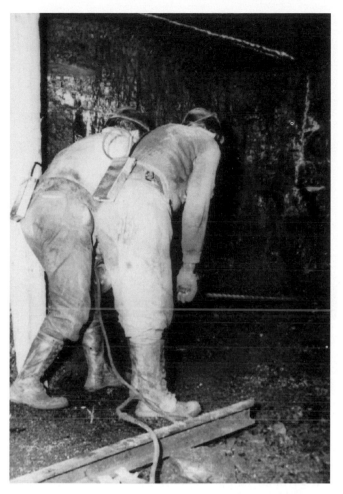

Fig. 38-3. Miners using a two-man coal machine to drill blasting holes into the coal face.

the mine floor. The coal is gathered onto a conveyor, which moves the coal into a waiting buggy.

The *loading machine helper* assists the loading machine operator to avoid becoming entangled in the electrical cable supplying the continuous miner. He assists in repairing and adjusting the loading machine. He also observes the roof for evidence of instability or imminent danger.

The *timberman* is one who cuts, fits, installs, and repairs supporting timbers and other framework in an underground mine, using carpentry tools. He measures and cuts timbers for roof supports and framing, such as ladders, chutes, walls, and ventilation doors, using a handsaw or power saw, square, and rule. He sets roof timbers and inserts wedges to hold them in place. He erects cribbing to increase support or control ventilation. He installs braces to repair or shore up loose timbering, using a hammer and spikes. He may set and wedge props (posts) in place as temporary support for the roof or the working face. He cuts timbers to size and loads them onto cars for haulage to the mine. He may build wooden forms and mix and pour concrete supports.

The *section foreman* supervises the activities of all workers engaged in a specified section of an underground mine. He coordinates such activities as timbering, roof bolting, track laying, undercutting, drilling, blasting, loading, and conveying of coal. He examines malfunctioning equipment and orders transfer of the faulty unit to a shop or orders repair at the work site. He inspects the section for hazards such as gas, falling rock, squeezes, and poor ventilation, using devices such as safety lamps, an anemometer, and a crowbar. He maintains records of production, area mined,

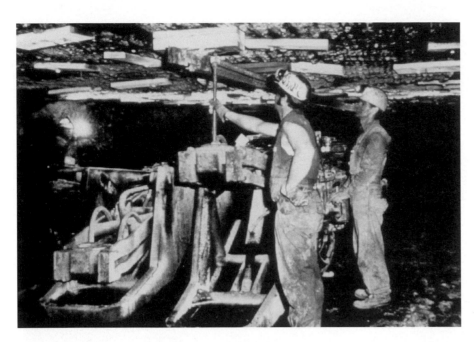

Fig. 38-4. A roof bolter and a helper drilling into the roof of a coal mine.

and location of personnel and equipment. He orders and distributes supplies, such as bits, wire, machine parts, bulbs, and chalk. He is responsible for ensuring the safety of the section team.

A *roof bolter* is one who operates a self-propelled machine to install roof support bolts in an underground mine. He positions a safety jack to support the roof until bolts can be installed. He drives the machine into position, inserts a bit into the drill chuck, and starts the drill. He moves a lever to advance the bit into the roof at specified distances from ribs or adjacent bolts. He removes the bit from the chuck and replaces it with a bolt and starts the hydraulic action that forces the bolt into the hole. He starts the rotation of the chuck to turn the bolt and open an expansion head to exert pressure on the rock formation. He tests the bolt for specified tension, using a torque wrench. He may install truss bolts traversing the entire ceiling span and tighten ends of the anchored truss bolts, using a turnbuckle. Since roof bolters drill into the rock strata above the coal seam, they are at risk of exposure to silica as well as coal dust from the face (Fig. 38-4).

The *longwall mining machine operator* tends equipment that plows across the face of coal strata in an underground mine. He monitors the electronic control panel that activates the machine. He observes indicator lights and gauges on the control panel to detect machine malfunction. He advances the plow blade through the coal strata by remote control on electronic or radio signals from a tailer. He listens for unusual sounds that would indicate equipment malfunctions. He may assist in the routine maintenance or repair of machinery (Fig. 38-5).

The *longwall mining machine helper (tailer)* works at the opposite end of the coal strata, assisting the longwall mining machine operator to advance a plow blade through the face of coal in an underground mine. He pulls levers to adjust the depth of penetration of the blade. He signals the longwall mining machine operator by an electronic buzzer or two-way radio when the machine plow blade is properly positioned. He adjusts and makes minor repairs to equipment, using hand tools. He may assist in positioning jacks, timbers, or roof supports to prevent cave-ins when working underground (Fig. 38-6).

Occupations with intermittent face exposure

These occupations are associated with dust levels that were generally one third to one half of the values measured in the mechanized face operations.[10]

A *brattice man* is one who builds doorways and brattices (ventilation walls or partitions) in underground passageways of various materials, such as canvas, wood, concrete, brick, or concrete block as specified, to construct partitions to control the circulation of air through passageways and working areas. He erects partitions to support the roof in areas unsuited to timbering or bolting. He may install rigid and flexible air ducts to transport air into work areas. He may drill and blast obstructing boulders to reopen ventilation shafts.

A *beltman* walks along the conveyor belt from inside an underground mine to the surface tipple. He inspects, monitors, and adjusts the length and tension of the conveyor (belt) during use to ensure the steady movement of coal. He checks transfer points for the proper transfer of coal and for malfunctions. He lubricates pulleys and bearings. In the event of malfunction, he notifies the conveyor attendant by buzzer or two-way radio. He replaces worn or damaged belting as needed. He shovels spills onto the conveyor belt as needed. He uses a chain and hoist as well as hand tools to make repairs on the belt.

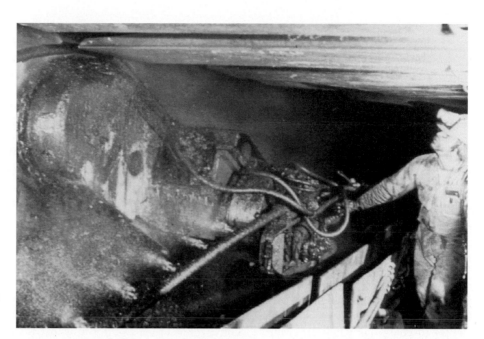

Fig. 38-5. A longwall mining machine operator directing the coal plow along the coal face. (Courtesy of Robert L. Grayson.)

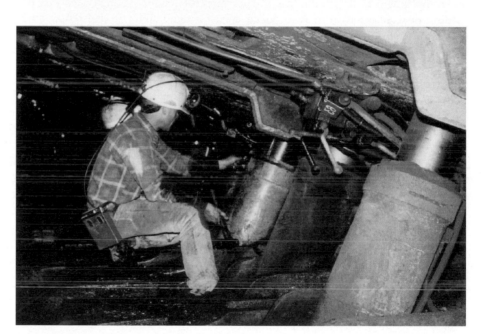

Fig. 38-6. A longwall helper preparing to move the hydraulic roof support of a longwall miner. (Courtesy of Robert L. Grayson.)

The *chute loader* is one who loads railroad cars or a conveyor with coal obtained from the face by the shuttle car. He pulls levers or presses buttons to open and close the chute of a storage bin to regulate the flow of the coal. He loosens clogged material, using a bar or compressed air. He may spray water on the materials to settle dust.

The *motorman* controls an electrically powered engine to transport and shunt cars at a coal mine. He controls the movement of an engine that transports coal out of the mine and supplies into the mine. He positions cars for loading or unloading according to the signals of the dumper. He may throw switches and couple or uncouple cars. He may trans-port personnel and equipment into and out of the mine. He uses abrasive material (sand) for traction on inclines.

Since motormen use sand to provide traction on the rails, particularly on inclines, they risk exposure to crystalline silica as well as the ambient coal mine dust in common with other miners. Anderson and colleagues[11] examined the question of whether motormen who used sand developed a different type of pneumoconiosis from that of miners working at the coal face. They compared 153 miners who worked exclusively as hand loaders to 53 miners who had worked exclusively as motormen. The loaders had predominantly *p* and *q* (less than 3-mm) opacities and the motormen had predominantly nodular *r* (greater than 3-mm) opacities on their chest radiographs.

A *rock duster* is one who sprays water and/or rock dust onto the walls, roof, and floor of underground mine workings to mix with coal dust deposits and prevent explosions. He uses a portable compressed-air pump and hose. He mixes rock dust with water and sprays the slurry during working hours to reduce the amount of suspended coal dust in the air while miners are present. During nonworking hours he may blow dry rock dust onto the ceilings, sides, and floors of the haulage way to reduce the explosive concentration of fine coal dust, using a compressed-air blower mounted on a railroad car (Fig. 38-7).

The *shuttle car operator* drives a diesel or electrically powered car in an underground mine to transport materials from the working face to mine cars or a conveyor. He positions the shuttle car under a discharge conveyor of the loading machine and observes that the materials are loaded properly. He maneuvers the shuttle car to keep its nose under the discharge conveyor. He controls a conveyor that runs the entire length of the shuttle car to apportion the load as loading progresses. He drives a loaded car to a ramp and moves the controls to discharge the load into mine cars or onto a conveyor. He may move mine cars into position to be loaded from a shuttle car. He may charge batteries when operating a battery-powered vehicle.

Occupations away from the face

These jobs are generally near to or at the surface and have a relatively low exposure to dust. They include the following.

The *dispatcher* coordinates the movements of haulage trips (trains) in an underground mine to or from the working face or dump area. He schedules the movements of trains hauling coal or supplies in accordance with the ca-

pacity of the system, the interval between trains, and the length and direction of trains. He directs the movements of emergency and repair rail cars, using telephone, radio, or track signals. Although the dispatcher may be physically located underground, he is often in a room or shack somewhat separated from the rest of the mining operations.

A *cager* pushes mine cars onto and off the mine shaft cage and informs workers when the cage is used to carry mine personnel. He pushes or pulls loaded cars off the cage at the surface and replaces them with cars that are empty or loaded with supplies. He pulls empty cars from the cage at the bottom or at intermediate levels and moves them onto sidings for distribution and loading.

The *mine inspector (fire boss)* inspects underground mines to ascertain compliance with contractual agreements and with health and safety laws. He inspects for rotted or incorrectly placed timbers, dangerously placed or defective electrical and mechanical equipment, improperly stored explosives, and other hazardous conditions. He tests air quality to detect toxic or explosive gas or dust, using portable gas analysis equipment, in order to control health hazards and reduce injuries and fatalities. He observes mine activities to detect violations of federal and state health and safety standards. He may instruct mine workers in safety and first-aid procedures.

Surface occupations at underground mines

A *coal washer* is one who operates equipment to size and wash the coal for shipment or further processing. He starts equipment, such as washers, tables, shakers, sizing screens, and conveyors. He regulates the flow of coal and water to separate coal from slate, rock, and other foreign material and transfers cleaned and sized coal to loading chutes or storage. He observes equipment and gauges, may lubricate and repair equipment, and may test refuse samples

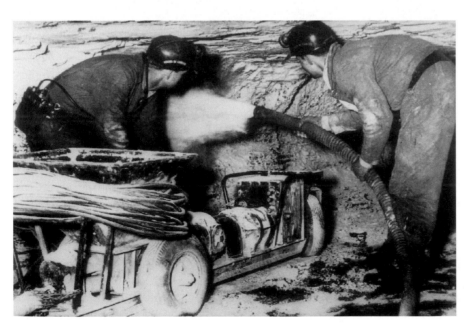

Fig. 38-7. A rock duster and a helper spreading rock dust (limestone) along the sides of an underground coal mine.

to determine coal content. Although measured dust levels at this operation are low, there is a small risk of exposure from escaping dust at belt transfer and chute-loading points.

MINE GASES

The gases encountered in underground mines may also be found in other industries. The unusual hazards they present in mining depend on the ventilation of underground workings.[12]

Methane is an odorless, tasteless gas found in virtually all undisturbed coal seams. Methane will cause asphyxiation only if the amount is so large that oxygen is diluted below respirable levels. This is likely to occur when there is a sudden, massive release or emission of this gas from the coal seam. The principal danger of methane is its ability to form an explosive mixture in certain concentrations with air.

The hazard of methane asphyxiation is largely confined to workers at the face operations, such as the hand loader, cutting machine operator, continuous miner operator, shot firer, drilling machine operator, continuous mining machine operator, and loading machine operator. Pockets of methane build-up can occur in relatively poorly ventilated rooms or entries even when the remainder of the mine receives adequate ventilation.

Oxygen deficiency may occur in unused and therefore unventilated areas of the mine as a consequence of the slow oxidation of the coal seam when exposed to air. Face workers, such as those listed above, are at little risk from this source. However, the fire boss, whose job is to inspect not only the working faces for evidence of oxygen deficiency and toxic atmospheres but also the poorly ventilated and unused "returns," is at risk for oxygen deficiency.

Carbon monoxide is produced by explosions of flammable gas or coal dust. It is also produced during underground fires and even a small amount by shot firing. The major risk during mining operations is to the shot firer and the hand loader, who return prematurely to the face before there has been adequate clearing of the gas by the mine ventilation. In the event of a coal mine explosion or fire, all workers in the underground work force are at risk for carbon monoxide poisoning. It is for this reason that regulations require all persons going underground to wear a "self-rescue" device that may permit escape in a carbon monoxide–containing atmosphere.[13] Carbon monoxide poisoning and roof falls have been the major sources of fatalities among coal miners throughout the history of mining.[12,13]

Nitrogen oxides occur in the fumes from shot firing and present a risk to the shot firer and the hand loader, especially if they return prematurely to the mine face after the explosion.[12] Nitrogen oxides also occur in the exhausts from diesel engines, which are utilized in some underground coal mines, primarily those located in Utah, Wyoming, Colorado, and Kentucky.[14]

Hydrogen sulfide may be found in underground coal mines as a result of reaction of acidic mine water with natu-

rally occurring pyrites in the coal seam. It is poisonous in concentrations as low as 100 ppm. It has, on occasion, caused the death of miners, but is rarely encountered in lethal concentrations in adequately ventilated mines. The miner most likely to encounter toxic concentrations of this gas is the fire boss, who enters a relatively poorly ventilated area. It is usually more of a nuisance than a hazard.[12]

Cable fires

The electric cable, providing high-voltage electricity to the cutting and continuous mining machines, contains polyvinylchloride sheathing. When the cable sheathing is cut or otherwise damaged, the resulting cable fire releases a number of toxic gases, which may include hydrochloric acid vapor, hydrogen cyanide, phosgene, and chlorine. These gases are not diluted in the underground mine as they would be on the surface.[12] The miners most likely to be affected by these gases are the face workers, particularly the cutting machine operator, the continuous miner operator, the loading machine operator, and their helpers.

Belt fires

The conveyor belts used to transport coal out of underground coal mines to the surface also contain polyvinylchloride materials. Excessive heating of bearings on which the belts ride may result in either fires or decomposition of the belting material. This, too, will result in the release of toxic gases such as hydrochloric acid vapor, hydrogen cyanide, phosgene and, chlorine. The beltman is the miner at highest risk for exposure to these toxic gases from belt fires.

SURFACE MINERS AT SPECIAL RISK

Relatively few of the miners who work at surface coal mines (strip mines) are at risk for intense dust exposures. The mine atmosphere is not enclosed and critically dependent on adequate ventilation as is the case in underground mines. However, several surveys, beginning in the early 1970s, have revealed an excessive exposure among drillers and driller helpers to high concentrations of crystalline silica. These miners have developed acute or accelerated silicosis with brief periods of exposure.[15-17]

The *surface driller* sets up and operates a self-propelled or truck-mounted drilling machine to bore blasting holes in overburden (rock) at a strip mine, open pit, or quarry. He positions and stabilizes the machine, using jacks, and lowers the drill shaft into position. He moves levers to start and advance the drill into the overburden or rock formation. He stops the drill to install additional drill stems, observes the operation to detect binding or stoppage of the drill, and removes the drill when a specified depth has been reached. He replaces worn or broken parts, and may charge and set off explosives in blasting holes (Fig. 38-8).

The *driller helper* bores or burns blast holes in overburden at a strip mine, open pit, or quarry as an assistant to the driller. He signals the driller to position the machine.

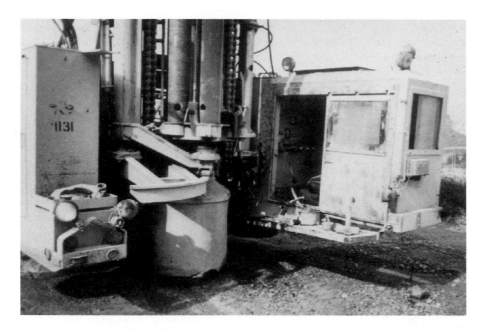

Fig. 38-8. A surface drill with its dust skirt. Note the proximity of the operator's cab to the drill. (Courtesy of Daniel Banks.)

He adds, positions, and replaces drill stems, burners, castings, cables, and hoses to assist in the drilling operation. He pulls electric cables and water hoses clear of machine treads and observes ground surface and machine operation for indications of unsafe conditions. He collects samples for laboratory analysis and lubricates and cleans equipment.

METAL AND NONMETAL MINING

A common type of underground mining method in the metal mines is referred to as *stoping*. In this method the ore is extracted via tunnels excavated in a series of vertical steps, or stopes, rather than in horizontally oriented tunnels.[18] This type of mining lends itself to block caving, in which the ore body is situated above the stopes, and either by blasting or by the effects of gravity, the ore body is fractured. The ore-containing rock is allowed to fall into chutes or grizzlies into mine cars or onto conveyors, or directly into crushers situated below the grizzlies.

A *stope miner* is one who works in an excavation from which ore is extracted via a series of vertical, steplike tunnels rather than horizontally situated tunnels. He shovels ore or rock into cars or onto conveyors, pushes loaded mine cars from the working face to the haulage road, and couples them together for transportation to the surface. He may position and adjust bits on drill shafts and place cables, jacks, roof bolts, and related equipment in specific locations (Fig. 38-9).

The *grizzly man* is a miner who works above and around the guardrails or coverings that protect the chutes in a metal mine. He observes the movement of the ore-containing rock from the ore body through the chute into the grizzly. He breaks up oversized lumps with a sledge hammer so they will pass through the grizzly or chute to storage, a crusher, or the loading station.[1]

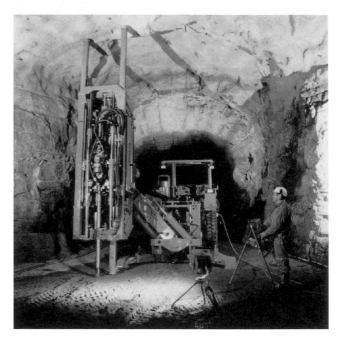

Fig. 38-9. A stope miner drilling into the roof of a metal mine. (Courtesy of Matti Pulkkinen.)

The term *slusher* or *slusher hoist operator* refers to a miner who operates a hoisting engine and a cable-drawn scraper or scoop, to load ore or rock into mine cars or onto conveyors in an underground metal mine.[19,20]

A *scraper* refers to a miner who uses a machine-mounted front-end blade to push or scoop ore-containing rock and load it into mine cars or onto conveyors.[20]

A *skip tender* is a miner who pushes mine cars onto and off the mine shaft cage and informs the workers when the cage is available to carry mine personnel.

The *diamond driller* is a miner who sets up and operates a diamond drill that is used to obtain solid cores of strata so that the character of the ground and the wealth of ore may be obtained. This operation can be done underground or at the surface.

The term *sampler* refers to one whose duty is to select the samples for an assay or to prepare the mineral to be assayed. This operation is generally done at the surface but may be done underground as well.

Mucker refers to the miner who, either by hand or with a machine, cleans the working areas and haulage track and digs and maintains drainage ditches or shovels muck, ore, or rock aside or into cars or onto conveyors. This job may be equivalent in the metal mines to the coal digger or hand loader in a coal mine.

The *breaker (crusher)* operates a panel board to control conveying, blending, washing, crushing, and sizing of ore to prepare it for commercial or industrial use or for further processing.

The miner who does *barring-down* removes, with a bar, loose rock from the sides and roof of mine workings.

Trammer refers to the miner who loads broken rock or ore into tram cars and pushes them along a track to deliver them to the shaft.

The *concreter* is a skilled worker who spreads and levels concrete with or without form work, shaping it into chambers over bowlike beams or girders or roof falls as required.

MINE GASES IN METAL AND NONMETAL MINES

The majority of metal and nonmetal mines do not contain high concentrations of methane, which is the explosive hazard in underground coal mines. As a result, there has been extensive use of diesel rather than electrically operated equipment in metal and nonmetal mines.

Miners who work underground in these mines may be exposed to *diesel exhaust,* which contains carbon monoxide, carbon dioxide, nitrogen dioxide, oxides of nitrogen, sulfur dioxide, and aldehydes in various concentrations depending on the type of engine and operating parameters (see Chapter 33).[21,22]

The special case of *radon gas* is largely confined to metal and nonmetal mines, although radon progeny are ubiquitous and exposure cannot be entirely eliminated, even in the nonoccupational setting (see Chapter 31). There were 22,499 workers employed in 427 metal and nonmetal mines in the United States in 1986.[23] The highest concentrations of radon were found in the uranium and uranium/vanadium mines. The number of uranium miners decreased from 9076 in 1979 to 448 in 1986. Workers in these mines are exposed not only to radon but also to dust from the rock-containing ore. They are at risk for developing silicosis as well as the consequences of inhaling radon. Uranium miners, like other metal miners, also use diesel equipment, and are exposed to diesel exhaust components.

REFERENCES

1. Thrush PW and the Staff of the Bureau of Mines: *A dictionary of mining, mineral and related terms,* Chicago, 1968, Maclean Hunter Publishing.
2. US Department of Labor: *Dictionary of occupational titles,* ed 4, Washington, DC, 1977, US Government Printing Office.
3. Morgan WKC: Coal workers' pneumoconiosis. In Morgan WKC and Seaton A, editors: *Occupational lung diseases,* pp 377-448, Philadelphia, 1984, WB Saunders.
4. Morgan WKC: The prevalence of coal workers' pneumoconiosis, *Am Rev Respir Dis* 98:306-310, 1968.
5. Morgan WKC, Burgess DB, Jacobsen G, et al: The prevalence of coal workers' pneumoconiosis in US coal miners, *Arch Environ Health* 27:221-226, 1973.
6. Attfield MD and Castellan RM: Epidemiological data on US coal miners' pneumoconiosis, 1960 to 1988, *Am J Public Health* 82:964-970, 1992.
7. Stefanko R: Room and pillar mining. In Bise CJ, editor: *Coal mining technology theory and practice,* pp 101-126, Littleton, Colo, 1983, Society of Mining Engineers of American Institute of Mining, Metallurgical, and Petroleum Engineers.
8. Stefanko R: Longwall and shortwall mining. In Bise CJ, editor: *Coal mining technology theory and practice,* pp 127-170, Littleton, Colo, 1983, Society of Mining Engineers of American Institute of Mining, Metallurgical, and Petroleum Engineers.
9. Wheeler HP Jr: The working environment: statement of the steps and rationale for action taken by the Department of the Interior. Papers and Proceedings of the National Conference on Medicine and the Federal Coal Mine Health and Safety Act of 1969, Public Law 91-173 1977 June 15-18, Washington, DC, 1982, US Bureau of Mines.
10. Jacobson M: Respirable dust in U.S. bituminous coal mines. Papers and Proceedings of the National Conference on Medicine and the Federal Coal Mine Health and Safety Act of 1969, Public Law 91-173 1977 June 15-18, Washington, DC, 1982, US Bureau of Mines.
11. Anderson WH, Hamilton GL, and Dossett RE Jr: A comparison of coal miners exposed to coal dust and those exposed to silica dust, *Arch Environ Health* 1:540-547, 1960.
12. Spencer TD and Lawther PJ: Mine gases. In Rogan JM, editor: *Medicine in the mining industries,* pp 224-235, Philadelphia, 1972, FA Davis.
13. Turner NL and Hodous TK: Respiratory protection in the mining industry. In Banks DE, editor: *The mining industry, state of the art reviews: occupational medicine,* pp 143-154, Philadelphia, 1993, Hanley & Belfus.
14. Reger R, Hancock J, Hankinson J, et al: Coal miners exposed to diesel exhaust emissions, *Ann Occup Hyg* 26:799-815, 1982.
15. Banks DE, Bauer MA, Castellan RM, et al: Silicosis in surface coalmine drillers, *Thorax* 38:275-278, 1983.
16. Amandus HE and Piacitelli G: Dust exposures at U.S. surface coal mines in 1982-1983, *Arch Environ Health* 42:374-381, 1987.
17. US Department of Health and Human Services (DHHS), Public Health Service, Centers for Disease Control, National Institute for Occupational Safety and Health (NIOSH) *Alert: request for assistance in preventing silicosis and deaths in rock drillers,* DHHS (NIOSH) Pub No 92-107.
18. Peele R and Church JA, editors. *Mining engineer's handbook,* Vol I, ed 3, New York, 1941, John Wiley & Sons.
19. Flinn RF, Brinton HP, Doyle HN, et al: *Silicosis in the metal mining industry. A revaluation 1958-1961,* pp 1-238, Washington, DC, 1963, US Government Printing Office.
20. US Department of Health and Human Services (DHHS), Public Health Service, Centers for Disease Control, National Institute for Occupational Safety and Health (NIOSH): *A recommended standard for occupational exposure to radon progeny in underground mines,* DHHS (NIOSH) Pub No 88-101.

21. Cummins AB and Given IA, editors: *SME engineering handbook,* New York, 1973, American Institute of Mining, Metallurgical, and Petroleum Engineers.

22. Ames RG, Attfield MD, Hankinson JL, et al: Acute respiratory effects of exposure to diesel emissions in coal miners, *Am Rev Respir Dis* 125:39-42, 1982.

23. US Department of Health and Human Services (DHHS), Public Health Service, Centers for Disease Control, National Institute for Occupational Safety and Health (NIOSH): *Proceedings of a workshop on the use of diesel equipment in underground mines,* DHHS (NIOSH) Pub No 82-122.

Chapter 39

FOUNDRIES AND STEEL MAKING

Sean R. Muldoon
David J. Tollerud

Evidence for the antiquity of humans' use of iron is provided by references to iron both in fragmentary writings and in inscriptions on monuments, palaces, and tombs that survived the collapse of such ancient civilizations as those of Assyria, Babylonia, Egypt, China, India, Greece, and Rome. In addition, archeologists have unearthed actual iron tools, weapons, and ornaments in many parts of the world that were occupied by prehistoric people. By the 20th century steel production had become a symbol of national economic strength, infrastructure growth, and quality of life in general among industrialized nations.

The perception that the American steel industry is "dying" is unfounded. This may be a result of well-publicized accounts of labor-management disputes and layoffs in the past several decades. However, according to the American Iron and Steel Institute, U.S. iron and steel production levels are only slightly lower than those of 25 years ago.[1] The dominant feature of modern steel production is that the employment requirements have drastically been reduced through improvements in efficiency and through automation (Fig. 39-1). Despite the downward trend in employment, as of 1990, 164,000 U.S. workers were employed in the direct manufacture and sale of iron and steel, as well as thousands more in mining, quarrying, shipping, warehousing, and other steel-related functions. As of 1986 over 300,000 workers were employed in U.S. foundry work.

THE STEEL AND FOUNDRY INDUSTRY

In any industry the occupational history forms the foundation of the inquiry into job-related illness and disease. Implicit in this inquiry is an understanding of potential health

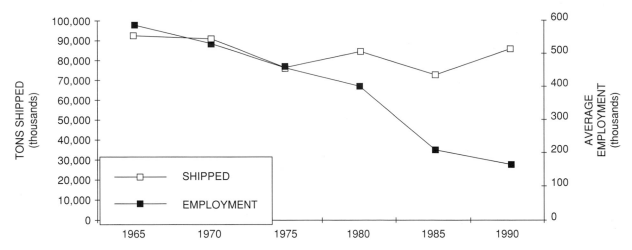

Fig. 39-1. Improvements in iron and steel industry productivity and recycling have led to a fall in employment out of proportion to a modest annual production decline. (Data provided by the American Iron and Steel Institute.)

hazards associated with that occupation; a working knowledge of a given occupation's tasks is prerequisite to effective occupational medicine practice. Therefore this chapter has three basic objectives: (1) to describe in some detail the steel-making process and to identify respiratory hazards at each step, (2) to review the epidemiologic data linking work in the steel industry and respiratory disease, and (3) to familiarize the reader with current preventive medicine strategies.

The steel-making process can be divided into four general phases:

1. The making of coke from coal.
2. The production of iron from iron ore and other raw materials.
3. The making of steel from iron.
4. Physically transforming crudely shaped steel into finished rods, beams, sheets, etc.

Each of these steps is reviewed in turn. This background information will facilitate reconstruction of a potential exposure history from a patient's description of past and present jobs in the steel-making industry.

The steel-making process

The basic ingredients of steel are iron ore, limestone, and coke. The steel-making process follows a well-defined series of steps (Fig. 39-2). In most steel-making facilities the foundry and melting processes are carried out on the same site. The melting process begins with iron ore, coke, and limestone moving up a conveyer system called a *skip hoist* and being dumped into the top of a large, insulated container called a *blast furnace* (Fig. 39-3). Preheated hot air is blown into the furnace, causing the coke to burn and bringing the furnace temperature to about 3000° F. The ore is melted into drops of molten *pig iron* that settle to the bottom of the blast furnace. The limestone joins with other impurities from the ore to form a material called *slag,* the

fused product formed by the action of a flux on the ore or on the oxidized impurities in any metal. Slag floats on top of the pool of liquid iron, is skimmed off, solidifies by cooling, and is hauled away to be stored in slag pits. Slag provides the means by which impurities are separated from the metal and removed from the furnace in both iron and steel-making processes. It has little use except potentially as landfill.

The iron produced from the blast furnaces is periodically drained from the bottom into a ladle and transported a short distance by crane, where it is transformed into steel by further removal of impurities in a second furnace, either electric arc or oxygen fueled, called a *converter.* Steel scrap is added along with any alloying metals and a *flux,* inorganic material added to help extract impurities. Fluxes are categorized as either acid fluxes (silica) or basic fluxes of limestone (calcium carbonate) or dolomite (primarily calcium or magnesium carbonate). The limestone and dolomite are mined in quarrying operations, crushed, and separated by size. They are then transported by ship or rail to the steel plant, where, along with scrap iron, molten iron from the blast furnace, and alloy additions, the flux is added to the converting furnace. Flux is used to neutralize acids and bases in the ore, forming a solid material, analogous to the salts formed in water solutions during ordinary chemical reactions.

Pure oxygen is added to the molten mix, and additional impurities are again removed as a limestone slag, consisting of oxides of silicon, manganese, phosphorus, and iron. Liquid steel from this step is poured into molds to form *ingots,* each weighing several tons. The ingots are hauled off to rectangular furnaces called *soaking pits,* where they are brought to a uniform temperature prior to transportation by rail to the rolling mill. There, the white hot steel ingots pass through rollers that form the desired crude shapes, called blooms, billets, or slabs, each a variation of a long slab of rectangular cross-sectional area. More modern plants utilize

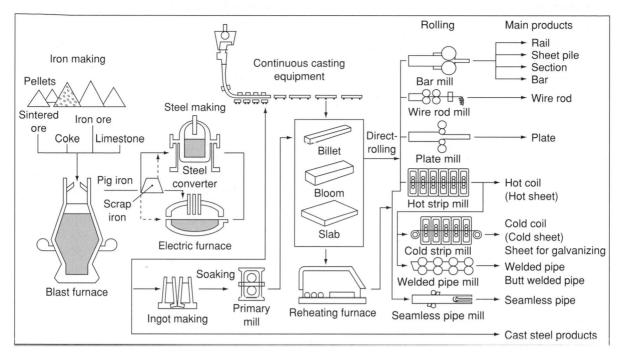

Fig. 39-2. A schematic representation of iron production. Raw steel in the form of billets, bloom, or slabs is formed into finished product in rolling mills of various configurations. (Adapted from Kawaguchi and Sugiyama: Steel industry I: manufacturing system, Yverdon, Switzerland, 1989, Gordon and Breach. With permission.)

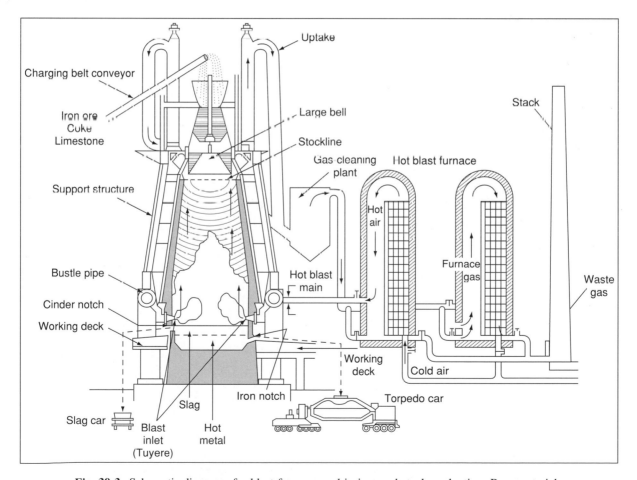

Fig. 39-3. Schematic diagram of a blast furnace used in iron and steel production. Raw materials enter the furnace through the top while molten iron leaves the furnace from below the surface. (Adapted from Kawaguchi and Sugiyama: Steel industry I: manufacturing system, Yverdon, Switzerland, 1989, Gordon and Breach. With permission.)

a *continuous caster* in which liquid steel from the converter is poured onto a moving production line, where it solidifies upon cooling and is shaped into a slab by a series of rollers (Fig. 39-4). Continuous casting was used for 61% of the U.S. steel production in 1988, an increase from 17% in 1980.[2] These semifinished slabs are then transported to a *finishing mill,* where they are rolled into their final forms, such as rods, pipes, beams, or sheets.

Coke oven operation

Production process. Coke, a highly purified coal, is an essential ingredient in steel making. Coke provides the high heat energy necessary to melt iron ore and other materials in the blast furnace. Coke is produced by heating bituminous coal in special facilities called coke ovens (Fig. 39-5).

A coke plant consists of one or more "batteries," each consisting of several dozen ovens, called slot ovens, arranged in parallel rows. A cross-section of a typical coke oven is shown in Fig. 39-6. Each slot oven consists of a coking chamber, a heating chamber, and a regenerative chamber. Typical dimensions for coking chambers are 3 to 6 m in height, 11 to 15 m in length, and 40 to 50 cm in width, although in more modern ovens they may be larger. The heating and coking chambers are lined up in a side-to-side alternating pattern such that a *heating chamber* is lo-

cated on each side of a coking chamber. A *regenerative chamber,* where fuel mixture is regulated and fuel flow is directed into each individual chamber, is located beneath the heating and coking chambers.

Coal is unloaded from railroad cars or river barges onto a conveyor belt and taken by belt to a coal *storage bunker* high above the coke oven battery. Coke production is run in cycles, beginning when the coal is dropped from the bunker into a transporting vehicle called a *larry car.* The larry car travels along the top of the battery on rails, and drops a measured amount of coal through charging holes into each oven. A worker known as a *lidman* manually removes the cover of the charging holes before each cycle begins. After the oven has been loaded, the lids are replaced and sealed in a process called luting. A *luterman* pours or paints on a refractory material around the lid to minimize the escape of emissions around the lid. Hot fuel gas is pumped into the heating chambers and burned, volatilizing impurities in a process called *destructive distillation,* creating what is now called coke. The heating cycle continues for about 24 hours.

Access to the coke chamber is provided by doors on both ends of the chamber, designated the "push" side and the "coke" side (Fig. 39-7). A worker called a *door man* operates the door on each side. On the push side a pushing ram sequentially enters each chamber and forces the coked coal

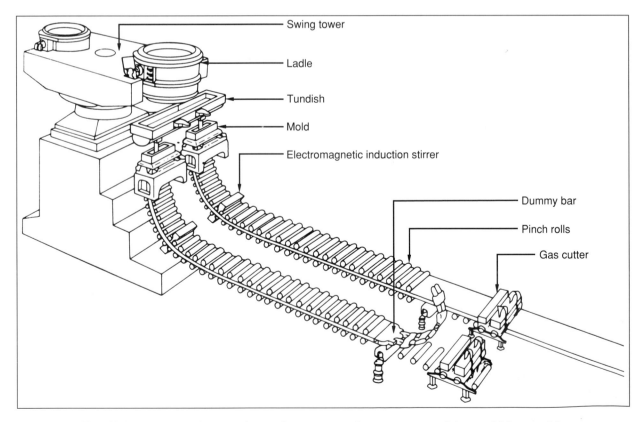

Fig. 39-4. Schematic diagram of a continuous caster, the current state of the art. Molten steel is poured from the ladle into parallel molds. The steel progressively hardens and is shaped as it travels between the rollers. (Adapted from Kawaguchi and Sugiyama: Steel industry I: manufacturing system, Yverdon, Switzerland, 1989, Gordon and Breach. With permission.)

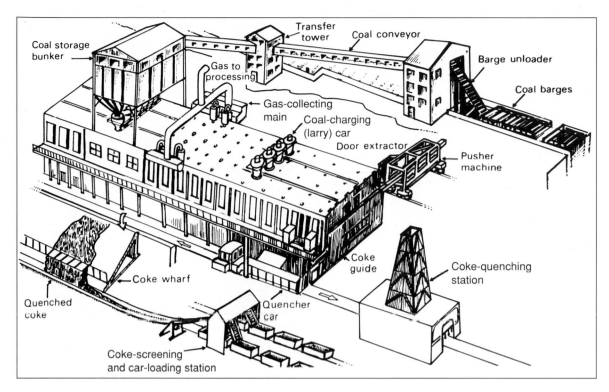

Fig. 39-5. View of a typical coke production plant. Coal is charged from the top of the battery from a larry car. A pusher machine pushes finished coke from each slot oven into a quencher car for cooling. (Adapted from McGannon HE: Metallurgical coke and coal chemicals. In McGannon HE, editor: Reprinted from the 10th edition of *Making, shaping, and treating of steel,* with the permission of the AISE, p 109, Pittsburgh, 1964, USX Corporation.)

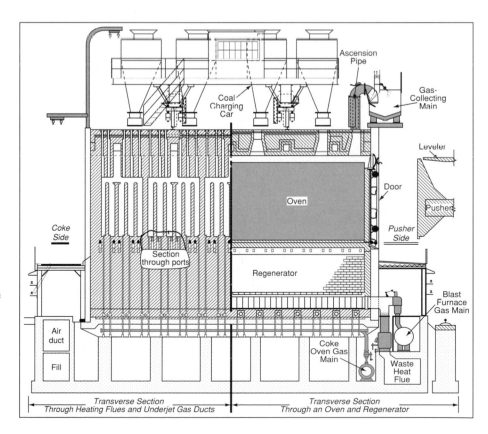

Fig. 39-6. Coking station overview. A cross-section through the ports of a single slot coke oven. The larry car rides above the oven and drops coal into each oven. (Adapted from McGannon HE: Metallurgical coke and coal chemicals. In McGannon HE, editor: Reprinted from the 10th edition of *Making, shaping, and treating of steel,* with the permission of the AISE, p 109, Pittsburgh, 1964, USX Corporation.)

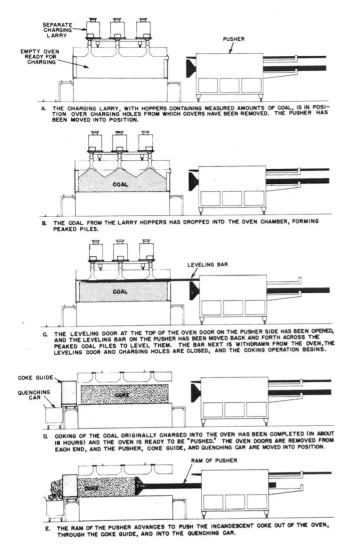

A. THE CHARGING LARRY, WITH HOPPERS CONTAINING MEASURED AMOUNTS OF COAL, IS IN POSITION OVER CHARGING HOLES FROM WHICH COVERS HAVE BEEN REMOVED. THE PUSHER HAS BEEN MOVED INTO POSITION.

B. THE COAL FROM THE LARRY HOPPERS HAS DROPPED INTO THE OVEN CHAMBER, FORMING PEAKED PILES.

C. THE LEVELING DOOR AT THE TOP OF THE OVEN DOOR ON THE PUSHER SIDE HAS BEEN OPENED, AND THE LEVELING BAR ON THE PUSHER HAS BEEN MOVED BACK AND FORTH ACROSS THE PEAKED COAL PILES TO LEVEL THEM. THE BAR NEXT IS WITHDRAWN FROM THE OVEN, THE LEVELING DOOR AND CHARGING HOLES ARE CLOSED, AND THE COKING OPERATION BEGINS.

D. COKING OF THE COAL ORIGINALLY CHARGED INTO THE OVEN HAS BEEN COMPLETED (IN ABOUT 18 HOURS) AND THE OVEN IS READY TO BE "PUSHED." THE OVEN DOORS ARE REMOVED FROM EACH END, AND THE PUSHER, COKE GUIDE, AND QUENCHING CAR ARE MOVED INTO POSITION.

E. THE RAM OF THE PUSHER ADVANCES TO PUSH THE INCANDESCENT COKE OUT OF THE OVEN, THROUGH THE COKE GUIDE, AND INTO THE QUENCHING CAR.

Fig. 39-7. Charging, leveling, and pushing operations in one coking cycle of a by-product coke oven. This process is repeated in dozens of ovens arranged in parallel banks. (Adapted from McGannon HE: Metallurgical coke and coal chemicals. In McGannon HE, editor: Reprinted from the 10th edition of *Making, shaping, and treating of steel,* with the permission of the AISE, p 109, Pittsburgh, 1964, USX Corporation.)

out the coke side, into *quenching cars,* where ambient air and water spray cool the coke. The quench car collects the hot coke and carries it by rail to a quenching station, where the coke is cooled to stop further combustion. After cooling, the coke is transported to a *screening station,* where it is sized in preparation for transport to a blast furnace.

Job descriptions. Work in a coke battery is divided into two basic areas: the top side and the bench side. Job classifications on the top side include the larry car operator, lidman, luterman, tar chaser (who makes sure no condensed tar clogs the exhaust ducts), reliever (who fills in for workers on break), and perhaps other titles specific to the facility. The bench side is divided into the push and coke sides. On the push side job titles include pusher machine operator, bench man (who cleans the door), oven patcher (who patches gas leaks), luterman, and reliever. Coke side job classifications include door machine operator, quench car operator, door cleaners, and relievers. Due to the likelihood of combustion gas exposure, all top- and bench-side workers must wear personal protective equipment (PPE). The job requirements of supervisory personnel and "heaters" necessitate that they move through all areas of the battery.[3,4]

Foundry operation

Production process. Foundry work involves pouring hot liquid metal into hollow cavities made in sand. Upon cooling, the sand is broken or shaken off, leaving a coarse casting of the desired shape. The metal can be simple steel, remelted scrap, or complex alloys. In general, foundries are geographically separate from iron and steel production facilities. A typical foundry is shown in Fig. 39-8 and includes the processes shown in Fig. 39-9.

Operations that make up iron and steel foundries are listed below. A worker's job title usually identifies his primary work station as one of the following:

1. Pattern making
2. Molding
3. Core making
4. Melting and pouring
5. Shake-out
6. Fettling

A typical foundry mold includes the basic components of a pattern, a cope (lower section), a drag (upper section), and the cores (Fig. 39-10). This section discusses the basic foundry process. For the interested reader, a more comprehensive discussion of foundry work can be found in the International Agency for Research on Cancer (IARC) monograph on polycyclic aromatic hydrocarbons (PAHs).[97]

Pattern making. The pattern shop makes the detailed, precise model of the final casting, from which the mold is made. Patterns have historically been constructed from wood or metal; therefore pattern shop equipment can include machines, saws, lathes, and planes. Patterns for special castings can be made from natural or synthetic waxes, polystyrene foam, or other single-use, expendable materials. More recently, patterns have been made from reinforced epoxy and polyurethane plastics, adding glues, paints, and solvents to the list of potential exposures. The pattern shop is usually located far from the foundry because of the necessity of keeping the machinery and patterns free of sand and dust.

Molding and core making. Foundry sand, the substance from which molds are made, passes through several processes, including preparation, distribution, shaking, and reclamation. Workers called *molders* make small molds on

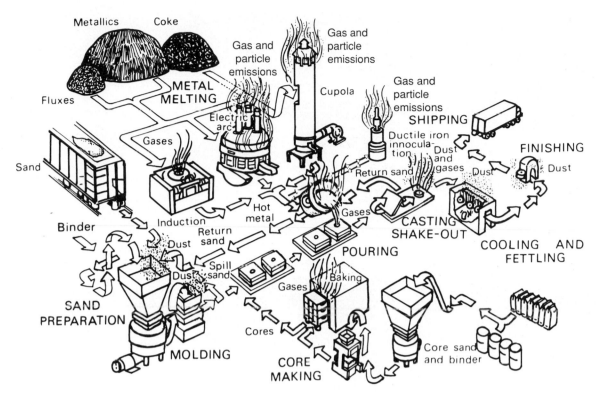

Fig. 39-8. Schematic of the iron foundry process, showing location of furnace and sand preparation, shake-out, and fettling areas. Note the numerous sources of emission, all of which must be controlled. (Adapted from Research Triangle Institute, 1980. With permission.)

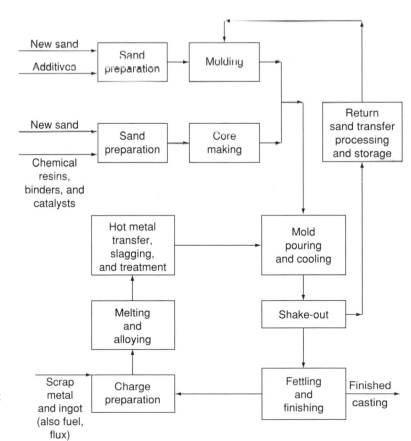

Fig. 39-9. Typical flow sheet of operation in a sand cast foundry. Most job titles can be identified with one of these steps. (Adapted from the National Institute for Occupational Safety and Health, 1978. With permission.)

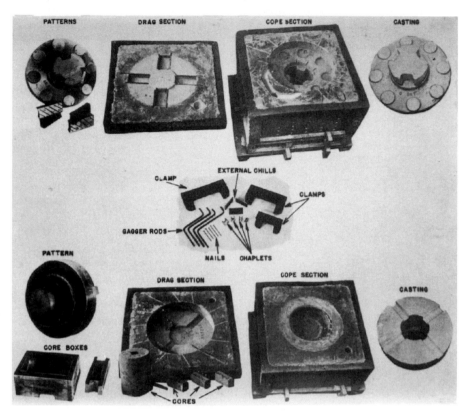

Fig. 39-10. Parts and accessories for preparing typical molds for two relatively small ferrous castings. The cope and drag sections of the mold make up the top and bottom of the casting. After the casting is removed from the mold, it must be fettled and finished to remove imperfections. (Adapted from McGannon HE: Metallurgical coke and coal chemicals. In McGannon HE, editor: *The making and shaping of steel,* vol 8, p 109, Pittsburgh, 1964, USX Corporation. With permission.)

a bench and large molds on the foundry floor or in a pit dug into the foundry floor. Workers pack the sand with hand-operated ramming tools or large molding machines, depending on the size of the mold. Pneumatic-powered vibrating hand tools are frequently used to compress the sand.

Cores are the heat-resistant inserts placed in the molds to form casting features such as cavities and holes. Alternatively, a tool called a *core blower* can be used to blow sand into the mold box to produce small and medium-sized cores.

Melting and pouring. Most of the cast iron produced in U.S. and Canadian foundries is melted in ovens called *cupolas*. The cupola is filled ("charged") through the top with pig iron, scrap iron, coke, limestone, and fluxes and is melted by the combustion of coke, in a process analogous to that of the blast furnace in steel making. Alternatives to coke-fired cupolas include electric induction furnaces and electric arc furnaces.

The molten metal is then transported by a manually operated overhead crane to the casting area in ladles equipped for bottom pouring. The metal is poured into the molds and solidified by cooling in ambient air.

Shake-out. The newly formed cast is separated from the mold and the core in an aptly named *"shake-out"* area. The core box is opened, the cast is pulled or falls out, and most of the hot, dry sand falls away. Mechanical aids such as hand-held pneumatic tools, hammers, or vibrating tables and grids shake the remaining sand from the casting. The sand is collected for recycling, although losses are inevi-

table. This is a step potentially high in silica exposure, and high-volume ventilation is needed to collect the dust and minimize exposure to silica dust.

Fettling. The surface of the cast is usually covered with casting imperfections due to irregularities in the sand mold. The cast is cleaned of sand residues and finished in the *fettling shop*. A rough cleaning is first done manually or mechanically with pneumatic picks or crowbars or by jets of abrasive particles. Hot sand, steel shot, cut wire, or slag pellets are commonly used as abrasives. The operator either wears full protective clothing, including enclosed air supply, or may operate fettling equipment from an isolated, air-supplied control booth.

Binders. Most molding sands are based on the mineral quartz, maintaining a crystalline structure up to temperatures of 1700° C (3100° F). Grain sizes of foundry sands are generally between 0.1 and 1 mm. However, sand dust generated in reclamation processes can be in the respirable size range (below 10 μm). *Binding materials* are added to silica-based sand to improve the adherence, strength, and heat durability required to maintain the cast form when the liquid metal is added.

Many sands are "naturally bonded" by naturally occurring clay contaminants. Artificially added binders may consist of coal dust, synthetic organic oils and resins, cereals, asphalts, and a variety of organic materials (Table 39-1). Urea-formaldehyde has been used as a core binder, sometimes blended with phenol-formaldehyde or with furfuryl alcohol, collectively referred to as furan resins.

Workers may report that they work with "green sand," implying that the binders contain organic additives such as dextrin, starch, wood flour pitch, or pulverized coal dust in addition to clay. During pouring contact with the hot metal causes these materials to partially decompose, emitting hydrogen, carbon monoxide, carbon dioxide, and volatile hydrocarbons.

Table 39-1. Some types of organic sand binders

Oils
  Core oils
  Oil-oxygen no-bake
Hot box
  Urea-formaldehyde
  Phenol-formaldehyde
  Furan
  Modified furan
    Urea-formaldehyde/furfuryl alcohol
    Phenol-formaldehyde/furfuryl alcohol
    Phenol-formaldehyde/urea-formaldehyde
Urethane no-bake
  Alkyd isocyanate
  Phenolic isocyanate
  Polyester urethane
Acid no-bake
  Furan with:
    Phosphoric acid
    Toluenesulfonic acid
    Benzenesulfonic acid
  Phenol-formaldehyde

From the International Agency for Research on Cancer, as adapted from Emory et al. (1978). With permission.

EXPOSURES IN FOUNDRIES AND IN STEEL MAKING (Table 39-2)
Coke production

Coke oven workers are exposed to respiratory hazards primarily in the form of *coke oven gas*. Gas is collected in ductwork above each coke oven and piped to the *"byproducts plant"* for scrubbing, purification, and recycling. Although this is designed as a closed system, there are numerous opportunities for emissions through leaks and from opening and closing ports and doors into the oven during operation and maintenance work. The focus of most research has been potentially carcinogenic substances, including benzene, arsenic, and PAHs. The studies by Masek,[6] Buonicore,[7] and Bjorseth and associates[8] have characterized many of the PAHs in coke oven gas, including benzo-[*a*]pyrene (B[*a*]P), chrysene, and 2-naphtylamine.

Polycyclic aromatic hydrocarbons, named for their multiple benzene rings, are ubiquitous in nature and are formed as by-products in the combustion of oil, coal, and coke. Numerous sites of methylation differentiate the classes of PAHs. After hepatic metabolism most PAHs are excreted in the urine or the bile.

The large number of PAHs preclude the monitoring of each agent. Benzo[*a*]pyrene is readily measured and is commonly used as a surrogate for PAHs in general. Coke oven emissions are also monitored by dissolving particulate emissions in benzene, from which a calculation of the benzene-soluble fraction of total particulate matter (BSFTPM) is made. BSFTPM and B[*a*]P form the basis of quantitative exposure assessment in coke oven workers.

Table 39-2. Exposure limits relevant to the steel-making industry

Substance	TLV (ACGIH, 1994) 8-Hr TWA[5]	PEL (OSHA) 8-hour TWA (CFR citation)
Crystalline silica		
Quartz	0.1 mg/m^3	0.1 mg/m^3
Tripoli	0.05 mg/m^3	0.1 mg/m^3
Cristobalite	N/A	0.05 mg/m^3
Tridymite	N/A	0.05 mg/m^3 (1910.1001)
Asbestos		0.2 fibers/cm^3 for all forms (1910.1001)
Amosite	0.5 fibers/cm^3	
Crysotile	2.0 fibers/cm^3	
Crocidolite	0.2 fibers/cm^3	
Other forms	2.0 fibers/cm^3	
	Proposed: 0.2 fibers/cm^3 for all forms	
Coal tar pitch volatiles (BSFTPM)	0.2 mg/m^3	N/A
Coke oven emissions	N/A	0.150 mg/m^3 (1910.1029)
Benzene	32 mg/m^3 or 10 ppm	1 ppm
	Proposed: 3 mg/m^3 or 0.1 ppm	Proposed: 0.1 ppm (1910.1028)
Sulfur dioxide	5.2 mg/m^3	N/A
Sulfuric acid	1.0 mg/m^3	N/A
Limestone ($CaCO_3$)	10 mg/m^3	N/A
Carbon monoxide	29 mg/m^3	N/A

Data are from the 1993 to 1994 threshold limit values (TLV) of the American Conference of Governmental Industrial Hygienists (ACGIH)[5] and the permissible exposure limits (PEL) of the Code of Federal Regulations (CFR), U.S. Occupational Safety and Health Administration (OSHA) Part 1910.
BSFTPM, Benzene-soluble fraction of total particulate matter; ***TWA,*** time-weighted average.

Breathing zone exposure varies greatly among different jobs, with a nearly 10-fold difference in BSFTPM (exposure limit, 0.150 mg/m^3) between pusher machine operators and tar chasers (Fig. 39-11). Area sampling of B[a]P also demonstrates large variations by work station and by country of operation.

Potentially irritating or asphyxiating noncarcinogenic respiratory hazards include sulfuric acid, carbon monoxide, aromatic hydrocarbons, methane, hydrogen, and nitrogen-containing pyrolysis products, including hydrogen cyanide and ammonia (Table 39-3). Coal itself is a heterogeneous mixture of metals and other compounds, many of which are known to cause disease when absorbed in sufficient quantity.

Foundries

There are numerous respiratory health hazards in iron and steel foundries. Crystalline silica is ubiquitous in foundries using quartz sand, particularly the molding and core-making facilities. Metallic fumes are present during melting, pouring, and welding operations. Metal dust is produced from abrasive grinding operations. Casting and metal operations may emit carbon monoxide. Organic binders in sand molds may contain formaldehyde, furfuryl alcohol, isocyanates, and amines.[9] Polynuclear aromatic hydrocarbons may be formed by pyrolysis of binder organic materials in contact with molten metal. The main airborne contaminants to which workers may be exposed are given in Table 39-4. As with most occupational exposures, risk is determined by dose, which in turn is estimated by a combination of exposure level and exposure duration.

Silica and other dusts. Hundreds of studies of silica dust exposure in various occupational settings have been carried out over the past 50 years. Those most pertinent to foundry work are discussed here.

A nationwide survey of exposure to silica was conducted in Swedish foundries in the late 1960s.[10] The average exposure for workers was 19.5 mg/m^3 in iron foundries and 10.6 mg/m^3 in steel foundries. Heaviest exposure to dust in the iron foundries was during furnace and ladle repair. In sand preparation areas in iron foundries total dust exposure was 16.5, 19.6, and 16.2 mg/m^3 in manual, mechanized, and automated operations, respectively. Dust exposure of individual workers was more severe in the automated plants. In core-making areas of iron foundries, the dust concentration averaged 4.4 and 6.2 mg/m^3 in area samples and personal breathing zone samples, respectively. In iron foundries the average dust exposure of fettlers grinding with portable and stationary machines was 20.8 and 17.2 mg/m^3, respectively. In small foundries an average of 126.9 mg/m^3 was recorded, suggesting that foundry size was a major determinant of dust levels.

The relationship between foundry size and dust exposure was further studied by Koponen et al.[11] As plant size increased from those with fewer than 25 employees to those with greater than 100 employees, dust exposure increased in the sand preparation and melting processes and decreased in shake-out and fettling. This stratification

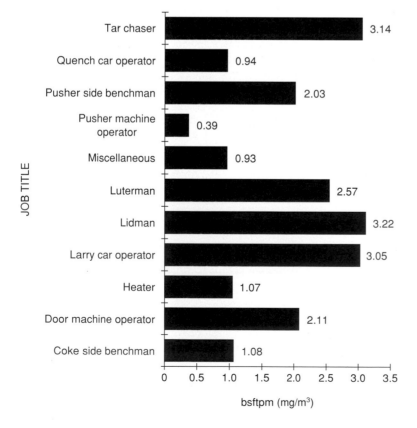

Fig. 39-11. Exposure to benzene-soluble fraction of total particulate matter (bsftpm). Lidman, tar chaser, larry car operator, and luterman were the job titles associated with the highest exposures. (Data from Fannick N, Gonshorit J, and Shockley J: Exposure to coal tar and pitch volatiles at coke oven, *Am Ind Hyg Assoc J* 33:461-468, 1972.

was roughly attributed to the degree of mechanization within the foundries. In automated factories workers were often assigned to the same work station for the entire shift, with little opportunity to be away from high-exposure areas. In small foundries workers often had a cycle of various consecutive tasks, not all with high dust concentration, resulting in a smaller time-weighted average exposure. This relationship was confirmed by a review of breathing zone measurements in U.S. foundries taken by the U.S. Occupational Safety and Health Administration (OSHA) between 1976 and 1981.[12] In this survey 40.6%

Table 39-3. Airborne substances (and classes of substances) found in the coke production industry*

Material	Principal uses or sources of emission
Aldehydes, aliphatic and aromatic	Coke oven operations
Amines, aliphatic and aromatic	Coke oven operations
Ammonia	Coke oven operations
Arsenic, oxides and salts (occurs infrequently)	Coke oven operations
Asbestos (occurs infrequently)	Thermal insulation or clothing
Carbon	Coal storage, transport, preparation and feeding, coke quenching and handling, or soot removal
Carbon dioxide	Coke oven operations
Carbon disulfide	Coke oven operations
Carbon monoxide	Coke oven operations
Carbonyl sulfide	Coke oven operations
Carboxylic acids	Coke oven operations
Hydrocarbons, aliphatic, cyclic, and aromatic	Coke oven operations and by-product handling
Hydrogen cyanide	Coke oven operations
Hydrogen sulfide	Coke oven operations
Mercaptans	Coke oven operations
Nitrogen heterocyclics	Coke oven operations
Oxygen heterocyclics	Coke oven operations
Phenols	Coke oven operations
Polynuclear aromatic hydrocarbons	Coke oven operations
Silica	Coal storage, transport, preparation and feeding, ash removal, or refractory materials
Sulfur dioxide	Coke oven operations
Sulfur heterocyclics	Coke oven operations
Thiocyanates	Coke oven operations

From the International Agency for Research on Cancer. (IARC): Ploynuclear aromatic compounds, part 3. Industrial exposures in aluminum production, coke production, and iron and steel founding, Lyon, France, 1984. With permission.

*This list includes chemicals or classes of chemicals used in or formed during coke production, and the processes during which they are used or formed or during which exposures are most likely to occur. It is not exhaustive.

of 1743 air samples were above 120% of the OSHA permissible exposure limit (PEL), with higher exposure in larger foundries (Figure 39-12) and in melting and cleaning operations (Figure 39-13).

Additional information on foundry silica exposure can be found in reports by Meyer,[13] Capodaglia,[14] and Zimmerman and Barry.[15]

Polycyclic aromatic hydrocarbons. Thermal decomposition of organic binders in foundry sand produces PAHs by way of free radical reactions. As in coke oven gas studies, measurement of a single compound, usually B[a]P or BSFTPM have been used in exposure assessments. The concentration of these materials is highly dependent on the type of binding system, as shown in Table 39-5. Benzene-soluble material varies by a factor of greater than 100 between the low-emitting phenolic urethane and high-emitting green sand systems. The data demonstrate that benzene-soluble material and B[a]P vary independently, complicating dose-response relationships.[9]

Predictably, exposure also varies by job title. Verma and colleagues measured airborne PAHs in 10 Canadian foundries using both area samples and breathing zone samples (Figure 39-14).[16] Total PAH levels were highest for the job titles of melt man, pourer, shake-out, and molder. These groups also had high levels of B[a]P and other specific PAHs.

Metal fumes. Foundry work also entails potential exposure to numerous metal fumes formed by condensation, oxidation, and evaporation (see Chapter 29). Welders in particular may be exposed to chromium, nickel, manganese, and iron. Most of the airborne chromium is water soluble and hexavalent, the carcinogenic form (see Chapter 42).[17] Arc welding of stainless steel can lead to chromium air levels of 0.06 to 0.2 mg/m^3 as (CrO_3) in areas with and without local exhaust ventilation, respectively.[18] Metal fumes in a Finnish survey of 25 foundries[19] showed the major compounds of metal fumes to be iron oxides, magnesium oxides, and zinc oxide, making siderosis a relevant consideration in these workers. There have been no foundry-based epidemiologic studies relating metal fume exposure to disease.

STUDIES OF MORTALITY
Coke oven workers

The association of work in coke ovens with malignancies, particularly lung cancer, has been the focus of numerous epidemiological studies over the last 50 years (see Chapter 34). Excess lung cancer in coke oven workers was first reported by Kuroda in 1937.[20] In a cross-sectional study of a Japanese coking operation, he found 61 cases of cancer, including 12 lung cancers, all occurring in workers in the gas generation works. There were no lung cancers among the 46 malignancies identified in the rest of the plant. Employment in the gas generating plant averaged 15.6 years.

Table 39-4. Airborne substances (and classes of substances) found in iron and steel foundries*

Material	Principal uses or sources of emission
Common airborne contaminants	
Amines, aliphatic and aromatic (e.g., hexamethylenetetramine triethylamine, dimethylethylamine, or aniline)	Urethane binders, amine gassing of urethane resins, or thermal decomposition of urea, urethane, or shell binders
Ammonia	Thermal decomposition of hexamethylenetetramine in shell molding or decomposition of urea or urethane binders
Bentonite	Foundry sand or refractory materials
Carbon	Coal powder, graphite, and soot in foundry sand, coke in cupola melting, core and mold coatings, constituent of ferrous alloys, or electrodes in arc melting and gouging
Carbon dioxide	Combustion of carbonaceous materials in foundry sand, cupola melting, fuel combustion in furnaces, ovens, heaters, and engines, carbon dioxide gassing of silicate binders, or inert gas welding
Carbon monoxide	Combustion of carbonaceous materials in foundry sand, cupola melting, fuel combustion in furnaces, ovens, heaters, and engines, or flame cutting and welding
Chromite	Foundry sand or refractory materials
Chromium and chromium oxides	Steel alloys or melting, pouring, cutting, grinding, and welding operations
Chlorinated hydrocarbons (e.g., 1,1,1-trichloroethane)	Solvents
Cristobalite	Refractory materials, high-temperature transformation of silicon dioxide
Fluorides	Melting, slagging, and welding
Formaldehyde	Urea, phenol, and furan resins or thermal decomposition of organic materials in core baking and casting
Furfuryl alcohol	Furan resins
Hydrocarbons, aliphatic and aromatic (e.g., benzene, toluene, xylene, or naphthalene)	Solvents for binders and paints, pattern resins and glues, core and mold dressings, metal primers, petroleum fuels, or thermal decomposition of organic materials in foundry sand
Hydrogen sulfide	Water quenching of furnace slag or thermal decomposition of sulfur compounds in foundry sand
Iron and iron oxides	Ferrous alloys or melting, pouring, cutting, grinding, and welding operations
Isocyanates (e.g., 4,4'-methylenediphenyl diisocyanate)	Urethane resins or thermal decomposition of urethane binders in foundry sands
Lead and lead oxides	Scrap melting or spray painting operations
Magnesium and magnesium oxide	Inoculation process in production of nodular iron
Manganese and manganese oxides	Ferrous alloys or melting, pouring, cutting, grinding and welding operations
Nickel and nickel oxides	Steel alloys or melting, pouring, cutting, grinding, and welding operations
Nitrogen oxides	Thermal decomposition of urea or urethane binders in foundry sand, flame cutting and welding, or internal combustion engines
Olivine	Foundry sand or refractory materials
Phenols (e.g., cresol, phenol, or xylenol)	Phenolic binders or thermal decomposition of organic materials in foundry sand
Polynuclear aromatic hydrocarbons	Coal tar pitch, thermal decomposition of carbonaceous materials in foundry sand, fuel combustion in furnaces, ovens, heaters, and engines
Silica, quartz	Foundry sand, refractory materials, or sandblasting
Sulfur dioxide	Combustion of sulfurous fuels, sulfur dioxide gassing, or decomposition of furan resins
Tridymite	Refractory materials or high-temperature phase transformation of quartz
Vanadium and vanadium oxides	Steel alloying
Zinc and zinc oxides	Scrap melting
Zircon	Foundry sand or refractory materials
Other airborne contaminants	
Acrolein	Thermal decomposition of vegetable oils in core baking and casting

Continued.

Table 39-4. Airborne substances (and classes of substances) found in iron and steel foundries*—cont'd

Material	Principal uses or sources of emission
Alcohols, aliphatic (e.g., isopropanol)	Solvents for binders and paints, carriers for core and mold dressings, or components of urethane resins
Asbestos	Thermal or electrical insulation in furnaces and ovens or coverings, troughs, and clothing in pouring areas
Cadmium and cadmium oxide	Scrap melting
Calcium carbide, calcium carbonate, calcium silicide, or calcium oxide	Melting, alloying, and slagging operations
Carbon disulfide	Decomposition of furan resins with sulfonic acid catalysts
Carbonyl disulfide	Decomposition of furan resins with sulfonic acid catalysts
Copper and copper oxides	Scrap melting or arc gouging with coated carbon electrodes
Cyanides (e.g., hydrogen cyanide)	Thermal decomposition of urea or urethane binders or heat treatment of special castings
Esters (e.g., glycerol diacetate or butyl acetate)	Ester silicate process or foundry solvents
Ethyl silicate	Silicate binders
Ferrochromium, ferromanganese, ferromolybdenum, ferrosilicon, or ferrovanadium	Melting and alloying
Methylethylketone peroxide	Sulfur dioxide gassing process
Nitrogen heterocyclics (e.g., pyridine)	Coal tar pitch or thermal decomposition of carbonaceous materials in foundry sand
Nitrosamines (e.g., N-nitrosodimethylamine or N-nitrosodiethylamine)	Reaction of nitrogen oxides with amines in foundry sand
Oxygen heterocyclics (e.g., furan or methylfuran)	Furan resins
Ozone	Inert gas welding
Phosphine	Reaction of water with phosphides in ferroalloys, decomposition of furan binder, or furan resins catalyzed with phosphoric acid
Phosphoric acid	Catalyst for furan resins
Radon	Zircon sands
Sulfonic acids (e.g., toluene/sulfonic acid)	Catalyst for furan resins
Sulfur heterocyclics (e.g., thiophene)	Decomposition of furan resins
Talc	Core and mold dressings

From the International Agency for Research on Cancer, (IARC): Polynuclear aromatic compounds, part 3. Industrial exposures in aluminum production, coal gasification, coke production, and iron and steel founding, Lyon, France, 1984. With permission

*This list includes chemicals (or classes of chemicals) used or formed in iron and steel founding operations, and the processes during which they are used or formed or during which exposures are most likely to occur. It is not exhaustive.

Table 39-5. Relative total weights of particulate matter, benzene-soluble materials, and benzo[a]pyrene recovered from emissions from approximately equal amounts of binder sands*

Binder system	Particulate matter (mg)	Benzene-soluble materials (mg)	Benzo[a]pyrene (mg)*
Green sand	1652	1021	1.2
Dry sand	430	405	2.5
Sodium silicate ester	17	13	0.01
Core oil	472	355	0.30
Alkyd isocyanate	74	21	0.02
Phenolic urethane	23	7	0.007
Phenolic no-bake	66	61	0.002
Zero-nitrogen furan	359	125	0.016
Medium-nitrogen furan	50	10	0.012
Furan hot box	211	181	0.002
Phenolic hot box	195	75	0.006
Shell phenolic	157	107	0.21

From the International Agency for Research on Cancer, (IARC): Polynuclear aromatic compounds, part 3. Industrial exposures in aluminum production, coal gasification, coke production, and iron and steel founding, Lyon, France, 1984, as adapted from the Southern Research Institute.[9] With permission from the American Foundrymen's Society.

*Amounts of benzo[a]pyrene analyzed are very small, and there could be a 20% error in analysis. They were calculated by assuming a carbon monoxide dilution of 50 ml/m^3.

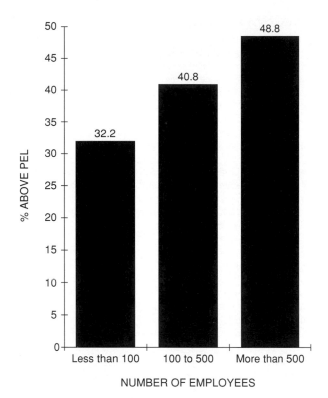

Fig. 39-12. Relationship between foundry size and exposure to silica. Larger foundries were associated with higher exposures, possibly due to higher production rates and single-job assignments. PEL, Permissible exposure limit. (Data from Oudiz J, Brown J, Ayer HE, et al: A report on silica exposure levels in United States foundries, *Am Ind Hyg Assoc J* 44:374-376, 1983.)

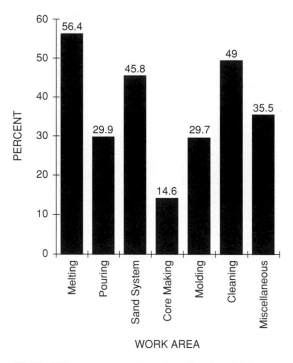

Fig. 39-13. Silica exposure. Samples showing high exposure (more than 120% of the permissible exposure limit) were most common in the melting, cleaning, and sand system areas of the foundry. (Data from Oudiz J, Brown J, Ayer HE, et al: A report on silica exposure levels in United States foundries, *Am Ind Hyg Assoc J* 44:374-376, 1983.)

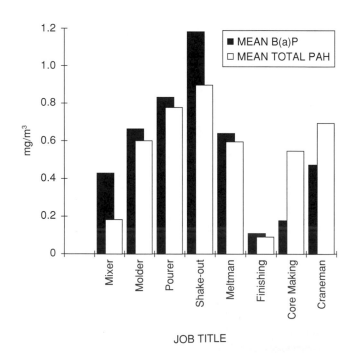

Fig. 39-14. Foundry exposure to polycyclic aromatic hydrocarbons (PAH) and benzo[*a*]pyrene [B(a)P] by job title. Shake-out, pourer, molder, and meltman were the job titles associated with the highest exposures. (Data from Verma DK, Muir DCF, Cunliffe S, et al: Polycyclic aromatic hydrocarbons in Ontario foundry environments, *Ann Occup Hyg* 25:17-25, 1982.)

This cohort formed the basis of several other studies. In 1938 Kawahata reported a total of 21 lung cancers among workers from the gas works.[21] An additional 6 lung cancer cases occurring between 1946 and 1953 were added by Kawai and coworkers[22] and 4 more cases occurring between 1954 and 1960. Kawai's group reported a follow-up study of 504 men working in the gas generating plant at the time of its closure in 1953.[23] Subjects were followed up through 1965 using plant records to identify death until the retirement age of 55. Compared with the remaining 25,000 workers in the steel plant, the relative risk of lung cancer for men over the age of 46 in the gas works was 44. Consistent with the concept of long latency periods for cancer, no case occurred in men younger than 45. These investigators also identified a dose-response rate with a relative risk of 18 for those employed less than 10 years, 33 for those with 10 to 19 years of employment, and 136 for those with more than 20 years of exposure. A significant limitation was that cigarette smoking was not controlled for in this study.

Cancer deaths in an English coking plant cohort were reported for the period of 1949 to 1954 by Reid and Buck.[24] Eight thousand workers identified from a plant census in 1952 were compared with a "large industrial population."

The authors concluded that there was no increase in the risk of lung cancer associated with work in the coke ovens. This study has been criticized because it was limited to workers active in 1949, with only 6 years of follow-up. In addition, death rates for retired workers were not adjusted for age.

The largest series of modern epidemiologic studies of the steel industry was done at the University of Pittsburgh Graduate School of Public Health by Lloyd, Ciocco, and Redmond. In 1962 the Department of Biostatistics, under contract with the National Cancer Institute and with the cooperation of Allegheny County (Pennsylvania) steel companies, assembled a cohort of almost 60,000 workers. The cohort consisted of men employed in seven steel plants in Allegheny County in 1953, approximately 62% of all men working in basic U.S. iron and steel production that year. Lloyd and Ciocco focused on coke oven workers in a 1969 study.[25] For males who had worked in the coke plant for 5 years or more, the standardized mortality ratio (SMR) for malignant neoplasms was 102 for whites and 204 for nonwhites. All of the cancer excess in nonwhites was due to respiratory tract cancers, with an SMR of 342. This cohort was further studied, comparing workers in oven and nonoven areas, employed through 1953.[26] The SMR for respiratory cancers was elevated among all workers in the coke plant, highest for coke oven workers (SMR, 248), and substantially greater than for nonoven workers (SMR, 47). Oven workers who had worked for at least 5 years full time on the top of the oven experienced a 10-fold excess risk of lung cancer.

In addition to the two coke oven plants studied by Lloyd and Ciocco, 10 additional plants from various parts of the United States or Canada were included for analyses by Redmond.[27] Follow-up to 1966 was approximately 13 years, with matched controls from nonoven portions of the plant. The combined population experienced significant excess relative risk of lung cancer both for white (2.06) and nonwhite (3.35) men. Workers who worked on the top side of the ovens throughout their employment experienced the highest relative risk of lung cancer, reported as 7.68. A dose-response relationship was also found on the basis of exposure, with full-time top-side workers having a relative risk of 7.24; part-time top-side workers, 2.14; and full-time side oven workers, 1.73. An update of this cohort was published in 1981, extending the follow-up through 1975.[28] Significant excess risk of lung cancer was again found, with a 2.6-fold excess risk for coke oven workers with 5 or more years of exposure.

Follow-up of the original population from Allegheny County steel plants was published by Lloyd in 1980.[29] The excess relative risk for lung cancer in men employed for at least 5 years and working full time on the top side was 6.94. The lung cancer deaths were skewed toward the earlier periods, suggesting a decreasing risk in more recent periods. It is not known whether this is due to decreased exposures with time or simply an aging phenomenon. Nonoven work-

ers also experienced an excess relative risk of 3.87 for buccal and pharyngeal cancers.[30] The control groups in these studies were also steel workers, a population at risk for lung cancer, perhaps leading to an underestimation of the risk for coke oven workers.

In a retrospective mortality study of coke oven workers from the Netherlands, Swaen and coworkers found higher death rates for lung cancer and a higher prevalence of nonmalignant respiratory disease.[31] Chau and collaborators found elevated SMRs for lung cancer (SMR, 238) and unspecified death for workers near the ovens (SMR, 252) and in the workshop (SMR, 433).[32] An unexpected SMR of 228 for unexposed and slightly exposed workers suggests that selection occurred at the time of hiring and makes interpretation of this study more difficult.

Other researchers have studied coke oven workers, using a variety of methodologies. These include a union-based, proportionate mortality ratio study with local controls by Radford,[33] a South Wales population by Davies,[34] a small Swedish population by Axelson et al.,[35] a short follow-up study of English, Scottish, and Welsh workers by Hurley and associates,[36] a smoking-controlled, whites-only study from eastern Pennsylvania by Blot's group,[37] and a study of French retirees.[38] Each had methodologic weaknesses that preclude confident interpretation.

Taken as a whole, epidemiologic studies provide strong evidence linking work in coke ovens to the development of lung cancer. Dose-response relationships have generally been observed, using both time of employment and working position on the coke oven battery, but not in the by-products plant.[39] Polycyclic aromatic hydrocarbons and coal tar pitch volatiles have been suggested as etiologic agents. Based on these studies, the IARC concluded that there is "sufficient evidence" that certain exposures in the coke production industry are carcinogenic to humans, giving rise to lung cancer. The American Conference of Governmental Industrial Hygienists (ACGIH) has classified benzene as a "suspected" human carcinogen and anticipates upgrading it to a "confirmed" human carcinogen in the near future. Other suspected or confirmed human carcinogens relevant to coke oven emission include benzidine, benz[a]anthracene, B[a]P, benzo[b]fluoranthene, and coal tar pitch volatiles.[5]

Foundry workers

Unlike coke oven workers, in whom the exposure of interest is a collective term ("coke oven emissions"), foundry work can involve several specific exposures, including silica, asbestos, metal fumes, and PAHs, each potentially carcinogenic. Therefore, the most one can expect from a PMR or SMR study is to associate lung cancer with foundry work per se or with a specific job title or work area. Defining the etiologic agent is not possible without quantitative dose reconstruction, a rare occurrence.

Mortality studies in foundry workers are particularly fraught with uncertainty due to methodologic problems because increases in overall mortality, when found, tend to be small. Often, analysis of small subcohorts is needed to find elevated rates of malignancy, making statistical significance difficult to achieve. Trends of increased mortality should be expected with increasing exposure, but rarely have they been demonstrated.

Studies finding no increase in lung cancer mortality include an extensive 1970 mortality study in seven steel plants in the United States by Lloyd and colleagues,[40] later updated by Lerer and co-workers.[41] Workers were later divided into groups by Breslin[42] based on extent of foundry work, showing a small but statistically significant excess lung cancer mortality (relative risk, 1.27), but a relative risk of 1.39 did not reach statistical significance in a follow-up by Redmond et al. using the same methodology.[28] No significant excess in respiratory cancers was found in workers employed between 1938 and 1967 in a U.S. study by Decoufle and Wood.[43]

Studies finding statistically significant excess lung cancer rates required subcohort analysis. In a study by Koskela's group, Finnish foundry workers employed between 1950 and 1972 in the subgroup exposed for more than 5 years had an SMR of 270 for lung cancer, but did not otherwise demonstrate a trend with exposure.[44] A statistically significant SMR of 144 for lung cancer was found in the same cohort by Tola and collaborators,[45] but only in jobs with heavy PAH coexposure, such as "floor molders" and "casters." In a Canadian study by Gibson,[46] lung cancer deaths were more frequent in foundry workers between 45 and 64 years of age, but not in those older than 65.

Studies of U.S. foundry workers by Egan[47] and Egan-Baum[48] and their co-workers demonstrated a significant relative risk for respiratory cancer of 1.4 for blacks and 1.8 for whites. However, only workers receiving union benefits (70% of those eligible) were included in the study, making interpretation difficult. Fletcher and Ades studied male British foundry workers employed between 1946 and 1965,[49] using job classification for exposure estimation. Statistically significant lung cancer SMRs were found for several groups, including furnace repairmen (SMR, 125), fettlers (SMR, 203), machinists and maintenance fitter's mates (SMR, 225), and grinders and heat treatment workers (SMR, 356), many of whom had asbestos coexposure. A study in eastern Pennsylvania for the period 1974 to 1977 assigned workers to a job category that he had held for at least 15 years.[37] The highest odds ratio for lung cancer was obtained for foundry workers and mold makers, with a statistically significant odds ratio of 7.1. A recent study of 21,013 foundry and engine manufacturing workers from Ohio found a positive trend between lung cancer and duration of employment, although the overall excess of lung cancer deaths was only 6% to 13%.[50]

In a 1990 review of all available studies of iron foundry workers, Andjelkovich and associates reported an overall lung cancer increase of 43%.[51] However, the lack of trend with time since hire and with duration of foundry employment weakens the association between lung cancer and foundry work. Studies finding increased mortality often found this only in selected groups of workers, usually foundry workers with coexposure to asbestos or to PAHs, such as molders, casters, and coremen, in whom two- to threefold increases in lung cancer mortality have been reported.[52] The IARC considers iron and steel foundry work to be industrial processes causally associated with lung cancer, the probable agents being PAHs, silica, and metal fumes. The IARC has classified crystalline silica as a "probable" occupational carcinogen with limited evidence of human carcinogenicity (see Chapters 24 and 34). The ACGIH considers crystalline silica to be a "suspected" human carcinogen (see Chapters 24 and 34).

MORBIDITY STUDIES
General respiratory morbidity

There are few studies of morbidity in any heavy industry, including the steel industry. However, morbidity was explored as a secondary outcome in several studies. Mayer et al. studied 354 French coke oven workers who retired between 1963 and 1982 for evidence of increased respiratory morbidity.[53] In this small sample of workers, no significant association was found between retrospectively estimated exposure and the frequency of respiratory symptoms. In a spirometric evaluation of 68% of this cohort studied by Chau et al., lung function was negatively correlated with smoking, the presence of a respiratory symptom, and discreet abnormalities on chest radiographs but not with estimated occupational exposure.[54]

Several studies have shown an excess in ventilatory function abnormality and chest symptoms in foundry workers. Obstructive and restrictive abnormalities were found in nearly half of a Vojvodina, Russia, cohort.[55] Marazzine and coworkers reported an increased prevalence of chest symptoms and obstructive ventilatory function in workers who used a binder containing phenol formaldehyde resin, a recognized sensitizer,[56] compared to control workers.[57]

Silicosis (see Chapter 24)

Although silicosis dates to antiquity, pneumoconiosis in foundry workers was first reported in a 1954 autopsy study by Ruttner.[58] The severity of pneumoconiosis was proportional to the length of exposure, estimated as the length of employment. Occupation within a foundry was also associated with pneumoconiosis due to silicosis or mixed-dust fibrosis in a 1956 series by McLaughlin and Harding.[59] Steel fettlers had a very high risk of silicosis and early death, as did sand- and shotblasters. Steel molding appeared to be one of the least hazardous occupations. The highest incidence of radiographic pneumoconiosis among foundry workers in the United Kingdom was also reported to occur among fettlers.[60]

McBain et al. found evidence of some chest abnormality in 14% of foundry workers.[61] The prevalence of pneumoconiosis in this cohort was about 4%, and over 10% in workers employed in the main foundry, fettling, and welding shops in a British survey from the 1950s.[62] In Finnish foundry workers employed between 1950 and 1972 with a mean exposure of 17 years, 3.8% had pneumoconiosis, and this rate increased to 5.5% among those with greater than 10 years' exposure.[63]

Chronic bronchitis

Although chronic bronchitis has been poorly studied for an occupational etiology, it has been widely reported in foundry workers (see Chapter 27). In Karava's study of Finnish foundry workers, the prevalence of chronic bronchitis was related to cigarette smoking, with rates of 11%, 24%, and 61% for nonsmokers, former smokers, and current smokers, respectively.[63]

Becklake has reviewed the epidemiologic evidence relating obstructive lung disease and occupational exposure, and concluded that the evidence probably supports an association,[64] although others disagree with this conclusion.[65]

Allergic lung disease

Although not systematically reported, symptoms consistent with occupational asthma have been described in foundry workers, and appear to have increased in prevalence with the introduction of new binders. Phenol-formaldehyde resin and hexamethylenetetramine and diphenylmethane diisocyanate have been implicated as causative agents.[66] Case studies of hypersensitivity pneumonitis were reported in one foundry worker exposed to PepSet, who also demonstrated IgG to diphenylmethane diisocyanate human serum albumin complex, and in another worker with apparent asthma after exposure to hexamethylene diisocyanate.[67] This remains an area of great potential for study.

Miscellaneous

Alveolar, septal, and perivascular deposits of iron oxide can lead to siderosis, a nonfibrotic pneumoconiosis. The chest radiograph is impressive for nodular shadows, which may be mistaken for fibrotic pneumoconiosis if a precise exposure history is not obtained. In pure iron oxide inhalation there is no restrictive lung disease and no respiratory impairment. However, in the presence of coexposure of a fibrogenic dust, fibrotic lung disease may develop.

Exposure to asbestos may occur in a variety of settings in the steel and foundry industry. Although recent efforts to educate workers about potential exposures have been successful in limiting exposures, workers from previous eras may not have been aware of their exposure. Almost any construction, production, and maintenance function has the potential for asbestos exposure. Ladle, converter, and blast furnace insulation contains asbestos, and repair operations carry a significant risk of exposure. Historically, any heated pipe was insulated with asbestos, and often friable due to inadequate maintenance and repair (see Chapter 20).

Although pure graphite is not fibrogenic, contamination with free silica is common in graphite mining. The manufacture of the carbon electrodes used in electric arc furnaces can lead to graphite exposure and chest radiographic findings consistent with pneumoconiosis.[68] In spite of no known silica coexposure, progressive massive fibrosis has been reported as a rare event in carbon electrode workers.[69]

PREVENTION

Efforts aimed at the prevention of respiratory disease in the steel industry have succeeded in markedly decreasing the elevated risk of lung disease. Through the combined efforts of labor unions, management, and government regulators, steel making has become considerably safer in the last 15 years than it was when most of the mortality studies were conducted. This is particularly true for coke oven operations, in which successful improvement in health and safety was symbolized by the coke oven emission standard enacted in 1976. Silicosis remains an important preventable cause of morbidity and mortality. Primary preventive measures have been made in the areas of engineering, administration, and PPE, whereas secondary preventive measures have been made in medical surveillance and biologic monitoring.

Engineering

The most effective form of primary disease prevention involves engineering changes to minimize exposure. In coke production the driving force for emission reduction was shared by increasingly stringent environmental (the Clean Air Act) and health regulations (the OSHA Act). These improvements have taken the form of gas by-product recycling plants, more reliable equipment with fewer breakdowns and subsequent shutdowns and repairs, and more efficient oven design. Improvements in ventilation, dust collection, and automation have occurred in foundry and furnace operations. Coke oven emissions have been dramatically reduced over the past 25 years (Fig. 39-15). Despite gains in emission reduction and exposure control in coke oven plants, Keimig et al. found that mean breathing zone samples of coke oven emission (BSFTPM) were above the OSHA PEL of 0.150 mg/m^3 for 90% of larry car drivers, 78% of lidmen, and 73% of door machine operators on the coke side during the period from 1979 to 1983.[70] Personal protection equipment is still a necessary component of prevention for these job activities.

Administrative

Administrative preventive programs related to work practices, operating procedures, preventive maintenance and patching of leaks, and safety precautions are now com-

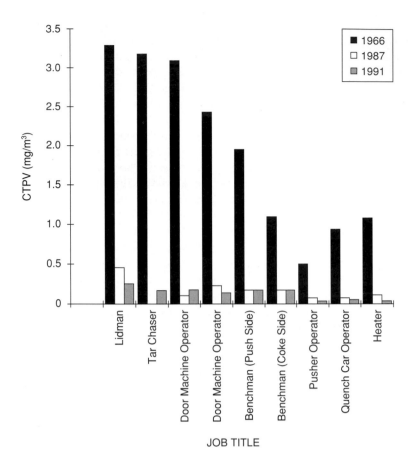

Fig. 39-15. Average exposure to coke oven emissions (CTPV) by job title. Across all job titles, exposure levels have dramatically dropped over the past 25 years. (Data from Black MH: The value of sputum cytology in the early detection of lung cancer in coke oven workers, thesis, Pittsburgh, 1992, University of Pittsburgh Graduate School of Public Health.)

mon. The practice of rotating workers to and from high-exposure assignments, while successful in reducing a worker's time-weighted average (TWA) exposure, remains an unacceptable long-term solution to exposure reduction, particularly those agents that are potentially carcinogenic.

Personal protective equipment

Respirators and supplied air are commonly used to reduce worker exposure. Although these are clearly inferior to engineering controls, in some situations there is little choice. Recognizing the additional cardiac stress and work of breathing involved with using PPE, OSHA issued a formal standard related to respirator use. Whereas much of the program is administrative, involving education, training, and respirator maintenance, a physician is often asked to declare a worker "fit" for respirator use (see Chapter 59).

Biologic monitoring

Although it is clearly inferior to effective primary prevention, biologic monitoring is being explored as a means of confirming exposure and, to a lesser extent, estimating the absorbed dose of PAHs as a means of secondary prevention. These techniques have been evaluated in coke oven workers, and fall into three categories: (1) those that test urine for mutagenicity, (2) those that look for secondary evidence of chromosomal damage in the form of deoxyribonucleic acid (DNA) adducts in peripheral blood cells,[71] and

(3) those that look for evidence of oncogene activation in serum.[72]

Urine mutagenicity. Mutagenicity studies are based on the Ames test, which evaluates the ability of a substance, in this case urinary metabolites, to cause a reverse mutation in *Salmonella* species. Preshift and postshift urine mutagenic activity with *S. typhimurium* strain TA98 was investigated in 7 battery workers, 10 truck drivers, and 3 shift foremen.[73] The exposed workers did not have mutagenic activity significantly different from those of the nonexposed workers. However, smokers demonstrated significantly higher mutagenic activity than nonsmokers. Kriebel compared 12 nonsmoking coke battery workers and 35 nonsmoking office and laboratory workers[74] and found significantly higher mutagenic activity with strain TA1538 but not strain TA100. In a study of top-side coke oven workers, urine mutagenicity was increased only in workers who smoked.[75]

Direct measure of PAHs in the urine of coke oven workers has been assessed by radioimmunoassay.[76] Stratifying workers by low, medium, or high exposure to PAHs and comparing them with unexposed controls showed a dose-response relationship to urinary PAH levels. The PAH urinary levels were about 30% higher during the summer months than in the winter months, consistent with the findings of VanRooij et al., who showed that the skin was the main route of uptake for PAHs, using a pyrene mass balance analysis.[77] The increase in urinary PAHs during the summer months could therefore be explained by a lack of skin covering associated with warm weather. At present, both urine mutagenicity and urinary PAH determinations remain research tools.

Deoxyribonucleic acid adducts. In a study comparing coke oven workers and graphite electrode–producing plant workers with a controlled population of maintenance workers in a blast furnace, Van Hummelen's group analyzed 13 PAHs in the work environment by personal air samplers and measured cytogenetic aberrations in lymphocytes.[78] Urine concentrations of hydroxypyrene was used as an index of exposure. Based on PAH measurements in the work environment and hydroxypyrene concentration in the urine, graphite electrode–producing plant workers were the most exposed. However, they were unable to consistently correlate biologic markers and airborne PAH levels.

In a 1993 community-based study of Chinese women with coal-burning home heating, Mumford and others compared DNA adducts in peripheral white blood cell samples and placental blood from women burning either smoky coal or wood and those using natural gas.[79] No dose-response relationship was observed between the air B[a]P concentration and DNA adduct levels. However, using a group analysis they found that adduct levels were significantly higher in women burning wood or coal than in those burning natural gas.

Kriek et al. analyzed white blood cell DNA from coke oven workers and from workers in an aluminum production plant and demonstrated the presence of PAH-DNA adducts.[80] Comparing coke oven workers and aluminum production workers, they found that, using enzyme-linked immunosorbent assay (ELISA), adducts were present in 47% of the coke oven workers and 27% of unexposed controls, but in none of the aluminum workers. However, using a more sensitive P32 postlabeling assay, the prevalence of PAH-DNA adducts in aluminum workers reached 91%. Therefore it appeared that the sensitivity of the assay is critical, and until the clinical epidemiology of the assays are defined, this remains a research tool.

Just as the mutagenicity assay could not separate smoking effects from occupational exposure effects, DNA adducts are not specific for occupational exposures. Rothman and others[81] measured PAH-DNA adducts by ELISA in California firefighters early and late in the firefighting season concomitant with administering a dietary questionnaire. They found that PAH-DNA adduct levels were not associated with recent firefighting activity but were positively associated with the frequency of charbroiled food consumption in the previous 2 weeks. Cigarette smoking contributes to PAH-DNA adduct formation to an unpredictable degree. However, by analyzing both the lymphocyte and monocyte fractions of blood, 77% of smokers and 22% of nonsmokers had detectable PAH-DNA adducts,[82] suggesting that some groupwise separation may be possible.

In a study of Finnish coke oven workers, Vahakanagas and collaborators[83] studied workers before and after beginning employment in a coke battery, accompanied by air sampling and a detailed questionnaire. There was a small increase in DNA adducts after work in the plant started. Contrary to some other studies, there was no difference between smokers and nonsmokers at any time during the study. Battery workers had slightly increased average levels of DNA adducts compared with nonbattery workers.

As an alternative to DNA adduct formation, cytochrome P-450 activity (measured by the urinary caffeine ratio) as well as urinary hydroxypyrene levels were measured in 45 foundry workers and 52 controls.[84] Air sampling determined total PAH and pyrene concentrations. Smokers in both the study and control groups had raised urinary caffeine ratios compared with nonsmokers. Foundry workers had urinary caffeine ratios similar to those of nonsmoking controls and smoking controls. Only smoking foundry workers had raised hydroxypyrene concentrations compared with smoking controls. It therefore appeared that these two measures were neither sensitive nor specific as determinants of internal dose.

Hemminki and co-workers attempted to establish a dose-response relationship between coke oven work and the presence of DNA adducts and peripheral white blood cells using coke workers, persons living in close proximity to the coke plant, and remote countryside controls.[85] Adducts levels were highest in the coke workers and lowest in the countryside controls.

Some studies have been able to demonstrate dose-response relationships between DNA adducts and exposure. Perera and associates stratified foundry workers by high, medium, and low exposures and found that both PAH-DNA adducts and genetic mutations at several loci increased with increasing exposure category.[86]

Adduct levels fall after a 3-week vacation in top-side workers,[87] as well as in foundry workers,[88] suggesting that workplace exposure was related to the adduct formation.

Serum oncogene protein activity. Using immunoblotting techniques, it is now possible to assay serum for protein products associated with the expression of oncogenes. Brandt-Rauf and colleagues have been able to show that oncogene expression and DNA adduct formation are correlated with exposure to PAH in foundry workers.[89] Oncogene expression may be a useful marker for earlier detection of malignancies in patients with pneumoconiosis.[90]

Sputum cytology. The elevated risk of lung cancer in certain subsegments in the steel industry, notably coke oven workers, has led to interest in screening workers for lung cancer by using sputum cytology.[91] This modern screening technique is based on a program of sequential cytologic examinations developed for Colorado uranium miners. That study led to the establishment of the Early Lung Cancer Cooperative Group in 1972, consisting of cohorts of cigarette smokers established at the Mayo Clinic (Rochester, Minnesota), Memorial Sloan-Kettering Cancer Center (New York), and the Johns Hopkins University (Baltimore), to evaluate sputum cytology and chest radiography for screening lung cancer.[92] The interim data published 2 years into the 5-year study supported the use of these techniques.[93] However, the final analysis failed to demonstrate an effect on survival, except perhaps for squamous cell carcinoma.[94] There was no effect of screening on the number of inoperative cases, the number of cases discovered in advanced stages, and most importantly the number of deaths from lung cancer. In fact, the death rate for the study group was slightly higher than that for the control group: 3.2 deaths versus 3.0 deaths per 100,000 person-years. The lack of effectiveness was largely due to the low sensitivity of the test, reported as 38%, 54%, and 57% in the Mayo Clinic, Johns Hopkins University, and Memorial Sloan-Kettering Cancer Center cohorts, respectively. The specificity was also poor, showing cellular atypia in 10.3% of the cases without lung cancer, primarily in patients with pulmonary infections and asthma.

Prior to final publication of the Cooperative Group's findings, OSHA established a coke oven emission standard and incorporated screening modalities of sputum cytology and chest radiographs into the 1976 standard.[95] The effectiveness of screening in accordance with the coke oven emission standard has not formally been studied. However, in a large coke plant in the United States, Black reviewed 23,000 sputum cytologies collected between 1977 and 1991.[96] As of 1992 only 1 case of lung cancer had been detected by cytology alone and another was detected by a combination of cytology and chest x-ray, leading to a positive yield of 2 cases per 23,143 tests, or 0.000086. The definition of a positive cytology in this study was class 4 atypia. Over the life of the project, the number of false-positive results for atypia of a lesser class was three and five for class 3 and class 2, respectively. These data, combined with the final results of the Early Lung Cancer Cooperative Group, cast serious doubt on the usefulness of this approach for early detection of lung cancer (see Chapter 51).

REGULATORY ENVIRONMENT
Coke oven standard

The OSHA Act of 1970 provides specific standards, with relevance to steel and foundry workers, in the areas of respirator use, coke oven emissions, and asbestos exposure. There is no explicit silica standard, although protection is implied by the General Duty Clause. Respiratory protection and the asbestos standard are covered in Chapters 20, 55, and 59. The coke oven standard contains the following major provisions:

- Worker training/education
- Industrial hygiene surveillance
- 0.150 mg/m^3 personal samples (BSFTPM)
- Engineering controls

- Protective clothing
- Work practices
- Signs and labels
- Personal hygiene facilites and practices
- Respiratory protection
- Medical surveillance

With the exception of occupational physicians, the effect of the coke oven standard on most practitioners falls under medical surveillance.

Medical surveillance and recordkeeping

For most practicing physicians, contact with the Occupational Safety and Health Act occurs in the context of medical surveillance examinations. The OSHA coke oven standard requires that employers make available to all coke oven workers a medical surveillance program. The employer's responsibilities are described in the OSHA Standard CFR 1910.1029, Section J. This document is available in any large library or through National Institute of Occupational Safety and Health– (NIOSH–) sponsored, university-based educational resource centers. Although the Act requires that the employer furnish the examining physician with a copy of the required components of the examination, the basic requirements of the Act are reviewed here.

The medical surveillance examination applies to any employee who is or was employed in a "regulated coke oven area" for a least 30 days in a given year. Identifying covered employees is the employer's responsibility. A regulated area is defined as the coke oven battery, including the top side and its machinery, the coke side and its machinery, the push side and its machinery, the battery ends, the wharf, and the screening station. According to the Act, preemployment examination is required, consisting of the components in Table 39-6. Under the U.S. Americans with Disabilities Act (ADA), enacted in July 1993, this examination is to occur postoffer, preplacement.

The coke oven standard requires a periodic physical examination, but not cytology, on an annual basis for employees younger than 45 years of age or with less than 5 years of employment in a regulated area. For those employees older than 45 or with 5 or more years of employment in a regulated area, examinations must be semiannual and must include cytologic examinations. Periodic examinations are

Table 39-6. Components of a medical examination for coke oven workers

1. Medical and occupational history, including respiratory symptoms and a smoking history
2. Postero/anterior chest radiograph
3. Simple spirometry
4. Weight measurement
5. Skin examination
6. Urinalysis for glucose, albumin, and occult blood
7. Cytologic examination of sputum and urinary sediment

also required when a worker older than 45 or with 5 or more years of employment in a regulated area transfers back into a regulated area. All employees are required to undergo periodic examinations upon termination of employment unless one had been performed within the previous 6 months.

The physician is required to provide the employer with a written opinion, including (1) the results of the examination, (2) any detected medical condition that would place the employee at increased risk of impairment from coke oven emissions, and (3) any recommended limitations on the employee's exposure to coke oven emissions and limitations on the use of protective clothing or respiratory equipment. The Act offers no guidance on what conditions place the worker at increased risk of impairment. However, current lung cancer or severe cardiovascular impairment are reasonable disqualifying conditions. Although the written opinion must also state that the physician has informed the employee of the results of the examination, it is the *employer's* responsibility to provide a copy of the written opinion to the affected employee. In keeping with the ADA, the physician may not reveal to the employer specific medical findings or diagnoses unrelated to occupational exposure or to his or her ability to perform that specific job.

The medical record generated as part of medical surveillance requires special handling, specifically described in CFR 1910.1029, Section M2. In keeping with long disease latency, medical records must be kept for at least *40* years or the duration of the employment plus *20* years, whichever is longer. In addition, the initial chest radiograph, those from the most recent 5 years, any abnormal radiograph and all subsequent x-rays must be maintained for *40* years. The initial sputum cytology slide with a written report, cytology slides from the most recent 10 years, any slide that demonstrated atypia persisting for at least 3 years, and all subsequent slides and written reports must be maintained for *40* years. These records may be kept by the employer in a confidential manner separate from other employment records. However, frequently, a physician is designated to maintain the medical records. It is therefore imperative that occupational records be separated from other medical records that may be routinely discarded.

CONCLUSION

The American steel industry is alive and surviving. Steel production has remained relatively stable over the last 20 years, even though efficiency improvements have drastically reduced required manpower needs by almost two thirds. The hazards of coke oven emissions and silica exposure are now recognized and have been reduced, but not eliminated, by primary preventive measures. In the case of coke oven emissions, the high exposures of the post–World War II era were clearly associated with increased lung cancer rates. Since that time a reduction in exposure to coke oven emissions has also been well documented. However, no epidemiologic studies comparable in size or depth to past studies have been done to quantify changes in lung cancer mortality.

Foundry work remains a potential respiratory hazard in the 1990s, particularly in two settings: those large enough to have full-time work at a single high-exposure work station and those in which engineering controls of dust exposure have not been made or are poorly maintained. Only through the combined efforts of industry, labor, and vigilant physicians can these hazards be recognized and the expectation of a healthy work environment be realized.

REFERENCES

1. American Iron and Steel Institute: 1992.
2. American Iron and Steel Institute: 1988.
3. Fannick N, Gonshorit J, and Shockley J: Exposure to coal tar pitch volatiles at coke ovens, *Am Ind Hyg Assoc J* 33:461-468, 1972.
4. National Institute for Occupational Safety and Health: *Criteria for a recommended standard. Occupational exposure to coke oven emission,* HSM-73-11016, Washington, DC, 1973, US Government Printing Office.
5. American Conference of Governmental Industrial Hygienists (ACGIH): *Threshold limit values and biologic exposure indices, 1993-1994,* Cincinnati, 1993, ACGIH.
6. Masek V: Benzo(*a*)pyrene in the workplace atmosphere of coal and pitch coking plants, *JOM, J Occup Med* 13:193-198, 1971.
7. Buonicore AJ: Analyzing organics in coke oven emissions, *Environ Sci Technol* 13:1340-1342, 1979.
8. Bjorseth A, Bjorseth O, and Fjeldsted PE: Polycyclic aromatic hydrocarbons in the work atmosphere II: Determination at a coke plant, *Scand J Work Environ Health* 4:224-230, 1978.
9. Southern Research Institute: Binder decomposition during pouring and solidification of foundry castings, part II: particulate emissions from foundry molds, *Am Foundrymen's Soc Int Cast Metals J* June 14-15, 1979.
10. Gerhardsson SS, Engman L, Andersson A, et al: Final report on silicosis project, section 2. Aim, scope, results, *Natl Bd Occup Safety Health* 165-183, 1974.
11. Koponen N, Siltanen E, Kokko A, et al: Effects of foundries size on the dust concentration of different work phases, *Scand J Work Environ Health* 2(suppl 1):32-36, 1976.
12. Oudiz J, Brown J, Ayer IIE, et al: A report on silica exposure levels in United States foundries, *Am Ind Hyg Assoc J* 44:374-376, 1983.
13. Meyer PB: Dust measurement in Dutch oven foundries, *Staub-Reinhalt Luft* 33:76-79, 1973. In German.
14. Capodaglia E, Pozzoli L, Massola A, et al: Environmental dust in foundries: risk of silicosis based on dust measurements, *Med Lav* 67:454-464, 1976.
15. Zimmerman RE and Barry JM: Determining crystalline silica compliance using respirable mass, *Am Foundrymen's Soc Trans* 84:15-20, 1976.
16. Verma DK, Muir DCF, Cunliffe S, et al: Polycyclic aromatic hydrocarbons in Ontario foundry environments, *Ann Occup Hyg* 25:17-25, 1982.
17. Tola S, Kilpio J, Virtamo M, et al: Urinary chromium as an indicator of the exposure of welders to chromium, *Scand J Work Environ Health* 3:192-202, 1977.
18. Ulfvarson U: Survey of air contaminants for welding, *Scand J Work Environ Health* 7(suppl 2):1-28, 1981.
19. Tossavainen A: Metal fumes in foundries, *Scand J Work Environ Health* 2(suppl 1):42-49, 1976.
20. Kuroda S: Occupational pulmonary cancer of generator gas workers, *Ind Med* 6:304-306, 1937.
21. Kawahata K: Occupational lung cancers occurring in gas generator workers in the steel industry, *Gann* 32:369-387, 1938. In German.

22. Kawai M, Matsuyama T, and Amamoto H: A study on occupational lung cancer of the gas producer workers in Yawata iron and steel works, *J Labor Hyg* 10:5-9, 1961. In Japanese.

23. Kawai M, Amamoto H, and Harada K: Epidemiologic study of occupational lung cancer, *Arch Environ Health* 14:859-864, 1967.

24. Reid DD and Buck C: Cancer in coking plant workers, *Br J Ind Med* 13:265-269, 1956.

25. Lloyd JW and Ciocco A: Long term mortality study of steel workers. I. Methodology, *JOM, J Occup Med* 11:299-310, 1969.

26. Lloyd JW: Long term mortality study of steel workers. V. Respiratory cancer in coke plant workers, *JOM, J Occup Med* 13:53-68, 1971.

27. Redmond CK, Ciocco A, Lloyd JW, et al: Long term mortality study of steel workers. VI. Mortality from malignant neoplasms among coke oven workers, *JOM, J Occup Med* 14:621-629, 1972.

28. Redmond CK, Wieand HS, Rockette HE, et al: Long term mortality experience of steel workers, National Institute for Occupational Safety and Health Pub No 81-120, Cincinnati, 1981.

29. Lloyd JW: Problems of lung cancer mortality in steel-workers. In: *Air pollution by polycyclic aromatic hydrocarbons: overview and estimation,* pp 237-244, Dusseldorf, Germany, 1980, Verlag des Vereins Deutscher Ingenieure.

30. Redmond CK, Strobino BR, and Cypess RH: Cancer experience among coke by-product workers, *Ann NY Acad Sci* 217:102-115, 1976.

31. Swaen GMH, Slangen JJM, Volovics A, et al: Mortality of coke plant workers in the Netherlands, *Br J Ind Med* 48:130-135, 1991.

32. Chau N, Bertand JP, Mur JM, et al: Mortality in retired coke plant workers, *Br J Ind Med* 50:127-135, 1993.

33. Radford EP: Cancer mortality in the steel industry, *Ann NY Acad Sci* 271:228-238, 1976.

34. Davies GM: A mortality study of coke oven workers in two South Wales integrated steel works, *Br J Ind Med* 34:291-297, 1977.

35. Axelson O, DeVerdier A, Sundell L, et al: The mortality pattern among employees in a Swedish coke oven works, *Nord Foret Halsov* 2:5-12, 1979. In Swedish.

36. Hurley JF, Archibald R, Callings PL, et al: The mortality of coke workers in Britain, *Am J Ind Med* 4:691-704, 1983.

37. Blot WJ, Brown LM, Pottern LM, et al: Lung cancer among long term steel workers, *Am J Epidemiol* 117:706-716, 1983.

38. Bertrand JP, Chau N, Patris A, et al: Mortality due to respiratory cancers in the coke oven plants of the Lorraine coal mining industries, *Br J Ind Med* 44:559-565, 1987.

39. Doll R, Vessey MP, Beasley RWR, et al: Mortality of gas workers—final report of a prospective study, *Br J Ind Med* 29:394-406, 1972.

40. Lloyd JW, Lundin FE, Redmond CK, et al: Long term mortality study of steel workers. IV. Mortality by work area, *JOM, J Occup Med* 12:151-157, 1970.

41. Lerer TJ, Redmond CK, Breslin PP, et al: Long term mortality study of steel workers VII: mortality among crane operators, *JOM, J Occup Med* 16:608-614, 1974.

42. Breslin PP: Mortality among foundrymen in steel mills. In Lemon R and Dement JR, editors: *Dust and disease,* pp 439-447, Park Forest South, Ill, 1979, Pathotox Publishers.

43. Decoufle P and Wood DJ: Mortality patterns among workers in a gray iron foundry, *Am J Epidemiol* 109:667-675, 1979.

44. Koskela RS, Hernberg S, Karava R, et al: A mortality study of foundry workers, *Scand J Work Environ Health* 2(suppl 1):73-89, 1976.

45. Tola S, Koskela RS, Hernberg S, et al: Lung cancer mortality among iron foundry workers, *JOM, J Occup Med* 21:753-760, 1979.

46. Gibson ES, Martin RH, and Lockington JN: Lung cancer mortality in a steel foundry, *JOM, J Occup Med* 19:807-812, 1977.

47. Egan B, Waxweiler RJ, Blade L, et al: A preliminary report of mortality patterns among foundry workers, *J Environ Pathol Toxicol* 2:259-272, 1979.

48. Egan-Baum E, Miller BA, and Waxweiler RJ: Lung cancer and other mortality patterns among foundrymen, *Scand J Work Environ Health* 7(suppl 4):147-155, 1981.

49. Fletcher AC and Ades A: Lung cancer mortality in a cohort of English foundry workers, *Scand J Work Environ Health* 10:7-16, 1984.

50. Rotimi C, Austin H, Delzell E, et al: Retrospective follow-up study of foundry and engine plant workers, *Am J Ind Med* 24:485-498, 1993.

51. Andjelkovich DA, Mathew RM, Richardson RB, et al: Mortality of iron foundry workers: I. Overall findings, *JOM, J Occup Med* 32:529-540, 1990.

52. Palmer WG and Scott WD: Lung cancer in ferrous foundry workers: a review, *Am Ind Hyg Assoc J* 42:329-340, 1981.

53. Mayer L, Chau N, Bertand JP, et al: Morbidity in retired coke oven plant workers, *Am J Ind Med* 22:347-361, 1992.

54. Chau N, Bertand JP, Guenzi M, et al: Lung function in retired coke plant workers, *Br J Ind Med* 49:316-325, 1992.

55. Mikov MI: Chronic bronchitis in foundry workers in Vojvodina: ventilatory capacity in foundry workers, *Arch Environ Health* 29:261-267, 1974.

56. Schoenberg JB and Mitchell CA: Airway disease caused by phenolic (phenol-formaldehyde) resin exposure, *Arch Environ Health* 30:574-577, 1975.

57. Marazzine L, Polosi V, Vezzoli F, et al: Prospective study of airway obstruction in a population with small airways disease, *Bull Eur Phisiopathol Respir* 13:219-229, 1977.

58. Ruttner JR: Foundry workers pneumoconiosis in Switzerland (anthracosilicosis), *Arch Ind Hyg* 9:297-305, 1954.

59. McLaughlin AIG and Harding HE: Pneumoconiosis and other causes of death in iron and steel foundry workers, *Arch Ind Health* 14:350-378, 1956.

60. McLaughlin AIG: Pneumoconiosis in foundry workers, *Br J Tuberc Dis Chest* 51:297-309, 1957.

61. McBain G, Cole CWD, and Shepherd RD: Pneumoconiosis in a group of large iron and light alloy foundries, *Trans Assoc Ind Med Off* 12:17-28, 1962.

62. Gregory J: A survey of pneunoconiosis in a Sheffield steel foundry, *Arch Environ Health* 20:385-399, 1970.

63. Karava R, Hernberg S, Koskela RS, et al: Prevalence of pneumoconiosis in chronic bronchitis in foundry workers, *Scand J Work Environ Health* 2(suppl 1):64-72, 1976.

64. Becklake MR: Chronic airflow limitation: its relationship to work industry occupations, *Chest* 88:608-617, 1985.

65. Morgan WKC: Industrial bronchitis, *Br J Ind Med* 35:285-291, 1978.

66. Low I and Mitchell C: Respiratory disease in foundry workers, *Br J Ind Med* 42:101-105, 1985.

67. Malo J-L and Zeiss CR: Occupational hypersensitivity pneumonitis after exposure to diphenylmethane diisocyanate, *Am Rev Respir Dis* 125:113-116, 1982.

68. Gaensler EA, Cadigan JB, Sasahara AA, et al: Graphite pneumoconiosis of electrotypers, *Am J Med* 41:864-882, 1966.

69. Watson AJ, Black J, Doig AT, et al: Graphite pneumoconiosis, *Br J Ind Med* 16:274-285, 1959.

70. Keimig DG, Slymen DJ, and White O: Occupational exposure to coke oven emissions from 1979 to 1983, *Arch Environ Health* 41:363-367, 1986.

71. dell'Omo M and Lauwerys RR: Adducts to macromolecules in the biological monitoring of workers exposed to polycyclic aromatic hydrocarbons, *Crit Rev Toxicol* 23:111-126, 1993.

72. Brandt-Rauf PW: Oncogenes and oncoproteins in occupational carcinogenesis, *Scand J Work Environ Health* 18(suppl 1):27-30, 1992.

73. Moller M and Dybing E: Mutagenicity studies with urine concentrates from coke oven workers, *Scand J Work Environ Health* 6:216-220, 1980.

74. Kriebel D, Commoner B, Bollinger D, et al: Detection of occupational exposure to genotoxic agents with urinary mutagens, *Mutat Res* 108:67-79, 1983.

75. Jongenellen FJ, Bos RP, Anzion RBM, et al: Biological monitoring of polycyclic aromatic hydrocarbons; metabolites in urine, *Scand J Work Environ Health* 12:137-143, 1986.

76. Herikstad BV, Ovrebo S, Haugen A, et al: Determination of polycyclic aromatic hydrocarbons in urine of coke oven workers with a radioimmunoassay, *Carcinogenesis* 14:307-309, 1993.

77. VanRooij JGM, Bodelier-Bade MM, and Jongeneelen FJ: Estimation of individual dermal and respiratory uptake of polycyclic aromatic hydrocarbons in twelve coke oven workers, *Br J Ind Med* 50:623-632, 1993.

78. Van Hummelen P, Gennart JP, Buchet JP, et al: Biological markers in PAH exposed workers and controls, *Mutat Res* 300:231-239, 1993.

79. Mumford JL, Lee X, Lewtas J, et al: DNA adducts as biomarkers for assessing exposure to polycyclic aromatic hydrocarbons in tissues from Xuan Wei women with high exposure to coal combustion emissions and high lung cancer mortality, *Environ Health Perspect* 99:83-87, 1993.

80. Kriek E, Ban Schooten FJ, Hillebrand MJ, et al: DNA adducts as a measure of lung cancer risk in humans exposed to polycyclic hydrocarbons, *Environ Health Perspect* 99:71-75, 1993.

81. Rothman N, Poirier MC, Haas RA, et al: Association of PAH-DNA adducts in peripheral white blood cells with dietary exposure to polyaromatic hydrocarbons, *Environ Health Perspect* 99:265-267, 1993.

82. Santella RM, Grinberg-Funes RA, Young TL, et al: Cigarette smoking related polycyclic aromatic hydrocarbon-DNA adducts in peripheral mononuclear cells, *Carcinogenesis* 13:2041 2045, 1992.

83. Vahakanagas K, Pyy L, and Yrjanheikki E: Assessment of PAH exposure among coke oven workers, *Pharmacogenetics* 2:304-308, 1992.

84. Sherson D, Sigsgaard T, Overgaard H, et al: Interaction of smoking, uptake of polycyclic aromatic hydrocarbons and cytochrome P450-IA2 activity in foundry workers, *Br J Ind Med* 49:197-202, 1992.

85. Hemminki K, Grzydowska E, Chorazy M, et al: Aromatic DNA adducts in white blood cells in coke workers, *Int Arch Occup Environ Health* 62:467-470, 1990.

86. Perera FP, Tang DL, O'Neill JP, et al: HPRT and glycoprotein A mutations in foundry workers: relationship to PAH exposure and to PAH-DNA adducts, *Carcinogenesis* 14:967-973, 1993.

87. Haugen A, Becher G, Benestad C, et al: Determination of polycyclic aromatic hydrocarbons in the urine, benzo(α)pyrene diol epoxide-DNA adducts in lymphocyte DNA and antibodies to the adducts in sera from coke oven workers exposed to measured amounts of polycyclic aromatic hydrocarbons in the work atmosphere, *Cancer Res* 46:4178-4183, 1986.

88. Lee BM, Yin BY, Herbert R, et al: Immunologic measurement of PAH-albumin adducts in foundry workers and roofers, *Scand J Work Environ Health* 17:190-4, 1991.

89. Brandt-Rauf PW, Smith S, Perera FP, et al: Serum oncogene protein in foundry workers, *J Soc Occup Med* 40:11-14, 1990.

90. Brandt-Rauf PW, Smith S, Hemminki K, et al: Serum oncoproteins and growth factors in asbestosis and silicosis patients, *Int J Cancer* 50:881-885, 1992.

91. Frost JK, Ball WC, Levin ML, et al: Spectum cytopathology: use and potential in monitoring the workplace environment by screening for biological effects of exposure, *JOM, J Occup Med* 28:692-703, 1986.

92. Early Lung Cancer Cooperative Study Group: Early lung cancer detection: summary and conclusions, *Am Rev Respir Dis* 130:565-570, 1984.

93. Berlin NI, Buncher CR, Fontana RS, et al: National Cancer Institute Cooperative Early Lung Cancer Detection Program; results of the initial screen (prevalence), early lung cancer detection: introduction, *Am Rev Respir Dis* 130:545-549, 1984.

94. Ball WC, Frost JK, Tockman MS, et al: Screening for lung cancer: the effects of five to seven days of periodic roentgenographic and cytologic examinations on detection, survival and mortality from lung cancer, *Am Rev Respir Dis* 131:A84, 1985.

95. US Occupational Safety and Health Administration: Occupational safety and health standards. Exposure to coke oven emissions, *Fed Regist* 41:46742-46790, 1976.

96. Black MH: The value of sputum cytology in the early detection of lung cancer in coke oven workers, thesis, Pittsburgh, 1992, University of Pittsburgh Graduate School of Public Health.

97. International Agency for Research on Cancer (IARC): Polycyclic aromatic compounds, part 3. Industrial exposures in aluminum production, coal gasification, and steel founding, Lyon, France, 1984.

Chapter 40

PETROLEUM

Peter J. Nigro
William B. Bunn

HISTORICAL BACKGROUND

Petroleum has been used for fuel and lubricants since the days of the ancient Egyptians; however, the modern oil industry began in the United States in 1859 with the successful completion of the Drake well near Titusville, Pennsylvania. The initial petroleum production leadership was in the state of Pennsylvania and the principal product was kerosene for lamps.

With the discovery of oil reserves in the early 1900s and the consequent reduction in oil prices, the use of oil in the railroad industry increased by more than 10 times and marine fuel sales rapidly increased. Subsequently, industry energy needs for oil and gas production increased exponentially. Shortly after 1900 worldwide expansion of oil exploration and production began in Europe, Asia, and South America.

Despite the conversion of existing energy needs to petroleum, the most economical fuel, the greatest impact was the invention of the combustion engine and its subsequent utilization in automobiles. Post–World War I petroleum sales skyrocketed as a 10-fold increase in consumption occurred. Currently, the petroleum refining industry produces more than 2500 products, including liquefied natural gas, propane, gasoline, aviation fuels, diesel fuels, home heating oils, industrial and marine fuel oils, lubricating oils, and feedstock for the petrochemical industry.

INTRODUCTION

The *petroleum industry* is often considered synonymous with the *petroleum refinery.* Although a significant fraction of the estimated 400,000 to 500,000 employees[1] in the industry work in refineries, many are engaged in other major areas, such as exploration, production, marketing, and distribution. The risks of the exposures of these employees to respiratory toxins vary not only by the area in which they work, but also by the characteristics of the material being handled, the procedures and refining processes used, and the effectiveness of the engineering controls in each process. The spectrum of work environments in the industry can be conveniently broken down into four areas: exploration, production, refining, and distribution.

SOURCES OF EXPOSURE—OCCUPATIONAL
Exploration

During the process of drilling for new oil and gas fields, pulmonary exposures are dependent, to a large degree, on the composition and physical characteristics of the raw material (crude oil or natural gas). These characteristics may vary not only among geographic locations but even by the hole depth. The exposures are primarily composed of four basic families of aliphatic/paraffin compounds, naphthenic structures, and the aromatics. Further characterization, important from a health and safety perspective, is the classification of crude oil as sweet or sour. Sweet crudes have less than 0.05 ft^3 of dissolved hydrogen sulfide (H$_2$S) per 100 gal of oil, equivalent to 5 to 6 ppm H$_2$S by weight. Sour crudes often contain much more, with concentrations up to 180,000 ppm. Due to the high morbidity and mortality rates associated with exposures at or above 1000-ppm concentrations of H$_2$S, drilling operations include monitoring systems to detect its presence in the drilling mud arising from the hole as well as a safety shutoff system. Although normal operations involving drilling seldom result in exposures above the American Conference of Governmental Industrial Hygienists threshold limit value of 10 ppm for H$_2$S, unexpected exposures are possible.[2]

Drilling muds play an integral part in the drilling process, serving to cool and lubricate the drill bit and to transfer rock, sand, and earth from the hole to the surface. Although the muds may provide an added safety feature by holding down subsurface gases such as H$_2$S, these complex mixtures may contain potential respiratory toxins to which the worker may be exposed while mixing and using them.[2] The wide variety and proprietary nature of the muds preclude exhaustive consideration of their role in pulmonary hazards.

Production

Once the well has been completed, the product is channeled to the gathering stations for separation, storage, and eventual transportation to a refinery, gas plant, or other processing facility. The more volatile fractions of the crude oil contained in the storage vessels at these stations provide opportunity for exposure to pulmonary toxins. Head space constituents for sour crude pose a serious risk of H$_2$S exposure to those peering into or sampling storage vessels, where concentrations of this hazardous gas up to 10,000 ppm can be found. Although it is not a primary respiratory toxin, benzene represents another exposure risk.[3]

Some production fields may contain elevated levels of radon.[2] Scale formation in oil field piping and equipment has been an issue for petroleum companies, but in the past these secondary deposits of mainly organic compounds caused by the flow of fluids have been considered nonhazardous. Recently, naturally occurring radioactive radon-226 has been discovered in some scale. Radon-226, an α-particle emitter, is a potential hazard to workers due to inhalation of the dust produced during descaling or pipe-cleaning operations. Also, a higher-than-normal background γ-exposure rate is seen where pipe cleaning is routinely performed. The primary γ-sources are the radon progeny bismuth-214 and lead-214. In surveys of pipe descaling areas at production sites, the highest exposure found by Wilson and Scott was a rate of 1800 μR/hr, compared to a background rate of 9 μR/hr.[4] Exposure to these dusts can be minimized by the use of personal protective equipment.

Transportation of crude and petroleum products by pipeline or ships to the refinery involves similar risks (i.e., H$_2$S and benzene exposures) to those encountered in drilling and production. Although modern vessels use superstructure vents that discharge vapors far above the breathing zones of dock and ship personnel, some exposure may occur when workers draw samples for quality control and assurance purposes.[5]

Figure 40-1 summarizes the major manufacturing processes used in a petroleum refining complex.[1]

The first step in petroleum refining is separation of the crude oil arriving via pipelines and ships to lighter hydrocarbons. The first process used in separation is distillation by heating at atmospheric pressures. The crude is separated into a number of fractions, the lighter fractions having the greatest utility. The lightest fractions from atmospheric distillation are transferred to the gas processing area for separation. The recovery process depends on the components of the mixture and commonly utilizes distillation and absorption processes. Gases are used in other processes such as alkylation to make more useful hydrocarbons. The heavy residue of atmospheric distillation (and other processes) may be separated by vacuum distillation. Vacuum distillation produces fuel and lubricant, oils, and fractions for further processing to gasoline.

After the crude separation stage light hydrocarbon processing consists of polymerization to high-octane gasolines or petrochemical feedstock. Alkylation increases the yield of highly branched high-octane paraffins. This process is catalyzed by hydrofluoric or sulfuric acid. Sulfur (and nitrogen) are removed by hydrodesulfurization. Isomerization and reforming of products catalytically produces gasoline.

Middle distillate processing includes sweetening processes to remove sulfur from low-sulfur (sweet) gases, desulfurization, and various forms of catalytic cracking. Heavy distillation processing includes deasphalting to separate asphalts from heavy oils. The products of deasphalting are bitumen and heavy oils for further processing (e.g., cracking). Heavy hydrocarbons are also broken apart by "visbreaking" (viscosity breaking) and coking (high-temperature, low-pressure cracking) to produce distillates and coke, or can be made into lubricants by various other processes.

Refining

Oil refineries present the appearance of a haphazard maze of pipes, storage tanks, and process vessels. This deceiving appearance belies their careful design to maintain proper processing conditions while minimizing the risk of explosion, fire, or toxic releases. Great effort must be made to ensure the safe and orderly confinement of the flammable materials as they pass through and are modified by each process unit. The number and type of process units found in any given refinery depend on a number of factors, including the characteristics of the crude to be processed, product demands, product economic values, and the avail-

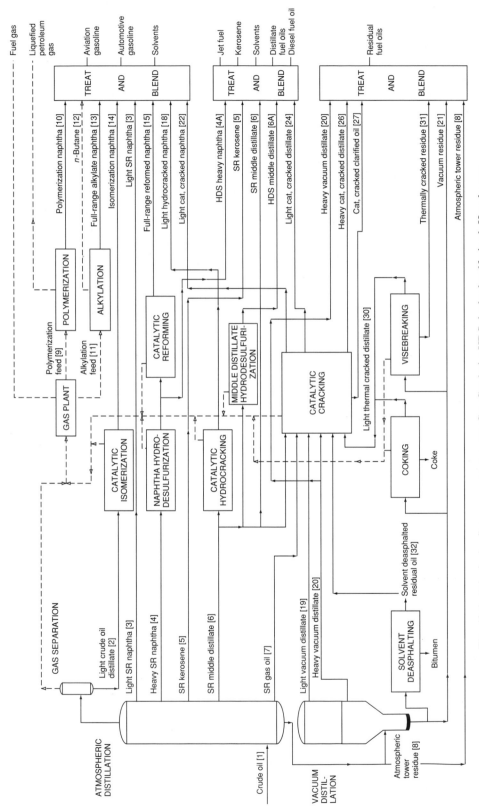

Fig. 40-1. Principal refinery process streams. Cat, Catalytic; HDS, hydrodesulfurized; Hvy, heavy; Lt, light; SR, straight run. (Adapted from the American Petroleum Institute.[1])

ability and cost of equipment and utilities. Thus the type and size of processing units in different refineries show wide variation. There are, however, potential respiratory toxins common to certain units (see Fig. 40-1).[6]

Crude oil must first be treated to remove inorganic impurities, including silt and sand, before it is introduced into the distillation process. Most refineries use desalters to remove these impurities. Depending on the character of the crude, H_2S may be present. The crude is then frac-tionated into various components, based on their boiling range. After the crude is separated into its major fractions, these fractions are converted to products of greater economic value through changes in size and structure of the hydrocarbon molecules. This is accomplished by several processes, such as desulfurization, cracking, alkylation, polymerization, catalytic reforming, and isomerization units.[6]

A major step in refining involves desulfurization. Mercaptans, H_2S, and a number of other sulfur-containing impurities must be eliminated from many petroleum materials in order to produce safe and environmentally friendly products (i.e., low-sulfur heating oils). Desulfurization is currently done in a process unit by treating the oil with hydrogen in the presence of a catalyst. The new catalyst is primarily composed of cobalt and as molybdenum oxides on aluminum. Handling spent catalyst and its dust in the newer units can expose workers to nickel, nickel subsulfide, cobalt, and molybdenum, of which at least nickel subsulfide has been identified as a potential lung carcinogen.[2] However, these materials are usually handled by closed systems. Hydrogen sulfide, concentrated in by-product streams as high as 300,000 ppm, is led to sulfur recovery units for reduction to elemental sulfur. Such high concentrations create exposure potentials, from chronic low-level leaks to immediately life-threatening situations, for the unwary worker performing such activities as manually drawing off accumulated water from a knockdown drum.[2] Workers may also be exposed to sulfur dioxide (SO_2) on or near sulfur recovery units.

The catalytic cracking process uses an alumina silicate–type catalyst, which permits the refinery to produce a high-octane gasoline, kerosene, and heating oils from heavier petroleum fractions. Hydrogen sulfide and carbon monoxide are the primary pulmonary toxins associated with this process. In catalytic reforming units, naphthalenes and paraffins are transformed into aromatics that serve as petrochemical base stocks and high-octane gasoline components. Carbon monoxide contamination of the hydrogen gas produced as a by-product on this type of unit can react with metal catalysts under certain conditions of temperature and pressure to form highly toxic metal carbonyl.[2] The acute and chronic toxicities of these carbonyl compounds, especially nickel, cobalt, and iron, are discussed under the section on specific toxic agents.

Polymerization and isomerization process steps potentially expose workers to catalyst dusts, including aluminum chloride, antimony chloride, nickel, cobalt, and silica-aluminum. The alkylation process that produces high-octane gasoline typically uses hydrogen fluoride or sulfuric acid to assist in the process.

The bottom fractions of the crude oil are commonly referred to as residuum. This material is frequently processed by coking, which involves thermal decomposition in reactors called coking drums, which convert the residuum into higher-value materials and petroleum coke. Polycyclic aromatic hydrocarbons (PAHs) are found in the high boiling fractions of petroleum. Refinery workers may be exposed to PAHs during heavy oil processing steps. This exposure is minimized by handling these materials in closed systems, thereby reducing exposure to these high molecular-weight compounds.[7]

Respiratory exposures to toxins are relatively rare in refineries due to the need for enclosure of the processes during normal operations. Exposures have the greatest potential to occur when the units are prepared for shutdown and personnel entry, as well as nonroutine maintenance, process flow interruptions, and emergencies.

Auxiliary operating facilities. Normal operating conditions are maintained at refineries through the action of a number of auxiliary units. These units function to improve the efficiency of other units, recover valuable products from waste streams, or enable the refinery to meet environmental standards. Units such as hydrogen production, light ends recovery, acid gas treatment, sulfur recovery, tail gas treatment, sour-water stripping, and wastewater treatment are considered auxiliary operating units. Other auxiliary systems include storage tanks, steam-generating facilities, flare and blowdown safety systems, cooling units, machine shops, laboratories, and distribution systems.[6] Respiratory toxins, when present in these units, are not specific to the petroleum industry.

Plant maintenance. A relatively recent change in refinery operations has led to an important change in both the level and types of workers with the greatest potential respiratory exposures. The increased use of automation in modern refineries has moved the process unit operators off the units into control rooms, often a substantial distance from their units. With the ability to monitor large amounts of data from remote sensors and modify process conditions from within the control rooms, operators spend much less time in the operating area. The result of this reduction is a dramatically decreased potential for respiratory exposure for unit operators, as well as a decrease in the number of operation personnel needed for control of the units.

Maintenance of the facility, however, has not experienced the same degree of automation. Unexpected failures, leaks, and changes in the systems are a part of maintenance, as are preventive and scheduled servicing. To a large extent, maintenance workers have assumed the primary "hands-on" role in refineries, and may have the greatest risk of potential exposure to respiratory toxins.

After 12 to 24 months of operation, large sections of a refinery are shut down for inspection, servicing, or refitting. This is known as a "turnaround." During turnaround outside contractors are often employed to supplement plant personnel and perform specialized jobs. As independent contractors, these individuals may perform tasks with significant potential exposure and may not be legally required to receive the medical and exposure monitoring or follow-up provided to regular employees by the refinery.

Servicing of units may involve shutting down and blanking off the unit piping from the remaining refinery process flows. After being cleared with solvent or purged with steam, piping is flooded with air to remove crude fractions, toxic liquids and gases, and wastes. Some catalyst beds are flushed with nitrogen or carbon dioxide. Gas checks are made to verify safe levels of hydrocarbons and H_2S, as well as an oxygen content of at least 19.5%. Despite these precautions compacted debris and sludges may remain accumulated within the process unit or storage tank floors. When physically removed, low levels of residual gases or vapors may be released in the breathing space of maintenance workers.[2]

Many trades are employed in refineries, performing activities such as welding, chipping, grinding, painting, sandblasting, and pipe fitting. The respiratory hazards associated with these activities are exacerbated by the presence of large amounts of insulation throughout the refinery. These activities often involve work on or near asbestos-insulated or refractory ceramic–insulated components. This potential for asbestos exposure is expected to continue for many years, since replacement with nonasbestos insulating material is, for the most part, carried out on an "as needed" basis.[2] However, this exposure is generally very low due to the protective equipment and respirators worn by the workers.[2,8-10]

Distribution

Distribution of petroleum products has the potential for pulmonary exposure to vapors, since bulk transfer of large quantities involves displacement of vapors by the liquid product. Vents on most ships direct vapors above the breathing zones of shipboard personnel, but barges have knee-high or waist-high deck vents rather than the elevated structures found on ships. Rail cars and trucks afforded significant exposures in the past with top-loading equipment. Current vapor recovery systems and bottom loading have nearly eliminated these exposures today.[2]

Summary of exposures

In summary, although respiratory exposure potentials consist primarily of hydrocarbons and contaminants found in crude oil and natural gas, these exposures are minimized during normal operating procedures at the exploration, production, refining, and distribution sites. Exposure potential

to dusts and fumes during maintenance procedures, the use of catalysts, and handling products such as bitumen and coke add to the potential respiratory hazards that may be encountered. Significant reductions in exposure have resulted in the past 30 years, with better control of fugitive emissions, minimization of benzene exposure, and automation of refinery operations. The current level of automation, along with the shifting of many duties to independent contractors, has resulted in the industry's reducing the work force, particularly process unit operators. Fugitive emissions from seals and valves in the vast network of pipes and columns provide low-level potential exposures. Heavier exposures may be encountered during routine maintenance and turnaround operations, from episodic emissions resulting from opening the system for construction and sampling, and in emergencies.[1]

SOURCES OF EXPOSURE—SPECIFIC AGENTS
Sulfur compounds

Sulfur compounds are the most important contaminant of petroleum products from both an economic and a health and safety perspective (Table 40-1). Their presence throughout most of the petroleum process flow, from drilling through refining, gives rise to their nearly ubiquitous exposure potential. Hydrogen sulfide has been historically the best known of the sulfur compounds due to its ability to cause death from respiratory arrest and tissue hypoxia even after a single breath at levels over 2000 ppm. The mecha

Table 40-1. Potential pulmonary toxicants of importance in the petroleum industry

Irritant gases	Particles
Ammonia	Diatomaceous earth
Chlorine	Aluminum compounds
Hydrazine	Cobalt
Nitrogen oxides	Chromium compounds
Phosgene	Nickel compounds
	Silica
	Vanadium compounds
	Drilling muds
Sulfur compounds	**Fibers**
Hydrogen sulfide	Asbestos
Sulfur dioxide	Refractory ceramics
	Mineral wool
Acids	**Sensitizers**
Hydrogen chloride	Platinum compounds
Hydrogen fluoride	Furfural
Phosphoric acid	
Sulfuric acid	
Carcinogens	
Polynuclear aromatics	
Metal carbonyl	
Radon	

nism of action of H_2S is similar to that of cyanide, producing tissue hypoxia through interference with the function of oxidative enzymes, primarily cytochrome oxidase. Although H_2S has an easily recognizable smell of rotten eggs, the use of the olfactory sense as an indicator of exposure is dangerous due to olfactory fatigue after prolonged exposure to concentrations greater than 150 ppm.[7] Compounding this risk is the tendency of H_2S to accumulate in depressions and low-lying areas, where the unwary worker may be exposed to lethal concentrations and quickly succumb with little or no warning or chance for escape. Although the hematologic effects of H_2S are not considered cumulative, since it is rapidly eliminated from the body, sublethal exposures have been shown in humans and animals[11] to result in interstitial (and alveolar pulmonary) edema, bronchitis, and pneumonia. No studies have been published showing long-term health effects from chronic low-level exposures to H_2S.[12]

Sulfur dioxide is a highly water-soluble gas with significant irritating properties that is predominantly absorbed by, and thus has its most significant effect in, the upper airways. The efficient removal of SO_2 by the nasal turbinates and mucosal surfaces prevents up to 98% of the inhaled gas from reaching the lungs, but during exertion, appreciable amounts may be found in the small airways and the alveoli. The airways of the lower lungs are at risk to SO_2 bound to respirable-sized particles in the form of acid aerosols. Sulfuric acid aerosols of particles smaller than 10 μm may be deposited in the tracheobronchial tree, and those that are 1 to 2 μm can reach the alveoli.[7] Although SO_2 and acid aerosols may be encountered throughout the refinery, the highest exposure potentials are found on alkylation and sulfur recovery units. Sulfur dioxide can be considered a primary irritant, capable of causing acute and chronic bronchospastic pulmonary disorders.

Acids

Hydrochloric and phosphoric acids can be found in significant quantities as process chemicals in refinery operations and have been associated with upper airway irritation. The more serious potential threat, however, lies in units using hydrogen fluoride (HF). Hydrogen fluoride is used in the alkylation process to chemically combine low-molecular-weight olefins with isoparaffins to produce gasoline components with high octane ratings.[13]

Although air containing as little as 5-ppm HF causes irritation of the eyes and the nose, serious exposure to HF fumes is rare. Hydrofluoric acid fumes from leaks or inadvertent releases in the alkylation unit may lead to severe and potentially fatal pulmonary complications. Burns from vapor or liquid contact to the oral mucosa or the upper airways may result in severe edema necessitating emergency tracheostomy.

Hydrofluoric acid releases usually involve explosions or accidents producing high concentrations of fumes or exposure of the skin and clothing of the upper body to high concentrations of HF (over 50%). Major and Guelich[31] reported in 1963 three cases of inhalation and skin exposure to 70% HF in which all three individuals developed pulmonary edema and died within 2 hours of exposure. Other cases of inhalation exposure have reported rapid hemorrhagic pulmonary edema, frank pulmonary hemorrhage, and death 30 to 150 minutes after exposure. Delayed effects have been reported up to days after a relatively small exposure, including tracheobronchitis, bronchopneumonia, and pulmonary edema. Systemic toxicity after inhalation of HF fumes is also a serious sequel.[14] Rapid absorption of HF into the bloodstream may lead to metabolic acidosis. The immediate threat to life, however, is the binding of the fluoride ion to serum calcium and the multiple system effects of the resultant precipitous decrease in serum calcium. While chronic exposure to low levels of HF may cause pulmonary symptoms or functional changes, studies have not shown evidence that it leads to chronic respiratory disease.[12] Hydrogen fluoride or hydrofluoric acid exposures should be rapidly treated with the appropriate form of calcium gluconate (i.e., gel, injection, or aerosol).

Irritant gases

Exposures to irritant gases such as ammonia, chlorine, and hydrazine are occasionally found in process units of refineries **(see Chapter 30).** The pulmonary effects of these irritant gases are well known and not specific to the petroleum industry.

Solid catalysts

Solid catalysts pose a respiratory hazard that includes several categories, including particles, sensitizers, and carcinogens. Current refinery technology involves widespread use of solid catalysts to improve the quality of products and meet market demand. Catalysts are used to improve the octane quality of naphthas, convert heavier petroleum fractions into gasoline, and remove contaminants. The form of each catalyst varies, depending on how the process unit achieves desired contact between the catalyst and the reactant. Catalytic cracking units use a variety of acid-function catalysts, including natural clays, alumina-silicates, and synthetic zeolites. Some zeolites are used for ion exchange and selective absorption capabilities. Some classes of naturally occurring zeolites may be fibrous, resulting in a risk for pleural mesothelioma similar to that with forms of asbestos. Refinery uses, however, do not require the fibrous types. Natural clays and alumina-silicate dust present inhalation risks for silica during the occasions of plant turnarounds, process upsets, and catalyst dumping and loading. Reforming and isomerization catalysts are generally alumina with low levels of platinum. Again, because of the closed nature of refinery processes, exposure of workers to catalysts is rare.

Sensitizers

Platinum contained in low levels in the reforming catalyst is the best-known sensitizer in petroleum refining. However, a pulmonary sensitizer with greater exposure potential than platinum is furfural. Furfural is an oily, relatively volatile liquid derived from various cellulosic waste materials, such as oats, rice hulls, and corn cobs. It is used to remove complex aromatics and resins from lube oil stocks that cause low viscosity indexes. Furfural vapors are a strong irritant to mucous membranes of the eyes and the respiratory tract, and it has been suggested by Tarlo[32] that this irritation of the respiratory tract resembles that of sensitizer-induced asthma. This supports a study in Poland in 1984[33] that revealed symptoms of chronic bronchitis in 25% of workers exposed to furfural. Due to studies released by the National Toxicology Program showing evidence of furfural carcinogenicity in animals, furfural exposures have been significantly decreased on furfural extraction units through improved seals and ventilation.

The presence of nickel compounds on process units provides several potential respiratory hazards. In addition to the carcinogenic effects of nickel, nickel sulfate exposure has been associated with asthma, as well as increased susceptibility to pulmonary infections and nasal septal perforation, chronic rhinitis, and anosmia (see Chapter 29).[7] The toxic effects of nickel may be immune mediated, and recent evidence of nickel-induced oxidative bursts in pulmonary macrophages exposed to nickel suggests that this mechanism is an important component in both the toxicology and carcinogenesis of nickel compounds.[7]

Particles

Drilling mud constituents provide potential exposure to respirable particles. Drilling muds are aqueous suspensions of clay, barite, and numerous other compounds. Muds are pumped into a well through the hollow drill stem, passing through the tip of the bit and back up the space between the stem and the walls of the hole. The mud is effective in lubricating and cooling the drill bit, sealing the walls to prevent caving of the hole, suspending the drill cuttings and carrying them to the surface, and restraining the release of toxic gases and fluids through creation of a weighted column. This reduces the tendency for blowouts.[15] Characterizing the inhalational risk from the powdered dry constituents of the drilling mud is difficult, since there is no patent on drilling mud additives, and they are treated by many petroleum production companies as proprietary.[16] In addition, drilling mud constituents vary almost with every site due to different rocks, depths of drilling, sulfur content of the crude or natural gas, and pressure of the well head. Commonly, drilling muds contain surface-active agents, weighing agents, lubricants, and antifungals/antimicrobials.[16] Specific constituents may also include the polyacrylamides used to control viscosity, benzoic acid for temporary plugging subterranean formations, and barium. Barium is a ma-

terial of choice because of its high density, chemical inertness, nonabrasiveness, and widespread availability at a reasonable cost. When used in drilling mud, barite is first pulverized into a fine powder, most of which is of respirable size. Barium for oil drilling contains approximately 92% barium sulfate. Barium sulfate has been known to cause a noncollagenous, nonfibrosing pulmonary picture similar to that of a pneumoconiosis. It has been shown that these findings are reversible with removal from exposure, and that the alveolar architecture remains intact. Many experts consider this condition of nodular granules throughout the interstitium, termed "baritosis," a benign pneumoconiosis because the particles are not fibrogenic and there is limited respiratory impairment.[17] Despite the fact that barite production has grown due to increased gas and oil drilling needs, baritosis is relatively uncommon.[18,19] Indeed, the lack of functional impairment or structural change suggests that this "pneumoconiosis" may be a radiographic finding due to retention of the radiopaque material in the lungs with no significant pulmonary pathology. Further studies are necessary to answer the question of pulmonary disease and barium exposure.

Metal carbonyl forms when carbon monoxide reacts with free metal under certain conditions of temperature and pressure. Hydrogen and nitrogen gases, which are extensively used throughout the refining process, may contain trace amounts of carbon monoxide contamination that may react with metal catalysts and form metal carbonyl. Nickel, cobalt, and iron carbonyls are the most common hazards of this kind in the petroleum industry. The operating conditions normally present during petroleum processing preclude the formation of metal carbonyl. However, circumstances such as initiation or termination of process operations may allow carbon monoxide to contact catalyst metals and form carbonyl. In addition, finely divided catalysts are capable of retaining a considerable amount of metal carbonyl by adsorption, which may result in a potential release.[20] Worker exposures to metal carbonyl are rare but can occur when process units are being shut down and prepared for personnel entry. High concentrations may also occur when the unit is improperly operated, allowing the presence of excess hydrogen with carbon monoxide contamination at abnormally reduced process temperatures.[2]

Since metal carbonyl remains as carbonyl only in the presence of carbon monoxide, it is relatively unstable in air and will dissociate rapidly into carbon monoxide and metal. Half-lives for nickel, cobalt, and iron carbonyls are thought to be 675 seconds, 15 seconds, and 1 to 2 hours, respectively. Nickel carbonyl is acutely toxic to humans by both the dermal and inhalational routes, although the latter is much more important in terms of risk and likelihood of occurrence.[20] Nickel carbonyl is the most toxic of the nickel compounds, with an estimated lethal human respiratory exposure level of 30 ppm. Initial symptoms of toxicity are shortness of breath and chest tightness, followed within 12

Chapter 41

ELECTRIC POWER GENERATION

Edward L. Petsonk

BACKGROUND

The first commercial generation and distribution system for electric power was described in Surrey, England in 1882.[1] Several other systems were established in the late 1800s, and in North America, major expansion of power system coverage took place in the early 1900s. Industrialization in the United States and elsewhere has been accompanied by growth in the electrical supply system, and a close correlation has been observed in developed countries between per capita income and per capita electric power consumption. In the United States, annual power consumption in 1990 was 3040.9 billion kilowatt-hours, and over 511,000 workers were employed by investor-owned electric utilities alone.

The major sources of energy for electrical power in the United States are coal, representing 56%, nuclear fission, 21%, and hydroelectric power, 9%. Certain power stations can utilize other fossil fuels, such as oil and natural gas. In recent years, natural gas utilization has increased somewhat, although since the early 1970s, oil has decreased as a source of power in the United States to an historic low of less than 5%. Some stations also burn refuse and other wastes, which may entail additional occupational considerations. Smaller proportions of commercial electrical energy are derived from geothermal, wind, solar, and biomass.

COAL- AND OIL-FIRED POWER STATIONS
Process description

The burning of coal and generation of steam for turbines represent the most widespread sources of energy used in the commercial generation of electrical power in the United States. Occupational hazards related to coal are dealt with in Chapter 23. After coal is processed at the mine, it is transported by railroad car, tired-vehicles, river barge, or conveyor belt to the power station. At the power station, prior to burning, coal is stored in silos, hoppers, bunkers, or open coal piles. Heavy equipment vehicles may be used to move the coal.

The primary function of all power stations is the efficient conversion of the chemical energy represented by the coal into electrical power available for transmission to customers. Control of boiler ventilation, for example, is generally addressed toward efficiency of boiler operation and control of general atmospheric releases, rather than power station interior air. Depending on actual specific conditions of operation, the various draft fans can either ameliorate or worsen workspace contaminant concentrations. Because these facilities may have a considerable adverse impact on the general environment, pollution controls are important components of their design and operation.

Coal combustion cycle

In newer power stations, coal is pulverized prior to injection into the boilers. The coal is transported via gravity feeds or conveyors to one or several coal mills, where it is pulverized into a fine particulate (approximate 200 mesh). The powdered coal is then blown through pipes into the burner. The operation of the boilers may result in a generally balanced draft (usually slightly negative) or a positive pressure within the combustion zone. A number of facilities have adopted a newer "fluidized-bed combustion" technique. In this technique, pulverized coal is mixed with limestone and then injected into the boiler. Burn efficiency is good, and acids are captured in the alkaline mixture within the boiler, thus reducing the release of acid particles and gases to the atmosphere.

During combustion, coal is transformed into a variety of combustion-related gases and vapors, and a particulate fraction termed *fly ash*. Larger particles settle out from the boiler emission stream in the economizer unit. Further techniques to reduce the release of particles into the atmosphere include the passage of emissions through electrostatically charged plates, which attract charged particles and precipitate them out of the stack emissions, and/or through fabric filters in "bag houses," which physically trap particles. Captured particulate is periodically cleaned from these devices using techniques such as reverse gas flow or "shake and deflate." Gases and particles that remain in the emission stream may be scrubbed before they are released to the stack, using limestone, magnesium oxide, sodium bisulfite, or catalytic (vanadium) oxidation.[2]

Power generation

To allow transfer of the combustion heat to create steam, water is carried through the burner in a series of pipes. The steam is regulated and directed through a series of turbines, losing pressure and temperature while transferring mechanical energy to the shaft of the electrical generator. The shaft rotates a coil within a magnetic field to generate the desired electrical current. Spent steam goes through a condenser, forming water, which is then recycled through the process. Cooling water for the condenser may be passed through a cooling tower prior to release or recycling.

Job activities

A variety of jobs are required for the operation of a coal-fired power station. A number of operators manage the control room and monitor all phases of the operation. Employees working in materials handling are required to unload and store coal. Additional exposures may occur in cleaning bag houses and precipitators and in storage and removal of waste materials, such as fly ash and klinker, which may be accumulated in hoppers or in ponds and transported off-site for landfill or use in construction materials. A variety of other supplies and materials are required. Many other jobs can be classified as maintenance work. Boiler makers and steamfitters repair and replace various components of the combustion and steam turbine systems. Insulation workers manage asbestos and nonasbestos insulation materials that are used throughout the facility. Mechanics adjust and repair instruments and other mechanical systems. Electricians maintain and repair electrical control systems, as well as power generation electrical components. Janitors perform housekeeping and other duties.

Potential respiratory health hazards

A typical 1000 MW coal-fueled plant uses 6400 tons of coal per day and releases 450 tons of particles, 100 tons of sulfur dioxide, 50 tons of NO_x, and smaller quantities of toxic metals and aromatic hydrocarbons. Important environmental releases include carbon dioxide and acid precipitation (SO_2, NO_x).[3] Several occupational exposures in power stations have received attention as representing potential lung hazards (Table 41-1). This section will review the recognized respiratory hazards. Other occupational risks in power stations (e.g., related to noise, systemic toxins, heat, or safety concerns) will not be considered.

Pulverized fuel ash (PFA) derived from coal burning is produced in large quantities. Particle sizes range from 2 to 50 μm.[4] PFA contains 60% to 80% glass particles (aluminosilicates), and 2% to 4% soluble materials. Insoluble crystalline materials total 15% to 30% and include mullite, magnetite, carbon, and quartz, with quartz generally from 1% to 9%.[5] Coal ash contains Al, Si, K, Ca, Fe, and lesser amounts of Li, Na, Mg, Ti, Pb, V, Cd, Cu, Ni, Hg, molybdenum, and tungsten. Enrichment of ash in volatile elements such as Hg, Se, Sb, As, Cl, F, and I occurs by condensation on the surface of small particles during cooling of combustion products in the stack. PFA may be enriched up to 20 times the amounts of these elements that would be predicted, based on levels in the unburned coal.[3] Beryllium, thallium, antimony, and vanadium have also been detected in PFA. Concerns regarding chronic lung injury in power generation have focused on quartz, silicates, and possibly mullite.

The toxicity of PFA has been studied extensively in animal and in-vitro studies. Direct toxicity to the lung of inhaled coal fuel ash appears to be less than that of quartz.[6] Animal inhalation studies have demonstrated an acute inflammatory response in the airspaces and interstitium after exposure to high levels of fuel ash, which tends to diminish several months after the exposure. Ash is noted to accumulate in the regional lymph nodes, and when tested after exposure to some fuel ashes, animals have shown abnormalities of certain immune responses.[7] The significance of these findings to human exposures is unclear.

Mutagenicity and carcinogenicity of PFA have also been concerns. Analyses of ash have revealed that some specimens contain polycyclic aromatic hydrocarbons (PAHs) that are recognized carcinogens.[8] These appear to condense on the surface of particles during cooling of the flue gases. Mu-

Table 41-1. Respiratory hazards in electric power generation

Fuel source	Exposure	Respiratory hazards	Comments
Coal	Coal dust	Pneumoconiosis Chronic bronchitis	Related to coal mining, processing, and handling
Coal, oil	Fuel ash	Pneumoconiosis Chronic bronchitis Asthma	Concurrent exposures to silica and heavy metals; variable mutagenic activity
Coal	Acid aerosols	Membrane irritation Exacerbation of asthma or COPD	
Various	Cooling water	Legionella pneumonia Flulike illness	Microbiologic contaminants implicated
Various	Asbestos	Lung cancer Pleural disorders, including malignant mesothelioma Lung fibrosis	Power plant exposure levels reportedly declining
Various	Welding fumes	Chronic bronchitis Membrane irritation Fume fever Siderosis Lung cancer	Special alloys often encountered
Oil	Welding	Acute bronchitis	Related to vanadium in fuel
Geothermal	Free silica	Silicosis	Drilling and development
Geothermal	Irritant gases	Asphyxiation Membrane irritation Exacerbation of asthma or COPD	

COPD, Chronic obstructive pulmonary disease.

tagenicity studies have shown variable results, with some suggesting a moderate mutagenic potential for the tested materials and others revealing minimal evidence in standard bacterial assays. The source of the tested ash in the facility may explain some of these differences, with materials obtained from the stack showing more activity than ash obtained from the electrostatic precipitators.[9] Other factors may influence the completeness of combustion and the concentration of the constituents of fuel ash, including residual genotoxic hydrocarbons, such as the specific type of coal burned, the presence of associated refuse being incinerated, the type of burner (e.g., fluidized bed), and the conditions of the burn.[10,11]

There has been little formal investigation into the effects of occupational exposures to fuel ash in humans. Bronchoalveolar lavage studies of nonsmoking power plant workers have reported an increase in inflammatory cells in the lung fluids from power plant workers compared with controls.[12] A health survey was performed in 268 current and former male power station workers in England.[5] Jobs held by the workers included boiler cleaners, ash plant attendants, fitters, unit adjusters, and turbine operators. Respiratory symptoms, including chronic cough, chronic phlegm, dyspnea, wheeze, and chest tightness, were increased in those

with over 20 years of tenure in the highest exposure category. After taking smoking into account, a significant exposure effect was found for peak expiratory flow (PEF), vital capacity (VC), and diffusing capacity, but not for forced expiratory volume in 1 second (FEV1) or flows at lower lung volumes. Pleural calcifications were noted on eight chest radiographs, most commonly in men who reported exposure to asbestos. Small opacities 1/0 or greater were found on the chest films of 19 workers. These changes were most prevalent in men with high dust exposure but tenure <20 years, suggesting to the authors a survivor phenomenon. Interpretation of the x-ray changes was complicated by the finding that several workers with small opacities had prior lung illnesses or had worked in other dusty trades.

Bonnell and co-workers[13] reviewed several chest radiographic surveys in a total of 1465 power plant workers that had been performed in 1951, 1954, 1957, and 1960. They reported several cases of radiographic pneumoconiosis, but felt the findings were due to prior employment in coal mines.[13] In 1974, an additional 246 workers were surveyed, and in four workers (1.5%) category 1 pneumoconiosis was felt to be related to power station work. In three of these four, pleural changes suggested that asbestos may have contributed.

A medical and environmental survey of power plant workers was performed by the U.S. National Institute for Occupational Safety and Health (NIOSH) in 1981, and indicated that 4 of 113 workers who received chest radiographs were interpreted as having pneumoconiosis. Three of these four were equipment operators. No exposures outside of the power station could be implicated, and the authors suggested that silica or asbestos exposure may have explained the findings.[14]

Golden and colleagues[15] reported on a 65-year-old man with a 5-year history of exertional dyspnea and restrictive lung impairment who subsequently died of lung cancer. He had worked in a steel mill that was fired by pulverized coal and also as a shipyard boilermaker. At autopsy, the lungs showed honeycombing, with an interstitial inflammatory and fibrotic process. There were asbestos fibers and a striking number of particles that were felt to be consistent with coal fly ash. Although the authors did not definitely attribute the fibrosis to fly ash, they indicated that the quantity of asbestos in the lungs was considerably less than in other cases of asbestosis.[15]

The onset of asthma in relation to fuel ash exposure has also been reported.[16] A 27-year-old man with a history of atopy developed symptoms of dyspnea and wheezing 9 months after beginning work as an attendant at a power station, cleaning filter bags. Peak flow recordings documented work-related airflow obstruction. Exposure to the fuel ash in a laboratory setting resulted in a late asthmatic reaction, with an exposure-associated increase in airway responsiveness to histamine. While working at the power station, severe attacks had precipitated hospital admissions on two occasions, but all symptoms and findings resolved after the man transferred to other work.

Other airborne exposures in coal-fired power plants may occasionally contribute to lung disease. Cooling water may become contaminated with *Legionella* and other microbial species. An outbreak of pneumonia in men working in a power station was attributed to *Legionella* contamination, on the basis of serologic testing and isolation of the organism from a cooling tower.[17] Febrile illnesses of undetermined origin have also been related to occupational exposures in power plant workers.[18,19] Outbreaks of an illness characterized by fever up to 40.6°C, headache, myalgia, nausea, sore throat, and cough, without lung infiltrates, have been reported at several power plants. Of 22 men who worked in cleaning steam condensers with compressed air jets, 21 became ill following an incubation time of 10 to 50 hours from initial exposure.[20] Sickness absence lasted an average of 4.6 days. Precipitating antibody to thermophilic organisms was absent, and the authors suggested that the illness may have been related to inhalation of aerosols containing microbial toxins from the condenser sludge. Although the plants in which these outbreaks occurred were oil-fired, potentially similar exposures to steam condensers occur in coal-fired plants.

An extensive IH survey of workers at 12 coal-fired power plants of the Tennessee Valley Authority was performed from 1974 to 1979.[21] The survey suggested that SO_2 levels above the U.S. Occupational Safety and Health Administration's (OSHA) permissible exposure limit (PEL) occurred in 2% to 8% of the samples. NO_2 levels were generally low or nondetectable, but personal NO levels ranged from 0.48 to 5.0 ppm, and area samples showed NO generally in the 30 to 40 ppm range, with the OSHA PEL of 25 ppm. Airborne mercury was generally low, with occasional higher levels attributed to spills. Airborne asbestos fibers were noted, but average levels declined during the years of the surveys and reached 0.05 fiber/ml in 1979. Vast amounts of asbestos were used in construction of many power stations, and exposures during maintenance and removal still occur. Asbestos-related diseases continue to be recognized in power plant workers.[22] Coal combustion may release small amounts of radioactive elements into the environment.[23] This has not generally been reported to be a significant occupational concern, although after the Chernobyl nuclear accident, ash from some Finnish peat fuels was reported to have important radioactive contamination (also see Nuclear fission power plants).[24] If appropriate controls are not in place, dust levels in coal storage and transfer areas may exceed the current (MSHA) standard of 2 mg/m^3.

The hazards of welding in coal-fired power plants are generally similar to those of other industries (see Chapter 42). To improve strength and resistance to degradation, stainless steel and chromium and molybdenum alloy steels are often used in construction. Additionally, a unique illness, labeled "boilermaker's bronchitis," has been described.

Oil- and wood-fired boilers

Respiratory hazards of oil-fired power plants are similar to those of coal, although ash particles derived from fuel oil are considerably smaller than those derived from coal. Concentrations of trace elements are generally lower, aside from vanadium, nickel, molybdenum, and mercury. Limited animal studies indicate the possibility of greater acute toxicity of oil versus coal fly ash.[3] An outbreak of respiratory illness in power plant workers has been attributed to vanadium pentoxide exposure during conversion of a boiler from oil- to coal-fired (see Chapter 29).[25] After several days to a few weeks of cutting and welding in an area with little ventilation, 74 of 100 workers became ill with symptoms of cough, sore throat, sputum production, dyspnea, and chest discomfort. Lung wheezes and crackles, as well as mild hypoxia, were documented in some cases. The illness lasted from 9 to 82 days. Vanadium is known to contaminate fuel oil, and during conversion work at this facility, VO_5 fumes were measured up to 100 times the OSHA PEL. It was hypothesized that the fumes were derived from a thin layer of fuel oil that had remained after washing of the boiler. Sulfur dioxide and other potential contaminants were not elevated.

Wood chips are also at times used as fuel in power generation, generally at smaller-scale facilities.[26] Health concerns have arisen related to ambient and indoor air pollution from domestic wood burning. Wood smoke is thought to contribute to particulate and PAH levels in homes and has been associated with respiratory illnesses in children and adults.[27] The potential risks from wood smoke or ash from commercial power uses are unknown. Although wood ash is considered less toxic than fossil fuel ash, burning of treated woods may involve exposure to metals and other toxics used in treatment. Additionally, handling of contaminated wood chips can lead to acute respiratory tract illnesses, probably related to bacterial contamination.[28-30] Handling of refuse-derived fuels may also represent a potential risk for exposure to airborne microbial contaminants.

NUCLEAR FISSION POWER PLANTS

The nuclear fuel cycle includes uranium mining and milling, fuel processing, power plant operation, fuel recycling, and disposal of high and low level radioactive wastes. Respiratory hazards in the mining and milling of uranium are discussed in Chapters 31, 34, and 38 and include increased risk of lung cancer, silicosis, and pulmonary fibrosis. In one study, work in a nuclear power station was associated with an increased risk of death from lymphatic and hematopoietic malignancies and bladder cancer, but not lung cancer.[31] Materials specific to the nuclear power stations include plutonium and uranium fuels, with a zirconium or magnesium alloy jacket, boron carbide, silver, indium, and cadmium. Water treatment may be more vigorous in nuclear compared with other power stations to minimize corrosive tendencies. The risks to workers during decommissioning nuclear plants and storage or disposal of radioactive wastes are not completely understood. In addition to the risks of the nuclear fuels and associated materials, the mechanical and electrical maintenance workers in nuclear power plants have many potential exposures similar to those in coal-fired plants.

GEOTHERMAL POWER PLANTS

Geothermal plants recover heat stored deep in the earth's crust. Although use of these sources dates back to the turn of the century, the proportion of current U.S. power production from this technology is small. Worldwide, a minority of geothermal energy sources is used for generating electricity, with the majority being domestic and commercial heat sources and direct power applications.[32] Previously, geothermal technologies relied on hydrothermal convection (water and steam) to transfer heat from the source to the surface location. New facilities may use other fluids to transfer heat, such as isobutane and propane, with attendant hazards. Relevant occupational exposures are greatest during development of the sources and during blowouts. Drillers may encounter high levels of airborne crystalline silica. Other releases include CO_2, H_2S, NH_3, radon gas, and heavy metals. Asphyxiant levels of gases may accumulate with inadequate ventilation. Abatement of environmental H_2S release involves use of caustics and metal catalysts. Maintenance workers may have exposure to welding fumes as well as gases from the wells.

SPECIFIC REGULATORY ISSUES

Electrical power generation is extensively regulated. The Federal Energy Regulatory Commission regulates the sale and interstate transfer of natural gas and oil, licenses certain hydroelectric plants, and controls wholesale rates charged for electricity. The Nuclear Regulatory Commission licenses and regulates construction and operation of nuclear power and other reactors and regulates the management of nuclear materials, radiation exposures, and employee conduct and communications. The Army Corps of Engineers regulates construction and use of projects involving the navigable waterways of the United States. Construction and operation, as well as environmental discharges from electrical power plants, are regulated by the U.S. Environmental Protection Agency (EPA). Limits on stack emissions of SO_2, NO_x, and particles are determined by permits directed at the prevention of significant deterioration in air quality, based on the National Ambient Air Quality Standards, stipulated in the U.S. Code of Federal Regulations (CFR) 40 CFR Part 60 (see Chapter 56). Operation of cogeneration facilities and small power plants is also regulated (18 CFR 292). As indicated, measures taken in compliance with these air pollution regulations may affect worker exposures to airborne hazardous substances. Management of toxic substances used during power plant operations, releases of process fluids to surface waters, and operation of landfills may also have regulatory considerations.

The working environment for power plant employees is chiefly regulated by the general and construction standards and reporting requirements promulgated under the Occupational Safety and Health Act, with regulations pertaining to specific exposures (see Chapter 55). For example, power plant respiratory protection programs must follow requirements of the Personal Protective Equipment standard (29 CFR 1910, Subpart I). Under both construction (29 CFR 1926 Subpart D, for asbestos removal) and general industry standards (29 CFR 1910.1001 Subpart Z), exposures to asbestos are extensively regulated. Worker fiber exposures, respiratory protection programs, use of protective clothing, decontamination, and training are stipulated. Welding exposures that occur during maintenance and repair work are also regulated (29 CFR 1926 Subpart J). Electrical hazards and electrical safety-related work practices are covered by standards (20 CFR 1910 Subpart S and 1926 Subpart K), for example, directed at preventing hazardous atmospheres from fumes during storage battery charging. Although not specifically related to respiratory hazards, many general safety regulations (e.g., walking surfaces, lifts, platforms, power tools, and guards) are clearly relevant to power station work.

HAZARD CONTROL APPROACHES

Strategies for controlling respiratory hazards in power generation are similar to the approaches used in other industries (Chapter 60). Studies reviewed previously highlight the exposures that are most likely to represent hazards. Strict management of exposures from the coal supply and ash disposal is important. To suppress dust, coal piles may be sprayed with polymer coatings, and gravity or conveyor feeds covered and ventilated. Worker exposures during cleaning of bag filters and precipitators should be carefully controlled using engineering controls. Personal protection programs (see Chapter 59) are an important and necessary addition to an overall power house safety and occupational exposure control strategy, to be used during unanticipated/upset conditions, and nonroutine maintenance and repair situations. Maintaining fuel ash in a slurry can limit worker exposures. Operation of boilers with a balanced/negative pressure draft should reduce exposures to oxides of sulfur and nitrogen. The probability of fugitive combustion emissions release into the working areas increases if pressures above atmospheric develop within the boiler. Careful management of asbestos and other insulation materials, including appropriate training of personnel, is of course imperative. Cooling towers and heat exchangers represent a potential source of Legionella and other biologic contaminants. The risk can be reduced or eliminated by monitoring the water temperature and conditions, periodic flushing and cleaning, and appropriate use of biocides. Personnel involved in welding and cutting should be trained in the increased hazards presented by the alloys present, and the potential contamination of surfaces (e.g., vanadium). A comprehensive program of safety and health hazard training is essential and should be integrated with the personal respiratory protection program targeted toward intermittent exposures, such as during cleaning and repair work, which are not amenable to engineering controls.

REFERENCES

1. Bonnel JA: The electricity supply industry. In Harrington JM, editor: *Recent advances in occupational health,* pp 37-54, Edinburgh, 1987, Churchill Livingston.
2. Hill PG: *Power generation,* Cambridge, MA, 1977, MIT Press.
3. Sanders CL: Coal and oil, In *Toxicological aspects of energy production,* pp 181-209, Columbus, OH, 1986, Battelle Press.
4. el-Mogazi D, Lisk DI, and Weinstein LH: A review of the physical, chemical, and biological properties of fly ash and effects on agricultural systems, *Sci Total Environ* 74:1-37, 1988.
5. Schilling CJ, et al: A survey into the respiratory effects of prolonged exposure to pulverised fuel ash, *Br J Ind Med* 45:810-817, 1988.
6. Benson J, Bice DE, Carpenter RC, et al: Comparative inhalation toxicity of quartz and coal combustion fly ash, In Goldsmith DF, Winn DW, and Shy CM, editors: *Silica, silicosis, and cancer,* New York, 1986, Praeger Publishers.
7. Bice DE, Hahn FF, Beason J, Carpenter RC, and Hubbs CH: Comparative immunotoxicity of inhaled quartz and coal combustion fly ash, *Environ Res* 43:374-389, 1987.
8. Srivastava VK, Chauhan SS, Srivastava PK, Kumar V, and Misra UK: Fetal translocation and metabolism of PAH obtained from coal fly ash given intratracheally to pregnant rats, *J Toxicol Environ Health* 18:159-169, 1986.
9. Fisher GL, Chrisp CE, and Raabe OG: Physical factors affecting the mutagenicity of fly ash from a coal-fired power plant, *Science* 204:879-881, 1979.
10. Mozzon D, Brown DA, and Smith JW: Occupational exposure to airborne dust, respirable quartz, and metals arising from refuse handling, burning, and landfilling, *J Am Ind Hyg Assoc* 48:111-116, 1987.
11. Victorin K, Jantunen MJ, Itkonen A, Ahlborg UG, Stahlberg M, and Honkasalo S: Mutagenic effluents from a coal-fired power plant: short-term variations and relation to power load and other load-dependent emissions, *Environ Sci Technology* 20:400-404, 1986.
12. Goodman G, Lapp N, Pailes WH, Lewis D, and Castranova V: Bronchoalveolar lavage in subjects exposed to occupational dusts. In *Proceedings: VIIth International Pneumoconiosis Conference,* pp 1351-1353, DHHS (NIOSH) Pub No 90-108, Part II, 1990.
13. Bonnell JA, Schilling CJ, and Massey PMO: Clinical and Experimental Studies of the effects of pulverized fuel ash—a review, *Ann Occup Hyg* 23:159-164, 1980.
14. Zey JN and Donohue M: *Health hazard evaluation report: Culley Generating Station, Yankeetown, IN.* Cincinnati, U.S. Dept. of Health and Human Services, Public Health Service, CDC, NIOSH: HETA 81-112-1372, 1983.
15. Golden EB, Warnock ML, Hulett LD, and Churg AM: Fly ash lung: a new pneumoconiosis? *Am Rev Respir Dis* 125:108-112, 1982.
16. Davison AG, Durham S, Newman-Taylor AJ, and Schilling CJ: Asthma caused by pulverised fuel ash, *Br Med J* 292:1561, 1986.
17. Morton S, Bartlett CLR, Bibby LF, Hutchinson DN, Dyer JV, and Dennis PJ: Outbreak of legionnaires' disease from a cooling water system in a power station, *Br J Ind Med* 43:630-635, 1986.
18. Lauderdale JF, and Johnson CC: An outbreak of acute fever among steam turbine condenser cleaners, *J Am Ind Hyg Assoc* 44:156-160, 1983.
19. Seifert HE: Illnesses among workers cleaning condensing tubes, *J Am Ind Hyg Assoc* 14:207-209, 1953.
20. Deubner DC and Gilliam DK: Fever of undetermined etiology after cleaning of steam turbine condensers, *Arch Environ Health* 34:116-119, 1977.
21. McFeters JJ: *Industrial hygiene study of TVA workers in coal-fired power plants,* Morgantown, WV, 1981, U.S. Dept. of Health and Human Services, Public Health Service, NIOSH: Report No. PB83-139295.
22. Lerman Y, Finkelstein A, Levo Y, Tupilsky M, Baratz M, Solomon A, and Sackstein G: Asbestos related health hazards among power plant workers, *Br J Ind Med* 47:281-282, 1990.
23. Nakaoka A, Takagi S, Fukushima M, and Ichikawa Y: Evaluation of radiation dose from a coal-fired power plant, *Health Phys* 48:215-220, 1985.
24. Mustonen RA, Reponen AR, and Jantunen MJ: Artificial radioactivity in fuel peat and peat ash in Finland after the Chernobyl accident, *Health Phys* 56:451-458, 1989.
25. Levy BS, Hoffman L, and Gottsegen S: Boilermakers' bronchitis. Respiratory tract irritation associated with vanadium pentoxide exposure during oil-to-coal conversion of a power plant, *J Occup Med* 26:567-570, 1984.
26. Birkhead G, Vogt RL, and Hudson PJ: Investigation of possible health effects of community exposure to fermenting wood chips, *Am J Public Health* 78:318-319, 1988.
27. Samet J, Marbury MC, and Spengler JD: Health effects and sources of indoor air pollution. Part I, *Amer Rev Respir Dis* 136:1486-1508, 1987.

28. Enarson DA and Chan-Yeung M: Characterization of health effects of wood dust exposures, *Am J Ind Med* 17:33-38, 1990.

29. Jappinen P, Haahtela T, and Liira J: Chip pile workers and mold exposure, *J Allergy* 42:545-548, 1987.

30. Weber S, Kullman G, Petsonk E, et al: Organic dust exposure from compost handling: case presentation and respiratory exposure assessment, *Am J Ind Med* 24:365-374, 1993.

31. Smith PG and Douglas AJ: Mortality of workers at the Sellafield plant of British nuclear fuels, *Br Med J* 293:845-854, 1986.

32. Anspaugh LR and Hahn JL: Human health implications of geothermal energy, In Rom WN and Archer VE, editors: *Health implications of new energy technologies,* pp 565-580, Ann Arbor, Ann Arbor Science Publishers, 1980.

Chapter 42

WELDING

William S. Beckett

Welding, a common occupation, has in recent decades become a highly skilled occupational specialty. It is estimated that over 100,000 individuals are employed full-time as welders in the United States, several hundred thousand worldwide, and many more if those who weld part-time are counted.

This chapter will address the diagnosis, treatment, and prevention of respiratory symptoms in welders. Differential diagnoses leading to appropriate therapeutic and preventive interventions will be emphasized.

Welding includes processes used to join pieces of material by heat, pressure, or both. Included in the discussion will be two closely allied processes: *cutting* uses a high temperature heat source, such as an acetylene gas torch and pure oxygen, to burn through metal (Fig. 42-1); *brazing* and *soldering* use a molten filler material introduced between two pieces of the base metal to form a bond without melting the base metal. All these processes involve the potential for inhalation exposures that may lead to acute or chronic respiratory disease.

The presence of oxygen or nitrogen in the molten weld may weaken the bond of many metals, so most welding processes involve an added "shielding" gas around the arc to exclude ambient air. Welders commonly grind or chip their work with power tools once the welding is completed, removing slag and irregularities from the welded surface and smoothing the surface with a high-speed abrasive wheel that may create an additional respiratory hazard in the form of fine metal particles. Welders may also be exposed to a variety of nonrespiratory hazards leading to common occupational injuries—electric current, high temperatures, noise, projected foreign bodies, and ultraviolet light (causing acute keratoconjunctivitis or "arc-eye"), mechanical trauma, and incidental exposures from the work environment such as asbestos and lead. They often work in confined spaces where the process can create a deficiency of oxygen. Although this chapter deals with the respiratory hazards, these other hazards cannot be overlooked when evaluating welders. A comprehensive bibliography of the health-effects literature on welding is published and updated regularly by the American Welding Society.[1] The proceedings of a major international conference on recent welding health-effects research also has been published.[2a]

SOURCES OF EXPOSURE

The primary source of inhaled particulate material in most welding jobs is a consumable electrode (stick) or filler metal electrode, which provides filler material for the pieces of base metal being joined and is partially volatilized in the welding plume in the process. The welding plume is made up primarily of this filler metal, and includes material from electrode coatings, shielding gases, fluxes added to the weld, gases formed by the high temperatures and light of the arc, base metal, and paint or coatings. (Fluxes are materials that form a protective liquid phase around the weld, help to carry impurities away, and may chemically scavenge oxygen from the weld.) Metal fume is formed when vaporized metal condenses in air as metal-oxide particles of respirable size. These particles often further coalesce in air to form chain aggregates.

Metal oxide fume is a particularly important component of the welding plume because of its size—it is small enough

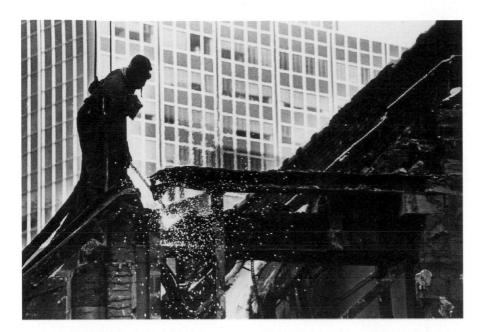

Fig. 42-1. A "burner" (using the oxy-acetylene cutting process) with an acetylene and oxygen fuel system to cut through steel structural beams in building demolition. Cutting and gouging are processes allied to welding, but the purpose is to sever or remove metal rather than join metal. Because materials are often coated with or contiguous with other materials such as paints, and asphalt, there is a risk of inhalation exposure to complex toxic pyrolysis products. This burner appropriately wears a full-face respirator while working. (Photograph by Steve Cagan, Cleveland, Ohio. With permission.)

to deposit in terminal bronchioles and alveoli, distal to the clearing action of the mucociliary system. Thus, when assessing the inhalation exposures of a welder, knowledge of the composition of the "stick" or "wire" electrode is as important as knowledge of the type of base metal used. This information is provided in Material Safety Data Sheets (MSDS) supplied by the welding products manufacturer. Alternatively, the number printed at the base of the electrode (Fig. 42-2) can be compared with Filler Metal Comparison Charts (Table 42-1) to identify the category of electrode,[2b] and the recommended uses for this category of electrode can then be determined from the corresponding American Welding Society Specifications Sheet for that category.

By far the most frequently used welding process is electric arc welding of steel. Over 90% of all welding is performed on carbon and low alloy steels with stainless steels, aluminum, titanium, nickel, and all other metals combined comprising less than 10% of all welding. Although much welding in industry is automated, manual arc welding is still widely practiced and requires the welder to closely observe the weld from a distance of less than 2 feet to assure optimum quality of the weld.

Two of the most common arc welding variants, shielded metal arc welding[2c] and gas metal arc (GMA) welding, are illustrated in Figs. 42-3 and 42-4. In shielded metal arc welding, a solid coating on the electrode, when heated by the arc, volatilizes and melts to form a local shielding gas and protective flux. In GMA welding, shielding gas is introduced over the arc through a nozzle from a tank of compressed gas. (The box includes a glossary of other common terms in welding and allied processes. Welders use a variety of additional terms that may differ from these.)

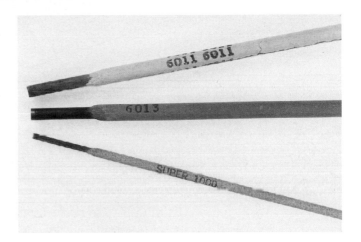

Fig. 42-2. Consumable electrodes used in shielded metal arc welding, composed of a metal core and coating materials that are vaporized by the arc as the core is consumed, and form a shielding gas to exclude ambient air from the weld. If Material Safety Data Sheets are not available, the numbers printed on the coating near the base of the electrodes can be used to identify the composition by using Filler Metal Comparison Charts (see Fig. 42-1 for example) available from the American Welding Society.

Chemical reactions in the gas phase of the welding processes occur not only from the heating of the welding materials, shielding gases, and ambient air, but also by photochemical processes driven by ultraviolet light emitted by the arc. In certain welding processes (such as gas tungsten arc welding of aluminum) the ultraviolet wavelength generated can create sufficient ozone (O_3) from ambient oxygen to create a respiratory hazard in a poorly ventilated area.

Because welding and allied processes encompass a number of different techniques performed on a wide variety of

Table 42-1. Carbon steel covered arc welding electrodes

| | AWS classification | | |
Manufacturer	E6010	E6011	E6012
AGA Venezolana, C.A.	AGA C-10	AGA C-11, C-11ELS	—
Airco Filler Metals	PIPE-CRAFT	EASY ARC 6011, 6011C	EASY ARC 6012
Alloy Rods Corporation	AP100, SW610	SW-14	SW-612
Arcrite Welding Consumables	E6010, E6010M	E6011, 6011P	E6012
Arctec Alloys Limited	—	—	—
Astrolite Alloys	Astrolite 6010	Astrolite 6011	Astrolite 6012
Bohler Bros. of America, Inc.	Fox CEL	—	—
CONARCO, S.A.	CONARCO 10, 10P	CONARCO 11	CONARCO 12, 12D

See AWS A5.1-91, Specification for Carbon Steel Electrodes for Shielded Metal Arc Welding, Filler Metal Comparison Charts, compiled by American Welding Society, AWS FMC-93.
AWS, American Welding Society.

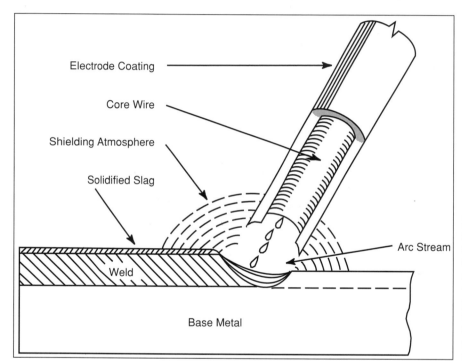

Fig. 42-3. Schematic of the shielded metal arc welding (stick welding) process. The arc stream consists of droplets of the molten electrode (or filler electrode) moving in the direction of the current from electrode to work. The electrode coating, when heated, produces a shielding atmosphere that excludes ambient oxygen and nitrogen. When the work is uncoated metal, most of the respirable particulate in the welding plume comes from the electrode and its coating.

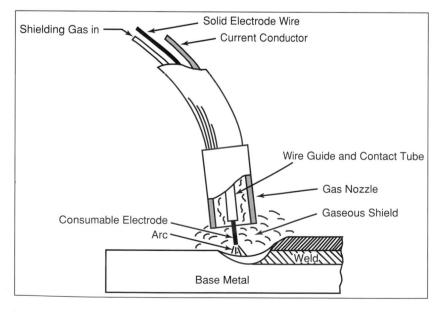

Fig. 42-4. Schematic of gas metal arc welding. Here a consumable electrode wire feeds through the wire guide. An inert shielding gas (usually argon, helium, or carbon dioxide) is flowed continuously over the weld through the gas nozzle, to exclude oxygen and nitrogen.

A glossary of terms used in welding and allied processes

Arc cutting

Cutting processes that melt the metals to be cut with the heat of an arc between an electrode and the base metal.

Arc welding

Welding processes that produce coalescence of metals by heating them with an arc with or without the application of pressure and with or without the use of inert gases or filler metal.

Carbon arc cutting

An arc cutting process in which metals are severed by melting them with the heat of an arc between a carbon electrode and the base metal.

Carbon arc welding

An arc welding process that produces fusion of metals by heating them with an arc between a carbon electrode and the work. No shielding is used. Pressure and filler metal may or may not be used.

Cold welding

A solid-state welding process in which pressure is used at room temperature to produce coalescence of metals with substantial deformation at the weld.

Electron beam welding

A welding process that produces coalescence of metals with the heat obtained from a concentrated beam composed primarily of high-velocity electrons impinging on the joint to be welded.

Flux-cored arc welding

An arc welding process that produces coalescence of metals by heating them with an arc between a continuous filler metal (consumable) electrode and the work. Shielding is provided by a flux contained within the tubular electrode. Additional shielding may or may not be obtained from an externally supplied gas or gas mixture.

Furnace brazing

A brazing process in which the parts to be joined are placed in a furnace heated to a suitable temperature.

Gas metal arc welding

An arc welding process that produces coalescence of metals by heating them with an arc between a continuous filler metal (consumable) electrode and the work. Shielding is obtained entirely from an externally supplied gas or gas mixture. Some variations of this process are called MIG or CO_2 welding (nonpreferred terms).

Gas tungsten arc welding

An arc welding process that produces coalescence of metals by heating them with an arc between a tungsten (nonconsumable) electrode and the work. Shielding is obtained from a gas or gas mixture. Pressure and filler metal may or may not be used.

Gouging

The forming of a bevel or groove by material removal.

Laser beam welding

A welding process that produces coalescence of materials with the heat obtained from the application of a concentrated coherent light beam impinging on the members to be joined.

MIG welding

See preferred terms—Gas metal arc welding and flux-cored arc welding.

Oxyacetylene welding

An oxyfuel gas welding process that produces coalescence of metals by heating them with a gas flame obtained from the combustion of acetylene with oxygen. The process may be used with or without the application of pressure and with or without the use of filler metal.

Oxyfuel gas welding

Welding processes that produce coalescence by heating materials with an oxyfuel gas flame with or without the application of pressure and with or without the use of filler metal.

Plasma arc cutting

An arc cutting process that severs metal by melting a localized area with a constricted arc and removing the molten material with a high-velocity jet of hot ionized gas issuing from the orifice.

Plasma arc welding

An arc welding process that produces coalescence of metals by heating them with a constricted arc between an electrode and the workpiece (transferred arc) or the electrode and the constricting nozzle (nontransferred arc). Shielding is obtained from the hot ionized gas issuing from the orifice, which may be supplemented by an auxiliary source of shielding gas. Shielding gas may be an inert gas or a mixture of gases. Pressure may or may not be used, and filler metal may or may not be supplied.

Continued.

A glossary of terms used in welding and allied processes—cont'd

Resistance welding

Welding processes that produce coalescence of metals with the application of pressure and with the heat obtained from resistance of the work to electric current in a circuit that includes the work.

Shielded metal arc welding

An arc welding process that produces coalescence of metals by heating them with an arc between a covered metal electrode and the work. Shielding is obtained from decomposition of the electrode covering. Pressure is not used, and filler metal is obtained from the electrode.

Submerged arc welding

An arc welding process that produces coalescence of metals by heating them with an arc or arcs between a bare metal electrode or electrodes and the work. The arc and molten metal are shielded by a blanket of granular fusible material on the work. Pressure is not used, and filler metal is obtained from the electrode or sometimes from a supplemental source (welding rod, flux, or metal granules).

TIG welding

See preferred term—gas tungsten arc welding.

Torch brazing

A brazing process in which the heat required is furnished by a fuel gas flame.

From *NIOSH criteria for a recommended standard: welding, brazing, and thermal cutting,* abridged edition, Cincinnati, 1988, U.S. Department of Health and Human Services, Public Health Service, Centers for Disease Control, National Institute for Occupational Safety and Health.[3]
MIG, Metal inert gas shielded arc welded; *TIG,* tungsten inert gas.

---

metals and alloys (and sometimes on nearby contaminants), the list of hazardous substances that can be associated with welding processes is long. Table 42-2 is a partial listing of gases, metals, minerals, and physical agents that may be encountered by welders or those working nearby, their toxic effects, and some of the laboratory tests that may be used to assess exposure or effects.

The rate of generation of these substances in the welder's immediate environment is specific to the welding process used, and is affected by such variables as the current applied, the shielding gas employed, and the welder's personal technique. The concentration of substances in air is also a function of the volume of the space in which welding is being done, and the number of air changes of that space per hour, or the rate of direct removal from the welder's breathing zone by the presence of ventilation. With proper work preparation and the provision of sufficient ventilation to keep the welding plume from the breathing zone of the welder, welding can be performed safely without apparent harm to the respiratory system. But without attention to local ventilation or the provision of a respiratory protective device, some welding processes in enclosed spaces can lead to the rapid buildup of irritant gases, metal fume, and particle.

Arc welding is characterized by the local generation of intensely high temperatures, up to 12,000° C, which can vaporize many metals and produce highly toxic pyrolysis reaction products from other relatively innocuous substances, such as the highly toxic gas, phosgene, from the common chlorinated hydrocarbon industrial solvents often used in metal degreasing. When welding or cutting is performed on metals coated with paints or on metal alloys containing cadmium, zinc, beryllium, or others, high concentrations of highly irritant and toxic substances may be generated leading to acute severe lung injury or death.

Some of the exposures previously measured in association with specific processes are listed in Table 42-3. Welding processes have changed with time, and the kind and amount of materials in the plume may change as processes change. One newer technique, pulsed gas metal arc welding, uses rapid on-off pulsing of the power source, which may reduce the rate of fume formation. Resistance spot welding, a partially automated form of welding using pressure as well as electricity but without the presence of anelectric arc, is usually associated with minimal production of plume.

CLINICAL MANIFESTATIONS

The respiratory effects known to be associated with the welding occupation are discussed here. Each of these is treated separately in other chapters. Emphasis will be placed here on their relationship to inhalation of the welding plume,[4] and the reader is referred to the other chapters for a more complete clinical description.

Metal fume fever

Metal fume fever (see Chapter 17) is the acute respiratory illness most frequently encountered by welders. Many if not most career welders experience at least one episode during their work life. Because the most common cause of this acute and self-limiting febrile illness is freshly generated zinc oxide fume, welders who work on galvanized sheet metal (usually steel coated with zinc) experience metal fume fever unless special precautions are taken to minimize inhalation exposures. Other metal oxide fumes have been reported to cause metal fume fever but not as frequently as zinc oxide. Most welders are familiar with its

Table 42-2. Hazardous agents associated with welding processes and their potential toxic effects

Hazardous agent	Toxic effects†		Supplemental tests‡
	Short-term	Long-term	
Gases			
Acetylene§	Anesthesia (at high concentration)	N/A	
Carbon monoxide	Headache, nausea, dizziness, collapse, death	Cardiovascular effects (cardiomyopathy, exacerbates existing coronary artery disease)	Carboxyhemoglobin (COHb)
Oxides of nitrogen	Pneumonitis, pulmonary edema	Chronic bronchitis, emphysema, pulmonary fibrosis	
Ozone	Respiratory tract irritation (cough, chest tightness), dryness of mucous membranes, headache, sleepiness, fatigue, pulmonary edema, wheezing	Pulmonary insufficiency	
Phosgene	Pneumonitis, pulmonary edema	Emphysema, pulmonary fibrosis	
Metals			
Arsenic	Dermatitis, gastrointestinal symptoms (nausea, vomiting, diarrhea)	Cancer (lung, lymphatic, skin), skin (hyperpigmentation, palmar and plantar warts, hyperkeratosis), anemia, leukopenia, cardiomyopathy, hepatic cirrhosis, peripheral neuritis (numbness, weakness, ataxia)	
Beryllium	Skin (ulcers, dermatitis); conjunctivitis; rhinitis, pharyngitis, tracheobronchitis, chemical pneumonitis	Cancer (lung), pulmonary symptoms (cough, chest pain, cyanosis), systemic weakness, enlargement of liver and spleen	
Cadmium	Pulmonary edema (cough, dyspnea, chest tightness), nasal irritation and ulceration	Cancer (prostate, lung); pulmonary fibrosis, emphysema, honeycomb lung; kidney (proteinuria-low molecular); hematopoietic disturbance (anemia); skeletal (suspected osteomalacia), prostate examination (for workers 40 years and older); anosmia (loss of sense of smell)	Blood urea nitrogen (BUN), complete blood count (CBC), low molecular weight (MW) protein in urine
Chromium(VI)*	Skin irritation (dermatitis, ulcer), respiratory tract irritation, and effects on nose (epistaxis, septal perforation), eyes (conjunctivitis), and ears (tympanic membrane perforation)	Cancer (lung), kidney and liver damage (suspected)	
Cobalt	Pulmonary sensitization (asthma-like reaction), skin sensitization and irritation	Pulmonary fibrosis, thyroid hyperplasia (possible), polycythemia (possible)	
Copper	Metal fume fever,†† nasal mucosa irritation	Not known	
Iron		Siderosis (pulmonary deposition of iron dust)	
Lead		Nervous system (neuropathy-extensor palsy), gastrointestinal symptoms (anorexia, constipation, abdominal colic), nephropathy, reproductive effects (on fetal brain), hematopoietic effects (porphyrin metabolism disturbance)	Zinc protoporphyrin (ZPP)
Magnesium	Irritation of nasal mucosa and conjunctiva, metal fume fever††	Not known	
Manganese	Chemical pneumonitis	Nervous system (irritability, drowsiness, impotence, muscular rigidity, spasmodic laughing/weeping, speech and gait disturbances)	
Molybdenum	Irritation of mucous membranes (eyes and nose)		

Continued.

Table 42-2. Hazardous agents associated with welding processes and their potential toxic effects*—cont'd

Hazardous agent	Toxic effects[†]		Supplemental tests[b]
	Short-term	**Long-term**	
Nickel	Dermatitis, asthma-like lung disease	Cancer (nose, larynx, and lung), upper and lower respiratory tract irritation (nose bleeding, ulcer and septal perforation), renal dysfunction	
Silver		Argyria or argyrosis (pigmentation of skin and eyes resulting from silver deposition)	
Tin		Stannosis (pneumoconiosis resulting from inhalation of tin oxide)	
Titanium		Pneumoconiosis	
Tungsten‡‡	Conjunctivitis, upper respiratory tract irritation (cough, dyspnea)	Extrinsic asthma, pneumoconiosis, diffuse interstitial pneumonitis, fibrosis	
Vanadium	Upper and lower respiratory tract irritation (nose bleeding, cough), conjunctivitis, dermatitis	Chronic bronchitis, emphysema, pneumonia, chronic eye irritation, dermatitis, possible skin and/or respiratory allergy	
Zinc	Metal fume fever,†† skin eruption (oxide pox)	Not known	
Other minerals			
Asbestos		Cancer (lung, mesothelium), asbestosis, pleural thickening	
Fluorides	Respiratory irritation, gastrointestinal symptoms	Osteosclerosis, pulmonary insufficiency, kidney dysfunctions§§	Postshift urinalysis for F; bone density on periodic chest x-ray; renal functions§§
Silica		Silicosis	
Physical agents			
Electricity	Electrocution, burns	Not known	
Hot environments	Heat rash, heat cramps, heat exhaustion (irritability, mental dullness, general weakness), heat stroke	Not known	
Noise	Temporary auditory threshold shift	Hearing loss	
Vibration		Vibration white finger syndrome, Raynaud's phenomenon resulting from localized vibration (tingling numbness, blanching of fingers)	
Ionizing radiation	Erythema, radiodermatitis, nausea, vomiting, diarrhea, weakness, bone marrow depression, shock, death	Cancer, cataracts, reproductive effects	Film badges or dosimeters
Ultraviolet radiation (200-400 nm)	Photokeratitis, conjunctivitis, skin erythema and burns	Cancer (skin), cataracts	
Visible light (400-760 nm)	Eye discomfort, fatigue, headache, retinal changes (retinal burn)	Eye discomfort, fatigue, headache, retinal changes (retinal burn)	

From *NIOSH criteria for a recommended standard: welding, brazing, and thermal cutting,* abridged edition, Cincinnati, 1988, U.S. Department of Health and Human Services, Public Health Service, Centers for Disease Control, National Institute for Occupational Safety and Health.[3]

†Distinction between short-term and long-term effects is not clear-cut and is somewhat arbitrary. Short-term effects are usually the result of acute exposure(s) and may appear immediately to several days or weeks after the exposure. Long-term effects are usually the result of chronic, repeated low-dose exposures extending from several months to many years. However, long-term effects may also include the aftereffects of single or repeated acute exposures.

‡Tests to be considered at the discretion of the attending physician.

§May contain toxic impurities such as arsine, carbon disulfide, carbon monoxide, hydrogen sulfide, and phosphine.

*Toxicity information is mostly from chromium plating operation and chromium pigment manufacturing.

††Metal fume fever is manifested by fever, chills, cough, joint and muscle pains, and general malaise.

‡‡Reports of health effects of tungsten come almost exclusively from the studies of workers exposed to tungsten carbide, which usually contains cobalt.

§§Renal functions should be evaluated because renal dysfunctions are known to hinder urinary excretion of fluorides.

Table 42-3. Welding processes associated with specific inhalation exposures

Welding process	Respiratory hazard
Shielded metal arc welding	
Of iron or steel	Iron oxide
Of stainless steel	Hexavalent chromium
Gas metal arc welding (MIG or CO_2 welding)	
Of aluminum or aluminum magnesium	Ozone
Of stainless steel	Nickel
CO_2 shielded arc welding	Carbon monoxide
Flame cutting, flame welding	Carbon monoxide
	Nitrogen oxide
	Nitrogen dioxide
Plasma cutting of aluminum	Ozone
Carbon arc gouging	
Brazing, cadmium filler	Cadmium
Brazing and gas welding, fluorine-containing fluxes	Fluorines
Tungsten inert gas shielded welding on aluminum	Oxides of nitrogen

Adapted from Sundin DS: National occupational exposure survey data base, 1981-83. In *NIOSH criteria for a recommended standard for welding, brazing, and thermal cutting,* DHHS (NIOSH) Pub No 88-10, Bethesda, 1988, U.S. Department of Health and Human Services, Centers for Disease Control.
MIG, Metal inert gas shielded arc welding.

symptoms and do not seek medical attention, aware that the illness usually passes within hours. Although occurring more frequently in welders than toxic or hypersensitivity pneumonitis, metal fume fever, early in its course, may be difficult to distinguish from these entities. All may have an onset delayed by a few hours, fever, and peripheral leukocytosis. In a patient with apparent metal fume fever, the presence of prominent crackles on chest exam, an increased alveolar-arterial gradient, or a pulmonary infiltrate, should raise suspicion of a more serious inhalation injury and lead to continuing observation.

Bronchitis

Acute or chronic airway symptoms are the most frequently detected abnormality in large controlled cross-sectional studies of active welders. Many, but not all studies, have noted an increased prevalence of cough and phlegm among welders compared with nonwelding controls, after adjusting for smoking. For example, Cotes et al. found that shipyard welders and caulker burners (who polish and burn completed welds and burn through metal plates) had a relative risk for chronic bronchitis of 2.8 (after adjustment for age and smoking), compared with shipyard controls. In the same study, cigarette smoking produced a relative risk of 3.2 (after adjusting for age and trade).[5] Welders more frequently experience work-related airway symptoms that do not fulfill criteria for chronic bronchitis. A recent prospective study of shipyard arc welders found increased reports of reversible cough, phlegm, wheeze, and chest tightness on workdays, with improvement on weekends and holidays. In the same group there was no significant increase in chronic bronchitis. In these welders, the prevalence of the airway symptoms declined over 3 years as welding exposure decreased.[6]

Asthma

There are relatively few case reports of occupational asthma in welders, and only a handful of studies have followed welders prospectively for incident asthma. Conversely, occupational asthma has been frequently reported in solderers, most often as a result of allergic sensitization to colophony, the pine-resin material used as a flux-core in many solders (see Chapters 26 and 43). Case reports of occupational asthma confirmed by specific challenge have been reported in welders of stainless steel and with exposure to chromium fume in steel welding.[7,8] Whether excessive acute or chronic exposure to irritant welding plume can cause or enhance nonallergic airway hyperresponsiveness is an area of research needing more investigation. A recent, prospective controlled study of 50 arc-welders working under relatively well controlled exposure conditions, detected no significant increase in mean methacholine challenge responsiveness over the 3 years of observation, although 1 of 50 welders appeared to develop new-onset occupational asthma, associated with a marked increase in airway responsiveness.[6]

Hypersensitivity pneumonitis and toxic pneumonitis

A diverse array of substances generated in the welding plume can cause hypersensitivity or toxic pneumonitis—usually under conditions of welding or cutting where unusual or unknown metals or coatings are being worked on. (Toxic pneumonitis is used synonymously here with the terms chemical pneumonitis, acute lung injury, pulmonary edema, the adult respiratory distress syndrome, and fatal lung injury.) (See Chapters 29 and 30.)

Table 42-4 is a partial listing of substances known to cause acute toxic or hypersensitivity pneumonitis in welding or the allied processes. Welding work practices have evolved over this century to prevent the occurrence of acute lung injury, and such occurrence is infrequent, although not rare. The potential for toxic inhalation exposures is greatest when the standard practice of removing paint and coatings from metal before working on it is disregarded (Fig. 42-5).

In an acutely ill welder who presents with respiratory symptoms after exposure to the plume, differentiation of hypersensitivity pneumonitis from toxic pneumonitis may be difficult, although there may be a therapeutic need (the use of systemic corticosteroids) to make this distinction.

Because hypersensitivity pneumonitis represents an anamnestic response of the immune system, it requires at least

Table 42-4. A partial listing of substances that have caused hypersensitivity or toxic pneumonitis in welding and allied processes*

Substance	Reference
Beryllium	Grier (1946)[9]
Cadmium	Barnhart and Rosenstock (1984)[10]
Manganese	Lloyd-Davies (1949)[11]
Nitrogen dioxide	Norwood et al. (1966)[12]
Ozone	Doig and Challen (1964)[13]
Phosgene	Doig and Challen (1964)[13]
Phosphine	Doig and Challen (1964)[13]

Adapted from Sferlazza S and Beckett W: The respiratory health of welders, *Am Rev Respir Dis* 143:1134-48, 1991. With permission.[4]

*The presence of these substances at toxic levels in welding plume is process dependent, and unusual in common welding processes. These substances are found only where certain base metals, base metal coatings, or electrode components are used.

one previous exposure to the antigenic substance. The welder with hypersensitivity pneumonitis usually gives a history of serial, and sometimes crescendo, episodes of cough, chest tightness, or chest pain, shortness of breath, and fever in association with repeated welding exposure, often occurring several hours after the start of exposure. Toxic pneumonitis is often an isolated event associated with unusual exposure. It also may have its onset delayed at 4 to 6 or more hours after exposure. (This delayed onset is particularly characteristic of the pulmonary edema caused by nitrogen dioxide.) Fever and rigors may be present in some cases of toxic pneumonitis, but are more suggestive of hypersensitivity pneumonitis. The peripheral white blood count may be elevated in both conditions. Information about others working in the same area may be helpful. The welder with hypersensitivity pneumonitis, once sensitized, may develop symptoms and pulmonary infiltrates with levels of exposure that have no apparent ill effect on others in the same workplace.

Pneumoconiosis

The term "welder's lung" is so nonspecific as to be almost useless; in most cases a much more specific diagnosis can and should be made by careful comparison of the exposure history with the clinical condition of the welder. Pneumoconiosis in a welder may represent any of several individual exposures, or the cumulative effect of mixed exposures. Exposures to asbestos or silica dust must be considered in the differential diagnosis. Repeated episodes of hypersensitivity pneumonitis may result in chronic pulmonary interstitial fibrosis, which may be mistaken for pneumoconiosis.

Early in this century, iron welders were found to develop an increased profusion of small opacities on chest x-ray from chronic inhalation of iron oxide fume. The iron oxide, in the form of ferric oxide (Fe_2O_3), is more radioopaque than most other occupationally encountered dusts but is minimally, if at all, fibrogenic so that the patient with purely iron oxide pneumoconiosis (usually called siderosis) may have a prominently abnormal chest film with no impairment of pulmonary function attributable to the welding exposure (see Chapter 15). Some follow-up studies of welders with siderosis have shown gradual clearing of the x-ray with removal from exposure. Follow-up of a group of active and retired shipyard welders with a technique for measuring magnetic ferrous content of the lungs using magnets (magnetopneumotography) has indicated an accumulation of about 70 mg of iron in the lungs per year in active younger welders, an average total lung burden of about 1 g of iron after 10 years of welding, and net clearance from the lung of about 20% of the accumulated burden per year in unexposed former welders.[4] Radiographically, evident siderosis is probably not a frequent occurrence in industry today. Its occurrence may be considered a Sentinel Health Event indicating the need to investigate the welder's work practices and exposures carefully. Siderosis does not have a radiographic appearance distinct from other forms of pneumoconiosis and so cannot easily be distinguished from mixed dust fibrosis, silicosis, or asbestosis on clinical grounds. Welders may also develop pneumoconiosis from tin oxide (stannosis), carbon dust (anthracosis), and aluminum oxide (aluminosis). In a survey of actively employed electric arc welders in Britain reported in 1978, 7% had some degree of pneumoconiosis, but none showed progressive massive fibrosis.[15]

The authors of case reports and case series of welders with functionally significant pulmonary fibrosis have proposed that silica dust, nitrogen dioxide gas, or other components of the welding plume may lead to this more severe form of fibrosis in welders, which has been likened to the complicated pneumoconiosis occurring in a minority of those with silicosis or coalworkers' pneumoconiosis.[16] Others have proposed that interstitial fibrosis in the absence of excess silica in lung tissue indicates that welding plume exposures in the absence of silica can lead to chronic interstitial pulmonary fibrosis,[17] and based on in vitro toxicology studies, hexavalent chromium (chromium VI) from stainless steel welding and nitrogen dioxide have been proposed as candidate causative substances.[18]

"Welding bodies" have been described in hematoxylin and eosin sections of lung specimens from welders. These iron-coated particles represent carbonaceous or metallic constituents of the welding plume, inhaled and deposited along the respiratory bronchioles.[18,19]

Chronic effects on lung function

As with other studies of occupation and lung function, epidemiologic studies of welding are complicated by smoking, which in the past has been more common among welders than those in the general U.S. population.[20] The dra-

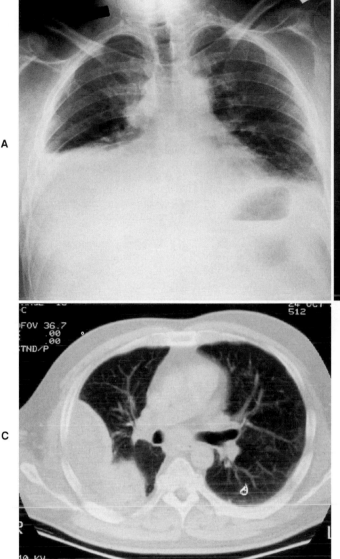

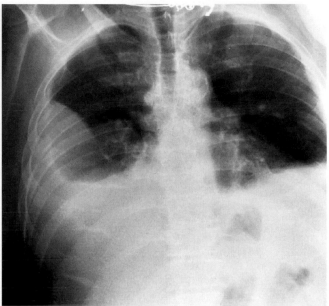

Fig. 42-5. Case report: acute lung injury in a "burner." A 49-year-old marine salvage company owner used an oxyacetylene torch to cut through an asphalt-covered steel hatch in the hold of a poorly ventilated barge. He used no local exhaust ventilation or respiratory protection. Although asymptomatic while at work, he had the onset of cough, dyspnea, nausea, and vomiting later that evening. **A,** His chest film the following day is shown with bilateral basilar densities; he was febrile with cough and chest pain and progressively hypoxic, requiring 95% oxygen by mask. Decubitus films showed air bronchograms at both lung bases and a small right pleural effusion. **B,** A left lateral decubitus film taken 8 days after admission shows bilateral infiltrates and a large right pleural-based mass. On the ninth day thoracentesis produced a thick exudate without growth on culture. **C,** A CT scan of the chest on the twelfth day with loculated pleural collections and dense consolidation of the right lower and middle lobes is shown. The discharge diagnosis was acute bilateral toxic pneumonitis complicated by pleural effusion from a mixed inhalational exposure of materials in cutting and burning.

matic appearance of welding plumes may be one of the factors that has led to many respiratory surveys of welders, testing for chronic effects on spirometry and other tests of lung mechanics and function. Most such studies have been cross-sectional in design, using workplace, nonwelder controls for comparison. Most have examined only actively working welders, who may represent a "survivor" population. Within these constraints, some studies have found no differences between groups, whereas others have found small differences only between welding and nonwelding cigarette smokers[21] or effects on mid-flows or closing volume without effects on forced expiratory volume in 1 second (FEV1).[22,23] Table 42-5 summarizes 11 studies of effects of welding occupation on lung function. One of the best-designed of these studies, because it included retirees and others who had left the work force, examined shipyard welders and caulker/burners from a British shipyard. After

adjusting for pack-years smoking, a small effect on FEV1 and forced vital capacity (FVC) annual decline was seen in welders and caulker-burners, and an interaction was seen between welding status and cigarette smoking.[24] Because of the complexity of welding exposure, the marked variation in level of exposure between welders, and the lack of individual exposure measurements in these studies, it is difficult to assume that the findings of one study are applicable to another exposed group.

Bronchogenic carcinoma

Bronchogenic carcinoma is the primary malignancy of concern in welding. Welding fumes have been categorized as "possibly carcinogenic to humans" by an expert committee of cancer epidemiologists and toxicologists of the International Agency for Research on Cancer (IARC) Working Group on the Evaluation of Carcinogenic Risks to Hu-

Table 42-5. Studies of the welding occupation and measures of chronic lung function

Country	Year	Welders/control subjects (n)	Selection method	Tests performed	Results, comments
USA	1954	100/100	>10 yr welding <60 yr old Shipyard welders	Spirometry	Statistically significant effects seen on occurrence of obstructive and restrictive abnormality; seen in smoking welders only
Denmark	1969	156/152	Unspecified	Spirometry	No difference in FEV1 (ex-smokers analyzed in nonsmoker (group)
USA	1973	61/63	Shipyard welders matched with pipe-fitters and (asbestos-exposed) pipe-coverers by age and employment	Spirometry Helium lung volume DLCO Airway resistance	No significant differences between welders and pipefitters; welders and shipyard controls all had lower lung function when compared with nonshipyard controls
Sweden	1979	119/20	Shipyard welders matched with controls by smoking status	Spirometry: SBN$_2$ Closing volume Closing capacity	No significant difference Significantly greater Significantly greater
Britain	1980	209/109	Shipyard welders	Spirometry: FEV1 FVC Transfer factor (DLCO)	 Significant Significant NS Statistically significant difference between group overall and nonsmokers alone but not smokers alone
USA	1983	91/80	Welders 25-49 yr old with >4 yr employment	Spirometry FVC FEV1 DLCO	 NS NS NS All employed in heavy equipment manufacturing
Britain	1984	135/135	Welders ≥45 yr old Random sample of total work force in shipyard; controls matched for age, sex, smoking	Spirometry DLCO Alveolar volume or helium volume	NS NS RV increased TLC decreased
Sweden	1985	258/180	Arc welders Aluminum Stainless steel Railroad track	Spirometry: FEV1 FVC	 NS NS
Britain	1989	526/81	All shipyard welders, and caulker/burners ≥45 yr old, random sample of 50% of those age <45, and 5% of remaining trades as controls	Spirometry	In current or ex-smokers, FEV1 reduced in relation to estimated fume exposure (mean, −0.25 L); no impairment in nonsmokers (survey performed in 1979)
Britain	1990	386/64	Shipyard welders and caulker/burners compared with shipyard controls matched for age, trade (same cohort as in reference 32); longitudinal follow-up	Spirometry	FEV1 and FVC annual rates of decline increased by 16 ml/yr in welders and caulker/burners; interaction between welding status and cigarette smoking; many retirees included
USA	1989	226/-	Male nonshipyard welders without radiographic asbestos is ILO < 1/0; compared with historical, population-based probability sample of population from same state, which included smokers and ex-smokers	Spirometry	Midflow and terminal flow reduced compared with historical controls, whereas FEV1 and FVC not significantly different

From Sferlazza S and Beckett W: The respiratory health of welders, *Am Rev Respir Dis* 143:1134-1148, 1991. With permission.[4]

FEV1, Forced expiratory volume in 1 second; *FVC,* forced vital capacity; *ILO,* International Labor Organization; *NS,* no statistically significant difference found between welders and control subjects; *RV,* residual volume, *TLC,* total lung capacity.

mans. This conclusion was based on "limited" evidence for the carcinogenicity of welding fumes and gases in humans, and inadequate evidence in animals. Among many epidemiologic studies of the relationship of welding occupation to lung cancer, some (but by no means all) have found a significant association. Six studies of welding occupation and lung cancer published since 1980 are summarized in Table 42-6. This association of welding occupation with excess lung cancer could be explained by (1) cigarette smoking, asbestos exposure, or exposure to other carcinogens not in the welding plume, (2) by an excess lung cancer risk associated only with certain welding processes, with the magnitude of the effect diluted among all welders, or (3) by an increase in welding risk caused by welding plume that is not apparent until 20 to 30 years after the first exposure.[25] In a recent study of occupational mortality in California from 1979 to 1981, a 33% excess of lung cancer was present in welders after adjustment for smoking and socioeconomic status.[26] The U.S. National Institute for Occupational Safety and Health (NIOSH) has recommended that welding on stainless steel with exposure to nickel and chromium be treated as an exposure to occupational carcinogens pending further research.[3]

SPECIAL DIAGNOSTIC CONSIDERATIONS

Immediately after an acute episode of pneumonitis, measurement of metals (such as cadmium, mercury, or zinc) in a 24-hour urine specimen can sometimes help confirm exposure. Analysis of lung tissue for metals and minerals has sometimes been useful in establishing etiologic factors in evaluating welders with interstitial lung disease, although such studies do not usually affect treatment decisions. Several new techniques to characterize and quantitate inorganic particulate matter in lung, including microprobe analysis, are available on a clinical basis at selected centers to quantitate the presence of a variety of metals in small specimens.[27,28]

SURVEILLANCE

Little research has been done on the effectiveness of surveillance for respiratory health in welders. Where surveillance is conducted, respiratory symptom questionnaires are often used in conjunction with spirometry. If administered at frequent enough intervals and reviewed by informed readers, these measures should be useful in identifying new cases of industrial bronchitis and occupational asthma at an early stage. Although not required by the U.S. Occupational Safety and Health Administration (OSHA) standards,

Table 42-6. Selected recent studies of welding occupation and lung cancer incidence or mortality

Country	Year	Selection of welders, control subjects	Results, comments
USA	1981	3,247 welders in western Washington who were union members for 3 yr between 1950 and 1973; compared with nonwelder union members and U.S. death rates	Deaths >20 yr after first employment showed 74% excess for lung cancer compared with U.S. statistics; no assessment of asbestos exposure, smoking, other factors
USA	1985	771 U.S. veterans with past occupation of welder or flamecutter, categorized as never smoked or ever smoked; compared with U.S. mortality rates by smoking status	No excess lung cancer occurred
Germany	1985	1,221 welders and a comparison group of 1,694 turners, cutters, and drillers working in 25 factories; smoking status of welders ascertained by interviews with foremen	No excess in lung cancer seen in welders compared with national rates; welders had slightly higher lung cancer rates than did turner control group, and welders using "coated electrodes" had slightly higher lung cancer rate than did those not using coated electrodes; overall cancer rate (not organ specific) significantly higher in welders than in turners or in national rate
USA	1987	506 patients with lung cancer and 771 controls with detailed smoking and occupational histories from New Mexico Tumor Registry	Increased odds ratio for lung cancer identified in welders (as well as in uranium miners, underground miners, painters)
USA	1989	90 white male welders with diagnosed lung cancer in Los Angeles County between 1972 and 1987; 116 controls were welders with a nonpulmonary malignancy, all identified from tumor registry	Significantly increased risk of lung cancer associated with shipyard welding with 10-yr latency period since first exposure; odds ratio, 1.7; conclusion: excess lung cancer in welders associated with excess smoking and probable asbestos exposure in shipyards; no association with specific welding process
USA	1989	Population-based study of occupational mortality patterns in California adjusted for estimated smoking, alcohol, socioeconomic status	Welders had significant 33% excess lung cancer mortality after adjusting for heavier than average smoking habits

From Sferlazza S and Beckett W: The respiratory health of welders, *Am Rev Respir Dis* 143:1134-1148, 1991. With permission.

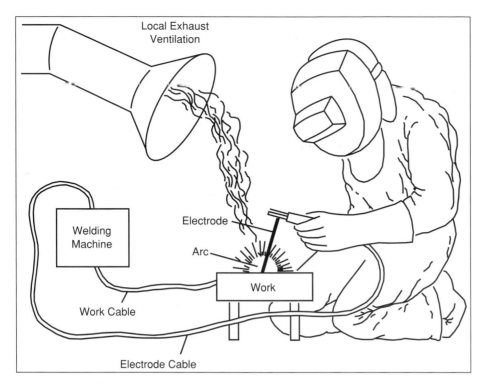

Fig. 42-6. The arc welding process. Energy from the AC or DC power source creates an electrical arc with intense heat in the small air gap between electrode and work. The pieces of base metal are fused with filler metal from a consumable electrode or a filler electrode fed into the arc. The welder must watch the weld from about 15 ft through ultraviolet-shielding glass. Industry standards for indoor welding advise local exhaust (duct) ventilation to draw welding plume away from the welder's breathing zone.

NIOSH has recommended a medical monitoring program for welders consisting of at least annual history and physical, ophthalmologic examination, chest radiograph, and audiogram.[3]

PREVENTION

Efforts to reduce health risks in welding include the development and use of processes that produce less plume. The arrangement of the welding environment to provide necessary ventilation and work practices that prevent the generation of either excessive amounts or highly toxic components of the plume are the mainstays of preventive practice. Preparation of the metal to be welded by the removal of cutting oils, paints, and other coatings is essential to safe welding practice. Where breathing zone levels of toxins cannot be kept at a safe level, respiratory protective devices are used, although the discomfort of some devices may lead to underuse. The welder's proximity to a source of heat and the increased discomfort of respirators in relationship to higher temperature within the mask[29] may make the use of negative pressure respirators less feasible in welding than in other occupations. A survey of skilled full-time welders who had negative pressure respirators available indicated that only a third used the respirator during a routine workday. Because welders must keep their faces close to the arc, the use of local exhaust ventilation to draw the plume away from the welder (Fig. 42-6) is the practical means to minimize exposure. Welders with asthma or other nonoccupational lung disease may need special accommodations to be able to weld safely.

REGULATORY ISSUES

Regulation of inhalation exposures in welding is accomplished through standards for the maximum inhaled concentration (permissible exposure limits) for each of the components that may be in the welding plume and a "dust" standard for mixed respirable particles of 5 mg/m[3]. In addition, the OSHA General Industry Standard contains a section of 25 pages in length with health and safety standards.[30] Manufacturers and suppliers of welding electrodes, filler metals, and fluxes are required to label all product containers with a general health warning that is to be passed on to the end-user (the welder). Materials containing cadmium and fluorine compounds require specific warnings about their health hazards.

ACKNOWLEDGMENTS

The contributions of Dr. Steven Sferlazza (who performed much of the initial literature search on which this chapter was based) and Professor Thomas Eagar of the Massachusetts Institute of Technology (who provided critical review of the manuscript) are very gratefully noted.

REFERENCES

1. American Welding Society: *Effects of welding on health,* vols I-VII (published 1979 through 1990) available from American Welding Society, 550 N.W. LeJeune Rd., P.O. Box 351040, Miami, Fla 33135 (Tel: 800-334-9353).
2a. Stern RM, Berlin A, Fletcher AC, et al (eds): *Health hazards and biological effects of welding fumes and gases,* Amsterdam, 1986, Excerpta Medica.
2b. American Welding Society: *Filler metal comparison charts,* AWS

FMC-93, available from American Welding Society, 550 N.W. Le-Jeune Rd., P.O. Box 351040, Miami, Fla 33135 (Tel: 800-334-9353).

2c. American Welding Society: *Specifications for arc welding electrodes,* available individually by kind of electrode from American Welding Society, 550 N.W. LeJeune Rd., P.O. Box 351040, Miami, Fla 33135 (Tel: 800-334-9353).

3. NIOSH: *Criteria for a recommended standard for welding, brazing, and thermal cutting* (abridged edition). DHHS (NIOSH) Pub No 88-110a, 1988.

4. Sferlazza S and Beckett W: The respiratory health of welders: state of the art, *Am Rev Respir Dis* 143:1134-1148, 1991.

5. Cotes JE, Feinman EL, Male VJ, et al: Respiratory symptoms and impairment in shipyard welders and caulker burners, *Br J Ind Med* 46:292-301, 1980.

6. Beckett WS, Pace PE, Sferlazza SJ, et al: Airway responsiveness, lung function and respiratory symptoms in welders: a controlled prospective cohort study. (Manuscript in review.)

7. Keskinen H, Kalliomaki P-L, and Alanko K: Occupational asthma due to stainless steel welding fumes, *Clin Allergy* 10:151-159, 1980.

8. Moller DR, Brooks SM, Bernstein DI, et al: Delayed anaphylactoid reaction in a worker exposed to chromium, *J Allergy Clin Immunol* 77:451-456, 1986.

9. Grier RS: Acute pulmonary beryllium poisoning, *Beryllium symposium,* Oak Ridge, Tenn, 1946, Atomic Energy Commission (AECD-1803), Office of Scientific and Technical Information.

10. Barnhart S and Rosenstock L: Cadmium chemical pneumonitis, *Chest* 86:789-791, 1984.

11. Lloyd-Davies TA: Manganese pneumonitis, *Br J Ind Med* 6:82-90, 1949.

12. Norwood WP, Wisehart DE, Earl CA, et al: Nitrogen dioxide poisoning due to metal cutting with an oxyacetylene torch, *J Occup Med* 8:301-306, 1966.

13. Doig AT and Challen PJR: Respiratory hazards of welding, *Ann Occup Hyg* 7:223-229, 1964.

14. Kalliomaki P-L, Kalliomaki K, Rahkonen E, et al: Lung retention of welding fumes and ventilatory lung functions. A follow-up study among shipyard welders, *Ann Occup Hyg* 24:449-452, 1983.

15. Attfield MD and Ross DS: Radiologic abnormalities in electric-arc welders, *Br J Ind Med* 35:117-122, 1978.

16. Guidotti TL, Abraham JL, DeNee PB, and Smith JB: Arc welders' pneumoconiosis: application of advanced scanning electron microscopy, *Arch Environ Health* 33:117-124, 1978.

17. Funahashi A, Schlueter D, Pintar K, et al: Welders' pneumoconiosis: tissue elemental microanalysis by energy dispersive x-ray analysis, *Br J Ind Med* 45:14-18, 1988.

18. Stern RM, Pigott GH, and Abraham JL: Fibrogenic potential of welding fumes, *J Appl Toxicol* 3:18-30, 1983.

19. Moatamed F and Johnson FB: Identification and significance of magnetite in human tissues, *Arch Pathol Lab Med* 110:618-621, 1986.

20. Sterling TD and Wenkham JJ: Smoking characteristics by type of employment, *J Occup Med* 18:797-801, 1976.

21. Hunnicut TN, Cracovaner DJ, and Myles JT: Spirometric measurements in welders, *Arch Environ Health* 8:661-669, 1954.

22. Kilburn K and Warshaw R: Pulmonary functional impairment from years of arc welding, *Am J Ind Med* 87:62-69, 1989.

23. Oxhoj H, Bake B, Wedel H, et al: Effects of electric arc welding on ventilatory function, *Arch Environ Health* 24:211-217, 1979.

24. Chinn D, Stevenson I, and Cotes J: Longitudinal respiratory survey of shipyard workers: effects of trade and atopic status, *Br J Ind Med* 47:83-90, 1990.

25. Peto J: Cancer morbidity and mortality studies of welders. In Stern RM, Berlin A, Fletcher AC et al, editors: *Health hazards and biological effects of welding fumes and gases,* pp 423-424. Amsterdam, 1986, Excerpta Medica.

26. Singleton JA and Beaumont JJ: *COMS II: California occupational mortality 1979-1981, adjusted for smoking, alcohol, and socioeconomic status,* Division of Occupational and Environmental Medicine, University of California, Davis, CA 95616. Prepared for the Health Demographics Section, Health Data and Statistics Branch, 1989, California Department of Health Services.

27. Abraham JL and Burnett BR: Quantitative *in situ* analysis of inorganic particulate burden in tissue sections—an update. In Ingram P, Shelburne JD, and Roggli VL, editors: *Microprobe analysis in medicine,* pp. 111-131, New York, 1989, Hemisphere.

28. Abraham JL, Burnett BR, and Hunt A: Development and use of a pneumoconiosis database of human pulmonary inorganic particulate burden in over 400 lungs, *Scanning Microsc* 5:95-108, 1991.

29. Nielsen R, Gwosdow AR, Berglund AG, and Dubois AG: The effect of temperature and humidity levels in a protective mask on user acceptability during exercise, *Am Ind Hyg Assoc J* 48:639-645, 1987.

30. 29 CFR (Code of Federal Regulations) 1910.252, Office of the Federal Regulations, U.S. Government Printing office.

Chapter 43

ELECTRONICS AND SEMICONDUCTORS

Marc B. Schenker

Sources of exposure
    Wafer manufacturing
    Semiconductor fabrication
        Electronic component assembly
        Solvents
Clinical manifestations
    Mucous membrane and respiratory tract irritation
    Asthma and airway hyperresponsiveness
Epidemiology
Prevention

The electronics industry has undergone dramatic development and evolution during the twentieth century and continues to be one of the most technologically intensive, rapidly changing, and economically important modern industries. In the United States there are over 250,000 people working in this industry, and large numbers of people work in manufacturing facilities in other parts of the world.[1] During the first half of this century electronic components consisted of electrical circuits often employing large and inefficient x-ray tubes. In about 1950, development of the transistor led to the second generation of electronic equipment, which was more compact and efficient. The third generation, or microelectronics, developed in the 1960s with the commercialization and mass production of integrated circuits using semiconductor technology. Semiconductors have now replaced older electronic components in numerous applications and are the basis of electronic signal transmission, reception, and manipulation in telecommunications, data processing, consumer electronics, medical science, automotive and military products, industrial control and measurement, and many other applications.

Semiconductor manufacturing or fabrication refers to the production of integrated circuits or "chips" that combine the function of thousands of electronic components onto a wafer that is millimeters in diameter. There are three steps in the manufacturing of electronics based on silicon wafers. The *first* step is production of the silicon wafer itself. *Second* is manufacturing of the integrated circuit or "chip." *Third* is the assembly of electronic components into various electronic devices, with semiconductor chips often serving as the "brains" of the devices. Silicon wafers are usually manufactured in specialized manufacturing facilities that make only the substrate wafers. The wafers are fabricated into semiconductor chips or integrated circuits in a wafer fabrication facility or "fab" (Fig. 43-1). Finally, chips are integrated into electronics components and other products in the various appropriate manufacturing facilities.

The production of silicon wafers and manufacturing of integrated circuits are relatively new and rapidly changing processes, and there are few data on actual respiratory hazards to workers in these industries. However, many agents with known respiratory toxicity are handled in semiconductor manufacturing, and these agents with their potential respiratory effects will be discussed. The fabrication of electronic components may involve soldering of circuit components, a process for which there are many data on occupational respiratory hazards. Other respiratory hazards may also exist such as insulating materials that use epoxy resin systems and capacitor coatings using chloronaphthalene.

Sources of exposure in semiconductor and electronics manufacturing are discussed in this chapter.[2] This discussion is followed by a description of clinical manifestations from exposures to these agents, and finally epidemiologic data on respiratory outcomes among workers in these industries is presented. The focus in this chapter is on subacute and chronic effects of exposure. The principles and specific examples of respiratory effects from acute, high level exposure to gases are covered in Chapter 30.

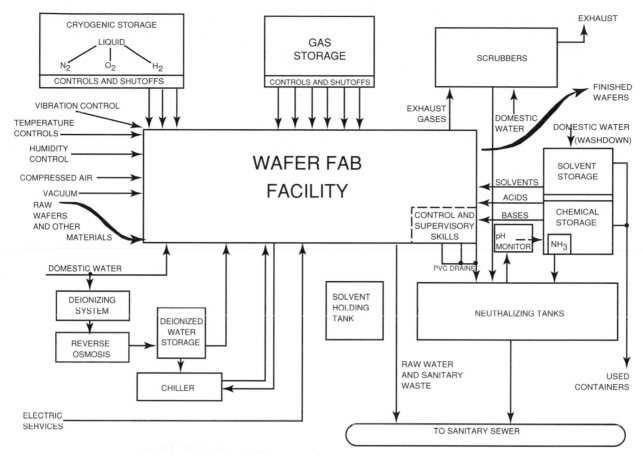

Fig. 43-1. Schematic of a wafer fabrication facility ("fab"). Total control of the fabrication facility is maintained to provide necessary substrate and chemicals for processing, control the environment in the facility (temperature, humidity, vibration, particle concentrations), remove used and contaminated materials, and prevent release of dangerous levels of toxic materials.

SOURCES OF EXPOSURE
Wafer manufacturing

Silicon is the most common material for wafer substrates, although some specialized chips use gallium arsenide, germanium, or other materials. The silicon must be of extremely high purity. Because silicon is a relatively poor electron conductor, precise amounts of impurities are introduced or doped into the crystalline matrix. These impurities or "dopants" are atoms from groups IIIa and Vb (Table 43-1) and provide the electrons that allow electricity to flow.

Silicon wafer production (Fig. 43-2) begins with the reduction of quartzite in an electric arc furnace. The silicon is removed from the furnace and blown with oxygen to remove impurities. It is then reacted with hydrochloric acid (HCl) to form a halide (SiX_4) or trichlorosilane ($SiHCl_3$),which is reconverted to polycrystalline silicon by reduction with hydrogen.

Single crystal silicon is manufactured by the Czochralski or the float zone techniques.[3] In the Czochralski method, the single crystal silicon is melted in a vessel with an argon atmosphere. A silicon seed crystal is drawn from the melt and rotated to form an ingot a few inches in diameter and several feet in length. Dopants are added to the molten silicon. The ingot is ground to a uniform diameter and then sliced into uniform wafers that are lapped in a grinding slurry of fine silica. After lapping the wafers are etched with a nitric/hydrofluoric/acetic acid mixture (HNO_3/HF/CH_3COOH), and one side is polished.

Gallium arsenide (GaAs) wafers require pure gallium and arsenic with the addition of various dopants. It is more difficult to form GaAs crystals because of the disparate melting points of Ga and As, and a furnace is required for the vaporization of the substrates, with the resulting GaAs having a melting point of 1238° C. A variety of methods for forming GaAs crystals and ingots have been developed. Once the ingot is formed, it is sandblasted in a glovebox with silicon carbide or calcined alumina. Wafers are cut and polished similarly to silicon-based wafers.

Most wafers used in semiconductor manufacturing are made by specialty companies in separate facilities from the production of integrated circuits. Potential exposures derive directly from the materials and processes used in wafer manufacturing. These exposures include various acids, gases, caustics, and solvents used in wafer production

Table 43-1. Agents with known or potential respiratory toxicity in electronics and semiconductor industries

Agent	Threshold limit values*	Effects
Dopants and dopant materials		
Antimony compounds		
$SbCl_3$	0.5	Forms HCl, corrosive
Sb_2O_3,	0.5	Respiratory irritant
SbH_3	0.5	Colorless gas, hemolysis similar to arsine
Arsenic compounds		
As_2O_3	0.01	Mucous membrane irritant
AsH_3	0.2	Nonirritating gas, hemolysis, renal failure
AsF_5		Decomposes to HF and As, corrosive
Boron compounds		
B_2O_3,	10.	Irritant
BBr_3	10.	Hydrolyzes to boric and bromic acids
BF_3	3.	Hydrolyzes to boric and HF acids
B_2H_6	0.1	Hydrolyzes to boric acid and hydrogen, metal fume feverlike syndrome
Cadmium compounds		
Cd, Cd_2O_3	0.05	Metal fume fever, pneumonitis, pulmonary edema Chronic exposure may cause emphysema
Indium compounds		
$InSb$	0.1	Pneumonitis
Phosphorus compounds		
$POCl_3$	0.6	Hydrolyzes to HCl and phosphoric acids, irritant
PCl_3	1.5	Similar to $POCl_3$
PH_3	0.4	Colorless gas, cough, dyspnea, pneumonitis, pulmonary edema; systemic symptoms nausea, headache, tremor, coma
Selenium compounds		
$SeO2$		Respiratory irritant
$SeOCl_2$		Respiratory irritant
H_2Se, SeF_6	0.2, 0.4	Gases, respiratory irritant, pulmonary edema
Silane (SiH_4)		Asphyxiant
Zinc compounds		
ZnO	5.0	Metal fume fever
$ZnCl_2$ (fume)	1.0	Hydrolyzes to hydrochloric acid, irritant
Acids and caustics		Mucous membrane, respiratory irritants
Ammonia		
Hydrochloric acid		
Hydrofluoric acid		
Sulfuric acid		
Solvents		Mucous membrane irritants
Aromatic hydrocarbons (toluene, xylene)		
Halogenated hydrocarbons (trichloroethylene, methylene chloride)		
Alcohols (isopropanol)		
Acetates (*n*-butyl acetate)		
Ketones (methyl ethyl ketone)		
Glycol ethers (ethylene glycol)		
Others		
Freons		Asthma
Other agents		
Trimellitic anhydride		Rhinitis and asthma, late systemic syndrome, irritant
Epoxy resins		Irritants, asthma
Soldering resins (colophony)		Asthma

*(mg/m^3), ACGIH.

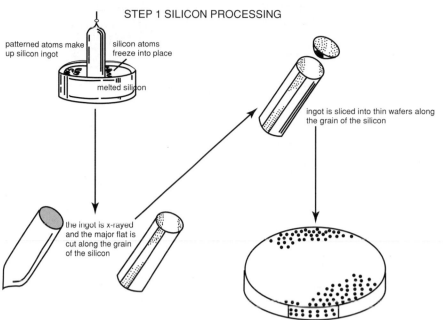

STEP 1 SILICON PROCESSING

patterned atoms make up silicon ingot

silicon atoms freeze into place

melted silicon

ingot is sliced into thin wafers along the grain of the silicon

the ingot is x-rayed and the major flat is cut along the grain of the silicon

The finished product is a silicon wafer with an oriented diamond lattice structure, the surface of which is smooth. The front side is so highly polished that it has a mirror finish.

Fig. 43-2. Silicon wafer manufacturing is usually done in separate facilities devoted exclusively to this process. The process requires the production of extremely pure crystalline silica to which impurities or "dopants" are added.

(Table 43-1). Probably the greatest potential respiratory hazard in silicon wafer manufacturing is from an uncontrolled release with resulting exposure to toxic gases. Gases used in silicon and GaAs wafer production include extremely toxic agents such as arsine and phosphine (Table 43-1). Exposure to elemental arsenic, or to arsenic trioxide, may occur in the preparation of materials for GaAs wafers, and exposure to particulate GaAs may occur during the sandblasting, lapping, cutting, or polishing of GaAs-based wafers. Exposure to GaAs dust may also occur during maintenance or other contact with the production equipment.[4]

Semiconductor fabrication

Integrated circuits or chip fabrication involves repeated steps of oxidation, photolithography, etching, and doping (Fig. 43-3 A). The processes, which may be repeated up to 15 times, build up precise circuits on the wafers, which are connected by metallization (Fig. 43-3 B). This work is done in a "clean room," a specialized environment with highly filtered air that has extremely low particle concentrations (Fig. 43-4). Air in the clean rooms is highly recirculated, leading to entrainment of chemical vapors or gases. Work is done in total body protective gear or "bunny suits," which are meant to protect the wafers from contaminant particles. The bunny suits, face masks, lighting, and "high technology" equipment may contribute to feelings of stress among employees working in the clean rooms.

Silicon wafers are first oxidized in a furnace to form a silicon dioxide coating of the surface (Fig. 43-5). The photolithography process involves coating a wafer with a photoresist solution and then baking on the solution. Photoresists may be positive or negative, and the solutions commonly contain a glycol ether, n-butyl acetate, and/or xylene. The wafer is then aligned with a mask, the photoresist is exposed, and it is developed in an organic solvent or caustic. Etching is next done with an acid, caustic, or solvent and nonprotected areas of photoresist are stripped off.

Impurities or dopants are also introduced into wafers during chip manufacturing, either by gas diffusion or ion implantation. In gas diffusion, wafers are placed into a furnace into which the dopant materials are introduced (Table 1, Fig. 43-5). Ion implantation involves the ionization of dopants that are accelerated into the wafers. Exposure may occur to dopant gases during ion implantation or during the offgassing of wafers when furnaces are opened and wafers removed.

Chips have a layer of metal applied, during a process called metallization, to form the necessary connection points. The circuits are then tested, and finally the silicon wafer is cut into hundreds of individual chips which are sealed in plastic or ceramic (Figs. 43-6, 43-7 on pages 724 and 725).

Potential exposures that may occur during the various stages of silicon wafer patterning include various dopant gases, acids, and solvents (Table 43-1). The greatest potential for respiratory exposures is from accidental releases or during equipment maintenance. Cutaneous exposures may occur from splashes or cleaning up spills. Lack of local exhaust in photolithography machines may increase exposure. Etching may involve exposure to acid or solvent vapors, particularly when these processes are not automated, and gaseous exposures may occur following the opening of diffusion furnaces.

Large quantities of many very toxic gases are used in

the semiconductor industry. In a 1979 California survey, over one million cubic feet of ammonia, arsine, diborane, hydrogen chloride, phosphine, and silane were reported to be consumed by 42 semiconductor manufacturing companies.[5] The use of such highly toxic materials has led to very stringent control measures, and normally measured concentrations of most materials are only a small fraction of the permissible exposure limits (PELs).[6] However, the possibility of acute toxicity to individuals or to larger numbers of workers from a gas release is an ever present danger in semiconductor manufacturing facilities.

Electronic component assembly. The assembly of electronic components involves the insertion of semiconductor chips as well as other electronic components into the entire range of commercial and consumer electronic products. The electronics industry uses standard fabrication materials such as aluminum, glass, and plastic, as well as more specialized materials such as soldering fluxes and germanium. Printed circuit boards are made by an offset printing process that uses etching to produce the circuit paths. Resin systems may be used in electronics equipment as protective or insulating material. For example, solid blocks of epoxy or polyester resins may be used to enclose electronic components or circuit boards. These resins are produced by a two-component catalyzed system, sometimes with silica flour added to the mixture. Epoxy compounds include propylene oxide, butylene oxides, epichlorohydrin, and trimellitic anhydride (TMA). Curing of epoxy resins is done by a variety of agents including formaldehyde. Generation of resins may also result in exposure to acidic and alkali fumes, in addition to various epoxy compounds.

Soldering is a fundamental operation for joining electronic component during assembly, often onto printed circuit boards. This is normally done with a lead-zinc solder, which may be contained in a molten solder tank. Many newer soldering operations are fully automated with local exhaust ventilation, but exposure to zinc and lead fumes may occur from some soldering operations. Exposures may also occur to the resins used in soldering fluxes. One flux in common use contains colophony, a pine resin derivative that consists of resin acid, stilbene derivatives, and hydrocarbons. Other fluxes are water based and contain cores of "phosphorous hexate" ($C_6H_8P_6O_{28}$) or other acids instead of colophony. Solderers may also be exposed to toluene diisocyanates fumes from polyurethane-coated wires and to organic solvents such as trichloroethylene and methyl alcohol that are used to clean circuit boards.[7]

Solvents. Organic solvents are used in many aspects of microelectronics manufacturing. In silicon wafer and integrated circuit manufacturing a wide range of organic solvents are used in many of the production processes. In the study of 42 California semiconductor manufacturing companies, over 500,000 gallons of organic solvent were used in a single year.[5] Isopropanol (2-propanol) was the most commonly used solvent, and solvents used in photoresist

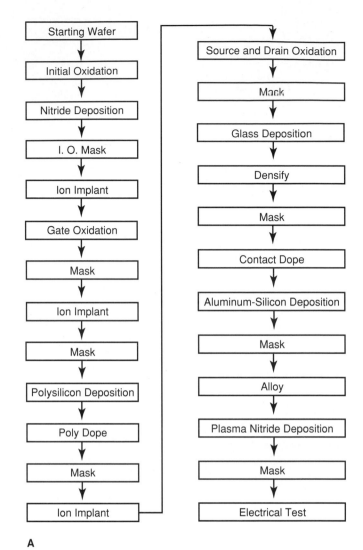

A

Fig. 43-3. A, The flow chart shows the processing steps of a silicon wafer to build an integrated circuit ("chip"). Upon completion each wafer will have from 200 to 2,900 integrated circuits on it, each capable of storing from 1,000 to 64,000 bits of information. The "chips" are manufactured in a wafer fabrication clean room facility (Fig. 43-1). **B,** The integrated circuit will have built-up layers that block electronic flow (insulate), semiconduct, or conduct electrons.

developers such as *n*-butyl acetate and xylene were also very commonly used. Other frequently reported agents included halogenated hydrocarbons (trichloroethylene, 1,1,1-trichloroethane, tetrachloroethylene), freons, glycol ethers, and ketones (methyl ethyl ketone).

Although there is concern about the recirculation of clean room air to reduce particle but not chemical vapor concentrations, most air concentrations of solvents in clean rooms are substantially below the threshold limit values (TLVs).[6] However, experimental studies with butyl glycol ether have demonstrated that dermal exposure may result in substantially more solvent uptake than does inhalation exposure.[8] Furthermore, substantial exposure of solvents

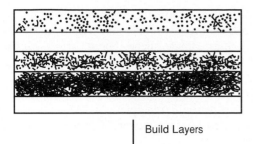

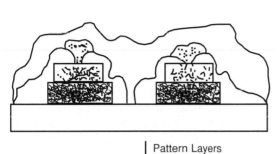

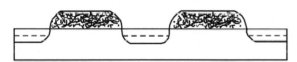

INSULATE
Some of the layers are insulation that will completely block electron flow.

Build Layers

SEMICONDUCT
Some layers are semiconductors, which can be doped to carry a specific amount of electron flow.

Pattern Layers

CONDUCT
Some layers are conductors, which guide and carry electricity throughout the integrated circuit.

Dope Regions

B

Fig. 43-3. Continued.

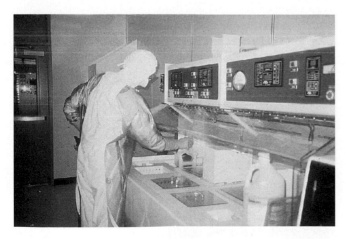

Fig. 43-4. Photograph of a wafer fabrication clean room. "Bunny suits" are worn by workers in the clean room to prevent particle release from skin and clothes or body secretions that could contaminate and harm the integrated circuits being fabricated. (Photo courtesy of Kathie S. Hammond and The Massachusetts Microelectronics Center.)

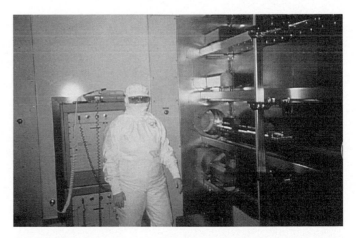

Fig. 43-5. Photographs of furnaces in a semiconductor fab. Furnaces are used at several steps in chip manufacturing, including oxidation of the silicon wafers, baking the photoresist solution onto the wafer, and diffusion of dopants into wafers. (Photo courtesy of Kathie S. Hammond and The Massachusetts Microelectronics Center.)

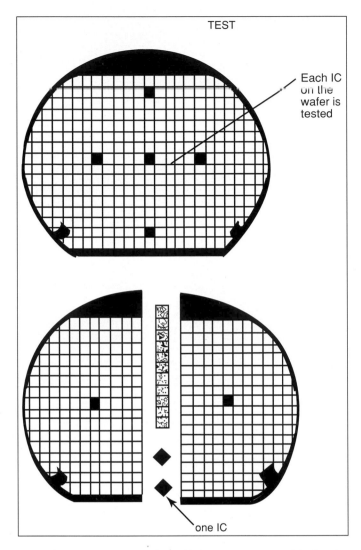

Fig. 43-6. The silicon wafer, which measures several inches in diameter, is cut into individual integrated circuit (IC) chips.

used in semiconductor manufacturing may occur through commonly used rubber gloves.[9]

Organic solvents are heavily used in electronic component manufacturing. Solvents uses include removing excess soldering flux after soldering, cleaning printed circuit boards, degreasing, and other processes. Commonly used solvents include alcohols, halogenated hydrocarbons, and petroleum distillates. Exposure will depend largely on the control of vapors from these processes. Local exhaust ventilation on automated soldering, printing, and washing machines for printed circuit boards will substantially reduce solvent vapor exposures.

CLINICAL MANIFESTATIONS

Gases used in semiconductor manufacturing have a wide range of acute toxicities including severe hemolytic anemia with renal failure from arsine exposure, pulmonary edema from phosphine and diborane, and mucous mem-

brane irritation from ammonia, hydrogen chloride, and other water-soluble irritants (Table 43-2). Other gases used in microelectronics include silane, boron, ozone, nitrogen oxides (NO_x), and carbon monoxide. Deaths from acute gas exposures in semiconductor manufacturing are rare. Two deaths of technicians from arsine exposure have been reported.[10] The general principles of acute toxic gas exposures are covered in Chapter 30, and will not be repeated here.

Mucous membrane and respiratory tract irritation

Several highly soluble irritant gases are commonly used in semiconductor manufacturing. Ammonia (NH_3) is an irritating, alkaline gas that reacts with water to form ammonium hydroxide (NH_4OH). It is highly soluble in water and reacts with conjunctiva, mucous membranes of the nose and mouth, and upper respiratory tract. The spectrum of manifestations depends on the concentration and duration of exposure, with an increasing dose associated with effects lower into the respiratory tract. Manifestations include redness, irritation, and pain in the eyes, nose, and mouth, laryngeal edema, and stridor. Very high concentrations may cause pulmonary edema, asphyxiation, and death. Acute or chronic exposures may result in ulcerations of the mucous membranes.

A similar spectrum of clinical manifestations may be seen with hydrochloric (HCl), sulfuric (H_2SO_4), hydrofluoric (HF), and other acid vapors, all of which are water-soluble irritant exposures that initially affect the mucous membranes. These agents are commonly used in the etching process that occurs during several steps of semiconductor chip manufacturing. Acid exposure is the most commonly reported cause of inhalation injury in the semiconductor industry.[5]

Several elements used in dopant materials may result in mucous membrane and respiratory tract irritation. Phosphorous oxychloride ($POCl_3$) is a commonly used liquid that hydrolyzes to form hydrochloric acid and phosphoric acid. Other phosphorous compounds that hydrolyze to form irritants include phosphorous trichloride (PCl_3) and phosphorous pentoxide (PO_5). Phosphine (PH_5) is a highly toxic colorless gas with the odor of decaying fish that ignites spontaneously in air. It is an irritant to exposed surfaces and in the respiratory tract causes cough, dyspnea, and pulmonary edema. Symptoms of poisoning may include headaches, nausea, vomiting, paresthesias, and tremors.

Antimony is another dopant material that is used in various compounds in chip manufacturing. Antimony trioxide (Sb_2O_3) is an irritant powder, and antimony trichloride ($SbCl_3$) is a liquid that oxidizes to hydrochloric acid. Hemolysis and multiorgan failure may result from exposure to the gas stibine (SbH_3), similar to the effects of arsine exposure.

Boron is another dopant material with a variety of compounds used in semiconductor manufacturing. Similar to

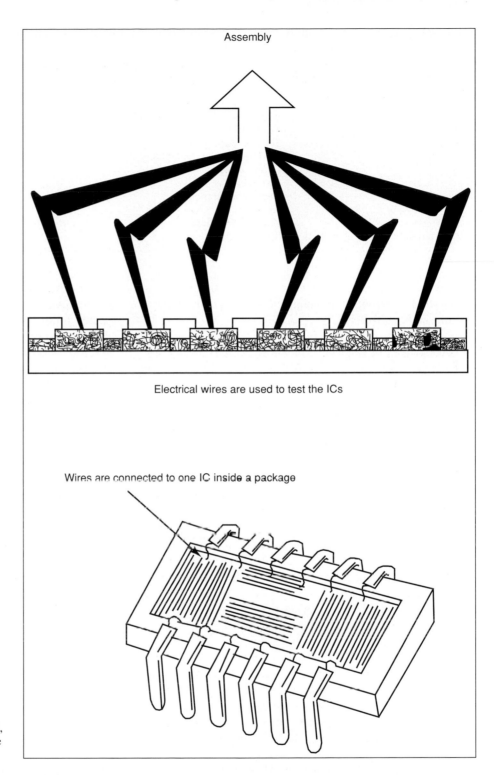

Assembly

Electrical wires are used to test the ICs

Wires are connected to one IC inside a package

Fig. 43-7. The individual integrated circuits (ICs) have metal connectors applied, are sealed into plastic or ceramic, and are individually tested.

phosphorous and antimony, halide compounds of boron may hydrolyze to form halogen acids that are irritants to the mucous membranes and respiratory tract. Diborane (B_2H_6) is a commonly used, flammable gas in semiconductor doping that hydrolyzes to boric acid and hydrogen. The boranes are potent irritants of the skin and mucous membranes, and may cause bronchopulmonary injury.

Asthma and airway hyperresponsiveness

The water-soluble irritants described above have their predominant effects on the mucous membranes and upper respiratory tract, and are generally not a cause of asthma or airway hyperresponsiveness, although exposures to high concentrations of these agents may cause acute inflammatory changes in the airways and asthmatic symptoms.[11]

Table 43-2. Respiratory health outcomes associated with exposures in electronics and semiconductor industries

Outcome	Exposures (examples)	Occurrence
Mucous membrane irritation	Mineral acids (HCl, H_2SO_4, HF), caustics (NaOH, HN_3)	Circuit board cleaning, etching
	Hexamethyldisilazane	Photolithography, semiconductor
Tracheobronchitis	Antimony, phosphorus, selenium compounds	Semiconductor dopants
Rhinitis	Trimellitic anhydride	Electronics
Asthma	Toluene diisocyanate	Wire and equipment insulation
	Soldering resins (colophony)	Soldering
	Epoxy resins	Insulation
	Platinum	Electrical equipment
Pneumonitis	Cadmium compounds	
Acute hemolysis	Arsine	Semiconductor dopant gas
Metal fume fever	Zinc oxide fumes	Electrical equipment
Asphyxiation	Silane, CO_2, N_2	Electronics, semiconductors

However, there are many known and suspect toxins in electronics and semiconductor manufacturing that cause asthma by allergic sensitization.

The best described specific asthma etiology in these industries is from flux exposure of solderers (see Chapter 26). Early studies had demonstrated that asthma resulted from fumes of aminoethyl-ethanolamine in aluminum soldering flux.[12] Asthma among electronics workers was subsequently demonstrated with exposure to electronic soldering flux.[13,14] The principal causal agent in soldering flux was found to be colophony, or pine resin, although specific antibodies to colophony or its conjugates have not been identified. Some sensitized workers further showed a specific response to abeitic acid, the principal resin acid in colophony. Reactions are of the immediate type, beginning within minutes after challenge exposure and with pulmonary function returning to normal within 90 minutes.[14] A latent period of months to 25 years has been observed before the onset of symptoms.[15] Other exposures in electronics manufacturing that may cause asthma include toluene diisocyanate and other isocyanates used in glues, adhesives, wire insulation, and packing materials.[7]

The epoxy compounds cause a variety of respiratory effects. Propylene (CH_2OCHCH_3) and butylene oxides (C_4H_8O) are highly reactive, low-molecular-weight compounds that cause irritation of the eyes and mucous membranes. Epichlorhydrin (CH_2OCHCH_2Cl) is also irritating to the skin, eyes, mucous membranes, and respiratory tract, and may increase the risk of respiratory cancer.[16]

Trimellitic anhydride ($HOCOC_6H_3(CO)_2O$) is a curing agent for epoxy and other resin systems. Several distinct clinical syndromes have been described following exposure to TMA.[17] The first is a sensitization that develops after weeks to years, resulting in allergic rhinitis or asthma. The symptoms recur rapidly upon exposure to TMA dust or fume. The syndrome is mediated by a specific IgE, and can be demonstrated in affected subjects by skin prick testing with a trimellityl-human serum albumin conjugate, or by

specific IgE binding of trimellityl-human serum albumin (TM-HSA).[17] Specific IgG to TMA has also been demonstrated following exposure. The second syndrome, termed the late respiratory systemic syndrome (LRSS), is also a specific sensitization resulting in delayed symptoms of cough, wheeze, and dyspnea. These symptoms may be accompanied by malaise, chills, fever, muscle, and joint aches. Symptoms usually begin 4 to 8 hours after a work shift. Immunologic mediation of this syndrome has been demonstrated.[17] A late onset asthma without systemic symptoms has also been observed. Finally, TMA may cause irritation of the respiratory tract from acute exposures. The spectrum of clinical effects varies with the exposure dose and may range from rhinitis and nosebleed to bronchitis, hemorrhagic pneumonitis, and pulmonary edema. Immunologic mediation may contribute to these effects with repeated lower level exposures.[18]

The positive and negative photoresist systems used in semiconductor chip production include a diverse variety of reactive chemicals.[19] These agents are a part of complex chemical systems developed to polymerize upon light activation. Photoresists include butadienes, isoprenes, nitroanilines, phenones, and quinones. There are few toxicologic data on these agents, but respiratory effects including allergic sensitization are possible.

EPIDEMIOLOGY

There are more epidemiologic studies of electronics workers than of workers in the comparatively newer semiconductor industry, although some recent studies have begun to investigate the prevalence of respiratory disease in semiconductor fabrication facilities. Studies in electronics factories have generally focused on soldering, the most completely described respiratory hazard in the electronics industry.[20-23] Respiratory effects of solvent exposure are specifically covered in Chapter 28.

A cross-sectional investigation of an electronics manufacturing facility found 22% of workers with exposure to soldering fumes had work-related wheezing or dyspnea, and exposed workers had lower forced expiratory volume in 1 second (FEV1) and forced vital capacity (FVC) than unexposed workers.[21] The suspected etiology in these cases was sensitivity to colophony fumes. Occupational rhinitis, eye irritation, and headaches were also common findings among the exposed workers. Atopy and a history of allergic disease, but not cigarette smoking, were weakly associated with soldering asthma in this population.[24]

A study of U.S. electronics workers observed no difference in respiratory symptom prevalence or pulmonary function between solderers using resin-core (colophony) and aqua-core ("phosphorous hexate") solders,[23] suggesting that the irritant effect of acidic fumes from aqua-core fluxes may be as potent as colophony fumes, although the aqua-core fumes are not known to cause a specific allergic reaction.

A cross-sectional study of 1,770 electronics workers in India found a higher prevalence of respiratory complaints (cough, breathlessness, coryza, and chest pain) among exposed workers than among controls.[25] Analysis by exposure categories found the increase only significant among the solderers. Pulmonary function was also decreased among the solderers, but not in the solvent or metal oxide groups. No data on exposure levels are provided for the population.

A cross-sectional study of nonsmoking Chinese female solderers found increased eye and nose irritation but no increase in respiratory symptoms compared to nonexposed controls.[26] The women used rosin-based solder (colophony core), but little information is given on actual exposures. There was no increase in cross-shift decline in peak expiratory flow among the solderers, although static pulmonary function tests showed increased airflow obstruction among the women who had been solderers for more than 5 years compared to those who had soldered for less than 5 years. As with other studies, this cross-sectional analysis is greatly limited by potential bias from a healthy-worker effect.

Although not all studies of electronics workers have demonstrated respiratory symptoms or functional changes from soldering, a clear picture of the "healthy worker effect" phenomena has been observed in this population. Ex-solderers[22] and employees who left an electronics factory[27] had higher rates of respiratory symptoms than those who were current solderers or employees, indicative of "healthier" workers remaining at work as solderers.

Many potential respiratory hazards exist in semiconductor manufacturing, but there have been few epidemiologic investigations of respiratory disease incidence or prevalence in this industrial sector.[28] An early study at a single manufacturing facility found no increase in respiratory symptoms among manufacturing groups,[28] but in a more recent study of 3200 U.S. semiconductor workers in several facilities, small but statistically significant increases in upper respiratory symptoms (eye, nose, or throat irritation) were present among current fabrication room workers compared to nonfabrication workers.[29] Symptom prevalence increased with time in the fabrication room. Persistent wheeze and any lower respiratory symptom (chronic cough, phlegm, or persistent wheeze) were also increased among fabrication workers, and the increased risks were present after adjustment for smoking and other risk factors. The greater prevalence and risk of respiratory symptoms, particularly of the upper respiratory tract, are consistent with the many soluble irritants in fabrication facilities. However, more research is necessary to identify specific agents and tasks associated with the observed effects.

PREVENTION

The general principles of respiratory symptom or disease prevention in electronics and semiconductor manufacturing are the same as in other industries. These are all directed at reducing exposure to toxic agents, either by localized exhaust ventilation, substitution for less hazardous materials, or other established industrial hygiene principles. A few issues specific to these industries will be mentioned.

In electronics manufacturing, printed circuit board wave soldering machines may generate large amounts of soldering fumes, and require localized exhaust. Area exhaust may result in the distribution of soldering fumes throughout the work area. While asthma has been shown to result from rosin-core (colophony) solder, aqua-core solder may also result in respiratory symptoms and cannot be considered a "safe" substitute.[23] In general, substitution of newer agents must be done with caution because they may have toxicities similar to the agents they are replacing.

In semiconductor manufacturing, the highly toxic gases used in manufacturing require exquisite attention to storage, use, and disposal to prevent accidental releases. This includes various engineering controls to protect gas cylinders from physical hazards, such as gas cabinets with local exhaust, interlock systems, and continuous monitoring for leaks in the cabinets and the general environment. Administrative controls should include standard handling procedures, special training of maintenance personnel and other workers who handle gas cylinders, adequate warnings, and emergency procedures for releases.[30,31]

REFERENCES

1. Schenker M: Occupational lung diseases in the industrializing and industrialized world due to modern industries and modern pollutants, *Tubercle Lung Disease* 73:27-32, 1992.
2. Wald PH and Jones JR: Semiconductor manufacturing: an introduction to processes and hazards, *Am J Ind Med* 11:203-221, 1987.
3. Oldham WG: The fabrication of microelectronic circuits, *Sci Am* 237(iii):237, 1977.
4. Sheehy JW and Jones JH: Assessment of arsenic exposures and controls in gallium arsenide production, *Am Ind Hyg Assoc J* 54(2):61-9, 1993.
5. Wade R and Williams M: Semiconductor industry study. In California Department of Industrial Relations, Division of Occupational Safety and Health, Taskforce on Electronics Industry, 1981.
6. Scarpace L, Williams M, Baldwin D, Stewart J, and Lassiter DV: Results of industrial hygiene sampling in semiconductor manufacturing. In ACGIH, editor: *Hazard assessment and control technology in semi-*

conductor manufacturing, pp 47-52. Chelsea, MI, 1989, Lewis Publishers.

7. Paisley DPG: Isocyanate hazard from wire insulation; an old hazard in new guise, *Br J Ind Med* 26:79-81, 1969.

8. Johanson G and Boman A: Percutaneous absorption of 2-butoxy-ethanol vapour in human subjects, *Br J Ind Med* 48:788-792, 1991.

9. Zellers ET, Ke HQ, Smigiel D, et al: Glove permeation by semiconductor processing mixtures containing glycol-ether derivatives, *Am Ind Hyg Assoc J* 53(2):105-16, 1992.

10. Wald PH and Becker CH: *Toxic gases used in the microelectronics industry.* In LaDou J, editor: Occupational Medicine: state of the art reviews, pp 105–117, vol 1. Philadelphia, 1986, Hanley & Belfus, Inc.

11. O'Neil C: Review: mechanisms of occupational airways diseases induced by exposure to organic and inorganic chemicals, *Am J Med Sci* 299(4):265-275, 1990.

12. Pepys J and Sterling CAC: Asthma due to inhaled chemical fumes-amino-ethyl ethanolamine in aluminium soldering flux, *Clin Allergy* 2:197, 1972.

13. Fawcett IW, Taylor AJN, and Pepys J: Asthma due to inhaled chemical agents—fumes from 'Multicore' soldering flux and colophony resin, *Clin Allergy* 6:577-585, 1976.

14. Burge PS, Harries MG, O'Brien I, and Pepys J: Bronchial provocation studies in workers exposed to the fumes of electronic soldering fluxes, *Clin Allergy* 10(2):137-149, 1980.

15. Burge PS, Harries MG, O'Brien IM, and Pepys J: Respiratory disease in workers exposed to solder flux fumes containing colophony (pine resin), *Clin Allergy* 8:1-14, 1978.

16. Enterline PE, Henderson V, and Marsh G: Mortality of workers potentially exposed to epichlorohydrin [see comments], *Br J Ind Med* 47(4):269-76, 1990.

17. Zeiss CR, Mitchell JH, Van PP, Harris J, and Levitz D: A twelve-year clinical and immunologic evaluation of workers involved in the manufacture of trimellitic anhydride (TMA), *Allergy Proc* 11(2):71-7, 1990.

18. Zeiss CR, Leach CL, Levitz D, Hatoum NS, Garvin PJ, and Patterson R: Lung injury induced by short-term intermittent trimellitic anhydride (TMA) inhalation, *J Allergy Clin Immunol* 84(2):219-23, 1989.

19. Wald PH and Becker CH: *Toxic gases used in the microelectronics industry.* In LaDou J, editor: Occupational Medicine: state of the art reviews, pp 105–117, vol 1. Philadelphia, 1986, Hanley & Belfus, Inc.

20. Gupta BN, Rastogi SK, Husain T, Mathur N, and Pangtey BS: A study of respiratory morbidity and pulmonary function among solderers in the electronics industry, *Am Ind Hyg Assoc J* 52:45-51, 1991.

21. Burge PS, Perks W, O'Brien IM, Hawkins R, and Green M: Occupational asthma in an electronics factory, *Thorax* 34:13-18, 1979.

22. Courtney D and Merrett JD: Respiratory symptoms and lung function in a group of solderers, *Br J Ind Med* 41:346-351, 1984.

23. Greaves IA, Wegman DH, Smith TJ, and Spiegelman DL: Respiratory effects of two types of solder flux used in the electronics industry, *JOM* 26:81-85, 1984.

24. Burge PS, Perks WH, O'Brien IM, et al: Occupational asthma in an electronics factory: a case control study to evaluate aetiological factors, *Thorax* 34:300-307, 1979.

25. Mathur N, Gupta BN, Rastogi SK, et al: Socioeconomic and health status of electronics workers employed in organized industry, *Am J Ind Med* 23(2):321-31, 1993.

26. Lee HS, Koh D, Chia HP, and Phoon WH: Symptoms, lung function and diurnal variation in peak expiratory flow rate among female solderers in the electronics industry, *Am J Ind Med* 26:613-619, 1994.

27. Perks WH, Burge PS, Rehahn M, and Green M: Work-related respiratory disease in employees leaving an electronics factory, *Thorax* 34:19-22, 1979.

28. Pastides H, Calabrese EJ, Hosmer DJ, and Harris DJ: Spontaneous abortion and general illness symptoms among semiconductor manufacturers, *J Occup Med* 30(7):543-51, 1988.

29. Schenker MB, Beaumont J, Eskenazi B, et al: Epidemiologic study of reproductive and other health effects among workers employed in the manufacture of semiconductors. Final report to the Semiconductor Industry Association, University of California at Davis, 1992.

30. Sherin BJ: Risk assessment and control of toxic gas releases. In *Hazard assessment and control technology in semiconductor manufacturing,* pp 115-133. Chelsea, MI, 1989, Lewis Publishers.

31. Varadi L: Process hazard reviews in the semiconductor industry. In *Hazard assessment and control technology in semiconductor manufacturing,* vol II, pp 145-157. Cincinnati, OH, 1993, American Conference of Governmental Industrial Hygienists, Inc.

Chapter 44

HOSPITALS AND LABORATORIES

Melissa McDiarmid
Virginia Weaver
Ellen R. Kessler

Hospital and laboratory environments have long been associated with infectious hazards causing a multiplicity of illness, including respiratory disease in exposed workers. Beyond biologics, however, hospitals and laboratories possess every type of hazard class capable of causing respiratory disease including chemical toxicants, physical hazards, and allergens. Hospitals and laboratories have not been considered part of a traditional industrial base, and, until recently, many of its hazards have gone unrecognized or underrecognized.

Probably the longest standing program of hospital hazard control concerns the control of hospital infections. Here the focus traditionally has been on preventing patient-to-patient spread, although workers and bystander exposure was of some concern as well. There continues to be a "tension," in fact, between Hospital Infection Control and Employee Health Units due to their differing missions and priorities. Infection Control Committees traditionally have not been concerned with worker health. Moreover, until recently many hospitals have not had Employee Health programs. There was no institutional unit responsible for worker health and safety.

Many myths contributed to this situation. First, the myth that, compared with the industrial setting, hospitals were safe, clean places to work implied no need for a worker health and safety function in the hospital institution. Then the myth that health care professionals are more aware of hazards than the average public and will "police their own" adds to the misconception. A third and most unsettling myth is that exposure to infectious patients or other hazards is "part of the job" in health care, so that prevention strategies, safe work practices, and health and safety programs do not belong in hospitals. Increasingly, hospitals are recognizing the need for an employee health and safety function.

Hospitals are estimated to employ greater than 5 million workers nationwide. In many municipalities, they are the principal employer. Thus, the impact hospital and laboratory exposures exert on a working population may be significant. Recent work has reflected this and has attempted to describe and catalogue hospital and laboratory hazards.[1,2] This chapter focuses on respiratory illness derived from this work and will discuss clinical manifestations of illnesses encountered as well as the common biologic agents, physical hazards, and chemical toxicants that must be considered.

SOURCES OF EXPOSURE

Employee health and safety functions increasingly are being established in the hospital and laboratory settings. These units may have varying configurations and include professionals from Infection Control, Industrial Hygiene and Engineering, Administration, and Clinicians from Employee Health Units. Beyond establishing standard operating procedures and safe work practices, this team performs the hazard identification function for the institution and locates exposure sources for various hazards.

Lewy has suggested that hospital hazards fall into three categories: the patient; the technology involved with the diagnosis, treatment, and research of a disease; and the institutional infrastructure or the environmental operations.[1] Given that paradigm, the major hazards associated with these three exposure sources are displayed in the box.

The principal potential hazard that patients pose to hospital workers is infection. This risk includes infectious diseases for which the patient is being hospitalized that might, if contracted by the worker, result in the disease. Addition-

ally, exposure to patients with undiagnosed illness, especially tuberculosis (TB), poses a significant hazard. The resurgence of TB is a major hazard for health care workers (HCWs) and are discussed further.

Sources of exposure to respiratory toxicants associated with patients' diagnosis and treatment and disease research are myriad. All hazard classes are represented here. Chemical toxicants such as laboratory reagents and disinfectants as well as pharmaceuticals, especially those agents classified as hazardous drugs,[3,4] and unique products such as methacrylate resins used in orthopedic surgical procedures are commonly encountered in today's hospital and laboratory environments. Radiation and radionuclide exposure, although possible, is extremely unlikely except in a mishap. However, laboratory exposures to infectious material and laboratory animal allergy (LAA) occur more commonly. Hospitals and laboratories pose many occupational hazards for workers; although those causing nonrespiratory insult are beyond the scope of this chapter.

Maintaining a clean environment requires hospital and laboratory staff to use industrial cleaners, detergents, and disinfectants that in themselves present potential respiratory toxicities when inhaled acutely or when inadequately diluted. Liquid sterilants such as formaldehyde and glutaraldehyde are well known respiratory irritants. Ethylene oxide (EtO), used in gas sterilization operations, may cause some respiratory irritation.

Industrial cooling systems required in large hospital complexes have had *Legionella* contamination with outbreaks of disease principally in immunocompromised patients but also in some workers.[5,6] Other indoor air quality problems related to mold or spore exposure are also a hazard in hospitals.

RESPIRATORY INFECTIONS

The major hospital-acquired infection concerning HCWs has been hepatitis B infection, which does not manifest as a respiratory illness. Among respiratory pathogens, bacterial agents including *Mycobacterium tuberculosis, Corynebacterium diphtheriae,* and *Legionella* and others have caused historical outbreaks. Many viral agents have also caused respiratory illness in workers including cytomegalovirus (CMV) influenza, measles, respiratory syncytial virus (RSV), rotovirus, rubella, and varicella (see Chapter 32). The major respiratory pathogens threatening HCWs are described in this chapter.

Tuberculosis

Tuberculosis, once a major cause of morbidity and mortality in HCWs and on the decline in the middle part of this century, is unfortunately again on the rise. Reports of cases among HCWs date to the last century.[7] Nonoccupational prevalence of disease has always been a significant factor in determining HCW exposure. In the 1930s, prior to the advances made in infection control and chemo-

---

Sources of exposure to respiratory hazards

Patient

Tuberculosis
Cytomegalovirus
Varicella
Meningococcus
Respiratory syncytial virus

Diagnosis, treatment, research

Radiation and radionuclides
Pharmaceuticals
Disinfectants
Laboratory animals
Methacrylate resins
Infectious agents
Chemical reagents
Compressed gas

Hygiene and environment

Ethylene oxide
Disinfectants and cleaners
Formaldehyde
Glutaraldehyde
Legionella
Molds and spores

therapy, a study of student nurses at Philadelphia General Hospital revealed positive tuberculosis skin tests for 28% of entering students but 100% for graduates 3 years later.[8] The 28% rate was presumed to be the background rate in the general population. Clearly, the opportunity for exposure was a reflection of the higher background prevalence and the lack of now recognized infection control techniques.

Classical public health and infection control measures, including early identification and isolation of patients, together with advances in antituberculosis chemotherapy in the middle part of this century, dramatically lowered the incidence of TB. In the mid-1980s, however, the declining rate of TB cases was halted. The increase in cases can be attributed to the classical risk factors for TB including poverty, overcrowding, homelessness, limited access to health care, poor nutritional status, and other recognized indicators of decline in the nation's social fabric.[9]

An important new factor in the current outbreak, however, is the increase in immunocompromised people exposed to TB. Tuberculosis is an opportunistic infection in immunocompromised persons, including those with human immunodeficiency virus (HIV) infection.[10-12] The convergence of populations who are immunocompromised and persons who possess the described other risk factors occurs in several congregational settings. Highly publicized nosocomial TB outbreaks have in several cases been attributed to infection transmitted from hospitals to prisons and the reverse, while rendering care to ill inmates.[13]

Epidemiology

The Centers for Disease Control and Prevention (CDC) in cooperation with the American Hospital Association (AHA) recently completed a survey of 729 medical institutions. They reported active TB in HCWs had occurred at 90(13.1%) of the responding institutions.[14] Additional institutions reported HCW skin test conversions but not active disease. Comprehensive data on work-related TB, even in a health care setting, have been difficult to acquire. One recent review documented historical employee pufiried protein derivative (PPD) conversion rates in annual HCW screening ranging from <1% to 5% in the 1960s to 1990.[15] Postexposure conversion rates, however, have been documented in the literature with much higher rates, ranging from 6% to 77% of those HCWs exposed.[15]

A significant barrier to obtaining occupational data regarding TB is that until recently the form used to report TB cases to the CDC did not collect occupational data. This caused lack of recognition of the disease's relation to work exposures. The U.S. Occupational Safety and Health Administration (OSHA), recognizing the significant work-related component to the current epidemic, has promulgated compliance guidelines for its inspectors, giving direction on elements to consider when investigating a TB complaint. OSHA may thus utilize recognized safety and health standards of practice recommended by consensus standard set-

ting bodies. These standards as published in the medical or professional literature can be seen as methods of abatement in citing exposure of employees to a recognized, serious hazard for which there is a feasible and useful method of control. Specific guidelines for controlling TB have been published by the CDC in its Morbidity and Mortality Weekly Reports (MMWRs).

Prevention

The regulatory approach to occupational TB control derives from the classical hierarchy of workplace controls, which employs engineering and administrative controls and personal protective equipment (PPE) to protect workers. OSHA derived the elements for TB exposure control for health care workers from the CDC document addressing the hospital work setting.[16] These elements (Table 44-1) include administrative controls such as developing an exposure control plan including timely identification and isolation of patients, employee TB skin testing and training, providing negative pressure TB isolation rooms, and use of respiratory protection by workers in some settings.

Respiratory syncytial virus

Respiratory syncytial virus is a single-stranded ribonucleic acid (RNA) organism that is a member of the paramyxoviridae family and *Pneumovirus* genus. RSV is the major cause of bronchiolitis and pneumonia in young children, particularly those under 2 years old. For premature infants, or young children afflicted with certain heart or lung diseases, the mortality rate can be high. For infants who develop bronchiolitis, asthma and chronic obstructive pulmonary disease (COPD) can occur in later life.[17,18] The mortality rate is also high in immunocompromised adults who develop RSV pneumonia.

Community outbreaks of RSV generally affect a large percentage of young children, many of whom are admitted to the hospital with lower respiratory infections. Studies have demonstrated that over 40% of the hospital personnel may become infected from the infants in their care.[19] Direct person-to-person contact is responsible for most of the

Table 44-1. Elements of a tuberculosis control program

Administration controls
    Identification and isolation of patients
    Skin test surveillance
    Respiratory isolation signs
    Controlling traffic in and out of respiratory isolation room
    High-hazard procedure practices
    Worker training and education
Engineering controls
    Negative pressure respiratory isolation
    Treatment booth and local exhaust ventilation
Personal protective equipment
    Particulate respirators

---

nosocomial spread; however, transmission of the virus has also occurred even when direct contact with infected persons did not take place. This implies that hospital personnel caring for these children can also be a vector in the spread of virus.[19] Similar patterns of nosocomial spread have been observed in a marrow transplant center where 16% of marrow transplant patients became infected despite the use of routine respiratory precautions.[20]

Respiratory syncytial virus harbored in the secretions of an infected patient may survive for over 24 hours on countertops, skin, hospital gowns, and paper for up to 1 hour.[21]

The frequency and severity of nosocomial spread involve several factors:

1. Natural immunity to RSV is incomplete, and virtually every person present is at risk for acquiring and transmitting the disease.[22]
2. Patients who have been hospitalized for RSV infection (i.e., infants with lower respiratory tract disease) shed virus in high titers over prolonged periods of time.[23]
3. Employees can carry contaminated secretions on hands and gowns.[19]
4. Employees can inoculate themselves by inadvertently touching their eyes and mouth with contaminated secretions.

Clinical manifestations in health care workers

The impact of RSV infection on the hospital and its employees is notable. Morbidity, economic loss, and decreases in a much needed workforce are significant consequences. Studies have shown that nearly half the HCWs who have become infected by close contact with patients become symptomatic enough to lose work time.[19] In addition, repeated infections occurring a few weeks apart can be caused by an inoculum that is large enough to overcome the host's natural but incomplete immunity. Some employees have had both persistently increased pulmonary resistance as measured by Pulmonary function tests (PFTs) and hyperreactive airway responses to cholinergic challenge for up to 8 weeks after developing the disease.[24]

Epidemiology

Hall et al. studied two separate outbreaks of RSV in an infant ward concurrent with two community outbreaks of RSV 1 year apart.[25] The magnitude of both outbreaks in the community was felt to be similar as well as the numbers of patients admitted with RSV infection. In the study of the first outbreak, 45% of infants who were hospitalized for ≥1 week developed nosocomial infection. In the study of the second outbreak, only 19% developed nosocomial infection—a statistically significant decrease. In contrast, the rate of RSV infection among hospital staff increased from 42% in the first study to 56% in the second study. Several changes took place after the first study including new procedures for handwashing, changing gowns between pa-

tients, and cohorting of staff to infected patients. A new infant ward was also built, but the procedural changes were postulated to play the greater role. The increased rate of infection of the staff in the second study was most likely the result of prolonged contact to infected infants and fomites.

Prevention

Careful handwashing by all hospital staff and visitors is by far the most important factor in preventing transmission. Studies show that gown and mask use have little benefit, but the use of eye–nose goggles is effective by decreasing self-inoculation. The combination of gown and glove use also appears to be effective.[19,26] Infected infants should be isolated, and symptomatic employees should avoid caring for patients at particular risk.

Influenza

Community epidemics of influenza type A or B viruses occur in the winter months at a rate of every 1 to 3 years. Yearly antigenic changes of the virus prevent natural immunity in individuals who have been previously infected with antigenically dissimilar strains. This helps to explain the epidemic nature of this infection. Outbreaks occur explosively; simultaneous infections occur suggesting that many susceptible people can be infected by one individual. School children have the highest attack rate (50%); it is generally considered a self-limited malady of fever and upper respiratory infection.[27] Mortality, however, is significant in the elderly and others with underlying medical conditions such as cardiac or pulmonary disease. Death is most often a consequence of primary viral or secondary bacterial pneumonia.

During epidemics, hospitalizations for influenza-related pneumonia increase dramatically. The pattern of nosocomial infection with influenza A or B virus is similar to RSV in that the HCW can be either the source of a person-to-person transmission or the vector. In contrast, dissemination of the influenza virus is potentially more efficient because small droplets of infected secretions become aerosolized during sneezing, coughing, or talking. Spread to hospitalized and nursing home patients has been well documented.[28,29] However, given the prevalence of the disease in the community, it is difficult to determine a nosocomial rate of spread to the patients and especially to the hospital staff.

Prevention is primarily attempted with an inactivated virus vaccine that is usually composed of 2 A subtypes and 1 B subtype of the influenza virus. The subtypes of virus from the previous year's outbreak go into the formulation of the vaccine for the upcoming year. The Immunization Practices Advisory Committee (ACIP) recommends that HCWs who have prolonged contact with increased-risk patients receive the vaccine yearly.[30] This recommendation is based on the assumption that HCWs are responsible for a significant portion of the nosocomial spread to these patients; however, the degree of efficacy of the vaccine in preventing nosocomial spread is not entirely clear.[31–33]

Amantadine prophylaxis, which must be taken for the entire influenza season, has been well studied and is considered to be effective against influenza A.[34] Unfortunately, its unpleasant side effects prevent it from being widely used for this purpose. Amantadine also minimizes the severity and duration of illness with influenza A and should be considered early in the course of the disease. This treatment may be especially applicable to increased-risk individuals and those caring for them.

Prevention can be further facilitated by isolating infected patients, restricting visitors with respiratory illnesses, and limiting elective surgery.

Measles (rubeola)

Measles, a paramyxovirus, has for the most part been regarded as a disease of childhood. It is highly contagious and is spread by direct contact with droplets of secretions from infected individuals. Airborne spread is well documented, particularly in low humidity where infected droplets remain in the air longer. The incidence of measles began to decrease in 1963 when the live-attenuated vaccine was introduced. This decrease was continued through 1983 when the number of cases reported reached an all time low of 1,497. However, since then, there has been a measurable increase in the number of reported cases.[35]

Uncomplicated measles generally lasts between 7 and 10 days. Preliminary symptoms may begin with cough, coryza, and fever, characteristically followed by a rash. Koplik spots appear in the buccal mucosa several days before the rash appears. Infectivity is greatest several days before the onset of the rash and continues for several days thereafter. In uncomplicated measles, individuals generally recover completely; when death does occur, it is caused by one of the two primary complications of measles—pneumonia or encephalitis. Although death occurs in 1 of every 1,000 reported cases, the greatest risk of death is for children under 2 years and individuals over 15 years.[22]

When the measles virus attacks the respiratory epithelium, possibly complicated by a bacterial superinfection, pneumonia will occur. Primary rubeola pneumonia is acute and occurs soon after the onset of the rash. Pneumonia caused by a bacterial superinfection generally develops 1 to 7 days after the onset of the rash. A severe, often fatal form of measles manifested by a giant cell pneumonia also occurs in individuals immunocompromised with cellular deficiencies. The typical rash is absent, which makes the diagnosis extremely difficult.[36]

Immunity following measles infection is considered lifelong. The ACIP has concluded that those at risk of contagion are individuals who never received the vaccine, were vaccinated once before 16 months of age, or were born in or after 1957 and received only one childhood vaccination. According to the ACIP, all these groups should be vaccinated unless contraindicated.[37]

Outbreaks in medical facilities have been a serious problem. Susceptible HCWs can contract the disease and pass it on to patients and other workers, resulting in potentially serious and fatal complications.[38]

The ACIP specifically addresses vaccination guidelines for medical facilities where the risk is higher than for the general population.[39] Hospitals should require staff members who were born after 1956 and have direct patient contact to supply evidence of two live vaccinations, documentation of physician diagnosed measles, or serologic evidence of immunity. The ACIP is less clear concerning those individuals born before 1957, recommending one dose during an outbreak in the hospital or in the community it serves.

Several studies support the claim that whereas age is the best predictor of immunity, many individuals born before 1957 are susceptible to measles. For example, Schwarcz et al. found that 5.3% of all employees in one California hospital had inadequate immunity by serologic testing.[40] Of that 5.3%, 45% were born before 1957. Other investigators also challenged the "1957 cutoff" for measles immunity determination. The results of one survey led Kim et al. to make a recommendation that individuals who were born between 1950 and 1957 should also be included in hospital vaccination programs.[41]

Hospital-wide vaccination programs can be extremely costly. In addition, contraindications such as pregnancy should be considered when designing an effective protection program for this employee population. Therefore, initial screening of all "susceptible" employees for immunity may be a choice to consider before administering the vaccine.

Varicella

Varicella zoster virus (VZV) is the responsible agent in varicella (chickenpox) and herpes zoster (shingles). Varicella, the primary infection, is extremely contagious but is generally considered a self-limited disease of childhood. Only 10% of individuals over the age of 15 are considered susceptible to varicella. Herpes zoster is the reactivation of a latent varicella infection and occurs in 10% of the population. It appears to attack the elderly most frequently but is seen in all age groups. Although herpes zoster can cause serious morbidity, particularly in the immunocompromised, it is rarely fatal. On the other hand, varicella is noted for its potentially serious and sometimes fatal manifestations in adults and immunocompromised individuals.[22]

Uncomplicated chickenpox presents with fever, malaise, and a characteristic vesicular rash. The rash develops over a period of 2 to 4 days and heals in various stages by scab formation. For adults, the complications most often seen are encephalitis and interstitial pneumonitis.

In varicella pneumonitis, symptoms range from a nonproductive cough to severe dyspnea, hemoptysis, and cyanosis. In advanced conditions, hypoxia results from marked impairment in diffusing capacity. Physical findings in the milder cases are usually limited to fine rales, but in severe cases, rhonchi, inspiratory and expiratory wheezing, as well as decreased breath sounds are heard. Diffuse nodular densities are seen on chest x-ray; a coalescent pattern is often noted in life-threatening cases. Occasionally, pleural effusions occur. One out of 400 infected adults is afflicted with pulmonary complications that are serious enough to require hospitalization.[42] Pregnant women are especially at risk for serious varicella pneumonitis. Varicella pneumonitis occurs more frequently than symptoms suggest. In one prospective study, 16% of adults had radiographic evidence of pneumonitis, however, only 6% of this study population had any accompanying respiratory symptoms.[43]

Varicella is transmitted by direct person-to-person contact and by airborne spread. The virus, however, is quite labile and thus contact with contaminant objects, such as countertops, does not appear to be a successful route of spread. Susceptible individuals coming into direct contact with herpes zoster lesion can also contract chickenpox. Disseminated herpes zoster and possibly localized zoster lesions also have an airborne mode of VZV spread.

Nosocomial transmission of VZV is problematic. Airborne spread by varicella and herpes zoster has been documented even when direct contact with susceptible individuals was not considered to have occurred.[44,45] Studies have implied that strict isolation without the implementation of negative pressure rooms may fail to prevent transmission of the virus to others.[46] In one report, airflow studies by using tracer gases demonstrated that air exchanges took place between the infected patients' rooms and the adjacent corridors.

Personnel without a positive history of varicella should be tested with an antibody assay such as fluorescent antibody to membrane antigen (FAMA), immune adherence hemagglutination (IAH), or enzyme-linked immunosorbent assay (ELISA). Testing is very important if varicella is prevalent in the institution or in areas of the hospital with increased-risk patients.

Susceptible personnel who have been exposed to varicella should be sent home during the incubation period of 10 to 21 days after exposure. If varicella develops, the employee is considered infectious until all lesions crust over.

Varicella immune globulin (VZIG) can prevent or modify the course of the illness when given soon after the exposure. The Committee of Infectious Disease and The American Academy of Pediatrics recommends that susceptible adults, especially pregnant women, should be considered for this treatment if significant exposure has occurred.[47]

Recently, a live varicella vaccine has been developed and licensed in the United States. However, it is unlikely that its applications will extend to use in healthy susceptible adults.

Legionnaires' disease

The bacterium *Legionella* pneumophilia was first identified in 1976 following an investigation of an outbreak of pneumonia in a Philadelphia hotel hosting an American Legion Convention.[48] It has been demonstrated that those at risk for developing the disease tend to be over 50 years of age, smokers, or have an underlying condition that impairs immunity such as diabetes or malignancy. A milder form of the disease called Pontiac fever is not associated with pneumonia.[22]

The natural habitat of this bacterium is aquatic; contaminated water systems including cooling towers, condensers, and air conditioning units are the ideal environment for proliferation. Transmission is by inhalation of infected aerosolized water and not by person-to-person contact.

Nosocomial spread has been well documented, but HCWs seem to be at little risk for developing the disease. Epidemiologic evidence suggests that exposed HCWs will develop antibodies to *Legionella*, whereas a small proportion may develop a mild flulike illness.[5,6] On the other hand, surgical patients, particularly transplant patients, are at greatest risk with a mortality rate that may approach 50%.[49,50]

Prevention of *Legionella* outbreaks in a hospital setting can be achieved by routine testing of the water supply. If bacteria are present, control means may include pasteurization (heat treatment), chlorination, UV light, ozonation, or metal ionization. Once in place the appropriate control system must be monitored for effectiveness with environmental cultures.

Laboratory workers

Laboratory associated infections were identified as early as the turn of this century. Since then, well over 6,000 cases, including 250 fatalities, have been reported in the medical literature.[51] Pulmonary infections represent a significant portion of these occupationally occurring contagions.

In 1974, a booklet entitled *Classification of Etiologic Agents on the Basis of Hazard* was published and served as a reference guide for classifying the risks of laboratory-acquired infections.[52] Four levels of safety measures were established in accordance with the hazards of the infectious agents and the specifics of the work practices. These guidelines became the framework for the first edition of *Biosafety in Microbiological and Biomedical Laboratories* (BMBL).

In the early 1980s, there was growing concern about transmission of the deadly etiologic agent of acquired immunodeficiency syndrome (AIDS) in the laboratory setting even before the HIV was actually identified. A formula for protecting against bloodborne pathogens was devised and in 1991, "Universal Precautions" became mandated. Now with the recent emergence of multiple drug-resistant strains of TB regulatory issues concerning the prevention of airborne transmission of TB and other infectious agents in the laboratory setting are necessarily being addressed.

Table 44-2. Hospital- and laboratory-acquired respiratory pathogens

Common name	Microorganism	Clinical signs	Mode of spread	Reservoir
Q fever[130,131]	*Coxiella burnetti*	Pneumonia	Airborne, contaminated clothing	Chick embryos
Psittacosis[53]	*Chlamydia psittaci*	Pneumonia	Airborne, contaminated clothing	Dried bird excreta
Histoplasmosis[132]	*Histoplasma capsulatum*	Bronchopneumonia	Airborne	Bird excreta, contaminated soil
Tuberculosis[133,134]	*Mycobacterium tuberculosis*	Cavitary pneumonia, pleural effusion	Airborne, skin inoculation	Infected specimens
Blastomycosis[135]	*Blastomyces dermatitidis*	Pneumonia	Airborne, skin inoculation	Not reported
Coccidiomycosis[136,137]	*Coccidiodes immitis*	Cavitary pneumonia, pneumonitis	Airborne, skin inoculation	Infected specimen, contaminated glassware
Glanders[138]	*Pseudomonas mallei*	Pneumonia	Skin inoculation	Culture material
Anthrax[138]	*Bacillus anthracis*	Pneumonia	Airborne	Vaccine preparation, smoking while handling culture
Tularemia[139]	*Francisella tularensis*	Pneumonia, lung abscess	Airborne	Culture material
Hemorrhagic fever with renal syndrome[140,141]	Hantaan virus	Pulmonary edema	Fomites	

The Bloodborne Pathogen Standard includes the only mandated methods for documenting laboratory-related infections *and* exposures. Without a national reporting system to encompass all laboratory-associated infections, reported cases will remain a significant underestimation of actual occurrences. Many exposures result in subclinical infection with only immunological evidence of transmission.

Epidemiology

Table 44-2 includes many of the respiratory infections that have been reported in the literature. Aerosol and percutaneous exposures represent the most frequent means of transmission. Aerosols can occur in several ways (i.e., as a result of a spill or while practicing normal laboratory techniques such as placing a loop into a flame). Airborne transmission has been implicated in most of the common source infections. For example, of the 11 cases of psittacosis that occurred at a laboratory facility in 1930, only two employees had direct exposure to infected birds.[53] The others worked elsewhere in the same building.

Prevention

A description of the different levels of biosafety recommendations as described in the third edition of BMBL are beyond the scope of this chapter. Limiting access, control of airflow, use of personal protection, and the strict adherence to work practices are integral for maintaining a safe working environment. Biologic safety cabinets (BSCs), such as the vertical laminar airflow system with a high-efficiency particulate air filter (HEPA), are an essential factor of worker protection. When absolute containment is essential, closed negative air pressure cabinets that are accessed by ports with attached rubber gloves are indicated.

CHEMICAL HAZARDS

The chemical hazards encountered in hospitals and laboratories are extremely varied, reflecting the diversity of occupations found in these environments. Toxicants range from unique chemicals, such as hazardous drugs, to those common in many workplaces, such as solvents. These chemicals have significant toxicities, ranging from sensitization to reproductive effects to human carcinogenesis. Table 44-3 contains a summary of the chemical and physical pulmonary toxicants discussed in this chapter with information on their clinical effects, diagnostic considerations, prevention strategies, and applicable OSHA regulations.

Acids and alkalis

Acid and base compounds are common in hospital and laboratory settings. Acids ranging from acetic to sulfuric and bases in the form of sodium hydroxide were noted in a recent study of chemical exposures in an academic medical center.[2] Laboratory workers, both clinical and research, are commonly exposed to such toxicants. Housekeeping staff may be exposed to bleach (sodium hypochlorite), ammonia, and caustic floor strippers.

Acute inhalational exposure can cause upper respiratory tract irritation and, if in high concentrations, chemical pneumonitis with pulmonary edema. Reactive airways dysfunction syndrome (RADS) has been reported in a group of hospital employees exposed to glacial acetic acid after a spill.[54] Mineral laboratory analysis employees exposed to several acid vapors, including hydrochloric, hydrofluoric, nitric,

Table 44-3. Chemical and physical hazards causing respiratory disease in hospitals and laboratory environments

Toxicant	Pulmonary effects		Diagnostic considerations	Specific preventions	OSHA regulations*
	Acute	Chronic			
Acids and bases	Irritation, pulmonary edema, bronchospasm	Bronchitis,† cancer†			1910.1000
Ethylene oxide	Irritation, pulmonary edema, RADS	Asthma	IgE antibodies, EtO in blood and expired air	Engineering controls for sterilizers	1910.1047
Formaldehyde	Irritation, pulmonary edema	Asthma, nasopharyngeal cancer in animals	IgE and IgG antibodies, specific inhalation challenges	Local exhaust ventilation, isolation	1010.1048
Glutaraldehyde	Irritation	Asthma	Specific inhalation challenges	Local exhaust ventilation	1010.1000
Hazardous drugs	Irritation	Rhinitis Asthma	IgE antibodies, skin testing, specific inhalation challenges	BSCs, administration booths	Guidelines
Latex		Asthma	IgE antibodies, skin testing, specific inhalation chalenges	Nonlatex gloves	
Mercury	Pneumonitis		Mercury in blood and urine	Local ventilation, spill management	1910.1000
Methyl methacrylate	Irritation	Asthma		Local ventilation	1910.1000
Solvents	Irritation, bronchospasm		Blood, urine, and expired air measures		1910.1000
Radiation		Pulmonary fibrosis	Dosimetry		1910.96
Asbestos		Asbestosis, cancer, pleural plaques		Removal of friable asbestos, encapsulation	1910.1001

*The 1989 PELs in 29 CFR 1910.1000 were recently rescinded, however they can still be cited under the General Duty Clause.
†Sulfuric acid.
BSCs, Biologic safety cabinets; ***OSHA,*** U.S. Occupational Safety and Health Administration; ***RADS,*** reactive airways dysfunction syndrome.

and sulfuric, were reported to have symptoms of dyspnea and chest tightness during a period of increased work.[53] Two of the affected workers were found to have a decrease in forced expiratory volume in 1 second (FEV1) during their workshift. Initial histamine challenge hyperreactivity was no longer present in two individuals several months after exposure ceased.

Toxic inhalations have been reported in hospital personnel after inadvertent mixing of bleach and acid solutions, resulting in the release of chlorine gas.[56] Bleach and ammonia combinations can also release toxic products. Such inhalations can be quite severe, with resultant pulmonary edema and chronic scarring. Other acute manifestations from acid or base exposure include chemical burns from skin contact and severe systemic and gastrointestinal (GI) effects following ingestion. Chronic exposure to sulfuric acid can lead to tracheobronchitis.[51]

Adverse outcomes can be prevented by measures to reduce exposure. These include the use of local ventilation (e.g., chemical fume hoods) and PPE when working with concentrated acids and bases. Worker education is essential for compliance with these measures.

Ethylene oxide

Ethylene oxide is a colorless gas with a sweet etherlike odor. It is used to sterilize heat-sensitive medical instruments. Exposed workers include employees in central supply who are responsible for the sterilization of this equipment as well as end-users such as operating room and dental staff.

Pulmonary effects from acute exposure include respiratory tract irritation with sore throat, rhinitis, cough, and shortness of breath. Questionnaire evaluation of sterilizer operators with a mean EtO exposure of 3.4 ppm per sterilizer cycle found the presence of these symptoms in 15% to 20%.[58] Systemic manifestations may result from inhalation and range from headache and nausea to decreased consciousness and pulmonary edema with extremely high exposures.[59] Bronchospasm following 4 days of acute high level exposure has been reported in a railway worker.[60] This individual developed persistent obstructive pulmonary function abnormalities and was diagnosed with RADS. Other acute effects include burns from skin contact.

Asthma and rhinitis can occur in renal dialysis patients exposed to EtO through equipment sterilization.[61] IgE antibodies to human albumin-EtO conjugates have been measured in these patients and their presence has shown an association with chronic asthma and anaphylaxis during dialysis.[62] Rarely, asthma in employees can occur.[63] In the last decade, EtO has been recognized as an animal and probable human carcinogen.[64,65] Exposure has also been associated with an increased risk of spontaneous abortion.[66] Other effects include peripheral neuropathy,[67] central nervous system (CNS) dysfunction,[68] and dermal sensitization.[59]

EtO-specific tests include IgE antibodies to the EtO-albumin conjugate, which have been used in studies of dialysis patients.[62] Researchers have reported measurements of EtO in blood and expired breath of exposed workers that correlated with environmental sampling.[69] Tests to monitor genetic damage are also receiving a great deal of attention. One study compared a number of markers of deoxyribonucleic acid (DNA) damage and found EtO-hemoglobin adducts and certain sister chromatid exchange measures to be correlated with exposures at or below the OSHA permissible exposure limit (PEL).[70] This information, although useful in research settings to identify groups of workers at higher risk and to determine no observable effect levels, cannot, at present, be used to predict individual risk.

Medical surveillance for EtO is required by OSHA for all employees exposed at or above the action level [0.5 ppm for an 8 hour time-weighted average (TWA) for 30 or more days per year].[71] Annual examinations are to be performed before exposure, and at the termination of exposure. In addition, employees should be evaluated if signs or symptoms of exposure develop, if the employee has questions regarding reproductive issues, after exposures in emergency situations, or if the physician believes more frequent examinations are warranted.

Specific requirements for surveillance are detailed in the Standard. Most are for nonpulmonary endpoints; however, in situations where exposure remains above the OSHA PEL of 1 ppm for an 8-hour TWA (i.e., maintenance activities or during installation of engineering controls), respiratory protection is mandated by the Standard. In such cases, workers need evaluation for fitness to use a respirator. The Standard recommends a chest x-ray every 5 years, PFTs every 3 years, and an annual evaluation of cardiovascular function.

Engineering controls and proper work techniques designed to reduce exposure are the cornerstones of prevention. Extensive air monitoring evaluations by the U.S. National Institute for Occupational Safety and Health (NIOSH) documents exposure reduction from changes made in the design and function of EtO sterilizers to comply with the current OSHA Standard. Isolation of sterilizers in a separate, well-ventilated room, local exhaust ventilation at the sterilizer door, aeration cabinets, and continuous monitoring for EtO constitute some of these changes.[72]

Formaldehyde

Formaldehyde (see Chapter 28) is used as a fixative in pathology and anatomy laboratories and as a sterilant, especially in renal dialysis units. It is often encountered as formalin, a solution of water, formaldehyde, and small amounts of alcohol. Airborne levels in this environment can be significant as evidenced by a study of personal breathing zone samples in anatomy laboratories that found 44% of samples to be in excess of 1 ppm.[73]

Acute effects include eye and upper respiratory tract irritation from exposure to low ambient air concentrations (0.1 to 5 ppm).[72] Inhalation of higher concentrations (10 to 20 ppm) can lead to lower respiratory tract irritation manifested by cough, chest tightness, and tachycardia. Exposures of 50 to 100 ppm can cause pulmonary edema and death. Eye contact with formalin solutions may result in severe corneal damage.[72]

Chronic exposure is a well known cause of irritant and allergic contact dermatitis. Less commonly, exposed individuals may develop bronchospasm. Hendrick and Lane reported the 5-year follow-up of two renal dialysis nurses with formaldehyde asthma following high-level exposure.[74] The individual whose exposure continued had persistent symptoms and remained responsive to formaldehyde inhalational challenge testing consisting of 3 ppm for 5 minutes. The worker who was no longer exposed was symptom free and had no response after 15 minutes at 6 ppm.[75] Whether formaldehyde asthma is due to an irritant or sensitizing mechanism is still controversial.[76]

Blood formaldehyde levels and urinary formate have been evaluated as biologic monitoring methods but due to the presence of formaldehyde normally in the body and rapid metabolism, these tests are of little value.[77] Antibodies to formaldehyde-albumin conjugates have been measured in studies of exposed, symptomatic individuals;[78,79] however, the prognostic value of these antibodies is currently unknown.[76]

Formaldehyde is an OSHA-regulated chemical.[80] Medical surveillance is mandated by the Standard and must be implemented for all workers exposed at or above the action level (0.5 ppm per 8 hour TWA) or above the short-term exposure limit (2.0 ppm for 15 minutes). Employees who experience potentially related signs and symptoms or who are exposed in emergencies are included as well.

Mandated surveillance includes a questionnaire eliciting information on occupational exposures, smoking, and medical history, especially allergies and symptoms of pulmonary or skin disease. An example is contained in Appendix D of the Standard. Examinations are to be performed prior to exposure, annually in those who will use respirators, and at the discretion of the reviewing physician based on information in the medical disease questionnaire. Respirator users are required to have baseline and annual PFTs.

Prevention includes substitution with less hazardous chemicals and engineering controls such as local exhaust ventilation in laboratories where formaldehyde is used. Isolation of the sterilization process is useful in dialysis units. Personal protective equipment and worker training are important as well.

Glutaraldehyde

Glutaraldehyde is a sterilizing agent for heat-sensitive medical equipment and has been used in the histology laboratory as a tissue fixative. Glutaraldehyde is commonly used as a 2% solution in hospitals; however, it is produced in as high as 50% solutions, that are volatile at room temperature.[81] Exposed workers include nurses and technicians responsible for the cleaning of equipment used in clinical procedures as well as laboratory employees.

Glutaraldehyde is chemically related to formaldehyde and has similar adverse effects, including irritation of the eyes, respiratory system, and skin.[81] It can cause sensitization resulting in allergic contact dermatitis,[82] asthma,[83] and asthmatic exacerbation.[84] Exposure resulting in recurrent epistaxis has also been reported.[85] Fetotoxic effects have been found in animal studies.[81]

Prevention is achieved by exposure reduction. Local exhaust ventilation, even in the form of simple plexiglass structures connected to duct ventilation, can be constructed over areas where glutaraldehyde is used. Dilution of stronger solutions should be performed in locally ventilated areas. Employees should be educated regarding potential adverse health outcomes and the protection provided by PPE.

Hazardous drugs

There are a number of medications that, although beneficial to patients, can pose risks to HCWs both acutely and/or through chronic, low-dose exposure. The nomenclature "hazardous drugs" is now used to describe these agents.[3] The chemotherapeutic drugs, with their carcinogenic potential, are the most commonly recognized examples in this category. However, there are a number of medications that can cause adverse pulmonary outcomes in HCWs. Pharmacists, physicians, and nurses are exposed to such drugs during preparation and administration. Laboratory personnel may also be exposed.

Although most often reported in manufacturing settings, occupational exposure to numerous medications can result in allergic manifestations, including asthma. Antibiotics and proteolytic enzymes, such as pancreatic extracts and papain, are commonly mentioned examples in this category.[86,87] Preparations that involve working with dusts are a particular problem, but even pill counting often leaves residual powder on the equipment.

Recent concerns have focused on pentamidine, a drug used to treat *Pneumocystis carinii* pneumonia. It is administered in aerosolized form, which easily leads to environmental contamination resulting in both occupational and bystander exposure. Patient coughing and removal of the nebulizer prior to turning it off have been shown to greatly increase the air levels of pentamidine.[88] Doll reported the onset of bronchospasm in a nurse during the administration of an aerosolized pentamidine treatment.[89] This individual had no history of asthma, and the symptoms resolved when exposure ceased. Bronchospasm has also been noted as a side effect in patients receiving these treatments.[90]

Gude reported the case of a respiratory technician who experienced a decrease in his carbon monoxide diffusion capacity from over 100% of predicted before he began administering pentamidine to 81% after 14 months of work.[91] Measurable urinary pentamidine levels have also been documented in HCWs involved in the administration of such treatments, thus showing absorption from this type of inhalational exposure.[88]

Psyllium, a component of bulk laxatives, has been shown to cause sensitization in exposed workers, which can lead to asthma. This problem is more common in chronic care settings, where dispensation of these laxatives is a routine practice. Questionnaire evaluations have found as high as 18% of HCWs reporting allergic reactions while handling psyllium, ranging from nasoconjunctival symptoms to shortness of breath or hives.[92] Malo et al. evaluated health personnel in four chronic care hospitals for evidence of respiratory effects due to psyllium.[93] Specific psyllium inhalation challenges were performed in individuals suspected of occupational asthma. Prevalence based on new cases found in this study and those diagnosed in this workforce in the preceding year was 4.1% for occupational asthma with immunologic sensitization of 5.1% (skin testing) to 14.6% (serum IgE levels). The asthmatic prevalence was similar to that found in a cross-sectional study of workers in psyllium manufacturing conducted by the same researchers.[94]

In addition to radioallergosorbent tests (RASTs) and specific inhalational challenges, several biologic monitoring tests have been used in research protocols. Examples include assays to measure various hazardous drugs and their metabolites in blood and urine, tests of urine mutagenicity, and measures of cytogenetic effects. Problems with intraindividual and interindividual variability and lack of prognostic value for adverse clinical outcomes currently limit the use of these tests to the research arena.

Medical surveillance for pulmonary endpoints is important for employees exposed to these drugs in a manner that could lead to inhalation, (e.g., aerosols or powders). Documenting the extent of exposure for the purposes of meaningful medical surveillance is somewhat problematic because environmental sampling data are not routinely available. This is due to the large number of these chemicals and the fact that they are handled periodically in varying amounts. However, the connection between exposure and medical outcomes is particularly important for these hazards since information on their toxicity profiles in the health care environment is often incomplete. Therefore, in the absence of air levels, records of specific drugs and quantities handled are useful, as is information on the use of PPE.

Prevention depends primarily on measures to reduce exposure, including engineering controls and PPE. The use of biologic safety cabinets (BSCs) with vertical flow has been widely adopted in pharmacies for the preparation of hazardous drugs. OSHA and the American Society of Hospital Pharmacists have both published guidelines for handling these agents.[3,95] Some institutions have installed administration booths or tents as a means of reducing exposure in employees giving aerosolized medications. A study to evaluate the effectiveness of such controls for pentamidine monitored air levels before and after booths and increased room ventilation were installed.[96] A postintervention decrease to levels below the limit of detection was found. Exposure to drugs known to cause sensitization in patients or manufacturing employees should be minimized. In addition, workers with occupational allergies to these medications should not receive them therapeutically.

Mercury

Mercury is commonly used in hospital equipment such as sphygmomanometers. HCWs can be exposed when equipment breakage occurs, resulting in spills, or during equipment repair. Mercury is also used as a fixative in histology labs. Dentists are exposed through the use of mercury in dental amalgams. The primary route of exposure is inhalation since mercury readily vaporizes at room temperature.

Acute inhalation of mercury vapor can lead to corrosive bronchitis and interstitial pneumonitis, which may be fatal.[97] Chronic effects are primarily neurologic including the classic triad of excitability (erethism), tremors, and gingivitis, noted in felt and hat industry workers.

Mercury can be measured in blood and urine. Biological exposure indices have been established for these assays.[98] Although affected by fish consumption, blood mercury appears to be a better measure for acute high level exposure, such as after a spill.[99] Urinary excretion of mercury is absent during the initial exposure period while the metal accumulates in the body. Treatment of symptomatic patients includes chelation.

Prevention strategies consist of local ventilation for equipment repair and training on hazards and spill management. The latter includes the use of special mercury vacuum cleaners, respirators, and decontaminants. Mercury must be disposed of as hazardous waste in accordance with federal, state, and local regulations.

Methyl methacrylate

Methacrylates are used as adhesives in orthopedic and dental procedures. Two components, a liquid and a powder, must be mixed to produce the adhesive. Employee exposure occurs during this process. In addition to dental and orthopedic staff, workers in prosthetics are also exposed.

Acute exposure leads to respiratory tract irritation and both irritant and allergic contact dermatitis. Occupational asthma in a dental assistant after several years exposure to the material has been reported.[100] Asthma has been reported in dental patients as well.[101] Prevention includes local exhaust ventilation during the mixing process, worker training, and the use of PPE.

Miscellaneous

Phenol is a disinfectant used on fomites such as glassware, instruments, and floors. It is extremely corrosive and skin contact may result in severe burns, ulcers, and hypopigmentation.[72] Inhalation causes respiratory tract irritation and, if exposure is high, serious systemic manifestations (convulsions, coma, death) can occur. Specific tests include a urinary assay for which the ACGIH has established a biological exposure determinant of 250 mg/g creatinine for an end of shift urine sample.[98]

Employees in research and clinical laboratories may be exposed to a wide variety of chemicals depending on the type of lab. Certain of these agents are known to be respiratory toxicants. Pauli's reagent, the sodium salt of diazobenzenesulfonic acid, is used to identify aryl amines and phenols. Hypersensitivity pneumonitis has been reported in a medical school laboratory technician after several years of exposure.[102]

Latex contact is increasingly common due to the use of gloves to prevent the spread of infectious agents. Occupational risk groups include housekeepers, laboratory personnel, and staff in direct patient care. Allergic reactions range from urticaria to asthma to anaphylaxis.[103]

Iodine is used as a disinfectant in hospitals and can cause respiratory tract irritation if exposure to concentrated solutions occurs. Prevention of adverse health outcomes from these miscellaneous chemicals includes proper ventilation, worker education, and the use of PPE. Nonlatex glove substitutes are available for those who develop allergies.

Organic solvents

Solvents are common industrial chemicals found in laboratories, print shops, and maintenance areas (see Chapter 28). Acute effects include CNS depression as well as headaches, nausea, and dizziness. Upper respiratory tract and dermal irritation can occur,[72] and bronchospasm has been reported following acute high level exposures.[104]

Prevention includes substitution, local exhaust ventilation, and the use of PPE. Employee training should include information on routine use and management of spills.

PHYSICAL HAZARDS
Ionizing radiation

Radiation exposure in health care personnel results from two main sources: (1) the scatter from x-ray beams and (2) beta or gamma emissions from patients who are treated with therapeutic implants or undergo nuclear medicine studies (see Chapter 31).[72] Personnel in radiology are at risk for exposure as are staff caring for patients who have had implants or recent radionuclide injections.

Effects from acute exposure are usually localized, resulting in erythema or radiodermatitis. Acute radiation syndrome, due to whole body exposure, is unlikely in this occupational setting. Chronic exposure can result in pulmonary fibrosis and a variety of other outcomes of which cancers are the most notable. However, the extent of risk from the low-dose exposure hospital workers may receive remains controversial.[105]

The OSHA standard for ionizing radiation does not discuss medical surveillance, but it does mandate limits for radiation exposure.[106] Prevention includes proper maintenance of radiation equipment, protective equipment in the form of leaded aprons, and monitoring with dosimeters.

Asbestos

Although asbestos is a well-known pulmonary toxicant (see Chapter 20), its presence in hospitals is less well appreciated. Hospitals, like most older buildings, had asbestos insulation installed when they were constructed. This material is still present in many buildings and is a hazard when it becomes friable. This situation leads to exposure of all personnel in the vicinity. Maintenance workers are at particular risk since they can easily be exposed during repair work on pipes or other insulated areas. Heat-resistant gloves used in laboratories and equipment sterilization may also be made of asbestos and can become a hazard as they age and become friable.

Asbestos can cause a number of adverse pulmonary effects. The OSHA Asbestos Standard mandates exposure monitoring and medical surveillance.[107] The latter includes a questionnaire, physical examination, PFTs, and chest x-rays on a schedule dependent on factors such as the employee's age and exposure and smoking histories. Prevention is similar to that in other settings; the emphasis in this particular workplace is on hazard recognition and management.

Medical surveillance

Surveillance for pulmonary endpoints in the health care industry is similar to that in other industries. The history should be complete but should emphasize the pulmonary system. Information of past respiratory disease and allergies should be elicited. An assessment of exposure, both routine and accidental, should be linked to medical outcome information to facilitate increased knowledge regarding the toxicities of many of the unique exposures found in this environment. The physical examination should also be complete with emphasis on the pulmonary system.

Baseline and periodic chest x-rays and PFTs are commonly used to follow workers exposed to pulmonary toxicants. Additional laboratory evaluation can be guided by the utility and availability of specialized testing as discussed under each individual hazard.

A variety of modalities are available for the evaluation of symptomatic workers or those with abnormalities on routine surveillance. Standardized American Thoracic Society questionnaires, preshift and postshift PFTs, and serial peak flow monitoring with an accompanying symptom log have all been used in assessment of hospital and laboratory workers. Methacholine inhalation challenge or specific provocation testing has been used for a variety of these toxicants including formaldehyde, glutaraldehyde, and psyllium. In addition, specific tests such as skin testing or RAST may also be of benefit in these work-ups. Employees who have evidence of occupational asthma should be removed from exposure.

ALLERGIC SENSITIZATION

Allergic sensitization is another principal mechanism causing respiratory injury in laboratory and hospital workers. The clinical spectrum of allergic sensitization includes rhinitis, nonspecific bronchial hyperreactivity (NSBH), and asthma. Mechanistic discussions of allergic sensitization have divided potential antigens into substances of high molecular weight—usually greater than 20,000—and low molecular weight—usually less than 5,000—daltons.[108-109] The high–molecular-weight antigens are largely animal and plant proteins, whereas the low–molecular-weight group usually comprises chemicals and drugs. Both classes of antigens play a role as potential sensitizers in laboratory and hospital workers.

The box displays substances associated with allergic sensitization found in hospitals and laboratories. Although the list includes chemically diverse agents, the majority of allergic sensitization in these work settings are due to laboratory animal allergy and pharmaceutical exposure. These examples are discussed in detail below.

Allergy caused by pharmacologic dusts

Allergy caused by pharmacologic dusts has been a long-recognized hazard in hospital pharmacology laboratory settings. In the 1920s separate reports of ipecac-induced asthma in pharmacists were made.[110,111] Other reports of allergy in pharmacists followed in the 1930s and beyond.

Scientific studies of exposed workers and epidemiologic surveys in the 1950s advanced knowledge of pharmacologic sensitization suggested in early case reports.

A 1955 study of penicillin-manufacturing workers found 19 of 156 workers (12.2%) had allergic symptoms.[112] Three of the 19 had asthma, and penicillin sensitization was postulated by the authors to be responsible for the symptoms.

A 1958 investigation of occupational allergy in nurses, pharmacists, and physicians described reactions to penicillin exposure in 3 of 19 asthmatic nurses; 9 of 13 allergic pharmacists reacted to penicillin and respiratory discomfort

Some causes of allergic sensitization in hospital and laboratory workers

Animal proteins

Dander, excreta, secretions, serum
Hamsters
Rabbits
Rats
Guinea pigs

Enzymes

Bacillus subtilis
Papain
Pepsin
Pancreatic extracts

Pharmaceuticals

Antibiotics and related compounds
Penicillin
Tetracycline
Sulfuramides

Other pharmaceuticals

Psyllium
Salbutamol
Methyldopa
Cimetadine
Enflurane
Piperazine
Chloramine
Isonicotine hydrazine

Sterilizing agents

Chloramine
Sulfone chloramide
Hexachlorophene
Formaldehyde
Glutaraldehyde

Organic chemicals

Acrylates
Amines
Colophony
Latex

Adapted from Salvaggio and O'Neil[109] and Montanaro.[142]

was reported in some members of the last group from penicillin drug handling.[113]

A epidemiologic survey of 1,176 pharmacists in 1959 revealed 364 (30.9%) reported allergic symptoms including rhinitis, asthma, and allergic dermatitis.[114]

More recently, in a Japanese investigation of 119 hospital pharmacists returning questionnaires, 54 (45.5%) reported allergic symptoms. Those same 54 respondents represent 17.8% of the total, 304 pharmacists (including nonrespondents) surveyed.[115]

In another Japanese investigation, which included physi-

cal examination and skin testing with drug allergens, 95 of 191 (49.7%) hospital pharmacists with allergy or allergy-like symptoms, in contrast to 5 of 33 (15.2%) institutes of hygiene workers (controls) were identified.[116] Stratified into groups by presence of family or personal allergy history, Honma et al. reported symptoms in 27 of 44 (61.4%) workers with such a history and in 27 of 67 (40.3%) in those not reporting such a history. The author suggested these data indicate the importance of atopy in drug allergy.[116]

Surveys have attempted to identify classes of agents more commonly observed to cause occupational sensitization. Mizano et al. reported "Central Nervous System Drugs" including chlorpromazine and oxazolodine as well as drugs used for treatment of gastrointestinal illness such as diastase and other synthetic enzymes were responsible for approximately 40% and 30% of cases, respectively, with antibiotics accounting for about 8% of cases.[117] Feuki's work has roughly corroborated these findings.[89]

Pathogenesis and presentation

As seen in LAA, the symptomatic presentation of drug allergies in workers includes a variety of symptoms including allergic rhinitis, contact dermatitis, upper respiratory irritation, conjunctivitis, and asthma.[115]

Feuki has discussed occupational drug allergy compared to drug allergy therapeutically derived.[86] He reflects that observed differences in incidence (occurring more commonly in workers than treated patients (18% to 45% vs. 3% to 4%), types of symptoms (allergic rhinitis and contact dermatitis versus urticaria, angioneurotic edema, and fixed eruption), and principal causitive agents (CNS and GI drugs versus pyrazonolone derivatives, penicillin, and others) may be attributed to route of sensitization. Allergy caused by pharmacologic dusts is usually due to skin contact or inhalation contrasted with an oral or injected route in treated patients. He attributed sensitization route as a major determinant in antigen distribution, thus influencing the target organ of response. The immunogenicity and molecular weight of the allergen are other well-described determinants of the immunologic mechanism.

Prevention may be achieved through workplace hygiene including the use of vertical laminar flow hoods and other efforts to contain drug dust generation. As with LAA, worker counselling regarding employment choices and safe work practices for sensitized workers should be implemented. The role of atopy is not sufficiently clear to use to screen workers for denial of employment. Such a history may, however, be used as a counseling tool.

Laboratory animal allergy

First identified in the mid-1970s, LAA has received increasing attention as a significant occupational hazard (see Chapter 26).[118-120] Laboratory animal allergy is defined as a Type I-IgE mediated hypersensitivity reaction due to skin or respiratory exposure to animal allergens.[121] Prevalence of the condition in exposed animal workers ranges from 11% to 30%.[118,122,123] Allergens from animal secretions (urine and saliva) and dander appear to affect symptom onset.[122] Risk factors for LAA development have been difficult to define. A history of atopy, for example, was not found to increase the risk of LAA by some authors[120,124] but was found to be a risk factor by others.[121,125] Varying results have also been observed relating skin prick and RAST results to LAA. Davies et al. found no correlation between such tests and symptom development.[124] However, significant differences in skin prick test results with environmental allergens were reported between subjects with LAA asthma and controls by several authors.[120,122,126]

Newill et al. found in 364 animal handlers, 168 had a history of allergic symptoms; 48 had positive immediate skin tests (29 to laboratory animals) and 18.4% had a positive methacholine challenge test.[127]

Authors note that LAA may first present as rhinitis, rather than asthma.[120] In fact, the majority of symptoms reported by affected workers are those of rhinitis, upper air way irritation, and skin rashes, not asthma.[120,126]

Environmental surveillance for airborne allergens may be considered to assist in hazard control. One group performed a prevalence survey of LAA and correlated this to airborne rat urinary allergen concentration by job task and found a significant association.[125]

One large study of over 500 animal handlers found that nearly one quarter of workers reported LAA symptoms and one third of those had to stop work either temporarily or permanently because of symptoms.[121] This study attempted to determine the effect of wearing PPE, but the results were unclear. The current approach of using gowns and gloves when the offending agent is like an airborne allergen seems of little use. These authors suggest keeping the allergen close to the cage by using dustless bedding, reducing use of bedding, or using local exhaust ventilation (hoods) when cleaning cages. The use of respiratory protection for workers might also be considered, especially for those with rhinitis, who have not yet developed asthma. In the study of Bland et al., 58% of workers reported some reduction of symptoms with the use of PPE.[121] They argue that the cost of stepped-up exposure prevention could be offset by reduction in lost work time and employee turnover.

One interest in studying risk factors for LAA is to assist in employment counseling. Even where trends exist suggesting risk, however, the predictive value of these tests does not allow ethical exclusion of workers from handling animals. For example, the consensus at present regarding a history of atopy is that it is not sufficiently sensitive to be used as a reliable indicator for LAA development and thus should not be used as a screening tool in the denial of employment requiring animal handling.[121,125]

Other authors who found a family or personal history of allergy, positive skin prick testing to environmental allergens, and total serum IgE were predictors of at-risk indi-viduals, that is those at risk of developing LAA asthma, suggest using such information in employment counseling.[126] A new hire with these criteria might be counseled to seek other work. Incumbents with asthmatic symptoms should be relocated regardless of the above criteria. Incumbents with only upper airway irritation symptoms, but with the above criteria, may be at risk to develop asthma and should be carefully followed. Follow-up of asymptomatic workers with these criteria is also recommended, but the predictive value of these criteria in an asymptomatic population is questionable.

REGULATORY CONSIDERATIONS

The Occupational Safety and Health Administration regulates many of the chemical and physical hazards, pharmaceuticals, and biologic agents discussed in this chapter.[128] Comprehensive standards for several agents exist including regulation of formaldehyde and ethylene oxide. Broader approaches to ensuring worker protection from pathogens found in patient blood and body fluids requiring a written exposure control plan, worker training, and hepatitis B vaccines for affected workers are required under the Bloodborne Pathogen Standard.

Although not as comprehensive as standards, OSHA also issues guidelines to the public indicating OSHA's opinion about certain hazards and encouraging voluntary acceptance. Such a guidance document was issued in 1986 on the Safe Handling of Anticancer or Cytotoxic Drugs.[95] It emphasizes the need for engineering controls in handling certain hazardous drugs (some of which may cause acute respiratory effects). The recent compliance directive issued to OSHA Compliance Officers describing elements to be reviewed in a TB inspection also provides employers with information regarding elements OSHA believes comprise a TB control program to protect HCWs.

Even more broadly, the Hazard Communication Standard[129] requires employers to inform workers about the chemical hazards to which they come in contact. This includes pharmaceuticals requiring preparation or reconstitution. It also requires employers to provide written documentation of the nature of the hazards these chemicals may cause. These written forms are termed material safety data and sheets (MSDS). Familiarizing workers on how to read an MSDS is part of the required hazard communication training.

A summary of specific OSHA Standards applicable to hospital and laboratory hazards is found in Table 44-3.

FUTURE CONSIDERATIONS

How do we prevent respiratory illness in hospital workers and laboratories? Perhaps first, attention must be paid to both work environments as potentially hazardous workplaces. Certainly the case has been made that many hazard classes, respiratory and otherwise, are encountered in these settings. Informed laboratory supervisors and hospital safety and infection control committees can do much to advance broader approaches to occupational safety and health, beyond traditional infection control goals that emphasize preventing patient-to-patient spread.

Critical lessons have been learned during the present resurgence of TB. For example, some hospitals that in the past year initiated campaigns requiring its employees, including physician staff, to have PPDs checked, included in the requisite visit to the employee health unit an opportunity to receive antibody screening for other biologic exposures and any vaccines that the employee required.

The concept of an "express lane" in the emergency room grew out of the experience of one midwest urban hospital that was hard hit by TB in its medical staff. They initiated a five-question screening program for patients presenting to the emergency room, focusing on classical symptoms of TB. If any of the questions were answered affirmatively the patient is removed from the communal waiting room, instructed to cover their mouths during cough, x-rayed immediately, and placed in TB isolation while awaiting disposition. This type of triage has been an approach used to decrease successfully the TST conversion rates in that institution. Such an approach, however, would be applicable to minimize exposure to other respiratory pathogens in congregational settings, especially in settings where engineering controls and personal respiratory protection are not fully feasible.

Reviewing grouped data of TB skin test conversions or any apparent outbreaks of respiratory disease may assist in identifying gaps in work practices or infection control that allowed exposure. This targets topics for worker training and may also suggest industrial hygiene or engineering interventions.

Although the complexities of hospital and laboratory environments pose a significant potential hazard to workers, many strategies exist to mitigate health risk. These include use of the classical industrial hygiene controls of engineering, administrative, and work practice controls and use of personal protective equipment. Additionally, sound infection control practices must be maintained with vigilance. Worker education about the hazards they may encounter is also crucial to a successful primary prevention program in these work settings. Taken together, these approaches serve to extend protection from unnecessary hazardous exposure to workers performing vital functions in health care and laboratory facilities.

REFERENCES

1. Lewy RM: *Employees at risk. Protecting the health of the health care worker.* New York, 1991, Van Nostrand Reinhold.
2. Weaver VM, McDiarmid MA, Guidera JA, Humphrey FE, and Schaefer JA: Occupational chemical exposures in an academic medical center, *J Occup Med* 35:701-706, 1993.
3. American Society of Hospital Pharmacists: ASHP technical assistance bulletin on handling cytotoxic and hazardous drugs, *Am J Hosp Pharm* 47:1033-1049, 1990.
4. McDiarmid MA, Gurley HT, and Arrington D: Pharmaceuticals as hospital hazards: managing the risks, *J Occup Med* 33:155-158, 1991.
5. Marrie TJ, George J, McDonald S, et al: Are health care workers at risk for infection during an outbreak of nosocomial Legionnaires' disease?, *Am J Infect Control* 14:209-213, 1986.
6. O'Mahony MC, Stanwell-Smith RE, Tillett HE, et al: The Stafford outbreak of Legionnaires' disease, *Epidemiol Infect* 104:361-380, 1990.
7. Geiseler PJ, Nelson KE, Crispen RG, and Moses VK: Tuberculosis in physicians: a continuing problem, *Am Rev Respir Dis* 133:773-778, 1986.
8. Catanzaro A: Nosocomial tuberculosis, *Am Rev Respir Dis* 125:559-562, 1982.
9. Joseph S: Editorial: tuberculosis, again, *Am J Pub Health* 83:647-648, 1993.
10. Barnes PF, Bloch AB, Davidson PT, and Snider DE Jr: Current concepts: tuberculosis in patients with human immunodeficiency virus infection, *N Engl J Med* 324:1644-1650, 1991.
11. Nolan CM: Human immunodeficiency syndrome—associated tuberculosis: a review with an emphasis on infection control issues, *Am J Infect Control* 20:30-34, 1992.
12. Pitchenik AE, Burr J, Suarez M, Fortel D, Gonzalez G, and Moas C: Human T-cell lymphotrophic virus-III (HTLV-III) seropositivity and related diseases among 71 consecutive patients in whom tuberculosis was diagnosed: a prospective study, *Am Rev Respir Dis* 135:875-879, 1987.
13. Centers for Disease Control: Nosocomial transmission of multidrug-resistant tuberculosis among HIV-infected persons—Florida and New York, 1988-1991, *MMWR* 40:585-591, 1991.
14. Rudnick J, Krock K, Manangan L, Banerjee S, Pugliese G, and Jarvis W: How prepared are U.S. hospitals to control nosocomial transmission of tuberculosis? Abstract, Society of Hospital Epidemiologists of America, Chicago, April, 1993.
15. Bowden K and McDiarmid MA: Occupationally-acquired tuberculosis: what's known, *J Occup Med* 36:302-325, 1994.
16. Centers for Disease Control: Guidelines for preventing the transmission of tuberculosis in health-care setting, with special focus on HIV-related issues, *MMWR* 39:(No. RR-17), 1990.
17. Gurwitz D, Mindorff C, and Levison H: Increased incidence of bronchial reactivity in children with a history of bronchiolitis, *J Pediatr* 98:551-555, 1981.
18. Stokes GM, Milner AD, Hodge IG, et al: Lung function abnormalities after acute bronchiolitis, *J Pediatr* 98:871-874, 1981.
19. Hall CB, Douglas RG, Geiman JM, and Messner MK: Nosocomial respiratory syncytial virus infections, *N Engl J Med* 293(26):1343-1346, 1975.
20. Harrington RD, Hooton TM, Hackman RC, et al: An outbreak of respiratory syncytial virus in a bone marrow transplant center, *J Infect Dis* 165:987-993, 1992.
21. Hall CB, Geiman JM, and Douglas RG Jr: Possible transmission by fomites of respiratory syncytial virus, *J Infect Dis* 141:98-102, 1980.
22. Mandell GL, Douglas RG, and Bennett JE, editors: *Principles and practice of infectious diseases,* ed 3, pp 1153-2205, New York, 1990, Churchill Livingstone.
23. Hall CB, Douglas RG Jr, and Geiman JN: Quantitative shedding patterns of respiratory syncytial virus in infants, *J Infect Dis* 132:151-156, 1975.
24. Hall WJ, Hall CB, and Speers DM: Respiratory syncytial virus infection in adults: clinical and physiologic manifestations, *Ann Intern Med* 88:203, 1978.
25. Hall CB, Geiman JM, Douglas RG, and Meagher MP: Control of nosocomial respiratory syncytial viral infections, *Pediatrics* 62(5):728-732, 1978.
26. Gala CL, Hall CB, Schnabel KC, et al: The use of eye-nose goggles to control nosocomial respiratory syncytial virus infection, *JAMA* 256:2706-2708, 1986.

27. Monto AS and Cavallaro JJ: The Tecumseh study of respiratory illness. Patterns of occurrence of infection with respiratory pathogens, 1965-1969, *Am J Epidemiol* 94:280-289, 1971.

28. Peters NL, Ebeler S, Hair C, et al: Treatment of an influenza A outbreak in a teaching nursing home, effectiveness of a protocol for prevention and control, *J Am Geriatr Soc* 37:210-218, 1989.

29. Weingarten S: Influenza surveillance in an acute-care hospital, *Arch Intern Med* 148:113-116, 1988.

30. Centers for Disease Control: Recommendations for prevention and control of influenza, *Ann Intern Med* 105:399-400, 1986.

31. Hammond GW and Cheang M: Absenteeism among hospital staff during an influenza epidemic: implications for immunoprophylaxis, *Can Med J* 131:449-452, 1984.

32. Hynes NA and Hinman AR: Influenza immunization of health care providers, *J Gen Intern Med* 3:94-95.

33. Weingarten S, Staniloff H, Ault M, et al: Do hospital employees benefit from the influenza vaccine?, *J Gen Intern Med* 3:32-37, 1988.

34. O'Donoghue JM, Ray CG, Terry DW Jr, et al: Prevention of nosocomial influenza infection with amantadine, *Am J Epidemiol* 39(97):276-282, 1973.

35. Centers for Disease Control: Measles—United States, first 26 weeks 1987, *MMWR* 37:527-531, 1988.

36. Baum GL and Wolinsky E, editors: *Textbook of pulmonary diseases,* ed 4, vol 1, pp 355-387, Boston, 1989, Little, Brown.

37. ACIP: Immunization Practices Advisory Committee. Measles prevention: supplementary statement, *MMWR* 38:1-18, 1989.

38. Freebeck PC, Clark S, and Fahey PJ: Hypoxemic respiratory failure complicating nosocomial measles in a healthy host, *Chest 102(2): 625-626, 1992.*

39. ACIP: Immunization Practices Advisory Committee. Update on adult immunization, *MMWR* 40:19-22, 1991.

40. Schwarcz S, McCaw B, and Fukushima P: Prevalence of measles susceptibility in hospital staff: evidence to support expanding the recommendations of the immunization practices advisory committee, *Arch Intern Med* 152:1481-1483, 1992.

41. Kim M, LaPointe J, and Liu FJG: Epidemiology of measles immunity in a population of healthcare workers, infect control hosp. *Epidemiology* 13:399-402, 1992.

42. Guess HA, Broughton DD, Melton LT 3rd, et al: Population-based studies of varicella compliances, *Pediatrics* 78:723-729, 1986.

43. Triebwasser JH, Harris RE, Bryant RE, et al: Varicella pneumonia in adults: report of seven cases and a review of the literature, *Medicine (Baltimore)* 46:409-423, 1967.

44. Josephson A and Gombert ME: Airborne transmission of nosocomial varicella from localized zoster, *J Infect Dis* 158(1):238-241, 1988.

45. Menkhaus NA, Lanphear B, and Linnemann CC: Airborne transmission of varicella-zoster virus in hospitals, *Lancet* 336:1315, 1990.

46. Gustafson TL, Lavely GB, Brawner ER, et al: An outbreak of airborne nosocomial varicella, *Pediatrics* 70(4):550-556, 1982.

47. Report of the Committee on Infectious Diseases: In Peter G, editor: American Academy of Pediatrics, ed 22, Elk Grove Village, IL, 1991.

48. Fraser DW, Tsai TR, Orenstein W, et al: Legionnaires' disease: description of an epidemic of pneumonia, *N Engl J Med* 297:1183-1197, 1977.

49. Fuller J, Levinson MM, Kline, JR, et al: Legionnaires' disease after heart transplantation, *Ann Thor Surg* 39:308-311, 1985.

50. Korvick J and Yu VL: Legionnaires' disease: an emerging surgical problem, *Ann Thorac Surg* 43:341-347, 1987.

51. Gantz, N: Hazardous workplace exposures. In Levy BS and Wegman DH, editors: Recognizing and preventing work-related disease, pp 235-249, 1983.

52. Centers for Disease Control: *Classification of etiologic agents on the basis of hazard,* US Dept HEW 13, 1974.

53. McCoy, G: Psittacosis amoung the personnel of the hygenic laboratory, *J Infect Dis* 55:156-167, 1934.

54. Kern DG: Outbreak of the reactive airways dysfunction syndrome after a spill of glacial acetic acid, *Am Rev Respir Dis* 144:1058-1064, 1991.

55. Musk AW, Peach S, and Ryan G: Occupational asthma in a mineral analysis laboratory, *Br J Ind Med* 45:381-386, 1988.

56. Hattis RP, Greer JR, Dietrich S, Olafsson S, and McAndrew KR: Chlorine gas toxicity from mixture of bleach with other cleaning products—California, *J Am Med Assoc* 266:2529-2534, 1991.

57. NIOSH/OSHA: *Occupational health guidelines for chemical hazards: sulfuric acid,* Cincinnati, OH, 1981, U.S. Department of Health and Human Services, Public Health Service, Centers for Disease Control, National Institute for Occupational Safety and Health, and U.S. Department of Labor, Occupational Safety and Health Administration. DHHS (NIOSH) Pub No 81-123.

58. Bryant HE, Visser ND, and Yoshida K: Ethylene oxide sterilizer use and short-term symptoms amongst workers, *Occup Med* 39:101-106, 1989.

59. Glaser ZR: Ethylene oxide: toxicology review and field study results of hospital use, *J Environ Pathol Toxicol* 2:173-208, 1979.

60. Deschamps D, Rosenberg N, Soler P, Maillard G, Fournier E, Salson D, et al: Persistent asthma after accidental exposure to ethylene oxide, *Br J Ind Med* 49:523-525, 1992.

61. Bousquet J and Michel F: Allergy to formaldehyde and ethylene-oxide, *Clin Rev Allergy* 9:357-370, 1991.

62. Rumpf KW, Seubert S, Seubert A, et al: Association of ethylene-oxide-induced IgE antibodies with symptoms in dialysis patients, *Lancet* ii:1385-1387, 1985.

63. Schepers GWH: Allergenic occupational air pollutants. In Frazier CA, editor: *Occupational asthma,* pp 307-356, New York, 1980, Van Nostrand Reinhold.

64. NIOSH: *Current intelligence bulletin 35: ethylene oxide,* Cincinnati, OH, 1981, U.S. Department of Health and Human Services, Public Health Service, Centers for Disease Control, National Institute for Occupational Safety and Health. DHHS (NIOSH) Pub No 81-130.

65. International Agency for Research on Cancer: *IARC monographs on the evaluation of the carcinogenic risk of chemicals to humans: allyl compounds, aldehydes, epoxides and peroxides,* Lyon, France, 36:189-226, 1985.

66. Hemminki K, Mutanen P, Saloniemi I, Niemi ML, and Vainio H: Spontaneous abortions in hospital staff engaged in sterilizing instruments with chemical agents, *Br Med J* 285:1461-1463, 1982.

67. Landrigan PJ, Meinhardt TJ, Gordon J, et al: Ethylene oxide: an overview of toxicologic and epidemiologic research, *Am J Ind Med* 6:103-115, 1984.

68. Estrin WJ, Cavalieri SA, Wald P, Becker CE, Jones JR, and Cone JE: Evidence of neurologic dysfunction related to long-term ethylene oxide exposure, *Arch Neurol* 44:1283-1286, 1987.

69. Brugnone F, Perbellini L, Faccini GB, Pasini F, Bartolucci GB, and DeRosa E: Ethylene oxide exposure: biological monitoring by analysis of alveolar air and blood, *Int Arch Occup Environ Health* 58:105-112, 1986.

70. Mayer J, Warburton D, Jeffrey AM, et al: Biologic markers in ethylene oxide-exposed workers and controls, *Mut Res* 248:163-176, 1991.

71. U.S. Department of Labor, Occupational Safety and Health Administration: *Ethylene oxide Standard 29 CFR 1910.1047,* 1989.

72. NIOSH: *Guidelines for protecting the safety and health of health care workers,* Washington, DC, 1988, U.S. Department of Health and Human Services, Public Health Service, Centers for Disease Control, National Institute for Occupational Safety and Health. DHHS (NIOSH) Pub No 88-119.

73. Skisak CM: Formaldehyde vapor exposures in anatomy laboratories, *Am Ind Hyg Assoc J* 44:948-950, 1983.

74. Hendrick DJ and Lane DJ: Occupational formalin asthma, *Br J Ind Med* 34:11-18, 1977.

75. Hendrick DJ, Rando RJ, Lane DJ, and Morris MJ: Formaldehyde asthma: challenge exposure levels and fate after five years, *J Occup Med* 24:893-897, 1982.

76. Bardana EJ: Formaldehyde asthma. In Bardana EJ, Montanaro A, and O'Hollaren MT, editors: *Occupational asthma*, pp 151-170, Philadelphia, 1992, Hanley & Belfus.

77. Clary JJ and Sullivan JB: Formaldehyde. In Sullivan JB and Krieger GR, editors: *Hazardous material toxicology: clinical principles of environmental health*, pp 973-980, Baltimore, 1992, Williams & Wilkins.

78. Thrasher JD, Madison R, Broughton A, and Gard Z: Building-related illness and antibodies to albumin conjugates of formaldehyde, toluene diisocyanate, and trimellitic anhydride, *Am J Ind Med* 15:187-195, 1989.

79. Salkie ML: The prevalence of atopy and hypersensitivity to formaldehyde in pathologists, *Arch Pathol Lab Med* 115:614-616, 1991.

80. U.S. Department of Labor, Occupational Safety and Health Administration: *Formaldehyde Standard 29 CFR 1910.1048*, 1990.

81. NIOSH: Symptoms of irritation associated with exposure to glutaraldehyde—Colorado, *MMWR* 36:190-191, 1987.

82. Nethercott JR, Holness DL, and Page E: Occupational contact dermatitis due to glutaraldehyde in health care workers, *Contact Dermatitis* 18:193-196, 1988.

83. Cullinan P, Hayes J, Cannon J, Madan I, Heap D, and Newman Taylor A: Occupational asthma in radiographers, *Lancet* 340:1477, 1992.

84. Corrado OJ, Osman J, and Davies RJ: Asthma and rhinitis after exposure to glutaraldehyde in endoscopy units, *Hum Toxicol* 5:325-327, 1986.

85. Wiggins P, McCurdy SA, and Zeidenberg W: Epistaxis due to glutaraldehyde exposure, *J Occup Med* 31:854-856, 1989.

86. Fueki R: Allergy due to pharmacologic dusts. In Frazier CA, editor: *Occupational asthma*, pp 245-256, New York, 1980, Van Nostrand Reinhold.

87. Tarlo SM, Shaikh W, Bell B, Cuff M, Davies GM, Dolovich J, et al: Papain induced allergic reactions, *Clin Allergy* 8:207-215, 1978.

88. O'Riordan TG and Smaldone GC: Exposure of health care workers to aerosolized pentamidine, *Chest* 101:1494-1499, 1992.

89. Doll DC: Aerosolized pentamidine (letter), *Lancet* ii:1284-1285, 1989.

90. Katzman M, Meade W, Iglar K, Rachlis A, Berger P, and Chan CK: High incidence of bronchospasm with regular administration of aerosolized pentamidine, *Chest* 101:79-81, 1992.

91. Gude JK: Selective delivery of pentamidine to the lung by aerosol (letter), *Am Rev Respir Dis* 139:1060, 1989.

92. Nelson WL: Allergic events among health care workers exposed to psyllium laxatives in the workplace, *J Occup Med* 29:497-499, 1987.

93. Malo J, Cartier A, L'Archeveque J, Ghezzo H, Lagier F, Trudeau C, et al: Prevalence of occupational asthma and immunologic sensitization to psyllium among health personnel in chronic care hospitals, *Am Rev Respir Dis* 142:1359-1366, 1990.

94. Bardy J, Malo J, Seguin P, Ghezzo H, Desjardins J, Dolovich J, et al: Occupational asthma and IgE sensitization in a pharmaceutical company processing psyllium, *Am Rev Respir Dis* 135:1033-1038, 1987.

95. U.S. Department of Labor, Occupational Safety and Health Administration: *Work practice guidelines for personnel dealing with cytotoxic (antineoplastic) drugs*, 1986, OSHA Pub No 8-1.1.

96. McDiarmid MA, Schaefer J, Richard CL, Chaisson RE, and Tepper BS: Efficacy of engineering controls in reducing occupational exposure to aerosolized pentamidine, *Chest* 102:1764-1766, 1992.

97. Goyer RA: Toxic effects of metals. In Klaassen CD, Amdur MO, and Doull J, editors: *Casarett and Doull's toxicology: the basic science of poisons*, ed 3, pp 582-635, New York, 1986, Macmillan.

98. American Conference of Governmental Industrial Hygienists: *Threshold limit values for chemical substances and physical agents and biological exposure indices*. Cincinnati, OH, 1992-1993, ACGIH.

99. Lauwerys RR and Hoet P: *Industrial chemical exposures: guidelines for biological monitoring*, ed 2, Boca Raton, 1993, Lewis Publishers.

100. Lozewicz S, Davison AG, Hopkirk A, Burge PS, Boldy D, Riordan JF, et al: Occupational asthma due to methyl methacrylate and cyanoacrylates, *Thorax* 40:836-839, 1985.

101. Basker RM and Hunter AM: A severe asthmatic reaction to poly (methyl methacrylate) denture base resin, *Br Dental J* 169:250-251, 1990.

102. Evans WV and Seaton A: Hypersensitivity pneumonitis in a technician using Pauli's reagent, *Thorax* 34:767-770, 1979.

103. Bardana EJ: Asthma associated with amine-based epoxy resins, latex, reactive dyes, and miscellaneous chemicals. In Bardana EJ, Montanaro A, and O'Hollaren editors: *Occupational asthma*, pp 189-204. Philadelphia, 1992, Hanley & Belfus.

104. Boulet L: Increases in airway responsiveness following acute exposure to respiratory irritants, *Chest* 94:476-481, 1988.

105. Patterson WB: Occupational hazards to hospital personnel, *Ann Intern Med* 102:658-680, 1985.

106. U.S. Department of Labor, Occupational Safety and Health Administration: *Ionizing Radiation Standard, 29 CFR 1910.96*, 1984.

107. U.S. Department of Labor, Occupational Safety and Health Administration: *Asbestos, tremolite, anthophyllite, and actinolite, 29 CFR 1910.1001*, 1990.

108. Chan-Yeung M and Lam S: Occupational asthma, *Am Rev Respir Dis* 133:686-703, 1986.

109. Salvaggio JE and O'Neil CE: Pathogenetic mechanisms in occupational hypersensitivity states in occupational asthma and allergies, *Immun Allergy Clin North Am* 12:711-729, 1992.

110. Peshkin MM: Ipecac sensitization and bronchial asthma, *JM Med* 32:1133, 1920.

111. Widal F, Abram P, and Joltrain, editors: Anaphyaxie a' l'ipec, *La Presse Med* 32:341, 1922.

112. Maffei R and Napolitane L: Allergic reaction to penicillin implant of the antibiotic's production, *Minerva Med* 46:1785, 1955.

113. Timal J and Tabort J: Respiratory allergy in the medical profession and its auxiliaries, *Occupational Allergy* 169 (lecture to Danish Allergy Associates), 1958.

114. Quarles WJ: *Occupational allergy*, Suppl 100, Leiden, 1959, Stenfert Krosse.

115. Fueki R: Allergy in pharmacy, *Farumacia* 6:364, 1970.

116. Honma S, Kondo T, Kobayashi T, Fueki R, Kobayashi S, and Aoshino N: Allergic symptoms observed in pharmacists, 23rd Congress of Japanese Society of Allergology, 1973.

117. Mizano K, Kanekubo Y, Miyaiye J, Tomonaga F, and Nakagawa F: Investigation on drug allergy in pharmacists, *Yakuzaigaku* 31:60, 1971.

118. Lincoln TA, Bolton NE, and Garrett AS: Occupational allergy to animal dander and sera, *J Occup Med* 16:465-469, 1974.

119. Lustsky II and Neuman I: Laboratory animal dander allergy: I. an occupational disease, *Ann Allergy* 35:201-205, 1975.

120. Cockcroft A, Edwards J, McCarthy P, and Anderson N: Allergy in laboratory animal workers, *Lancet* ii:827-830, 1981.

121. Bland SM, Levine MS, Wilson PD, Fox NL, and Rivera JC: Occupational allergy to laboratory animals: an epidemiologic study, *J Occup Med* 28:1151-1157, 1986.

122. Seovak AJM and Hill RN: Laboratory animal allergy: a clinical survey of an exposed population, *Br J Ind Med* 38:38-41, 1981.

123. Agrup G, Belin L, Sjostedt L, and Skerfving S: Allergy to laboratory animals in laboratory technicians and animal keepers, *Br J Ind Med* 43:192-198, 1986.

124. Davies GE, Thompson AV, Niewola Z, Burrows GE, Teasdale EL, Bird DJ, and Phillips DA: Allergy to laboratory animals: a retrospective and a prospective study, *Br J Ind Med* 40:442-449, 1983.

125. Kibby T, Powell G, and Cromer J: Allergy to laboratory animals: a prospective and cross-sectional study, *J Occup Med* 31:842-846, 1989.

126. Sjostedt L and Willers S: Predisposing factors in laboratory animal allergy: a study of atopy and environmental factors, *Am J Ind Med* 16:199-208, 1989.

127. Newill CA, Prenger VL, Fish JE, Evan R, Diamond EL, Wei Q, and Eggleston PA: Risk factors for increased airway responsiveness to methachloride challenge among laboratory workers, *Am Rev Respir Dis* 146:1494-1500, 1992.

128. U.S. Department of Labor, Occupational Safety and Health Administration: *Air contaminants—permissible exposure limits, 29 CFR 1910.1000,* 1989.

129. U.S. Department of Labor, Occupational Safety and Health Administration: *Hazard Communication Standard, 29 CFR 1910.1200,* 1989.

130. Burnet FM and Freeman M: Note on a series of laboratory infections with the rickettsia of Q fever, *Med J Aust.* 7:11-12, 1939.

131. Huebner RJ: Report of an outbreak of Q fever at the National Institute of Health, *Am J Public Health* 37:431-440, 1947.

132. Dickie HA and Murphy ME: Laboratory infection with histoplasma capsulations, *Am Rev Tuberculosis* 72:690-692, 1955.

133. Carbonelle B, et al: Épidémiologie et prévention des contaminations tuberculeuses dous les laboratoriens de bactériologie, *Rev Epidem Méd Soc et Santé Publ* 23:417-428, 1975.

134. Long E: The hazard of acquiring tuberculosis in the laboratory, *Am J of Public Health* 1:782-787, 1951.

135. Ramsey FK and Carter GR: *J Am Vet Med Assoc* 120:93-98, 1952.

136. Smith D and Harrell ER: *Am Rev Tuberculosis,* 57:368-374, 1948.

137. Smith CE: Coccidioidmycosis In Alello L, editors: *XIII-XXII,* p 434, Tucson, Arizona, 1967.

138. Pike R: Laboratory-associated infections: incidence, fatalities, causes, and prevention. *Ann Rev Microbio* 33:42-66, 1979.

139. Asburn LL and Miller SE: *Arch Pathol* 39:388-392, 1945.

140. Lee HW and Johnson KM: Laboratory-acquired infections with Haantan virus; the etiologic agent of Korean haemorrhagic fever, *J Infect Dis* 146:645-651, 1982.

141. Umenai T, Lee HW, and Lee PW: Korean haemorrhagic fever in staff in an animal laboratory, *Lancet* 1(8130): 1314-1316, 1979.

142. Montanaro A: Occupational asthma associated with low molecular weight antigens in: occupational asthma and allergies, *Immun Allergy Clinics North Am* 12:779-793, 1992.

Chapter 45

DIVING

Kenneth W. Kizer

Approximately three fourths of the earth is covered by water; this underwater world has begun to be extensively explored in recent decades. Much of this exploration has occurred consequent to developments in compressed air diving, and the advent of scuba diving in particular.

Human beings did not evolve for an aquatic existence and are not well-adapted for functioning in the aquatic environment. Among the intrinsic hazards of the aquatic environment that confront the human diver are cold, lack of air to breathe, changes in light and sound conduction, increased density of the surrounding medium, dangerous marine life, and increased atmospheric pressure. In addition, various problems caused by the diver's breathing medium can occur as a consequence of the higher environmental pressure found underwater. Not surprisingly, many diverse medical problems are related to diving (box).

The ears, paranasal sinuses, and central nervous system (CNS) are most often the site of medical problems associated with compressed air diving. The lungs also can be affected in a number of ways. This chapter focuses primarily on the pulmonary disorders associated with compressed air diving, and the reader is referred to standard reference texts for more information on the nonpulmonary problems associated with diving.

HISTORICAL PERSPECTIVE

Human beings have been breathhold diving to gather food and other natural resources from the sea for thousands of years.[1] Some archeological evidence indicates that even Neanderthal man breathhold dived 10,000 years ago. Written records of diving for military and salvage purposes go back to ancient Greece. However, man's underwater activities remained limited to breathhold diving until the late seventeenth century, at which time various types of external air supply began to be used to prolong submergence time.

A number of diving technological developments occurred in the early and mid-nineteenth century, but diving remained an esoteric activity having limited utility until the 1930s. During the late 1930s and World War II, however, the importance of undersea military operations became evident to navies throughout the world. Likewise, it was during World War II that scuba diving was developed, and this ultimately led to widescale opening up of the underwater environment.

The "demand regulator"—a device that can supply air on demand at ambient pressures other than sea level—had been invented in 1865 and was later modified for use in aviation so that pilots could breath oxygen at high altitude. However, it was not until 1943 that Jacques-Yves Cousteau and Emile Gagnon mated a demand valve regulator with a compressed air tank, giving rise to what they called Self-Contained Underwater Breathing Apparatus, or "scuba" for short.

After World War II, scuba equipment was developed and marketed for the general public, making the underwater world accessible as never before. Since the first scuba tanks were imported into the United States in 1951, it is estimated that over 7 million Americans have been certified as recreational or sport divers. Scuba should now be viewed as a basic tool having many different applications for commercial, military, scientific, and recreational purposes.

THE UNDERWATER HIGH-PRESSURE ENVIRONMENT

Of the various environmental factors affecting divers, pressure is by far the single most important, with its effects either directly or indirectly accounting for the majority of serious diving medical problems.

Pressure is defined as force per unit area, and *atmospheric pressure* is the pressure exerted by the air above the earth's surface. Atmospheric pressure varies with alti-

---

tude, and at sea level it is 760 millimeters of mercury (mm Hg), or 14.7 pounds per square inch (psi). Sea level pressure is generally referred to as 1 *atmosphere* (atm).

Absolute pressure is the total barometric pressure at any point. With pressure gauges calibrated to read zero at sea level, *gauge pressure* is the amount of pressure greater than atmospheric pressure. Gauge pressure is typically 1 atm less than absolute atmospheric pressure.

Except in situations that require laboratory precision, the units most often used to express water pressure are pounds per square inch (psi), feet of sea water (fsw), feet of fresh water (ffw), or atmospheres absolute (ata). Psi may be either gauge or absolute (i.e., psig or psia) (Table 45-1).

As a diver descends underwater, absolute pressure increases much faster than in air because of the greater density of water. Each foot of sea water exerts a force of 0.445 psig. At 33 fsw, the absolute pressure is double that of sea level, and each 33 feet of depth in the ocean adds an additional atmosphere of pressure. Because sea water contains more solutes, it is slightly heavier than freshwater. In freshwater, atmospheric pressure increases by 1 ata each 34 feet.

Pressure change with increasing depth is linear, although, importantly, *the greatest relative change in pressure per unit of depth change occurs nearest the surface.* This is why most barotrauma occurs at relatively shallow depths.

When a diver submerges, the force of the weight of the water is exerted over the entire body. Except for air-containing spaces like the lungs, paranasal sinuses, intestines, and middle ears, the body behaves as a liquid. Pascal's law describes the behavior of pressure in liquids and states that a pressure applied to any part of a fluid is transmitted equally throughout the fluid. Thus, when a diver reaches 33 fsw, the pressure on the surface of the skin and throughout the body tissues is 29.4 psia or 1,520 mm Hg.

Medical problems of divers

Environmental exposure problems

Motion sickness
Near drowning and other immersion syndromes
Hypothermia
Heat illness
Sunburn, phototoxic and photoallergic reactions
Contact, irritant and other dermatitides
Infectious diseases
Physical trauma

Dysbarism

Barotrauma
Dysbaric air embolism
Decompression sickness
Dysbaric osteonecrosis
Dysbaric retinopathy

Breathing gas-related problems

Inert gas narcosis (e.g., nitrogen narcosis)
Hypoxia
Oxygen toxicity
Hypercapnia
Carbon monoxide poisoning
Lipoid pneumonitis

Hazardous marine life

Miscellaneous

Hyperventilation
Hyperbaric cephalgia
Hearing loss
Carotid-compression syncope
Panic and anxiety reactions

Table 45-1. Common units of pressure measurement in the underwater environment

Depth (fsw)	psig	psia	ata	mm Hg
Sea level	0	14.7	1	760
33	14.7	29.4	2	1,520
66	29.4	44.1	3	2,280
99	44.1	58.8	4	3,040
132	58.8	73.5		
165	73.5	88.2	5	3,800
198	88.2	102.9	6	4,560
231	102.9	117.6	7	5,320
264	117.6	132.3	8	6,080
297	132.2	147.0	10	7,600

ata, Atmospheres absolute; *fsw,* feet of sea water; *mmHg,* millimeters of mercury; *psia,* pounds per square inch—absolute, *psig,* pounds per square inch—gauge.

The diver is generally unaware of this pressure, except in the air-containing spaces of the body. The gases in these spaces obey Boyle's law (Table 45-2), which states that the pressure of a given quantity of gas varies inversely with its volume (when temperature remains constant). Hence, air in the middle ear, paranasal sinuses, lungs, and gastrointestinal tract is reduced in volume during descent underwater. Inability to maintain gas pressure in these body spaces equal to the surrounding water pressure leads to various mechanical traumas known as barotrauma.

Because of the weight of the water exerting pressure over the chest wall, humans can breathe surface air through a snorkel or tube connected to the surface for only a short distance underwater—typically only to a depth of 1 to 2 feet. Attempts to breathe at greater depths through the tube are dangerous because the respiratory effort greatly augments the already physiologic negative-pressure breathing. In other words, when the respiratory muscles are relaxed at sea level alveolar pressure is equal to surrounding air pressure. At a depth of 1 foot, the total water pressure on the chest wall is nearly 200 pounds. Because of the loss of normal chest expansion and the pressurization of intraalveolar air, the diver has to "suck" or use negative-pressure breathing to draw surface air into the lungs through the tube. Even at a depth of 1 foot, the great respiratory effort required is rapidly fatiguing. Additional work is created by the added dead space of the tube. Respiration becomes impossible at only minimally deeper depths. Forced negative-pressure breathing will ultimately result in pulmonary capillary damage, with intraalveolar edema or hemorrhage. Symptoms of this include dyspnea and hemoptysis. Should this occur, there is no specific treatment; therapy is purely supportive.

DIVING SYNDROMES

Diving medical problems are due to the intrinsic hazards of the aquatic environment (e.g., near drowning, hypothermia, aquatic skin disorders, water-borne infectious diseases, and hazardous marine life, to name some), and the breathing of air at increased atmospheric pressure. This chapter will focus only on pulmonary-related diving syndromes.

Dysbarism is a general term that encompasses the pathologic changes that result from altered environmental pressure. It is primarily a disorder of divers and compressed air workers exposed to increased atmospheric pressure, but dysbaric problems also occur in aviators, astronauts, and some industrial workers as a result of exposures to the reduced pressure found at actual or simulated high altitude.

Dysbarism most often presents acutely due to problems caused by the mechanical effects of pressure on closed air spaces (i.e., barotrauma) or problems caused by breathing gasses at elevated partial pressure (e.g., nitrogen narcosis or decompression sickness). Less often, it may present after a delay of months or years, such as with dysbaric osteonecrosis (a form of aseptic necrosis associated with inadequate decompression).

BAROTRAUMA

The gas pressure in the air-filled spaces of the body is normally in equilibrium with the environment. If anything should obstruct the passageways of gas exchange for these spaces when there is a change in ambient pressure, then a pressure disequilibrium will develop. The tissue damage resulting from such pressure imbalance is known as barotrauma.

Barotrauma is the most common medical problem affecting divers, potentially involving any structure or combination of structures that leads to entrapment of gas in a closed space. This may include skin trapped under a fold in a dry suit, the portion of the face under a face mask, or the ears, paranasal sinuses, lungs, or gastrointestinal tract. The middle ears, however, are by far the organs most often affected by barotrauma, with middle ear barotrauma, or barotitis media, affecting more than 80% of divers at one time or another.[2,3]

Lung squeeze

A very unusual form of barotrauma known as lung squeeze has been occasionally observed in breathhold diving. Persons having this syndrome typically complain of shortness of breath and dyspnea after surfacing from a deep (i.e., greater than 100 fsw) breathhold dive. The diver may have hemoptysis, hypoxemia, and pulmonary edema on chest x-ray. It is treated with supplemental oxygen and respiratory support, as needed, typically with complete resolution of symptoms within a few days.

The classic pathophysiologic understanding of lung squeeze is that it occurs when a diver descends to a depth at which total lung volume (TLV) is reduced to less than residual volume (RV). At this point transpulmonic pressure exceeds intraalveolar pressure, causing transudation of fluid or blood into the alveolae (from rupture of pulmonary capillaries).

Table 45-2. Boyle's law*

	Depth (fsw)	Gauge pressure (atm)	Absolute pressure (atm)	Gas bubble volume (%)	Gas bubble diameter (%)
Air					
Sea level	0	0	1	100	100
Sea water	33	1	2	50	79
	66	2	3	33	69
	99	3	4	25	63
	132	4	5	20	58
	165	5	6	17	54

*Boyle's law states that the volume of a given quantity of gas at constant temperature varies inversely with its pressure or $P_1V_1 = P_2V_2$.

atm, Atmosphere; *fsw,* feet of sea water.

According to this scenario, a breathhold diver with a TLV of 6,000 ml and a RV of 1,200 ml could dive to only 6,000/1,200 or 5 ata (equal to 132 fsw) before lung squeeze would occur. However, breathhold divers are known to go much deeper than this without apparent problem.

In 1968, Schaefer et al. reported that breathhold divers pool their blood centrally,[4] accumulating a central volume increase of as much as 1,047 ml at 90 fsw. This adjustment in pulmonary blood volume reduces the RV, and theoretically it should be possible for the diver with a TLV of 6,000 ml to breathhold to 6,000/(1,200 − 1,047), or to almost 40 ata. And although Jacques Mayol's world record breathhold dive to 316 fsw seems to support this concept, there continue to be cases of lung squeeze at much shallower depths. The exact pathophysiology of this condition remains unclear. Fortunately, it occurs very infrequently.

Underwater blast injury

Another unusual form of barotrauma can be caused by underwater explosions. Shock waves from a blast are propagated farther in the dense water medium than in air. Underwater explosions may result from ordnance or ignition of explosive gases during cutting or welding operations.

Underwater blasts can cause serious injuries to divers. Air-containing body cavities such as the lungs, intestines, ears, and paranasal sinuses are most vulnerable. Pneumothorax, pneumomediastinum, and air embolism may result from laceration of the lung and pleura.[5] There may be intestinal perforation, subserosal hemorrhage, and subsequent peritonitis. The occurrence of air embolism at depth, which will worsen with ascent to the surface, would require treatment by recompression. Otherwise, management of underwater blast injuries is similar to that for terrestrial blast injuries.

Pulmonary barotrauma of ascent or the pulmonary overpressurization syndrome

The most serious type of barotrauma is pulmonary barotrauma of ascent resulting from expansion of entrapped gas in the lungs. If the expanding gas cannot escape from the lungs it will rupture the alveolae or terminal bronchioles, producing a spectrum of injuries that the author has collectively dubbed the *pulmonary overpressurization syndrome* (POPS) or "burst lung." In essence, the POPS is a dramatic clinical demonstration of Boyle's law.

Divers suffering from the POPS typically give a history of rapid and uncontrolled ascent to the surface prior to the onset of symptoms. Such may occur as a result of running out of air while submerged, panic, sudden development of uncontrolled positive bouyancy (e.g., loss of weight belt or inadvertent inflation of a bouyancy compensator), or some similar circumstance. However, localized overinflation of the lungs from focally increased elastic recoil may also occur in divers who ascend at a proper rate.[6]

If a given intrapulmonic gas volume is trapped by forcible breathholding or a closed glottis, or even a small portion of the lung by bronchospasm or a mucous plug, during ascent then intrapulmonic volume increases (according to Boyle's law) until the elastic limit of the chest wall is reached. After that, intrapulmonic pressure rises until, at a positive differential pressure of about 80 mm Hg, air is forced across the pulmonary capillary membrane. This air enters either the pulmonary interstitial spaces or the pulmonary capillaries.

The diagnosis of the POPS is based on the development of characteristic symptoms and signs after diving. The actual clinical manifestations may take several forms, including pneumomediastinum, subcutaneous emphysema, pneumopericardium, pneumothorax, pneumoperitoneum, and pulmonary interstitial emphysema. Recently, diffuse alveolar hemorrhage has been described as a manifestation of pulmonary barotrauma.[7] Systemic arterial gas embolism (AGE) resulting from gas leaking into ruptured pulmonary veins is the most feared complication of the POPS.

The specific clinical manifestations of the POPS will depend on the location and amount of air that escapes into an extraalveolar location.

Mediastinal emphysema is the most common form of the POPS, resulting from pulmonary interstitial air dissecting along bronchi back to the mediastinum. In these cases, the diver usually presents several hours after diving with gradually increasing hoarseness, neck fullness, and substernal chest pain. Subcutaneous emphysema may be present. In severe cases the diver may complain of marked chest pain, dyspnea, and dysphagia. Syncope may occur. Radiographs will usually show extraalveolar air in the neck or mediastinum.

Treatment of mediastinal emphysema, as well as most other strictly pulmonary forms of the POPS, is conservative, consisting of rest, avoidance of further pressure exposure (including flying in commercial aircraft), and observation. Supplemental oxygen administration may be useful in severe cases. Recompression is indicated in only extraordinarily severe cases, since it carries a risk of causing further lung injury.

Pneumothorax is another manifestation of diving-related POPS. This occurs less frequently than mediastinal emphysema since this requires that air be vented through the visceral pleura, a route having greater resistance than the interstitium.

In cases of diving-related pneumothorax, the diver usually complains of pleuritic chest pain, breathlessness, and dyspnea, just as in cases of pneumothorax due to other causes. Radiographs may confirm the diagnosis. It is treated in the standard fashion with tube thoracostomy in all but trivial cases.

Importantly, a diver with an untreated pneumothorax should have a tube thoracostomy before recompression treatment begins. Since the intrapleural gas of a pneumothorax cannot be vented to the environment, it may convert to a lethal tension pneumothorax during depressurization from the hyperbaric treatment.

ARTERIAL GAS EMBOLISM

Arterial gas embolism —also known as "dysbaric air embolism" or "cerebral air embolism"—is the most feared complication of pulmonary overpressurization. It is a major cause of death and disability among sport divers and is one of the most dramatic maladies associated with compressed air diving.[8]

Arterial gas embolism results from air bubbles entering the pulmonary venous circulation from ruptured alveolae or bronchioles. As air enters the pulmonary capillaries, the gas bubbles rapidly travel to the heart and then into the aorta, where they may then enter the coronary arteries and produce myocardial infarction or cardiac arrest secondary to vessel occlusion.[9] Gas embolization to the coronary arteries may induce arrhythmias, which may be exacerbated or independently generated by cerebral air embolism.[10,11]

Most of the bubbles entering the aorta will pass into the systemic circulation, lodging in small arteries and occluding the more distal circulation. Bubbles most often pass up the carotid arteries to embolize the brain. They may also embolize the vertebral arteries, causing sudden cardiopulmonary arrest from brain stem ischemia.

The clinical manifestations of cerebral air embolism are dramatic and often life-threatening. Depending on the site(s) of circulatory occlusion, the specific neurologic consequences vary. The neurologic pattern may be confusing, as showers of bubbles randomly embolize the brain's circulation, producing ischemia and infarction of diverse brain regions. Combined carotid and vertebral artery embolization may produce severe diffuse brain injury.[8]

The neurologic manifestations of AGE are typical of an acute stroke, although hemiplegia and other purely unilateral brain syndromes are infrequent. Most often observed are loss of consciousness, monoplegia or asymmetric multiplegia, focal paralysis, paresthesias or other sensory disturbances, convulsions, aphasia, confusion, blindness or visual field defects, vertigo, dizziness, or headache.[3,8,12] Physical findings are extremely variable. Specific pulmonary manifestations of the POPS (e.g., subcutaneous or mediastinal emphysema) may or may not be present in AGE patients.

All cases of suspected arterial gas embolism must be referred for recompression treatment (i.e., hyperbaric oxygen treatment) as rapidly as possible. This is the primary and essential treatment for this condition. Space restraints here do not allow for a discussion of hyperbaric treatment.

INDIRECT EFFECTS OF PRESSURE

Several diving-related problems may develop as a result of breathing gases at higher than normal atmospheric pressure. Chief among these conditions are nitrogen narcosis, oxygen toxicity, and decompression sickness (DCS). The behavior and physiologic effects of gases at elevated pressure is based upon Dalton's law of partial pressures. This fundamental gas law states that the total pressure exerted by a mixture of gases is the sum of the pressures that would be exerted by each individual gas if it alone occupied the same volume. Said differently, the partial pressure of a gas in a mixture is the pressure exerted by that gas alone. Dalton's law states that in an air mixture, combining nitrogen, oxygen, carbon dioxide and water vapor, the total pressure $(PT) = P_{N_2} + P_{O_2} + P_{CO_2} + P_{H_2O}$. The partial pressure of each gas in the mixture is found by multiplying the percentage of that gas present by the total pressure.

The partial pressures of inspired gases, not their percentages, are of prime importance in diving. For example, it has been shown that in hyperbaric chamber treatment of decompression sickness, 100% oxygen can be safely used at depths up to 60 fsw (2.8 ata) for 20-minute periods with the subject at rest in the dry chamber. On the other hand, if a diver breathed 20% oxygen in a helium–oxygen mixture at 600 fsw (20 ata), this would be equivalent to breathing 4.2 ata of oxygen, which would rapidly produce central nervous system oxygen poisoning.

Breathing gas-related problems

The diver who breathes compressed air is subject to the effects of the component gases in the air according to their partial pressures. Although the gas mixture is simply air with normal percentages of oxygen and nitrogen, the increases in partial pressures of these gases may create various problems. If there are contaminants in the breathing gas these can become toxic when breathed at pressure.

Nitrogen narcosis. Most notable among the breathing medium-related problems is nitrogen narcosis, also known as "rapture of the deep," "inert gas narcosis," or "the narks." This condition results from the increasing development of anesthesia or intoxication as the partial pressure of nitrogen increases at depth. Nitrogen narcosis is important to divers because it causes a deterioration in judgment and cognition, euphoria, and overconfidence, all of which can lead to serious errors in diving techniques, accidents, and drowning.

Typically, a diver breathing compressed air develops symptoms of nitrogen narcosis at depths between 70 and 100 feet. These symptoms include lightheadedness, loss of fine sensory discrimination, giddiness, and euphoria. Symptoms progressively worsen with deeper depth. At depths over 200 fsw most divers are severely intoxicated, manifesting poor judgment, impaired reasoning, overconfidence, and slowed reflexes. At a depth of 300 fsw, auditory and visual hallucinations may occur, along with feelings of impending blackout. Most divers will lose consciousness by 400 fsw.

There is both individual and daily variability in the depth at which symptoms of nitrogen narcosis will occur, as well as the severity of symptoms. Some degree of acclimatization allows experienced divers to work more safely at greater depths. Nonetheless, nitrogen narcosis is a major problem for all compressed air divers at depths greater than 100 fsw.

Treatment of nitrogen narcosis simply requires ascent to a shallower depth, where symptoms promptly clear. Of course, the condition can be prevented by avoiding deep dives. In commercial diving, where there may be reason to dive deeper than 100 fsw, the problem is prevented by substituting helium–oxygen for compressed air.

Oxygen toxicity. Although oxygen is essential for most life forms on earth, it becomes a poison at elevated partial pressures. Oxygen toxicity in divers can affect the central nervous or pulmonary systems.

Pulmonary oxygen toxicity. Retrolental fibroplasia in premature infants and pulmonary oxygen toxicity in adults are well known problems associated with the use of therapeutic oxygen. Pulmonary oxygen toxicity is induced by breathing a relatively low P_{O_2} for prolonged periods. It is generally considered that the limit for indefinite exposure without demonstrable lung damage is a P_{O_2} of about 0.5 ata, and that on a time–dose curve it is safe to breathe 100% oxygen at 1 ata for up to about 20 hours or at 2 ata for up to 6 hours. This time can be lengthened significantly by using intermittent exposures, e.g., interspersing a 5-minute air break between every 20 minutes of oxygen breathing.[13] At 2.8 to 3.0 ata (60 to 66 fsw), where 100% oxygen is used to treat decompression sickness, gas gangrene, and carbon monoxide poisoning, pulmonary oxygen toxicity is rarely a problem because CNS toxicity usually manifests before sufficient time elapses to induce pulmonary damage. A complete review of this subject has been provided by Clark and Lambertsen.[14] Use of hyperbaric oxygen according to standard treatment tables (e.g., as used in treating decompression sickness) does not produce clinical manifestations of pulmonary oxygen toxicity.

The most common clinical manifestation of pulmonary oxygen toxicity is substernal discomfort on inhalation. If exposure continues, this can progress to severe burning substernal pain and persistent coughing. Reduction of inspired oxygen partial pressure between 0.21 and 0.50 ata usually results in prompt relief. Severe cases of pulmonary oxygen toxicity may require endotracheal intubation and positive end-expiratory pressure (PEEP) ventilation to achieve adequate arterial oxygenation at the required lower partial pressures of inspired oxygen.

Central nervous system oxygen toxicity. During the 1880s, the French physiologist Paul Bert described convulsions in animals breathing 100% oxygen at elevated chamber pressures. This work was confirmed in human studies during the 1930s. The classic human observations on divers by Donald in the 1940s provided much of our current knowledge about predisposing factors and clinical manifestations of CNS oxygen toxicity.[15,16]

Common symptoms and signs of CNS oxygen poisoning are feelings of apprehension or anxiety, sweating, nausea and vomiting, muscle twitching, tinnitus, tunnel vision, and convulsions. In some persons there may be no early warning symptoms, and the first manifestation of CNS oxygen toxicity may be a generalized seizure.

Treatment for CNS oxygen toxicity in a hyperbaric chamber involves removal of the oxygen mask, maintenance of the airway, and keeping the patient from injuring himself. Chamber pressure should be maintained constant until any seizing is over so as to avoid a pulmonary overpressure accident.

After a postictal period, the CNS toxic patient should recover without sequelae. Recurrent seizures are rare. Although anticonvulsants used in seizure treatment theoretically should suppress oxygen-induced seizures, none has been tested to determine doses needed to suppress oxygen seizures. Anticonvulsant drug therapy is not usually necessary, in any case, because termination of oxygen breathing routinely stops the seizure. Removing oxygen at the first sign of CNS toxicity has to date prevented any documented permanent central nervous system damage after an oxygen-induced seizure.

Contaminated breathing gas. As a diver descends under water, the sea level partial pressure of each gaseous component in the breathing medium increases. Should the breathing gas be contaminated, then various problems can occur. The most common problem in this regard is *carbon monoxide poisoning* from engine exhaust contamination of the compressed air supply. Another problem that can occur if the compressor motor is not free of oil, because this oil can be pumped into the scuba tanks or air supply system, is lipoid pneumonitis.

Lipoid pneumonitis is a complication of oil aspiration of any kind and is a well described occupational hazard in industries involving exposure to oil sprays. The potentiality of introducing oil vapor into the conpressed air has been of concern in diving for decades; however, there is only one report in the literature of this actually occurring.[17] Historically, this condition probably has occurred but was not reported in the literature. Fortunately, procedural and technical developments in modern diving have minimized the likelihood of this occurring.

Lipoid pneumonitis may lead to pulmonary fibrosis and restrictive lung disease with resultant reduced lung volumes, increased alveolar to arterial oxygen tension difference, and reduced exercise tolerance.

Decompression sickness

In the mid-nineteenth century, tunnel and bridge workers who labored in caissons pressurized with compressed air were sometimes observed to suffer joint pains, paralysis, and various other medical problems after decompressing from the caisson. The condition was not understood and was dubbed "caisson disease" or "compressed air illness."

For many decades "caisson's disease" remained a medical curiosity, but because of its occurrence in diving, aviation, and a few other important areas of activity in the twentieth century, there was considerable research into its causes and treatment. We now know that these early high-pressure workers were experiencing symptoms of DCS.

Today, we know that DCS is caused by the formation of inert gas (e.g., nitrogen) bubbles within the intravascular and extravascular spaces following a reduction in ambient pressure. This may occur during or following decompression after being underwater or in a caisson or hyperbaric chamber in which pressures are greater than sea level, as well as in aviators, astronauts, or hypobaric (high altitude) chamber workers who rapidly travel from sea level to pressures less than 0.5 ata.

Etiology. To understand the etiology of DCS one must understand the temporal uptake and elimination of inert gases in the diver's breathing medium.

If it were possible for a diver to breathe 100% oxygen while underwater then there would be no problems with decompression, since oxygen is rapidly metabolized by the body and, for practical purposes, does not contribute to bubble formation on ascent from depth. Unfortunately, pure oxygen breathing at increased atmospheric pressure causes CNS toxicity, as already discussed. The need for an inert gas diluent (e.g., nitrogen) in the diver's breathing medium is at the crux of the problem in decompression sickness.

As pressure increases underwater, the partial pressures of inspired gases increase. For example, at 99 fsw (4 ata) the absolute pressure is 3,040 mm Hg. Seventy-nine percent of this pressure is caused by nitrogen (i.e., 2,400 mm Hg, as compared with 600 mm Hg P_{N_2} at sea level). Accounting for water vapor and carbon dioxide, this results in an alveolar partial pressure of nitrogen ($P_A N_2$) of about 2,360 mm Hg. This $P_A N_2$ is rapidly reflected across the alveolar–capillary membrane to the arterial blood, where, according to Henry's law, nitrogen becomes physically dissolved in the blood. (Henry's law states that the amount of gas dissolved in a liquid at any given temperature is a function of the partial pressure of the gas in contact with the liquid and the solubility coefficient of the gas in the particular liquid.) As this nitrogen-laden blood is presented to tissues at the capillary level, a complex set of variables, dictated by perfusion, diffusion, and inert gas solubility, results in a family of nitrogen uptake curves similar to the pharmacokinetic drug uptake curves commonly displayed for medications.

Navies and commercial diving companies around the world have developed various decompression schedules based on theoretical calculations and actual testing (animal and human) that will allow divers to avoid exceeding safe rates of decompression after specified depth–time dive profiles, so as to prevent the occurrence of decompression sickness. These listings of "safe" depth-time diving profiles are generally referred to as *decompression tables*. Many different sets of decompression tables exist, with the U.S. Navy Standard Air Decompression Tables being the most widely used.[18] Decompression tables are the subject of considerable scientific controversy, however, resulting in periodic revision and continual search for improved safety.

Clinical manifestations. Decompression sickness is a multisystem disorder caused by a rapid decrease in ambient atmospheric pressure such that inert gas comes out of solution, causing the formation of bubbles in tissue and venous blood. Conceptually, DCS is the same illness whether it occurs in high altitude aviators or deep sea divers, although there are some differences in the specific clinical manifestations of the disease depending on whether it is due to hyperbaric or hypobaric exposure (see Chapter 46).

The specific physiologic sequelae of bubble formation in tissue and venous blood are myriad. These effects include cellular distention and rupture, mechanical stretching of tendons or ligaments producing pain, and intravascular or intralymphatic occlusion, resulting in congestive ischemia and infarction or lymphedema.

Intravascular bubbles also cause multiple biophysical effects at the blood–bubble surface interface. In brief, bubbles are viewed by the immune system as foreign matter and incite an inflammatory reaction. The key step in the process is activation of Hageman factor, which in turn activates the intrinsic clotting, kinin and complement systems, producing platelet activation, cellular clumping, lipid embolization, increased vascular permeability, interstitial edema, and microvascular sludging. The overall effect is decreased tissue perfusion and ischemia.

As with AGE, the diagnosis of DCS is a clinical diagnosis based on the history of diving with compressed air and the subsequent development of characteristic symptoms and signs.

The majority of patients having DCS will become symptomatic in the first hour after surfacing from a dive, with most of the rest noticing symptoms within 6 hours after diving. One to two percent of DCS patients may not note their symptoms until 24 to 48 hours after diving.

The clinical manifestations of DCS are protean, with the neurologic and musculoskeletal systems being most often affected.

Periarticular joint pain is the most common symptom of DCS, being found in about 70% of patients. This form of DCS is often referred to as "limb bends," "joint bends," or "pain only bends." The shoulders and elbows are the joints most often affected by DCS in scuba divers, but any joint may be involved. The pain may radiate to surrounding areas. This pain is usually described as a dull ache deep within the joint but may also be characterized as sharp or throbbing. It is sometimes described as feeling like tendinitis or bursitis. Movement of the joint typically worsens the pain.

Profound fatigue that is out of proportion to the activity performed may be an early manifestation of DCS. Although its etiology is unknown, a feeling of severe fatigue after diving demands careful evaluation for other manifestations of DCS.

Decompression sickness also may present a variety of cutaneous manifestations, including scarlatiniform, erysipeloid, or mottled rashes, pruritus, and formication. Localized swelling or peau d'orange may result from lymphatic obstruction. Skin manifestations are relatively uncommon, though, and in and of themselves are usually not serious. However, they are often a harbinger of more severe DCS. Mottling or marbling of the skin (cutis marmorata) is considered especially important, since it often heralds the delayed onset of neurologic problems. The exact physiologic basis of cutis marmorata is unknown.

The "chokes" or *pulmonary decompression sickness* is a serious form of DCS characterized by dyspnea, burning substernal pain, cyanosis, and nonproductive cough. Animal studies have demonstrated gas bubbles or foam in the pulmonary arteries, right atrium, and right ventricle following unsafe decompression. Most likely, chokes represents massive pulmonary gas embolism with mechanical obstruction of the pulmonary vascular bed by bubbles. Typically, symptoms of pulmonary venous air embolization begin when 10% or more of the pulmonary vascular bed is obstructed. Chokes patients can progress rapidly to profound shock or neurologic DCS. The specific clinical and radiologic manifestations of the chokes are similar to those seen with venous gas embolism (VGE) from other causes.[19]

Symptoms of VGE include air hunger, dyspnea, cough, and chest pain. Findings may include tachypnea, tachycardia, hypotension, cyanosis, expiratory wheezing, neurologic signs, and a "mill wheel" heart murmur. Victims may also exhibit increased central venous or pulmonary artery pressure, ischemic electrocardiographic changes or cor pulmonale, decreased end-tidal CO_2 fraction, and precordial Doppler sounds of circulating gas bubbles. Visualization of air in the main pulmonary artery is pathognomonic of pulmonary air embolism.[5,19]

Neurologic impairment may occur as the sole manifestation of DCS or as part of a progressive dysbaric syndrome. Neurologic DCS is manifested by a myriad of symptoms and signs because of the unpredictable and random nature by which DCS affects the nervous system. Whereas any level of the CNS may be affected, the most commonly involved site in compressed air divers is the spinal cord, and specifically the lower thoracic and lumbar regions of the cord.

Historically, neurologic DCS was believed to occur in only 10 to 20% of DCS cases, based on military experience,[20] but neurologic manifestations of DCS have been found in 50% to 60% of scuba diving casualties treated in Hawaii[21] and have been reported in alarmingly high frequencies in other populations of sports divers as well.[22,23]

Classically, dysbaric spinal cord injury occurs in the lower thoracic, lumbar, and sacral portions of the cord, producing low back pain, subjective "heaviness" in the legs, paraplegia or paraparesis, lower extremity paresthesias, and possible bladder or anal sphincter dysfunction.

Decompression sickness of the brain produces a variety of symptoms, most of which are indistinguishable from AGE. Involvement of the cerebellum or inner ear may produce a condition known as the "staggers" because of the resultant ataxia.

Vasomotor decompression sickness or "decompression shock" is an extremely rare, and life threatening, form of DCS. The pathogenesis of this shock syndrome is poorly understood, but it is believed to be due to a rapid shift of fluid from intravascular to extravascular spaces secondary to diffuse bubble embolization, ischemia, and hypoxia.[24] Hypotension also may result from massive venous air embolization of the lungs. This condition is highly lethal, and many patients do not survive to undergo recompression unless a hyperbaric chamber is immediately available.

Treatment. All patients suspected of having decompression sickness must be referred to a hyperbaric treatment facility as quickly as possible, since recompression is the primary and essential treatment for this condition. One must have a high index of suspicion for the often diverse and confusing clinical manifestations of decompression sickness. The history of the dive profile is helpful if the diver knowingly violated decompression procedures, but decompression sickness may occur on dives that should be safe according to current decompression schedules. Likewise, the reported depth and time of the dive may be erroneous for a number of reasons.

Management of DCS must be commenced as soon as the condition is suspected.[22] Sport divers are usually far from a recompression chamber when their symptoms develop, so treatment will often be initiated in the field or at an outpatient acute care facility. One hundred percent oxygen should be administered by a tight oronasal mask to provide a favorable gradient for nitrogen washout. Of equal importance is maintenance of intravascular volume to ensure capillary perfusion for elimination of microvascular inert gas bubbles and for tissue oxygenation. An intravenous infusion of isotonic solution should be started and run at a flow rate sufficient to maintain urine output at 1 to 2 ml/kg/hour. With spinal cord involvement, an indwelling urinary catheter may be needed because of sacral nerve root dysfunction. Intractable vomiting or vertigo should be treated with appropriate parenteral agents. Advanced life support measures should be undertaken appropriate to the patient's clinical condition.

Although these measures are undertaken, emergency transportation to the nearest recompression chamber should be arranged. There are a large number of recompression chambers in the United States, and their operational status frequently changes. Thus, the reader is referred to the National Divers Alert Network (DAN) located at Duke University for help identifying the location of the nearest recompression chamber, as well as help with the treatment of dive-related incidents. DAN may be accessed 24-hours a day at 1-919-684-8111.

MEDICAL FITNESS FOR DIVING

Persons wishing to learn to scuba dive should be medically cleared before taking up the sport. The diving examination should especially focus on the pulmonary, otolaryngologic, cardiac, neurologic, and integumentary systems, as well as the person's psychologic stability.

Because of the changes in pressure that occur with excursions underwater and the physical and sometimes psychologic factors associated with diving, and because of the stress of diving, the potential for nitrogen narcosis, altered sensory stimulation, and other factors that interact with pharmaceuticals, as well as the inherent nature of being underwater, many medical conditions are contraindications for diving. In general, these things can be divided into five categories. People falling into any one of the following categories are at increased risk of incurring a diving-related problem:

1. Persons who are unable to equalize pressure in one or more of the body's air spaces (e.g., ears, paranasal sinuses, or lungs) and, thus, are at increased risk of barotrauma
2. Persons who have a medical or psychiatric condition that may become manifest underwater or at a remote diving site and endanger the life of the diver because of the condition itself, because it occurs in the water, or because there is inadequate medical help available
3. Persons who have impaired tissue perfusion or diffusion of inert gases and, thus, have an increased risk of DCS
4. Persons who are in poor physical condition and, thus, are at increased risk of DCS or exertion-related medical problems; of note, the compromised physical condition may be physiologic or pharmacologic
5. Women who are or think they might be pregnant because the fetus may be at increased risk of suffering dysbaric injury

In accordance with the likelihood of causing a diving problem, as well as the potential seriousness of the problem, conditions falling into one of these five categories may be absolutely, relatively, or temporarily disqualifying for scuba diving.

The primary pulmonary problems of concern for diving are as follows:

1. *Bullous or obstructive lung disease.* Air-containing pulmonary blebs or cysts can trap air and lead to local pulmonary overpressure accidents during decompression. If a ball-valve or flutter-valve effect allows a bleb or cyst to equalize with the elevated breathing pressure during compression or descent but blocks the escape of air during decompression, rupture could cause the POPS and air embolism.

2. *Hyperresponsive airways disease or asthma.* Because of the risk of local air trapping and consequent pulmonary overpressure accidents, persons having asthma should not dive. It is generally true that scuba air is free of pollens, but other stresses in diving (e.g., cold, heavy exertion, or emotional stress) could precipitate bronchospasm at depth, with resultant local air trapping during ascent. If there is any suggestion of bronchospastic tendencies, pulmonary function studies should be performed. Even minimal air trapping at sea level takes on great significance at depth.

Given the prevalence of asthma in the population and the popularity of diving, the question of whether asthmatics can dive safely comes up frequently. The consensus of diving medicine experts is that persons with active or symptomatic asthma absolutely should not dive. This includes persons who have ever had bronchospasm as a result of exercise (i.e., exercise induced asthma) or inhalation of cold air. The risk is too great that such persons will suffer pulmonary barotrauma when scuba diving, endangering their lives and the lives of others. Even so, it is generally difficult to deny these typically young, eager, enthusiastic, and overtly healthy appearing persons the right to dive.

Expert opinion varies on the question of diving clearance for the asymptomatic asthmatic. Unfortunately there are insufficient data on which to base useful risk determinations. Asthmatics are invariably banned from commercial or military diving, and a history of asthma on a medical form is generally grounds for exclusion from recreational diving courses. Thus, there are no useful denominator data to assess the risk of diving for individuals with childhood or inactive asthma. Individuals with inactive asthma who wish to dive should have a complete pulmonary evaluation including exercise and bronchial challenge testing. Any determination of fitness for diving must be made on the basis of such examination and testing, and will ultimately be a clinical judgment.

3. *Spontaneous pneumothorax.* Even without the pressure variations of diving, a history of previous spontaneous pneumothorax carries a significant incidence of recurrence, and the candidate must be advised against compressed gas diving. A pneumothorax that occurs while still at increased pressure underwater or in a recompression chamber can become a life-threatening tension pneumothorax as the pleural cavity air expands (Boyle's law) during ascent. Persons having had traumatic or surgical pneumothorax may be cleared for diving depending on the specific circumstances.

4. *History of overpressure accident in previous diving.* The circumstances of the offending dive are especially important in these cases. For instance, if a diver suffers a "physiologically undeserved" or unexplained episode of the POPS (i.e., the diver breathes normally to the sur-

face, yet suffers an air embolism) there would be concern about the risk of recurrence. On the other hand, a diver who suffers a pulmonary overpressure accident that is considered "physiologically deserved" (e.g., rapid ascent following inadvertent inflation of a buoyancy compensator) could be considered for a return to diving after full neurologic recovery and with the determination of normal pulmonary function. However, some experts argue that even this diver is at greater risk because of potential pulmonary scarring and the inability to detect small airway air trapping.

5. *Coryza or bronchitis.* These conditions may cause inability to equalize pressure in the ears, sinuses, or lungs due to mucosal edema, mucus plugs, or bronchospasm, and thus are temporarily disqualifying for diving.

REFERENCES

1. Bayne CG: Breath-hold diving. In Davis JC, editor: *Hyperbaric and undersea medicine,* vol 1, San Antonio, 1981, Medical Seminars Publishing.
2. Edmonds C, Freeman P, Thomas R, et al: *Otological aspects of diving,* pp 29-34, Glebe, NSW, Australia, 1973, Australasian Medical Publishing Company Limited.
3. Green SM, Rothrock SG, Hummel CB, and Green EA: Incidence and severity of middle ear barotrauma in recreational scuba diving, *J Wilderness Med* 4:270-280, 1993.
4. Schaefer KE, et al: Pulmonary and circulatory adjustments determining the limits of depths in breath-hold diving, *Science* 162:1020, 1968.
5. Huller T and Buzini Y: Blast injuries of the chest and abdomen, *Arch Surg* 100:24, 1970.
6. Colebatch HJH, Smith MM, and Ng CKY: Increased elastic recoil as a determinant of pulmonary barotrauma in divers, *Respir Physiol* 55:64, 1976.
7. Balk M and Goldman JM: Alveolar hemorrhage as a manifestation of pulmonary barotrauma after scuba diving. *Ann Emerg Med* 19:930-934, 1990.
8. Kizer KW: Dysbaric cerebral air embolism in Hawaii, *Ann Emerg Med* 16:535, 1987.
9. Cales RH, et al: Cardiac arrest from gas embolism in scuba diving, *Ann Emerg Med* 10:589-592, 1981.
10. Evans DE, Kobrine AI, Weathersby PK, and Bradley ME: Cardiovascular effects of cerebral air embolism, *Stroke* 12:338-344, 1981.
11. Kizer KW: Ventricular dysrhythmia associated with serious decompression sickness, *Ann Emerg Med* 9:580-584, 1980.
12. Dutka AJ: A review of the pathophysiology and potential application of experimental therapies for cerebral ischemia to the treatment of cerebral gas embolism, *Undersea Biomed Res* 12:403-421, 1985.
13. Hendricks PL, et al: Extension of pulmonary oxygen tolerance in man at 2 ATA by intermittent oxygen exposure, *J Appl Physiol* 42:593, 1977.
14. Clark JM and Sambertsen CJ: Pulmonary oxygen toxicity: a review, *Pharmacol Rev* 23:37, 1971.
15. Donald K: *Oxygen and the diver,* Worcester, United Kingdom, 1992, Kenneth Donald in conjunction with The Self Publishing Association, Ltd.
16. Donald KW: Oxygen poisoning in man, *Br Med J* 1:667, 1947.
17. Kizer KW and Golden JA: Lipoid pneumonitis in a commercial abalone diver, *Undersea Biomed Res* 14:545, 1987.
18. Department of the Navy. *U.S. Navy Diving Manual,* vol 1, rev 2, Flagstaff, Arizona, 1988, Best Publishing.
19. Kizer KW and Goodman PG: Radiographic manifestations of venous air embolism, *Radiology* 144:35, 1982.
20. Rivera JC: Decompression sickness among divers: an analysis of 935 cases, *Milit Med* 129:314-334, 1964.
21. Kizer KW: Dysbarism in paradise, *Hawaii Med J* 39:109-116, 1980.
22. Davis JC, editor: *Treatment of serious decompression sickness and arterial gas embolism,* Bethesda, MD, 1979, Undersea Medical Society Pub No 34, WS (SDS).
23. Dick APK and Massey EW: Neurological presentation of decompression sickness and air embolism in sport divers, *Neurology* 35:667-671, 1985.
24. Chryssanthou C, et al: Studies on dysbarism, II: influences of bradykinin and "bradykinin-antagonists" on decompression sickness in mice, *Aerospace Med* 35:741, 1964.

Chapter 46

AEROSPACE

Roy DeHart

In clinical medicine, the physician is most often concerned for the ill or abnormal patient in the terrestrial or normal environment. In aerospace medicine, the flight surgeon is concerned for the crew member or normal patient in the aerospace or abnormal environment. Understanding this juxtaposition of individual and environment between clinical and aerospace medicine is important in understanding the challenges that aerospace brings to pulmonary medicine.

THE ENVIRONMENT

To understand the aerospace environment it is necessary to understand something of the atmosphere, both its chemical composition and its physical properties.

The composition of the atmosphere remains relatively constant from sea level until the physiologic equivalent of space altitude is attained. The vast amount of air commerce occurs in the region between sea level and 70,000 ft (22,000 m). Table 46-1 provides a listing of the major constituents of a dry atmosphere.

Another characteristic of the atmosphere is its pressure. Unlike its constituents, the atmospheric pressure is nonconstant and decreases with altitude ascent. The atmospheric pressure is an expression of the weight of the column of air extending from one's position upward for approximately 60 miles (100 km), where the atmosphere becomes so thin that its weight can be ignored physiologically. The density of the atmosphere is greatest at sea level and rapidly thins with increasing altitude. The sea level atmospheric pressure is approximately 760 mm Hg, 760 Torr, or 1013.2 mbar. The density of the atmosphere at this altitude is 1.225 kg/m^3. With increasing altitude, density should decrease in a near exponential manner; however, temperature is not constant as it decreases with altitude. As a rule, one half of the atmosphere is below the altitude of 18,000 ft (6650 m) and the other half extends to the edge of space. Table 46-2 presents the relationship of altitude and pressure.

The gas laws

To better understand the characteristics of the atmosphere and the physiologic impact of changes in these char-

Table 46-1. Composition of the atmosphere

Gas	Concentration in dry air (% by volume)
Nitrogen	78.09
Oxygen	20.95
Argon	0.93
Carbon dioxide	0.03
Neon	0.18×10^{-2}
Helium	0.52×10^{-3}
Krypton	0.11×10^{-3}
Hydrogen	0.50×10^{-4}
Xenon	0.87×10^{-5}

Table 46-2. Altitude–pressure relationships

Altitude (m)	Pressure	
	mbar	Torr
Sea level	1,013	760
100	1,001	751
200	989	742
300	977	733
400	966	724
500	954	716
1,000	898	674
2,000	795	596
3,000	701	525
4,000	616	462
5,000	540	405
10,000	264	198
15,000	121	90
20,000	55	41
25,000	25	19
30,000	11	8
40,000	2	2
50,000	0.8	0.6

acteristics, it is helpful to be familiar with a number of the gas laws.

Dalton's law. In our atmosphere there is a mixture of gases; this law addresses the pressure of each gas. The law states that the total pressure of a gas mixture is the sum of the partial pressures of each gas in that mixture. It is expressed as

$$P_T = P_1 + P_2 + P_3 \ldots P_n$$

where P_T is the total pressure of the mixture, and P_1, P_2, $\ldots P_n$ are the partial pressures of each individual gas in the mixture.

Boyle's law. This addresses the relationship of a gas's volume and pressure. Given constant temperature, the volume of a given mass of gas varies inversely as its pressure. It is expressed as

$$\frac{V_1}{V_2} = \frac{P_2}{P_1}$$

where V_1 is the initial volume, V_2 is the resultant volume, P_1 is the initial pressure, and P_2 is the final pressure.

Charles' law. It is recognized that as a gas is heated, it expands or increases in volume. When pressure is constant, the volume of the gas is proportional to its absolute temperature. It is expressed by

$$\frac{V_1}{V_2} = \frac{T_1}{T_2}$$

where V_1 is the initial volume, V_2 is the resultant volume, T_1 is the initial absolute temperature in degrees Kelvin (Celsius + 273°), and T_2 is the final absolute temperature. Within physiologic parameters, the narrow temperature change on the absolute temperature scale means that this law has little practical effect.

Henry's law. This is important as it deals with the solubility of gases in liquids. The quantity of gas dissolved in 1 cm^3 of a liquid is proportional to the partial pressure of the gas in contact with the liquid. A chemical reaction would void the law. The volume of gas dissolved in the fluid can be increased by increasing the pressure of the gas and by the same law reducing the pressure of the gas will result in the fluid releasing gas, provided equilibrium had been attained.

Space-equivalent altitudes

In 1952 Dr. Hubertus Strughold, the "Father of Space Medicine," described the atmospheric equivalency of space.[1] He did not consider space to be a set boundary but rather a continuum that, for specific situations, moves from terrestrial to celestial.

Zone 1. At 9.6 miles (15 km), the pressure of the atmosphere is reduced to 87 mm Hg. This is equivalent to the combined pressure for off gassing of water vapor and carbon dioxide from the lungs. Thus the astronaut would be unable to establish a respiratory gas exchange.

Zone 2. At 12 miles (20 km), the atmospheric pressure is down to 47 mm Hg. This is the vapor pressure of body fluids generated by normal body temperature. Fluids, including blood, would begin vaporizing resulting in the same desiccating process evident in deep space.

Zone 3. Above this altitude, 12 miles, the atmosphere becomes too thin to effectively be mechanically compressed to maintain cabin pressurization. Thus the cabin must be sealed to maintain a shirt sleeve environment—a space cabin.

Zone 4. At 18 miles (30 km), there is little ozone and thus minimal filtering of ultraviolet radiation. The astronaut must now be protected from such nonionizing radiation.

Zone 5. At 60 miles (100 km), the atmospheric blanket is too thin to protect from the full impact force of meteorites.

Zone 6. At 90 miles (150 km), the light scattering effect of the atmosphere is lost, and the astronaut has reached the black void of space. Illumination is direct from the light source.

Zone 7. Beyond 96 miles (160 km) the spacecraft has attained orbital altitude. For the first time, the astronaut has attained the microgravity of space flight.

Exposure

Although approximately 100 astronauts and cosmonauts have been exposed to the environment of space, tens of millions have traveled the nearer aviation environment. Aviation is a major component of international commerce with one of the nations' largest industries serving the traveling public. Additionally, hundreds of thousands of private pilots fly for business and recreation. Military aviators are the ones who challenge the extremes of this aerospace environment.

In 1992, approximately 500 million revenue passengers enplaned aboard U.S. scheduled airlines. Nearly 80% of American adults have flown at least once. These airlines have approximately 45,000 flight deck personnel and 65,000 flight attendants. There are 675,000 active civilian pilots and student pilots licensed in the United States upon whom 490,000 periodic flight physical examinations are performed by 6,500 aviation medical examiners.[2] Any of these individuals could be exposed to the hazards of the flight environment should mechanical failure occur in today's modern aircraft.

HAZARDS OF THE AEROSPACE ENVIRONMENT

In reality, the flight environment can be extremely hazardous and unforgiving. Humans are not physiologically equipped to engage routinely in aerial flight even with machines. Within this environment one can become exposed to low pressure, low oxygen, high accelerative forces, three-dimensional movement, noise, cold, and vibration. These stressors, singularly or in combination, may lead to hypoxia, dysbarism, "G"-loss of consciousness, spatial disorientation, hypothermia, noise-induced neurosensory hearing loss, and motion sickness. For the purposes of this chapter, the focus will be on the respiratory system.

Hypoxia

Hypoxia can occur when there is a deficiency of alveolar oxygen. In the aerospace environment, the deficiency is not due to pulmonary pathology but rather inadequate atmospheric oxygen. The alveolar partial pressure is the determining factor in this environment as the atmospheric partial pressure is reduced.

Symptoms may appear at altitudes as low as 5,000 ft (1520 m) when night vision is the critical function. This is due to the high metabolic oxygen requirements of the central nervous system and, particularly, the retina. As one climbs to a higher altitude the percentage of available oxygen remains constant; however, the overall atmospheric pressure falls and thus there is a concomitant fall in the O_2 partial pressure.

As a pilot climbs from 5,000 ft (1520 m) to 10,000 ft (3100 m), there are compensatory mechanisms that will come into action to reduce the adverse effects of lowered alveolar oxygen partial pressure (Po_2). Respiration will first increase in depth followed by an increase in rate. These effects are produced by the aortic and carotid chemoreceptors responding to the reduced arterial Po_2 and signal the respiratory center to initiate compensatory effort. Maximum response is achieved by 22,000 ft (6,700 m) where the respiratory minute volume is nearly double.

Once the cardiovascular system senses hypoxic changes, reflex responses act to increase heart rate, systolic blood pressure, and cardiac output, and is redistributed blood flow to the heart and brain.

With the respiratory system response to the decreased arterial Po_2, the increased breathing rate produces a fall in the carbon dioxide (CO_2) tension, leading to cerebral vasoconstriction and reduced blood flow. Once the arterial Po_2 falls to 16 mm Hg, hypoxia becomes the stronger influence and produces cerebral vasodilatation with increased blood flow.

Hypoxic effects on performance. It has been traditional to stage the effects of hypoxia into four categories. Table 46-3 defines the stages in terms of altitude and arterial oxygen saturation while breathing air and 100% oxygen. In the indifferent stage, dark adaptation is compromised. Performance of new tasks becomes difficult as the central nervous system is affected. Increases in both pulmonary and cardiac rates occur.

During the compensatory stage, physiologic reserve is able to provide some protection. The central nervous system effects are drowsiness, indifference, compromised judgment, faulty memory, and poor performance for mental tasks and discrete motor skills. The pilot is entering the envelope of "time of useful consciousness" or "effective performance time." This is the time the pilot is able to perform important flight duties without compromise to flying safety. Prolonged stays at the limit of this altitude or ascent

Table 46-3. Stages of hypoxia

Stage	Altitude breathing air (m)	Altitude breathing 100% oxygen (m)	Arterial oxygen saturation (%)
Indifferent	0-3,050	10,400-11,900	98-87
Compensatory	3,050-4,550	11,900-13,000	87-80
Disturbance	4,550-6,100	13,000-13,700	80-65
Critical	6,100-7,000	13,700-13,900	65-60

to the next stage without oxygen will compromise flying safety. Average effective performance times are provided in Table 46-4.

Physiologic compensatory mechanisms no longer are sufficient as a pilot enters the disturbance stage. Symptoms include shortness of breath, confusion, fatigue, euphoria, headache, loss of peripheral and color vision. Mental performance deteriorates and loss of consciousness occurs.

In the critical stage incapacity and unconsciousness have a rapid onset.

Management of Hypoxia. Increasing the alveolar Po_2 level to normal is the sine qua non for hypoxia management. There are a variety of oxygen delivery systems available and several will be described later in this chapter.

Prevention is the best protection, by using oxygen when flying at ambient altitudes exceeding the indifferent stage (10,000 ft, 3050 m). As will be discussed, higher altitudes may require positive pressure or pressure suit systems to ensure appropriate delivery of oxygen. In commercial aircraft, the cabin is typically maintained at an altitude of 8,000 ft (2,600 m), which provides a comfortable environment for most passengers.

Recovering from hypoxia occurs within seconds. Inhalation of 100% O_2 typically clears most symptoms within the heart–brain circulating time. On occasion an individual will experience a magnification of symptoms when initiating oxygen breathing. This phenomenon is known as the "oxygen paradox." This paradox occurs because of pulmonary vasodilatation responding to the high alveolar Po_2 with resulting hypotension leading to decreased cerebral profusion.[3]

Hyperventilation

Within the aerospace environment, hyperventilation is a concern for two reasons. First, the psychologic stress of flying with resulting anxiety, fear, and apprehension may lead to rapid respiration similar to a mild panic attack. Second, many of the symptoms of hyperventilation are similar to those experienced with hypoxia. Should hyperventilation occur, the resultant hypocapnia and alkalosis can produce a cascade of symptoms. Table 46-5 provides a comparison of hyperventilation and hypoxia symptoms.

An inexperienced aviator may be confused by the symptoms and unable to determine the cause. The initial response may be opposite to that required to correct the symptoms; for example, breath holding in an attempt to manage hyperventilation while actually experiencing hypoxia or increasing the breathing rate and depth to correct hypoxia when hyperventilation is the cause of the symptoms. In such a predicament the "rule of thumb" is to go on 100% oxygen and breathe slowly and deeply. Near instant improvement will occur if symptoms are due to hypoxia. But the same corrective action will also gradually correct the symptoms associated with hypocapnia from hyperventilation.

Pulmonary dysbarism

Dysbarism is a term that has been used over the years to refer to the adverse affects of pressure changes on the body. Such changes may be as common as an ear block while flying or the tragic consequences of alveolar rupture with rapid decompression.

The body has a number of cavities that communicate with varying ease with the ambient environment. Examples are the middle ear, sinuses, lungs, and the gastrointestinal tract. Under normal circumstances the gradual pressure changes that occur with the passage of weather systems are readily accommodated. Even changes associated with terrestrial travel up and down, by foot, automobile, or rail, are gradual enough to permit accommodation. With aviation, the rate of change in pressure may be too rapid for adjustment to occur especially when tissues are swollen from an

Table 46-4. Effective performance time at altitude

| Approximate altitude | | Effective performance time |
m	ft	
5,490	18,000	20 to 30 min
6,700	22,000	10 min
7,600	25,000	3 to 5 min
8,500	28,000	2.5 to 3 min
9,100	30,000	1 to 2 min
19,700	35,000	0.5 to 1 min
12,200	40,000	15 to 20 sec
13,100	43,000	9 to 12 sec

Table 46-5. Comparison of hyperventilation and hypoxia syndromes

Signs and symptoms	Hyperventilation	Hypoxia
Muscle activity	+	−
Cyanosis	−	+
Tetany	+	−
Breathlessness	+	+
Dizziness	+	+
Drowsiness	+	+
Euphoria	+	+
Fatigue	+	+
Headache	+	+
Judgment poor	+	+
Lightheadedness	+	+
Memory faulty	+	+
Muscle incoordination	+	+
Numbness	+	+
Performance deterioration	+	+
Respiratory rate increased	+	+
Reaction time delayed	+	+
Tingling	+	+
Vision blurred	+	+
Unconsciousness	+	+

allergy or infection. This is evident when one experiences sinus or ear "block."

The lungs are able to equilibrate with the ambient pressure except in the potentially catastrophic circumstance of rapid decompression. The lungs contain a large gas volume distributed among the alveoli. The bronchial passages become so fine that with near instantaneous pressure change over a high gradient, air flow is not adequate and gas expansion according to Boyle's law results. The thin wall alveoli are subject to disruption from overpressure. Should such damage occur, tissue tears and blood vessels are severed. Free air passes along the tissue plains producing a surgical type emphysema. Air may also enter the circulatory system with resultant gas embolism. Fortunately, such events have been rare and limited to altitude chamber instruction when an individual fails to maintain an open glottis during rapid decompression training resulting in pulmonary overpressure and lung damage.

Decompression sickness

Another form of dysbarism is the evolution of gas bubbles from the circulation when there is a drop in ambient pressure and gas has achieved near saturation at higher pressure. For Henry's law to apply, a differentiated pressure produced by gas supersaturation must occur. This phenomenon was first described by Haldane in 1906. He suggested that a supersaturation ratio of 2:1 is required for gas to come out of solution and form bubbles.

At sea level, breathing atmospheric air, the dissolved P_{N_2} is 573 mm Hg in body fluids. Supersaturation occurs at an altitude of 7,500 feet (2,290 m). The lowest altitude for a sea level acclimatized individual to encounter decompression symptoms is reported to be 18,600 feet (5,600 m).[2] The ratio for P_{N_2} at sea level and at atmospheric pressure for the new altitude can be expressed:

$$R = P_{N_2}/P_B$$

where P_{N_2} is 573 mm Hg and P_B for the attained altitude is 375 mm Hg, and R is then 573/375 or 1.52. This approaches the critical ratio described by Haldane for gas to evolve forming bubbles from a supersaturated solution. More typically, decompression sickness becomes evident at altitudes of 25,000 ft (7,620 m) or higher.

When gas bubbles form in body tissue or fluids, they produce two effects. As the bubble has structure and can exert pressure it has a mechanical effect, which disrupts tissue and can block circulation. This can lead to pain, hypoxia, and infarction. The blood–bubble interface produces the second effect causing platelet aggregation and initiating a clotting cascade.

Bubble formation may originate in the lungs or bubbles may be transported into the pulmonary microcirculation from elsewhere. When this rare event occurs, approximately 2% of decompression sickness, a potentially fatal situation, exists. This syndrome is known as "chokes" due to the non-productive, coughing spasm generated by the microemboli formed by the evolved gas. In addition to the cough, there is substernal pain and dyspnea. This condition may rapidly progress to circulatory collapse unless immediate and rapid descent occurs. Once on the ground, the victim should be placed in a hyperbaric unit.

Flying after diving

When a pilot engages in recreational pressure diving, a new factor enters the equation in considering the risk of decompression sickness. When diving, there is an increase in ambient pressure due to the weight of the water. Pressure breathing delivers air including 78% nitrogen at increased pressure to the diver. Depending on the depth, duration, and repetitiveness of the dive, the nitrogen tissue saturation increases. Once returned to the surface, there will be some degree of tissue supersaturation. If proper diving discipline has been observed, there should be no adverse effect.

However, if the diver now ascends from sea level by driving into the mountains or in flying home after an enjoyable vacation, there is a further reduction in ambient pressure and decompression sickness may occur. Several crew members of a commercial flight experienced symptoms at a cabin altitude of only 7,000 ft (2,100 m) after scuba diving.[4]

To avoid decompression problems, the Federal Aviation Administration recommends these simple guidelines:[5]

When the cabin altitude does not exceed 8,000 ft:
    Wait 4 hours if nondecompression dive;
    Wait 24 hours if decompression dive.
When the cabin altitude will exceed 8,000 ft:
    Wait for at least 24 hours following any scuba diving.

Hyperbaric treatment

Any of the manifestations of decompression sickness including bends, chokes, neurologic effects, and circulatory collapse may benefit from hyperbaric treatment. Such therapy helps to mechanically compress the bubble and raises the partial pressure of inspired gases. This results in diminished bubble size, a positive nitrogen pressure gradient, improved tissue profusion, and reduced tissue hypoxia.[6]

Until the victim is in a hyperbaric unit on a prescribed treatment regimen, 100% O_2 should be administered and transport should occur at minimal altitude. If it is necessary to transfer the patient, time can be critical, thus air transport may be preferred. Helicopter transport is the form most commonly available, and the flight plan can usually maintain a minimal altitude. Increased altitude should be avoided because of the decreased partial pressure of the ambient atmosphere. On the occasion when a helicopter may not be available or the flight plan dictates another form of air transport, the military's C-130 Hercules Turbo prop transport is ideal. This aircraft has a pressurization system capable of maintaining or even surpassing the pressure of takeoff altitude, thus minimizing the potential of adverse effects of decreased atmospheric pressure.

ADDITIONAL PULMONARY CONCERNS IN THE AVIATION ENVIRONMENT

In addition to the problems already discussed with hypoxia and pressure changes impacting the pulmonary system, other stressors within the flight environment can present additional pulmonary challenges to the clinician.

Pulmonary atelectasis

A pilot who has been flying for several hours on 100% oxygen, which may at times be under increased pressure, has been exposed to the drying effects of a very low humidity gas. In response to this irritation, the bronchi may become swollen with increased fluid secretions . Oxygen is absorbed preferentially to other ambient gases, and as the pilot had been breathing 100% oxygen rapid absorption can be expected. This bronchial swelling can be sufficient to interfere with gas exchange and lead to alveolar O_2 trapping. Because of the rapid absorption of oxygen, mild blockage of the alveoli and minimal off gassing of water vapor and CO_2, alveolar collapse can occur. This pattern is relatively common with military pilots returning from extended high altitude missions who subsequently develop plate-like atelectasis principally in the upper lobes, compromising pulmonary function. Symptoms are principally shortness of breath, and cough. The condition is self-limited and resolves in 24 to 48 hours.

Acceleration-induced perfusion changes

During high-speed maneuvers, the pilot is frequently exposed to accelerative changes that are expressed as "G." Sustained acceleration will affect the lungs and alter the perfusion patterns. A large pressure gradient is noted to occur from the apex to the base when exposed to $+G_z$, stress, an acceleration vector pressing the pilot downward into the seat. This is the positive G most commonly experienced in aviation and is referred to as "eyeballs-down." During $+G_z$ acceleration, the plural pressure increases accentuating the expansion between the apex and the base of the lung. The distribution of pulmonary blood flow results from the balance of the hydrostatic forces and the driving pressure of the heart. Sustained acceleration results in both a posterior and caudal shift in blood flow. Various training maneuvers known as the M-1 and the L-1, used to increase "G" tolerance, increase intrathoracic pressure.

PULMONARY PROTECTION IN THE AEROSPACE ENVIRONMENT

With the development and advancement of aviation technology, engineering solutions were necessary to overcome man's frailty in performing at high altitude.

Oxygen systems

The type of aircraft, the number of persons requiring oxygen, the altitude ceiling of the aircraft, and the reliability of the aircraft pressurization system are factors that dictate the type of oxygen system on board. The most common oxygen supply system for aircraft is gaseous. Military specifications for oxygen require 99.5% purity by volume and no more than 0.005 ml/L of water vapor at 761 mm Hg and 20° C.[7] The water vapor content in the oxygen is important because at the very low ambient temperatures at altitude water vapor would freeze and thus compromise the oxygen supply.

Gaseous oxygen. The storage system may either be low pressure operating at 450 pounds per square inch (psi) or high pressure with an operational pressure of 1,800 to 2,200 psi. Given the same space the higher pressure system stores the larger space of oxygen.

Liquid oxygen. For the majority of aircraft in use today, the liquid oxygen (LOX) system is preferable to the gaseous system. A single 25-L container of liquid oxygen equals approximately 105 large bottles of high-pressure gaseous oxygen. In addition, LOX has a 3.5 : 1 weight advantage.

Solid chemical source. Many small private aircraft are not equipped with an onboard oxygen system. A self-contained unit can quickly be fitted into the aircraft and when oxygen is needed a sodium chlorate candle or other oxygen-producing chemical device can be activated. The system normally generates about 95% pure oxygen. The amount of available oxygen is dependent upon the size and burning rate of the chemical system.

Continuous generation systems. For over a decade, several oxygen supply systems have been under development that generate their own supply of oxygen and thus are not dependent on a separate logistics source.

The fuel cell common to space flight is an electrochemical concentration system for oxygen generation. An electrical current is supplied to a cell containing dry air. Oxygen is collected at the anode and hydrogen at the cathode. The hydrogen is then oxidized to water by combining with oxygen in the air flowing over the cathode. The oxygen is collected from the anode, concentrated, and stored.

A reversible absorption system uses fluomine to capture oxygen, then releases it. Compressed air is passed over an absorbate bed and then the pressure is reduced and oxygen is released. Two absorbate beds can be used alternately and provide a continuous oxygen supply.

A molecular sieve has been developed to selectively pass oxygen and absorb nitrogen. Pressurized air from the engine turbine is passed over a bed of crystalline aluminosilicate or zeolites and the atmosphere is divided into its major components. The oxygen-enriched portion is then supplied to the crew. A major disadvantage of this system is the potential for contamination as the system is only 95% effective in concentrating oxygen.

An oxygen-permeable membrane has been developed as a concentrator system. As air flows over the membrane, oxygen molecules dissolve on the surface. The opposite surface of the membrane is at a lower pressure pulling oxygen through because of the selective solubility coefficient of the membrane. The oxygen is collected and concentrated from the low-pressure side.

Delivery systems

Between the user and the oxygen supply is a delivery system. The systems in general are designed to meet air crew and passenger needs based on the cabin or flight deck environment at the time oxygen is required.

Continuous flow. This is the delivery system most common in civilian aircraft. It will provide protection up to a cabin altitude of 25,000 ft (7,620 m). It provides an emergency "get me down" capability to 30,000 ft (9,140 m). The regulator provides a continuous flow of 100% oxygen. This system is commonly used for emergency breathing by passengers in airline jet aircraft.

Dilutor demand. When the flight altitude exceeds 25,000 ft, the continuous flow oxygen system is unable to provide the necessary physiologic protection. Further, at lower altitudes 100% oxygen from the continuous flow system may not be required and the supply is not efficiently used. The demand system has an altitude sensor that meters the proper ambient air/oxygen mixture adjusted for altitude to meet physiologic requirements. Once 35,000 ft (10,360 m) is attained, the system provides 100% oxygen.

Positive pressure. At an altitude above 40,000 ft (12,200 m), 100% oxygen can no longer provide physiologically adequate oxygen blood levels. The regulator and mask are designed to provide oxygen at positve pressure to the lungs. This reverses the normal breathing mechanism as the lungs fill with relaxation and require forced exhalation. Pressures of up to 100 mm Hg can be delivered without mask-fit leakage. However, the maximum breathing pressure tolerated using only a mask is approximately 30 mm Hg. To maintain an alveolar oxygen tension of 60 mm Hg, the positive pressure system has a 45,000 ft (17,700 m) altitude limitation. If some degree of hypoxia can be tolerated then cabin altitudes of 50,000 ft (15,200 m) can be permitted for a limited time. With a 100% oxygen pressure of 30 mm Hg at this altitude, there is an absolute lung pressure of 117 mm Hg and an alveolar oxygen partial pressure of 45 mm Hg. Altitude protection under these circumstances is measured in minutes, and thus the oxygen delivery system is only satisfactory for emergency "get me down" when cabin pressure is lost.

Without support for the chest wall, the lungs will rupture if inflated to 40 to 50 mm Hg. At 40 mm Hg, the expiratory reserve volume is greatly increased and forced expiration becomes a tiring process. Positive pressure breathing increases minute ventilation with a fall in arterial partial pressure of CO_2. The increased interthoracic pressure

alters the pressure in the vascular system with blood volume displacement to the limbs, reduced venus return, a fall in cardiac output, and possible pressure breathing syncope.

The military aerospace medical community has designed a chest counterpressure device that allows positive pressure of up to 70 mm Hg. Provided all protection systems are working as designed, including regulator, mask, chest counterpressure vests, and "G" suit to prevent vascular pooling, an altitude of 60,000 ft can be tolerated for a few minutes.

PRESSURE PROTECTION
Cabin and cockpit pressurization

Small private aircraft may have a maximum altitude capability or ceiling up to 25,000 ft (7,620 m) without a pressurized cabin.[8] However, most aircraft routinely flying above 15,000 ft (4,570 m) are pressurized. Certainly this applies to commercial aircraft. Pressurization provides patient comfort and protects from hypoxia without the use of augmented oxygen systems. Pressurization is controlled by an isobaric differential system. The take off ambient pressure is maintained in the cabin until a preset altitude is reached. Pressure differentiation between cabin pressure and outside altitude pressure determines the activation of the pressure system. As the aircraft continues to climb, the system maintains the pressure differential. In most cases, the cabin altitude on commercial jet aircraft rarely exceeds 8,000 ft (2,430 m) or 545 mm Hg.

Individual pressure protection

For an aviator to reach altitudes safely beyond that allowed by partial pressure breathing, even with counterpressure, the individual must have some form of total body protection. The partial-pressure suit is form-fitted with external bladders or capstans. As these capstans are inflated, the increased pressure is transferred to the garment creating a counterpressure. The head is covered by a pressure helmet as the face mask can no longer provide the necessary pressure without leaking. This type of pressure protection suit was used with the U-2 aircraft high-altitude flights.

The full pressure suit or spacesuit provides the aviator or astronaut a microenvironment. The entire body is surrounded in a pressurized gas envelope. A typical suit pressure is 3.5 psi or 180 mm Hg.

Space cabins are designed as completely closed environments. Initially, in the United States, the cabin was designed to operate at a lower pressure, but with an oxygen atmosphere. Modern spacecraft, such as the space shuttle, have a shirt sleeve mixed gas, 760 mm pressure environment. Because it is a closed system, the environmental control system must maintain humidity, CO_2, and trace contaminates at an acceptable level while filtering the air and maintaining a balance between nitrogen and oxygen.

REGULATIONS

In aerospace operations, regulations, directives, orders, and policies direct most activities whether originating from the Federal Aviation Administration, Department of Defense, or the National Aeronautics and Space Administration. These directives touch pulmonology in two areas: medical qualifications of pilots and astronauts and maintenance of physiologic function under the stresses of flight.

Medical qualifications

Minimal medical standards have been established to qualify as a pilot. These standards are established to maintain flying safety. Respiratory disease that interferes with oxygen exchange may be incompatible with the lower oxygen partial pressure of altitude. Further, medications that are used to control respiratory system disease may be incompatible with alertness, cognition, and reflex response required in flight.

Diseases of concern include asthma, chronic obstructive pulmonary disease, sarcoidosis, pulmonary bullae, and lung cancer. There are few absolute prohibitions regarding respiratory disease and flight. Functional testing is able to demonstrate that a pilot with early sarcoidosis may be able to continue flying. An individual who has survived a spontaneous pneumothorax may be able to demonstrate in a low-pressure (altitude) chamber with chest x-ray that there are no bullae, and thus minimal risk for return to flight. A collaboration between the pulmonologist and the aerospace medical specialist represents the best case for the pilot seeking administrative review of a medical disqualification.

Altitude protection

The Federal Aviation Administration regulations prescribe when oxygen will be available to passengers and crew.

When flying at cabin altitudes between 12,500 ft and 14,000 ft for greater than 30 minutes at least one pilot will use oxygen. Both altitude and time are factors in applying this rule. Regardless of flight duration, one pilot will use oxygen when flying above 14,000 ft. Once cabin altitude exceeds 15,000 ft all persons, crew and passengers, must use oxygen. The rules are most applicable for unpressurized aircraft.

For pressurized aircraft, the rule addresses the availability of oxygen and is based on the possibility of sudden loss of cabin pressurization. Rather than addressing the cabin altitude, the rule applies to the flight level or ambient outside altitude.

When flying above 25,000 ft, sufficient oxygen must be available to all for 10 minutes. The rules as described above for cabin altitude of 12,500 to 15,000 ft apply. Above 35,000 ft, if there is only one pilot, he or she will wear and use an oxygen mask. If two pilots are available on the flight deck, each must have available a quick-donning mask up to 41,000 ft. The mask need not be worn on the face.

Perhaps more than any other occupation, aerospace is sensitive to pulmonary physiology and respiratory disease. Although the occupation is rarely the source of pulmonary pathology, it is dependent on worker selection and health maintenance.

REFERENCES

1. Strughold H: Atmospheric space equivalence, *J Aviat Med* 25:420, 1952.
2. Federal Aviation Administration. *Aviat Safety J* 2(2):6-8, 1992.
3. Harding RM: Oxygen equipment and pressure clothing. In Erasting J and King P, editors: *Aviat Medicine*, 2nd ed., pp 72-111. London, 1988, Butterworths.
4. Sheffield MS: Flying after diving guidelines: a review, *Aviat Space Environ Med* 61:1130-1138, 1990.
5. Federal Aviation Administration. Decompression sickness after scuba diving. In *Airman's information manual*, Washington, D.C., 1988, US Government Printing Office.
6. Grim PS, Gottliev LJ, Boddie A, and Batson E: Hyperbaric oxygen therapy, *JAMA* 263:2216-2220, 1990.
7. Heinbach RD and Sheffield JP: Protection in the pressure environment. In DeHart RL, editor: *Fundamentals of aerospace medicine*, pp 110-131, Philadelphia, 1985, Lea & Febiger.
8. Black WR and DeHart RL: Decompression sickness: an increasing risk for the private pilot, *Aviat Space Environ Med* 63:200-203, 1992.

Environmental Health Effects

JOHN R. BALMES

This section covers several major categories of environmental exposures that can cause or contribute to respiratory tract illness. The respiratory effects of exposure to environmental tobacco smoke, in children as well as adults, are discussed in Chapter 47. Despite the considerable strides that have been made to reduce the levels of outdoor air pollutants in North America and Europe, these pollutants remain a significant source of respiratory morbidity and even mortality. Chapter 49 provides a concise overview of the respiratory health effects associated with the primary outdoor air pollutants. As the outdoor air quality has improved in much of the developed world and with the introduction of energy-efficient buildings that tend to recirculate air, increased attention has been directed toward the indoor environment. By now, most pulmonary and occupational and environmental medicine physicians have encountered individual patients or clusters of workers in nonindustrial settings who attribute respiratory and other symptoms to the indoor air quality of their homes or workplaces. Chapter 48 distills the experience of two experts in this often vexing but important area. Unfortunately, individuals who are exposed to occupational and environmental toxins often also smoke tobacco products. Chapter 50 discusses the potential for interactive effects of toxic exposures and smoking on the respiratory tract.

Chapter 47

ENVIRONMENTAL TOBACCO SMOKE

John P. Hanrahan
Scott T. Weiss

"Youk'n hide the fier, but w'at you gwine do wid de smoke?" Uncle Remus "plantation proverbs"

JOEL CHANDLER HARRIS

Long accepted by nonsmokers as an unavoidable nuisance or annoyance, exposure to environmental tobacco smoke (ETS) in the indoor environment, or "passive smoking," has come under extensive public health scrutiny in the past decades. Measures to limit exposure to ETS in public indoor environments has evolved from first ignoring its presence, to then segregating smokers from nonsmokers, and most recently to banning smoking entirely in many, if not most, public indoor environments. The impetus for this change derives from accumulating evidence that the same serious adverse health effects caused by active cigarette smoking are also associated with passive smoking, albeit with lower frequency or more protracted exposure. In particular, passive smoking exposure is now known to increase risk of lung cancer and coronary heart disease among adult nonsmokers and is associated with a variety of respiratory conditions, particularly in young children.

Three publications serve as landmark summaries of the effects of ETS on human health. In 1986, the U.S. Surgeon General's Report[1] and a report of the National Research Council[2] both comprehensively detailed the emerging knowledge of the health risks of passive smoking. In 1992, the Environmental Protection Agency (EPA) released an extensive report that causally linked passive smoking with lung cancer and classified ETS as a Group A carcinogen, a category restricted for substances for which extensive and compelling evidence exists linking exposure to human cancer.[3] The same document compiled and summarized reports examining the association of ETS with nonmalignant respiratory illnesses. The report concluded that ETS was a substantial contributor to acute respiratory illnesses, chronic respiratory symptoms, and exacerbations of asthma. The report further concluded the association between ETS and respiratory morbidity was particularly strong for infants and young children.

In this chapter, the authors have attempted to summarize salient points related to the adverse health effects of ETS exposure in the indoor environment. Wherever possible, we have highlighted issues that remain unresolved or controversies related to ETS exposure.

ETS COMPOSITION AND MEASURES OF EXPOSURE

ETS composition

There are in excess of 4000 compounds[4,5] that comprise environmental tobacco smoke, present in both particulate[6] and vapor phases.[7] Many of these constituents are known carcinogens or mitogens, whereas the impact of many other chemical compounds present in ETS on human health is unknown. ETS is comprised of a mix of sidestream (SS) smoke, the products emitted from the burning end of the cigarette between puffs, and exhaled mainstream (MS) smoke, the product of combustion first inhaled into the smoker's lung and then exhaled. The composition of MS and SS smoke is roughly similar in the number of compounds they contain, but they can differ substantially in the concentration of compounds or other physical or chemical properties. Sidestream smoke is generated at lower temperatures, is slightly more alkaline, and has a smaller particle size distribution than mainstream smoke.[4,7] Known human mutagens and carcinogens in general are present in higher concentrations in SS than in MS, sometimes by a factor of 10 or more. Among the classes of toxic compounds present in SS are nitrosamines, polycyclic aromatic hydrocarbons, formaldehyde, toluene, and benzene derivatives.[2-4] The composition of sidestream smoke does not vary substantially by brand, a situation that is quite different for mainstream smoke, owing to differences in filters from one brand to the next.

Despite its relatively stable composition of toxic constituents, the effective exposure dose of toxins is complicated and impacted by a number of factors, including the size and ventilation of the room in which the exposure takes place, number of cigarettes burning within the room, and variations in absorbent surfaces within the room. Despite differences in concentration of ETS from one indoor environment to the next, measurable quantities of the components of sidestream smoke are usually found in indoor environments, frequently in concentrations substantially higher than background.[1] Therefore, it is a reasonable inference that persons spending time in indoor environments where ETS is present have exposure to the same substances present in mainstream smoke. Since low-level active smoking of even several cigarettes per day increases the risk of most respiratory outcomes associated with smoking, the possibility of an augmented risk of such outcomes with ETS exposure is biologically plausible.

ETS exposure assessment

There are numerous difficulties in identifying valid instruments to assess an individual's exposure to ETS. First, for all the adverse health outcomes associated with ETS, the biologically relevant compound (or compounds) from the more than 4000 chemical constituents of ETS is unknown. Second, as with most exposure–response relationships, variability in exposure is introduced by differences in time spent indoors and other features of behavior, physical properties of the indoor environment, and susceptibility differences from one individual to the next. Most exposure assessment is based either on subjective reporting of cumulative exposure or objective measurements of exposure at one point in time or over a brief interval.

Most epidemiologic studies of ETS and health have utilized subjective exposure assessment by questionnaire. A minority have employed measurement of a constituent of ETS in an indoor environment or biologic fluid. In these latter studies, a surrogate exposure marker is selected because it is known to be present in ETS and the technical ability to measure it exists at relatively low cost. Although this yields a quantitative exposure estimate, this method cannot characterize cumulative exposure nor can it estimate dose during potentially critical time windows in the past, where host susceptibility factors (e.g., periods of allergic illness, growth) may make the exposures most critical. In the sections that follow, the authors summarize the advantages and disadvantages of the three most wisely used methods of ETS exposure assessment.

Questionnaire. Questionnaires have been and remain the most frequent exposure assessment tool in epidemiologic studies of ETS and human health. Questionnaire exposure assessment affords several distinct advantages over other methods.[8] First, they are inexpensive, simple to administer, and require no measuring devices or technical expertise. Second, they are, at present, the only assessment tool that can estimate the timing, duration, and intensity of past exposures. Most questionnaires are developed individually for specific studies. As such, few have been externally validated. Several studies have verified that the questionnaire-reported magnitude of ETS exposure is correlated with cotinine, a metabolite of nicotine measured in biologic fluids.[8-11] Most studies, however, show wide variability of levels of nicotine by-products within questionnaire-derived exposure categories.

The assessment of ETS exposure by questionnaire has two compelling advantages over other assessment methods. First, self-reporting better accounts for biologically relevant exposures than measurement of a single ETS constituent. Second, the impressive and consistent data collected to date in many epidemiologic studies linking ETS to human outcomes used questionnaires as the sole exposure measurement tool. Optimal exposure assessment will probably involve both a questionnaire assessment of overall and past exposure and a biomarker or environmental sampling measure that better quantitates recent exposure and allows identification of persons with unreported active smoking.

Environmental sampling. Environmental sampling in an indoor environment is another method that has been employed in studies of ETS health effects. Although many of the components of ETS can be measured in the indoor environment,[3] vapor phase nicotine and respirable suspended particulates (RSP) have been the two environmental sampling measures most widely used to date in ETS exposure assessment. Both have been demonstrated to be associated with questionnaire reports of ETS exposure.[4,7,12,13] Nicotine has the advantage of being a specific constituent of ETS. RSP can be present in the indoor environment from non-ETS sources. However, several compounds of known direct human health concerns have concentrations in ETS that are directly correlated with RSP levels.[3,4,13] Two strategies have been employed using environmental sampling to measure ETS exposure. The first is fixed or stationary sampling in an indoor environment where exposure is known to occur. This exposure assessment method is frequently combined with questionnaire assessment of time–activity patterns to estimate cumulative exposure in this environment over an extended time period. The second environmental sampling strategy involves the use of personal monitors.[14-17] Passive personal exposure devices such as nicotine dosimeters have been recently developed and demonstrated to be valid exposure measures.[17] These have the advantage of summating exposure over multiple microenvironments for an individual. Active personal air sampling devices have also been used but are not well suited to large-scale epidemiologic studies.

Biomarkers. Biomarkers of exposure are chemical substances that are measurable in human biologic tissue or fluid that both verify that an exposure has taken place and provides a quantitative estimate of the extent of exposure. An ideal biomarker for ETS exposure would have a relatively long half-life in biologic tissue, be easily measured at relatively low expense, be specific for tobacco smoke, and have concentrations both in ETS and in human tissues or fluids in concentrations that are strongly associated with the compound(s) adversely affecting human health.

In theory, biomarkers offer some distinctive advantage over questionnaire or environmental sampling measures of exposure assessment. First, they are the only exposure methodology that provides biologic proof of exposure, as well as an index of an individual's summated exposure over multiple microenvironments. They are also the only exposure methodology that reliably identifies persons who are covert active smokers, an important potential confounder.

Unfortunately, there is no ideal single biomarker available to assess ETS exposure. Alveolar carbon monoxide concentrations or carboxyhemoglobin and thiocyanate levels have been useful in identifying active smokers[18] but are either not specific for tobacco smoke or may not be sensitive enough to identify passive exposure. One protein adduct, the 4-aminobiphenyl adduct of hemoglobin, is specific for tobacco exposure and has a long half-life, a property offering distinct advantage over other biomarkers.[19] However, it has not yet been used in any large study of health outcomes related to ETS.

The biomarkers that have gained most widespread use and acceptance in studies of ETS are nicotine and especially its metabolite cotinine. These have been measured in most biologic fluids including blood, urine, and saliva, and have been shown in a number of studies to correlate with subjective estimates of ETS exposure.[9-11,20,21] The elimination half-life of cotinine is between 20 and 37 hours,[3] making it a useful marker of exposure over a period of 1 to 2 days. The presence of nicotine in some foods, such as tomatoes, eggplant, and tea, challenges the specificity of this marker for ETS,[22] although in all likelihood levels for most individuals are predominantly determined by tobacco exposure. Cotinine also affords a good ability to discriminate active smoking from passive exposure. Nonetheless, there is considerable variability of cotinine levels due to individual differences in uptake, metabolism, and elimination of nicotine. Like all other biomarkers, direct links between nicotine or cotinine and human health outcomes are not known, emphasizing its probable role as a surrogate marker for meaningful biological exposures.

Summary. Exposure assessment in studies of health effects of ETS is difficult and complicated by lack of knowledge of the specific compounds in ETS responsible for adverse health outcomes. Optimal exposure assessment should attempt to estimate long-term exposure, in addition to an objective quantitative estimate of recent exposure. Optimally, exposure estimation in studies of health outcomes associated with long-term ETS exposure will require both a subjective estimation of such exposure solicited by questionnaire and an objective quantitative measure of recent exposure, as provided by cotinine or another biomarker. This combined approach can allow characterization of exposure–response relationships for ETS and allow for identification of misreported active smoking.

ETS AND LUNG CANCER

The biologic plausibility of ETS increasing risk of lung cancer was suggested by two features of the epidemiologic association of lung cancer with active smoking. First, there appears to be no safe or threshold level of active smoking; smoking as little as one or two cigarettes a day confers increased risk. Second, as indicated previously, the chemical and physical composition of sidestream smoke contains the same compounds as mainstream smoke, frequently in higher concentrations.

Verification of an increased risk of lung cancer in nonsmokers exposed to ETS first came in the early 1980s. Two studies, one a large prospective study of Japanese women[23] and the second a case-control design among Greek women,[24] suggested that nonsmoking women married to smokers had a 40% to twofold excess risk of lung cancer over female nonsmokers whose spouses did not smoke. These two reports engendered a storm of controversy and spawned more than 30 additional studies examining this issue in the 12 years subsequent to their publication.

A number of methodologic issues are important in considering epidemiologic studies of ETS and lung cancer. The vast majority of studies are case control in their design, with exposure assessment occurring after the development of disease. This poses some specific difficulties in obtaining reliable exposure information, as case persons with lung cancer have often expired at the time exposure information is collected, necessitating that this be obtained from spouses or other survivors with knowledge of the case person's exposure status. Some, but not all, studies have attempted to control this potential source of information bias by collecting exposure information from surrogates or proxies in a comparable number of cases and controls. Another potential source of confounding for these studies could be introduced by misreporting of active smoking, either at the time of diagnosis or in the past by case patients. Because active or exsmokers are more likely to have spouses who smoke, misclassified current or former smokers would falsely elevate risk attributable to ETS. The vast majority of studies also classify exposure based simply on the dichotomy of whether a spouse or household member smokes, frequently with an estimate of the spouses' duration of smoking and the number of cigarettes smoked per day. These are crude exposure estimates, as differences in home size, ventilation, and amount of time spent in the home could all affect actual biologic dose.

Studies also differ substantially in outcome ascertainment. Most studies do not distinguish among cell types of lung cancer, and some accept diagnoses based on radiographic, clinical, or other criteria without histologic confirmation. Finally, studies from different geographic areas or that include persons of different ethnic or economic backgrounds could have additional features, such as the particulars of the indoor environment, diet, or genetic predisposition that could affect the magnitude of risk.

Despite these potential pitfalls, the collective data obtained from the vast majority of the studies examining this issue over the past decade have yielded both consistent and compelling evidence that prolonged ETS exposure in the home environment increases the risk of lung cancer in nonsmokers. Table 47-1 lists 15 studies that have examined household ETS exposure and lung cancer risks among nonsmoking women.[23-36] These were selected as the most convincing studies based on their methodologic rigor or the number of cases that they contained or both. A more comprehensive summary of a larger number of studies is included in the 1992 Environmental Protection Agency (EPA) report.[3] These studies support a 20% to 50% overall excess risk of lung cancer occurrence in nonsmoking women with smoking spouses when compared with women whose husbands do not smoke. The excess risk may be as high as twofold or greater among nonsmoking women with the highest exposure levels. The EPA report estimates that this degree of increased risk translates to approximately 3000 cases of lung cancer in nonsmokers per year in the United States caused by ETS exposure in the home.[3]

Evidence of the causal association between ETS exposure in the home and lung cancer is provided by the consistency of the risk estimates in different studies, as well as the fact that in many of these studies an exposure–response relationship is evident between the degree of household exposure and the magnitude of excess risk. Elevated risks are found in different cultures and in disparate geographic localities. It is unlikely that unmeasured or unexplained confounding is responsible for this result.

There remain, nonetheless, many issues related to risk of lung cancer from ETS that require further clarification. Among these are whether a certain threshold dose must be reached to augment risk, the relative importance of intensity of exposure versus the duration of exposure, and

Table 47-1. Passive smoking and lung cancer in adult nonsmokers

Reference	Country	Design	Cases/controls	Exposure source	Overall estimated relative risk		Dose-response	Relative risk—highest exposure group	
Hirayama (1981)[23]	Japan	Cohort	174 (91,540)	Spouse	1.38	(1.03, 1.87)	Yes	1.93	(≥20 cg/day)
Trichopoulos et al. (1981, 1983)[24,26]	Greece	CC	40/149	Spouse	2.08	(1.31, 3.29)	Yes	2.55	(≥21 cg/day)
Garfinkel (1981)[25]	U.S.	Cohort	153 (176,739)	Spouse	1.17	(0.85, 1.61)	No	1.1	(≥20 cg/day)
Correa et al. (1983)[27]	U.S.	CC	22/133	Spouse	2.07	(0.94, 4.52)	Yes	3.5	(≥41 pk yr.)
Garfinkel et al. (1985)[28]	U.S.	CC	134/402	Spouse	1.31	(0.93, 1.85)	Yes	2.1	(≥21 cg/day)
Koo et al. (1987)[29]	Hong Kong	CC	86/136	Spouse	1.55	(0.98, 2.44)	No	1.2	(>20 cg/day)
Lam et al. (1987)[30]	Hong Kong	CC	199/335	Spouse	1.65	(1.21, 2.21)	No	2.1	(≥20 cg/day)
Pershagen et al. (1987)[124]	Sweden	CC	67/368	Spouse	1.2	(0.7, 2.1)	Yes	3.2	(≥16 cg/day)
Hole et al. (1989)[31]	U.K.	Cohort	6 (1784)	All household	1.99	(0.24, 16.7)	Yes	1.8	(≥15 cg/day)
Kalandidi et al. (1990)[32]	Greece	CC	90/116	Spouse	1.92	(1.13, 3.23)	Yes	1.9	(≥40 yr.)
Janerich et al. (1990)[33]	U.S.	CC	191/191	Spouse	0.86	(0.57, 1.29)	Yes	1.1	(≥50 pk yr.)
Fontham et al. (1991)[34]	U.S.	CC	420/780	Spouse	1.29	(1.03, 1.62)	Yes	1.33	(≥80 pk yr.)
Stockwell et al. (1991)[35]	U.S.	CC	210/301	All household	1.6	(0.8, 3.0)	Yes	2.4	(≥40 pk yr.)
Brownson et al. (1992)[36]	U.S.	CC	431/1166	All household	1.1	(0.8, 1.3)	No	1.3	(≥40 pk yr.)

CC, Case control.

whether a critical time window of exposure is associated with increased risk. At least one study[33] found that increased risk of lung cancer in nonsmoking adult women was associated with high ETS exposure levels during childhood and adolescence. Correa et al.[27] also found increased risk among nonsmokers whose mothers smoked during childhood, whereas no risk elevation occurred among persons whose fathers smoked. A more recent study[36] among 421 nonsmoking women with lung cancer identified in a tumor registry found no association with parental smoking in childhood. Thus, the possible importance of early childhood ETS exposure and/or prenatal maternal smoking in the later development of lung cancer among nonsmokers remains open to question.

Moreover, it is likely that differences in family history or genetic predisposition to lung disease, diet, occupational exposure, and other indoor exposures such as products of combustion from cooking fuels comprise important risk modifiers for ETS and lung cancer. A recent study from China bears on this last point. Liu et al.[37] conducted a case-control comparison of 326 incident cases of lung cancer, of whom 38 were nonsmoking women. In addition to verifying an increased risk among women with high levels of ETS exposure at home, the study also found that living in a dwelling without a separate kitchen and a dwelling with poor air circulation was associated with increased risk, especially for women. This study underscores the probable importance of many features of the indoor environment, including the adequacy of ventilation, in determining actual risk posed to nonsmokers occupying the same dwelling with smokers.

ETS AND CANCERS OTHER THAN LUNG

In general, there are sparse data available examining the risk posed by ETS on the development of neoplasms other than lung cancer. On theoretic grounds, cancer sites of greatest interest are those known to be associated with active smoking, such as cancers of the sinuses or oral pharynx, larynx, and esophagus, or cancers with high incidence and mortality, such as breast cancer, where even small increments in risk could translate to high population attributable risks for ETS exposure. In the same cohort of Japanese women cited previously, Hirayama reported an increased relative risk of developing both brain and nasal sinus cancer in nonsmoking women who lived with smoking spouses.[23] There appear to be dose–response relationships for both sites, odds ratios ranging from 1.7 to 2.6 for nasal cancer and 3.0 to 4.3 for brain neoplasms in the low to high exposure strata. There has been speculation about the role of passive smoking as an initiator of breast cancer in women, based on temporal time trend associations of cigarette consumption with breast cancer incidence.[38] However, there is no body of convincing data linking passive smoking exposure to any nonrespiratory cancer that has been developed to date.

ETS AND HEART DISEASE

In the last decade, an emerging body of evidence has suggested that household exposure to ETS is associated with augmented risk of death from ischemic heart disease. As is the case with exposure to ETS and lung cancer, the outcome examined in a majority of the studies is death from ischemic heart disease among nonsmoking persons whose spouse smokes. Risk ratios in these investigations generally range between a 20% and twofold excess risk of cardiac death in ETS-exposed nonsmokers (Table 47-2).[31,39-46] This epidemiologic relationship is supported by a positive exposure–response association in studies where this has been examined. As was the case with lung cancer and ETS, exposure over a prolonged period of years or even in childhood may be associated with increased risk.

The pathophysiologic mechanism by which ETS exposure accelerates atherogenesis and risk of cardiac death has been speculated to involve a number of pathways. Passive smoking exposure elevates carboxyhemoglobin levels, which in turn has been associated with decreased exercise performance in both healthy persons and persons with ischemic heart disease.[46] Time on a treadmill until onset of angina also decreases with increasing concentrations of carboxyhemoglobin,[47] as does the frequency of arrhythmias during exercise.[48] ETS has also been proposed to damage the vascular endothelium,[46] to lower levels of high-density lipoprotein cholesterol, and to increase levels of fibrinogen, which may be associated with fibrinogenesis.[41]

Although both the consistency of increased risk of coronary heart disease death in ETS-exposed nonsmokers and the dose–response relationships observed in these studies support a casual role for ETS, the possibility remains that some part of the observed increased risk may be due to unexplained or uncontrolled confounding. For example, nonsmokers with smoking spouses may have more atherogenic diets or more sedentary lifestyles than households where all members are nonsmokers, both of which are risk factors for ischemic cardiac events. However, it is unlikely that these confounders explain all of the increased risk demonstrated in studies to date. Even with risk ratios as low as 1.2, the American Heart Association[49] estimates that the excess cardiac mortality in the United States attributable to household ETS exposure is likely to be between 30,000 and 40,000 deaths per year. If correct, this means that ETS-related cardiac death exceeds those of lung cancer by an order of magnitude, making it a much more important public health issue than deaths due to respiratory neoplasms.

ETS AND RESPIRATORY CONDITIONS IN CHILDREN

From the standpoint of overall morbidity, the largest impact of ETS exposure is undoubtedly attributable to the increased frequency and severity of respiratory illnesses and respiratory symptoms caused in children, particularly young children and infants. The 1992 report of the EPA estimated

Table 47–2. Passive smoking and ischemic heart disease: risk among nonsmokers living with smokers

Reference	Country	Design	Outcome	Cases/controls	Exposure source		Relative risk (95% CI)		Dose-response
Hirayama (1984)[39]	Japan	Cohort (women)	Death	494 (91,540)	Spouse		1.2	(0.9-1.4)	Yes
Garland et al. (1985)[40]	U.S.	Cohort (women)	Death	19 (695)	Spouse		2.3	Husband current smoker	NR
							3.0	Husband former smoker	
Svendsen et al. (1987)[41]	U.S.	Cohort (men)	Death	18 (1245)	Spouse		2.1	(0.7-6.5)	Yes
			Coronary event	90 (1245)			1.5	(0.9-2.5)	Yes
Lee et al. (1986)[42]	U.K.	CC	Death	48/182	Spouse	Men	1.2		No
						Women	0.9		No
Helsing et al. (1988)[43]	U.S.	Cohort	Death		Household	Men	1.3	(1.1-1.6)	No
			Men	370 (3454)		Women	1.2	(1.1-1.4)	No
			Women	988 (12,345)					
Hole et al. (1989)[31]	Scotland	Cohort	Death	84 (2455)	Household		2.0	(1.2-3.4)	Yes
Humble et al. (1990)[44]	U.S.	Cohort (women)	Death	76 (513)	Household		1.6	(1.0-2.6)	Yes
Dobson et al. (1991)[45]	Australia	CC	Death		Household	Men	0.97	(0.5-1.9)	NR
			Men	183/293		Women	2.46	(1.5-4.1)	
			Women	160/532					

CC, Case-control; *NR,* not recorded.

that between 150,000 and 300,000 cases per year of lower respiratory illnesses were caused by household exposure to ETS in the United States, resulting in 7500 to 15,000 hospitalizations.[3] ETS was also judged to play a significant role in exacerbations of wheezing in asthmatic children and was an important independent risk factor in the development of asthma in childhood. Taken together, lower respiratory infections and asthma are by far the leading cause of hospitalization for children and are responsible for several billion dollars in annual costs.

In the past 20 years, more than 50 studies have examined the impact of household ETS exposure on acute respiratory illness, chronic respiratory symptoms, and exacerbations of asthma in children. In general, these reports have supported an increased risk of each of these outcomes in children exposed to ETS in the home, particularly children whose mothers smoke. A majority of reports have suggested that susceptibility for children is greatest in infancy and early childhood.

Several factors may explain the heightened risk of respiratory illness associated with ETS exposure in younger children. These include (1) more intense exposures in infancy due to closer proximity with mothers, (2) residual effects of maternal smoking during pregnancy, (3) augmented susceptibility of a rapidly growing respiratory system in infancy, (4) smaller airway geometry in infants, making respiratory irritants or insults to the respiratory epithelium more critical, and (5) dysmaturity in the immunologic and/or other systems, making the airway response to ETS and other inhaled stimulants qualitatively different during early life.

The consistency of findings from different populations and widely separate geographic locales of an increased risk of ETS-associated respiratory illness in the younger children and infants, coupled with the findings from most studies that a maternal source of ETS exposure is the most influential, has led to speculation that in utero exposure of infants to active maternal smoking during pregnancy may explain a portion of the excess respiratory morbidity observed in young children who are exposed to maternal ETS. The role of active smoking by mothers during pregnancy and mechanisms by which it may impact respiratory illness outcomes independent of ETS are also examined in this section.

The results of studies that have chronicled the risks of respiratory illness and symptoms in ETS-exposed children, once again, have been summarized in the reports of the Surgeon General,[1] National Research Council,[2] and, most recently, the EPA.[3] In the following sections and tables, the authors will summarize the evidence implicating ETS in these respiratory outcomes, estimate the magnitude of the excess risk attributable to passive smoking, and describe other factors that may be important in modifying or influencing this risk.

ETS and acute respiratory illness in children

There is now strong and consistent evidence that children residing in households with smokers have an increased risk of acute respiratory illnesses in childhood. Once again, pertinent features of the larger or more recent studies addressing this issue are listed in Table 47-3.[50-63] In general, associations of household ETS exposure with acute respi-

Table 47-3. Passive smoking and acute respiratory illness in children

Reference	Number of subjects and country	Age (yr)	Design	Exposure assessment	Outcome	Result	ETS source
Harlap and Davies (1974)[50]	10,672 Israel	0-1	L	Q	Resp. hosp.	RR 1.4	M only
Leeder et al. (1976)[51]	2149 England	0-1	L	Q	Bronchitis and pneumonia	RR 2.0 (DR)	Parents
Fergusson et al. (1981)[52]	1265 New Zealand	0-3	L	Q	Bronchitis and pneumonia	RR 2.04 (DR)	M only
Schenker et al. (1983)[53]	4071 U.S.	5-14	X-CC	Q	Resp. illness in last year and ages 0-2	DR based on number of smoking parents	M > F
Ware et al. (1984)[55]	8528 U.S.	5-8	Retrospective cohort	Q	Respiratory illness ages 0-2	OR 1.0-2.7 (DR)	M only
Fergusson et al. (1985)[54]	1265 New Zealand	0-3	L	Q	Bronchitis and pneumonia	RR 2.04 (DR)	M only
McConnochie et al. (1986)[56]	53 U.S.	0-2	CC	Q	Bronchitis	OR 2.4 (1.2, 4.8)	M only
Chen et al. (1986)[57]	1058 China	0-1.5	Retrospective cohort	Q	Resp. hosp.	1-9 cig/day OR 1.2 > 9 cig/day OR 1.9	Family
Ogston et al. (1987)[58]	1565 New Zealand	0-1	L	Q	URI/LRI	OR 1.4 (1.1-2.0) 1.8 (1.3-3.6)	F M
Taylor and Wadsworth (1987)[59]	12,743 England	0-5	Retrospective cohort	Q	Hosp. for LRI	≤12 mo: RR 2.2 12-31 mo: RR 1.6	M only
Chen et al. (1988)[60]	2227 China	0-1.5	Retrospective cohort	Q	Resp. hosp.	0-6 mo OR 3.0 7-18 mo OR 1.8	Family
Woodward et al. (1990)[61]	2125 Australia	1.5-3	CC - Retrospective cohort	Q - first year of life	Increase resp. sx. score	OR 2.0 (1.3, 3.4)	M
Wright et al. (1991)[62]	847 U.S.	0-1	L	Q	LRI	OR 1.5 (1.1-2.2) first 6 months only	M only
Reese et al. (1992)[63]	471 Australia	0-1.5	X-CC	Urine cotinine	Hospital for bronchiolitis vs. other diagnoses	Cotinine sign. higher in infants with bronchiolitis	All

CC, Case control; *DR,* dose-response; *F,* female; *L,* longitudinal; *LRI,* lower respiratory illness; *M,* male; *OR,* odds ratio; *Q,* questionnaire; *RR,* relative risk; *URI,* upper respiratory illness; *X,* cross-sectional.

ratory infants in children are strongest for young infants, especially those less than 1 year of age. Most of the studies that have examined the source of ETS in the home have found that smoking by the child's mother is most closely aligned with increases in a child's respiratory illness risk. In general, smoking by fathers or other household members has been found to pose lower or no additional increased risk when smoking by mothers is taken into account. Nonetheless, the studies of Chen et al.,[57,60] which examine respiratory hospitalization for infants 18 months of age or younger in Shanghai, China, indicate that any source of household ETS exposure can be associated with increased risk. These investigators report that among more than 3000 infants studied, those from smoking households have a 20% to 300% increased risk of hospitalization for a respiratory illness. This increased risk was greatest for infants less than 6 months of age. Of interest, the authors report that none of the more than 3000 infants had smoking mothers, and po-

tentially important confounders or modifiers such as infant gender, birth weight, and infant feeding practices were accounted for in the analysis. These studies in particular suggest that the effects of ETS from nonmaternal sources may have the same detrimental effects as has been shown for maternal smoking. However, the nonsmoking status of mothers in these and most other studies was not verified by objective exposure assessment.

Wright and colleagues[62] found a 50% increase in the incidence of lower respiratory illness in the first 6 months of life among infants with smoking mothers taken from a cohort of 840 infants enrolled at birth in Tucson, Arizona. These same researchers found no effect of paternal smoking in this age range nor any increased risk in respiratory illness incidence in infants 6 to 12 months of age. This study also controlled for important covariates such as child's gender, maternal feeding practices, education, and parental respiratory symptoms in childhood. The authors further found that among a subsample of 133 infant cord bloods tested for cotinine, that 7 (7%) of 100 samples had detectable cotinine levels despite mothers reporting being nonsmokers. These authors could not conclusively distinguish the relative importance of prenatal versus postnatal maternal smoking on acute respiratory disease risk but concluded that both were likely to be important, particularly the amount smoked by mothers.

Several studies found the risk of respiratory illness was accentuated for ETS-exposed infants who were bottle fed versus breast fed,[60,61] but other studies have failed to identify such an association.[62]

In summary, children born to parents who smoke have an increased risk of acute respiratory illness in the first 1 to 2 years of life. The available evidence suggests that this increase in risk may be as high as twofold and is principally related to smoking by mothers. Among the areas of controversy requiring further clarification are the extent to which in utero smoking by mothers explains the augmented risk early in life, the degree to which smoking by fathers or other household members may increase risk, and the extent to which household ETS exposure contributes to acute respiratory illness incidence in older children. Furthermore, a more thorough understanding is needed of how other host or environmental factors, including gender of the child, feeding practices early in life, ethnicity, and allergic predisposition modify the risk posed by ETS exposure.

ETS and chronic respiratory symptoms in children

Studies of the contribution of ETS in the home environment to chronic, persistent, or recurrent respiratory symptoms in children have paralleled those examining the impact on acute respiratory illness. Once again, summary compilations of relevant studies have been presented in the 1986 Surgeon General's Report,[1] the report of the National Research Council,[2] and, most recently, in an extensive report by the EPA.[3] In general, a majority of these studies support an association between ETS exposure in the household and increased risk of several respiratory symptoms in children. Among these are cough, persistent or recurrent episodes of bronchitis, and recurrent wheezing. These studies estimate that the extent of elevated risk from ETS exposure ranges from a low odds ratio of 1.2 to a high of approximately 2.5, depending on the symptom outcome under scrutiny. The consistency of these findings among different studies from different geographic areas and the presence in many of a dose–response relationship based on number of smokers or amount smoked in the home argues that the observed association is not due to unmeasured confounding. The larger and/or more recent studies not covered in the three reports cited previously are presented in Table 47-4.[55,64-75] Other smaller cohort or case-control studies, most of which have similar findings, are summarized in the EPA report.[3] Included in the study cited in Table 47-4 are two from Italy that add snoring to

Table 47-4. Passive smoking and chronic respiratory symptoms in children

References	Number of subjects and country	Age (yr)	Design	Exposure assessment	Outcome	Result	ETS source
Weiss et al. (1980)[64]	650 U.S.	5-9	L	Q	Persistent wheeze	DR	P
Ware et al. (1984)[55]	10,106 U.S.	6-9	L	Q	Cough, wheeze, bronchitis	OR 1.3, DR	M > F
Charlton (1984)[65]	15,000 U.K.	8-19	X	Q	Cough	DR	M > F
Park and Kim (1986)[66]	3651 Korea	0-14	X	Q	Cough in last 3 mo	≤14 cig/day OR 2.4 (1.4, 4.3) >14 cig/day OR 3.2 (1.9, 5.5)	P
Bisgaard et al. (1987)[67]	5953 Denmark	0-1	R-cohort	Q	Wheezing	OR 2.7 (1.8, 4.0)	M
Andrae et al. (1988)[68]	4990 Sweden	0.5-16	X	Q	Exercise ind. cough	OR 1.4 (1.1, 1.8)	P
Somerville et al. (1988)[69]	7144 Scotland	5-11	X	Q	Wheezing	>20 cig/day OR 1.6 (1.2, 2.2)	P
Strachan (1988)[70]	1012 Scotland	7	X	Q	Nocturnal cough Chesty colds	One smoker OR 1.6 Two smokers OR 2.5 One smoker OR 1.3 Two smokers OR 1.9	P P
Neuspiel et al. (1989)[71]	9670 U.K.	0-10	L	Q	Wheezing	RR 1.11 (1.02, 1.21) (DR)	M
Corbo et al. (1989)[72]	1615 Italy	6-13	X	Q	Snoring	OR 1.9 (1.2, 2.8)	P
Ugnat et al. (1990)[73]	6529 Canada	0-14	X	Q	Chronic bronchitis	OR 3.0 (1.6, 5.7)	M
Dijkstra et al. (1990)[74]	1051 Netherlands	6-12	X	Q	Cough > 3 mo Wheeze	OR 2.5 (1.1, 5.1) OR 1.9 (1.0, 3.5)	P
Forastiere et al. (1992)[75]	2929 Italy	7-11	X	Q	Night cough Snoring	OR 1.8 (1.2, 2.7) OR 1.4 (1.1, 1.7)	M > F M > F

DR, Dose-response; *F,* female; *L,* longitudinal; *M,* male; *OR,* odds ratio; *P,* parents; *Q,* questionnaire; *R,* retrospective; *X,* cross-sectional.

the list of chronic symptoms that are observed more frequently in ETS-exposed children.[72,75]

Several points warrant emphasis in considering the association of ETS with chronic respiratory symptoms in children. Most of the studies cited base the presence of symptoms in children on parental reports. Several studies have suggested that parents who are themselves symptomatic are more likely to report symptoms in their children. Since active smoking causes these symptoms in parents, ascertainment bias may be inherent in parental reports of children's symptoms. However, adjustment for parental reports of symptoms may result in overadjustment and in an underestimation of the true effect of ETS, if it does cause symptoms in children. As was the case for acute respiratory illnesses, the risk of chronic respiratory symptoms appears greatest in infants and for household smoking by mothers. Thus, a possible contributing role of maternal smoking during pregnancy to the observed increased risk of chronic respiratory symptoms cannot be excluded, although studies that control for prenatal smoking continued to show risk associated with postnatal ETS. ETS-associated risks among schoolchildren are, in general, lower than for younger children. In addition, active smoking among school-aged children may explain some symptoms, and this may be difficult to control as it is often covert.

Especially in older children, it is possible that an augmented risk of ETS-associated respiratory symptoms is limited to susceptible individuals. These susceptible subtypes may include persons with a history of atopy,[76] respiratory illness early in childhood, or children with low birth weight[77] or low levels of pulmonary function[78] early in life.

ETS and asthma

Environmental tobacco smoke has been postulated to affect the asthmatic condition in two ways: (1) to exacerbate the frequency and severity of attacks in existing asthmatics, and (2) to predispose the development of new cases of asthma in previously unaffected children.

There is now ample evidence to support the role of ETS in exacerbations of asthma. Evans and co-workers[79] demonstrated in a group of 191 asthmatic children from New York City that children from low income households with smoking parents had a greater frequency of annual emergency room visits for asthma than children from nonsmoking households. Similarly, Ehrlich et al.[80] found that 107 asthmatic children recruited from both an emergency room and asthma clinic were more likely to have smoking mothers and were themselves more likely to have high urinary cotinine levels than control children. O'Connor et al.[81] found that cold air bronchial challenge testing caused a greater decline in forced expiratory volume in 1 second (FEV1) among asthmatic or wheezing children with smoking mothers than among similar children whose mothers did not smoke. Investigators from Vancouver, Canada[82] who studied 415 children referred to an allergy clinic for asthma,

found that asthma severity scores were higher, forced expiratory volume in 1 second (FEV1) was lower, and degree of responsiveness to histamine challenge was increased in asthmatic children with smoking mothers. Severity of asthma increased in parallel with the duration of ETS exposure. In a later publication, these same investigators[83] report a decrease in asthma severity scores of children when ETS exposure in the home is reduced. Most recently, investigators from Maine have documented in 199 asthmatic children that urinary cotinine levels and parental estimates of ETS exposure correlate with number of asthma exacerbations in the previous year.[84]

More controversial is the role of ETS in the development of new cases of asthma in children and adults (Table 47-5).[75,85-92] Several large cohort studies have suggested that prevalent cases of asthma occur more frequently in children in smoking households, particularly in households with smoking mothers. Odds ratios for ETS exposure in the home have generally been in the range of 1.5 to 2.5, with several studies[89,92] suggesting a possible threshold effect, with risk becoming substantial if mothers smoke more than one-half pack per day. In two large longitudinal studies,[86,90] incident cases of asthma were not associated with home ETS exposure. However, in one case-control study[88] and an additional longitudinal study,[92] new cases of asthma in children were 2.5-fold more frequent in households with smoking mothers. In the latter study, risk elevation was evident only for children whose mothers did not complete high school and who smoked greater than one half pack per day.

These studies confirm the importance of ETS in increasing the severity of asthma in affected children and support a contributing role of household ETS exposures, especially maternal smoking, in the development of asthma. As was the case for acute respiratory illness and chronic symptoms, the separate influences of preexisting level of lung function, maternal smoking during pregnancy, and allergic predisposition remain incompletely defined. The findings in some studies that asthma incidence is increased only for ETS exposures in the home of certain magnitude and for persons of lower socioeconomic level suggest that a threshold level (both in duration and intensity) and other cofactors may be necessary to confer increased risk of asthma.

ETS and airway responsiveness

Studies examining the relationship of ETS to airway responsiveness are compiled in Table 47-6. The most plausible mechanism by which passive cigarette smoke exposure is related to airway responsiveness is airway inflammation. It is also possible, however, that the influence of ETS on airway responsiveness is mediated via its effect on the atopic state. A number of epidemiologic and clinical studies have considered ETS exposure and its relationship to airway responsiveness. The earliest study was performed in a population-based sample in East Boston, Massachusetts.[93] These investigators found no association between

Table 47–5. Passive smoking and asthma in children

References	Number of subjects and country	Ages (yr)	Design	Exposure assessment	Outcome	Result	ETS source
Gortmaker et al. (1982)[85]	3966 U.S.	0-17	X-cohort	Q	Asthma prevalence	OR 1.5-1.8	M
Horwood et al. (1985)[86]	1056 New Zealand	0-6	L	Q	Asthma incidence	OR 0.9 (NS)	P
Burchfield et al. (1986)[87]	3482 U.S.	0-19	X-cohort	Q	Asthma prevalence	OR 1.7 (1.2, 2.5) boys 1.2 (0.8, 1.9) girls	P
Willers et al. (1991)[88]	129 Sweden	3-15	CC	Q and urine cotinine	Asthma incidence	OR 2.6 (1.2-5.3) Cotinine >20: 4.2 (1.8-9.9)	M only
Weitzman et al. (1990)[89]	4331 U.S.	0-5	X-cohort	Q	Asthma prevalence	OR 2.1 for > 0.5 PPD	M
Sherman et al. (1990)[90]	770 U.S.	5-9	L	Q	Asthma prevalence and incidence	OR 1.1 (0.7, 1.7)	M
Dekker et al. (1991)[91]	13,495 Canada	5-8	X	Q	Asthma prevalence	1 smoker: OR 1.4 (1.1, 1.7) >1 smoker: OR 1.6 (1.3, 2.0)	House-hold
Martinez et al. (1992)[92]	774 U.S.	0-5	L	Q	Asthma incidence	OR 2.5 for > 0.5 PPD*	M
Forastiere et al. (1992)[75]	2992 Italy	7-11	X	Q	Asthma prevalence	OR 1.5 (1.0, 2.2)	M only

CC, Case-control; *HS,* high school; *L,* longitudinal; *M,* male; *OR,* odds ratio; *P,* parents; *PPD,* packs per day; *Q,* questionnaire; *X,* cross-sectional.
*Only for children whose mothers did not complete high school.

Table 47-6. Passive smoking and airway responsiveness

Reference	Number of subjects	Age (yr)	Exposure assessment	Outcome	Result	ETS source
Weiss et al. (1985)[93]	173	12-16	Q	Cold air	No association	M
Murray and Morrison (1986)[94]	41	7-17	Q	Histamine $PC_{20}FEV1$	Significant association	M
O'Connor et al. (1987)[81]	286	6-21	Q	Cold air	Significant association among asthmatics	M
Corbo et al. (1987)[95]	255	11-14	Q	Methacholine $PC_{20}FEV1$	No association	M
Martinez et al. (1988)[97]	166	9	Q	Carbachol $PC_{20}FEV1$	Significant association males > females	M
Murray and Morrison (1989)[82]	104	7-17	Q	Histamine $PC_{20}FEV1$	Significant association males only	M
Strachan et al. (1990)[96]	770	7	Cotinine	Exercise	No association	P
Young et al. (1991)[99]	63	1 month	Q	$PC_{40}V_{max}FRC$	Significant association	P
Forastiere et al. (1991)[98]	1777	7-11	Q	Methacholine $PC_{20}FEV1$	Significant association females > males	P

FEV1, Forced expiratory volume in 1 second; *FRC,* functional residual capacity; *M,* male; *P,* parents; *PC,* provocative concentration; *Q,* questionnaire; *V,* flow.

airway responsiveness to cold air and maternal cigarette smoking. Clinical studies with small numbers of subjects selected from allergy clinics have noted an association between maternal cigarette smoking and histamine-induced airway responsiveness.[82,94] This is consistent with population-based studies that have found an association between airway responsiveness to cold air and maternal cigarette smoking among asthmatic subjects.[81] Unfortunately, these clinical studies do not establish whether the relationship is simply an exacerbation of airway responsiveness in subjects with preexisting disease or whether the association precedes disease development.

At least two relatively large studies have examined the relationship of maternal cigarette smoking to airway responsiveness and have found no effect,[95,96] although one study[96] used a precise measurement of cigarette smoking exposure (cotinine) but a relatively imprecise measurement of airway responsiveness (exercise). Two additional studies utilizing a questionnaire assessment of smoking status and carbachol[97] or methacholine[98] as the measure of airway responsiveness have found significant associations between maternal and parental report of cigarette smoking and airway reactivity. These studies differ in that the association was more significant in men in one study,[97] and in women in the other.[98]

Of interest is the study of Young et al., who examined the provocative concentration of histamine that caused a

Table 47-7. Passive smoking and pulmonary function in children

References	Number of subjects and country	Age (yr)	Design	Exposure assessment	Outcome	Result	ETS source
Tager et al. (1983)[100]	1156 U.S.	5-10	L	Q	FEV1, FEF25-75	↓Growth 3-5% by adulthood	M only
Vedal et al. (1984)[101]	3175 U.S.	5-14	X	Q	FEF25-75	↓4% Girls	M only
Berkey et al. (1986)[102]	7834 U.S.	6-10	L	Q	FVC, FEV1	↓Growth 3% by adulthood	M > F
Burchfield et al. (1986)[87]	3482 U.S.	0-10	L	Q	FVC, FEV1	↓FEV1, FVC growth 5-10% boys only DR	P
Kauffmann et al. (1989)[103]	1160 France	6-10	X	Q	FEV1, FEF25-75	FEV1: ↓10 ml/sec/g tobacco/day FEF25-75: ↓15 ml/sec/g tobacco/day	M only
Strachan et al. (1990)[96]	757 U.K.	7	X	Salivary cotinine	FEF25-75	↓7% between high and low quintiles	All
Dijkstra et al. (1990)[74]	634 Netherlands	6-12	X	Q	FEV1, FEF25-75	↓1.8% FEV1 ↓5.2% FEF25-75	M only
Sherrill et al. (1992)[104]	634 New Zealand	9-15	L	Q age 3-15	FEV1/FVC	↓3.9% boys, ↓2.3% for girls who wheeze by age 15; no effect in nonwheezing children	P
Martinez et al. (1992)[92]	316 U.S.	6-10	Cohort	Q age 0-5	FEF25-75, FVC	FVC: ↑7% girls; FEF25-75 ↓10% for >1/2 PPD	M

DR, Dose-response; *F,* female; *FEF,* forced expiratory flow; *FEV1,* forced expiratory volume in 1 second; *FVC,* forced vital capacity; *L,* longitudinal; *M,* male; *P,* parents; *PPD,* packs per day; *Q,* questionnaire; *X,* cross-sectional.

40% decrease in maximum flow at functional residual capacity (PC40 VMAX FRC) as a measure of airway responsiveness in 1-month-old infants, and its relationship to maternal cigarette smoking in utero.[99] These investigators found a significant relationship between maternal cigarette smoking and airway responsiveness at birth. This provocative study raises important questions as to whether maternal smoking during pregnancy may be related to airway responsiveness early in life. Studies examining this association using conventional challenge techniques will be difficult to perform. Given the known association between maternal cigarette smoking and the occurrence of asthma early in life, it seems highly likely that an association between ETS exposure and airway responsiveness would also be present, but additional studies are necessary to confirm this hypothesis.

ETS and pulmonary function

As has been the case with studies examining ETS and respiratory symptoms, the past decades have seen the emergence of numerous studies that have examined the impact of ETS on pulmonary function in children. Interest in a possible deleterious impact of ETS on pulmonary function stems from knowledge in adults that obstructive pulmonary deficits are associated with an increased incidence of wheezing and respiratory illnesses, suggesting that this may represent the physiologic mechanism by which ETS causes

increased risk of these conditions in children. In addition, reduced growth of pulmonary function parameters in childhood, particularly those that relate to airway function, are postulated to correlate with steeper declines and earlier impairment of pulmonary function in adult life.

A majority of the studies that have explored ETS and lung function in children have found a small but consistent reduction in measures of airway function in exposed children, particularly attainable flow rates during forced expiratory maneuvers. Table 47-7 compiles some of the larger and more recent studies addressing this issue.[74,87,92,96,100-104] Most studies suggest modest declines in FEV1 in the range of 1% to 5%, and larger decrements (5% to 10%) of measures of flow at moderate to low lung volumes such as forced expiratory flow of 25% to 75% of vital capacity (FEF25-75). Some studies suggest that boys are more significantly affected than girls. Three longitudinal studies of lung function[87,100,102] predict deficits of 3% to 5% in ETS-exposed children by the time the adult level of pulmonary function is attained. An additional recent longitudinal study among New Zealand children,[104] however, found that impaired growth of measures of airway function was limited to children with wheeze symptoms. In addition to the findings of flow impairment suggesting small airway dysfunction, several of the studies have reported mild increases in forced vital capacity (FVC) in ETS-exposed children.[55,92,101]

These findings of mild degrees of small airways impairment in ETS-exposed children are compatible with persistent or protracted ETS exposure inducing a condition of mild airway inflammation and/or bronchoconstriction, which results in narrowing of small airways. This narrowing could, in turn, lead to the increase in obstructive symptoms of wheezing and cough and the heightened degree of airway responsiveness observed in ETS-exposed children. Even greater degrees of airway narrowing could occur with acute respiratory infections, causing the more severe profile of respiratory illnesses seen in ETS-exposed children, especially those less than 2 years of age.

In very young infants, measures of maximal flow rates and airway size are likely to be closely associated with the severity and frequency of respiratory illness. At least three studies[78,97,99] have demonstrated that either a measure of forced expiratory flow in infants induced by rapid thoraco-abdominal compression (V_{FRC}) or a measure of airway conductance during passive title breathing (ratio of the time-to-peak tidal flow in exhalation to the total time for exhalation, T_{ME}/T_E) are reduced in young infants who later experience wheezing respiratory illnesses in the first year of life. Significantly, a separate study examining infant pulmonary function in the first 10 weeks of life has demonstrated 40% reductions in V_{FRC} in healthy infants born to mothers who smoked during pregnancy when compared with infants born to nonsmoking mothers.[105] This finding, coupled with the exclusive or predominant effect in most studies of maternal smoking on infant pulmonary function, suggests that active smoking by mothers during pregnancy may underlie some or most of the observed decrease in pulmonary function previously ascribed to ETS exposure. This may be particularly relevant to the increased risk of respiratory illness and symptoms conferred by lower levels of pulmonary function early in life.

OTHER EFFECTS OF ETS IN CHILDREN
ETS, atopy, and the immune system

Cigarette smoke is known to have important effects on the human immune system. Specifically, active cigarette smoking is known to be associated with (1) increases in peripheral blood neutrophils, monocytes, and eosinophils, (2) increases in serum IgE, (3) activation of natural killer T cells and alveolar macrophages, and (4) decreases in serum IgG and IgM.[106] It has been postulated that passive cigarette smoking may be related to atopy in either of two ways. First, passive cigarette smoking may induce airway inflammation, which may alter the permeability characteristics of the airway epithelium with regard to antigen. This may lead to the presentation of a greater concentration or a greater number of antigens to effector cells. Second, ETS may also lead to nonspecific immune system activation, independent of antigen, causing the host to have heightened response to foreign antigen.

Several studies have examined the role of ETS in allergy (Table 47-8). Early studies focused on the relationship of ETS to skin test reactivity. Weiss and co-workers studied 173 subjects between the ages of 12 and 16 drawn from a random population sample in East Boston, Massachusetts.[93] Maternal cigarette smoking was related to skin test reactivity in these children. However, current smoking status was less important than smoking status in the past. These data suggested that early life exposure might be important for sensitization. These results were not examined by the gender of the child. Martinez and co-workers studied 172 subjects, all 9 years of age, from a suburban community outside of Rome, Italy.[107] These investigators demonstrated a dose–response relationship in males between parental cigarette smoke exposure and a skin test index. Again, this report does not clearly differentiate between current and past exposure and leaves unanswered at which stage in life ex-

Table 47-8. Passive smoking, atopy, and IgE

References	Number of subjects	Age (yr)	Exposure assessment	Outcome	Result	ETS source
Weiss et al. (1985)[93]	173	12-16	Q	Any positive skin test	43% in exposed vs. 25%	M
Kjellman (1981)[110]	46	0-3	Q	IgE growth after birth	Steeper rise in exposed	P
Osaka et al. (1985)[109]	766	Elementary school	Q	Mite IgE	42% in exposed vs. 30%	M not F
Martinez et al. (1988)[97]	172	9	Q	Skin test index	↑in boys only dose-response	P
Ronchetti et al. (1990)[108]	159	9	Q	IgE, eosinophil count	↑in boys only dose-response	P
Halonen et al. (1991)[113]	679	Birth	Q	Cord blood IgE 9 month IgE	No difference in exposed vs. nonexposed	M
Ownby et al. (1991)[111]	847	Birth	Q with cotinine validation	Cord blood IgE	No difference in exposed vs. nonexposed	M and F
Oryszczyn et al. (1991)[112]	132	Birth	Q	Cord blood IgE	No difference in exposed vs. nonexposed	P

F, Female; *M,* male; *P,* parents; *Q,* questionnaire.

posure may influence sensitization. Using a subsample of the same population, Ronchetti et al. confirmed the skin test data with serum IgE levels. Importantly, the skin test and IgE data do correlate with an inflammatory marker (peripheral blood eosinophil count), suggesting that there may be a relationship between ETS-induced atopy and inflammation.[108]

Relatively few data are available concerning the possibility that cigarette smoke may act as a hapten for other antigens. Osaka et al. studied 766 elementary school children in Japan and found that ETS exposure was associated with a higher prevalence of allergy to house dust mite.[109] This research raises the possibility that passive smoke exposure may increase allergic sensitivity in those genetically predisposed. This hypothesis has not been formally tested.

Finally, Kjellman published a small study on 46 subjects between birth and 3 years old, examining cord blood IgE and its relationship to parental cigarette smoke exposure.[110] These data initially suggested that passive smoke exposure might be related to cord blood IgE level. However, at least three subsequent reports have suggested that these findings could not be confirmed.[111-113]

In summary, it appears that there is a suggestion that passive smoke exposure is related to sensitization and, potentially, to the development of the atopic state. What remains unclear is at what age and what individuals are specifically susceptible to these effects and whether ETS exposure can influence sensitization to other environmental antigens.

ETS and middle ear conditions

Passive smoking by parents has also been implicated in several other common or serious conditions of infancy and childhood. Prominent among these is the finding of several studies that exposed children have higher incidence of acute otitis media and chronic middle ear effusions. Table 47-9 summarizes the larger studies examining this issue, which suggest a 20% to 60% increase in these outcomes among ETS-exposed children.[114-121] The studies of Strachan et al.[118] and Etzel et al.[120] are particularly convincing, the former reporting of exposure-response relationship with respect to level of salivary cotinine, the latter due to its longitudinal prospective design. A more recent longitudinal study in Sweden,[121] however, failed to find an excess of tympanotomy procedures among children exposed to maternal ETS in a birth cohort of over 1300 children. The pathophysiologic mechanism whereby ETS increases risk of middle ear conditions may be related to impaired patency of the eustachian tubes, either by persistent inflammation, impaired mucociliary function, or enlargement of the adenoids or tonsils tissues impeding their drainage. The public health implications of even a small increase in risk of middle ear disease due to ETS are significant, as otitis represents the most frequent childhood diagnosis requiring antibiotics and myringotomy the most frequent surgical procedure in children.

ETS and sudden infant death syndrome

Perhaps the most serious consequence of maternal smoking in young children is the increase in sudden infant death syndrome (SIDS). This condition affects approximately two of every thousand live born infants and is responsible for more than 5000 deaths each year in the United States.[122] First, reported by Steele and Langworth in 1966,[123] many subsequent studies have confirmed a 50% to fourfold increased risk of SIDS in infants born to mothers who smoke.[124-131] Studies that have examined potential confounders suggest that the increased risk associated with maternal smoking is independent of other risk factors for SIDS, including maternal birthweight, maternal age and socioeconomic status, breast-feeding, ethnicity, or race. The evidence for a causal association with maternal smoking is further supported by the presence of a dose–response relation-

Table 47-9. ETS and middle ear conditions in children

References	Number of subjects and country	Age (yr)	Design	Exposure assessment	Outcome	Result	ETS source
Iversen et al. (1985)[114]	337 Denmark	5-7	X-Cohort	Q	MEE	OR 1.6 (1.0, 2.6)	P
Black (1985)[115]	150 U.K.	4-9	CC	Q	Hosp. MEE	OR 1.6 (1.0-2.6)	P
Pukander et al. (1985)[116]	264 Finland	2-3	CC	Q	Acute OM	↑60%	P
Teale et al. (1989)[117]	877 U.S.	0-7	L	Q	Acute OM	↑13% yr 1 only	P
Strachan et al. (1989)[118]	736 U.K.	7	X	Salivary cotinine	MEE	OR 1.3 (1.1-1.3) for 2-fold ↑ in cotinine	All
Rowe-Jones and Brockbank (1992)[119]	100 U.K.	2-12	CC	Q	OM with effusion	NS	P
Etzel et al. (1992)[120]	132 U.S.	0-3	L	Salivary cotinine	AOM	↑Incid. density 1.4 (1.2, 1.6)	All
Rasmussen (1993)[121]	130 Sweden	0-7	L	Q	Tympanostomy for OM	NS	M

AOM, Acute otitis media; *CC*, case-control; *L*, longitudinal; *M*, male; *MEE*, middle ear effusions; *NS*, not significant; *OR*, odds ratio; *P*, parents; *Q*, questionnaire; *X*, cross-sectional.

ship with amount of maternal smoking,[123-125,128-131] particularly when smoking exceeds one pack per day.

An issue that remains unresolved is the relative importance of maternal smoking during pregnancy versus postnatal smoking by mothers. One recent large survey[131] found a risk of SIDS to be elevated twofold in children exposed to passive smoking by mothers and threefold for children exposed to both active maternal smoking in utero and passive smoking from a maternal source after birth. Thus, both prenatal and postnatal maternal smoking probably contribute to the elevated risk of SIDS in exposed infants. Unclear, too, is the role of other smokers in the household. One study suggested an increase in risk of SIDS for infants exposed to paternal ETS when the mother also smokes but no increase in risk if fathers are the sole smoker in the home.[130]

SUMMARY AND CONCLUSION

The evidence is now unequivocal that prolonged exposure to ETS in the indoor environment is associated with numerous significant health risks. The composition of ETS is complex and contains several thousand substances. In general, the concentration of most of these substances is at least as great and sometimes many times greater in sidestream smoke compared with mainstream smoke. Exposure assessment is likewise complex, and optimally should rely on questionnaire reporting of cumulative exposure over long periods of time, coupled with objective determination of more recent exposure as is provided by biomarkers.

In adults, ETS exposure in the household is associated with a 1.2- to twofold increase of lung cancer, and most studies suggest a similar magnitude of increase in risk of coronary death and other coronary events. The latter finding is particularly significant, owing to the prevalence of coronary disease in the developed world. Unresolved issues in adults include the extent of risk increase accompanying shorter exposure periods to ETS, such as what would occur in the work environment and the identification of other cofactors important in conferring increased risk from ETS.

In children, exposure to ETS is associated with an increased incidence of acute lower respiratory tract illnesses, particularly in children less than 18 months of age. This has been estimated to account for 150,000 to 300,000 cases per year in the United States alone.[3] In addition, ETS causes more frequent and severe exacerbations of asthma, estimated to affect 200,000 to 1,000,000 children per year. Maternal smoking during pregnancy is likely to be an important contributor to the risk of these outcomes. Exposure to ETS in the household is associated with a 20% to 60% increase in the incidence of acute and chronic middle ear conditions in children, and maternal smoking during pregnancy and early infancy is associated with a two- to fourfold increased risk of SIDS.

To date, the vast majority of the adverse outcomes associated with ETS are related to protracted exposure of family members in the home. Risk of these or other outcomes by shorter term exposure at work or in other indoor environments has not been adequately studied. It is important to remember, however, that the risk for most, if not all, of these outcomes engendered by active smoking is many times greater than that associated with passive ETS exposure. Therefore, preventive strategies designed to avoid ETS exposure and all of its attendant health risks should include a focus on quitting, especially for mothers contemplating pregnancy or with young children, and to dissuade young women and men from starting this hazardous habit.

Acknowledgments

The authors thank Darlene Bramble and Daniel Barrows for assistance in preparation of this chapter.

REFERENCES

1. U.S. Department of Health and Human Services: *The health consequences of involuntary smoking.* A report of the Surgeon General. U.S. DHHS, Public Health Service, Office of the Assistant Secretary for Health, Office of Smoking and Health, DHHS Pub No (PHS) 87-8398, Washington, DC, 1986.
2. National Research Council: *Environmental tobacco smoke: measuring exposures and assessing health effects,* Washington, DC, 1986, National Academy Press.
3. U.S. Environmental Protection Agency: *Respiratory health effects of passive smoking: lung cancer and other disorders,* Office of Health and Environmental Assessment, Office of Research and Development, Washington, DC, 1992.
4. Guerin MR, Jenkins RA, and Tomkins BA: *The chemistry of environmental tobacco smoke: composition and measurement,* Chelsea, MI, 1992, Lewis Publishers.
5. International Agency for Research on Cancer: In O'Neill IK, Brunneman KD, Dodet B, Hoffmann D, editors: *Environmental carcinogens—methods of analysis and exposure measurement,* vol 9, *Passive smoking,* Lyon, France; 1987, IARC Sci Publ. No. 81.
6. Benner CL, Bayona JM, Caka FM, et al: Chemical composition of environmental tobacco smoke. 2. Particulate-phase compounds, *Environ Sci Technol* 23:688-699, 1989.
7. Eatough DJ, Benner CL, Bayona JM, Richards G, Lamb JD, Lee ML, Lewis EA, and Hansen L: Chemical composition of environmental tobacco smoke. 1. Gas-phase acids and bases, *Environ Sci Technol* 23:679-687, 1989.
8. Coultas DB, Peake GT, and Samet JM: Questionnaire assessment of lifetime and recent exposure to environmental tobacco smoke, *Am J Epidemiol* 130:338-347, 1989.
9. Cummings KM, Markello SJ, Mahoney M, Bhargave AK, McElroy PD, and Marshall JR: Measurement of current exposure to environmental tobacco smoke, *Arch Environ Health* 45(2):74-79, 1990.
10. Jarvis MJ and Russell MH: Passive exposure to tobacco smoke, *Br Med J* 291:1646, 1985.
11. Riboli E, Preston-Martin S, Saracci R, Haley NJ, et al: Exposure of nonsmoking women to environmental tobacco smoke: a 10-country collaborative study, *Cancer Causes Control* 1:243-252, 1990.
12. Henderson FW, Holly FR, Morris R, et al: Home air nicotine levels and urinary cotinine excretion in preschool children, *Am Rev Respir Dis* 140:197-201, 1989.
13. Leaderer BP: Assessing exposures to environmental tobacco smoke, *Risk Anal* 10(1):19-26, 1990.
14. Spengler JP, Treitman RD, Tosteson TD, Mage DJ, and Soczek ML: Personal exposures to respirable particulates and implications for air pollution epidemiology, *Environ Sci Technol* 19:700-707, 1985.

15. Sexton R, Spengler JD, and Treitman RD: Personal exposure to respirable particulates: a case-study in Waterbury, Vermont, *Atmos Environ* 18:1385-1398, 1984.

16. Muramatsu M, Umemura S, Okada T, and Tomita H: Estimation of personal exposure to tobacco smoke with a newly developed nicotine personal monitor, *Environ Res* 35:218-227, 1984.

17. Hammond SK and Leaderer BP: A diffusion monitor to measure exposure to passive smoking, *Environ Sci Technol* 31:494-497, 1987.

18. Jarvis MJ, Tunstall-Pedoe H, Feyerabend C, Vesey C, and Saloojee Y: Comparison of tests used to distinguish smokers from nonsmokers, *Am J Public Health* 77:1435-1438, 1987.

19. Hammond SK, Gann PH, Coughlin J, Tannenbaum SR, and Skipper PL: Tobacco smoke exposure and carcinogen-hemoglobin adducts, In *Indoor air '90: proceedings of the 5th international conference on indoor air quality and climate,* vol. 2, *Characteristics of indoor air,* pp 157-161, Ottawa, Ontario, Canada, 1990, Canada Mortgage and Housing Corporation.

20. Coultas DB, Howard CA, Peake GT, Skipper BJ, and Samet JM: Salivary cotinine levels and involuntary tobacco smoke exposure in children and adults in New Mexico, *Am Rev Respir Dis* 136:305-309, 1987.

21. Greenberg RA, Bauman KE, Glover LH, et al: Ecology of passive smoking by young infants, *J Pediatr* 114:774-780, 1989.

22. Idle JR: Titrating exposure to tobacco smoke using cotinine: a minefield of misunderstandings, *J Clin Epidemiol* 43:313-317, 1990.

23. Hirayama T: Non-smoking wives of heavy smokers have a higher risk of lung cancer: A study from Japan, *Br Med J* 282:183-185, 1981.

24. Trichopoulos D, Kalandidi A, Sparros L, and MacMahon B: Lung cancer and passive smoking, *Int J Cancer* 27:1-4, 1981.

25. Garfinkel L: Time trends in lung cancer mortality among nonsmokers and a note on passive smoking, *J Natl Cancer Inst* 6:1061-1066, 1981.

26. Trichopoulos D, Kalandidi A, and Sparros L: Lung cancer and passive smoking: conclusion of Greek study (letter), *Lancet* 667-668, 1983.

27. Correa P, Fontham E, Pickle L, Lin Y, and Haenszel W: Passive smoking and lung cancer, *Lancet* 2:595-597, 1983.

28. Garfinkel L, Auerbach O, and Joubert L: Involuntary smoking and lung cancer: a case-control study, *J Natl Cancer Inst* 75:463-469, 1985.

29. Koo LC, Ho JH, Saw D, and Ho CY: Measurements of passive smoking and estimates of lung cancer risk among non-smoking Chinese females, *Int J Cancer* 39:162-169, 1987.

30. Lam TH, Kung ITM, Wong CM, Lam WK, Kleevens JWL, Saw D, Hsu C, Seneviratne S, Lam SY, Lo KK, and Chan WC: Smoking, passive smoking and histological types in lung cancer in Hong Kong Chinese women, *Br J Cancer* 6:673-678, 1987.

31. Hole DJ, Gillis CR, Chopra C, and Hawthorne VM: Passive smoking and cardiorespiratory health in a general population in the west of Scotland, *Br Med J* 299:423-427, 1989.

32. Kalandidi A, Katsouyanni K, Voropoulou N, et al: Passive smoking and diet in the etiology of lung cancer among nonsmokers, *Cancer Causes Control* 1:15-21, 1990.

33. Janerich DT, Thompson WD, Varela LR, et al: Lung cancer and exposure to tobacco smoke in the household, *N Engl J Med* 323:632-636, 1990.

34. Fontham ETH, Correa P, Wu-Williams A, Reynolds P, Greenberg RS, Buffler PA, Chen VW, Boyd P, Alterman T, Austin DF, Liff J, and Greenberg SD: Lung cancer in nonsmoking women: a multicenter case-control study, *Cancer Epidemiol Biomarkers Prev* 1(1):35-334, 1991.

35. Stockwell HG, Candelora EC, Armstrong AW, and Pinkham PA: Environmental tobacco smoke and lung cancer in never smoking women. Presented at the annual meeting abstract forum: Society for Epidemiologic Research, Buffalo, New York, 1991.

36. Brownson RC, Alavanja MCR, Hock ET, and Loy TS: Passive smoking and lung cancer in nonsmoking women, *Am J Public Health* 82:1525-1530, 1992.

37. Liu Q, Sasco AJ, Riboli E, and Hu MX: Indoor air pollution and lung cancer in Guangzhou, People's Republic of China, *Am J Epidemiol* 137:145-154, 1993.

38. Horten AW: Epidemiologic evidence for the role of indoor tobacco smoke as an initiator of human breast carcinogenesis, *Cancer Detect Prevent* 16:119-127, 1992.

39. Hirayama T: Lung cancer in Japan: effects of nutrition and passive smoking, In Mizell M and Correa P, editors: *Lung cancer: cause and prevention,* pp 175-195, New York, 1984, Verlay Chemie International.

40. Garland C, Barrett-Connor F, Suarez L, Criqui MH, and Wingard DL: Effects of passive smoking on ischemic heart disease mortality of nonsmokers, *Am J Epidemiol* 121:645-650, 1985.

41. Svendsen KH, Kuller LM, Marten MJ, and Ockene JK: Effects of passive smoking in the multiple risk factor intervention trial, *Am J Epidemiol* 126:783-795, 1987.

42. Lee P, Chamberlain J, and Alderson M: Relationship of passive smoking to risk of lung cancer and other smoking-associated diseases, *Br J Cancer* 54:97-105, 1986.

43. Helsing KJ, Sandler DP, Comstock GW, and Chee E: Heart disease mortality in nonsmokers living with smokers, *Am J Epidemiol* 127:915-922, 1988.

44. Humble C, Croft J, Gerber A, Casper M, Haines C, and Tyroler H: Passive smoking and twenty year cardiovascular disease mortality among nonsmoking wives in Evans County, Georgia, *Am J Public Health* 80:599-601, 1990.

45. Dobson AJ, Alexander HM, Heller RF, and Lloyd DM: Passive smoking and the risk of heart attack or coronary death, *Med J Aust* 154:793-797, 1991.

46. Glantz SA and Parmley WW: Passive smoking and heart disease: epidemiology, physiology, and biochemistry, *Circulation* 83:1-12, 1991.

47. Altred E, Bleecker E, Chaitman B, Dahms TE, Gottlieb SO, Hackney JD, Pagano M, Selevester RH, Walden SM, and Warren J: Short-term effects of carbon monoxide exposure on the exercise performance of subjects with coronary artery disease, *N Engl J Med* 321:1426-1432, 1989.

48. Sheps D, Herbst M, Hunderliter AL, Adams KF, Ekelund LG, O'Neil JJ, Goldstein GM, Brombert PA, Dalton JL, Ballenger MN, et al: Production of arrhythmias by elevated carboxyhemoglobin in patients with coronary artery disease, *Ann Intern Med* 113:343-351, 1990.

49. Taylor AF, Johnson DC, and Kazemi H: Environmental tobacco smoke and cardiovascular disease. Position paper from the Council on Cardiopulmonary and Critical Care, American Heart Association. *Circulation* 86:699-702, 1992.

50. Harlop S and Davies AM: Infant admissions to hospital and maternal smoking, *Lancet* 1(7857):529-532, 1974.

51. Leeder SR, Corkhill RT, Irwig LM, and Holland WW: Influence of family factors on the incidence of lower respiratory illness during the first year of life, *Br J Prevent Social Med* 30(4):203-212, 1976.

52. Fergusson DM, Horwood LJ, Shannon FT, and Taylor B: Parental smoking and lower respiratory illness in the first three years of life, *Epidemiol Comm Health* 35(3):180-184, 1981.

53. Schenker MB, Samet JM, and Speizer FE: Risk factors for childhood respiratory disease: the effect of host factors and home environmental exposures, *Am Rev Respir Dis* 128(6):1038-1043, 1983.

54. Fergusson D, Hons BA, and Horwood LJ: Parental smoking and respiratory illness during early childhood: a six-year longitudinal study, *Pediatr Pulmonol* 1:99-106, 1985.

55. Ware JH, Dockery DW, Spiro A III, Speizer FE, and Ferris BG Jr: Passive smoking, gas cooking, and respiratory health of children living in six cities, *Am Rev Respir Dis* 129(3):366-374, 1984.

56. McConnochie KM and Roghmann KJ: Breast feeding and maternal smoking as predictors of wheezing in children age 6 to 10 years, *Pediatr Pulmonol* 2:260-268, 1986.

57. Chen Y, Li W-X, and Yu S: Influence of passive smoking on admissions for respiratory illness in early childhood, *Br Med J* 293:303-306, 1986.

58. Ogston SA, Florey C, Du V, and Walker CHM: Association of infant alimentary and respiratory illness with parental smoking and other environmental factors, *J Epidemiol Comm Health* 41:21-25, 1987.

59. Taylor B and Wordsworth J: Maternal smoking during pregnancy and lower respiratory tract illness in early life, *Arch Dis Childhood* 62:786-791, 1987.

60. Chen Y, Li W-X, Yu S, and Qian W. Chang-Ning epidemiological study of children's health: I: passive smoking and children's respiratory diseases, *Int J Epidemiol* 17(2):348-355, 1988.

61. Woodward A, Douglas RM, Graham NM, and Miles H: Acute respiratory illness in Adelaide children: breast feeding modifies the effect of passive smoking, *J Epidemiol Comm Health* 44(3):224-230, 1990.

62. Wright AL, Holberg C, Martinez FD, and Taussig LM: Relationship of parental smoking to wheezing and nonwheezing lower respiratory tract illnesses in infancy. Group Health Medical Associates, *J Pediatr* 118(2):207-214, 1991.

63. Reese AC, James IR, Landau LI, and Lesouef PN: Relationship between urinary cotinine level and diagnosis in children admitted to hospital, *Am Rev Respir Dis* 146(1):66-70, 1992.

64. Weiss ST, Tager IB, Speizer FE, and Rosner B: Persistent wheeze: its relation to respiratory illness, cigarette smoking and level of pulmonary function in a population sample of children, *Am Rev Respir Dis* 122:697-707, 1980.

65. Charlton A: Children's coughs related to parental smoking, *Br Med J* 288:1647-1649, 1984.

66. Park JK and Kim IS: Effects of family smoking on acute respiratory disease in children, *Yonsei Med J* 27(4):261-270, 1986.

67. Bisgaard H, Dalgaard P, and Nyboe J: Risk factors for wheezing during infancy: a study of 5953 infants, *Acta Paediatr Scand* 76:719-726, 1987.

68. Andrae S, Axelson O, Bjorksten B, Fredriksson M, and Ljellman N-IM: Symptoms of bronchial hyperreactivity and asthma in relation to environmental factors, *Arch Dis Child* 63:473-478, 1988.

69. Somerville SM, Rona RJ, and Chinn S: Passive smoking and respiratory conditions in primary school children, *J Epidemiol Comm Health* 42(2):105-110, 1988.

70. Strachan DP: Damp housing and childhood asthma: validation of reporting of symptoms, *Br Med J* 297:1223-1226, 1988.

71. Neuspiel DR, Rush D, Butler NR, Golding J, Bijur PE, and Kurzon M: Parental smoking and post-infancy wheezing in children: a prospective cohort study, *Am J Public Health* 79(2):168-171, 1989.

72. Corbo GM, Fuciarelli F, Fousi A, and DeBenedetto F: Smoking in children: association with respiratory symptoms and passive smoking, *Br Med J* 299:1491-1494, 1989.

73. Ugnat AM, Mao Y, Miller AB, and Wigle DT: Effects of residential exposure to environmental tobacco smoke on Candian children, *Can J Pub Health* 81:345-349, 1990.

74. Dijkstra L, Houthuijs D, Brunekreef B, Akkerman I, and Boleij JSM: Respiratory health effects of the indoor environment in a population of Dutch children, *Am Rev Respir Dis* 142:1172-1178, 1990.

75. Forastiere F, Corbo GM, Michelozzi P, Pistelli R, Brancato G, Ciappi G, and Perucci CA: Effects of environment and passive smoking on the respiratory health of children, *Int J Epidemiol* 21:66-73, 1992.

76. Murray AB and Morrison BJ: It is children with atopic dermatitis who develop asthma more frequently if the mother smokes, *J Allergy Clin Immunol* 86:732-739, 1990.

77. Chan KN, Elliman A, Bryan E, and Silverman M: Respiratory symptoms in children of low birthweight, *Arch Dis Child* 64:1294-1304, 1989.

78. Tager IB, Hanrahan JP, Tosteson TD, Castile RG, Brown RW, Weiss ST, and Speizer FE: Lung function, pre- and post-natal smoke exposure, and wheezing in the first year of life, *Am Rev Respir Dis* 147:811-817, 1993.

79. Evans D, Levison J, Feldman CH, et al: The impact of passive smoking on emergency room visits of urban children with asthma, *Am Rev Respir Dis* 135:567-572, 1987.

80. Ehrlich R, Kattan M, Godbold J, Saltzberg DS, Grimm KT, Landrigan PJ, and Lilienfield DE: Childhood asthma and passive smoking. Urinary cotinine as a biomarker of exposure, *Am Rev Respir Dis* 145:594-599, 1992.

81. O'Connor GT, Weiss ST, Tager IB, and Speizer FE. The effect of passive smoking on pulmonary function and non-specific bronchial responsiveness in a population based sample of children and young adults, *Am Rev Respir Dis* 135:800-804, 1987.

82. Murray AB and Morrison BJ: Passive smoking by asthmatics: its greater effect on boys than on girls and on older than on younger children, *Pediatrics* 84:451-459, 1989.

83. Murray AB and Morrison BJ: The decrease in severity of asthma in children of parents who smoke since the parents have been exposing them to less cigarette smoke, *J Allergy Clin Immunol* 91:102-110, 1993.

84. Chilmonczyk BA, Salmon LM, Megathn KK, Neveux LM, Palomaki GE, Knight GJ, Polkkinen AJ, and Haddon JE: Association between exposure to environmental tobacco smoke and exacerbations of asthma in children, *N Engl J Med* 328:1665-1669, 1993.

85. Gortmaker SL, Walker DK, Jacobs FH, and Ruch-Ross H: Parental smoking and the risk of childhood asthma, *Am J Public Health* 72:572-579, 1992.

86. Horwood LJ, Fergusson DM, and Shannon FT: Social and familial factors in the development of early childhood asthma, *Pediatrics* 75:859-868, 1985.

87. Burchfield CM, Higgins MW, Keller MW, Howatt WF, Butler WJ, and Higgins ITT: Passive smoking in childhood - Respiratory conditions and pulmonary function in Tecumseh, Michigan, *Am Rev Respir Dis* 133:966-973, 1986.

88. Willers S, Svenonius E, and Skarping G: Passive smoking and childhood asthma, *Allergy* 46:330-334, 1991.

89. Weitzman M, Gortmaker S, Walker DK, and Sobol A: Maternal smoking and childhood asthma, *Pediatrics* 83:505-511, 1990.

90. Sherman CB, Tosteson TD, Tager IB, Speizer FE, and Weiss ST: Early childhood predictors of asthma, *Am J Epidemiol* 132:83-95, 1990.

91. Dekker C, Doles R, Bartlett S, Brunekreef B, and Zwanenberg H: Childhood asthma and the indoor environment, *Chest* 100:922-926, 1991.

92. Martinez FD, Cline M, and Burrows B: Increased incidence of asthma in children of smoking mothers, *Pediatrics* 89:21-26, 1992.

93. Weiss ST, Tager IB, Munoz A, and Speizer FE: The relationship of respiratory infections in early childhood to the occurrence of increased levels of bronchial responsiveness and atopy, *Am Rev Respir Dis* 131:573-578, 1985.

94. Murray AB and Morrison BJ: The effect of cigarette smoke from the mother on bronchial hyperresponsiveness and severity of symptoms in children with asthma, *J Allergy Clin Immunol* 77:575-581, 1986.

95. Corbo GM, Foresi A, Valente S, and Bustacchini S. Maternal smoking and bronchial responsiveness in children, *Am Rev Respir Dis* 127(suppl:245), 1987.

96. Strachan DP, Jarvis MJ, and Feyerabend C: The relationship of salivary cotinine to respiratory symptoms, spirometry, and exercise-induced bronchospasm in seven-year old children, *Am Rev Respir Dis* 142:147-151, 1990.

97. Martinez FD, Morgan WJ, Wright AL, Holberg CJ, and Taussig LM: Diminished lung function as a predisposing factor for wheezing lower respiratory tract illness in infants, *N Engl J Med* 319:1112-1117, 1988.

98. Forastiere F, Pistelli R, Michelozzi P, Corbo GM, Agabiti N, Bertillini R, Ciappi G, and Perucci CA: Indices of non-specific bronchial responsiveness in a pediatric population, *Chest* 100:927-934, 1991.

99. Young S, Arnott J, Stick SM, LeSoeuf PN, and Landau LI: The relationship between various measures of lung function and their association with lower respiratory symptoms in the first 12 months of life, *Am Rev Respir Dis* 145(4 pt 2):A660, 1992.

100. Tager IB, Weiss ST, Munoz A, Rosner B, and Speizer FE: Longitudinal study of the effects of maternal smoking on pulmonary function in children, *N Engl J Med* 309:699-703, 1983.

101. Vedal SE, Schenker MB, Samet JM, and Speizer FE: Risk factors for childhood respiratory disease, *Am Rev Respir Dis* 130:187-192, 1984.

102. Berkey CS, Dockery DW, Ferris BG Jr, Speizer FE, and Ware JH: Indoor air pollution and pulmonary function growth in preadolescent children, *Am J Epidemiol* 123(2):250-260, 1986.

103. Kauffmann F, Tager IB, Munoz A, and Speizer FE: Familial factors related to lung function in children aged 6-10 years: Results from the PAARC epidemiologic study, *Am J Epidemiol* 129(6):1289-1299, 1989.

104. Sherrill DL, Martinez FD, Lebowitz MD, et al: Longitudinal effects of passive smoking on pulmonary function in New Zealand children, *Am Rev Respir Dis* 45:1136-1141, 1992.

105. Hanrahan JP, Tager IB, Segal MR, Castile RG, Van Vunakis H, Weiss ST, and Speizer FE: The effect of maternal smoking during pregnancy on early infant lung function, *Am Rev Respir Dis* 145:1129-1135, 1992.

106. Holt PG: Immune and inflammatory function in cigarette smokers, *Thorax* 42:241-249, 1987.

107. Martinez FD, Antognoni G, Macri F, Bonci E, Midulla F, DeCastro G, and Ronchetti R: Parental smoking enhances bronchial responsiveness in nine-year old children, *Am Rev Respir Dis* 138:518-523, 1988.

108. Ronchetti R, Macri F, Ciofetta G, Indinnimeo L, Cutrera R, Bonci E, Antognoni G, and Martinez FD: Increased serum IgE and increased prevalence of eosinophilia in 9-year old children of smoking parents, *J Allergy Clin Immunol* 86:400-407, 1990.

109. Osaka F, Kasuga H, Sugita M, Matsuki H, and Miyake T: A study of the relationship between mite IgE in the serum of school children and smoking habits in mothers, *Nippon Eiseigaku Zasshi* 40(4):789-795, 1985.

110. Kjellman NI: Effect of parental smoking on IgE levels in children, *Lancet* 1(8227):993-934, 1981.

111. Ownby DR, Johnson CC, and Peterson EL: Maternal smoking does not influence cord serum IgE or IgD concentrations, *J Allergy Clin Immunol* 88:555-560, 1991.

112. Oryszczyn MP, Godin J, Annesi I, Hellier G, and Kauffmann F: In utero exposure to parental smoking, cotinine measurements, and cord blood IgE, *J Allergy Clin Immunol* 87:1169-1174, 1991.

113. Halonen M, Stern D, Lyle S, Wright A, Taussig L, and Martinez FD: Relationship of total serum IgE levels in cord and 9-month sera of infants, *Clin Exp Allergy* 21:235-241, 1991.

114. Iversen M, Birch L, Lundqvist GR, and Elbrond O: Middle ear effusion and the indoor environment, *Arch Environ Health* 40:74-79, 1985.

115. Black N: The etiology of glue ear — a case-control study, *Int J Pediatr Otorhinolaryngol* 9:121-133, 1985.

116. Pukander J, Luotonen J, Timinen J, and Karma P: Risk factors affecting the occurrence of acute otitis media among 2-3 year old urban children, *Acta Otolaryngol* 100:260-265, 1985.

117. Teale DW, Klein JO, and Rosner B: Epidemiology of otitis media during the first seven years of life in children in greater Boston: a prospective cohort study, *J Infect Dis* 160:83-94, 1989.

118. Strachan DP, Jarvis MJ, and Feyerabend C: Passive smoking, salivary cotinine concentrations, and middle ear effusion in 7 year old children, *Br Med J* 298:1549-1552, 1989.

119. Rowe-Jones JM and Brockbank MJ: Parental smoking and persistent otitis media with effusion in children, *Int J Pediatr Otorhinolaryngol* 24:19-24, 1992.

120. Etzel RA, Pattishall EN, Haley NJ, Fletcher RM, and Henderson FW: Passive smoking and middle ear effusion among children in day care, *Pediatrics* 90:228-232, 1992.

121. Rasmussen F: Protracted secretory otitis media. The impact of familial factors and day-care center attendance, *Int J Pediatr Otorhinolaryngol* 26:29-37, 1993.

122. Centers for Disease Control: Years of potential life lost before age 65 — United States, 1987, *MMWR* 38:27-28, 1989.

123. Steele R and Langworth JT: The relationship of antenatal and postnatal factors to sudden unexpected death in infancy, *Can Med Assoc J* 94:1165-1171, 1966.

124. Pershagen G, Hrubec Z, and Svensson C: Passive smoking and lung cancer in Swedish women. *Am J Epidemiol* 125:17-24, 1987.

125. Naeye RL, Ladis B, and Drage JS: Sudden infant death syndrome: a prospective study, *Am J Dis Child* 130:1207-1210, 1976.

126. Bergman AB and Wiesner BA: Relationship of passive cigarette smoking to sudden infant death syndrome, *Pediatrics* 58:665-668, 1976.

127. Malloy MH, Kleinman JC, Land GH, and Schramm WF: The association of maternal smoking with age and cause of infant death, *Am J Epidemiol* 128:46-55, 1988.

128. Hoffman HJ, Damus K, Hillman L, and Krongrad E: Risk factors for SIDS. Results of the National Institute of Child Health and Human Development SIDS Cooperative Epidemiological Study, *Ann NY Acad Sci* 533:13-30, 1988.

129. Haglund B and Cnattingius S: Cigarette smoking as a risk factor for sudden infant death syndrome: a population based study, *Am J Public Health* 80:29-32, 1990.

130. Mitchell EA, Scragg R, Stewart AW, et al: Results from the first year of the New Zealand cot death study, *N Z Med J* 104:71-76, 1991.

131. Schoendorf KC and Kiley JL: Relationship of sudden infant death syndrome to maternal smoking during and after pregnancy, *Pediatrics* 90:905-908, 1992.

Chapter 48

INDOOR AIR POLLUTION

William E. Lambert
Jonathan M. Samet

INDOOR AIR POLLUTION
The scope of the problem

Indoor air quality has been widely recognized as a public health concern only within the past 20 years.[1,2] This recognition followed the reduction of concentrations of outdoor air pollutants in many developed countries and research showing the dominant contribution of indoor exposures to total personal exposures for many pollutants.[1,2] Concurrently, rising energy costs prompted shifts in approaches to building design and operations to reduce air exchange rates, new synthetic materials became more widely used in construction, and new types of processes and equipment were introduced into nonindustrial workplaces. The recognition of indoor air pollution as a threat to public health soon extended to less developed countries where reliance on biomass fuels for heating and cooking leads to widespread exposure to smoke.[3]

The common presence of indoor pollution sources causes nearly everyone to be exposed to air pollutants in residences, public and commercial buildings, and transportation environments. Indoor pollution sources include combustion-driven appliances, such as gas-fueled cooking ranges and furnaces, tobacco smoking, furnishings and construction materials that emit organic gases and vapors, and asbestos-containing and other types of fibrous materials that release fibers into the air when they are disturbed or inadequately maintained. Radon gas present in soils can enter buildings through the foundation. Allergens and biologic agents in indoor air include animal dander, fecal material from house dust mites and other insects, fungal spores, and bacteria. In addition to these indoor sources, pollutants in outdoor air are brought into the indoor environment by natural and mechanical ventilation.

The responses of the respiratory system to indoor air pollution are diverse, ranging from acute irritation and bronchoconstriction to chronic inflammation, fibrosis, and cancer. The impact of these responses can range from slight but measurable physiologic impairment to frank disability and disease, depending on the agent, the level of exposure, and the inherent susceptibility of the exposed person. The effects of air pollutants have been characterized through multidisciplinary approaches, typically involving in vitro and in vivo laboratory studies, controlled human exposure studies, and epidemiologic investigations.

Risk assessment has been increasingly applied to estimate the burden of disease associated with indoor air pollution, particularly for respiratory carcinogens—environmental tobacco smoke (ETS), radon, and asbestos. The process of *quantitative risk assessment* was defined by a National Research Council committee as the "quantitative characterization of the potential health effects of particular substances on individuals or populations."[4] Risk assessments performed on radon, asbestos, and ETS have followed the general four-step process outlined by the National Research Council. The first step is hazard identification; that is, agents posing risks are identified through animal bioassays, controlled human studies, and epidemiologic investigations. Mechanisms of toxicity and factors placing particular groups at special risk for adverse health effects are also identified. Second, the dose–response relation is established to quantify the risk per unit of exposure. Third, the magnitude and frequency of population exposures are determined. In the fourth step, the dose–response relation is combined with the exposure data to estimate the magnitude and distribution of health effects in the population. As will be made clear by the risk assessments reviewed in this chapter, uncertainties are inherent in this process. Quantitative risk assessment requires systematic consideration of uncertainties and attendant assumptions; nevertheless, it offers a guide to the relative magnitudes of environmental pollutants.

This chapter reviews the evidence on health effects for the principal indoor pollutants: the two combustion-related pollutants, carbon monoxide (CO) and nitrogen dioxide (NO_2), ETS, wood smoke, volatile organic compounds (VOCs), asbestos and man-made mineral fibers, radon, and biologic agents. This chapter begins by addressing the concept of total personal exposure and establishing a framework within which to consider the health effects associated with exposure to indoor air pollution. Next the authors review the sources and typical concentrations of indoor pollutants, their health effects, clinical manifestations, and the opportunities for their control. Finally, the authors consider the implications of the evidence for clinicians whose concern is the care of individual patients and, on a broader level, for readers concerned with the public health.

The scope of this chapter is necessarily limited; however, more comprehensive treatments of some of these pollutants are given in several recent books[5-7] and reviews.[8]

Total personal exposure

Patterns of activity and time use throughout the day place individuals in diverse indoor and outdoor environments, each of which may have its particular set of air contaminants. The total personal exposure to the pollutants can be conceptualized as representing the time-weighted average pollutant concentration in each of these settings, termed microenvironments,[9] in the "microenvironmental model,"

$$E = \sum c_i t_i$$

where E, the total integrated exposure of an individual to a particular pollutant, is the sum of the products of c_i, the average concentration in the ith "microenvironment" (or setting), and t_i, the time spent in the ith microenvironment. The principal microenvironments contributing to total exposure are those with relatively high concentrations or in which relatively large amounts of time are spent. For an office worker, the key microenvironments contributing to total personal exposure might be home, office, and car; for a child, they may be home, school, and outdoor settings.

Studies of time–activity patterns show that residents of more developed countries spend more time indoors than outdoors, and their personal exposure to many pollutants occurs predominantly indoors. Data from the benchmark study of time use conducted by Alexander Szalai and colleagues in 12 countries during the late 1960s indicated that people spend an average of 65% to 70% of their time inside their residences, and more than 90% of their time indoors, either at home, work, or elsewhere.[10] Patterns of time use do not appear to have changed substantially during the past 20 years. A population-based survey of California residents conducted in 1987 and 1988 estimated that employed adults averaged 15 hours per day indoors at home and an additional 6 hours per day in other indoor settings, primarily commercial and institutional buildings.[11] School-age children (ages 2 to 11 years) averaged more time outdoors each day, but still spent an average of 18 hours indoors at home and 2 hours indoors at school or in child care.[12] The survey also considered time spent in proximity to sources of indoor air pollution. Of nonsmoking respondents to the survey, 61% of adults and 64% of youths aged 12 to 17 years reported exposure to ETS at some time during the day. For respondents of all ages, 39% were reported as being in a room with an operating gas stove, and 30% in a room heated by a gas furnace; 27% of adults reported using cleaning agents, 12% reported using solvents, 7% reported using pesticides, 5% reported using latex paints, and 5% reported using oil-based paints. These data clearly demonstrate that individuals are frequently in close proximity indoors to appliances or products that generate pollution.

Outdoor air pollution. Although indoor sources are mainly responsible for the concentrations of some indoor pollutants, outdoor air pollution can also impact the quality of indoor air. Through the processes of infiltration and ventilation, mass air movements from outdoors can carry pollutants indoors. Infiltration may occur naturally as a consequence of the flow of outdoor air through windows, doors, vents, and unintentional openings (e.g., joints and cracks). This movement of air is caused by the dynamic pressure of the wind and the buoyant forces resulting from indoor and outdoor temperature differences (i.e., stack effect). In residences, opened windows and doors are the usual sources of ventilation. Mechanical ventilation may also be used in residences and is the most common means for supplying fresh air and heating and cooling in commercial and institutional buildings.

Indoor levels of nonreactive pollutants, such as CO and fine particles, are essentially at equilibrium with outdoor levels.[13] However, many outdoor pollutants, such as ozone (O_3), sulfur dioxide (SO_2), NO_2, and coarse suspended particles (including pollen and spores) are reactive, and their concentrations fall when they enter indoor spaces from outside because of chemical and physical interaction with building surfaces and ventilation systems. For example, levels of NO_2 due to outdoor sources in a residence are approximately one-half of levels outdoors,[14] O_3 levels range from 10% to 80% of outdoor levels,[15,16] and concentrations of particles of aerodynamic diameter 2 to 10 μm range from 10% to 50% of outdoor levels.[13] Findings of indoor–outdoor ratios higher than unity for these latter pollutants can be explained by the presence of indoor sources. Because outdoor air is the source for ventilation to dilute the emissions of indoor pollution sources, outdoor air with pollutant concentrations above acceptable levels for indoor air quality must be cleaned before it can be used for ventilation. Although the number of areas that are not in attainment of National Ambient Air Quality Standards has declined dramatically since the mid-1970s, many heavily populated areas remain in "nonattainment" for one or more pollutants. In 1987, 98 counties (representing 107 communities and 135 million people) were classified by the U.S. Environmental Protection Agency (EPA) as nonattainment areas for O_3.[17]

Adverse effects of indoor air pollution

The spectrum of adverse responses to indoor air pollution is broad, ranging from acute and dramatic exposures that may lead to death to far more subtle responses that may affect well-being. Judgment as to the adversity of these responses is societal and is likely to vary as it reflects prevalent views. Concepts of health have been variable across history, changing in response to societal expectations and understanding of the nature and causes of disease. The World Health Organization (WHO) has described health as "a state of complete physical, mental, and social well-being, and not merely the absence of disease or infirmity." If the broad construct of health explicit in this definition is accepted, then adverse effects of air pollution include not only clinically evident disease but also more subtle symptomatic and physiologic responses that compromise well-being and increase risk of disease.

Any definition of an "adverse health effect" is also made in the context of prevalent societal values. The need to define this context has been made clear in interpreting the language of the Clean Air Act in the United States. Although the Clean Air Act uses the term, "adverse health effect," its failure to offer an explicit definition and the boundary between "adverse" and "nonadverse" has been a subject of controversy. A committee of the American Thoracic Society (ATS)[18] offered guidelines in a 1985 report on what constitutes an adverse respiratory health effect in epidemiologic data and implicitly focused on outdoor air pollution. The committee defined adverse respiratory health effects as "medically significant physiologic or pathologic changes generally evidenced by one or more of the following: (1) interference with the normal activity of the affected person or persons, (2) episodic respiratory illness, (3) incapacitating illness, (4) permanent respiratory injury, and (5) progressive respiratory dysfunction." The committee report noted that all changes are not adverse, and described a spectrum of response extending from pollution exposure through mortality. In this continuum, the boundary between adverse and nonadverse effects was placed between "physiologic changes of uncertain significance" and "pathophysiologic changes."

Increased risk for cancer estimated by risk assessment methods has not been addressed in defining an adverse health effect. The increased risks for cancer estimated for individuals exposed to carcinogens have no detectable correlates at present and the ultimate manifestation, malignancy, is discrete. Varying susceptibility to indoor pollutants further complicates any schema for classifying adverse health effects. Responses to indoor air pollutants are not uniform within populations. The term "susceptible" has most often been applied to groups of people who share one or more characteristics that place them at increased risk compared with people without these characteristics. Even within a susceptible group, a range of susceptibility can be assumed for many determinants of susceptibility and environmental agents. Many susceptibility factors are potentially relevant to indoor air pollution; for example, the underlying degree of airways responsiveness or the presence of asthma, the presence of cardiac or vascular disease, abnormal lung function and the presence of chronic obstructive pulmonary disease, the presence of atopy, and inherently increased risk for respiratory cancer.

A spectrum of health responses to indoor air pollution can be identified. The box on the next page provides a classification of these responses that can be applied by clinicians and researchers to bring a conceptual structure for ap-

---

A classification of the adverse effects of indoor air pollution

Clinically evident diseases: Diseases for which the usual methods of clinical evaluation can establish a causal link to an indoor air pollutant.

Exacerbation of disease: The clinical status of already established disease is exacerbated by indoor air pollution.

Increased risk for diseases: Diseases for which epidemiologic or other evidence establishes increased risk in exposed individuals. However, the usual clinical methods indicative of injury typically cannot establish the causal link in an individual patient.

Physiological impairment: Transient or persistent effects on a measure of physiologic functioning that are of insufficient magnitude to cause clinical disease.

Symptom responses: Subjectively reported responses that can be linked to indoor pollutants or are attributed to indoor pollutants.

Perception of unacceptable indoor air quality: Sensing of indoor air quality as uncomfortable to an unacceptable degree.

Perception of exposure to indoor air pollutants: Awareness of exposure to one or more pollutants with an unacceptable level of concern about exposure.

Adapted from Samet (1993).[169]

proaching the general problem of indoor air pollution and health. The categories include disease, impairment, symptoms, increased risk, and perceptions.

Clinically evident disease. In the case of a clinically evident disease, such as CO poisoning, hypersensitivity pneumonitis, *Legionella* pneumonia, and cat- and mite-induced asthma, a link can be established to an indoor pollutant by specific diagnostic tests. Although exposures to indoor air pollutants associated with these illnesses are universal, clinically evident cases of pollution-related disease appear to be relatively infrequent. For example, an appropriate clinical picture and an elevated serum precipitin titer are sufficient to document hypersensitivity pneumonitis due to thermophilic actinomycetes contaminating an air conditioning system.[19] In a classification of illnesses associated with public and commercial building environments, the category of hypersensitivity pneumonitis has been referred to as specific building-related illnesses.[20,21] However, the distinction between specific building-related illnesses and the nonspecific syndrome referred to as sick (or tight) building syndrome rests only on the ability to establish a clinical diagnosis. The occurrence of building-related illnesses is not limited to commercial environments.

Exacerbation of established disease. Conditions that may be exacerbated by indoor air pollution are common in the general population. Asthma, for example, affects approximately 5% to 10% of children and adults. The estab-

lished diseases of concern include asthma, chronic obstructive pulmonary disease, cystic fibrosis, and cardiovascular disease.

Increased risk for disease. Many pollutants in indoor air are associated with increased risk for a variety of malignant and nonmalignant diseases. The evidence supporting the relationships between exposures to these agents and increased risk comes from epidemiologic studies, short-term exposures of volunteer subjects, animal studies, and in vitro toxicologic studies. The population burden of disease attributable to such agents is often estimated using quantitative risk assessment. The problem of indoor radon and lung cancer, discussed subsequently, is illustrative.

Physiologic impairment. Exposures to indoor pollutants can impair physiologic functioning, although not to a degree necessarily associated with disability or disease. For example, exposure to ETS during childhood reduces the rate of lung growth and the maximum level of lung function,[22,23] but the average estimated effect would not be clinically detectable or associated with reduced functional capacity.[24] Similarly, low levels of CO exposure transiently impair oxygen delivery to tissues, but their impact on exercise capacity in healthy individuals is limited and would be manifest only during maximal activity[25]; on the other hand, reduced oxygen transport in individuals with coronary artery disease may increase the likelihood of clinically significant myocardial ischemia.[26]

Symptom responses. Epidemiologic evidence links specific indoor air pollutants to a variety of symptoms. Environmental tobacco smoke exposure is associated with increased risk of respiratory symptoms in children.[22] The sick-building syndrome is a nonspecific constellation of symptoms characteristically affecting several occupants of a building.[27]

Perception of unacceptable indoor air quality. To the extent that unacceptable indoor air quality reduces wellbeing, the perception of indoor air quality as unacceptable should be classified as an adverse health effect in the context of current concepts of health. Judgments of the acceptability of indoor air quality presumably integrate several characteristics of the air, including the presence of odor and irritants, humidity, air movement, and temperature.[28,29] Undoubtedly, there are ranges of responses and of expectations across the population. Physical and psychological aspects of the environment not directly related to indoor air quality may also influence judgments as to the acceptability of indoor air quality.

Perception of exposure to indoor air pollutants. The perception of exposure to indoor pollutants should also be regarded as an adverse health effect if it reduces well-being. The range of responses to the perception of exposure is broad, extending from annoyance because of an odor to cases of the often disabling symptom complex now frequently referred to as "multiple chemical sensitivity."

INDOOR POLLUTANTS AND HEALTH EFFECTS
Carbon monoxide

Sources and concentrations. Carbon monoxide is a by-product of the combustion of carbonaceous fuels, including gasoline, natural gas, oil, coal, wood, and tobacco. The principal outdoor sources of CO in the urban environment are automobiles. Surveys of urban population exposures conducted by the U.S. EPA in Denver, Colorado, and Washington, D.C., indicate that residential exposures to CO are generally low, ranging from 2 to 4 ppm during the winter when homes are closed up and heating is necessary.[30] Although these levels are low, the effects of indoor sources are still detectable. In Denver, living in homes with gas cooking ranges was associated with slightly higher levels of personal exposure (34% increase), as was living with smokers (84% increase). Measurements of CO in commercial and institutional buildings in the Denver and Washington, D.C. surveys indicated mean concentrations of 3.0 and 1.9 ppm, respectively. These levels are typical of offices without smoking activity, but during smoking the levels may reach 10 ppm.[22] The presence of CO in residences and public buildings that do not have unvented sources of combustion is largely due to motor vehicle exhaust in outdoor air entering the building through natural and mechanical ventilation. Because CO is nonreactive, indoor–outdoor ratios are generally near one. Although CO levels are generally low in residential and public buildings, elevated levels are sometimes found in commercial buildings with drive-up operations (e.g., banks), buildings with underground parking garages,[31] and enclosed ice rinks with propane-powered ice resurfacing machines.[32] The use of charcoal briquettes for indoor heating has been associated with accidental CO poisonings.[33]

Health effects. Odorless, colorless, and tasteless, carbon monoxide gas is a particularly insidious toxicant. About 900 accidental deaths in the United States are attributed annually to asphyxiation by CO inhalation.[34] Although the majority of these deaths occur from the operation of motor vehicles, some deaths occur in residences and a small proportion occur in public buildings having faulty or unvented or improperly ventilated combustion sources like charcoal briquettes.[33]

Inhaled CO avidly binds to hemoglobin, with affinity more than 200 times greater than oxygen, to form carboxyhemoglobin (COHb). The COHb complex is very stable; depending on ambient levels of CO, the half life of CO in the body ranges from 2.5 to 4 hours. The rate of accumulation of CO in the body above endogenous levels is influenced by ambient CO concentrations, alveolar ventilation, lung diffusivity, total hemoglobin mass, and COHb level.[35] Breathing rates and temporal patterns of ambient CO exposure dominate the flux of CO in the body. For these physiologic reasons, anemic individuals will tend to develop elevated COHb levels more rapidly than normal, and people with impaired gas exchange (e.g., persons with chronic ob-

structive pulmonary disease) have compromised capability of eliminating vascular stores of CO.

The binding of CO to hemoglobin reduces oxygen transport by red blood cells to tissues. The binding of CO to hemoglobin directly displaces oxygen and further induces an allosteric change in the hemoglobin molecule that impedes the dissociation of oxygen carried by adjacent heme groups on the hemoglobin molecule.[36] Other mechanisms of toxicity have been postulated and include the binding of CO to heme proteins such as myoglobin and cytochrome oxidase.[37,38] It is not known whether the binding of CO to these intracellular heme proteins could be significant enough to reduce oxygen transport in sensitive tissues, such as the heart and brain, or to interfere with electron transport and phosphorylation of adenosine diphosphate. The tissue hypoxia induced by COHb is presently the most widely accepted mechanism of toxic action.

It follows that the level of CO in the blood is a valid biomarker of dose, and the health effects of exposure to CO can be described relative to COHb levels. In nonsmoking individuals not exposed to environmental CO, COHb levels are approximately 0.5%. This endogenous level of COHb results from the catabolism of hemoglobin and heme-containing enzymes of the liver. In comparison, COHb levels of cigarette smokers range from 4% to 10%. Frank carbon monoxide poisoning, as manifest in headache, loss of motor control, and coma, generally occurs with COHb levels above 20%.

Clinicians have recently advanced the concept of "occult" CO poisoning, which results from persistent exposure to low levels of CO in indoor environments. Headache and dizziness, early symptoms of CO poisoning, have been associated with COHb levels greater than 10%, with self-reports of problems with gas furnaces in residences and with the use of gas stoves for heating.[39,40] These studies suggest that occult CO poisoning explains 3% to 5% of emergency room patient complaints of headache and dizziness during the winter season. The prevalence of occult CO poisoning from public access buildings is unknown, but due to the smaller proportion of time spent in this type of building, it should be lower. The clinician should be alert to the possibility of CO poisoning at COHb levels lower than those often presented in tables that describe the spectrum of symptoms.

Health effects have been demonstrated at levels of exposure much lower than those causing frank poisoning. Elevated COHb levels resulting from indoor exposures may at times extend into the range where clinical testing has demonstrated cardiovascular and neurobehavioral effects. Reductions in maximal oxygen consumption and exercise time occur in normal young men at COHb levels near 5%.[41] Individuals with cardiovascular disease are generally considered to be at greatest risk for CO exposure. Standard exercise tests on subjects with ischemic heart disease have demonstrated a decreased time interval to the onset of angina at COHb levels ranging from 2% to 6%.[26,42] In addition to myocardial ischemia, aggravation of ventricular arrhythmias has been investigated in controlled human exposure studies. Experimental elevation of COHb levels in patients with ischemic heart disease and chronic ventricular ectopy has not increased the rate of single or repetitive ventricular ectopic beats.[43,44] The 1-hour 35 ppm and 8-hour 9 ppm federal standards for outdoor air were selected to prevent COHb levels from rising above 1.5%, thereby protecting individuals with ischemic heart disease from aggravation of myocardial ischemia and loss of exercise capacity. Epidemiologic evidence on the relationship between CO exposure and incidence of cardiorespiratory complaints including angina is limited and is potentially biased by inaccurate measures of personal exposure. Some evidence also suggests prenatal effects at low levels of COHb.[45]

Nitrogen dioxide

Sources and concentrations. NO_2 is produced by high-temperature combustion processes, in which elemental nitrogen, present in air, is oxidized. Sources of NO_2 include the automobile, gasoline engines, and in the home, gas-fueled appliances. In the United States, with the exception of a few urban areas where outdoor NO_2 levels are high, indoor environments are the predominant determinant of total personal exposure.[46,47] In particular, residential exposures from unvented gas cooking stoves and kerosene space heaters are the key contributors to total personal exposure. Approximately 60% of the 90 million residences in the United States have gas-fueled cooking stoves (U.S. Census, 1990) and over 10 million or more households were estimated to use kerosene space heaters for heating in 1985.[48] Although vented, gas furnaces and water heaters may pollute residences because of flue-gas spillage and backdrafting caused by improper installation, maintenance, and weather conditions.[48] Residential NO_2 levels have been characterized in many regions of the United States. Indoor NO_2 levels are generally increased during the winter periods when ventilation is reduced to conserve heating energy. During the winter, average indoor concentrations of NO_2 in homes with gas cooking stoves are one-half to two times higher than outdoor levels. For example, in Albuquerque, New Mexico, indoor levels averaged 24 ppb in the bedroom and 34 ppb in the kitchen, and outdoor levels averaged 15 ppb.[49] In homes with electric cooking stoves, indoor levels averaged 7 ppb, reflecting the penetration of outdoor NO_2 and reaction with structural surfaces. During cooking, transient elevations on the order of 1000 ppb and lasting for 20 to 60 minutes have been documented by continuous monitoring.[50] Some of the highest indoor NO_2 concentrations have been measured in small city apartments and in residences where the oven was used for space heating. Limited data are available on NO_2 levels associated with unvented kerosene and gas-fired space heaters. Concentrations vary with the home air space volume, air exchange rate, operat-ing time, and number of heaters in use. In homes monitored in New Haven, Connecticut, NO_2 levels averaged 20 ppb in homes with one kerosene space heater and 37 ppb in those with two. Nitrogen dioxide and other flue gas may spill or backdraft into living spaces. Data on NO_2 levels in commercial and institutional buildings are very limited, reflecting the lack of indoor sources and low potential for induction of symptoms and illness. In 44 offices assessed by Weber and Fischer[51] under varied smoking conditions, NO_2 levels averaged 10 ppb. Several studies of buildings show that high outdoor levels of NO_2 may be reflected indoors.[52] In several descriptions of diagnostic evaluations of public buildings, high concentrations of NO_2 have not been found.[53] However, elevated NO_2 levels have been repeatedly observed in enclosed ice skating rinks, which are contaminated by emissions from diesel-powered resurfacing machines.[54]

Health effects (see Chapter 49). Nitrogen dioxide is an oxidant gas that is soluble in tissues. Studies of the uptake of this gas in the respiratory system show that most inhaled NO_2 is retained in the lungs and deposited primarily in the large and small airways, with little deposition in the alveoli. Because of its degree of tissue solubility, NO_2 reacts not only with the alveolar epithelium but with the interstitium and endothelium of the pulmonary capillaries. Inhaled NO_2 is thought to combine with water in the lung to form nitric (HNO_3) and nitrous (HNO_2) acids, although substantial uncertainty remains concerning the reactions of tissue with NO_2.[55]

Oxidant injury has been postulated to be the principal mechanism by which NO_2 damages the lung. At high concentrations, NO_2 causes extensive lung injury in animals and in humans. Fatal pulmonary edema and bronchopneumonia have been reported at extremely high concentrations; lower concentrations are associated with bronchitis, bronchiolitis, and pneumonia.

Experimental evidence indicates that NO_2 exposure adversely affects lung defense mechanisms.[56] Lung defense mechanisms against inhaled particles and gases include aerodynamic filtration, mucociliary clearance, particle transport and detoxification by alveolar macrophages, and local and systemic immunity. In experimental models, NO_2 reduces the efficacy of several of these lung defense mechanisms; effects on mucociliary clearance, the alveolar macrophage, and the immune system have been demonstrated. The findings in some experimental models, however, do not imply adverse effects of NO_2 on lung defenses.

In animal experiments involving challenge with respiratory pathogens, exposure to NO_2 reduces clearance of infecting organisms and increases the mortality of the experimental animals. In these infectivity models, the pathogens have most often been bacteria, although viruses have also been used. The viral exposure studies have generally, but not uniformly, suggested an adverse effect of NO_2 exposure on the outcome of infection.[57] Adverse effects in these animal experiments have been demonstrated at concentrations an order of magnitude greater than those typically found in indoor environments.

The health effects of NO_2 have been investigated using controlled exposures of volunteers in the laboratory and with epidemiologic approaches in the community setting, largely directed at the consequences of exposures indoors for children. The toxicology of NO_2 implies that a wide variety of health effects are of potential concern including reduced efficiency of host defenses against infectious organisms, exacerbation of asthma and chronic obstructive pulmonary disease, and respiratory tract inflammation with manifestations of respiratory symptoms and lung function. In spite of extensive investigation using laboratory and epidemiological approaches, the evidence remains inconclusive in regard to each of these health outcomes.

The hypothesis that NO_2 increases risk for respiratory infection has been tested primarily with epidemiologic studies, but laboratory approaches have also been devised. A number of epidemiologic studies have compared the occurrence of respiratory infection in children in homes having gas stoves and higher concentrations of NO_2 with that in children in homes with electric stoves and lower concentrations of NO_2.[58,59] The findings of these studies have been inconsistent—the inconsistency largely reflecting the methodologic complexities of investigating this association.[59] A recent prospective study involved over 1200 infants who were followed from birth through 18 months of age with monitoring for illnesses and exposure to NO_2.[49] Neither incidence of lower respiratory illnesses nor the duration of the illnesses was associated with exposure to NO_2. Experimental exposures have also failed to provide consistent evidence that NO_2 increases infectivity in humans.[60]

Inflammation of the airways by NO_2 could plausibly be associated with increased respiratory symptoms and reduced lung function. These potential adverse effects of NO_2 have been examined using data from epidemiologic studies of children and adults.[59,61] Many of these studies have included large numbers of participants studied cross-sectionally. The health outcome measures (e.g., reports of symptoms and levels of spirometric lung function) have been compared for participants living in homes with NO_2 sources such as gas stoves and space heaters and participants living in homes without such sources. In spite of the multiplicity of such studies, there has not been a clear pattern of effect; the evidence has been similarly inconsistent from brief experimental exposures, although high levels of NO_2 can cause clinically significant lung damage.[59]

The deposition of NO_2 in the airways of persons with lung disease might worsen clinical status by inducing inflammation or invoking irritant responses. Persons with asthma have a chronic inflammatory process associated with increased responsiveness of the airways to environmental stimuli, and NO_2 could plausibly worsen this process. Short-term effects of NO_2 exposures on asthmatics have been studied by exposing volunteers and measuring pulmonary function and nonspecific airways responsiveness. An important early study[62] showed that some asthmatics had increased airways responsiveness following experimental exposure to NO_2 at concentrations found in some urban and indoor environments. However, subsequent evidence has been conflicting[59] and the findings are limited because of the selection of relatively mild asthmatics in most studies. Only a few studies have addressed NO_2 exposure and the status of persons with chronic obstructive pulmonary disease. At this time, the NO_2 exposures typically found in indoor and outdoor environments have minimal clinical implications for most persons with asthma.

Environmental tobacco smoke

Sources and concentrations. Although the prevalence of smoking has decreased to approximately 26% in the United States,[63] smoking remains a common activity in public places and homes. The available data on ETS exposure for nonsmokers and children are very limited but suggest widespread exposures to ETS. For example, nationally based survey data indicate approximately 42% of children, 5 years of age and younger, live in households with smokers.[64] If smokers are present in the home, exposures received indoors at home may dominate total personal exposures of involuntary smokers for particles and some gaseous pollutants, such as benzene.[65] Environmental tobacco smoke is a term now widely used to refer to the combination of sidestream smoke that is released from the cigarette's burning end and the mainstream smoke exhaled by the smoker. Hundreds of chemical compounds have been identified in cigarette smoke and the indicators most often used to quantify its presence in the environment are respirable suspended particles (RSP) (particles of mean aerodynamic diameter of less than 2.5 μm), CO, and nicotine, which is in the vapor phase of ETS.[23,66] Nicotine is a highly specific marker for the presence of tobacco smoke; it can be monitored using both active and passive techniques. Largely because RSP can be readily monitored with area and personal sampling methods, level of RSP has been widely used as a marker for ETS. Data on RSP levels in households in six U.S. cities indicated that a one-pack-a-day smoker contributes approximately 20 μg/m³ to 24-hour average indoor RSP concentrations.[67] The personal exposures of nonsmokers living with smokers is raised to an average of 64 μg/m³ per 24 hours from 36 μg/m³ per 24 hours[68] by the presence of smokers. Higher short-term exposures must occur in homes when smoking is taking place that are not reflected in these longer-term integrated measurements. Limited data are available on ETS levels in public buildings.[66] Short-term measurements, integrated over 15-minute intervals in bowling alleys, cocktail parties, and a bar, indicate that RSP concentrations can be as high as 200 to 350 μg/m³.[69] In the smoking and no-smoking sections of seven restaurants in Albuquerque, median concentrations of RSP were 53 and 28 μg/m³, respectively, averaged over two lunch and dinner periods.[70] Peak concentrations as high as 1000 μg/m³ have been observed in the smoking sections of airliners.[71]

Health effects. The adverse effects of ETS have been assessed in the context of the voluminous evidence on active smoking and health and of the detailed characterizations that have been made of the composition and toxicology of mainstream and sidestream cigarette smoke (see Chapter 47). Diverse associations of ETS with disease and other adverse outcomes have been demonstrated (see box). The evidence has now been reviewed by a number of expert panels with the repeated finding that ETS causes both malignant and nonmalignant diseases in nonsmokers.[22,23,72,73]

Studies of the children of smoking parents provided the first warning of the adverse effects of ETS on nonsmokers. Maternal smoking was found to increase risk of infants for lower respiratory tract illnesses, and smoking by household members, particularly the mother, was shown to increase the incidence of chronic respiratory symptoms and reduce the rate of lung growth in children.[22,23] More recently, additional adverse effects of ETS on children have been found. Children with asthma whose parents smoke have heightened airways responsiveness[74] and increased morbidity, as documented by indexes of medical care utilization.[23] Exposure to ETS is also a suspect cause of asthma,[23,75] and infants of smoking parents have increased airways responsiveness shortly after birth.[76] Epidemiologic studies also show that parental smoking is associated with persistent middle ear effusions.[23]

Exposure to ETS was first linked to lung cancer in nonsmokers in two reports published in 1981.[77,78] Subsequently, numerous epidemiologic studies of either case-control or cohort design have addressed this association.[23,79] Living with a cigarette-smoking spouse has been the principal exposure variable in these studies, although exposure to ETS in the workplace has been addressed in some studies. Inevitably, exposure measures based on such simple contrasts as spouses of smokers versus spouses of nonsmokers introduce misclassification, but these measures do define groups with greater and lesser exposures. Nevertheless, the weight of the evidence shows a positive association between living with a smoker and risk of lung cancer. In a 1992 risk assessment published by the U.S. EPA,[23] 30 epidemiologic studies were reviewed. The number of studies showing a positive association exceeded the expectation based on chance, and pooled estimates by country of study indicated increased risk for all regions except China (Fig. 48-1). The positive association could not be completely explained by potential sources of bias including confounding and differential misclassification of smoking status (never or ever smoking). It has been argued that the association could reflect misclassification of smoking status in the context of aggregation of spouses by smoking,[80] but assessments of this potential bias have shown that it cannot account for the observed association.[23,73]

Based on review of the epidemiologic evidence as well as the supporting toxicological data, the Environmental Protection Agency classified ETS as a class A carcinogen, a designation applied to agents causally linked to cancer.[23] This designation mirrored the earlier conclusions of the International Agency for Research on Cancer (1986), the U.S. Surgeon General,[22] and the U.S. National Research Council.[73] The U.S. EPA estimated that ETS exposure causes approximately 2000 lung cancer deaths annually in never smokers.[23]

Additional health effects of ETS remain under investigation. A number of epidemiologic studies have shown that

---

Established and potential health effects of involuntary exposure to tobacco smoke

Established

    Increased lower respiratory infections in children
    Increased respiratory symptoms in children
    Reduced lung growth in children
    Increased lung cancer risk in nonsmokers
    Irritation of the eyes, nose, throat, and lower respiratory tract

Potential

    Increased respiratory symptoms in adults
    Reduced lung function in adults
    Increased risk for asthma
    Exacerbation of asthma
    Increased risk for cardiovascular disease
    Increased risk for nonrespiratory cancers
    Earlier age at menopause
    Increased risk for sudden infant death
    Reduced birth weight

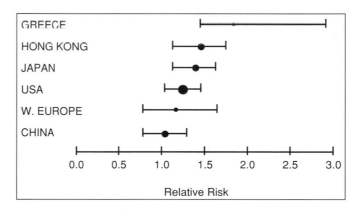

Fig. 48-1. Relative risks of lung cancer and living with a smoker by country. Point estimates of relative risk and 90% confidence intervals. (From U.S. Environmental Protection Agency: *Respiratory health effects of passive smoking: lung cancer and other disorders* [EPA/600/6-90/006F], Washington, DC, 1992, U.S. Environmental Protection Agency.)

marriage to a smoker increases risk for ischemic heart disease.[81,82] Although the evidence is not so extensive as for the respiratory consequences of ETS exposure, the American Heart Association has concluded that ETS exposure is a major preventable cause of cardiovascular disease and death.[83] The Council on Cardiopulmonary and Critical Care of the American Heart Association offered the estimate that 35,000 to 40,000 cardiovascular disease-related deaths occur annually due to ETS exposure. Cited mechanisms include promotion of atherosclerosis, increased platelet aggregation, endothelial cell damage, and the consequences of carbon monoxide exposure. ETS exposure at home and in the workplace has been linked to reduced lung function in some studies.[84] Other proposed associations of ETS with disease include increased risk for cancers at sites other than the lung, younger age at menopause, increased risk for sudden infant death syndrome, reduced birth weight, and worsening of cystic fibrosis.[84]

Wood smoke

Sources and concentrations. Measurements of wood smoke in indoor settings are very limited. The presence of wood smoke indoors can be assessed by measurements of particles, organic compounds, and CO. Moschandreas and co-workers[85] measured total and respirable-sized particle levels in two homes with fireplaces and one home with a wood-burning stove. Indoor levels of total suspended particles and RSP were four times as high on days when wood burning occurred. Concentrations of RSP ranged from 14 to 72 $\mu g/m^3$ in the home with the wood stove and averaged 68 and 160 $\mu g/m^3$ in the two homes with fireplaces. In the home with the wood stove, benzo[a]pyrene concentrations averaged 5 ng/m^3 on a day with wood burning, representing a fivefold increase over days when the stove was not used; higher concentrations were observed in one of the homes with a fireplace, averaging 11.4 ng/m^3. During starting, stoking, and reloading the wood stove, CO levels increased from 1 to 5 ppm indoors. In a study of indoor air quality in a Vermont community where wood burning is the most common means of residential heating, measurements of RSP were made in 19 homes with wood-burning appliances and 5 homes without.[86] No statistical difference was observed comparing 24-hour average RSP levels in homes where wood was burned and homes with other types of heating. These findings suggest that the operations of a wood stove do not directly affect indoor air quality and that outdoor air contaminated with wood smoke of neighbors can enter and pollute the interior air of homes without wood stoves.

Health effects. Wood smoke is an extremely complex mixture, both in its physical and chemical characteristics and in its toxicologic properties. The toxicology of some components of wood smoke, such as benzo[a]pyrene, other polycyclic organic compounds, and nitrogen oxides, has been extensively studied. Little research, however, has addressed the toxicology of wood smoke as a complex mixture.

In vitro experiments demonstrate that emissions from a wood stove induce sister chromatid exchange and are mutagenic,[87] as assessed by the Ames *Salmonella* assay.[88,89] A few studies with animal models indicate respiratory effects of wood smoke. Fick and colleagues[90] exposed rabbits to Douglas fir wood smoke and then obtained respiratory tract cells by bronchoalveolar lavage. Significantly more cells were recovered on lavage of exposed rabbits, compared with unexposed controls, and defects in macrophage phagocytic activity, bacterial uptake, and surface adherence were found. Cell differential counts and macrophage viability and bactericidal processing were not affected by the wood smoke.

Most of the available epidemiologic evidence on the health effects of wood smoke is derived from investigations in developing countries, where intense smoke exposure results from the use of cooking fires in poorly ventilated dwellings.[3] The studies from less developed countries suggest that smoke exposure adversely affects children and adults, increasing the occurrence of acute respiratory illness in children and chronic respiratory morbidity in children and adults.[91-93] Data from more developed countries are sparse[94-96] and do not clearly indicate adverse effects at the lower concentrations of wood smoke generally present.

Organic compounds

Sources and concentrations. Organic compounds are ubiquitous in indoor environments where they are released from furnishings and equipment, construction materials, and consumer and office products (Table 48-1). The organic compounds found in indoor air can be grouped by boiling point range as volatile (0°C to 240°C), semivolatile (240°C to 380°C), and particulate (>380°C).[97] Volatile organic compounds exist as vapors over the normal range of air temperatures and pressures, whereas semivolatile organic compounds are liquids or solids but also evaporate. For example, termiticides such as chlordane and heptachlor are injected into the ground beneath homes as liquids but are effective against termites because the liquid form releases vapors. Some higher-molecular-weight organic molecules occur as particulate matter in air.

Hundreds of organic compounds have been identified in indoor air.[65,97] Although many of these agents are also released by outdoor sources, indoor concentrations and sources have been shown to drive personal exposures to most of the organic compounds.[65] The Total Exposure Assessment Methodology (TEAM) Study conducted by the U.S. EPA showed the dominant contributions of indoor sources to personal exposures, even in locations with outdoor air polluted by industry.[98] For example, benzene, a human carcinogen, may be released outdoors from industry and from gasoline. However, the TEAM study showed that the main source of personal exposure for cigarette smokers

Table 48-1. Common organic chemicals and their sources

Chemicals	Measured peak nonoccupational exposure (μg/m^3)	Major sources of exposure
Volatile chemicals		
Benzene	1,000	Smoking, auto exhaust, passive smoking, driving, pumping gas
Tetrachloroethylene	1,000	Wearing or storing dry-cleaned clothes; visiting dry cleaners
p-Dichlorobenzene	1,000	Room deodorizers, moth cakes
Chloroform	250	Showering (10-min average)
	50	Washing clothes, dishes
Methylene chloride	500,000	Paint stripping, solvent usage
1,1,1-Trichloroethane	1,000	Wearing or storing dry-cleaned clothes, aerosol sprays, fabric protectors
Trichloroethylene	100	Unknown (cosmetics, electronic parts)
Carbon tetrachloride	100	Industrial-strength cleansers
Aromatic hydrocarbons (toluene, xylenes, ethylbenzene, trimethylbenzenes)	1,000	Paints, adhesives, gasoline, combustion sources
Aliphatic hydrocarbons (octane, decane, undecane)	1,000	Paints, adhesives, gasoline, combustion sources
Terpenes (limonene, α-pinene)	1,000	Scented deodorizers, polishes, fabrics, fabric softeners, cigarettes, food, and beverages
Semivolatile chemicals		
Chlorpyrifos (Dursban)	10	Insecticide
Chlordane, heptachlor	100	Termiticide
Diazinon	100	Insecticide
Polychlorinated biphenyls (PCBs)		Transformers, fluorescent ballasts, ceiling tiles
Polycyclic aromatic hydrocarbons (PAHs)	1	Combustion products (smoking, wood burning, kerosene heaters)

Adapted from Wallace LA: Volatile organic compounds. In Samet JM and Spengler JD, editors. *Indoor air pollution. A health perspective*, pp 252-272, Baltimore, 1991, Johns Hopkins University Press. With permission.

was benzene in mainstream cigarette smoke; passive smokers are also exposed to benzene.[99]

Formaldehyde, used in hundreds of products, is one of the most ubiquitous indoor organic compounds.[100] The largest use of formaldehyde is in urea and phenolformaldehyde resins, which are used to bond laminated wood products and to bind the wood chips in particle board. Formaldehyde-containing wood products are used as shelving, counters, bookcases, cabinets, floors, and wall coverings in homes, offices, and public buildings. Formaldehyde resins are also used to treat paper products and fabrics and are also constituents of numerous other consumer products. In the mid-1970s, urea formaldehyde foam insulation (UFFI) became a popular insulation material. Sustained release of formaldehyde from improperly installed or formulated UFFI can elevate indoor formaldehyde concentrations; because of the potential for sustained release, UFFI is no longer used in North America.

Health effects. The health risks of the organic compounds are diverse; the organics found in indoor air include several dozen carcinogens and mutagens (e.g., benzene), irritants (e.g., formaldehyde and terpenes), and neurotoxins (e.g., aromatic compounds).[65] In spite of the potential risks of the organic compounds in indoor air, few studies have shown specific exposure-disease associations, largely because of the difficulty of characterizing exposures and identifying effects of components of complex mixtures in indoor air. Published sources on the toxicology of individual volatile organic compounds found in indoor air are available.[101,101a] Indoor exposures to organics may contribute to the risks for several cancers, although few epidemiologic studies have been directed specifically at assessing cancer risk in relation to indoor exposures to organics.[102]

Irritation of mucosal surfaces and neurotoxic effects may contribute to the symptom complex widely referred to as "sick-building syndrome" (see page 800).[97] Harving and colleagues[103] investigated the effects of a mixture of volatile organic compounds on lung function of 11 subjects with bronchial hyperreactivity. At the highest concentration studied, 25 mg/m^3, there was evidence of a significant decline of forced expiratory volume in 1 second (FEV1) following exposure, although histamine responsiveness was unchanged.

Radon

Sources and concentrations. Radon-222, a noble gas, is produced in the decay of naturally occurring uranium-238. It decays with a half-life of 3.8 days into a series of short-lived progeny: polonium-218, lead-214, bismuth-214, and polonium-214, all with half-lives less than 30 minutes (Fig. 48-2).[104] The principal source of radon in buildings is naturally occurring gas in soil.[105] The driving pressure for entry of soil gas into a building is the pressure gradient established by a structure across the soil; the gradient varies with atmospheric pressure, wind flow over the structure, and buoyancy of air within the structure. The soil gas penetrates through openings such as sump pump wells, drains, cracks, and utility access holes. In most locales, building materials and water used in the home do not contribute significantly to concentrations of radon indoors. However, potable water drawn from wells in areas where soils and rocks are enriched in radium may be a significant source of radon.[106]

Extensive data are now available on radon concentrations in U.S. homes, confirming early estimates that the average value in U.S. homes is about 1.5 pico-Curies per liter (pCi/L).[107] The EPA has surveyed samples of homes in most states, using a screening protocol and short-term measurements that yield upwardly biased concentrations. These data indicate that homes with high concentrations can be identified in all states, although the proportion exceeding the Agency's action guideline of 4 pCi/L is variable among the states. In a national survey conducted from 1988 through 1991, the U.S. EPA measured radon concentration in 6000 randomly selected homes in the United States using alpha track detectors.[108] This National Residential Radon Survey yielded an estimated annual average indoor radon concentration in U.S. homes of 1.25 pCi/L. About 4% of homes were estimated to exceed the guideline of 4 pCi/L annual average.

Health effects. Exposure to radon progeny, the short-lived decay products of radon, has been causally linked to increased risk of lung cancer in uranium and other underground miners.[109] Measurements made since the 1970s showed that radon was present in most homes and could reach high concentrations, as high as those in underground mines with documented excess lung cancer. Many homes throughout the United States have been found to have high levels of radon, and current risk models imply that even the values under current guidelines cause a significant number of lung cancer cases.[110,111]

The hazard posed by radon progeny exposure in indoor air has been addressed primarily through risk estimation procedures,[109,112] although ecologic and case-control studies more directly examining indoor radon and lung cancer have been published. In the most widely applied risk assessment approach, the risks for the general population are projected by extrapolating risks observed in the studies of miners to the general population. A number of risk models have now been developed; these risk projection models differ in the underlying assumptions and in the quantitative conclusions, and their results are subject to diverse uncertainties.[109] Nevertheless, use of each of the models leads to the conclusion that radon contributes significantly to the burden of lung cancer in the population, causing an estimated 10,000 to 20,000 cases annually in the United States.[113] The burden of radon-related lung cancer in the general population reflects in part the synergism between radon and cigarette smoking, assumed in several of the models on the basis of the data from underground miners.[109,111,112]

The most recent risk model is based on a pooled analysis of data from 11 studies of male underground miners.[114] The combined data set included 68,000 miners who experienced over 2700 lung cancer deaths during nearly 1.2 mil-

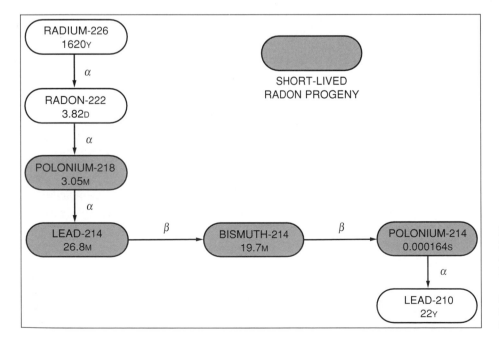

Fig. 48-2. Decay series from radium-226 to lead-210 showing the emission of α, β, and γ radiation and the half-lives for radon progeny. Half-life units = Y, year; D, day; M, minute; S, seconds. (Adapted from Samet JM: Radon and lung cancer, *J Natl Cancer Inst* 81:745-757, 1989.)

lion person-years of observation. Lung cancer risk was found to decline with attained age and time since exposure as in the model published in 1988 by the Biological Effects of Ionizing Radiation (BEIR) IV Alpha Committee of the National Research Council[109]; the risk was also found to increase as the rate of exposure decreased, the so-called "inverse-dose rate effect." Applying the model to the U.S. population, indoor exposure to radon at home was estimated to be responsible for about 12% of U.S. lung cancer deaths. Of the 18,200 lung cancer deaths attributed to radon in 1993, 12,400 were in smokers and 5800 in never smokers.

Epidemiologic studies of the general population provide an alternative approach for confirming that indoor radon is a cause of cancer and estimating the associated risk. To date, however, the findings of epidemiologic investigations of indoor radon and lung cancer have been limited by the methodologic difficulties of studying this exposure.[115,116] A number of descriptive or "ecologic" studies have been reported, but this design is uninformative for characterizing the lung cancer risk associated with indoor radon.[116]

The case-control design is a more appropriate epidemiologic approach for addressing the risks of indoor radon, and a number of studies are now in progress in the United States and other countries.[117] The findings of several studies have already been reported.[79,118,119] The published studies compare radon concentrations in current and previous residences of lung cancer cases with those of appropriate controls. The findings are potentially limited by the difficulty of estimating the past exposures and other, methodological, problems.[115] Because of the error inherent in estimating lifetime exposure to indoor radon, extremely large studies including thousands of cases and controls are needed to estimate the risk with sufficient precision for risk assessment and policy needs. The most informative assessment of the risk of indoor radon from the studies in the general population may be gained by a pooled analysis of data from the individual case-control studies.

Asbestos and man-made fibers

Sources and concentrations. Asbestos comprises several fibrous inorganic materials characterized by chemical formulation and crystalline structure (see Chapter 20). Asbestos minerals are grouped on the basis of configuration as serpentine or amphibole, curved and straight, respectively; the former group includes chrysotile asbestos and the latter includes primarily crocidolite, anthophyllite, amosite, actinolite, and tremolite. Because of its high tensile strength and thermal properties, asbestos has been extensively used in building materials since the beginning of this century.[120] The broad categories of use are thermal and acoustical insulation, fire protection, and the reinforcement of building products. In addition to its use in acoustic ceiling tiles and vinyl floor tiles, asbestos has been used in paints and wall and ceiling plaster. Until banned in the late 1970s, asbestos

materials were used to coat pipes, boilers, and steel structural beams.

The use of asbestos in the United States has decreased since 1973, coincident with the banning of certain applications by the U.S. Environmental Protection Agency. However, asbestos-containing materials are still present in homes, offices, and schools. The U.S. EPA has estimated that 20% of the nation's buildings, about 733,000 not including schools and residential buildings with less than 10 units, contain some asbestos materials.[121]

Asbestos has been widely used in ceiling tiles, pipe wrap, plaster, floor tiles, shingles, and sprayed-on insulation, among other applications. Release of fibers from these materials may result from impact, abrasion, fallout, vibration, air erosion, and fire damage.[120] Water damage and the normal aging of binders leading to friability of the material increase the likelihood of release. Asbestos-contaminated surface dust may contribute to airborne concentrations in buildings. The episodic nature of fiber release and gravitational settling reduce the likelihood that elevated concentrations will be detected with area-integrated monitoring.

Man-made mineral fibers are now used increasingly as substitutes for asbestos in building materials. These are fibrous inorganic substances made primarily from rock, clay, slag, or glass; the three principal types include glass fibers (comprising glass wool and glass filaments), rock wool, and slag wool and ceramic fibers.[120] Fiberglass and glass wool refer to silica-based vitreous fibers manufactured by a number of different processes. Mineral, rock, and slag wools are made by remelting the precursor materials and then applying a process that generates fibers. The different types of fibers vary in their chemistry and dimensions, as well as in their durability in vivo.[120]

An enlarging data base on airborne asbestos concentrations in buildings demonstrates extremely low average values under the conditions of normal building use.[120,122] Occupant risk is determined by exposures to airborne fibers rather than the presence of asbestos-containing materials in the building. Results of monitoring buildings for asbestos cannot be readily compared across studies because different sampling, analysis, and counting criteria have been used.[120] Phase-contrast microscopy (PCM), the most widely used method, identifies fibers with a length to aspect ratio of 3. Because it is typically used at 400 power, this method underestimates thin fibers (diameters less than 0.25 μm). On the other hand, transmission electron microscopy (TEM) is used at a magnification of 20,000× and can classify asbestos fibers by type. Typically, TEM counts five times the number of fibers detected by PCM. Further, some investigators use an indirect method for TEM that transfers fibers to a counting stage. This method tends to further fracture fiber bundles and hence yields higher counts. Furthermore, interlab comparison studies indicate that not only do results vary among laboratories but even the technicians handling, preparing, and counting TEM-analyzed fibers may introduce important variations.

Surveys of asbestos concentrations in commercial buildings demonstrate very low fiber concentrations under normal conditions.[120] The Literature Review Panel Report published by the Health Effects Institute—Asbestos Research[120] compiled all published data as well as previously unpublished information on buildings sampled for litigation and for other purposes. The total data set included 1377 measurements made by TEM in 198 buildings. For fibers greater than 5 μm in length, which are considered most relevant to disease risk,[123] the mean and median concentrations were low, as were the 90th percentile values (see Fig. 20-2-1). The report acknowledged that these data cannot be considered representative of U.S. buildings and that buildings with deteriorated asbestos-containing materials may have been subjected to remediation rather than sampling.

Individual buildings with levels much higher than the typical values in the data assembled by the Health Effects Institute—Asbestos Research have been reported. For example, one of the first reports to draw attention to the problem of indoor asbestos described the Art and Architecture building at Yale University.[124] The interior of this building was coated with a highly friable material containing chrysotile asbestos. Shortly after the application of this material, it began to deteriorate, visibly contaminating surfaces. Levels measured by PCM were 0.02 fibers per cubic centimeter (f/cm^3) under quiet conditions and normal use and as high as 4 f/cm^3 after direct impact or during sweeping. A pioneering operations and maintenance program was put in place to control the problem.[124]

A limited number of measurements of concentrations of man-made mineral fibers in indoor environments have been reported.[120] These data indicate extremely low concentrations of respirable fibers. Fiber concentrations are thought to decay rapidly because of the large size of the fibers.

Health effects. Epidemiologic investigations in occupationally exposed populations and the supporting toxicologic evidence have convincingly demonstrated that asbestos exposure causes asbestosis, pleural and peritoneal mesothelioma, lung cancer, larynx cancer, and, possibly, gastrointestinal cancers.[120,125] However, the occupational risks have been demonstrated at levels of exposure that are orders of magnitude greater than the levels considered to be prevalent indoors. For office workers, visitors to buildings, and schoolchildren and teachers, mesothelioma and lung cancer are the principal health effects of concern; asbestosis would not be expected at exposures arising from buildings for these classes of building occupants.[120] The risks of indoor asbestos for the general population have been estimated by extrapolating risks for occupationally exposed persons. Uncertainty is inherent in this approach, but the risks cannot be directly investigated by epidemiologic methods. The Literature Review Panel Report of the Health Effects Institute—Asbestos Research estimated risks for various scenarios of exposure (see box). These levels of risk are far lower than the risks associated with many voluntarily assumed risks.[122]

Custodial and maintenance workers in buildings with asbestos-containing materials may be exposed to higher levels of asbestos than other building occupants if their activities disturb the materials and release fibers. The workers may be at particular risk if they are unaware that asbestos-containing materials are present or are untrained in dealing with these materials. Several studies have shown that custodial and maintenance workers may have pleural plaques and possibly asbestosis,[126-128] and concern has been expressed that a "third wave" of asbestos-caused disease could occur in custodial and maintenance workers.[129] We have few data, however, on the exposures sustained by custodial and maintenance workers in buildings with asbestos-containing materials.

Because of the morphologic and toxicologic comparability of asbestos and man-made mineral fibers, there has been concern that exposure to man-made mineral fibers could produce the same diseases caused by asbestos.[123] The relevant epidemiologic data from exposed workers are less extensive than for asbestos. There is an indication of increased lung cancer risk in workers who produced rock and slag wool in the early years of the industry; however, data on levels of exposure are unavailable and other carcinogens may have contributed to the increased risk.[123,130] Animal studies have shown the fibers that are long and thin to be carcinogenic.[120] Lippmann[123] concluded from the epidemiologic evidence and toxicologic properties of the materials that the health risk of man-made mineral fibers is likely to be negligible for exposures of building occupants.

Classification of potential exposure to indoor asbestos

C1: Bystanders or nonoccupationally exposed building occupants (e.g., office workers, visitors, students, and teachers)

C2: Housekeeping or custodial employees who may disturb materials in the course of routine cleaning and service functions

C3: Maintenance or skilled workers who may disturb asbestos-containing material (ACM) in the course of making repairs, installing new equipment, or during minor renovation activity

C4: Abatement workers or others involved in the removal or renovation of structures with ACM

C5: Firefighters and other emergency personnel who may be present during or after the fabric of the building has been extensively damaged by fire, wind, water, or earthquake

Adapted from Health Effects Institute—Asbestos Research Literature Review Panel: *Asbestos in public and commercial buildings,* Cambridge, MA, 1991, Health Effects Institute—Asbestos Research.

Biologic agents

Sources and concentrations. Until recently, indoor biologic pollution received less attention than other types of indoor air pollution, although it had long been known that infectious diseases were transmitted through indoor air. However, advances in sampling methodology and analysis have now made possible more detailed characterization of biologic agents in indoor air, particularly a number of the major allergenic proteins.[131] Indoor allergens and microbes have diverse sources, both indoors and outdoors (see box). Indoor levels of allergens and microbes may be elevated as the result of material accumulating indoors, such as human and animal dander, and the growth of fungi and bacteria on interior surfaces or in air conditioning systems. Indoor pollen is almost entirely derived from outdoor plants, and fungus spores from outdoors may also enter the indoor environment through air infiltration and on the surfaces of people, animals, or objects.

The most severe indoor biologic pollution problems result from the growth of microorganisms on interior surfaces. Virtually any substrate providing a source of both carbon and water can support the growth of microorganisms. Wood

---

Sources of biologic air pollutants

Acarids

Dust mites and spiders

Insects

Cockroaches, crickets, beetles, fleas, moths, flies, and midges

Domestic animals

Cats, dogs, other mammals, and birds

Rodents

WILD

Mice and rats

PETS

Mice, gerbils, and guinea pigs

Fungi

Indoors (growing on interior surfaces or in air conditioning system)

Penicillium, Aspergillus, Rhizopus, and Cladosporium

Outdoors

Multiple species entering with incoming air

Pollens

Derived from outdoor plants or plant materials brought inside

Bacteria

Legionella (introduced to ventilation systems by cooling towers and standing water reservoirs)

---

and cellulose-based materials (e.g., paper) can support the growth of fungi, as can hydrocarbon films on surfaces, including paint, soap, grease, and skin oils. The presence of water is essential for growth of microorganisms. High relative humidity, in excess of 70%, provides conditions for condensation on interior surfaces (e.g., cool exterior walls or window sills).[48] Small leaks from water pipes and roofs can also provide a consistent source of moisture. Other moisture sources include humidifiers, vaporizers, and air conditioners, and when contaminated, these devices can disperse fungal fragments, spores, and dissolved allergens into room air.[132] Improper venting of the exhaust of clothes dryers to interior spaces can add moisture and substrate (i.e., lint) for microbial growth to indoor spaces.

Airborne levels of microbial particles in indoor environments are not yet well-characterized and multiple methods for measurement are in use.[131] Volumetric air samples are collected by pumping air through filters, impactors, or impingers, and the samples are usually analyzed by culture, microscopy, and immunological assays. In general, levels of biologic particles are low in rooms with little air movement or human activity.[133] Indoor levels, and hence personal exposures, are highly variable and are probably affected by activities such as vacuuming, sweeping, dusting, bed making, scrubbing contaminated surfaces, and using electric fans. Further, airborne and dust concentrations of allergens probably have limited value for assessing the contribution of a particular allergen in causing disease. Factors such as aerodynamic behavior, respirability, solubility, and cross-reactivity with other allergens are also important in the process of immunologic sensitization and the development of allergic disease.[131] Therefore, the *potential* for exposure is estimated through the use of questionnaires (e.g., time-activity) in combination with data on bulk or reservoir samples (e.g., swabbing of surfaces and vacuuming of floors and bedding). The following paragraphs give selected data on the occurrence of biologic agents in indoor environments; a more detailed treatment can be found in Pope et al.[131]

Dust mites (*Dematophagoides pteronyssinus, D. farinae,* and *Euroglyphus maynei*) are commonly found in houses and are an important source of allergens. These mites are approximately 0.3 mm in length and live in carpets, upholstered furniture, mattresses, and bedding, where they eat skin scales. Two major dust mite allergens have been identified, *Der p* I and *Der p* II. These proteins are derived from digestive enzymes in the gut of the mite and are found in high concentrations in the fecal pellets. Vacuum sampling and immunologic assay indicate that in the home, the highest levels of allergen occur in the bedroom in carpeting, mattresses, and bedding.

Domestic cockroaches, including the German cockroach *Blattella germanica,* are commonly found indoors and represent another important source of allergen in the home. Fecal material and saliva contain large amounts of the allergen *Bla g* I and *Bla g* II. The highest levels of this allergen in house dust are generally found in kitchens.

Cats and dogs are common household pets and prevalent sources of allergen exposures. *Fel d* I is the most important allergen associated with cats, and high levels of this protein are found in cat dander and fur and also in saliva and urine. The median level of *Fel d* I in samples of settled household dust in homes with a cat are reported to range from 2 to 130,000 ng/g of dust, with a median level of 90 ng *Fel d* I/g of dust.[134] In homes without a cat, much lower levels are observed, ranging from 2 to 7500 ng *Fel d* I/g of dust. The presence of the allergen in the dust of homes and buildings in which cats are not kept suggests that the allergen can be transported on clothing. The major dog allergen, *Can f* I, is present in dog fur and saliva and is a relatively stable protein that may persist in dust for long periods of time. The content of *Can f* I in household dust from homes with a dog range from 10 to 10,000 µg/g of dust and 0.3 to 23 µg/g of dust in homes without a dog.[135]

Fungi are present in the air of virtually all homes and public buildings. Commonly isolated genera include *Cladosporium, Pennicillium, Alternaria, Epicoccum, Aspergillus,* and *Drechslera.*[131,136-138] Although the factors influencing indoor levels have not been adequately characterized, evidence suggests that dampness, water damage, ambient winds, and gardening and agricultural activities near a building can increase indoor levels of fungi and molds.

Health effects. Biologic agents in indoor air may cause disease through multiple mechanisms including direct toxicity, infections, and immune hyperresponsiveness. A complete review of these diverse effects is beyond the scope of this chapter. The following paragraphs give selected examples of diseases caused by biologic agents; more extensive information is available in recently published reviews.[131]

Home dampness and mold, determined by questionnaire, have been associated with upper respiratory symptoms and eye irritation in large studies in the United States[139] and Canada.[140] These associations were adjusted for known determinants of respiratory symptoms, including maternal smoking, city, child age and gender, and parent education. Because the exposure and outcome variables were based on parental report, the findings are limited by the subjective nature of the study designs.

Hypersensitivity reactions are classified by the major immune mechanisms involved.[141] For indoor allergens, the principal types of reactions are Type I, IgE-mediated reactions, and Type IV, IgG- and lymphocyte-mediated reactions. Biologic pollutants are associated with several immunologically mediated respiratory diseases, including allergic rhinitis, asthma, and hypersensitivity pneumonitis. The allergic diseases mediated by Type I hypersensitivity occur with increased frequency in individuals with an inherited tendency (atopy) to form immunoglobulin E against antigens encountered in the environment. Atopic individuals

constitute between 5% and 22% of the population.[142] Hypersensitivity pneumonitis may be classified as a Type IV immunologic reaction that is mediated by the action of sensitized T-lymphocytes. In this process, tissue damage occurs as the result of the killing of target cells, the production of lymphokines, and interaction and activation of natural killer cells and macrophages.[19] Hypersensitivity pneumonitis has been associated with the contamination of air handling systems of office buildings.[143-145]

Allergic rhinitis or "hay fever" is manifest as nasal congestion and rhinorrhea, and may be accompanied by allergic conjunctivitis and allergic sinusitis. Identification of the specific indoor allergen associated with the symptoms may be accomplished by skin testing and in vitro measurement of antibody (radioallergosorbent test [RAST]). Estimates of the prevalence of hay fever in the United States range from 3% to 19%.[142] Nasal provocation tests with cockroach allergen have elicited acute rhinitis responses.[146] Environmental exposures also have been demonstrated to induce rhinitis; in a room containing living cats, acute rhinitis and asthma attacks occurred in all 10 exposed cat-allergic subjects.[147]

Asthma occurs commonly among atopic individuals. Many of these individuals may have multiple sensitivity to specific antigens from pollens, animal fur, fungi spores, and house dust. Data from population surveys indicate that the prevalence of asthma in the United States ranges from 4% to 8%.[148] The risk of acute or severe attacks of asthma is increased in residences with levels of *Der p* I in excess of 10 µg/g of house dust,[149] and asthmatic patients have been reported to show a 25% prevalence of skin test positively to cat or dog allergen extracts.[150] Building-related allergic respiratory disease and epidemic asthma have been reported for office buildings in association with air handling systems and humidifiers contaminated with bacteria and fungi.[145,151]

Avian proteins present in bird excreta (e.g., the droppings of pet birds such as parakeets), and fungal spores from thermophylic actinomycetes, *Aspergillus* species, and *Aureobasidium* species may contaminate the indoor environment and cause hypersensitivity pneumonitis. This disease is characterized by inflammation of the lung parenchyma and may present in a range of forms (see Chapter 14). In the acute form, the exposed person may experience fever, chills, and shortness of breath, and chest x-ray may show radiodensities mimicking acute pneumonia. In the chronic form, recurrent illness with flulike symptoms occurs. Pulmonary function testing may show a restrictive pattern of ventilatory impairment and chest x-ray may show an interstitial pattern of lung disease. In the chronic form, irreversible lung damage may occur with gas exchange impairment. Diagnosis of the chronic form is often difficult because of the nonspecific physical findings and the nonspecificity of precipitins as a marker of exposure. Hypersensitivity pneumonitis occurs infrequently in the general population[152] and its occurrence has been difficult to quantify.[144]

The bacterium *Legionella pneumophila* is the agent of Legionnaire's disease, an often fatal pneumonia associated with exposure to the bacterium in aerosols of cooling towers and air handling systems[153] and humidifiers and spas.[154] It exemplifies a respiratory pathogen primarily associated with indoor environments, both with regard to source and transmission. Of course, indoor environments are the locus of transmission of many infectious respiratory diseases including influenza and tuberculosis. The disease was first discovered among attendees of an American Legion convention in a Philadelphia hotel in 1976. Legionnaire's disease has a relatively high mortality rate but a low attack rate; predisposing factors for infection include cigarette smoking, existing respiratory disease, use of immunosuppressing drugs, and older age. The cardinal symptoms appear 2 to 10 days after exposure and include malaise, headache, and high fever. Pneumonia-like symptoms of lung consolidation and respiratory failure may follow. *L. pneumophila* also causes a nonpneumonic disease, Pontiac Fever, which has a high attack rate but is usually not fatal. Symptoms associated with this disease syndrome include fever, malaise, myalgia, and headaches.

CLINICAL IMPLICATIONS
General considerations

The health consequences of exposure to indoor air pollution have clinically relevant dimensions (see box). Indoor exposures to some pollutants may cause severe disease and even death. For example, deaths still occur in the United States from carbon monoxide, and hypersensitivity pneumonitis can result from exposures in homes and offices. Indoor air pollution undoubtedly contributes to respiratory morbidity by causing symptoms and exacerbating chronic respiratory diseases such as asthma. Indoor air pollution is now widely known to contain carcinogens, such as radon and ETS, and health care providers are frequently asked to advise on the risks of such agents and how to control them. Clinicians are also becoming increasingly involved in the evaluation of patients affected by sick-building syndrome or "multiple chemical sensitivity," both of which are complex clinical syndromes apparently linked, at least in part, to indoor air pollution.

Clinicians should have knowledge of the common indoor air pollutants that affect health and of the illnesses that have specific and nonspecific relationships to indoor air pollution.[27] Specific-building-related illnesses are caused by a specific agent in indoor air and conform to a single diagnostic entity (see top box in column 2). For example, hypersensitivity pneumonitis caused by thermophilic actinomycetes is classified as a specific building-related illness. By contrast, sick-building syndrome is nonspecific in its clinical picture, and most cases cannot be linked to a specific agent.[27]

In evaluating patients who may have a building-related illness, whether specific or nonspecific, the history should

---

Selected examples of exposure–disease associations for indoor air pollution

Radon: Lung cancer
Environmental tobacco smoke: Lung cancer, increased lower respiratory illness in infants
Benzene: Leukemia
Asbestos: Lung cancer and mesothelioma
Formaldehyde: Nasal cancer

Selected examples of clinically evident disease linked to indoor air pollution[97]

Carbon monoxide poisoning
Hemorrhagic pneumonitis from high levels of NO_2
Hypersensitivity pneumonitis and humidifier fever
Legionella pneumonia
Cat- and mite induced asthma

---

cover all relevant microenvironments and address sources of pollutants and activities. Information on the characteristics of the building, including its age, location, cleanliness, and whether the ventilation is natural or mechanical, may also be relevant.

Sick-building syndrome

Nonspecific symptoms attributed to the indoor environment are a frequent complaint among occupants of buildings.[155,156] The spectrum of building-related symptoms is broad, including symptoms related to effects on the skin, eyes, and respiratory tract, and neuropsychologic effects. Factors determining the occurrence of building-related symptoms have not been readily identified, presumably because of multifactorial causation in most instances.[21,156] Low ventilation rates alone do not explain the development of symptoms in building occupants; in fact, the widely applied ventilation standard of the American Society of Heating, Refrigerating, and Air Conditioning Engineers (ASHRAE) is intended to assure comfort for most (80%) of building occupants.[157] Organic compounds are suspect causes of symptoms because of their presence in indoor air and their diverse effects.[97]

"Sick-" or "tight-building syndrome" refers to the occurrence of nonspecific symptoms among either a substantial proportion of a building's occupants or among occupants of a specific space within a building.[27] An international working group of the World Health Organization proposed five broad groups of symptoms reflective of sick-building syndrome (see bottom box in this column).[97] Characteristically, the symptoms occur on entering the building and are relieved when leaving. In making the diagnosis of sick-building syndrome, a clinician should exclude alternative diagnoses and establish the dimensions of the complaints to

---

Five categories of symptoms exemplified by some complaints reported by occupants supposed to suffer from the sick-building syndrome

Sensory irritation in eyes, nose, and throat

Pain, sensation of dryness, smarting feeling, stinging, irritation, hoarseness, voice problems

Neurologic or general health symptoms

Headache, sluggishness, mental fatigue, reduced memory, reduced capability to concentrate, dizziness, intoxication, nausea and vomiting, tiredness

Skin irritation

Pain, reddening, smarting or itching sensations, dry skin

Nonspecific hypersensitivity reactions

Running nose and eyes, asthmalike symptoms among nonasthmatics, sounds from the respiratory system

Odor and taste symptoms

Changed sensitivity of olfactory or gustatory sense, unpleasant olfactory or gustatory perceptions

---

Adapted from Molhave L: Volatile organic compounds and the sick building syndrome. In Lippmann M, editor: *Environmental toxicants: human exposures and their health effects*, pp 633-646, New York, 1992, Van Nostrand Reinhold.

determine whether the diagnosis is tenable. Characteristic symptom complexes bearing an appropriate temporal relationship to being in the building and occurring in several building occupants are compatible with sick-building syndrome. The information available from a single patient may be insufficient to establish a diagnosis, in which case the patient or physician must obtain additional data. If the patient does not draw the physician's attention to the possibility of work-related symptoms, alternative diagnoses are likely to be made.

To date, research on the sick-building syndrome has primarily consisted of case studies. These studies have identified many factors that may be associated with symptoms, but no single factor appears to be responsible for most of the outbreaks of the syndrome.[21,156] Management of patients with sick-building syndrome may, therefore, be difficult, and physicians may need to contact the building operator or management for a solution to a patient's problem.[27] The American Thoracic Society[27] has outlined clinical approaches to patients with suspected sick-building syndrome.

Multiple chemical sensitivity

This symptom-defined entity is as complex and controversial as sick-building syndrome. Although a standardized definition is lacking, the term is applied to patients with diverse symptom manifestations considered to be associated with environmental agents.[158,159] Indoor air pollutants have been considered to be involved in the etiology of multiple chemical sensitivity. The pathophysiologic basis of multiple chemical sensitivity is controversial. Current concepts of pathogenesis have their roots in the writings of Randolph in the 1950s.[158,160] The physicians who accept this pathogenetic model are now referred to as clinical ecologists. However, the committees of traditional medical organizations have considered the diagnostic and therapeutic approaches of clinical ecology to be inadequately supported.[161] Patients with multiple chemical sensitivity often consult allergists and pulmonologists. Several reviews of the subject have recently been published.[158,159]

GENERAL CONSIDERATIONS
Control strategies

Methods of control. The broad approaches to limiting the health effects of indoor air pollution include removal and control of sources, increased rate of exchange of indoor with outdoor air, and air cleaning (Table 48-2).[27] Sources may be removed, relocated, or controlled; for many pollutants source removal or control represents the most effective and economic approach. For example, tobacco smoking can be restricted or eliminated in indoor spaces, and household products that release VOCs can be stored outside an occupied area and their indoor use minimized. Building materials and furnishings can be selected for low emission rates. Ventilation may be increased throughout a structure or in a specific area that has inadequate ventilation or particularly strong sources. ASHRAE publishes consensus guidelines for ventilation requirements.[157] A wide variety of air-cleaning devices are available; these operate by filtration, adsorption, absorption, electrostatic precipitation, or on other principles. The devices have not yet been shown to be effective for specific health conditions such as asthma and allergic rhinitis.

Radon is a widespread pollutant of indoor air, and as such merits special consideration; the level of radon in a home can be measured inexpensively, and effective mitigation techniques are available. As recommended by the U.S. EPA,[162] homeowners should be encouraged to test the radon level in their homes, particularly in regions where some homes are known to have high concentrations. In the event of a high concentration, a variety of mitigation strategies can be followed. An effective and cost-efficient approach is to seal all cracks in the foundation and then depressurize the subslab area, venting the subslab away from the house.

Regulatory approaches. It is now clear that the protection of public health requires satisfactory outdoor and indoor air quality. Moreover, the public expects a degree of indoor air quality that ensures comfort. The elements of comfort include, among other factors, temperature, temperature gradients, draftiness, humidity, noise, odors, and lighting. We do not yet have comprehensive data on or criteria for acceptable indoor air quality.

Table 48-2. Pollutant control measures

Pollutant	Measures and materials	Ventilation and design
Respirable particles	Install high-efficiency filters, tight sealing doors and grates; properly draft chimney; provide electrostatic precipitators	Zone and ventilate for smoking; supply outside combustion air to heater and fireplace; relocate air intakes; maintain filter system
Nitric oxide, nitrogen dioxide	Remove gasoline engines; install pilotless ignition	Use effective hood vent over source; isolate garage from living space
Carbon monoxide	Install pilotless ignition; restrict heater use to uninhabited space; use catalytic converter; replace indoor gasoline engines with electric	Supply outside combustion air; vent emission outside; use kitchen hood vents; relocate vents; provide smoking zones; isolate garage from living space
Carbon dioxide	Check static pressure in return air ducts to make sure return is not overriding fresh-air intake	Isolate garage from indoor space
Agents from biologic sources	Insulate to prevent condensation; dampproof foundation, ducts; install proper drainage of drip pans under condenser coils; add bactericides to steam and water for humidifiers and cooling towers; schedule proper maintenance of filters and ducts; routinely clean; discard water damaged floor covering; do not use cool-mist humidifiers and vaporizers	Maintain inside relative humidity of 35% to 50%; exhaust bath and kitchen; vent crawl spaces
Formaldehyde	Substitute products such as phenolic resin plywood; seal sources; remove materials	Increase air exchange to house or office
Radon and radon progeny	Vapor barrier around foundation; dampproof basement and crawl space; seal cracks and holes in floor traps and drains; install charcoal waterscrubber for well water; seal foundation completely	Vent crawl space; vent sumphole to exterior; depressurize subslab; vent bathroom and laundry to exterior
Volatile organic compounds	Substitute products; isolate storage area; apply only according to specifications; do not locate transformers indoors	Use only with adequate ventilation; ventilate laundry, shop; provide separate ventilation to storage area
Asbestos	Remove; use injection sealant; wrap pipes with plastic and duct tape	Ventilation does not provide adequate protection

The Clean Air Act provides a regulatory framework for the United States that is designed to achieve and maintain lower pollutant levels in outdoor air, meeting standards established to prevent adverse health effects. However, we lack a comparable comprehensive legal, regulatory, administrative, and technical framework for approaching the problem of indoor air pollution. Indoor air pollution has diverse sources, and may result from poor building design, inadequate building maintenance, structural components and furnishings, consumer products, and occupant activities. The standards and guidelines developed for outdoor air or for the workplace are not appropriate for direct application to indoor environments.

The government has various options for controlling an indoor air pollution problem, ranging from taking no action to implementing specific rules and regulations. However, the U.S. Government has not yet established a framework for policy on indoor air. Sexton published a report in 1986[163] that addresses the sequence of steps needed to develop responsible and effective control strategies (see box). The federal government has so far pursued voluntary industry codes and standards for kerosene space heaters and has offered "action guidelines" for radon; it has also pro-

vided guidance on handling asbestos in schools and has eliminated most uses of asbestos. Some states and municipalities have moved to restrict indoor air pollution by ETS,[164] and public education to alter smoking behavior has been undertaken by various government agencies.

Existing statutory authorities in the United States do not provide a single federal agency with jurisdiction over indoor air (see box).[165] Under the provisions of Title IV of the Superfund Amendments and Reauthorization Act of 1986, Radon and Indoor Air Quality Research, Congress directed the U.S. EPA to establish a research program to address radon and other indoor pollutants. The research program was mandated to address data gathering, to coordinate research activities, and to assess federal actions on mitigation of environmental and health risks associated with indoor air.

In its 1987 report to Congress on indoor air quality, as mandated by Title IV of the Superfund Amendments and Reauthorization Act, the EPA outlined policy objectives and strategy.[165] Research was proposed to refine understanding of health effects, with emphasis placed on obtaining data for risk assessment. The EPA also planned to identify and assess methods for mitigating high-priority problems. The

---

Summary of the major steps in addressing indoor air quality problems

Problem definition

Emission sources
Dilution
Indoor concentrations
Activity patterns
Exposures
Health consequences

Health risk assessment

Number of people exposed
Severity of exposure
Dose–response relationship

Applicability of mitigating measures

Ventilation
Source removal
Source modification
Air cleaning behavior adjustment
Air cleaning

Resolution of policy issues

Building "publicness"
Conservation benefits
Voluntary versus involuntary risks
Importance of short- and long-term health effects
Public versus private responsibility
Local, state, or federal intervention
Appropriate government responses

Alternative government responses

No action
More research
Public information
Economic incentives
Moral suasion
Legal liability
Guidelines
Rules and regulations

---

proposed strategy for control was multifaceted and included regulation under existing authorities, augmenting government and private capabilities to manage indoor air quality problems, referring problems to other federal agencies with regulatory authority, and requesting regulatory authority from Congress. The Agency stated a clear preference for avoiding regulation and for achieving its goals through research and development, dissemination of information, and technical assistance and training.

In addition to the EPA, other federal agencies are also involved in ensuring indoor air quality. The U.S. National Institute for Occupational Safety and Health (NIOSH) conducts health hazard evaluations of workplaces considered to be unhealthy; many evaluations have been conducted in nonindustrial settings to evaluate problems related to indoor air quality. The Department of Energy oversees energy conservation activities and is charged with considering the health consequences of energy conservation programs. The Department of Energy also has its own program of research in several areas, including radon. Under the Consumer Product Safety Act, the Consumer Product Safety Commission has authority to regulate injurious products. The Commission has addressed asbestos, urea formaldehyde foam insulation, biologic dissemination from humidifiers, and unvented combustion appliances. The Department of Housing and Urban Development sets building standards for agency-funded projects and standards for materials for mobile homes. Federal activities on indoor air are coordinated through the congressionally mandated Interagency Committee on Indoor Air Quality.

Nonregulatory approaches. Several alternative approaches have been employed to achieve acceptable indoor air quality in residences and public access buildings. Implementation of these approaches is generally less cumbersome than conventional regulations and the air quality standard setting process, and allows more flexibility to the public and industry. These alternative strategies include (1) voluntary industry codes and standards (e.g., kerosene space heaters), (2) consumer warnings (e.g., label requirements for kerosene space heaters and pesticides), (3) health guidelines (e.g., 4 pCi/L "action level" for radon), (4) public information programs (e.g., radon, asbestos in schools, indoor air quality information clearinghouse), (5) encouraging professional organizations to develop guidelines, statements, and recommendations (e.g., ASHRAE, ATS).

Implications for public health and control

The broad spectrum of health effects associated with exposure to indoor air pollution makes clear the potential scope of the public health problem and the difficulty of fully estimating the magnitude of adverse effects (see box). Some adverse effects have clear definitions (e.g., death from carbon monoxide poisoning) whereas others are defined on the basis of subjective responses, and any criteria for placing responses into a particular category require the assumption of a societal framework for separating adverse from nonadverse responses. Risk assessment has been used to quantify the hazard associated with some carcinogens of current concern and a few exposures associated with nonmalignant respiratory effects. However, symptom and perceptual responses to indoor air pollutants can be addressed only by directly investigating exposed populations. To date, few studies have addressed these responses in population-based samples, and we lack a comprehensive and population-based assessment of the full scope of the public health consequences of indoor air pollution.

Nevertheless, both the government and the public consider indoor air pollution to be an important public health problem. An expert committee assembled by the EPA at-

Federal laws potentially applicable to indoor air

National Environmental Policy Act: A broad act that establishes a national goal "to assure for all Americans safe, healthful, productive, and aesthetically and culturally pleasing surroundings."

Clean Air Act: Gives the Environmental Protection Agency (EPA) regulatory authority over outdoor air.

Toxic Substances Control Act: Provides EPA with authority to collect and develop data on the risks of chemicals and to restrict manufacturing, distribution, and use of toxic chemicals, including indoor air contaminants.

Federal Insecticide, Fungicide, and Rodenticide Act: Provides EPA with authority to collect data, to monitor, and to regulate use of pesticides, including those used indoors.

Asbestos Hazard Emergency Response Act and the Asbestos School Hazard Detection and Control Act: Requires EPA to develop regulation detailing methods for handling asbestos in schools.

Superfund Amendments and Reauthorization Act, Title IV: Radon Gas and Indoor Air Quality Research Act: Requires EPA to establish a research program.

Safe Drinking Water Act: Authorizes EPA to perform research on contaminants of drinking water. The regulatory authority extends to contaminants in public water supplies that have adverse effects through indoor air pollution.

Consumer Product Safety Act: Provides Consumer Product Safety Commission with authority to regulate consumer products that cause injury.

Federal Hazardous Substance Act: Authorizes Consumer Product Safety Commission to require labeling for hazardous household products.

Occupational Safety and Health Act: As a national policy, "to assure as far as possible every working man and woman in the nation safe and healthy working conditions."

National Manufactured Housing Construction and Safety Standards Act of 1974: This state directs the Department of Housing and Urban Development to establish standards for construction and safety of manufactured housing (e.g., mobile homes). Features related to indoor air pollution have been regulated.

Department of Energy Organization Act of 1977: Requires integration of national environmental protection goals in developing energy programs. Mandates research on energy technologies and programs.

Energy Conservation and Production Act: Has the goal of reducing energy demand, but Department of Energy must consider potential health consequences.

posures to chemicals. This prominent ranking reflects the high prevalence of exposure and the severity of the morbidity and mortality associated with exposure to indoor air pollution.

However, we still need societal guidelines for describing the scope of the problem. In the United States, for example, public policy has evolved for single pollutants without broader consideration of more fundamental principles. Even for single agents, such as radon, conflicting views among involved regulators, the Congress, and scientists have led to persistent controversy.[167] Without any firm guidelines, the scope of the problem of indoor air pollution can be readily manipulated as underlying assumptions in risk assessments are varied or certain types of effects are dismissed. A process is needed for establishing a conceptual framework for interpreting the adverse effects of indoor air pollution and for putting a set of principles in place for managing them.[7,168]

REFERENCES

1. National Research Council, Committee on Indoor Pollutants: *Indoor pollutants,* Washington, DC, 1981, National Academy Press.
2. Spengler JD and Sexton K: Indoor air pollution: A public health perspective, *Science* 221:9-17, 1983.
3. Smith KR: *Biofuels, air pollution, and health: a global review,* New York, 1987, Plenum Press.
4. National Research Council, Committee on the Institutional Means for Assessment of Risks to Public Health: *Risk assessment in the Federal Government: managing the process,* Washington, DC, 1983, National Academy Press.
5. Lippmann M, editor: *Environmental toxicants: human exposures and their health effects,* New York, 1992, Van Nostrand Reinhold.
6. Watson AY, Bates RR, and Kennedy D, editors: *Air pollution, the automobile and public health,* Washington, DC, 1988, National Academy Press.
7. Samet JM and Spengler JD, editors: *Indoor air pollution: a health perspective,* Baltimore, 1991, Johns Hopkins University Press.
8. Bascom R, Bromberg P, Costa DA, et al: Health effects of outdoor air pollution, *Am J Resp Crit Care Med,* in press.
9. Duan N: Models for human exposure to air pollution, *Environ Int* 8:305-309, 1982.
10. Szalai A: *The use of time: daily activities of urban and suburban populations in twelve countries,* The Hague, 1972, Mouton.
11. Jenkins PL, Phillips TJ, Mulberg EJ, and Hui SP: Activity patterns of Californians: Use of and proximity to indoor pollutant sources, *Atmos Environ* 26:2141-2148, 1992.
12. Wiley JA: *Study of children's activity patterns. Final report,* Sacramento, CA, 1991, California Air Resources Board.
13. Ligocki MP, Salmon LG, Fall T, Jones MC, Nazaroff WW, and Cass GR: Characteristics of airborne particles inside southern California museums, *Atmos Environ* 27A(5):697-711, 1993.
14. Drye EE, Ozkaynak H, Burbank B, et al: Development of models for predicting the distribution of indoor nitrogen dioxide concentrations, *J Air Pollut Control Assoc* 39:1169-1177, 1989.
15. Weschler CJ, Shields HC, and Naik DV: Indoor ozone exposures, *J Air Pollut Control Assoc* 39:1562-1568, 1989.
16. Hayes SR: Use of an indoor air quality model (IAQM) to estimate indoor ozone levels, *J Air Waste Manage Assoc* 41(2):161-170, 1991.
17. Office of Technology Assessment: *Catching our breath: next steps to reducing urban ozone,* Washington, DC, 1989, Government Printing Office.

tempted in 1990 to place the risks of various classes of pollutants in a relative order.[166] In this ranking, indoor radon ranked behind outdoor air pollution (the so-called "criteria" air pollutants and hazardous air pollutants), but ahead of drinking water pollution, pesticides, and occupational ex-

18. American Thoracic Society: Guidelines as to what constitutes an adverse respiratory health effect, with special reference to epidemiologic studies of air pollution, *Am Rev Respir Dis* 131:666-669, 1985.

19. Weissman DN and Schuyler MR: Biological agents and allergic diseases, In Samet JM and Spengler JD, editors: *Indoor air pollution: a health perspective*, pp 285-305, Baltimore, 1991, Johns Hopkins University Press.

20. American Thoracic Society: Report of the ATS workshop on the health effects of atmospheric acids and their precursors, *Am Rev Respir Dis* 144:464-467, 1991.

21. Marbury MC and Woods JEJ: Building-related illness, In Samet JM and Spengler JD, editors: *Indoor air pollution: a health perspective*, pp 306-322, Baltimore, 1991, Johns Hopkins University Press.

22. U.S. Department of Health and Human Services: *The health consequences of involuntary smoking. A report of the surgeon general*, Washington, DC, 1986, U.S. Government Printing Office.

23. U.S. Environmental Protection Agency: *Respiratory health effects of passive smoking: lung cancer and other disorders* (EPA/600/6-90/006F), Washington, DC, 1992, U.S. Environmental Protection Agency.

24. Samet JM: Environmental tobacco smoke, In Lippmann M, editor: *Environmental toxicants: human exposures and their health effects*, pp 231-265, New York, 1991, Van Nostrand Reinhold.

25. Coultas DB and Lambert WE: Carbon monoxide, In Samet JM and Spengler JD, editors: *Indoor air pollution: a health perspective*, pp 187-208, Baltimore, 1991, Johns Hopkins University Press.

26. Allred EN, Bleecker ER, Chaitman BR, et al: Short-term effects of carbon monoxide exposure on the exercise performance of subjects with coronary artery disease, *N Engl J Med* 321:1426-1432, 1989.

27. American Thoracic Society: Environmental controls and lung disease, *Am Rev Respir Dis* 142:915-939, 1990.

28. Berglund B and Lindvall T: Sensory criteria for healthy buildings. In *Indoor air '90, Proceedings of the 5th international conference on indoor air quality and climate*, vol 5, pp 65-79, Toronto, Ottawa, 1990, Canada Mortgage and Housing Corporation.

29. Spengler JD and Samet JM: A perspective on indoor and outdoor air pollution, In Samet JM and Spengler JD, editors: *Indoor air pollution: a health perspective*, Baltimore, 1991, Johns Hopkins University Press.

30. Akland GG, Hartwell TD, Johnson TR, and Whitmore RW: Measuring human exposure to carbon monoxide in Washington, D.C., and Denver, Colorado, during the winter of 1982-1983, *Environ Sci Technol* 19:911-918, 1985.

31. Wallace L: Carbon monoxide in air and breath of employees in an underground office, *J Air Pollut Control Assoc* 33:678-682, 1983.

32. Levesque B, Dewailly E, Lavoie R, Prudhomme D, and Allaire S: Carbon monoxide in indoor ice skating rinks: evaluation of absorption by adult hockey players, *Am J Public Health* 80:594-598, 1990.

33. Hampson NB, Kramer CC, Donford RG, and Norkool DM: Carbon monoxide poisoning from indoor burning charcoal briquettes, *JAMA* 271(1):52-53, 1994.

34. Cobb N and Etzel RA: Unintentional carbon monoxide-related deaths in the United States, 1979 through 1988, *JAMA* 266:659-663, 1991.

35. Coburn RF, Forster RE, and Kane PB: Considerations of the physiological variables that determine blood carboxyhemoglobin concentration in man, *J Clin Invest* 44:1899-1910, 1965.

36. Stryer L: *Biochemistry*, San Francisco, 1975, W.H. Freeman.

37. Coburn RF: Mechanisms of carbon monoxide toxicity, *Prevent Med* 8:310-322, 1979.

38. Wittenberg BA: *Effects of carbon monoxide on isolated heart muscle cells*, Health Effects Institute, Cambridge, MA, 1993.

39. Heckerling PS, Leikin JB, Maturen A, and Perkins JT: Predictors of occult carbon monoxide poisoning in patients with headache and dizziness, *Ann Intern Med* 107:174-176, 1987.

40. Kirkpatrick JN: Occult carbon monoxide poisoning, *West J Med* 146:52-56, 1987.

41. Ekblom B and Huot R: Response to submaximal and maximal exercise at different levels of carboxyhemoglobin, *Acta Physiol Scand* 86:474-482, 1972.

42. Kleinman MT, Davidson DM, Vandagriff RB, Caiozzo VJ, and Whittenberger JL: Effects of short-term exposure to carbon monoxide in subjects with coronary artery disease, *Arch Environ Health* 44:361-369, 1989.

43. Hinderliter AL, Adams KF, Price CJ, Herbst MC, Koch G, and Sheps DS: Effects of low-level carbon monoxide exposure on resting and exercise induced ventricular arrhythmias in patients with coronary artery disease and no baseline ectopy, *Arch Environ Health* 44:89-93, 1990.

44. Dahms TE, Younis LT, Wiens RD, Zarnegar S, Byers SL, and Chaitman BR: Effects of carbon monoxide exposure in patients with documented cardiac arrhythmias, *J Am Coll Cardiol* 21:442-450, 1993.

45. Longo LD: The biological effects of carbon monoxide on the pregnant woman, fetus, and newborn infant, *Am J Obstet Gynecol* 129:69-103, 1977.

46. Quackenboss JJ, Spengler JD, Kanarek MS, Letz R, and Duffy CP: Personal exposure to nitrogen dioxide: relationship to indoor/outdoor air quality and activity patterns, *Environ Sci Technol* 20:775-783, 1986.

47. Ryan PB, Soczec ML, Treitman RD, and Spengler JD: The Boston residential NO_2 characterization study. II. Survey methodology and population concentration estimates, *Atmos Environ* 22:2115-2125, 1988.

48. Godish T: *Indoor air pollution control*, Chelsea, MI, 1989, Lewis Publishers.

49. Samet JM, Lambert WE, Skipper BJ, et al: Nitrogen dioxide and respiratory illnesses in infants, *Am Rev Respir Dis* 148:1258-1265, 1993.

50. Harlos DP: *Acute exposure to nitrogen dioxide during cooking or commuting*, dissertation, Boston, 1988, Harvard School of Public Health.

51. Weber A and Fischer T: Passive smoking at work, *Int Arch Occup Environ Health* 47:209-221, 1980.

52. Turiel I, Hollowell CD, Miksch RR, Rudy JV, Young RA, and Coye MJ: The effects of reduced ventilation on indoor air quality in an office building, *Atmos Environ* 17:51-64, 1983.

53. Melius J, Wallingford K, Keenlyside R, and Carpenter J: Indoor air quality—the NIOSH experience, *Ann Am Conf Government Ind Hyg* 10:3-7, 1984.

54. Lee K, Yanagisawa Y, and Spengler JD: Carbon monoxide and nitrogen dioxide levels in an indoor ice skating rink with mitigation methods, *J Air Waste Manage Assoc* 43:769-771, 1993.

55. Bresnitz ED and Rest KM: Epidemiologic studies of effects of oxidant exposure on human populations, In Watson AY, Bates DR, and Kennedy D, editors: *Air pollution, the automobile and public health*, Washington, DC, 1988, National Academy Press.

56. Morrow PE: Toxicological data on NO_2: An overview, *J Toxicol Environ Health* 13:205-227, 1984.

57. Schlesinger RB: Nitrogen oxides, In Lippmann ML, editor: *Environmental toxicants: exposures and their health effects*, pp 412-453, New York, 1992, Van Nostrand Reinhold.

58. Samet JM, Marbury MC, and Spengler JD: Health effects and sources of indoor air pollution. Part II, *Am Rev Respir Dis* 137:221-242, 1988.

59. Samet JM and Utell MJ: The risk of nitrogen dioxide: what have we learned from epidemiological and clinical studies? *Toxicol Indust Health* 6:247-262, 1990.

60. Goings SAJ, Kulle TJ, Bascom R, et al: Effect of nitrogen dioxide exposure on susceptibility to influenza A virus infection in healthy adults, *Am Rev Respir Dis* 139:1075-1081, 1989.

61. Samet JM: Nitrogen dioxide, In Samet JM and Spengler JD, editors:

Indoor air pollution: a health perspective, pp 170-186, Baltimore, 1991, Johns Hopkins University Press.

62. Orehek J, Massari JP, Gayrard P, Grimaud C, and Charpin J: Effect of short-term, low level nitrogen dioxide exposure on bronchial sensitivity of asthmatic patients, *J Clin Invest* 57:301-307, 1976.

63. U.S. Environmental Protection Agency: *Respiratory health effects of passive smoking: lung cancer and other disorders,* Smoking and Tobacco Control Monograph 4 (NIH Pub No 93-3605), Washington, DC, 1993, National Institutes of Health.

64. Overpeck MD and Moss AJ: *Children's exposure to environmental cigarette smoke before and after birth,* Hyattsville, MD, 1991, U.S. Department of Health and Human Services.

65. Wallace LA: Volatile organic compounds, In Samet JM and Spengler JD, editors: *Indoor air pollution. A health perspective,* pp 252-272, Baltimore, 1991, Johns Hopkins University Press.

66. Guerin MR, Jenkins RA, and Tomkins BA: *The chemistry of environmental tobacco smoke: composition and measurement,* Chelsea, MI, 1992, Lewis Publishers.

67. Spengler JD, Dockery DW, Turner WA, et al: Long-term measurements of respirable sulfates and particles inside and outside homes, *Atmos Environ* 15:23-30, 1981.

68. Spengler JD, Treitman RD, Tosteson T, Mage DT, and Soczek ML: Personal exposures to respirable particulates and implications for air pollution epidemiology, *Environ Sci Technol* 19:700-707, 1985.

69. Repace JL and Lowrey AH: Indoor air pollution, tobacco smoke, and public health, *Science* 208:464-472, 1980.

70. Lambert WE, Samet JM, and Spengler JD: Environmental tobacco smoke concentrations in no-smoking and smoking sections of restaurants, *Am J Public Health* 83:1339-1341, 1993, and (Errata) 83:1399, 1993.

71. National Research Council: *The airliner cabin environment: air quality and safety,* Washington, DC, 1986, National Academy Press.

72. International Agency for Research on Cancer: *IARC monographs on the evaluation of the carcinogenic risk of chemicals to humans: tobacco smoking,* Monograph 38, Lyon, France, 1986, World Health Organization, IARC.

73. National Research Council, Committee on Passive Smoking: *Environmental tobacco smoke: measuring exposures and assessing health effects,* Washington, DC, 1986, National Academy Press.

74. Murray AB and Morrison BJ: The effect of cigarette smoke from the mother on bronchial responsiveness and severity of symptoms in children with asthma, *J Allergy Clin Immunol* 77:575-581, 1986.

75. Coultas DB and Samet JM: Epidemiology and Natural History of Childhood Asthma, In Tinkelman DG, Falliers CJ, and Naspitz CK, editors: *Childhood asthma,* pp 71-114, New York, 1993 Marcel Dekker.

76. Stick SM, Turnbull S, Chua HL, Landau LI, and Lesouef PN: Bronchial responsiveness to histamine in infants and older children, *Am Rev Respir Dis* 142:1143-1146, 1990.

77. Hirayama T: Nonsmoking wives of heavy smokers have a higher risk of lung cancer: a study from Japan, *Br Med J* 282:183-185, 1981.

78. Trichopoulos D, Kalandidi A, Sparros L, and MacMahon B: Lung cancer and passive smoking, *Int J Cancer* 27:1-4, 1981.

79. Pershagen G: Passive Smoking and Lung Cancer, In Samet JM, editor: *Epidemiology of lung cancer,* pp 109-130, New York, 1994, Marcel Dekker.

80. Lee PN: *Environmental tobacco smoke and mortality,* New York, 1992, Karger.

81. Glantz SA and Parmley WW: Passive smoking and heart disease: epidemiology, physiology, and biochemistry, *Circulation* 83:1-12, 1991.

82. Steenland K: Passive smoking and the risk of heart disease, *JAMA* 267:94-99, 1992.

83. Taylor AE, Johnson DC, and Kazemi H: Environmental tobacco smoke and cardiovascular disease: A position paper from the council on cardiopulmonary and critical care, American Heart Association, *Circulation* 86:1-4, 1992.

84. Samet JM and Utell MJ: The environment and the lung: changing perspectives, *JAMA* 266:670-675, 1992.

85. Moschandreas DJ, Zabransky J, and Rector HE: The effects of wood-burning on the indoor residential environment, *Environ Int* 4:463-468, 1980.

86. Sexton K, Spengler JD, and Treitman RD: Effects of residential wood combustion on indoor air quality: a case study in Waterbury, Vermont, *Atmos Environ* 18:1371-1383, 1984.

87. Hytonen S, Alfheim I, and Sorsa M: Effect of emissions from residential wood stoves on SCE induction in CHO cells, *Mutat Res* 118:69-75, 1983.

88. Alfeim I and Ramdahl T: Contribution of wood combustion to indoor air pollution as measured by mutagenicity in *Salmonella* and polycyclic aromatic hydrocarbon concentration, *Environ Mutagen* 6:121-130, 1984.

89. Van Houdt JJ, Daenen CMJ, Boleij JJM, and Alink AGM: Contribution of wood stoves and fire places to mutagenic activity of airborne particulate matter inside homes, *Mutat Res* 171:91-98, 1986.

90. Fick RB, Paul ES, Merrill WW, Reynolds HY, and Loke JSO: Alterations in the antibacterial properties of rabbit pulmonary macrophages exposed to wood smoke, *Am Rev Respir Dis* 129:76-81, 1984.

91. Pandey MR, Neupane RP, and Gautam A: Domestic smoke pollution and acute respiratory infection in Nepal. In Seifert B, Esdorn H, Fischer M, and Ruden H, editors: *Indoor air '87. Proceedings of the 4th international conference on indoor air quality and climate,* vol 3, pp 25-29, Berlin, 1987, Institute for Water, Soil and Air Hygiene.

92. Mumford JL, Hw XZ, Chapman RS, et al: Lung cancer and indoor air pollution in Xuan Wei, China, *Science* 235:217-220, 1987.

93. Dekoning HW, Smith KR, and Last JM: Biomass fuel combustion and health, *Bull WHO* 63:11-26, 1985.

94. Honicky RE, Osborne JS, and Akpom CA: Symptoms of respiratory illness in young children and the use of wood-burning stoves for indoor heating, *Pediatrics* 75:587-593, 1985.

95. Osborne JS and Honicky RE: Chronic respiratory symptoms in young children and indoor heating with a woodburning stove, *Am Rev Respir Dis* 133:A300, 1986.

96. Dockery DW, Spengler JD, Speizer FE, Ferris Jr BG, Ware JH, and Brunekreef B: Associations of health status with indicators of indoor air pollution from an epidemiologic study in six U.S. cities, In Seifert B, Esdorn H, Fischer M, Ruden H, and Wegner J, editors: *Indoor air '87. Proceedings of the 4th international conference on Indoor air quality and climate,* Vol 2, pp 203-207, Berlin, 1987, Institute for Water, Soil and Air Hygiene.

97. Molhave L: Volatile organic compounds and the sick building syndrome, In Lippmann M, editor: *Environmental toxicants: human exposures and their health effects,* pp 633-646, New York, 1992, Van Nostrand Reinhold.

98. Wallace LA: *The total exposure assessment methodology (TEAM) study: summary and analysis,* Vol. 1, Washington, D.C., 1987, Office of Research and Development, U.S. Environmental Protection Agency.

99. Wallace L, Pellizzari E, Hartwell T, Perritt K, and Ziegenfus R: Exposures to benzene and other volatile compounds from active and passive smoking, *Arch Environ Health* 42:272-279, 1987.

100. Marbury MC and Krieger RA: Formaldehyde, In Samet JM and Spengler JD, editors: *Indoor air pollution: a health perspective,* pp 223-252, Baltimore, 1991, Johns Hopkins University Press.

101. Rom WN: *Environmental and occupational medicine,* Boston, 1992, Little, Brown.

101a. Sullivan JB and Krieger GR: *Hazardous materials toxicology: clinical principles of environmental health,* Baltimore, 1992, Williams & Wilkins.

102. Tancrede M, Wilson R, Zeize L, and Crouch EAC: The carcinogenic risk of some organic vapors indoors: a theoretical survey, *Atmos Environ* 10:2187-2205, 1987.

103. Harving H, Dahl R, and Molhave L: Lung function and bronchial

reactivity in asthmatics during exposure to volatile organic compounds, *Am Rev Respir Dis* 143:751-754, 1991.

104. Evans RD: Engineers' guide to the elementary behavior of radon daughters, *Health Phys* 17:229-252, 1969.

105. Nero AV Jr: Radon and its decay products in indoor air: an overview, In Nazaroff WW and Nero AV Jr, editors: *Radon and its decay products in indoor air,* pp 1-53, New York, 1988, John Wiley.

106. Nazaroff WW, Doyle SM, Nero AV Jr, and Sextro RG: Radon entry via potable water, In Nazaroff WW and Nero AV Jr., editors: *Radon and its decay products in indoor air,* pp 131-157, New York, 1988, John Wiley.

107. Nero AV, Schwehr MB, Nazaroff WW, and Revzan KL: Distribution of airborne radon-222 concentrations in U.S. homes, *Science* 234:992-997, 1986.

108. U.S. Environmental Protection Agency: *National residential radon survey: summary report,* Washington, DC, 1992, U.S. Environmental Protection Agency.

109. National Research Council, Committee on the Biological Effects of Ionizing Radiation: *Health risks of radon and other internally deposited alpha-emitters: BEIR IV,* Washington, DC, 1988, National Academy Press.

110. U.S. Environmental Protection Agency: *Technical support document for the 1992 citizen's guide to radon* (EPA/400-R-92-011), Washington, DC, 1992, U.S. Environmental Protection Agency.

111. Lubin JH, Boice JD, Edling C, et al: *Radon and lung cancer risk: a joint analysis of 11 underground miner studies* (NIH Pub No 94-3644), Washington, DC, 1994, U.S. Department of Health and Human Services.

112. Samet JM: Radon and lung cancer, *J Natl Cancer Inst* 81:745-757, 1989.

113. Darby SC and Samet JM: Radon, In Samet JM, editor: *Epidemiology of lung cancer,* pp 219-243, New York, 1994, Marcel Dekker.

114. Lubin JH, Liang Z, Hrubec Z, et al: Radon exposure in residences and lung cancer among women: combined analysis of three studies, In *Cancer causes and control,* 5:114-128, 1994.

115. Lubin JH, Samet JM, and Weinberg C: Design issues in epidemiologic studies of indoor exposure to radon and risk of lung cancer, *Health Phys* 59:807-817, 1990.

116. Stidley CA and Samet JM: A review of ecological studies of lung cancer and indoor radon, *Health Phys* 65:234-251, 1993.

117. Samet JM, Stolwijk J, and Rose SL: Summary: international workshop on residential radon epidemiology, *Health Phys* 60:223-227, 1991.

118. Blot WJ, Xu Z-Y, Boice JD, et al: Indoor radon and lung cancer in China, *J Natl Cancer Inst* 82:1025-1030, 1990.

119. Pershagen G, Liang ZH, Hrubec Z, Svensson C, and Boice JD: Residential radon exposure and lung cancer in women, *Health Phys* 63:179-186, 1992.

120. Health Effects Institute—Asbestos Research Literature Review Panel: *asbestos in public and commercial buildings,* Cambridge, MA, 1991, Health Effects Institute—Asbestos Research.

121. U.S. Environmental Protection Agency: *Study of asbestos-containing materials in public buildings: a report to Congress,* Washington, DC, 1988, United States Environmental Protection Agency.

122. Mossman BT, Bignon J, Corn M, Seaton A, and Gee JBL: Asbestos: Scientific developments and implications for public policy, *Science* 247:294-301, 1990.

123. Lippmann M: Asbestos and other mineral fibers, In Lippmann M, editor: *Environmental toxicants: human exposures and their health effects,* pp 30-75, New York, 1992, Van Nostrand Reinhold.

124. Sawyer RN: Yale art and architecture building asbestos management revisited, *Appl Occup Environ Hyg,* 9:781-4, 1994.

125. Becklake MR: Asbestos and other fiber-related diseases of the lungs and pleura: distribution and determinants in exposed populations, *Chest* 100:248-254, 1991.

126. Oliver LC, Sprince NL, and Greene R: Asbestos-related abnormalities in school maintenance personnel, In Landrigan PJ and Kazemi H, editors: *The third wave of asbestos disease: exposure to asbestos in place. Public health control,* pp 521-529, New York, 1991, The New York Academy of Sciences.

127. Balmes JR, Daponte A, and Cone JE: Asbestos-related disease in custodial and building maintenance workers from a large municipal school district, In Landrigan PJ and Kazemi H, editors: *The third wave of asbestos disease: exposure to asbestos in place. Public health control,* pp 540-549, New York, 1991, The New York Academy of Sciences.

128. Levin SM and Selikoff IJ: Radiological abnormalities and asbestos exposure among custodians of the New York City Board of Education, In Landrigan PJ and Kazemi H, editors: *The third wave of asbestos disease: exposure to asbestos in place. Public health control,* pp 530-539, New York, 1991, The New York Academy of Sciences.

129. Landrigan PJ and Kazemi H, editors: *The third wave of asbestos disease: exposure to asbestos in place. Public health control,* New York, 1991, The New York Academy of Sciences.

130. International Agency for Research on Cancer: *IARC monographs on the evaluation of carcinogenic risks to humans. Man-made mineral fibers and radon,* Monograph 43, Lyon, France, 1986, World Health Organization, IARC.

131. Pope AM, Patterson R, and Burge H: *Indoor allergens: assessing and controlling adverse health effects,* Washington, DC, 1993, National Academy Press.

132. Burge H, Solomon WR, and Boise JR: Microbial prevalence in domestic humidifiers, *Appl Environ Microbiol* 39:840-844, 1980.

133. O'Rourke MK, Quackenboss JJ, and Lebowitz MD: Indoor pollen and mold characterization in homes in Tucson, Arizona, U.S.A. In *Indoor air '90. Proceedings of the 5th international conference on indoor air quality and climate,* vol 2, pp 9-14, Toronto, Ottawa, 1990, Canada Mortgage and Housing Corporation.

134. Wood RA, Eggleston PA, Lind P, et al: Antigenic analysis of household dust samples, *Am Rev Respir Dis* 137:358-363, 1988.

135. Schou C, Hansen GN, Linter T, and Lowenstein H: Assay for major dog allergen. Conf I: Investigation of house dust samples and commercial dog extracts, *J Allergy Clin Immunol* 88:847-853, 1991.

136. Kozak P, Gallup J, Cummins LH, and Gilman SA: Currently available methods for home mold surveys. II. Example problem homes surveyed, *Ann Allergy* 45:167-176, 1980.

137. Brunekreef B, de Rijk L, Verhoeff AP, and Samson R: Classification of dampness in homes. In *Indoor air '90. Proceedings of the 5th international conference on indoor air quality and climate,* vol 2, pp 15-20, Toronto, Ottawa, 1990, Canada Mortgage and Housing Corporation.

138. Su HJ and Burge HA: Examination of microbiological concentrations and association with childhood respiratory health. In *Indoor air '90. Proceedings of the 5th international conference on indoor air quality and climate,* vol 2, pp 21-26, Toronto, Ottawa, 1990, Canada Mortgage and Housing Corporation.

139. Brunekreef B, Dockery DW, Speizer FE, et al: Home dampness and respiratory morbidity in children, *Am Rev Respir Dis* 140:1363-1367, 1989.

140. Dales R, Burnett R, and Zwanenburg H: Adverse health effect in adults exposed to home dampness and molds, *Am Rev Respir Dis* 143:505-509, 1991.

141. Gell PGH and Coombs RRA: *Clinical Aspects of Immunology,* Philadelphia, 1964, F.A. Davis.

142. Smith JM: Epidemiology and natural history of asthma, allergic rhinitis, and atopic dermatitis (eczema), In Middleton E Jr and Reed CE, editors: *Allergy, principles and practice,* St. Louis, 1983, C.V. Mosby.

143. Banaszak EF, Thiede WH, and Fink JN: Hypersensitivity pneumonitis due to contamination of an air conditioner, *N Engl J Med* 283:271-276, 1970.

144. Fink JN: Hypersensitivity pneumonitis, In Middleton E and Reed CE, editors: *Allergy principles and practice,* St. Louis, 1983, C.V. Mosby.

145. Hoffman RE, Wood RC, and Kreiss K: Building-related asthma in Denver office workers, *Am J Public Health* 83:89-93, 1993.

146. Steinberg DR, Bernstein DI, Gallagher JS, Arlian L, and Bernstein IL: Cockroach sensitization in laboratory workers, *J Allergy Clin Immunol* 80:586-590, 1987.

147. Van Metre TE, Marsh DG, Adkinson NF, et al: Dose of cat (Felis domesticus) allergen I (*Fel d* I) that induces asthma, *J Allergy Clin Immunol* 78:62-75, 1986.

148. National Asthma Education Program: *Guidelines for the diagnosis and management of asthma* (Pub No 91-3042), Bethesda, MD, 1991, Department of Health and Human Services.

149. Platts-Mills TAE: The importance of indoor allergens in the treatment of asthma, In *The American Academy of Allergy and Immunology postgraduate course syllabus,* 44th Annual Meeting, March, pp 158-175, Milwaukee, WI, 1988, The American Academy of Allergy and Immunology.

150. Mathison DA, Stevenson DD, and Simon RA: Asthma and the home environment, *Ann Intern Med* 97:128-130, 1982.

151. Finnegan MJ and Pickering CAC: Building related illness, *Clin Allergy* 6:389-405, 1986.

152. Coultas DB, Zumwalt MD, Black WC, and Sobonya RE: The epidemiology of interstitial lung diseases (ILDs), *Am J Respir Crit Care Med* 150:967-972, 1994.

153. Hung L-L, Copperthite DC, Yang CS, Lewis FA, and Zampiello FA: Environmental *Legionella* assessment in office buildings of the continental United States, *Indoor Air* 3:349-353, 1993.

154. Hlady WG, Mullen RC, Mintz CS, Shelton BG, Hopkins RS, and Daikos GL: Outbreak of legionnaire's disease linked to a decorative fountain by molecular epidemiology, *Am J Epidemiol* 138:555-562, 1993.

155. Woods JE, Drewry GM, and Morey PR: Office worker perceptions of indoor air quality effects on discomfort and performance, In Seifert B, Esdorn H, Fischer M, Ruden H, and Wegner J, editors: *Indoor air '87. Proceedings of the 4th international conference on indoor air and climate,* vol 2, pp 464-468, Berlin (West), 1987, Institute for Water, Soil and Air Hygiene.

156. Mendell MJ: Non-specific symptoms in office workers: a review and summary of the epidemiologic literature, *Indoor Air* 3:227-336, 1993.

157. ASHRAE Standard 62-1989: *Ventilation for acceptable indoor air quality,* Atlanta, GA, 1989, American Society of Heating, Refrigerating and Air Conditioning Engineers.

158. Ashford NA and Miller CS: *Chemical exposures,* New York, 1991, Van Nostrand Reinhold.

159. National Research Council: *Multiple chemical sensitivities: addendum to biologic markers in immunotoxicology,* Washington, DC, 1992, National Academy Press.

160. American College of Physicians: Clinical ecology, *Ann Intern Med* 111:168-178, 1989.

161. DeHart RL: Multiple chemical sensitivity—What is it? In *Multiple chemical sensitivities: addendeum to biologic markers in immunotoxicology,* pp 35-39, Washington, DC, 1992, National Academy Press.

162. U.S. Environmental Protection Agency: *A citizen's guide to radon: the guide to protecting yourself and your family from radon,* Washington, DC, 1992, U.S. Government Printing Office.

163. Sexton K: Indoor air quality: an overview of policy and regulatory issues, *Sci Technol Human Values* II:53-67, 1986.

164. U.S. Department of Health and Human Services: *Major local tobacco control ordinances in the United States,* Monograph 3, Washington, DC, 1993, National Institutes of Health.

165. U.S. Environmental Protection Agency: *EPA indoor air quality implementation plan,* Washington, DC, 1987, U.S. Government Printing Office.

166. U.S. Environmental Protection Agency: *Reducing risk: setting priorities and strategies for environmental protection* (SAB-EC-90-021), Washington, DC, 1990, U.S. Environmental Protection Agency.

167. Cole LA: *Elements of risk: the politics of radon,* Washington, DC, 1993, AAAS Press.

168. Nero AV: Developing a conceptual framework for evaluating environmental risks and control strategies: The case of indoor air, In Jantunen M, Kalliokoski P, Kukkonen E, Saarela K, Seppanen O, and Vuorelma H, editors: *Indoor air '93. Proceedings of the 6th international conference on indoor air quality and climate,* vol 3, pp 447-482, Helsinki, Finland, 1993, Indoor Air '93.

169. Samet J: Indoor air pollution: A public health perspective, *Indoor Air* 3:219-226, © 1993, Munksgaard International Publishers Ltd., Copenhagen, Denmark.

Chapter 49

OUTDOOR AIR POLLUTION

John R. Balmes

Sources of exposure
Deposition and clearance of inhaled pollutants
Specific pollutants
    Ozone
    Nitrogen dioxide
    Sulfur dioxide
    Particulate matter
    Atmospheric acidity

The potential for severe health effects due to the inhalation of outdoor air pollutants was made dramatically clear by several pollution episodes associated with increased mortality earlier in this century, in Belgium's Meuse Valley in 1930, in Donora, PA in 1948, and in London in 1952. These episodes were due to the large-scale combustion of coal in the presence of certain meteorologic conditions (i.e., an atmospheric inversion leading to a regionally stagnant, moist air mass). The deaths that occurred during these episodes typically were in elderly persons with preexisting chronic respiratory or cardiac disease. Although current air quality in North America precludes the development of pollution episodes of this historic magnitude, the combustion of high-sulfur-content coal in Ohio River Valley power plants fitted with tall stacks to reduce local pollution continues to cause the emission of sulfur dioxide (SO_2), acid aerosols, and particulate matter (PM) into the upper atmosphere where these pollutants can then be transported by prevailing winds to the northeastern United States and southeastern Canada. Even at currently attained levels in North America, certain pollutants, such as ozone and respirable particles, may be responsible for acute and chronic respiratory morbidity. In countries where sulfur-containing fuels are burned without adequate air quality regulation, such as in eastern Europe, Russia, and China, atmospheric conditions may approach those associated with deaths in the past.

A large body of research has been conducted over the past three decades on the effects of various air pollutants on respiratory health. Since the initial Clean Air Act was passed by the U.S. Congress in 1970, the U.S. Environmental Protection Agency (EPA) has been required to list those pollutants for which there is sufficient scientific evidence documenting the risk to public health from unregulated exposure. The EPA produces criteria documents that compile the available epidemiologic, controlled human exposure, and animal toxicologic studies on the adverse health effects of such pollutants. Each document is intended to provide a critical review of the existing scientific data base regarding a pollutant that will allow the rational design of an air quality standard. By this process of review, a National Ambient Air Quality Standard (NAAQS) has been developed for each so-called criteria pollutant. The current list of EPA criteria pollutants is shown in the box on the next page.

Regulation of highly toxic air pollutants that are emitted from point sources and that are present in extremely low concentrations, so-called "air toxics," is a feature of the 1990 Clean Air Act amendments. These pollutants typically do not cause respiratory toxicity and will not be discussed in this chapter.

SOURCES OF EXPOSURE

The sources of outdoor air pollution are usually categorized as stationary or mobile. Stationary sources are primarily power or manufacturing plants and are responsible for most SO_2 emissions as well as considerable amounts of nitrogen oxides (NO_x) and particulate matter. In the eastern United States and Canada, atmospheric acidity is largely due to the oxidation of SO_2 to sulfuric acid (H_2SO_4) and other acid sulfate species. The combustion of fossil fuel is the most important cause of stationary source emissions, although release of volatile organic compounds (VOCs) by various industrial facilities can contribute to the generation of ozone (O_3) in the atmosphere.

In contrast to the pollution from stationary sources that characterizes eastern North America, southern California

---

Criteria air pollutants (U.S. EPA)

Ozone
Nitrogen dioxide
Sulfur dioxide
Particulate matter
Carbon monoxide
Lead

"smog" is primarily derived from automotive or mobile source emissions. A large fraction of ambient O_3 is the product of complex photochemical reactions involving NO_x and VOCs emitted from automotive tailpipes. Nitric acid (HNO_3) is a more important contributor to atmospheric acidity than H_2SO_4 in southern California and is formed in the atmosphere from the reaction of NO_x with the hydroxyl radical (OH^-). Motor vehicles are also responsible for much carbon monoxide and particulate pollution. A major success story in the control of the criteria pollutants involves the markedly decreased concentrations of lead in the ambient air of U.S. cities achieved as a result of the required use of unleaded gasoline.

Monitoring of ambient air for concentrations of the criteria pollutants is performed at central stations. The regional average concentrations measured at such stations may not adequately characterize personal exposures. For example, local conditions will affect O_3 concentration such that areas downwind from major traffic congestion may have higher levels than those in the immediate vicinity of the congestion. How much time is spent outdoors is an important determinant of personal exposure. Most people spend most of their time indoors, where the concentrations of pollutants are generally lower than in the outdoor air. The concentration of NO_2, however, may be higher in indoor air, largely as a result of natural gas-burning stoves. Individuals who spend a lot of time outdoors, especially if they are increasing their effective dose by means of increased minute ventilation from exercise, may sustain relatively high exposures to pollutants such as O_3 and particulate matter.

DEPOSITION AND CLEARANCE OF INHALED POLLUTANTS

Pollutants in inhaled air are either gases or aerosols. Aerosols are droplets of liquid or particles suspended in gas.

The site of deposition for inhaled gases is largely determined by their water solubility. Gases that are extremely water soluble, such as sulfur dioxide and nitric acid vapor, will be deposited and removed primarily by the upper respiratory tract. These water-soluble gases will thus mainly induce toxic effects on the proximal airways and will damage the distal lung only when inhaled in high concentrations. In contrast, gases that are of relatively low water solubility, such as oxides of nitrogen and ozone, may predominantly injure the distal lung. The less soluble the gas, the greater the potential for damage at the level of the terminal respiratory unit.

The deposition of aerosols is determined by a number of factors, including the size and chemical characteristics of the aerosol, the anatomy of the respiratory tract, and the breathing pattern of the exposed person. The size of the droplet or particle is usually the primary factor affecting deposition, although the chemical nature of the inhaled pollutant can be important, especially if it is a water-soluble acid aerosol that can be neutralized by oral ammonia, such as a sulfuric acid mist. The majority of inhaled particles with a mass median aerodynamic diameter (MMAD) ≥ 10 μm are deposited in the nasopharynx and will not penetrate below the larynx. Particles in the range of 2.5 to 6 μm will deposit primarily in the conducting airways below the larynx and particles in the range of 0.5 to 2.5 μm will deposit primarily in the distal airways and alveoli. Particles with an MMAD <0.5 μm are exhaled without significant deposition. The site of particle deposition is also influenced by hygroscopic growth in the environment of the airways, the shape and dimensions of the respiratory tree, ventilatory pattern (respiratory rate and tidal volume), oral versus nasal breathing, and the amount and nature of respiratory tract secretions. Respiratory tract disease can affect particle deposition by altering airway dimension, airflow pattern, or respiratory secretions. Exercise increases oral breathing, bypassing the nasal scrubbing mechanism, and increases minute ventilation, thereby increasing particle velocity and inertial impaction. Both of these changes result in greater particle deposition in the lower airways.

Clearance of inhaled pollutants occurs by several mechanisms. In general, highly water-soluble particles and gases are absorbed through the epithelial layer into the bloodstream near where they have been deposited. The clearance of insoluble particles is dependent on where they impact. Those deposited in the anterior nasal cavity are expelled by sneezing or rhinorrhea, whereas the remainder of particles deposited in the nose are cleared posteriorly to the pharynx. Particles deposited in the trachea, bronchi, or bronchioles where there is ciliated epithelium and a layer of mucus are transported up the mucociliary escalator to be expelled by coughing or swallowing. Particles deposited distal to the terminal bronchioles are cleared by alveolar macrophages and/or dissolution. Alveolar macrophages will ingest particles and migrate to the mucociliary escalator or into lymphatics. A small fraction of particles deposited in the alveoli will migrate through the alveolar epithelial layer directly into the lymphatic circulation.

SPECIFIC POLLUTANTS
Ozone

Although O_3 has long been associated with southern California smog, many other areas of North America also experience high concentrations of this pollutant, especially Mexico City and cities in the eastern United States and

Table 49-1. Selected national ambient air quality standards (U.S. EPA)

Pollutant	NAAQS
Ozone	0.12 ppm as a 1-hour maximum concentration not to be exceeded more than 3 times in a 3-year period
Nitrogen dioxide	0.053 ppm as an annual arithmetic mean concentration
Sulfur dioxide	Primary: 0.03 ppm as an annual arithmetic mean concentration and 0.14 ppm as a 24-hour maximum concentration
	Secondary: 0.5 ppm as a 3-hour maximum concentration
Particulate matter ($\leq$10 μm in diameter, PM)	50 μg/m^3 as an annual geometric mean concentration and 150 μg/m^3 as a 24-hour maximum concentration

Canada during the summer months. In 1991, 69 million people in the United States resided in counties where the current NAAQS for O$_3$ (see Table 49-1) was not attained.[1] In some southern California communities, there were over 90 days in 1993 during which the standard was exceeded.[2] Thus, the adequacy of the current NAAQS for O$_3$ for the prevention of adverse respiratory effects is of considerable public health importance.

Atmospheric concentrations of the O$_3$-precursors, NO$_x$ and VOCs, have been rising for decades throughout the United States because of continuously increasing combustion of fossil-derived fuels, much of which occurs in automotive vehicles. The meteorologic conditions that tend to foster the generation of ozone are typically present from late spring to early fall. Peak concentrations of O$_3$ typically occur in midafternoon, after both the morning rush hour and several hours of bright sunlight. Because of its highly reactive nature, locally generated O$_3$ is rapidly consumed, and thus its concentration tends to diminish in evening air. This classic daily pattern of afternoon peak concentrations has become less common over much of the United States in recent years. More frequently seen now is a pattern in which the local generation of O$_3$ is less important than the contribution of upwind sources and a large reservoir of atmospheric O$_3$ above the mixing layer.[3] Rather than a sharp daily peak in the afternoon, local generation often appears as a small wave on a broad increase in O$_3$ concentration that may last for several days, especially during the summer months. The implication of this new pattern of O$_3$ concentration is that effective control of this pollutant requires cooperation over wide geographic areas.

Ozone is a highly reactive oxidant that can damage a variety of biomolecules.[4] In particular, O$_3$ reacts with unsaturated intracellular and extracellular lipids to generate free radicals and other toxic products such as hydrogen peroxide and aldehydes. Although direct cytoxicity is clearly a necessary mechanism of O$_3$-induced tissue injury, secondary damage from the inflammatory response may also play a role.

Dosimetric studies of the fate of inhaled O$_3$ indicate that much is deposited in the upper and proximal lower airways.[5] However, because of its relative water insolubility, a considerable fraction does penetrate to the alveoli. Increased inspiratory flow, such as with exercise, causes greater deposition of O$_3$ in the distal lung.

Most of the research on the health effects of O$_3$ has focused on short-term exposure (i.e., <8 hours), probably because the NAAQS is based on a 1-hour maximum concentration. Multiple controlled human exposure studies have demonstrated that O$_3$ inhalation by healthy subjects causes mean decrements in forced expiratory volume in 1 second (FEV1) and forced vital capacity (FVC) that correlate with concentration, exposure duration, and minute ventilation.[6-8] Figure 49-1 shows the mean decrement in FEV1 over time in a population of healthy volunteers exposed to 0.2 ppm O$_3$ for 4 hours during moderate exercise. These decrements in lung function are due primarily to decreased inspiratory capacity rather than to airways obstruction. The mechanism of the decreased inspiratory capacity appears to be neurally mediated involuntary inhibition of inspiratory effort involving stimulation of airway C-fibers.[9] Pretreatment with indomethacin or ibuprofen reduces O$_3$-induced decrements in pulmonary function, suggesting that this response is at least partially mediated by the release of cyclooxygenase products.[10] There is considerable interindividual variability in the magnitude of the lung function response to O$_3$; only 10% to 25% of subjects tested at 0.12 ppm will develop decrements in FEV1 of $\geq$10% after 1 to 2 hours of exposure, although a greater fraction of subjects will respond at higher concentrations.[11] Somewhat surprisingly, subjects who are cigarette smokers,[12] older,[13] asthmatic,[14] or have chronic obstructive pulmonary disease (COPD)[15] do not typically demonstrate greater O$_3$-induced decrements in pulmonary function than healthy subjects. The acute decrements in pulmonary function induced by O$_3$ usually resolve within 24 hours.

Respiratory symptoms appear to be associated with the mean decrements in pulmonary function observed in controlled exposure studies of adult subjects. A meta-analysis of the results from multiple studies showed a correlation between change in FEV1 and the probability of developing lower respiratory tract symptoms (e.g., substernal chest discomfort, cough, wheeze, and dyspnea).[16] Such symptoms have been reported by adult subjects engaged in exercise while exposed to O$_3$ in concentrations at or below the current NAAQS. In contrast, children do not generally report respiratory symptoms to the same extent as adults for a given effective dose or a given decrement in FEV1.[17] Their relative lack of symptomatic responsiveness may place chil-

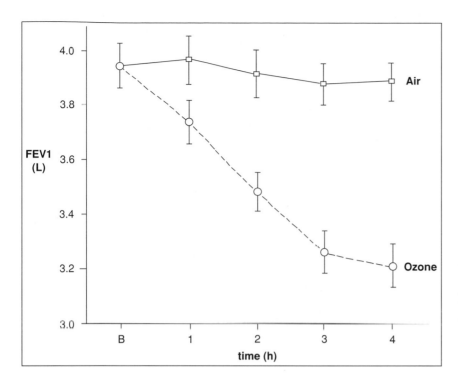

Fig. 49-1. Mean ± SEM FEV1 at baseline and at hourly levels for 66 healthy subjects who completed 4-hour exposure to both O_3 (0.2 ppm) and air. Solid line, air; dashed line, O_3. (Modified from Aris R, Tager I, Christian D, et al: Methacholine responsiveness is not associated with O_3-induced decreases in FEV1, *Chest* 107:621-628, 1995. With permission.)

dren at greater risk for adverse health effects, because they may be less likely to curtail their exposures.

Several field studies of children and young adults have yielded results that parallel those of controlled exposure studies.[18-20] Associations between ambient O_3 concentrations and both respiratory symptoms and lung function decrements have been documented in subjects spending considerable time exercising in outdoor settings such as summer camps. The slopes of the exposure–response relationships in field studies are often higher than those from controlled exposure studies, suggesting interactive effects as a consequence of coexposure to other pollutants. Studies of competitive athletes have also documented reduced performance during exposure to O_3 at or near the current NAAQS.[21,22]

Another adverse effect of short-term exposure to O_3 is enhanced airway responsiveness to nonspecific stimuli such as methacholine and histamine.[24,25] This effect may persist longer than the acute decrements in lung function. Ozone-induced increases in airway responsiveness have not correlated with postexposure decreases in FEV1.[11] There is also both in vitro and in vivo evidence from animal toxicologic studies that confirms the effect of O_3 to increase nonspecific airway responsiveness.[26,27]

Inflammation of the respiratory tract after O_3 exposure occurs in all species that have been studied. In animals exposed to O_3, the following acute changes have been demonstrated: Type I alveolar and ciliated airway epithelial cell injury, infiltration of the airway mucosa by neutrophils, and increased bronchoalveolar lavage (BAL) fluid neutrophils, histamine, eicosanoids, total protein, interleukin-6 (IL-6), and fibronectin.[28-30] The use of BAL in controlled human

exposure studies has documented O_3-induced inflammation of the lower respiratory tract in healthy adult volunteers.[24,30-32] Figure 49-2 shows the effect of 4-hour exposure to 0.2 ppm during moderate exercise on a number of inflammatory endpoints in BAL fluid obtained 18 hours after exposure. In addition, this study demonstrated evidence of proximal airway inflammation in isolated left mainstem bronchial lavage fluid and on endobronchial biopsy specimens.[32] Nasal inflammatory changes have also been reported in human subjects after relatively low-level exposure to O_3, and, in one study, neutrophils in nasal lavage fluid were correlated with neutrophils in BAL fluid.[33]

In experimental animals, the acute physiologic responses that are induced by a single short-term exposure to O_3 are blunted with subsequent exposures over time.[34] Multiple studies of human subjects have also shown that over 4 to 5 days of repeated short-term exposures to O_3, the greatest decrements in FEV1 and FVC occur on the second day with progressive diminution of these decrements on subsequent days.[35,36] This phenomenon has been called "tolerance" or "adaptation." In the absence of further exposure, adaptation persists for 4 to 7 days and then begins to wane. The mechanism of adaptation to O_3 remains unclear, although it has been suggested that increased levels of antioxidants play a role. A key question is whether adaptation of the acute physiologic responses to O_3 reflects a similar adaptation of the respiratory tract injury or inflammatory response. In both rats and humans, the increase in BAL neutrophils that is observed after a single, short-term exposure appears to diminish after 5 consecutive days of such exposure.[37,38] Although adaptation as measured by pulmonary function and BAL neutrophils may occur, there is animal experimental

Fig. 49-2. Bronchoalveolar lavage endpoints (mean ± scanning electron mircoscopy [SEM]) after exposure to air (dark striped) and 0.2 ppm O_3 (lightly stippled) for 4 hours. The mean for each endpoint is equal to the product of the ordinate value and the units displayed in parentheses below each endpoint. Neutrophils are expressed as a fraction of total cells. PMNs, neutrophils; LDH, lactate dehydrogenase; ALB, albumin; FN, fibronectin; IL-8, interleukin 8; GM-CSF, granulocyte-monocyte colony-stimulating factor; a-1-AT, α_1-antitrypsin. The asterisks indicate significant differences between air and O_3 at the $p < 0.05$ level. (Modified from Aris RM, Christian D, Hearne PQ, et al: Ozone-induced airway inflammation in human subjects as determined by airway lavage and biopsy, *Am Rev Respir Dis* 148:1363-1372, 1993. With permission.)

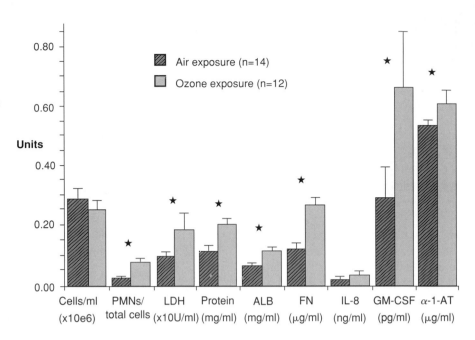

evidence that tissue injury may progress.[34] The attenuation of O_3-induced functional responses may actually be somewhat "maladaptive" because it could serve to prevent individuals from curtailing their exposure to concentrations of O_3 that may lead to lung injury. There is, in fact, limited evidence to support the existence of functional adaptation among southern California residents during the summer O_3 season.[39]

The effects of chronic exposure to O_3 in residents of southern California or Mexico City are obviously of considerable public health significance. It is clear from animal toxicologic studies that chronic exposure to O_3 at concentrations higher than the ambient range can cause morphologic changes from the nose to the distal lung. Loss of ciliated cells and metaplastic changes have been demonstrated in the nasal epithelium, and replacement of proximal alveolar Type I and Type II epithelial cells by airway cells (so-called "bronchiolarization") has been repeatedly documented in terminal lung units.[40,41] A mild peribronchiolar inflammatory reaction, localized deposition of collagen, and remodeling of the peribronchiolar airspace also occur. Primates appear to be significantly more susceptible to these effects of O_3 inhalation than rodents.[42] Because the site of greatest O_3-induced morphologic alteration in the lung is the terminal airway, similar to what is observed with cigarette smoking, it has been hypothesized that emphysema might be a consequence of chronic exposure. However, the changes described in chronically exposed animals are focal, confined to the centriacinar region, and not associated with the diffuse alveolar septal destruction characteristic of emphysema.[43] The functional impact of these changes has usually been relatively mild and, not infrequently, in a more restrictive- than obstructive-type pattern. Although higher-level exposures appear to cause collagen accumulation

and/or altered metabolism,[44] chronic exposures to near-ambient concentrations of O_3 have not always elicited this response.

Although most chronic animal studies have used experimental designs that involve stable long-term exposures, a few studies have looked at intermittent exposures to O_3 alternating with periods of nonexposure in an effort to mimic the diurnal or seasonal patterns of human exposure. The results of these intermittent exposure studies tend to suggest that cumulative exposure is not the sole determinant of lung structural remodeling; the pattern of exposure may also be relevant. For example, in one study of monkeys, exposure to 0.25 ppm O_3 for 8 hours per day during alternate months over an 18-month period was associated with greater morphologic and lung functional changes than was continuous exposure for the same period.[40] It appears that mechanisms of adaptation and repair may cause structural damage that is superimposed on that caused directly by O_3. The evidence concerning the reversibility of lung structural remodeling after animals have been removed from further O_3 exposure is mixed, with the data from some studies suggesting progression[45] and that from others indicating significant recovery.[46]

The effects of chronic exposure to pollutants can be investigated in humans only by means of epidemiologic studies. There are limited epidemiologic data available to answer the question of whether chronic exposure to ambient levels of O_3 can cause permanent damage to the lungs. As part of a prospective study of COPD, spirometry was obtained at baseline and then 5 years later on never-smokers in two communities in southern California with frequent high O_3 concentrations, Lancaster and Glendora.[47] The annual rate of decline in FEV1 among the Lancaster and Glendora residents was almost twice that observed in Tucson,[48] where levels of O_3 are generally much lower. Impaired single-breath nitrogen washout was present in the youngest age group, 7 to 10 years, and worsened with age. This pulmonary function abnormality is consistent with the changes in small airway morphology seen in the animal studies described above. A cross-sectional study comparing wives of Long Beach shipyard workers who were never or former smokers with a previous study of women from Michigan reported that the Long Beach subjects had significantly lower values for FEV1 and a number of other parameters of pulmonary function.[49] Although the data from both of these studies of southern California residents suggest a chronic effect of air pollution on lung function, the lack of exposure information and inadequate control of potential confounding factors complicate their interpretation.

Other evidence of chronic effects of O_3 on lung function comes from an analysis of data from the second National Health and Nutrition Examination Survey (NHANES II).[50] In this study, ambient O_3 concentration was associated with reduced lung function in residents of areas where the annual average concentration exceeded 0.04 ppm. The contribution of peak exposures to this association was not reported, but the effect seen for the annual average supports the hypothesis that chronic O_3 exposure leads to cumulative lung injury. Preliminary but highly provocative data from an autopsy study of accidental deaths in young Los Angeles residents referred to the coroner's office showed the presence of respiratory bronchiolitis in a high proportion of the cases.[51] The pathologic changes noted in this study were similar to those demonstrated in animal toxicologic studies of chronic O_3 inhalation, but the interpretation of the results as showing an O_3 effect is again limited by the lack of information about potentially confounding exposures such as cigarette smoking.

There is considerable animal toxicologic evidence that short-term exposure to O_3 can increase susceptibility to bacterial pneumonia. Exposure to as little as 0.08 ppm for 3 hours was associated with increased mortality in rodents subsequently challenged with bacteria either by aerosolization or tracheal instillation.[52] The presumed mechanism for the increased susceptibility to bacterial pneumonia after O_3 inhalation is impaired alveolar macrophage (AM) function since these cells play a critical role in the initial host defense against bacteria in the respiratory tract. Both in vivo and in vitro studies (including those using human cells) have confirmed that O_3 can depress AM function.[53,54] Evidence of increased respiratory tract infection in humans following O_3 exposure, however, is lacking.

Unlike the mandate of the U.S. Occupational Safety and Health Administration (OSHA) to protect the "average" worker from adverse health effects, the EPA is required by the Clean Air Act to protect sensitive subgroups, such as the very young, the elderly, and individuals with preexisting respiratory or cardiac disease. Because of their tendency to experience bronchoconstriction on inhalation of noxious

stimuli, persons with asthma are a frequently studied subgroup. With O_3 in particular, it is reasonable to expect that asthmatic persons would be more sensitive, given that two characteristic features of asthma, airway inflammation and increased nonspecific airway responsiveness, are acute responses induced by its inhalation. Several controlled exposure studies of asthmatic and atopic subjects have failed to show enhanced spirometric responses to short-term O_3 inhalation.[14,55] This result is not as surprising as it might seem when one considers that the primary mechanism for O_3-induced decrements in FEV1 is decreased inspiratory capacity rather than airways obstruction. One study involving a high concentration (0.4 ppm) and relatively heavy exercise did show enhanced responses in asthmatic subjects compared with normal controls.[56]

In contrast to the results of the controlled exposure studies of asthmatic subjects described previously, several epidemiologic studies have provided evidence that high ambient O_3 concentrations are associated with an increased rate of asthma attacks.[57,58] Other studies have documented increased hospital admissions or emergency department visits for respiratory disease, including asthma, after high O_3 days.[59] A recent controlled exposure study has provided a possible explanation for the apparent disparity between the results of chamber studies, which tend not to show enhanced responses of asthmatic subjects to O_3, and epidemiologic studies, which show an O_3-related increase in asthma attacks.[60] In this study, a 1-hour exposure to 0.12 ppm while at rest caused a twofold reduction in the provocative concentration of inhaled antigen required to cause immediate bronchoconstriction in specifically sensitized asthmatic subjects. Although there are animal experimental data that support enhanced responsiveness to antigen after O_3 inhalation,[61] there are also data that suggest O_3-related blunting of responses to antigen.[62] The question of the effect of O_3 inhalation on asthma remains one of intense research interest.

Ozone is rarely the sole pollutant of concern in urban smog. It has long been suspected that O_3 toxicity may be enhanced by coexposure to other pollutants. As noted, the results of field studies involving exposure of human subjects in the ambient environment have added to this suspicion. In general, the effect of O_3 on FEV1 in field studies is greater than that in chamber studies. Thus, it appears likely that environmental cofactors can potentiate the toxicity of O_3. There is considerable animal toxicity evidence to support synergism between O_3 and H_2SO_4 aerosols.[63] The identification of the specific environmental cofactors that are responsible for the enhancement of O_3 toxicity is of obvious regulatory significance, so further research in this area will be required.

In summary, tens of millions of persons in the United States are exposed to levels of O_3 above the current NAAQS that are capable of inducing both acute decrements in lung function and respiratory symptoms. Although these effects are transient, acute respiratory tract inflammation can also be induced by short-term exposure to ambient concentrations of O_3 with exercise. The long-term consequences of this type of acute inflammatory response are not well understood. Chronic exposure of experimental animals at higher than ambient levels is not associated with emphysema or diffuse fibrosis. However, chronic exposure to near-ambient concentrations has been demonstrated to cause morphologic changes in the terminal bronchioles in which metaplastic airway epithelium extends into the proximal acinar regions accompanied by a mild inflammatory reaction, localized deposition of collagen, and remodeling of the peribronchiolar airspace. Whether such pathologic changes occur in residents of areas with persistent O_3 pollution such as southern California or Mexico City is not known. Because O_3 inhalation can induce both airway inflammation and enhanced airway responsiveness, it is reasonable to expect persons with asthma to have greater susceptibility to this pollutant. There is both animal toxicologic and epidemiologic evidence to support this expectation. Ozone is rarely the sole pollutant of concern in urban smog, and again there are animal and human field study data that suggest that environmental cofactors enhance the toxicity of O_3.

Nitrogen dioxide

Most ambient NO_2 is generated by the burning of fossil-derived fuels, during which oxygen and nitrogen react to form nitrogen oxide (NO), which further reacts to form NO_2 and other NO_x. The principal source of NO_2 in outdoor air is motor vehicle emissions, but power plants and fossil-fuel-burning industrial facilities also contribute. In most U.S. urban areas, ambient levels of NO_2 vary with traffic intensity. Annual average concentrations range from 0.015 to 0.035 ppm.[1] Of all regions in the United States reporting NO_2 monitoring data in recent years, only the Los Angeles Basin exceeded the current NAAQS (see Table 49-1).

In contrast to other criteria pollutants, NO_2 is a common contaminant of indoor air, and indoor levels often exceed those found outdoors. Indoor sources of NO_2 include gas cooking stoves, gas furnaces, and kerosene space heaters. Because the majority of homes in the United States have gas cooking stoves and Americans spend a large proportion of time in their homes, the home environment is usually the most important contributor to total NO_2 exposure. Concentrations as high as 0.5 ppm may persist for as long as 45 minutes in a kitchen with a gas stove in use, and peak levels may exceed this by several-fold.[64] Nitrous acid (HNO_2) and other NO_x are emitted by gas stoves so that health effects associated with the use of such appliances may not be due to NO_2 alone.

While both NO_2 and O_3 are oxidant pollutants, NO_2 is less chemically reactive and thus is usually considered less potent. Although both pollutants are relatively insoluble in water, the solubility of NO_2 is somewhat higher. When NO_2 is absorbed onto the moist surfaces of the respiratory tract,

it can be hydrolyzed to evolve acidic species such as HNO_2 and nitric acid (HNO_3). The potential for NO_2 to cause the local generation of hydrogen ions in the airways may be an important feature of its toxicity, especially if the animal toxicologic data that indicate synergism between O_3 and acidity are confirmed in humans. Nitrogen dioxide and O_3 are frequent copollutants in southern California smog, where the 1-hour NO_2 concentration may occasionally exceed 0.25 ppm.

The annual averaging time of the NAAQS for NO_2 (as opposed to the 1-hour maximum for O_3) reflects an assessment that the health effects of this pollutant are determined more by chronic, low-level exposure than by transient, high-level exposures. Whether this assessment is correct or not has important consequences for individuals in the population with preexisting respiratory disease, such as those with asthma or COPD, who are susceptible to the development of acute exacerbations. The lack of a short-term averaging time in the current NAAQS means that asthmatic persons are not felt to be at risk of developing acute exacerbations after brief exposures to NO_2.

The results of multiple controlled human exposure studies have demonstrated no significant decrements in pulmonary function in normal, healthy subjects after exposure to NO_2 at concentrations below 1.5 ppm for 2 hours or less.[65] Controlled exposure studies of subjects with asthma, however, have produced inconsistent results. In the earliest study to demonstrate an increased sensitivity of asthmatic subjects to low-level NO_2 exposure, 13 of 20 subjects were reported to have enhanced airway responsiveness to carbachol after inhalation of 0.1 ppm NO_2 for 1 hour while at rest.[66] Unfortunately, two subsequent studies attempting to confirm the earlier report of enhanced airway responsiveness produced conflicting results.[67,68]

Perhaps the best evidence that short-term exposure to ambient levels of NO_2 can cause adverse respiratory effects in subjects with asthma came from a University of Rochester study that included exercise during exposure.[69] In this study, a 20-minute exposure via mouthpiece during rest caused no effects, but the addition of a 10-minute exposure with moderate exercise potentiated exercise-induced bronchospasm and enhanced airway responsiveness to cold air 1 hour later. Unfortunately, a follow-up study by the Rochester investigators involving exposure to 0.3 ppm NO_2 for 4 hours in a chamber during exercise failed to confirm their earlier findings, although subjects who participated in both studies remained consistent in their responses.[70]

The most recent reports of low-level NO_2 exposure in subjects with asthma continue to be inconsistent. Two studies with relatively large numbers of asthmatic subjects showed no significant effects on pulmonary function or airway responsiveness after exposure in a chamber with exercise for as long as 2 hours to concentrations of NO_2 as high as 3.0 ppm.[71,72] In contrast, another study involving exposure of asthmatic subjects to 0.5 ppm NO_2 for 1 hour while at rest demonstrated a significant increase in airway responsiveness to methacholine (measured using partial expiratory flow at 40% of the vital capacity as the response endpoint).[73] One possible explanation for the inconsistent results from controlled NO_2 exposure studies of asthmatic subjects is that only a subgroup are "responders." Unfortunately, there appears to be no obvious way to identify such responders before NO_2 exposure, as neither baseline pulmonary function nor airway responsiveness has predicted responses to NO_2.

In a pilot field study, continuous monitoring of NO_2 levels in 11 asthmatic subjects for 5 days was combined with periodic spirometry.[64] The limited data suggested that at NO_2 concentrations >0.3 ppm, most of the subjects developed decreased spirometric function, while at concentrations <0.3 ppm there were no consistent effects. Another epidemiologic study has linked indoor NO_2 exposure to the development of respiratory symptoms and decrements in peak expiratory flow in subjects with asthma (but not in normal subjects).[74]

There are abundant animal toxicologic data and reports of accidental human exposure that indicate that short-term inhalation of high concentrations of NO_2 can produce terminal bronchiolar and diffuse alveolar injury; exposure of humans to concentrations >150 ppm NO_2 typically results in death.[75] The relevance of such acute effects to ambient exposures has been questioned. In contrast to what is seen with O_3, short-term exposure to NO_2 at concentrations in the ambient range does not induce neutrophil migration into the airways and alveoli. However, multihour exposure to 2.0 ppm NO_2, a concentration considerably higher than what occurs even transiently in Los Angeles, does appear to be associated with mild increases in BAL neutrophils in human subjects.[76] Of interest given the evidence that NO_2 increases the susceptibility to respiratory tract infections, there is both animal and human study evidence that it may also alter lymphocyte subsets in the lung and possibly the blood as well.[77,78]

Chronic exposure of animals to high concentrations of NO_2 has been shown to cause structural damage to alveoli with airspace enlargement that is somewhat analogous to human emphysema.[79] It is more controversial whether chronic exposure to lower concentrations can lead to such structural damage. There is some similarity in the morphologic changes induced by NO_2 and O_3. The terminal lung unit is the site of greatest NO_2-induced injury. The ciliated cells of the terminal bronchioles undergo hypertrophy and hyperplasia with loss of secretory granules in Clara cells, and loss of cilia.[80] Type I alveolar cells also undergo hypertrophy and hyperplasia followed by cell death and desquamation and replacement by Type II cells. As is the case with O_3, intermittent exposure with short-term peaks appears to induce more structural lung damage than continuous exposure to the same concentration.[81] Again similar to what has been observed with O_3, there is evidence of inter-

species variability in susceptibility to the injury and inflammatory effects of NO_2 inhalation; rats are much less susceptible than monkeys.[82] Evidence of age-related effects on susceptibility to NO_2 has also been found.[83] Neonates seem to be relatively resistant to NO_2, and susceptibility increases with age until adulthood.

Animal infectivity studies after NO_2 exposure have generally shown that concentrations approximately an order of magnitude above the ambient range may impair respiratory tract defenses against some bacteria and viruses. Exposure to NO_2, usually in mice, is followed by inhalational innoculation of bacteria or viruses. Nitrogen dioxide exposure increases mortality from a subsequent bacterial challenge, and concentration seems to be a more important factor than exposure duration. Increased mortality has been demonstrated in mice exposed to as low as 0.5 ppm NO_2 for 3 months.[84] The mechanism(s) of NO_2-induced enhanced microbial infectivity is not clearly understood but is likely due to AM dysfunction. Both impaired phagocytic ability and decreased antibacterial superoxide production of AMs have been shown in vitro after NO_2 exposure.[85,86]

One human experimental study was designed to test the hypothesis that exposure to NO_2 increases susceptibility to viral infections.[87] Healthy volunteers were exposed to either 1.0 to 3.0 ppm NO_2 or filtered air for 2 hours per day for 3 consecutive days and innoculated with a live, attenuated influenza A virus on the second day. The study involved annual reexposure and reinnoculations over a 3-year period. Viral infection was monitored by recovery of virus from nasal washings and by specific antibody titers in nasal washings and serum. Because of the experimental design of this study, it was hoped that a definitive answer to the question of whether NO_2 exposure decreases resistance to viral infection would be forthcoming. Unfortunately, the results of the study were ambiguous, allowing either an interpretation that an insufficient number of subjects was responsible for the failure to observe a more significant NO_2 effect or an interpretation that ambient NO_2 exposure is unlikely to exert a strong effect on resistance to viral infection. Another approach has been to obtain AMs from NO_2-exposed human subjects by BAL and to investigate the in vitro responses of these cells to influenza virus. The limited data available to date utilizing this approach suggest that an exposure to NO_2 as low as 0.6 ppm for 3 hours has the potential to alter AM responses to influenza virus.[88]

Epidemiologic studies that have assessed the role of ambient NO_2 exposure as a risk factor for respiratory infection have been limited by the inability to isolate the effects of NO_2 from those of copollutants. However, numerous studies have focused on NO_2 in the indoor environment. Many of these studies were cross-sectional surveys of schoolchildren. Early reports from cross-sectional surveys indicated that children from homes with gas stoves had an increased prevalence of respiratory symptoms and illnesses compared with children from homes with electric stoves.[89,90] Unfortunately, subsequent surveys have often failed to confirm the initial findings.[91,92] Prospective studies of the effect of stove type and indoor NO_2 exposures on respiratory morbidity also have produced conflicting results.[93,94] The methodologic problems that complicate the interpretation of epidemiologic studies on the risk of respiratory illness from indoor exposure to NO_2 include small sample size, inadequate quantification of exposure, inability to control potential confounding variables (e.g., exposure to environmental tobacco smoke, socioeconomic status, the presence of other children in the home, day care attendance), and lack of objective endpoints. A recent meta-analysis pooled the data from 11 studies with various outcome measures of lower respiratory illness.[95] The pooled analysis showed a significant association between estimated NO_2 exposure and respiratory illness that implied that a 15-ppb increase in exposure (roughly the effect of living in a home with a gas stove) was correlated with a 20% increase in illness risk.

As was noted for O_3, environmental exposures to NO_2 do not occur without coexposure to other pollutants. Somewhat surprisingly, given that both pollutants are oxidants, studies of combined exposure to NO_2 and O_3 in human subjects generally have not demonstrated enhanced toxicity; the effects on pulmonary function have been those seen with exposure to O_3 alone. A recent study, however, showed that preexposure of healthy women to 0.6 ppm NO_2 for 2 hours enhanced the effect of a subsequent exposure to 0.3 ppm O_3 on nonspecific airway responsiveness.[96] Two studies that have investigated the effects of NO_2 exposure on subsequent SO_2-induced bronchoconstriction have produced conflicting results; one study showed increased responsiveness to SO_2[97] and the other showed no change.[98]

In summary, NO_2 is a pollutant that is a ubiquitous component of urban smog that is generated by combustion of fossil-derived fuels from both mobile and stationary sources. Indoor concentrations often exceed those outdoors, however, primarily due to the use of gas stoves. Inhaled NO_2 penetrates to the deep lung because of the relatively low water solubility of the gas. The toxicity of NO_2 is probably due to its oxidative properties. Controlled exposure studies of normal, healthy subjects have shown no effects of low-level exposure on pulmonary function. Controlled studies of subjects with asthma have been inconsistent, with some evidence of a subgroup with increased sensitivity. The data from epidemiologic studies of the effect of indoor NO_2 exposure on risk of respiratory illness in children are also inconsistent. Chronic exposure of experimental animals to high concentrations of NO_2 has caused emphysema-like changes, and mice exposed to concentrations approximately an order of magnitude higher than the ambient range have decreased resistance to bacterial infection. The applicability of these results to ambient exposure of humans is not straightforward, however. Based on the available evidence, indoor NO_2 exposure is of greater concern regarding po-tential adverse respiratory health effects than outdoor exposure. Nevertheless, NO_2 emissions remain an important regulatory target in terms of ambient air quality because of their role in the generation of tropospheric O_3.

Sulfur dioxide

Sulfur dioxide is a major air pollutant in many urban areas and is produced by the combustion of sulfur-containing fuels at stationary sources. Perhaps the most important cause of SO_2 emissions is the burning of sulfur-containing coal at electric power plants. Because high-sulfur-content coal has remained a relatively cheap fuel in regions where it is mined, SO_2 emissions generally have been more of a problem in the eastern United States than in southern California, where smog is primarily a result of photochemical reactions involving motor vehicle emissions. Unfortunately, the building of tall smokestacks to reduce the local concentrations of SO_2 around midwestern and eastern U.S. power plants has led to the long-distance transport of sulfur oxide pollutants and their progeny, acid sulfates, to New England and Canada (so-called "acid rain").

Sulfur oxide emissions in the United States increased steadily during the twentieth century to a peak of 32 million tons in 1970.[99] After the enactment of the Clean Air Act in 1970, SO_2 emissions did decrease. Prior to the passage of the Clean Air Act amendments of 1990, SO_2 emissions were projected to increase as a consequence of population growth. The 1990 amendments, however, mandate a 50% reduction in SO_2 emissions over time. Exposure to high concentrations of SO_2 is highly localized to the vicinity (within 20 km) of major stationary sources. Away from such sources, urban SO_2 concentrations do not often exceed 0.2 to 0.3 ppm as a 1-hour average.[100]

The current primary NAAQS for SO_2 consists of an annual arithmetic mean concentration and a 24-hour maximum concentration; the secondary standard is a 3-hour maximum concentration (see Table 49-1). Similar to the discussion for NO_2 above, the lack of a 1-hour averaging time in the current NAAQS for SO_2 indicates that persons with asthma are not thought to be at risk for developing acute exacerbations after brief exposures. Although the data on responses of subjects with asthma to NO_2 exposure are inconsistent, there is no question that brief (i.e., <1 hour) exposures to low concentrations of SO_2 can induce bronchoconstriction in such subjects.

The initial clues that SO_2 might be an air pollutant capable of causing adverse respiratory effects came from the severe pollution episodes described in the introduction to this chapter that were associated with exacerbations of preexisting respiratory disease and excess mortality. Although exposure information for these episodes is not usually available, significantly elevated concentrations of SO_2 were probably present. Until about 15 years ago, however, the results of both animal toxicologic and controlled human exposure studies had suggested that only concentrations of

SO$_2$ likely to occur after industrial accidents were capable of causing respiratory tract injury.

Morphologic evidence of injury typically has not been demonstrated in experimental animals unless exposure has been to concentrations >25 ppm.[101] Even at high concentrations, chronic exposure conditions are often required to cause structural lung damage. However, exposure to lower concentrations of SO$_2$ (but usually >5 ppm) has been shown to cause pulmonary function changes in animals.[102] The results of early controlled human exposure studies involving normal, healthy subjects confirmed that inhalation of concentrations <5 ppm did not cause significant decrements in pulmonary function.[103] Because ambient levels are usually <1 ppm, SO$_2$ was deemed unlikely to be an important contributor to respiratory morbidity due to air pollution.

Since 1980, multiple studies from different laboratories have documented that concentrations of SO$_2$ that have no effect on normal subjects can induce bronchoconstriction in subjects with asthma. The first investigators to demonstrate the bronchoconstrictor potential of SO$_2$ administered the gas via mouthpiece, thereby bypassing the scrubbing mechanism of the nasal passages.[104] Because of the relative water solubility of the gas, the nose is effective at removing most inspired SO$_2$ during resting breathing. Subsequent studies have demonstrated, however, that freely breathing subjects with asthma will develop bronchoconstriction during moderate exercise (i.e., at workloads calibrated to achieve minute ventilations ≥40 L/min).[105,106] Figure 49-3 shows the results of one such study. In addition to allowing delivery of a larger dose over a given period, high ventilatory rates require a greater component of oral breathing, which is associated with decreased warming and humidification of inspired air. Breathing cold and/or dry air can induce bronchoconstriction in subjects with asthma in the absence of SO$_2$. Airway cooling and/or drying enhance the effects of inhaled SO$_2$,[107] and it is clear that this pollutant has greater bronchoconstrictor potency when exposure is via the oral route or during exercise. Under these conditions, concentrations as low as 0.4 ppm have been demonstrated to induce significant decrements in FEV1 in subjects with asthma.[108]

The bronchoconstrictor response to inhaled SO$_2$ occurs early, within minutes of onset of exposure. The response increases for only a relatively short time (i.e., 5 to 10 minutes) as exposure duration increases and then tends to plateau. The induced bronchoconstriction tends to resolve spontaneously within 1 hour after the end of exposure but can be reversed more rapidly with administration of inhaled β-adrenergic bronchodilator medications.[109] There also appears to be a refractory period after SO$_2$ inhalation during which the bronchoconstrictor response to a repeat exposure will be of lesser magnitude; this period may last up to several hours.[110] Sulfur dioxide-induced bronchoconstriction can be partially blocked by pretreatment with antimuscarinic agents or cromolyn sodium.[111] The effect of antimus-

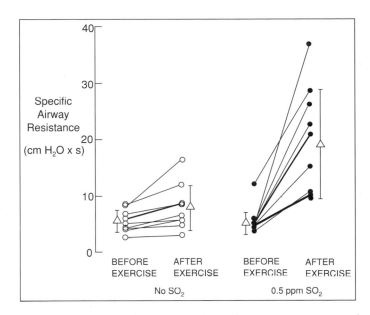

Fig. 49-3. Increase in specific airway resistance from before to after 5 minutes of heavy exercise in 10 asthmatic subjects breathing filtered air containing no SO$_2$ (open circles) or containing 0.5 ppm SO$_2$ (closed circles). Means are indicated by a triangle beside the individual data points and SD by extensions from the means. (Modified from Bethel RA, Epstein J, Sheppard D, et al: Sulfur dioxide-induced bronchoconstriction in freely-breathing, exercising, asthmatic subjects, *Am Rev Respir Dis* 128:987-990, 1983. With permission.)

carinic agents suggests that a reflex mechanism involving parasympathetic pathways is an important component of the bronchoconstrictor response to SO$_2$. Rapidly adapting irritant receptors in the larynx and trachea may initiate the response.

The bronchoconstrictor effect of inhaled SO$_2$ in individuals with asthma will occur after extremely brief periods of exposure. Several studies have demonstrated that brief exposure of asthmatic subjects to concentrations as low as 0.25 ppm is capable of causing increases in airway resistance as compared with control exposures, especially with oral breathing and high ventilatory rates.[105,106,112] Some individuals clearly responded with symptomatic bronchoconstriction requiring bronchodilator after even 1-minute exposure to 0.5 to 1.0 ppm SO$_2$.[113] The implications of these results with regard to the current NAAQS are obvious. Although SO$_2$ concentrations in excess of 0.5 ppm are unlikely to occur for prolonged periods, 5- to 10-minute peaks exceeding this level do occur in the vicinity of sources such as smelters, oil refineries, and power plants.[114]

There is also animal experimental evidence for another potential effect of SO$_2$ in subjects with asthma. Guinea pigs exposed to SO$_2$ for 8 hours per day for 5 consecutive days also were exposed to an aerosol of ovalbumin on days 3 to 5.[115] Exposure to as little as 0.1 ppm SO$_2$ in this protocol enhanced allergic sensitization to inhaled ovalbumin as measured by the development of bronchoconstriction during specific inhalation challenge testing and increased concentrations of specific antibodies in both BAL fluid and serum.

As previously noted and in contrast to O_3, near-ambient concentrations of SO_2 have not been found to cause lung injury in animal toxicologic studies even after chronic exposures. Investigators from Sweden, however, have demonstrated the presence of an inflammatory reaction in BAL fluid in normal human subjects exposed to 0.4 ppm SO_2 for 20 minutes.[116] These results again suggest that short-term exposure to relatively low concentrations of SO_2 is potentially harmful to the respiratory tract.

In summary, a critical review of the data base on the health effects of SO_2 reveals that the current NAAQS may not protect the most susceptible members of the population, i.e., individuals with asthma. In contrast to the animal toxicologic data for O_3 and NO_2, there is no definitive evidence that chronic exposure to near-ambient concentrations of SO_2 causes structural lung damage. However, although the current standard may provide an adequate margin of safety to prevent chronic lung injury in normal subjects, its 24-hour (primary) and 3-hour (secondary) averaging times allow short-term peaks to occur that will induce symptomatic bronchoconstriction in some individuals with asthma.

Particulate matter

The NAAQS for PM was revised in 1987. Previously, the primary standards for PM were 75 $\mu g/m^3$ as an annual geometric mean concentration (and 260 $\mu g/m^3$ as a 24-hour maximum concentration) of total suspended particulates (TSP). In the revised standard, the EPA replaced TSP with a new measure of particulate pollution (PM), or that fraction of the TSP with an aerodynamic diameter ≤ 10 μm. After a long period of review, PM was selected because particles >10 μm in diameter are unlikely to be deposited in the lower respiratory tract. Extrathoracic deposition of PM was deemed of little consequence to public health. The primary standards for PM are shown in Table 49-1.

Particulate matter is always a mixture of substances, often including both solid and liquid particles, particles of biologic origin such as fungal spores and pollens, as well as particles of varying size. The size distribution of atmospheric PM is often bimodal with so-called coarse (2.5 to 30 μm in aerodynamic diameter) and fine (≤ 2.5 μm) fractions. Coarse particles are primarily derived from soil and rock. Particles derived from combustion processes, which are frequently acidic, constitute the largest fraction of fine particles by mass. The PM standard does not refer to any specific chemical composition of particles.

The primary sources of fine PM are power plants, heavy industrial plants (e.g., steel mills, smelters), wood-burning stoves, and diesel-fueled motor vehicles. Although substantial progress has been made across the nation in reducing PM since the passage of the Clean Air Act in 1970, there are still many communities in which the PM standard is ex-

ceeded. The American Lung Association has estimated that nearly 23,000,000 people resided in areas where this standard was exceeded in 1992.[117] Emission controls, relocation of facilities, and changes in fuel use have resulted in a reduction in TSP, but concentrations of fine particles have not been correspondingly reduced.

Most of the evidence supporting the need for a NAAQS for PM comes from epidemiologic studies. Extensive analysis of exposure data from the severe pollution episodes in London in the 1950s and 1960s has suggested that the concentration of particles, so-called "British Smoke" (a measure of the blackness of particles in comparison with a standard sample of a specific mass concentration), correlated better with excess mortality than the concentration of SO_2.[118] Early studies using U.S. data showed some association between daily total mortality and coefficient of haze, a measure of the light-scattering effect of particles that reflects the concentration of very fine particles, (i.e., those <1 μm in diameter).[119,120] More recently, daily total mortality has been reported to be associated with TSP concentration in several cities, including Steubenville, Ohio, and Philadelphia.[121,122] A meta-analysis of time-series studies of this association in nine U.S. cities and London indicated that for every 100 $\mu g/m^3$ increase in TSP, there was an approximately 6% increase in daily mortality.[123]

Because PM levels have only been routinely measured since 1987, there are limited data available regarding the association of this parameter of PM and mortality. One study from Utah Valley, Utah, reported that daily mortality was 11% higher on days when the PM concentration was >100 $\mu g/m^3$ than on days when it was <50 $\mu g/m^3$.[124] In a prospective cohort study of air pollution and mortality involving participants from six cities in the eastern United States, mortality was most strongly associated with fine particulates.[125] The adjusted mortality-rate ratio for the most polluted city as compared with the least polluted city was 1.26, using fine PM as the index (see Fig. 49-4). A strength of this study was that the investigators were able to adjust the analysis for the effects of cigarette smoking, occupational exposure to respiratory irritants, and several chronic diseases (hypertension and diabetes mellitus).

Most of the time-series studies involving data from single cities have not had sufficient power to address associations between PM and cause-specific mortality. Where such associations have been found, however, deaths due to cardiovascular disease appear to be the primary contributor to the observed association between PM and total mortality.[122,124] The specific biologic mechanism linking relatively low-level PM and acute cardiovascular effects sufficiently severe to cause death is not apparent. Nonetheless, the consistent results across studies from multiple cities suggest that the reported association is real.

The association of PM and a number of acute morbidity endpoints has been investigated in epidemiologic studies in the United States. In the Utah Valley, a strong corre-

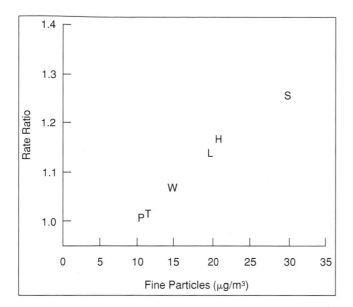

Fig. 49-4. Estimated adjusted mortality-rate ratios and respirable particulate pollution (PM) in six cities. The PM concentrations are mean values. P, Portage, WI; T, Topeka; W, Watertown, MA; L, St. Louis; H, Harriman, TN; S, Steubenville, OH. (Modified from Dockery DW, Pope CA, Xu X, et al: An association between air pollution and mortality in six U.S. cities. Reprinted, by permission of *The New England Journal of Medicine,* 329; 1757, 1993.)

lation between PM levels measured from 1985 to 1988 and hospital admissions for respiratory illnesses (pneumonia, pleurisy, bronchitis, and asthma) was observed.[126] During months when 24-hour PM concentrations exceeded 150 μg/m³, the current NAAQS, mean respiratory admissions for children nearly tripled; in adults the increase in admissions was 44%. There also were increased rates of admission for respiratory illness for both children and adults during months when the mean PM concentration was ≥50 μg/m³, the annual arithmetic mean component of the current NAAQS. The strength of the association between PM and respiratory morbidity observed in this study may be a function of lack of confounding exposure to photochemical pollution and cigarette smoke in the Utah population that was used.

Particulate pollution has been convincingly shown to cause acute respiratory symptoms. Several studies analyzing data collected through the National Health Interview Survey have demonstrated an association between PM and acute respiratory symptoms severe enough to result in restricted activity, including missed work days.[127] A diary study of schoolchildren participating in the Harvard Six Cities Study documented an association between PM concentration and lower respiratory symptoms despite the fact that all PM measurements were below the current NAAQS.[128] Studies using panels of schoolchildren in the Utah Valley also documented an association between PM concentration and lower respiratory symptoms; daily peak expiratory flow measurements also were decreased on days with elevated

PM levels.[129] In another Utah Valley study, increased use of asthma medications by a panel of asthmatic subjects was correlated with PM concentration.[130]

There are also considerable epidemiologic data to support an association between PM and chronic respiratory health. A 1986 report from the Harvard Six Cities Study reported strong associations between frequencies of chronic cough, bronchitis, and lower respiratory illness in preadolescent schoolchildren and concentrations of TSP and the sulfate fraction of TSP.[131] An exposure-respiratory morbidity gradient across the six cities was noted, with the cities characterized by the highest TSP and sulfate concentrations having symptom and illness rates approximately twofold higher than cities with the lowest concentrations. No association was found, however, between TSP, sulfate, or SO$_2$ concentrations and the pulmonary function of the schoolchildren in the study. A later report from the Six Cities Study presented the results of a second cross-sectional assessment of the effects of air pollution on chronic respiratory health.[132] In this report, exposure measurements included TSP, PM with an aerodynamic diameter of <15 μm (PM$_{15}$), PM with an aerodynamic diameter of <2.5 μm, fine particulate sulfate, SO$_2$, O$_3$, and NO$_2$. In general, frequencies of chronic cough, bronchitis, and chest illness were better correlated with measures of PM than with the gaseous pollutants measured. The only statistically significant association, however, was between PM$_{15}$ and bronchitis. As in the previous report, no associations were found between pollutant concentrations and pulmonary function. The results of this second Six Cities Study report provided additional evidence that rates of chronic respiratory symptoms and lower respiratory illness are elevated among children living in areas with high levels of PM. Nonetheless, the consistent lack of association between PM concentrations and pulmonary function suggests that particulate-related respiratory morbidity does not lead to structural lung damage.

Because of the high levels of oxidant pollutants that are present in southern California smog, it is often believed that PM is not a major problem in that region. On the contrary, a study among Seventh Day Adventists (who are nonsmokers by religious stricture) residing in California demonstrated a strongly significant association between "symptoms of COPD" (i.e., chronic bronchitis, history of asthma and wheezing, or history of emphysema and dyspnea on exertion) and hours of exposure to TSP above 200 μg/m³.[133] The association between chronic respiratory symptoms and TSP persisted even when the confounding effects of exposures to other pollutants were controlled in a multiple logistic regression model.

Although there are some animal toxicologic data that demonstrate adverse health effects from the inhalation of high concentrations of PM alone, animal studies involving exposure to particles generated from combustion processes are perhaps the most relevant to ambient exposures. A series of studies has documented that ultrafine zinc oxide particles that carry a layer of H_2SO_4 are considerably more potent than H_2SO_4 mist of similar particle size.[134,135] Significant enhancement of the effects of H_2SO_4 exposure on functional, histologic, and BAL inflammatory responses of guinea pigs occurs when acid-coated particles are administered. The experimentally generated acid-coated, zinc oxide particles have been carefully characterized and considered analogous to primary emissions from smelters and coal combustion processes. In vitro studies of the cytotoxicity of particles collected from polluted urban air have also demonstrated that such particles can be highly toxic to AMs.[136] The relative toxicity of the particles studied was dependent on both the metal and combustion-derived organic content of the particles. Smoke particles derived from various types of combustion also have been documented to cause inflammatory changes in guinea pig lungs when administered by inhalation or tracheal instillation.[137]

No controlled human exposure studies of PM have been reported that are relevant to the effects of ambient air pollution.

In summary, epidemiologic evidence is accumulating that even the revised NAAQS using PM as the measure of particulate pollution may offer an inadequate margin of safety to protect the most susceptible members of the general population such as children and adults with preexisting cardiovascular or respiratory diseases. Concentrations of respirable particulate at levels below the current standard have been associated with increased respiratory morbidity and total daily mortality. Unfortunately, it is difficult to link the effects of low-level exposure observed in epidemiologic studies to any biologic mechanism based on the available animal toxicologic data. Further research will be needed to resolve this issue.

Atmospheric acidity

Because atmospheric acidity is not listed by the EPA as a criteria pollutant, there is no NAAQS for this form of pollution at the present time. However, the EPA's Clean Air Scientific Advisory Committee has recommended that the agency consider developing an air quality standard for acid aerosols.[138] This recommendation was based on an evaluation of the animal toxicologic, controlled human exposure, and epidemiologic data concerning the potential adverse health effects of acid aerosols.

Sulfuric acid is the acidic air pollutant most commonly found across the nation and, as such, has been the focus of most health effects studies. In the atmosphere of the northeastern United States, H_2SO_4 is primarily in the form of fine aerosols. The tall stacks designed to reduce local pollution in the vicinity of Ohio River Valley power plants release SO_2 and PM into the upper atmosphere where these emissions mix with strong oxidizing agents generated by photochemical reactions involving NO_x, VOCs, and O_3. Under these conditions, SO_2 is slowly oxidized to H_2SO_4 and acid sulfate aerosols may remain aloft for days, traveling for hundreds of miles. In the northeastern United States and southeastern Canada (downwind from the Ohio River Valley), the highest levels of atmospheric acidity occur in the summer months, so-called "acid haze." In most studies of the health effects of inhaled H_2SO_4, it has been administered as an aerosol of small, respirable-size particles and low liquid water content in an attempt to model acid haze conditions. In contrast to the relatively slow generation of acid haze, when foggy air masses are present in the vicinity of SO_2 sources, the SO_2 can be rapidly oxidized to H_2SO_4, giving rise to so-called "acid fogs." The particle size and liquid water content are both greater in acid fogs as compared to acid haze.

Sulfuric acid is not the only acidic species of concern. Nitric acid is a common constituent of ambient urban air in sunny areas where mobile sources that emit NO_x generate the bulk of the air pollution. As noted previously, HNO_3 is formed in the atmosphere from the reaction of NO_x with OH^-. Because of its low vapor pressure, HNO_3 is normally in the gaseous state at typical ambient conditions. In the presence of foggy conditions, however, it is completely scavenged by water droplets. The differences between the atmospheric chemistry of H_2SO_4 and HNO_3 suggest that a single measure of exposure of atmospheric acidity relevant to conditions across the country may prove difficult to develop for use in a future NAAQS.

Exposure to atmospheric acidity may be substantially reduced as a result of neutralization from ammonia (NH_3) near ground level, particularly in agricultural regions. Much of the sulfate in atmospheric aerosols is usually found in the form of partially or fully neutralized salts such as ammonium sulfate (NH_4SO_4) or ammonium bisulfate [$(NH_4)_2SO_4$]. The irritant potential of these sulfate salts is less than H_2SO_4.[139] Gaseous NH_3 present in the mouth can also neutralize inhaled H_2SO_4, thereby reducing deposition in the lower respiratory tract.

The best evidence for an association of exposure to acidic pollutants and adverse health effects comes from epidemiologic studies. Although specific measurements of atmospheric acidity are not available, it seems likely that high levels of aerosol acidity were present during the severe pollution episodes associated with high mortality described above. One analysis of London air pollution data from 1958 to 1972, including daily measurements of British smoke, SO_2, and aerosol acidity (most of which was probably H_2SO_4), showed aerosol acidity to be more predictive of daily mortality than either British smoke or SO_2.[140] Several studies in Ontario and New York have also shown levels of atmospheric acidity or sulfate to correlate with rates of hospital admissions for acute respiratory diseases during summer months when acid hazes occur.[59,141] In the Harvard Six Cities Study, chronic cough and bronchitis were more closely correlated with hydrogen ion (H^+) concentration than with particle concentration.[142] Daily ambient concentrations of H^+ in Denver were associated with reports of cough and shortness of breath from a large panel of adult subjects with asthma.[143]

Although H^+ has been proposed as the agent responsible for the acute health effects associated with summer pollution in the northeastern United States and southeastern Canada, there are some data that suggest otherwise. For example, daily mortality in St. Louis and Knoxville, Tennessee was associated with PM but not aerosol acidity.[144]

Because the endpoints that have been most clearly associated with atmospheric acidity (deaths and hospital admissions for respiratory diseases) occur during or soon after pollution episodes, most of the animal toxicologic and controlled human exposure studies of H_2SO_4 and HNO_3 have investigated acute effects. There is no question that strong acids can cause severe chemical injury to cells and tissues. The issue is whether ambient concentrations of these acid species can cause injury to the respiratory tract when inhaled. Acidic sulfate aerosols induce lung function changes in guinea pigs only at high concentrations.[145] Concentrations of H_2SO_4 many times greater than those currently encountered during air pollution episodes have failed to cause normal, healthy subjects to develop significant decrements in lung function in a number of studies.[146] Because subjects with asthma are known to be more sensitive to SO_2, however, the response of these subjects to inhalation of H_2SO_4 has been the focus of considerable research interest.

Statistically significant changes in pulmonary function in subjects with asthma have been observed after brief exposure to 100 to 1000 $\mu g/m^3$ H_2SO_4 aerosol[147,148]; no such changes have been reported for normal subjects exposed to concentrations below 900 $\mu g/m^3$. Although concentrations approaching this level occurred in London in the past, the highest H_2SO_4 concentrations in North America in recent years have been <50 $\mu g/m^3$.[149]

The lowest concentration of H_2SO_4 in a submicronic aerosol that has been demonstrated to cause decrements in pulmonary function is 100 $\mu g/m^3$ in a study of adolescents with both allergic asthma and exercise-induced bronchospasm.[147] Duration of exposure was 30 minutes at rest followed by 10 minutes of exercise (minute ventilation ~40 L/min). There was no significant difference from the baseline value after exposure at rest, but immediately after exposure during exercise, the mean FEV1 was significantly reduced. This reduction, however, was slight (8%) and transient (no longer than 5 minutes). A second team of investigators attempted to replicate this study and could not confirm an effect of this low concentration of H_2SO_4.[150] In a study of adult subjects with asthma that demonstrated statistically significant changes in lung function after 16-minute exposure during rest to submicronic aerosols containing 450 and 1000 $\mu g/m^3$ H_2SO_4, the mean decreases in specific airway conductance were small (19% and 21%, respectively).[148] Other investigators, including the author, have failed to find significant changes in lung function in

subjects with asthma after exposure to submicronic aerosols of H_2SO_4 in concentrations as high as 1000 $\mu g/m^3$.[151] If the particle size of the aerosol is larger (i.e., >5 μm in mass median aerodynamic diameter), as in fogs, then even higher concentrations of H_2SO_4 are required to elicit bronchoconstriction in subjects with asthma.[152]

There are limited data from asthmatic subjects that suggest that short-term inhalation of an H_2SO_4 aerosol can cause an increase in nonspecific airway hyperresponsiveness 24 hours after the exposure.[153] In rabbits, daily exposure to 250 $\mu g/m^3$ H_2SO_4 was associated with increased responsiveness to acetylcholine after 4 months.[154]

Another endpoint that has been extensively studied in both animals and humans after acid aerosol inhalation is mucociliary clearance. Tracheobronchial clearance of labeled particles has been consistently observed to be altered by inhalation of acid sulfates. Brief (i.e., <1 hour) exposures to relatively low concentrations of H_2SO_4 (<250 $\mu g/m^3$) tend to induce faster clearance and more prolonged exposures or higher concentrations will cause slower clearance.[155] However, repeated exposure to relatively low concentrations can also lead to delayed clearance. In rabbits, chronic intermittent exposure to submicronic H_2SO_4 aerosols at 250 $\mu g/m^3$ (1 hour per day, 5 days per week) for 12 months induced a marked slowing of bronchial clearance that persisted at least 3 months after the cessation of exposure.[156] The magnitude of the effect of an acidic aerosol on mucociliary clearance appears to be associated with the acidity of the aerosol.[157] Daily exposure to H_2SO_4 aerosols in rabbits and donkeys for weeks to months has resulted in persistent slowing of mucociliary clearance even after exposure ceased, suggesting that prolonged exposure may lead to chronic airway injury.[156,158] Airway secretory cell hyperplasia, altered mucus glycoprotein secretion, and decreased dynamic lung compliance were additional persistent responses observed in the rabbit study. Although the H_2SO_4 concentration used in this study was an order of magnitude higher than ambient levels during most acid haze conditions in North America, the demonstration of chronic structural and functional changes provides strong evidence of the potential for acid aerosols to cause lung injury.

Daily exposures to 500 $\mu g/m^3$ H_2SO_4 also have been shown to affect AM function in rabbits.[159] Phagocytic activity increased after 3 days but decreased after 14 days. Human AM function was not appreciably affected by a single, 2-hour, in vivo exposure to 1000 $\mu g/m^3$ H_2SO_4.[160] There was also no evidence of an inflammatory response in BAL fluid.

Compared with the relative wealth of information about the effects of H_2SO_4, the available data on HNO_3 are sparse. Several controlled human exposure studies of both HNO_3 fogs and vapor have been conducted, however. A study involving nine allergic adolescents with exercise-induced bronchospasm demonstrated a 4% decrease in FEV1 after a 40-minute exposure to 126 $\mu g/m^3$ HNO_3 vapor compared with a 2% decrease after air.[161] A 2-hour exposure to 500 $\mu g/m^3$ HNO$_3$ fog (MMAD of ~6.5 μm) caused no change in lung function in 10 healthy, exercising subjects.[162] Similarly, exposure to 500 $\mu g/m^3$ HNO$_3$ as a vapor for 4 hours during moderate exercise caused no changes in lung function or lavage fluid cellular and biochemical constituents in normal subjects.[163] Another study in which normal subjects were exposed to 200 $\mu g/m^3$ HNO$_3$ vapor also showed no evidence of injury or inflammation in BAL fluid analysis.[164]

Although the controlled human exposure studies described above have demonstrated little toxicity of HNO$_3$ in the 100 to 500 $\mu g/m^3$ range, these studies all used a single, short-term exposure. Subchronic exposure (i.e., 4 hours per day, 3 days per week, for 4 weeks) of both rats and rabbits to 50 to 450 $\mu g/m^3$ HNO$_3$ vapor was associated with dose-dependent changes in lung morphometry consistent with alveolar wall remodeling.[165] These results are somewhat surprising given the high water solubility and reactivity of HNO$_3$ vapor, characteristics favoring upper airway deposition. If confirmed, however, these animal toxicologic data do suggest that subchronic exposure to relatively low concentrations of HNO$_3$ vapor can penetrate to the deep lung and cause alteration of lung parenchymal structure.

Because atmospheric acidity and O$_3$ frequently coexist in relatively high concentrations, the issue of whether acid sulfate aerosols and/or HNO$_3$ vapor can enhance the toxicity of O$_3$ is an important one. The results of a series of animal toxicologic studies have demonstrated synergistic effects of acid sulfate aerosol and O$_3$ on lavageable protein, tissue protein content, lung collagen synthesis rate, tracheal mucus glycoprotein secretion, and bacterial infectivity.[63,166] Combined exposure to an acidic pollutant and O$_3$ in studies of human subjects, on the other hand, has provided conflicting results. A study of adolescent subjects with allergic asthma and exercise-induced bronchospasm found greater decrements in FEV1 when a low concentration of an acidic pollutant (either H$_2$SO$_4$ aerosol or HNO$_3$ vapor) was added to an oxidant (O$_3$ plus NO$_2$) atmosphere compared to those induced by the oxidants alone.[161]

In contrast, two studies of normal subjects found no evidence that preexposure to HNO$_3$ fog or coexposure with HNO$_3$ vapor enhanced the lung function responses to O$_3$.[162,163] No evidence of HNO$_3$ vapor enhancement of O$_3$-induced injury and inflammation was demonstrated either.[163] Again, all of the controlled human exposure studies of combinations of acidic and oxidant pollutants have involved single, short-term exposures. Given the animal toxicologic data suggesting synergistic effects of acid sulfate aerosols and O$_3$ as well as a lung remodeling effect of subchronic exposure to HNO$_3$ vapor, there must still be concern that atmospheric acidity has the potential to enhance O$_3$ toxicity in humans with repeated daily exposures.

In summary, a critical review of the data base on the health effects of atmospheric acidity provides somewhat

conflicting information regarding the need to establish a new NAAQS for this type of pollution. Although there is substantial epidemiologic evidence to support an association between exposure to acid sulfate aerosols at high-ambient concentrations and exacerbation of preexisting respiratory disease, the results of controlled human exposure studies suggest that concentrations much higher than those currently encountered in North America are required to produce significant changes in lung function in individuals with asthma. The available animal toxicologic evidence also indicates that chronic exposure to acid sulfate aerosols at relatively high concentrations is required to produce structural lung injury. The evidence that acid aerosols and O$_3$ may have synergistic effects on lung remodeling in rodents is also compelling. The data base on the effects of HNO$_3$ is inadequate for standard setting. On balance, it seems premature to establish an NAAQS for atmospheric acidity at the present time.

REFERENCES

1. Office of Air Quality Planning and Standards: *National air quality and emissions trends report* (EPA Pub No 450-R-92-001), Research Triangle Park, NC, 1991, United States Environmental Protection Agency.
2. South Coast Air Quality Management District: *1993 air quality,* Diamond Bar, CA, 1994, South Coast Air Quality Management District.
3. Lippman M: Health effects of ozone: a critical review, *J Air Pollut Control Assoc* 39:672-695, 1989.
4. Pryor WC: Free radical reactions in biology: initiation of lipid autooxidation by ozone and nitrogen dioxide, *Environ Health Perspect* 16:180-181, 1976.
5. Hu S-C, Ben-Jebria A, and Ultman JS: Longitudinal distribution of ozone absorption in the lung: quiet respiration in healthy subjects, *J Appl Physiol* 73:1655-1661, 1992.
6. Kulle TJ, Sauder LR, Hebel JR, and Chatham MD: Ozone response relationships in healthy nonsmokers, *Am Rev Respir Dis* 132:36-41, 1985.
7. McDonnell WF, Horstman DH, Hazucha MJ, Seal E, Haak ED, Abdul-Salaam S, and House DE: Pulmonary effects of ozone exposure during exercise: dose-response characteristics, *J Appl Physiol* 54:1345-1352, 1983.
8. Hazucha MJ: Relationship between ozone exposure and pulmonary function changes, *J Appl Physiol* 62:1671-1680, 1987.
9. Coleridge JCG, Coleridge HM, Schelegle ES, and Green JF: Acute inhalation of ozone stimulates bronchial C-fibers and rapidly adapting receptors in dogs, *J Appl Physiol* 74:2345-2352, 1993.
10. Schelegle ES, Adams WC, and Siefkin AD: Indomethacin pretreatment reduces ozone-induced pulmonary function decrements in human subjects, *Am Rev Respir Dis* 136:1350-1354, 1987.
11. McDonnell WF: Individual variability in the magnitude of acute respiratory response to ozone, In Utell MJ and Frank R, editors: *Susceptibility to inhaled pollutants,* pp 75-88, Philadelphia, 1989, ASTM.
12. Shepard RJ, Urch B, Silverman F, and Corey PN: Interaction of ozone and cigarette smoke exposure, *Environ Res* 31:125-137, 1983.
13. Dreschler-Parks DM, Bedi JF, and Horvath SM: Pulmonary function responses of older men and women to ozone exposure, *Exp Gerontol* 22:91-101, 1987.
14. Linn WS, Buckley RD, Spier CE, Blessey RL, Jones MP, Fischer DA, and Hackney JD: Health effects of ozone exposure in asthmatics, *Am Rev Respir Dis* 117:835-843, 1978.
15. Solic JJ, Hazucha MJ, and Bromberg PA: The acute effects of 0.2

ppm ozone in patients with chronic obstructive pulmonary disease, *Am Rev Respir Dis* 125:664-669, 1982.

16. Ostro BD, Lipsett MJ, and Jewell NP: Predicting respiratory morbidity from pulmonary function tests: a reanalysis of ozone chamber studies, *J Air Pollut Control Assoc* 39:1313-1318, 1989.

17. McDonnell WF, Chapmann RS, Leigh MW, Strope GL, and Collier AM. Respiratory responses of vigorously exercising children to 0.12 ppm ozone exposure, *Am Rev Respir Dis* 132:875-879, 1985.

18. Spektor DM, Thurston GD, Mao J, He D, Hayes C, and Lippman M: Effects of single- and multi-day ozone exposures on respiratory function in active normal children, *Environ Res* 55:107-122, 1991.

19. Spektor DM, Lippman M, Thurston GD, Lioy PJ, Stecko J, O'Connor G, Garschick E, Speizer FE, and Hayes C: Effects of ambient ozone on respiratory function in healthy adults exercising outdoors, *Am Rev Respir Dis* 138:832-838, 1988.

20. Kinney PL, Ware JH, Spengler JD, Dockery DW, Speizer FE, and Ferris BG: Short term pulmonary function change in association with ozone levels, *Am Rev Respir Dis* 139:56-61, 1989.

21. Adams WC and Schelegle ES: Ozone and high ventilation effects on pulmonary function and endurance performance, *J Appl Physiol* 55:805-812, 1983.

22. Gong H, Bradley PW, Simmons MS, and Tashkin DP: Impaired exercise performance and pulmonary function in elite cyclists during low-level ozone exposure in a hot environment, *Am Rev Respir Dis* 134:726-733, 1986.

23. Golden JA, Nadel JA, and Boushey HA: Bronchial hyperirritability in healthy subjects after exposure to ozone, *Am Rev Respir Dis* 118:287-294, 1978.

24. Seltzer J, Bigby BG, Stulbarg M, Holtzman MJ, Nadel JA, Ueki IF, Leikauf GD, Goetzl EJ, and Boushey HA: O₃ induced change in bronchial reactivity to methacholine and airway inflammation in humans, *J Appl Physiol* 60:1321-1326, 1986.

25. Janssen LJ, O'Byrne PM, and Daniel EE: Mechanism underlying ozone-induced in vitro hyperresponsiveness in canine bronchi, *Am J Physiol* 261(5):L55-L72, 1991.

26. Walters EH, O'Byrne PM, Graf PD, Fabbri LM, and Nadel JA: The responsiveness of airway smooth muscle in vitro from dogs with airway hyperresponsiveness in vivo, *Clin Sci* 71:605-611, 1986.

27. Stevens RJ, Sloan MF, Evans MJ, and Freeman G: Early response of lung to low levels of ozone, *Am J Pathol* 74:31-58, 1974.

28. Holtzman MJ, Fabbri LM, O'Byrne PM, Gold WM, Aizawa H, Walters EH, Alpert SE, and Nadel JA: Importance of airway inflammation for hyperresponsiveness induced by ozone, *Am Rev Respir Dis* 127:686-690, 1983.

29. Guth DJ, Warren DL, and Last JA: Comparative sensitivity of measurements of lung damage made by bronchoalveolar lavage after short-term exposure of rats to ozone, *Toxicology* 40:131-143, 1986.

30. Koren HS, Devlin RB, Graham DE, Mann R, McGee MP, Horstman DH, Kozumbo WJ, Becker S, House DE, McDonnell WF, and Bromberg PA: Ozone-induced inflammation in the lower airways of human subjects, *Am Rev Respir Dis* 139:407-415, 1989.

31. Devlin RB, McDonell WF, Mann R, Becker S, House DE, Schreinemachers D, and Koren HS: Exposure of humans to ambient levels of ozone for 6.6 hours causes cellular and biochemical changes in the lung, *Am J Respir Cell Mol Biol* 4:72-81, 1991.

32. Aris RM, Christian D, Hearne PQ, Kerr K, Finkbeiner W, and Balmes JR: Ozone-induced airway inflammation in human subjects as determined by airway lavage and biopsy, *Am Rev Respir Dis* 148:1363-1372, 1993.

33. Graham DE and Koren HS: Biomarkers of inflammation in ozone-exposed humans, *Am Rev Respir Dis* 142:152-156, 1990.

34. Tepper JS, Costa DL, Lehmann JR, Weber MF, and Hatch GE: Unattenuated structural and biochemical alteration in the rat lung during functional adaptation to ozone, *Am Rev Respir Dis* 140:493-501, 1989.

35. Hackney JD, Linn WS, Mohler JG, and Collier CR: Adaptation to short-term respiratory effects of ozone in men exposed repeatedly, *J Appl Physiol* 43:82-85, 1977.

36. Farrell BP, Kerr HD, Kulle TJ, Sauder LR, and Young JL: Adaptation in human subjects to the effects of inhaled ozone after repeated exposures, *Am Rev Respir Dis* 119:725-730, 1979.

37. Devlin RB, Folinsbee LJ, Biscardi F, Becker S, Madden M, Robins M, and Koren HS: Attenuation of cellular and biochemical changes in the lungs of humans exposed to ozone for five consecutive days, *Am Rev Respir Dis* 147:A71, 1993.

38. Van Bree L, Koren HS, Devlin RB, and Rombout PJA: Recovery from attenuated inflammation in lower airways of rats following repeated exposure to ozone, *Am Rev Respir Dis* 147:A633, 1993.

39. Linn WS, Avol EL, Shamoo DA, Peng R-C, Valencia LM, Little DE, and Hackney JD: Repeated laboratory ozone exposures of volunteer Los Angeles residents: apparent seasonal variation in response, *Toxicol Ind Health* 4:505-520, 1988.

40. Tyler WS, Tyler NK, Last JA, Gillespie MJ, and Barstow T: Comparison of daily and seasonal exposures of young monkeys to ozone, *Toxicology* 50:131-144, 1989.

41. Barr BC, Hyde DM, Plopper CG, and Dungworth DL: A comparison of terminal airway remodeling in chronic versus episodic ozone exposure, *Toxicol Appl Pharmacol* 106:384-407, 1990.

42. Plopper CG, Harkema JR, Last JA, Pinkerton KE, Tyler WS, George JAS, Wong VJ, Nishio SJ, Weir AS, Dungworth DL, Barry BE, and Hyde DM: The respiratory system of nonhuman primates responds more to ambient concentrations of ozone than does that of rats, In Berglund RL, Lawson DR, and McKee DJ, editors: *Tropospheric ozone and the environment,* pp 137-150, Pittsburgh, 1991, Air and Waste Management Association.

43. Chang L, Huang Y, Stockstill BL, Graham J, Grose E, Menache M, Miller FJ, Costa DL, and Crapo JD: Epithelial injury and interstitial fibrosis in the proximal alveolar regions of rats chronically exposed to a simulated pattern of urban ambient ozone, *Toxicol Appl Pharmacol* 115:241-252, 1992.

44. Last JA, Greenberg DB, and Castleman WL: Ozone-induced alterations in collagen metabolism of rat lungs, *Toxicol Appl Pharmacol* 51:247-258, 1979.

45. Last JA, Reiser KM, Tyler WS, and Rucher RB: Long-term consequences of exposure to ozone: I. Lung collagen content, *Toxicol Appl Pharmacol* 72:111-118, 1984.

46. Gross KB and White HJ: Functional and pathologic consequences of a 52-week exposure to 0.5 ppm ozone followed by a clean air recovery period, *Lung* 165:283-295, 1987.

47. Detels R, Tashkin DP, Sayre JW, Rokaw SN, Coulson AH, Massey FJ, and Wegman DH: The UCLA population studies of chronic obstructive respiratory disease: 9. Lung function changes associated with chronic exposure to photochemical oxidants; a cohort study among never-smokers, *Chest* 92:594-603, 1987.

48. Knudson RJ, Lebowitz MD, Holberg CJ, and Burrows B: Changes in the maximum expiratory flow-volume curve with growth and aging, *Am Rev Respir Dis* 127:725-734, 1983.

49. Kilburn KH, Warshaw R, and Thornton JC: Pulmonary functional impairment and symptoms in women in the Los Angeles harbor area, *Am J Med* 79:23-28, 1985.

50. Schwartz J: Lung function and chronic exposure to air pollution: a cross-sectional analysis of NHANES II, *Environ Res* 50:309-321, 1989.

51. Sherwin RP and Richters V: Centriacinar region (CAR) disease in the lungs of young adults: a preliminary report, In Berglund RL, Lawson DR, and McKee DJ, editors: *Tropospheric ozone and the environment,* pp 178-196, Pittsburgh, 1991, Air and Waste Management Association.

52. Van Louveren HS, Wagenaar S, Walvoort HC, and Vos JG: Effect of ozone on the defense to a respiratory Listeria monocytogenes infection in the rat, *Toxicol Appl Pharmacol* 94:374-393, 1988.

53. Gardner DE: Use of experimental airborne infections for monitoring altered host defenses, *Environ Health Perspect* 43:99-107, 1982.

54. Oosting RS, Van-Golde LM, and Van-Bree L: Species differences in impairment and recovery of alveolar macrophage function following single and repeated ozone exposures, *Toxicol Appl Pharmacol* 110:170-178, 1991.

55. McDonnell WF, Horstman DH, Abdul-Salaam S, Raggio LJ, and Green JA: The respiratory responses of subjects with allergic rhinitis to ozone exposure and their relationship to nonspecific airway reactivity, *Toxicol Ind Health* 3:507-517, 1987.

56. Kreit JW, Gross KB, Moore TB, Lorenzen TJ, D'Arcy J, and Eschenbacher WL: Ozone-induced changes in pulmonary function and bronchial hyperresponsiveness in asthmatics, *J Appl Physiol* 66:217-222, 1989.

57. Whittemore AS and Korn EL: Asthma and air pollution in the Los Angeles area, *Am J Public Health* 70:687-696, 1980.

58. Holguin AH, Buffler P, Contant CF, Stock TH, Hsi BP, Jenkins DE, Gehan BM, Noel LM, and Mei M: The effect of ozone on asthmatics in the Houston area, In Lee SD, editor: *Evaluation of the scientific basis for ozone/oxidants standards,* pp 262-280, Pittsburgh, 1985, Air Pollution Control Association.

59. Bates DV and Sizto R: Relationship between air pollution levels and hospital admissions in southern Ontario, *Can J Public Health* 74:117-133, 1983.

60. Molfino NA, Wright SC, Katz I, Tarlo S, Silverman F, McClean PA, Szalai JP, Raizenne M, Slutsky AS, and Zamel N: Effect of low concentrations of ozone on inhaled allergen responses in asthmatic subjects, *Lancet* 338:199-203, 1991.

61. Yanai M, Ohrui T, Aikawa T, Okayama H, Sekizawa K, Maeyama K, Sasaki H, and Takishima T: Ozone increases susceptibility to antigen inhalation in allergic dogs, *J Appl Physiol* 68:2267-2273, 1990.

62. Turner CR, Kleeberger SR, and Spannhake EW: Preexposure to ozone blocks the antigen-induced late asthmatic response of the canine peripheral airways, *J Toxicol Environ Health* 28:363-371, 1989.

63. Warren DL and Last JA: Synergistic interaction of ozone and respirable aerosols on rat lungs: III. Ozone and sulfuric acid aerosol, *Toxicol Appl Pharmacol* 88:203-216, 1987.

64. Goldstein IF, Lieber K, Andrews LR, Foutrakis G, Kazembe F, Huange P, and Hayes C: Acute respiratory effects of short-term exposures to nitrogen dioxide, *Arch Environ Health* 43:138-142, 1988.

65. Shy CM and Love GJ: Recent evidence on the human health effects of nitrogen oxides, In Lee SD, editor: *Nitrogen oxides and their effects on health,* pp 291-305, Ann Arbor, 1980, Ann Arbor Science.

66. Orehek J, Massari JP, Gayrard P, Grimaud C, and Charpin J: Effect of short-term, low-level nitrogen dioxide exposure on bronchial sensitivity of asthmatic patients, *J Clin Invest* 57:301-307, 1976.

67. Ahmed T, Marchette B, Danta I, Birch S, Dougherty RL, Schreck R, and Sackner MA: Effect of 0.1 ppm NO_2 on bronchial reactivity in normals and subjects with asthma, *Am Rev Respir Dis* 125:A152, 1982.

68. Hazucha MJ, Ginsberg JF, McDonnell WF, Haak ED, Pimmel RL, Abdul-Salaam S, House DE, and Bromberg PA: Effects of 0.1 ppm nitrogen dioxide on airways of normal and asthmatic subjects, *J Appl Physiol* 54:730-739, 1983.

69. Bauer MA, Utell MJ, Morrow PE, Speers DM, and Gibb FR: Inhalation of 0.30 ppm nitrogen dioxide potentiates exercise-induced bronchoconstriction in asthmatics, *Am Rev Respir Dis* 134:1203-1208, 1986.

70. Bauer MA, Utell MJ, Morrow PE, Speers DM, and Gibb FR: Route of inhalation influences airway response to 0.30 ppm nitrogen dioxide in asthmatic subjects, *Am Rev Respir Dis* 133:A171, 1985.

71. Roger LJ, Horstman DH, McDonnell WF, Kehrl H, Ives PJ, Seal E, Chapman R, and Massaro EJ: Pulmonary function, airway responsiveness, and respiratory symptoms in asthmatics following exercise in NO_2, *Toxicol Ind Health* 6:155-171, 1990.

72. Linn WS, Shamoo DA, Avol EL, Whynot JD, Anderson KR, Venet TG, and Hackney JD: Dose-response study of asthmatic volunteers exposed to nitrogen dioxide during intermittent exercise, *Arch Environ Health* 41:292-296, 1986.

73. Moshenin V: Airway responses to nitrogen dioxide in asthmatic subjects, *J Toxicol Environ Health* 22:371-380, 1987.

74. Lebowitz MD, Holberg CJ, Boyer B, and Hayes C: Respiratory symptoms and peak flow associated with indoor and outdoor air pollutants in the southwest, *J Air Pollut Control Assoc* 35:1154-1158, 1985.

75. Morrow PE: Toxicological data on NO_x: an overview, *J Toxicol Environ Health* 13:205-227, 1984.

76. Frampton MW, Finkelstein JN, Roberts NJ, Gavras JB, and Utell MJ: Effects of NO_2 exposure on bronchoalveolar lavage proteins in humans, *Am J Respir Cell Mol Biol* 1:499-505, 1989.

77. Richters A and Damji KS: Changes in T-lymphocyte subpopulations and natural killer cells following exposure to ambient levels of nitrogen dioxide, *J Toxicol Environ Health* 25:247-256, 1988.

78. Sandstrom T, Ledin M-C, Thomasson L, Helleday R, and Stjernberg N: Reductions in lymphocyte subpopulations after repeated exposure to 1.5 ppm nitrogen dioxide, *Br J Ind Med* 49:850-854, 1992.

79. Kleinerman J, Gordon RE, Ip MPC, and Collins A: Structure and function of airways in experimental chronic nitrogen dioxide exposure, In Gammage RB and Kaye SV, editors: *Indoor air and human health,* Chelsea, MI, 1985, Lewis Publishers.

80. Stephens RJ, Freeman G, Crane SC, and Furiosi NJ: Ultrastructural changes in the terminal bronchiole of the rat during continuous, low-level exposure to nitrogen dioxide, *Exp Mol Pathol* 141:1-19, 1971.

81. Rombout PJA, Dormans J, Marra M, and Van Esch FJ: Influence of exposure regimen on nitrogen dioxide-induced morphological changes in the rat lung, *Environ Res* 41:466-480, 1986.

82. Furiosi NJ, Crane SC, and Freeman G: Mixed sodium chloride and nitrogen dioxide in air: biological effects on monkeys and rats, *Arch Environ Health* 27:405-408, 1973.

83. Azoulay-Dupuis E, Torres M, Soler P, and Moreau J: Pulmonary NO_2 toxicity in neonate and adult guinea pigs and rats, *Environ Res* 30:322-339, 1983.

84. Erlich R, Findlay J, and Gardner DE: Effects of repeated exposures to peak concentrations of nitrogen dioxide and ozone on resistance to streptococcal pneumonia, *J Toxicol Environ Health* 5:631-642, 1979.

85. Schlesinger RB: Intermittent inhalation of nitrogen dioxide: effects on rabbit alveolar macrophages, *J Toxicol Environ Health* 21:127-139, 1987.

86. Amoruso MA, Witz G, and Goldstein BD: Decreased superoxide anion radical production by rat alveolar macrophages following inhalation of ozone or nitrogen dioxide, *Life Sci* 28:2215-2221, 1981.

87. Goings SAJ, Kulle TJ, Bascom R, Sauder LR, Green DJ, Hebel JR, and Clements ML: Effect of nitrogen dioxide exposure on susceptibility to influenza A virus infection in healthy adults, *Am Rev Respir Dis* 139:1075-1081, 1989.

88. Frampton MW, Smeglin AM, Roberts NJ, Finkelstein JN, Morrow PE, and Utell MJ: Nitrogen dioxide exposure in vivo and human alveolar macrophage inactivation of influenza virus in vitro, *Environ Res* 48:179-192, 1989.

89. Melia RJ, Florey CV, Altman DG, and Swan AV: Association between gas cooking and respiratory disease in children, *Br Med J* 2:149-152, 1977.

90. Speizer FE, Ferris B, Bishop YM, and Spengler J: Respiratory disease rates and pulmonary function in children associated with NO_2 exposure, *Am Rev Respir Dis* 121:3-10, 1980.

91. Melia RJ, Florey CV, Morris RW, Goldstein BD, John HH, Clark D, and MacKinlay JC: Childhood respiratory illness and nitrogen dioxide, temperature, and relative humidity, *Int J Epidemiol* 11:164-169, 1982.

92. Schenker MB, Samet JM, and Speizer FE: Risk factors for childhood respiratory disease: the effect of host factors and home environmental exposures, *Am Rev Respir Dis* 28:1038-1043, 1983.

93. Ware JH, Dockery DW, Spiro A, Speizer FE, and Ferris BG: Passive smoking, gas cooking, and respiratory health of children living in six cities, *Am Rev Respir Dis* 129:366-374, 1984.

94. Neas LM, Dockery DW, Ware JH, Spengler JD, Speizer FE, and Ferris BG: Association of indoor nitrogen dioxide with respiratory symptoms and pulmonary function in children, *Am J Epidemiol* 134:204-209, 1991.

95. Hasselbad V, Kotchmar DJ, and Eddy DM: Synthesis of environmental evidence: nitrogen dioxide epidemiology studies, *J Air Waste Management Assoc* 42:662-671, 1992.

96. Hazucha MJ, Folinsbee LJ, Seal E, and Bromberg PA: Lung function response of healthy women after sequential exposures to NO_2 and O_3, *Am J Respir Crit Care Med* 150:642-647, 1994.

97. Jorres R and Magnussen H: Airways response of asthmatics after a 30 min exposure, resting ventilation, to 0.25 ppm NO_2 or 0.5 ppm SO_2, *Eur Respir J* 3:132-137, 1990.

98. Rubenstein I, Bigby BG, Reiss TF, and Boushey HA: Short-term exposure to 0.3 ppm nitrogen dioxide does not potentiate airway responsiveness to sulfur dioxide in asthmatic subjects, *Am Rev Respir Dis* 141:381-385, 1990.

99. Gschwandtner G, Gschwandtner K, Elridge K, Mann C, and Mobley D: Historic emissions of sulfur and nitrogen oxides in the United States from 1900 to 1980, *J Air Pollut Control Assoc* 36:139-149, 1986.

100. Office of Health and Environmental Assessment: *Air quality criteria for particulate matter and sulfur oxides* (EPA Pub No 600/8-82-029), Research Triangle Park, NC, 1987, United States Environmental Protection Agency.

101. Sheppard D: Sulfur dioxide and asthma: a double-edged sword? *J Allergy Clin Immunol* 82:961-964, 1988.

102. Frank NR and Speizer FE: SO_2 effects on the respiratory system in dogs: changes in mechanical behavior at different levels of the respiratory system during acute exposure to the gas, *Arch Environ Health* 11:625-634, 1965.

103. Frank NR, Amdur MO, Worchester J, and Whittenberger JL: Effects of acute controlled exposure to SO_2 on respiratory mechanics in healthy male adults, *J Appl Physiol* 17:252-258, 1962.

104. Sheppard D, Wong SC, Uehara CD, Nadel JA, and Boushey HA: Lower threshold and greater bronchomotor responsiveness of asthmatic subjects to sulfur dioxide, *Am Rev Respir Dis* 122:873-878, 1980.

105. Bethel RA, Erle DJ, Epstein J, Sheppard D, Nadel JA, and Boushey HA: Effects of exercise rate and route of inhalation on sulfur dioxide-induced bronchoconstriction in asthmatic subjects, *Am Rev Respir Dis* 128:592-596, 1983.

106. Linn WS, Venet TG, Shamoo DA, Valencia LM, Venet TG, and Hackney JD: Respiratory effects of sulfur dioxide in heavily exercising asthmatic subjects: a dose-response study, *Am Rev Respir Dis* 127:278-283, 1983.

107. Sheppard D, Eschenbacher WL, Boushey HA, and Bethel RA: Magnitude of the interaction between the bronchomotor effects of sulfur dioxide and those of cold (dry) air, *Am Rev Respir Dis* 130:52-55, 1984.

108. Linn WS, Avol EL, Peng R-C, Shamoo DA, and Hackney JD: Replicated dose-response study of sulfur dioxide in normal, atopic, and asthmatic volunteers, *Am Rev Respir Dis* 136:1127-1134, 1987.

109. Linn WS, Avol EL, Shamoo DA, Peng R-C, Spier C, Smith MN, and Hackney JD: Effect of metaproterenol sulfate on mild asthmatics' response to sulfur dioxide exposure and exercise, *Arch Environ Health* 43:399-406, 1988.

110. Sheppard D, Epstein J, Bethel RA, Nadel JA, and Boushey HA: Tolerance to sulfur dioxide-induced bronchoconstriction in subjects with asthma, *Environ Res* 30:412-419, 1983.

111. Myers DJ, Bigby BG, Calvayrac C, Sheppard D, and Boushey HA: Interaction of cromolyn and a muscarinic antagonist in inhibiting bronchial reactivity to sulfur dioxide to eucapneic hyperpnea alone, *Am Rev Respir Dis* 133:1154-1158, 1986.

112. Horstman D, Roger LJ, Kehrl H, and Hazucha MJ: Airway sensitivity of asthmatics to sulfur dioxide, *Toxicol Ind Health* 2:289-298, 1986.

113. Balmes JR, Fine JM, and Sheppard D: Symptomatic bronchoconstriction after short-term inhalation of sulfur dioxide, *Am Rev Respir Dis* 136:1117-1121, 1987.

114. Lott RA: SO_2 concentrations near tall stacks, *Atmos Environ* 19:1589-1599, 1985.

115. Reidel F, Kramer M, Scheibenbogen C, and Rieger CHL: Effects of SO_2 exposure on allergic sensitization in the guinea pig, *J Allergy Clin Immunol* 82:527-534, 1988.

116. Sandstrom T, Stjernberg N, Andersson M-C, Kolmodin-Hedman B, Lundgren R, and Angstrom T: Is the short-term limit value for sulphur dioxide safe? Effects of controlled chamber exposure investigated with bronchoalveolar lavage, *Br J Ind Med* 46:200-203, 1989.

117. American Lung Association: *The perils of particulates*, New York, 1994, American Lung Association.

118. Mazumdar S, Schimmel H, and Higgins ITT: Relation of daily mortality to air pollution: an analysis of 14 London winters, 1958/59-1971/72, *Arch Environ Health* 37:213-220, 1982.

119. Schimmel H: Evidence for possible acute health effects of ambient air pollution from time series analysis: methodological questions and some new results based on New York City daily mortality, 1963-1976, *Bull NY Acad Med* 54:1052-1108, 1978.

120. Fairley D: The relationship of daily mortality to suspended particulates in Santa Clara County, 1980-1986, *Environ Health Perspect* 89:159-168, 1990.

121. Schwartz J and Dockery DW: Particulate air pollution and daily mortality in Steubenville, Ohio, *Am J Epidemiol* 135:12-19, 1992.

122. Schwartz J and Dockery DW: Increased mortality in Philadelphia associated with daily air pollution concentrations, *Am Rev Respir Dis* 145:600-604, 1992.

123. Schwartz J: Air pollution and daily mortality: a review and meta-analysis, *Environ Res* 64:36-52, 1994.

124. Pope CA, Schwartz J, and Ransom MR: Daily mortality and PM pollution in Utah Valley, *Arch Environ Health* 47:211-217, 1992.

125. Dockery DW, Pope CA, Xu X, Spengler JD, Ware JH, Fay ME, Ferris BG, and Speizer FE: An association between air pollution and mortality in six U.S. cities, *N Engl J Med* 329:1753-1759, 1993.

126. Pope CA: Respiratory disease associated with community air pollution and a steel mill, Utah Valley, *Am J Public Health* 79:623-628, 1989.

127. Ostro BD: Associations between morbidity and alternative measures of particulate matter, *Risk Anal* 10:421-427, 1990.

128. Schwartz J, Dockery DW, Neas LM, Wypji D, Ware JH, Spengler JD, Koutrakis P, Speizer FE, and Ferris BGJ: Acute effects of summer air pollution on respiratory symptom reporting in children, *Am J Respir Crit Care Med* 150:1234-1242, 1994.

129. Pope CA, Dockery DW, Spengler JD, and Raizenne ME: Respiratory health and PM pollution, *Am Rev Respir Dis* 144:668-674, 1991.

130. Pope CA and Dockery DW: Acute health effects of PM pollution on symptomatic and asymptomatic children, *Am Rev Respir Dis* 145:1123-1128, 1992.

131. Ware JH, Ferris BG, Dockery DW, Spengler J, Stram D, and Speizer F: Effects of ambient sulfur oxides and suspended particles on respiratory health of children, *Am Rev Respir Dis* 133:834-842, 1986.

132. Dockery DW, Speizer FE, Stram DO, Ware JH, and Spengler JD: Effects of inhalable particles on respiratory health of children, *Am Rev Respir Dis* 139:587-594, 1989.

133. Euler GL, Abbey DE, Magie AR, and Hodgkin JE: Chronic obstructive pulmonary disease symptom effects of long term cumulative ex-

posure to ambient levels of total suspended particulates and sulfur dioxide in California Seventh-Day Adventist residents, *Arch Environ Health* 42:213-222, 1987.

134. Amdur MO and Chen LC: Furnace-generated acid aerosols: speciation and pulmonary effects, *Environ Health Perspect* 79:147-150, 1989.

135. Chen LC, Miller PD, Amdur MO, and Gordon T: Airway hyperresponsiveness in guinea pigs exposed to acid-coated ultrafine particles, *J Toxicol Environ Health* 35:165-174, 1992.

136. Hatch GE, Boykin E, Graham JA, Lewtas J, Pott F, Loud K, and Mumford JS: Inhalable particles and pulmonary host defense: *in vitro* and *in vivo* effects of ambient air and combustion particles, *Environ Res* 36:67-80, 1985.

137. Beck BD, Brain JD, and Wolfthal SF: Assessment of lung injury produced by particulate emissions of space heaters burning automotive waste oil, *Ann Occup Hyg* 32:257-265, 1988.

138. Sun M: Acid aerosols called health hazard, *Science* 240:1727, 1988.

139. Amdur MO, Bayles J, Ugro V, and Underhill DW: Comparative irritant potency of sulfate salts, *Environ Res* 16:1-8, 1978.

140. Thurston GD, Ito K, Lippman M, and Hayes C: Re-examination of London, England mortality in relation to exposure to acidic aerosols during 1963-1972 winters, *Environ Health Perspect* 79:73-82, 1989.

141. Thurston GD, Ito K, Hayes CG, Bates DV, and Lippmann M: Respiratory hospital admissions and summertime haze air pollution in Toronto, Ontario: consideration of the role of acid aerosols, *Environ Res* 65:271-290, 1994.

142. Speizer FE: Studies of acid aerosols in six cities and in a new multicity investigation: design issues, *Environ Health Perspect* 79:61-67, 1989.

143. Ostro BD, Lipsett MJ, Wiener MB, and Selner JC: Asthmatic responses to airborne acid aerosols, *Am J Public Health* 81:694-702, 1991.

144. Dockery DW, Schwartz J, and Spengler JD: Air pollution and daily mortality associations with particulates and acid aerosols, *Environ Res* 59:362-373, 1992.

145. Amdur MO, Dubriel M, and Creasia DA: Respiratory response of guinea pigs to low levels of sulfuric acid, *Environ Res* 15:418-423, 1978.

146. Utell MJ: Effects of inhaled acid aerosols on lung mechanics: an analysis of human exposure studies, *Environ Health Perspect* 63:39-44, 1985.

147. Koenig JQ, Pierson WF, and Horike M: The effects of inhaled sulfuric acid on pulmonary function in adolescent asthmatics, *Am Rev Respir Dis* 128:221-225, 1983.

148. Utell MJ, Morrow PE, Speers DM, Darling J, and Hyde RW: Airway responses to sulfate and sulfuric acid aerosols in asthmatics, *Am Rev Respir Dis* 128:444-450, 1983.

149. Lioy PJ and Waldman JM: Acidic sulfate aerosols: characterization and exposure, *Environ Health Perspect* 79:15-34, 1989.

150. Avol EL, Linn WS, Shamoo DA, Anderson KR, Peng R-C, and Hackney JD: Respiratory responses of young asthmatic volunteers in controlled exposures to sulfuric acid aerosol, *Am Rev Respir Dis* 142:343-348, 1990.

151. Aris R, Christian D, Sheppard D, and Balmes JR: Lack of bronchoconstrictor response to sulfuric acid aerosols and fogs, *Am Rev Respir Dis* 143:744-750, 1991.

152. Linn WS, Avol EL, Anderson KR, Shamoo DA, Peng R-C, and Hackney JD: Effect of droplet size on respiratory responses to inhaled sulfuric acid in normal and asthmatic volunteers, *Am Rev Respir Dis* 140:161-166, 1989.

153. Utell MJ, Morrow PE, and Hyde RW: Airway reactivity to sulfate and sulfuric acid aerosols in normal and asthmatic subjects, *J Air Pollut Control Assoc* 34:931-935, 1984.

154. Gearhart JM and Schlesinger RB: Sulfuric acid-induced airway hyperresponsiveness, *Fundam Appl Toxicol* 7:681-689, 1986.

155. Leikauf GD, Yeates DB, Wales KA, Spektor DM, Albert RE, and Lippmann M: Effects of sulfuric acid aerosol on respiratory mechanics and mucociliary particle clearance in healthy nonsmoking adults, *Am Ind Hyg Assoc J* 42:273-282, 1981.

156. Gearhart JM and Schlesinger RB: Response of the tracheobronchial mucociliary clearance system to repeated irritant exposure: the effect of sulfuric acid mist on function and structure, *Exp Lung Res* 14:587-605, 1988.

157. Schlesinger RB: Comparative irritant potency of inhaled sulfate aerosol: effects on bronchial mucociliary clearance, *Environ Res* 34:268-279, 1984.

158. Schlesinger RB, Halpern M, Albert RE, and Lippmann M: Effect of chronic inhalation of sulfuric acid mist upon mucociliary clearance from the lungs of donkeys, *J Environ Pathol Toxicol* 2:1351-1367, 1979.

159. Schlesinger RB: Functional assessment of rabbit alveolar macrophages following intermittent inhalation exposures to sulfuric acid mist, *Fund Appl Toxicol* 8:328-334, 1987.

160. Frampton MW, Voter KZ, Morrow PE, Roberts NJ, Culp DJ, Cox C, and Utell MJ: Sulfuric acid aerosol exposure in humans assessed by bronchoalveolar lavage, *Am Rev Respir Dis* 146:626-632, 1992.

161. Koenig JQ, Covert DS, and Pierson WE: Effects of inhalation of acidic components on pulmonary function in allergic adolescent subjects, *Environ Health Perspect* 79:173-178, 1989.

162. Aris R, Christian D, Sheppard D, and Balmes JR: The effects of sequential exposure to acidic fog and ozone on pulmonary function in exercising subjects, *Am Rev Respir Dis* 143:85-91, 1991.

163. Aris R, Christian D, Tager I, Ngo L, Finkbeiner WE, and Balmes JR: Effects of nitric acid gas alone or in combination with ozone on healthy volunteers, *Am Rev Respir Dis* 148:965-973, 1993.

164. Becker S, Roger LJ, Devlin RB, and Koren HS: Increased phagocytosis and antiviral activity of alveolar macrophages from humans exposed to nitric acid, *Am Rev Respir Dis* 145:A429, 1992.

165. Mautz WJ, Nadziejko CE, and Schlesinger RB: Effects of subchronic exposure to nitric acid vapor on alveolar structure in the rat and rabbit, *Am Rev Respir Dis* 147:A382, 1993.

166. Grose EC, Richards JH, Illing JW, Miller FJ, Davies DW, Graham JA, and Gardner DE: Pulmonary host defense responses to inhalation of sulfuric acid and ozone, *J Toxicol Environ Health* 10:351-362, 1982.

Chapter 50

INTERACTION OF TOBACCO SMOKING WITH OCCUPATIONAL AND ENVIRONMENTAL FACTORS

Kent E. Pinkerton
Stacy H. Grimes
Marc B. Schenker

Cigarette smoking is the best described external cause of lung disease, but its interaction with various occupational and environmental causes of lung disease is not well characterized. This chapter examines occupational and environmental exposures and tobacco smoking. Diseases of the respiratory tract range from mild airway irritation to advanced forms of emphysema and lung cancer. A number of occupational and environmental factors may interact with tobacco in an additive or synergistic manner to increase the risk of respiratory disease. However, those mechanisms involved have not been clearly elucidated, and models based on actual epidemiologic data that demonstrate the nature of these interactions are limited.

This chapter reviews epidemiologic studies that address relationships between occupation, cigarette smoking, and respiratory illness. Environmental factors that may interact with cigarette smoking to produce increased levels of disease in the respiratory tract are addressed. Biologic principles regulating the function of the respiratory tract and the diversity of epithelial cells that populate the airways and alveoli are examined. Other cell types that play a role in lung immunity and defense, and exposure conditions that impact directly on these cells to impair clearance or alter the normal function of the respiratory tract are also considered. All of these factors are likely to play an important role in the consequences of interplay between occupational or environmental exposures and tobacco smoking and, ultimately, in the multifactorial etiology of respiratory disease.

The interaction of environmental, occupational, and smoking exposures may act in an additive, greater than additive (synergistic), or less than additive (antagonistic) manner.[1] The nature of the interaction is complex and does not always follow obvious assumptions. For example, there is consistent evidence that allergic alveolitis is reduced among cigarette smokers, although the mechanism for this effect is not known.[2,3] Some studies have shown that workers who smoke, in addition to being exposed to pollutants, tend to have greater amounts of mucus present in the airways. This may serve as an initial protection against disease in smokers versus the nonsmokers who were exposed under the same conditions.[4] On the other hand, numerous studies have demonstrated additive or greater than additive effects of smoking and occupational exposures on both respiratory symptoms and pulmonary function as well as lung cancer. Findings also suggest that once cancer is established, the disease proceeds at a much greater rate in smokers than in nonsmokers.[4]

TOBACCO USE: SOCIETAL AND GENDER IMPLICATIONS FOR LUNG DISEASE ETIOLOGY

The use of tobacco and tobacco products is still a prevalent practice in the United States today, and the prevalence is even greater in many other countries of the world. Numerous epidemiologic studies have noted that occupation is a significant correlate of tobacco use.[5] Workers in "blue-collar" occupations are more likely to smoke than those in "white-collar" work environments. Smoking is more prevalent among occupational groups and social strata that are more likely to be exposed to hazards in the workplace. Consequently, studies of the interaction of smoking and occupational exposures must carefully control for the nonrandom distribution of smoking and hazardous exposures in the workplace.[6]

Tobacco usage may also be a significant means to cope with psychologic and physiologic stresses induced by specific occupations.[5] This implies that workers with more physical and cognitive demands have higher levels of tobacco use. Conversely, men in white-collar occupations, particularly those in professions, are less likely to have ever smoked. One study found that the three highest rates for current smoking men were among handlers or cleaners, transportation or material movers, and machinists.[7] Among those who do smoke, men in white-collar occupations are more likely to quit or to smoke cigarettes with lower levels of nicotine. Overall, professional men are less likely to have ever smoked than those in other occupational groups. In addition, men in professional occupations consistently have the highest cessation rates, whereas those in blue-collar occupations have the lowest.[8] This pattern has not changed over time and appears to be most pronounced among men.[5]

Among women a similar inverse association between cigarette smoking with higher socioeconomic status or white-collar occupations is also present.[9] Smoking among adolescent girls is associated with lower socioeconomic status of the parents and among adults with downward mobility. Numerous studies have found an association of lower scholastic achievement and smoking.[9] The three highest rates of current smoking women were found among protective service workers, which was by far the highest proportion with 79% being smokers; handlers and cleaners; and machinists.[7] However, smoking has been found to be less related to occupation among women than among men.[8] Further, rates of smoking cessation among women are significantly lower than for men in similar occupational categories. For example, the rate of quitting among managers, officials, and proprietors for men is almost twice the rate for women in these occupations.

The interaction of occupational exposures, smoking, and gender may be further complicated by the nonrandom distribution of occupational exposures. For example, in a study from Finland, it was noted that men and women working in the laundry industry have different jobs (and exposures). Women who were washers were more often exposed to soaps, detergents, and other chemicals, whereas men were involved in the service aspect of this industry. Little information was available regarding specific work tasks or exposures in this study, which made the analysis of the interaction of workplace exposures with smoking and gender difficult because of the diverse job nature of men and women in this industry.[10]

Both laboratory and epidemiologic studies have provided strong evidence that cigarette smoking and exposure to other substances may have a synergistic effect on disease risk or severity. Analysis of a potential synergistic effect exemplifies the difficulties that may arise when two agents both act as causes of a particular outcome. The greater than additive effects may result from the possibility that either of the two agents modifies the extent to which the other produces the effect. If the risk attributable to a combined exposure exceeds the sum of the risks attributable to each exposure separately, this is referred to as synergy.[11] Because of the clinical and public health importance of a synergistic effect, it is important for epidemiologists to examine the various types and amounts of occupational and environmental exposures and their potential interaction with tobacco smoking, and for clinicians to be aware of the nature of this interaction when diagnosing and advising patients.

Certain industries, such as lead smelting, metal working, chemical processing, grain storage, and mining, monitor more extensively for occupational exposures than others. The use of individual monitoring data in large surveys of specific occupations may provide unique insights for epidemiologic studies on smoking and occupationally related diseases, including cancer among workers who handle substances that are potential carcinogens in occupational environments.[10] However, there are several factors that prevent careful modeling of the interaction of smoking and workplace exposures. Historical cohort investigations may use less reliable indicators of cigarette smoking among subjects who died years before the data collection. Furthermore, there may be subjects in historical cohort investigations without either the toxic exposure or cigarette smoking history, thus limiting the ability to model the interaction of these two factors. This is the case in most investigations of cigarette smoking and asbestos exposure.[12] In studies of current workers and in some historical studies, the "healthy worker" or "healthy smoker" effect may be another factor limiting the analysis of risk factor interactions.[13,14] Specifically, smokers who are less affected by smoking (or the interaction of smoking and workplace exposures) may be more likely to continue smoking than those more affected.

There is little question that smoking and smoking-related disease occurrence is associated with gender. Most respiratory diseases directly related to cigarette smoking, such as chronic bronchitis, emphysema, and lung cancer, have higher morbidity and mortality rates among men, reflecting the historically greater prevalence of smoking among men.[15] However, the pattern of cigarette smoking and occupational exposures has changed dramatically over the past few decades, and a current question of scientific interest is whether equivalent exposure to cigarette smoke, occupational exposures, or both results in an equivalent risk of disease in men and women. This remains an important question because about one in three adult men and one in four adult women in the United States continue to smoke despite public health efforts to encourage cessation.[16]

TOBACCO AND TRACE CONTAMINANTS

Tobacco smoke contains more than 3500 compounds found in three phases: gaseous, vapor, and particulate. These represent a complex mixture of carcinogenic, cytotoxic, and tumor-promoting agents.[17] Tobacco also contains a number of inorganic metals in addition to its numerous organic constituents. These metals found in the tobacco plant are derived from the soil, fertilizer, mulch, agricultural sprays, and polluted rainfall. Many of the metals in tobacco such as chromium, nickel, cadmium, lead, and arsenic are toxic and some are suspected of being human carcinogens (see Chapter 34). Traces of these metals that have been detected in human lung tissue could be derived from a variety of environmental sources.[18] It is clear that there may be some relationship between metal exposure and the practice of cigarette smoking. It is known that the concentration of cadmium, for example, in tobacco leaves is about 10 times higher than that in dried soil.[18] Again, these additional factors contribute to the potential risk of increased respiratory toxicity associated with the combination of cigarette smoking and occupational and environmental exposures.

RESPIRATORY MORBIDITY

Although smoking is the most important cause of chronic obstructive pulmonary disease (COPD) including emphysema, occupational and environmental factors may be important independent causes or may interact with the effects of cigarette smoking. The effects of workplace exposures on COPD are described in Chapter 27, and this chapter will focus only on the interactions with cigarette smoking.

Population-based studies have demonstrated an additive effect of smoking and dust exposure on the risk (relative odds) of chronic cough, chronic phlegm, persistent wheeze, and breathlessness.[19] Similar independent effects of smoking and occupational exposure were observed in a cross-sectional survey of men in Tucson.[20]

Numerous epidemiologic studies have evaluated the interaction of smoking and occupational exposures on respiratory symptoms or function in working population, often with mixed results. For example, some studies have suggested that asbestos and smoking have a greater than additive effect on pulmonary fibrosis, while others have ob-

served a simple additive effect of these two exposures.[21] Among workers exposed to cotton dust, epidemiologic studies have suggested that cotton dust and smoking have a greater than additive effect on risk of byssinosis symptoms, but interact only additively on the reduction in lung function.[21] Similarly, among workers exposed to grain dust the interaction with cigarette smoking appears to be synergistic for respiratory symptoms but additive or less than additive for the effect on pulmonary function.

Early cross-sectional studies among miners who were exposed to dust found an excess of bronchitic symptoms such as mucus hypersecretion beyond rates attributable to smoking alone. One study showed that nonsmoking miners had more chronic bronchitis than nonminers at all ages in both smokers and nonsmokers. Among current smokers, 27.3% of the nonminers had chronic bronchitis compared to 35.6% of the miners. The prevalence of reported chronic bronchitis was roughly an additive effect in exposed miners who also smoked.[22] In addition, among nonsmoking U.S. miners, workers at the coal face, or the mine location with the highest concentration of respirable particles, had the highest prevalence of chronic bronchitis. In a cross-sectional survey of British miners, the effects of cigarette smoking and dust exposure on decrement in forced expiratory volume in 1 second (FEV1) were roughly additive.[23] Another study of Utah miners also found additive effects of smoking and dust exposure on expiratory flow.[24] Prospective studies of coal miners have also demonstrated additive effects of dust exposure and smoking on decline in FEV1.[25,26]

Autopsy studies of miners exposed to silica have clearly shown independent effects of dust exposure and cigarette smoking on the risk of histologic evidence of chronic obstructive pulmonary disease[27] (see Chapter 20). The interaction is at least additive, and recent data suggest that there may be a multiplicative interaction of the two factors.

LUNG CANCER

In recent years, exposure to environmental carcinogens including radon and environmental tobacco smoke and radon (see Chapters 34 and 47) has been of growing concern within the United States. The nature of the interaction of cigarette smoking and occupational or environmental carcinogen exposure is particularly important because of the large proportion of the population that continues to smoke, and the even larger proportion of the population exposed to environmental tobacco smoke. Further, a synergistic interaction will greatly increase the individual risk of those subjects with both exposures, as well as substantially increase the population attributable risks.

Asbestos

Asbestos is arguably the occupational agent with the most research on risks of lung cancer following exposure.[28] However, although there are ample data on the risks of lung cancer following occupational exposure to asbestos, remarkably few studies have characterized the interaction of cigarette smoking and asbestos on lung cancer risk.[12] Analysis of this interaction, as with the interaction of smoking and other occupational carcinogens, is difficult because of inaccuracies in obtaining historical smoking histories and the low incidence of lung cancer among nonsmokers with occupational exposure. In a review of over 2100 lung cancer cases from studies that have evaluated the interaction of smoking and asbestos exposure, Saracci found only 34 cases of lung cancer among nonsmoking asbestos workers plus 53 cases in a "mixed" category that included nonsmokers and light smokers.[29] This small number of cases among nonsmokers plus misclassification of prior cigarette smoking limits the sensitivity of interaction analyses. Overall a multiplicative (i.e., greater than additive) model best explained the interaction of smoking and asbestos exposure, although there was great variability among studies with some suggesting a greater than multiplicative interaction and others finding something closer to an additive effect. In general, none of the studies provided data allowing a statistical rejection (i.e., $p > 0.05$) of a multiplicative interaction, and this synergistic model remains the best explanation of the phenomena. Variations in the observed strength and nature of the interaction also are thought to reflect multiple stages of carcinogenesis at which both asbestos and cigarette smoking can act.

In studies that have characterized the interaction of smoking and asbestos it is also possible to calculate the percent of excess risk due to the interaction, i.e., the percent of excess cancers over those that would have occurred with a simple additive model. For most studies of asbestos and smoking, this percent excess risk due to interaction is between 25% and 50%.[29] The nature of a greater than additive interaction (synergism) is such that the risks attributable to individual agents will total greater than 100%, which should be kept in mind when considering the risk attributable to individual agents such as smoking.[1]

Radon and radon progeny

Radon and radon progeny are naturally occurring forms of radiation found within the soil and emitted to the air (see Chapters 31 and 34). Numerous studies have demonstrated the increased risk of lung cancer in occupationally exposed cohorts.[30] Analysis of studies that have permitted characterization of the smoking–radon interaction have most commonly found a multiplicative interaction among uranium miners, but other mining populations have found an additive or less than additive interactions of these two factors.[29,31] The reasons for this difference are unknown, and may include lower dose-rate of exposure, differences in mining practices (e.g., interaction with dust exposure), and length of follow-up. Few studies have adequately characterized cigarette smoking characteristics (e.g., cigarette type, smoke inhalation) to fully understand this interaction.

Interestingly, the magnitude of the excess risk due to the interaction in studies of radon exposure is commonly over 50%, but this value must be viewed with caution. If the interaction is less than multiplicative, the excess risk due to interaction will be reduced, as will the risk associated with radon exposure for smokers.[32] In summary, while the carcinogenicity of cigarette smoke and radon exposure has been established, the exact nature and mechanism of the interaction as well as the underlying cellular and molecular mechanisms of their combined carcinogenic effects are not fully characterized.[17]

Recent concern about exposure to radon and its progeny has centered on residential settings, where the accumulation of radon progeny in homes presents an increased risk of lung cancer (see Chapter 48). Most data on the nature of the interaction of smoking and radon progeny in this setting are inferred from analyses of the studies analyzing interactions in mining cohorts. However, many characteristics of exposure to radon progeny in the home are different from the mining environment, such as lower dust levels, different ages of exposure, and different breathing patterns, and the nature of this interaction remains to be characterized. As in occupational cohorts, the low risk of lung cancer in lifetime nonsmokers makes investigation of this interaction more difficult.

Particulate matter

Many studies have reported associations between particulate air pollution and daily mortality rates in metropolitan areas of the United States.[33,34] This association was first observed in time-series studies but has more recently been observed in the prospective data of the Six-Cities study.[34] Particulate air pollution is a mixture of solid particles and liquid droplets that varies in size, composition, and origin. U.S. national health standards for the quality of ambient air are based on the mass concentration of inhalable particles defined to include particles with an aerodynamic diameter less than 10 μm (see Chapter 49). Fine particulate pollution typically contains a mixture of particles including soot, acid condensates, and sulfate and nitrate particles. These are thought to pose a particularly greater risk to health because they are more likely to be toxic than larger particles, and they can be breathed more deeply into the lungs.

The recent observation of an association of ambient particle concentration (PM) and mortality from lung cancer and cardiopulmonary diseases is noteworthy, but requires further replication and laboratory corroboration before it can be accepted as causal in nature.[35] It also raises many questions about the nature of the interaction with cigarette smoking, a known cause of these outcomes. Although limited data suggest an independent (and possibly multiplicative) contribution of these factors on lung cancer (and overall mortality) risk, the complex nature of this interaction requires further investigation in epidemiologic studies and laboratory models.

MECHANISMS OF INTERACTION

Although smoking is the most prominent cause of several chronic lung diseases, including emphysema and chronic bronchitis, other environmental factors may also be important contributors.[31] Numerous studies have demonstrated an association of occupational dust exposure and COPD (see Chapter 27), although the nature of the interaction between smoking and occupational exposures on the risk of chronic airflow obstruction is less well defined.[36,37] As noted, epidemiologic studies have not always been able to accurately characterize the nature of the interaction of smoking and occupational or environmental exposures on respiratory outcomes. For example, there is controversy as to whether focal emphysema in coal miners is due to the dust accumulating within the lungs or whether the dust has accumulated in the emphysematous lesions caused by other factors such as smoking.[38] It is also important to note that exposure of rats and hamsters to cigarette smoke has not consistently produced emphysema.[38]

Laboratory studies have also been inconsistent in characterizing the nature of the smoking–occupational-environmental exposure interaction. Air pollutants cause lung cell damage, inflammatory responses, and impairment of pulmonary host defenses in addition to other types of responses. Acute changes in lung function and respiratory symptoms as well as chronic changes in lung cells and airways may be important factors in the interaction between environmental and occupational exposures and the use of tobacco products.

An interesting finding has been the presence of cadmium within emphysematous lungs in direct proportion to the severity of the disease.[38] The persistent presence of neutrophils has been shown to be related to the development of emphysema. Chalon and colleagues[39] found that epithelial cytomorphologic changes caused by smoking substantially preceded any alteration in lung function tests.[40] The induction of airway epithelial inflammation has been an area of great interest, particularly due to the production of cytokines, which may be important in the recruitment of inflammation to other areas of the lungs.[40]

To better understand the pathogenesis of emphysema, it is important to note that there are differences in susceptibility within the smoking population.[41] The accurate diagnosis of emphysema in pathologic specimens has been difficult because although normal airspace size is thought to be in the region of 250 μm, until recently the limits of normality of airspaces have been undefined in the human.[41] There has also been some indication that smoking is not the only factor responsible for the onset of microscopically excessive emphysema. Those individuals with this pathology may have an inherent susceptibility to the disease. It has been suggested that susceptibility is sex and dose related with respect to smoking habit. A large number of heavy smokers have not developed microscopic emphysema so variations of susceptibility to disease cannot be accounted for by smoking habit alone.[41]

Cigarette smoking has been found to increase permeability of the airways and mucosa, which allows for greater or increased penetration of a variety of substances. These substances may include irritants or allergens. In the workplace, the risk of sensitization depends, in many instances, on the relationship between smoking status of an individual and the degree of exposure to occupational allergens.[42] Enhanced risk of sensitization may represent the most compelling human evidence for direct effect of cigarette smoking to increase the incidence of nonmalignant respiratory conditions associated with exposure to other agents. A number of studies using animal models have shown that exposure to cigarette smoke will significantly alter the epithelial barrier of the airways and deep lung. In addition, these studies have shown that prior exposure to cigarette smoke, followed by the injection of a bolus of asbestos fibers by intratracheal installation, leads to a significantly greater retention of these fibers within the lungs themselves. Studies that have looked at the deposition of these fibers have demonstrated their penetration through the epithelium to the interstitial wall of the airways.[43]

Studies that have examined the experimental effect of environmental pollutants on the clearance of particles from the lungs have suggested that an interaction is occurring. For example, one study investigated the effect of ozone on the clearance of asbestos fibers. Fischer 344 rats were exposed over a 6-week period to ozone delivered in a cyclic pattern to mimic that of the Los Angles air basin. Baseline levels of ozone were maintained at 0.06 ppm during nonexposure periods. Over a 9-hour period five times each week, the ozone concentrations were increased to a peak of 0.25 ppm and subsequently decreased to the baseline level of 0.06 ppm. Three days after the end of this exposure, animals were exposed to aerosolized asbestos fibers for a single 5-hour period and examined immediately after, or 30 days after the exposure test. It was found that there was no difference in the number of asbestos fibers found in the lungs of animals immediately after exposure to either air or ozone. However, 30 days after the end of exposure, those animals that had been preexposed to ozone contained twice as many asbestos fibers as those animals which had only been exposed to filtered air.[44] The cause for this marked disparity in asbestos fiber clearance of the lungs of rats is not immediately known. However, this enhanced retention of asbestos after exposure to ozone may be due to alterations in macrophage function and/or changes in lung epithelial permeability. Exposure to a variety of substances other than ozone or asbestos fibers may lead to similar consequences. It is logical to speculate that any particle that may be covered with a toxic or irritating substance, particularly carcinogenic compounds, will have a greater potential to elicit a lasting or debilitating process if the retention of the particle is enhanced in the respiratory tract. Although not proven, this may be one of the major factors responsible for interaction of occupational or environmental exposures with tobacco smoking leading to increased risks for a variety of diseases in humans.

Cellular basis of disease

Most of our discussion to this point has dealt with the more global aspects of occupational and environmental factors and their interaction with tobacco smoking. The effects of gases, vapors, and particles in the respiratory tract are initiated primarily at the cellular level. The endpoints of exposure to occupational agents or to tobacco smoke are those diseases that have already been touched on, including bronchitis, emphysema, fibrosis, and cancer. Although the initiation of the disease process in each instance is an active area of research today, the precise mechanisms leading to the final disease endpoint are not clear.

Two primary cell types that play an important role in each of these diseases include epithelial cells and macrophages.[45] Cigarette smoke affects alveolar macrophages, which, in turn, may affect the immune system. The risk of lung cancer may be directly influenced by macrophages, because these cells can release products that can suppress lymphocyte proliferation and thereby decrease anti-tumor cell surveillance activity.[21] Pulmonary macrophages are primarily responsible for protecting the lung from environmental pollutants and maintaining the sterility of the environment within the respiratory system. This is accomplished in part by phagocytosing particles, which are degraded by lysosomal enzymes. However, this process may also damage the lungs by releasing hydrolytic enzymes and metabolites into the lung milieu and tissue compartments.[46] Adverse reactions due to interactions with alveolar macrophages include a variety of pneumoconioses such as asbestosis and silicosis, which are characterized by inflammation and fibrosis throughout the parenchyma. In turn, these changes may also lead to emphysematous changes in the lungs.

Many studies have demonstrated that stimulation of alveolar macrophages and other phagocytic cells results in the release of a variety of inflammatory mediators. These mediators stimulate the influx of other inflammatory cells. The release of growth factors may also result in the proliferation of cells, particularly epithelial cells lining the respiratory tract. Chronic stimulation of epithelial cells to proliferate due to the presence of particles or irritating stimuli within the lungs could be a critical factor in the evolution of tumors in the lung.[47]

Alveolar macrophages are also capable of cell replication and division in response to inflammatory stimuli. Studies have suggested that tobacco smoke contains substances that will promote alveolar macrophage activation and proliferation.[48] The ultrastructural appearance of macrophages from the lungs of smokers clearly shows marked increases in size and surface ruffling in contrast to macrophages from nonsmokers.[40] Alveolar macrophages can also change in number and ultrastructural appearance with exposure to a variety of environmental pollutants.[49] Since these cells are present along the epithelial lining of the lungs and come into direct contact with inhaled air, it is natural to expect that they play a critical role in the overall response to factors found in the environment and different occupational settings.[50] Thus, alveolar macrophage number and activity may represent an important means of measuring the extent or degree of exposure to a variety of pollutants. Since macrophages clear a variety of inhaled substances through phagocytosis, the interaction of inhaled foreign particles and gases with macrophages is key to the expression of a variety of mediators in the lungs.[51] Alveolar macrophages are one of the primary cell types present in the lung that contain isozymes of the cytochrome P-450 monoxygenase system. The P-450 system is responsible for the metabolism of a variety of inhaled substances. In general, xenobiotics that are metabolized become less toxic. However, there are a variety of constituents, particularly within cigarette smoke, that become activated to their proximate carcinogenic form when metabolized through the cytochrome P-450 system. Therefore, some cellular interactions with inhaled compounds may actually lead to adverse health consequences.

More than 40 different cell types are found within the respiratory system.[52] Epithelial cells represent a significant proportion of the cell types found in the lungs. The diversity and distribution of epithelial cell types in the lungs are based on site and location. Epithelial cells are present from the nasal cavity to the alveolus. Since these cells are at the direct interface with the environment, they are also highly susceptible to injury by inhaled pollutants. These cells may react in a variety of ways to inhaled substances.[47] A number of nonspecific irritants within tobacco smoke such as hydrogen cyanide, acrolein, formaldehyde, and nitrogen oxides may result in a loss of ciliated cells. If this irritation is chronic, it is possible that these cells may become more susceptible to squamous cell differentiation and other potentially premalignant conditions.

Significant associations have been observed between smoking and mucous gland alterations.[21] As a part of bronchitis, more mucus will be present within the airway walls and the lumina with exposure to cigarette smoke. Potent irritants, such as the oxidant gases ozone and sulfur dioxide, will also increase the permeability of the airway epithelium. With the loss of ciliated epithelium, it is likely that mucociliary transport would also be reduced.[21] Each of these factors may lead to a reduced clearance of particles from the lung and enhanced uptake through the epithelium into the interstitial wall where clearance will be delayed.

In both allergic and nonallergic individuals, tobacco smoke may simply irritate the respiratory tract. The mucosal lining of the airway can be particularly susceptible to the irritating effects of exposure to tobacco smoke.[53] Cigarette smoking is thought to initiate a multistep process in terms of mutagenesis and carcinogenesis in the tracheobronchial epithelium. This begins with early mutational events that may evolve into bronchial metaplasia or dysplasia, a potential forerunner of squamous cell carcinomas.[54] A number of recent studies have examined the deoxyribonucleic acid isolated from human bronchial epithelium by ^{32}P postlabeling for the presence of aromatic adducts.[55] This may be a particularly and potentially useful predictor of lung tumors or early lung cancer detection due to the fact that most smoking-related tumors arise from the bronchial epithelium in humans.

CONCLUSIONS

It is clear that the potential risks and interactions with exposure to environmental or occupational agents and tobacco smoking are complex. Exposure to tobacco smoke and exposure to environmental agents such as radon and asbestos may act independently, additively, or, in many cases, synergistically with one another. The interactions of these exposures may speed up the process of a number of respiratory diseases. In studying the effects of occupational and environmental exposures, smoking habits must clearly be taken into account. Similarly, when studying the effects of tobacco smoke, the potential for interactions with occupational and environmental exposures must be considered.

REFERENCES

1. Rothman KJ, Greenland S, and Walker AM: Concepts of interaction, *Am J Epidemiol* 112(4):467-470, 1980.
2. Warren C: Extrinsic allergic alveolitis: a disease commoner in nonsmokers, *Thorax* 32:567-569, 1977.
3. Cormier Y, Gagnon L, Bérubé F, and Furnier M: Influence of cigarette smoking on experimental extrinsic allergic alveolitis, *Am Rev Resp Dis* 137:1104-1109, 1988.
4. Blackwood MJ: Health risks of smoking increased by exposure to workplace chemicals, *Occup Health Saf* 23-28, 81, 1985.
5. Serxner S, Catalano R, Dooley D, and Mishra S: Tobacco use: selection, stress, or culture? *J Occup Med* 33(10):1035-1039, 1991.
6. Sterling T and Weinkam J: The confounding of occupation and smoking and its consequences, *Soc Sci Med* 30(4):457-467, 1990.
7. Statistical Bulletin: *Metropolitan Insurance Companies* 73(4):12-19, 1992.
8. Covey LS, Zang EA, and Wynder EL: Cigarette smoking and occupational status: 1977 to 1990, *Am J Public Health* 82:1230-1234, 1992.
9. Health consequences of smoking for women: a report of the Surgeon General, 1980.
10. Anttila A, Sallmén M, and Hemminki K: Carcinogenic chemicals in the occupational environment, *Pharmacol Toxicol* 72(Suppl 1):69-76, 1993.
11. Rothman K: Causes, *Am J Epidemiol* 104:587-592, 1976.
12. Saracci R: Asbestos and lung cancer: an analysis of the epidemiological evidence on the asbestos-smoking interaction, *Int J Cancer* 20:323-331, 1977.
13. Becklake MR and Lalloo U: The 'healthy smoker': a phenomenon of health selection? *Respiration* 57(3):137-144, 1990.
14. Choi BC: Definition, sources, magnitude, effect modifiers, and strategies of reduction of the healthy worker effect, *J Occup Med* 34(10):979-988, 1992.
15. The Surgeon General's 1989 report on reducing the health consequences of smoking: 25 years of progress (abstract), 1989.
16. Simon JA, Browner WS, and Mangano DT: Predictors of smoking relapse after noncardiac surgery, *Am J Public Health* 82(9):1235-1237, 1992.
17. Piao CQ and Hei TK: The biological effectiveness of radon daughter alpha particles I. Radon, cigarette smoke and oncogenic transformation, *Carcinogenesis* 14(3):497-501, 1993.
18. Pääkkö P, Kokkonen P, Anttila S, and Kalliomäxi PL: Cadmium and chromium as markers of smoking in human lung tissue, *Environ Res* 49:197-207, 1989.
19. Korn RJ, Dockery DW, Speizer FE, Ware JH, and Ferris BG Jr: Occupational exposure and chronic respiratory symptoms. A population based study, *Am Rev Respir Dis* 136:298-304, 1987.
20. Lebowitz MD: Occupational exposures in relation to symptomatology and lung function in a community population, *Environ Res* 14:59-67, 1977.
21. Greaves IA and Schenker M: Tobacco smoking, In Brain JD, Beck BD, Warren J, and Shaikh R, editors: *Variations in susceptibility to toxic agents in the air: identification, mechanisms and policy implications*, pp 182-203, Baltimore, 1988, The Johns Hopkins University Press.
22. Lowe CR and Khosla T: Chronic bronchitis in ex-coal miners working in the steel industry, *Br J Ind Med* 29:45-49, 1972.
23. Rogan JM, Attfield MD, Jacobsen M, Rae S, Walker DD, and Walton WH: Role of dust in the working environment in the development of chronic bronchitis in British coal miners, *Br J Ind Med* 30:217-226, 1973.
24. Rom WN, Kanner RE, Renzetti AD, Shigeoka JW, Barkman HW, Nichols M, et al: Respiratory disease in Utah coal miners, *Am Rev Respir Dis* 123:372-377, 1981.
25. Love RG and Miller BG: Longitudinal study of lung function in coal miners, *Thorax* 37:193-197, 1982.
26. Attfield MD: Longitudinal decline in FEV$_1$ in United States coal miners, *Thorax* 40:132-137, 1985.
27. Hnizdo E: Combined effect of silica dust and tobacco smoking on mortality from chronic obstructive lung disease in gold miners, *Br J Ind Med* 47:656-664, 1990.
28. Becklake MR, Irwig L, Kielkowski D, Webster I, de Beer M, and Landau S: The predictors of emphysema in South African gold miners, *Am Rev Respir Dis* 135(6):1234-1241, 1987.
29. Saracci R: The interactions of tobacco smoking and other agents in cancer etiology, *Epidemiol Rev* 9:175-193, 1987.
30. Lubin JH, Boice JD, Edling C, Hornung RW, Howe G, Kunz E, et al: *Radon and lung cancer risk: a joint analysis of 11 underground miners studies*, NIH Pub 94-3644, Washington, DC, 1994, National Institutes of Health.
31. The health consequences of smoking, cancer and chronic lung disease in the workplace. A report of the Surgeon General, 1985.
32. NRC: *Health risks of radon and other internally deposited alpha-emitters (BEIR IV)*, Washington, DC, 1988, National Academy Press.
33. Schwartz J: Particulate air pollution and daily mortality: a synthesis, *Public Health Rev* 19:39-60, 1991/92.
34. Dockery DW, Pope CA III, Xu X, Spengler JD, Ware JH, Fay ME, et al: An association between air pollution and mortality in six U.S. cities, *N Engl J Med* 329:1753-1759, 1993.
35. Schenker M: Air pollution and mortality [editorial], *N Engl J Med* 329(24):1807-1808, 1993.
36. Becklake MR: Occupational exposures: evidence for a causal association with chronic obstructive pulmonary disease, *Am Rev Respir Dis* 140:S85-S91, 1989.
37. Garshick E and Schenker M: Occupation and chronic airflow limitation, In Hensley MJ and Saunders NA, editors: *Clinical epidemiology of chronic obstructive pulmonary disease*, vol 43, pp 227-258, New York, 1989, Marcel Dekker.

38. Snider GL: Chronic obstructive pulmonary disease: risk factors, pathophysiology and pathogenesis, *Ann Rev Med* 40:411-429, 1989.

39. Chalon J, Tayyab MA, and Ramanathan S: Cytology of respiratory epithelium as a predictor of respiratory complications after operation, *Chest* 67:32-35, 1975.

40. Roby TJ, Swan GE, Sorensen KW, Hubbard GA, and Schumann GB: Discriminant analysis of lower respiratory tract components associated with cigarette smoking, based on quantitative sputum cytology, *Acta Cytol* 34(2):147-154, 1990.

41. Gillooly M and Lamb D: Microscopic emphysema in relation to age and smoking habit, *Thorax* 48:491-495, 1993.

42. Shirakawa T, Kusaka Y, and Morimoto K: Combined effect of smoking habits and occupational exposure to hard metal on total IgE antibodies, *Chest* 101:1569-1576, 1992.

43. Tron V, Wright JL, Harrison N, Wiggs B, and Churg A: Cigarette smoke makes airway and early parenchymal asbestos-induced lung disease worse in the guinea pig, *Am Rev Respir Dis* 136:271-275, 1987.

44. Pinkerton KE, Brody AR, Miller FJ, and Crapo JD: Exposure to low levels of ozone results in enhanced pulmonary retention of inhaled asbestos fibers, *Am Rev Respir Dis* 140:1075-1081, 1989.

45. Collins M and Schenker M: Susceptibility to neoplasia altered by tobacco smoke exposure, In Brain JD, Beck BD, Warren J, and Shaikh R, editors: *Variations in susceptibility to toxic agents in the air: identification, mechanisms and policy implications,* pp 269-294, Baltimore, 1988, The Johns Hopkins University Press.

46. Malmberg P, Hedenström H, and Sundblad BM: Changes in lung function of granite crushers exposed to moderately high silica concentrations: a 12 year follow up, *Br J Ind Med* 50:726-731, 1993.

47. Dungworth DL, Mohr U, Heinrich U, Ernst H, and Kittel B: Pathological effects of inhaled particles in rat lungs: associations between inflammatory and neoplastic processes, In Dungworth DL, Mauderly JL, and Oberdörster, editors: *Toxic and carcinogenic effects of solid particles in the respiratory tract,* pp 75-98, Washington, DC, 1994, ILSI Press.

48. Barbers RG, Evans MJ, Gong H, and Tashkin DP: Enhanced alveolar monocytic phagocyte (macrophage) proliferation in tobacco and marijuana smokers, *Am Rev Respir Dis* 143:1092-1095, 1991.

49. Sköld CM, Forslid J, Eklund A, and Hed J: Metabolic activity in human alveolar macrophages increases after cessation of smoking, *Inflammation* 17(3):345-352, 1993.

50. Rylander R: Environmental exposures with decreased risks for lung cancer? *Int J Epidemiol* 19(3) Suppl 1:S67-S72, 1990.

51. Adler KB, Fischer BM, Wright DT, Cohn LA, and Becker S: Interactions between respiratory epithelial cells and cytokines: relationships to inflammation, *Ann NY Acad Sci* 725:128-145, 1994.

52. Plopper CG, Weir A, St. George J, Tyler N, Mariassy A, Wilson D, et al: Cell populations of the respiratory system: interspecies diversity in composition, distribution, and morphology, In Mohr U, Dungworth D, Kimmerle G, Lewkowski J, McClellan R, and Stober W, editors: *Inhalation toxicology,* pp 25-40, New York, 1988, Springer-Verlag.

53. Cummings KM, Zaki A, and Markello S: Variation in sensitivity to environmental tobacco smoke among adult non-smokers, *Int J Epidemiol* 20(1):121-125, 1991.

54. Lippman SM, Peters EJ, Wargovich MJ, Stadnyk AN, Dixon SD, Dekmezian RH, et al: Bronchila micronuclei as a marker of an early stage of carcinogenesis in the human tracheobronchial epithelium, *Int J Cancer* 45:811-815, 1990.

55. Phillips DH, Schoket B, Hewer A, Bailey E, Kostic S, and Vincze I: Influence of cigarette smoking on the levels of DNA adducts in human bronchial epithelium and white blood cells, *Int J Cancer* 46:569-575, 1990.

Clinical Programs

PHILIP HARBER

Systematic approaches may be used for the prevention and control of occupational and environmental respiratory disease. Chapters in this section describe methods that focus upon exposed at-risk persons, and Section XI discusses environmental control approaches. Primary prevention methods seek to prevent illness, such as preplacement evaluation to optimize job assignment. Secondary prevention seeks to detect and treat disease in an early state; screening programs fall in this category. Tertiary prevention includes the management of existing disease, and relevant areas of interest include pulmonary rehabilitation, work site accommodation of impaired workers, and compensation for occupational illness.

Chapter 51

SURVEILLANCE AND SCREENING OF RESPIRATORY DISEASE

Philip Harber

The prevention of occupational and environmental respiratory disease depends upon timely and accurate data. Sur

veillance systems are organized, planned systems for the purpose of collecting and utilizing data to *prevent* disease. This chapter will provide an overview of respiratory surveillance methods and general principles. Specific methodologic details are covered in other chapters.

The definition of surveillance implies many different components. An individual constituent standing alone does not constitute a surveillance program. The ultimate goal of surveillance is *prevention of disease*. For this reason, data collection and analysis that do not ultimately lead to prevention are not considered a surveillance activity. For example, an epidemiologic study of mesothelioma incidence in a formerly asbestos-exposed cohort is unlikely to lead to prevention of future disease and, therefore, should not be considered a surveillance activity. This chapter has two parts. In the first part, general principles are reviewed. In the second part, specific applications of surveillance and screening methods are discussed.

GENERAL PRINCIPLES OF SURVEILLANCE
Categories of surveillance programs

Surveillance programs may be categorized in several ways. The design of a program should consider the nature of the disease as well as available resources.

Health versus hazard surveillance. A surveillance system may be based on collecting data about health outcomes or about exposures. Furthermore, hybrid systems may collect both types of information.

Surveillance systems based upon health outcomes ascertain the frequency of health effects in population *groups*. When excesses are detected, preventive interventions may then be targeted at the members of the group or at the exposures.

Although there is an a priori assumption that determining disease frequency is a useful guide to targeting prevention, several conditions must be present for this to be useful.

First, the health outcome must be specifically defined, and there must be a clear mechanism for assuring consistency in its ascertainment. The pathologic diagnosis of mesothelioma or carefully defined criteria for pneumoconiosis (e.g., using the International Labor Organization (ILO) radiographic system) are relatively specified. Conversely, nonspecific health outcomes are generally less useful (e.g., "cough").

Second, consistency in use of these criteria by those generating the primary data is requisite. To the extent that radiograph interpreters use a standardized system, such as the ILO scheme (see Chapter 7), the data can be meaningfully utilized to reflect disease prevalence. Conversely, if the definition of the outcome is vague and subject to marked interobserver variability, the data may be less useful.

Third, health outcome surveillance is generally most effective when there is a specific association between the health effect and the exposure of interest. Small rounded opacities in the upper lung zones on chest radiography are closely linked to silica and coal dust exposure, and the presence of this would trigger investigative and preventive efforts. Nonspecific symptoms such as cough or dyspnea, however, are only nonspecifically linked to specific exposures. In addition, there are numerous causes for such symptoms, and, therefore, their presence does not directly point to a locus for intervention.

Relatively nonspecific symptoms (which do not in themselves constitute a specific clinical entity) still may be useful for health-based surveillance. Under such circumstances, a larger population must be employed, and formal statistical analysis becomes crucial. Although a single case of de novo asthma with a clear temporal relationship to work indicates the need for intervention, the occurrence of a single case of lung cancer, a common and multifactorial disorder, would not itself warrant such concern.

Fourth, the time course determines the utility of health-based surveillance. If the health effect typically occurs in clear temporal relationship to the exposure, surveillance is facilitated. This makes detecting the relationship easier. Even for a relatively non–cause-specific effect (such as asthma), a close temporal relationship between onset of symptoms and work with a particular agent leads to strong suspicion. In addition, long delays between exposure and disease make the causal link to a particular worksite more difficult to detect. When a health effect might be a consequence of several job sites, it may be difficult to determine which actually led to the problem.

Fifth, the opportunity for preventive interventions may have been missed with long latencies. For example, asbestos exposure at high levels was much more ubiquitous in the past than it is currently. For this reason, currently detected asbestos-related disease actually reflects work practices from 20 to 30 years ago. Hence, this information will not affect preventive interventions in current workplaces.

Sixth, health-based surveillance requires systematic access to health data. If health services are provided in numerous locations, health data may be difficult to acquire in uniform formats. However, in some instances, the situation can be remedied if there is a single payer, even if the services are provided diffusely.

Finally, the health problem must be one for which individuals are likely to enter the health care system. Thus, severe asthma or bronchogenic carcinoma will be detected using health-based surveillance, but chronic bronchitis or premature air flow obstruction may be more difficult to detect.

There are many advantages to health-based surveillance. The significance of the outcome is obvious in most cases. There are extensive health care systems in place, and these may be utilized for the purpose of preventive surveillance. In addition, worker cooperation may be relatively easy to develop if there is a perceived health benefit.

Hazard surveillance has a different focus—it is based upon measuring exposure factors, typically air levels of agents capable of producing respiratory disease. Methods of determining such exposure levels are discussed in Chapter 11.

Exposure-based methods are effective when the agent causing the disease is well characterized, and there is reasonable consensus about "acceptable" exposure levels. Exposure-based surveillance cannot be employed when the specific causative agent is not well identified. Thus, measurement of airborne silica is much more useful than is environmental measurement for surveillance for "sick building syndrome."

Hazard-based surveillance is particularly useful for long latency diseases. Waiting for detection of excess cases of pneumoconiosis inherently leads to a 20 to 30 year delay in instituting preventive measures, but measurement of airborne silica levels can lead to immediate prevention. One can be confident that controlling silica levels will reduce silicosis, and it is therefore not necessary to wait for disease to develop.

Hazard surveillance is most effective when the exposure levels are relatively constant over time. In situations where there are frequent process changes, measurement of levels at one particular time may not provide useful information about the overall extent of exposure and risk. For agents that require a significant *cumulative* dose for health impact, there is a clear assumption that risk is related to the product of level measured times duration of exposure. Thus, while one day of exposure to 1 fiber/cm^3 of asbestos would not imply high risk, if extended over a working lifetime, this is important. Biases in air level measurements are discussed in Chapter 11.

Short-term excursions and variability are often significant but make hazard-based surveillance more difficult. For example, isocyanate asthma is closely related to the peaks of exposure rather than average or cumulative exposure.

Thus, intermittent measurement of air levels of isocyanates may have only limited ability to detect worksite areas requiring intervention because samples are unlikely on a statistical basis to find the peaks. (See Chapter 11 for discussion of sampling strategies.)

Conversely, exposure-based surveillance is particularly useful when there is variability of the relationship of the worker to the worksite. Thus, if it is not feasible to identify a specific cohort of workers for health surveillance, measurement of the worksite exposure can be useful in assessing risk.

Exposure-based surveillance is also often less subject to reporting biases than is health-based surveillance. Fiber counts can generally be accomplished with more interobserver consistency than can the clinical diagnosis of early asbestosis or asthma.

Often, the measurements to be performed are already mandated (e.g., by the U.S. Occupational and Safety Health Administration [OSHA]). In such circumstances, the data are likely to be already available and do not require incremental effort.

There are situations in which hazard-based surveillance is ineffective. It is difficult when there is a multiplicity of agents in the workplace or if the causative agent is not specifically identified or measurable.

Hazard surveillance is also not useful for identifying new hazards. When a new chemical agent is introduced, measuring exposure will not provide useful information about whether it actually represents a health hazard (this can be determined only by measuring health outcomes).

Although hazard surveillance for respiratory disease prevention usually entails measurement of air levels, other methods may also be employed. For example, ongoing review of purchase orders to screen for the ordering of respiratory toxins can be of use, as can periodic review of material safety and data sheets (MSDS) (see Chapter 10). Furthermore, walk through surveys (Chapter 10, Part II) without actual measurement of air levels can frequently be of benefit in detecting hazards.

In summary, surveillance programs may be characterized as either health-based or hazard-based. Table 51-1 compares the relative benefits and limits of these methods. Of course, a hybrid approach may also be used. Indeed, a joint hazard and health surveillance approach is necessary when investigating new previously unknown hazards or for quantifying the exposure–effect relationship. Health-based surveillance is a necessity for detecting the effects of new agents; exposure surveillance requires the a priori knowledge of the agent–disease relationship.

Active versus passive surveillance. Surveillance programs may be designed to employ data that are routinely collected (i.e., not specifically for surveillance purposes); such surveillance programs are considered "passive." For example, systematic analysis of Workers' Compensation

Table 51-1. General categories of health versus exposure surveillance

	Health	Hazard
Outcome	Health effects	Exposure data
Examples	Anemia	Air levels
	FEV1	Biologic levels of toxicants
	Cancers	Workplace ergonomic survey
Latency	Short	Long
Effect immediacy	Immediate	Delayed
Causative agents	Uncertain	Definite
Health effect specificity	Clear	Vague
At-risk population	Defined	Difficult to ascertain
Possible intervention	Health care	Environmental control
Stability of work environment	Variable	Consistent

FEV1, Forced expiratory volume in 1 second.

claims for respiratory disease can provide useful information. Analysis of death certificates, employee health records that include routine periodic medical examination results (often including spirometry), or sickness absence records also constitute passive data sources.

An *active* surveillance system requires that the data collection system be instituted specifically for the purpose of surveillance. For example, a specific targeted spirometry or radiographic program may be instituted solely for the purpose of respiratory surveillance. Many hazard surveillance systems are active in nature, specifically determining exposure factors for the purpose of surveillance.

Passive systems offer several advantages and disadvantages. A major advantage is cost—the incremental cost of data acquisition and analysis is small in comparison with establishing a de novo data collection system. Furthermore, such systems can avoid subjecting workers to duplicate testing if procedures such as spirometry or radiography are already being performed. In addition, passive surveillance methods can produce data relatively quickly when retrospective analysis is employed. Thus, if there is current concern that a particular material may be a respiratory carcinogen, retrospective analysis of death certificates can be effected more quickly than a prospective cohort study in which incident cases are delineated.

There are, however, significant disadvantages to passive methods. First, they are only rarely of direct benefit to the involved individuals, whereas an active health or exposure surveillance program will frequently provide information of direct benefit. Furthermore, the quality of data from passive programs may be suboptimal. Because they were not designed for surveillance purposes, the consistency of methodology (e.g., standardization of spirometry) may not be adequate to foster meaningful aggregate interpretation. In addition, necessary passive data sources may not exist. Worker or community populations may not have had the opportunity to have testing performed.

Ethical concerns are also occasionally present; individuals may give consent to their physicians to acquire data for personal benefit, but such permission may not extend to outside agencies that desire to incorporate this information. This is a particular problem when an individual might be personally identified as an index case.

Passive data sources are subject to many potential biases. For example, individuals at greatest risk may have inadequate access to routine health care and therefore not have data available. The opposite bias may occur, such that the a priori belief that a particular material is hazardous may lead to a positive diagnostic bias. For example, pathologists may be more likely to diagnose malignant mesothelioma if they are in an area where asbestos exposure is a well-known problem. Systematic biases may also be introduced by the methodology by which the data were acquired. It is well known that worker's compensation evaluations are not always free from bias. Claim incidence rates would therefore be higher than in a reference population even in the absence of a significant respiratory effect. Contravening effects may be seen in employer-provided health data, wherein there may be a subtle tendency to underreport respiratory effects as work related unless they are well documented.

Active surveillance programs can therefore overcome many of these limitations. They are specifically designed for the purpose of respiratory surveillance, and they therefore may try to avoid the biases. The at-risk population may be defined carefully and particular efforts instituted to ensure adequate participation. Where spirometry or chest radiography are employed, careful standardization of techniques (see Chapters 4 and 7) must be instituted. Data collection forms must be designed and pilot tested carefully. Active surveillance systems may also directly link exposure to health outcome data.

Active surveillance may be designed in a cost-effective manner. Wasted data can be minimized, whereas in passive programs, many of the data collected may not be useful. Wasted data occur in two fashions. First, test quality may be so poor or undocumented for many individuals that the test results cannot be employed. Second, unnecessary information may be routinely acquired. Thus, if surveillance is designed to detect airway effects, spirometry alone should be employed without collecting numerous irrelevant data such as radiographic findings.

Active respiratory health surveillance is generally more narrowly focused than passive systems. This comprises both benefits and limitations. The benefits include higher data quality, and, in some instances, more cost effectiveness because the program is designed for a specific class of respiratory effects. This requires very clear a priori hypotheses about exposure–effect relationships. Hence, active surveillance is generally not useful for hypothesis generation, looking for heretofore unsuspected associations or opportunities for prevention. Furthermore, since the size of data sets for passive surveillance systems is often considerably larger, there is greater likelihood of detecting statistical associations or by chance finding a "sentinel case," pointing to a new prevention strategy.

Relationship of population studied to population benefiting from surveillance. There is no a priori reason that the subjects, worksites, or communities that serve as data sources must be those that will benefit. In some situations (such as classic disease screening programs), the benefit focuses solely on those who participate; in many surveillance systems, however, information collected is much more generalizable. The detection of adverse respiratory health effects in a small sample of exposed persons may have direct implications for a much wider population. Similarly, the determination that a new work process leads to hazardous levels of exposures may have implications that will benefit more than the particular sites studied. For example, a study of a small member of dental laboratories showed that a new alloy[1] led to beryllium exposure; this benefited the entire dental industry, not just the small number of locations tested.

From a statistical study design standpoint, the marginal benefit of increasing sample size decreases as more subjects or sites are added. Thus, in many situations, resources can be most optimally employed to obtain high quality data from a relatively small subset of exposed individuals. Nevertheless, exposed workers or community members often do not wish to be excluded from testing solely on the basis of statistical power calculations. Surveillance program designers must carefully determine whether the program is fundamentally a research project or a survey of exposed individuals. Often, there is a tradeoff between political expediency and scientific rigor in designing surveillance programs that are seeking new generalizable data. Figure 51-1 shows the results of statistical power calculations as a function of sample size. The figure illustrates that the shape of the curve relating probability of detecting a significant effect (vertical axis) in relation to sample size (horizontal axis) becomes quite flat as the sample size increases. This implies that the marginal benefits of adding additional subjects become quite low.

What surveillance is not. Although there are many overlaps between surveillance and other occupational and environmental endeavors, they should not be considered synonymous. A research project is not a surveillance activity unless it will lead to prevention. Similarly, clinical evaluations of individual workers on an ad hoc basis are not surveillance; however, a systematic program to collect and analyze results of such evaluations may be useful for surveillance purposes.

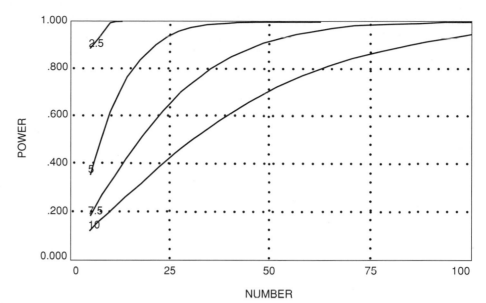

Fig. 51-1. Statistical power. The graph shows statistical power (probability of finding a true difference of 5% predicted between two groups) as a function of the number in each group tested. The graphs are shown for four different standard deviations (2.5% to 10% predicted). Graph was generated based on *t* test with $p = 0.05$, using Solo Statistical System power analysis (BMDP Statistical Software Inc., Los Angeles, CA).

BIOLOGIC MONITORING FOR EXPOSURE

Surveillance programs may occasionally utilize biologic samples derived from exposed persons as indicators of exposure. Such methods are termed "biologic monitoring." They fall into three classes[2]:

1. Biologic monitoring for exposure: The goal is to use the human subject as "a transducer" to reflect the workplace or environmental exposures.
2. Biologic monitoring for effect: The human subject's physiologic response can serve as an early indicator that an environmental agent is producing effects.
3. Biologic monitoring for susceptibility: The biologic test serves to identify individuals who have increased risk of an adverse health outcome from the exposure.

Measurement of lead concentration in workplace air may not adequately describe the exposure of workers because it does not reflect ingestion of lead from surface contamination. A biologic analyte, such as the blood or urine lead concentration, however, is sensitive to the integrated dose from *all* routes of exposure. The use of such forms of biologic monitoring has been more limited for the respiratory system than for many other target organs. Because of the primary importance of inhalation as the exposure route for respiratory effects, measurement of air levels is often more adequate for pulmonary problems than for those of other organ systems.

Nevertheless, there are applications of biologic-based exposure measures in respiratory surveillance programs. For example, exposure to beryllium can lead to chronic beryllium disease (CBD) (see Chapter 29). Beryllium may be measured in the urine, and this can serve as a reflection of exposure. Significantly elevated levels in an individual might indicate that he or she is at increased risk of developing CBD. Similarly, if the average level of urine beryllium concentration in a *group* of workers is more elevated than in a reference group, one may surmise that exposure is occurring.

The counting of asbestos fibers and ferruginous bodies in sputum has also been used as indirect surrogate measures of exposure[3]; bronchoalveolar lavage is much more accurate but not feasible on a population basis.[4] However, in this instance, air levels are much more likely to reflect current exposures.

A potentially useful form of biologic monitoring for respiratory hazards is the measurement of plutonium in exposed workers.[5] Because of its long half-life and the high sensitivity of measurement systems, this may be very useful as a surveillance measure of exposure (albeit applicable to a very small population of workers).

In the future, measurement of exposure by biologic surveillance methods may increase. Determination of deoxyribonucleic acid (DNA)- adducts (chemical agents bound to DNA) and hemoglobin adducts may be useful as indicators of exposure to respiratory carcinogens.[6] Furthermore, novel imaging techniques may allow determination of materials within the lung. Magnetopneumography has had limited application in reflecting the content of ferromagnetic materials in the lung. This technique is performed noninvasively, placing the subject in a varying magnetic field. This method has been applied to assessment of the *exposure* to several mineral dusts.[7,8] It has considerable future potential.

Finally, there has been extensive application of biologic monitoring based on autopsy material of coal miners. Extensive programs have been implemented in the United States to acquire the lungs of deceased miners in a consistent fashion.[9] Tissue analysis (see Chapters 8 and 12) very effectively describes trends in exposures. In addition, pathologic examination has been shown to be a highly sensitive method for detecting silicosis.[10]

In actuality, there is considerable semantic overlap among the three biologic measures (susceptibility, effect, exposure). For example, should a serologic survey of the presence of antibodies to coccidioidomycosis be considered a measure of exposure, effect, or past disease? At what point does an effect become so severe as to be considered a disease? Despite these unclarities, it is strongly advisable to understand the purpose of the outcome measures before initiating a program. In this manner, participants will not be misled, and clear communication of results will be assisted.

SCREENING PROGRAMS

Screening is one particular form of surveillance activity with several unique characteristics. Screening is the application of testing procedures to members of an at-risk population group to detect disease in *individuals* at an early stage. In the United States, much of the activity described by OSHA as "medical surveillance" is actually screening. Two criteria define "early." First, the screening test must detect the disease earlier in its course than the time at which symptoms would naturally bring the individual to medical attention. For example, due to the progressive nature of lung cancer, essentially all patients will ultimately be seen by physicians even in the absence of a screening program. Second, the case must be detected sufficiently early that treatment is more beneficial than if it had not been instituted until symptoms led to medical care.

Thus, determining the value of a screening program depends upon both the quality of treatment as well as the efficacy of the diagnostic maneuvers.[11] Changes in available therapy may make a formerly useless screening program worthwhile.

Figure 51-2 shows a conceptual model of the natural course of a disease. In screening theory, the disease progresses in an ordered, sequential fashion rather than on a sudden basis. Screening theory of this sort is particularly useful for understanding malignancy. The box illustrates the stages of a bronchogenic carcinoma (lung cancer).

Thus, the disease progresses through a series of discrete stages. This theory implies monotonic progression in a relentless, one-way manner. However, even this simple model notes that in some instances, the tumor will become symptomatic yet still curable (e.g., a squamous cell carcinoma producing early hemoptysis), whereas in other cases, it progresses directly to being incurable before becoming symptomatic.

The early-detectable stage exists only if there is a test that can find cases in the presymptomatic stage. Efficacy of a screening test depends upon the length of the early-detectable stage relative to the natural history of the disease. Thus, if there is only a very brief sojourn in this stage, it is unlikely that the prevalence will be high in this stage if a population is screened on a periodic basis. Short sojourn times occur either because the disease rapidly changes its characteristics, becoming metastatic early in its course as in small cell lung carcinoma, or because the screening test can detect only relatively large tumors. Under such circumstances, screening is unlikely to be effective.

If treatment is uniformly useful even when the patient seeks care due to advanced symptoms, then screening is also not needed. Theoretically, as treatment for an illness becomes more efficacious, screening might become less useful.

Often, screening is a *two-stage process*. A relatively simple test (e.g., chest radiography, sputum cytology examination) is applied to a large number of individuals. A first stage screening test should be highly sensitive (likely to detect as "positive" those who truly have the disease), but it often need not be exceedingly specific (likely to be negative if the disease is truly absent). Then, a second stage test

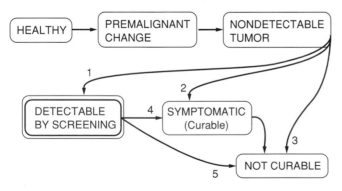

Fig. 51-2. Screening model of disease progression. The conceptual model for cancer screening is shown. The proportion of cases that follow path 1 rather than paths 2 or 3 sets the theoretical maximum benefit of screening. The rates of paths 4 and 5 determine how long the case is in the "asymptomatic detectable" stage.

> ### Stages of lung cancer from screening theory perspective
>
> 1. Completely *healthy.*
> 2. *Premalignancy:* Early premalignant change, such as genetic damage, occurs.
> 3. *Nondetectable* malignancy is present but is so small that it is completely undetectable by any method.
> 4. *Detectable* by screening–presymptomatic: The tumor has now enlarged so that special screening methods, but not symptoms, will lead to its detection. It is still curable.
> 5A. *Symptomatic—curable:* The tumor is now sufficiently large that it produces symptoms that would bring the patient to medical attention. At this stage, the tumor is still curable.
> 5B. *Symptomatic—incurable:* The tumor is sufficiently large (or metastatic) and leads to symptoms; however, it is not curable.
> 6. Death.

is applied only to those who are detected as positive in the first stage. Such a second stage test need not be as easy to apply since it will be used in a relatively small number of individuals, but it should be specific, avoiding false positives. For example, although chest radiographic abnormalities are relatively common, fiber optic bronchoscopy with biopsy can be applied to delineate those who truly have lung cancer.

Another example of a two-stage screening test is the application of the cotton dust spirometry screening method recommended by OSHA (see Chapter 25). A highly sensitive criterion for detecting a cross-shift change in forced expiratory volume in 1 second (FEV1) is applied to cotton workers, looking for only a 5% drop in this value over the course of a work shift. Persons who are detected as positive, however, will then be subjected to more detailed, confirmatory testing. As a result, use of a highly sensitive but nonspecific first stage screening test will not lead to a high number of false-positive diagnoses.

The acceptable mix of characteristics between a first and second stage screening test must be determined for each individual situation. Not all individuals who are labeled as "positive" in a screening program will actually benefit. For example, even if a second stage specific test is found to be negative, the individual may have had considerable anxiety. One can imagine the feelings of a patient in the period between being told that an x-ray examination was "positive" and receiving the final report of a lung biopsy.

Only some individuals who receive treatment, even for early disease, will be cured or have prolonged remissions. For example, even with the best available therapy, the prognosis for stage 2 lung carcinoma is generally poor, and the prognosis for malignant mesothelioma is worse. The treatment itself can often produce adverse effects or even death. A thoracotomy with resection has a significant associated mortality, and, therefore, an individual with a small detectable-asymptomatic lung cancer may actually have his life shortened. Diagnostic testing itself (e.g., bronchoscopy) also may be associated with morbidity or mortality.

On the average, however, the screening test must be beneficial to the *individuals* screened. Thus, although some screened persons with false positives may actually suffer, the *average* individual must benefit. To determine the average effect, one must consider the utility (cost or "benefit") of a false positive and of a true positive result. One must also factor in the actual prevalence of the disease in the screened population. A one in one thousand adverse effect rate for false positives would be totally unacceptable in a population in which the disease incidence is very low, but it would be reasonable in populations with 1:100 cancer risks.

The importance of the net benefit to the *individual* also distinguishes screening from other forms of surveillance. In screening, the person screened must expect a useful outcome. Thus, screening cannot be justified solely if it will provide information that can be generalized to protect other populations of workers or even members of the same population.

Another adverse effect of participation in a screening program is the potential for false "reassurance" in individuals with negative test results.[12] The presence of a screening program might also divert resources from primary prevention.

Screening programs must be *evaluated* carefully. Often, the decision of whether and how to institute a program is very context dependent. The "gold standard" for evaluating a screening method is a clinical trial. Large populations are generally necessary, and the population is randomly divided into individuals who receive the screening test and those who do not. In some clinical trials, several different screening tests may be utilized for different population groups.

Finally, some clinical trials have compared "usual care" versus "special care"; in such instances, the test is not withheld from the controls; rather, it simply is not offered in an organized manner. Because participation in a large organized trial may be beneficial even if the test itself is not of value, the control population should be treated similarly to the screened group. For example, educational programs emphasizing stopping smoking are often associated with screening trials for cancer. Even if the test procedure itself is not beneficial, screened persons would appear to achieve benefit.

Unfortunately, clinical trials are often extremely expensive and take a long time to complete. A very large multi-center clinical trial for evaluating the value of sputum cytology screening for lung cancer cost over 25 million dollars and lasted a decade.[13] The results, are generally interpreted as negative, but there is still disagreement among interpreters about the true meaning. Furthermore, because of the length of the study, changes in cytologic techniques and tumor localization methods had occurred, thereby indicating that the clinical trial used an "outmoded" technology. A very large ongoing clinical trial of screening smokers for airway hyperreactivity and lung function changes has required modification mid-course as the value of inhaled corticosteroid therapy gained acceptance.

For these reasons, program planners and clinicians must often rely on good judgment rather than formal clinical trials to guide screening programs. This is particularly true because local population and exposure factors may differ from those of clinical trials. For example, high technology, complex treatment methods may be unavailable or unaffordable for certain populations. Conversely, many clinical trials are conducted in populations at lower risk than that of selected occupational cohorts. The large National Cancer Institute clinical trial of sputum cytology cancer screening[13] was conducted among middle-aged smokers, a population at lower risk than shipyard workers who smoke. Such a group are at much higher risk and might have greater marginal benefit than the general population of smokers.

Several theoretical and practical considerations are necessary in interpreting screening trials.[12] Some of these are biases, whereas others represent unique characteristics of populations studied. Some of these factors relate to questions about the fundamental assumptions of the simple model. These considerations include the following:

1. Volunteer bias: Individuals who choose to participate in screening programs on a voluntary basis are often more health conscious than individuals who do not. Hence, they may have better mortality expectation than nonparticipants. Thus, even subjects randomized to the unscreened group would have a better than average prognosis.

2. Nonprogressive disease: The traditional screening model assumes that disease is progressive and that in time, every case will progress to a more advanced stage. However, it is possible that screening tests may find abnormalities that may be cytologically or histologically interpreted as malignant but that do not have a progressive nature. For example, carcinoma in situ is a relatively common finding in autopsies, and non-clinically significant adenocarcinomas may be seen in breast and prostate at autopsy. Similar considerations apply to the thyroid gland. As a result, if a screening test detects such nonprogressive tumors, those detected as positive would artifactually appear to have a good prognosis (i.e., they would not have come to medical attention otherwise and would have lived their lives without the effect of the malignancy). Assuming that the treatment in itself is not extremely harmful, this will lead to the false belief that screening is a benefit.

   Similar considerations apply even more strongly to many nonmalignant conditions. "Abnormality" does not necessarily imply that the treatment will be of benefit for an individual with a minor abnormality of FEV1. Such considerations are important when the screening test really measures exposure rather than disease.

3. Lead time bias: A screening test may detect a disease earlier in its course than would occur by strict reliance on clinical symptoms. Hence, even if treatment were of no benefit in prolonging life, there would be an apparent increase in survival time from diagnosis to death. For example, in conjunction with a research project, the author found a plumber with a malignant mesothelioma appearing as a very small pleural effusion. He lived for 2½ years. The only (questionable) benefit of having been detected early was that he knew that he had a terminal illness for 2½ years rather than only 6 months. The "lead time" is the time by which the diagnosis is accelerated.

4. Length biased sampling: Malignancies are heterogeneous in their growth rates. Some are likely to move rapidly from the present-nondetectable stage through the detectable-curable stage and on to the incurable stages; however, others progress through the stages much more slowly. If the population is subjected to screening tests on a regular interval (e.g., once a year), the testing procedure has a much greater likelihood of finding long sojourn time tumors rather than short (i.e., a tumor that remains in the detectable-curable stage for a year will almost inevitably be found by an annual screening, whereas, there is only 1 in 12 chance that a tumor with an average of 1 month in the detectable-curable sojourn will happen to be at that stage when the testing is performed).

   In general, tumors that rapidly progress through the stages are associated with worse prognoses than those that move slowly and have longer detectable-curable sojourn times. As a result, sampling over time is biased toward finding those with longer sojourn lengths and better prognoses (and hence the term, "length biased sampling").

5. "Will Rogers Effect": A final potential bias is related to the process of staging. Reportedly, Will Rogers stated that when the "Okies" moved from Oklahoma to California, they raised the average I.Q. of both states. A similar phenomenon may affect the staging of malignancies in carefully conducted clinical trials of screening. If there is more extensive and careful staging evaluation performed as part of a clinical trial than in usual practice, many individuals may be "upgraded" in stage. Thus, someone who by routine care would be considered to have a stage 1 tumor might have a lymph node detected in the mediastinum, making the tumor a stage 2 case. Removal of such an individual from the stage 1 group will improve the overall prognosis for that group. Similarly, including this person who is "minimally" into stage 2 in the stage 2 group would improve the overall average prognosis in that group. Thus, use of special staging techniques in association with the screening program may lead to the appearance of improved prognosis in each stage even in the absence of any true benefit.

6. Competing cause mortality: A screening program may be effective in decreasing mortality due to one particular respiratory disorder (e.g., lung cancer), but the net effect on the population may be obviated by an increase in other causes of death. (Eventually, everyone dies of something.) This effect may be particularly pronounced when the cause of the screened disease also causes other disorders. Cigarette smoking causes lung cancer, but it also causes coronary artery disease. Therefore, it is likely to increase the number of deaths due to emphysema and myocardial infarctions. As a result, analysis must focus on the net lives saved.

7. Quality of life as well as quantity of life must be considered in measuring the efficacy. Increasingly, adjustment for the quality of life is included in outcome determination. A screening and treatment program that markedly diminishes quality for minimal quantity of life benefit may not be worthwhile.

In summary, screening programs need to be carefully evaluated. Unfortunately, accurate and complete clinical trials are only rarely available as a guide to such programs. Even randomized clinical trials are subject to many biases as discussed above, and, therefore, the best measure of efficacy is the effect on overall population mortality. Such a measure, however, is difficult to acquire.

Screening for noncancer conditions

Although screening theory is most immediately applicable to malignant conditions, screening programs are also often of potential use for nonmalignant conditions as well. For example, in some situations, pulmonary morbidity or symptoms may be used as the endpoint for screening. When screening for nonmalignant disease, there are special considerations:

1. The definition of "abnormal or diseased" is often less clear than for malignancies. Thus, there is a gradual continuum from clearly normal to clearly abnormal when the diagnosis of concern is chronic obstructive pulmonary disease (COPD). The apparent sensitivity of a screening modality may differ depending upon the case definition.

2. Furthermore, the screening test itself may be related to the definition of the disease rather than representing an independent criterion. Thus, whereas the true presence or absence of bronchogenic carcinoma is defined independent of a chest radiograph, the presence of COPD is determined to a large extent based upon the screening test (spirometry) itself. Hence, the presence of concordance between the "screening test" and the disease is not itself an indicator of the value of the screening.

3. The definitions of normal may depend upon the purpose of the screening program.[14] Thus, while in a clinical practice, a rigid definition for separating normal from abnormal is used, in a screening context, there may be benefits to using a more flexible approach. For example, the OSHA cotton dust standard in the United States employs a criterion that is likely to lead to many "false positives." However, there is limited adverse implication of this since this is viewed only as a first stage screening, only committing the "positive" to more detailed, appropriate follow-through.

When using a lung function test as a screening modality, a cutoff must be used to determine those individuals who require additional attention (the "positives"). There is a tradeoff between sensitivity and specificity, such that a cutoff that is lax will include many individuals who require a follow-up but will also include many who do not.

PERIODICITY OF SCREENING

Generally, screening should be periodically repeated for persons at risk. Often, this is done on a regularly scheduled basis with the same interval applied to all possible subjects. However, in some situations, the frequency can be adjusted dependent on either the results of the initial screen or personal characteristics. For example, individuals with borderline results at the initial evaluation may be offered screening tests at more frequent intervals than those whose initial results were clearly negative. Personal characteristics can also stratify risk, and, hence, the optimal frequency of screening. For example, when screening for lung cancer, age and smoking status clearly affect the risk.

Periodicity is very dependent upon the natural course of the illness. When there is a long sojourn in the preclinical detectable phase, frequency of testing may be less often than if this phase is relatively brief.

APPLICATIONS OF SURVEILLANCE METHODS
Screening methods for lung cancer

As discussed earlier, many screening efforts have been directed at the early detection of lung cancer. This is an extremely common problem (see Chapter 18) with a poor prognosis. Furthermore, a large number of environmental agents are causally associated with lung cancer, thereby defining exposed high risk populations for targeted screening programs. In the United States, lung cancer screening is mandated for certain worker populations (e.g., coke oven workers).

Lung cancer is felt to develop in a sequential fashion. Nevertheless, there is still no proof that screening is of value for populations at risk of occupational and environmental lung cancer. Chest radiography and sputum cytology testing have been employed, and two additional measures have been suggested (tumor antigen screening and oncogene product screening). The latter two methods will be discussed subsequently.

Chest radiography is an effective means of finding bronchogenic carcinoma. Because of the high radiographic contrast between tumor density and the surrounding air density, neoplasms can be imaged more easily in the chest than in other body areas. The Philadelphia Neoplasm Project (PNP) was an early attempt to detect cancers early, utilizing regularly scheduled radiographic examinations.[15] Unfortunately, the radiographic technique employed small film size, and there was no evident benefit of chest radiography.

A more recent, extensive, and expensive trial of screening utilized sputum cytology methods.[13] In this trial, three clinical centers (Johns Hopkins, Mayo Clinic, and Memorial Sloan-Kettering) enrolled 10,000 subjects each in a trial using sputum cytology and chest radiography screening. The latter two centers randomized subjects into radiography alone versus dual screen testing (radiography plus cytology). The Mayo study compared dual screening to "usual care," which for some subjects may actually have included cytology and/or radiographic testing. Overall, it appeared that there was little evident benefit to the screening testing.[11,12]

Population mortality was not affected. Lung cancer mortality also was not significantly affected. For example, in the Hopkins study, the rate was 3.4 per 1,000 person-years versus 3.8 in the reference group. For Mayo, the lung cancer death rates are 3.2 in the screened group versus 3.0 per 1,000 person-years in the controls.[12]

The screening modalities did lead to diagnosis of malignancy. At Hopkins,[16] the initial screening yielded 39 cases among the 5,000 subjects who received dual testing. Eleven of the 39 were detectable only by cytology; 5 of these 11 were found to be at the in situ state. A large proportion of the cancers were surgically resectable (69% of the dual screened group and 42% of the x-ray only controls; these are well above the 18% resectability rate seen in the general population). The absence of survival benefit despite diagnosis earlier in the course of the disease illustrates lead time bias.

"False positive" tests were relatively common for radiography but not for cytology. Sloan-Kettering reported that 10% of subjects required further studies following radiographic examination, and Hopkins reported 18% had "suspicious" radiographs.[12]

However, there were some positive aspects of the trial. As might be expected, the screened population had a larger number of early stage neoplasms than the control population. If treatment becomes more efficacious, there may be benefit to detection at this stage.

Interpretation of this clinical trial is also limited by the control group selected. In two of the three centers, those screened with sputum cytology and radiography were compared to a population screened by radiography alone rather than to an unscreened population. In other words, the trial was really aimed at assessing the incremental value of sputum cytology. As the trial progressed, it became evident that a large number of peripheral early cancers (particularly adenocarcinoma) were being detected by radiography. Thus, even if sputum cytology were better than no screening at all, comparison with the radiography group might have led to underestimating its effectiveness.

It is also notable that these three screening trials were not focused in occupational cohorts. From 9% to 21% reported ever having had exposure to an occupational carcinogen.[13] In occupational cohorts the risk may have been greater. In addition to higher risk, lung cancer may occur at earlier ages in some occupationally exposed groups.

Screening efforts in occupational groups have been tried, but these limited efforts have not been demonstrated to be of benefit,[17,18] although cancers were detected.

Overall, the studies have led to the general recommendation that routine screening for lung cancer cannot currently be regularly justified in the general population.[19] The trials of particularly high risk occupational groups are not adequate to assess efficacy.

Based upon the hope that sputum cytology might be useful for at-risk exposed workers, OSHA mandated that coke oven workers have periodic sputum cytology testing. Because this is done on an ad hoc local basis, it is not possible to determine if there is efficacy.

FUTURE POSSIBILITIES FOR LUNG CANCER SCREENING

There are several promising avenues for screening for lung cancer. These include improving current methods, application of molecular biologic techniques, and preventive interventions based on screening.

Improved cytological techniques may allow earlier detection. Furthermore, the second stage testing procedures have markedly improved since the earlier multicenter National Cancer Institute (NCI) trial. Unfortunately, many individuals had positive cytology results, but the source of the tumor could not be localized. Improved bronchoscopic technique, including the use of protoporphyrin imaging and other fluorescent techniques, now can facilitate finding small areas of in situ or microinvasive malignancy.

A particularly promising method is the detection of tumor-associated surface antigens. Rather than relying on morphologic criteria alone for ascertainment of malignancy, such techniques may permit detection of much earlier tumors. Preliminary trials only, however, have been reported using immunoperoxide-labeled monoclonal antibody for tumor surface antigens that can be determined in sputum samples. Specimens obtained from the Hopkins studies were tested with antibody to small cell and non-small cell cancers. Sputum samples from subjects who subsequently developed malignancy were tested. Preliminary data suggest a sensitivity of 91% and specificity of 88%.[20] Qualitative interpretation has been complemented by quantitative partially automated interpretation,[21] increasing the potential for more widespread implementation. Other new methods rely upon the detection of DNA adducts.[22] Finding binding of the carcinogen to DNA suggests genetic damage and a greater likelihood of subsequent tumor. Testing for adducts may be particularly useful as indicators of the biologically effective dose (BED) and would therefore be useful for defining exposure-based risk cohorts. Relationships between quantity of cigarette smoking and DNA adducts have been found,[23] suggesting that this may be applicable to other inhaled carcinogens.

In theory, approaches based upon molecular biologic principles may also prove useful in the future. These methods rely upon detecting a change that occurs considerably earlier than the development of a morphologically visible tumor that might be detected by bronchoscopy or radiography, or from expectorated cells shed from its surface. Earlier events occur, involving changes in genetic regulation. Oncogenes control cell differentiation and may serve important roles during embryogenesis and growth. Normally, certain protooncogenes (e.g., *ras, myc*) are suppressed. Should they become activated or amplified, unrestricted cell growth can occur, ultimately producing a detectable and evident malignancy.

Molecular biologic-related methods may be feasible in the future that depend upon either recognition of the oncogene itself or a protein product that is produced as a consequence of its activation (i.e., an oncoprotein[24]).

A family of oncogenes known as *ras* has received particular attention.[25] This protooncogene can be activated by transferring viruses, point mutations in DNA, or larger scale DNA effects (e.g., translocations). Amplification of *ras* genes also occurs. Activation of *ras* is observed in a high proportion of pulmonary adenocarcinomas. A specific single codon mutation is detectable in many such lung tumors.

Activation of *ras* leads to expression of a group of proteins that is known as p21. These bind guanine nucleotides (e.g., guanosine diphosphate [GDP]), probably serving as a regulatory signal.[25]

Other groups of oncogenes (e.g., *myc, jun*) are associated with lung cancers. For example, L-*myc* is associated with small cell lung cancers. At present, there are multiple candidate oncogenes, growth factors, and proteins that might be used. One pilot study found that over 50% of the exposed population had at least one elevated level.[26]

Theoretically, oncogene activation could be subjected to screening tests focused at the gene itself (determining DNA), the messenger ribonucleic acid (mRNA), or the oncoprotein product. Measurement of the p21 protein in serum or urine provides a potentially useful method for occupationally exposed cohorts.[26]

Theoretically, a screening program that detects the oncogene or the products of oncogene derepression could lead to very early diagnosis. Even if the tumor could not be visualized and treated at that early stage, such individuals might be subjected to extremely careful periodic testing. Thus, although semiannual fluorescence bronchoscopy[27] could hardly be recommended on a regular basis for most individuals, it might prove justifiable in the future for a selected subset of extraordinarily high-risk persons with evidence of pulmonary oncogene activation.

The third avenue of potential benefit for screening persons at very high risk of environmental and occupational lung cancer is improvement in the interventions instituted if there is a "positive" test. The earlier cytology and radiographic screening programs relied upon "traditional" surgical resection as the primary treatment intervention. However, other responses to test results, particularly for tests relying on earlier stages of the oncogenic process, might make screening useful.

There are several trials of chemoprevention.[28] If they show benefits in humans, then screening for adducts or early evidence of genetic damage might select individuals for chemopreventive therapy. Retinoids are vitamin A derivatives that may be of benefit even after cells have dedifferentiated. Carotenoids may function by trapping free radicals and are better tolerated than retinoids. Other agents, such as ornithine decarboxylase (ODC) inhibitors, may also be of theoretical benefit.

Very intensive and invasive screening techniques might be justified in individuals with high levels of DNA adducts or elevated p21 levels. For example, periodic photofluorescent bronchoscopy and perhaps even laser photodynamic killing of in situ tumors might theoretically be employed.

In summary, all prior studies of lung cancer screening have not shown it to be of any benefit. There is *hope* that screening might decrease the risk of lung cancer death in environmentally exposed persons in the future for three reasons:

1. There have been improvements in cytologic and radiographic techniques.
2. Screening based on genetic effect ascertainment might find tumors at much earlier stages or at least define subcohorts of persons at extraordinarily high risk for intensive screening.
3. Interventions other than surgical resection may be applicable to cases detected *very* early.

The repeated failure of all prior screening efforts, however, warrants caution. Careful studies are needed before widespread implementation of any method, no matter how ostensibly attractive it is.

SPECIAL SURVEILLANCE TECHNIQUES

In many instances, methods that are utilized in routine, single patient oriented clinical situations are applicable to surveillance. Frequently, they must be modified to be optimally employed.

QUESTIONNAIRES

Questionnaires can play a vital role in surveillance. Respiratory health questionnaires have several potential uses. For example, the definition of chronic bronchitis, including industrial bronchitis, is based on symptoms of cough and sputum production. Therefore, standardized respiratory questionnaires provide the most effective means of determining the prevalence of such conditions and relating disease prevalence to exposures.

Questionnaires may also be effectively used for finding individual cases of occupational and environmental lung disease for early intervention purposes. For example, periodic administration of questionnaires to workers at risk of occupational asthma (see below) can detect those who have symptoms of wheezing or dyspnea that are temporally related to work. Such individuals may then be offered more detailed medical evaluations.

There are several standardized respiratory questionnaires available. In the United States, the American Thoracic Society Division of Lung Diseases (ATS)/(DLD) questionnaire is widely employed.[29] This questionnaire may be self-administered or administered by an interviewer, and it has been well standardized. There are several limitations, however, on its utility for occupational and environmental respiratory surveillance. It focuses on COPD and asthma. It therefore is not directly applicable to surveillance for respiratory problems related to releases of agents on an intermittent basis. Second, it assesses dyspnea, a critically important respiratory symptom, with a range of responses oriented to a level of symptoms greater than that typically found in an active work force. The dyspnea questions are shown in the box.

A third major limitation is that the ATS/DLD Questionnaire essentially ignores the occupational history. It does not collect adequate exposure information in any fashion.

The utilization of questionnaires in occupational and environmental disease surveillance requires special care to avoid external biases. Studies have compared self-administration versus interviewer administration, generally finding comparability.[30]

Breathlessness questions

Breathlessness

12. If disabled from walking by any condition other than heart or lung disease, please describe and proceed to Question 14A. Nature of condition(s):

_____

_____

13A. Are you troubled by shortness of breath when hurrying on the level or walking up a slight hill?
1. Yes _____ 2. No _____
If "YES" to 13A:
B. Do you have to walk slower than people of your age on the level because of breathlessness?
1. Yes _____ 2. No _____ 8. Does not apply
C. Do you ever have to stop for breath when walking at your own pace on the level?
1. Yes _____ 2. No _____ 8. Does not apply
D. Do you ever have to stop for breath after walking about 100 yards (or after a few minutes) on the level?
1. Yes _____ 2. No _____ 8. Does not apply
E. Are you too breathless to leave the house or breathless on dressing or undressing?
1. Yes _____ 2. No _____ 8. Does not apply

Derived from the Epidemiology Standardization Project.[29]

Questionnaires may also be employed to assess exposures. Individuals may be asked to provide an occupational history, including job title, industry, and employer. Alternatively, the questionnaire may be agent based, asking individuals about exposures to specified agents. Data suggest that subjects tend to underestimate exposures[31] and that more recent jobs are described more accurately than those in the past.[30] Nevertheless, standardized questionnaires provide a useful tool for determining exposures. An effort to develop an adequate occupationally oriented questionnaire has been initiated.[32] In addition to use in worker group surveillance, they are also potentially useful in surveillance for assessing exposures in more general population groups. Several studies have shown that potentially significant exposures are common in general populations (e.g., 31% reported occupational dust exposure in one study[33]), and 50% reported at least one exposure in another.[34] Even broad exposure categories such as "dust" and "fumes" have been related to respiratory health.[33,34] Of course, it is possible that the apparent relationships between broad categories and respiratory health may be confounded by education and income effects,[35] such that low education leads to poorer respiratory health.

HEALTH CARE SYSTEM-BASED SURVEILLANCE

Many persons with respiratory disease due to occupational or community-based environmental exposures enter the general health care system. Thus, clinic and hospital data are potential valuable sources of surveillance information. Approaches have ranged from using anecdotal information from poison control centers[36] to systematic studies based on hospital discharge data. With increased computerization of the records, information will facilitate this in the future.

Several factors currently limit the utility of these approaches. Misdiagnosis—both over- and underdiagnosis—are common problems. Only 6% of cases coded on discharge records as extrinsic allergic alveolitis were confirmed on detailed record review.[37] In addition, exposure data may be limited or inaccurate in routine hospital data sets. Comparisons of routine cancer registry data with interviews showed agreement in only 33% of cases.[38] Only 50% of hospital records had useful industry and occupation data in another study.[39]

Larger scale hospital discharge analyses have also been employed for surveillance. The National Hospital Discharge Survey (NHDS) is a large U.S. sample of discharge diagnoses. It is useful in showing trends and geographic distributions; but since NHDS is based on discharges, rather than persons, multiple admissions of the same person could lead to overestimation.[40] Another database is based on Medicare patients only (MEDPAR) and provides more accurate information,[40,41] but excludes many younger patients; it is therefore useful mainly for long latency diseases (e.g., cancer, silicosis).

RADIOLOGIC TECHNIQUES

Radiography is a primary component of respiratory surveillance for interstitial lung disease. It is useful for both case finding and for broad-based surveillance seeking relationships between exposures and health effects on an aggregate basis.

Standardization is important in surveillance. The ILO system for classifying chest radiographs for pneumoconiosis provides a standardized methodology. It has been discussed in detail in Chapter 7. For example, it assigns a numeric score to the profusion of radiographic opacities consistent with pneumoconiosis using a 12-point scale.

Findings at the very low end of the scale (e.g., 0/1, 1/1) are often equivocal, inconsistent, and nonspecific. For this reason, such results are often not useful for case finding (diagnosing disease in individual workers). Nevertheless, the low level profusion results may be extremely useful when considered on a group basis. A consistent finding of statistically significant excesses of subjects with 1/0 findings in an exposed versus a control population (particularly when adjusted for potential confounders) is a strong indication that further, detailed investigation may be warranted.

Standardization in interpretation is fostered by periodic retesting and recertification of readers; in the United States, "B-readers" (certified in the ILO system) must be recertified every 4 years. Regular exchange of films by mail and continual monitoring and feedback have been used in Canadian efforts.[42]

When used for surveillance purposes, including epidemiologic studies, an a priori plan for interpreting the radiographs is necessary. Generally, readers who are thoroughly familiar with the ILO system should interpret the radiographs. Often, the results for each radiograph are interpreted by several trained interpreters. A means for integrating these results should be established in advance. For example, the average score of the readers may be used. Alternatively, when there is a significant disagreement among interpreters (e.g., greater than two minor categories), films may be sent to two additional interpreters, and the overall average utilized. In some instances, "consensus readings" are employed, wherein the interpreters jointly review films for which scores differ significantly.

Individual radiograph interpreters may tend to read higher than or lower than the overall average. In some circumstances, an adjustment for the interpreter's tendency is incorporated into the analysis as a covariate. Other techniques may be used to foster consistency. Radiographs from an unexposed population (i.e., a control group) may be included, although this increases the cost of such a program. In addition, this implies that routine radiographs will be obtained on individuals for whom there is not a clear indication for such testing and (low dose) radiation exposure. Known positive radiographs and known negatives may be included as positive and negative controls for the radiographic interpreter. Internal consistency in interpretation is important, and, therefore, the same radiograph may be included several times to measure the interpreter's consistency. To detect if a secular drift in interpretation (over time) has occurred, a series of reference radiographs may be included intermittently to determine if there is a systematic trend over time.

Often, surveillance programs include obtaining radiographs on the same subjects over time (for example annually). Whether for individual or aggregate analysis, it is often useful to directly consider the change in profusion score in addition to the absolute score. Thus, while the score "1/0" might be considered equivocal, it is less equivocal if it is known that prior radiographs for this individual were interpreted as completely negative. To accomplish such evaluations for trends, several techniques may be used. The current films may be interpreted routinely, and the numeric scores compared. Alternatively, the interpreter may perform side by side interpretation, seeing the prior film and the current film. There is some debate about whether the interpreter should be told which film is older.[43]

A number of other radiographic techniques have been suggested for application to diagnosis and perhaps to surveillance of occupational lung disease. Such methods have included gallium scanning, computerized radiographic interpretation, radiographic estimation of lung volume, computerized tomography (CT) scanning, and high-resolution CT (HRCT) scanning. Several, particularly HRCT scanning, show promise but have not yet been demonstrated to be efficacious on a surveillance basis.[44] These techniques are discussed further in Chapter 7.

Pulmonary function testing

Similar concerns apply to the utilization of lung function testing, particularly spirometry.[45] Standardized testing is critically important when early changes are sought and when changes between groups or statistical associations between level of exposure and results are sought.

Standardization of efforts must be focused on both equipment and personnel. As discussed in Chapter 4, proper equipment must be purchased, and regular maintenance and calibration are essential.[46] Both volume and flow-based spirometers can be effectively used for these purposes. Personnel training is also requisite. In the United States, the National Institute for Occupational Safety and Health (NIOSH) certifies courses that may be attended by spirometrists. Periodic retraining and recertification may also be useful.[47] Quality control criteria for lung function tests other than spirometry are less well established, although there are guidelines available. Quality control efforts for multisite surveillance programs utilizing nonspirometric testing such as determination of the diffusing capacity of the lung for carbon monoxide are difficult. Unlike spirometry, there is no simple hard copy tracing that can facilitate external review of methodology.

Surveillance of asbestos-exposed subjects. The widespread use of asbestos has created a large number of persons who have had exposure. The health effects of asbestos are described in Chapter 20. This section will discuss implications for surveillance, illustrating several program design considerations.

Targeted health disorders. Surveillance for asbestos-related disease may serve two fundamentally different purposes; the first is to identify populations and/or worksites at risk and the second is to detect disease in specific individuals (either for screening/prevention or possibly for compensation).

For the former purpose—identifying populations at risk—surveillance for mesothelioma is useful because of the relative specificity of this disorder. Hence, if mesotheliomas are detected in a worker or in a community population, it is quite likely that there has been significant asbestos exposure in the past. Thereafter, source exposures could be controlled, or the individuals might be offered screening (if effective).

However, screening for asbestos-related disease with the goal of earlier intervention for prevention purposes in an individual should be based on disorders other than mesothelioma (for which there is little or no effective treatment). Bronchogenic carcinoma and asbestosis may be useful targets for screening. Unfortunately, as discussed elsewhere in this chapter, it is still moot whether screening for lung cancer actually is beneficial at the current time. Asbestosis screening might prove useful if treatment could be instituted to control symptoms or if knowing that an individual has asbestosis would change treatment for other causes of pulmonary fibrosis (i.e., affect the differential diagnosis). In addition, increasing data[48,49] suggest that the risk of lung cancer is focused largely in individuals with asbestosis; hence, asbestosis screening might define any extremely high-risk subgroup. Such identified individuals might be subjected to very intensive antismoking efforts, periodic intensive screening for lung cancer, and possibly chemoprevention (e.g., with oral retinoids if they prove effective).

Other disorders such as laryngeal or gastrointestinal cancer have been suggested as having increased risk in asbestos exposed individuals. If this is proven, then a strong case could be made for intensive screening for these disorders, for which treatment is particularly effective in the early stages.

Targeting of surveillance groups. Surveillance efforts, particularly screening, should be focused in individuals at significantly elevated risk and provided at the most useful time in the person's life. Therefore, since many of the asbestos-related disorders (e.g., lung cancer, asbestosis) have relatively long latencies, screening efforts are best conducted well after exposure has begun (and often long after exposure has ceased). Hence, for many individuals, the best time to screen is twenty or more years after exposure has started (often after the individual has retired). Despite this

logic, many governmental screening programs (such as OSHA) focus on current workers and largely ignore retirees, the group at highest risk.

In addition, the intensity of screening efforts should be related to the risk of the individual. Two factors affect the risk: the dose of asbestos is a major factor, there being clear dose–effect relationships for asbestos-related diseases. In addition, personal characteristics affect risk. Cigarette smokers are at much higher risk of asbestos-related lung cancers than are nonsmokers with comparable doses or latencies. Persons with early asbestosis are much more likely to progress to physiologically significant asbestosis than individuals with similar exposures but no evident effect; this is particularly true if the signs of fibrosis developed relatively quickly.[50] Furthermore, persons with fibrosis are much more likely to develop lung cancer than comparably exposed individuals without fibrosis.

Thus, these characteristics can determine the optimal target population and the adjustment of screening intensity based upon personal and dose factors.

Optimal screening modalities. Numerous test procedures are available to detect asbestos-related disease (see Chapter 20). They differ considerably in their general availability, cost, and risk.

Radiographic screening methods can be well standardized utilizing the ILO system (see Chapter 7), are widely available, relatively cheap, and noninvasive. They are sensitive for asbestos-related lung fibrosis. Similarly, diffusing capacity for carbon monoxide has been shown to be a sensitive (but not necessarily specific) test for early asbestosis. Spirometry has also been shown to be effective, and spirometry is more generally available and applicable in worksites. However, automated diffusing capacity determination systems are increasingly available. Thus, from the physiologic standpoint, although regulation and common practice have largely emphasized determination of the force vital capacity by spirometry, a role for diffusing capacity testing may be evolving.

Other test procedures, notably HRCT scans are highly sensitive for asbestos-related disease of the interstitium and of the pleura. Such tests are, however, still relatively expensive, and they are not standardized. In addition, the implications of an "abnormal" HRCT are not clear; one study found that almost two thirds of a worker group (which was probably not a representative group) had abnormal or possibly abnormal HRCT scans. The implications of this are unclear for the individual worker or for preventive benefit.

There are numerous diagnostic tests that are used to establish the diagnosis of asbestosis, to assess the degree of inflammation in the lung, or to carefully characterize the physiologic status. Many of these are discussed in Chapter 20. These tests are quite useful in carefully selected individual cases but do not in themselves have an essential role in surveillance according to many workers.

Exposure-based surveillance. There is a particular need for exposure-, rather than health- effect-, based surveillance. Asbestos is still in place in many buildings. Even if it is not currently friable or leading to significant exposures, currently there is a possibility of producing fiber aerosol if the building is subjected to reconstruction. Therefore, identifying vocations where asbestos is in place can lead to specific precautions (such as enclosure and ventilation) when construction or other activities with potential for creating airborne asbestos are conducted. This concept, which relies upon identifying physical locations with asbestos in place is discussed in more detail in Chapter 20, Part II.

Surveillance for occupational asthma. Surveillance plays a particularly important role in limiting the morbidity and mortality due to occupational asthma.[51,52] Unlike the situation for many environmentally related malignancies and most pneumoconioses, there is a very close temporal relationship between exposure and symptoms. It is thus often easier for workers to suspect an association.

In addition, the opportunities for prevention are often quite significant. Detection of lung cancers in a population group generally reflects exposures that have occurred decades ago. In many instances (e.g., for asbestos exposures), working conditions have changed markedly in the interim, and information gained from ascertaining current illness may not be useful in guiding controls for environmental conditions. This is not the case for occupational asthma. Because of the short latency and the close symptom-exposure relationships, detection of single cases or elevated rates will usually reflect recent exposure.

From the standpoint of the individual, participation in surveillance activities for occupational asthma is beneficial. Several studies have shown that early case detection can improve the long-term prognosis in the individual. A longer duration of symptoms prior to establishing the diagnosis or continued exposure after diagnosis adversely affects the prognosis. Interventions are available (e.g., process change, avoidance of specific inciting agents) to protect individuals who have been sensitized.

Due to the relatively low levels of exposures that can produce severe attacks in those who are sensitized, reliance upon governmental-mandated exposure levels would not be fully protective. Hence, surveillance to detect individual cases becomes important. Additionally, intermittent peaks of exposure appear to be important as factors in increasing the likelihood of development of sensitization, yet such peaks are much more difficult to detect by exposure assessment than are average exposures. Thus, routine industrial hygiene monitoring generally must be complemented by health-based surveillance where asthma hazards exist.

There are several methods applicable to surveillance for occupational asthma; they will be briefly reviewed here and are discussed in more detail in other chapters. *Symptom surveillance* depends upon the reporting of symptoms of shortness of breath with wheezing or allied symptom complexes

in exposed individuals. Recognizing such symptoms can then lead to more specific medical diagnostic and environmental assessment efforts. To foster symptom surveillance, exposed individuals must be trained that symptoms are important, and there must be a system in place for medical follow-up evaluation. Symptom-based surveillance is relatively simple and without extensive costs except for follow-up. Furthermore, because it relies upon the workers themselves, cases will not be missed in time gaps between application of periodic testing. Several studies have shown only limited correlation between symptoms and airway hyperresponsiveness.[53,54] However, since airway hyperresponsiveness does not in itself define asthma in the absence of symptoms, this may not be a major shortcoming. It suffers from nonspecificity and reliance upon worker reporting. While questionnaires relying on reports of physician-diagnosed asthma may be more specific than utilization of symptoms (e.g., wheeze), it is likely to be much less sensitive and subject to diagnostic bias.[55]

The use of *peak flow meters* in the workplace or in community settings has proved to be quite useful. Such devices are relatively cheap and are capable of moderately accurate measurement of peak expiratory flow rates. Their use must be coupled to a diary in which the individual logs exposures, symptoms, and recorded flow rates on a regular basis. In this manner, it is possible to delineate the interrelationships among exposures and respiratory function. It is particularly useful because workers themselves can perform the testing, and the lung function tests are performed at a time close to the inciting exposures. Practical considerations (worker compliance with proper testing, workplace access, etc.) may limit the applicability; one study found that only 14 of 70 possible cases could obtain useful data.[56] To be useful, a formal method of collecting and analyzing the results from the individuals is necessary.

Cross shift spirometry is also useful for case detection. FEV1 is measured before a work shift with exposure and following such a work shift. A significant pattern of change therefore indicates a possibility of work causal factor. To be useful, it is necessary that the exposure of interest actually occur on the day the spirometry testing is performed. Furthermore, this method presumes that affected individuals will have recovered from prior exposures before the beginning of a new work shift. However, if the baseline remains low because of the prior day's exposures, a decrement may not be found. For this reason, it is often preferable to perform this testing following a period of absence (for example, testing on Mondays).

Cross shift spirometry is the fundamental method of medical surveillance employed in the cotton industry according to OSHA regulation. A 5% decrement is considered sufficient to warrant more detailed monitoring and evaluation of the individual.

In addition to case detection for the benefit of the individual, cross shift spirometry may also be used for epidemiologic surveillance. A consistent pattern of cross shift change in FEV1 may indicate a strong possibility of exposure to an asthma inducing agent. However, caution is needed. If the agent affects only a small minority of workers (e.g., 5%), a significant change in the affected proportion may be missed because of the noise of measurement of the large number of unaffected individuals. Furthermore, natural tendencies of affected workers to leave such exposures may selectively bias the results toward negativity. Circadian rhythms must also be considered under such circumstances. Typically, average lung function is better in the afternoon than in the morning. Hence, a smaller decrement in lung function may be significant in a worker across a day shift than when assessed across a night shift.

Measurement of bronchial responsiveness (see Chapter 5) may also be useful in asthma surveillance. Airway hyperresponsiveness is found in most but not all cases of occupational asthma. Airway responsiveness can be measured with a variety of provocative agents, including methacholine, histamine, cold air, exercise, and hyperventilation. Methacholine inhalation is most commonly employed; an abbreviated version has been developed for research and surveillance use.[57] Means of summarizing results for epidemiologic purposes optimally should characterize the dose–response slope, rather than simply classifying each person as "positive" or "negative" based on responsiveness to a single arbitrary dose.[58]

The major limitation of these methods is logistic. They require considerable effort, and some subjects may consider inhalation of a drug unacceptable as part of a screening or surveillance test.

Other methods of asthma surveillance show promise. A case definition of occupational asthma suitable for surveillance, as opposed to definitive diagnosis in an individual patient, has been developed.[59] For certain agents, preliminary data suggest that rhinitis often precedes asthma. Hence, surveillance for asthma may be aided by surveillance for rhinitis. In addition, there has been extensive research effort expended in trying to develop *immunologic tests* (e.g., antibody assays, skin tests) that would be of use in asthma diagnosis and surveillance. Unfortunately, such efforts have not yet yielded uniformly useful methods. However, there are promising suggestions that for some agents, immunologic surveillance may have a role. For example, platinum-exposed workers with evidence of skin test reactivity show an increased likelihood of subsequently developing platinum asthma.[60] Blood tests (e.g., radioallergosorbent test [RAST]) may also have a role, although there is not uniform correlation of antibody assays with bronchoprovocation tests.[61]

Because of the close temporal association between exposure and symptoms, surveillance for occupational asthma in populations must consider those who have left the job. Only evaluating those who remain at work (the survivors) will lead to a considerable survivor bias, significantly underestimating the actual disease rates.

For evaluating *environmental asthma,* as opposed to occupational asthma, additional techniques may be useful for delineating links between exposure and asthma. In general, assessment of community (environmental) asthma is more difficult because the exposures are less well characterized, and the population is less clearly delineated. Nevertheless, environmentally affected asthma may be particularly important because of the large size of exposed populations and because community populations include many particularly susceptible persons. Environmentally affected asthma is a broad rubric, including asthma that is directly caused by environmental agents and asthma that is worsened either transiently or permanently by such agents.

Generally, epidemiologic methods (see Chapter 2) are used for these purposes. Exposure assessment is particularly challenging because of its diversity and geographic inhomogeneity. Often, community-based air monitoring stations are used, and extrapolation of results over time and between geographic monitoring sites becomes necessary. Several types of health outcome data may be utilized. Emergency room visits and hospital admissions for respiratory conditions (such as asthma) have proven particularly useful in the community setting.[62] Short-term correlations between exposure variation and such use of medical care have been demonstrated.

In addition to examining long-term relationships between variations and exposure (e.g., air pollutants) and use of medical services for respiratory conditions, single episodes of exposure have been demonstrated to be causally related to such health outcomes.

Cross-sectional population studies are also utilized to demonstrate relationships between community levels of air pollution and indices of lung function. Particular care is needed in interpreting such studies because lung function is also affected by socioeconomic factors, smoking, and the type of cooking performed in residences. Increasingly, community air pollution surveillance and epidemiologic studies are ascertaining such factors as well.

Exposure unique to specific geographic areas also affects the community dwellers, (e.g., exposures from effects of industrial operations such as the release of soybean dust from ship loading operations in Spain).[63] Under such circumstances, the unique aspects of the exposure can affect risk and severity of illness.

OLFACTORY EFFECTS

Surveillance programs, particularly in community settings, are also subject to measures of olfactory effect. For example, residents near waste disposal sites may have intermittent olfactory exposures. These lead to reporting to a variety of symptoms, including many respiratory symptoms. Epidemiologic surveys and analyses of community residents near such sites have shown an increase in the frequency of respiratory symptoms. It has been suggested that such symptoms may be related to the olfactory load itself rather than to directly toxic materials for which the olfactory sensation is simply a marker.[64,65]

RESPIRATORY INFECTION SURVEILLANCE PROGRAMS

Respiratory infection surveillance is facilitated by immunologic indicators of exposure and infection. Tuberculosis is an increasingly important problem in many communities and occupational settings. The use of purified protein derivative (PPD) skin testing is useful on both an individual and group basis. For exposed individuals, monitoring skin test reactivity to PPD provides an extremely useful indicator of early infection. There is definitive evidence that treatment of individuals who have converted from negative to positive skin test status is of net benefit to them. Such skin testing is easily accomplished.

Monitoring of the prevalence of positive skin tests and the frequency of conversions of populations (whether it is defined by occupational or other criteria) provides a major public health tool for assessing the need for preventive interventions. For hospital workers, a rise of PPD positive rates in one setting must sound an alarm that tuberculosis (TB) exposure controls are failing (see Chapter 44).

Other immunologic techniques, particularly serologic, may also be of considerable benefit for other infections. Monitoring antibody status in individuals with potential exposure to respiratory pathogens, particularly if they are unique to the workplace, may be quite effective. For example, antibodies to Q fever *(Coxiella burnetti)* can indicate uncontrolled exposures even in individuals who are asymptomatic themselves.

SURVEILLANCE SYSTEMS

Surveillance is useful only if it can lead to prevention and only if it is used in a systematic, planned fashion. This section will briefly describe several large-scale systems in which the surveillance tools may be implemented.

In the United States, the SENSOR program (Sentinel Event Notification System for Occupational Risks) is a national program for occupational disease surveillance based on state and county health departments. Such departments develop relationships with health care providers to determine the trends in occupational disease. The case definition utilized is often less specific[59] than that typically employed in clinical settings in order to increase the sensitivity of the surveillance methodology. Several of the local SENSOR programs have initiated efforts in the area of occupational asthma surveillance.[59,66]

The Surveillance of Work-Related Occupational Respiratory Disease (SWORD) program in the United Kingdom employs a different approach.[67] Pulmonary physicians are largely employed in governmental geographic based programs. A formal program exists in which such clinicians

provide case reports of possible occupational respiratory disease to a central coordinating unit, which then collates the information. To maintain the support of the participants, the central unit provides feedback, including newsletters and case specific information, to participants. An initial evaluation of reported cases showed that 222 of the 282 reports did qualify for work-related disability benefits when assessed carefully.[68]

Mandatory case reporting is employed with variable success. For diseases such as tuberculosis, mandatory reporting of cases to health departments is traditional and often effective. However, although several states legally mandate reporting of other occupational respiratory diseases, the illnesses are rarely reported.

Worker's compensation data are often available but are difficult to utilize because of the nonspecificity of many diagnoses. Furthermore, it is likely that many cases of occupational respiratory disease do not enter the worker's compensation system and would therefore be underreported.

Assessment of occupational and environmental respiratory disease also may be facilitated by standardized analysis of death certificate data. Such methods have been utilized in the United States, which now has a national death index, to gain insight into the frequency of certain occupational diseases. Such methods, however, are subject to diagnostic basis and are of use only in diseases that are fatal.

Sentinel physicians, who practice in community settings, have played pivotal roles in other surveillance systems. A small number of community-based physicians whose practices are typical of the geographic area they serve can show early trends in occupational and environmental respiratory disease. Thus, the frequency of certain respiratory disorders in their practices can be viewed as a sample to reflect the frequency in the larger population. Under such circumstances, the sentinel physician may provide data about the rates of nonspecific respiratory disease (which can have either environmental or nonenvironmental causes) and can also detect disorders relatable to specific exposure agents (e.g., asbestos, isocyanates). In addition, physicians in communities with relatively frequent exposures of a particular type may be recruited to offer preventive services in conjunction with surveillance data collection.[69]

Health care providers in community settings may also play pivotal roles in respiratory communicable disease surveillance. Routine culture of patients seen can reflect the trends of such agents in the general population. Changes in the pattern in influenza virus antigen types can presage major epidemics.

To be most useful for either communicable or noncommunicable respiratory disease surveillance, the sentinel health care provider must be representative of the general community. Furthermore, where establishment of a specific diagnosis and suspicion of occupational or environmental causation is necessary, these physicians must have adequate knowledge and experience to make such links in a mean-

---

Additional large scale data sources (U.S.)

National hospital discharge survey

Discharge diagnoses of a large sample of short stay hospitals.

Multiple cause of death data

Codes all conditions listed on death certificates. Exposure information is limited.

Annual reports of occupational injuries and illnesses—Bureau of Labor Statistics

Based upon large annual mail survey of employers. Misses long latency diseases.

Supplemental data systems (SDS)

Based on workers compensation reports from participating states.

Medicare provider analysis and review file

Summarizes hospital stays of Medicare beneficiaries.

Social Security Administration disability awards

Based on awards to persons less than age 65 years.

National occupational exposure survey

1981 to 1983 survey of a large sample of workplaces. Limited by its age and lack of quantitative data.

---

ingful manner. Thus, university-based clinics are rarely representative of general populations.

Specialized large-scale surveillance programs have been developed for particular settings. An individual employer can develop morbidity or mortality surveillance for its employees.[70] In the United States, coal miners participate in several surveillance programs; the National Coal Workers Autopsy Study has performed 5,500 autopsies, representing 10% of miner deaths for the covered period.[9] Although unlikely to be completely representative, it shows trends in disease and dust content. The Coal Workers X-Ray Surveillance program[71] is a systematic effort to obtain periodic radiographs on miners, and it has performed over a quarter million radiographs. It is linked to a specific preventive intervention—miners with positive results may elect transfer to less dusty locations. Despite this legal right, very few actually chose to exercise this option (only 2,026 of 10,467 eligible miners chose this).[71] This illustrates that data collection alone does not automatically constitute an effective surveillance program.

Several additional data sources, reflecting large numbers of subjects, are summarized in the box.[40,41] They provide large volumes of data, but many lack specificity, and not all are truly representative.

There are two very large population (rather than occupation) health surveys in the United States. The National

Health and Nutrition Examination Survey (NHANES) includes both interview and examination data,[72] whereas the National Health Interview Survey (NHIS) is based upon interview data.[73] Community-based surveillance on a smaller scale is applicable to investigation of potential case clusters in the community.[74]

There are many potential data sources for large-scale surveillance. However, there is a tradeoff between sample size and data quality (accuracy, representation) in many instances.

CONCLUSION

In summary, surveillance for occupational and environmental respiratory disease is an essential function. In many instances, it may be a benefit to the individual worker or community member who participates (in screening programs). In other situations, however, the surveillance program is designed to be of more general benefit.

Surveillance may either be based on health or on exposure. Optimally, both aspects of surveillance are linked together.

The ability to act upon the results of data that are collected and analyzed for prevention is a requirement. Careful planning and regular, standardized effort are essential components of successful surveillance programs.

REFERENCES

1. Rom WN, Lockey JE, Lee JS, Kimball AC, Bang KM, Leaman H, et al: Pneumoconiosis and exposures of dental laboratory technicians. *Am J Public Health* 74(11):1252-1257, 1984.
2. Committee on Biological Markers of the National Research Council: Biological markers in environmental health research. *Environ Health Perspect* 74:3-9, 1987.
3. McDonald JC, Sebastien P, Case B, McDonald AD, and Dufresne A: Ferruginous body counts in sputum as an index of past exposure to mineral fibres, *Ann Occup Hygiene* 36(3):271-282, 1992.
4. Dodson RF, Garcia JGN, O'Sullivan M, Corn C, Levin JL, Griffith DE, et al: The usefulness of bronchoalveolar lavage in identifying past occupational exposure to asbestos: a light and electron microscopy study, *Am J Ind Med* 19(5):619-628, 1991.
5. Voelz GL and Lawrence JNP: A 42-yr medical follow-up of Manhattan Project plutonium workers, *Health Phys* 61(2):181-190, 1991.
6. Perea FP, Santella RM, Brenner D, et al: DNA adducts, protein adducts, and sister chromatid exchange in cigarette smokers and non-smokers, *J Natl Cancer Inst* 79:449-456, 1987.
7. Le Gros V, Lemaigre D, Suon C, Pozzi JP, and Liot F: Magnetopneumography: a general review, *Eur Respir J* 2(2):149-159, 1989.
8. Weng X, Yao J, Wang Y, Hu T, Yu Z, Lu Z, et al: A study of magnetic field in the lung of workers in an asbestos factory, *Ind Health* 27(1):9-15, 1989.
9. Cassidy EP: The National Coal Workers' Autopsy Study. The development and implementation of an occupational necropsy study, *Arch Pathol* 94:133-136, 1972.
10. Hnizdo E, Murray J, Sluis-Cremer GK, and Thomas RG: Correlation between radiological and pathological diagnosis of silicosis: an autopsy population based study, *Am J Ind Med* 24:427-445, 1993.
11. Marfin AA and Schenker M: Screening for lung cancer: effective tests awaiting effective treatment, *Occup Med: State Art Rev* 6(1):111-131, 1991.
12. Eddy DM: Screening for lung cancer, *Ann Intern Med* 111:232-237, 1989.

13. Bailar JC: Screening for lung cancer—where are we now? *Am Rev Respir Dis* 130:542-543, 1984.

14. Harber P and Rappaport S: Clinical decision analysis in occupational medicine, *J Occup Med* 27(9):651-658, 1985.

15. Boucot KR, Seidman H, and Weiss W: The Philadelphia Pulmonary Neoplasm Research Project. The risk of lung cancer in relation to symptoms and roentgenographic abnormalities, *Environ Res* 13(3):451-469, 1977.

16. Frost JK, Ball WC, Levin JL, Tockman MS, Bake RR, and Carter D: Early lung cancer detection: results of the initial (prevalence) radiologic and cytologic screening in the Johns Hopkins Study, *Am Rev Respir Dis* 1308:549-554, 1984.

17. Lemen RA, Johnson WM, Wagoner JK, Archer VE, and Saccomanno G: Cytologic observations and cancer incidence following exposure to BCME, *Ann NY Acad Sci* 271:71-80, 1976.

18. Figueroa WG, Raszkowski R, and Weiss W: Lung cancer in chloromethyl methyl ether workers, *N Engl J Med* 288(21):1096-1097, 1973.

19. American Cancer Society: Guidelines for the cancer related checkup, *CA* 30:199-207, 1980.

20. Tockman MS, Gupta PK, Myers JD, et al: Sensitive and specific monoclonal antibody recognition of human lung cancer antigen on preserved sputum cells: a new approach to early lung cancer detection, *J Clin Oncol* 6:1685-1693, 1988.

21. Tuckman M, Pressman N, Gill G, Piantadosi S, Gupta P, and Mulshine J: Quantification of molecular markers for pre-neo plastic lung cancer, *Am Rev Respir Dis* 143 Suppl:A203, 1991.

22. Santella RM: Application of new techniques for the detection of carcinogen adducts to human population monitoring, *Mutat Res* 505:271-282, 1988.

23. Phillips DH, Hewer A, Martin CN, Garner RC, and King MM: Correlation of DNA adduct levels in human lung with cigarette smoking, *Nature (London)* 366:790-792, 1988.

24. Brandt-Rauf PW: The molecular epidemiology of oncoproteins, *Scand J Work Environ Health* 18(1 Suppl):46-49, 1992.

25. Anderson NW, Reynolds SH, You M, and Maronpot RM: Role of proto-oncogene activation in carcinogenesis, *Environ Health Perspect* 98:13-24, 1992.

26. Brandt Rauf PW, Smith S, Hemminki K, Koskinen H, Vainio H, Niman II, et al: Serum oncoproteins and growth factors in asbestosis and silicosis patients, *Int J Cancer* 50(6):881-885, 1992.

27. Edell ES and Cortese DA: Bronchoscopic phototherapy with hematoporphyrin derivative for treatment of localized bronchogenic carcinoma: a 5-year experience, *Mayo Clin Proc* 62:8-14, 1987.

28. Greenwald P, Cullen JW, Kelloff G, and Pierson HF: Chemoprevention of lung cancer; problems and progress, *Chest* 96(1 Suppl):14S-16S, 1989.

29. Ferris BG: Epidemiology standardization project, *Am Rev Respir Dis* 118(6 Part 2):1-120, 1978.

30. Rona RJ and Mosbech J: Validity and repeatability of self-reported occupational and industrial history from patients in EEC countries, *Int J Epidemiol* 18(3):674-679, 1989.

31. Holmes E and Garshick E: The reproducibility of the self-report of occupational exposure to asbestos and dust, *J Occup Med* 33(2):134-138, 1991.

32. Ehrenberg RL and Sniezek JE III: Development of a standard questionnaire for occupational health research, *Am J Public Health* 79 Suppl:15-17, 1989.

33. Korn RJ, Dockery DW, Speizer FE, Ware JH, and Ferris BG, Jr: Occupational exposures and chronic respiratory symptoms. A population-based study, *Am Rev Respir Dis* 136(2):298-304, 1987.

34. Lebowitz MD: Occupational exposures in relation to symptomatology and lung function in a community population, *Environ Res* 14(1):59-67, 1977.

35. Lebowitz MD: The relationship of socio-environmental factors to the prevalence of obstructive lung diseases and other chronic conditions, *J Chronic Dis* 30(9):599-611, 1977.

36. Blanc PD, Rempel D, Maizlish N, Hiatt P, and Olson KR: Occupational illness: case detection by poison control surveillance, *Ann Intern Med* 111(3):238-244, 1989.

37. Kipen HM, Tepper A, Rosenman K, and Weinrib D: Limitations of hospital discharge diagnoses for surveillance of extrinsic allergic alveolitis, *Am J Ind Med* 17(6):701-709, 1990.

38. McDiarmid MA, Bonanni R, and Finocchiaro M: Poor agreement of occupational data between a hospital-based cancer registry and interview, *J Occup Med* 33(6):726-729, 1991.

39. Balmes J, Rempel D, Alexander M, Reiter R, Harrison R, Bernard B, et al: Hospital records as a data source for occupational disease surveillance: a feasibility study, *Am J Ind Med* 21(3):341-351, 1992.

40. Althouse RB, Castellan RM, and Wagner GR: Pneumoconioses in the United States: highlights of surveillance data from NIOSH and other federal sources, *Occup Med: State Art Rev* 7(2):197-208, 1992.

41. NIOSH: *Work related lung disease surveillance report,* Pub No DHHS (NIOSH) 91-113, Cincinnati (OH), 1991, Division of Respiratory Disease Studies, NIOSH, Department of Health and Human Services.

42. Muir DCF, Julian JA, Roos JO, Maehle WM, Chan J, Mountain W, et al: Classification of radiographs for pneumoconiosis: The Canadian pneumoconiosis reading panel, *Am J Ind Med* 24:139-147, 1993.

43. Liddel FDK and Morgan WKC: Methods of assessing serial films of the pneumoconioses: A review, *J Soc Occup Med* 28:6-15, 1978.

44. Harber P and Smitherman J: Asbestosis: diagnostic dilution, *J Occup Med* 33(7):786-793, 1991.

45. Lewinsohn HC, Bresnitz EA, Gould Jr KG, Hatfield TR, Holthouser MG, Kent DC, et al: Spirometry in the occupational setting: notes for guidance, *J Occup Med* 34(5):559-561, 1992.

46. Hankinson JL: Pulmonary function testing in the screening of workers: guidelines for instrumentation, performance, interpretation, *J Occup Med* 28(10):1081-1092, 1986.

47. Enright PL: Surveillance for lung disease: quality assurance using computers and a team approach, *Occup Med: State Art Rev* 7(2):209-225, 1992.

48. Kipen HM, Lilis R, Suzuki Y, Valciukas JA, and Selikoff IJ: Pulmonary fibrosis in asbestos insulation workers with lung cancer: a radiological and histopathological evaluation, *Br J Ind Med* 44(2):96-100, 1987.

49. Hughes JM and Weill H: Asbestosis as a precursor of asbestos related lung cancer: results of a prospective mortality study, *Br J Ind Med* 48(4):229-233, 1991.

50. Cookson W, De Klerk N, Musk AW, Glancy JJ, Armstrong B, and Hobbs M: The natural history of asbestosis in former crocidolite workers of Wittenoom Gorge, *Am Rev Respir Dis* 133(6):994-998, 1986.

51. Smith AB, Castellan RM, Lewis D, and Matte T: Guidelines for the epidemiologic assessment of occupational asthma, *J Aller Clin Immun* 84(5 Part 2):794-805, 1989.

52. Balmes JR: Surveillance for occupational asthma, *Occup Med: State Art Rev* 6(1):101-110, 1991.

53. Enarson DA, Vedal S, Schulzer M, Dybuncios A, and Chan-Yeung M: Asthma, asthmalike symptoms, chronic bronchitis, and the degree of bronchial hyperresponsiveness in epidemiologic surveys, *Am Rev Respir Dis* B6:613-617, 1987.

54. Dales RE, Ernest P, Hanley JA, Pattista RN, and Becklake MR: Prediction of airway reactivity from responses to a standardized respiratory symptom questionnaire, *Am Rev Respir Dis* 135:817-821, 1987.

55. Burney P and Chinn S: Developing a new questionnaire for measuring the prevalence and distribution of asthma, *Chest* 91:795-835, 1987.

56. Henneberger PK, Stanbury MJ, Trimbath LS, and Kipen HM: The use of portable peak flowmeters in the surveillance of occupational asthma, *Chest* 100(6):1515-1521, 1991.

57. Hendrick D, Fabbri LM, Hughes JM, Banks DE, Barkman HW Jr, Connolly MJ, et al: Modification of the methacholine inhalation test and its epidemiologic use in polyurethane workers, *Am Rev Respir Dis* 133(4):600-604, 1986.

58. Rijcken B and Schouten JP: Measuring bronchial responsiveness in epidemiology, *Eur Respir J* 6:617-618, 1993.

59. Klees JE, Alexander M, Rempel D, Beckett W, Rubin R, Barnhart S, et al: Evaluation of a proposed NIOSH surveillance: case definition for occupational asthma, *Chest* 98(5 Suppl):212S-215S, 1990.

60. Brooks SM, Baker DB, Gann PH, Jarabek AM, Hertzberg V, Gallagher J, et al: Cold air challenge and platinum skin reactivity in platinum refinery workers. Bronchial reactivity precedes skin prick response, *Chest* 97(6):1401-1407.

61. Cartier A, Grammer L, Malo J-L, Lagier F, Ghezzo H, Harris K, et al: Specific serum antibodies against isocyanates: association with occupational asthma, *J Allergy Clin Immun* 84(4, Part 1): 507-514, 1989.

62. Weiss KB and Wagener DK: Asthma surveillance in the United States. A review of current trends and knowledge gaps, *Chest* 98(5 Suppl):179S-184S, 1990.

63. Anto JM, Sunyer J, Rodriguez-Roisin R, Suarez-Cervera M, and Vazquez L: Community outbreaks of asthma associated with inhalation of soybean dust, *N Engl J Med* 320(17):1097-1102, 1989.

64. Shusterman DJ and Dager SR: Prevention of psychological disability after occupational respiratory exposures, *Occup Med: State Art Rev* 6(1):11-27, 1991.

65. Neutra R, Lipscomb J, Satin K, and Shusterman D: Hypotheses to explain the higher symptom rates observed around hazardous waste sites, *Environ Health Perspect* 94:31-38, 1991.

66. Matte TD, Hoffman RE, Rosenman KD, and Stanbury M: Surveillance of occupational asthma under the SENSOR model, *Chest* 98(5 Suppl):173S-178S, 1990.

67. Meredith SK, Taylor VM, and McDonald JC: Occupational respiratory disease in the United Kingdom 1989: a report to the British Thoracic Society and the Society of Occupational Medicine by the SWORD Project Group, *Br J Ind Med* 48(5):292-298, 1991.

68. Jones DJ: Prescribed respiratory diseases in the 1990s. *Respir Med* 86(4):283-287, 1992.

69. Wagner GR and Spieler EA: Disease surveillance and health promotion for coal miners utilizing independent community health care centers, *Ann Am Conf Gov Ind Hyg* 14:285-291, 1986.

70. Teta MJ, Ott MG, and Schnatter AR: Population based mortality surveillance in carbon products manufacturing plants, *Br J Ind Med* 44(5):344-350, 1987.

71. Hoffman JM: X-ray surveillance and miner transfer programs—efforts to prevent progression of coal workers' pneumoconiosis, *Ann Am Conf Gov Ind Hyg* 14:293-297, 1986.

72. Hankinson JL and Bang KM: Acceptability and reproducibility criteria of the American Thoracic Society as observed in a sample of the general population, *Am Rev Respir Dis* 143(3):516-521, 1991.

73. Sterling TD and Weinkam JJ: Comparison of smoking-related risk factors among black and white males, *Am J Ind Med* 15(3):319-333, 1989.

74. Elliott P, Westlake AJ, Hills M, Kleinschmidt I, Rodrigues L, McGale P, et al: The small area health statistics unit: a national facility for investigating health around point sources of environmental pollution in the United Kingdom, *J Epidemiol Community Health* 46(4):345-349, 1992.

Chapter 52

JOB DEMAND, PREPLACEMENT EVALUATION, AND ACCOMMODATION

Philip Harber
M. Joseph Fedoruk

This chapter describes the principles for determining the ability of a worker with a respiratory impairment to do a specific job and potential methods for accommodating persons with respiratory handicaps. Accommodation is the process of making specific changes (generally to the workplace) for the purpose of enabling a disabled individual to be able to safely and effectively perform a job that he or she otherwise would be unable to perform. In addition, methods for quantifying the physical demands of jobs are discussed. Regulations governing work-related medical evaluations and the criteria upon which medical decisions concerning employability are made in the United States are also described.

In the United States, federal[1] and in some instances state laws mandate that individuals with disabilities who are otherwise qualified to perform a job must be provided "reasonable accommodation." Reasonable accommodation refers to a change in the work environment or in the manner that work is performed that enables an otherwise qualified disabled person to be offered equal employment opportunities. This chapter identifies the categories of accommodation that should be considered for individuals with respiratory conditions and how such accommodations differ from those that have been traditionally provided for persons with other physical disabilities.

REASONS FOR WORK ABILITY EVALUATION

There are several clinical situations in which physicians may be required to assess an individual's ability to perform a job. These include:

1. *Preplacement medical evaluations.* Preplacement examinations are commonly performed on behalf of employers for the purpose of determining whether a job applicant has any medical conditions that would preclude him or her from safely performing a job.
2. *Fitness for duty examinations.* Fitness for duty examinations are commonly performed to determine if an employee has any medical problems that would preclude him or her from continuing to work in a job. These examinations are often requested because an employee demonstrates impaired work performance

that the employer or employee suspects could be potentially related to a medical problem. Fitness for duty examinations can also be performed before an employee returns to work after a serious illness or a prolonged absence when there is concern that the employee's condition could interfere with performing a job safely.

3. *Workers' compensation evaluation.* A person's ability to work following an industrial illness involving the respiratory system must often be assessed as part of the compensation evaluation process.

4. *Evaluation of "reasonable accommodation."* The physician may be requested to determine if a proposed accommodation is necessary or likely to be successful for a new hire or in the event that an employee is being considered for transfer to a new job.

5. *Following medical surveillance examinations.* In the course of routine medical surveillance examinations (e.g., as required by the U.S. Occupational Safety and Health Administration [OSHA], Mine Safety and Health Administration [MSHA], and the Department of Transportation) employees may be discovered to have underlying medical conditions that require further assessment to determine if continued employment constitutes a substantial risk of harm.

There are three categories of limitations that may preclude persons with respiratory disorders from being able to perform a job:

1. *Physical limitations.* A respiratory condition may prevent a person from performing a job because a critical work task(s) requires a level of exertion that the individual cannot achieve due to ventilatory or gas exchange limitation. This assessment is achieved by comparing the person's exercise or work capacity against the critical job demands. For example, an individual with smoking-related chronic obstructive pulmonary disease (COPD) might have insufficient aerobic capacity due to ventilatory limitation to perform certain critical fire-fighting tasks, such as being able to pull an unconscious victim out of a burning building while wearing heavy turn-out gear and a 65-pound self-contained breathing apparatus. Methods of assessing physiologic capacity are discussed in Chapter 4.

2. *Working condition limitations.* A respiratory medical condition may preclude a person from performing a job if the working conditions (including exposure to physical, chemical, or biological agents) could lead to a worsening of the person's respiratory condition or impair the person's ability to safely perform the job. For example, a person with a recurrent pneumothorax may not be qualified to work as a deep sea commercial diver because barometric pressure changes would place him or her at substantial risk of experiencing an incapacitating and/or potentially fatal pneumothorax in a deep sea environment.

3. *Episodic incapacitation.* A respiratory condition may result in a person being frequently incapacitated because of acute intermittent exacerbations of an underlying respiratory illness. Although such an individual may have no physical or working condition limitations from performing a specific job at the time of medical evaluation, he or she would be expected to continue to experience significant episodes of incapacitation due to the natural course of the condition. These episodic incapacitations would preclude normal work attendance and effective overall job performance. For example, a person with cystic fibrosis might be expected to have recurrent episodes of respiratory infections that would likely result in regular absences at work.

ASSESSMENT OF WORK CONDITIONS FOR PLACEMENT ADVICE

Determining whether a person with a respiratory condition requires work limitations or preclusions is based upon an assessment of the interaction of the person's respiratory disorder with the physical demands and working conditions of the job. When there is uncertainty about the physical demands and/or working conditions of a job, medical evaluators should request this information from the employer. Four types of information may be acquired:

1. Physical demand of the job;
2. Workplace chemical exposures;
3. Likelihood of accidental uncontrolled exposures; and
4. Capability of job modification to accommodate the impaired worker.

ASSESSMENT OF PHYSICAL DEMANDS

Traditionally, physical demand is described via job analyses that are commonly performed by rehabilitation counselors, physical therapists, industrial nurses, or industrial psychologists. The amount of information contained in a job analysis can vary greatly since the types of investigation required to assess job demands have not been standardized.

The job should be identified as specifically as possible. Some jobs are uniform, composed of repetitive conduct of the same physical task (e.g., assembly line work or some ambulatory medical practices). In others, however, a job is composed of many distinct subtasks with very different physical workloads. For example, a study of coal mining work found wide variation in heart rate throughout the workday in individual miners[2]; similarly, peak work rates of fishermen were found to be markedly higher than average values.[3] For jobs composed of many different tasks, two alternative approaches may be applied: description of all tasks or development of summary indices. For the former approach, tasks are enumerated and then individually evaluated for physical demand. Then, the relative frequency and duration of each task are described. Alternatively, the overall physical demand of the job can be described by the "typical" task and its imposed workload and by describing the most demanding task.

Some job tasks are a fundamental part of the job (so called "essential job functions"), whereas inability to do others does not preclude a worker from doing a job. Determining whether a task is "essential" is typically the responsibility of the employer, not of the medical practitioner. In the United States, the U.S. Americans with Disabilities Act (ADA) mandates that only "essential" job duties be considered in placement decisions.[1,4]

METHODS FOR ASSESSING JOB DEMAND

Several techniques may be used to measure the physical demands of the job. These are summarized in the box.

Direct physiologic assessment of jobs

The most direct method is to directly measure the job demands at the worksite. To accomplish this, the appropriate physiologic parameter should be assessed. Measurement of oxygen consumption or ventilation is appropriate. This may then be compared with the oxygen consumption an individual can attain in a clinical laboratory test.

The obvious strength of the physiologic validation method is the potential direct link between a clinical measure and the job demand. For example, oxygen consumption can be measured in both the clinical and worksite settings.

The major limitation of this method is the technical requirement. It mandates a high level of technical capability to make the measurements. Furthermore, measurement must be done under field conditions and must be performed on an adequate number of subjects to provide a statistically valid description. Measurement techniques themselves (e.g., use of bags to collect exhaled air or use of masks)[5] may interfere with work performance. Nevertheless such methods have been successfully and extensively used without a mask or mouthpiece. Use of the respiratory inductive ple-

thysmography[6,7] permits measuring ventilation noninvasively but is very complex and may not be applicable to all work situations. This method is based upon determining ventilation from changes in the chest and abdominal circumference.

Another potential limitation of this technique is its limitation to describing the current state, not directly predicting future conditions. Thus, if an individual can meet the job demands currently, he or she may not be able to do so in the future. Also, the oxygen consumption required to do a job may vary considerably with body weight[8] and efficiency. Thus, measurement of oxygen consumption by an obese person performing a job may overestimate the demand of the job for persons of normal weight.

Estimation from heart rate

Heart rate generally correlates with both oxygen consumption and ventilation,[9] and therefore this relatively simple measure has often been used as an indirect measure of the respiratory demands of a job.[10,11] Heart rate may be easily determined, and it may be continuously measured by tape recording devices or telemetry, even in difficult worksite settings.

Several factors must be considered in interpreting the heart rate as an indicator of pulmonary demand. First, the relationship between heart rate (HR) and oxygen consumption ($\dot{V}O_2$) varies considerably among persons. Well-conditioned persons typically have a lower heart rate at a given $\dot{V}O_2$ than less fit persons. Furthermore, body fat affects this relationship.[7] Hence, while there is generally a linear HR–$\dot{V}O_2$ relationship within an individual, the slope may differ considerably among different persons. It is therefore advisable to determine the relationship of $\dot{V}O_2$ to HR in each subject before using HR as a general measure of job demand. The HR–$\dot{V}O_2$ relationship can often be determined by a simple two-stage exercise test.[12] The relationship between HR and $\dot{V}O_2$ is determined by a simple laboratory test in a laboratory setting; HR may be measured in a field setting and directly interconverted to $\dot{V}O_2$.[2]

A second consideration is that even within an individual the $\dot{V}O_2$–HR relationship is affected by many factors besides the job's respiratory demand. Ambient conditions, such as heat, nutrition, and hydration, can affect the HR. Stress can also affect the HR, and indeed deviation from the expected HR–$\dot{V}O_2$ relationship has been used as an indirect indicator of psychological activation.[13] Such factors confound the use of HR as an indicator of $\dot{V}O_2$.

Third, the relationship between HR and $\dot{V}O_2$ is dependent upon the type of workload. The heart rate tends to be higher for any $\dot{V}O_2$ with static rather than dynamic workloads.[14] Arm work and leg work lead to different $\dot{V}O_2$–HR relationships,[15] and therefore the relationship should optimally be determined in a test that is comparable to the actual work. For example, a study of manual postal delivery showed that accuracy was best when the regressions rela-

---

Methods of assessing overall job demand

1. Direct physiologic measures (e.g., oxygen consumption)
2. Heart rate measurement
3. Work simulation
4. Work sampling
5. Worker rating methods (relative perceived exertion)
6. Prospective predictive validity
7. Industrial psychology—global ratings
8. Consensus of experts
9. Reference data

tionship between $\dot{V}O_2$ and HR was determined by a treadmill test in which a mailbag was carried.[16]

Fourth, the linear relationships between HR and $\dot{V}O_2$, between HR and ventilation, and between ventilation and $\dot{V}O_2$ are not uniformly maintained of real low or very high exertion levels. At low level exertion, the influence of other factors such as psychologic activation or body position may be large in comparison with the influence of exertion level changes. At very high exertion levels, the relationships change due to crossing the anaerobic threshold.

Work simulation

In some instances, actual measurement of the physiologic demands in the *field (worksite)* setting is impractical or infeasible. Under such circumstances, work simulation methods may be employed. The technique allows the critical aspects of the job to be tested in the laboratory setting. This can greatly facilitate the utilization of physiologic equipment that might not be sufficiently rugged for field use.

To use simulation properly, a field study (methods discussed below) must be employed initially to identify those tasks that should be simulated. It is essential that the conditions in the laboratory setting be as comparable as possible to worksite conditions.

The advantage of the simulation method, similar to the physiologic method, is that it has an inherent degree of validity. It also is generally less technically demanding than field physiologic measurements. Finally, similar to the field physiology technique, it allows a common measurement technique to be used in the clinical setting and in the job descriptive setting.

There are several limitations to this method. Many job sites cannot be easily simulated in a laboratory. Jobs that are highly varied are also difficult to simulate because of the many distinct tasks involved. Even in simulation studies, it is advisable to have actual workers perform the task simulation rather than relying upon naive volunteer subjects (e.g., graduate students). Actual workers typically develop efficient ways to accomplish tasks, thereby potentially decreasing overall demand, whereas volunteer subjects may be more physically fit than many workers. Thus, simulation methods may be limited by difficulty in recruiting actual workers to come to laboratories for testing.

Work sampling

Some jobs consist of repetitive performance of the same task, whereas others are highly varied. When there are only a few tasks, each may be evaluated. Moreover, when there are very many tasks, a work sampling technique is needed to assume an adequate description of job demands. A probability sampling approach may be employed. For a work sampling analysis, a statistically valid sample of the work is recorded, generally by videotape or by direct on-site coding. Such samples must be chosen with due regard to the variety of locations and tasks within a job category. Often, work sampling is performed for a relatively brief period of time for each sampling frame, but a valid analysis becomes feasible based upon having an adequate number of samples.

The major strength of work sampling is that it can provide a well-rounded, valid description of the work required. It directly utilizes statistical sampling methods to determine the length and intensity of sampling. It can describe the extreme, the mean, and the degree of variation effectively.

Two limitations apply to this technique. First, it is personnel intensive. Second, there is no direct link between the work site analysis and the clinical evaluations. That is, while the oxygen consumption is measured in the clinical setting, motions and forces typically are determined in the field. "Judgment" is needed rather than allowing dependence upon an objective measure.

Worker rating methods

Rating methods rely on ratings provided by workers. Ratings are done at the time a work task is performed, rather than by memory. Borg[17] or similar ratings may be applied to each of several job tasks.

Relative perceived exertion (RPE) scales typically use a series of ordered categories to describe exertion. The method developed by Borg[17] is most commonly used. Theoretically, there is a logarithmic relationship between categories.

Visual analog scales (VAS) may also be employed. These provide a continuous variable measure. The subject chooses a point on a line representing a continuum from very light to very heavy exertion. The ends of the line are anchored by descriptions, but there are no intermediate descriptions.

The accompanying box illustrates a Borg type and a VAS type scale. In using rating methods to assess job demand, it is important to clearly state the question. The subjects must understand that exertion and not dyspnea is being measured. Dyspnea is a complex sensation and is affected by many distinct mechanisms.[18] Dyspnea is discussed further in Chapter 53.

RPE methods have shown surprisingly excellent correlation with physiologic measures when applied to work performed by large muscle groups (e.g., lifting) or to overall physical exertion.[19,20] However, the major muscle groups and type of activity involved affect the ratings; for example, ratings tend to be higher with a bike ergometer than treadmill exercise at the same level of oxygen consumption.[21] Furthermore, there is some evidence that ratings are affected by psychologic factors. Short-term anxiety and more characterologic features (e.g., extroversion) affect ratings.[22] Therefore, anxiety-inducing experimental conditions must be avoided.

RPE methods are relatively easy to apply and may be task specific. They depend on documentable ratings, and they may be validated by direct physiologic measures if

---

Rating methods

Relative perceived exertion (RPE) scale

2 Very very light
3
4 Very light
5
6 Fairly light
7
8 Somewhat hard
9
10 Hard
11
12 Very hard
13
14 Very very hard

Visual analog scale (VAS)

Very light		Very heavy

---

needed. The scientific literature and much practical experience support their use.

Prospective predictive validity test

A particularly powerful, but rarely used, method is predictive validity testing. Here, a group of workers is tested clinically for exercise capacity. They are then followed over a period of time to determine who can successfully remain on the job. Those who leave are characterized into three categories: voluntary departure unrelated to work or clinical concerns, inability to do the work, and adverse health effect of the work. From this, it is possible to determine outcomes—which clinical findings adequately predict with reasonable certainty that an individual will not be able to continue working?

This method has obvious inherent validity, but it is also difficult to utilize.

Industrial psychology—global ratings

Industrial psychologists frequently estimate job demands using a different form of worker ratings.[23,14] Typically, a group of "subject matter experts" (experienced workers) meets to develop the work description. First, they list all the individual tasks associated with a job. Then, they assign ratings to each task for typical prolonged and greatest exertion. Unlike the RPE method described above, the ratings are usually not done at the time the task is actually performed.

These methods are particularly useful when the job tasks are highly varied. Unlike measures with extensive physiologic observations, they are limited by reliance on subjective assessments; nevertheless, correlation with objective physiologic measures has been shown.[24]

Consensus of experts

In this method, a consensus panel of experts makes recommendations according to formal decision-making methodology. Unlike committees in which conclusions may be inappropriately influenced by a single individual, formal consensus methods provide a structured approach.

Such methods have many advantages. In particular, they do not require extensive field investigations. Nevertheless, they are more "objective" than simply collecting the "opinions" of experts. Furthermore, because there is a formal process for reaching the conclusions, the process is documentable.

There are three possible weaknesses to this method. First, this is somewhat cumbersome, occasionally requiring multiple rounds until convergence of opinion can be achieved. Another disadvantage of this method is that it can apply only to a limited number of situations. Finally, if the questions are complex, it would not work effectively.

Reference data

There are several reference sources that list exertion levels associated with a very large number of jobs. Unfortunately, much of the information may be outdated[25,26] or extremely nonspecific. There may be very large differences in the exertion levels associated with a job title depending upon the location, use of mechanical assist devices, and work organization.

Nevertheless, the widely used *Dictionary of Job Titles*[27] provides a good qualitative description of physical demand.

ASSESSMENT OF CHEMICAL EXPOSURES FOR PLACEMENT DECISIONS

In many instances, the information provided on the working conditions is cursory. Qualitative descriptions, such as "dusty environment or fume exposure," are insufficient for determining whether the job exposures must be avoided for the person with the respiratory condition. Chapter 10 describes industrial hygiene methods applicable to worksites. Such methods may often be helpful in obtaining adequate information.

ASSESSMENT OF LIKELIHOOD OF "ACCIDENTAL" EXPOSURES

Unanticipated events may occur in some work settings. Such events may potentially lead to chemical exposures and/or very high physical exertion demands. For example, a fire in a chemical plant might impose a high ventilatory demand (to run to the exit) as well as uncontrolled exposure to a chemical agent (e.g., chlorine gas).

The likelihood of such occurrences can often be estimated based upon the past history of the industry or facility. In addition, specific process controls may be evaluated.

The consequences of such an event for the specific individual may be considered as well.

INTEGRATION OF DATA

Worksite factors, personal susceptibilities, and personal respiratory impairments all must be integrated into a final recommendation regarding placement. The placement decision may be viewed from several perspectives. The worker may wish to avoid all possible risk or, alternatively, may be strongly motivated by financial or other considerations to work even in the presence of risk. Similarly, employers may feel pressured to encourage employment or to avoid any possible liability.

The final recommendation whether a person should perform a job is based upon whether the magnitude of risk that an individual would incur to him or herself or others by performing the job is acceptable. In the past, physicians were often asked to determine whether a candidate was considered "acceptable" for employment or "passed" a physical examination. Historically, physicians have used inconsistent criteria to assess the ability and risk of an applicant or an employee's ability to work in a given position. To the extent possible, available chemical and other workplace data should guide such decisions.

LEGAL CONSIDERATIONS

With the advent of the U.S. Americans with Disabilities Act in 1992, the medical examination process and the medical criteria upon which medically related decisions concerning employability are based are now subject to federal law. In addition, other industrial nations may also have regulations that protect the rights of disabled or handicapped persons that could impact how physicians conduct employment-related medical examinations and make decisions concerning employability. Violations of ADA regulations can result in considerable penalties. Physicians performing employment-related medical examinations cannot continue to perform such assessments without an understanding of the impact of these regulations on this medical process. These considerations have been discussed in a recent review, from which this section has been derived.*

Individuals are protected by the ADA if they have a disability, had a disability, or are *perceived* to have a disability. A disability is defined as a physical or mental impairment that substantially limits one or more major life activities. Major life activities include those that a person can usually perform with little difficulty such as breathing, walking, hearing, seeing, performing manual tasks, etc. If a person's condition significantly restricts ability to be employed in a class or broad range of jobs compared to an average person with similar training and experience, such a condition

*This section reprinted with permission from Harber P, Fedoruk M, and Goldberg L: Accomodating respiratory handicaps, *Semin Respir Med* 14:240–249. 1993. © Thieme Medical Publishers, Inc.[28]

could be viewed as being "substantially limiting" from performing major life activities.[10] Therefore, a wide range of conditions and persons potentially qualify for protection under the umbrella of the ADA.

The ADA identifies how medical examinations are to be integrated into the hiring process and for other employment-related examinations. For preplacement medical evaluations, the ADA precludes the employer from making any inquiries concerning whether an applicant has any unusual medical conditions prior to making a job offer. The employer cannot inquire about an applicant's specific medical condition or ask for diagnoses, medication use, or past medical history. However, the employer may inquire about the ability of the applicant to perform specific job tasks. Thus, the employer cannot ask, "Do you have obstructive lung disease or asthma?," but *could* ask, "Are you able to walk for four hours?"

Once an employment offer has been made, employment can be contingent on the applicant passing a postemployment offer medical examination. The preplacement medical examination can also serve as a baseline medical evaluation. However, only information from medical tests that are related to the ability of an individual to perform work tasks may be used for making decisions concerning employability.

The ADA prohibits excluding workers with a disability that interferes only with the performance of a task that is not an essential aspect of the job. Thus, an individual cannot be considered disabled for a job if he or she cannot perform all the job duties since only essential tasks should be considered.

An employer is not required to hire an applicant or retain an employee if a person's job performance would pose a direct threat to the health and safety of the individual, coworkers, or the public. A direct threat means a significant risk to health and safety that cannot be eliminated by reasonable accommodation. The determination of what constitutes a direct threat is not a typical component of clinical decision making and is subject to varying interpretation. The criteria by which such a determination can be made have been defined in broad terms by ADA regulations.

The ADA identifies four criteria to assess direct threat:

1. *Duration of risk.* Duration refers to the length of time that the risk of substantial harm due to respiratory impairment will last (e.g., is it treatable and/or reversible, such as an infection, or irreversible such as a terminal malignancy or severe COPD? A teacher with active tuberculosis may represent a substantial risk to others, but this risk is brief since chemotherapy will rapidly make the individual noncontagious.)
2. *Nature and severity of potential harm.* Severity does not refer to the illness itself, but rather refers to an adverse *event* that is a *consequence* of the interaction between the medical illness and the work condition.

Severity must consider both the impact on the individual and the impact on others (public safety, coworkers, etc.). Exercise-induced asthma could significantly impair an urban law enforcement officer who may have to chase and restrain a felon, but may not severely affect a delivery person who may occasionally have to climb stairs to deliver packaged goods.

3. *Likelihood.* Likelihood is the estimated probability that this adverse event or harm will actually occur. Risks that are considered remote or speculative should not be considered.

4. *Imminence.* Imminence describes how soon the adverse health event or consequence is likely to occur.

The assessment of risk cannot be made solely on the opinion or belief of the physician, but has to be established on current medical information including data in the medical literature and objective evidence from the individual concerning his or her medical condition and the past and future affects from the specific job. This could include information concerning the individual's ability to perform similar tasks in other positions. In general, a risk of harm that is likely to be of long duration, cause severe outcome events with a high probability, and cause these in a short time frame is particularly likely to constitute a substantial direct threat.

The ADA specifically mandates that "reasonable" accommodation be provided by the employer to an otherwise qualified individual with a disability. A qualified individual with a disability is a person who has a disability as defined by ADA and can perform the essential functions of the job with or without reasonable accommodation.

The definition of "reasonable" is open to interpretation, but the factors that must be considered in determining what is a reasonable accommodation are defined by the ADA. In general, the extent of effort required is proportional to the employer's available resources. Greater resources must be expended by major employers than by small business owners where an accommodation could result in a substantial business hardship. Furthermore, the expected duration of the employee's tenure may be considered in determining the extensiveness of the required accommodation.

It is the responsibility of the employer and not the physician to make a final decision concerning whether a reasonable accommodation can be provided to an otherwise qualified applicant. However, in some select cases, the physician may be required to suggest what specific accommodation methods could be offered to enable an employee to work without posing a significant direct threat. The physician may also be requested to comment on whether a proposed accommodation would reasonably be expected to mitigate the health threat associated with the worker's performance of a task or work in a select environment. For example, an air-purifying negative pressure respirator may not eliminate all irritant exposures in a job for which a person with irritant-induced asthma is applying. However, the reduction in exposure level that may be achieved, assuming the applicant can effectively use a respirator, may be sufficient to reduce the exposure to a concentration that would not trigger an asthma attack and, consequently, enable the individual to safely perform the job.

ACCOMMODATION

The accommodation process for persons with respiratory disease can include several different types of potential accommodations. Measures can be taken to modify the physical demands for individuals who have exercise limitations. Working conditions can be modified through engineering controls primarily by limiting exposures. Administrative methods that involve limiting the time spent at performing a task can also be considered to be part of the accommodation process. Since denial of employment has to be based upon conditions that pose a direct threat, methods of improving the ability of the worker to perform the critical tasks or eliminating such tasks can be successful in addressing this concern. In some cases an iterative approach could theoretically be taken, especially with an existing employer where there are no clear-cut answers concerning whether a specific accommodation or effort will be successful. These approaches are summarized in the box, and each is described.

Modifications of physical demands

The physical demands associated with performance of critical job tasks can be potentially modified through *physical modification* of the workplace. The success of any

---

Approaches to accommodation

Physical demands

· Job redesign with task modification
· Mechanical assistance devices

Working conditions

· Engineering controls
· Hazard elimination
· Ventilation (local or dilutional)
· Substitution
· Enclosure
· Work practice modification
· Personal protective equipment
· Exposure control monitoring
· Emergency plan procedures

Administrative controls

· Work schedule
· Job rotation

Individual considerations

· Medical monitoring
· Worker training

physical modification is dependent upon several factors, including the individual's exercise or functional capacity. In addition to determining the practicality of implementing any proposed physical modification, the impact of the modification on lowering the job demands to a level that would enable the disabled person to perform the job must be assessed.

There are several methods by which the physical demands of the job can potentially be changed. Changing the process of the job can foster accommodation. For example, a job may require the applicant to move 50 pound drums to different locations as part of an industrial process. Purchase of smaller size containers may result in a diminution of the job demands. In other situations, *assistance devices* can be particularly useful in lessening the physical demands of critical tasks. Overhead hoists, power lift assistors, motorized conveyors, motorized carts, and other devices can decrease the work requirements of a job. In some instances the reduction of job demands can be sufficient to allow a patient with COPD or other lung disease to work. For example, a patient considered for an assembly job could be accommodated by providing a lift assist device or conveyor to eliminate the need for the applicant to lift and carry heavy metal parts.

The assessment of what measures can be used to successfully modify a job may require a multidisciplinary effort that includes health professionals who are familiar with assistance devices such as physical therapists, physical medicine and rehabilitation specialists, occupational medicine specialists, and plant industrial or process engineers who are familiar with the job tasks and work processes.

Modification of workplace exposures

Working conditions can include physical, chemical, and biological agents that are present in the work environment. Several approaches can be taken to limit or manage these hazards for the purpose of enabling a worker to be accommodated in the workplace.

Engineering controls provide the best method of reducing exposure to airborne contaminants. Engineering controls involve physical modifications of the work environment that result in changes in exposure. The consideration of whether such controls would be reasonable for a single individual should be based upon how easily such changes can be implemented and their impact on business operations. Implementation of the engineering controls could have benefit to other workers by reducing the overall hazards to which the plant personnel are exposed.

Ideally, the best approach to eliminating a potential hazardous working condition is to eliminate it *(hazard elimination)*. For chemical substances, product substitution or a chemical process change using a less hazardous material may not always be achievable. There may be no acceptable product substitute or such a substitution might represent an unacceptable business hardship. Furthermore, prior to substituting a product, it is essential to determine that the product substitute does introduce a new and potentially more significant hazard.

As an alternative, complete *enclosure* of a manufacturing or other process can essentially eliminate exposures by preventing the employee from having any direct contact with the chemical agent involved. However, this may not always be practical and may be difficult to achieve in many work environments, especially as a method of accommodating a single individual.

Improving *ventilation* to reduce airborne concentrations of chemical contaminants is another principal engineering control method. There are two principal categories of ventilation changes. Local exhaust ventilation involves the use of a hood, slot, or vent at the source or point where the airborne contaminant is generated. For example, a hood over a chemical mixing area is a local exhaust ventilation control measure. Increases in the general ventilation to an area can also lessen contaminants to an area, but this is often less effective than local exhaust ventilation and cannot be relied upon as a method of controlling exposures to agents that are very hazardous. Chapter 60 describes engineering controls in more detail.

The clinical characteristics of the individual must be carefully evaluated in conjunction with evaluation of the proposed worksite ventilation controls. Lowering levels of nonspecific irritant gases or fumes may be adequate for someone with asthma and nonspecific responses to workplace irritants, but may not be adequate to protect a person with asthma due to allergic sensitization to a workplace agent (who may react, even fatally, to levels in the parts per billion range).

Engineering controls can also include the *modification of work practices*. For example, implementing the use of vacuuming for cleaning floors instead of sweeping can reduce ambient dust exposure levels. Wetting of powders or other dusts prior to handling or as part of a general process change can reduce ambient dust exposures, e.g., conversion of a dry chemical mixing process to wet process can result in a major reduction of ambient dust exposures.

Respiratory *personal protective equipment* (respirators) can also decrease exposures. In general for persons with respiratory problems, this involves the use of *respiratory protection* (respirators). Respirators can effectively decrease exposures, and they may be used by a single individual (e.g., one with an impairment). However, respirator use requires excellent compliance by the worker. In addition, respirators may themselves interfere with work performance or produce adverse physiologic effects. Respirators are discussed in more detail in Chapter 59. Respirators may be used on a regular basis or may be provided for emergency use only. Their use as an accommodation measure requires answering two questions: "Is the worker likely to use it regularly" and "will it *reliably* provide adequate protection?"

There are several situations in which the use of respirators can be considered an accommodation method. First, asthmatics with nonspecific irritant-affected asthma may potentially utilize respirators to decrease inhaled exposure levels of irritants to a level that would not be expected to produce adverse effects. A respirator with a high protection factor, such as an air-supplied respirator, may theoretically allow accommodation of a sensitized individual, especially if the time of potential exposure to the particular agent is brief and predictable. However, this must be used with great caution because of the possibility of malfunction. The individual's past response to similar exposures needs to be considered in this type of evaluation.

Exposure or environmental control monitoring, which involves the measurement of a chemical or agent in environmental specimens, can be an integral component of a respiratory accommodation program. This type of monitoring provides a mechanism to determine if an engineering control has been successfully implemented. Although it is generally obvious whether an appropriate wheelchair lift has been placed, compliance with environmental modifications for inhalation exposures may not be as self-evident, especially when an agent has limited warning properties, such as a strong odor, to rapidly identify exposure. It is important to not only initiate exposure control measures for the specific worker, but also to assure that they remain effective. To assure continued efficacy of the exposure controls, several forms of monitoring may be employed.

Direct reading instruments can be used to perform real time monitoring of ambient air in general work areas (area monitoring) for many air pollutants, including toxic gases such as phosphine, aerosols, dusts, and mists that can produce significant respiratory injury.

Direct reading instruments can be linked to alarms (visual and sound) that can alert plant personnel that there is a build-up of contaminants. Chemical leaks can be detected at an early stage and theoretically allow a sensitized individual to leave early. This may be practical only when an individual does not work directly with the sensitizing agent but the agent is present in other parts of the same building.

Personal monitoring on a periodic basis also may be useful in assuring compliance with the accommodation plan.

An *individualized emergency plan* for protecting the impaired individual may be considered as part of an accommodation program for a person with a respiratory disability. For example, an individual may be capable of working as a chemical plant operator or even in a mine under normal operating conditions. However, should a chemical leak or fire develop, the individual may not be able to use routine escape methods from the worksite (e.g., the plant elevator may become nonfunctional). An accommodation method should consider an emergency escape plan for the individual by incorporating a personal escape system. This may include planned assistance by designated co-workers or even mechanical devices to assist in building or work area evacuation.

Decreasing the criticality of an individual's role in the event of an emergency may avoid endangering public safety. For example, a refinery operator or peace officer might theoretically endanger public health and safety should he or she be unable to perform optimally in an unlikely emergency situation.

Administrative controls

Administrative controls may also facilitate respiratory accommodation and may include limiting the time a worker performs a task by *job rotation* or shortening the work period. The tasks may be subdivided among employees in a different manner to avoid the highest exertion components of the impaired individual's jobs. *Work scheduling* may be modified to allow periodic breaks and self-pacing may be substituted for machine pacing so that the exertion impaired individual (e.g., with COPD or idiopathic pulmonary fibrosis) may adopt an appropriate pattern. In some instances, a pulmonary patient may be subject to periodic absences due to the natural waxing and waning of the disease (exacerbations of cystic fibrosis, COPD variation, etc.). Cross training of co-workers may allow such absences to be tolerated.

Administrative controls may be successful in controlling responses to adverse working conditions such as exposures to airborne irritants. Whether an individual will develop an adverse response is dependent upon several factors, including both the duration and magnitude of an exposure concentration and individual sensitivity. Studies involving experimental challenges with TDI have revealed that reactions are dependent upon the dose received by an individual, which is dependent upon both concentration and duration of exposure.[11]

Individual considerations

The accommodation process may include *medical monitoring* in situations where the physician cannot determine if a proposed work modification will be sufficient to reduce the probability of substantial harm.

The types of monitoring that could be considered have to be based upon the likelihood of detecting the adverse outcome at an early stage, which may not be recognized by the individual, and the availability of resources to achieve the monitoring. Medical monitoring could range from performing on-site pre- and postshift spirometry tests to periodic medical evaluation by an independent physician. In worksites with an occupational health staff, a physician or trained nurse can perform spirometry and other evaluations either in response to symptoms or on a scheduled periodic basis. Even though there may be no occupational health department in the company, an employee may be taught to utilize medical monitoring techniques to determine early adverse effects. Asthmatics may be taught to measure peak flow rates using a peak flow meter to assess their lung function throughout the day. This information can provide key data to determine if an exposure is adversely impacting an individual. Significant decrements in peak flow should be further evaluated to determine whether they represent failures of the exposure control measures or individual variability.

Workers, their co-workers, and supervisors should have adequate *training* to understand and effectively use the accommodation methods. This does not imply that the individual's medical confidentiality has to be broken since functional status information can be released without any disclosure of information concerning the identity of the underlying medical condition. Paternalism in communicating the need for special accommodation should be avoided.

SUMMARY

Placement recommendations require thorough understanding of exposures and attendant tasks, not only for the "average" worker, but for the *specific* individual being considered.[29] Exposure levels that are "safe" for most persons may not be acceptable for an individual with respiratory impairment. Persons with respiratory conditions often can be successfully accommodated in the workplace.

The determination of what represents an appropriate pulmonary accommodation can involve several disciplines including occupational and pulmonary medicine specialists, ergonomic specialists including industrial engineers, and other related specialists. The determination of whether a working condition can be successfully mitigated can involve other select specialists including industrial hygienists who routinely recognize, evaluate, and control industrial hazards. For several respiratory conditions there can be uncertainty concerning the response an individual will have to a work environment and there can be considerable divergence of medical opinion concerning the likely impact of a work environment on an applicant's condition. An iterative approach to accommodation provides an opportunity to determine whether an individual is capable of performing a job in situations where there is little likelihood that such an approach could result in significant potential for personal or public harm.

The recent regulatory changes will decrease the probability that persons with select conditions will be unfairly stigmatized and denied opportunities afforded the general public. The goal of avoidance of discrimination is accompanied by another challenge of protecting both the worker's health and public safety. The right of a disabled person to perform a job may also be perceived by a member of the general public as a potential public safety risk if the applicant may be unable to effectively perform his or her job. There are no clear guidelines for physicians to follow concerning what level of risk is acceptable, although factors such as duration, severity, likelihood, and imminence of risk have to be considered. For respiratory conditions, the decisions regarding whether accommodation can be success-

fully achieved will not be clearly obvious as for other physical handicaps, such as loss of limb or sight.

REFERENCES

1. Equal employment opportunity for individuals with disabilities. 29 CFR 1630. *Fed Register* 56:35726-35756, 1991.
2. Harber P, Tamimie J, Emory J, Bhattacharya A, and Barber M: Effects of exercise using industrial respirators. *Am Ind Hyg Assoc J* 45:603-609, 1984.
3. Rodahl K, Vokac Z, Fugelli P, Vaage O, Maehlum S: Circulatory strain, estimated energy output and catecholamine excretion in Norwegian coastal fishermen, *Ergonomics* 17:585-602, 1974.
4. Equal Employment Opportunity Commission: *A technical assistance manual on employment provisions (Title 1) of the Americans with Disabilities Act,* Washington DC, 1992, U.S. Government Printing Office.
5. Louhevaara V, Ilmarinen J, and Oja P: Comparison of three field methods for measuring oxygen consumption, *Ergonomics* 28:463-470, 1985.
6. Hodous TK, Hankinson JL, and Stark GP: Workplace measurement of respirator effects using respiratory inductive plethysmography, *Am Ind Hyg Assoc J* 50:372-378, 1989.
7. Harber P, Lew M, Shimozaki S, and Thomas B: Noninvasive measurement of respirator effect at rest and during exercise, *Am Ind Hyg Assoc J* 50:428-433, 1989.
8. Wasserman K: Dyspnea on exertion, *J Am Med Assoc* 248:2039-2043, 1982.
9. Donald KW, Bishop JM, Cumming C, and Wade CL: The effects of exercise on the cardiac output and central dynamics of normal subjects, *Clin Sci* 14:37-73, 1955.
10. Payne PR, Wheeler EF, and Salvosa CB: Prediction of daily energy expenditure from average pulse rate, *Am J Clin Nutr* 24:1164-1170, 1971.
11. Malhotra MS, Gupta JS, and Rao RM: Pulse count as a measure of energy expenditure, *J Appl Physiol* 18:999-1006, 1963.
12. Margaria R, Aghemo P, and Rovelli E: Indirect determination of maximal O_2 consumption in man, *J Appl Physiol* 20:1070-1073, 1965.
13. Blix AS, Stromme SB, and Ursin H: Additional heart rate—An indicator of psychological activation, *Aerospace Med* 45:1219-1222, 1974.
14. Maas S, Kok MLJ, Westra HG, and Kemper HCG: The validity of the use of heart rate in estimating oxygen consumption in static and in combined static/dynamic exercise, *Ergonomics* 32:141-148, 1989.
15. Vokac Z, Bell H, Bautz-Holter E, and Rodahl K: Oxygen uptake/heart rate relationship in leg and arm exercise, sitting and standing, *J Appl Physiol* 39:54-59, 1975.
16. Oja P, Ilmarinen J, and Louhevaara V: Heart rate as an estimator of oxygen consumption during manual postal delivery, *Scand J Work Environ Health* 8:29-36, 1982.
17. Borg G: Perceived exertion: A note on 'history' and methods, *Med Sci Sports* 5:90-93, 1973.
18. Simon PM, Schwartzstein RM, Weiss JW, Fencl U, Teghtsoonian M, and Weinberger SE: Distinguishable types of dyspnea in patients with shortness of breath, *Am Rev Respir Dis* 142:1009-1014, 1990.
19. Pandolf KB, and Noble BJ: The effect of pedalling speed and resistance changes on perceived exertion for equivalent power outputs on the bicycle ergometer, *Med Sci Sports* 5:132-136, 1973.
20. Skinner JS, Hutsler R, Bergsteinova V, and Buskirk ER: The validity and reliability of a rating scale of perceived exertion, *Med Sci Sports* 5:94-96, 1973.
21. Skinner JS, Hutsler R, Bergsteinova V, and Buskirk ER: Perception of effort during different types of exercise and under different environmental conditions, *Med Sci Sports* 5:110-115, 1973.
22. Morgan WP: Psychological factors influencing perceived exertion, *Med Sci Sports* 5:97-103, 1973.

23. Hogan JC, Ogden GD, Gebhardt DL, and Fleishman EA: Reliability and validity of method for evaluating perceived physical effort, *J Appl Psychol* 65:672-679, 1980.

24. Fleishman EA, Gebhardt DL, and Hogan JC: The measurement of effort, *Ergonomics* 27:947-954, 1984.

25. Passmore R, and Durnin JVGA: Human energy expenditure, *Physiol Rev* 35:801-840, 1955.

26. U.S. Department of Labor, Bureau of Employment Security, U.S. Employment Service. Estimates of worker trait requirements for 4,000 jobs as defined in the *Dictionary of Occupational Titles,* Washington, DC, 1957, U.S. Department of Labor.

27. U.S. Department of Labor: *Dictionary of Occupational Titles: Revised 4th Edition,* Washington, DC, 1991, U.S. Government Printing Office.

28. Harber P, Fedoruk M, and Goldberg L: Accommodating respiratory handicaps, *Semin Respir Med* 14:240-249, 1993.

29. Harber P, and Fedoruk M: Work placement and worker fitness: implications of the Americans with Disabilities Act for pulmonary medicine, *Chest* 105:1564-1571, 1994.

Chapter 53

RESPIRATORY IMPAIRMENT AND DISABILITY

Scott Barnhart
John R. Balmes

The evaluation of respiratory impairment and disability seeks to address three questions: Do subjective respiratory symptoms, most commonly dyspnea, correlate with objective measures in the form of decrements in lung function? Has a patient sustained a loss of lung function at a rate greater than expected? Does the degree of impairment prevent the patient from performing the activities of daily living, including gainful employment? In addressing these questions there are a number of uncertainties, but careful attention to a rational approach can usually lead to providing the patient with a clear understanding of the cause of the dyspnea and the limits to which respiratory impairment may adversely affect his or her life.

Frequently, the evaluation of impairment and disability is done in the context of a patient being evaluated for benefits under a disability or entitlement program. These programs will provide benefits to individuals who meet program-specific criteria for the degree of impairment, and in the case of workers' compensation, criteria for attributing the cause of impairment to a workplace exposure. To aid in these evaluations, professional organizations such as the American Thoracic Society (ATS) and the American Medical Association (AMA) have developed detailed guidelines for the evaluation of impairment and disability.[1-3] A knowledge of the detailed requirements of the entitlement system, as well as any rating system required by the entitlement system, is important if a good evaluation is to take place. It is equally important to note that the physician usually does not make the determination as to whether a patient is entitled to benefits. The physician's role is usually to evaluate the patient in a standard format, to make a judgment about the presence or absence of medical diagnoses, and, in the case of workers' compensation, to assess the work-relatedness of the impairment. These results are then provided in a summary report to the administrative agency, and the administrative agency will decide whether the patient is entitled to benefits.

ETHICAL CONSIDERATIONS

The role of the physician in evaluating impairment and disability is often unique. Many patients ask their physicians for assistance in filling out workers' compensation or disability forms. In addition, many entitlement systems require the patient to consult a physician other than his or her own for an independent medical examination (IME). Evaluation of impairment and disability poses several ethical challenges that are best addressed by ensuring that the patient is well informed about the role of the physician in the process.[4]

For physicians who are treating their own patients, it is important to clearly state that their job is to acquire the data in a standard format required by the entitlement system and to review, interpret, and summarize the data objectively in offering their opinions. It is also appropriate for a patient's personal physician who has special knowledge of the unique aspects of his or her condition or care to make information available to the adjudicating agency if it is germane to the patient's level of impairment or disability. By ensuring that patients fully understand their personal physician's role, the risk of significant misunderstanding or future jeopardizing of the physician–patient relationship is minimized.

Physicians who perform IMEs are in a unique relationship with patients, which is often unprecedented in the patient's interaction with the medical system, and may be similarly new to the performing physician. The unique characteristics of an independent medical examiner are that he or she is often selected by the entitlement system rather than the patient, he or she often is not paid by the patient, he or she does not enter a physician–patient relationship, and he or she does not treat the patient beyond making recommendations to the patient's provider or to the requestor of the IME for further care and follow-up. It is extremely important that the patient understand the nature of this relationship: that the physician is required to make a fair and objective assessment. Independent medical examiners, in reviewing their status should also make clear that the results of their reports are available to the patient. This latter aspect may be problematic due to medical–legal constraints but has important ethical implications for physicians who choose to see patients and then do not make the results of their evaluation known to them.

Often, the opinions of independent medical examiners and treating physicians will be contradictory. In this situation, it is important first to recognize that the potential for bias on all sides may exist. For this reason, no single opinion should be treated as final without a very careful review of the data on all sides.

MEDICAL–LEGAL CONSIDERATIONS

The results of evaluations of impairment and disability must often be translated into a format used by an administrative agency or a legal proceeding.[5] A detailed review of the differences between the medical and legal systems is beyond the scope of this section. However, it is important to note that the standard of proof that is commonly accepted is one of "more probable than not." This is quite different from the usual standard of 95% certainty that is applied in medical research. "More probable than not" simply sets a level of proof greater than 50%.

DEFINITIONS

The vocabulary used in impairment and disability is different from that used in everyday medical terminology and often has important implications inherent to the evaluation process. Commonly used definitions include the following:

Dyspnea is the sensation of undue and/or uncomfortable shortness of breath.[6]

Impairment is the reduction of body organ function.[6]

Disability is the inability to engage in any substantial gainful activity by reason of any medically determinable mental or physical impairment or impairments.[6]

Handicap is the disadvantage for a given individual, resulting from impairment or disability, that limits or prevents fulfillment of a role that is normal (depending upon age, sex, and social and cultural factors) for that individual.[7]

Subjective refers to symptoms perceived by the patient only and not evident to the examiner.[8]

Objective refers to findings evident to the examiner in a reproducible manner and not dependent only on the patient's perceptions.

Preexisting refers to any impairment or disease that existed prior to the onset of another disease or impairment (see *Coexisting*).

Coexisting refers to any impairment or disease that exists concurrently with another disease or impairment (see *Preexisting*).

Organic impairment is an impairment explained on the basis of demonstrable abnormality, dysfunction or disease.[6]

Functional impairment is an impairment not explained on the basis of demonstrable abnormality, dysfunction or disease.[6]

Permanent partial disability is a disability at a level less than total disability that is not expected to improve.

Permanent total disability is a disability that prevents gainful employment that is not expected to improve.

Temporary disability is either total or partial disability that is thought to have a high probability of being short-term and thus can be expected to improve to a higher level of function.

CLINICAL CONSIDERATIONS

When the sensation of undue dyspnea becomes the rate-limiting factor for an individual to perform exertionally related activities, particularly gainful employment, the patient will seek medical evaluation. It is important to recognize that the patient's perception of dyspnea means much more to him or her than objective measures in either the respiratory system or other organ system. Patients care about being short of breath, not about a reduction in their forced expiratory volume in 1 second (FEV1). Entitlement systems, however, almost uniformly rely upon objective measures to base determination of disability. It is important for the physician to recognize the distinction between the subjective symptoms perceived by a patient and the objective measures required by entitlement systems, and to seek to reconcile the subjective with the objective to the greatest extent possible. When these cannot be reconciled, it is important also to recognize that the genesis of dyspnea is a complicated process incorporating both physiologic and psychologic inputs. For this reason, the inability to fully explain dyspnea on the basis of objective measures does not necessarily invalidate the symptom, even though that symptom may not meet the test required for compensation under an entitlement system.

Turning briefly to the physiologic underpinnings of dyspnea, there are several key inputs to consider in defining the clinical approach. Dyspnea can be elicited by stimulation of central chemoreceptors to arterial P_{CO_2} and, to a far lesser degree, changes in arterial P_{O_2}.[9,10] Stimulation of peripheral chemoreceptors may also result in dyspnea. Alterations in lung volume may stimulate stretch receptors, and changes in vascular pressure may stimulate C-receptor fibers. Additionally, mechanical receptors within the respiratory muscles may result in dyspnea when stimulated. The above inputs in the setting of increased minute ventilation are integrated to produce the sensation of dyspnea.

There are many disease processes within the upper and lower airways, as well as the pulmonary vasculature, that may contribute to the symptoms of dyspnea.[11,12] The measurement of dyspnea poses a substantial challenge to the clinician. It is crucial that the clinician recognize that the correlation of dyspnea with objective measures of impairment is modest.[13,14] Furthermore, mild dyspnea, which may be correlated with mild respiratory impairment, often does not represent disability with respect to the patient's current employment. For example, most white-collar jobs could be performed by patients with moderate respiratory impairment. However, jobs that require high exertion, such as performing heavy labor at a construction site, require sufficiently high cardiopulmonary capacity to not permit workers with impairment in either organ system to perform adequately.

Some reasons behind the lack of correlation between dyspnea and objective measures include the limitations in measuring dyspnea using dyspnea scales, the multiple physiologic inputs and organ systems that are integrated to cause dyspnea, the presence or absence of anxiety or other physiologic factors, and, rarely, the presence of malingering.

Dyspnea scales

The attempt to develop scales to characterize dyspnea has met with limited success.[3,11,14-18] The major utility of dyspnea scales is to provide an indication of whether the extent of dyspnea may be explained by the available objective measures. When the dyspnea cannot be sufficiently explained, it is important to proceed with further evaluation.

Dyspnea usually arises from limitations in either the respiratory or the cardiac system. Whereas acknowledging the important role of the cardiovascular system in the genesis of dyspnea, a discussion of those factors is beyond the scope of this chapter. The main pulmonary function tests used for categorizing dyspnea include spirometry, maximal voluntary ventilation (MVV), single breath diffusing capacity, and exercise capacity. None of these tests is a strong predictor of dyspnea.[13]

When assessing dyspnea scales, it is important to remember that subjective estimates of dyspnea occurring during or at the end of exertion are better correlated with measures of physiologic impairment than dyspnea recorded when the subject was at rest.[13] In addition, patient estimates of their maximal exercise capacity measured by exercise testing are relatively poor.[12,14] Similarly, neither spirometry, diffusion capacity of the lung for carbon monoxide (DLCO), nor MVV are strong predictors of oxygen consumption ($\dot{V}O_2$) max.

Malingering

Respiratory impairment has been characterized as resulting from physiologic and/or psychologic factors or, respectively, organic versus functional factors.[19] Because the evaluation of impairment and disability frequently involves potential for secondary gain, the issue of a patient malingering need always be considered. Organic impairment is defined by the presence of objective measures indicating respiratory impairment or disease. These physiologic or organic factors may include both respiratory diseases and nonrespiratory diseases, as seen with reduced oxygen delivery in the setting of cardiac failure or anemia. Where the dyspnea cannot be measured objectively, the possibility that it is based on psychologic factors must be entertained. Functional impairment is impairment that cannot be objectively measured. There are several explanations. Clearly, dyspnea is multifactorial, representing the integration of psychologic factors (e.g., anxiety) as well as physiologic factors. Objective measures are not able to fully explain all cases of dyspnea and are potentially insensitive as tests. Dyspnea may be falsely reported, as in the case of outright fraud, although in the author's experience this is quite rare. It is also possible that subconscious factors may result in amplification of dyspnea.[20]

In one important study of patients applying for compensation, it was noted that for a given level of dyspnea, those who were applying for compensation had higher levels of

FEV1.[21] These patients were also noted to have higher body masses. Although it would be incorrect to interpret that these patients applying for workers' compensation were malingering or committing fraud, medical examiners must acknowledge the potential for dyspnea to be consciously or unconsciously overestimated.

Given the inability for pulmonary function tests to fully predict dyspnea, most entitlement systems make an arbitrary decision to base ratings of impairment solely on results of objective measures.

There are several steps that may be of help when malingering is a concern. It is crucial to ensure the patient understands the goals of the evaluation so that a lack of understanding of the purpose or the performance of pulmonary function tests is not misclassified as malingering. Next, the careful review of tests to ensure that the patient has made a good effort will help assess the validity of the results. In addition, exercise testing, including a comparison of ventilatory rate, heart rate, ventilatory reserves, and work rate at maximal exercise period may aid in determining the level of effort. There is no perfect test, however, to identify malingering. Fortunately, frank malingering is rare, and a careful evaluation can usually provide the examiner with a good estimate of a patient's capabilities.

THE CLASSIFICATION OF IMPAIRMENT AND DISABILITY

The classification of impairment and disability depends upon the goal of the evaluation period. If it is simply to evaluate a patient's dyspnea and whether it may be explained by objective measures of physiologic impairment and related diagnoses, then simple scales of dyspnea and an understanding of the range of pulmonary function tests that correlate with that level of dyspnea will suffice. Often, however, the nature of the evaluation depends upon the requirements of an entitlement system. The examiner is required to meet the specifications of the entitlement system. Many entitlement programs recommend that respiratory impairment be classified according to guidelines provided by professional organizations such as the AMA, the ATS, the Canadian Medical Association (CMA), or the European Society for Clinical Respiratory Physiology.[1-3,22,23]

There are many entitlement programs, including social security disability insurance, workers' compensation, and state-based eligibility programs. Under the heading of workers' compensation, there are multiple systems, including state-based workers' compensation, federal Office of Workers' Compensation Programs, specific programs for shipyard and railway workers, and the Veteran's Administration. Under all workers' compensation systems there is a necessary requirement that impairment be attributed, usually on a "more probable than not" basis, to a workplace illness or injury.

Another program that requires impairment and disability evaluations is third-party litigation under the tort system. In addition, many individuals carry their own personal disability insurance, or employers may offer disability insurance. Finally, there may be state and municipal programs, such as eligibility for bus passes or disabled parking license plates, that depend on an impairment and disability evaluation. As is apparent from the preceding discussion, the evaluation of impairment and disability truly represents the intersection between medical evaluations and legal and administrative rules. Furthermore, the passage of the Americans with Disabilities Act (ADA) is changing the nature of what is recognized as impairment and disability and the accommodation offered to those with impairments.

Although the systems for the evaluation of impairment and disability are many, the most widely recognized and accepted system is the Guides to Evaluation of Permanent Impairment published by the AMA.[3]

The American Medical Association's Guides to Evaluation of Permanent Impairment

The AMA's *Guides to Evaluation of Permanent Impairment* represents a comprehensive system for evaluating impairment in all organ systems. Where impairment exists in more than one organ system, a method is provided to determine the percentage of total bodily impairment.

For the purpose of evaluating respiratory impairment, the guides make specific recommendations with respect to the medical history, physical examination, and laboratory tests. Under the guides, there are four classes of respiratory impairment, as shown in Table 53-1.[3] The four classes of respiratory impairment are normal, mild, moderate, and severe. Each of these impairment categories is linked to specific ranges of results from spirometry, DLCO, or $\dot{V}O_2$ max derived from exercise testing. Minimal laboratory evaluation under the guides includes spirometry and diffusing capacity. Subjective levels of dyspnea, chest radiographs, and routine arterial blood gas testing are not recommended. Resting hypoxemia with Pao_2 of less than 50 mm Hg, or a Pao_2 of less than 60 mm Hg along with either pulmonary hypertension or cor pulmonale, represents severe impairment.

Exercise testing is primarily reserved for those cases where subjective symptoms, such as dyspnea, are out of proportion to the objective tests. Of note, the DLCO is largely beneficial in the setting of interstitial lung disease, and corroboration with exercise testing is recommended. The ATS approaches exercise testing and maximal oxygen consumption somewhat differently.[2] Under the ATS guidelines, workers are judged able to perform their jobs comfortably when the $\dot{V}O_2$ requirements of a specific job are less than 40% of the patient's $\dot{V}O_2$ max. However, it is important to note the purpose of the disability evaluation. This "rule of thumb" is quite useful when the purpose of the im-

Table 53-1. AMA classes of respiratory impairment

Class 1: 0% no impairment of the whole person	Class 2: mild impairment of the whole person	Class 3: moderate impairment of the whole person	Class 4: severe impairment of the whole person
FVC ≥ 80% of predicted and	FVC between 60% and 79% of predicted or	FVC between 51% and 59% of predicted or	FVC ≤ 50% of predicted or
FEV1 ≥ 80% of predicted and	FEV1 between 60% and 79% of predicted or	FEV1 between 41% and 59% of predicted or	FEV1 ≤ 40% of predicted or
FEV1/FVC ≥ 70% and DLCO ≥ 70% of predicted or	FEV1/FVC between 60% and 69% or	FEV1/FVC between 41% and 59% or	FEV1/FVC ≤ 40% or
	DLCO between 60% and 79% of predicted or	DLCO between 41% and 59% of predicted or	DLCO ≤ 40% of predicted or
$\dot{V}O_2$ max > 25 ml/(kg-min)	$\dot{V}O_2$ max between 20 and 25 ml/(kg-min)	$\dot{V}O_2$ max between 15 and 20 ml/(kg-min)	$\dot{V}O_2$ max < 15 ml/(kg-min) or <1.05 L/min

DLCO, Diffusion capacity of the lung for carbon monoxide; *FEV1,* forced expiratory volume in 1 second; *FVC,* forced vital capacity; $\dot{V}O_2$, oxygen consumption.

pairment and disability evaluation is to identify whether a patient can perform a specific job. Often, however, the question posed to the examiner is whether a specific loss of function has occurred, regardless of whether the patient can perform the job. If the latter is the question to be addressed, then this "rule of thumb" of performing a job with a $\dot{V}O_2$ requirement at 40% of the patient's $\dot{V}O_2$ max is not relevant.

The ATS has made recommendations for the evaluation of impairment and disability due to asthma.[24] These recommendations provide important information and are probably more in line with modern day practice and care of patients with asthma than the more limited guidelines provided by the AMA. The ATS protocol for evaluating asthma incorporates data from three categories to determine the level of impairment among five classes. The three categories of data considered include the postbronchodilator FEV1, a measure of airway responsiveness based upon the reversibility of FEV1 following inhalation of a bronchodilator or the provocative concentration of methacholine or histamine that results in a 20% decline in FEV1, and, finally, the medication requirements when the patient is receiving optimal therapy. Each of these major categories receives a weighted score that is summed to determine the final level, as shown in Table 53-2.

The selection of the impairment level is usually performed by seeking the best fit between the levels of impairment and the results of pulmonary function tests. This does permit some freedom for the examiner, who must use good judgment in making the final determination. For example, in the setting of interstitial lung disease, it is very possible that the FEV1, forced vital capacity (FVC), and DLCO will all be reduced proportionally. In the case of diseases characterized by an obstructive defect, it is very possible to have a substantially reduced FEV1 and a normal FVC. In this setting, it would be inappropriate to look to the FVC and use that to determine the level of impairment.

Timing and use of predicted normals under the American Medical Association's Guides

Evaluations for impairment should occur when the patient is at a fixed and stable point, and not in an exacerbation of his or her illness. Protocols for spirometry and DLCO developed by the ATS set the standards for these tests. In addition, spirometry should be performed after bronchodilator.

The AMA Guides recommend using percent of predicted normal for the assessment of abnormality of the FEV1, FVC, and DLCO. The ratio of the FEV1 to the FVC is assessed as an absolute value. Predicted normal equations provided by Crapo for spirometric values and for DLCO form the basis of the AMA rating.[25,26] For the evaluation of patients who are of African or Asian descent, the Guides recommend that the predicted normal value be multiplied by 0.9. Although this recommendation is based on population-based studies, the lumping of multiple ethnicities under these broad categories as well as the issue of mixed race descent leave this area open to questions. Some examiners may prefer to use one set of predicted normals for all patients while openly acknowledging the difficulties of generalizing from predicted normals to the assessment of abnormality in a single patient.

Evaluation of specific diseases

Several disease processes are singled out for individual recommendations. Under the Guides, asthma is characterized as severe if three successive measures each spaced 1 week apart are at a level of Class Four, or severe impairment. Where sensitizers are a factor, the importance of preventing further exposure to those sensitizers is also noted. Similarly, those patients who are felt to have hypersensitivity pneumonitis are not recommended to have further exposure to the likely antigen. In the case of a pneumoconioses diagnosis, regardless of the level of impairment, further exposure to the culpable dust is not recommended. Noting

Table 53-2. ATS asthma impairment rating scheme

2a: Postbronchodilator FEV1*

FEV1 (% predicted)

>lower limit of normal
70–lower limit of normal
60-69
50-59
<50

2b: Reversibility of FEV1 or degree of airway hyperresponsiveness*

% FEV1 change	PC_{20} mg/ml
<10	>8
10-19	8->0.5
20-29	0.5->0.125
≥30	≤0.125

2c: Minimum medication needed†

Score	Medication
0	No medication
1	Occasional bronchodilator, not daily, and/or occasional cromolyn, not daily
2	Daily bronchodilator, and/or daily cromolyn, and/or daily low-dose inhaled steroid (<800 μg beclomethasone or equivalent)
3	Bronchodilator on demand and daily high-dose inhaled steroid (>800 μg beclomethsone or equivalent), or occasional course systemic steroid
4	Bronchodilator on demand, daily high-dose inhaled steroid (>1000 μg beclomethasone or equivalent), and daily systemic steroid

2d: Summary impairment rating classes (the impairment rating is calculated as the sum of the patient's scores from 2a, 2b, and 2c)

Impairment class	Total score
0	0
I	1-3
II	4-6
III	7-9
IV	10-11
V	Asthma not controlled despite maximal treatment (i.e., FEV1 remaining <50% despite use of ≥20 mg prednisone/day)

*When postbronchodilator forced expiratory volume in 1 second (FEV1) is above the lower limit of normal, PC_{20} should be determined and used for rating of impairment; when postbronchodilator FEV1 is <70% predicted, the degree of reversibility should be used; when FEV1 is between 70% predicted and the lower limit of normal, either reversibility or PC_{20} can be used.

†The need for minimum medication should be demonstrated by the treating physician (e.g., previous records of exacerbation when medications have been reduced).

the multiorgan effects of sleep apnea syndrome, the Guides recommend that impairments in each of the systems affected (e.g., nervous system, cardiovascular system, respiratory system, and mental or behavioral disorders) be assessed and combined under the formula noted in the Guide for impairment in multiple organ systems. Patients with lung cancer also receive special consideration. At the time of diagnosis, those with lung cancer are considered severely impaired. If, following treatment, at 1 year the patient is noted to be free of disease, respiratory impairment is rated based on the four classes. If the cancer recurs, the patient is again categorized as severely impaired.

Disability systems

Disability assessment is performed under several distinct administrative systems. The system employed affects the type of data collected and the manner in which they are used.

Some systems (e.g., the U.S. Social Security Disability Insurance System) do not require determination of causation of the respiratory disease; assessment is made only of its physiologic impact. Conversely, most workers' compensation systems in the United States require explicit assessment of the specific medical diagnosis and also of the degree to which it is work related.

When causation is an issue to be resolved, some systems allow disability compensation only if the putative causative agent is on a prescribed list, whereas others consider each case individually. To a large degree, British systems depend upon scheduled lists, whereas American systems tend to be less structured. Furthermore, certain respiratory disability assessment systems are limited to diseases due to a specific agent (e.g., coal-related disease).

Some systems seek to determine the presence or absence of only complete and total impairment, whereas others mandate considering the full range of impairment. Generally, workers' compensation requires rating of the degree of partial disability.

The flexibility of assessment varies among systems. Some are nearly completely prescriptive, describing in detail which tests are to be performed as well as the criteria for their interpretation. For example, under Social Security, the patient's test results are compared with specific criteria values in tables. Other systems, such as tort evaluations in the United States, have no preset criteria. In such circumstances, there may be conflicts of opinion about the significance of minor deviations from average values for parameters such as midexpiratory flow rates. In some settings, scheduled awards are made, in which the amount of compensation is determined from tables based solely on lung function tests, whereas in other situations, physician or patient opinion very much influences the degree of compensation.

To facilitate processing, some systems employ presumptions. These are rules that define work relatedness on administrative rather than medical basis. For example, in the United States, lung function abnormalities in individuals in the coal industry covered by the Black Lung laws are automatically presumed to be work related. Such presumptions are occasionally rebuttable if one or another side of a case can demonstrate that the presumption is inaccurate.

Systems differ administratively. Pneumoconiosis Medical Panels may be employed, in which a predesignated panel of expert physicians (occasionally government employees) examines each case and jointly reaches conclusions about causation and degree of disability. Such methods are rarely used in the United States, in which individual physicians evaluate cases. This leads to more controversy. The efficiency and consistency of the Panel approach have led many to favor it. In addition, these also (theoretically) ensure that the examiner has the necessary expertise. However, evaluation by individual physicians is felt by many to be essential to ensure fairness to both workers and their employers. The possibility of undue political influence on Panels raises concerns; in addition, Panels may become fixed in thought patterns and slow to adapt new information. Many in the United States quote the Black Lung regulations as an example of a compensation system in which political motives have superseded scientific considerations. Hybrid systems also exist, in which government evaluators (occasionally physicians) review records and may request an examination by an independent physician if needed; the U.S. Railroad Retirement Board illustrates this method.

In summary, there are very significant differences in how respiratory disability assessments are conducted. These range from rigid government-based systems in which a small number of designated "experts" evaluate each case using predesignated criteria for disease due to agents on a specific list to highly adversarial systems with few if any agreed-upon criteria.

Specific entitlement systems: Social Security disability insurance

The Social Security Disability Insurance Program and the Supplemental Security Income (SSI) program are both administered by the Federal Social Security Administration.[27] The Social Security Disability Insurance Program provides disability benefits to patients who have made regular contributions to Social Security. In addition, to prevent disabled persons from becoming destitute, the Social Security Supplemental Income Program provides benefits to persons who have severe impairment and meet specific criteria with respect to fiscal assets. Eligibility for either program is based upon the presence of severe impairment for a period of at least 1 year.

Social Security provides specific criteria for three broad categories of respiratory impairment. These are chronic obstructive pulmonary disease, chronic restrictive ventilatory disorders, and chronic impairment of gas exchange. As shown in Tables 53-3, 53-4, and 53-5, the criteria for eligi-

Table 53-3. Social Security disability rating scheme for COPD

Height without shoes (inches)	FEV1 equal to or less than	MVV equal to or less than (L/min)
60 or less	1.0	40
61-63	1.1	44
64-65	1.2	48
66-67	1.3	52
68-69	1.4	56
70-71	1.5	60
72 or more	1.6	64

COPD, Chronic obstructive pulmonary disease; *FEV1,* forced expiratory volume in 1 second; *MVV,* maximal voluntary ventilation.

Table 53-4. Social Security disability rating scheme for restrictive disorders

Height without shoes (inches)	VC equal to or less than
60 or less	1.2
61-63	1.3
64-65	1.4
66-67	1.5
68-69	1.6
70-71	1.7
72 or more	1.8

VC, Vital capacity.

bility for each category are quite strict. Moreover, the lack of adjustment for age or sex biases these criteria against males and those of younger age groups. Another specific disorder considered under Social Security is asthma. Criteria for severe asthma impairment may be met either under the criteria for obstructive disorders or by noting the presence of severe asthmatic attacks an average of six times per year with wheezing present in the interval periods. This strict criterion should be reviewed against the graduated spectrum of impairment provided under the more recently defined ATS guidelines, which require that the patient receive optimal therapy and consider several parameters in determining impairment. It should be noted that there are few asthmatics who, when optimally treated, would meet the SSI criteria, and those who do likely deserve a second opinion to determine whether medical therapy is optimal. Patients with pneumoconiosis, bronchiectasis, or mycobacterial disease also receive special consideration but generally should be reviewed under the criteria for restrictive or obstructive diseases.

There are specific criteria provided for evaluating patients with cor pulmonale. Finally, many patients have multiple diseases contributing to their total impairment, and these should all be considered in the report documenting

Table 53-5. Social Security disability rating schemes for disorders of gas exchange*,†

Arterial P_{CO_2} (mm Hg) and	Arterial P_{O_2} equal to or less than (mm Hg)
Applicable at test sites less than 3,000 feet above sea level	
37	58
38	57
39	56
40 or above	55
Applicable at test sites 3,000 to 5,000 feet above sea level	
37	53
38	52
39	51
40 or above	50
Applicable at test sites over 6,000 feet above sea level	
30 or below	55
31	54
32	53
33	52
34	51
35	50
36	49
37	48
38	47
39	46
40 or above	45

*Steady-state exercise blood gases demonstrating values of Pa_{O_2} and simultaneously determined Pa_{CO_2}, measured at a workload of approximately 17 ml O_2/kg/min or less of exercise, equal to or less than the values specified in the table.

†Diffusing capacity for the lungs for carbon monoxide less than 6 ml/mm Hg/min (steady-state methods) or less than 9 ml/mm Hg/min (single breath method) or less than 30% of predicted normal. All methods, actual values, and predicted normal values for the methods used should be reported.

impairment. Providers and patients should also be aware that an initial rejection of a claim for benefits under Social Security leaves open the door for an appeal, which may substantially increase the patient's chance of receiving benefits.[28,29]

Workers' compensation

Workers' compensation covers a broad range of, but not all, occupations. Central to workers' compensation is attributing a disease and impairment related to that disease on a "more probable than not" basis to an occupational exposure.[5,30] Understanding the broad range of workers' compensation systems and multiple different requirements under each system for both the provider and the patient can be likened to obtaining health benefits in the current era of health care reform—too many requirements with too little coverage. There are separate workers' compensation systems in each state; within states not all workers may be covered, and there may be state insurance funds, self insurance

by large companies, and third party insurance provided by large insurance companies. Shipyard workers, railway workers, federal workers, veterans, and seafarers all operate under different systems. It is essential that the patient and provider determine under which system a claim for benefits may be filed and also the specific requirements of the system. It is also important to note that railway workers and merchant mariners are covered under liability acts where the worker must obtain the services of an attorney to file a claim.

As mentioned earlier, the key criterion for receiving benefits is attribution of the illness and impairment on a "more probable than not" basis to a workplace exposure. Given limitations in the current knowledge of occupational illnesses, the multifactorial nature of disease causation and the frequent long latency between exposure and disease, attribution is a difficult task that often requires balancing a number of uncertainties. For this reason claims for occupational illnesses are frequently contested.[28] It is also important for physicians to note their role in workers' compensation claims. Physicians are obligated to diagnose and treat work-related illness, and when attributing illness to an occupational exposure, to inform the patient, and to assist with the appropriate documentation to file claims for benefits. The awarding of benefits, however, is an administrative matter that is out of the control of the physician. An especially important point to be aware of is that the physician must be clear of the level of certainty at which an attribution to workplace exposure is made. As noted above, the test is on a "more probable than not" basis; thus, indicating that a disease is possibly related (less than 50% probability) will, in most situations, result in no benefit being awarded. On the other hand, a level of certainty higher than "more probable than not" (e.g., 95% certainty) is not required. Often, physicians are faced with situations where further exposure may result in immediate or long-term harm to the patient. For example, patients with occupational asthma who continue to be reexposed may have an immediate risk due to a severe asthmatic reaction, or may also risk greater long-term impairment as a result of their continued exposure. In this situation physicians may need to discuss in detail with the patients early removal from work and placement on temporary total disability. Ideally, one would have a workers' compensation system that would adjudicate such matters and approve benefits, including the time loss for temporary total disability, without delay. Many workers' compensation cases, however, drag on for weeks, months, and sometimes years, and thus the physician and patient often need to make a decision about removal from work on the best available evidence prior to adjudication of the claim. Given these real life situations, it is important for the physician to explain the process carefully to the patient, including who determines the awarding of benefits, as well as the medical facts for consideration and the extent to which the physician is able to support the claim. A physician should be extremely careful about removing a patient from work, especially if he or she is not willing to strongly support the patient for benefits under workers' compensation. To do less is potentially to jeopardize the patient's livelihood.

Department of Veterans Affairs

The Veterans Administration provides disability to those veterans who have service-connected injuries or illnesses. Under the Veterans Administration there is a highly codified rating system for impairment where specific diseases are rated on a 0% to 100% basis.[31] Ratings are based on both clinical symptoms and objective measures of lung function. However, because specific levels of pulmonary function are not tied directly to levels of impairment, there is ample opportunity for the evaluating physician to interpret the results. Provided in Table 53-6 are rating schedules for common respiratory diseases.

Black Lung Benefits Act

The Black Lung Act is designed to provide benefits for disability among coal miners. The basic evaluation includes chest roentgenograms, physical examination, and pulmonary function tests (including arterial blood gas measurement).[32] Chest radiographs are classified under the International Labor Office system.[33] There are also alternative methods under which one may become eligible. These include histologic evidence of pneumoconiosis, or, in the face a negative chest radiograph, a finding by a physician that the miner suffers impairment attributable to a pneumoconiosis. Miners may be eligible by presumption if they have been employed for a minimum of 15 years and have a totally disabling respiratory impairment, regardless of cause.

Benefits are provided to eligible miners or dependents who are considered totally disabled. Those who cannot perform usual coal mine work or other gainful employment available in their immediate area of residence are considered totally disabled.[32] Specific criteria for pulmonary function tests are also included based on the regression equations of Knudsen et al.[34] When compared with the reference values used by the ATS and the AMA, total disability is defined as an FEV1 of approximately 58% of predicted.[2,3,25] It should be emphasized that there is opportunity for physicians to provide input.

CLINICAL APPROACH TO THE EVALUATION OF RESPIRATORY IMPAIRMENT

The approach to evaluating patients for respiratory impairment follows the standard medical history and physical and laboratory evaluation. There are, however, several caveats. As noted, the specific requirements of the system under which benefits may be sought should be reviewed and addressed. Where workers' compensation may be a consideration, attribution to a workplace exposure becomes an important point in the evaluation. Finally, the approach should seek to explain fully the physiologic underpinnings of dyspnea and resort to attributing dyspnea to functional factors as a last resort.

Medical history

The medical history should be a comprehensive history with additional specific attention to respiratory symptoms, including dyspnea, cough, production of phlegm, chest tightness, and wheezing. The usual characterization of intensity, onset, duration, and progression should be noted. It may be beneficial to try to categorize the extent of dyspnea according to either the questions of the ATS Epidemiology Standardization Project[17] or those provided by the AMA (see Table 53-7).

The medical history should also assess symptoms related to the cardiovascular system in detail and include the usual review of systems and past medical history.

The occupational history should focus on a detailed description of the current job, including exposures and use of personal protective equipment. Where there are questions regarding the exposures, the patient should be asked to bring in material safety data sheets (MSDS) for each exposure. The use of personal protective equipment, the availability of facilities for personal hygiene, and a separate area to eat meals should also be ascertained. A detailed listing of all prior jobs should also be made.

The work history should review whether there is a temporal association between symptoms and exposures. The examiner should keep in mind that important points for attributing a disease to a workplace exposure include the following steps: (1) obtaining a diagnosis, (2) identifying a potential exposure that could be a plausible cause of the disease, (3) excluding other potential causes of the disease, and (4) identifying whether there is an appropriate temporal relationship between the exposure and disease, as well as an appropriate dose and duration of the exposure.

Avocational activities should be reviewed in the history. Some patients may have hobbies that expose them to high levels of fumes, dust, or chemicals. A detailed smoking history should be obtained. Additionally, a review of other habits, including ethanol usage and inhaled substance abuse, should be made. The patient and the physician should keep in mind that the medical record may not be kept fully confidential in workers' compensation cases and other medical legal matters, and it may become available to the insurance company, employer, or other party. For this reason, while it is important that appropriate pertinent medical information be part of the file, the inclusion of material not relevent to the evaluation should be approached with the limits of confidentiality under workers' compensation in mind.

Physical examination

Physical examinations should include a thorough physical examination with a strong emphasis on the respiratory and cardiovascular systems. The pertinent positives and negatives should be included in the report.

Table 53-6. Veterans Administration rating schedule for chronic obstructive pulmonary disease, asthma, and pneumoconiosis

	Rating
Chronic bronchitis	
Pronounced—With copious productive cough and dyspnea at rest; pulmonary function testing showing a severe degree of chronic airway obstruction; with symptoms of associated severe emphysema or cyanosis and findings of right-sided heart involvement	100
Severe—With severe productive cough and dyspnea on slight exertion and pulmonary function tests indicative of severe ventilatory impairment	60
Moderately severe—Persistent cough at intervals throughout the day, considerable expectoration, considerable dyspnea on exercise, rales throughout the chest, beginning chronic airway obstruction	30
Moderate—Considerable night or morning cough, slight dyspnea on exercise, scattered bilateral rales	10
Mild—Slight cough, no dyspnea, few rales	0
Bronchiectasis	
Pronounced—Symptoms in aggravated form, marked emphysema, dyspnea at rest or on slight exertion, cyanosis, marked loss of weight or other evidence of severe impairment of general health	100
Severe—With considerable emphysema, impairment in general health manifested by loss of weight, anemia, or occasional pulmonary hemorrhages; occasional exacerbations of a few days duration, with fever, are to be expected; demonstrated by lipoidol injection and layer sputum test	60
Moderate—Persistent paroxysmal cough at intervals throughout the day, abundant purulent and fetid expectoration, slight, if any, emphysema or loss of weight	30
Asthma	
Pronounced—Asthmatic attacks very frequently with severe dyspnea on slight exertion between attacks and with marked loss of weight or other evidence of severe impairment of health	100
Severe—Frequent attacks of asthma (one or more attacks weekly), marked dyspnea on exertion between attacks with only temporary relief by medication; more than light manual labor precluded	60
Moderate—Asthmatic attacks rather frequent (separated by only 10-14 day intervals) with moderate dyspnea on exertion between attacks	30
Mild—Paroxysms of asthmatic type breathing (high pitched expiratory wheezing and dyspnea) occurring several times a year with no clinical findings between attacks	10
NOTE: In the absence of clinical findings at time of examination, a verified history of asthmatic attacks must be of record.	
Emphysema	
Pronounced—Intractable and totally incapacitating; with dyspnea at rest, or marked dyspnea and cyanosis on mild exertion; severity of emphysema confirmed by chest x-rays and pulmonary function tests	100
Severe—Exertional dyspnea sufficient to prevent climbing one flight of steps or walking one block without stopping; ventilatory impairment of severe degree confirmed by pulmonary function tests with marked impairment of health	60
Moderate—With moderate dyspnea occurring after climbing one flight of steps or walking more than one block on level surface; pulmonary function tests consistent with findings of moderate emphysema	30
Mild—With evidence of ventilatory impairment on pulmonary function tests and/or defined dyspnea on prolonged exertion	10
Pneumoconiosis	
Pronounced—With extent of lesions comparable with far advanced pulmonary tuberculosis or pulmonary function tests confirming a markedly severe degree of ventilatory deficit; with dyspnea at rest and other evidence of severe impairment of bodily vigor producing total incapacity	100
Severe—Extensive fibrosis, severe dyspnea on slight exertion with corresponding ventilatory deficit confirmed by pulmonary function tests with marked impairment of health	60
Moderate—With considerable pulmonary fibrosis and moderate dyspnea on slight exertion, confirmed by pulmonary function tests	30
Definitely symptomatic with pulmonary fibrosis and moderate dyspnea on extended exertion	10

Table 53-7. AMA classification of dyspnea

Mild	Dyspnea is present with fast walking on level ground or walking up a slight hill; the person can keep pace with other persons of same age and body build on level ground but not on hills or stairs
Moderate	Dyspnea is present while walking on level ground with persons of the same age and body build or walking up one flight of stairs
Severe	Dyspnea is present after the person walks more than 4 to 5 minutes at own pace on level ground; the person may be short of breath with less exertion, or even at rest

Laboratory tests

Chest radiographs are of limited use in assessing impairment. They are, however, an important component in assessing the presence of pulmonary, as well as extrapulmonary, disease. In the vast majority of cases, a chest radiograph should be obtained. Where pneumoconiosis is suspected, the film should be read by a physician trained in the classification of pneumoconioses according to the system of the International Labor Office.[33]

Pulmonary function tests

Spirometry forms the cornerstone of the impairment evaluation based on pulmonary function tests. Lung volumes, arterial blood gas, single breath diffusion capacity, and exercise play important roles as well. Spirometry and diffusing capacity measurements should be performed according to the ATS recommended standards.[35-37] One should note, however, that there are limitations in the predictive value of spirometry and the other tests, including DLCO, in predicting exercise capacity as measured by $\dot{V}O_2$ max.[38-41] Of measurements of lung volume, FVC provides the best measure in conjunction with FEV1. Of additional importance is the use of predictive equations. The ATS and the AMA recommend the use of predictive equations by Crapo and colleagues.[25,26] Of note, however, the Black Lung Act is based on the use of regression equations by Knudsen et al.[34] Although the use of specific predictive equations may or may not be required by a particular entitlement system, it is important for the examiner to recognize that there are some relatively small variations among predictive equations when used for spirometry and that they are much larger with DLCO.[42]

As noted above, the AMA also recommends a correction factor for patients of African or Asian descent. The correction factor involves multiplying the predicted value for Caucasians by 0.9.[3] Although there is substantial documentation in the literature for the occurrence of ethnic variations and variations based on gender, the use of correction factors should be approached with caution. It should be recognized that the aggregation of all Africans and all Asians into a single ethnic group and the issue of mixed racial descent limit the generalizability of this adjustment.

Finally, the single breath diffusion capacity frequently has marked intralaboratory variability. For this reason it is recommended that careful attention be directed at test performance according to the ATS criteria.[36] In reporting results, the ATS recommends that laboratories use the regression equations of Crapo and Morris.[26] These results should be adjusted to a standard hemoglobin ratio of 12.8 g/dl for women, and 14.6 g/dl for men. When corrected for severe anemia or erythrocytosis, uncorrected values should be reported as well. In addition to respiratory diseases, other factors may affect the DLCO, including hemoglobin concentration and altitude. Most important, however, is the performance of the test, which requires inspiration of 90% of the vital capacity and a standardized breathholding time. Of these two factors, diminished inspiratory volume is by far the most important.

Arterial blood gas measurement

There is relatively poor correlation between resting arterial Pa_{O_2} and exercise capacity. The ATS statement recommends that the Pa_{O_2} be considered only in cases that straddle two classes of impairment.[2] Because arterial hypoxemia shows great variability, it is recommended that at least two measurements at least 4 weeks apart be obtained.

Exercise testing

When the purpose of loss of function is the goal of the evaluation, there is frequently little need for exercise testing. On the other hand, when the goal is to determine whether a patient can perform a job with a known energy requirement, then exercise testing has great utility if the answer is not obvious from spirometry and DLCO, or from the patient's history. However, there are limitations to directly tying maximal oxygen consumption with work.[43] For example, if the patient describes an active occupational and avocational lifestyle, has no respiratory complaints, and has normal spirometry and DLCO, there is likely little to be gained by exercise testing. On the other hand, patients may have modest impairments in spirometry or DLCO and still be capable of performing a wide variety of jobs with substantial energy requirements. For these latter patients, exercise testing provides a valuable tool to overcome the recognized limitations in spirometry and DLCO in predicting exercise tolerance.[39,40,44] Along these lines, the ATS recommends using exercise testing in those situations where the static pulmonary function tests, such as spirometry and DLCO, may underestimate the level of the patient's impairment.[2] In summary, exercise testing is useful to determine a worker's exercise capacity, but it is not useful in situations where the goal is to determine objectively the loss of function, in situations where the patient clearly has a severe respiratory impairment, or in those instances where history, physical examination, and static lung function test demonstrate normal respiratory function.[40]

An advantage of exercise testing is that it does give, in a standardized fashion, a measure of oxygen consumption that may be related to a patient's job. Additionally, patients may be directly observed, and there are several parameters to examine that may indicate both the extent of patient effort and other causes of dyspnea. In particular, examination of the work rate, $\dot{V}O_2$ max, heart rate, oxygen pulse, anaerobic threshold, and V_d/V_t all are of use. Direct measurements of arterial blood gas, oxygen concentration in mixed expired gas, and total minute ventilation are preferred over extrapolations from work rate, heart rate, and submaximal test results.

There has been considerable controversy over whether exercise tests should be maximal, symptom limited tests or submaximal tests.[1,2,40,44,45] While substantial information may be derived from submaximal tests, determination of maximal work capacity is by extrapolation. This may result in underestimation of $\dot{V}O_2$ max.[45] Given the controversy, it is reasonable to follow the ATS recommendation for maximal exercise tests.[2]

Whether $\dot{V}O_2$ max has been estimated or directly measured, the value may be used to determine the patient's ability to perform a job based on the energy requirements for that work.[46-50] Exercise physiologists generally feel that a patient can work for an 8-hour shift at a level of energy expenditure that is 40% of his or her $\dot{V}O_2$ max. In general, a patient whose $\dot{V}O_2$ max is 25 ml/kg/min or greater is capable of performing all but the most physically demanding jobs. Between 15 and 25 ml/kg/min, the energy requirements of the specific jobs should be estimated. Where the patient's $\dot{V}O_2$ max is less than 15 ml/kg/min, he or she is considered generally unable to perform most jobs. Table 53-8 provides a rough guide for energy requirements for some jobs.

A critical limitation in the application of exercise testing to estimate a patient's capacity to perform a job is the lack of specific information about job demands or energy requirements.[46-50] For this reason, examiners should pay particular attention to characterizing the work requirements of current jobs. Further research is definitely needed in this area.[51] Methods of assessing job demands are discussed in Chapter 52.

EVALUATION OF SPECIFIC RESPIRATORY IMPAIRMENTS
Chronic airflow obstruction

There are several considerations for evaluating patients with chronic airflow obstruction. As mentioned earlier, spirometry, in particular FEV1, shows a fairly high correlation with exercise limitation.[14,52,53] Whereas on a population basis there is a high correlation between spirometry and $\dot{V}O_2$ max, prediction of exercise tolerance for an individual

Table 53-8. Energy requirements of various types of work

	$\dot{V}O_2$ (approximate)		
	ml/kg/min	L/min	METS
Light to moderate work (sitting)			
Clerical	5.6	0.42	1.6
Using repair tools	6.3	0.47	1.8
Operating heavy equipment	8.8	0.66	2.5
Heavy truck driving	12.6	0.95	3.6
Moderate work (standing)			
Light work, own pace	8.8	0.66	2.5
Janitorial work	10.5	0.79	3.0
Assembly line (lifts 45 lb+)	12.3	0.92	3.5
Paper hanging	14.0	1.05	4.0
Standing and/or walking (arm work)			
General heavy labor	15.8	1.19	4.5
Using heavy tools	21.0	1.58	6.0
Lift and carry 60-80 lb	26.2	1.97	7.5

METS, 3.5 ml O_2/kg/min; $\dot{V}O_2$, oxygen consumption.

worker using spirometry is relatively limited. Patients with chronic bronchitis who may have only modest decrements in their FEV1 and relatively modest impairment with respect to $\dot{V}O_2$ max may, due to their heavy production of sputum, be unable to wear a respirator. In addition, concomitant disorders such as cor pulmonale may compound the degree of impairment.

Asthma

As noted previously, ATS has provided recent recommendations on the evaluation of asthma. As with chronic airflow obstruction, individuals with asthma, regardless of cost, are subject to aggravation when exposed to inhaled irritants such as dust fumes, gases, or smoke. For this reason, asthma should be evaluated not only with respect to impairment, but also when establishing whether a patient can return to work. The absence of triggers should be assessed.[24] For patients whose asthma is caused by a specific sensitizer as with exposure to isocyanates, the relative contraindication of exposure to inhaled irritants becomes much more of an absolute contraindication. In addition, it is important for those identified with asthma induced by a sensitizer to be removed fairly quickly after exposure, as this will lessen the likelihood of long-term impairment disability.[54] In addition, a patient's failure to improve dramatically after cessation of exposure is by no means an argument that the asthma was not caused by the potential offending agent.[55]

The ATS statement places patients with asthma induced by sensitizers in a unique category and considers them totally impaired for any job involving exposure to the causative agent.[2,3] In addition, attention should be directed to whether the impairment or disability is permanent or temporary.[24] In those cases where the asthma is recently diagnosed or treatment is considered inadequate, the asthma should be rated as temporary. In these situations a temporary rating should be given and specific recommendations provided to the treating physician. Evaluation should occur in 6 months or whenever the treatment objectives are obtained. When the asthma appears to be stable, symptoms appear to be minimal, pulmonary function is at a maximum on the least extent of medications to achieve this control, and no further improvement is likely, then a permanent rating should be performed.

Interstitial lung disease

In a landmark study by Epler and co-workers, DLCO and resting spirometry were good predictors of the extent of dyspnea.[13] Histologic severity of disease did not correlate well with resting lung function. With occupationally induced interstitial lung diseases, the diagnosis of pneumoconiosis in the setting of normal respiratory function may still represent an impairment in that the patient should no longer be exposed to that dust. An absolute contraindication to exposure as with occupational asthma due to sensitizers, however, does not exist. With the appropriate use of personal protective equipment and adequate administrative and engineering controls, individuals with pneumoconiosis can work provided that further exposure, except at the most minimal level, does not continue.[2,3] Hypersensitivity pneumonitis, however, should be viewed in a fashion similar to occupational asthma and further exposure cannot be recommended.[2] The evaluator must recognize, however, that for some workers, this is not possible. For example, farmers who develop hypersensitivity pneumonitis may be encouraged to prevent further exposure by giving up their farm. For obvious reasons, many are reluctant to comply. In these less optimal situations, an emphasis on ventilation, avoidance, and use of personal protective equipment may provide a middle ground as long as all parties recognize the risks.

Sleep apnea

Sleep apnea is associated with impairment in two ways. The first is the presence of hypoxemia resulting in cor pulmonale, which when present represents a severe impairment. The second is that day time hypersomnolence may result in sufficient inattention to make working in certain jobs, such as driving, contraindicated.[2] Similarly, if the patient has a history of cough resulting in syncope, this too represents an impairment.[2] Finally, patients with severe bullae or airflow obstruction are not recommended to work as divers. In addition, if high altitude flying in unpressurized cabins is a concern, the risks of barotrauma should also be taken into consideration.

CLINICAL ASSESSMENT OF IMPAIRMENT AND DISABILITY AND REQUIREMENTS FOR REPORTS

In general, most evaluations require a comprehensive report. This need not be overly burdensome but should include the pertinent positives and negatives on history, physical examinations, and laboratory tests. Certain entitlement systems will also require that the actual pulmonary function test results, including tracings of spirometry, be included.

The discussion section should begin with a very brief summary of the problem or question being addressed, the diagnosis, and the degree of impairment. For workers' compensation claims, it is important that there be a discussion on attribution. Attribution is a process whereby a disease is caused or aggravated by a workplace exposure.[28] Attribution is generally done on a "more probable than not," or 51% probability, basis. Frequently, examiners will have to rely upon the detailed occupational history and generalize to the epidemiologic literature, as well as to literature on mechanisms, to decide whether a disease may be attributed to a workplace exposure. This is especially challenging where there is multifactorial causation. It is important to recognize that many factors may be additive or synergistic. Important considerations for attribution include the extent or certainty with which the diagnosis is established: Is it plausible that the diagnosed disease was caused by the exposure? Was the intensity and duration of the exposure sufficient to cause or aggravate the disorder? Finally, was there an appropriate temporal association? This latter point should take into consideration that some diseases, such as an acute inhalation injury, should have a very close temporal relationship, whereas others, such as asbestosis, may have 20 or more years latency between first exposure and the development of the disease.

Many workers' compensation systems will ask the examiner also to address the challenging issue of apportionment.[56] Apportionment is used to assess the relative contributions of multiple factors in the genesis of a disease or impairment. Although it is theoretically possible to apportion among cases when excellent data on expected contributions are available and when these contributions are additive, for the most part, the interaction of multiple factors in causing disease, whether additive or synergistic, and the difficulties of exposure assessment make apportionment extremely problematic. For this reason, apportionment should be approached with great caution. When examiners must apportion, they should do so recognizing the pitfalls that may occur due to uncertainties of exposure assessment or failure to recognize that the synergistic interaction of factors is much more important than the contribution of either single factor alone. For example, among asbestos insulators the risk of cigarette smoking has been noted to increase the risk of lung cancer tenfold. Asbestos exposure was shown in this group to increase the risk of lung cancer fivefold. When both factors were present together, the risk of lung cancer increased fiftyfold. Clearly, the synergistic interaction of asbestos and cigarette smoking is the most powerful risk factor. In this setting it is obvious that apportionment based on relative contributions is not possible because taking cigarettes away would eliminate 90% of the cancers, and taking asbestos away would eliminate 80% of the cancers. In summary, while apportionment may well be a fact of life, it should be approached with great caution, and one should remember that the apportionment is more often precise than accurate.

SUMMARY

The evaluation of impairment and disability represents the intersection between medicine and the administrative and legal system. Although much of what needs to be done requires following a cookbook approach to meet the specific requirements of an entitlement system, there are also substantial challenges to the medical practitioner. The medical practitioner must use careful judgment in making a diagnosis and obtaining the appropriate laboratory tests to characterize the extent of impairment, as well as the presence and contribution of other nonrespiratory diagnoses. Many of the entitlement systems rely heavily upon the judgment and input from the evaluators, and care must be taken to provide the most unbiased account possible. The process also requires substantial skill in working with patients, a process that works best when the patient is well informed of the purpose of the evaluation and has an opportunity at the close to have full access to his or her report.

REFERENCES

1. American Thoracic Society: Evaluation of impairment/disability secondary to respiratory disease, *Am Rev Respir Dis* 126:945-951, 1982.
2. American Thoracic Society: Evaluation of impairment/disability secondary to respiratory disorders, *Am Rev Respir Dis* 133:1205-1209, 1986.
3. American Medical Association: *Guides to the evaluation of permanent impairment,* ed 4, Chicago, 1993, American Medical Association.
4. Rosenstock L: Ethical dilemmas in providing health care to workers, *Ann Intern Med* 107:575-580, 1987.
5. Bascom R: Occupational and environmental diseases. A medicolegal primer for physicians, *Occup Med* 7:331-345, 1992.
6. Richman SI: Meanings of impairment and disability, *Chest 78* (Suppl.2):367-371, 1980.
7. World Health Organization: *International classification of impairments, disabilities, and handicaps,* Geneva, 1980, World Health Organization.
8. Carrieri V: The sensation of dyspnea: a review, *Heart Lung* 13:436-446, 1984.
9. Cherniak N, and Altose M: Mechanisms of dyspnea, *Clin Chest Med* 8:207-214, 1987.
10. Killian K, and Jones N: Respiratory muscles and dyspnea, *Clin Chest Med* 9:237-248, 1988.
11. Fishman AP, and Ledlie JF: Dyspnea, *Bull Eur Physiopathol Respir* 15:789-804, 1979.
12. Killian KJ, and Jones NL: The use of exercise testing and other methods in the investigation of dyspnea, *Clin Chest Med* 5:99-108, 1984.
13. Epler G, Saber F, and Gaensler E: Determination of severe impairment (disability) in interstitial lung disease, *Am Rev Respir Dis* 121:647-659, 1980.
14. McGavin FR, Artvinli M, Naoe H, and McHardy GJR: Dyspnea, disability, and distance walked: comparison of estimates of exercise performance in respiratory disease, *Br Med J* 241-243, 1978.
15. Fletcher CM: The clinical diagnosis of pulmonary emphysema—an experimental study, *Proc R Soc Med* 577-584, 1953.
16. Borg G: Perceived exertion as an indicator of somatic stress, *Scand J Rehab* 2-3:92-98, 1970.
17. Ferris BG: Recommended standardized procedures for pulmonary function testing, *Am Rev Respir Dis* 118(Part 2):55-88, 1978.
18. Stoller JK, Ferranti R, and Feinstein AR: Further specification and evaluation of a new clinical index for dyspnea, *Am Rev Respir Dis* 134:1129-1134, 1986.
19. Becklake M: Organic or functional impairment, *Am Rev Respir Dis* 129:S96-S100, 1984.
20. Robertson AJ: Malingering, occupational medicine, and the law, *Lancet* 2:828-831, 1978.
21. Cotes J: Assessment of disablement due to impaired respiratory function, *Bull Physiopathol Respir* 11:210-217, 1975.
22. Ostiguy GL: Summary of task force report on occupational respiratory disease (pneumoconiosis), *Can Med Assoc J* 121:414-421, 1979.
23. Cotes JE: Rating respiratory disability: a report on behalf of a working group of the European society for clinical respiratory physiology, *Eur Respir J* 3:1074-1077, 1990.
24. American Thoracic Society: Guidelines for the evaluation of impairment/disability in patients with asthma, *Am Rev Respir Dis* 147:1056-1061, 1993.
25. Crapo RO, Morris AH, and Gardner RM: Reference spirometric values using techniques and equipment that meet ATS recommendations, *Am Rev Respir Dis* 123:659-664, 1981.
26. Crapo RO and Morris AH: Standardized single breath normal values for carbon monoxide diffusing capacity, *Am Rev Respir Dis* 123:185-190, 1981.
27. Social Security Administration: Disability evaluation under Social Security: a handbook for physicians. DHEW Pub No (SSA)79-10089, Washington, DC, 1979, Department of Health, Education, and Welfare.
28. Barnhart S: Evaluation of impairment and disability in occupational lung disease, *Occup Med* 2:227-241, 1987.
29. Hadler NM: Medical ramifications of the federal regulation of the social security disability insurance program, *Ann Intern Med* 96:665-669, 1982.
30. Edwards LS: Workers' compensation insurance, *Ortho Clin North Am* 14:661-668, 1983.
31. Veterans Administration: Code of federal regulations: pensions, bonuses, and veterans relief, vol 38, pp 346-398, Washington, DC, 1991, US Government Printing Office.
32. Department of Labor: Standards for determining coal miners' total disability of death due to pneumoconiosis, *Fed Register* 45:13678-13712, 1980.
33. International Labour Office: Guidelines for the use of the ILO International Classification of Radiographs and Pneumoconioses. Geneva, 1980, International Labour Office.
34. Knudson RJ, Lebowitz MD, Holberg CV, and Burrows B: Changes in the normal maximal expiratory flow-volume curve with growth and aging, *Am Rev Respir Dis* 128:413-418, 1983.
35. American Thoracic Society: Standardization of spirometry—1987 update, *Am Rev Respir Dis* 136:1285-1298, 1987.
36. American Thoracic Society: Single breath carbon monoxide diffusing capacity (transfer factor): recommendations for a standard technique, *Am Rev Respir Dis* 136:1299-1307, 1987.
37. American Thoracic Society: Lung function testing: selection of reference values and interpretative strategies, *Am Rev Respir Dis* 144:1202-1218, 1991.

38. Cotes J, Zejda J, and King B: Lung function impairment as a guide to exercise limitation in work-related lung disorders, *Am Rev Respir Dis* 137:1089-1093, 1988.

39. Wasserman K, Hansen J, Sue D, and Whipp B: *Principles of exercise testing and interpretation,* Philadelphia, 1987, Lea & Febiger.

40. Wiedemann HP, Gee BL, Balmes JR, and Loke J: Exercise testing in occupational lung diseases, *Clin Chest Med* 5:157-171, 1984.

41. Harber P and Rothenberg LS: Controversial aspects of respiratory disability determination, *Semin Respir Med* 7:257-269, 1986.

42. Harber P, Schnur R, Emergy J, Brooks S, and Ploy-Song-Sang Y: Statistical "biases" in respiratory disability determinations, *Am Rev Respir Dis* 128:413-418, 1983.

43. Harber P: Respiratory disability. The uncoupling of oxygen consumption and disability, *Clin Chest Med* 13:367-376, 1992.

44. Jones NL and Campbell EJ: Clinical exercise testing, 2nd ed, pp. 94, 119, 139-141, 248-251, Philadelphia, 1982, W.B. Saunders.

45. Weller JJ, El-Gamal FM, Parker L, Reed JW, and Cotes JE: Indirect estimation of maximal oxygen uptake for study of working populations, *Br J Ind Med* 45:532-537, 1988.

46. Astrand PO and Rodahl K: Textbook of work physiology, ed 3, 354-390, New York, 1986, McGraw-Hill.

47. Passmore R and Durnin JVGA: Human energy expenditure, *Physiol Rev* 35:801-840, 1955.

48. Gordon EE: Energy costs of activities in health and disease, *Arch Intern Med* 101:702-713, 1958.

49. Tennessee Heart Association: Physician's handbook for evaluation of cardiovascular and physical fitness, Nashville, 1972, Tennessee Heart Association.

50. Karvonen MJ: Work and activity classification. In Larson LA, editor: *Fitness, health and work capacity,* New York, 1974, Macmillan.

51. Becklake MR, Rodarte J, and Kalica AR: Scientific issues in the assessment of respiratory impairment, *Am Rev Respir Dis* 137:1505-1510, 1988.

52. Jones NL, Jones G, and Edwards RHT: Exercise tolerance in chronic airway obstruction, *Am Rev Respir Dis* 103:477-491, 1971.

53. Gilbert R, Keighley J, and Auchinloss JH: Disability in patients with obstructive pulmonary disease, *Am Rev Respir Dis* 90:383-394, 1964.

54. Chan-Yeung M: State of the Art Reviews-Occupational asthma, *Chest* 98:148s-161s, 1990.

55. Chan-Yeung M: Evaluation of impairment/disabilities in patients with occupational asthma, *Am Rev Respir Dis* 135:950-951, 1987.

56. Harber P: Alternative partial respiratory disability rating schemes, *Am Rev Respir Dis* 134:481-487, 1986.

Chapter 54

PULMONARY REHABILITATION PROGRAMS

Bertrand Shapiro
Maureen A. Finnerty

Pulmonary rehabilitation is an effective, established therapy. Improved exercise tolerance, better self-image, diminished despondency, more optimal utilization of medications, and better quality of life are some of the documented benefits.[1,2] By improving functional status, participation in pulmonary rehabilitation programs can help many persons with lung disease remain in the work force, particularly when combined with reasonable workplace accommodation changes (see Chapter 52). The benefit most pervasive to "third-party payers" is the repeated demonstration that hospitalization days decrease after participation in a pulmonary rehabilitation program.[2] There are suggestive data that longevity may be improved as shown in Fig. 54-1.[3] Standard pulmonary function tests that reflect pulmonary mechanics and gas exchange, such as spirometry, lung volumes, diffusing capacity, and arterial blood gases, are not significantly improved by pulmonary rehabilitation, nor do they predict the level of improvement to be expected.[4,5] Failure of pulmonary mechanics and gas exchange to improve must not be taken as evidence that rehabilitation is not effective. The beneficial outcomes mentioned above are more than enough to justify effectiveness.

Studies reviewing the outcome of pulmonary rehabilitation have focused upon patients with asthma or obstructive lung disease secondary to cigarette smoking. There are no specific studies of outcome in occupationally related lung disease, which range across the spectrum of the obstructive to restrictive lung impairment. However, some relevant information has been published on the benefit of pulmonary rehabilitation in diseases other than chronic obstructive pulmonary disease (COPD). For instance, non-COPD patients have good outcomes in Foster's experience, and preoperative lung transplant patients, many of whom have restrictive impairment, do better with pulmonary rehabilitation.[7,8] Most persons who run programs will relate that the outcome for pulmonary rehabilitation is good across a broad spectrum of pulmonary diseases. Based upon information presently available, persons with occupational lung disease are not adequately cared for unless they are evaluated for and appropriately treated with rehabilitation.

There are patients who should be excluded from formal rehabilitation programs. Patients who do not participate voluntarily are likely to fail and are frequently disruptive to others. Patients with very low intelligence or severe psychiatric disorders will not benefit. Patients with significant comorbidity that will lead to their demise generally are not considered suitable, but occasionally patients with unresectable lung cancer have participated in rehabilitation with a very successful outcome. Improved symptom control, diminished use of the hospital, and fewer demands on family and physicians are the benefits.

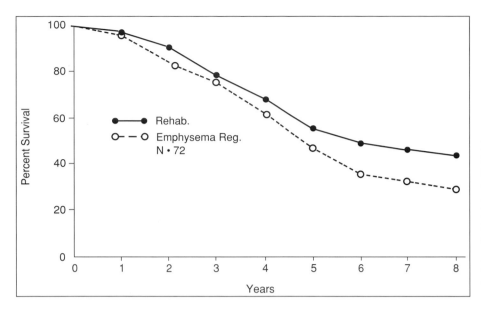

Fig. 54-1. Cumulative survival of 72 men following participation in a Denver, Colorado, pulmonary rehabilitation program (Rehab.) and a historical control group (Emphysema Reg.) matched for age, height, FEV1, oxygen saturation, and living in Denver. At 8 years the survival difference obtained borderline statistical significance ($p = 0.08$). (Adapted from Petty TL: Pulmonary rehabilitation, *Am Rev Respir Dis* 122(Pt 2):159-161, 1980. With permission.)

A reasonable definition of rehabilitation goals is "restoration of the individual to the fullest physical, medical, mental, emotional, economic, social, and vocational potential of which he is capable." In particular, pulmonary rehabilitation is "an art of medical practice wherein an individually tailored, multidisciplinary program is formulated through which accurate diagnosis, therapy, emotional support, and education stabilizes or reverses the physiopathology and psychopathology of pulmonary diseases."[6] Although this definition is intimidating, time, experience, and a growing body of scientific literature have produced a relatively uniform approach to rehabilitating the pulmonary patient.

MEDICATIONS

Before a patient is referred to a pulmonary rehabilitation program, the patient should be receiving optimal medication therapy. The common medications for the treatment of outpatient chronic pulmonary impairment are shown in the box.

The approach to prescribing medication is driven by current information, experience, and style. For instance, in the 1960s, inhaled β-agonists were criticized because of an association between their usage and mortality in England .[9] This concern was not confirmed in other countries, and the issue as to whether large doses of inhaled β-agonists increase asthma mortality continues.[10-12] On the other hand, high dose-inhaled β-agonists may be used in the severely ill patient.[13] In the late 1980s, theophylline was criticized because of its low therapeutic-to-toxic ratio and its lack of demonstrable therapeutic effect in the acute emergency treatment of asthma.[14] Time and thoughtful experience have restored theophylline to the therapeutic armamentarium.[15,16]

The pharmacologic approach to asthma has changed to suppression of the inflammatory pathways that lead to bronchospasm, mucus plugging, increased work of breathing, and hypoxia.[17,18] Suppression of the inflammatory pathways often requires the use of inhaled steroids and antibi-

---

Common medications for treatment of outpatient chronic pulmonary impairment

Inhaled

Anticholinergic bronchodilators, such as ipratropium bromide

β-Agonist bronchodilators, such as isoproterenol, metaproterenol, isoetharine, albuterol, terbutaline, bitolterol, pirbuterol, salmeterol

Steroid antiinflammatories, such as beclomethasone, triamcinolone, flunisolide

Nonsteroid antiinflammatories, such as cromolyn, nedocromil

Mucolytics, such as acetylcysteine, dornase-α

Oral

Methylxanthine bronchodilators (usually in sustained release form), such as theophylline, dyphylline, oxtriphylline

β-Agonist bronchodilators, such as albuterol, terbutaline

Steroid antiinflammatories, such as prednisone, methylprednisolone, prednisolone

---

otics if infection is present. This principle of inflammation suppression applies to the treatment of occupationally acquired asthma when control of exposure is not in itself adequate.

Since many pulmonary drugs are preferentially delivered by inhalation, proper patient technique and good inhalation delivery systems are important.[19] Many studies have revealed the difficulty patients have in using metered-dose inhalers (MDIs). The technique, which is outlined in Table 54-1, is complex. Spacers are devices to improve drug delivery by making technique easier (Fig. 54-2). The devices are usually tube-shaped chambers. In general the larger the spacer, the better the delivery of the drug. Upon activation

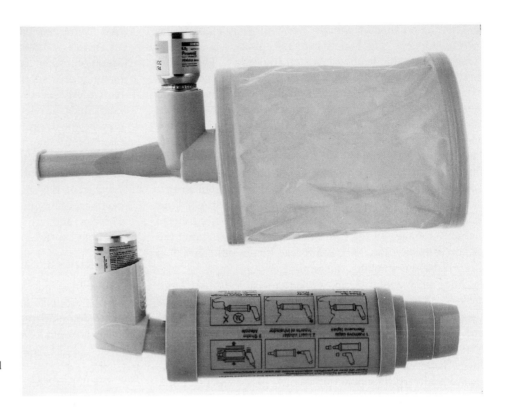

Fig. 54-2. Two widely available spacers that improve drug delivery from metered dose inhalers (MDIs). *Top,* collapsible bag spacer; *Bottom,* rigid tube spacer.

Table 54-1. Proper use of metered-dose inhalers (MDI)

Predose stage

1. Remove cap from MDI
2. Shake canister three or four times
3. Hold MDI upright and exhale normally (to functional residual capacity)
4. Close lips around mouthpiece of MDI (closed-mouth technique) or preferably hold mouthpiece two finger-breadths in front of open mouth (open mouth technique)

Dosing stage

5. Begin to inhale slowly; after 1 to 2 sec, discharge 1 puff from the MDI
6. Continue to inhale slowly for 5 to 10 sec; count the seconds while inhaling
7. Hold breath for 5 to 10 sec
8. Exhale

Follow-up

9. Wait 5 min before inhaling the next puff (if prescribed); then repeat steps 2 through 8
10. If the inhaled drug is a corticosteroid, rinse mouth with tap water when finished; spit the water out; do not swallow it

Adapted from Toogood JH: Helping your patients make better use of MDIs and spacers, *J Respir Dis* 15:151-166, 1994. With permission.

of the MDI, the aerosolized drug is released into the chamber. Only aerosol particles most likely to deposit into the lung remain suspended in the chamber. The patient then inhales the suspended particles. With spacers, timing of the inhalation is considerably less critical. Unfortunately spacers are cumbersome and do not easily fit into a pocket or purse. Breath-activated inhalers are effective and easiest to use but are available for only a few drugs. There are dry powder, breath-activated inhalers in which a capsule containing the powdered drug is punctured and the patient inhales the powder.[20] Breath-activated MDIs are also available, making coordination easier.[21]

SMOKING CESSATION

Smoking cessation is an essential step in the rehabilitation of the pulmonary-impaired patient and in decreasing mortality.[22] The relative risk of dying from lung cancer decreases as the length of time from smoking cessation increases. For instance, data suggest that men who smoke cigarettes have a 15.8 higher rate of dying from lung cancer than nonsmoking men. Following cessation of cigarette smoking for 5 to 9 years, the chance of dying from lung cancer decreases to 5.9 times the rate of nonsmokers, and after 15 years the chance decreases to 2 times.[23]

Yet cancer is only part of the smoking problem. Patients with lung cancer are usually dead or cured within 5 years. The morbidity and impairment from cigarette smoking due to chronic lung disease can last for decades. Thus, the importance of smoking cessation must be considered not only in relation to cancer mortality but in relation to chronic lung disease morbidity. The data regarding smoking cessation and decrease in pulmonary morbidity are not as striking as the data regarding cancer death. Nonetheless, morbidity does decrease after cessation of cigarette smoking. Forced expiratory volume in 1 second (FEV1) decreases 53 ml per year in the typical male patient with COPD. After cigarette smoking cessation the annual decline improves to 34 ml per year.[24,25]

There is no single technique that uniformly causes a patient to stop smoking. Ninety percent of those who quit stop "cold turkey;" that is, they just stop smoking.[26] The factors that go into this decision are difficult to define, but a positive educational approach by the physician with support in the workplace and home are definitely helpful.[27] Most patients realize that smoking is unhealthful but many do not understand how the unhealthfulness directly affects them. The physician should specifically advise the patient to stop smoking and relate the necessity to the patient's situation. For instance, there might be an early morning cough that the patient considers trivial. The physician should point out that the cough is not normal and almost certainly reflects cigarette damage to the lung. After smoking cessation the patient's success should be reinforced by periodic physician inquiries about smoking status.

Since only about 7% of smokers are able to quit "cold turkey," more interventional techniques have a role. Specific focus upon nicotine withdrawal is one approach. Nicotine has the qualities of an addictive drug, psychologic and physiologic dependence, withdrawal syndrome, and tolerance. Because of nicotine addiction, many cigarette smokers smoke in a fashion that titrates their blood nicotine level. Pharmacologic approaches are available to supply nicotine while the patient stops smoking; these approaches then withdraw the nicotine.[28] Nicotine gum can be chewed. The rate of chewing adjusts the rate of transbuccal nicotine absorption. Many smokers find that the gum does not relieve their craving and that it tastes bad. Nicotine dermal patches are currently popular and are marketed in the United States with a "starter kit" that includes patient information about patch usage and information on smoking cessation. The daily applied patches release a constant amount of nicotine, which is transcutaneously absorbed. The nicotine dosage is reduced at several week intervals until the patient is weaned from nicotine. Patients must not smoke while using the patches; the combined nicotine from both the patches and the cigarettes can lead to absorption of toxic nicotine quantities. Nicotine nasal sprays have been developed, but their role in smoking cessation is still being explored. It must be remembered that these pharmacologic approaches to nicotine withdrawal are only adjuvant to the physician's role in assisting the patient to stop smoking.

In the United States smoking cessation programs are offered by both nonprofit and profit-making organizations. These programs are combinations of counseling, education, support therapy, and a formal approach to smoking cessation. A few include an aversive approach, such as having the patient smoke so much that they become ill, minor electrical shocks when smoking a cigarette, or something as simple as putting an elastic band around the wrist that the patient snaps painfully when seeking a cigarette. Local chapters of the American Lung Association or the American Cancer Society can provide a list of smoking cessation programs in the area served by the chapter. Workplace-based programs have been successfuly established.

There is a broad range of other approaches to smoking cessation, such as psychotherapy, biofeedback, and acupuncture. No single interventional technique or program is particularly successful. Outcome data from a particular program must be viewed with caution. The follow-up period may be too short, or the data may not provide a true picture. If only one program was successful, others would no longer exist, and there would not be fifty million smokers in the United States, because most people would take advantage of the successful program. However, these interventional techniques add about 1% to the population of ex-smokers and are worthwhile since the consequences of smoking can be so devastating.

CONROL OF AIR POLLUTION

Common indoor air pollutants are cigarette smoke, combustion products such as carbon monoxide and nitrogen dioxide, biologic agents such as mites and molds, formaldehyde, and other volatile organic compounds.[29] These are discussed in Chapter 48. Control measures are described in Chapter 61.

Outdoor pollutants[30] are for the most part not under the control of the individual patient. Avoidance is the patient's major option. In most metropolitan areas in the United States, local officials will report the community level of outdoor air pollution with an index usually called the Air Quality Index (AQI) or Pollutant Standards Index (PSI). The index reflects the ratio of community pollutants to the national Ambient Air Quality Standards (NAAQS). An index greater than 100 is considered unhealthful. The higher the index, the more imperative it is for patients to avoid outdoor pollution.

To avoid the short-term effects of air pollution, patients should exercise early in the morning before the pollutants increase in concentration or, less preferably, in the evening when the concentrations are declining. When the index is high, patients should remain indoors with an air conditioner operating in the air recirculation mode. Many physicians believe that an air conditioner with filter and activated charcoal will provide even more protection.

The long-term consequences of air pollution are more difficult to characterize than the short-term consequences. Morbidity and even mortality have been demonstrated for many community air pollutants.[31] Whether patients living in communities with high concentrations of pollutants should be advised to move to another community is conjectural. Physicians should consider advising patients to move away from major roadways.

OXYGEN THERAPY

Cotes and Gilson demonstrated that patients with COPD improved in exercise ability when breathing oxygen.[32] Petty demonstrated that hypoxia caused polycythemia and that pulmonary hypertension improved with continuous oxygen therapy.[33] However, oxygen therapy is expensive, and the number of potential candidates for oxygen therapy is enormous. Therefore, to better delineate the cost benefit of long-term oxygen therapy, the U.S. National Institutes of Health and the British Medical Research Council set out to determine whether oxygen prolongs life and, if so, whether using oxygen only in the evening and at night was as effective as around the clock.[34,35] Figure 54-3 shows the results of the combined U.S. and British studies.[36] At 3 years, approximately 30% of persons not using oxygen were alive, 45% using oxygen for 15 hours a day were alive, and 65% using oxygen nearly round-the-clock were alive. The data from these studies are the basis for selecting those specific patients who will benefit with oxygen therapy. Table 54-2 lists the criteria established in the United States by Medicare and in other countries for prescribing continuous oxygen therapy.[37] Logical extrapolation has extended the same criteria for continuous oxygen therapy to patients with restrictive disease, but no similar studies have been done on those persons.

The method of providing continuous low flow oxygen has profound effects on the patient's quality of life and work status. In most cases oxygen is administered by a nasal cannula that is connected directly to an oxygen source. How-

ever, oxygen is wasted with that technique, since during the patient's expiration, oxygen flowing through the cannula is discharged into the surrounding environment and not administered to the patient. Oxygen conserver devices either stop oxygen flow or store flowing oxygen during expiration and deliver oxygen only during inspiration.[38] These devices decrease oxygen utilization more than 30%, but they may not provide adequate oxygen in patients with weak respiratory efforts, mouth breathing, or shallow breathing. Conservers also may not work effectively during exercise, if the conserver response characteristics do not keep up with the patient's exercise breathing pattern.

Transtracheal oxygen (TTO) for continuous oxygen therapy was first demonstrated by Heimlich.[39] He inserted a small catheter percutaneously through the neck into the trachea and fed oxygen continuously through the catheter. Oxygen flowing during expiration is stored in the trachea and pharynx. Upon the next inspiration the stored oxygen is inspired into the alveoli. Christopher and Spofford refined the technique and subjected the technique to significant clinical trials.[40] (see Fig. 54-4) In addition to conserving oxygen, TTO improves patient self-image since the transtracheal catheter can easily be hidden. Skin irritation from the nasal cannula, particularly around the

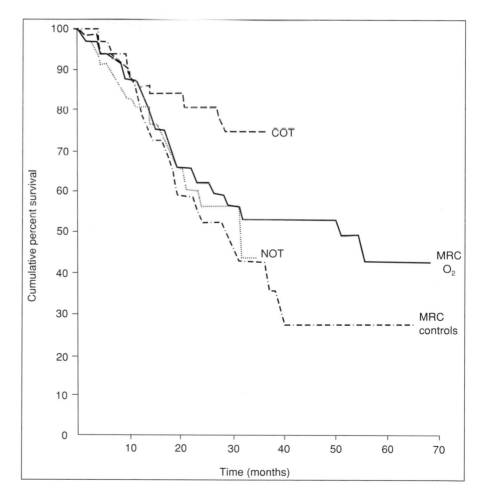

Fig. 54-3. Cumulative survival of hypoxic men with chronic obstructive pulmonary disease who did not use supplemental oxygen (MRC controls), used low flow oxygen an average of 12 hours per day (NOT), used low flow oxygen an average of 15 hours per day (MRC O_2), and used low flow oxygen nearly 24 hours per day (COT). The more hours of oxygen use, the better is the survival. (Adapted from Flenley DC: Long-term home oxygen therapy, *Chest* 87:99-103, 1985. With permission.)

Table 54-2. Prescribing criteria for long-term oxygen therapy

---

United States: CMN Form HCFA-484

1. $Pao_2 \leq 55$ mm Hg or $Sao_2 \leq 88\%$ (breathing room air)
2. $Pao_2 \leq 59$ mm Hg and evidence of at least one of the following: pulmonary hypertension (P wave > 3 mm in leads 11, 111, or aVF), cor pulmonale (dependent edema), or erythrocytosis (HCT > 56%)

United Kingdom: DHSS Drug Tariff, 1986

1. Absolute indications: COPD (FEV < 1.5 L, FVC < 2.0 L), hypoxemia (Pao_2 < 55 mm Hg), hypercapnia ($Paco_2$ > 45 mm Hg), and edema; stability demonstrated over 3 weeks
2. As in 1, but without edema or $Paco_2$ > 45 mm Hg
3. Palliative therapy may be prescribed

Europe: Report of an SEP Task Group, 1989

1. Pao_2 < 55 mm Hg; "steady-stage COPD"
2. Pao_2 55-65 mm Hg with additional features as on United States CMN Form HCFA-484
3. Restrictive disease with Pao_2 < 55 mm Hg

Australia: Thoracic Society of Australia, 1985

1. Pao_2 < 56 mm Hg, COPD, RVH, polycythemia, and edema
2. Desaturation < 90% on exercise
3. Refractory dyspnea associated with cardiac failure

From Cooper CB: Long-term oxygen therapy. In Casaburi R and Petty TL, editors: *Principles and practice of pulmonary rehabilitation*, pp 183-203, Philadelphia, 1993, Saunders. With permission.
CMN, Certificate of Medical Necessity; *COPD,* chronic obstructive pulmonary disease; *DHSS,* Department of Health and Social Security; *FEV,* forced expiratory volume; *FVC,* forced vital capacity; *HCT,* hematocrit; *RVH,* right ventricular hypertrophy; *SEP,* European Society of Pneumology.

nares and ears, is gone, and surprisingly dyspnea is diminished.[41] TTO is not for patients who are psychologically unsuited to manipulate a tube that penetrates their body, have poor eye-to-hand coordination, or have a large volume of sputum. Sputum can obstruct the catheter or can use the catheter as a nidus to form a large mucus plug that obstructs the trachea.

Oxygen can be supplied to nasal cannulas or transtracheal catheters from liquified gas stored in Dewar-style containers, compressed gas stored in thick, heavy metal cylinders, and extracted gas from the surrounding environment. Liquid oxygen, which is the most portable because a large quantity of gas can be stored in light, easily movable storage vessels, is best suited for the active patient, but its cost is relatively high. Vendors, when left to their own preference, will usually supply active patients with more profitable but less portable compressed gas. For the patient who is essentially house bound, oxygen extracted by a molecular sieve (commonly called an oxygen concentrator) is a relatively inexpensive oxygen source. A major positive feature is that periodic oxygen deliveries are not required to replenish the oxygen supply.

ALTITUDE

Millions of people work at or visit an altitude considerably higher than where they reside. For most this poses no problem, but for people with pulmonary impairment altitude can have serious adverse physiologic effects. These effects are related to the rate and duration of ascent, which determine the pace at which physiologic adaptation occurs, and to the final altitude reached, which determines barometric pressure and consequentially partial pressure of inspired oxygen. Patients with pulmonary disease may be unable to adapt to altitude for several reasons. Their ability to hyperventilate and partially compensate for hypoxemia may be mechanically impaired or limited by diminished ventilatory hypoxic drive. Concomitant cardiac dysfunction and pulmonary hypertension may prevent appropriate increase in cardiac output necessary for adequate oxygen delivery, particularly during stress, such as anemia and/or exercise. Alcohol and sedating medications may worsen adaptation.

Expansion of gases in body cavities due to lower barometric pressure can cause problems. Principles applied to normal persons are discussed in Chapter 46. Gastrointestinal gas may bloat the abdomen and restrict lung expansion. This is usually transient because the expanded gastrointestinal gas is expelled and the gas volume returns to normal. Pneumothorax or pneumomediastinum from a ruptured bleb or bullous can occur. Patients who have had this in the past are more susceptible. There are no data as to the incidence of assent to altitude-caused pneumothorax or pneumomediastinum, but it must be relatively low since there are so few reports of it happening. Gas in bullae or blebs may expand without rupture and compress the surrounding lung parenchyma causing further pulmonary impairment. High altitude or mountain sickness, which consists of a spectrum of symptoms, including insomnia, headache, nausea, and poor appetite, can affect patients, but this problem can just as easily occur in normal persons.

Altitude exposure is often neglected in assessing patients with pulmonary impairment. For example, a patient was hospitalized for pulmonary impairment evaluation. All testing was done at sea level. The patient lived in Las Vegas, which has an altitude reasonably close to sea level. When arranging for discharge, the use of nocturnal oxygen was being discussed when the patient stated that the oxygen might also help him at work. Unknown was that the patient worked at an altitude of 6,000 feet.

Protocols have been developed to predict how patients with obstructive pulmonary impairment will function at high altitudes. These protocols are useful but must be interpreted with caution. The protocols are based upon the study of small numbers of patients who had eucapnic, obstructive pulmonary impairment and no other major medical problem. Evaluation time was short, and there were no other hypoxic stresses, such as sleep or exercise during the testing. Further, most of the subjects were patients living at sea

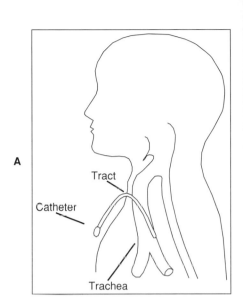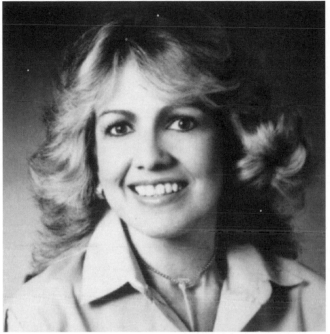

Fig. 54-4. A, Diagram depicting the path of a transtracheal oxygen catheter. (Adapted from training manual, The Institute for Transtracheal Oxygen Therapy. With permission.) **B,** Photograph of a patient with a transtracheal catheter in place. (From advertising brochure, The Institute for Transtraheal Oxygen Therapy. With permission.)

level. Patients not living at sea level and ascending or descending to another altitude may have different responses.

Dillard et al. measured the magnitude of hypoxemia during hypobaria in 18 patients with COPD.[42] The barometric pressure obtained was equivalent to 8,000 feet. They found that the greatest predictors for determining the Pao_2 at that altitude was the Pao_2 at ground level and the FEV1. Gong et al. studied 22 pulmonary disease patients using a hypoxic altitude stimulation test (HAST).[43] This was not truly an altitude test since only the hypoxic but not the hypobaric components of altitude were simulated. Dillard subjected data from his research, Gong's study, and three other studies on the effects of low inspired oxygen concentration on arterial oxygenation to meta-analysis.[44] The meta-analysis reinforced Dillard's position that in COPD both the initial Pao_2 and the FEV1 predict the response to altitude. Dillard's and Gong's equations for predicting Pao_2 at altitude are given in Table 54-3. Dillard's equation is more predictive, but Gong's equation is easier to use.

These equations do not allow for variability in individual patient response and, as noted previously, are based upon eucapnic patients with COPD. They should be used only when there are constraints on testing the patient's individual response. A true simulation test that involves both a decrease in barometric pressure and a partial pressure of oxygen requires complex and expensive equipment such as a hypobaric chamber. Vohra and Klocke have described a simplified version of the HAST in which a venturi-type oxygen mask is used to create hypoxic gas mixtures.[45] Nitrogen is bled into the venturi causing a low inspired partial pressure of oxygen. Selection of the appropriate venturi and flow rate of nitrogen adjusts the inspired oxygen concentration to the equivalent altitude being studied.

The most accurate approach, if feasible, is to assess oxygenation in the patient's usual living or working environment. For example, this proved useful for a patient who lived at 5,800 feet was sent home with a portable oximeter. Oxygen saturation ranged from 73% to 87% while the patient was doing his house chores including lifting and transporting his disabled daughter and wife.

EXERCISE TRAINING

More than 1,000 studies have been published regarding exercise training in chronic lung disease.[46] These studies have ranged from analyzing the basic physiology of exercise to studies on training techniques. In summary, it is clear that exercise training improves exercise tolerance. This improvement occurs despite no significant improvement in pulmonary functions, indicating that exercise improvement is secondary to cardiovascular conditioning and general improvement in the musculoskeletal system.

Table 54-4 shows the results of a treadmill test for two patients referred for pulmonary rehabilitation. Patients are considered pulmonary limited if they stop exercising when their minute ventilation exceeds 80% of their predicted maximum exercise ventilation. Patients are considered deconditioned if they do not achieve 80% of their predicted maximum exercise ventilation and age-predicted maximum heart rate and if there is no confounding factor that causes the test to be prematurely stopped, such as angina pectoralis or exercise limitation caused by arthritis. Patients achieving 80% of the predicted maximum heart rate, but not 80% of the predicted maximum exercise ventilation, could have intrinsic heart disease or be deconditioned. In Table 54-4, patient 1 is deconditioned since she achieved only 27% of her predicted maximum exercise ventilation and 48% of her

Table 54-3. Formulas for predicting arterial oxygenation at altitude in eucapnic patients with chronic obstructive pulmonary disease

Dillard's equations[44]

$\ln \dfrac{Pao_2 \text{ altitude}}{Pao_2 \text{ ground}} = k \times (PIo_2 \text{ altitude} - PIo_2 \text{ ground})$

$k = 0.01731 - 0.00019 \times \%$ predicted FEV1 where %FEV1 does not exceed 60%

$PIo_2 = 0.209 \times (\text{barometric pressure} - 47)$

Gong's equation[43]

Pao_2 altitude $= 22.8 - 2.74 \times$ altitude in thousands of feet $+ 0.68 \times Pao_2$ ground

Example

Patient with chronic bronchitis ascending from sea level to 8,000 feet (barometric presses = 565 mm Hg) who has an FEV1 of 31% of predicted and a Pao_2 of 72 mm Hg at sea level

According to Dillard's equations

$k = 0.01731 - 0.00019 \times 31 = 0.01141$

PIo_2 altitude $= 0.209 (565 - 47) = 108$

PIo_2 ground $= 0.209 (760 - 47) = 149$

$\ln \dfrac{Pao_2 \text{ altitude}}{72} = 0.01142 \times (108 - 149)$

Pao_2 altitude $= 45$mm Hg

According to Gong's equation

Pao_2 altitude $= 22.8 - 2.74 \times 8 + 0.68 \times 72$

Pao_2 altitude $= 50$ mm Hg

FEV1, Forced expiratory volume in 1 second.

maximum predicted heart rate. Patient 2 is pulmonary limited since she attained 101% of her predicted maximum exercise ventilation.

Many patients with pulmonary impairment are deconditioned and are not pulmonary or cardiac limited despite their severe pulmonary disease and shortness of breath. With exercise training, deconditioned patients improve exercise ability particularly well; almost all patients improve exercise ability to some extent.

Exercise training is a major component of pulmonary rehabilitation programs. Rapid floor or track walking has advantages over treadmill walking or bicycling since walking does not require special equipment and is more readily adaptable by the patient to other daily activities. The 12-minute walk test has been used as a monitor of changing exercise tolerance.[47] It is simple, can be repeated at frequent intervals, and does not require special equipment. A predetermined pathway or course is measured for length. A patient then walks as far as he can in 12 minutes. The distance achieved is recorded as a result. A 6-minute walk achieves similar information and is even easier to do repeatedly but may not reflect maximum exercise capacity as well as a 12-minute walk.[48]

Specific training of respiratory muscles is an area of active research. Generally the technique for respiratory muscle training is placement of a resistive load upon the respiratory system by having the patient breathe through a constricting orifice. Respiratory muscle training does improve respiratory muscle strength, but at present there is no consensus that training of respiratory muscles improves clinical outcome.[49] Therefore, specific respiratory muscle training is not uniformly a part of rehabilitation programs. However, respiratory muscle maneuvers that accompany exercise, stair climbing, getting in and out of a chair, and bending over, are stressed.

Pursed lip breathing, that is, breathing through constricted lips, is a traditional technique taught to patients with COPD when they feel particularly short of breath. This technique is believed to improve symptoms by preventing dynamic collapse of airways during expiration and by reminding the patient to control the panic associated with dyspnea. The physiologic consequences are decreased respiratory rate, minute ventilation, oxygen consumption, and $Paco_2$

Table 54-4. Examples of exercise limitation caused by deconditioning (patient 1) and pulmonary impairment (patient 2)

Patient	Age	Diagnosis	Pred max ex $\dot{V}_E$ 1/min	Actual $\dot{V}_E$ 1/min	%Pred max ex $\dot{V}_E$	Pred max HR	Actual max HR	%Pred HR
1	86	Emphysema	66	17.5	27	154	74	48
2	61	Chronic bronchitis	35.5	36	101	170	122	72

Predicted maximum (pred max ex $\dot{V}_E$), exercise minute ventilation = forced expiratory volume in 1 second (FEV1) $\times$ 35. Actual $\dot{V}_E$ = the minute ventilation achieved at maximum exercise. Predicted maximum heart rate (pred max HR) = $210 - 0.65 \times$ age. Actual HR = the heart rate achieved at maximum exercise.

and increased oxygen saturation and tidal volume.[50-52] Also, there is a shift of inspiratory muscle effort from the diaphragm and abdominal muscles to the rib cage muscles, which may allow the diaphragm muscles to recover from fatigue.[53] Most patients feel that pursed lip breathing controls their shortness of breath and contributes significantly to their coping practices. Interestingly patients with restrictive lung disease, in which dynamic collapse is not a significant component of the pathophysiology, believe that pursed lip breathing improves their dyspnea.

Assuming the leaning forward position, sometimes called positional breathing, is associated with less dyspnea and diminished use of the neck muscles as accessory muscles of respiration.[54-56] Diaphragmatic breathing, a technique that emphasizes motion of the diaphragm and abdominal muscles, is taught in many rehabilitation programs but has unproven value.

POSTURAL DRAINAGE WITH PERCUSSION AND INTERMITTENT POSITIVE PRESSURE BREATHING TREATMENTS

Postural drainage with percussion, sometimes called chest physiotherapy, is taught to patients with sputum production in most pulmonary rehabilitation programs. The purpose is to clear secretions from the tracheobronchial tree, which decreases airway obstruction, interrupts the inflammatory cycle, and diminishes bacterial burden within the bronchi. The technique has been likened to getting ketchup out of a bottle.[57] The patient assumes positions that promote gravity flow of mucus from the bronchial tubes while the patient's chest is vibrated with the use of a mechanical device called a percussor or with rapid hand motion. Transient improvements in sputum production and pulmonary functions have been reported, but there is no proven long-term effect on morbidity or mortality.[58] There may be select patients with large volumes of sputum production that improve, such as patients with cystic fibrosis or severe bronchiectasis. The former is not an occupationally related disease, and the latter is only occasionally an occupationally related disease.

Intermittent positive pressure breathing (IPPB) was a widely used therapy beginning in the 1950s. By the late 1970s its efficacy was questioned. In 1982, a multicenter study involving over 985 patients with COPD compared IPPB with simple nebulizer treatment.[59,60] Although the study had flaws, IPPB treatments were no more effective than simple nebulizer treatments, and IPPB may have been detrimental since the IPPB group of patients became more hyperinflated. Since that study, IPPB is rarely used in rehabilitation of patients with COPD.

NUTRITION

Weight loss in pulmonary disease had detrimental effects on respiratory muscle strength, ventilatory response to hypoxia, lung mechanics, and lung water hemostasis, and im-

pairs respiratory defense mechanisms to infection.[61] Further, weight loss is a poor prognostic sign.[62] Positive nitrogen balance improves respiratory muscle strength and presumably improves prognosis, although this latter point has not been established.[63] Body weight, triceps skin fold thickness, arm muscle circumference, and serum protein, such as prealbumin or retinol binding protein or transferrin, combined with an overall clinical impression are easily obtained markers of nutritional status. These markers can be determined serially for assessment of the success or failure of the patient's nutritional program. Albumin is also a serum protein marker of nutritional status, but its 21-day half life makes it insensitive to rapid changes in nutritional status. Therefore, an effective or failing nutritional program would not be recognized for several weeks if albumin is the nutritional status marker.

Patients' nutrition should be maintained by counseling and, if necessary, supplemental feeding. Total nutritional requirements can be estimated from the traditional Harris–Benedict basal metabolic rate (BMR) formulas and by multiplying the predicated BMR by 1.5, which compensates for such items as activity above the basal level and increased work of breathing.[64] Except for the Harris–Benedict formulas, other estimates of caloric consumption at rest are called the resting energy expenditure (REE), since they are not estimates from the basal state but from the resting state. Moore and Angelillo have developed less complex REE formulas than the Harris–Benedict equations as shown in Table 54-5. These formulas are based specifically upon ambula-

Table 54-5. Resting energy expenditure in ambulatory patients with chronic obstructive pulmonary disease

---

Male REE = $11.5 \times$ weight, kg + 952
Female REE = $14.1 \times$ weight, kg + 515
Example: The 24-hr caloric requirement for a 70 kg man with
  COPD can be estimated as follows:
  REE = $11.5 \times 70 + 952 = 1757$ kcal/24 hr
1757 kcal $\times$ 1.3 (normal activity factor) = 2284 kcal/day
  The Harris–Benedict equations below are harder to
    use and are not based upon patients with chronic
    obstructive lung disease[64]
  Male REE (BMR) = 66.4 + 13.7 $\times$
                      weight (kg) + 5 $\times$
                      height (cm) − 6.75 $\times$ age
  Female REE (BMR) = 655 + 9.5 $\times$
                       weight (kg) + 1.8 $\times$
                       height (cm) − 4.67 $\times$ age
  The normal activity factor is approximately 1.5

From Moore JA and Angelillo VA: Equations for the prediction of resting energy expenditure in chronic obstructive lung disease, *Chest* 94:1260-1263, 1988, and from Harris JA and Benedict FG: Biometric studies of basal metabolism in man, publication no. 279, Carnegie Institute of Washington, 1919.
BMR, Basal metabolic rate, **COPD**, chronic obstructive pulmonary disease; **REE**, resting energy expenditure.

tory persons with COPD.[65] Because the elevated work of breathing is already taken into consideration in the characteristic of the population, the activity multiplier to estimate daily caloric need is smaller, about 1.3.

The patient's diet prescription should specify as to the total number of calories. The problems of underfeeding are serious as described previously, but overfeeding also has problems. The consequences of obesity are long term and well known, but an immediate problem in patients with pulmonary disease is that excess calories overload the respiratory system with increased carbon dioxide production. This is particularly true with a high carbohydrate diet because carbohydrates in excess of caloric needs will be used in liponeogenesis, a metabolic pathway particularly rich in the production of carbon dioxide.[66] Even if the number of calories is not in excess, carbohydrate metabolism generates higher carbon dioxide production per unit of energy than lipids. Supplemental feedings, which are relatively high in fat and low in carbohydrate content, are designed to minimize carbon dioxide production.

In the anorectic pulmonary patient, feeding by mouth may be impossible. Percutaneous-endoscopic placement of a gastrostomy or jejunostomy feeding tube and feeding through the tube even when the patient has no appetite have become accepted therapy in patients with cystic fibrosis.[67] Whether acceptance spreads to other patients with pulmonary diseases remains to be seen.

VOCATIONAL AND OCCUPATIONAL THERAPY

Vocational and occupational therapists have a vital role in pulmonary rehabilitation programs. Patients with COPD who have significant pulmonary impairment need help in modifying their activities for optimal functioning. These modifications range from the simple to the complex. An example of a simple modification is conserving energy by showering while sitting on a stool and then drying by putting on a terry cloth robe as opposed to toweling. Total rearrangement of the kitchen, installation of low cabinets, and training in the usage of special cooking tools allow the patient to prepare meals while sitting. The patient's life-style should be individually analyzed by the vocational therapist and pulmonary clinical nurse specialist. Problems that physicians tend not to explore in depth will become obvious. For instance, few physicians discuss the details of how the patient will cope with shopping, but vocational therapists and nurses are aware of the problems and frequently have significant solutions. Occupational therapists can provide select patients with "work hardening" or new skills that make the patient eligible for jobs removed from their occupational hazard.

SEXUALITY

Sex is a universal activity, the performance of which is influenced by an exceptionally large number of factors, including social and religious values, natural desire, age, op-

portunity, relationships between people, emotional state, presence of illness, and side effects of medication. Sex therapy begins with the realization by the physician that for many patients, sex is part of the rehabilitation process. Yet there is frequently a reluctance to discuss the matter. It is the physician's role to inquire in an appropriate manner and setting as to whether sex is a concern to the patient. If the patient expresses concern, the range of therapies is as broad as the causes of sexual dysfunction. Occasionally, a simple suggestion is the necessary therapy. Examples include suggesting no heavy meal or alcohol before sex or assurance that it is permissible to use a bronchodilator in preparation for sex or oxygen for the hypoxic patient during sex. More often the development of a dialogue between the patient and the sexual partner to improve intimacy, express desires and limitations, and develop technique is important. If feasible, drugs with impotence as a side effect may have to be eliminated. Beyond these points, consultation and therapy with sex therapists, psychiatrists, or urologists who specialize in male impotence or gynecologists who specialize in female sexual dysfunction are indicated. Kravetz has developed slide and tape presentations about sex and COPD that are frequently shown in pulmonary rehabilitation programs.[68] These presentations followed by sensitive individual counseling can be very useful to patients.

PSYCHOSOCIAL ADJUSTMENTS

Psychosocial issues must not be underestimated in patients with chronic lung disease. For instance, dyspnea and psychosocial problems are better correlated with disability than lung function.[69] Strauss and Glaser have developed a framework shown in Table 54-6 for dealing with the psychosocial problems of chronic illness, which can be effectively applied to COPD.[70] Dudley et al. have more specifically examined the psychosocial concomitants of COPD.[71-73] Pulmonary rehabilitation programs have the personnel to provide individually tailored, multidisciplinary approaches that address patients' psychosocial problems.

Depression and anxiety frequently accompany COPD. McSweeny et al. found that 42% of patients with moderately advanced to advanced COPD had depression, and Yellowees el al. found that 34% had panic or anxiety disorders.[74,75] Depression or anxiety may be so severe that antidepressant and anxiolytic drugs are necessary adjuvants to treatment.

STRUCTURE OF PULMONARY REHABILITATION PROGRAMS

The specific structure of rehabilitation programs is driven mostly by experience, resources available, and reimbursement constraints. Although there are many variations in detail, rehabilitation programs are remarkably similar. First, rehabilitation programs are multidisciplinary in that a body of expertise is derived from physicians, nurses, respiratory therapists, nutritionists, physical therapists, vo-

Table 54-6. Framework for analyzing psychosocial needs of patients with chronic illness

1. Prevention of medical crises and their management once they occur
   Examples: Educating patients to contact their physicians soon after the development of respiratory infection; ensuring patient knows the most proficient method of getting to the nearest emergency room
2. Control of symptoms
   Examples: Education pursed-lip breathing; relaxation techniques
3. Carrying out of prescribed regimens and the management of problems attendant upon carrying out the regimens
   Examples: Ensuring patients understand their medication program; providing a low flow oxygen system that is appropriate for the patient's ambulation needs
4. Prevention of, or living with, social isolation caused by lessened contact with others
   Examples: Patient's participation in support groups such as "Better Breathers Clubs"; providing information to the patient's family and friends so that they understand the needs of the patient
5. Adjustment to changes in the course of the diseases, whether it moves downward or has remissions
   Examples: Education about the usual progression of the patient's disease; individual advice on how the progression will effect the patient's life and the plan for those changes
6. Attempts at normalizing both interaction with others and style of life
   Examples: Providing the patient with information and techniques of carrying out the activities of daily living such as shopping or cleaning house; moving the bedroom from the second floor to the first floor so there are no stairs to climb
7. Funding   finding the necessary money to pay for treatments or to survive despite partial or complete loss of employment
   Examples: Retraining for less physically demanding employment; ensuring that the patient has explored all financial resources to support living and health care expenses

From Strauss AL and Glaser BG: *Chronic illness and the quality of life,* St. Louis, 1975, Mosby.

cational therapists, clinical social workers, and psychologists. Most programs do not have staff from all these disciplines but have staff cross trained in these disciplines. Second, a patient-oriented, enthusiastic, attentive-to-detail program coordinator is essential to successful programs. Knowledge of pulmonary rehabilitation and organizational skills are necessary but alone are insufficient.

Pulmonary rehabilitation programs are generally divided into two types, inpatient and outpatient. Inpatient programs are mostly populated with persons who have been transferred from an acute care hospital where the patient was in respiratory failure. Initially the patients are bedbound and may even be ventilator dependent. Outpatient programs are populated with patients who are in the home environment. Patients with chronic pulmonary impairment should be evaluated for outpatient rehabilitation long before severe respiratory failure occurs. If there is an option for the patient to participate in either an outpatient or inpatient program, the outpatient program is the selection of choice since the patient is immediately capable of applying his new knowledge and skill to the home environment and to normal activities of daily living. Further, the lesser cost of an outpatient program is clearly an advantage.

Rehabilitation for the asthmatic patient is almost a separate discipline. In contrast to most other pulmonary-impaired patients these individuals are younger, many are fully employed, and their impairment is episodic. Their rehabilitation needs are more in the realm of education than training. Based upon data derived from a large health maintenance organization, Wilson et al. have concluded that asthma education in groups of six to eight people is best.[76] The National Asthma Education Program, a project of the National Heart, Lung, and Blood Institute of the United

States Public Health Service, has excellent teaching materials for professionals and patients.[77] It is reasonable that patients with occupationally derived asthma will benefit with asthma education programs.

TRAVEL

Aircraft travel poses special problems because, at cruising altitude, commercial aircraft cabin pressure is considerably lower than sea level barometric pressure and may cause significant hypoxemia in patients with pulmonary impairment. Predicting the cabin pressure is difficult but is chiefly dependent upon flight altitude. The pilot can regulate cabin pressure only by altering flight altitude because the maximum pressure differential between the outside and the cabin is fixed by aircraft design. New aircraft have approximately the same pressure differential as old aircraft but fly at higher altitudes and, thus, have lower cabin pressures at cruising altitude. For example, Cottrell found the mean cabin altitude of Boeing 767s and Aerobus 310s was 7,004 feet, whereas the cabin altitude was 5,480 feet in older aircraft.[78] Further complicating the prediction of cabin pressure is that flight altitude may change abruptly because of weather conditions or air traffic. In general, cabin altitude rarely exceeds 9,000 feet and most typically is between 6,000 and 8,000 feet.[79]

Prevalence of in-flight hypoxemia and related morbidity and mortality is unknown. The information available is probably an underestimate, since until recently there has been no systematic process for reporting in-flight medical emergencies and essentially no reporting of delayed illness. Fortunately, even taking into consideration underestimation, the data that are available suggest that the prevalence is low. Speizer et al. reported that 260 (0.003%) of 8,700,000 passengers arriving at Los Angeles International Airport had recognized in-flight medical complications.[80] Twenty passengers complained of dyspnea. Not all the patients were taken to an emergency room, but, of those who were taken, 12 had an exacerbation of COPD . Two of the patients were admitted to a hospital. Mortality from all causes was 1 in 1,300,000. Cummins et al. identified 577 in-flight deaths in 245,000,000 passengers carried aboard 42 international carriers from 1977 to 1984.[81] The mortality rate was 1 in 425,000. Thirty-five deaths were respiratory related.

Because of the low pulmonary morbidity and mortality from air travel, it is rare that a patient that should be advised not to fly following appropriate evaluation. Table 54-7 outlines the specific considerations for the physician and Table 54-8 details the responsibilities of the patient. These guidelines are not only applicable to air travel but travel in general.

Land travel by automobile or recreational vehicle may be the best option for some patients, because transfers are not as harried, the patient can more easily control his or her immediate environment, and acclimatization to varying altitudes is slower. Train service varies among countries and rail lines. In the United States, Amtrack will provide a sleeping room to accommodate the patient's oxygen equipment, deliver meals to the room, and provide assistance for inter-train transfer. Commercial bus travel is cumbersome for long distances, but, for short distances, it may be the best commercial travel means. Ocean cruises can provide an ideal vacation for pulmonary-impaired patients.[82] Regulations, policies, and procedures vary according to cruise line, country of vessel registration, and in some cases rules of the territory in which the vessel is cruising. All cruise lines require the permission of the ship's captain to place oxygen on board.

EMPLOYMENT

Diener analyzed the work status of 99 men younger than age 65 with COPD.[83] Few, if any, had occupationally acquired lung disease. If the work was sedentary, patients continued to work until their FEV1 was below 0.75 L. If work was mild to moderately physically demanding, the patients continued to work until the FEV1 fell below 1 L. Such data are poor predictors to whether patients with occupationally acquired lung disease will continue to work since there are many factors that discourage continued working or encourage continued working under unreasonable circumstances. Among the discouraging factors are an adversarial relationship between the employee and the employer, an inability to employ the patient within the patient's physical capabilities or skills, and a lack of employment opportunities at a site removed from agents that aggravate the lung disease.[84] On the other hand, patients will return to work that is detrimental to their health because of socioeconomic pressures or other factors not predicted by their degree of lung impairment. For instance, Maraini et al. found that young

Table 54-7. Pretravel medical evaluation of respiratory patients

Overall medical stability
  History and physical examination
  Electrocardiogram
  Chest radiographs
  Blood studies (e.g., hemoglobin and serum electrolytes)
  Medications

Travel considerations
  Previous experience at altitude (aircraft or other)
  Expected altitude to be reached or cabin pressure if flying
  Duration of trip
  Number of transfers
  Amount of time between transfers
  Duration and altitude of intermediate and final destinations
  Ability to travel alone or with companion

Physiologic status
  Pulmonary function tests, including spirometry, bronchodilator response, lung volumes, and carbon monoxide transfer factor
  Arterial blood gas on room air
  Exercise study (optional)
  Prediction of altitude Pa_{O_2} and tolerance with formula or hypoxia-altitude simulation test

Adapted from Finnerty M and Gong H: Advising patients with respiratory disorders about air travel, *Travel Med Int* 9:99-105, 1991. With permission.

workers with red cedar asthma who had a large number of dependents continued working in red cedar exposure jobs despite declining pulmonary functions and worsening respiratory symptoms more frequently than older patients with less dependents presumably because of greater economic need.[85] Despite the problems in predicting which patients will successfully return to work, employment is a goal of rehabilitation and should be explored with each patient. Even patients with advanced lung disease who require continuous low flow oxygen can be accommodated in some jobs.

MECHANICAL VENTILATION

For some patients with advanced pulmonary impairment, the only means of prolonging life is mechanical ventilatory support. This therapy must not be undertaken casually. Quality of life, patient's goals, resource availability, and support systems are some of the major considerations. If the decision is made to provide mechanical ventilatory support, selection of a durable medical equipment supplier and home nursing agency that have experience in mechanical ventilation is essential.

Some patients require mechanical ventilatory support with devices that can be applied without the need for tracheostomy. The rocking bed and Pneumobelt (a bladder that rhythmically inflates over the abdomen) assist diaphragmatic excursion. Negative pressure ventilators, such as the

Table 54-8. Patient's responsibility for travel

1. Plan ahead for all aspects and phases of travel.
2. Use wheelchair during transfers and at any time when walking will exceed the patient's usual ability.
3. Arrange seating priority in a nonsmoking area and near a lavatory.
4. Personally carry all medications, and do not leave medications in difficult-to-access luggage; have adequate amounts available for entire trip.
5. Avoid overeating, alcohol, sedating medications; do not smoke.
6. Drink ample fluids to provide adequate hydration and to prevent drying of pulmonary secretions, especially when traveling long distances.
7. Travel with a companion who knows your needs.
8. Exercise leg muscles while seated or standing, and take short walks to reduce venous stasis.
9. Plan ahead for climate, weather, and temperature changes.
10. When arranging for hotel or other accommodations, ask about elevators, number of stairs, heating and air conditioning, and luggage assistance.
11. Pack lightly, and use a luggage carrier with sturdy wheels.
12. If traveling with a tour group choose one that is paced appropriately for your needs.
13. Frequent fliers should obtain a Frequent Traveler Medical Card (FREMEC) from the airline.
14. Regardless of the type of transportation, always carry a summary of medical conditions and the latest pertinent laboratory results, as well as the name, address, and telephone number of the primary care physician.
15. Electrically powered equipment such as hand-held nebulizers, chest percussors, and suction units may need current converters or other adaptors for operation in cars, trains, aircraft, and while staying in foreign countries.
16. If low flow oxygen is necessary, arrange ahead with an oxygen vendor to have oxygen available at destination and at any transfer points.
17. If traveling by aircraft, arrange for inflight oxygen in advance by contacting the carrier; if traveling by boat, train, or bus, contact the carrier to ensure that they will allow the use of oxygen.

Adapted from Finnerty M and Gong H: Advising patients with respiratory disorders about air travel, *Travel Med Int* 9:99-105, 1991. With permission.

iron lung and chest cuirass, support inspiration by applying a cyclic negative pressure about the body or chest. Positive pressure ventilation has been successfully applied to the airway by a tight-fitting nose or mouth mask, particularly in patients with respiratory failure caused by neuromuscular disease and, on occasion, to patients with COPD [86,87]

With the exception of the iron lung, all of the above ventilatory techniques are useful only for partial mechanical ventilatory support, and the iron lung is rarely used in the home. Patients who need full mechanical ventilatory support almost always require a tracheostomy for positive pressure ventilation. There is a good range of mechanical ventilators that can provide home mechanical ventilation, including some that are battery operated and small enough to fit under a wheelchair.

SUMMARY

This chapter has reviewed the facets of pulmonary rehabilitation, beginning with drug therapy and culminating, at one extreme, with the patient returning to employment or at the other extreme, becoming dependent on a mechanical ventilator. At both extremes "restoration of the individual to the fullest physical, medical, mental, emotional, economic, social, and vocational potential of which he is capable" is the goal. Rehabilitation of the patient with occupationally acquired pulmonary disease has not been studied as an independent discipline, but it is reasonable that the positive experiences acquired in other chronic pulmonary diseases can be extrapolated to the patient with occupationally acquired lung disease.

REFERENCES

1. Reis AL: Position paper of the American Association of Cardiovascular and Pulmonary Rehabilitation: scientific basis of pulmonary rehabilitation, *J Cardiopul Rehab* 10:418-441, 1990.
2. Petty TL: Pulmonary rehabilitation, *Am Rev Respir Dis* 122(Pt 2):159-161, 1980.
3. Sahn SA, Nett LM, and Petty TL: Ten-year follow-up of a comprehensive rehabilitation program for severe COPD, *Chest* 77 (Suppl):311-314, 1980.
4. Unger KM, Moser KM, and Hansen P: Selection of an exercise program for COPD patients, *Heart Lung* 9:68-76, 1980.
5. Niederman MS, Clemente PH, Fein AM, et al: Benefits of a multidisciplinary pulmonary rehabilitation program: improvements are independent of lung function, *Chest* 99:798-804, 1919.
6. American Thoracic Society. Pulmonary rehabilitation: ATS official statement, *Am Rev Respir Dis* 124:663-666, 1981.
7. Foster S and Thomas HM III: Pulmonary rehabilitation in lung disease other than chronic obstructive pulmonary disease, *Am Rev Respir Dis* 141:601-604, 1990.
8. Bigger DG, Malen JF, Trulock EP, and Cooper JD: Pulmonary rehabilitation before and after lung transplantation, In Casaburi R and Petty TL, editors: *Principles and practice of pulmonary rehabilitation,* pp 459-467, Philadelphia, 1993, Saunders.
9. Inman WHW and Adelstein AM: Rise and fall of asthma mortality in England and Wales in relation to use of pressurized aerosols, *Lancet* 2:279-285, 1969.
10. Ziment I: Beta-adrenergic agonist toxicity: less of a problem, more of a perception, *Chest* 103:1591-1597, 1993.
11. Skorodin MS: Response, *Chest* 103:1597-1598, 1993.
12. Sears MR: β-agonists and bronchial asthma, *Chest* 104:652, 1993.
13. Kelly HW and Murphy S: Beta-adrenergic agonists for acute, severe asthma, *Ann Pharmacother* 26:81-91, 1992.
14. Lam A and Newhouse MT. Management of asthma and chronic airflow limitation: are methylxanthines obsolete? *Chest* 98:44-52, 1990.
15. Milgrom H and Bender B: Current issues in the use of theophylline, *Am Rev Respir Dis* 147 (Suppl):s33-s39, 1993.

16. Vaz Fragoso CA and Miller MA: Review of the clinical efficacy of theophylline in the treatment of chronic obstructive pulmonary disease, *Am Rev Respir Dis* 147 (Suppl):s40-s47, 1993.

17. Jackson R, Sears MR, Beaglehole R, and Rea HH: International trends in asthma mortality: 1970 to 1985, *Chest* 94:914-919, 1988.

18. Hargreave FE, Dolovich J, and Newhouse MT: The assessment and treatment of asthma: a conference report, *J Allergy Clin Immunol* 85:1098-1111, 1990.

19. Toogood JH: Helping your patients make better use of MDIs and spacers, *J Respir Dis* 15:151-166, 1994.

20. Newman SP, Moren F, Trofast E, Talaee N, and Clarke SW: Deposition and clinical efficacy of terbutaline sulphate from Turbuhaler, a new multi-dose powder inhaler, *Eur Respir J* 2:247-252, 1989.

21. Newman SP, Weisz AWB, Talace N, and Clarke SW: Improvement of drug delivery with a breath actuated pressurized aerosol for patients with poor inhaler technique, *Thorax* 46:712-716, 1991.

22. Baily WC and Foshee LM: Reasons to quit smoking: update for 1993, *J Respir Dis* 14:626-638, 1993.

23. Doll R, and Peto R: Mortality in relation to smoking: 20 years' observation on male British doctors, *Br Med J* 2:1525-1536, 1976.

24. Xu X, Dockery DW, Ware JH, et al: Effects of cigarette smoking on the rate of loss on pulmonary function in adults: a longitudinal assessment, *Am Rev Respir Dis* 146:1345-1348, 1992.

25. Fletcher C and Peto R: The natural history of chronic airflow obstruction, *Br Med J* 1645-1648, 1977.

26. Report of the Surgeon General: Self motivated quitting. In *The health consequences of smoking, cancer,* pp 257-270, Washington, DC, 1982, Superintendent of Documents, U.S. Government Printing Office.

27. Owens GR: How to help your patients stop smoking, *J Respir Dis* 14:641-656, 1993.

28. Lee EW and D'Alonzo GE: Cigarette smoking, nicotine addiction, and its pharmacologic treatment, *Arch Intern Med* 153:34-48, 1993.

29. Gold DR: Indoor air pollution, *Clin Chest Med* 13:215-229, 1992.

30. Gong H Jr: Health effects of air pollution: a review of clinical studies, *Clin Chest Med* 13:201-214, 1992.

31. Dockery DW, Pope CA, Xu X, et al: An association between air pollution and mortality in six U.S. cities, *N Engl J Med* 329:1753-1759, 1993.

32. Cotes JE and Gilson JC: Effect of oxygen on exercise ability in chronic respiratory insufficiency, *Lancet* 1:872-876, 1956.

33. Levine BE, Biglow DB, Hamstra RD, et al: The role of long-term continuous oxygen administration in patients with chronic airway obstruction with hypoxemia, *Ann Intern Med* 66:639-650, 1967.

34. Nocturnal Oxygen Therapy Trial Group: Continuous or nocturnal oxygen therapy in hypoxemic chronic obstructive lung disease, *Ann Intern Med* 93;391-398, 1980.

35. Medical Research Council Working Party: Long-term domiciliary oxygen therapy in chronic hypoxic cor pulmonale complicating chronic bronchitis and emphysema, *Lancet* 1:681-686, 1981.

36. Flenley DC: Long-term home oxygen therapy, *Chest* 87:99-103, 1985.

37. Cooper CB: Long-term oxygen therapy. In Casaburi R and Petty TL, editors: *Principles and practice of pulmonary rehabilitation,* pp 183-203, Philadelphia, 1993, Saunders.

38. Barker AF, Burgher LW, and Plummer AL: Oxygen conserving methods in adults, *Chest* 105:248-252, 1994.

39. Heimlich HJ: Respiratory rehabilitation with transtracheal oxygen system, *Ann Otol Rhinol Laryngol* 91:643-647, 1982.

40. Christopher KL, Spofford BT, Petrun MD, McCarty DC, Goodman JR, and Petty TL: A program for transtracheal oxygen delivery, *Ann Intern Med* 107:802-808, 1987.

41. Scott GC, Hinson JM, Scott RP, Quigley PR, Christopher KL, and Metzler M: The effects of transtracheal gas delivery on central inspiratory neuromuscular drive, *Chest* 104:1199-1202, 1993.

42. Dillard TA, Berg BW, Rajagopal KR, Dooley JW, and Mehm WJ: Hypoxemia during air travel in patients with chronic airway obstruction, *Ann Intern Med* 111;362-367, 1989.

43. Gong H Jr, Tashkin DP, Lee EY, and Simmons MS: Hypoxia-altitude stimulation test: evaluation of patients with chronic obstruction, *Am Rev Respir Dis* 130:980-986, 1984.

44. Dillard TA, Rosenberg AP, and Berg BW: Hypoxemia during altitude exposure: a meta-analysis of chronic obstructive pulmonary disease, *Chest* 103:422-425, 1993.

45. Vohra PK and Klocke RA: Detection and correction of hypoxemia associated with air travel, *Am Rev Respir Dis* 148:1215-1219, 1993.

46. Smith K, Cook D, Guyatt GH, Madhavan J, and Oxman AD: Respiratory muscle training in chronic airflow limitation: a meta-analysis, *Am Rev Respir Dis* 145:533-539, 1992.

47. McGavin CR, Gupta SP, and McHardy GJR: Twelve minute walking test for assessing disability in chronic bronchitis, *Br Med J* 1:822-823, 1976.

48. Bernstein ML, Despars JA, Singh NP, Avalos K, Stansbury DW, and Light RW: Reanalysis of the 12-minute walk in patients with chronic obstructive pulmonary disease, *Chest* 105:163-167, 1994.

49. Belman ML and Shadmehr R: Targeted resistive ventilatory muscle training in chronic obstructive pulmonary disease, *J Appl Physiol* 65;2726-2735, 1988.

50. Thoman RL, Stoker GL, and Ross JC: The efficacy of pursed-lip breathing in patients with chronic obstructive pulmonary disease, *Am Rev Respir Dis* 93:100-106, 1966.

51. Mueller RE, Petty TL, and Filley GF: Ventilation and arterial gas changes induced by pursed lip breathing, *J Appl Physiol* 28:784-789, 1970.

52. Tiep BL, Burns M, Kao D, et al: Pursed lips breathing training using ear oximetry, *Chest* 90:218-221, 1986.

53. Roa J, Epstein S, Breslin E, Shannon T, and Celli B: Work of breathing and ventilatory muscle recruitment during pursed lip breathing in patients with chronic airway obstruction, *Am Rev Respir Dis* 143:A77, 1991.

54. Barach AL: Chronic obstructive lung disease: postural relief of dyspnea, *Arch Phys Med Rehabil* 55:494-50, 1974.

55. Druz WS and Sharp JT: Electrical and mechanical activity of the diaphragm accompanying body position in severe chronic obstructive pulmonary disease, *Am Rev Respir Dis* 125:275-280, 1982.

56. Sharp JT, Drutz WS, Moisan T, Foster J, and Machnach W: Postural relief of dyspnea in severe chronic obstructive pulmonary disease, *Am Rev Respir Dis* 122:201-211, 1980.

57. Murray JF: The ketchup-bottle method, *N Engl J Med* 300:1155, 1979.

58. Rochester DF and Goldberg SK: Techniques of respiratory physical therapy, *Am Rev Respir Dis* 122(5 pt 2):133-146, 1980.

59. Intermittent Positive Pressure Breathing Trial Group: Intermittent positive pressure breathing therapy of chronic obstructive pulmonary disease: a clinical trial, *Ann Intern Med* 99:612-620, 1983.

60. Shapiro BJ, Welch MA Jr, and Mercurio P: The IPPB trial, *Ann Intern Med* 100:457-458, 1984.

61. Memsic L, Silberman AW, and Silberman H: Malnutrition and respiratory distress: who's at risk? *J Respir Dis* 11:529-535, 1990.

62. Wilson DO, Rogers RM, Wright EC, and Anthonisen NR: Body weight in chronic pulmonary disease. The National Institutes of Health intermittent positive-pressure breathing trial, *Am Rev Respir Dis* 139:1435-1438, 1989.

63. Knowles JB, Fairbarn MS, Wiggs BJ, Clan-Yan C, and Pardy RL: Dietary supplementation and respiratory muscle performance in patients with COPD, *Chest* 93:977-983, 1988.

64. Harris JA and Benedict FG: Biometric studies of basal metabolism in man. Carnegie Institute of Washington, 1919 Pub No 279.

65. Moore JA and Angelillo VA: Equations for the prediction of resting energy expenditure in chronic obstructive lung disease, *Chest* 94:1260-1263, 1988.

66. Silberman H and Silberman AW: Parenteral nutrition, biochemistry and respiratory gas exchange, *J Parent Enteral Nutr* 10:151-154, 1986.

67. Bowser EK: Criteria to initiate and use supplemental gastrostomy feedings in patients with cystic fibrosis, *Top Clin Nutr* 5;62-73, 1990.

68. Kravetz HM: A visit with Harry. A visit with Helen. Sexual counseling for the COPD patient (slide and tape presentation). Available from 1011 Ruth St., Prescott, AZ 86301.

69. Williams SJ and Bury MR: Impairment, disability and handicap in chronic respiratory illness, *Soc Sci Med* 29:606-616, 1989.

70. Strauss AL and Glaser BG: *Chronic illness and the quality of life,* St. Louis, 1975, Mosby.

71. Dudley DL, Glaser EM, Jorgenson BN, and Logan DL: Psychosocial concomitants to rehabilitation in chronic obstructive pulmonary disease: Part 1. Psychosocial and psychological considerations, *Chest* 77:413-420, 1980.

72. Dudley DL, Glaser EM, Jorgenson BN, and Logan DL: Psychosocial concomitants to rehabilitation in chronic obstructive pulmonary disease: Part 2. Psychosocial treatment, *Chest* 77:544-551, 1980.

73. Dudley DL, Glaser EM, Jorgenson BN, and Logan DL: Psychosocial concomitants to rehabilitation in chronic obstructive pulmonary disease: Part 3. Dealing with psychiatric disease (as distinguished from psychosocial or psychophysiologic problems), *Chest* 77:677-684, 1980.

74. McSweeny AJ, Grant I, Heaton RK, Adams KM, and Timms RM: Life quality of patients with chronic obstructive pulmonary disease, *Arch Intern Med* 142:473-478, 1982.

75. Yellowees PM, Alpers JH, Bowden JJ, et al: Psychiatric morbidity in subjects with chronic airflow obstruction, *Med J Aust* 146:305-307, 1987.

76. Wilson SR, Scamagas P, German DF, et al: A controlled trial of two forms of self-management education for adults with asthma, *Am J Med* 94:564-576, 1993.

77. National Asthma Education Program: *Teach your patients about asthma: a clinician's guide,* Bethesda, MD, 1992, National Institutes of Health, National Heart, Lung, and Blood Institute, Pub No 92-2737.

78. Cottrell JJ: Altitude exposures during aircraft flight: flying higher, *Chest* 93:81-84, 1988.

79. Finnerty M and Gong H: Advising patients with respiratory disorders about air travel, *Travel Med Int* 9:99-105, 1991.

80. Speizer C, Rennie CJ III, and Breton H: Prevalence of inflight medical emergencies on commercial airlines, *Ann Emerg Med* 18;26-29, 1989.

81. Cummins RO, Chapman PJ, Chamberlain DA, Schuback JA, and Litwin PE: In-flight deaths during commercial air travel: how big is the problem? *JAMA* 259:1983-1988, 1988.

82. Burns MR: Cruising with COPD, *Am J Nurs* 87:479-482, 1987.

83. Diener CF and Burrows B: Occupational disability in patients with chronic airway obstruction, *Am Rev Respir Dis* 96:35-42, 1967.

84. Harber P: Assessing disability from occupational asthma: a perspective on the AMA guides, *Chest* 98(suppl):232s-235s, 1990.

85. Maraini A, Dimich-Ward H, Kwan SYL, Kennedy SM, Waxler-Morrison N, and Chan-Yeung M: Clinical and socioeconomic features of subjects with red cedar asthma, *Chest* 104:821-824, 1993.

86. Bach JR, Alba AS, and Saporito LR: Intermittent positive pressure ventilation via the mouth as an alternative to tracheostomy for 257 ventilator users, *Chest* 103:174-182, 1993.

87. Hill NS: Noninvasive positive pressure ventilation in neuromuscular disease, *Chest* 105:337-338, 1994.

Section **XI**

Regulatory and Policy Issues

MARC B. SCHENKER

Treating and preventing occupational and environmental respiratory diseases often require a knowledge of the responsible regulatory agencies and standards or statutes for the workplace and the ambient environment. These topics are covered in this section in chapters on occupational and environmental regulatory approaches. With increasing concern about occupational and environmental hazards, particularly those due to low level exposures, the topic of hazard communication has become increasingly important for the physician or the public official who must communicate concepts of disease risk to individuals or to community groups. Finally, this section includes a chapter on the approaches to occupational and environmental respiratory hazards in the developing countries of the world. Whereas the pathology of disease may be the same around the world, the diagnostic tools and resources for addressing these problems may be quite different. Chapter 58 highlights some of the different approaches to these problems in countries with less resources and very different regulatory and administrative structures.

Chapter 55

OCCUPATIONAL REGULATORY APPROACHES

John R. Froines

As a result of exposure to silica dust during the construction of the Hawk's Nest Tunnel at Gauley Bridge, West Virginia between 1930 and 1932, 764 workers died from silicosis.[1] The Gauley Bridge disaster, as it has become known, represents one of the greatest tragedies in U.S. industrial history. Even the death toll does not begin to describe the depth of human suffering nor did it reflect an exposure to a substance with previously unknown toxicity. The toxicity of silica and silicosis had been recognized by writers such as Hippocrates in the fifth century B.C. and Ramazzini in the eighteenth century.[2]

The relevance of Gauley Bridge to this chapter is the state of regulatory policy with respect to occupational respiratory disease in the early 1930s versus the status of social legislation enacted in more recent years to prevent occupational respiratory disease or compensate its victims. In the period 1900 to 1936, legislation that addressed the safety and health of workers was enacted at the state level and focused on the compensation of workers for occupational injuries, amputations, or death as a result of workplace accidents. Little attention was given to prevention of occupational disease even though the effects of lead, silica, and other chemical agents were recognized. Congressional hearings held as a result of the Gauley Bridge disaster focused not on prevention of silicosis through social legislation but more on the adequacy of worker's compensation. At the 1936 hearings then Congressman Jennings Randolph stated that only 11 States in the United States had laws in which silicosis was compensable.[3] By the end of 1937, 46 states had enacted compensation laws covering workers with silicosis.[1]

The first workers' compensation laws had been passed at the state level in 1911, and the first laws that addressed compensation of occupational disease were enacted by California and Massachusetts in 1917, but it was not until 1976 that all states provided coverage of occupational disease.

The first occupational safety and health legislation that was enacted in the United States occurred at the state level and began in the nineteenth century. Massachusetts passed legislation in 1852 and 1877, and by 1890, 22 states had promulgated regulations of safety in mining, and 14 states had enacted legislation providing for industrial workplace inspections.[4] The Office of Technology Assessment[4] has pointed out that, on average, there was only one occupational health staff member at the state level for every 108,000 workers. Overall state safety and health programs were underfunded, lacked authority, and in many states were nonexistent even into the 1960s.[5]

The first federal legislation providing protection of workers was the Walsh–Healy Act of 1936, which was later supplemented by the McNamara–O'Hara Act of 1966 and the Construction Safety Act of 1969. These laws covered employees working for employers who had contracts with the federal government and required employers to comply with Walsh–Healy safety and health standards. These standards were recommended by the Bureau of Labor Standards of the U.S. Department of Labor.[4] Inspections were conducted by the Bureau of Labor Standards, and penalties included "blacklisting," the prohibition of bidding on Federal contracts for up to 3 years. These Acts clearly impacted workplace conditions, but overall the performance of these agencies indicated a need for more comprehensive federal legislation. A study conducted by the Department of Labor itself described the nation's health and safety laws as being inadequate and fragmented.[6] In 1968, President Lyndon Johnson proposed federal legislation to establish safety and health regulatory programs that provided for setting and enforcing occupational standards. Unfortunately, there was significant opposition to the legislation and it never reached the floor of Congress, but it set the stage for legislation that was to follow.

THE OCCUPATIONAL SAFETY AND HEALTH ACT OF 1970

As the 1960s came to a close, it was apparent that at long last the U.S. Congress was prepared to enact legislation to address health and safety in the 5 million workplaces that employed approximately 90 million workers in jobs ranging from service and clerical work to high technology professional employment to heavy industry with its myriad of recognized health and safety hazards. At that time it was estimated that 14,000 employees were dying annually in accidental deaths; there were 2 million lost workday injuries each year and an estimated 100,000 new cases of occupational disease yearly. Although these numbers may have had questionable validity, they did indicate a need for legislation to protect the health and safety of employees in the workplace. The legislation itself was broad in scope and included a number of provisions that have required subsequent judicial review, but overall the law represented a major step forward in providing protection for the tens of millions of American workers. The overall Congressional intent is summarized in the box. A review of some of the Congressional findings and purpose will illuminate the un

---

Congressional findings and purpose: Occupational Safety and Health Act of 1970

Sec. (2) The Congress finds that personal injuries and illnesses arising out of work situations impose a substantial burden upon, and are a hindrance to, interstate commerce in terms of lost production, wage loss, medical expenses, and disability compensation payments.

(b) The Congress declares it to be its purpose and policy, through the exercise of its powers to regulate commerce among the several States and with foreign nations and to provide for the general welfare, to assure so far as possible every working man and woman in the Nation safe and healthful working conditions and to preserve our human resources—

(1) by encouraging employers and employees in their efforts to reduce the number of occupational safety and health hazards at their places of employment, and to stimulate employers and employees to institute new and to perfect existing programs for providing safe and healthful working conditions;

(2) by providing that employers and employees have separate but dependent responsibilities and rights with respect to achieving safe and healthful working conditions;

(3) by authorizing the Secretary of Labor to set mandatory occupational safety and health standards applicable to businesses affecting interstate commerce, and by creating an Occupational Safety and Health Review Commission for carrying out adjudicatory functions under the Act;

(4) by building upon advances already made through employer and employee initiative for providing safe and healthful working conditions;

(5) by providing for research in the field of occupational safety and health, including the psychological factors involved, and by developing innovative methods, techniques, and approaches for dealing with occupational safety and health problems;

(6) by exploring ways to discover latent diseases, establishing causal connections between diseases and work in environmental conditions, and conducting other research relating to health problems, in recognition of the fact that occupational health standards present problems often different from those involved in occupational safety;

(7) by providing medical criteria which will assure insofar as practicable that no employee will suffer diminished health, functional capacity, or life expectancy as a result of his work experience;

(8) by providing for training programs to increase the number and competence of personnel engaged in the field of occupational safety and health;

(9) by providing for the development and promulgation of occupational safety and health standards;

(10) by providing an effective enforcement program which shall include a prohibition against giving advance notice of any inspection and sanctions for any individual violating this prohibition;

(11) by encouraging the States to assume the fullest responsibility for the administration and enforcement of their

Continued.

> **Congressional findings and purpose: Occupational Safety and Health Act of 1970—cont'd**
>
> occupational safety and health laws by providing grants to the States to assist in identifying their needs and responsibilities in the area of occupational safety and health, to develop plans in accordance with the provisions of this Act, to improve the administration and enforcement of State occupational safety and health laws, and to conduct experimental and demonstration projects in connection therewith;
>
> (12) by providing for appropriate reporting procedures with respect to occupational safety and health which procedures will help achieve the objectives of this Act and accurately describe the nature of the occupational safety and health problem;
>
> (13) by encouraging joint labor-management efforts to reduce injuries and disease arising out of employment.

derlying philosophy of the Occupational Safety and Health Act (OSHAct).

Research, standards, and enforcement

Sections 3 and 9 of the Congressional findings emphasized the primary importance of standards within the OSHAct. Establishing appropriate health and safety standards represented the central theme of the Act. Research was to be conducted to provide the basis for standards. Those standards were to be the foundation of the enforcement program as well as being the basis for education and training and voluntary compliance. The central role of the administrative agency established by the Act, the U.S. Occupational Safety and Health Administration (OSHA), which was located in the Department of Labor, was the promulgation and enforcement of standards in businesses and industries within the jurisdiction of the OSHAct. Standards are crucial because they define the minimum level of health and safety practice that industry must meet. They formed the basis around which a business may plan its health and safety program, and they provided information for workers on what are the appropriate conditions for the work environment.

The OSHAct established three types of standards: (1) interim standards, (2) permanent standards, and (3) temporary emergency standards. Interim standards are defined under Section 6(a) of the Act: "the Secretary (of Labor) shall, as soon as practicable during the period beginning with the effective date of this Act and ending two years after such date, by rule promulgate as an occupational safety and health standard any national consensus standard, and any established Federal standard, unless he determines that the promulgation of such a standard would not result in improved safety or health for specifically designated employees." This decision by Congress to permit the Agency to adopt existing national consensus standards has implica-

tions for health and safety practices today and will be discussed further below.

Section 10 of the findings emphasized the need for an effective enforcement program. The OSHAct established procedures for enforcement that included the right to enter establishments covered by the act for the purpose of conducting inspections to determine compliance with existing health and safety standards. Inspections were to be conducted at reasonable times and prior notification of the intent to conduct an inspection was prohibited.

The legislation emphasized the need for research that would lead to "innovative methods, techniques and approaches for dealing with occupational safety and health problems"[5] and "by exploring ways to discover latent diseases, establishing causal connections between diseases and work in environmental conditions and conducting other research relating to health problems, in recognition of the fact that occupational health standards present problems often different from those involved in occupational safety."[6] This latter finding has direct relevance to occupational respiratory disease. To meet this challenge for increased research Congress established a research agency, the U.S. National Institute for Occupational Safety and Health (NIOSH), whose mission included "development and establishment of recommended occupational safety and health standards and conducting research to enable the Agency to make recommendations for standards." NIOSH is located in the Department of Health and Human Services (HHS).

Other findings of importance in the OSHAct included provision 11, which established the right of states to establish state OSHA programs that would be funded in part by the federal program.

The Congressional findings in section 7 required that medical criteria be established that would ensure that employees would not suffer diminished health, functional capacity, or life expectancy as a result of their work experience. This provision is quite important in the context of occupational respiratory disease, and it has received considerable attention by NIOSH in its research efforts and by OSHA in the setting of occupational health standards.

The Congressional findings provided the framework for the Act. The specific provisions will now be discussed in greater detail, particularly in the context of policy decisions that have emerged during the history of the Act's implementation.

OCCUPATIONAL SAFETY AND HEALTH STANDARDS
Interim standards

Following passage of the Act an immediate issue concerned how the Agency would proceed to establish standards to begin an enforcement effort. The Congress addressed this issue in the OSHAct by providing 2 years during which OSHA could adopt existing standards developed by consensus standards bodies or already promulgated applicable Federal standards. These standards would be exempt from the rulemaking procedures required by the Administrative Procedure Act, and they would be immediately effective.

In the health area OSHA adopted recommendations developed by two "consensus" standards organizations, the American Conference of Governmental Industrial Hygienists (ACGIH) and the American National Standards Institute (ANSI). ACGIH is an organization that was founded in 1938 by industrial hygienists employed in government agencies. Today the organization includes governmental and academic industrial hygienists.

ACGIH is noteworthy because of its development of threshold limit values (TLVs). TLVs refer to the airborne concentrations of chemical substances and physical agents to which nearly all workers may be repeatedly exposed day after day without adverse health effects. These limits are intended for use in industrial hygiene as guidelines or recommendations in the control of potential workplace health hazards. TLVs are partially updated on an annual basis. Using their authority under Section 6(a) of the Act, OSHA adopted the 1968 TLVs, which had previously been incorporated in 1969 by the Bureau of Labor Standards using the authority in the Walsh–Healy Act. Approximately 400 chemicals were included in this list. Since 1971 OSHA has adopted 24 permanent standards, but the 1968 TLVs remain the operative standards for most of the chemicals regulated by OSHA.

In 1971 OSHA adopted as standards for a few chemicals the recommendations developed by another consensus organization, the American National Standards Institute (ANSI), which also develops recommendations for improvement of workplace safety and health conditions. ANSI was originally formed in 1918, and its membership primarily consists of companies, trade associations, government agencies, some unions, and private groups. ANSI established a Board of Standards Review in 1969 that was composed of 15 persons, 9 from industry, 2 from the federal government, 1 from municipal government, 2 academic representatives, and 1 member from a consumer organization.

Permanent standards

Under Section 6(b) of the OSHAct the Secretary of Labor may promulgate, modify, or revoke any occupational safety and health standard. The decision of the Secretary to promulgate a standard was to be based on information submitted by interested persons, a representative of any organization of employers or employees, a nationally recognized standards-producing organization, the Secretary of HHS, NIOSH, or a State or political subdivision. The Agency then publishes a proposed rule in the *Federal Register* generally after having requested comments from interested parties on the substance in question. Following publication of the proposed standard OSHA holds public hearings to obtain written and oral comment on the proposed standard. The Secretary must issue the standard within 30 days of the close of the comment period. Persons who are adversely affected by the standard may challenge its validity by petitioning the appropriate U.S. Circuit Court of Appeals within 60 days.

Emergency temporary standards

If the Secretary determines that employees are exposed to grave danger from exposure to substances or agents determined to be toxic or physically harmful or from new hazards, he may promulgate an emergency temporary standard that takes immediate effect upon publication in the *Federal Register* providing the emergency temporary standard is necessary to protect employees from such danger. The emergency temporary standard remains in effect for 6 months after which the Secretary must promulgate a permanent standard.

Criteria for permanent standards that address toxic materials

Establishing permanent occupational safety and health standards was envisioned by Congress as being central to achieving the goals of the OSHAct. For the Agency to establish permanent standards, it was necessary for Congress to define the criteria that OSHA would use in promulgating standards. In general the criteria for health standards must address two general issues:

1. What is the level of scientific evidence required to support and justify a standard that seeks to limit exposure to a toxic chemical?
2. How are the costs and technological requirements of a standard to be considered?

What is the level of evidence required to justify a standard that addresses toxic chemicals.

First, it is important to recognize that the level of evidence on chemical toxicity and exposure required for action is not absolute. In addressing the level of scientific evidence required for the development and justification of a standard, the principal factors that must be evaluated include the scope of the evidence required to establish a causal and quantitative relationship between adverse health consequences and exposure to a chemical toxicant, and how the uncertainty in the scientific information should be evaluated and considered. For example, when considering the scope of the evidence for setting a standard for a carcinogen, one extreme argument would require epidemiologic evidence as an absolute requirement because it is based on human studies. However, this approach is slow, expensive, and insensitive with respect to the need to provide an adequate level of protection. By contrast, the use of short-term tests for genetic toxicity or analysis of the chemical structure to define a substance as a potential toxicant may result in false positive conclusions with significant cost impacts on an affected industry.

Qualitative and quantitative evaluation of scientific uncertainty is a crucial concept that has direct relevance to decision making. For example, animal evidence may yield important information on toxicity that has application to humans. Or there may be factors associated with animal testing that bias the end result, such as the testing of chemicals in animals at high doses with a potential toxicant. How we view the uncertainties associated with animal experiments may influence our decision that data derived from this source are adequate for regulatory purposes. Another level of uncertainty concerns the absolute definition of a disease or illness. The criteria used for a standard will likely differ markedly from the criteria for compensation insofar as standards are intended to prevent the development of an occupational disease. For example, should OSHA establish standards based on a respiratory irritation that is non–life-threatening or should standards seek to control only those exposures that result in chronic, debilitating disease.

Congress established limited criteria in the initial legislation, and during the past two decades judicial decisions on standards promulgated by OSHA have further refined the criteria for standard setting. A review of the more important decisions will illuminate our current understanding of the basis for standard setting. Questions of economics and technology will be addressed in the context of those decisions.

Section 6(b)(5) addresses the criteria that the Secretary must meet in promulgating permanent standards for toxic materials or harmful physical agents. "The Secretary, in promulgating standards dealing with toxic materials or harmful physical agents shall set the standard which most adequately assures, to the extent feasible, on the basis of the best available evidence, that no employee will suffer material impairment of health or functional capacity even if such employee has regular exposure to the hazard dealt with by such standard for the period of his working life." The key terms that require further analysis are *feasibility* and *material impairment*. The former term has particular relevance when the Agency attempts to address the issue of what types of controls are appropriate to limit exposure to safe levels. The concept of material impairment has direct relevance to occupational respiratory disease. For example, the respiratory disease byssinosis is associated with exposure to cotton dust (see Chapter 25). There is evidence that the disease may progress from an acute, apparently reversible phase to a chronic irreversible stage. What stage constitutes material impairment is a health and a scientific policy issue that has been litigated in the appellate courts.

In promulgating standards the Secretary must make a finding that a particular standard is feasible. What constitutes feasibility is a matter of interpretation, and there has been significant debate over the meaning of the term. Some of the pertinent issues include the following:

1. Does feasibility mean technological feasibility or are economic considerations to be considered?

2. Does the term feasibility imply that the Agency can require controls not yet in actual use?
3. Is the time required to come into compliance with the standard to be considered within the context of defining feasibility?
4. Can OSHA require a more expensive technology such as automated processes or ventilation that may be more costly than rudimentary controls such as respiratory protection?
5. Can a standard be so strict that an entire industry or sectors of an industry, for example, small facilities, are forced out of business?

What is a permanent standard?

OSHA has promulgated 26 permanent health standards for specific chemical agents since passage of the OSHAct in 1970. The standards developed under Section 6(b) of the Act are listed in Table 55-1 and include the permissible exposure limits (PELs). These standards can be subdivided into two categories of regulations: (1) standards for individual chemicals such as cotton dust or asbestos, and (2) generic standards that address broad issues such as a carcinogen policy or access to medical records.

Table 55-1. Chemical toxicants for which the Occupational Safety and Health Administration has promulgated permanent health standards: 1972-1994.

Chemical	Current PEL (8-hour time weighted average)
Acrylonitrile	2 ppm
Arsenic (inorganic)	10 μg/m^3
Asbestos	0.2 fiber/cm^3 of air
Benzene	1 ppm
Cadmium	5 μg/m^3
Coke oven emissions	150 μg/m^3
Cotton dust	200 μg/m^3
1,2-Dibromochloropropane	1 ppb
Ethylene oxide	1 ppm
Formaldehyde	0.75 ppm
Lead	50 μg/m^3
Methylenedianiline	10 ppb
Vinyl chloride	1 ppm

Carcinogens with permanent standards but no PEL

2-Acetylaminofluorine
4-Aminodiphenyl
Benzidine
Bis-Chloromethyl ether
3,3'-Dichlorobenzidene
4-Dimethylaminoazobenzene
Ethyleneimine
Methyl chloromethyl ether
α-Naphthylamine
β-Naphthylamine
4-Nitrobiphenyl
N-Nitrosodimethylamine
β-Propiolactone

Standards for individual chemicals

There are important distinctions between an ACGIH TLV including the 1968 TLVs adopted by OSHA in 1971 and an OSHA permanent standard for a single chemical substance. The ACGIH TLVs are specific numerical limits below which most workers may be exposed with a reasonable anticipation that a worker will not suffer harm if exposed to the substance in the work environment at or below the prescribed level. For example, the TLV for cotton dust is 0.2 mg/m^3 for lint-free dust averaged over an 8-hour workday. It is important to emphasize that ACGIH acknowledges that the TLV is not protective of all workers. "Because of the wide variation in individual susceptibility, a small percentage of workers may experience discomfort, and a smaller number may develop an occupational illness" (TLV 1994-1995).

In contrast to the ACGIH TLV, the standard promulgated by OSHA to control workplace exposure to cotton dust is not a single number but rather a comprehensive strategy to protect workers from byssinosis associated with exposure to cotton dust in the textile industry. The specific provisions of the standard include specific numeric limits, the PEL, which is 0.2 mg/m^3 in opening through spinning and 0.75 mg/m^3 for weaving in the textile industry, but there are also provisions that require (1) establishment of workpractices to reduce exposure to cotton dust, (2) environmental monitoring, (3) medical surveillance, (4) a respirator program, (5) employee education and training, (6) signs, and (7) recordkeeping. Other standards also include provisions for hygiene facilities and practices, regulated areas, protective clothing, housekeeping, and biologic monitoring. These provisions, taken as a whole, provide much greater protection than would occur through enforcement solely of a specific limit. The multiple provisions represent a strategy for protecting workers as completely as feasible and provide a comprehensive approach to controlling workplace exposures. Also included in any standard is an explanation of the basis for the standard and a discussion of the issues of technologic feasibility and the costs of compliance with the standard. This approach is characteristic of all the permanent standards promulgated since the passage of the OSHAct.

Generic standards

OSHA became interested in the concept of generic standards when the Agency recognized that the standard-setting process was slow at best, and there were many unregulated workplace hazards. There was also a series of workplace issues requiring attention that were not unique to a specific substance, but were relevant to the protection of workers' health on a broad basis. To address some of these issues OSHA has adopted the following generic standards: the generic cancer standard, access to medical records standard, and the hazard communication standard. The Agency is currently considering adoption of a generic standard that will mandate environmental monitoring of workplace exposure across a wide range of industries and chemical agents.

The general duty clause

Section 5(a) of the OSHAct describes the general duties of employers and employees within the Act. Section 5(a)(1) states that an employer "shall furnish to each of his employees employment and a place of employment which are free from recognized hazards that are causing or likely to cause death or serious physical harm to his employees." Sections 5(a)(2) and 5(b) state that employers and employees, respectively, must comply with health and safety standards promulgated under the legislation.

Section 5(a)(1) is generally referred to as the "general duty clause" and it is the requirement used for enforcement purposes where no standard exists to cover exposure to a hazard. Citations have been issued to employers for violation of the general duty clause where workers have been exposed to chemicals for which no standard has been promulgated. There are legal issues that require interpretation where the general duty clause is used including the question of what constitutes "serious" physical harm and what is meant by the term "recognized hazards."

THE HISTORY OF OCCUPATIONAL HEALTH STANDARD SETTING AND LEGAL REVIEW: POLICY ISSUES

This section reviews selected permanent standards promulgated by OSHA, in particular those that have specific legal and policy implications for the overall implementation of the Act. Some substances will be addressed that do not produce respiratory disease but for which the legal decisions surrounding promulgation have wider implications than the specific substance itself.

Asbestos

OSHA's first permanent standard was asbestos. A PEL of 5 fibers/cm^3 was established for the first 4 years (1972 to 1976), and the PEL was then reduced to 2 fibers/cm^3. A new PEL of 0.2 fibers/cm^3 as an 8-hour time-weighted average (TWA) was established in 1986. A fiber means a particulate form of asbestos, 5 μm or longer, with a length-to-diameter ratio of at least 3:1. This standard applies to all forms of asbestos including chrysotile, amosite, crocidilite, tremolite asbestos, anthophyllite asbestos, and actinolite asbestos. An action level of 0.1 fibers/cm^3 calculated as an 8-hour TWA was also established. This action level has relevance to specific requirements of the standard including environmental monitoring and medical surveillance, because these provisions are required to be initiated when airborne asbestos concentrations exceed this level, not when the PEL is exceeded.

Benzene

OSHA promulgated a permanent standard for benzene in 1978, which reduced the PEL from 10 parts per million (ppm) averaged over an 8-hour workday to 1 ppm to reduce the risk of leukemia from exposure to benzene in the work environment. The evidence in the record for benzene firmly established a causal relationship between benzene exposure and leukemia. The permanent OSHA standard was first litigated before the Fifth Circuit Court of Appeals, which invalidated the standard and later the U.S. Supreme Court upheld the invalidation of the standard.

The principal issue in the benzene decision concerned an often overlooked section of the Act, "Definitions." In this Section the term occupational safety and health standard is defined as meaning "a standard which requires conditions, or the adoption or use of one or more practices, means, methods, operations, or processes, *reasonably necessary* or appropriate to provide safe or healthful employment and places of employment." In the benzene decision the U.S. Supreme Court ruled that OSHA had a duty to show that the toxic substance poses a significant health risk in the workplace and that a new, lower standard is "reasonably necessary." In other words, the Agency has an affirmative duty to demonstrate in a rulemaking for a toxic substance that a stricter standard is reasonably necessary; there is an incremental benefit in terms of lives saved, disease avoided, or some other criteria in reducing the standard from one level to another.

What then constitutes "significant risk" in chemical carcinogenesis? Since there is often no threshold for carcinogenesis, there is risk at any level of exposure. In an environmental setting the risk of one excess cancer in a million persons has generally been considered the standard for significant risk. The U.S. Environmental Protection Agency (EPA) has adopted a general policy that a lifetime cancer risk of 1 in 10,000 for the most exposed person might constitute acceptable risk and that the margin of safety should reduce the risk for the greatest possible number of persons to an individual lifetime risk of no higher than 1 in 1 million. The Supreme Court was not explicit in its findings. It stated that a risk of one excess cancer in a billion persons is not significant, but that a risk of one in a thousand would be considered significant, which leaves six orders of magnitude between those two values. Subsequent to the benzene decision, OSHA has used the one in a thousand risk as the defining criteria for significant risk. There is clearly no "gold standard" for risk, and the selection of a one in a thousand risk is controversial since it results in a less protective posture for occupational exposures than is used for environmental risks. This issue of what constitutes significant risk or, conversely, an acceptable risk will continue to be debated, but the benzene decision has been one of the important decisions that has led to an emphasis on quantitative risk assessment, which is defined as a process whereby relevant biologic, dose–response, and exposure data are combined to produce a qualitative or quantitative estimate of adverse outcome from a defined activity or chemical agent.[7] This emphasis on quantitative risk assessment has been a central feature of environmental and occupational health regulation for more than a decade.

Cotton dust

OSHA promulgated a standard to limit exposure to cotton dust in 1978. The previous standard had been 1 mg/m^3 total dust (an ACGIH TLV that had been previously adopted as a Walsh–Healy standard), and the new standard was 0.2 mg/m^3 in opening through spinning and 0.75 mg/m^3 in weaving in the textile industry. These values are for respirable not total dust, and they are determined by measurement with a vertical elutriator, an instrument that measures the concentration of cotton dust aerosol with a mass median diameter 15 μm or less. Other requirements were established for other nontextile industries such as mattress and bedspring manufacture, warehousing, classing offices, knitting, waste processing, garnetting, nonwoven fabric and surgical dressings, spun yarn, and cottonseed oil production, but those industries are not addressed here.

The standard was primarily adopted to reduce the incidence of byssinosis in the textile industry. Cotton dust was described as an airborne particle by-product of the preparation and manufacture of cotton products that produces a "constellation of respiratory effects" known as "byssinosis."[7a] The cotton dust standard is one of two permanent standards developed by OSHA in its history that addresses noncarcinogens. There are a large number of noncarcinogens that produce respiratory disease that have not been addressed in any rulemaking by the Agency. The standard for cotton dust was challenged by the courts by labor and industry. The U.S. Supreme Court addressed both the question of material impairment and feasibility in its decision on cotton dust.

The American Textile Manufacturer's Institute, who was one of the petitioners in the appellate court review of the cotton dust standard, argued that the Act requires OSHA to demonstrate that a standard reflects a reasonable relationship between the costs and benefits associated with the standard. The term "to the extent feasible" is the key language in Section 6(b) for resolution of the issue of whether cost–benefit analysis is a required criterion for standard setting in cotton dust and any other occupational health standard. The Supreme Court went to the dictionary to determine the meaning of the term "feasible" since Congress had not given a specific definition of the term. Feasible means literally "capable of being done," and the Court ruled that Section 6(b)(5) directs the Secretary to issue the standard that "most adequately assures . . . that no employee will suffer material impairment of health" limited only by the extent to which this is "capable of being done." Any standard that is based on the explicit balancing of costs and benefits would be inconsistent with this command, and cost–benefit analysis by OSHA is not required by the statute because feasibility is required. The Supreme Court therefore rejected the argument that Congress intended to require cost–benefit analysis as a basis for establishing the PEL in occupational health standards.

Overall, the U.S. Supreme Court upheld the OSHA cotton dust standard.[8] In complying with the standard the textile industry introduced more advanced engineering controls than were anticipated by OSHA or NIOSH. These controls also increased productivity and reduced energy costs, and were significantly less costly than estimated during the rulemaking process. The information from these studies illustrates that the standard was not only feasible but resulted in improved technology and at far less cost than anticipated.

During the promulgation of the cotton dust standard an important issue that was debated concerned the use of engineering controls versus respiratory protection to reduce worker's exposure to cotton dust.

Occupational health professionals have established a hierarchy of controls according to their efficacy in reducing exposure to hazardous agents. For example, in 1963 ACGIH and the American Industrial Hygiene Association jointly issued a comprehensive guide to respiratory protection in industrial settings. They concluded: "In the control of those occupational diseases caused by breathing air contaminated with harmful dusts, fumes, mists, gases, or vapors, the primary objective should be to prevent the air from becoming contaminated. This is accomplished as far as possible by accepted engineering control measures."[9] This hierarchy represents the preferred order that should be followed when selecting between options for controlling hazards.

As recently as 1985 the Office of Technology Assessment (OTA) of the U.S. Congress reviewed the issue of the hierarchy of controls and concluded that engineering controls are most likely to meet the essential requirements for hazard control.[4] OTA also concluded that respiratory protection was limited in its efficacy because of (1) limitations in performance, (2) difficulties in evaluating their performance, (3) problems associated with their use, (4) the physical and other burdens they create, and that policy changes (at OSHA) that would allow greater use of personal protective equipment could endanger the health and well-being of many American workers.

During the promulgation of the cotton dust standard OSHA's policy with respect to this hierarchy of controls stated that respirators were acceptable only during the period that engineering controls were being implemented. Respirators could not be considered a permanent method of protecting workers but were always to be viewed as an interim method of control.

Feasibility: other considerations

Three major decisions on feasibility arose in the Court of Appeals decision on the coke oven emission standard and the Supreme Court decision on lead. Coke oven emissions have been associated causally in epidemiologic studies with increased risks of lung cancer, and OSHA moved to regulate these exposures in the latter 1970s. In its decision, the District Court of Appeals ruled that OSHA can impose a standard that requires an employer to implement technology "looming on today's horizon" and is not limited to issuing a standard solely based upon technology that is fully developed today.

The Court also clarified the meaning of economic feasibility in this standard. It determined that a standard is not economically infeasible because it is financially burdensome or even because it threatens the survival of some companies within an industry. "Nor does the concept of economic feasibility necessarily guarantee the continued existence of individual employers." It would appear consistent with the Act to envisage economic demise of an employer who has lagged behind the rest of the industry in protecting the health and safety of employees and is consequently financially unable to comply with new standards as quickly as other employers. However, a standard could be considered economically infeasible if an entire industry were dislocated, that is, if it affected the competitive stability of an industry or led to undue concentration.

Material impairment: cotton dust and lead

A key regulatory issue with direct relevance to occupational respiratory disease is what constitutes "material impairment" in light of the Act's requirement that OSHA promulgate permanent standards so "that no employee will suffer material impairment of health or functional capacity." The precise question is what is the meaning of the term "material." The legislative history of the Act shows that the term "material impairment" was substituted for "any impairment." The Courts addressed the issue of material impairment in their review of two standards promulgated by OSHA in 1978, the cotton dust standard. Cotton dust and lead have a continuum of effects. For example, OSHA[7a] argued in the cotton dust standard that byssinosis is a continuum: "it is axiomatic that the chronic, irreversible stage is preceded, at the opposite end of the disease progression, by an acute, relatively mild, apparently reversible stage of disease."

OSHA found that although the earliest stages of the disease are characterized by varying subjective or objective symptoms that do not impair the individual, these stages represent a pathologic state. OSHA concluded that a standard should be promulgated that protected workers from the acute consequences of cotton dust exposure. In contrast, the textile industry argued that OSHA need not establish a standard to protect against the acute but reversible symptoms of byssinosis because they themselves do not constitute a "material impairment of health." The U.S. District Court of Appeals in Washington, D.C.[10] ruled that this claim by the industry could not be sustained, and the U.S. Supreme Court upheld the reasoning of the District Court. The District Court ruled that OSHA is not restrained from acting to prevent irreversible health damage until workers actually suffer the early symptoms of byssinosis. The Court upheld OSHA's decision to reduce the prevalence of chronic byssinosis by establishing a standard that would reduce the occurrence of the reversible, acute stage of the disease.

The decision by the U.S. Supreme Court on the cotton dust standard has important relevance to occupational respiratory disease associated with chemical exposure because it defines the level of protection that may be afforded to workers. For example, loss of pulmonary function associated with exposure to chemical agents such as silica and asthma symptoms associated with agents such as toluene diisocyanate (TDI) and organic dusts would fall within the limits of the court decisions. Thus in developing standards in the future for respiratory toxicants, OSHA will be guided by the definitions outlined in the two court decisions.

Formaldehyde

A permanent 6(b) standard for formaldehyde was promulgated by OSHA in 1987[13] and the standard was modified in 1992.[14] The final standard establishes a permissible exposure limit of 0.75 ppm with additional provisions for training of workers and hazard labeling requirements where workplace levels exceed 0.1 ppm. Formaldehyde is a major industrial chemical in the United States where it is ranked 24th in production volume.[13] Formaldehyde has four primary uses: as a chemical intermediate, in resin production, as a component in end-use consumer items, and as a bacteriocide and fungicide.[13]

As required under the Supreme Court decision on benzene OSHA conducted an evaluation of the significance of the risk associated with workplace formaldehyde exposure. The Agency evaluated the health risks associated with formaldehyde on both a qualitative and quantitative basis. The PEL of 0.75 ppm was considered both technologically and economically feasible by OSHA.

In determining the risk of cancer associated with exposure to formaldehyde OSHA noted that these risks are "in addition to the risk of other, non–life threatening but potentially materially impairing risks to the workers's health posed by formaldehyde's irritating and sensitizing properties." As previously cited, OSHA recognized the significance of the noncarcinogenic effects associated with formaldehyde exposure but did not incorporate these considerations into the establishment of a PEL.

To comply with the Court's remand OSHA reduced the PEL from 1 to 0.75 ppm. It justified this selection as being a point within the continuum defined by the MLE and UCL risk estimates.

This standard raises a number of policy issues in standard setting for chemical carcinogens including mathematical model selection, the use of ancillary provisions for standard setting, questions concerning the statistical characterization of risk, and the problems of defining a standard based on irritant or other noncarcinogenic effects. To date, OSHA has not developed a clearly defined policy for quantitative risk assessment, preferring to approach each standard on a chemical-by-chemical basis. In contrast, the EPA has defined a reasonably consistent policy on quantitative risk assessment methodology. The problems with the form-aldehyde standard indicate the need for a better defined policy if the Agency's ability to promulgate standards in a timely fashion is to be improved.

Noncarcinogen endpoints in standard setting

More recent standards for the carcinogens formaldehyde and cadmium have also addressed noncarcinogenic endpoints in the context of risk assessment. There are significant differences in the issues associated with the development of standards for noncarcinogens versus substances that are carcinogenic. As a matter of regulatory policy these include the following: (1) noncarcinogens are assumed to have a "threshold," a dose below which the probability of an individual response is zero; (2) cancer is a well-defined endpoint; data indicate that a subject has or does not have cancer, that is, the data are dichotomous; noncarcinogen endpoints are generally not dichotomous, but are represented by continuous variables, for example, loss of pulmonary function; and (3) there are well-defined albeit sometimes controversial procedures for determining "acceptable risk" for carcinogens, but the approaches for risk assessment for noncarcinogens are limited and often inadequate.

The standard for cotton dust developed by OSHA have neither attempted to protect the entire working population exposed to those toxicants nor have they defined a threshold. The ability to protect workers was limited by consideration of feasibility. For example, the PEL for cotton dust was 0.2 mg/m^3 for opening through spinning in the textile industry. Merchant et al.[11] predicted the prevalence of byssinosis (all grades) of 12.7% at the PEL. The prevalence at a median dust level of 0.1 mg/m^3 was 6.5%, but with this level of predicted effect the standard was considered technologically infeasible.

Respiratory effects, which range from acute and reversible conditions to chronic and irreversible, are often difficult to characterize, and there may be no clear delineation between stages. It is not apparent, for example, when the loss of lung function associated with exposure to silica dust produces a "disease," silicosis. Radiographic identification of pulmonary changes may be sufficient for worker's compensation purposes, but the issue is less clear for regulatory purposes.

OSHA attempted to address acceptable risk for noncarcinogenic effects in its standards for cadmium and formaldehyde. In formaldehyde, OSHA determined that in addition to cancer there is also a risk of acute irritant effects, which are not easily measured by a quantitative clinical test. Acute irritant effects depend more on the subjective perceptions of the individual, which may vary. OSHA also acknowledged additional factors that make identification of acute irritant effects difficult, including (1) the inherent genetic variability in susceptibility in a heterogeneous species such as humans, (2) the acquisition of tolerance to exposure, and (3) the fact that as the concentration of formaldehyde increases, both the number of different biologic effects and their severity increases. Because of these factors OSHA chose not to conduct a quantitative assessment of risk of irritant effects from formaldehyde, but it did develop a quantified estimate of effects as a function of exposure concentration (Table 55-2).

OSHA concluded that the cumulative experience of workers and volunteer subjects suggests that at concentrations below 0.5 ppm, the 20% response is a combination of odor detection with approximately half of these individuals showing more severe but transient effects of slight eye irritation and dry throat. At 1 ppm nearly all persons would be aware of the formaldehyde odor and mild irritation of the eyes, nose, and throat would probably occur in about half of these persons. OSHA also stated from case studies, worker surveillance, and human volunteers that the evidence is sufficient to conclude that formaldehyde either causes asthma or exacerbates existing asthmatic conditions.

Since OSHA developed its PEL primarily on the basis of the carcinogenesis of formaldehyde, the issue of how a PEL would be established for a compound that produces noncarcinogenic effects such as asthma and irritant effects has not been finally addressed. In cotton dust the Supreme Court ruled that a PEL that reduced the acute, reversible effects of exposure to cotton dust to prevent the development of chronic obstructive pulmonary disease was appropriate. In the case of lead the court ruled that a PEL could be established to limit biochemical and subjective central nervous system (CNS) effects associated with this compound. Therefore, it would appear acceptable for OSHA to establish a standard based solely on the irritant effects or asthma producing concentrations within the context of the requirement for a standard preventing material impairment or functional capacity.

There is to date no well-developed methodology for conducting risk assessments associated with noncarcinogenic chemicals and OSHA has not yet established an approach to defining what constitutes an acceptable risk for a noncarcinogen. This issue has particular relevance to occupational respiratory disease. For example, Kennedy[12] re-

Table 55-2. Predicted irritation responses of humans exposed to airborne formaldehyde

Concentration (ppm)	Percent of population giving indicated response	Degree of irritation*
1.5-3.0	10-20	7-10
	30	5-7
0.5-1.5	10-20	5-7
	30	3-5
0.25-0.5	20	3
Less than 0.25	20	1-3

From OSHA formaldehyde standard.
*Irritation Index: 10 = strong irritation, great discomfort; 7 = moderate irritation, discomfort; 5 = mild irritation, mild discomfort; 1 = minimal irritation, minimal discomfort; 0 = no effects.

viewed the question of whether nonallergic airway hyperresponsiveness is an acquired or an inherent phenomenon. In particular, she reviewed the evidence for irritant workplace exposures, gases, fumes, or vapors, that are capable of inducing tissue injury via nonimmunologic pathways, and suggests that if exposures in the workplace may cause hyperresponsiveness, that the same exposures may be responsible for the initiation of adult-onset asthma. Kennedy concludes that the data are very limited, and no prospective studies have been conducted that would further illuminate these issues, but she does ultimately conclude that the answer of whether nonallergic airway hyperresponsiveness is an acquired phenomenon is at present a "qualified yes." How OSHA would use data of this nature in establishing standards to prevent untoward respiratory effects is unclear.

Medical removal protection

Medical removal protection is an extremely critical conceptual and policy issue in standard setting in occupational health and has direct relevance to occupational respiratory disease. Before discussing the history of MRP in OSHA rulemaking it is necessary to define the concept. The provisions in the standard for formaldehyde are illustrative.

The formaldehyde standard included MRP provisions. It required medical surveillance, such as completion of an annual medical questionaire, coupled with employees' reports of signs and symptoms and medical examinations where necessary. As OSHA noted, this approach requires a high degree of employee participation and cooperation to determine if employee health is being adversely affected by exposure to formaldehyde. On the basis of the medical surveillance program, a physician may recommend that an employee be removed from continued exposure to formaldehyde. To maximize employee participation and cooperation with the medical surveillance program, employees must be assured that their earnings, seniority, and other employment rights and benefits will be maintained during their medical removal. This type of provision is known as medical removal protection. An MRP provision has been incorporated into three permanent standards by OSHA: cotton dust, lead, and formaldehyde.

In the formaldehyde standard the conditions that are covered by MRP include significant irritation of the mucosa of the eyes and of the upper airway, respiratory sensitization, dermal irritation, or dermal sensitization. The standard gives the physician broad discretion in selecting appropriate tests to evaluate the employee's report of signs or symptoms. If, in the examining physician's professional judgment, certain restrictions or removal are required to alleviate the symptoms of formaldehyde exposure, then medical removal with its intended protections is an option that may be exercised. The employee may be transferred to a job with lower formaldehyde exposure or may be removed entirely for up to 6 months or until a physician determines either that the employee is able to return to work or that the employee will never be able to return to work.

The standard also provides for multiple physician review to address differences of opinion between the initial examining physician and the employee. Multiple physician review enables an employee to have a medical opinion by a second physician if the first decision is considered questionable, to ensure confidence in the soundness of medical determinations.

Industry representatives argued that MRP was not necessary in the formaldehyde standard since, in contrast to lead, there are no objective criteria for determining when a worker should be removed. Most symptoms of formaldehyde exposure are transient and minor including reversible irritation, but workers who are sensitized will likely not recover even after the initial reactions cease and will not be able to work with formaldehyde in the future. In the latter circumstance the worker may require some other financial protection than that provided by MRP, which could include worker's compensation. In the formaldehyde standard OSHA decided that the need for worker protection outweighed these arguments. These issues concerning MRP will be important in future standards that address chemicals that produce respiratory disease. For example, pulmonary function testing represents an objective criterion that OSHA might consider for an MRP provision. How OSHA and the scientific community will address chemicals with chronic cumulative toxicity, such as crystalline silica, or chemicals, such as toluene diisocyanate, which are sensitizers, is yet to be defined.

Generic standards

OSHA has promulgated generic standards including the air contaminants standard, the generic cancer policy, access to medical records, hazard communication, blood-borne pathogens, occupational exposure to hazardous chemicals in laboratories, and a hazardous waste workers standard. Two standards, the air contaminants standard and the generic cancer policy, will be discussed here.

The air contaminant standards. During the period from 1970 when the OSHAct was adopted to the mid 1980s OSHA adopted only 24 permanent standards although they had promulgated standards for approximately 400 chemicals soon after passage of the Act. These latter standards were derived from the 1968 ACGIH TLVs and a small number of ANSI standards. Many of the 1968 TLVs were recognized as being inadequate, and there were a large number of chemicals for which no standards had been promulgated. In 1987 OSHA concluded that a generic approach was required for the promulgation of permissible exposure limits for airborne chemical contaminants to more rapidly address the regulation of chemicals in the workplace. This resulted in the 1987 "air contaminants project" in which OSHA reduced the PEL for 212 substances, raised the PEL for one substance, set PELs for 164 substances not previ-

ously regulated, added or changed STELs for 70 substances and, as appropriate, set skin, short-term, or ceiling limits.

OSHA primarily used the 1987-88 ACGIH TLVs for establishing the new PELs. OSHA claimed that the ACGIH TLVs were the sole readily available recommendations available for establishing standards. As an example of the approach taken, Table 55-3 lists the standards adopted by OSHA for which the proposed limits are based on avoidance of respiratory effects. This air contaminants project was an attempt by OSHA to address a large number of substances more quickly and to develop a generic process for updating PELs. OSHA, by and large, selected ACGIH recommendations over those of NIOSH. The OSHAct specifically defines a role for NIOSH in the standard setting process. Section 22 (c) of the Act states "The Institute *(NIOSH)* is authorized to (1) develop and establish recommended occupational safety and health standards;" and Section 22 (d) states "the Director *(of NIOSH)* is authorized to (1) conduct such research and experimental programs as he determines are necessary for the development of criteria for new and improved occupational safety and health standards, and (2) after consideration of the results of such research and experimental programs make recommendations concerning new or improved occupational safety and health standards. Any occupational safety and health standard recommended pursuant to this section shall immediately be forwarded to the Secretary of Labor, and to the Secretary of Health, Education and Welfare *(now Health and Human Services).*" NIOSH has historically focused significant research and resources on the development of recommended exposure limits (RELs). At public hearings NIOSH presented more than 4,000 pages of written testimony and supporting documents that in part criticized the use of TLVs as a basis for the standards and pointed out that it had developed RELs for approximately 50 of the toxic substances. In addition, NIOSH had developed RELs on 42 substances that were excluded from the Air Contaminants Standard due to the absence of TLVs.[15]

Robinson[15] pointed out that 67 of the substances with PELs based on noncancer health effects were identified as confirmed or probable human carcinogens by NIOSH, the National Toxicology Program (NTP), or the International Agency for Research on Cancer (IARC), and an additional 68 substances previously identified as occupational carcinogens by NIOSH or NTP were completely excluded from the Air Contaminants Standard due to OSHA's reliance on TLVs. Robinson et al.[16] provide examples of substance TLVs adopted by OSHA considered inadequately protective by NIOSH.

Other critics have questioned the quality of the TLVs themselves.[17,18] In particular, questions have been raised about the adequacy of the documentation of the TLVs and the overall consistency and quality of the scientific review leading to the TLVs. The ACGIH TLVs provide useful guidance for practitioners of occupational safety and health and

Table 55-3. Summary of dose–response evidence for adverse respiratory effects

H.S. number/ chemical name	CAS No.	Current PEL*	ACGIH TLV†	NIOSH REL‡	Dose/duration associated with observed effects	Species	Comments
1034 Bismuth telluride (Se-Doped)	1304-82-1	5 mg/m³ TWA	5 mg/m³ TWA	—	15 mg/m³, 1 year	Dogs, rats, rabbits	Granulomatous lesions in lungs seen after 6 months of exposure
1096 Coal dust, <5% quartz	None	2.4 mg/m³ TWA	2 mg/m³ TWA	—	4 mg/m³, 35 years	Humans	Calculated estimate of 10% probability of developing pneumoconiosis with fibrosis after 35 years of exposure to coal dust (quartz content not identified)
1097 Coal dust, >5% quartz	None	10 mg/m³ % SiO₂+2	0.1 mg/m³ TWA	—			
1190 Grain dust (oat, wheat, barley)	None		4 mg/m³ TWA	—	20 mg/m³	Humans	Chronic bronchitis, shortness of breath, reduced pulmonary function
					13.9 mg/m³	Humans	Increased incidence of respiratory symptoms
					4 mg/m³	Humans	No increased incidence of respiratory symptoms
						Humans	Fibrosis and mottling, pneumoconiosis
1191 Graphite, natural, respirable	7782-42-5	15 mppcf TWA	2.5 mg/m³ TWA	—	NA§	Humans	Anthracosilicosis, similar to that seen in coal miners
1213 Indium and compounds	7440-74-6		0.1 mg/m³ TWA	—	24-97 mg/m³	Rats	Widespread alveolar edema following exposure to In₂O₂
1276 Mica§	12003-38-2	20 mppcf TWA	3 mg/m³ TWA	—	NA	Humans	Signs and symptoms resembling silicosis and pneumoconiosis in 8 of 57 workers
1289 Nitrogen dioxide**	10102-44-0	5 ppm ceiling	3 ppm TWA, 5 ppm STEL	1 ppm ceiling (15 min)	NA 0.4-2.7 ppm, chronic	Humans Humans	Fatal pulmonary edema Change in pulmonary vital capacity
1300 Oxygen difluoride	7783-41-7	0.05 ppm TWA	0.05 ppm, ceiling	—	0.5 ppm, two 7 hr exposures	Laboratory animals	Lethal to a wide variety of laboratory species, causing pulmonary edema and hemorrhage after several hours of exposure

Continued.

Table 55-3. Summary of dose–response evidence for adverse respiratory effects—cont'd

H.S. number/ chemical name	CAS No.	Current PEL*	ACGIH TLV†	NIOSH REL‡	Dose–response data		
					Dose/duration associated with observed effects	Species	Comments
1301 Ozone	10028-15-6	0.1 ppm TWA	0.1 ppm TWA, 0.3 ppm STEL	—	1.5 ppm, 3 hr/day	Humans	Significant reduction in pulmonary vital capacity
					1 ppm, 1 day	Mice	Damage to alveolar tissue
					NA	Humans	69 accidental deaths from pulmonary injury reported through 1972
1303 Paraquat, respirable dust	4685-14-7	0.5 mg/m^3 TWA, skin	0.1 mg/m^3 TWA	—			
1354 Silica, crystalline cristobalite	14464-46-1	½ value for quartz	0.05 mg/m^3 TWA	50 µg/m^3 TWA	0.5 mg/m^3 (as total dust) 2.5 years	Dogs	Cellular infiltration of lung and fibrotic nodules in pulmonary lymph nodes
1355 Silica, crystalline quartz, respirable	14808-60-7	10 mg/m^3 % SiO$_2$+2	0.1 mg/m^3 TWA	50 µg/m^3 TWA	0.1 mg/m^3, chronic	Humans	Accelerated loss of pulmonary function over effects of aging alone
1356 Silica, crystalline tridymite	15468-32-3	½ value for quartz	0.05 mg/m^3 TWA	50 µg/m^3 TWA	NA	Rats	Most active form of free silica when administered by intratracheal injections
1357 Silica, crystalline tripoli (as quartz dust)	1317-95-9	10 mg/m^3 % SiO$_2$+2	0.1 mg/m^3 TWA	50 µg/m^3 TWA	NA	Laboratory animals	Progressive nodular fibrosis
1375 Sulfur dioxide	7446-09-5	5 ppm TWA	2 ppm TWA, 5 ppm STEL	0.5 ppm TWA	1 ppm	Humans	Accelerated loss of pulmonary function predicted based on data in smelter workers
1378 Sulfur tetrafluoride	7783-60-0	—	0.1 ppm, ceiling	—	4 ppm, 4 hr/day/10 days	Rats	Emphysema, marked clinical signs of respiratory impairment
1409 Trimellitic anhydride	552-30-7	—	0.005 ppm TWA	—	NA	Rats	Intraalveolar hemorrhage (no exposure duration indicated)

*OSHA's TWA limits are for 8-hour exposures, its STELs are for the durations specified, and its ceilings are peaks not to be exceeded for any period of time.
†The ACGIH TWA-TLV is for an 8-hour exposure, its STELs are 15-minute limits not to be exceeded more than 4 times per day with a minimum of 60 minutes between successive STEL exposures, and its ceilings are peaks not to be exceeded for any period of time.
‡NIOSH TWA limits are for 10-hour exposures unless otherwise specified, and its ceilings are peaks not to be exceeded for any period of time unless a duration is specified in parentheses.
§Measured as total dust.
**Proposed limit is the NIOSH REL.

ACGIH, American Conference of Governmental Industrial Hygienists; *NA*, not available; *NIOSH*, U.S. National Institute for Occupational Safety and Health; *OSHA*, U.S. Occupational Safety and Health Administration; *REL*, recommended exposure limit; *STEL*, Short-term exposure limit; *TLV*, threshold limit value; *TWA*, time-weighted average.

the appropriateness of the TLVs has improved in recent years, but it is important to recognize the limitations of earlier TLVs.

The air contaminants standard was litigated in the U.S. Court of Appeals for the Eleventh Circuit (AFL-CIO v. OSHA, CA 11, No. 89-7185, 7/7/92), which vacated the standard. The Court concluded that OSHA had failed to establish a significant risk of material health impairment for each regulated substance and had not determined whether the new exposure limit for each substance was feasible for the affected industries. The court determined that the "generic" rulemaking was not appropriate and the air contaminants standard was an attempt to promulgate a set of 428 individual exposure limits without addressing feasibility, significant risk, and material impairment. The Court determined that the exposure limit for each substance must be based on substantial evidence in the record, and there must be an adequate explanation of the reasons for the PEL change. In particular, OSHA had failed to determine that each new standard was "reasonably necessary" or appropriate as required by the Supreme Court's benzene decision.

It would appear that OSHA should request that NIOSH proceed to update its RELs in a manner that would meet the requirements of court decisions on the key issues of material impairment and feasibility, and whether the standards are reasonably necessary. Future NIOSH RELs will need to incorporate the requirements that court decisions have placed on OSHA. The NIOSH RELs have historically been based on a careful review of the scientific literature, and this level of review will facilitate acceptance of proposed changes in requirements.

Generic cancer policy. The objective of the generic cancer policy was similar to that of the air contaminants standards, namely that OSHA sought to increase the pace of standard setting for chemical carcinogens. Although hundreds of chemical compounds have been identified as human or animal carcinogens, only 24 compounds have been regulated as carcinogens, and only 11 carcinogen standards were comprehensive in nature. Standards were promulgated for 13 carcinogens in 1974, but many of these chemicals have no current industrial use, and no PELs were established for the substances.

The generic cancer policy standard was promulgated in 1980, with the objective of establishing a policy definition of what is the level of evidence required to classify a substance as a carcinogen. More specifically the standard (1) established criteria for identifying and classifying potential occupational carcinogens, (2) set out procedures and timetables for the identification and classification process, and (3) established model standards as guidelines for the standard setting process. It was OSHA's intent to resolve the scientific issues surrounding the definition of a chemical carcinogen as a matter of OSHA policy, thereby standardizing carcinogen regulation, improving the pace of standard setting, and more effectively regulating carcinogens.

Although the generic cancer standard has not been withdrawn, it has never been implemented in part because the policy did not address the requirements defined by the U.S. Supreme Court in the benzene decision. There are still a large number of identified chemical carcinogens that have not been regulated, and the agency has no consistent policy with respect to the regulation of chemical carcinogens. The regulation of chemical carcinogens is addressed on a case-by-case basis, at a very slow pace.

Identification of carcinogens by other agencies

In addition to OSHA there are three agencies with particular responsibility for carcinogen identification. They include two U.S. federal agencies, EPA and NTP, and the international agency, IARC. A brief review of the criteria they use for carcinogen identification will be of value in considering the scope of evidence required for identification by these agencies. Quantitative risk assessment to define carcinogenic potency is not within the scope of this chapter. In the benzene decision the Court held that animal evidence could be used to define a substance as a carcinogen and to determine potency. However, to date OSHA has not regulated a carcinogen strictly on the basis of animal data preferring to promulgate standards for which there is human as well as animal data. There are a large number of substances that have been designated as animal carcinogens, but that have inadequate epidemiologic information. How OSHA will address those compounds in the future is not readily apparent given their history.

International Agency for Research on Cancer and U.S. Environmental Protection Agency

IARC and EPA have developed similar classification schemes for categorizing evidence of carcinogenicity. Under both schemes, the relevant data are evaluated in a series of sequential steps. First, separate evaluations are made of the degree of evidence of carcinogenicity in humans and the degree of evidence of carcinogenicity in experimental animals. These evaluations are made on the basis of results from epidemiologic studies and chronic animal bioassays. Under the IARC classification scheme, the evidence in humans and animals is judged to fall into one of the four categories: sufficient, limited, or inadequate evidence of carcinogenicity, or evidence suggesting lack of carcinogenicity. IARC then states that "other data relevant to an evaluation of carcinogenicity" are then considered. In particular, data relevant to the mechanism of the carcinogenic action of an agent, such as mutagenicity, are evaluated and the strength of the evidence that any carcinogenic effect is due to a particular mechanism is assessed. In the final step of the IARC evaluation the evidence is considered as a whole, and the toxic agent is then placed in one of the following categories: Group 1, agent is carcinogenic to humans; Group 2A, the agent is probably carcinogenic to humans; Group 2B, the agent is possibly carcinogenic to humans; Group 3, the agent is not classifiable as to its carcinogenicity to humans; and Group 4, the agent is probably not carcinogenic to humans. The criteria for placing an agent in these categories are defined in the IARC guidelines (Table 55-4). EPA has a similar classification scheme (Table 55-4). The IARC criteria were most recently revised in 1991. The primary change made was with respect to the use of "other data relevant to an evaluation of carcinogenicity." Such data now include preneoplastic lesions, tumor pathology, genetic and related effects, structure–activity relationships, metabolism and toxicokinetics, and physicochemical parameters. These criteria are also used by EPA.

To date, OSHA has not established a carcinogen identification scheme similar to those developed by IARC or EPA. Although they take notice of the classifications of these Agencies, there is no ongoing effort to define which substances should be classified as carcinogens as a basis for subsequent regulation.

The National Toxicology Program

The NTP is located in the HHS and participating agencies include the National Cancer Institute, National Institute of Environmental Health Sciences, National Center for Toxicologic Research, NIOSH and the Agency for Toxic Substances and Disease Registry. In addition the Consumer Product Safety Commission, EPA, OSHA, and Food and Drug Administration (FDA), agencies responsible for regulating hazardous substances, also participate in the NTP. Section 301 (b) (4) of the Public Health Service Act requires the Secretary of the Department of HHS to publish an annual report that contains (1) a list of all substances (a) that either are known to be carcinogens or may reasonably be anticipated to be carcinogens, and (b) to which a significant number of persons residing in the United States are exposed, and (2) information concerning the nature of such exposure and the estimated number of persons exposed to such substances. Other requirements are detailed in the annual reports. These reports are available from HHS and NTP.

Table 55-4. U.S. EPA and IARC carcinogen classification schemes

Level of evidence	U.S. EPA category*	IARC category*
1. Sufficient evidence from epi studies	A—Human carcinogen	1—Agent is carcinogenic to humans
2. In exceptional cases, less than sufficient evidence in humans, with sufficient evidence in animals and strong evidence in humans that the agent acts through a relevant mechanism of carcinogenicity	B1 or B2—Probable human carcinogen	1—Agent is carcinogenic to humans
3. Limited evidence from epi studies with sufficient evidence from animal studies	B1—Probable human carcinogen	2A—Agent is probably carcinogenic to humans
4. Sufficient evidence from animal studies with strongly supportive evidence from other relevant studies	B2—Probable human carcinogen	2A—In some cases, classified as probably carcinogenic to humans
5. Limited evidence from epi studies with other supporting data	B1—Probable human carcinogen	2A—In exceptional cases, classified as probably carcinogenic to humans
6. Sufficient evidence from animal studies	B2—Probable human carcinogen	2B—Agent is possibly carcinogenic to humans
7. Limited evidence from animal studies with strongly supportive evidence from other relevant studies	C—Possible human carcinogen	2B—Agent is possibly carcinogenic to humans
8. Limited evidence from epi studies with no or inadequate supporting data	B1—Probable human carcinogen	2B—Agent is possibly carcinogenic to humans
9. Limited evidence from animal studies with no or inadequate supporting data	C—Possible human carcinogen	3—Agent is not classifiable as to its carcinogenicity to humans
10. Inadequate evidence from epi animal or other relevant studies	D—Not classifiable as to human carcinogenicity	3—Agent is not classifiable as to its carcinogenicity to humans
11. Sufficient evidence from animal studies, with sufficient data to show that these studies are not relevant to humans	Currently not classified	3—Agent is not classifiable as to its carcinogenicity to humans
12. All available evidence suggests lack of carcinogenicity	E—Evidence of noncarcinogenicity for humans	4—Agent is probably not carcinogenic to humans

*These categories have recently been added in the IARC (1993) guidelines. Both U.S. EPA and Cal/EPA are revising their guide data. Chemicals falling into these categories will likely require in-depth review by the SAB Carcinogen Identification Commission.
EPA, U.S. Environmental Protection Agency; *IARC,* International Agency for Research on Cancer.

ENFORCEMENT

The Congress clearly intended that enforcement of occupational safety and health standards was central to achieving the goals of the OSHAct. The Act states that it is the intent of Congress to provide "an effective enforcement program."

In carrying out its enforcement program the Department of Labor has divided the United States into 10 federal regions, each of which contains four to nine area offices. Within regions, certain states conduct their own occupational safety and health programs, whereas in others there is primarily federal enforcement. Each region is headed by a regional administrator and each area by an area director. Compliance officers conduct enforcement inspections from area offices.

The enforcement program is intended to ensure that employers have recognized, adopted, and are in compliance with promulgated safety and health standards. The enforcement program consists primarily of workplace inspections conducted by compliance officers who determine whether the affected facility is in compliance with relevant occupational safety and health standards. The OSHAct as drafted gave permission for inspectors to enter workplaces to conduct inspections in establishments covered by the Act at reasonable times, without delay, and without prior notification to inspect the premises. There is a specific prohibition against giving advance notice of any inspection in the Act. In 1978 the Supreme Court held that the provision guaranteeing access at the discretion of the agency was a violation of the Fourth Amendment. Inspectors may now be required to obtain a search warrant before an inspection may be conducted.

Companies that are not in compliance with OSHA standards may be given civil penalties that are in relation to the severity of the violation, and they must come into compliance within a reasonable period of time. The OSHA inspection serves two purposes if carried out effectively: (1) the inspection has a direct impact on an inspected firm by requiring the facility to come into compliance with existing standards, and (2) the inspection represents a "threat" to firms not yet inspected.

In conducting an inspection the Act provides for an inspector questioning privately any employer, owner, operator, agent, or employee. A representative of the employer and a representative authorized by the employees shall be given the opportunity to accompany the OSHA compliance officer on the inspection. Where there is no authorized representative of the employees, the inspector is required to consult with a reasonable number of employees concerning matters of health and safety in the workplace.

Where a compliance officer has determined there has been a violation of safety or health standards a determination is made by an area director whether a citation should be issued for the identified violations. The citation issued to an employer will list the specific standards violated, a determination of severity of the violations, and a reasonable time for abatement will be established. The citation must be placed at or near the place of violation. A citation must be issued with reasonable promptness but within 6 months of the inspection.

The citation will generally include notification of any proposed penalties. The employer has 15 days from the receipt of the notice in which to contest the proposed penalties or citation. The appellate process is described in detail in Section 11 of the OSHAct.

The Act requires that the citation specify a reasonable period for abatement of a hazard. Representatives of employees may contest the abatement period, but they may not contest other aspects of the citation. If an employer fails to correct a violation for which a citation has been issued within the period permitted for abatement a civil penalty of not more than $1,000 a day may be levied for the period the violation continues.

The Act establishes different severities for each violation. Violations may be considered "other than serious," "serious," "willful," "failure to abate," and "repeated." A willful violation may be issued to an employer who is aware of a hazardous condition in a facility but makes no reasonable attempt to eliminate the condition. An employer who commits a willful violation is liable upon conviction for a penalty of up to $10,000 per violation. A repeat violation may include a similar penalty. An employer who receives a serious violation may be assessed a civil penalty of not more than $1,000 per violation. Penalties for "other than serious" violations are discretionary but mandatory for serious violations. Violations of standards for controlling exposure to toxic substances are considered serious. A person giving unauthorized advance notice of an inspection can be fined up to $1,000 and may be liable for imprisonment of up to 6 months.

Overlapping jurisdictions

There are other agencies of the federal government with statutory responsibilities for occupational safety and health. These agencies include the Department of Transportation, and its constituent agencies, such as the Federal Railroad Administration and the Federal Aviation Administration, the EPA, the Department of Defense, Department of Energy, and, to a lesser extent, the FDA and the Consumer Product Safety Commission. There is currently no ongoing coordinating body for interagency cooperation.

One example of the problems of coordination is in the regulation and enforcement of pesticide standards. OSHA has authority for the enforcement of standards relating to pesticide manufacture and formulation, but EPA has authority for pesticide regulation as it concerns application of pesticides in field operations. This dichotomy exists at the State level as well.

EMPLOYEE RIGHTS UNDER THE OCCUPATIONAL SAFETY AND HEALTH ACT

The most important employee right defined by the Act is the right of any employee "who believes that a violation of a safety or health standard exists that threatens physical harm, or that an imminent danger exists, to request an inspection by giving notice of such violation or danger." Any complaint shall be reduced to writing, and a copy shall be provided to the employer at the time of inspection. The employee's name on the written complaint may be withheld if requested by the employee. No employee may be discharged or discriminated against as a result of having filed a complaint. Procedures for addressing termination of employment or discrimination are defined in Section 11(c) of the OSHAct.

The United Steelworkers of America have developed a comprehensive list of employee rights under the OSHAct.[19] These include the following:

1. The right to petition the Secretary to commence the procedure for promulgating standards [Section 6(b)1)].
2. The right to standards that most adequately and *feasibly* assure that no employee will suffer any impairment of health or functional capacity, or diminished life expectancy, even if such employee has regular exposure to toxic or harmful materials [Section 6(b)(5)].
3. The right to standards that prescribe, where necessary, the labeling of hazardous substances, protective equipment, and monitoring [Section 6(b)(7)].
4. The right to medical examinations so as to determine whether exposure is adversely affecting health [Section 6(b)(7)].
5. The right to have the results of one's medical examination transmitted to an employee's physician [Section 6(b)(7)].
6. The right to notification of an employer's request for variance and to participate in the hearing called to evaluate the request [Section 6(d)].
7. The right to employee representation on the standard-setting advisory committees and on coalitions of occupational safety and health (COSH) groups.
8. The right to have employers keep them informed of their rights under the Act [Section 8(c)(1)].
9. The right to observe the monitoring equipment and have access to the records thereof [Section 8(c)(3)].
10. The right to be notified when concentration levels are being exceeded, and to be informed of measures being taken to correct such a situation [Section 8(c)(3)].
11. The right to accompany the OSHA inspector [Section 8(e)].
12. The right to request a special inspection, to be able to inform the inspector of any alleged violation, and to receive written explanation of failure by the inspector to issue a citation of violation and to receive an informal review thereof [Section 8(f)(1-2)].
13. The right to demand a hearing if an unreasonable (long) time is set for the abatement of a hazardous situation by the Secretary [Section 10(c)].
14. The right to participate in hearings to determine whether an employer should receive a modification of the original abatement order [Section 10(c)].
15. The right to protection against disciplinary action for exercising rights under the Act [Section 11(c)(1-3)].
16. The right to request HHS determination of the toxicity of any substance normally found in the workplace [Section 20(a)(6)].

STATE PLANS

One of the principal reasons underlying the passage of the OSHAct was the failure of the states to develop effective health and safety programs. Although states had developed worker safety laws as early as 1877 in Massachusetts the record of state activities was dismal at best.[4,5] For example, a survey conducted in 1968 found that only 20 states had occupational health programs and that most states had more game wardens than safety inspectors.[4]

The Act in Section 18 describes the procedures and requirements for a state to develop its own occupational safety and health plan, which must then be approved by the U.S. Secretary of Labor (see the box). The Secretary shall continue to enforce regulations in a given state until which time the state meets the criteria established in the Act whereupon the state will then have sole responsibility for carrying out the provisions of the Act. The safety and health plan estab-

---

States with state OSHA programs

Alaska
Arizona
California
Hawaii
Maryland
Michigan
Nevada
New Mexico
North Carolina
Oregon
South Carolina
Rhode Island
Tennessee
Utah
Vermont
Virginia
Washington

lished by the state must be "at least as effective" as the Federal program. Even after approval of the plan the Secretary is required to carry out a continuing evaluation of the State's performance.

THE NATIONAL INSTITUTE FOR OCCUPATIONAL SAFETY AND HEALTH

The OSHAct established seven major responsibilities for the Secretary of Health, Education and Welfare (now HHS) in the area of occupational safety and health. These requirements include (1) the conduct of research in occupational safety and health, (2) establishing criteria for the identification of toxic substances, (3) develop criteria dealing with toxic materials and harmful physical agents that describe safe exposure levels, (4) conduct research on new problems including research on motivational and behavioral factors relating to the field of occupational safety and health, (5) setting requirements for recordkeeping and establishing programs of medical examinations and tests necessary for determining the incidence of occupational illness, (6) publication of a list of all known toxic substances by generic family and the concentrations at which such toxicity occurs, and (7) the conduct of industrywide studies on the effects of chronic or low-level exposure to industrial materials, processes, and stresses on the potential for illness, disease, or loss of functional capacity in aging adults. To carry out these functions Congress established the NIOSH.

The Institute is an element within the Centers for Disease Control and Prevention (CDC). Overall, NIOSH's plans are integrated with the CDC's strategy for preventing premature mortality, reducing unnecessary morbidity, and improving the quality of life.[19a] NIOSH has organized its strategies into five tactical areas that constitute a system for defining and solving occupational safety and health problems.[19a]

1. Identify occupational safety and health problems so as to detect and define epidemiologically significant changes in the status of occupational safety and health.
2. Evaluate occupational safety and health hazards so as to understand their causes and to detect their vulnerabilities to prevention.
3. Control occupational safety and health problems through discovering, assessing, and improving measures to reduce occupational hazards, especially through control technology, protective equipment, workpractices, and hazard-detection devices.
4. Disseminate scientific findings and appropriate recommendations to all organizations and individuals with the need to know to assist them in acting to reduce occupationally related health problems; training and developing personnel for the field are essential elements of this program.

5. Administer these programs with a sense of total commitment to the highest principles of public stewardship.

There are research facilities in Cincinnati, Ohio, and Morgantown, West Virginia. The Institute is subdivided into seven divisions (Fig. 55-1). The Institute is headed by a Director who is appointed to a term of 6 years.

There are two NIOSH divisions that have special relevance to occupational respiratory disease, the Division of Surveillance, Hazard Evaluations and Field Studies (DSHEFS) and the Division of Respiratory Disease Studies (DRDS). DSHEFS has responsibility for surveillance of occupational hazards, disease, and illness within NIOSH. In keeping with this mandate, DSHEFS has developed a number of surveillance projects that focus on both chemical exposure and illness surveillance.

An example of a surveillance program developed by NIOSH with particular relevance to health care providers who have a direct interest in occupational respiratory disease is the Sentinel Event Notification System for Occupational Risks (SENSOR). This system is operative in approximately 10 states and consists of a network of sentinel health care providers with direct linkages to state health departments. A *sentinel health event* has been defined by Rutstein et al.[20] as a case of unnecessary disease, unnecessary disability, or untimely death whose occurrence is a warning signal that the quality of preventive or medical care may need to be improved. Rutstein's sentinel health event concept has been adapted to occupational health surveillance by NIOSH in its SENSOR program. A network of sentinel health care providers is linked to a state health department. The conditions requiring reporting include carpal tunnel syndrome, lead poisoning, noise-induced hearing loss, pesticide poisoning, and, most notably for this text, silicosis and occupational asthma. A response is triggered in a state health department as a result of the reports received from the sentinel health care providers. The actions that may subsequently take place include (1) management of the individual case, (2) screening of other workers with similar exposures, or (3) investigation of the particular worksite. These data could be used more broadly to define priorities for intervention, research, and education/training in industries with identified problems. The SENSOR system is one example of NIOSH's attempt to address the problem described by former NIOSH Director, Donald Millar: "in the practice of epidemiologic surveillance, the field of occupational safety and health is at least 70 years behind the field of communicable disease control."

The objective of the overall NIOSH surveillance program is the early detection and continuous assessment of the magnitude and extent of occupational illnesses, disabilities, deaths, and exposures to hazardous agents using new and existing data sources from federal, state, and local agen-

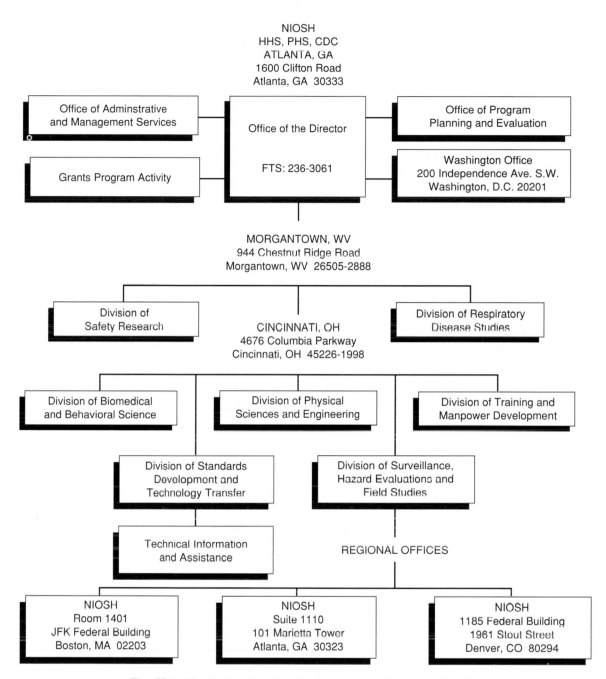

Fig. 55-1. The National Institute for Occupational Safety and Health.

cies, labor, industry, tumor registries, physicians, and medical centers.

DSHEFS is also responsible for the health hazard evaluation (HHE) and health evaluation and technical assistance (HETA) programs, which are field investigations of potential workplace problems and often involve both a medical and an industrial hygiene evaluation. An employee, union, or an employer can request a NIOSH HHE, and the employee may request anonymity if desired. These investigations or consultative services are conducted without cost to the requestor, and the final reports are available to the public. NIOSH has the same right of entry as OSHA, but they may be required to obtain a court order if the employer denies entry. HHEs have been conducted for a wide range of respiratory complaints and illnesses. The reports of these specific evaluations may be requested from NIOSH. More than 7,000 HHEs have been completed since the inception of the program.

The industrywide studies program seeks to (1) identify the occupational causes of disease in the working population and their offspring; (2) conduct studies that form the basis for intervention to reduce occupational disease, (3) collect information on exposure to chemical and physical agents in the workplace, (4) develop information to be used by OSHA in standard setting, and (5) provide information on risk to subjects of epidemiologic investigations.

DRDS can be described as a multidisciplinary center for research and public health activities directed toward the prevention of occupational respiratory diseases. In contrast to DSHEFS, whose primary focus is epidemiologic investigation, DRDS combines epidemiologic, environmental, clinical, and laboratory research to investigate the causes and scope of occupational respiratory disease.

DRDS currently centers its activities around eight program areas:

1. Silicosis prevention: NIOSH has extensive research activities in the area of silicosis and silicosis-related disease prevention. This includes an eradication strategy that focuses on communication, education, screening, and surveillance, and scientific research.
2. Prevention of lung disease in agricultural workers:
   - Determination of the extent of agricultural lung disease.
   - Identification of etiologic agents and mechanisms of agricultural lung disease.
   - Recommendation of effective work practices and other lung disease prevention strategies.
3. Development of techniques and approaches for evaluating fiber toxicity:
   - To evaluate the toxicity and carcinogenic potential of natural and synthetic fibers, including asbestos substitutes.
   - To determine the relationships between a fibers physical and chemical properties and its toxicity.
   - To develop a technique for defining fiber durability.
4. Development of biologic markers for identifying genotoxic and carcinogenic substances.
5. Reduction of the incidence of lung disease in miners:
   - To assess the extent and severity of lung disease in miners.
   - To explore relationships between dust exposure and indicators of lung disease.
   - To explore the role of particle composition and size in lung disease, action of particles in the lung, relationships between radiologic and pathologic findings, nature of disease progression, and its implications.
   - To improve health surveillance of and intervention programs for miners.
6. Identification of workers at high risk of occupational lung disease:
   - To identify trends in the extent and severity of occupational lung disease.
   - To develop and test methods for identifying early signs of lung diseases.
7. Improvement of methods for detecting and preventing occupational asthma:
   - Improve medical monitoring and hazard surveillance methods for occupational asthma.
   - Identify and improve medical screening techniques for workers at risk.
   - Refine current systems for monitoring trends.
   - Develop and validate in vitro and animal models of occupational asthma, to screen materials for asthmogenic potential and define pathogenic mechanisms of disease.
8. Support for extramural research in the prevention of occupational illness and injury in agricultural settings:
   - Develop and conduct applied preventive research.
   - Develop and conduct education and training programs.

During much of its early history NIOSH had a very active program to "develop and establish recommended occupational safety and health standards" as required by the Act. The RELs were developed in their Criteria Documents Division, and many RELs were defined.

The NIOSH RELs do represent the most thorough evaluation of chemical toxicity available to investigators, although NIOSH stopped developing criterial documents more than a decade ago, and some of the recommendations may now be somewhat dated. New approaches to the development of criteria for standards by NIOSH are a priority, particularly in the area of occupational respiratory disease with particular emphasis on toxic substances that produce noncarcinogenic effects.

One of the approaches taken by NIOSH to identify areas for priority research was to identify the leading work-related diseases and injuries in the United States. NIOSH developed a list of the 10 leading work-related diseases and injuries based on the following criteria: (1) the disease's or injury's frequency of occurrence, its severity in the individual case, and its amenability to prevention.[21] The leading work-related disease and injury is occupational lung disease, including asbestosis, byssinosis, silicosis, coal workers pneumoconiosis, lung cancer, and asthma.

FEDERAL MINE SAFETY AND HEALTH ACT OF 1977

With the exception of coal mine safety and health issues, mining has received less public attention in the United States, and the regulatory activities of the federal agency established to address health and safety issues, the Mine Safety and Health Administration (MSHA) are not widely described. Congress passed the first federal statute covering mine safety in 1891 and the Bureau of Mines was established in the Department of the Interior in 1910. Unfor tunately, the authority of this agency was limited and the bureau inspectors were not given the right of entry to conduct inspections of mines. It was not until 1941 that Congress gave authority for inspectors to enter mines to conduct inspections. The Federal Coal Mine Safety Act of 1952 provided for annual inspections in certain underground coal mines and gave limited enforcement authority to issue violation notices, imminent danger withdrawal orders, and assessment of civil penalties, although there was no provision for monetary penalties for noncompliance with safety standards.

The Federal Coal Mine Health and Safety Act of 1969 was passed after a disastrous explosion in 1968 killed 78 miners in Farmington, WV. This Act was later followed by the Federal Mine Safety and Health Act of 1977, which encompassed all miners, millers, and ancillary personnel. The regulatory agency, MSHA, established by the Act was moved from the Department of the Interior to the Department of Labor, and it is headed by an Assistant Secretary of Labor, which is consistent with the administrative structure of OSHA.

The Mine Act requires MSHA inspectors to inspect each underground mine at least four times a year and each surface mine two times per year to determine whether an imminent danger exists and whether a mine is in compliance with safety and health standards or with any citation, order, or decision issued under the Act. MSHA has a warrantless right of entry to mine sites, in contrast to OSHA. MSHA investigates mine accidents, complaints of retaliatory discrimination filed by miners, and knowing or willful criminal violations. Under MSHA there are no state programs as with OSHA, and all enforcement activities are carried out by MSHA inspectors. The Agency has authority to develop improved mandatory standards for both health and safety. It may assess and collect civil monetary penalties for violations of applicable standards.

During fiscal year 1992, MSHA conducted 26,863 regular mandatory inspections at the 15,000 surface and underground mines in the United States. To provide similar coverage of the nation's general industry, OSHA would have to employ approximately 750,000 compliance officers instead of the less than 2,000 inspectors employed by OSHA and state plan states. Under OSHA each workplace is likely to receive an inspection every 70 years in contrast to four per year for each underground mine under MSHA. As a result of this intensive inspection program, mine fatalities have decreased from a high of 4,192 in 1907 to 97 in 1992 in all types of mining both metal and nonmetal.[22] Fatality rates declined markedly following the passage of the 1969 Act and have continued to drop even to the present. Injury rates have also decreased in mining. Mining continues to be a dangerous occupation, but the recent Acts of 1969 and 1977 have clearly led to improvements in working conditions for employees.

Mine Safety and Health Administration and respiratory disease

Weeks[22] evaluated estimates of the prevalence of pneumoconiosis from NIOSH, which conducts the National Study of Coal Workers' Pneumoconiosis (NSCWP). NIOSH[23] concluded that "the prevalence of [coal workers' pneumoconiosis] appears to have declined over the three rounds [from 1970 to 1981] of the [surveillance program] and the NSCWP. He states that the main cause of the decline in coal worker's pneumoconiosis (CWP), seen between rounds 1 and 3, lies more with population changes than with the effects of preventive measures." Therefore, the Act has had a significant impact on fatalities and injury rates in the mining industry, but the problem of respiratory disease in the mines remains unresolved.

The current exposure standard for respirable coal mine dust is 2.0 mg/m^3. This standard was derived from the British Pneumoconiosis Field Research Program and was based on a dose–response evaluation that predicted that the risk of developing CWP (of grade 2 or higher) was zero at this limit. Employers are required by MSHA to collect a minimum of five samples in each section of a coal mine six times per year. The highest exposed miners are monitored most frequently and every individual miner is monitored at least two times per year. These samples are sent to MSHA for weighing and calculation of the airborne dust concentration. Thus industry is required to determine compliance with the standard by its own environmental monitoring program, and the data are collected and evaluated by MSHA. MSHA inspectors periodically inspect mines to determine the accuracy of the employers' monitoring strategy and to assure its validity. The MSHA inspectors conduct their own sampling of respirable dust for comparative purposes. This program resulted in approximately 100,000 samples being collected by mine operators and 20,000 by MSHA in 1987.

OSHA has no program comparable with these environmental monitoring requirements under MSHA. Many of the 6(b) standards cited earlier require employers to conduct environmental monitoring to determine compliance with the standard, but no standard requires the employer to submit the results to OSHA or NIOSH for evaluation. A program of this nature with spot checks by OSHA inspectors would represent an important innovation in how OSHA determines compliance with its standards. OSHA is currently considering the promulgation of a generic environmental monitoring standard, but whether it will contain features similar to those required by MSHA remains to be seen.

The 2.0 mg/m^3 standard for respirable coal dust appears to be appropriate and scientifically sound, but there have been allegations that the employers have falsified environmental samples. MSHA compared mine operator data with inspector generated information and found the mean exposure concentrations collected by the employers were 0.2 to 0.3 mg/m^3 lower than those collected by the inspectors.[23a] Seixas and his co-workers[25] reported similar findings with a 13% underestimate of mean exposures. As a result of these and other studies MSHA issued 4,710 citations to mine companies for tampering with environmental monitoring samples, and by 1995, 33 mine operators and contractors pleaded guilty to criminal charges of conspiring to submit tampered or fraudulent samples. This issue has been discussed in greater detail by Seixas,[26] and it is apparent that although the strategy for employer collected measurements of airborne concentration is an important approach to achieving regulatory compliance with standards for limiting exposure to respirable coal dust, there is a clear need for safeguards designed to prevent tampering and fraud to assure the accuracy of sampling results.

Many of the metal and nonmetal commodities mined in the United States are toxic and have particular effects on the lung. MSHA has historically focused its health activities on coal mining and the risk of coal workers pneumoconiosis with some attention being given to silica. NIOSH and MSHA have jointly developed efforts to prevent silicosis from exposure to respirable crystalline silica. MSHA has focused its attention on the risk of rock drillers in coal mines, quarries, and metal mining. Rock drillers are at particular risk of exposure to respirable silica in their jobs, and MSHA in 1993 identified at least 23 cases of silicosis. The silicosis associated with rock drilling may be a result of chronic exposure, accelerated silicosis from exposure to high concentrations, and acute silicosis, which occurs from the highest levels of exposure and may manifest symptoms and signs as early as a few weeks to 4 or 5 years after initial exposure. MSHA has also been concerned with the health risks associated with exposure to diesel exhaust in underground mines in recent years. In the future, MSHA will doubtlessly focus additional attention on the issue of preventing silicosis and silica-related respiratory disease in the mines, and they will need to work closely with NIOSH to identify and regulate other exposures to chemical toxicants that produce respiratory disease in mining.

NIOSH has an important role in both research and epidemiologic surveillance in mining. DRDS administers the National Coal Worker's X-ray Surveillance Program and the National Coal Workers Autopsy Study under the Federal Mine and Safety and Health Act of 1969, as amended in 1977. Mandated activities include certification of x-ray facilities, Mine Plan approvals, B-Reader Examinations, and coordination of processing, storage, and retrieval of files and records from medical examinations. Data are analyzed for trends in the prevalence of miner lung diseases.

CURRENT ISSUES IN OCCUPATIONAL SAFETY AND HEALTH REGULATORY POLICY

The principal issues concerning OSHA at present include: how to address generic standards within the context of the Supreme Court decisions cited earlier; the specific problem of indoor air pollution; notification of high risk individuals (notification of workers at high risk of serious disease as a result of past exposures to toxic substances); improved recordkeeping for occupational injuries, illnesses, disease, and mortality; construction health and safety; development of a generic standard requiring exposure monitoring in the workplace; the "right to act"; the right to refuse work that would expose an individual to serious injury or illness; how OSHA should set inspection priorities and evaluate the effectiveness of its own enforcement effort; how OSHA should conduct risk assessment; and whether Congress will amend the legislation to require cost-benefit analysis.

These policy debates are of great concern and will represent the fundamental policy debates in the latter half of the 1990s and the early twenty-first century, but there is an additional feature that confounds OSHA's ability to meet the highly laudable goals of the Act. OSHA has approximately 1,000 inspectors to address 6 million workplaces, and the budgets of both OSHA and NIOSH are inadequate to meet the demands of the problems that the Agencies confront, and the scope of the problems that the Agencies are required to address continues to expand. For example, indoor air pollution and smoking in the workplace are each major issues that already require significant resources from each Agency, but these problems were never envisioned in the original OSHAct.

REFERENCES

1. Cherniak M: *The Hawks Nest incident,* New Haven, 1986, Yale University Press.
2. Corn JK: Historical aspects of industrial hygiene: II. Silicosis, *Am Ind Hyg Assoc J* 41:125, 1980.
3. U.S. Congress: House Committee on Labor: *An investigation relating to health conditions of workers employed in the construction and maintenance of public utilities,* Hearings on H.R. 4973, 96th Congress, 1st session, 1936.
4. Office of Technology Assessment: *Preventing illness and injury in the workplace,* Washington D.C., 1985, U.S. Congress, OTA-H256.
5. Page JA and O'Brien MW: *Bitter wages,* New York, 1973, Grossman.
6. MacLaury J: The job safety law of 1970: its passage was perilous, *Monthly Labor Rev* 104(3):18-24, 1981.
7. Scala RA: In Amdur MO, Doull J, and Klaassen CD, editors: *Casarett and Doull's toxicology: the Basic Science of Poisons,* pp 985-996, New York, 1991, Pergamon Press.
7a. OSHA: *Standard for occupational exposure to cotton dust,* 43 Fed. Reg. 27350-99, 1978.
8. U.S. Supreme Court, 452U.S.490, 1981.
9. American Industrial Hygiene Association and American Conference of Governmental Industrial Hygienists: *Respiratory protective devices manual,* Ann Arbor, MI, 1963, Braun and Brumfield.
10. U.S. District Court of Appeals, D.C., 617F.2d, 1979.
11. Merchant JA, Halprin GM, Hudson AR, et al: Responses to cotton dust, *Arch Environ Health* 30:222, 1975.
12. Kennedy SM: Acquired airway hyperresponsiveness from nonimmunogenic irritant exposure, *Occup Med State Art Rev* 7(2):287, 1992.
13. OSHA: *Occupational exposure to formaldehyde,* 52FR46168, 1987.
14. OSHA, *Occupational exposure to formaldehyde,* 57FR22290, 1992.
15. Robinson JC: *Toil and toxics,* pp 160-161, Berkeley, 1991, University of California Press.
16. Robinson JC, Paxman DG, and Rappaport SM: Implications of OSHA's reliance on TLVs in developing the air contaminants standard, *Am J Ind Med* 19(1):3–13, 1991.

17. Roach SA and Rappaport SM: But they are not thresholds: a critical analysis of the documentation of threshold limit values, *Am J Ind Med* 17:727-753, 1990.

18. Castleman BI and Ziem GE: Corporate influence on threshold limit values, *Am J Ind Med* 13:531-559, 1988.

19. Ashford, NA and Caldart CC: *Technology, law and the working environment,* New York, 1991, Van Nostrand Reinhold.

20. Rutstein DD, Berenberg W, Chalmers TC, Child CG, Fishman AP, and Perrin EB: Measuring the quality of medical care: a clinical method, *N Engl J Med* 294:582-588, 1976.

21. NIOSH: Prevention of leading work-related diseases and injuries, *MMWR* 32(2), 1983.

22. Weeks JL: Is regulation effective: a case study of underground coal mining, *Ann NY Acad Sci* 572:189-199, 1989.

23. Attfield M: *Past, present and predicted future levels of coal workers pneumoconiosis in working U.S. coal miners,* Morgantown, WV, 1987, National Institute for Occupational Safety and Health.

24. Boden and Gold 1984.

25. Seixas NS, Robins TG, Rice CH, and Moulton LH: Assessment of potential biases in the application of MSHA respirable coal mine dust data to an epidemiologic study, *Am Ind Hyg Assoc J* 5:534-540, 1990.

26. Seixas NS: Exposure assessment and public health, *New Solutions* 4(2):34-42, 1994.

Chapter 56

ENVIRONMENTAL
REGULATORY APPROACHES

Michael P. Kenny
Leslie M. Krinsk

In 1990, Congress substantially amended the Clean Air Act (the "Act") for the fourth time.[1] The amendments entailed 11 chapters—called Titles—that reflect specific subject matter. (Originally adopted in 1963, the Act was previously amended in substantial fashion in 1970, 1975, and 1977.) With the latest amendments, Congress maintained the course it had previously established for achieving healthful air quality in the United States, but provided new time frames for accomplishing the goal.

That goal requires not only a substantial effort from the U.S. Environmental Protection Agency (EPA), the primary federal agency with responsibility for carrying out the mandates of the Act, but also from state and local authorities. Consequently, the control of air pollution is a multitiered regulatory effort, including not only the federal statutes and regulations but also state and local statutes and regulations. Each of these fits within a unified framework designed to achieve emission reductions in as comprehensive and expeditious a manner as possible.

That framework is unified by the federal statutory process, which requires that states bear the primary responsibility for achieving the necessary emission reductions to attain clean air.[2] To the extent any state fails in this effort, the EPA will substitute itself in place of the state to ensure that the air quality objectives are achieved.[3] To understand how this framework is implemented is best explained by approaching it from the top down. Thus, an understanding of the requirements of the federal Clean Air Act is primary to this discussion. Subsequently, one can view the state and local effort to obtain the complete view of the overall regulatory approach.

THE CLEAN AIR ACT
National Ambient Air Quality Standards

At the heart of the Act is the requirement that the EPA establish National Ambient Air Quality Standards (NAAQS).[4] The standards (initially required and adopted pursuant to earlier versions of the Act) are subject to routine review and exist for specified pollutants (referred to as criteria pollutants). The primary standards reflect the maximum ambient concentrations of criteria pollutants that can be present in the air without causing harm to the public.[5]

Table 56-1. National Ambient Air Quality Standards

| Pollutant | Averaging time | Ambient standard | |
		Primary	Secondary
Ozone	1 hour	0.12 ppm	Same
Carbon monoxide	8 hours	9 ppm	—
	1 hour	35 ppm	—
Nitrogen dioxide	Annual average	0.053 ppm	Same
Sulfur dioxide	Annual average	80 $\mu g/m^3$	—
	24 hours	365 $\mu g/m^3$	—
	3 hours		1300 $\mu g/m^3$
Suspended particulate matter (PM)	24 hours	150 $\mu g/m^3$	Same
	Annual arithmetic mean	50 $\mu g/m^3$	Same
Lead	Calendar quarter	1.5 $\mu g/m^3$	Same

ppm, Parts per million.

Secondary standards exist to protect the public welfare from any known or anticipated adverse effects associated with the presence of such pollutants (i.e., secondary standards are set to provide a measure of protection for plants and animals).[6] Table 56-1 identifies the criteria pollutants and the relevant national ambient air quality standards.

Attainment designations

With the NAAQS as a guide, all areas of the country are designated as being in attainment, nonattainment, or unclassifiable of the standards. The designations are then used as the basis for determining the statutorily required effort that will be assigned to each of the areas to achieve and maintain the NAAQS. The primary emphasis in the Act is on those areas that are nonattainment for the standards, particularly the ozone standard.

For an area that is in attainment, the Act requires less but does demand that measures be undertaken in the prevention of significant deterioration (PSD). These measures are known as PSD requirements.[7]

Attainment classifications

For areas that are nonattainment for certain criteria pollutants, a further inquiry occurs. The historical severity of the air pollution for the area (defined as Standard Metropolitan Statistical Areas [SMSAs] as determined by the U.S. Census Bureau) is used to determine the degree of air pollution control that will be required. The determination of severity of nonattainment in an area is referred to as its classification. Classification structures are not the same for each of the criteria pollutants. Ozone has a classification structure that reflects five levels of severity,[8] carbon monoxide and particulate matter (PM) have only two levels,[9] whereas sulfur dioxide, nitrogen dioxide, and lead do not rely upon classifications, but simply require control strategies to achieve attainment.[10]

Table 56-2. Ozone classifications

Classification	Design value (ppm)	Attainment required
Marginal	0.121-0.137	11/15/93
Moderate	0.138-0.159	11/15/96
Serious	0.160-0.179	11/15/99
Severe	0.180-0.190	11/15/05
Severe	0.191-0.279	11/15/07
Extreme	0.280 or above	11/15/10

ppm, Parts per million.

Ozone. Table 56-2 lists the applicable time frames associated with areas that are nonattainment for the ozone NAAQS. Areas are classified as marginal, moderate, serious, severe, or extreme based upon a "design value" that reflects an area's history of ozone violations. Areas with the most severe pollution problems are provided with the most time for achieving attainment of the ozone NAAQS. However, in return for the additional time to achieve the NAAQS, such areas are required to impose more severe control requirements on their sources of emissions. As an example, the only extreme area—Los Angeles—is not required to show attainment until the year 2010. The time frame recognizes the severity of the problem in Los Angeles and the substantial effort that will be required to eradicate it. There is a price to be paid for the severity of the problem and the amount of time granted for its resolution: controls that are more daunting than those imposed on lesser classified areas. Consequently, there is no benefit in being granted more time to attain; instead, there is only unhealthful air for a longer period of time and more stringent and costly controls imposed to clean up that air. (In viewing the design values, one should remember that ozone attainment exists at 0.12 parts per million [ppm].)

Carbon monoxide. Table 56-3 identifies the applicable time frames assigned by the Act for attainment of the car-

Table 56-3. Carbon monoxide classifications

Classification	Design value (ppm)	Attainment required
Moderate	9.1-16.4	12/31/95
Serious	16.5 and above	12/31/01

ppm, Parts per million.

bon monoxide NAAQS. As with ozone, the carbon monoxide classifications reflect a recognition that more time is necessary for those areas with greater historical problems.

Particulate matter. For areas that have been designated as nonattainment for the particulate matter (PM$_{10}$) standard, a classification of moderate is presumptively assigned. The Act then required that such areas attain the standard as expeditiously as possible but no later than December 31, 1994. For areas that are subsequently designated as nonattainment, a classification of moderate will be assigned and attainment is required within 6 years of the designation as nonattainment. If an area that is classified as moderate fails to attain the standard within the applicable time frame, the area is reclassified as serious. A serious classification requires additional statutory efforts to attain and provides for additional time to demonstrate attainment—until December 31, 2001.

Sulfur dioxide, nitrogen dioxide, and lead. The Act requires States with existing areas designated as nonattainment for sulfur dioxide, nitrogen dioxide, or lead to submit a State Implementation Plan (SIP) that demonstrates attainment within 5 years of the date of adoption of the 1990 Amendments (i.e., November 15, 1995). The SIP submission must be made within 18 months of the Act's adoption. For those areas that are subsequently designated nonattainment, SIP submissions must be made within 18 months of the designation, and attainment must be demonstrated within 5 years of the nonattainment designation.

State Implementation Plans

Although it might seem as if SIP submissions that demonstrate attainment would be sufficient to carry out the purpose of the Act, several other types of SIP submissions are also required. Consequently, attainment SIPs are not the only SIP submissions required of the states. The essence of any SIP submission, however, is the same: it is a state plan with associated enforceable measures—generally statutes and regulations—designed to reduce air pollution or to meet other requirements specified in the Act.

Before reviewing the variety of SIP submissions that are required of the states, it is appropriate to review in more detail what a SIP is, what is required for its adoption, and the consequences of a failure to adopt.

The SIP is a federally enforceable document that reflects a state's air pollution control strategies for achieving attainment or for meeting a specific requirement of the Act. Those

strategies must be given life through statutes or regulations that reduce air pollution in a measurable fashion. It is the state's obligation to put forth that strategy with measures that will achieve necessary emission reductions. In adopting its strategy, the state must provide the opportunity for public participation. Once the state has completed its effort, it submits the SIP with its attendant air pollution reduction measures to the EPA for consideration. (At this point, the SIP is not a federally enforceable document since it has not been approved by the EPA.)

It is important to note that the SIP is a constantly evolving document. Although specific deadlines are required to be met for submission of particular SIP requirements, the reality of the situation is that SIPs and SIP amendments are generated continuously and from the bottom up in many instances. What is meant by the "bottom up" is that local authorities often provide ordinances or regulations that limit the emissions of air pollution. Those ordinances or regulations are then provided to the state for review and submission to the EPA. This process is constantly ongoing as a result of the many SIP submissions required by the EPA. Additionally, states must respond to EPA disapprovals by modifying and resubmitting prior SIP submissions. Finally, as a result of continuing efforts by state and local authorities to achieve emission reductions, regulations are continually modified to reflect more effective emission control technologies. Those modified regulations are then forwarded to the EPA as SIP revisions to substantiate additional emission reductions over what prior submissions were expected to achieve.

The EPA begins its review by assessing whether the submitted SIP is a complete document (i.e., whether all the required components are present in the submission).[11] The Act provides the EPA with a limited time frame within which to make this determination (a maximum of 6 months). To assist states in passing this initial completeness review, the EPA has published "Completeness Criteria" for the states' use in adopting SIPs.[12] These criteria identify the scope of EPA's consideration during its completeness review. If the SIP submission is determined to be complete, the EPA then reviews the submission for approveability. If a submission is approved, it then becomes a part of the federally approved SIP and is enforceable under federal law.

If a submission is disapproved, a notification of disapproval is provided to the state. The consequences of disapproval include the initiation of a sanctions process and the ultimate promulgation of a Federal Implementation Plan (FIP). The EPA has a mandatory obligation to impose specific sanctions 18 months after a state's failure to make a required SIP submission.[13] Sanctions are defined in the Act as being a cutoff of federal funds for highway projects and/or the imposition of a requirement on new and modified sources that they offset their stationary source emissions by a ratio of at least 2 to 1. The impact of this second sanction is that it makes business expansion more expensive than it would otherwise be. The EPA also has the authority under its discretionary sanctions authority to impose either of these sanctions in less than 18 months if it believes it is necessary.[14]

Finally, if sanctions fail to elicit an approveable SIP from the state, the EPA must undertake the responsibility itself. The Act requires that the EPA promulgate a FIP within 2 years after a state has failed to make a required SIP submission.[15] In promulgating a FIP, the EPA is placed in the same role that the state would otherwise have occupied. As such, the EPA is required to step into the state's shoes and fulfill the SIP requirement of that state.

State Implementation Plan submittals—stationary sources. As noted, attainment SIPs for the criteria pollutants must be submitted to the EPA within specific time frames. In addition to these submittals, however, the Act also requires states to make a large number of other SIP submittals. These submittals include both the control of specific types of sources and other actions to enhance the states' understanding of pollution control. The actions and the control of sources—both mobile and stationary—are specifically mandated by Congress. As to how these SIP requirements fit within the context of the attainment SIPs, one can view the attainment SIPs as providing the overall strategy and emission reductions necessary to achieve attainment, while viewing the other required SIP submittals as being necessary to meet certain requirements that Congress has specifically identified as necessary to assist in moving areas toward attainment.

To fully understand the nature of the additional SIP requirements imposed by the Act on the states, it is useful to view the SIP requirements as either pertaining to stationary sources or mobile sources. Since the control of air pollution essentially follows this distinct line, it is helpful to recognize the manner in which the federal statutory scheme treats each of these substantial sources of emissions.

Stationary sources primarily subject to the requirements of the Act are those that are considered to be "major." Major sources are defined differently depending upon whether one is referring to criteria or toxic pollutants. For now, our review will be limited to criteria pollutants. For purposes of controlling criteria pollutants, sources that constitute major sources can vary depending on the classification that exists for the nonattainment area in which the source is located.

The general rule is that a source is considered "major" and subject to stationary source control requirements if it has the potential to emit 100 tons of volatile organic compounds (VOCs) per year.[16] However, in ozone nonattainment areas, the thresholds are lowered to reflect the need to obtain greater emission reductions in areas that have suffered from more severe air pollution problems. A source is considered major if it has the potential to emit 50 tons per year of VOCs in serious areas, 25 tons per year in severe areas, and 10 tons per year in extreme areas.[17] These same thresholds are applicable to sources in ozone nonattainment areas with emissions not only of VOCs, but also of oxides of nitrogen. The major source definition remains consistent with the general rule for areas that are nonattainment with the other criteria pollutants. In areas that are nonattainment for multiple pollutants including ozone, the ozone nonattainment major source definitions apply.

There are several required SIP submittals that must be made by the states to the EPA. The following is a list of some of the more significant SIP submittals required under the Act but is in no way exhaustive.

Emissions inventory. This SIP submittal is required to have been submitted to the EPA by November 15, 1992.[18] It must include a comprehensive, accurate, current inventory of actual emissions from all sources of the relevant pollutant or pollutants in nonattainment areas.

Trip reductions. For severe and extreme ozone nonattainment areas, the Act required states to submit an SIP revision that both quantifies the vehicle miles traveled (VMT) and includes specific enforceable transportation control strategies to offset the growth in emissions from vehicle miles traveled or the growth in the number of trips.[19] Additionally, the SIP submission was required to include a program that at a minimum imposed upon employers of 100 or more persons the requirement to reduce work-related trips and miles traveled by employees. The reduction to be achieved under this requirement is at least 25% from the number in existence at the time of the submission.

Employers are obligated to submit their compliance plans for achieving these reductions within 2 years of the SIP submission. The plans must "convincingly demonstrate compliance" within 4 years of the SIP submission.

Enhanced monitoring. For serious, severe, or extreme ozone nonattainment areas, the Act required that the EPA promulgate rules within 18 months of enactment for the enhanced monitoring of ozone, oxides of nitrogen, and VOCs.[20] The stated purpose of this requirement was to obtain more comprehensive and representative data on ozone air pollution. Following promulgation by the EPA, the states were obligated to commence whatever actions were necessary to adopt and implement a program based on the federal rules. An SIP submission reflecting the enhanced monitoring by the state must then be submitted for review to the EPA.

Reasonable further progress demonstration. States with ozone nonattainment areas that are moderate or worse were required to make a SIP submission by November 15, 1993 that provided for a 15% reduction in VOCs from baseline emissions by November 15, 1996.[21] Furthermore, the SIP submission was required to provide for specific annual reductions in emissions of VOCs and oxides of nitrogen sufficient to attain the primary NAAQS by the date applicable under the Act.

Reasonably available control technology. States with ozone nonattainment areas were required to make a SIP submission by November 15, 1992 that required the application of "reasonably available control technology" (RACT) to all VOC sources covered by EPA issued guidance for such sources and also for all major sources of VOCs.[22]

Operating permit program. The Act imposed upon the EPA and the states the obligation to adopt and implement an operating permit program for all sources, both major and minor.[23] The EPA's obligation was to adopt by regulation the minimum requirements for such a program within 12 months of the Act's adoption. Although the EPA failed to meet this timetable, the regulations as ultimately promulgated reflected the EPA's decision to exercise its discretion to initially limit the program to only major sources. This choice reflected a clear recognition of the difficulties that would be associated with the implementation of this new program. Although many states had state operating permit programs in place prior to the adoption of the Act, a substantial number of states did not.

The states' obligation was to make a SIP submittal showing compliance with the specific requirements of the Act and the EPA regulations by November 15, 1993. Pursuant to the Act, upon submission of the operating permit program, the EPA is provided 1 year to approve, approve conditionally, or disapprove a state's submittal.

In reviewing the submittal, the EPA must determine that the specific criteria identified in both the Act and the federal operating permit regulations have been satisfied. Those requirements include but are not limited to standardized applications and permits, monitoring and reporting requirements, minimum fees, requirements for adequate personnel and funding, the extent of applicable legal authority, streamlined procedures, the ability to incorporate changes to the permits, public participation, and enforcement.

State Implementation Plan submittals—mobile sources. Mobile sources are treated substantially differently than stationary sources under the Act. Whereas stationary sources are regulated by the states through either their own power or through that of local authorities, the primary regulation of mobile sources is accomplished at the federal level.[24] With a single exception that will be discussed, states are not permitted to regulate the emissions from motor vehicles. Instead, the EPA is charged by Congress with regulating the levels to which new vehicles may cause emissions from tailpipes and through evaporative losses.[25] The EPA has utilized this authority to establish national tailpipe and evaporative standards for all new vehicles sold in the country. Those standards are not all identical since varying standards are necessary to accommodate different classes of vehicles (i.e., heavy duty truck standards differ from passenger car standards). However, no new vehicle may be sold in the country that fails to comply with these standards. This has not prevented Congress from requiring several mobile source-related SIP submissions, but those submissions are not directed at the tailpipe or evaporative emissions from vehicles; instead, the control require-

ments associated with the SIP submissions are in the nature of operational limitations on fuels, vapor recovery from refueling, and the establishment of fleet standards. Additionally, for areas that are nonattainment for the ozone standard, the Act requires routine inspection and maintenance of the existing vehicle fleet.

Before reviewing the specific SIP submittal requirements, it would be useful at this point to briefly discuss one further aspect of vehicle regulation. As mentioned, the Act preempts the regulation of on-road vehicle emissions by the states with one exception. That exception allows the state of California to establish emission limitations for vehicles.[26] California's emission limitations are then submitted to the EPA for review pursuant to specific criteria established in the Act. California was provided this special authority by Congress in the 1970 amendments to the Act in recognition of its already existing program and the extraordinary air pollution problems present in California. Other states may not promulgate their own vehicle emission standards, but they may adopt the California standards if they choose to do so.[27] Thus, only two types of vehicles are permitted in the United States—federal and California vehicles.

The 1990 amendments to the Act continued to recognize California's unique authority with regard to the regulation of motor vehicles. In addition, a provision was added to the Act that recognized California's ability to regulate off-road vehicles while preempting other states from regulating these sources.[28] Again though, as with on-road vehicles, Congress provided that other states could adopt the California standards. In the area of off-road vehicle controls, however, even California was preempted in part. California may not regulate emission standards for new locomotives or locomotive engines or for new construction and farm equipment or new construction and farm equipment engines.[29]

State Implementation Plan submittals—motor vehicle fuels. As with motor vehicles, the states (with two exceptions) are generally preempted from regulating the components or characteristics of motor vehicle fuels—provided the EPA has prescribed such components or characteristics.[30] The first exception is that California may regulate the content of motor vehicle fuels. The second is that the EPA may approve a state's regulation of fuel components or characteristics if the state demonstrates it is necessary for the attainment of a national primary or secondary standard.

The result of this preemption in the area of fuels is that the primary obligation for achieving emission reductions in the United States (outside California) lies with the EPA. For that reason Congress placed the burden on the EPA to develop a reformulated gasoline.[31] Reformulated gasoline—an ozone control strategy—must be designed to achieve the greatest emissions reduction possible of both VOCs and toxic air contaminants in comparison with existing gasoline. Specific reformulated gasoline formula components were also identified by Congress to achieve this goal.

Three other major fuel-related emission reduction control strategies were mandated by the Act. Each is a strategy that is implemented through the SIP submission process. Consequently, the burden is on the states to adopt the requisite statutes or regulations and provide them to the EPA as an SIP submission.

Oxygenated fuels. To address carbon monoxide, the Act recognized that the EPA had not acted on oxygenated fuels (increased oxygen content of fuels has been shown to decrease carbon monoxide emissions) and required states to provide SIP submissions by November 15, 1992 that reflected the implementation of an oxygenated fuels requirement in carbon monoxide nonattainment areas.[32] The specific requirement mandated an oxygen content of not less than 2.7% oxygen by weight. If a state could demonstrate that this oxygen content would prevent or interfere with the attainment of a primary or secondary standard for any pollutant other than carbon monoxide, the EPA was then directed to waive application of the 2.7% minimum standard.

Inspection and maintenance. The Act required serious, severe, and extreme ozone and carbon monoxide nonattainment areas with urban populations greater than 200,000 to enhance their inspection and maintenance programs to meet specific performance criteria established by the EPA.[33] (Such a program is commonly referred to as "Enhanced I & M.") In establishing those criteria, the EPA promulgated regulations identifying the specific manner through which the performance criteria could be satisfied. In general, those criteria required states to adopt programs that required centralized testing of vehicles to ensure that they met in-use emission limits. If repairs were necessary for the vehicles to meet the limits, those repairs could not be performed at the testing station. This design was intended to avoid the potential for fraud that EPA presumed to exist if testing and repair were accomplished at a single location.

Additionally, for those nonattainment areas classified as moderate, the Act also required SIP submissions establishing an inspection and maintenance program. This program differed from that required in serious, severe, and extreme areas in that its requirements for emission reductions are not as stringent as those required in areas subject to Enhanced I & M. (This type of program is commonly referred to as "Basic I & M.")

Centrally fueled fleets. The Act identifies an emissions standard for heavy-duty vehicles or engines manufactured after 1997.[34] This standard is a clean-fuel vehicle standard that is equivalent to 50% (or a less stringent standard if the EPA determines that the 50% standard is not feasible) of the combined emissions standards for oxides of nitrogen and nonmethane hydrocarbons for 1994 heavy-duty diesel-fueled vehicles or engines. To implement this requirement, the Act further requires for specified ozone and carbon monoxide nonattainment areas that an SIP submission be made within 42 months of enactment of the Act to establish a clean-fuel vehicle fleet program.

The SIP submission must reflect a requirement that specified percentages of new fleet vehicles purchased in model year 1998 and thereafter be clean-fuel vehicles and that they shall operate on clean alternative fuels. A "fleet" is defined in the Act as 10 or more motor vehicles owned or operated by a single person.

Other federal requirements pursuant to the Act

Toxics. The 1990 Amendments substantially modified the manner in which toxic air substances were regulated. Prior to the amendments, toxics (referred to in the Act as hazardous air pollutants [HAPs]) were regulated through a cumbersome process that required an initial determination that a substance was toxic; only then was it regulated. This process, because of its cumbersomeness, had resulted in the regulation of very few toxic substances. As a result, Congress expressed its dissatisfaction by revamping the process of regulating toxic air substances.

Instead of a process for identifying HAPs, Congress simply identified 189 substances in the Act.[35] Since the HAPs were now identified by the Act, Congress instructed the EPA to regulate the emissions of these substances from major sources and area sources. Major sources were defined as any source or group of sources within a contiguous area and under common control that emit or have the potential to emit 10 tons or more per year of any HAP or 25 tons per year of a combination of HAPs.[36] An area source is any source of HAPs that is not a major source.[37]

In controlling the HAPs, the EPA must promulgate emission standards for categories of sources within specified periods of time.[38] The degree of reduction for new or modified sources must be equivalent to that achieved in practice by the best controlled similar source. For existing sources, the degree of reduction must be equivalent to the average emission limitation achieved by the best performing 12% of the existing sources.[39] These reduction requirements are commonly referred to as "Maximum available control technology" (MACT) standards. After the EPA has identified an MACT standard for a particular category of sources, sources in that category must generally comply within 3 years.[40]

Within this general framework for the control of toxic air substances, the Congress also provided for additional requirements and for flexibility. The additional requirements are in the nature of protection from residual risk after controls, work practice standards, and protection from accidental releases.[41] The flexibility lies in Congress' recognition that states may develop alternative approaches that may achieve equivalent public health protection.

Acid deposition. Acid deposition from the use of sulfur-containing fossil fuels has been a recognized problem in the United States for several years. The Act attempts to reduce acid deposition by imposing an innovative control strategy on its primary source of generation—utility power generators.[42] That control strategy requires approximately a 50% reduction in sulfur dioxide and oxides of nitrogen emissions by the year 2000. The program is structured into two phases. Phase 1, which began January 1, 1995, requires specified power plants to reduce emissions of sulfur dioxide and oxides of nitrogen to a specified level. Phase 2, beginning January 1, 2000, requires that annual emissions of sulfur dioxide be limited to 8.9 million tons (less than half of the identified emissions in 1990).

The acid deposition control strategy is particularly unique in that it relies upon a market-based approach to achieve reductions. It establishes allowances (a license to emit one ton of sulfur dioxide) for the affected sources that can be traded. The market-based approach is intended to achieve emissions reductions by providing flexibility to the sources to achieve those reductions. Sources may buy, sell, or trade the allowances, but a source must have sufficient allowances to cover its emissions. The Act specifies the sources that are included within the program and also identifies the allowances that are to be provided to the sources for the duration of Phase 1.

Enforcement. The Act provides the EPA with extensive authority to enforce its provisions.[43] In addition to providing the EPA with authority to undertake action against a state for failure to enforce SIP requirements, the Act authorizes the EPA to institute administrative, civil, and criminal actions against specific sources for violations of the provisions of the Act. The Act provides for penalties for source violations up to $25,000 per day of violation.

The EPA's national goal is to ensure that all federal, state, and local enforcement actions for violations of the Act assess a penalty sufficient to achieve effective deterrence for the source subject to enforcement and for the regulated community as a whole. The EPA's policy is to assess penalties that remove the economic benefit of noncompliance and include a gravity component that reflects the severity of the violation.

In addition to the enforcement authority provided to the EPA, the Act provides the public with a means of ensuring compliance with, and enforcement of, the Act's provisions—citizen suits.[44] The Act provides that any person, after providing notice to the EPA, may commence an action against the United States, another governmental entity, or a person alleged to have violated the Act. However, such an action is precluded if the EPA is diligently prosecuting the action. If a person brings such an action, the federal court may award the costs of litigation and attorneys fees whenever the court deems it appropriate.

Finally, actions may also be commenced by citizens against the EPA for its failure to perform a nondiscretionary duty required by the Act.[45] Historically, this provision has been used extensively to compel the EPA to take required actions or to challenge improper actions by the EPA.

STATE AND LOCAL REQUIREMENTS

Whereas the blueprint for air pollution control is generated at the federal level by means of the Clean Air Act, the daily work of adopting, implementing, and enforcing clean air requirements occurs at the state and local levels. Moreover, many states go beyond Clean Air Act requirements in one or more program areas,[46] and most states have developed implementation approaches that respond to their individual needs and philosophies[47] while meeting the minimum federal requirements. This section sets forth an illustrative model of state and local air pollution control based on the California program; although other state programs will vary from the model to some degree and generally are less comprehensive, basic program components are equivalent. Major differences will be noted.

In California, the state Air Resources Board[48] divides the state into air basins and adopts state ambient air quality standards that are generally more stringent than the corresponding national standards.[49] The agency also coordinates, encourages, and reviews the activities of all levels of government relating to air quality, and particularly oversees the efforts of 34 separate local and regional air pollution control districts[50] to ensure attainment of the state and national ambient standards and to carry out their statutory responsibilities. These responsibilities are set forth in a separate Division 26, "Air Resources," of the California Health and Safety Code. The Air Resources Board (ARB), in turn, adopts rules, regulations, and standards to clarify, implement, and enforce the air pollution control laws that it is directed to administer; these rules are set forth in Titles 13 and 17, respectively, of the California Code of Regulations.[51]

Regional and local districts also adopt numerous rules and regulations necessary to implement their statutory responsibilities.[52] The primary responsibility of an air pollution control district is to adopt, implement, and enforce emission standards and limitations[53] that limit the type and quantity of pollution emitted from various categories of sources: industrial facilities such as powerplants, oil refineries, and manufacturing plants; area sources such as gas stations and dry cleaners; indirect sources such as shopping centers and sports complexes that do not directly pollute but that attract motor vehicles; and transportation sources. Each type of source is subject to more or less stringent emission limitations, depending upon such factors as the technologic availability of controls, the cost of control, the nature and degree of pollution, public acceptability, and so forth.[54]

With regard to the criteria pollutants, the purpose of setting emission standards is to ensure that, in the aggregate, pollution from all regulated source categories will not exceed the threshold expressed by the ambient air quality standard. For toxic air pollutants, which generally are emitted more locally and operate more discreetly than the ubiquitous criteria pollutants, the objective of an emission limit is to ensure that pollutants that may cause or contribute to an increase in mortality or in serious illness, either acutely or chronically, are not emitted in quantities that may endanger public health.

Emission standards reduce, avoid, or eliminate emissions of a pollutant through the use of add-on control technology (e.g., scrubbers, electrostatic precipitators, catalytic converters, and baghouses), the specification of process inputs (e.g., sulfur content of fuel), the imposition of operational and maintenance conditions (e.g., minimum combustion temperatures, filter replacement, hours of operation), design, equipment, or work practice standards, and specification of process changes or substitution of materials (e.g., use of less toxic solvents or prohibition of ozone-depleting compounds). Since planning and implementation of control measures are different for criteria pollutants and toxic pollutants, we will discuss them separately, beginning with criteria pollutants, where efforts to control air pollution began.

As long as the minimum requirements and interim milestones of the federal Clean Air Act are met, states are free to develop any mix of control strategies that will accomplish attainment of the national ambient standards, by the specified dates, and may develop additional or more stringent requirements than those set forth in federal law. To ensure that the controls on individual sources will all add up to attainment of the ambient standards, elaborate air quality predictive models are used and plans are developed and continually refined based on current information about population, growth rates, source mix, emission factors, meteorology, availability of technology, and chemical transformation of pollutants. In California, plans must be developed and revised every 3 years to demonstrate how the state standards will be attained; these plans are in addition to the SIP required under federal law.[55] The plans are adopted at the local level after public comment and hearings, and they specify what control measures need to be adopted during what time frames to ensure attainment.

Each control measure, in turn, is again subject to public comment prior to adoption by the policy or governing board of the local district,[56] which performs the district's legislative function, and is then set forth in the district's comprehensive book of rules and regulations. The rules are available to the public at district offices and often in public libraries. Once reviewed, approved, and compiled by the state agency, some or all of these rules comprise the SIP and are forwarded to the federal EPA. Upon EPA approval by notice in the Federal Register, these SIP components are set forth in 40 Code of Federal Regulations (CFR) Part 52.[57] In California, the districts are authorized to adopt requirements that are more stringent than state law requires, with specified exceptions; cities and counties also are specifically authorized to control air pollution, although most are content with district rules and regulations.[58]

In states that are not large enough or industrial enough to need local districts, or where the pollution problem can be adequately handled statewide, or where the legislature prefers a more centralized approach, a state air pollution control agency performs the function ascribed above to local districts, generally through a state policy board of commissioners. In these states, the control measures may be implemented at the state level or through regional offices, or by contract with counties or public health offices, with the state retaining ultimate control and responsibility.

After rules are established for specific source categories, they are generally implemented and enforced through a permit system whereby the owner or operator of any facility or piece of equipment that may emit air pollutants must obtain both a permit to construct and, subsequently, to operate[59] the source from the air pollution control officer of the district or a similar executive of the state.[60] The air pollution control officer (or director, as the case may be), who, along with his or her staff of rule developers, inspectors, modelers, planners, and engineers, performs the executive function of the district, reviews the application completed by the source, and may issue a permit only if she or he determines that the source will comply with the provisions of state law, with the rules, regulations, and orders of the district and of the state air agency, and with applicable federal requirements. The permit generally references applicable rules and sets forth specific conditions with which each source must comply. Once the federal EPA approves the Title V Operating Permit Program submitted by every state, the operating permits will be issued by the state or local permitting agency after receiving input from the public, and will contain every requirement to which the source is subject. Once it is issued, any person can inspect the permit and in a single document be apprised of exactly what standards and conditions the particular facility must meet.

In all states, construction permits issued to major sources are subject to public comment prior to issuance. Minor source construction permits, as well as minor source operating permits, may also be subject to public review and comment.[61] Once issued, the permit is available for public inspection and copying at the office or agency that issued it. The Title V operating permit will clearly indicate whether any of the requirements are imposed for state law purposes only; all other requirements in the Title V operating permit may be enforced against the source by any citizen pursuant to section 304 of the Federal Clean Air Act. (By contrast, states do not generally authorize so-called "citizen suits," although citizen complaints often lead to investigations and enforcement actions by state or local government officials such as the Attorney General or District Attorney.)

The primary enforcer of the permit conditions is the air pollution control officer, or similar state or local official. The control officer and his or her staff periodically inspect and test most industrial and area sources, review the records the sources are required to keep by the state or district, analyze any monitoring data required to be provided by the source, and respond to public complaints pertaining to source operations that may cause air pollution. Most states and districts inspect sources periodically, such as once a year for major sources and every 2 years for nonmajor sources.[62] Citizen complaints also trigger inspections.

If a violation of any rule, regulation, permit condition, or other applicable requirement is detected, an elaborate enforcement and penalty scheme is triggered. The range of options available to the control officer spans office conferences and administrative penalty assessments all the way up to major enforcement actions in state or federal court, where both the state and the federal EPA may also be parties to the litigation. A panoply of civil and criminal penalties is set forth in the state statute. In California, penalties range from $1,000 per violation per day up to $50,000 per day per willful violation of an emissions limit, depending upon the specific penalty statute and the circumstances of the violation.[63] The general penalty philosophy of both the EPA and the states is to deter violators by making the cost of violations significantly higher than the cost of compliance.

Although the permits discussed will generally contain requirements and conditions to ensure compliance with rules pertaining to toxic air contaminants as well as to criteria pollutants, most state programs for regulating air toxics were developed several years after the criteria pollutant program[64] and operate somewhat differently because of this and the nature of the pollution. The purpose of state air toxics programs is to reduce the risk of harm, both chronic and acute, from toxic substances.

Many toxic air pollutants are chemical components of the criteria pollutant categories but merit individual regulatory attention. For example, hydrocarbons, or VOCs, are a vast class of chemicals that is regulated as a precursor to ozone, or photochemical smog, to attain the ozone ambient standard; many hydrocarbons are also more or less toxic and may be individually regulated to reduce harmful emissions and risk of harm from discreet sources. The same is true of PM, whose toxicity is dependent on such factors as particle size and chemical composition. Facilities emitting toxic air contaminants create "hot spots" of pollution that may expose people who live and work in the vicinity to elevated levels of substances that may cause cancer, birth defects, lung function impairment, nerve damage, skin and eye irritation, and other adverse health effects.

There are generally two approaches to controlling hazardous, or toxic, air pollutants that do not have an identifiable threshold below which adverse health effects can be expected not to occur (e.g., carcinogens and teratogens). One approach, such as the federal Clean Air Act §112 approach, is technology based; it imposes a specified control technology or performance standard to each source category[65] and concerns itself with the harmful effects that may remain after the technology is in place ("residual risk")

later. The other approach is risk based, and control requirements are based upon the decisionmaker's determination of "acceptable risk" to the exposed public, generally anywhere from 1 cancer per million to 100 cancers per million.[66] Sometimes technology is specified that will result in an acceptable level of emissions, but if the risk is still above the acceptable level once the technology is applied, more must be done, such as limiting operation of the facility or using substitute compounds.[67]

If a "no significant effects" threshold can be identified for a toxic air pollutant, an emission limit will be established to keep emissions below that threshold, usually with a margin of safety. This would eliminate the difficulty and controversy of establishing an "acceptable risk" level, but most toxic air pollutants are not amenable to "no effects" levels.

In California, the state ARB, acting pursuant to statute, has identified all of the §112 pollutants as toxic air contaminants and has developed a number of control measures for several of these, including benzene, chromium, dioxins, and perchloroethylene. In some cases there is no corresponding federal control measure and in other cases the state requirements are more stringent.[68] Once adopted by the state agency, each district must adopt the ARB measure or an equally or more stringent measure. For most of the 189 hazardous air pollutants listed by Congress, however, no specific federal or state control standards have yet been developed, either for new or existing sources. Some districts have used their independent authority to regulate toxics by requiring each source to conduct a risk assessment prior to construction and imposing permit requirements accordingly on a case by case basis.[69]

To date, the treatment of toxics is by no means uniform or comprehensive. Once the Title V operating permit programs are in effect, every major source operating permit must set forth requirements to ensure compliance with every toxic control measure (i.e., every MACT) promulgated by the EPA. That agency is working at a feverish pace to develop and propose MACT standards; however, to date only about eight have been promulgated and several more proposed.[70] The toxic air contaminant control gap has also been filled to some extent by the hydrocarbon control measures adopted by states to help attain the ozone standard. For example, the vapor recovery systems at gas stations in nonattainment areas also control benzene, a potent toxic air contaminant. Moreover, a number of states have community "right to know" laws[71] that not only require facilities to quantify and report emissions of specified air toxics, but also have had the salutary effect of inducing companies to greatly reduce emissions on a voluntary basis for "good neighbor" reasons.

In California, the Air Toxics "Hot Spots" Assessment and Information Act requires companies that manufacture, formulate, use, or release any of several hundred chemicals in specified amounts, which vary based upon the potency of the substance, to perform exacting emission inventories and submit reports of emissions to the local air pollution control district. These reports are available to the public. The districts prioritize each facility based on the nature and quantity of the toxic substance released, its proximity to susceptible receptors, and other factors, and may require a risk assessment to be performed. Based on the results of the risk assessment and a public notification level determined by the district policy board, some of the facilities must notify exposed persons of the specific, significant health risks attributable to the facility. The stigma of notification has encouraged numerous facilities to reduce their emissions below the notification thresholds, which generally are 10 additional cancers per million people.

Moreover, new legislation in California requires existing facilities to reduce toxic emissions over a 5- to 10-year period to below the significant risk level. The key issue in public workshops and hearings to determine the risk notification and emission reduction requirements is the threshold level of significant risk. Since controlling toxic emissions is often costly at best, and sometimes not technologically feasible, industry consistently advocates higher thresholds than environmental groups and the general public.

Regardless of the nuances of each state's program, most of the debate and decision making regarding toxic air contaminants occurs in a public forum, and the final regulations and permits are uniformly available for public inspection and copying at the regulatory agency's offices. All of the states take pains to respond in some way to citizen inquiries, although it will often take several telephone calls to reach the appropriate official and perhaps more to achieve a satisfactory and expeditious resolution.

In addition to their specific prohibitory rules and permit programs, many states also have a general air pollution nuisance law, which provides in essence that no source may emit such quantities of air pollutants as may endanger the health, safety, or welfare of the public or any significant number of persons or that may cause damage to property.[72] Although this type of statute does not provide a private citizen a cause of action against a facility, citizen complaints are a key factor in inducing the air pollution authority to investigate the facility and determine whether the evidence indicates the existence of a nuisance. Often states or districts will have a minimum number of complainants necessary to establish a sufficient basis for a nuisance, but even one complaint, if substantial, should suffice to alert the agency of a problem that could rise to the level of nuisance and supports investigation and possible enforcement.

All of the states regulate other sources of pollution that do not fit into the general pattern of source regulation and permitting described above. These other sources fall into several discreet categories, with the nature and extent of control determined by the environmental circumstances, source category inventory, and regulatory philosophy of each state.[73] Core source categories include architectural

coatings, which emit VOCs, consumer products such as deodorants, hair sprays, room fresheners, charcoal lighter fluids, and windshield washer fluids, which contain VOCs, pesticides, which emit VOCs as well as toxic air contaminants, and vehicle fuels, which emit VOCs and toxic pollutants. Some states also regulate agricultural operations, lawn and garden equipment, marine vessel and terminal operations, and off-road vehicles.

In addition, all states that have nonattainment areas are developing, adopting, and implementing transportation control measures to reduce the length and number of motor vehicle trips and to mitigate emissions of oxides of nitrogen, VOCs, PM, carbon monoxide, and toxic air contaminants. Indirect source control programs, which require facilities that do not directly emit pollutants but that attract motor vehicles to mitigate or offset these emissions, are designed to accomplish the same objectives, but have run into difficulty due to the perception that they are "land use control," which usurps the traditional and jealously guarded authority of city and county land use planning agencies.

In larger and more populous states where local and regional agencies take direction from the state air agency but retain primary responsibility for stationary source pollution control, the state agency, nevertheless, guides and, in some cases, directs the activities of the local agencies, coordinates their efforts to attain and maintain the ambient air quality standards, and may assume the powers of these agencies, or cancel their contracts and grants, if they are not carrying out their legal responsibilities. In such cases, the state agency may be amenable to citizen input if efforts to motivate the local or regional districts fail. In California, for example, the state agency can assume district planning, rulemaking, and enforcement authority, after notice and hearing, and can directly enforce district rules and regulations against violators.[74] Often the specter of state involvement is sufficient to motivate would-be polluters to comply with air pollution requirements.

A discussion of air pollution control at the state level would not be complete without some mention of the control of emissions from motor vehicles and fuels. Whereas transportation control measures reduce pollution by altering driving patterns and vehicular use, they do not directly affect tailpipe or evaporative emissions from individual vehicles; this occurs at the national, or in limited instances, a statewide level. Because it would not be practical to have separate emission standards for vehicles in all 50 states, Congress has required the federal EPA to adopt and implement nationwide standards. However, because California has historically regulated motor vehicles, the federal Clean Air Act permits California to adopt and enforce its own standards if they "will be, in the aggregate, at least as protective of public health and welfare as applicable Federal standards" (Clean Air Act section 209 (b)(1)) and if the Administrator of the EPA grants a waiver of the prohibition against individual state standards. Section 177 of the Clean

Air Act, in turn, allows states that have areas where the NAAQS are not attained to adopt the California standards. Currently, California has a robust program to drastically reduce emissions from both light- and heavy-duty vehicles and fuels, including requirements for reformulated gasoline and diesel fuels and penetration of vehicle fleets by zero emission vehicles (i.e., electric cars) by 1998, increasing in future years. The Northeast States for Coordinated Air Use Management (NESCAUM) states have decided to adopt the California vehicle (but not fuel) standards and other states may follow. Since motor vehicles contribute about 50% of the NO_x and VOC emissions (and 90% of CO emissions) in urban nonattainment areas, programs that reduce vehicular emissions are expected to have a major beneficial impact on air quality.

An active and informed citizenry is essential for an effective air pollution control program, either at the state or local level. Table 56-4 presents the names, addresses, and phone numbers of the members of the State and Territorial Air Pollution Program Administrators (STAPPA). Detailed information about each state's program and contacts can be obtained from the agencies listed. As indicated above, many states also have local agencies that are directly involved in air pollution control. The Association of Local Air Pollution Control Officials (ALAPCO) is comprised of these agencies, which are too numerous to set forth here. However, a copy of the STAPPA and ALAPCO membership directory can be obtained for a fee from their combined office at 444 N. Capitol Street, N.W., Washington D.C. 20001, (202) 624-7864.

Table 56-4. Directory of state and territorial air pollution programs

Alabama: Department of Environmental Management—Air Division
1751 Cong. W.L. Dickenson Drive, Montgomery, AL 36130
Telephone: (205) 271-7950
Alaska: Department of Environmental Conservation—Air Quality Management Section
P.O. Box 0, Juneau, AK 99811-1800
Telephone: (907) 465-5100
Arizona: Department of Environmental Quality—Office of Air Quality
P.O. Box 600, Phoenix, AZ 85001-0600
Telephone: (602) 207-2308
Arkansas: Department of Pollution Control and Ecology—Air Division
8001 National Drive, P.O. Box 9583, Little Rock, AR 72209
Telephone: (501) 562-7444
California: Air Resources Board
P.O. Box 2815, Sacramento, CA 95812
Telephone: (916) 445-4383
Colorado: Department of Health Air Pollution Control Division B-1
4300 Cherry Creek Drive South, Denver, CO 80222-1530
Telephone: (303) 692-3100
Connecticut: Department of Environmental Protection—Bureau of Air Management
79 Elm Street, Hartford, CT 06106
Telephone: (203) 566-7854
Delaware: Department of Natural Resources and Environmental Control—Division of Air and Waste Management—Air Quality Management Section
89 Kings Highway, P.O. Box 1401, Dover, DE 19903
Telephone: (302) 739-4791
Washington, D.C.: Department of Consumer and Regulatory Affairs—Environmental Control Division—Air Quality Control and Monitoring Branch
2100 Martin Luther King Avenue, SE, Washington, D.C. 20020
Telephone: (202) 404-1180, Ext 3073
Florida: Department of Environmental Protection—Air Resources Management
2600 Blair Stone Road, Twin Towers Office Building, Tallahassee, FL 32399-2400
Telephone: (904) 488-0114
Georgia: Department of Natural Resources—Environmental Protection Division—Air Protection Branch
4244 International Parkway, Suite 120, Atlanta, GA 3054
Telephone: (404) 363-7000
Hawaii: State Department of Health—Clean Air Branch
P.O. Box 3378, Honolulu, HI 96801
Telephone: (808) 586-4200
Idaho: Division of Environmental Quality—Permits and Enforcement Division
1410 North Hilton, 3rd Floor, Boise, ID 83706
Telephone: (208) 334-5898
Illinois: Environmental Protection Agency—Bureau of Air
2200 Churchill Road, P.O. Box 19276, Springfield, IL 62794-9276
Telephone: (217) 782-7326

Continued.

Table 56-4. Directory of state and territorial air pollution programs—cont'd

Indiana: Department of Environmental Management—Office of Air Management
  P.O. Box 6015, 105 South Meridian Street, Indianapolis, IN
  46206-6015
  Telephone: (317) 232-8384
Iowa: Department of Natural Resources—Air Quality Bureau
  Henry Wallace Building, 900 East Grand, Des Moines, IA 50319
  Telephone: (515) 281-8895
Kansas: Department of Health and Environment—Bureau of Air and Radiation
  Forbes Field, Building 740, Topeka, KS 66620
  Telephone: (913) 296-1593
Kentucky: Department for Environmental Protection—Division for Air Quality
  316 St. Clair Mall, Frankfort, KY 40601
  Telephone: (502) 564-3787
Louisiana: Department of Environmental Quality—Office of Air Quality and Radiation Protection: Air Quality Division
  P.O. Box 82135, Baton Rouge, LA 70884-2135
  Telephone: (504) 765-0219
Maine: Department of Environmental Protection—Bureau of Air Quality Control
  State House, Station 17, Augusta, ME 04333
  Telephone: (207) 289-2437
Maryland: Department of the Environment—Air Management Administration
  2500 Broening Highway, Baltimore, MD 21224
  Telephone: (410) 631-3255
Massachusetts: Department of Environmental Protection—Division of Air Quality Control
  One Winter Street, 7th Floor, Boston, MA 02108
  Telephone: (617) 292-5630
Michigan: Department of Natural Resources—Air Quality Division
  P.O. Box 30028, Lansing, MI 48909
  Telephone: (517) 373-7023
Minnesota: Pollution Control Agency—Air Quality Division
  520 Lafayette Road North, St. Paul, MN 55155
  Telephone: (612) 296-7331
Mississippi: Department of Environmental Quality   Office of Pollution Control—Air Division
  P.O. Box 10385, Jackson, MS 39289
  Telephone: (601) 961-5171
Missouri: Department of Natural Resources—Division of Environmental Quality   Air Pollution Control Program
  P.O. Box 176, Jefferson City, MO 65102
  Telephone: (314) 751-4817
Montana: Department of Health and Environmental Sciences—Air Quality Bureau
  Cogswell Building, Room A116, Helena, MT 59620
  Telephone: (406) 444-3454
Nebraska: Department of Environmental Quality—Air Quality Division
  301 Centennial Mall South, Box 98922, Lincoln, NE 68509-8922
  Telephone: (402) 471-2189
Nevada: Division of Environmental Protection—Bureau of Air Quality
  123 West Nye Lane, Carson City, NV 89710
  Telephone: (702) 687-4670
New Hampshire: Air Resources Division
  64 North Main Street, Caller Box 2033, Concord, NH 03301
  Telephone: (603) 271-1370
New Jersey: Department of Environmental Protection and Energy—Office of Air Quality Management
  401 East State Street, 7th Floor West, Trenton, NJ 08625
  Telephone: (609) 292-6710
New Mexico: Environment Department—Air Quality Bureau
  Harold Runnels Building, Room S2100, P.O. Box 26110, Santa Fe, NM 87502
  Telephone: (505) 827-0070
New York: Department of Environmental Conservation—Division of Air Resources
  50 Wolf Road, Albany NY 12233-3250
  Telephone: (518) 457-7230
North Carolina: Department of Environment, Health, and Natural Resources—Air Quality Section
  P.O. Box 29535, Raleigh, NC 27626
  Telephone: (919) 733-3340
North Dakota: Department of Health—Division of Environmental Engineering
  1200 Missouri Avenue, Room 304, P.O. Box 5520, Bismarck, ND 58502-5520
  Telephone: (701) 221-5188

Continued.

Table 56-4. Directory of state and territorial air pollution programs—cont'd

---

Ohio: Environmental Protection Agency—Division of Air Pollution Control
1800 Watermark Drive, Columbus, OH 43266-0149
Telephone: (614) 644-2270
Oklahoma: Department of Environmental Quality—Air Quality Program
4545 North Lincoln Boulevard, Suite 250, Oklahoma City, OK 73105-3483
Telephone: (405) 271-5220
Oregon: Department of Environmental Quality—Air Quality Control Division
811 SW 6th Avenue, Portland, OR 97203
Telephone: (503) 229-5359
Pennsylvania: Department of Environmental Resources—Bureau of Air Quality Control
400 Market Street, P.O. Box 8468, Harrisburg, PA 17105-5468
Telephone: (717) 787-9702
Rhode Island: Department of Environmental Management—Division of Air Resources
291 Promenade Street, Providence, RI 02908-5767
Telephone: (401) 277-2808
South Carolina: Department of Health and Environmental Control Bureau of Air Quality Control
2600 Bull Street, Columbia, SC 29201
Telephone: (803) 734-4750
South Dakota: Department of Environment and Natural Resources—Point Source Control Program
523 East Capital Avenue, Joe Foss Building, Pierre, SD 57501
Telephone: (605) 773-3351
Tennessee: Department of Environment and Conservation—Division of Air Pollution Control
401 Church Street, 9th Floor, L & C Annex, Nashville, TN 37243-1531
Telephone: (615) 532-0554
Texas: Texas Natural Resource Conservation Commission—Office of Air Quality Management
12124 Park 35 Circle, Austin, TX 78753
Telephone: (512) 239-1000
Utah: Department of Environmental Quality—Division of Air Quality
1950 West North Temple, Salt Lake City, UT 84114-4820
Telephone: (801) 536-4000
Vermont: Agency of Natural Resources—Air Pollution Control Division
103 South Main Street, Building 3 South, Waterbury, VT 05671-0402
Telephone: (802) 241-3840
Virginia: Department of Environmental Quality—Air Division
P.O. Box 10089, Richmond, VA 23240
Telephone: (804) 786-2378
Washington: Department of Ecology—Air Program
P.O. Box 47600, Olympia, WA 98504-7600
Telephone: (206) 407-6800
West Virginia: Department of Labor, Commerce and Environmental Resources—Division of Environmental Protection—Office of Air Quality
1558 Washington Street, East, Charleston, WV 25311
Telephone: (304) 558-3286

NOTES

1. The 1990 Amendments were enacted by Public Law 101-549, which was signed by the President on November 15, 1990. The Clean Air Act and amendments are codified in Title 42 of the United States Code (USC). All references to Clean Air Act sections are to Title 42 of the USC unless otherwise specified.

2. See section 7410 (a) (1).

3. See section 7410 (c).

4. See section 7409.

5. See section 7409 (b) (1).

6. See section 7409 (b) (2).

7. See sections 7470 et seq.

8. See section 7511.

9. See sections 7512 and 7513.

10. See section 7514.

11. Section 7410 (k) establishes the statutory requirements for completeness. See also 40 CFR Part 51, Appendix V.

12. See 40 CFR Part 51, Appendix V.

13. See section 7509.

14. See section 7410 (m).

15. See section 7410 (c).

16. See section 7602 (j).

17. See section 7511a.

18. See section 7511a.

19. See section 7511a.

20. See section 7511a.

21. See section 7511a.

22. See section 7511a.

23. See section 7661a.

24. See section 7543.

25. See section 7521.

26. See section 7543.

27. See section 7507.

28. See section 7543 (e).

29. See section 7543 (e) (1).

30. See section 7545.

31. See section 7545.

32. See section 7545 (m).

33. See section 7511a (c) (3).

34. See section 7585.

35. See section 7412 (b).

36. See section 7412 (a) (1).

37. See section 7412 (a) (2).

38. See section 7412 (c).

39. See section 7412 (d).

40. See section 7412 (i).

41. See sections 7412 (f), 7412 (h) and 7412 (l) respectively.

42. See sections 7651 et seq.

43. See section 7413.

44. See section 7604.

45. See section 7604.

46. Most states, for example, require new and modified sources of pollution to go through a preconstruction review process and receive a permit to construct, even for minor sources whose emissions are below federal Clean Air Act thresholds.

47. Some states, including Michigan, Washington, and South Dakota, have or are exploring a multimedia approach to permitting and source inspection; others, such as California and North Carolina, are initiating voluntary or mandatory pollution prevention programs.

48. The ARB is an independent regulatory agency within an umbrella agency, the California EPA, which maintains loose control over the state's air, water, pesticide, solid waste, hazardous waste, and toxics programs. Most other states have a state air agency that is a division of a larger statewide environmental regulatory agency; usually air pollution regulations are adopted by the larger multimedia agency (e.g., Oregon, Maine, Michigan, and North Carolina), although some states follow the California approach and have the air agency adopt its own regulations (e.g., Colorado). Others have a unique approach—in South Dakota, for example, a citizens board appointed by the Governor adopts air quality regulations.

49. Many states use the national ambient air quality standards (e.g., Texas, Oregon, Michigan, South Dakota, and North Carolina). Others adopt different or more stringent state ambient standards for one or more pollutants. Maine, for example, has a state PM standard and an ambient standard for hexavalent chromium; Washington has a short-term SO_2 standard and a state fluoride standard.

50. Most states have regional offices that are not independent of the state air quality agency (e.g., Texas, North Carolina, Oregon, and South Dakota). Others, such as Washington and California, have county or regional districts that operate fairly autonomously. Many states, such as Michigan and Colorado, execute contracts with counties to carry out one or more pollution control activities. Some states, such as California, authorize local governments to go beyond state air pollution requirements.

51. All state air pollution programs are carried out pursuant to state law. The citation to the applicable statute(s) can be obtained by calling the state air pollution control office (see Table 56-4) or by visiting a law library. A state agency official can also indicate where the regulations that implement the statutory provisions are codified. A computer program published by the Bureau for National Affairs also has this information.

52. In states without local districts, the state agency adopts rules and regulations pertaining to air pollution. The rule adoption process may be done by a commission after a public hearing (Oregon, North Carolina, Texas, and Colorado), by a director after public notice and written comment (Washington), by a citizen board appointed by the Governor (South Dakota), or by a hybrid approach. The regulations are always accessible and available to the public.

53. In addition to emission standards, there are rules that may pertain to permit applications, the construction and operation of new sources (called "new source review" rules), variances and abatement orders, source testing and monitoring, obtaining information from sources and providing it to the public, the conduct of public hearings, and other substantive and administrative components of an air pollution control program.

54. The federal EPA publishes information regarding the availability of control technology for both existing and new or modified sources, called "reasonable available control technology" (RACT) and "best available control technology" (BACT), respectively. Although BACT is the presumptive minimum for use to control criteria pollutants in clean areas subject to PSD requirements, a performance standard, called "lowest available emission rate" (LAER), must be used in nonattainment areas. Other minimum technology standards apply to toxics, "maximum available control technology" (MACT), and certain large source categories "new source performance standards" (NSPS). Some states do not go beyond federal minimum standards (e.g., Colorado, South Dakota, North Carolina), whereas others do so frequently (e.g., California, Washington, Texas, Michigan), and others occasionally (e.g., Oregon, Maine).

55. The vast majority of other states do not require separate state plans.

56. In states with centralized air pollution control, the control measures are adopted by a commission, director, or similar body, and are subject to public comment as a matter of due process.

57. Rules incorporated into the SIP become "federally enforceable" by the EPA and by citizens. Many states that adopt rules that go beyond federal requirements do not put them into the SIP, although they apply to sources within the state and are enforceable by the state (and local) agency. Unlike federal law, very few states have a law authorizing citizens to sue sources directly for violations of air pollution requirements (Maine has a civil citizens suit provision).

58. In some cases a particular pollutant or source category is of such local interest that a local government agency will be induced to control emissions to a greater extent than the state or a district, often as a requirement of a conditional use permit, issued pursuant to a local entity's authority to control land use.

59. Although many states require separate permits, or licenses, to construct and to operate (North Carolina, California), a number provide a combined permit (Oregon, Maine, Colorado), and others require only a construction permit (Texas, Michigan) or only an operating permit (South Dakota). Many state permit programs are in transition due to the requirement in Title V of the 1990 Clean Air Act Amendments that all major sources have operating permits. In some states the Title V operating permit program will be entirely new, whereas other states are attempting to graft the Title V program onto their existing permit programs.

60. In centralized state programs, the director or commission of the combined environmental management program may issue permits, or this function may be delegated to the air quality office.

61. Some states solicit public input on all permits (South Dakota, Washington), and others only for permits for sources that emit specified quantities of a pollutant (for example, in Colorado comments are accepted for sources over 25 tons per year). Many states offer a public hearing on permit applications if specified criteria are met (Texas, Oregon), and some states periodically review permits and accept comment on the proposal to renew (Maine).

62. All states respond more or less promptly and more or less thoroughly (often depending upon resources available) to citizen complaints about individual facilities. Most states or districts also inspect major sources at least annually, and others at least every 2 years or more often, depending upon the source's compliance history, available resources, and citizen complaints.

63. Although some states employ in-house attorneys or contract with outside counsel to pursue enforcement litigation, others are required to use the Attorney General's Office for litigation (Michigan, Washington) and in some cases for settlement negotiations as well (Maine). Most cases are settled before they go to court.

64. The California program was initiated in 1983, although the general air quality nuisance law was used in some districts to curb toxic polluters before them. Texas is currently developing its formal toxics program, although for years sources applying for permits were reviewed for toxic emissions through the use of an "effects screening level" and required to control emissions found to "significantly" affect public health. The toxics air program in Maine began in 1992, and many other states are initiating their programs as this text is written (Oregon, Washington for existing sources, Colorado, South Dakota). As with the Title V operating permits program, many states will take their lead from the EPA program, which was greatly expanded by Congress in the 1990 Clean Air Act Amendments.

65. Many states plan to use the EPA approach by applying the federal MACT standard to each new and existing source of hazardous air pollutants as it is promulgated by EPA (Washington, South Dakota, Oregon). Some states, such as Maine and North Carolina, plan to begin with MACT standards but may consider residual risk sooner than required by federal law.

66. There are two distinct stages in toxic substance control. First, during the risk assessment process, scientific methodology is applied to available data and assumptions on the nature and extent of exposure to the substance to determine its potency and the resultant health risk; second, during the risk management phase, policy makers must determine how to manage this risk in consideration of such factors as the types and numbers of sources that emit the substance, the cost and technologic feasibility of controlling emissions, the magnitude of the risk and the number of people exposed, the availability and efficacy of less hazardous substitute compounds, public awareness and interest, industry participation, and other factors both scientific and nonscientific.

67. Michigan, for example, considers residual risk after imposing "toxics best available control technology" (T-BACT). Risk management can be a highly negotiative process, with varying degrees of public participation (Texas, for example, performs a case-by-case analysis of facilities whose residual risk is above the level determined to be significant to reach agreement with the source on the degree of emission control that is feasible).

68. Several other states may go beyond the federal MACT standards, but generally considerable administrative effort must be expended to demonstrate the necessity for greater stringency (e.g., Colorado, Michigan).

69. A number of states have also been using this approach (e.g., Texas, North Carolina, Washington).

70. MACTs have been promulgated to reduce emissions of perchloroethylene from dry cleaners, for example, to regulate emissions of hazardous organic compounds by the synthetic organic chemical manufacturing industry, and to control emissions of HAPs from coke ovens. Some source categories to which MACTs will apply emit more than one

toxic pollutant, and for some of the HAPs, separate MACTs will be proposed for different source categories. It is a long complex regulatory process, and extensive comment is usually received from the industry about to be regulated.

71. Colorado, for example, requires companies to report specified toxic substance emissions of greater than 50 pounds per year. Most states have no "right to know" reporting requirements of their own but rely on the provisions of the federal SARA Title III to inform the public of toxic emissions.

72. Texas has a nuisance law for odor and dust, Oregon for backyard burning, Maine for PM, Colorado for odor and dust, and North Carolina for odor. The California statute is very general and has been used to require permit applicants to perform risk assessments and to impose emission limitations on toxic air contaminants in individual permits, as well as to curb odor and dust problems. In Washington, the nuisance law is used by the state air agency to impose case-by-case technology requirements on existing sources.

73. States that are attaining all of the federal standards, such as South Dakota, have little need for additional regulation beyond that necessary to maintain the NAAQS, whereas others, like California, must go beyond the realm of what is currently technologically feasible (i.e., "technology forcing") if extremely polluted areas are ever to attain.

74. Thus, in addition to encouraging, coordinating, and reviewing the efforts of all levels of government as they affect air quality, the state agency may undertake control activities in any area where the local agencies are failing to carry out their responsibilities to develop, implement, or enforce adequate control programs. This is rarely done, though occasionally threatened, and must be preceded with notice and public hearings where witnesses may question the staff of the state agency and where detailed findings and response to comments must be prepared.

Chapter 57

HAZARD AND RISK COMMUNICATION AND PUBLIC POLICY

Eddy A. Bresnitz
Kathleen M. Rest
Harriet L. Rubenstein

EMERGING IMPORTANCE OF HAZARD AND RISK COMMUNICATION

The public is increasingly concerned about the potential adverse health effects of toxic agents in the environment.[1,2] They encounter potential health hazards in their communities, schools, homes, and workplaces, as well as in the food they eat, the air they breathe, and the products they use. As concerned citizens become aware of or experience health effects attributed to hazardous occupational and environmental agents, their interest in information about exposure sources and routes, acute and chronic health effects, and remediation, prevention, and control strategies increases.[3]

Hazard and risk communication roles have been assumed by or delegated to a variety of different actors. In addition to their traditional public education activities, federal, state, and local governments frequently are involved in hazard and risk communication activities, often in the context of specific disease clusters, exposure situations, or community concerns.[4,5] Chemical manufacturers are required to compile material safety data sheets (MSDS) and make them available to users. Employers are required to provide "Hazcom" education and training to their workers exposed to hazardous substances. Unions, environmental groups, and public interest organizations often conduct organizing campaigns and educational programs to provide information and action strategies to workers and citizens. And increasingly, concerned citizens seek information and advice from physicians and other health care providers.[6]

There are important reasons for growing physician involvement in hazard and risk communication activities. First, physicians are credible and trusted sources of information about health risk.[7] With the steady erosion of public trust in government and industry experts, physicians and other health professionals—along with environmental groups—continue to enjoy the trust and confidence of the public. Second, physicians have easy access to information about toxic substances and their health effects, even when such information is protected by the mantle of trade secrecy. Third, physicians have ample opportunity to engage in dialogue with individual patients, their families, and other groups. And finally, physicians have experience in educating and counseling patients about risk, disease, behavior, and prevention.

The importance of hazard and risk communication in the national health strategy is underscored by the inclusion of several related health promotion and disease prevention objectives in the Healthy People 2000 report of the U.S. Public Health Service.[8] This report is intended to serve as a guidepost for health providers and private and public health agencies to reduce the nation's burden of morbidity and mortality through the development of health promotion and disease prevention programs. The underlying tasks to achieve many of these objectives include hazard and risk communication.

REGULATORY BASIS FOR HAZARD AND RISK COMMUNICATION

The need and demand for knowledge about hazards and risks by the public have been generated, in part, by the passage of federal, state, and local laws and regulations to transfer information about hazardous exposures and their potential effects in the workplace and community. Prior to the promulgation of the Hazard Communication Standard (29 U.S. Code of Federal Regulations [CFR] 1910.1200) (also called the "right to know" law) by the U.S. Occupational Safety and Health Administration (OSHA) in 1983, many states and localities already had their own right-to-know laws that were broad in mandating hazard and risk communication within both the manufacturing and nonmanufacturing sectors and the community.[9] However, these local and state laws were preempted by the federal standard that, after its extension in 1987, require all employers to educate their employees about chemical hazards in their workplace. Employers must develop a written communication plan that outlines how they will comply with the standard's requirements on hazard labeling, provision of MSDS, and worker training programs. An important provision of the standard is the ability of physicians to obtain information on chemical hazards from the manufacturer in cases when the information is needed to care for the patient.

The major impetus for providing community residents with similar information about the storage, use, and release of toxic substances in their area was the passage of the Superfund Amendments and Reauthorization Act (SARA) of 1986.[10] Title III of SARA, known as the Emergency Planning and Community Right-to-Know Act, has many provisions that make such information available to communities and their emergency response organizations. Title III's Section 304 on emergency notification, Sections 311-312 on chemical inventories and community right-to-know reporting, and Section 313 on toxic chemical release reporting are all designed to facilitate the public's awareness of hazardous substances in their communities as well as their associated health effects.[10]

ELEMENTS OF HAZARD AND RISK COMMUNICATION

Although risk and hazard communication share common approaches and purposes, they are not precisely the same. The National Research Council defines a hazard as "an act or phenomenon posing potential harm to some person or thing."[11] Risk is the quantification of a hazard in terms of the probability that the harm will occur. Both hazard and risk communication cover a variety of parameters. Hazard information covers such factors as the agent's physical properties (e.g., flammability, volatility), routes of exposure, toxicity, first aid measures, acute and chronic health effects, exposure limits, handling and storage, and recommendations for prevention and control of exposure. Risk communication, on the other hand, adds notions of probability to the transfer of information about the nature, magnitude, significance, acceptability, and control of a hazard—in this case, the risk of an adverse health effect caused by exposure to an environmental agent.[6,12]

These different parameters begin to suggest some of the difficulties in both hazard and risk communication. In addition to the technical language, statistical and probabilistic concepts, and uncertainty that pervade attempts to communicate information about hazard and risk, there may be significant differences in values, perceptions, and expectations among those involved in the communication process.

A key feature of both hazard and risk communication derives from the word "communication" itself. Early risk communication activities were conceived as the unidirectional conveyance of technical information and expert opinion about health risk to a public often characterized as irrational and uninformed. The public often perceived this as a "public reassurance" campaign in which experts attempt to decrease or deflect community concern.[13] More recent conceptions emphasize the symmetrical nature of effective communication—i.e., communication as an exchange of information, which necessarily includes both listening and responding[11]—and place risk communication in a social and cultural context in which explicit goals or purposes of the communication may be varied and ill-defined.[14] The public is a diverse entity whose segments have different needs, perceptions, and channels for risk information.

Within this context, risk perception is a critical factor. It has been noted that expert and public opinion about the nature and magnitude of risk often vary.[5] Although this divergence has been cited as evidence of the public's tendency to distort risk information, it is more instructive to consider the nonstatistical (but not irrational) factors that are part of the public's (and experts') understanding of risk.[15,16] These factors, shown in Table 57-1, modify risk perception and have been described as characterizing the "outrage" dimension of risk. These factors—addressing issues of voluntariness, controllability, familiarity,

Table 57-1. Factors important in risk perception and evaluation

Factor	Conditions associated with increased public concern	Conditions associated with decreased public concern
Catastrophic potential	Facilities and injuries grouped in time and space	Facilities and injuries scattered and random
Familiarity	Unfamiliar	Familiar
Understanding	Mechanisms or process not understood	Mechanisms or process understood
Uncertainty	Risk scientifically unknown or uncertain	Risk known to science
Controllability (personal)	Uncontrollable	Controllable
Voluntariness of exposure	Involuntary	Voluntary
Effects on children	Children specifically at risk	Children not specifically at risk
Effects on future generations	Risk to future generations	No risk to future generations
Effects manifestation	Delayed effects	Immediate effects
Effects on future generations	Risk to future generations	No risk to future generations
Victim identity	Identifiable victims	Statistical victims
Dread	Effects dreaded	Effects not dreaded
Trust in institutions	Lack of trust in responsible institutions	Trust in responsible institutions
Media attention	Much media attention	Little media attention
Accident history	Major and sometimes minor accidents	No major or minor accidents
Equity	Inequitable distribution of risks and benefits	Equitable distribution of risks and benefits
Benefits	Unclear benefits	Clear benefits
Reversibility	Effects irreversible	Effects reversible
Origin	Caused by human actions or failures	Caused by acts of nature or God

Source: Covello VT, Sandman PM, and Slovic P: *Risk communication, risk statistics, and risk comparisons: a manual for plant managers,* p. 54, Washington, D.C., 1988, Chemical Manufacturers Association. With permission.

fairness, and alternatives—influence acceptability of risk and must be appreciated by those engaged in the risk communication process, be it in the physician's office or in a public forum.

TOWARD EFFECTIVE HAZARD AND RISK COMMUNICATION

It is important to understand the theoretical and philosophic basis of hazard and risk communication activities and requirements in order to design and conduct effective communication programs. Underpinning federal and state requirements to transfer information about hazardous substances is the assumption that people need and are entitled to knowledge about the hazards they face at work and in their other environments to make informed decisions and take appropriate action to protect themselves from the potential adverse effects of these hazards.[17] On the individual level, patients approach health care providers with questions and concerns about environmental risk for similar reasons—they seek understanding so they can make decisions about the need for treatment and the steps they can take to prevent, mitigate, or address potential or actual threats to their health. Thus conceived, effective communication embodies two essential elements—information and opportunities for action. Those engaged in hazard and risk communication activities must address both.

Although the above discussion has highlighted theoretic and conceptual issues relating to risk and risk communication, they suggest very practical guidelines for communicating with patients and members of the public about environmental risks.[18] These can be summarized as follows:

- Be sensitive to the nonstatistical or "outrage" factors that influence the patients' concerns, perceptions, and expectations.
- Appreciate and nurture the trust that patients have in their health care providers; do not dismiss their concerns. If trust is lost, it is almost impossible to regain.
- Speak plainly; as in all other forms of patient–provider communication, avoid technical terms and jargon.
- Do not make assumptions about what the patient knows, thinks, or wants done about the hazard or risk. Take time to identify *all* the patients' concerns.
- Be aware of and take steps to address language barriers or other cross-cultural factors that may influence expectations and/or hamper the patient's understanding or ability to take follow-up action.
- Acknowledge uncertainty, whether it reflects your own or the status of current scientific knowledge.
- Use risk comparisons very cautiously. You will not engender trust by comparing the environmental risk with lifestyle risks (e.g., by comparing the risks of breathing industrial pollutants with smoking). The latter is, in large measure, a voluntary risk.
- Identify opportunities for the patient to assert some control over or take some action regarding the issue of concern. This may be as simple as encouraging

and supporting the patient to follow-up for additional help or information or providing the patient with names and telephone numbers of relevant government or community resources. Other pieces of advice may also help the patient assume some measure of control (e.g., guidance on how to reduce exposure until the problem is resolved, such as by using bottled water).

- Read the papers, listen to news reports, and listen to patients, colleagues, friends, and family. The media, friends, and family are among the most frequent sources of people's information about environmental risk. It will help to be prepared for the kinds of questions that patients will bring to their health care providers.

OPPORTUNITIES FOR HAZARD AND RISK COMMUNICATION

With an increasing demand from a public thirsty for knowledge on how to reduce disease risk, the health practitioner must seize all available opportunities to provide information on occupational and environmental hazards and risks. The potential settings are diverse and include occupational medical screening and surveillance programs, community meetings, and the evaluation of individual patients.

Medical screening programs

Medical screening in the workplace refers to the cross-sectional testing of a population of workers for evidence of excessive exposure or early stages of disease that may or may not be related to work and that may or may not influence the ability to tolerate or perform work. For example, over the past decade, screening of cohorts of asbestos-exposed workers has provided many opportunities for group education on the risks of asbestos-related diseases and how to reduce those risks.[19,20] The educational sessions often include the presentation of a brief videotape, the distribution of literature on asbestos-related diseases, and information on the risks of smoking and its interaction with asbestos. A facilitator or educator then heads a discussion on the material presented and responds to questions and concerns about asbestos.

The major strength of this approach is the opportunity it provides for open expression and discussion by workers of their concerns about their health, and about possible strategies for preventing or controlling further exposures to reduce health risks. The session may serve as the first step on the road to abstinence among those workers who smoke. The concept of interaction between an occupational hazard (asbestos) and a personal risk factor (smoking) can be explored and information given on how the reduction of overall disease risk may be accomplished by modification of an important risk factor that may be of less concern to the worker.

Medical surveillance programs

Medical surveillance in the workplace refers to the longitudinal evaluation, by means of periodic examinations, of high risk individuals or potentially exposed workers in order to detect early pathophysiologic changes indicative of significant exposure. Surveillance programs may be voluntary or mandated by specific regulations, and may have a specific educational component. For example, under the Comprehensive Environmental Response, Compensation, and Liability Act (CERCLA) of 1980,[21] employers of hazardous waste workers are required to develop and implement a safety and health program for their employees involved in hazardous waste operations. Two key elements of this program are worker training and medical surveillance. Training requirements include the provision of information on safety, health, and other hazards present at a work site, including health effects, appropriate work practices, and use of personal protective equipment. Workers must receive a minimum of 40 hours of instruction off-site and then 3 days of field training. A baseline medical examination must be done and repeated annually and again upon termination of employment.

Although education about job site hazards takes place during the training program, the health provider has an opportunity to reinforce workplace risk reduction practices during the medical examination. For example, despite the chemical hazards encountered on a hazardous waste site, other hazards such as heat exposure, contact with poisonous plants, and insect bites and stings also pose significant risks, for example, heat stress, contact dermatitis, and Lyme disease, respectively. The physician can review the worker's knowledge of these risks during the examination, clarify any misconceptions, reinforce protective steps the worker can take to reduce exposures, and provide additional written literature at the end of the patient encounter. In this setting, the health provider often reinforces the information on hazards and risks previously provided in a group setting.

Community settings

Physicians are frequently called upon to address community groups on the potential health risks of exposures from hazardous waste sites, incinerators, burning landfills, and other sources of exposure to toxic agents. The circumstances vary and may occur during the process of siting a hazardous facility, after discovery of a toxic dump site, during a crisis situation, and following the release of a study of a toxic site by a government agency. Adherence to many of the principles outlined earlier in this chapter are essential when addressing public concerns and providing information to a large group of individuals about potential hazards and risks.

At times, one or more individuals in the group may appear to be hostile, unreasonable, or unwilling to hear the message on what is known about actual risks. It is crucial in these situations to appreciate the source of these emotions: fear, uncertainty, anger with the perpetrators, unfamiliarity with technical language, and mistrust of authorities. Ideally, the physician should be viewed as an independent expert and resource and not as the representative of the agency responsible for studying, remediating, or proposing the hazardous site. Some states have approached these sensitive situations by empaneling a group of experts consisting of individuals chosen by both the responsible government agency and the community at risk. New Jersey's Department of Health has taken this approach recently in the case of a burning landfill and a Superfund site.[22,23]

Evaluation of the individual patient

Physicians and other health providers frequently encounter patients who are concerned about the hazards and risks of an exposure situation in the workplace or environment. The key to effective hazard and risk assessment and communication is to take a comprehensive exposure history[24-28] (see Chapter 3). Exposure history forms are helpful in determining current and past exposures that may pose health risks to the patient's current or future health.[24] In addition to influencing diagnostic and treatment decisions the exposure history should be utilized to counsel the patient on appropriate measures for reducing their risk of disease.

The prevention of respiratory disease is based on the timing, focus, and modality of intervention of risk reducing measures.[29] The timing of a preventive intervention may be primary (before disease onset), secondary (in an asymptomatic state of disease), or tertiary (after clinical disease has developed). The focus of an intervention may be environmental (engineering controls), targeted at groups (screening programs), or targeted at the individual (case finding). The intervention may be administrative (regulatory policy or mandated actions), information-based (education of individuals), or behavior-based (directed at the patient).

A risk reduction program in the workplace should be comprehensive and involve the health provider, employer, and patient/worker. An important element of effective risk reduction is hazard and risk communication. Table 57-2 is an example of a prevention matrix for a cohort of sandblasters, some of whom have evidence of obstructive airway impairment caused by smoking.[30] The matrix highlights several opportunities for physician–patient communication in both the clinical and work settings.

HAZARD AND RISK COMMUNICATION RESOURCES*

Physicians and other health care professionals require information on hazards and risks in most of the settings outlined in the previous section. Written materials in the form of textbooks, journal articles, treatment manuals, and protocols are the most familiar and easily used resources available to health professionals.

Clinicians also require information on the process of risk communication, including how to design, implement, and evaluate education programs for groups of workers or community members that will promote action in response to information. Working with low-literacy or non-English-speaking participants can also present special challenges. Most physicians lack training or experience in participatory adult education. Resources are available to assist clinicians with these efforts.[31]

Print resources

The box lists books and other resources that offer practitioners information on various substances. These resources provide concise information on toxicology, acute and chronic health effects, diagnosis, and treatment. The books can also assist in establishing screening and surveillance programs, and provide information on groups at risk, product uses, and sources of further information. The use of printed or computerized information resources depends on the proper identification of the substance in question. The practitioner should take a logical approach to seeking information about hazardous substances. First, the substance must be identified by its generic name. To do this, the practitioner can begin by reviewing the MSDS if available or by contacting poison control centers, employers, manufacturers, unions, and government agencies. The practitioner must be sure to obtain the patient's consent before contacting the employer or the union. Once the generic name is known, the physician can research the toxicologic characteristics of the substance using resources shown in the box.

Material safety data sheets

The OSHAct requires chemical manufacturers to create MSDS for each chemical they produce, and employers who use these chemicals must retain these MSDS in the workplace.[32] Required information includes chemical and common names, physical, safety, and health hazard data, exposure limits, precautions for safe handling and use, generally applicable control measures, and emergency and first aid procedures[33] (Fig. 57-1). Individual employers are required to provide employees with information on the chemical agents used in their own workplaces. With the patient's permission, a call to the plant manager, foreman, or safety officer may be all that is necessary to determine the name of the substance in question. The OSHA medical access rule (29 CFR Sec. 1910.20) also required employers to provide employees with information on exposure levels in the patient's work environment, where these measurements have been made.

Material safety data sheets vary in their quality: some are excellent and others are incomplete and inadequate.[33]

---

*Adapted and modified from Bresnitz EA, Rubenstein H, and Rest KM: Recognition and follow-up of workplace poisonings. In Goldfrank LR, Florenbaum NE, Lewin NA, et al, editors: *Goldfrank's Toxicologic Emergencies,* pp 1153-1167, Norwalk, CT, 1994, Appleton & Lange. With permission.

Table 57-2. Prevention matrix for a cohort of sandblasters

Focus	Primary intervention	Secondary intervention	Tertiary intervention
Environmental			
Administrative	Test for and maintain below OSHA permissible exposure level for silica	Reevaluate engineering after elevated silica levels detected	Reevaluate engineering controls after silicosis case detected
Information-based	Provide material safety data sheet for workers	Post periodic information on environmental silica levels	Post new work practice guidelines
Directed at patient	Provide exhaust ventilation; HEPA filters	Make engineering changes after elevated silica levels detected	Make engineering changes after silicosis case detected
Group			
Administrative	Enforce no-smoking policy at work	**Enact mandated medical surveillance for early silicosis** (OSHA regulations)	Reduce total work hours for each worker
Information-based	**Provide group education on hazards of silica and smoking**	**Teach workers about symptoms of silicosis, tuberculosis, bronchitis**	**Provide educational sessions on reasons for excessive exposure and new cases**
Directed at patient	**Carry out influenza vaccination program**	**Obtain screening chest film, spirometry, PPD test**	Provide educational sessions on need to change work practices
Individual			
Administrative	Provide personal protective equipment; **preplacement screening for respiratory disease**	Remove worker when changes detected on chest film obtained during medical surveillance	**Counsel ill worker about workers' compensation**
Information-based	**Counsel individual on health hazards of silica and smoking;** proper use of personal protective equipment	**Note respiratory symptoms on history**	**Educate worker about silicosis and tuberculosis risks**
Directed at patient	**Provide nicotine substitute or other help in smoking cessation;** test fit of personal protective equipment	**Provide isoniazid prophylaxis for worker with positive PPD test**	Train patient for different job

From Bresnitz EA: Environmental respiratory disease: reducing the risks, *J Respir Dis* 14(11):1261, 1993. Adapted from Harber P: Pulmonary prevention: programmatic characterization, *Occup Med State Art Rev* 6:133-143, 1991. With permission.[29]
OSHA, U.S. Occupational Safety and Health Administration; *HEPA,* high-efficiency particulate air filter; *PPD,* purified protein derivative.
Bold type indicates responsibility of a physician.

Resource books on chemical hazards

Burgess WA: *Recognition of health hazards in industry,* ed 2 New York, 1995, John Wiley.
This book provides excellent descriptions of industrial processes and the general types of exposures you would find. This book should not be used when you already know the chemical name(s).
Clayton GD, and Clayton FE, editors: *Patty's industrial hygiene and toxicology,* ed 5, New York, 1995, John Wiley.
A compendium of three volumes of excellent reference value containing information on occupational health and general toxicologic data.
Gosselin RE, Smith RP, and Hodge HC: *Clinical toxicology of commercial products,* ed 5, Baltimore, 1984, Williams & Wilkins.
This text is useful as a first step for identifying trade name products and their ingredients, the addresses and telephone numbers of companies, and estimates of relative toxicities of various chemicals.

Hamilton A, Hardy HL, and Finkel AJ: *Hamilton and Hardy's industrial toxicology,* ed 4, Boston, 1983, John Wright PSG.
A classic textbook describing occupational diseases secondary to known exposures.
Key MM: *Occupational diseases: a guide to their recognition,* DHEW Pub No (NIOSH) 79-116, Washington, DC, 1977, US Department of Health, Education, and Welfare.
A classic manual helpful in identifying chemicals associated with various occupations and routes of entry (e.g., airway diseases). It is not comprehensive in term of the vast number of chemical substances.
Levy B, and Wegman D, editors: *Occupational health,* ed 3, Boston, 1995, Little, Brown.
An excellent general reference text on occupational health. This is not a compendium of chemical substances, but it does present a good overall approach. Good for more common hazardous substances.

Continued.

Resource books on chemical hazards—cont'd

Lewis RJ: *Hazardous chemicals desk reference,* ed 3, New York, 1993, Van Nostrand Reinhold.

Another compendium of over 20,000 chemicals listing all types of information including specific health hazards, chemical and physical properties, relevant regulations, and more. A good first book to use if you know the specific chemical(s).

Lewis RS, and Sweet D, editors: *Registry of toxic effects of chemical substances 1983-1984: cumulative supplement to the 1981-1982 edition,* 2 vol, Cincinnati, Ohio, 1985, US-GPO (Department of Health and Human Services).

RTECS is a complication that provides brief descriptions of substances for which acute or other toxic effects have been reported in the literature, as well as references to government regulations and standards. Also on-line at National Library of Medicine.

Mackison FW, Stricoff RS, and Partridge LJ Jr, editors: *Occupational health guidelines for chemical hazards,* DHHS Pub No (NIOSH) 81-123, Washington, DC, 1985, Department of Health and Human Services and Department of Labor.

A loose leaf, 3-volume compendium of chemicals describing their properties, health hazard information, recommended medical practices, monitoring and measurement procedures, personal protective equipment, and waste removal and disposal. Although the exposure limits may be out of date for some substances, this is a good resource for identifying the health effects for several hundred chemicals.

Mackison FW, Stricoff RS, and Partridge LJ Jr, editors: *NIOSH pocket guide to chemical hazards,* DHHS (NIOSH) Pub No 90-117, Cincinnati, Ohio, 1990, US Department of Health and Human Services, Public Health Service, Centers for Disease Control, National Institute for Occupational Safety and Health.

"The information is presented in tabular form to provide a quick, convenient source of information on general industrial hygiene and medical monitoring practices. The information in the Pocket Guide includes chemical structures or formulas, identification codes, synonyms, exposure limits, chemical and physical properties, incompatibilities and reactivities, measurement methods, respirator selections, signs and symptoms of exposure, and procedures for emergency treatment."

Plunkett ER: *Occupational diseases: a syllabus of signs and symptoms,* Stamford, Conn, 1977, Barrett Book Co.

This compendium is useful in suggesting potential chemical exposures when your patient has one or more signs or symptoms, and you have no idea what their exposure(s) may be.

Plunkett ER: *Handbook of industrial toxicology,* New York, 1987, Chemical Publishing Company.

This compendium is useful in suggesting potential chemical exposures when your patient has one or more signs or symptoms, and you have no idea what their exposure(s) may be.

Poisindex: Rocky Mountain Poison and Drug Center, Emergency Information Center, and University of Colorado Health Sciences Center.

This is not really a bookshelf resource. It is a microfiche or CD-ROM data bank that is available in most Emergency Departments or poison control centers (PCCs). It contains extensive files listing chemicals and trade names as well as detailed treatment and management protocols.

Proctor NH: *Chemical hazards of the workplace,* ed 3, New York, 1991, Van Nostrand Reinhold.

A handbook that consists mainly of monographs on chemical substances with entries on nomenclature, physical form of substance uses, means of exposure, toxicology, and treatment and medical control. A reasonable book to consult initially.

Rom W, editor: *Environmental and occupational medicine,* ed 2, Boston, 1992, Little, Brown.

An excellent general textbook on occupational medicine. Not comprehensive for many specific chemicals but excellent discussions of pathophysiologic mechanisms.

Rosenstock L, and Cullen MR: *Textbook of Occupational and Environmental Medicine,* Philadelphia, 1994, Saunders.

A comprehensive general reference textbook, with an excellent overall approach.

Sullivan JB, and Krieger GR: *Hazardous materials toxicology: clinical principles in environmental health,* Baltimore, Md, 1992, Williams & Wilkins.

An excellent reference text with sections on (1) basic science and clinical principles of hazardous materials toxicology, (2) organ system toxicity with principles of immediate treatment and evaluation, (3) specific hazardous substances and general industries, and (4) regulatory, health, and safety aspects of hazardous materials.

Wexler P: *Information resources in toxicology,* ed 2, New York, 1988, Elsevier.

This book does not give specific information on exposures. However, it is the best compendium of ALL the information resources available in toxicology, including print, audiovisual, government documents, journals, books, data bases, newsletters, organization, and international resources.

Zenz C, Dickerson B, and Horvath EP, editors: *Occupational medicine,* ed 3, St. Louis, 1994, Mosby.

A major reference book in occupational health. Good for broad and detailed overview of occupational health issues. This is not the first book to use to find out the hazardous effects of a specific substance.

From Ref. 30.

Health providers should not rely on these sheets as the sole source of information on disease risk, especially as they relate to effects of exposure to carcinogens, teratogens, and developmental toxins. Although some information may be easily obtained from large companies, smaller employers may have little written information for the health care provider. Chemical manufacturers generate much scientific and health data in the course of seeking approval from the Environmental Protection Agency (EPA) to manufacture chemical substances and mixtures. In addition, Section 8(c) of the Toxic Substances Control Act (TSCA) (15 United States Code [USC] 2601) requires chemical manufacturers

Material Safety Data Sheet

May be used to comply with
OSHA's Hazard Communication Standard,
29 CFR 1910.1200. Standard must be
consulted for specific requirements.

U.S. Department of Labor

Occupational Safety and Health Administration
(Non-Mandatory Form)
Form Approved
OMB No. 1218-0072

IDENTITY *(As Used on Label and List)* Lead Chromate; Yellow-34	Note: *Blank spaces are not permitted. If any item is not applicable, or no information is available, the space must be marked fo indicate that.*

Section I

Manufacturer's Name
  ABC Chemical Corporation
	Emergency Telephone Number
	  1-800-424-9300 (CHEMTREC)

Address *(Number, Street, City, State, and ZIP Code)*	Telephone Number for Information
	Date Prepared
	Signature of Preparer *(optional)*

Section II – Hazardous Ingredients/Identity Information

Hazardous Components (Specific Chemical Identity; Common Name(s))	OSHA PEL	ACGIH TLV	Other Limits Recommended	% *(optional)*
Lead as Pb	0.05 mg/m³			60
Chromate as Cr O₃	0.1 mg/m³			30

Section III – Physical/Chemical Characteristics

Boiling Point	N/A	Specific Gravity (H₂O – 1)	5.52
Vapor Pressure (mm Hg.)	N/A	Melting Point	1.0
Vapor Density (AIR = 1)	N/A	Evaporation Rate (Butyl Acetate = 1)	N/A
Solubility in Water Slight			
Appearance and Odor Fine yellow powder; Odorless			

Section IV – Fire and Explosion Hazard Data

Flash Point (Method Used) N/A	Flammable Limits	LEL	LEL
Extinguishing Media Water			
Special Fire Fighting Procedures N/A			
Unusual Fire and Explosion Hazards N/A			

(Reproduce locally)

OSHA 174, Sept. 1985

Fig. 57-1. Material safety data sheet for lead chromate. *Continued on page 946.*

Section V – Reactivity Data

Stability	Unstable		Conditions to Avoid
	Stable	X	

Incompatibility *(Materials to Avoid)*

Hazardous Decomposition or Byproducts

Hazardous Polymerization	May Occur		Conditions to Avoid
	Will Not Occur	X	

Section VI – Health Hazard Data

Route(s) of Entry:	Inhalation? Yes	Skin? Yes	Ingestion? Yes

Health Hazards *(Acute and Chronic)*
No immediate harmful effects. Repeated breathing of excessive concentrations can cause minor irritation of skin and mucous membranes.

Carcinogenicity:	NTP? Yes	IARC Monographs? Yes	OSHA Regulated? Yes

Signs and Symptoms of Exposure
Respiratory system irritation, nasal septum perforation, skin ulcer

Medical Conditions
Generally Aggravated by Exposure   Kidney disease

Emergency and First Aid Procedures
Wash thoroughly with soap and water, especially when exposed to open cuts. Consult physician if ingested.

Section VII – Precautions for Safe Handling and Use

Steps to Be Taken in Case Material Is Released or Spilled
Wear appropriate respirator; vacuum into receptacle for disposal. Wash area with water.

Waste Disposal Method
Sanitary landfill in accordance with local, state, and federal regulations.

Precautions to Be Taken in Handling and Storing
Store in dry area; keep containers tightly closed; protect from physical damage; avoid dust.

Other Precautions
Perform periodic blood tests according to OSHA [1910.1025].

Section VIII – Control Measures

Respiratory Protection *(Specify Type)*
NIOSH; supplied air respirator or self-contained breathing apparatus

Ventilation	Local Exhaust Required	Special
	Mechanical *(General)*	Other

Protective Gloves Leather gloves	Eye Protection Safety goggles

Other Protective Clothing or Equipment
Throw away plastic inserts in leather gloves.

Work/Hygienic Practices
Change clothes, wash face and hands before eating.

Fig. 57-1. Continued.

to report records of significant adverse reactions to human health or the environment. In contacting chemical manufacturers, physicians should ask to speak with a toxicologist, chemist, or someone in the products information department.

Poison control centers

Regional poison control centers (PCCs) may provide the quickest access to toxicologic information. These centers can provide assistance even when the exact chemical name is unknown because information on toxic substances and their management may be cross-referenced by trade name and manufacturer. Moreover, the health professionals in these centers are usually adept at suggesting additional resources.[34]

Most PCCs (and some hospital pharmacies) have microfiche listings of poisons that are updated regularly. The best known system is Poisindex® (Micromedex, Inc., Englewood, Col.). Subscribers to this system receive quarterly updates of an alphabetically organized listing of approximately 400,000 industrial and nonindustrial chemicals and compounds. The system includes trade names. The components of each industrial compound are listed along with their concentrations when available; these are cross-referenced to management protocols. The name of the manufacturer is also listed. Poisindex® is also available on a compact digital disc that allows for easier information retrieval and hard copy printout for dissemination to others.

Employers and manufacturers

As discussed earlier, many state and federal laws require employers and manufacturers to generate, retain, and disclose information that may help physicians care for persons with work- or environmentally-related health problems. Scientific information, exposure data, information on health effects, and collected medical data are included in the types of information that must be retained.

The Chemical Transportation Emergency Center (CHEMTREC) is sponsored by the Chemical Manufacturers Association. CHEMTREC's primary responsibility is to provide information to health care practitioners responding to hazardous spills. A health care provider, however, may also obtain information on the risks of commercial products found in his or her patient's workplace.

Unions

Labor unions should not be overlooked as sources of information on toxic exposures. At the local level, union officers, health and safety committee members, and shop stewards may be able to provide material safety data sheets, exposure data, medical and epidemiologic information, and reports of incidents or cases of interest in a particular plant. The health and safety department of the American Federation of Labor and Congress of Industrial

Organizations (AFL-CIO) in Washington, D.C. can provide information on labor's occupational health and safety activities as well as advice on which member unions may be of specific help. At the international level, unions often have well-trained health and safety professionals who may be able to provide or suggest sources of helpful information. In addition, some cities have coalitions of occupational safety and health (COSH) groups that may provide information about other known exposed or affected workers.

Government agencies

Several federal agencies have information services that can assist the practitioner in discovering the potential risks of toxic agents (box). These agencies include the U.S. National Institute for Occupational Safety and Health (NIOSH), the EPA, the National Toxicology Program (NTP), and the Agency for Toxic Substances and Disease Registry (ATSDR).

As part of the process of recommending exposure standards to OSHA, NIOSH develops comprehensive documents that critically evaluate all available scientific data on particular chemicals. These "criteria documents" review the particular chemical's properties, production methods, uses, and workers at risk, as well as studies of exposure effects in humans and animals. Methods of screening, surveillance, and control are also presented. The agency periodically issues technical reports and special occupational hazard reviews of specific occupations. In conjunction with OSHA, NIOSH develops and disseminates health hazard alerts to inform employers, employees, and health professionals of serious health effects of particular chemicals. Through its computerized databank of trade name ingredients gathered from the National Occupational Hazard Survey, NIOSH also provides information by telephone, free-of-charge, when only a trade name is known.

National contacts for information on toxic substances

Agency	Telephone number
Agency for Toxic Substances and Disease Registry, Division of Toxicology	404-639-6300
National Institute for Occupational Safety and Health	513-841-4491 800-35N-IOSH
National Toxicology Program Public Information Office	919-541-3991 919-541-3665
Toxic Substance Control Act Assistance Office	202-554-1404
Chemical Transportation Emergency Center	800-424-9300

The EPA is charged with protecting the nation's land, air, and water. The agency administers a number of laws designed to preserve the public health and environment, including the TSCA. This act authorizes the EPA to collect information on chemical risks from manufacturers and processors. The act requires the agency to review information on new chemicals and new uses of chemicals before they are manufactured. Unless designated a trade secret, this information is subject to disclosure and is, therefore, available. The TSCA Assistance Office may be most useful when resource materials listed in the box (Resource Books) and government documents contain no information about the chemicals or processes in question.

The NTP is a federal program established in 1978 to develop scientific information on exposure to toxic chemicals. The Public Information Office will respond to requests for information on specific chemicals.

The ATSDR is part of the Public Health Service. It was created by Congress to implement the health-related sections of laws that protect the public from hazardous wastes and environmental spills of hazardous substances. In 1986, the Superfund Amendments and Reauthorization Act made amendments to the initial enabling legislation of 1980 and broadened ATSDR's responsibilities in the areas of health assessment, toxicologic data bases, information dissemination, and medical education.[10] One of its offices, the Office of Health Assessment, provides the emergency response for toxic and environmental disasters, gives health consultations in public health emergencies, makes health assessments of hazardous waste sites, provides technical assistance to agencies and organizations, and estimates health risks to humans from exposure to hazardous substances. The Division of Toxicology can provide information on chemical hazards and their potential risks.

Telecommunications and online data bases

Often, print material is adequate to determine the adverse health effects of chemical exposures. Yet, some of the resources described in the preceding sections may be unavailable to physicians, and textbook publication usually lags 2 years or more behind new information. As a result, up-to-date findings and reports may be missed if the practitioner relies solely on printed material in books or government documents.

Table 57-3 shows the computerized data bases most likely to provide useful information to practitioners interested in all aspects of toxic exposures. Unfortunately, not all of these data bases are readily available to the practitioner, and different on-line data base vendors may not provide all of the data bases listed. As a result, comprehensive access requires having an account with several vendors, a potentially expensive proposition.

In summary, health practitioners needing information on hazards and their health risks have a broad-spectrum of resources to consult. Despite their availability, physicians and health practitioners may not have the knowledge and skills required to appropriately access and utilize this information.[35]

POLICY IMPLICATIONS OF HAZARD AND RISK COMMUNICATION

Delineating the physician's role in communicating with individual patients and the public about environmental health risks underscores deficiencies in the teaching of both environmental medicine and physician–patient communication at all levels of medical education. Effective environmental risk communication requires that clinicians acquire knowledge, skills, and attitudes, many of which are traditionally overlooked in undergraduate and graduate medical education curricula and continuing medical education programs.[27,36] Specifically, physicians need to be able to understand the complex relationships between environment and health. Students, residents, and practitioners need training in toxicology and epidemiology as they relate to exposures to chemical and physical agents in the environment. They need to be able to understand and explain concepts of "risk" and "risk assessment."

Since a key element in fostering and practicing preventive medicine is risk communication in the broadest sense, increasing emphasis of national health plans on preventive services may, indirectly, motivate medical and nursing schools to improve their teaching programs for current and future health providers in this area, providing them with the knowledge and skills needed to effectively communicate with their patients and the public about chemical hazards and their potential health risks.

The paucity of toxicologic and epidemiologic data for most environmental agents means that medical education must develop the physician's ability to cope with scientific uncertainty, to make decisions with limited data, and to help patients and the public to do so as well. Furthermore, to assist individual patients and communities in understanding and responding to environmental risks, clinicians need to know how to elicit and accommodate health-related beliefs, values, and preferences different from their own. Finally, because so much of environmental risk communication occurs in a politically and emotionally charged atmosphere, medical education should also prepare physicians to work effectively under these conditions.

Enhancing physicians' ability to communicate about environmental risks is only one aspect of the larger mandate to graduate physicians who are competent to address environmental health issues in the context of both personal and public health services delivery. The Institute of Medicine of the National Academy of Sciences has begun the process of curriculum development in environmental medicine and has articulated specific competencies in this area for medical school graduates.[27] Implementation of strategies to teach these competencies will go a long way toward creat-

Table 57-3. Data bases with information on industrial toxic exposures

Data base	Producer	Description
CA Search	CA Service	Chemical reference
Chemical Carcinogenesis Research Information System	NIH National Cancer Institute	Records of bibliographic references/data on test conditions and results of cocarcinogenicity, mutagenicity
Chemical Exposure	Science Applications Internat. Corp. Health/Environmental Information	Citations to chemicals that have been identified in human biologic media
Chemtox Online	Resource Consultants, Inc.	Integrates toxicologic and regulatory information on more than 6,400 chemicals
Chemical Regulations and Guidelines System (CRGS)	CRC Systems, Inc.	U.S. regulations on chemical substances
Chemical Safety Newsbase	Royal Society of Chemistry	Information on hazardous effects of chemicals and processes in industry and laboratories
Clinical Toxicology of Commercial Products (CTCP)	Dartmouth Medical School, University of Rochester	Corresponds to Gosselin's *Clinical toxicology of commercial products*
Dermal Absorpt Data Base	Office of Pesticides and Toxic Substances (EPA)	Information on health effects related to approximately 655 chemical substances entering via a dermal route
EMBASE	Elsevier Science Publisher	Biomedical literature related to human medicine
Environmental Bibliography	Environmental Studies Institute	Environmental hazards (including health hazards)
Hazardline	Occupational Health Services, Inc.	Data on over 78,000 hazardous chemicals
Hazardous Substances Data Bank	NLM—Toxicology Info Program	Data on over 4,100 known toxic substances
HEALSAFE	Cambridge Scientific Abstracts	Worldwide literature relating to public health, safety, and industrial hygiene
Laboratory Hazards Bulletin	Royal Society of Chemistry	Over 5,000 citations on hazards encountered in chemistry lab
Medical Science Research	Elsevier Applied Science Publishers Ltd.	Full text research papers in field of medicine
MEDLINE[R]	NLM	Worldwide biomedical literature
MSDS-CCOHS	Canadian Centre for Occupational Health and Safety	Material safety data sheets in the workplace
NIOSHTIC[R]	NIOSH	Over 138,000 citations since 1973 on all aspects of OS&H
NTIS	National Technical Info Service	Technical reports in biologic and other sciences
Occupational Safety & Health Reporter (OS&H)	Bureau of National Affairs, Inc.	Full text of OS&H Reporter—recent developments in OS&H
Registry of Toxic Effects of Chemical Substances (RTECS)	NIOSH	Toxicologic evaluation of chemical substances
SCI Search	Institute for Scientific Information	Wide range of scientific technologic disciplines (corresponds to coverage in Science Citation Index and Current Contents)
TOXLINE[R]	NLM Toxicology Info Programs	15 discrete files relating to all areas of toxicology
TSCA Chemical Substances Inventory	DIALOG and EPA	Dictionary listing of all chemical substances in commercial use in the U.S. since 1979

Adapted and reproduced with permission, from Bresnitz E. Clinical Industrial Toxicology. *Ann Intern Med.* 1985; 103:967-972.
EPA, Environmental Protection Agency; *NIOSH,* National Institute for Occupational Safety and Health; *NIH,* National Institutes of Health; *NLM,* National Library of Medicine.[41]

ing effective environmental risk communicators among medical school graduates.[37]

At the same time, the medical literature increasingly calls attention to the need to improve the communication skills of graduating and practicing physicians, and efforts to improve these skills are underway at all three levels of medical education.[38,39] The serious lack of information and training available to physicians on the general topic of health risk communication will hopefully be addressed by these efforts, and will enhance the clinician's ability to communicate about environmental health risks.

Practicing physicians also need timely updates on environmental exposures of sudden concern to the public. Federal agencies and state or local health departments need to develop mechanisms for rapidly disseminating reliable information to clinicians on the nature and extent of emergent hazards and possible measures for limiting exposure or adverse effects.

Although individuals can take steps to limit their exposure to many environmental risks, such as radon or those relating to the use of consumer products, reducing exposure to workplace or community hazards is generally far more difficult. Although right-to-know laws have fueled much of the public's interest in and concern about workplace and community environmental risks, these laws have not given either workers or community members the right to *act* upon that information to prevent or reduce their hazardous exposures. In some instances, unions and community activists have won the right to inspect workplaces for hazards and to make recommendations to management for their elimination or control. Efforts to secure the "right to act" are a logical follow-up to the right to know.[40] Beyond communicating with their patients and the public about specific risks, physicians can also lend their expertise to these risk reduction activities and, at a minimum, can direct their patients to appropriate organizations.

REFERENCES

1. Baxter RH: Some public attitudes about health and the environment, *Environ Health Perspect* 86:261-269, 1990.
2. Roper Organization, Inc: *The environment: public attitudes and individual behavior,* Report Commissioned by S.C. Johnson and Son, New York, 1990, The Roper Organization.
3. Hadden SG: *A citizen's right to know—risk communication and public policy,* Boulder, 1989, Westview Press.
4. Cardinal EA: Risky business-communicating risk for the government, *Environ Sci Technol* 25:1982-1983, 1991.
5. Chess C, Hance BJ, and Sandman PM: *Improving dialogue with communities: a short guide for government risk communication,* Trenton, NJ, 1988, Division of Science and Research, New Jersey Department of Environmental Protection.
6. Covello VT: Risk communication and occupational medicine, *J Occup Med* 35(1):16-19, 1993.
7. McCallum DB, Hammond SL, and Covello VT: Communicating about environmental risks: how the public uses and perceives information sources, *Health Educ Q* 18(3):349-361, 1991.
8. U.S. Department of Health and Human Services, Public Health Service: *Healthy people 2000: national health promotion and disease pre-*
vention objectives, DHHS Pub No (PHS)91-50212, Washington, DC, 1990, US Department of Health and Human Services.
9. Baram MS: The right to know and the duty to disclose hazard information, *AJPH* 74:385-390, 1984.
10. Superfund Amendments and Reauthorization Act (SARA) (42 U.S.C. Sec. 11001, et seq.).
11. National Research Council: *Improving risk communication,* Washington, DC, 1989, National Academy Press.
12. Covello VT, von Winterfeldt D, and Slovic P: Communicating risk information to the public, In Davies JC, Covello VT, and Allen F, editors: *Risk communication,* pp 109-134, Washington, DC, 1987, The Conservation Foundation.
13. Ozonoff D and Boden LI: Truth and consequences: health agency responses to environmental health problems, *Sci Technol Human Values* 12:70-77, 1987.
14. Krimsky S and Plough A: *Environmental hazards — communicating risks as a social process,* Dover, 1988, Auburn House Publishing Company.
15. Covello VT, Sandman PM, and Slovic P: *Risk communication, risk statistics, and risk comparisons: a manual for plant managers,* Washington, DC, 1988, Chemical Manufacturers Association.
16. Slovic P, Fischoff B, and Lichtenstein S: Facts and fears: understanding perceived risk. In Schwing RC, and Alberts WA, editors: *Societal risk assessment: how safe is safe enough?* New York, 1980, Plenum.
17. Ashford NA and Caldart CC: The right to know: toxics information transfer in the workplace, *Annu Rev Public Health* 6:383-401, 1985.
18. McNeil C, Arkin E, and McCallum D: *Toxic and hazardous substances, title III, and communities: an outreach manual for community groups,* Washington, DC, 1989, Environmental Protection Agency.
19. Bresnitz EA, Gilman MJ, Gracely E, et al: Asbestos-related radiographic abnormalities in elevator construction workers, *Am Rev Respir Dis* 147:1341-1344, 1993.
20. Tillet S and Sullivan P: Asbestos screening and education programs for building and construction trade unions, *Am J Med* 23:143-152, 1993.
21. Comprehensive Environmental Response, Compensation, and Liability Act (CERCLA), PL 96-510.
22. New Jersey Department of Health, Division of Occupational and Environmental Health: *A report on the health study of residents living near the Lipari landfill,* 1989.
23. New Jersey Department of Health, Division of Occupational and Environmental Health: *Report of the Health Effects Advisory Committee. PJP landfill,* 1987.
24. Agency for Toxic Substances and Disease Registry: *Case studies in environmental medicine: taking an exposure history,* Washington DC, 1992, US Department of Health and Human Services. Public Health Service.
25. American Lung Association of San Diego and Imperial Counties: Taking the occupational history, *Ann Intern Med* 99:641-651, 1983.
26. Goldman RH and Peters JM: The occupational and environmental health history, *JAMA* 246:2831-2836, 1981.
27. Institute of Medicine: *Environmental medicine and the medical school curriculum,* Washington, DC, 1993, National Academy Press.
28. Rest KM, Hake JC, and Cordes DH: *The occupational and environmental history,* Tucson, 1983, Center for Occupational Safety and Health.
29. Harber P: Pulmonary prevention: programmatic characterization, *Occup Med State Art Rev* 6:133-143, 1991.
30. Bresnitz EA: Environmental respiratory disease: reducing the risks, *J Respir Dis* 14(11):1261-1278, 1993.
31. Wallerstein N and Rubenstein HL: *Teaching about job hazards: a guide for workers and their health providers,* Washington, DC, 1993, American Public Health Association.
32. Occupational Safety and Health Act: Public Law 91-596. 19 U.S.C. Sec. 651 et seq.

33. Himmelstein JS and Frumkin H: The right to know about toxic exposures. Implications for physicians, *N Engl J Med* 312:687-690, 1985.

34. Litovitz L, Oderda G, White JD, and Sheridan MJ: Occupational and environmental exposures reported to poison centers, *Am J Public Health* 83(5):739-743, 1993.

35. Institute of Medicine: *Meeting physicians' needs for medical information on occupations and environments,* Washington, DC, 1990, National Academy Press.

36. Burstein JM and Levy BS: The teaching of occupational health in U.S. medical schools: little improvement in 9 years, *Am J Public Health* 84:846-849, 1994.

37. Institute of Medicine: Environmental medicine: integrating a missing element into medical education, Washington, DC, 1995, National Academy Press.

38. Levinson W and Roter D: The effects of two continuing medical education programs on communication skills of practicing primary care physicians, *J Gen Int Med* 8:318-324, 1993.

39. Novack DH, Volk G, Drossman DA, and Lipkin Jr M: Medical interviewing and medical skills teaching in U.S. medical schools, *JAMA* 269:2102-2105, 1993.

40. Lewis SJ: Community safety inspection and audit programs and policies, *New Solutions* 4(1):81-93, 1993.

41. Bresnitz EA, Rubenstein H, and Rest KM: Recognition and follow-up of workplace poisonings. In Goldfrank LR, Florenbaum NE, Lewin NA, et al, editors: *Goldfrank's Toxicologic Emergencies,* pp 1153-1167, Norwalk, CT, 1994, Appleton & Lange.

Chapter 58

OCCUPATIONAL LUNG DISEASE—POLICY IMPLICATIONS

International Issues

Q.T. Pham
Nicole Massin
Neil Walton White
Fran DuMelle
Don Enarson

The global economy is becoming increasingly integrated, with the result that national boundaries are more and more irrelevant to the production, marketing, and consumption of goods. The mobility of producers has been consequently increased by the increased efficiency and reduced hardware needs of production processes. The development of powerful regional trading blocs promotes this mobility within a wider range than national boundaries and is now making regulation and control of processes antiquated. The implications of these changes for occupational health are obvious, and some dramatic disasters, such as the industrial accident in Bhopal, India, illustrate the cost of ignoring such issues.

The formulation of policies to deal with occupational health will need to take note of these changes. The development of international consensus in terms of regulation, compensation, and disability evaluation, the process of enforcement of regulations and guidelines, and the provision of occupational health services will need careful thought. The increasing mobility of production is being met with an increasing atomization of national political jurisdictions and a trend to decentralization of administration, whereas the mechanism for consensus on issues in occupational health lags behind. Moreover, the infrastructure to deal with such issues is woefully inadequate in many jurisdictions. Some simple examples are Peru with a population over 20 million, 20,000 physicians but only 20 occupational health physicians, or Mozambique, with a population greater than 15 million but where the total number of Mozambican physicians is less than 200.

Although most industrial production takes place in the market economies and the former socialist states, an important and growing segment is occurring in developing countries. By 1982, one-sixth of world manufacturing output was coming from developing countries.[1] Moreover, although industrial growth had stagnated or declined in the market economies, falling from 5.1% to 1.8% over the previous two decades, industrial growth continued to rise in low income countries of the world, relative to that in industrialized countries, falling only slightly from 8.9% to 7.4% over the period. Thus, the gap between market economies and some low income countries is continuing to narrow and will likely do so into the next few decades as an increasing amount of the manufactured goods consumed in the market economies is produced in the low income countries. The manufacturing output of the low income countries is presently highly concentrated with 37% in Brazil and Mexico and a further 32% in India, Korea, Argentina, Turkey, Indonesia, Philippines, Venezuela, and Hong Kong. Indeed, the number of developing countries in which manufacturing as a proportion of gross domestic product equals or exceeds that of the United States (20% in 1992)[2] includes only the Philippines, Korea, Mexico, Brazil, Peru, and Venezuela, but no countries in Africa.

The mobility and internationalization of manufacturing capital are important developments promoting the extension of manufacturing throughout the countries of the world. A relatively small number of very large multinational corporations contributes most to the development of manufacturing in the low income countries.[3] One half of the parent corporations have their headquarters in the United States with the other half mainly in the United Kingdom, Germany, and Japan. The greatest proportion of the overseas branches of these multinational concerns is in Brazil, Mexico, Argentina, Indonesia, and Hong Kong. The corporations General Motors, Exxon, and Shell have a higher gross product than any country of sub-Saharan Africa; another 84 corporations have greater balance sheets than any country of sub-Saharan Africa except Nigeria and the Republic of South Africa. The jurisdiction under which regulations are developed and enforced for such large corporations is not entirely clear. Obviously, some influence over policy may be exerted within the country of origin of the parent corporation, and policies established by the regulatory bodies or suggested by the academic communities within these countries of origin need to reflect some responsibility for the impact of their activities on the branch plants that such parent corporations support in developing countries.

In this chapter, the authors review the current mechanisms for dealing with international issues in occupational health, including the regulatory bodies and academic communities, and identify outstanding issues in the area of occupational health policy.

INTERNATIONAL CONSENSUS ON REGULATION OF HAZARDOUS EXPOSURE IN THE WORKPLACE

Presently, more than 20 countries publish threshold limit values (TLVs) as guidelines for good industrial practice.[4-8] These TLVs are determined principally from studies carried out in only a very few countries.[9-11] The values recommended by three key sources form the basis for regulations adopted by many national and international bodies (Table 58-1). These sources are

American Convention of Government Industrial Hygienists of the United States

The American Convention of Government Industrial Hygienists (ACGIH) is a nongovernmental professional body that defines three categories of TLV:

1. TLV–time-weighted average (TLV-TWA). These are the estimated levels of exposure to which nearly all workers may be exposed without adverse effects, over an 8-hour work day for a 40-hour work week.
2. TLV–short-term exposure limit (TLV-STEL). This limit is defined as a 15-minute exposure that should not be exceeded at any time during a work day, even if the 8-hour TWA is within the TLV-TWA. The exposure should be no longer than 15 minutes and should occur no more than four times per day. There must be at least 60 minutes between successive exposures at this level. An averaging period other than 15 minutes may be used when warranted by the observed biologic effects.
3. TLV–ceiling (TLV-C). This is the concentration that should never be exceeded during any part of the work day.

Hygiieniska Gransvarden of Sweden

Two different types of TLVs are defined by the Hygiieniska Gransvarden:

1. The Nivagransvarde (NVG) corresponds to the TLV-TWA of the ACGIH.
2. The Tarkgrandvarden (TGV) corresponds to the TLV-C of the ACGIH.

Maximale Arbeitsplatz Konzentrationen Gesundheidschad-licher Arbeit Stoffe of Germany

Recommended values published by the Ministry of Labour of the Federal Republic of Germany indicate the TLV for an 8-hour working day and 40-hour work week. One of the unique features of this list is the technical reference to concentrations of gases, vapors, or acrosols that have no scientific basis for determination of regulations but for which recommended permissible concentrations for the protection and monitoring of the working atmosphere are provided. These values are statutory. Many of the latter substances are carcinogens and technical, social, and economic considerations are incorporated into the recommendations.

Risks of exposure to carcinogenic agents (published annually by Maximale Arbeitsplatz Konzentrationen Gesundheidschad-licher Arbeit Stoffe [MAK Commission], ACGIH, and the Hygiieniska Gransvarden) are included along with other workplace hazards. The identification of these hazards is usually based upon the work published by

Table 58-1. Organization and structure of the main committees for determination of exposure limits

Name of the committee	Date of creation	Frequency of publications	Composition	Decision criteria	Status	Characteristics of statements
TLV Committee of ACGIH (USA)	1938	Annual	Industrial hygienists, government or industry	Scientific, technicoeconomic	Nongovernmental	Recommendation
MAK Commission (Germany)	1955	Annual	Scientists, industrial hygienists from industry	Scientific	Section of the National Committee of Research (DFG)	Recommendation (published by Ministry of Labour)
AGA Committee (Arbeit Goverbe Aufsicht) (Germany)	1972	Indeterminate	Labor, management, scientists, regulators	Technicoeconomic	Committee, Ministry of Labour	Statutory (for carcinogens)
Reference Group, National Board of Occupational Safety and Health (Sweden)	1974	Biennial	Labor, management, scientists, regulators	Scientific, technicoeconomic	Government committee	Statutory
Advisory Committee on Toxic Substances (UK)	1980	Annual	Labor, management, health and safety executive	Scientific, technicoeconomic	Government committee	Statutory, recommendations

TLV, Threshold limit value; *ACGIH,* American Conference of Governmental Industrial Hygienists; *MAK,* Maximale Arbeitsplatz Konzentrationen.

the International Agency for Research on Cancer (IARC) located in Lyon, France.[12]

INTERNATIONAL COMPARISON OF OCCUPATIONAL HEALTH REGULATION: THE EXAMPLE OF ASBESTOS

The history and current situation of measures to control asbestos exposure are illustrative of policy development at the international level.[13] The first recommendations for control of exposure (TLV-TWA) were elaborated in 1946 and remained unchanged (5 million particles per cubic foot, mppcf) until 1973. In 1968, a reduction to 12 fibers/ml >5 μm in length (2 mppcf) was proposed. In 1970, this was changed to 5 fibers/ml and in 1972 asbestos was designated an A1a human carcinogen. This was revised in 1978 when different levels of TLV-TWA were proposed, depending upon the type of fiber (with concern for fibers of >5 μm in length with an aspect ratio equal to or greater than 3:1 as determined by the membrane filter method at 400 to 450 × magnification, using a 4-mm objective, phase contrast illumination): 0.2 fibers/ml for crocidolite, 0.5 fibers/ml for amosite and tremolite, and 2 fibers/ml for chrysotile and other fibers. These recommendations were adopted in 1980 and remained in effect until 1991 at which time a level of 0.2 fibers/ml has been proposed for all forms. Tables 58-2a and 58-2b give a summary of asbestos regulations prepared by the European Economic Community (EEC) with a comparison with regulations in effect in Denmark, France, Germany, the United Kingdom, Norway, Sweden, Poland, Canada, Japan, the United States, the Republic of South Africa, and Peru. The regulations adopted by the EEC con-

cern restrictions on use, labeling requirements, allowable exposure levels, medical surveillance, and environmental protection requirements. The allowable TLVs for crocidolite are higher (0.3 fibers/ml) and for amosite (0.3 fibers/ml) and chrysotile (0.6 fibers/ml) lower than those in the ACGIH document.

Regulations in all European countries and in Japan are considerably closer to those adopted by the EEC than are those in Canada, the USA, South Africa and Peru. It is of particular note that Canada, the United States, and South Africa are major producers of asbestos and the summary (Table 58-2b) indicates no restriction on its use for spraying, use of amphiboles, and control of import/export. Moreover, the TLV is higher in some instances than in the countries of Europe or than the EEC has adopted. Finally, the aspects of environmental protection are much less rigorous.

In another major producer of asbestos, the former Soviet Union, regulatory officials had espoused the position that, as far as they were concerned, the only acceptable value for exposure is zero (as an aim). If this level cannot be attained, the exposure must remain at a level at which no adverse effect of any kind can be observed. In spite of this official position, the actual situation is much different. In a recent visit to a university clinic in Estonia, at the site of a large former soviet military base, serving a total population of around 500,000 persons, a large number of cases of mesothelioma were observed to have occurred in the year prior to the visit. When asked the source of the asbestos to which the patients had been exposed, it was noted that, in former times, it was not permissible to enquire concerning such matters or to report such cases.

INTERNATIONAL COMPARISON OF STRUCTURES FOR ENFORCEMENT OF REGULATIONS

Table 58-3 provides a comparison of the structure for enforcement of regulations on occupational safety and health in some industrialized countries. As can be seen, although there is a similarity in the qualification and activities of the organizations, there is a large discrepancy among these countries concerning the "density" of inspectors in the various countries, varying from over 10 times in Sweden, with the highest coverage, to the United States with the lowest level of coverage among the countries compared. Many low income countries have considerably lower coverage (for example, Nigeria with 30 inspectors in a population of 99 million persons) or none at all.

In each of the regulatory agencies, the personnel consist primarily of engineers and technicians. However, in France, a second regulatory agency contains lawyers and economists as well. Little information is available concerning such regulatory bodies and their operations in most developing countries.

ISSUES IN OCCUPATIONAL HEALTH IN DEVELOPING COUNTRIES: THE EXAMPLE OF AFRICA

A survey of the services, structures, and activities associated with occupational health and specifically with occupational lung disease in selected African countries has been carried out (Table 58-4). The survey included the countries of Nigeria, Côte d'Ivoire, South Africa, and Zimbabwe. All countries had occupational health legislation. However, specific regulations governing occupational health practice were not well developed in any of the countries and were absent in Nigeria, the largest country in Africa. There were occupational health inspectors in each of the countries but, for example, in the case of Nigeria, there were a total of only 30 such individuals for the whole country. Labor was organized in three of the four countries, although this organization is rudimentary and only recently has improved in most. Although all countries have specific compensation for occupational injury, only two have a semblance of compensation for occupational disease. Of the four countries, only South Africa has a formal training program in occupational health (Algeria also has such a formal training program).

Whereas the dose–response relationship of ambient exposures and occupational lung diseases appears to be similar to that reported from other sites, the measured levels of ambient pollutants (for example, cotton dust) are considerably higher than is usual in studies from industrialized countries and (in the case of cotton dust) far exceed the recommended levels of the organizations noted above. The characteristics of the workforce are also considerably different, leading to bias in comparing the results of investigations or of reports of occupational health in the workforce in Africa

as compared to that in industrialized countries. The workforce in Africa, on the whole, is considerably younger and has a much reduced level of seniority as compared with that in industrialized countries. Moreover, in the case of large firms in South Africa, the workforce is frequently migrant, consisting to an important extent of citizens of surrounding countries, who have only short-term contracts and who, in some cases, may not be allowed to renew their contract should they show any evidence of disability or impairment.

Table 58-2a. Summary of asbestos regulations

Activity	Regulation
Restrictions	
Spraying	Directive 83/447/EEC
Amphiboles	Directive 91/659/EEC
Import/export	Regulation 2455/92/EEC
Labeling	Directive 83/478/EEC: all asbestos products
	Directive 91/325/EEC: logo and safety phrases
Regulations	
Chrysotile	
TLV	0.6 fibers/ml
Action level	0.1 fibers/ml
Crocidolite	
TLV	0.3 fibers/ml
Action level	0.1 fibers/ml
Amosite:	
TLV	0.3 fibers/ml
Action level	0.1 fibers/ml
Mixtures	
TLV	0.3 fibers/ml
Action level	0.1 fibers/ml
Surveillance	
Responsible	According to national regulation
Examinations	
x-ray	Yes
PFT	Yes
Frequency	q 3 years
Environmental protection	
Air	Directive 87/217/EEC
Asbestos	0.1 mg/ml
Mixed	
Waste	Directive 78/319/EEC [52],84/631/EEC,85/469/EEC,86/279/EEC P [53],
	Proposal for Council Directive COM (90) final 415-/Oc, 289/05
Type	Fibers and dust
Licensed transport	Yes
Dumping site	Yes
Import/export	Yes

EEC, European Economic Community; *TLV*, threshold limit value; *PFT*, pulmonary function test.

Table 58-2b. Summary of asbestos regulations: European economic community in comparison with individual countries

Activity	Denmark	France	Germany	UK	Norway	Sweden	Poland	Canada	Japan	United States	South Africa	Peru
Restrictions												
Spraying	Banned 1988	EEC directive	Banned 1990	Banned 1993	Banned 1986	Banned	Banned 2000	None	Banned	None	None	None
Amphiboles	Banned 1988		Banned 1990	Banned 1985	Banned 1986	Banned	Banned	None	Banned	None	None	None
Import/export	Banned 1988			Controlled 1992	Controlled 1986	Controlled	Banned 2000	None		None	None	None
Labelling	Yes 1986	EEC directive	Asbestos products	Directive 1984	All	NA	NA	Voluntary	As much as 5% asbestos	Most products	All	None
Regulations (fibers/ml)												
Chrysotile												
TLV	0.3	0.6	0.25	0.5	NA	0.5	0.5	2.0	0.5	0.2	2.0	NA
Action level	NA	0.2	NA	0.2	NA	NA	NA	NA	NA	NA	1.0	NA
Crocidolite												
TLV	0.3	0.3	NA	0.2	NA	NA	NA	0.2	NA	0.2	2.0	NA
Action level	NA	0.1	NA	0.1	NA	NA	NA	NA	NA	NA	1.0	NA
Amosite												
TLV	0.3	0.3	NA	0.2	NA	NA	0.5	0.5	0.2	0.2	2.0	NA
Action level	NA	0.1	NA	0.1	NA	NA	NA	NA	NA	NA	1.0	NA
Mixtures												
TLV	NA	0.3	NA	NA	NA	NA	NA	NA	NA	NA	NA	NA
Action level	NA	0.1	NA	NA	NA	NA	NA	NA	NA	NA	NA	NA

Continued.

Table 58-2b. Summary of asbestos regulations: European economic community in comparison with individual countries—cont'd

Activity	Denmark	France	Germany	UK	Norway	Sweden	Poland	Canada	Japan	United States	South Africa	Peru
Surveillance												
Responsible	Industry	Industry, any physician	Industry, any physician	Industry, government	NA	Industry	Industry	Industry, approved physician	Industry	Industry	Industry	Industry, approved physicians
Examinations												
x-ray	Yes	Yes	Yes	Yes	NA	Yes	Yes	Yes	Yes	Yes	Yes	NA
PFT	Yes	Yes	Yes	Yes	NA	Yes	Yes	Yes	No	Yes	Yes	NA
Frequency	q 2 years	Annual	NA	q 2 years	NA	q 5 years	Annual	Annual	q 6 years	NA		NA
Environmental protection												
Air (mg/ml)												
Asbestos	0.1	0.1	0.1	0.1	NA	NA	Limited		10 fibers/ml	Nonvisible	NA	NA
Mixed	NA	0.5	2.0	NA	NA	NA	Limited	NA	NA	NA	NA	NA
Waste												
Type	All	All	All	Special	NA	NA	Bound form	All	Demolition	>1% Asbestos	NA	NA
Transport	No	Yes	Yes	Yes	NA	NA	Yes	No	Yes	No	NA	NA
Dumping	Yes	Yes	Yes	Yes	NA	NA	Yes	No	Yes	Yes	NA	NA
Import/export	No	Yes	Yes	No	NA	NA	Yes	Yes	NA	NA	NA	NA

EEC, European Economic Community; *NA*, data not available; *TLV*, threshold limit value; *PFT*, pulmonary function test.

Table 58-3. Structure for enforcement of regulations on occupational safety and health in some industrialized countries

Country	Administration	Qualification	Time devoted (%)	Other activities	Inspectors/million population
Sweden	Arbetarskydds Styrelsen	Engineers, technicians/ equivalents	80	Length of working period	43.4
Germany	Bunderministerium fur Arbeit Bewerbeaufsicht	Engineers, technicians/ equivalents	20	Atmospheric pollution, length of working period	9.7
	Berufgenossen	Engineers, technicians	100	Major risk areas	19.4
France	Ministère du Travail	Lawyers, economists, engineers	15	Employment, length of working period, disputes	5.5
	Sécurité Sociale	Engineers, technicians	100		10.1
United Kingdom	Health and Safety Executive	Engineers, technicians/ equivalents	80	Major risk areas	12.2
United States	Occupational Safety and Health Administration	Engineers, technicians/ equivalents	100		4.3

Table 58-4. Summary of components related to occupational health in a selection of countries in Africa.

Component	Country			
	Nigeria	Côte d'Ivoire	South Africa	Zimbabwe
Legislation	Yes	Yes	Yes	Yes
Regulations	No	+/−	+/−	+/−
Inspectors	Yes	Yes	Yes	Yes
Organized labor	+/−	No	Yes	Yes
Compensation				
Injury	Yes	Yes	Yes	Yes
Disease	No	No	+/−	+/−
Formal training	No	No	Yes	No

Another important difference in the workforce in Africa as compared with that in many industrialized countries is the background sociology of work. Where the workforce is large and the industry concentrated geographically (such as in the mines in South Africa), the nature of the living conditions (often communal living of large numbers of single men) may result in the occurrence and transmission of diseases such as tuberculosis and human immunodeficiency virus, which have important consequences on the health of the workers and which are obvious in the context of occupational health assessments. For example, tuberculosis was the most important illness identified in a study of cotton mill workers in South Africa.[14]

Occupational health research, which provides the basis for policy formation, is not well developed in Africa. Most research into occupational lung diseases in Africa has been in relation to inorganic dust exposure in the mining industry in South Africa[15-21] and Zimbabwe.[22] Research into other types of exposure effects has been quite scanty and the majority of the work reported has come from South Af-

rica and Nigeria.[23-25] After inorganic dust exposure, investigations into the effects of exposure to cotton dust are the most frequent, having been reported from Cameroon,[26] Ethiopia,[27] South Africa,[14] Sudan,[28] and Tanzania.[29] The absence of an active research program is a reflection of the weakness of the structure of occupational health services in the region and particularly of formal training programs within the context of which most scientific investigation is carried out.

THE ROLE OF NONGOVERNMENTAL ACADEMIC ORGANIZATIONS IN INTERNATIONAL ISSUES IN OCCUPATIONAL HEALTH POLICY

The nongovernmental academic sector plays a role in determining public policy:

1. by producing scientific statements that reflect consensus in the scientific community that are meant to influence public policy,
2. through basic research upon which public policy is determined, and
3. through representation before policy-making bodies to ensure that public policy is cognizant of the concerns of the academic community.

The role of each of these components in relation to the development of international and especially developing country policy in relation to occupational lung diseases will be addressed in this section.

Consensus statements

In considering this issue, the example of the American Thoracic Society and American Lung Association (ATS-ALA) will be used as it is the largest nongovernmental academic body dealing with lung diseases in the world. A total of six current Statements and Position Papers are available from the American Thoracic Society concerning issues dealing with occupational lung diseases. These include statements on Disability Legislation for Occupational Lung Diseases,[30] Surveillance for Respiratory Hazards in the Occupational Setting,[31] Evaluation of Impairment/Disability Secondary to Respiratory Disorders,[32] The Diagnosis of Nonmalignant Diseases Related to Asbestos,[33] Public Responsibility in Asbestos-Associated Diseases,[34] and Health Effects of Tremolite.[35] Each of the statements contained general technical aspects that could be applied under a wide variety of circumstances, two dealt with issues related to public policy, one referred to issues in developing countries and only two dealt (to some degree) with variability associated with race or ethnic group.

International aspects of research into occupational lung diseases

A review of the official position papers and statements of the ATS noted above indicates that of a total of 196 cited references, 50 refer to work outside the United States, and, of these, 10 refer to work carried out in developing countries (all in relation to asbestos or tremolite exposure). Moreover, in a review of the *Index Medicus* entries from 1988 to 1993, of 2,322 references cited for research concerning occupational lung diseases, only six were recorded as having to do specifically with developing countries.

In recent years, three organizations have held symposia concerning occupational health in relation to developing countries: the International Union Against Tuberculosis and Lung Disease (IUATLD) held sessions at its World Conferences in Singapore in 1986 and in Boston in May 1990, a workshop of the subcommittee on Occupational health in Developing Countries was held at the International Congress on Occupational Health meeting in Singapore in September 1991, and the International Symposium on Epidemiology in Occupational Health was held in Paris in September 1991.

One of the earliest activities of the (then) newly formed Committee on Respiratory Disease of the IUATLD in 1978 was to carry out a survey of legislation for worker protection against occupational lung disease[36] with a particular focus on developing countries. The response to this survey from developing countries was very poor, thought to reflect the inadequate state of development of occupational health services. In a paper presented to the Respiratory Disease Committee of the IUATLD in 1986,[37] W.O. Phoon of Singapore noted that mineral dust-related lung diseases were at that time among the three most common causes of occupational health problems in Eastern Asia.[38,39] The impact of export of hazardous processes to developing countries due to tightening of regulations in industrialized countries was already apparent.[40]

A review of the 1991 conference of the International Congress on Occupational Health (ICOH)[41] indicated that no invited lecturers came from developing countries, there were no plenary communications from a speaker from a de-

veloping country, although one paper did deal with issues in developing countries, and 7 of 119 papers presented at the conference came from developing countries, 2 from Latin America, 1 from Africa, and 4 from Asia.

The workshop in Paris (summarized by Loewenson and Pham[41]) also identified important considerations in research in occupational health in developing countries. Important aspects of the background for research include the differing characteristics of labor (the informal and rural sectors, living environment), the work environment and technologies used (nature of work organization, limited information, export of hazardous processes), and the characteristics of production relations (foreign ownership, level of regulatory and enforcement activity). The priority tasks in occupational health research were suggested to be determination of the relationship between occupational and nonoccupational ill health, a focus on appropriate and cost-effective interventions, determination of the validity of standards, development of a low technology method of exposure and outcome measurement, and development of intervention approaches appropriate to the health services structure.

The workshop then considered a number of international strategies for communication and collaboration including the International Labour Organization (ILO) African Regional Occupational Health Project, the World Health Organization (WHO), Global Environmental and Health Network, the Swedish Agency for Research Cooperation with Developing Countries (SAREC) Pesticide Research Network, IARC program for development of skills in cancer epidemiology, and the ICOH subcommittee on occupational health. The IUATLD Committee on Respiratory Disease including the occupational health task groups and the network of training courses in pulmonary epidemiology has been an additional group with a focus on occupational lung disease with emphasis on developing countries.

The organization of labor in developing countries was considered within the IUATLD symposium in Boston in 1990[42] and varies considerably from that in industrialized countries with the greatest proportion of workers at risk of exposure to agricultural hazards, cotton dust,[43] and inorganic dust.[44] The number of workers exposed to mineral dust in metal mines was noted to be greatest in Africa,[45] over three times greater than in the Americas, the next highest number. The estimated prevalence of pneumoconiosis among metal miners in various developing countries (Mexico, El Salvador, Peru, Ghana, and Morocco) was 45 per 1,000 as compared with various countries of Europe (France, Germany, and the United Kingdom), which was 22. These differences are more likely to represent differences in levels of exposure than to host factors.

The development and evaluation of appropriate measurement technologies have received a certain amount of attention. The comparability of subjective responses elicited by a questionnaire, in various languages and cultural settings, has been demonstrated by comparing "dose–response" relationships between chronic bronchitis as determined from the ATS-ALA questionnaire and the average number of cigarettes smoked per day[46] and in a community setting in which the same questionnaire was translated into the various languages used in the same community.[47] Moreover, the utility and validity of subjective evaluation (based upon responses to a questionnaire) of breathlessness[48] and of exposures to harmful substances[49] have also been shown.

The health setting clearly influences the view of causation of disease in patients in the industrial setting. The similarity in appearance and close association between mineral dust diseases and tuberculosis[50] led to confusion of the two conditions well into the present century. It is likely that a similar confusion was associated with the initial observations of the health effects of grain dust exposure[51] and, in present settings in some developing countries, it is likely that the same confusion between tuberculosis (and possibly also AIDS-related illnesses) and occupational lung disease is presently observed when diagnostic facilities are not well developed.

Representation before policy makers

It is a truism that the pharmacy of the preventive health specialist is the parliament. Finally, to implement preventive strategies (the focus of an occupational health program), it is necessary to effect laws and regulations and these can be accomplished only through the political structure. Thus, one of the important activities of a nongovernmental, academic organization is to influence the decision makers in the political sphere. At the international level, the political body is the United Nations and its related organizations such as the WHO and the ILO. International policy issues may also be addressed at the national level, particularly in those countries that are the headquarters of multinational corporations. Using the example of the ATS-ALA noted previously, two of the current statements concerning occupational health issues relate to political representation, one summarizing an appearance before the U.S. Congress and the other to provide the basis for community level representation to local legislators.

Within the voluntary agency, political representation may be undertaken in various ways. The ALA maintains an office in Washington, D.C. to provide, in addition to other reasons, advice and direction to federal legislators and civil servants as related to issues of lung health. This may be initiated at the request of the political body itself, it may be initiated by the community that the ALA represents, or it may be initiated by the academic body represented by the ATS. Such activities provide the basis for framing legislation, regulations, and directives to deal with occupational health issues as well as other lung health concerns. To date, all representational activities of the ALA concerning occupational health have had essentially a national scope without specific reference to the international sphere. However, the Association has a record of effective intervention and

representation concerning other international lung health issues (most notably tuberculosis) and is an established vehicle through which such activities (concerning occupational health) might be undertaken.

REFERENCES

1. Griffin K: *Alternative strategies for economic development,* New York, 1989, St. Martin's Press.
2. Todaro MP: *Economic development in the third world,* ed 4, New York, 1992, Longman.
3. Todaro MP: *Economic development in the third world,* ed 4, New York, 1992, Longman, 469.
4. Rappaport SM: Threshold limit values, permissible exposure limits and feasibility: the bases for exposure limits in the United States, *Am J Ind Med* 23:683-684, 1993.
5. Roach SA and Rappaport SM: But they are not threshold: a critical analysis of the documentation of threshold limit values, *Am J Ind Med* 17:727-753, 1990.
6. Robinson JC and Paxman DG: The role of threshold limit values in US air pollution policy, *Am J Ind Med* 21:383-396, 1992.
7. Le Ricousse G: L'établissement de valeurs limites d'exposition aux substances toxiques dans les atmosphères de travail: un tounant dans la prévention des maladies professionelles en France? Les notes scientifiques et techniques de l'INRS no édit NS0058, Oct 1985.
8. International Labour Office: *Occupational exposure limits for airborne toxic substances: values of selected countries,* Occupational Safety and Health Series No 37, International Labour Office, Geneva, 1987.
9. American Conference of Government Industrial Hygienists: *Guide to occupational exposure values,* 1990.
10. National Swedish Board of Safety and Health: *Occupational exposure limit values,* Ordinance AFS 1987; 12: issued 5 June 1987.
11. INRS: Valeurs limites d'exposition professionnelle aux substances dangereuses de l'ACGIH et de l'Allemagne, *Cahier notes documenaire INRS* 144:419-449, 1991.
12. Spirtas R, Steinberg M, Wands RC, and Weisburger EK: Identification and classification of carcinogens: procedures of the chemical substances threshold limit values. Committee ACGIH, *Am J Public Health* 76:1232-1235, 1986.
13. American Conference of Governmental Industrial Hygienists Inc.: *Documentation on the threshold limit values and biological exposure indices,* ed 6, pp. 89-94, Cincinnati, Ohio, 1991.
14. White NW: Byssinosis in South Africa; a survey of 2,311 textile workers, *S Afr Med J* 75:435-442, 1989.
15. Cowie RL: Silica dust exposed miners with scleroderma (systemic sclerosis), *Chest* 92:260-262, 1987.
16. Sluis-Cremer GK, Hessel PA, Hnizdo E, Churchill AR, and Zeiss EA: Silica, silicoses and systemic sclerosis, *Br J Ind Med* 46:364-369, 1989.
17. Sluis-Cremer GK and Maier G: HLA antigens of the A and B locus in relation to the development of silicosis, *Br J Ind Med* 41:417-418, 1984.
18. Cowie RL and van Schalkwyk MG: The prevalence of silicosis in Orange Free State gold miners, *J Occup Med* 29:44-46, 1987.
19. Cowie RL and Mabena SK: Silicosis, chronic airflow limitation and chronic bronchitis in South African gold miners, *Am Rev Respir Dis* 143:80-84, 1991.
20. Cowie RL: Pulmonary dysfunction in gold miners with reactive airways, *Br J Ind Med* 46:873-876, 1989.
21. Irwig LM, du Toit RSJ, Sluis-Cremer GK, et al: Risk of asbestosis in crocidolite and amosite miners in South Africa, *Ann NY Acad Sci* 330:34-52, 1979.
22. Cullen MR, Lopez-Carillo L, Alli B, Pace PE, Shalat SL, and Baloyi RS: Chrysotile asbestos and health in Zimbabwe: II. Health status survey of active miners and millers, *Am J Ind Med* 19:171-182, 1991.

23. Oleru UG and Onyekwere C: Exposures to polyvinyl chloride, methyl ketone and other chemicals. The pulmonary and non-pulmonary effect, *Int Arch Occup Environ Health* 63:503-510, 1992.

24. Oleru UG: Pulmonary function of exposed and control workers in a Nigerian non-soapy detergent factory, *Arch Environ Health* 39:101-106, 1984.

25. Oleru UG: Pulmonary function and symptoms of Nigerian workers exposed to cement dust, *Environ Res* 33:379-385, 1984.

26. Takaui J and Nemery B: Byssinosis in a textile factory in Cameroon: a preliminary study, *Br J Ind Med* 45:803-809, 1988.

27. Woldejohannes M, Bergerin Y, Mgeni AY and Theriault G: Respiratory problems among cotton textile mill workers in Ethiopia, *Br J Ind Med* 48:110-115, 1991.

28. El Karim MAA and Ousa SH: Prevalence of byssinosis and respiratory symptoms among spinners in Sudanese cotton mills, *Am J Ind Med* 12:281-289, 1987.

29. Mustafa KY, Lakha AS, and Dahoma U: Byssinosis, respiratory symptoms and spirometric lung function tests in Tanzanian sisal workers, *Br J Ind Med* 35:123-128, 1978.

30. American Thoracic Society: Disability legislation for occupational lung diseases, *ATS News* 1981.

31. American Thoracic Society: Surveillance for respiratory hazards in the occupational setting, *Am Rev Respir Dis* 126:952-956, 1982.

32. American Thoracic Society: Evaluation of impairment/disability secondary to respiratory disorders, *Am Rev Respir Dis* 133:1205-1209, 1986.

33. American Thoracic Society: The diagnosis of nonmalignant diseases related to asbestos, *Am Rev Respir Dis* 134:363-368, 1986.

34. American Thoracic Society: Public responsibility in asbestos-associated diseases, *ATS News* Fall 1983.

35. American Thoracic Society: Health effects of tremolite, *Am Rev Respir Dis* 142:1453-1458, 1990.

36. International Union Against Tuberculosis: *Questionnaire on legislation for worker protection against occupational lung disease,* Committee on Respiratory Disease, 1978 (unpublished).

37. Phoon WO: *The geographical epidemiology of occupational lung disease,* IUATLD Committee on Respiratory Disease, Singapore, 1986 (unpublished).

38. Phoon WO: Occupational lung disease in southeast Asia, *Bronchus* 1:10-14, 1986.

39. Phoon WO and Ong CN: *Occupational health in developing countries in Asia,* p 141, Tokyo, 1985, Southeast Asia Medical Information Centre.

40. Phoon WO: Occupational health in developing countries: a simple case of neglect, *World Health Forum* 4:340-343, 1983.

41. Loewenson R and Pham QT: *Report of the workshop on occupational health epidemiology in developing countries,* Paris, France, 1991 (unpublished report).

42. Schenker M: Occupational lung disease: a worldwide problem in a changing world, *Tubercle Lung Dis* 73:4-6, 1992.

43. Rylander R: Diseases associated with exposure to plant dusts: focus on cotton dust, *Tubercle Lung Dis* 73:21-26, 1992.

44. Becklake MR: The mineral dust diseases, *Tubercle Lung Dis* 73:13-20, 1992.

45. International Labour Office: *Sixth international report on the prevention and suppression of dust in mining, tunnelling, and quarrying 1973-1977,* No. 48, pp 1-152, Occupational Safety and Health series, Geneva, 1987, ILO.

46. Enarson DA, Christiani DC, Ernst P, et al: The prevalence of chronic bronchitis: an international comparison, *Am Rev Respir Dis* 141:A327, 1990.

47. Becklake MR, Freeman S, Goldsmith C, et al: Respiratory questionnaires in occupational studies: their use in multilingual workforces on the Witwatersrand, *Int J Epidemiol* 16:606-611, 1987.

48. Vestbo J, Knudsen KM, and Rasmussen FV: Should we continue using questionnaires on breathlessness in epidemiologic surveys?, *Am Rev Respir Dis* 137:1114-1118, 1988.

49. Fonn S: *Exposure to grain dust and respiratory health in a South African grain mill,* PhD thesis, Johannesburg, 1989, University of Witwatersrand.

50. Meiklejohn A: History of lung diseases of coalminers in Great Britain. Part III. 1920-1952, *Br J Ind Med* 9:208-220, 1952.

51. Rammazzini B: *De Morbis artificum diatriba,* Chicago, 1940, University of Chicago Press.

52. Asbestos International Association: *Summary of main features of asbestos regulations (and other fibres when appropriate),* AIA Information Memorandum A/M 1/91.

53. Atis A, Becking G, Berlin A, Bernard A, Foa V, Kello D, Krug F, Leonard A, and Nordberg G: *Indicateurs pour l'évaluation de l'exposition aux produits chimiques génotoxiques et leurs effets biologiques,* Commission des Communautés Européennes, Hygiène et Sécurité du Travail, Direction Générale Emploi, Affaires Sociales et Education, 1988, EUR. 11659 Fr.

Environmental Control Strategies

PHILIP HARBER

This section describes methods for controlling potentially adverse exposures. More detail is found in standard textbooks of industrial ventilation and industrial hygiene controls. Methods for controlling point source and mobile source community air pollution range from regulation limiting industrial processes to control technology for capturing pollutants at the source; these methods are not discussed in detail in this book. Personal protective equipment such as respirators are used by individuals to decrease inhaled dose.

By analogy to clinical medicine, Section II, which discusses methods of measuring exposures in workplace and community settings, represents "diagnostic methods." This section is analogous to "treatment," describing principles for controlling exposures.

Chapter 59

RESPIRATORS

Brian A. Boehlecke

Types of respirators
Respiratory protection program
Physiologic effects and medical considerations
Worker tolerance of respirators
Medical evaluation for respirator use
Summary

Personal respiratory protective devices (respirators) may be necessary when adequate control of airborne contaminants in the workplace is not feasible, an individual has an increased risk for adverse effects from exposure, or the potential for accidental release of toxic agents is present. Respirators should be considered a secondary means of protection with reduction of the general environmental levels of toxic materials through engineering controls and work practices or substitution of less toxic materials as the primary measures.[1] Whenever feasible a reduction in airborne contaminants through enclosure of processes, increases in exhaust ventilation, or institution of work practices that reduce the generation of toxic aerosols should be attempted to decrease dependence on personal respiratory protective devices. Detailed discussions of the components of comprehensive respiratory protection programs can be found elsewhere.[2-5] This chapter will provide an overview with an emphasis on the aspects most relevant for health professionals.

TYPES OF RESPIRATORS

Respirators can either remove contaminants from the surrounding air, supply breathable air from another source, or utilize a combination of both methods.

Air-purifying respirators pass ambient air through fibrous filters to remove particulates or through chemical sorbents to remove gases. Particulate removal depends on physical deposition of the particles on the filter by impaction, interception, or diffusion. The efficiency of entrapment is dependent upon the composition of the filter and the size distribution of the particles. Small densely packed fibers in the filter material increase the efficiency of the filter but also increase resistance to airflow. As the entrapped particle load on the filter increases, deposition efficiency and resistance increase. The higher the ambient concentration of particulates and the greater the volume of air inhaled per minute through the respirator, the more quickly the filter becomes heavily loaded and requires replacement. Disposable respirators or dust masks are designed to be discarded when heavily loaded. The efficiency of filters for contaminant removal is measured as part of the certification testing of respirators performed by the U.S. National Institute for Occupational Safety and Health (NIOSH). Filters designed to provide protection from dusts of relatively low toxicity must remove 99% of the mass of suspended particles from 2.88 m^3 of air that contains 50 mg/m^3 of silica dust averaging 0.5 μm in aerodynamic diameter. A high-efficiency particulate air filter (HEPA) must remove 99.97% of a 0.3-μm-diameter aerosol at 100 mg/m^3 concentration.

Gases can be removed by absorption, adsorption, or a chemical reaction with material contained in a cartridge or cannister. Activated charcoal is a commonly used general sorbent, but other materials may be added to increase removal of contaminants with specific properties. Therefore, only respirators with sorbents certified by NIOSH or the Mine Safety and Health Administration (MSHA) for protection from the types of contaminants present should be used. Cartridges used to remove organic vapors must reduce penetration of carbon tetrachloride to less than 5 parts per million (ppm) from air containing 1,000 ppm passing through the cartridge at 32 L/min for at least 50 minutes. The ability of sorbents to remove gases and vapors decreases as the sorbent becomes saturated with the contaminant(s). If the sorbent is not replaced, "breakthrough" occurs, and protection is diminished. The wearer may sense an odor, taste, or irritation from the contaminant(s) penetrating the sorbent, but this warning may not occur for some substances until undesirable concentrations have been reached in the inhaled air. Warning properties are considered fully adequate only if they allow detection of the contaminant at concentrations at or below the permissible exposure limit (PEL). U.S. federal regulations prohibit the use of air-purifying respirators for protection from organic vapors if the detectable concentration is greater than three times the PEL.[6] They are considered acceptable for protection from substances with warning threshold concentrations between one and three times the PEL only if it has been determined that no serious or irreversible adverse health effects will occur from undetected short-term exposures at these levels. Certification ensures a minimum standard of performance under controlled conditions but does not guarantee acceptable efficiency under all conditions of use; high temperatures or humidity may adversely affect contaminant removal. Possible problems arising from an assumption of equal effectiveness under varying conditions and limitations of the federal testing program have been discussed.[7]

Air-purifying respirators use facepieces of varying types to prevent nonfiltered air from reaching the wearer's breathing zone. Quarter masks cover only the nose and mouth, half masks extend below the chin, and full masks also cover the eyes. Exhaled air leaves the mask through a one-way exhalation valve. Unless a powered blower is used to push air through the respirator's filter or cartridge, negative pressure is developed inside the mask when the wearer inhales. This creates the potential for leakage of unfiltered ambient air through the exhalation valve or between the skin and facepiece. Therefore, fit testing is required to determine the effectiveness of the mask-to-face seal for an individual. This aspect will be discussed.

If exposure to workplace air is considered to be immediately dangerous to life or health (IDLH) or the ambient air is deficient in oxygen, air-purifying respirators do not provide adequate protection. Respirators that provide breathable air from a separate source are then required. An atmosphere is considered IDLH if an acute exposure poses a risk for immediate loss of life, immediate or delayed irreversible adverse health effects, or acute eye or respiratory tract irritation that might prevent escape.[6] Oxygen deficiency requiring an atmosphere-supplying respirator has been defined by NIOSH as an oxygen content of less than 19.5% at sea level.[8] The American National Standards Institute (ANSI) considers a content of 16% at sea level to be the threshold.[9] Therefore, health professionals involved in medical certification for respirator use must be alert to the possibility that in some cases workers may be assigned to work areas with reduced oxygen content atmospheres without atmosphere-supplying respirators.

Atmosphere-supplying respirators may deliver air from a noncontaminated source through an airline or hose (supplied air respirator) or from a self-contained source (self-contained breathing apparatus, SCBA). This source may be compressed or liquid oxygen or an oxygen-generating substance. Flow from the source may be continuous or on demand through a valve that opens only when pressure inside the mask drops with inspiration. If the valve opens at a pressure above ambient (pressure-demand mode), positive pressure could be maintained inside the mask throughout the breathing cycle reducing the possibility of inward leakage of ambient air. Maintaining a positive pressure inside the mask requires that the flow rate from the source exceed the inspiratory flow of the wearer at all times. Heavy exertion may result in high inspiratory flow rates that exceed the system's capacity to maintain a positive pressure and thereby create the potential for penetration of contaminated air.[10] The additional flow required to maintain positive pressure also reduces the useful life of the oxygen source for SCBA.

To conserve oxygen, a closed circuit system may be used whereby expired gas is recirculated to retrieve its oxygen content while carbon dioxide is removed by absorption. Only the amount of oxygen absorbed by the wearer need be replenished from the source. A SCBA provides the advantage of freedom of mobility in highly toxic environments, but add considerable stress to the wearer due to their weight, which may exceed 30 lb. Self-rescuer respirators are lighter devices that contain a limited source of oxygen suitable for escape in emergencies. A procedure to ensure selection of the appropriate-type respirator is one component of an overall respiratory protection program.

RESPIRATORY PROTECTION PROGRAM

U.S. federal regulations require the employer to provide respirators when such equipment is required to protect the health of the employee.[1] The employer is also responsible for establishing and maintaining a respiratory protective program that meets the minimum requirements listed in the box. Exposure standards for various substances promulgated by the Occupational Safety and Health Administra-

---

Components of a minimal acceptable respiratory protective program adapted from U.S. Code of Federal Regulations (CFR) 1910.134

1. Written standard operating procedures governing section and use of respirators
2. Respirator selection based on hazards to which workers are exposed
3. Use of approved respirators when available
4. Instruction and training of users for proper use and limitations of respirators
5. Regular cleaning and disinfection of respirators
6. Adequate storage of respirators
7. Routine inspection and replacement of worn parts
8. Appropriate surveillance of work area conditions
9. Regular inspection and evaluation of the effectiveness of the program
10. Medical certification of the worker's ability to perform the work and use the equipment

tion (OSHA) may also establish specific requirements (e.g., those applicable to exposure to asbestos, benzene, formaldehyde, lead, and hazardous waste).[11] A draft generic respiratory protection standard has been prepared by OSHA but has not yet been promulgated.

Selection of an appropriate respirator should be based on the hazards present, current understanding of the capabilities and limitations of available respirators, the conditions of use, and individual characteristics of the user. NIOSH and ANSI have developed guidelines for decision logic for selection of respirators.[8,9] NIOSH also indicates recommended respirators for various air contaminants in its *Pocket-guide to chemical hazards.*[12] Generally, this aspect of the program is beyond the scope of responsibility of the medical personnel and requires detailed knowledge about conditions in the workplace and job duties while wearing the respirator as well as respirator characteristics. Nevertheless, individual medical considerations may favor one type of respirator when acceptable alternative selections are available. The health professional responsible for determining that the workers can safely use the equipment may need to request information concerning whether possible alternative selections can be considered before making a judgment.

Respirators are assigned protection factors (APFs) based on quantitative fit testing.[8,9] This requires laboratory measurement of the concentration inside the mask of the respirator of a test aerosol such as sodium chloride present in known concentrations in the atmosphere surrounding the respirator. This is usually done in a test chamber using a mask with a specially fitted probe. The ratio of the concentration inside the mask to the concentration outside is the protection factor. NIOSH conducts certification testing and publishes lists of respirators that meet the criteria. Assigned protection factors are based on the minimum anticipated workplace level of respiratory protection that would be provided a specified percentage of workers using a properly functioning and fitted respirator. The box at right shows representative protection factors for selected respirator types. However, these values should be considered only approximate guidelines for protection afforded an individual using a given respirator in the workplace. When tested in a laboratory setting on panels of individuals, some respirators achieved the target protection factors in only 22% of women and 60% of men.[13] Although the data are limited, studies suggest a poor correlation of protection factors measured in the laboratory with those attained in actual workplace settings.[14-16] Even atmosphere supplying types may achieve protection factors below 5 in some individuals when operated in the demand mode.[17] Recently, the validity of the standard method for quantitative fit testing used as the basis for assigning protection factors has been questioned, further reinforcing the need for caution in basing judgments about the effectiveness of respirators on APFs.[18]

Qualitative fit testing is usually performed to determine if an acceptable seal can be achieved for an individual with the mask selected. The wearer is exposed in a chamber or hood to an atmosphere containing a nontoxic aerosol or vapor that can be easily detected if it penetrates the respirator, e.g., saccharin aerosols, isoamyl acetate (banana oil) vapors, or irritant smoke. If the substance is detected, the fit is inadequate. The wearer should make movements during the test simulating those that might occur during work. Reading a standard paragraph aloud is a commonly used maneuver. The presence of facial hair is likely to interfere with a proper seal and therefore usually must be removed.[19] Special eyeglasses without temples that would disrupt the seal of full face pieces are available. If an adequate fit can be achieved, the worker should be instructed to perform a rapid fit test each time the respirator is worn by inhaling gently with the inlet occluded while observing for leaks. This allows detection of gross leaks, which may be alleviated by readjustment of the mask and straps.

Respirators are also used for protection against inhaled bioaerosols of infectious organisms (e.g., tuberculosis). Unfortunately, the standard methods of assigning protection factors may not be applicable to bioaerosols. Furthermore, there is generally only limited agreement on the specific air concentration of organisms that is acceptable. Thus, it is

---

Assigned protection factors (APFs) for selected respirator types

Type of respirator	*APF*
I. Air-purifying	
A. For protection against particulates	
1. Single-use or quarter mask	5
2. Half mask including disposable	10
3. Powered air equipped with hood or helmet	25
4. Full facepiece with high efficiency filter	50
B. For protection against gases and vapors	
1. Half mask including disposable	10
2. Powered air with loose fitting hood or helmet	25
3. Full facepiece with appropriate cartridges or cannisters	50
II. Atmosphere-Supplying	
1. SCBA in demand mode with full facepiece	50
2. Supplied air respirator in pressure demand mode with half mask	1,000
3. Supplied air respirator in pressure demand mode with full facepiece	2,000
4. SCBA in pressure demand mode with full facepiece	10,000

Adapted from NIOSH Respirator Decision Logic.[8]
SCBA, Self-contained breathing apparatus.

more difficult to evaluate adequacy of protection factors for biologic than for chemical hazards. (Special considerations for health care workers are discussed in Chapter 44).

Lack of worker adherence to appropriate use of respirators when indicated is likely to be a major factor in reducing the effectiveness of a respirator program. Workers must receive training regarding the need for respirators as well as their proper use. This training should include the nature of the respiratory hazard, the reasons why environmental controls are inadequate, the risks to health if respiratory protection is not used properly, and specific instructions regarding when respirators are to be worn. Not unexpectedly, the proportion of workers who use respirators is low when the health risk is associated with a cumulative effect of exposure and thereby perceived as remote.[20] However, use may also be intermittent when the threat is more immediate.[21] The amount of discomfort experienced or expected by the worker is likely to be an important determinant of use. The perception of discomfort may be strongly influenced by thermal effects of the mask. The rating of discomfort has been shown to be linearly related to skin temperature[22] with temperatures above 34.5°C increasingly uncomfortable.[23] Evaporative cooling of the mask increased the comfort rating.[24] Thermal conditions under the respirator also affected judgments about the acceptability of the room temperature. The worker's beliefs about the potential for discomfort or inconvenience and the attitude of co-workers are also important determinants of the intention to use a respirator.[25] These factors affect the relationship between the worker's ability to tolerate a respirator and the physiologic stress imposed by its use. This makes the clinical prediction of a worker's ability to tolerate respirator use more difficult and increases the importance of monitoring the worker's experience under conditions of actual use. Therefore administrative measures to ensure reporting and evaluation of any difficulties experienced are an important component of the respiratory protection program.

PHYSIOLOGIC EFFECTS AND MEDICAL CONSIDERATIONS

OSHA regulations require that a worker not be assigned to a task requiring a respirator unless he or she is physically able to perform the work and use the equipment.[1] The responsible physician must determine what health and physical conditions are pertinent and the criteria for acceptable fitness. Researchers have attempted to provide a basis for the medical judgment on fitness by determining the stress imposed by respirators. Detailed reviews of physiologic effects have been presented elsewhere.[26,27] A basic understanding of these effects is useful to the clinician who must assess whether the added stress of the respirator poses a medically unacceptable risk for the worker. The importance of considering the conditions of work (e.g., exertion level, flexibility for pacing of work, thermal environment, and severity of hazard present) as well as the medical con-

dition and physical capacity of the worker and the direct effects of the respirator has been emphasized.[28]

Air-purifying respirators increase resistance to airflow and thereby alter the pattern of breathing. Generally the obstructed phase of respiration is prolonged and the total minute ventilation is reduced.[29-34] These effects are present both at rest and during exercise. Whether a clinically significant gas exchange abnormality results depends on the user's ventilatory capacity and respiratory control system as well as the magnitude of the added resistance.[35-43] If ventilatory efficiency can be increased, significant hypoventilation may not be present.[44] Reduction in arterial blood oxygen content and elevations in carbon dioxide content have been noted in healthy persons during exercise with external added resistance to breathing. However, no clinically significant effect on blood lactate at peak exertion or during recovery was found in healthy young men doing progressive exercise to exhaustion wearing three different types of air-purifying canisters.[45] The investigators did indicate that prolonged work at high work intensities would likely be impaired given the 21% reduction in ventilation noted. Acceptable respirator resistances under the NIOSH certification criteria are measured as pressures at a steady air flow of 85 L/min.[6] Inspiratory pressure must be less than 5.0 cm H_2O for dust respirators and 8.5 cm H_2O for pesticide respirators. However, the pressure-flow characteristics of respirators are nonlinear such that resistance to flow increases steeply as flow is increased. During heavy exertion respiratory rate increases, time for inspiration is shortened, and therefore inspiratory peak flow must be increased. A significant increase in inspiratory pressure will be necessary to overcome the higher respirator resistance at these higher flows. The resulting higher pleural pressure swings may be sensed as uncomfortable by the wearer and cause intolerance to the respirator.[46] Also, persons with diseases such as emphysema that cause expiratory airflow obstruction require a greater portion of the total respiratory cycle for expiration, thereby further shortening the time for inspiration. This could result in a more pronounced effect of inspiratory resistance than would occur in a healthy individual at the same level of ventilation. Subjects with mild obstructive ventilatory impairment (mean forced expiratory volume in 1 second to forced vital capacity ratio of 0.60) showed small but statistically significant reductions in minute ventilation and elevations in end-tidal carbon dioxide concentration while walking at a moderate pace (oxygen consumption 3 to 4 times resting level) breathing through an external resistance of 5.6 cm H_2O measured at 85 L/min.[47] None of these persons reported respiratory discomfort during the exercise however. Women with mild restrictive lung disease showed no difference in heart rate or end-tidal P_{CO_2} between exercise with and without added external resistance of 5 cm H_2O on inspiration and 1.5 cm H_2O on expiration.[48] These subjects did show higher respiratory rates and lower tidal volumes than normal controls, indicating that their restrictive impairment was sufficient to influence the respiratory pattern, but adequate gas exchange was maintained.

Expiratory resistance of air-purifying respirators is generally lower than inspiratory since once the opening pressure of the expiratory valve is overcome, the airflow is relatively unimpeded. Allowable expiratory resistance is less than 2 cm H_2O. Pressure-demand atmosphere-supplying respirators may have expiratory resistances of up to 5.1 cm H_2O. The resulting increased intrathoracic pressure during expiration could impede blood return to the heart thereby reducing cardiac output. However, invasive monitoring did not show impairment of cardiac output during heavy exertion while wearing a positive pressure respirator so this consideration may not be of practical importance.[49] Thus, although the added resistance of certified respirators can produce a change in ventilatory pattern and some alteration in gas exchange, these effects are generally small at mild to moderate levels of exertion even for persons with mild obstructive or restrictive ventilatory impairment.

Respirator face masks increase the deadspace of the respiratory tract (i.e., the amount of the previously exhaled gas that is rebreathed on the subsequent inhalation). Because deadspace gas has the composition of mixed alveolar gas with a lower oxygen content and higher carbon dioxide content than fresh air, an increase in the deadspace necessitates an increase in total ventilation to maintain the same alveolar ventilation. Thus, the added deadspace of respirators could magnify the effect of added resistance by causing an increase in the total ventilation. However, not all the gas inside the face mask is rebreathed so that the effective deadspace is less than the measured volume inside the mask when in place. The effect of added deadspace will also diminish as exertion level increases with the usual concomitant increase in tidal volume. This has been demonstrated in normal volunteers exercised with 300 ml of added deadspace.[50] Also added deadspace produced little subjective response during moderate treadmill exercise in healthy volunteers.[51] Discomfort and perceived limitation of exercise duration were correlated with added resistance, especially inspiratory. Thus, deadspace effects appear to be of minor clinical significance for persons who can increase tidal volume during exertion.

Although less extensively studied than respiratory effects, cardiovascular responses to respirators have been measured during submaximal and maximal exertion. In most studies heart rates during submaximal exercise wearing a respirator or breathing through added external resistance to airflow have been similar to those during unloaded breathing.[47,48,50,52-54] Some studies have shown an increase in pulse rate during heavy exertion wearing a respirator[55] and progressive exercise to a moderate level of exertion (40% to 57% of previously measured maximal oxygen uptake) wearing a SCBA did show an increase in pulse relative to unloaded exercise at all stages.[56] The increase was approximately 18 beats per minute at the highest level of

exertion. Another study of SCBAs during exercise at 30% and 60% of maximal capacity found a heart rate increase of approximately 15 beats per minute over control exercise values and the addition of protective clothing caused a faster rise in heart rate than use of the SCBA alone.[57]

Small increases in blood pressure have been observed during respirator wear at rest and during exercise. One study reported systolic pressure increases of approximately 12 mm Hg with a smaller rise in diastolic pressure.[52] Wearing a disposable respirator did not affect blood pressure at light or moderate exertion (up to 50% of maximal oxygen consumption) but was associated with an approximately 20 mm Hg average rise in systolic pressure and 10 mm Hg rise in diastolic pressure at higher work rates.[55] These elevations were not sustained during recovery from exercise. Another study showed no significant effect on blood pressure of wearing an SCBA in healthy young men exercised to maximal capacity.[54] Thus, the direct effect of respirator wear on blood pressure is generally small, but the combined effects of high exertion or protective clothing while wearing a respirator could induce a clinically important increase in blood pressure.

Despite the lack of major effects on gas exchange or cardiovascular response to exercise, added resistance to breathing or use of SCBAs generally reduces maximal work performance of healthy individuals.[33,54,58,59] Respirator wear decreases the duration that very strenuous exertion can be maintained and reduces the maximal oxygen consumption attainable. This does not appear to be due to a reduction in cardiac output.[49] Maximal lactate levels and those at 2 minutes postexercise for progressive work to exhaustion were unaffected by use of 3 types of air-purifying cannisters indicating no significant impairment of oxygen delivery.[45] The subjective discomfort and increased work of breathing caused by the added resistance are likely the major factors for air-purifying respirators. For SCBA the restrictive effect of the chest harness[56] and the added weight are felt to be important in reducing maximal performance by up to 20%.[54]

Respirators may also impede the worker's ability to perform certain psychomotor tasks, e.g., movements requiring accurate control for positioning of objects or steadiness of work.[60] Performance was adversely affected by wearing a disposable dust mask or half-mask air-purifying respirator as well as by a full-face airline mask. There was no significant effect on cognitive tasks. Field testing of a full-face gas mask showed it interfered with performance of a digit-marking task by impeding vision and coordination but not with memory or concentration.[45] The performance decrement did not change over a 22.5-hour period in these military personnel who had had no prior experience with respirator use. Postural sway was also increased by use of a full facepiece respirator when measured after light to heavy exertion.[61] Thus, the potential hazard of interference with vision and motor skills must be considered when evaluating the risk of respirator use in the workplace. Reduction in auditory acuity and interference with speech may also be important considerations if the respirator is to be used in emergency situations.

WORKER TOLERANCE OF RESPIRATORS

A worker's ability to tolerate a respirator depends on the interaction between the psychophysiologic effects of the respirator and the physical and psychologic characteristics of the individual.[62] Federal regulations require that a respirator user "shall not experience undue discomfort because of airflow restriction"[6] and physiologic research has centered on investigation of which effects appear to correlate with intolerable discomfort. Added resistance to breathing will increase the intrapleural and intraairway pressure swings during breathing if flow rates and total ventilation are maintained near unloaded levels. When a certain threshold pressure is exceeded, the individual may experience an unpleasant sensation sufficient to cause an inability to tolerate the respirator. Approximately 10% of men exercising with added inspiratory resistance experienced an unpleasant awareness of breathing when peak inspiratory pressure exceeded 14 cm H_2O.[63] Breathing patterns adopted during exercise with resistive loads may vary between individuals depending on load sensitivity but limitation of peak pressure may be an important determinant.[64,65] Persons with a limited ability to alter their breathing pattern or with high load sensitivity may experience greater subjective discomfort and thereby be less capable of tolerating the resistive load of respirators.[46,66] At higher levels of exertion, respiratory pattern adjustment is more limited due to the need for increasing ventilation, and this may further decrease tolerance for persons with high load sensitivity. Interpersonal differences in load sensitivity are relatively large and thus may account for some of the variability in respirator tolerance among healthy persons.[67] Powered air-purifying respirators can theoretically decrease the resistive effects of the filter but may not effectively lower the magnitude of negative inspiratory pressures during exercise[68] or improve subjective comfort compared with nonpowered cartridge type respirators.[69]

Individual psychologic characteristics have also been implicated as predictors of respirator tolerance.[70] A sense of claustrophobia may lead to severe hyperventilation and intolerance. Behavioral modification therapy has been successful in alleviating this problem.[71] Trait anxiety, a measure of proneness to develop anxiety when stressed, was found to be highly predictive of distress while exercising with a respirator in a study of six subjects.[72] However, other personal characteristics that might confound the association were not discussed and trait anxiety was not correlated with degree of respiratory discomfort during actual work wearing air-purifying or airline respirators.[73] The most bothersome aspects of the respirators reported by the users were thermal effects and the added weight. As noted above, discomfort

from local thermal effects of the facepiece as well as increased overall heat stress may be important factors in respirator tolerance in addition to resistive loading effects.[22-24]

Added external resistance reduces the maximal voluntary ventilation (MVV) measured at rest in healthy persons and more so in individuals with conditions causing airflow limitation.[74] Reductions of 18% to 32% in MVV were demonstrated with resistances of 8.5 cm H_2O on inspiration and 2.5 cm H_2O on expiration at 85 L/min flow rate. The proportional reduction in ventilation during exercise with resistance was similar.[37] An individual's MVV with a respirator has been suggested as a measure that would be helpful in predicting the person's capacity for use of the respirator.[75] However, subjective effects are not necessarily closely correlated with objective physiologic changes[46,69] and thus measures of the physiologic response to added loads may not be highly predictive of tolerance. In one study reduction in physiologic effects by using a powered air-purifying respirator did not produce significant subjective benefit measured on visual analog scales.[69] Also, adaption to respirators allowing increased tolerance may occur without changes in objective physiologic measures. Young physically fit men were able to increase their running time to exhaustion while wearing a respirator by approximately 50% over a 6-day period but physiologic variables including heart rate and ventilatory measures were either unchanged or minimally altered.[76] Indeed, MVV with the respirator at rest was only weakly predictive of maximal work performance,[77] and thus this measure is not likely to be sufficient to judge a worker's capacity for respirator use.

Because many factors influence the ability to tolerate a respirator no single test is likely to be sufficiently predictive. As discussed, relevant considerations include the direct effects of the respirator (cardiopulmonary, local thermal, and interference with sensations and skilled motor functions) as well as the worker's psychologic sensitivity and response to these effects. His or her beliefs and motivation concerning respirator use are also important. Formal testing of individual workers in each of these areas is not feasible nor would it produce a reliable index of tolerance given the uncertainties in our current understanding of the interaction of these factors. Therefore, use of overall clinical judgment is still necessary. A practical approach is to perform basic medical screening to rule out the presence of clear contraindications to the proposed use and to identify the need for any restrictions during a trial of use. Follow-up of any difficulties that occur during the trial period is then a necessary component of the overall evaluation process.

MEDICAL EVALUATION FOR RESPIRATOR USE

The purpose of medical evaluation is to identify individuals for whom respirator use may pose an unacceptable risk to health or safety. General principles regarding evaluation for placement are discussed in Chapter 52. As discussed above, this risk may be caused by the additional stresses imposed by the respirator itself or by the working conditions requiring respirator use. The interaction between these two factors must be considered in assessing the overall stress for the worker.[28] Detailed discussions and recommendations of professional medical and safety organizations have been published.[78-82] However, substantial uncertainty regarding the necessary medical evaluation and criteria for authorization of a trial of use is still present. Although respirators do impose additional stresses, with certain exceptions these stresses are not likely to result in an unacceptable risk if the worker is otherwise medically qualified to perform the job. If the work to be done while wearing the respirator is significantly more stressful than other aspects of the job, the evaluating physician must consider the worker's fitness for this activity, not just for the ability to safely tolerate the respirator.

A screening questionnaire can be used to identify known medical conditions or symptoms that may necessitate restrictions or require further evaluation. Any previous difficulty using a respirator or worker concerns about his or her ability to tolerate the proposed use should be identified and evaluated. Feelings of claustrophobia or hyperventilation while wearing a facemask should be specifically queried. Also, skin conditions or sensitivities to the facepiece materials that may pose difficulties wearing tight fitting masks should be identified.

Breathlessness with exertion equivalent to that proposed during respirator use should be identified. For respirator use in IDLH environments or for emergency and rescue operations where even brief removal might be hazardous, questions on cough, phlegm, and episodic wheezing are relevant. Information concerning known cardiovascular impairments and symptoms suggestive of ischemic heart disease such as exertional chest pain should be obtained. More detailed questions are appropriate for use of SCBAs and when strenuous exertion or heat stress is to be present while wearing the respirator. Musculoskeletal impairments may be important factors if SCBAs are to be used or the work requires a high degree of agility. Queries about visual and auditory impairments may be relevant if these senses are critical for safety on the job, but use of glasses or contact lenses can usually be accommodated. General medical problems such as hypertension, diabetes, or seizure disorders should be identified. By themselves they are not absolute contraindications for respirator use,[81] but they may be relevant to the consideration of capacity for tolerating overall job stress or for fitness for certain tasks.

Clinical judgment should be applied to determine if a physical examination is required. Measurement of blood pressure and pulse is a basic health screen that is useful, especially if the job may require moderate or greater exertion. However, except for use of SCBAs, work in highly stressful conditions or with strenuous exertion, or the presence of responses on the screening questionnaire indicating possible pertinent abnormalities, a direct examination by a physician may not be necessary.

Pulmonary function testing is useful in estimating a worker's overall fitness for the demands of work requiring a respirator, but by itself is not predictive of respirator tolerance. Resting electrocardiograms are of little value in identifying ischemic heart disease and exercise testing is probably necessary only for older workers using SCBAs or performing strenuous work. The predictive power of this test for identifying workers at risk has, however, not been validated.[79] If the worker has demonstrated the ability to tolerate similar levels of exertion in other job situations, formal exercise will probably be of marginal value. Clinicians will need to apply individual judgment for workers with risk factors such as a family history of ischemic heart disease.

Hearing and visual acuity should be measured if these senses are especially critical to the work situation, e.g., for members of rescue teams.

After the initial evaluation workers can be categorized as unfit for any use of respirators, fit for all proposed uses, or restricted in some way. With the exception of SCBAs with the attendant cardiovascular stress of added weight, a trial of respirator use will seldom be completely contraindicated if the worker is otherwise fit for the work. Certain findings such as history of a pneumothorax or a perforated tympanic membrane are no longer felt to be contraindications for respirator use.[79,83] In most instances a trial of respirator use can be authorized if adequate provisions are made for detecting and evaluating any difficulties experienced by the worker. Use of the respirator in simulated working conditions under direct observation may be useful if the possibility of significant risk is present but not definite.

Periodic reevaluation is necessary, but the optimal frequency has not been determined. For younger workers without significant health problems, reassessment each 2 to 5 years may be adequate depending on conditions of use. For older workers or for use of SCBA, yearly reevaluation may be prudent. An update of the screening questionnaire with further examination only if significant changes in symptoms or medical status are noted may be sufficient. Overall, although many uncertainties are present, certification for a trial of respirator use should not require complex testing and should be based on a clinical judgment of whether the worker would be at risk for serious or irreversible harm if any difficulties were to be encountered during use. If not, a trial is warranted with procedures in place to ensure identification and evaluation of any problems that do arise.

SUMMARY

Respirators are often a necessary component of respiratory protection, but should be considered only when reduction of exposure through other means is not feasible. Administrative procedures must be established to ensure proper selection and maintenance of respirators as well as worker fitness evaluation and training. The added physiologic and psychologic stress of work requiring respirator use must be considered in determining the worker's fitness for a trial of use. However, because of the multiple factors influencing tolerance, no absolute criteria for fitness are available, and overall clinical judgment must be used.

REFERENCES

1. U.S. Code of Federal Regulations, Title 29, Part 1910.134(A) (1), Respiratory Protection.
2. Pritchard JA: *A guide to industrial respiratory protection,* NIOSH, 76-189, Washington, DC, 1976, U.S. Department of Health, Education, and Welfare.
3. Douglas D: Respiratory protective devices. In Clayton GD and Clayton FE, editors: *Patty's industrial hygiene and toxicology,* New York, 1985, John Wiley.
4. Lundin A: Respiratory protective equipment, In Olishifski JB, editor: *Fundamentals of industrial hygiene,* Chicago, 1979, National Safety Council.
5. Olishifiski JB: Elements of respiratory protection. In Zenz C, ed: *Occupational medicine: principles and practical applications,* ed 2, pp 53-58, Chicago, 1988, Year Book Medical Publishers.
6. U.S. code of Federal Regulations, Title 30, Part II, Respiratory Protective Devices; Tests for Permissibility; Fees.
7. Moyer ES: Review of influential factors affecting the performance of organic vapor air-purifying respirator cartridges, *Am Ind Hyg Assoc J* 44:45, 1983.
8. NIOSH Respirator Decision Logic—DHHS (NIOSH) Pub No 87-108, US Dept Health and Human Services, Centers for Disease Control, 1987.
9. American National Standard Practices for Respiratory Protection, Z88.2-1992, American National Standards Institute, New York, 1992.
10. Dahlback GO and Novak L: Do pressure-demand breathing systems safeguard against inward leakage? *Am Ind Hyg Assoc J* 44(5):336-340, 1983.
11. 29 CFR 1910.1001(g) Asbestos; 29 CFR 1910.1028(g) Benzene; 29 CFR 1910.1048(g) Formaldehyde; 29 CFR 1910.120(5) Hazardous waste; 29 CFR 1910.1025(f) Lead.
12. NIOSH: *Pocket guide to chemical hazards,* U.S. Dept Health & Human Services, 1985.
13. Hyatt EC: Respirator protection factors. Los Alamos Scientific Laboratory Report, 1976 Jan, #LA-6084-MS.
14. Myers WR, Peach MJ, Cutright K, and Iskander W: Workplace protection factor measurements on powered air-purifying respirators at a secondary lead smelter—results and discussion, *Am Ind Hyg Assoc J* 45(10):681-688, 1984.
15. Dixon SW and Nelson TJ: Workplace protection factors for negative pressure half-mask facepiece respirators, *J Int Soc Respir Protect* 2(4):347-361, 1984.
16. Henry M, Villa M, Hubert G, and Martin P: Assessment of the performance of respirators in the workplace, *Ann Occup Hyg* 35(2):181-7, 1991.
17. Hack AL, Bradley OD, and Trujillo A: Respirator protection factors: part II—protection factors of supplied air respirators, *Am Ind Hyg Assoc J* 41:376, 1980.
18. Crutchfield CD and VanErt MD: An examination of issues affecting the current state of quantitative respirator fit testing, *J Int Soc Respir Protect* Summer 5-18, 1993.
19. Stobbe TJ, daRoza RA, and Watkins MA: Facial hair and respirator fit: a review of the literature, *Am Ind Hyg Assoc J* 49(4):199-204, 1988.
20. Cotes JE: Advances in respiratory protection (conference report), *Ann Occup Hyg* 22:189, 1979.
21. Leving M: Respirator use and protection from exposure to carbon monoxide, *Am Ind Hyg Assoc J* 40:832, 1979.
22. Gwosdow AR, Nielsen R, Berglund LG, DuBois AB, and Tremml PG: Effect of thermal conditions in the acceptability of respiratory protective devices on humans at rest, *Am Ind Hyg Assoc J* 50(4):188-195, 1989.
23. DuBois AB, Harb ZF, and Fox SH: Thermal discomfort of respiratory protective devices, *Am Ind Hyg Assoc J* 51(10):550-554, 1990.
24. Fox SH and Du Bois AB: The effect of evaporative cooling of respiratory protective devices on skin temperature, thermal sensation, and comfort, *Am Ind Hyg Assoc J* 54(12):705-710, 1993.
25. White MC, Baker EL, Larson MB, and Wolford R: The role of personal beliefs and social influences as determinants of respirator use among construction painters, *Scand J Work Environ Health* 14(4):239-245, 1988.
26. Raven PB, Dodson AT, and Davis TO: The physiologic consequences of wearing industrial respirators: a review, *Am Ind Hyg Assoc J* 40:517, 1979.
27. Harber P, Brown CL, and Beck JG: Respirator physiology research: answers in search of the question, *J Occup Med* 33(1):38-44, 1991.
28. Louhevaara V: Respirator wearer's strain: a complex problem, *Am J Ind Med* 10:3-6, 1986.
29. Zechman F, Hall FG, and Hull WE: Effects of graded resistance to tracheal air flow in man, *J Appl Physiol* 10:356, 1957.
30. Gee JB, L Burton G, Vassallo C, and Gregg J: Effects of external airway obstruction on work capacity and pulmonary gas exchange, *Am Rev Respir Dis* 98:1003, 1968.
31. Cerretelli P, Sikand RS, and Farhi LE: Effect of increased airway resistance on ventilation and gas exchange during exercise, *J Appl Physiol* 27:597, 1969.
32. Tabakin BS and Hanson JS: Lung volume and ventilatory response to airway obstruction during treadmill exercise, *J Appl Physiol* 20:168, 1965.
33. Louhevarra V, Tuomi T, Kornhonen O, and Jaakkola J: Cardiorespiratory effects of respiratory protective devices during exercise in well-trained men, *Eur J Appl Phys* 52:340-345, 1984.
34. Lerman Y, Sherfer A, Epstein Y, et al: External inspiratory resistance of protective respiratory devices: effects on physical performance and respiratory function, *Am J Ind Med* 4:733-740, 1983.
35. Tabakin BS and Hanson JS: Response to ventilatory obstruction during steady-state exercise, *J Appl Physiol* 15:579, 1960.
36. Demedts M and Anthonisen NR: Effects of increased external airway resistance during steady-state exercise, *J Appl Physiol* 35:361, 1973.
37. Flook V and Kelman GR: Submaximal exercise with increased inspiratory resistance to breathing, *J Appl Physiol* 35:379, 1973.
38. Silverman L and Billings CE: Pattern of airflow in the respiratory tract. In Davis CN editor: *Inhaled particles and vapours,* pp 9-46, New York, 1961, Pergamon Press.
39. Thompson SH and Sharkey BJ: Physiological cost and air flow resistance of respiratory protective devices, *Ergonomics* 9:495, 1966.
40. Cherniack RM and Snidal DP: The effect of obstruction of breathing on the ventilatory response to CO_2, *J Clin Invest* 35:1286, 1956.
41. Milic-Emili J and Tyler JM: Relation between work output of respiratory muscles and end-tidal CO_2 tension, *J Appl Physiol* 18:497, 1963.
42. Clark TJH and Cochrane GM: Effect of mechanical loading on ventilatory response to CO_2 and CO_2 excretion, *Br Med J* 1:351, 1972.
43. Flenley DC, Pengelly LD, and Milic-Emili J: Immediate effects of positive-pressure breathing on the ventilatory response to CO_2, *J Appl Physiol* 30:7, 1971.
44. Deno NS, Kamon E, and Kiser DM: Physiological responses to resistance breathing during short and prolonged exercise, *Am Ind Hyg Assoc J* 42:616-623, 1981.
45. Jette M, Thoden J, and Livingstone S: Physiological effects of inspiratory resistance on progressive aerobic work, *Eur J Appl Physiol* 60(1):65-70, 1990.
46. Harber P, Shimozaki S, Barrett T, and Loisides P: Relationship of sub-

jective tolerance of respirator loads to physiologic effects and psychophysiological load sensitivity, *J Occup Med* 31(8):681-686, 1989.

47. Hodous T, Petsonk EL, Boyles C, et al: Effects of added resistance to breathing during exercise in obstructive lung disease, *Am Rev Respir Dis* 128:943, 1983.

48. Hodous TK, Boyles C, and Hankinson J: Effects of industrial respiratory wear during exercise in subjects with restrictive lung disease, *Am Ind Hyg Assoc J* 47(3):176-180, 1986.

49. Arborelius M, Dahlback GO, and Data PC: Cardiac output and gas exchange during heavy exercise with a positive pressure respiratory protective apparatus, *Scand J Work Environ Health* 9:471-477, 1983.

50. Harber P, Shimozaki S, Barrett T, Losides P, and Fine G: Effects of respirator dead space, inspiratory resistance, and expiratory resistance ventilatory loads, *Am J Ind Med* 16:189-198, 1989.

51. Shimozaki S, Harber P, Barrett T, and Loisides P: Subjective tolerance of respirator loads and its relationship to physiological effects, *Am Ind Hyg Assoc J* 49(3):108-16, 1988.

52. Raven PB, Jackson AW, Page K, et al: The physiologic responses of mild pulmonary impaired subjects while using a "demand" respirator during rest and work, *Am Ind Hyg Assoc J* 42:247, 1981.

53. Harber P, Tamimie J, Emory J, Bhattacharya A, and Barber M: Effects of exercise using industrial respirators, *Am Ind Hyg Assoc J* 45(9):603-609, 1984.

54. Raven PB, Davis TO, Shafer CL, and Linnebur AC: Maximal stress test performance while wearing a self-contained breathing apparatus, *J Occup Med* 19(2):803-806, 1977.

55. Jones JG: The physiological cost of wearing a disposable respirator, *Am Ind Hyg Assoc J* 52(6):219-225, 1991.

56. Louhevaara V, Smolander J, Tuomi T, Korhonew O, and Jaakkola J: Effects of an SCBA on breathing pattern, gas exchange, and heart rate during exercise, *J Occup Med* 27(3):213-216, 1985.

57. White MK, Vercruyssen M, and Hodous TK: Work tolerance and subjective responses to wearing protective clothing and respirators during physical work, *Ergonomics* 32(9):1111-1123, 1989.

58. Wilson JR, Raven PB, Morgan WP, Zinkgraf SA, and Garmon RG: Jackson AW. Effects of pressure-demand respirator wear on physiological and perceptual variables during progressive exercise to maximal levels, *Am Ind Hyg Assoc J* 50:85-94, 1989.

59. Louheevaara V, Smolander J, Korhonen O, and Tuomi T: Maximal working times with a self-contained breathing apparatus, *Ergonomics* 29:77-85, 1986.

60. Zimmerman NG, Eberts C, Salvendy G, and McCabe G: Effects of respirators on performance of physical, psychomotor and cognitive tasks, *Ergonomics* 34(3):321-334, 1991.

61. Seliga R, Bhattacharya A, Succop P, Wickstrom R, Smith D, and Willeke K: Effect of work load and respirator wear on postural stability, heart rate, and perceived exertion, *Am Ind Hyg Assoc J* 52(10):417-422, 1991.

62. Beckett WS and Billings CE: Individual factors in the choice of respiratory protective devices, *Am Ind Hyg Assoc J* 46:274-276, 1985.

63. Bentley RA, Griffin OG, Love RG, et al: Acceptable levels for breathing resistance of respiratory apparatus, *Arch Environ Health* 27:273, 1973.

64. Harber P, Shimozaki S, Barrette T, and Fine G: Determinants of pattern of breathing during respirator use, *Am J Ind Med* 13(2):253-262, 1988.

65. Yasukouchi A: Breathing pattern and subjective responses to small inspiratory resistance during submaximal exercise, *Ann Physiol Anthropol* 11(3):191-201, 1992.

66. Harber P, Shimozaki S, Barrett T, and Fine G: Effect of exercise level on ventilatory adaptation to respirator use, *J Occup Med* 32(10):1042-1046, 1990.

67. Harber P, SooHoo K, and Lew M: Effects of industrial respirators on respiratory timing and psychophysiologic load sensitivity, *J Occup Med* 30(3):256-262, 1988.

68. Arad M, Heruti R, Shaham E, Atsmon J, and Epstein Y: The effects of powered air supply to the respiratory protective device on respiration parameters during rest and exercise, *Chest* 102(6):1800-1804, 1992.

69. Harber P, Beck J, Brown C, and Luo J: Physiologic and subjective effects of respirator mask type, *Am Ind Hyg Assoc J* 52(9):357-362, 1991.

70. Morgan WP: Psychological problems associated with the wearing of industrial respirators: a review, *Am Ind Hyg Assoc J* 44:671-676, 1983.

71. Ritchie EC: Treatment of gas mask phobia, *Mil Med* 157(2):104-106, 1992.

72. Morgan WP and Raven PB: Prediction of distress for individuals wearing industrial respirators, *Am Ind Hyg Assoc J* 46(7)363-368, 1985.

73. Hodous TK, Hankinson JL, and Stark GP: Workplace measurement of respirator effects using respiratory inductive plethysmography, *Am Ind Hyg Assoc J* 50(7):372-378, 1989.

74. Awi S, Theron JC, McGregor M, and Becklake MR: The influence of instrumental resistance on the maximum breathing capacity, *Dis Chest* 36:361, 1959.

75. Raven PB, Moss RF, Page K, et al: Clinical pulmonary function and industrial respirator wear, *Am Ind Hyg Assoc J* 42:897, 1981.

76. Epstein J, Keren G, Lerman Y, and Shefer A: Physiological & psychological adaptation to respiratory protective devices, *Aviat Space Environ Med* 53(7):663-665, 1982.

77. Wilson JR and Raven PB: Clinical pulmonary function tests as predictors of work performance during respirator wear, *Am Ind Hyg Assoc J* 50(1):51-57, 1989.

78. Harber P: Medical evaluation for respirator use, *J Occup Med* 26:496-502, 1984.

79. Hodous TK: Screening prospective workers for the ability to use respirators, *J Occup Med* 28:1074-1080, 1986.

80. Beckett WS: Certifying the worker for respirator use, *Sem Occup Med* 1(2):119-124, 1986.

81. Committee on Occupational Medical Practice-American Occupational Medicine Association: Guidelines for respirator users, *J Occup Med* 28(1):72-72, 1986.

82. Kraut A: Industrial respirators: certifying the worker, *Am Fam Phys* 37:117-126, 1988.

83. Ronk R and White MK: Hydrogen sulfide and the probabilities of "inhalation" through a tympanic membrane defect, *J Occup Med* 27(2):337-340, 1985.

Chapter 60

EXPOSURE CONTROLS IN WORKPLACES

Paul A. Jensen
Dennis M. O'Brien

Prevention of occupational exposure to hazards and potential hazards should be considered at the early stages of process design. Certain basic principles of control apply in every case, but the optimum practice of these principles varies from case to case. In principle, controls may be applied at the source of the hazard, to the general workplace environment, and at the point of exposure of the individual employee. Adjunct control principles include monitoring of processes, controls and workplace and exposure levels, education, and effective management. In practice the selection of an optimum control strategy involves a system of interrelated control measures. Factors that dictate the selection of an optimum occupational health control strategy include economics, product parameters, and environmental pollution constraints. Major decisions must often be made between retrofitting existing plants and building new ones in developing a control strategy. The latter option often offers unique opportunities to design around hazards in a cost-effective manner.

Most basic to the control of any hazard is the concept that it can be controlled. Once the hazard is defined properly and the need for and the degree of necessary controls are determined, then the only requirements are imagination, trained personnel, and money to put the control methods to work.[1] The basic engineering principles for controlling the occupational environment consist of substitution, isolation, and ventilation. Not all control principles are applicable to every form of hazard, but all occupational hazards can be controlled by the use of at least one of these principles. Ingenuity, experience, and a complete understanding of the circumstances surrounding the control problem are required in choosing methods that will not only provide adequate control but that will consider installation, operating and maintenance costs, and personal factors such as employee acceptance, comfort, and convenience. Furthermore, hazards, costs, and benefits can change with time; hence, hazard control systems need continuous review and updating. The aim, then, must be not only to devise efficient hazard control methods but to evaluate the effectiveness of those methods at regular intervals.

PREREQUISITES TO CONTROL

The objective of a business involved in providing goods or services is to produce a product that meets certain quality requirements in such a way as to produce an acceptable return on the resources invested for production. A business must also do this in a manner that is safe from an occupational and environmental viewpoint. Decisions regarding control technology for safeguarding worker health cannot be made outside of the context of product parameters, environmental effects, and cost. Although these factors are not discussed in detail in this chapter, their importance is implicit in selecting optimum control strategies for preventing or controlling occupational exposure problems. In general, these factors will dictate the extent to which major investments are made for constructing new plants, for developing new or substantially modified process technology, and for providing "add-on" controls.

Industrial hygiene focuses upon the recognition, evaluation, and control of occupational health hazards. Industrial hygiene is discussed in more detail in Chapters 10 and 11. Proper recognition and evaluation are prerequisites to control. For example, it is very important to consider not only materials that are present as major raw materials but also chemical intermediates and by-products of the process. The formation of by-product nitrosamines through reaction of nitrates and organic amines,[2] the emission of pyrolysis products from metal casting operations,[3] the production of excessive carbon monoxide by diesel engines from rebreathing CO_2-laden exhaust,[4] and the production of nickel carbonyl in nickel-containing process equipment under reducing conditions are all examples of "nonobvious" hazards.[5] Hazards such as these may be overlooked either because of difficulty in predicting their presence at all or difficulty in analyzing for specific components.

Other factors that are important in recognizing and evaluating hazards include the inherent toxicity, route of exposure, physical state of both pure components and mixtures, and other related properties (vapor pressure, solubility in water and lipid tissues, and stability). Numerous resources are available in evaluating hazards,[6-10] but the essential ingredient in this process is the judgment of an experienced professional industrial hygienist. Some attempts have been made to develop a quantified hazard index using a variety of factors.[11]

Sentinel markers to identify sites at high risk for a catastrophic leak, explosion, or other disaster can be classified as administrative, information, technology and systems, transportation, and community emergency response in nature. Typical administrative sentinel markers include weak occupational safety and health programs, nonavailability or nonaccessibility of first aid stations, back up and hospital referral systems, and evacuation systems; lack of information concerning near accidents, low level exposures, or maintenance deterioration; lack of written disaster plans, punishment of troublesome individuals who report problems (whistleblowers), and not taking responsibility for subcontractors. Typical information sentinel markers include the absence of worker and community "right to know" programs about potential hazards associated with the processes, products, and technology used, nonuse of data on earlier accidents using similar technologies, and failure to provide hospitals, clinics, and other medical facilities with toxico-

logic data. Technology and systems sentinel markers consist of a lack of fail safe hazard controls and interlock systems and computerized early warning systems and nonuse of risk minimization principles such as substituting toxic substances in process lines with less toxic substances. Transportation sentinel markers include suboptimal vehicle standards and lack of programs for identifying drivers at high risk for accidents because of drug or alcohol use, driving long hours, or driving at high speeds. Community emergency response sentinel markers consist of a lack of preparation for disasters and an absence of a hospital and regional medical network for treating injuries and evaluating exposed persons.

PRINCIPLES OF CONTROL

Occupational exposures can be controlled by the application of a number of well-known principles.[1] These principles may be applied at or near the hazard source, to the general workplace environment, or at the point of occupational exposure to individual workers. Controls applied at the source of the hazard, including material substitution, process and equipment modification, isolation of processes, local exhaust ventilation, work practices, or any combination thereof, are generally the preferred and most effective means of control both in terms of occupational and environmental concerns. Controls applied to hazards that have escaped into the general workplace environment include general dilution ventilation and housekeeping. Control measures applied near or by individual workers include worker isolation, work practices, and personal protective equipment.

These principles apply to all situations, although the optimum application of the principles varies from case to case. Existing processes can be roughly categorized by degree of automation or labor intensity. In general, processes that are continuous and automated involve fewer employees with less uncontrolled exposures. For example, high volume organic and petrochemical manufacturing represent highly automated continuous processes. Metal casting, meat processing, and paint pigment packaging and formulating are typically more labor-intensive, less automated, and often batch processes and operators with associated higher exposure potential.

In typical bulk organic or petrochemical processes, emissions or exposure points occur as materials are added at the "front end" of the process, taken out at the "back end" of the process, at process leak points, and during maintenance procedures in between.[12] In general, small jobbing foundries are often near the other end of the spectrum in terms of degree of automation and intensity of labor interaction with the process.[13]

CONTROL AT THE SOURCE

Prevention of occupational exposure by control at the source of the hazard is generally preferred. The following discussion describes six approaches to controlling exposure at the source.

Substitution

Substitution of less hazardous materials or process equipment, or even of a less hazardous process, may be the least expensive as well as the most positive method of controlling an occupational hazard. However, when one thinks of controlling a hazard, often the first thing to come to mind is adding something to do the controlling. For example, some engineers may be more likely to think of controlling a vapor hazard by ventilation than by substituting a less hazardous material for the one that is causing the problem.

One method of prevention at the source involves substitution of a nonhazardous or less hazardous material for the substance of concern. Material substitution offers the intrinsic advantage of completely removing a more hazardous material from the workplace and replacing it with a less hazardous material. However, the ability to find suitable substitutes for a given material is by no means certain, and the substitute materials will also present a certain degree of hazard. The application of control measures may, therefore, be necessary even after a safer substitute has been found. Thorough testing for a variety of toxic effects is extremely important in selecting substitute materials that are indeed of low toxicity.

Selection of substitution as a control option can depend on the importance of the final product under question as well as the availability, substitutability, and cost of alternatives. Occupational exposure to highly toxic product ingredients or solvents is commonly controlled by substitution. A classic example of the substitution of a relatively inert substance for a highly toxic material is the use of titanium dioxide in place of white lead pigments in paints. Titanium dioxide has the additional advantage of lower cost. To compensate for increased costs associated with exactly matching lead-containing colored pigments with lead-free pigments, product color may be changed to browns, blues, violets, whites, grays, blacks, or certain shades of gray that can be made economically with lead-free pigments.[14] Several alternatives also exist for either the reduction or elimination of organic solvents in industrial finishing by the use of water-based finishes, nonaqueous dispersions, and changes in coating techniques such as high solids or powder coating techniques. Each of these options possesses a unique set of advantages and disadvantages. In general, the greater the deviation from the original formulation, the more other product parameters (such as polymer chain length in paint formulations) must be varied to compensate. Powder coating technology, which omits solvents altogether, is a sufficiently great deviation from standard solvent-based coating so as to be essentially an altogether different coating procedure. In general, the more critical the product performance characteristics, the more challenging substitution becomes as a control option.

Process modification

Process modification is a second method of controlling hazards at the source. Older processes often were not designed to meet existing or proposed occupational health standards. A reevaluation of process options with occupational health requirements included as a constraint will often identify process modifications as effective control measures, particularly with the additional option of varying the relative amounts of labor (or capital) in light of current labor or capital costs. In general, processes that are continuous, as opposed to intermittent or batch, are likely to be less hazardous from an occupational exposure standpoint. Processes should be designed to contain hazardous materials within sealed or enclosed equipment to the greatest extent possible, and to minimize the potential for emissions to the workplace.

Process modification can range from large-scale, expensive development of fundamental new process technology such as hydrometallurgy to much smaller scale process modification such as changes to powder coating or submerged arc welding. In many cases, changes in process chemistry can minimize the presence of unwanted toxic by-products. For example, a runaway chemical reaction occurred in Bhopal, India resulting in the release of methyl isocyanate, which killed and injured thousands of people, animals, and plants. Methyl isocyanate was an intermediate product (manufactured and stored in large quantities) that was later processed into carbaryl pesticide. Risk of catastrophic incident could have been reduced by either modifying the batch process to a continuous process without the production of methyl isocyanate *or* minimizing the quantity of methyl isocyanate on site.[15-17]

Another effective control measure by process modification involves the use of additives to furniture stripping solutions to reduce the rate of evaporation. The addition of parafin wax, disolved in xylene, to a mixture of methylene chloride and methanol significantly reduces the workers' exposure to these solvent vapors.[18]

Equipment modification

Equipment modification or substitution is a commonly used means of control. Modification of pieces of process equipment that present particularly serious exposure problems is usually a less drastic change than modifying an entire process. Clearly, the requirements for efficient equipment substitution or modification include an awareness of alternatives as well as a thorough understanding of the existing equipment. Modifications are often made on a trial-and-error basis. Equipment should be redesigned to contain hazardous materials within the equipment, to avoid the introduction of material or energy hazards to the workplace, and to require minimal maintenance. When maintenance is required, the equipment design should permit its performance with minimal hazard to the workers involved (e.g., the design might permit remote decontamination prior to disassembly for maintenance).

In spray finishing operations, airless or electrostatic spray guns can often be substituted for conventional compressed air spray equipment. Airless spray coating equipment produces much less fine spray than conventional compressed air equipment. Other advantages of airless or high pressure spraying include high capacity, compatibility with high solids coating, and adequate coverage of awkward shapes. The chief advantage of electrostatic spraying is the improved working environment and the paint economy achieved. Electrostatic systems usually permit use of substantially less exhaust and make-up air than conventional compressed air spraying for the same painted surface area due to the reduced overspray. This technique also provides significant wrap around, coats sharp edges, and can be automated.[19]

Isolation of process

Isolation of stored materials, of equipment, and of the process is a fourth means of controlling hazards at the source. Isolation involves the use of a barrier between a hazard source and those who might be affected by the hazard. The barrier may be provided by a physical structure or by distance. Physical enclosure normally requires ventilation of the enclosed area to avoid buildup of toxic and/or explosive materials. Limiting employee access to certain areas during hazardous operations may also be an effective means of isolation. Computerized process control, automation of various production and maintenance procedures, and the general concept of remote processing also help to isolate processes and equipment. Potential problems involved with isolation include remote measurement of process parameters for the purpose of process control, accessibility of equipment for maintenance, and the potential for exposure of workers during maintenance operations.

Process automation and isolation are often objectives that are achieved through process modification. Automated submerged arc welding or automated dip-painting operations are examples of process modification that also achieve isolation of the worker from the hazard.

Processes or equipment are isolated through a number of techniques in many bulk organic or petrochemical processes. One technique is the use of computers for process control. This technique allows a reduction in employee exposure because (1) the number of operators required to run the process is decreased, (2) the operators spend a significant amount of time in an enclosed control room (where exposure is essentially zero), and (3) operators do not have extensive interaction with the process, which eliminates errors and the concomitant exposures. Thus, the number of exposed employees, the amount of time spent in a potentially hazardous area, and the likelihood of a significant release of toxic chemicals are all reduced.

A second isolation technique is the use of physical barriers or distance to isolate equipment that is particularly likely to develop leaks or normally emit material. Limiting employee access to certain areas during particularly hazardous operation may also be used. Pumps, compressors, or other failure-prone pieces of process equipment are often located outdoors or isolated in ventilated enclosures.

Automation of high production gray iron melting operations has permitted isolation of the operators in booths during the majority of the workshift and control of air contaminants at the source. Exhaust hoods are used on charge bucket filling, preheating, and furnace operations. The combination of exhaust ventilation controls and worker isolation may be sufficient to control dust and metal fume exposures to below the allowable limits. Heat stress may be reduced and worker comfort improved by the use of remotely controlled mechanisms for slagging of large ladles. This method isolates the worker at a distance from the heat source and shortens the time to complete the process.[7]

The finish on the furniture (e.g., paint, varnish, lacquer, or polyurethane) is normally manually stripped in an uncontrolled or minimally controlled environment, using organic solvents. A unique enclosed, automated furniture stripping spray system allowed exposures to methylene chloride to be reduced using this equipment by an order of magnitude compared to conventional stripping processes.[20]

Local exhaust ventilation

A fifth means of controlling the source of emissions is local exhaust ventilation. Local exhaust ventilation involves a directed flow of air across an emission point and into a capture hood and ductwork system. Hood design depends on the physical configuration of the process equipment and emissions characteristics. Designs may range from exterior (free standing) hoods to complete process enclosure. Sufficient air flow is necessary to capture and convey the material of concern into the hood and through the ventilation system and to overcome the extraneous air patterns in the workplace. An adequate supply of air must be provided to replace the air that is exhausted. The make-up air may in some cases be used to assist in the local exhaust control. A recent review of local exhaust ventilation gives numerous examples of this control method.[21] More detailed guidelines are given in the American Conference of Governmental Industrial Hygienists (ACGIH) *Industrial Ventilation—A Manual of recommended practice* and *Heinsohn's Industrial Ventilation: Engineering Principles.*[22,23]

Local exhaust ventilation is probably the most commonly used and certainly one of the most versatile controls available. Uses range from standard fixed hoods or booths for welding, spray painting, sand shakeout in foundries, and process sampling stations to low volume–high velocity ventilation of power hand tools or welding guns. Local ventilation has the advantage of generally being divorced from process operating parameters or product quality. Disadvantages of local ventilation include moderately rigorous design, fabrication and maintenance requirements for hoods, associated ductwork, and air movers, cleaning requirements for the exhausted air to meet environmental constraints, and energy requirements for treating makeup air.

Local exhaust systems generally require much less air flow than do other systems. For example, a local exhaust ventilation system to control the exposure of embalmers to formaldehyde vapors was developed for an embalming room containing a single embalming table. When the local exhaust ventilation system was compared with the dilution ventilation rate required to achieve the same control over formaldehyde emissions, it was found that the local ventilation system would result in lower operating costs.[24] Such systems with exhaust hoods near the patient's mouth are also useful in dental offices to control nitrous oxide exposure.[25]

Work practices

Work practices are an essential adjunct to the "engineering" control measures that have been discussed thus far. Good work practices include structuring of standard operating and maintenance procedures that will minimize exposures and emissions as well as application of good judgment by individual workers during the performance of required production and maintenance functions.

For example, work practice modifications were successfully implemented in a pottery producing sanitary ware to reduce silica exposures.[26] Ceramic castings are allowed to dry for a few hours before removal from the molds before being smoothed and trimmed. Pieces that have been allowed to dry for a few hours are known as "green" castings. Parts that have dried for 2 or more days are known as "white" castings. Measurements indicated that a worker's exposure was about 4.5 times greater when cleaning "white" castings than cleaning "green" castings. Although it was not possible to completely eliminate cleaning white castings, the worker now wets "white" castings with a damp, nonabrasive sponge prior to cleaning.

The optimum use of work practices as a method of control for relatively automated process such as bulk organic or petrochemical plants requires a substantial degree of process–worker interaction. Automatic control devices have the advantage of being programmed to perform a given task in exactly the same manner each time, with the associated disadvantage of inflexibility in exercising judgment to respond to particular situations. Trained operators can exercise judgment, but are sometimes subject to inadvertent errors. Ideally, reliability of mechanical control devices should be used to back up the operators, and the judgment of the operators should supplement the mechanical control devices.

In many cases, stepping switches are used to control valve operations, pressure switches, weight set points, analog controller set points, and other sequential operations. The mechanical sequencer will not proceed until clearance is received from process condition sensors or from a switch triggered by the operator. The operators are thus required to interact with the control system in certain critical process steps. The potential for large releases of toxic chemicals is minimized by avoiding manual operation of process equipment.

The importance of considering human factors engineering is illustrated by the accident at the Three Mile Island (TMI) nuclear reactor. The three types of human error involved in the TMI accident included operator error, inadequate training, and inadequate instrumentation and display. The findings of the President's Commission on the causes of the TMI accident included inadequate training of operators and supervisors, divided management responsibilities, and lack of communication among regulatory agency officials, operators, and owners of the facility.[27] The methyl isocyanate leak at Bhopal, India has been cited as a major example of a large-scale industrial disaster that occurred because the sentinel markers of poor work practices were ignored.[28]

There are many other examples of work practices for control of emissions at the source. These include periodic leak-detection surveys with hand-held quick-response instruments and monitoring of airflows in ventilation systems with hand-held instruments. A good preventive maintenance program is an extremely important work practice measure for controlling exposures. Virtually all moving equipment is subject to wear and eventual failure. Regularly scheduled maintenance can both reduce the frequency of this failure and permit repairs to be made before the failure results in a large-scale release of hazardous materials. When piping, ductwork, or equipment has to be taken apart for maintenance, effective cleaning, flushing, or chemical decontamination procedures are often used prior to the disassembly.

CONTROL IN THE WORKPLACE

If a hazardous agent is introduced into the general workplace, control may still be achieved. Control at this stage, however, is generally more difficult and less effective than controls applied at the point of origin.

General ventilation

General or dilution ventilation is applied nearly universally as an adjunct to control at the source. Geographic location of the plant (possibly permitting open construction) and environmental pollution standards will affect the applicability of ventilation as a control method. Intake air for ventilation systems should be drawn from an uncontaminated atmosphere so as to avoid the recirculation of contaminated exhaust air from the plant itself or other sources of contamination outside the plant, such as auto exhaust gasses in a parking lot.[29]

Dilution ventilation can be successfully applied to the control of gases, vapors, and other materials if they are of low toxicity, their generation rate is known and relatively constant, and the workers are far enough away from the point of generation that they will not have an exposure exceeding a specific occupational exposure limit.[30] The calculation for determining the ventilation flow rate is straightforward, involving the generation rate of the contaminant, the degree of mixing in the workroom, and the desired concentration. Unfortunately, many times the generation rate and the mixing factor are unknown or may be only crudely estimated.

Assuming that the initial concentration is zero, the concentration build up of an air contaminant can be described by the following equation:

$$C = \frac{KG}{Q}\left[1 - \exp^{\frac{-Q}{kv}\,\Delta t}\right]$$

where

V = Volume of room or enclosure (m^3)
C = Concentration of gas or vapor at time t (mg/m^3)
G = Rate of generation of gas or vapor (mg/hr)
t = Time (hr)
Q = Rate of ventilation (m^3/hr)
K = Design distribution constant or mixing factor ranging from 1 to 10.

Air changes per hour (Q/V) is the ratio of the ventilation flow rate of the room (Q) divided by the volume of the room (V). The exponential term in the equation contains not only Q/V, but also the mixing factor (K). This mixing factor adjusts for the incomplete mixing of the ventilation air in the room.

Over the years, the term "air changes per hour" has been more often employed incorrectly than correctly. Inspection of the equation reveals that, at equilibrium, the above equation reduces to

$$C_{t_2} = \frac{KG}{Q}$$

Thus, it can be seen that the "number of air changes," Q/V, has no effect on the equilibrium concentration but only the rate at which that concentration is reached. Like the ratio Q/V, K affects the rate at which an equilibrium concentration is reached. Unlike Q/V, K appears in this equation, affecting the equilibrium concentration that is reached.

Typical air change rates in plants under a roof range from a few to 30 or more air changes per hour. Partial recirculation of air is commonly encountered (especially in conditioned air), but safeguards must be built into such systems at the design stage to avoid unacceptable exposure.[31] Good practice dictates that general ventilation airflow patterns should be directed so as to minimize the cross-contamination of work areas from emission sources.

Housekeeping

Good housekeeping also must be used nearly universally as a necessary adjunct to controls that are applied to the source of emissions. Relatively nonvolatile liquids such as certain pesticides or toxic materials containing polynuclear hydrocarbons found in coal conversion operations may present relatively smaller respiratory hazards in comparison with the hazard of dermal exposures associated with poor work practices and housekeeping.

In general, housekeeping procedures such as chemical decontamination, wet sweeping, and vacuuming are preferred over techniques such as dry sweeping, which result in a redispersion of airborne dust. The objective of housekeeping should be to reduce exposures from secondary sources to hygienically insignificant levels. One practical problem that arises in determining the significance of skin exposures is the roughly quantitative wipe testing. Ultraviolet fluorescence for polynuclear aromatics (PNAs) has been proposed for qualitative screening for surface contamination in coal conversion processes, and for oil or solvent spillage.

CONTROL BY THE WORKER

Controls may also be applied near or worn by the individual worker to prevent exposures to workplace hazards.

Worker isolation

Isolation of workers can be an important control measure. Many automated plants in the chemical process industries permit production employees to spend substantial amounts of time in enclosed control rooms that are positively pressurized with clean air. This time allocation results in substantially reduced time-weighted average exposures. Booths in production areas that are equipped with a positively pressurized clean air supply serve similar purposes (both in reducing exposures to material hazards and to noise) in cases where production requirements are intermittent. Crane cabs that are enclosed and air conditioned have been effective in reducing fume exposures when transferring metals in iron foundries.[32] Filtered (or supplied) air cabs are applicable to a variety of types of equipment, including earthmovers, and tractors used in pesticide spraying.

The applicability of worker isolation depends on the degree of process automation, which in turn depends on the scale of production and the complexity of the tasks. Many types of intermittent or complex operations do not lend well to worker isolation due to a loss of sensitivity in control of process or product parameters.

Work practices

Ultimately, the individual worker shares a great deal of personal responsibility in preventing exposures through good practices. Carelessness and operator error can circumvent the best of control systems. These concerns are particularly critical in maintenance operations, where exposure potentials are relatively high and a substantial amount of judgment may be necessary in dealing with unusual situations. Personal hygiene is another important area in which individual worker acceptance of responsibility is paramount.[33]

Administrative controls

The rotation of worker schedules can also help reduce exposures of individual workers. This method is effective in cases where a definite "safe" exposure level can be established or in the case of heat, cold, or physical stress. In general this method is less desirable for the population of workers than is control by reducing hazard levels.

Personal protective equipment

Personal protective equipment (PPE) is another means of isolating the worker from the potential exposure source. Instead of physically isolating the source from the surrounding work environment, the worker is isolated from the work area. One of the major drawbacks to this type of control is that less emphasis is often placed on maintaining the general workplace free from contamination and, as an easy and inexpensive solution, placing the main responsibility for safety on the workers themselves. Exposure can then occur during lapses in standard operating procedures, failure of PPE, removal of PPE at the end of work periods, or use of improper or damaged PPE. However, a properly administered PPE program can offer an effective means of control as a supplement or backup to controls at the source of hazards. When technical feasibility of controls is limited, the program becomes an important interim element in a control system. The U.S. Occupational Safety and Health Administration (OSHA) regulations provide legal requirements for PPE programs.[34]

Protective clothing. The importance of PPE is related to the hazard offered by the particular compound. The four principal types of hazards include dermal absorption or contact, eye contact, inhalation, and ingestion. With dermal absorption, protective clothing, gloves, boots, face shields, and head wear are the major personal protective measures required. The choice of clothing to be used should be based on the exposure hazards, the amount of body coverage required, and material used in construction of clothing. To protect the wearer from exposure, the clothing material should be impermeable or at least resistant to the particular hazardous agent encountered.

Preliminary decontamination of protective clothing may be required before removal. Again, both the type and degree of hazard and the properties of the clothing being considered deserve careful consideration.

Respiratory protection. Respiratory protection is used to reduce exposures at some point in many situations involving inhalation hazards. Cost effectiveness, acceptability, ease of use, and ability of the worker to wear devices are considerations in determining the proper use of respiratory protection. However, an effective respiratory protection program is not necessarily inexpensive.

In the United States, the minimum requirements of an acceptable respirator program are set forth in Title 29 U.S. Code of Federal Regulations (CFR) 1910.134.[33] The program should include proper equipment selection, training program, fit testing, employee evaluation, supervision and enforcement, and an adequate maintenance program.[35,36] Chapter 59 discusses the use of respirators in detail.

Respiratory protection is generally used during the period necessary to install or implement engineering or work practice controls, during plant maintenance, during emergencies or nonroutine operation, or in situations where complete control is not achievable through feasible engineering measures. Also, if the engineering controls are not able to reduce exposure to the permissible limit with the necessary degree of confidence, then respiratory protection can be implemented, in addition to engineering controls, to further reduce the possibility of exposure. This type of situation is often encountered with extremely toxic and hazardous materials. When it is necessary to minimize the possibility of all contact with the toxic material, a combination of engineering controls and protective equipment must be used. Standard operating procedures should be prepared, detailing types of protective equipment required for entry into certain plant areas.

In general, respiratory protection is most effectively employed in a control system as a backup to engineering controls. In event of engineering control failure, respiratory protection can be used to keep exposure to a minimum during repair. In an area equipped with monitoring devices, alarms can signal equipment or process failure and trigger use of respiratory protection.

THE CONTROL SYSTEM

A system of controls based on the previously described principles is adequate to prevent occupational exposures in all situations, subject to constraints of cost, product parameters, and environmental concerns. There are often a number of alternative control strategies for a given problem. One of the major decisions to be made is often between retrofitting existing plants, constructing new plants using modern process technology, or simply ceasing to do business. Many nonferrous smelters are currently faced with difficult decisions of this nature. Each time a substantial reduction in permissible exposure limits (PELs) is made for a material of economic importance, companies that use that material must select an optimum strategy within the given set of economic and market constraints.

Construction of new facilities using modern process technology is often one of the most expensive control options. However, long-term productivity improvements, energy efficiency gains, and competitive market advantages through product improvements can often help compensate for the initial investment. The development of new process technology and the subsequent construction of new facilities thus offer a unique opportunity to design around many occupational problems and actually improve the cost structure in the process.

The importance of plant layout, predictive design techniques for new process equipment, and the incorporation of adequate flexibility to permit relatively easy compliance with anticipated occupational and environmental health standards and other constraints (such as energy) cannot be overemphasized. Failure to adequately consider these factors during design stages is perhaps the most serious problem in existing plants. Predictive design methods are still in their infancy in the context of preventing occupational health hazards, and companies continue to experience difficulties in the layout and design of new plants.

There is no substitute for experienced, competent industrial hygienists and engineers working closely in designing and maintaining control systems both in existing and in new plants and processes. A cooperative, enlightened working relationship between the public and private sectors will also be necessary to achieve processes that are both productive and safe to the worker.

REFERENCES

1. Peterson JE: Principles for controlling the occupational environment. In *The industrial environment—its evaluation & control.* DHEW/NIOSH Pub No 74-117, NTIS No PB88-240106. Washington, DC, 1973, U.S. Department of Health, Education, and Welfare, Public Health Service, Center for Disease Control, National Institute for Occupational Safety and Health.
2. Shapley D: Nitrosamines: Scientists on the trail of prime suspect in urban cancer, *Science* 191(4224):268-270, 1976.
3. Moorman WJ, Palmer WJ, and Mulligan LT: Carcinogenic potential of condensed pyrolysis of effluents from iron foundry casting operations. In *Proceedings of the second NCI/EPA/NIOSH collaborative workshop: progress on joint environmental and occupational cancer studies,* September 9-11, 1981, Rockville, Md, pp 445-462, Contract No. 210-78-0033, 1982.
4. Marshall WF and Hurn RW: *Hazards from engines: rebreathing exhaust in confined space,* Pittsburgh, PA, 1973, Bureau of Mines. Report of Investigation 7757.
5. Antonsen DH and Springer DB: Nickel compounds. In *Kirk-Othmer encyclopedia of chemical technology,* ed 2, vol 13, pp 753-765, New York, 1967, John Wiley.
6. Eller PM and Cassinelli ME, editors: *NIOSH manual of analytical methods,* ed 4, DHHS (NIOSH) Publication No 94-113, NTIS No PB95-154191, Cincinnati, OH, 1994, U.S. Department of Health and Human Services, Public Health Service, Centers for Disease Control and Prevention, National Institute for Occupational Safety and Health.
7. National Institute for Occupational Safety and Health: *The industrial environment—its evaluation & control,* DHEW/NIOSH Pub No 74-117, NTIS No PB88-240106, Washington, DC, 1973, U.S. Department of Health, Education, and Welfare, Public Health Service, Center for Disease Control, NIOSH.
8. Clayton GD and Clayton FE, editors: *Patty's industrial hygiene and toxicology,* third edition, New York, NY, 1978, Wiley Interscience.
9. Peterson JE: *Industrial health,* Englewood Cliffs, NJ, 1977, Prentice Hall.
10. Gressel MG and Heitbrink WA, editors: *Analyzing workplace exposures using direct reading instruments and video exposure monitoring techniques,* DHHS/NIOSH Pub No 92-104, NTIS No PB93-137057, Cincinnati, OH, 1992, U.S. Department of Health and Human Services, Public Health Service, Centers for Disease Control, National Institute for Occupational Safety and Health.
11. Gillett JE: Preventing emissions from manufacturing processes by suitable process design, *Ann Occup Hyg* 19(3/4):301-308, 1976.
12. Haastrup P: Design error in the chemical industry: case studies. In *4th international symposium on loss prevention and safety promotion in the process industries,* vol 1, *Safety in Operations and Processes,* pp J15-J27, European Federation of Chemical Engineering Pub Series No 33, 1983.
13. National Institute for Occupational Safety and Health: *Proceedings of the symposium on occupational health hazard control technology in the foundry and secondary non-ferrous smelting industries,* DHEW/NIOSH Pub No 81-114, NTIS No PB81-167-710/A20, Washington, DC, 1981, U.S. Department of Health, Education, and Welfare, Public Health Service, Center for Disease Control, NIOSH.
14. Webb RJ: How to hold down costs with lead-free coatings, *Mat Eng* 90-91, 1976.
15. Kendall R: Bhopal: its implications for American industry, *Occup Hazards* 47(5):67-70, 1985.
16. Kalelkar AS: Investigation of large-magnitude incidents: Bhopal as a case study. In *Preventing major chemical and related process accidents,* IChemE Symposium Series No 110, EFCO Pub Series No 70, pp 553-575. Rugby, UK, 1988, The Institution of Chemical Engineers.
17. Bowonder B, Kasperson JX, and Kasperson RE: Avoiding future Bhopals, *Environment* 27(7):6-13, 31-37, 1985.
18. Jensen PA, Todd WF, and Fischbach TJ: *Walk-through survey report: control of methylene chloride in furniture stripping at Ronald Alsip Furniture Refinishing, Cincinnati, OH,* DHHS/NIOSH/DPSE/ECTB Report No CT 170-12A, NTIS No PB91-116533, Cincinnati, OH, 1989, U.S. Department of Health and Human Services, Public Health Service, Centers for Disease Control, National Institute for Occupational Safety and Health.
19. Norin M: The needs of the working environment, *Product Finishing* 24-28, 1976.
20. Hall RM and Sheehy JW: *Walk-through survey report: control of methylene chloride in furniture stripping at Jet Strip, Boulder, Colorado,* DHHS/NIOSH/DPSE/ECTB Report No CT 170-19A, NTIS No PB93-160927, Cincinnati, OH, 1992, U.S. Department of Health and Human Services, Public Health Service, Centers for Disease Control, National Institute for Occupational Safety and Health.
21. Socha GE: Local exhaust ventilation principles, *Am Ind Hyg Assoc J* 40(1):1-10, 1979.
22. American Conference of Governmental Industrial Hygienists: *Industrial ventilation—a manual of recommended practice,* ed 21, Cincinnati, OH, 1992, ACGIH.
23. Heinsohn RJ: *Industrial ventilation: engineering principles,* New York, 1991, John Wiley.
24. Gressel MG and Hughes R: Effective local exhaust ventilation for controlling formaldehyde exposures during embalming, *Appl Occup Environ Hyg* 7(12):840-845, 1992.
25. Mickelsen RL, Jacobs DE, Jensen PA, et al: Auxiliary ventilation for the control of nitrous oxide in a dental clinic, *Appl Occup Environ Hyg* 8(6):564-570, 1993.
26. Cooper TC, Gressel MG, Froehlich PA, Caplan PE, Mickelsen RL, Valiante D, and Bost P: successful reduction of silica exposures at a sanitary ware pottery, *Am Ind Hyg Assoc J* 54(10):600-606, 1993.
27. Hagen EW and Mays GT: Human factors engineering in the U.S. nuclear arena, *Nucl Safety* 22(3):337-346, 1981.
28. Deutsch PV, Adler J, and Richter ED: Sentinel markers for industrial disasters, *Israel J Med Sci* 28(8/9):526-533, 1992.
29. National Institute for Occupational Safety and Health: *Recirculation of exhaust air,* DHEW (NIOSH) Pub No 76-186, NTIS No PB267-396/A18, Washington, DC, 1976, U.S. Department of Health, Education, and Welfare, Public Health Service, Centers for Disease Control, NIOSH.
30. Hemeon WCL: *Plant and process ventilation,* New York, 1963, Industrial Press.

31. National Institute for Occupational Safety and Health: *Recommended approach to recirculation of exhaust air,* DHEW (NIOSH) Pub No 78-124, NTIS No PB83-142-729/A09, Washington, DC, 1978, U.S. Department of Health, Education, and Welfare, Public Health Service, Centers for Disease Control, NIOSH.

32. National Institute for Occupational Safety and Health: *An evaluation of occupational health hazard control technology for the foundry industry,* DHEW/NIOSH Pub No 79-114, Washington, DC, 1978, U.S. Department of Health, Education, and Welfare, Public Health Service, Center for Disease Control, NIOSH.

33. Vasikaran SD, Patel S, and O'Gorman PTI: Zinc and copper status of lead workers, *Trace Elements Med* 9(2):103-104, 1992.

34. Code of Federal Regulations: U.S. Department of Labor, Occupational Safety and Health Administration, 29 CFR 1910, Rev. July 1, 1990.

35. Bollinger NJ and Schutz RH: *NIOSH guide to industrial respiratory protection,* DHEW (NIOSH) Pub No 87-116, NTIS No PB88-188347, Cincinnati, OH, 1987, U.S. Department of Health and Human Services, Public Health Service, Centers for Disease Control, National Institute for Occupational Safety and Health.

36. National Institute for Occupational Safety and Health: *NIOSH respirator decision logic,* DHEW (NIOSH) Pub No 87-108, NTIS No PB88-149612, Cincinnati, OH, 1987, U.S. Department of Health and Human Services, Public Health Service, Centers for Disease Control, NIOSH.

Chapter 61

CONTROL OF INDOOR AIR POLLUTION

Philip R. Morey

The intent of indoor air pollution control is to reduce occupant exposure that results in adverse health effects, annoyance, and discomfort. Control is generally achieved through two approaches: (1) *source control*, which involves removal of the pollutant, and (2) *exposure control*, which may include actions such as dilution with relatively pollutant-free outdoor air, filtration, and cleaning. Source control, which is usually pollutant specific, is the most effective control strategy since occupant exposure is eliminated. However, source control is not always feasible, especially in existing buildings. Exposure control through dilution, filtration, or cleaning is generally nonspecific with regard to the pollutant removed and is performed with the realization that some occupant exposure will continue. The ventilation rate procedure of American Society of Heating, Refrigerating, and Air-Conditioning Engineers (ASHRAE) Standard 62-1989,[1] which recommends specific minimum amounts of ventilation for occupied spaces by clean outdoor air, is an example of exposure control achieved by reducing the concentrations of indoor air contaminants to levels that are acceptable to the majority of occupants. The next ASHRAE 62 standard will likely place much greater emphasis on source control.[2]

Approaches to control of indoor air pollutants may also be *reactive* or *proactive*. In the reactive approach recommendations are made to control the causes of sick building syndrome (SBS) or building-related illness (BRI). Proactive approaches to control are embodied in design and commissioning procedures for buildings and their heating, ventilation, and air-conditioning (HVAC) systems. Proactive approaches to control of indoor pollutants emphasize source management, whereas reactive evaluations tend to emphasize exposure control.

This review begins with a general discussion of control measures used both in reactive evaluations of problem buildings and in proactive evaluation of new buildings. The importance of source control for microbial and nonmicrobial pollutants in building design and construction is illustrated by examples in the third section. The fourth and fifth sections discuss the control of indoor pollution in the HVAC system and occupied spaces, respectively.

The topic of control of indoor pollution has been a focus of ASHRAE indoor air quality (IAQ) symposia[3,4] as well as other extensive reviews.[5,6] The intent of this review is to provide the reader with practical information drawn from case studies showing how the success and failure of source and exposure control affect indoor environmental quality. The box defines some common abbreviations used in this chapter.

APPROACHES TO INDOOR POLLUTANT CONTROL
Reactive evaluations in problem buildings

The ventilation rate procedure of ASHRAE Standard 62-1989[1] provides a method commonly recommended to control indoor air pollution. Relatively clean outdoor air is delivered in specific amounts [generally at least 15 or 20 cubic feet per minute (cfm) per occupant] to occupied spaces. The provision of minimum outdoor ventilation rates on a per person basis assumes that the occupant is the primary source of indoor air pollutants.

However, the work of Fanger et al.[7] has shown that the provision of more outdoor air to interior spaces will not necessarily ameliorate IAQ problems. Thus, occupant perception of poor IAQ can occur when the outdoor air ventilation rate is 50 cfm per person or even greater. The work of Fanger et al.[7] shows that the quality of air provided to occupants is more important than the actual outdoor ventilation rate. The HVAC system itself as well as emissions from interior finishing and construction materials can be more

significant sources of contaminants that degrade IAQ than contaminants produced by occupants or occupant activities.

The focus of HVAC corrective actions has in recent years been directed not only toward improvement in dilution ventilation but also on maintenance and cleaning strategies for the mechanical system itself. Inadequate maintenance of HVAC system components—especially air handling units (AHUs), fan coil units (FCUs), and induction units—is probably the most important factor responsible for poor IAQ in many buildings.[8] Thus, plenums in AHUs may be dirty, filters can be overloaded with dirt, insulation along the air stream surfaces in AHUs and FCUs encrusted with debris, and access into HVAC system components may be so restricted that cleaning is difficult or impossible. Although remedial actions based on upgrading maintenance and cleaning are straightforward, these actions so important for exposure control are often overlooked by building operators because of perceived lack of return on investment.

Recommendations to control indoor air pollutants and to reduce IAQ problems may be based on inadequate building and HVAC system design and operation. Some pollutant control actions based on design or operation deficiencies are easy to achieve. For example, damper linkages in AHUs can be reconnected and abandoned control systems can be made operative. Office equipment emitting copious quantities of volatile organic compounds (VOCs) can be replaced by products with low emissions.

Other recommendations to control indoor air pollutants based on inadequate building design may be very difficult and costly to implement. Thus, the location of the HVAC system outdoor air intake at ground level in an area easily contaminated by emissions from vehicular traffic may not be rectified by the operator of a large building because of the great cost of the retrofit. Control of occupant exposure to combustion products in the building may take the form of attempts to limit vehicular traffic near the outdoor air intake (exposure control) rather than the more effective relocation of the intake to the roof or side of the building where higher quality outdoor air is found (source control).

In some buildings significant IAQ problems may not be rectified because operators of the HVAC system and various equipment in the building fail to appreciate the potential effects of indoor pollutants on occupants. For example, a neonatal intensive care unit (ICU) in a major medical center experienced significant patient morbidity and mortality. The compressors supplying air to the respirators used by patients were located in a mechanical equipment room that also housed AHUs, workbench activities such as paint spraying and welding, and exhaust vents from various laboratories. Although the air entering respirator units was highly filtered for particulate contaminants, hospital facilities personnel did not realize that VOCs and combustion products that may have been emitted in the mechanical equipment room would be passed directly through filters to the patients by the ICU respirator system. In this example, source control by reloca-

---

Abbreviations in this chapter

AHU: Air handling unit
ASHRAE: American Society of Heating, Refrigerating, and Air-Conditioning Engineers
BRI: Building-related illness
cfm: Cubic feet per minute
ETS: Environmental tobacco smoke
HEPA: High-efficiency particulate air (filter)
HVAC: Heating, ventilation, and air-conditioning (system)
IAQ: Indoor air quality
SBS: Sick building syndrome
TVOC: Total volatile organic compound
VOC: Volatile organic compound

tion of the compressor air inlets to a zone of high quality outdoor air was the only remedial option. Exposure control by restricting or reducing work activities resulting in reduced emission of gaseous contaminants in the vicinity of compressor air inlets was unacceptable.

Proactive control of indoor air pollutants (especially in new buildings)

Buildings where exposure to indoor air pollutants is kept to the lowest feasible levels can be constructed if IAQ issues are addressed during design, construction, commissioning, and initial occupancy.[9,10] During the design phase for a new building or the retrofit of an existing building, IAQ pollution control options can be defined by both the architect and owner. If cigarette smoking is to be permitted, provision for containment and exhaust of environmental tobacco smoke (ETS) from smoking areas (lounges) should be made during design planning. In speculative buildings where the end use of the building is unknown, the architect can recommend a flexible HVAC system design to provide for control of indoor pollutants for a variety of potential users. Major potential IAQ problems are avoided at the design stage by careful attention to actions such as the prevention of entrainment of combustion products and bioaerosols associated with the location of the outdoor air inlet, provision of adequate outdoor air ventilation to meet the current and anticipated ASHRAE 62 standards, and the necessity based on ambient air pollution data of HVAC filtration to remove air contaminants such as ozone and combustion products that may be present in outdoor air at the building site. One of the most important actions made during construction is the specification and selection of carpet, wall, ceiling, and insulation systems with the lowest feasible VOC emissions.[9] The State of Washington has developed specifications for minimum VOC emission rates for finishing and furnishing materials used in new construction.[11]

Commissioning is the process of verifying the performance of HVAC and other building systems prior to occupancy. Training of facilities personnel in HVAC system operation and maintenance and building housekeeping is one of the most important and often overlooked components of commissioning.

The initial occupancy phase is probably the most critical aspect of a building's IAQ history. Premature occupancy of a building before HVAC system commissioning and completion of construction will likely result in exposure of occupants to VOCs, dusts, and other air contaminants. A preoccupancy flush-out period of 90 days during which time the HVAC system provides a continuous flow of 100% outdoor air is part of the State of Washington's compliance program intended to allow VOC emission rates from interior finishing materials to reach acceptable rates.[11] This kind and length of preoccupancy outdoor air ventilation, however, are probably inappropriate for most buildings in hot-humid or cold climatic regions.

SOURCE CONTROL CONSIDERATIONS DURING BUILDING CONSTRUCTION AND DESIGN
Condensation in hot-humid and cold climates

The primary environmental factor controlling the growth of microorganisms, especially fungi, in buildings is moisture availability. Condensation will occur on walls, ceilings, and floors when their surface temperatures are below the dew point temperature of the surrounding air. Condensation and control of potential fungal contamination are prevented by different design considerations for cold and hot-humid climates.

In hot-humid climates, condensation will occur on walls of air-conditioned buildings when warm moist outdoor air infiltrates through the building envelope and encounters a cold surface (with a temperature below that of the dew point temperature of the infiltrating outdoor air) on the "occupied" side of the wall. Fig. 61-1 shows the occupied side of a perimeter wall from which a small piece of gypsum board has been removed. A layer of polyethylene was placed over the hole in the gypsum board. Water droplets are forming on the wall cavity side of the polyethylene as moist warm air infiltrates through the wall and condenses on the relatively cold polyethylene surface. Fig. 61-2 shows the kind of fungal contamination that can occur in walls such as that illustrated in Fig. 61-1 where the moisture content of the gypsum board approaches or reaches the saturation point. The fungi present at the wall covering–gypsum board surface (Fig. 61-2) are mostly toxigenic species including *Aspergillus versicolor*, *Stachybotrys atra*, and various *Penicillium* species.

Table 61-1 shows the kind of fungal contamination that can occur in a building when design features to prevent condensation are neglected. *Aspergillus versicolor* was the dominant fungus present in the room before disruption of the wall covering (concentration about 10^2 cfu/m^3, see Table 61-1) and its concentration increased enormously coincident with the activity seen in Fig. 61-2. Phylloplane fungi (for example, *Cladosporium* and *Epicoccum*) would normally be

Table 61-1. Airborne fungi present in a building where condensation occurred in walls.*

Sampling location and description	cfu/m^3	Taxa
Sample collected 2 m away from wall with condensation damage	10^2	*Aspergillus versicolor* group
Same as above except wall covering removal as in Fig. 61-2	$>10^5$	Mostly *Aspergillus versicolor* group; some *Penicillium*
Outdoor air control	10^3	*Cladosporium, Epicoccum,* and other phylloplane species

*Samples collected on malt extract agar with Andersen Sampler. cfu/m^3, colony-forming units per cubic meter of air.

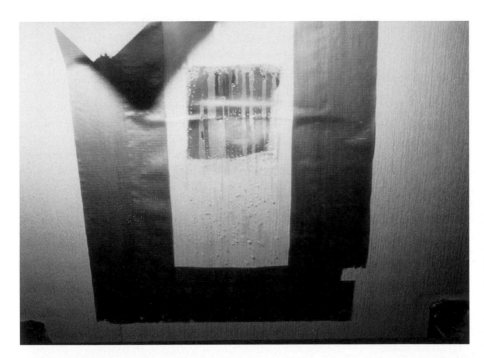

Fig. 61-1. Condensation on occupied side of the perimeter wall of a building in a hot-humid climate. The dew point temperature of the outdoor air infiltrating through the perimeter wall is higher than the surface temperature at the gypsum board surface. Condensation occurs in the gypsum board and on a small piece of polyethylene placed over a hole cut in the gypsum board.

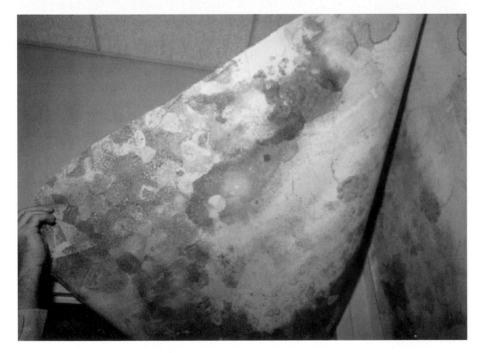

Fig. 61-2. Fungal contamination that occurs in a vinyl-covered gypsum board as a result of condensation.

expected to dominate the fungal taxa in the room if strong indoor sources were absent.

To reduce condensation, a layer of material with low moisture and air permanence (known as a vapor retarder) is conventionally installed in the envelope of buildings. The vapor retarder is usually located in the wall near or at the surface exposed to the higher water vapor pressure. In hot-humid climates, vapor retarders are located on or near the exterior surface of air-conditioned buildings because the higher water vapor pressure occurs in the outdoor air.

The following actions are recommended to control condensation and fungal contamination for buildings in hot-humid climates:[12]

• Minimize the infiltration of outdoor air into construction by installation of an external vapor retarder and by elimination of negative pressurization of the building.

• Do not use wet or moist materials (for example, wet concrete block) in construction.

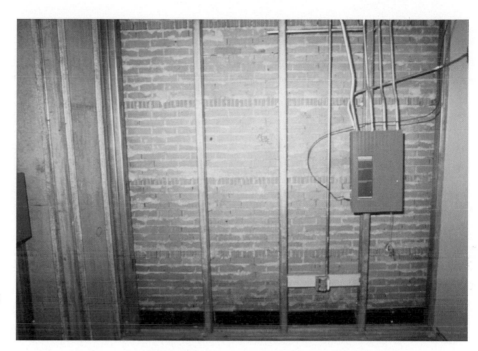

Fig. 61-3. Interior surface of brick facing of a building photographed from a room after gypsum board was removed from metal studs.

- Use permeable materials (permeance greater than 5 perms) on interior surfaces.
- Avoid cooling the indoor space below the design set-point temperature or the mean monthly outdoor dew point temperature.

In hot-humid climates condensation can occur on any interior surface whose temperature is less than the dew point temperature of room air. For example, condensation and the growth of *Cladosporium* and *Flavobacterium* species occur on cold painted surfaces and panels near air-conditioning supply vents.[13]

In cold climates, condensation is especially evident in residences in corners of walls, at the junction of the ceiling and the external wall, and at corners of the building that have little or no protective insulation.[14] Condensation can occur in the wall or building envelope itself when moist indoor air flows out through porous construction and encounters cold surfaces on the "weather side" of the building.

The following actions are recommended to control condensation and fungal contamination in buildings in cold climates:[15,16]

- Place the vapor retarder on the side of the insulation facing the occupied space.
- Prevent leakage of indoor air into wall and insulation cavities.
- Keep the moisture level of building materials significantly below their maximum sorption content (true for buildings in all climates).

Entry of water and microbial contaminants into buildings

Moisture can also enter buildings because of primarily climatic reasons. Wind-driven snow can enter HVAC system outdoor air inlets, especially those located at grade level or flush with horizontal roof surfaces. Wind-driven rain can enter the envelope and saturate construction materials, especially when roof and window flashing is inadequate. Moisture that enters walls and roofs must be removed by drainage to the outside or by indoor air-conditioning or ventilation.

Figures 61-3 and 61-4 show the wall cavity surface of an exterior brick wall where mortar did not seal all the joints around bricks. This construction defect led to the entry of large quantities of rainwater into the wall cavity (water could not drain out of walls because weep holes at the base of the wall were sealed) and chronic flooding of the carpet in the room in Fig. 61-3. *Stachybotrys*, a fungus that grows on very wet surfaces, dominated the viable spores present in the carpet (concentration about 10^5 per g of dust in the carpet).

The site where a building is constructed and the location of the HVAC system outdoor air intake have important bioaerosol consequences if there are nearby industrial facilities such as sewage, waste water treatment, and composting plants. For example, the concentration of endotoxin at the outside air intake of a building constructed about 100 m down wind from a sewage treatment facility was about 1 order of magnitude less than that in the facility but 1 order of magnitude greater than that at remote sites. An important design consideration for the building in this example

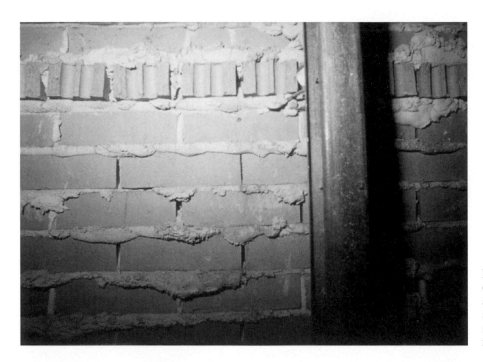

Fig. 61-4. In the building shown in Fig. 61-3, the spaces between bricks were not adequately sealed. This construction resulted in chronic flooding in occupied spaces and growth of *Stachybotrys* in room carpet.

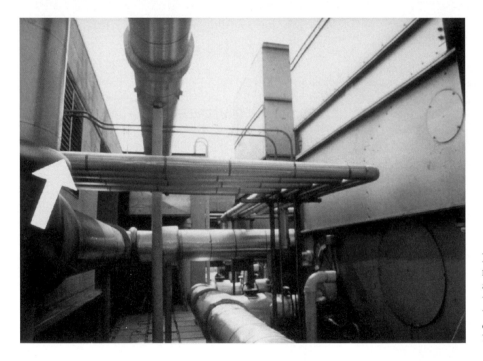

Fig. 61-5. Outdoor air inlet (arrow) for a new office building located within 3 m of a cooling tower reservoir. The area shown within the photograph was enclosed within an architectural fence, which encouraged entrainment of cooling tower bioaerosol into the outdoor air inlet.

is to provide for highly efficient filtration of outdoor air entering the HVAC system so as to remove particulate and possibly gaseous air contaminants being entrained from the sewage plant.

Placement of cooling towers on or around buildings and design of hot water service systems in buildings affect the potential risk of Legionnaires' disease. Thus, airflow patterns around a building should be considered before construction so as to maximally protect HVAC system outdoor air inlets and areas where people may congregate outdoors

from cooling tower aerosols. The hot water service system should be designed and built to avoid conditions of stagnation of tepid water.

Figure 61-5 shows a major defect in new construction, namely the location of a cooling tower less than 3 m from an HVAC system outdoor air inlet (Fig. 61-5, arrow). While dose–response data between *Legionella* concentrations in tower water reservoirs and risk of legionellosis do not exist, the close spatial proximity of a potential *Legionella* reservoir (tower reservoirs in Fig. 61-5 contained approximately 10^3 *L. pneumophila* serogroup 1 per ml) and a building inlet increases the chance that aerosol may enter interior spaces. The Health and Safety Executive in the UK[17] provides information on the control of legionellosis including design and construction guidelines, some of which are enumerated below:

- Use hot water tanks with a capacity that meets the needs of users. Excessive demand on undersized tanks can result in delivery of insufficiently heated lukewarm water. Use of oversized tanks can, however, result in water stagnation and poor mixing.
- Hot water tanks should be designed so that their contents can be heated to 60° C throughout.
- Install highly efficient drift eliminators on cooling towers to intercept water droplets where air is discharged.
- Cooling towers should be constructed of materials that can be readily disinfected and will not support microbial growth (for example, avoid the use of wood).

Special design considerations to prevent fungal contamination in medical centers

Respiratory hazards of health care facilities are discussed in Chapter 44. Fungal contamination in organ transplant facilities is a special risk because of the extreme susceptibility of immunosuppressed patients. The air supplied to patient areas must be of the highest quality[18] with the concentration of 37° C *Aspergillus* kept as low as possible but certainly below 1 cfu/m^3. One major source of *Aspergillus* in medical centers is soil disturbance associated with construction and entrainment of fungal aerosols into HVAC systems where germination, growth, and sporulation may subsequently occur on wet niches in AHUs. HVAC system design considerations thus are especially important for prevention of nosocomial aspergillosis.

Table 61-2 shows the type of fungal contamination found in one transplant facility with design defects in the HVAC system. All filters in the AHUs serving transplant patient areas were wet and heavily contaminated by *Aspergillus fumigatus*. This fungus was also present in settled dusts throughout the AHUs and was detected consistently in air samples collected in patient areas (Table 61-2). Significant morbidity and mortality occurred among transplant patients in this facility.

Table 61-2. Concentration of 37° C *Aspergillus fumigatus* in organ transplant center and its HVAC system

Location	Concentration
Rooms housing transplant patients	2–20 cfm/m^3
Corridor near nursing station	50 cfu/m^3
95% efficient filter in air handling unit; wet filter	>100 cfu /in.^{2} of filter surface
Settled dust in air handling unit	10^1–10^3 cfu /g

HVAC, Heating, ventilation, and air-conditioning

Control actions that can limit entrainment and dispersion of fungal spores to patient areas include the following:

- Protect outdoor air inlets from construction dusts by special filtration.
- Prevent outdoor sources of water such as wind-driven rain or fog from entering outdoor air inlets.
- Provide redundancy in AHU design so that while one unit is operating the other may be "offline" for thorough cleaning and maintenance.
- Protect patient rooms with terminal or point of discharge high-efficiency particulate air (HEPA) filters and by positive air pressurization.

Construction and finishing practices associated with microbial contamination

Unusual construction and finishing materials can be direct sources of microbial contaminants. Some natural building materials such as cork when used new in wall and floor covering may be heavily contaminated by microorganisms such as *Streptomyces*[19] and *Aureobasidium.* The occurrence of *Aspergillus* infections in cancer patients in a new hospital was causally associated with fireproofing materials present above the ceiling in patient rooms.[20] The cellulose-based fireproofing was applied wet to the beams on the underside of floor decks and this provided a niche for the growth of fungi including *Aspergillus* species.

Casein-based self-leveling compounds used in concrete provide an unusual substrate to support the putrefactive fermentation of various microorganisms including *Clostridia* species.[21,22] Ammonia and various malodorous amines can be detected beneath floor coverings when this kind of concrete is damp.

Certain indoor finishing and construction practices make it difficult to control microbial contaminants. For example, fleecy materials such as carpet often become reservoirs for fungal spores, soil bacteria, and mite and cat allergens. Xerophilic fungi can grow in dirty porous niches where moisture levels reach a water activity of 0.65 to 0.70. Mites optimally reproduce in environments where the relative humidity is 75% to 80% (range is 45% to 80%) and where human skin scales accumulate.[23] Techniques useful for control of microbial contamination in interior environments include the following:

- Restrict the use of fleecy, extended surface finishing materials to the greatest extent possible. Control of microbial contamination in these materials is difficult, especially when they become dirty and moist.
- Cover fleecy materials with impervious sheeting especially for control of dust mites.
- Use tacky floor strips or air curtains to reduce tracking of outdoor contaminants into buildings.
- Incorporate highly efficient vacuum cleaning into a central system so that contaminants physically exit the occupied spaces during cleaning.

- Avoid use of construction materials that have a high probability for containing or supporting the growth of microorganisms.

Specification of low volatile organic compound emissions in finishing materials

Control of VOC emissions from finishing materials being installed in new buildings or being used in the retrofit of an existing building is best accomplished through source reduction or elimination during planning and construction. The U.S. Carpet and Rug Institute has established a voluntary "Green Label" program to reduce contaminant emissions to rates below certain guidelines[24] as follows:

- Total volatile organic compounds (TVOCs) < 0.6 mg/m$^2 \cdot$ hr
- Styrene < 0.4 mg/m$^2 \cdot$ hr
- Formaldehyde < 0.05 mg/m$^2 \cdot$ hr
- 4-Phenylcyclohexene < 0.1 mg/m$^2 \cdot$ hr

The State of Washington has developed guidelines[11] requiring that products installed in new buildings not contribute emissions resulting in increase in indoor contaminant concentrations above levels as follows:

- TVOCs 0.5 mg/m^3
- Formaldehyde 0.05 ppm
- 4-Phenylcyclohexene 1 ppb

Compliance with these source control guidelines assumes a 30- to 90-day flush-out period with continuous 100% outdoor air ventilation.[11] Although ventilation with 100% outdoor air may be acceptable at certain periods of the year in temperate areas in the State of Washington, this kind of flush-out will not be achievable for most buildings in cold or hot-humid climates. Compliance with the above VOC concentration guidelines after 30 days of continuous preoccupancy ventilation at a rate of 20 cfm of outdoor air per "design" occupant or per 140 square feet of occupied space should currently be achievable for material selection in new construction.

Success of preoccupancy flush-out of finishing materials selected for low VOC emission depends highly upon the ability of the HVAC system to provide the recommended rate of outdoor air ventilation during preoccupancy. Table 61-3 illustrates the kind of HVAC system deficiency often associated with variable air volume (VAV) systems[25] that can confound the material selection protocol described by Black et al.[11] In VAV systems, the flow of supply air and often the flow of outdoor air delivered to the occupied space change to meet the temperature requirements dictated by the zone thermostat. In properly operated systems, when the thermostat controlling airflow to the occupied zone is thermally satisfied, the amount of outdoor air ventilation does not fall below 20 cfm per occupant or 20 cfm per 140 square feet of occupied space.

In Table 61-3, if the occupied zone being served by the VAV terminal was about 500 square feet and was designed to have four occupants, then at least 80 cfm of outdoor air ventilation should be provided at all times even when the thermostat does not call for cooling. Flush-out of VOCs is difficult or impossible to achieve when minimum air flow from VAV terminals is too low or in some very poor designs zero (no airflow whatsoever) when the thermostat is thermally satisfied.

The following general principles of VOC source control should be used during design planning and construction:

- Avoid the use of design materials, furnishings, and substances used in construction that contain carcinogens, toxins, or teratogenic agents.
- Avoid the use of materials with VOC emissions that result in indoor air concentrations of pollutants rising above the guidelines described by Black et al.[11] assuming continuous preoccupancy, outdoor air ventilation flush-out at a rate of 20 cfm per occupant or 20 cfm per 140 square feet of occupied space.
- Reduce to the lowest feasible amount the use of adhesives, paints, sealants, caulks, and other "wet" materials and provide alternatives for high-emitting products.[26]
- Plan and provide for adequate outdoor air ventilation or temporary ventilation[26] for a sufficient period of time to flush-out VOC emissions from new finishing and construction materials. For office buildings with VAV systems, ensure that terminals provide at least a continuous minimum of 20 cfm of outdoor air per occupant or 20 cfm of outdoor air per 140 square feet of floor space under all cooling load conditions.[27]

Table 61-3. Ventilation deficiency preventing outdoor air flush-out of volatile organic compounds during preoccupancy in new building

Variable air volume (VAV) terminal operation	Total airflow from ceiling diffusers (cfm)	Amount of outdoor air supplied to zone (cfm)
Maximum design airflow	700	210*
Measured maximum airflow†	680	204
Measured minimum airflow‡	70	21

*Assure outdoor air contributes 30% to total airflow.
†Maximum flow rate measured with VAV terminal thermostat set to minimum temperature thus calling for maximum supply of cool air.
‡Minimum flow rate measured with VAV terminal thermostat set to maximum temperature thus calling for minimum supply of cool air.

Heating, ventilation, and air-conditioning system outdoor air inlets and building pressurization

An obvious consideration for prevention of entrainment of vehicular combustion products during building design is to locate HVAC system outdoor air inlets as remote as possible from loading docks and highways or parking areas around the building. Less obvious, but still necessary during building and HVAC system design is the prevention of combustion product infiltration through building openings other than outdoor air inlets.

Figure 61-6 shows doors in a first floor corridor located approximately 10 m from the entrance to a tuck-under loading dock (note roll-up doors to dock and hospital laundry carts at dock entrance in Fig. 61-6). Stack effect in tall buildings during cold climatic periods creates a positive pressure at the top of a building and a negative pressure on the lower floors. Airborne contaminants can enter doors and other openings (for example, through loose construction) unless controls are initiated to prevent negative pressurization on lower floors. In the example illustrated in Fig. 61-6 airflow into the first floor corridor through the double doors was 28,000 cfm (negative pressurization of the first floor relative to the outdoor air was 0.05 to 0.10 in., water gauge). Carbon monoxide concentrations in interior (core) areas on the first floor ranged from 12 to 20 ppm (Table 61-4). Actions during building design and planning that can control the entrainment of combustion products include the following:

- Evaluate building design to ensure that locations with the highest quality of outdoor air are chosen for HVAC system outdoor air inlets.

- Avoid designs where potential sources of combustion products are located beneath or within the building. If this design feature cannot be avoided (for example, hotel with in-building parking garage) ensure that control systems are installed that keep occupied spaces positively pressurized relative to potential combustion sources.

- Eliminate stack effect in tall buildings by designing compartmentalized HVAC systems (one AHU for each floor) or for large centralized HVAC systems provide more return air volume for the lower floors.[28] Provide conditioned outdoor air from a separate AHU at first floor entrances such as that shown in Fig. 61-6.

Separate ventilation system for control of environmental tobacco smoke

Because ETS contains carcinogenic compounds, exposure control through dilution is not an option. Source control whereby exposure of nonsmokers to ETS is eliminated

Table 61-4. Carbon monoxide concentration in and around building with first floor tuck-under loading dock.*

Location	Carbon monoxide concentration (ppm)
Loading dock area	25–50
First floor rooms and corridor located 50 m from dock	12–20
Outdoor air	None detected

*Long-term (4 hours) length-of-stain colorimetric indicator tubes, limit of detection 10 ppm.

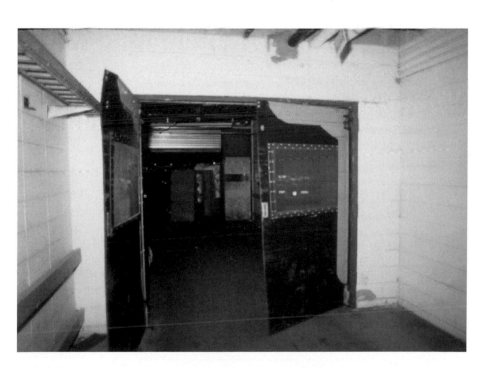

Fig. 61-6. Double doors swing open in corridor leading to loading dock (laundry carts at dock entrance) because of inrush of approximately 28,000 cfm of dock air into corridor. Loading dock air containing carbon monoxide and other combustion products enters the first floor of the building because of negative pressurization caused by stack effect.

can be achieved by smoke cessation or by restricting smoking to designated areas that are negatively pressurized (relative to indoor nonsmoking areas), well ventilated,[1] and directly exhausted outdoors (zero recirculation).

Table 61-5 illustrates sampling data for nicotine (a chemical marker for ETS) in an office building where the operator attempted to control ETS (one third of occupants smoke) through exposure control alone. Occupant density was initially one person per 70 square feet or approximately twice the ASHRAE Standard 62-1989 design density for offices (140 square feet per occupant or 7 people per 1,000 square feet). The operator initially attempted to control ETS exposure by changing occupant density to 100 square feet per occupant and by improving outdoor air ventilation. On the day when nicotine measurements were made only 40% of indoor air was being recirculated (60% outdoor air ventilation) and yet nicotine concentrations as a marker for ETS in indoor air were 12 to 14 μg/m³ (Table 61-5), a level comparable to those found in some designated smoking areas in other buildings.[29] Clearly, the only option for eliminating exposure of nonsmokers to ETS in the building in Table 61-5 is source control through smoke cessation or by restricting smoking and smokers to designated areas.

IMPORTANCE OF THE HEATING, VENTILATION, AND AIR-CONDITIONING SYSTEM FOR SOURCE AND EXPOSURE CONTROL

HVAC systems should be designed, operated, and maintained to provide building occupants with both acceptable thermal conditions and acceptable IAQ. Although a cursory review of NIOSH[10] studies suggests that more ventilation alone can control IAQ problems, the work of Fanger et al.[7] has demonstrated that HVAC systems are generally the primary source of pollutants that are associated with the perception of poor air quality. HVAC system components have long been recognized as important sources of bioaerosols.[8] The presence of contaminants in mechanical system components is almost always associated with inadequate HVAC system maintenance, operation, and design.

Table 61-5. Nicotine exposure in building where operator initiated exposure but not source control for environmental tobacco smoke

Location	Nicotine concentration (ppm)
Mailroom (approximately 1/3 occupants smoking)	12–14
Restroom (no smokers)	1
Outdoor air	None detected*

*Limit of detection 0.2 μg/m³; XAD-4 sorbent.

Outdoor air intake

Microbiologic contaminants from cooling towers and sanitary vents or emissions from exhaust vents can contaminate poorly located outdoor air intakes.

The protection of outdoor air intakes from microbial as well as from nonmicrobial (for example, combustion products) contaminants is unfortunately given only minor and inadequate attention in ventilation codes and standards. Section 5.12 of ASHRAE Standard 62-1989 states that care should be taken to avoid entrainment of water droplets from cooling towers.[1] Mechanical codes, such as the Southern Building Code Congress International, provide guidance that it is acceptable to locate chimneys or sanitary sewers up to 10 feet away and 2 feet above HVAC system outdoor air intakes.[30] Guidelines used for construction of hospital and medical facilities state that outdoor air intakes shall be located at least 25 feet from exhaust outlets and vents.[31]

Outdoor air intakes of some HVAC systems in some buildings may be at grade or below grade levels (see section "Entry of water and microbial contaminants into buildings"). These outdoor air intakes and passageways connecting to HVAC system AHUs can collect leaves and other debris. Water and debris that collect in poorly maintained and drained outdoor air pits and passageways can become reservoirs and amplification sites for microorganisms.

Source and exposure control guidelines for outdoor air intakes in addition to those previously given include the following:

- Keep the area around the outdoor air intake and connecting passageways clean and dry.
- Locate outdoor air intakes, at a minimum, 8 m (25 feet) from cooling towers (16 m or 50 feet is better) and preferably upwind from the predominant direction in which cooling tower emissions drift.
- Locate outdoor air intakes at least 8 m or 25 feet from sanitary vents and other relief and exhaust vents.
- Protect outdoor air intakes with bird screens.
- Avoid placement of outdoor air intakes within an architectural fence together with cooling towers and building relief and exhaust vents.

Mixed air plenum and other air handling unit plenums

The outdoor air entering a building's HVAC system passes from the outdoor air inlet into one or more AHUs. In the mixing plenum of the AHU outdoor air is usually mixed with return air. In many large HVAC systems, the amount of outdoor air entering the mixed air plenum varies automatically up to 100% (economizer operation).

Excessive moisture and consequent fungal contamination can occur indoors when large amounts of moist outdoor air are utilized by the HVAC system. HVAC systems with dry bulb temperature-based economizer operation often utilize large amounts (up to 100%) of outdoor air when the dry bulb temperature of the outdoor air is moderate (between 30° and 60° F) and low cost cooling is then available to control sensible heat loads (but not moisture heat loads because the AHU cooling coil does not operate in economizer cycles). Thus, when the outdoor air under economizer operation is cool and humid, indoor moisture levels can become excessive.

The use of air-to-air heat exchangers in moist coastal regions provides another example where the HVAC system can introduce elevated moisture indoors.[32] These devices are not designed to remove large amounts of moisture from incoming outdoor air.

The mixed air plenum should be devoid of debris such as leaves and feathers that, if present, indicate that the bird or leaf screen on the upstream outdoor air inlet is missing or defective. The occurrence of water or rust in the mixed air plenum indicates carryover of rain or snow into HVAC system AHUs or defective drain pans in upstream locations.

In large central HVAC systems the mixed air plenum of AHUs may be used by maintenance personnel for storage of supplies and equipment, which can have a negative impact on IAQ. Figure 61-7 shows an example where paints and adhesives (obvious sources of VOCs) have been stored in the mixed air plenum.

Source and exposure control guidelines for mixed air plenums and other AHU plenums include the following:

- Keep plenums clean and dry.
- Avoid storage of pesticides, cleaning materials, paints (see Fig. 61-7), HVAC system filters, and other maintenance equipment and supplies in plenums.
- Prohibit open floor drains in plenums unless trap seals are protected by automatic trap primers.

- Access to all plenums should be possible through hinged panels or doors. The size of doors and panels must be sufficient so that maintenance personnel can physically enter plenums to perform cleaning. Plenum access doors and panels should be unobstructed internally and externally.

Filters

Air from the mixed air plenum enters an AHU plenum, which may contain one or more sets of filters. Filters that capture particles in the airstream are classified in terms of arrestance (capacity of filter to capture a coarse synthetic dust) and dust spot efficiency (ability of filter to remove fine atmospheric dusts that can visually discolor interior surfaces).[33] In most office buildings prefilters have an arrestance of about 50% to 90% and no rated (less than 20%) efficiency.[25] The function of the prefilter or coarse filter is to prevent dirt and debris from depositing on downstream mechanical equipment. Prefilters remove only a limited amount of respirable particles from air moving through the AHU.

Some AHUs may contain high-efficiency filters in addition to prefilters. Bag filters generally have an efficiency of 60% to 90% with an arrestance greater than 98%. These filters effectively capture most fungal spores and some of the particulate fraction of ETS.

Prefilters remove 10% to 60% of bacteria particles from the airstream, while medium and high-efficiency filters remove 60% to 99% of bacterial particles.[34] The ability of filters in AHUs to capture bioaerosols has recently been reviewed.[35]

In AHUs that contain fabric filters, all ventilation air passes through a filter dust cake. The dust cake contains

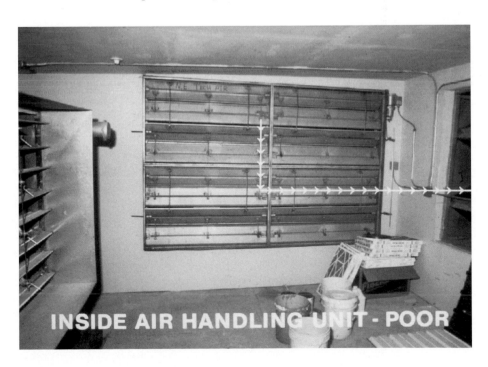

Fig. 61-7. Mixed air plenum inside air handling unit. Recycled (return) air enters at left. Outdoor air enters through almost closed dampers in background (following path of arrows). Paints, adhesives, and spare filters are stored in this ventilation space—an obvious poor source control practice.

contaminants such as human skin scales, phylloplane fungi, pollen, ETS, and atmospheric dust and debris. Filter dust cakes are secondary emission sources (reservoirs) of phylloplane fungi, VOCs, and ETS.

Fungi may grow on the nutrients in the dust cake when the relative humidity exceeds 70% or when the filter becomes physically wet.[36-38] The protection of filters from moisture and periodic replacement of the filter and its dust cake are essential for controlling potential fungal contamination in the HVAC system (see section "Special design considerations to prevent fungal contamination in medical centers").

Weschler et al.[39] showed that charcoal filters installed in AHUs serving cleanrooms were effective in removing pollutants such as ozone, sulfur dioxide, and certain VOCs such as toluene from the ventilation airstream. For example, the concentration of toluene decreased by approximately 1 order of magnitude from locations upstream ($1.4 \mu g/m^3$) to downstream ($0.1 \mu g/m^3$) of the filter. Filter performance did not show deterioration after 20 months of continuous usage, suggesting potential utility for this kind of filtration for IAQ exposure control.[39]

Exposure control guidelines for AHU filters include the following:

- Keep filters dry. Discard filters that become wet such as during economizer operation when moisture from outdoor air is absorbed in filter dirt and debris.
- Change fabric roughing filters approximately six times per year. Change bag or other high-efficiency fabric filters several times during the year to minimize the build-up of dust cake.
- Filters should fit tightly into holding frames so as to prevent bypass of unfiltered air through the AHU.

Heat exchangers

The air mixture next enters the heat exchanger section where heat is either added to or removed from the airstream in order to maintain thermally acceptable conditions in the occupied spaces. During the air-conditioning season, most coils in the heat exchanger use chilled water or halocarbon refrigerants and occasionally water from the cooling tower as the medium to remove heat from the airstream.

Air-conditioning has been associated with occupant complaints such as headache, lethargy, and upper respiratory/mucus membrane irritation.[40] During the air-conditioning process, moisture is removed from the airstream as it passes over the cooling coils in the AHU heat exchanger.[25] This occurs if the dew point temperature of the airstream is greater than the surface temperature of the cooling coil. Water from cooling coil surfaces collects in drain pans and should immediately exit the AHU through deep sealed traps.

Microorganisms, especially gram-negative bacteria[41] and yeasts, can amplify in the heat exchanger section because of the presence of wet surfaces and stagnant water. A slime on pan or coil surfaces is an indicator of bacterial amplification. Moisture that promotes the growth of microorganisms in downstream AHU locations can originate from water droplets being blown off coil surfaces when the air velocity around the coils is too great.

Water spray systems with recirculated chilled water (in place of cooling coils) were introduced for air-conditioning purposes in the 1930s. These systems, which are found in some older office buildings[42] and in industrial operations,[43] become strong microbiologic amplifiers because the dirt and debris that are also extracted or scrubbed from the airstream serve as nutrients, especially for bacteria present in the sumps of these systems. Water spray systems were originally designed to use sterile water or water that was treated with biocides.[44] The aerosolization of biocidal chemicals into the ventilation airstream of office buildings is generally considered unacceptable because of potential adverse health effects on occupants and also because it is (in the United States) a likely violation of the Hazard Communication Standard.[45]

Evaporative cooling is another form of air-conditioning where ventilation air passes through a mat that is continuously wetted by water from a recirculating sump. The dry bulb temperature of the air entering the unit may be reduced to its wet bulb temperature and the air exiting the unit thus becomes saturated with moisture. Microorganisms can grow in the evaporative mats or in the sumps of these units, and one case of hypersensitivity pneumonitis has been attributed to the growth of thermophilic actinomycetes in this type of unit.[46]

Source and exposure control measures for HVAC system heat exchangers include the following:

- Design drain pans for self-drainage.
- Prevent the build-up of biofilm through frequent cleaning.[47,48] Cleaning should be performed in such a manner that microbiocidal chemicals are never aerosolized into occupied spaces.
- Avoid the use of water spray systems in heat exchanger design.[48] If water spray systems are utilized, rigorous precautions must be taken to ensure that water droplets are not transported into downstream HVAC system components.
- Prohibit the use of odor maskers, pesticides, and rodenticides in heat exchanger plenums and in other portions of the HVAC system.
- Ensure that heat exchanger coils with direct connections to cooling tower water never leak.
- Install deep sealed-water filled traps for drains originating in the vicinity of cooling coils.[48]
- Ensure that air velocity through cooling coils is insufficient to result in aerosolization of water droplets from wet surfaces into downstream HVAC system components.

Air supply plenum and ductwork

After passing through the heat exchanger, conditioned air is distributed by a system of ducts to the occupied spaces. The main supply air ductwork immediately downstream of the heat exchanger is usually constructed of sheetmetal and can be externally or internally insulated.

Air from the main air supply plenum and ducts enters branch ducts that in buildings constructed since the 1970s often contain VAV terminals. The VAV terminals vary the amount of supply air in the branch duct (see section "Specification of low VOC emissions in finishing materials"). In constant air volume systems, the temperature in occupied spaces is maintained by varying the temperature of a consistent volumetric flow rate of air continuously supplied to the occupied zone.

Dirt and debris can be expected to accumulate in AHU plenums and in ductwork, especially in HVAC systems with inefficient filters, with filters that do not fit properly in filter frames, or with poorly designed filter banks where significant volumes of air can bypass the filter bank. Fungal spores from the outdoor air can be expected to accumulate in air supply ducts of HVAC systems with inadequate filtration characteristics. Pollen may also accumulate in supply air ducts.[49] Dust and debris in ductwork can be expected to be most abundant near elbows, turning vanes, and other locations where airflow restrictions occur, for example, near reheat coils. Toxigenic fungi have been found in duct systems subject to moisture damage.[50]

Protocols for the cleaning of air conveyance systems[51] involve physical removal of dust and debris using vacuum systems with HEPA filters. However, the mere presence of microorganisms in ductwork or AHUs is not an adequate basis for the initiation of duct cleaning. The presence of dust and debris sufficient to restrict airflow or to result in dissemination of visible particulate through diffusers into occupied spaces is a valid reason for cleaning air supply ducts.[52] In occupied buildings, the use of duct cleaning procedures using biocides in place of physical removal of dust or using encapsulation of dust and debris that may contain microorganisms has not been scientifically validated and should be avoided.[53]

Exposure control guidelines for HVAC system air supply ductwork include the following:

- Remove dirt and debris in air supply ductwork especially when airflow becomes restricted or when visible particulate from ductwork is being dispersed onto environmental surfaces in occupied spaces. The National Air Duct Cleaners Association (NADCA) provides an arbitrary gravimetric guideline of 1 mg of dust per 100 cm^2 for deciding if a duct surface is "clean."
- Determine why dust and debris are accumulating in ductwork and take appropriate corrective actions such as enhancing filtration (see section "Filters").

- Ensure that dusts aerosolized during duct cleaning are not dispersed into occupied spaces.
- Avoid the use of biocides, disinfectants, and encapsulants whose use cannot be scientifically justified.

Humidifiers in heating, ventilation, and air-conditioning systems

Humidifiers, if used in HVAC systems of large buildings, are usually incorporated into AHUs or main air supply ducts. Injection nozzles of humidifiers should be located in areas of AHUs or ductwork that is devoid of porous insulation that can provide a niche for fungal growth (see section "Porous insulation in HVAC systems"). Water from humidifiers should never wet nearby filters. Water spray humidifiers if used in AHUs must be fitted with effective downstream demisters or eliminator plates to remove carryover of water droplets.[54]

Maintenance of water sumps in cold water humidifiers must be fastidious to prevent the amplification of microorganisms.[18] Although the temperature of moisture emitted by steam humidifiers is biocidal, the steam itself may contain corrosion inhibitors such as volatile amines that can be nitrosated and are potentially toxic to occupants in humidified zones.[55]

Humidifiers that emit water droplets may discharge all water from a potable supply line or a portion of the water from a recirculation system. The potential for microbial contaminant emission from these humidifiers is directly related to the contamination in the water supply that is aerosolized. The temperature of the water in humidifiers that emit water droplets and are devoid of heating elements is usually too low (about 20° C) to support growth of *Legionella*, partially because of the evaporative cooling associated with the humidification process. Potential for microbiologic amplification in HVAC system humidifiers that emit droplets from sumps containing recirculated water is reduced by installation of highly efficient upstream filters that remove dusts that would otherwise enter the humidifier sump and serve as growth nutrient.

The Nordic Committee on Building Regulations[56] provides guidance with regard to humidification of the air. Section 4.6.6 of this guideline recommends as a general principle that where humidification is required, a type of device "which does not involve the risk of microorganisms being released into the air shall be chosen."

Porous insulation in heating, ventilation, and air-conditioning systems

Porous insulation is often installed on the inside surface of HVAC system components such as AHU plenums and the sheetmetal covers of fan coil units, induction units, and unit ventilators (see section "Peripheral HVAC system"). Internal insulation in these HVAC components reduces the transmission of fan noise and prevents the formation of condensation on exterior metal surfaces.

Insulation in the HVAC system is usually composed of fiberglass. Fiberglass insulation is porous but varies in density from the very rigid duct board to soft insulation mats.

New fiberglass insulation installed in HVAC systems is hydrophobic. Airborne particulate readily passes through the inefficient filters characteristic of many commercial buildings and accumulates in the porosities of insulation. Unlike smooth sheetmetal surfaces that may be subjected to vigorous cleaning processes, it is impossible to remove dirt and debris that has become entrained in insulation porosities. Dirt and debris are hydrophilic, and dirty insulation can absorb moisture from the ventilation airstream up to an equilibrium moisture content of about 50%.[57] Dirty insulation readily absorbs moisture because the relative humidity of ventilation air leaving the cooling coils approaches 100% as a result of the air-conditioning process and then becomes a growth site for microorganisms, especially fungi. The kinds of fungi that may grow in insulation often differ from those found in the outdoor air or normally present in indoor air.[58,59] Xerophilic fungi have been reported to be growing on surfaces of relatively new fiberglass insulation installed in residential HVAC systems.[58] Once fungi have grown in dirty porous HVAC insulation, remediation short of insulation removal is difficult if not impossible.[59]

Figure 61-8 shows fungi (mostly *Cladosporium* and *Penicillium,* concentration approximately 10^5 to 10^6 cfu/cm^2) covering the surface of porous insulation in the main air supply plenum of a large AHU. When an attempt was made to clean the insulation with an HEPA vacuum (AHU fan off; polyethylene sheeting placed across the main air supply duct; absence of negative air machines), the spore concentration in a room served by ductwork approximately 50 m downstream from the site of cleaning activities increased from 10^2 or 10^3 per m^3 to more than 10^5 per m^2 (Table 61-6). Spore concentrations in room air remained elevated only for a short period after the AHU fan was turned on presumably because of removal of spores by AHU filters and settling of spores in occupied space.

Porous insulation or fleecy surfaces in components of ventilation systems that remain dry such as forced air heating ducts (without air-conditioning) can become reservoirs

Table 61-6. Airborne fungi dispersed into occupied spaces during vacuum cleaning of contaminated insulation in AHU

Location and description	Concentration (spores/m^3) and taxa
Outdoor air	10^2 to 10^4; mostly *Cladosporium*
Room served by AHU (location approximately 50 m downstream from AHU), background conditions	10^2 to 10^3; mostly *Cladosporium*
Same as above, except during cleaning of AHU insulation (fan off)	$>10^5$; *Cladosporium* and hyphal fragments
Same as above, except 20 minutes after cleaning of AHU insulation stopped (fan on for 20 minutes to flush-out building)	$>10^4$; *Cladosporium* and hyphal fragments
Same as above, except 8 hours after cleaning of AHU insulation stopped (fan on for 8 hours to flush-out building)	10^2 to 10^3; mostly *Cladosporium;* rare hyphal fragments

AHU, Air handling unit.

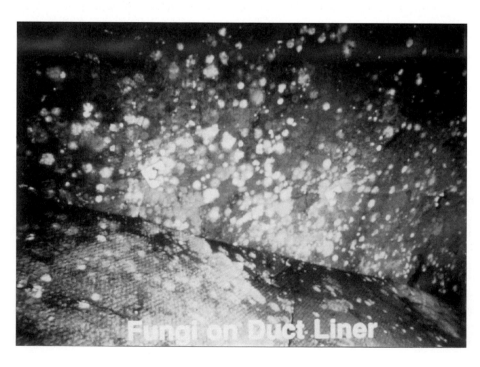

Fig. 61-8. Fungi, mostly *Cladosporium* and *Penicillium,* growing on dirty insulation in main supply air duct (see Table 61-6).

for outdoor-sourced bioaerosols such as common atmospheric fungi as well as for dust and debris containing nonmicrobiologic contaminants such as lead and ETS. The insulation then becomes a secondary emission source of outdoor-sourced fungal spores and other contaminants when HVAC system components are disturbed such as during maintenance activities.

Source and exposure control guidelines for porous insulation in HVAC systems include the following:

- Avoid the use of porous insulation on the airstream surfaces of plenums and ducts probably for a distance of 25 feet (8 m) downstream of sources of water or moisture (for example, cooling coils and water spray systems, humidifier nozzle outlets).
- Avoid the use of porous insulation on the airstream surfaces of plenums and ducts where moisture levels in the insulation can support the growth of xerophilic fungi.
- Upgrade the efficiency of AHU filter banks so that less dirt and debris (generally hydrophilic in nature) are entrained in insulation porosities.
- Follow the general principles used for the containment of asbestos when HVAC insulation contaminated with fungal growth is cleaned or remediated.[45] In general, it is better to remove insulation contaminated by fungal growth rather than to attempt to clean it.[59]

Peripheral heating, ventilation, and air-conditioning systems

In some buildings the HVAC system components previously described provide conditioned air to both interior and perimeter zones. In many buildings, however, a separate system of FCUs and induction units is used to heat and cool peripheral zones that are strongly affected by outdoor climatic conditions. In epidemiologic studies in the United Kingdom, HVAC systems containing induction or FCUs were associated with the highest index of building sickness.[60]

FCUs contain fans, low-efficiency filters, and heat exchangers and drain pans. FCUs condition and recirculate room air (often without any outdoor air) in peripheral zones. Sheetmetal enclosures of FCUs are often lined along interior surfaces with porous insulation. The maintenance of FCUs is often neglected because of the large number of units and difficulty with access. Dirt and debris accumulate in FCUs, which then can become a source of fungi during the air-conditioning season when the heat exchanger actively contributes moisture into each unit's enclosure.[48] Water from drain pan overflows and from pipe leaks can accumulate beneath units and support the growth of fungi.

Induction units receive conditioned outdoor air from a central AHU. Conditioned air exits each induction unit through a series of nozzles and mixes with room air. Induction units contain low-efficiency filters, a cooling coil that removes some sensible heat but little moisture, and drain pans that are not connected to drain lines. Because induction units contain little if any water, they are less likely to be sites for microbiologic amplification. These units are more likely to be reservoirs for pollen and phylloplane fungi assuming low-efficiency filtration in the primary AHU, and secondary sources of other contaminants such as ETS.

Operators of some buildings have used induction units for primary moisture removal with consequent massive flooding of perimeter zones because drain pans are not plumbed for drainage. Evidence of chronic flooding in perimeter zones in a building may therefore be indicative of inadequate operation or maintenance of the peripheral HVAC system.

Source and exposure control principles for peripheral HVAC system components include the following:

- Provide access into and beneath units for cleaning. If access cannot be provided, the units will become direct sources of microbial components and secondary emission sources of ETS and VOCs.
- Avoid using peripheral components during HVAC system design if maintenance cannot be guaranteed.
- Discourage occupants from blocking access panels, air inlets, and air outlets of peripheral units with furnishings, plants, or books.

Return air system

In most modern buildings, the space above the ceiling is utilized as an unducted passageway (common return air plenum) for air from the occupied space to return to main return ducts or shafts.[25] Return air then enters the mixed air plenum of HVAC system AHUs. In some large buildings fans are used in main return air passageways to move air back to AHUs. In these buildings it is important that return air and supply air fans be synchronized to avoid overall negative pressurization of the occupied spaces and to avoid positive pressurization of the mixed air plenum. The overall negative pressurization of portions of the building results in infiltration of unconditioned and unfiltered outdoor air through openings in the building envelope (see section "HVAC system outdoor air inlets and building pressurization"). The positive pressurization of the mixed air plenum (return air fan provides more air than supply fan) results in the transformation of the outdoor air intake into an exhaust air vent; consequently no outdoor air enters the AHU.

In some buildings, especially in medical centers, air from occupied spaces is returned to AHUs through a system of return air ducts. Contaminants that may be present in the space above the ceiling are thus physically isolated from the return airstream.

In the above ceiling return air plenum or in ducted return systems the space above the ceiling can become a source (amplification site) of microorganisms when fire and acoustic insulation and ceiling tiles become wet. Roof and pipe leaks resulting in high relative humidity in above ceiling cavities can result in microbiologic amplification on wood and gypsum board, and condensation of water (with subsequent microbial growth) on poorly insulated chilled water lines or on supply air ductwork (during air-conditioning season). Fire and acoustic insulation, ceiling tiles, and other extended surface materials can also be emission sources for contaminants such as VOCs.

Source and emission control principles for the HVAC return air system include the following:

- Avoid the use of materials that cannot be easily cleaned and materials with high surface areas. These materials can be strong sources of VOC emissions and when dirty and moist can be strong microbial growth sites.
- Use ducted returns in place of common return plenums.
- Replace high surface area materials such as ceiling tiles immediately after they become wet.
- Discourage the placement of AHUs and fan coil units in common return air plenums or in above ceiling spaces because access for preventive maintenance is usually difficult or impossible.

IMPORTANCE OF OPERATION AND MAINTENANCE FOR CONTAMINANT CONTROL IN OCCUPIED SPACES
Moisture and relative humidity

Chronic flooding or leaks in interior environments will result in the amplification of microorganisms indoors. For example, carpet that has been periodically flooded can function as a significant reservoir for fungal spores long after drying has occurred.[36,61] Carpet backing that is difficult to dry after a flood may be a strong fungal reservoir.

Devices such as hot tubs or saunas in indoor environments can provide the moisture needed to support the growth of microorganisms. *Cladosporium* was the cause of an outbreak of hypersensitivity pneumonitis in a residence because the fungus grew on the ceiling above the hot tub where the relative humidity was high and the ventilation was poor.[62]

The boiling of foods, activities such as showering, and even the use of water-based latex paints can be significant moisture sources in indoor environments, especially under conditions of low air exchange rates.[14]

Performance criteria for acceptable moisture levels, based primarily on comfort considerations, have been published by ASHRAE. ASHRAE Standard 55-1981[63] and the most recent interpretation of ASHRAE Standard 55-1992[64] recognize an acceptable range of relative humidity (depending on operative temperature) from over 70% to less than 30%.

It is widely recognized that fungi will grow in interior environments when the relative humidity in room air exceeds the 65% to 70% range.[48,65,66] Fungi, of course, do not grow in room air, but rather on or in finishing and construction materials. The moisture level (equilibrium relative humidity or water activity) in the substrate is the critical limiting factor that permits spores to germinate, grow, and sporulate.[67] Thus, fungal growth can occur in a room on a cold surface where the equilibrium relative humidity exceeds 70% while at the same time the relative humidity in room air at breathing height (or in the return airstream) is considerably less than 60% or 50% (see section "Condensation in hot-humid and cold climates").

Ventilation provides the only effective way for removing moisture that may be present in an interior environment. Moisture is removed from ventilation air by the dehumidification process that occurs at the surface of cooling coils in the heat exchanger (see section "Heat exchangers"). Moisture, however, cannot be removed by ventilation from an interior surface such as a wall if the surface is covered by an impermeable material (see section "Condensation in hot-humid and cold climates").

While ventilation (air-conditioning) is generally useful in reducing moisture found in interior spaces, under certain operational conditions (for example, economizer, see section "Mixed air plenum and other AHU plenums") ventilation air can actually add moisture to indoor air and promote fungal growth. Table 61-7 shows results of air sampling performed in an interior room of a large building in a hot-humid climate where the operator did not condition (dehumidify) outdoor air supplied to the occupied spaces at night and on weekends. Relative humidity was often in the 70% to 80% range; water leaks and condensation did not occur in the same room. Fungi in the room were dominated by *Aspergillus versicolor* (Table 61-7). This is a xerophilic fungus capable of growing at lower levels of moisture (water activity about 0.85) than most other fungi. *Aspergillus versicolor* also dominated the fungi present in clothes that the

Table 61-7. Xerophilic fungus grows in room when relative humidity was in the 70% to 80% range for months*

Sample location and description	Concentration of fungi	Kinds of fungi
Interior room in large building	120–190 cfu/m^3	*Aspergillus versicolor* (55% to 85% of total count), some *Cladosporium*
Clothing left for several weeks in room	>10^6 cfu/g	All *Aspergillus versicolor*
Outdoor air control	120–375 cfu/m^3	*Cladosporium* most common, some *Penicillium* and nonsporulating fungi, a few *Aspergillus ochraceous*

*Malt extract agar plus 20% sucrose culture medium; air sampling performed using a single stage volumetric impactor with 219 jets.

occupants had left in the room (Table 61-7). In this example, improper operation of the HVAC system (provision of unconditioned humid outdoor air to the occupied space) was the primary cause of fungal contamination.

The primary reason for fungal contamination in buildings is the availability of moisture levels sufficient to support growth. Although biocides have an important role in the control of bacterial growth in cooling towers that are present outside the building, a consensus has developed that biocides should generally not be used indoors for promotion of environmental quality.[52,53] Furthermore, the use of biocides in buildings can be obviated in most situations by proper attention to design, operation, maintenance, and cleaning.[68]

In recent years, several immobilized biostatic agents have been developed that can be added into the structure of interior finishing materials for the purpose of retarding potential microbial growth.[69,70] Although these products will not prevent fungal contamination associated with chronic floods, leaks, condensation, and elevated relative humidity, they may be useful in protecting interior finishing materials from biodeterioration associated with sporadic product wetting or periodic exposure to elevated relative humidity.

The presence of dirt and debris on interior surfaces such as in floors, ceilings, and walls affects the ability of the surface to support fungal growth. Dirt and debris that accumulate in or on surfaces are generally hydrophilic (see section "Porous insulation in HVAC systems") and soiled surfaces do not need to be as damp as clean surfaces to support fungal growth.[71]

Exposure control principles for occupied spaces include the following:

- Prevent floods and leaks. Dry out materials that have been flooded as fast as possible but preferably in less than 24 hours.
- Prevent the relative humidity in occupied spaces for rising above 60%. Realize that moisture in room air does not promote microbial growth. Rather, moisture in substrates (wall, ceiling, and floor systems) is what controls fungal growth. Keep the water activity in substrate below 0.65 (equilibrium relative humidity 65%).
- Keep surfaces in buildings free of dust and debris.

Human activity and exposure control

Repair work such as replacing windows generally results in increased concentrations of fungi detectable in occupied spaces.[72] The disturbance of finishing materials visually contaminated by fungi generally results in a 2 to 4 order of magnitude increase in airborne fungi, generally of a single taxon, at various distances from the disturbance.[72,73]

Studies in medical centers housing immunosuppressed patients show how easily fungal spores are dispersed by routine work and maintenance activities. In one hospital, renovation work on a floor above a renal transplant ward was associated with an outbreak of aspergillosis.[74] Vibration associated with movement of equipment on the floor above the transplant ward probably aerosolized dusts containing *Aspergillus* from the ceiling space to the patient breathing zone.

Fleecy materials such as carpet in interior spaces are strong reservoirs for fungi, bacteria, and various allergens such as those from mites and cats. The physical process of vacuum cleaning of carpet with instruments without HEPA filters leads to about an order of magnitude increase in airborne fungi such as *Cladosporium* and *Penicillium* species[72] as well as cat allergen.[75] A recent article in *Indoor Air Quality Update*[76] reviews the efficiency of various vacuum cleaners in removal of cat allergen particles from interior environments.

Humans shed bacteria and viruses, some of which may be infective, especially in poorly ventilated indoor environments.[77] The earliest ventilation standards in the nineteenth century in North America recommended a minimum of 30 to 60 cfm of outdoor air per person to dilute infectious bioaerosols to acceptable levels.[78] During the twentieth century up to the present time the concept of an acceptable minimum outdoor air ventilation rate generally from 10 to 30 cfm per occupant has been retained primarily to dilute human bioeffluent to acceptable levels. The current ASHRAE standard[1] recommends a minimum outdoor ventilation rate of 15 cfm per occupant primarily to control odor annoyance. In addition, there is some recent evidence that the incidence of respiratory infection (the common cold) among a population increases when the outdoor air ventilation rate drops below 15 cfm per occupant.[79,80]

Control of human sourced bioaerosols such as those that cause the common cold by source elimination or source reduction is not an option in most large buildings. Dilution ventilation is often the only practical control action. The outdoor air used in dilution ventilation is relatively clean and generally free of human shed bioaerosols. Filters of medium efficiency (50% to 70% dust spot efficiency; see section "Filters") will remove most human shed bacteria and viruses from recirculated air. Providing greater amounts of adequately filtered recirculated air (in addition to outdoor air) is probably more important than previously recognized for control of human-shed microorganisms in buildings.[81]

Highly infective human-sourced bioaerosols such as *Mycobacterium tuberculosis* may be controlled by the intervention techniques traditionally used in healthcare facilities to control other infectious diseases such as chickenpox and measles. These include source isolation, negative pressurization of patient rooms, and HEPA filtration of air exhausted from the patient areas. For *Mycobacterium tuberculosis,* special intervention techniques such as filtration[81] and ultraviolet light inactivation,[82] which provide the equivalent of supplemental outdoor air ventilation, are also useful exposure control techniques. In the case of tuberculosis, however, immediate recognition of the source (patient) and possibly use of personal protective equipment (respirators) by those who may be exposed to droplet nuclei provide the best control strategy. Additional information on this topic is in Chapter 59.

Principles of exposure control relative to human activity in occupied spaces include the following:

- Use care not to disturb and disperse microbial reservoirs including settled dusts that may be present in occupied spaces.
- Remove microbial reservoirs including allergens with highly efficient cleaning devices or techniques that do not recirculate or disperse bioaerosols.
- Provide as much outdoor air ventilation or equivalent outdoor ventilation[81] as possible to occupied spaces.
- Control the spread of highly infective droplet nuclei by source isolation procedures commonly used in hospital environments to contain airborne infectious disease.

Use of portable devices for enhancement of indoor air quality in occupied spaces

Humidifiers used primarily in residential environments have recently been evaluated for microbiologic emission potential.[83] Cool mist devices emit water droplets that are often contaminated by bacteria and hydrophobic fungal spores. Ultrasonic humidifiers that emit smaller size droplets often contain fragments of cells and primarily bacterial contaminants. To prevent microbiologic growth, cleaning and maintenance of all humidifiers must be thorough.[83] Scale and debris that accumulate on wet surfaces must be removed. Humidifiers containing water sumps near furnace hot air plenums have been associated with emission of thermophilic bacteria causing hypersensitivity pneumonitis.[84,85]

Portable air cleaning devices that contain HEPA or extended surface fabric filters or electrostatic precipitators are more effective than devices that rely on ionization or ozone generation.[86,87] Several air cleaners including a device with an antimicrobial component have been shown to be without effect on airborne fungi or bacterial contamination in rooms.[88,89]

One air cleaner that incorporates a HEPA filter was found to have little or no effect on mite allergen levels partly because the particle size of the allergen is such (size greater than 10 μm) that it will not remain airborne for long and thus will not be affected by any air filtration device.[90] The same type of air cleaner was effective in reducing airborne cat allergen only if surface reservoirs in the room were undisturbed and only at a very high air exchange rate (for example, 20 air changes per hour).[75] There is a consensus that portable air cleaners offer little or no additional cleaning ability over that achievable by central air conditioning alone.[91] The failure of most portable air cleaners to provide significant IAQ improvement is largely due to the small volume of air filtered in combination with strong emission rates of pollutants present in occupied spaces.

The placement of air filtration or purification devices in residential or commercial building HVAC systems can have positive effects on exposure control. For example, placement of electrostatic air cleaner in the return air system in a residence was found useful for controlling exposure to *Aspergillus* where source avoidance was not possible.[92] Charcoal filters in HVAC systems appear capable of removing significant amounts of gaseous air pollutants such as ozone, sulfur dioxide, and VOCs.[39,93]

Some air-purifying devices can degrade IAQ. Ozone generators are not only generally ineffective in terms of particle removal but also may emit ozone at rates that result in concentrations that exceed safe tolerances for humans.[94] The benefit of killing viable microorganisms by germicidal levels of ozone in occupied spaces in absence of physical removal of the microorganism is questionable at least for allergens where viability is of little importance.

Portable air cleaning devices are ineffective for exposure control in most occupied spaces because the rate of air filtration provided by the device is too low and the rate of contaminant emission from indoor reservoirs is too high. Incorporation of air-purifying devices into HVAC systems that are characterized by greater volumetric airflow is a better approach to exposure control.

Principles of exposure control for portable devices intended to enhance IAQ include the following:

- Consider contaminant source avoidance or source removal before using portable air-purifying devices.
- Incorporate air purification components into the HVAC system for maximum exposure control.
- Avoid use of air purifiers that generate ozone at levels exceeding safe tolerances for humans. Avoid use of portable devices that emit water droplets into the indoor environment.

Volatile organic compounds in occupied spaces

The sources of VOCs in occupied spaces are numerous and diverse, ranging from emissions of cleaning chemicals and products brought into a building to periodic interior renovation that is an ongoing process in most large buildings. Control of VOC emissions in occupied buildings often relies on dilution ventilation rather than source elimination or reduction. Several examples illustrate the limited value of IAQ exposure control through dilution ventilation alone.

Air sampling for VOCs in the same locations in a problem building before and 2 years after upgrading of outdoor air ventilation was performed. The building was at least 5 years old, contained moderate VOC emission sources such as paints used in a graphics department and fluids used in hydraulic elevator hoists, and was characterized initially by an outdoor air ventilation rate of approximately 5 to 10 cfm per occupant. The ventilation rate was enhanced to 15 cfm per occupant and limited source reduction measures (for example, local exhaust added to graphics department and exhaust vents added to elevator hoistways) were implemented. This resulted in only an approximate 50% decline in VOC concentrations in occupied spaces (Table 61-8). Further reduction in VOC levels will likely by achieved only through implementation of a vigorous source control policy.

Building bakeout that involves heating interior spaces and construction and finishing materials to a temperature of 90° F or more for several days in combination with some outdoor ventilation to remove VOCs has been performed in several new buildings to accelerate the emission of residual solvents from building materials.[96] Table 61-9 shows results of sampling for VOCs performed just prior to the commencement of bakeout and 1 week after bakeout completion. Sampling was performed under conditions of outdoor air ventilation at rates slightly higher than 50 cfm per occupant and at least this amount of outdoor air ventilation was continuously provided to occupied spaces between the end of bakeout and VOC sampling. The success of bakeout in this example was mixed, with TVOC concentrations declining in two locations but doubling in a third area (Table 61-9).

Building bakeout is not always successful. Although bakeout conditions accelerate the emission of VOCs ad-sorbed secondarily on extended surfaces such as carpet and ceiling tile, emissions from primary sources are only minimally affected.[97] Thus VOC emission rates may rebound to original prebakeout values several weeks after bakeout.[97]

Principles useful for controlling VOCs in occupied spaces include the following:

- Control of VOCs by source elimination or reduction during planning and construction (including renovations) is always preferred over exposure control through dilution ventilation and bakeout.
- Reduce the volatile chemicals used, for example, in cleaning agents and work processes in occupied spaces to the lowest feasible degree.
- Provide local exhaust ventilation or separate ventilation for equipment (for example, for spirit duplicating machines and printers using large amounts of solvent) or processes that are strong VOC sources.
- Provide exposure control for occupants when renovation occurs in other portions of the building.[98] Isolation of the construction area by physical barriers, negative pressurization of the work area relative to occupied spaces, and exhaust of contaminants directly outdoors (not through the HVAC system) are the most important aspects of exposure control.
- Provide maximum outdoor air ventilation continuously to dilute existing VOC emissions. Sheldon et al.[99] found that 3 to 12 months of aging with outdoor air ventilation is required in some buildings for indoor VOC concentrations to approximate outdoor concentrations. Outdoor air used to dilute indoor VOCs must be thermally acceptable and must not be elevated in moisture content (see section "Moisture and relative humidity").

Particulate in occupied spaces

Dusts present in buildings may play a role in the etiology of SBS.[100] In a building in a medical complex, SBS complaints were reported by office staff immediately adjacent to zones on the same floor undergoing wall demolition in preparation for renovation. Respirable dust concentrations in demolition zones exceeded 1,000 μg/m³ whereas those in the corridor outside closed office doors exceeded

Table 61-8. Control of VOCs in problem building primarily through upgrading outdoor air ventilation*

Sampling location	Concentration before upgrade		Concentration after upgrade	
	TVOC	Alkanes	TVOC	Alkanes
Printing/graphics	700	340	310	80
Office No. 1	710	560	340	130
Office No. 2	350	200	140	50

*Concentrations in μg/m³. Sampling and analytic method after Shields and Weschler.[95]
VOCs, Volatile organic compounds; *TVOC,* total volatile organic compound.

Table 61-9. VOC concentrations before and after bakeout*

Sample location	Before			After		
	TVOC	Alkanes	Halocarbons	TVOC	Alkanes	Halocarbons
Office No. 1	280	150	60	180	120	30
Office No. 2	300	190	60	240	160	40
Office No. 3	200	100	40	400	260	60

*Analysis by EPA TO-1 using gas chromatography/mass spectrometry. Tenax sorbent. Concentrations in μg/m³.
VOC, Volatile organic compound; *TVOC,* total volatile organic compounds; *EPA,* U.S. Environmental Protection Agency.

70 $\mu g/m^3$. Demolition dusts likely entered offices when doors were open and when offices were negatively pressurized to corridors.

Principles of exposure control for particulate in occupied spaces include the following:

- Avoid activities that generate particulate contaminants such as smoking or demolition. Avoid activities that stir-up settled dusts (dry mopping).
- Contain demolition dusts by floor to ceiling slab barriers, by negative pressurization of the work area, and by exhausting contaminant-laden air outdoors through appropriate filters (see section "VOCs in occupied spaces").
- Restrict the use of fleecy, extended surface furnishings in areas where dust control is most important.
- Use HEPA-filtered vacuums or other highly efficient cleaning devices to remove settled dusts from surfaces in occupied spaces.
- Provide highly filtered conditioned air at a sufficient air exchange rate to dilute particles that may be suspended in room air.

CONTAMINANT TRANSPORT TO THE OCCUPANT

Contaminants that can adversely affect building occupants may be found outdoors, for example, combustion products at a loading dock, or indoors, for example, on water-damaged gypsum board. For SBS or BRI to occur, the contaminant must be transported to the breathing zone of the susceptible occupant. A key aspect of indoor pollution contaminant control involves identifying pathways through which particulate and gaseous pollutants are transported to the occupant.

The outdoor air can be a significant source of air contaminants. Cases of aspergillosis decreased when patients in an old hospital with natural ventilation were moved to a new hospital with a central HVAC system.[101] Filters in AHUs of the new hospital now removed spores from outdoor air that had previously been infiltrating through open windows in the old naturally ventilated facility.

Soil excavation, road construction, and demolition of nearby buildings[102] are always associated with massive dust emissions, including dispersion of *Aspergillus* spores to patient areas. Under these conditions, outdoor air must be specially filtered or the outdoor air intake can be temporarily shut to protect highly susceptible patients from spores. For gaseous air contaminants, it would be far better to turn off an outdoor air intake for a few hours than to massively contaminate indoor air from vapors from a nearby asphalt paving operation or from carbon monoxide of an idling tractor trailer.

The HVAC system itself can be a significant source of air contaminants. *Aspergillus* spores from pigeon droppings in the relief or exhaust air portion of an HVAC system with a missing bird screen (at exhaust outlet) was the likely source of *Aspergillus* spores that caused aspergillosis in renal transplant patients.[103] Spores were transported through the HVAC system to patients when the exhaust fan malfunctioned and air from the exhaust outlet was transported to occupied spaces.

AHU filters that were moist and had not been changed were implicated as the source of *Aspergillus* spores that caused prosthetic value endocarditis.[104] Infection occurred even after cleaning the air conveyance system between the AHU and the patients. This study shows that viable spores are easily transported from a dirty filter through many meters of ductwork to patient rooms.

The most significant source of contaminants may occur in occupied spaces. Rotting wood in a sink was the source of thermophilic *Penicillium* species found in a corridor in a bone marrow transport ward that was supplied with air that was HEPA filtered.[105] A baseline thermophilic fungi concentration of 812 cfu/m^3 was present when doors to a rotted cabinet were open even though a portable HEPA filter air cleaner was operating at 20 air changes per hour.[105] This shows that emissions from microbiologic reservoirs can overwhelm even the best possible ventilation devices. In like manner strong contaminant sources including ETS from smokers and VOCs from solvent-based adhesives used in installation of new carpet can overwhelm the dilution ventilation capacity of any HVAC system.

REFERENCES

1. ASHRAE 62-1989. *Ventilation for acceptable indoor air quality. Standard 62-1989,* Atlanta, 1989, American Society of Heating, Refrigerating, and Air-Conditioning Engineers.
2. Tucker G: Status of ASHRAE standard 62-ventilation for acceptable indoor air quality, *Proc 6th Int Conf Indoor Air Quality Climate* 3:525-530, 1993.
3. ASHRAE. *IAQ 91 healthy Buildings,* Atalnta, 1991, American Society of Heating, Refrigerating, and Air-Conditioning Engineers.
4. ASHRAE. IAQ 92 *Environments for people,* Atlanta, 1992, American Society of Heating, Refrigerating, and Air-Conditioning Engineers.
5. Godish T: *Indoor air pollution control,* Chelsea, 1989, Lewis Publishers.
6. Samet JM and Spengler JD, editors: *Indoor air pollution a health perspective,* Baltimore, 1990, Johns Hopkins University Press.
7. Fanger O, Lauridsen J, Bluyssen P, et al: Air pollution sources in offices and assembly halls, quantified by the olf unit, *Energy Buildings,* 12:7-19, 1988.
8. Morey P: Experience on the contribution of structure to environmental pollution. In Kundsin R, editor: *Architectural design and indoor microbial pollution,* pp. 40-80, New York, 1988, Oxford University Press.
9. Levin H: Protocols to improve indoor environmental quality in new construction. In IAQ 87 *Practical control of indoor air problems,* pp. 157-170, Atlanta, 1987, American Society of Heating, Refrigerating, and Air-Conditioning Engineers.
10. Morey P and Singh J: Indoor air quality in nonindustrial occupational environments. In *Patty's industrial hygiene and toxicology,* ed 4, vol 1A, pp. 531-594, New York, 1991, John Wiley.
11. Black M, Pearson W, Brown J, et al: Material selection for controlling IAQ in new construction, *Proc 6th Int Conf Indoor Air Quality Climate* 2:611-616, 1993.

12. Burch D: An analysis of moisture accumulation in walls subjected to hot and humid climates, *ASHRAE Trans*, 99 (pt 2):10, 1993.

13. Odunfa S: Microorganisms associated with paint films in cold rooms and air-conditioning vent panels in Nigeria, *Int Biodeterior* 22:91-94, 1986.

14. White J: Solving moisture and mould problems, *Fifth Int Indoor Air Quality Climate* 4:589-594, 1990.

15. Burch D and Thomas W: An analysis of moisture accumulation in a wood frame wall subjected to winter climate. National Institute of Standards and Technology publication, *NISTIR 4674*, 1991.

16. Richards R, Burch D, and Thomas W: Water vapor sorption measurements of common building materials, *ASHRAE Tech Data Bull* 8(3):58-68, 1992.

17. Health and safety booklet HS (G) 70. *The control of legionellosis including legionnaires' disease.* London, 1991, Health and Safety Executive.

18. Rhame F: Prevention of nosocomial aspergillosis, *J Hosp Infect* 18 suppl A:466-472, 1991.

19. Strom G, Palmgren U, Wessen B, et al: The sick building syndrome: an effect of microbial growth in building constructions? *Fifth Int Conf Indoor Air Quality Climate*, 1:173-178, 1990.

20. Aisner J, Schimpff S, Bennett JE, et al: *Aspergillus* infections in cancer patients: Association with fireproofing materials in a new hospital, *J Am Med Assoc* 235:411-412, 1976.

21. Bornehag C-G: Problems associated with the replacement of casein-based self-leveling compound. In *IAQ 91 healthy buildings*, pp 273-275, Atlanta, 1991, American Society of Heating, Refrigerating, and Air-Conditioning Engineers.

22. Karlsson S, Banhidi F, Banhidi Z, et al: Accumulation of malodorous amines and polyamines due to clostridial putrefaction indoors, *Proc 3rd Int Conf Indoor Air Quality Climate* 3:287-293, 1984.

23. Andersen I and Korsgaard J: Asthma and the indoor environment: assessment of the health implications of high indoor air humidity, *Environ Int* 12:121-127, 1986.

24. Maryland state board of education technical bulletin. *Carpet and indoor air quality in schools.* Baltimore, 1993.

25. Morey P and Shattuck D: Role of ventilation in the causation of building-associated illness, *Occup Med State Art Rev* 4(4):625-642, 1989.

26. Levin H: Building materials and indoor air quality, *Occup Med State Air Rev* 4(4):667-693, 1989.

27. Cohen T: Providing constant ventilation in VAV systems. In *IAQ 93 Operating and maintaining buildings for health, comfort, and productivity*, pp 65-66, Atlanta, 1993, American Society of Heating, Refrigerating, and Air-Conditioning Engineers.

28. Tamblyn R: HVAC system effects for tall buildings, *ASHRAE transaction paper* DE-93-10-1, 1993.

29. Sterling T and Mueller B: Concentrations of nicotine, RSP, CO, and CO$_2$ in nonsmoking office areas under different conditions of recirculation of air from smoking designated areas, *Air pollution control association paper* 88-76.5, 1988.

30. SBCCI: *1988 standard mechanical code,* 1989/1990 revisions, section 514, Southern Building Code Congress International, 1990.

31. American Institute of Architects: *Guidelines for construction and equipment of hospital and medical facilities,* Committee on Architecture for Health, section 7.31D, 1993.

32. Tsongas G: A field study of indoor moisture problems and damage in new Pacific northwest homes. In *IAQ 91 healthy buildings,* pp 202-209, Atlanta, 1991, American Society of Heating, Refrigerating, and Air-Conditioning Engineers.

33. ASHRAE. 1992 *Systems and equipment handbook.* In *Air cleaners for particulate contaminants,* Chap 25, Atlanta, 1992, American Society of Heating, Refrigerating, and Air-Conditioning Engineers.

34. Decker H, Buchanan L, Hall L, et al: Air Filtration of microbial particles, *Am J Public Health* 53:1982-1988, 1963.

35. Kuehn T, Pui D, Vesley D, et al: Matching filtration to health requirements, *ASHRAE transactions paper* 3505, 1991.

36. Morey P: Case presentations: Problems caused by moisture in occupied spaces of office buildings, *Ann Am Conf Gov Ind Hyg* 10:121-127, 1984.

37. Pasanen P, Hujanen M, Kalliokoski P, et al: Criteria for changing ventilation filters. In *IAQ 91 healthy buildings,* pp 383-385, Atlanta, 1991, American Society of Heating, Refrigerating, and Air-Conditioning Engineers.

38. Schicht H: The diffusion of micro-organisms by air-conditioning installations, *Steam Heating Eng* 6-13, 1972.

39. Weschler C, Shields H, and Naik D: An evaluation of activated carbon filters for control of ozone, sulfur dioxide, and selected volatile organic compounds. In *IAQ 92 environments for people,* pp 233-241, Atlanta, 1992, American Society of Heating, Refrigerating, and Air-Conditioning Engineers.

40. Mendell M and Smith A: Consistent pattern of elevated symptoms in air-conditioned office buildings: A reanalysis of epidemiologic studies, *Am J Public Health* 80:1193-1199, 1990.

41. Hugenholtz P and Fuerst J: Heterotrophic bacteria in an air-handling system, *Appl Environ Microbiol* 58:3914-3920, 1992.

42. Hodgson M, Morey P, Simon T, et al: An outbreak of recurrent acute and chronic hypersensitivity pneumonitis of office workers, *Am J Epidemiol* 125:631-638, 1987.

43. Reed C, Swanson M, Lopez M, et al: Measurement of IgG antibody and airborne antigen to control an industrial outbreak of hypersensitivity pneumonitis, *J Occup Med* 25:207-210, 1983.

44. Yaglou C and Wilson U: Disinfection of air by air-conditioning processes, *Am Assoc Adv Sci Pub No 17* 129-132, 1942.

45. Morey P: Microbiological contamination in buildings: Precautions during remediation activities. In *IAQ 92 environments for people,* pp 171-177, Atlanta, 1992, American Society of Heating, Refrigerating, and Air-Conditioning Engineers.

46. Marinkovich V and Hill A: Hypersensitivity alveolitis, *J Am Med Assoc* 231:944-947, 1975.

47. Brundrett G, Collins J, DaCosta G, et al: Humidifier fever, *J Chart Inst Build Serv* 3:35-36, 1981.

48. Morey P, Hodgson M, Sorenson W, et al: Environmental studies in moldy office buildings, *ASHRAE Trans* 92(1):399-419, 1986.

49. Laatikainen T, Pasanen P, Korhonen L, et al: Methods for evaluating dust accumulation in ventilation ducts. In *IAQ 91 healthy buildings,* pp 379-382, Atlanta, 1991, American Society of Heating, Refrigerating, and Air-Conditioning Engineers.

50. Croft W, Jarvis B, and Yatawara C: Airborne outbreak of trichothecene toxicosis, *Atmos Environ* 20:549-552, 1986.

51. NADCA-01: *Mechanical cleaning of non-porous air conveyance system components,* Washington DC, 1992, National Air Duct Cleaners Association.

52. Girman J, Truter R, and McCarthy J: Maintaining clean HVAC systems, *Proc 6th Int Conf Indoor Air Quality Climate. Workshop Summaries* W4: 7-8, 1993.

53. Nevalainen N: Microbial contamination in buildings, *Proc 6th Int Conf Indoor Air Quality Climate* 4:3-13, 1993.

54. Ager B and Tickner J: The control of microbiological hazards associated with air-conditioning and ventilation systems, *Ann Occup Hyg* 27:341-358, 1983.

55. NRC: *An Assessment of the health risks of morpholine and diethylaminoethanol,* National Research Council, Washington, DC, 1983, National Academy Press.

56. NKB: *Indoor climate-air quality,* Nordic Committee on Building Regulations, Pub No 61E, section 4.6.6, 1991.

57. West M and Hansen E: Determination of material hygroscopic properties that affect indoor air quality. In *IAQ 89 the human equation: health and comfort,* pp 60-63, Atlanta, 1989, American Society of Heating, Refrigerating and Air-Conditioning Engineers.

58. Ahearn D, Price D, Simmons R, et al: Colonization studies of various HVAC insulation materials. In *IAQ 92 environments for people*, pp 179-183, Atlanta, 1991, American Society of Heating, Refrigerating, and Air-Conditioning Engineers.

59. Morey P and Williams C: Is porous insulation inside a HVAC system compatible with a healthy building? In *IAQ 91 healthy buildings*, pp 128-135, Atlanta, 1991, American Society of Heating, Refrigerating, and Air-Conditioning Engineers.

60. Burge S, Hodge A, Wilson S, et al: Sick building syndrome: a study of 4373 office workers, *Ann Occup Hyg* 31:493-504, 1987.

61. Kozak P, Gallup J, Cummins L, et al: Currently available methods for home mold surveys. II. Examples of problem homes surveyed, *Ann Allergy* 45:167-176, 1989.

62. Jacobs R, Thorner R, Holcomb J, et al: Hypersensitivity pneumonitis caused by *Cladosporium* in an enclosed hot-tub area, *Ann Intern Med* 105:204-206, 1986.

63. ASHRAE 55-1981: *Thermal environmental conditions for human occupancy, Standard 55-1981*, Atlanta, 1981, American Society of Heating, Refrigerating, and Air-Conditioning Engineers.

64. ASHRAE 55-1992: *Thermal environmental conditions for human occupancy, Standard 55-1992*, Atlanta 1992, American Society of Heating, Refrigerating, and Air-Conditioning Engineers.

65. Block S: Humidity requirements for mold growth, *Appl Microbiol* 1:287-293, 1953.

66. Lim G, Tan T, and Toh A: The fungal problem in buildings in the humid tropics, *Int Biodeterior*, 25:27-37, 1989.

67. Flannigan B: Approaches to assessment of the microbial flora of buildings. In *IAQ 92 environments for people*, pp 139-145, Atlanta, 1992, American Society of Heating, Refrigerating, and Air-Conditioning Engineers.

68. Flannigan B and Morey P: Control of moisture problems affecting indoor air quality, *Proc 6th Int Conf Indoor Air Quality Climate. Workshop summaries* W18:35-36, 1993.

69. Price D, Sawant A, and Ahearn D: Activity of an insoluble antimicrobial quaternary amine complex in plastics, *J Ind Microbiol* 8:83-90, 1991.

70. Speier J and Malek J: Destruction of microorganisms by contact with solid surfaces, *J Colloid Interface Sci* 89(1):68-76, 1982.

71. Grant C, Hunter C, Flannigan B, et al: The moisture requirements of moulds isolated from domestic dwellings, *Int Biodeterior* 25:259-284, 1989.

72. Hunter C, Grant C, Flannigan B, et al: Mould in buildings: The air spora of domestic buildings, *Int Biodeterior* 24:81-101, 1988.

73. Morey P: Bioaerosols in the indoor environment: Current practices and approaches. In: Gammage R and Weeks D, editors: *Indoor air quality international symposium*, pp 51-72, Akron, OH, 1990, American Industrial Hygiene Assoc.

74. Arnow P, Andersen R, Matinous D, et al: Pulmonary aspergillosis during hospital renovation, *Am Rev Respir Dis* 118:49-53, 1978.

75. Luczynska, C, Li Y, Chapman M, et al: Airborne concentrations and particle size distribution of allergen derived from domestic cats *(Felis domesticus)*, *Am Rev Respir Dis* 141:361-367, 1990.

76. Indoor air quality update: Vacuum cleaners vary in their ability to capture allergens, *IAQ Update* 6(8):5-7, 1993.

77. Burge H: Indoor air and infectious disease, *Occup Med State Art Rev* 4(4):713-721, 1989.

78. Woods J, Morey P, and Stolwijk J: Indoor air quality and the sick building syndrome: a view from the United States, *Conference on advances in air conditioning*, pp 10-15, Chartered Institute of Building Services Engineers, October 7, 1988.

79. Brundage J, Scott R, Lednar W, et al: Building-associated risk of febrile acute respiratory disease in army trainees, *J Am Med Assoc* 259:2108-2112, 1988.

80. Janssen J: Ventilation for acceptable indoor air quality, *ASHRAE J* 40-48, Oct. 1989.

81. Wheeler A: Better filtration: a prescription for healthier buildings. In *IAQ 93 operating and maintaining buildings for health, comfort, and productivity*, pp 131-136, Atlanta, 1993, American Society of Heating, Refrigerating, and Air-Conditioning Engineers.

82. Nardell E, Keegan J, Cheney S, et al: Airborne infection: theoretical limits of protection achievable by building ventilation, *Am Rev Respir Dis* 144:302-306, 1991.

83. Tyndall R, Dudney C, Katz D, et al: Characterization of microbial content and dispersion from home humidifiers, *Report to consumer product safety commission on project no. 86-1283*, January 25, 1989.

84. Fink J, Banaszak E, Thiede W, et al: Interstitial pneumonitis due to hypersensitivity of an organism contaminating a heating system, *Ann Int Med* 74:80-83, 1971.

85. Sweet L, Anderson J, Callies Q, et al: Hypersensitivity pneumonitis related to a home furnace humidifier, *J Allergy Clin Immunol* 48:171-178, 1971.

86. Offermann F, Sextro R, Fisk W, et al: Control of respirable particles in indoor air with portable air cleaners, *Atmos Environ* 19:1761-1771, 1985.

87. Shaughnessy R, Levetin E, and Sublette K: Effectiveness of portable indoor air cleaners in particulate and gaseous contaminant removal, *Proc 6th Int Conf Indoor Air Quality Climate* 6:381-386, 1993.

88. Edwards J, Trotman D, and Mason D: Methods for reducing particle concentrations of *Aspergillus fumigatus* conidia and mouldy hay dust, *Sabouraudia: J Med Vet Mycol* 23:237-243, 1985.

89. Nelson H and Skufca R: Double-blind study of suppression of indoor fungi and bacteria by the PuriDyne biogenic air purifier, *Ann Allergy* 66:263-266, 1991.

90. Antonicelli L, Bilo M, Pucci S, et al: Efficacy of an air-cleaning device equipped with a high efficiency particulate air filter in house dust mite respiratory allergy, *Allergy* 46:594-600, 1991.

91. Nelson H, Hirsch R, Ohman J, et al: Recommendations for the use of residential air-cleaning devices in the treatment of allergic respiratory diseases, *J Allergy Clin Immunol* 82:661-669, 1988.

92. Jacobs R, Andrews C, and Jacobs F: Hypersensitivity pneumonitis treated with an elecrostatic dust filter, *Ann Intern Med* 110:115-118, 1989.

93. Liu R: Use of activated carbon adsorbers in HVAC applications. In *IAQ 93 operating and maintaining buildings for health, comfort, and productivity*, pp 137-143, Atlanta, 1993, American Society of Heating, Refrigerating, and Air-Conditioning Engineers.

94. Shaughnessy R and Oatman L: The use of ozone generators for the control of indoor air contaminants in an occupied environment. In *IAQ 91 healthy buildings*, pp 318-324, Atlanta, 1991, American Society of Heating, Refrigerating, and Air-Conditioning Engineers.

95. Shields H and Weschler C: Analysis of ambient concentrations of organic vapors with a passive sampler, *J Air Poll Control Assoc* 37:1039-1045, 1987.

96. Girman J: Volatile organic compounds and building bake-out, *Occup Med State Art Rev* 4(4):695-712, 1989.

97. Offermann F, Loiselle S, Ander G, et al: Indoor contaminant emission rates before and after a building bake-out, *Proc 6th Intern Conf Indoor Air Quality Climate* 6:687-691, 1993.

98. Morey P, Eisenstein H, Girman J, et al: Construction and renovation during partial occupancy. In *IAQ 91 healthy buildings postconference proc*, pp 54-55, 1991 American Society of Heating, Refrigerating, and Air-Conditioning Engineers.

99. Sheldon L, Handy R, Hartwell T, et al: *Indoor air quality in public buildings: volume 1. Project summary*, EPA report no. 600/S6-88/009a, 1988.

100. Gravesen S, Ipsen H, and Skov P: Partial characterization of the components in the macromolecular organic dust (MOD) fraction and their

possible role in the sick-building-syndrome (SBS), *Proc 6th Intern Conf Indoor Air Quality Climate* 4:33-35, 1993.

101. Rose H: Mechanical control of hospital ventilation and *Aspergillus* infections, *Am Rev Respir Dis* 105:306-307, 1972.
102. Walsh T and Dixon D: Nosocomial aspergillosis: environmental microbiology, hospital epidemiology, diagnosis and treatment, *Eur J Epidemiol* 5:131-142, 1989.
103. Kyriakides G, Zimmerman H, Hall W, et al: Immunologic monitoring and aspergillosis in renal transplant patients, *Am J Surg* 131:246-252, 1976.
104. Petheram I and Seal R: *Aspergillus* prosthetic valve endocarditis, *Thorax* 31:380-390, 1976.
105. Streifel A, Stevens P, and Rhame F: In-hospital source of airborne *Penicillium* spores, *J Clin Microbiol* 25:1-4, 1987.

Appendix A

RESOURCES

Elizabeth A. Jennison
Gregory J. Kullman
John E. Parker

U.S. NATIONAL INSTITUTE FOR OCCUPATIONAL SAFETY AND HEALTH (NiOSH) PUBLICATIONS

NIOSH Bookshelf

NIOSH Bookshelf, a listing of basic reference publications of NIOSH, is available from

> Division of Standards Development and Technology Transfer
> National Institute for Occupational Safety and Health
> ATTN: Publications, C-13
> 4676 Columbia Parkway
> Cincinnati, OH 45226-1998
> Phone: (800) 35-NIOSH
> FAX: 513-533-8573

NIOSH Health Hazard Evaluation Program

> To request a Health Hazard Evaluation, contact:
> Hazard Evaluations and Technical Assistance Branch
> National Institute for Occupational Safety and Health
> 4676 Columbia Parkway, Mail Stop R-9
> Cincinnati, OH 45226
> Phone: (513) 841-4382

NIOSHTIC Database

NIOSHTIC Database is commercially available on-line from the following database vendors:

> Marketing Department
> DIALOG Information Services, Inc.
> 3460 Hillview Avenue
> Palo Alto, CA 94304
> Phone: (415) 858-3785 or (800) 334-2564

> Orbit Search Service
> 8000 Westpark Drive
> McLean, VA 22101
> Phone: (703) 442-0900 or (800) 421-7229

> Information Retrieval Service
> European Space Agency
> Via Galileo Galilei
> 00044 Frascati
> Rome, Italy
> Phone: 011-39-6-941801
> FAX: 011-39-6-94180361

NIOSHTIC CD-ROM

NIOSHTIC is commercially available on CD-ROM from the following vendors:

> SilverPlatter Information, Ltd.
> 100 River Ridge Drive
> Norwood, MA 02062-5026
> Phone: (617) 769-2599 or (800) 343-0064

> Inquiries Service
> Canadian Centre for Occupational Health and Safety
> 250 Main Street East
> Hamilton, Ontario, Canada L8N 1H6
> Phone: (416) 572-2981

U.S. OCCUPATIONAL SAFETY AND HEALTH ADMINISTRATION (OSHA) REGIONAL OFFICES

Region I (Connecticut, Maine, Massachusetts, New Hampshire, Rhode Island, and Vermont)
> 133 Portland Street, 1st Floor
> Boston, MA 02114
> Phone: (617) 565-7164

Region II (New Jersey, New York, and Puerto Rico)
> 201 Varick Street, Room 670
> New York, NY 10014
> Phone: (212) 337-2325

Region III (Delaware, District of Columbia, Maryland, Pennsylvania, Virginia, and West Virginia)
   Gateway Building, Suite 2100
   3535 Market Street
   Philadelphia, PA 19104
   Phone: (215) 596-1201

Region IV (Alabama, Florida, Georgia, Kentucky, Mississippi, North Carolina, South Carolina, and Tennessee)
   1375 Peachtree Street NE, Suite 587
   Atlanta, GA 30367
   Phone: (404) 347-3573

Region V (Illinois, Indiana, Michigan, Minnesota, Ohio, and Wisconsin)
   230 South Dearborn Street
   32nd Floor, Room 3244
   Chicago, IL 60604
   Phone: (312) 353-2220

Region VI (Arkansas, Louisiana, New Mexico, Oklahoma, and Texas)
   525 Griffin Street, Room 602
   Dallas, TX 75202
   Phone: (214) 767-4731

Region VII (Iowa, Kansas, Missouri, and Nebraska)
   911 Walnut Street, Room 406
   Kansas City, Missouri 64106
   Phone: (816) 426-5861

Region VIII (Colorado, Montana, North Dakota, South Dakota, Utah, and Wyoming)
   Federal Building, Room 1576

1961 Stout Street
Denver, CO 80204
Phone: (303) 844-3061

Region IX (American Samoa, Arizona, California, Guam, Hawaii, Nevada, and Trust Territory of the Pacific Islands)
   71 Stevenson Street, Suite 415
   San Francisco, CA 94105
   Phone: (415) 744-6670

Region X (Alaska, Idaho, Oregon, and Washington)
   1111 Third Avenue, Suite 715
   Seattle, WA 98101-3212
   Phone: (206) 442 5930

OTHER SOURCES

American College of Occupational and Environmental Medicine
55 West Seegers Road
Arlington Heights, IL 60005
Phone: (708) 228-6850
Publishes an annual directory of member physicians, including information about board certification, location, and type of practice.

Association of Environmental and Occupational Clinics (AOEC)
1010 Vermont Avenue NW, #513
Washington, DC 20005
Phone: (202) 347-4976
Publishes a directory of member clinics and physicians, including information about special interests, services, and location.

KEY REFERENCES IN
OCCUPATIONAL ASTHMA

Jean-Luc Malo
André Cartier

Appendix B. Key references in occupational asthma*

Agent	Occupation or industry	Reference	Subjects (n)	Prevalence (%)	Skin test	Specific IgE	Other immunologic tests	Broncho-provocation test	Other evidence
High–molecular-weight agents									
Animal-derived antigens									
Laboratory animal	Laboratory worker	1	296	13	17% +	34% of 255 +	ND	ND	
		2	5	NA	100% +	100% +	– Precipitin	100% +	
Cow dander	Agricultural worker	3	49	NA	100%	ND	Immunoblotting	ND	
Chicken	Poultry worker	4, 5	14	NA	79% +	79% +	ND	1 of 1 +	+ PEFR monitoring
Pig	Butcher	6	1	NA	ND	+	ND	ND	
Frog	Frog catcher	7	1	NA	+	+	– Precipitin	ND	
Lactoserum	Dairy industry	8	1	NA	+	ND	+ Basophil degranulation	+	
Casein (cow's milk)	Tanner	9	1	NA	ND	+	ND	+	
Bat guano	Various	10	7	NA	+	+	RAST inhibition	ND	
Insects									
Grain mite	Farmer	11	290	12	21% +	19% of 219 +	ND	ND	
	Grain storage worker	12	133	33	25% +	23% of 128 +	ND	1 of 1 +	21% of 116 with + PC20
Locust	Laboratory worker	13	118	26	32% of 113 +	Done	Specific IgG	ND	Reduced FEV1
Screw worm fly	Flight crew	14	15	60	77% +	53%+	RAST inhibition	ND	
Cricket	Laboratory worker	15	182	25	91% of 11 +	ND	ND	ND	
Bee moth	Fish bait breeder	16	2	NA	+	+	Passive transfer	+	
		17	1	NA	+	ND	Passive transfer / Histamine release	ND / +	
Moth, butterfly	Entomologist	18	2	NA	+	ND	ND	ND	
Mexican bean weevil	Seed house worker	19	2	NA	+	ND	Passive transfer	ND	
Fruit fly	Laboratory worker	20	22	32	27% +	27% +	RAST inhibition	21% of 14 +	
Honeybee	Honey processor	21	1	NA	+	+	ND	ND	
L. caesar larvae	Angler	22	5	NA	75% of 4 +	80% of 5 +	RAST inhibition	1 of 1 +	
Lesser mealworm	Grain and poultry worker	23	3	NA	–	100% of 3 +	RAST inhibition	ND	
Fowl mite	Poultry worker	24	13	NA	77% +	60%	ND	1 of 1 +	
Barn mite	Farmer	25	38	NA	100% +	~100%	ND	ND	
Mites and parasites	Flour handler	26	12	NA	ND	+	ND	ND	
Acarian	Apple grower	27	4	NA	+	ND	– Precipitin	ND	
Daphnia	Fish food storage worker	28	2	NA	+	+	ND	2 of 2 +	
Weeping fig	Plant keeper	29	84	7	21% +	21%	ND	100% of 6 +	PC20
Sheep blowfly	Technician	30	53	24	ND	67% of 15 +	ND	ND	
Silkworm	Silk worker	31	53	34	ND	ND	ND	ND	

Continued.

Appendix B. Key references in occupational asthma—cont'd

Agent	Occupation or industry	Reference	Subjects (n)	Prevalence (%)	Skin test	Specific IgE	Other immunologic tests	Broncho-provocation test	Other evidence
Plants									
Grain dust	Grain elevator worker	32	610	~40	9% +	ND	– Precipitin	ND	Spirometry preshift and postshift
		33, 34	502	47	~50% of 51 exposed +	ND	ND	ND	FEV1, volumes
Wheat, rye, and soya flour	Baker or miller	35	22	NA	0% +	ND	– Precipitin	27% +	50% PC20 +
		36	279	35	9% + (cereals)	ND	ND	ND	FEV1 and PC20
Lathyrus sativus	Flour handler	37	7	100	100% +	100% +	100% –	57% +	
Vicia sativa		38	9	100		100% +	Western blotting	ND	
	Farmer	39	1	NA	+	ND	+ Precipitin	+	
		40	1	NA	+	+	+ Precipitin and passive transfer	+	
Buckwheat	Baker	41	3	NA	100% +	ND	ND	ND	
Gluten	Baker	42	1	NA	+	+	RAST inhibition	+	
Coffee bean	Food processor	43	372	34	24% +	12% +	ND	ND	Function tests
		44	45	9	9%–40% +	ND	ND	ND	Spirometry
		45	22	NA	82% +	50% +	ND	67% of 12+	PC20 + in 14
Castor bean	Oil industry	46	14	NA	100% +	100% +	ND	ND	
Tea	Tea processor	47	3	NA	100% –	–	ND	100% of 3 +	
Herbal tea	Herbal tea processor	48	1	NA	ND	ND	ND	+	
Tobacco leaf	Tobacco manufacturer	49	1	NA	+	+	ND	+	
		50	16	69	ND	ND	ND	ND	+PEFR monitoring
Hops	Brewery chemist	51	1	NA	+	+	ND	ND	
Baby's breath	Florist	52	1	NA	+	+	Histamine release	+	
Freesia and paprika	Horticulturist	53	2	NA	+	+	Histamine release	ND	
Mushroom	Mushroom soup processor	54	8	NA	+	ND	ND	50% of 8 +	
Cacoon seed	Decorator	55	1	NA	+	ND	ND	ND	
Chicory	Chicory grower	56	1	NA	–	ND	ND	ND	
Rose hips	Pharmaceutical	57	9	NA	67% +	67% +	ND	50% of 4 +	FEV1 and PC20
Sunflower	Laboratory worker	58	1	NA	+	+	RAST inhibition	+	
Garlic dust	Food packager	59	1	NA	+	+	RAST inhibition	+	
		60	1	NA	+	+	RAST inhibition	+	
Lycopodium	Powder	61	30	7	ND	ND	ND	2 of 2 +	
Sericin	Hairdresser	62	2	NA	1 of 1 +	ND	ND	ND	
Nacre dust	Nacre (mother-of-pearl) button maker	63	1	NA	+	ND	– Precipitin	+	
Pectin	Christmas candy maker	64	1	NA	+	–	Specific IgG4	+	
Henna (conchiolin?)	Hairdresser	65	2	NA	+	+	ND	1 of 2 +	
Neurospora	Plywood factory worker	66	1	NA	+	+	ND	+	

Allergen	Occupation	Ref							
Biologic enzymes									
Bacillus subtilis	Detergent industry	67	1642	3.2 (over 7 years)	4.5%-75% +	26% of 248 +	ND	ND	Lung function
		58	38	NA	66% +	ND	Passive transfer, 100% of 5 +	90% +	Lung function
Trypsin	Plastic and pharmaceutical	59	667	NA	ND	5%	ND	ND	
			14	29	+	+	ND	75% of 4 +	
Papain	Pharmaceutical	70	29	45	34% +	34% +	ND	89% of 9 +	
Pepsin	Pharmaceutical	71	1	NA	+	+		+	
Pancreatin	Pharmaceutical	72	14	NA	93% +	100% of 3 +	+ Precipitin	100% of 8 +	Lung function
Flaviastase	Pharmaceutical	73	3	NA	+	+	ND	ND	
Bromelin	Pharmaceutical	74	76	11	25% +	ND	ND	ND	
	Pharmaceutical	75	2	NA	+	ND	ND	2 of 2 +	
Egg lysosyme	Pharmaceutical	76	1	NA	+	+	ND	+	+ PEFR monitoring
Fungal amylase	Baker	77	118	NA	100% of 13 +	2% exposed +, 34% with occupational asthma -	ND	ND	
Fungal amyloglucosidase and hemicellulase	Baker	78	1	NA	+	+	ND	+	
	Baker	79	140	NA	ND	5%-24%	ND	ND	
Esperase	Detergent industry	80	667	NA	ND	5%	ND	ND	
Vegetable gums									
Acacia	Printer	81	63	19% of 31 (selection)	ND	ND	ND	ND	
	Printer	82	10	NA	+	ND	Passive transfer (3 +)	ND	
Tragacanth	Gum importer	83	1	NA	+	ND	ND	ND	
Karaya	Hairdresser	84	9	4	+	ND	Passive transfer	ND	
Guar	Carpet manufacturer	85	162	2	5% +	8% +	ND	67% of 3 +	PC20
Other									
Crab	Snow crab processor	86	303	16	22% +	ND	ND	72% of 46 +	PEFR +, PC20 monitoring
Prawn	Prawn processor	87	50	36	26% +	16% +	ND	2 of 2 +	
Hoya	Oyster farm worker	88	1413	29	82% of ≤11 with asthma +	89% of ~180 with asthma +	ND	ND	
Cuttlefish	Deep-sea fisher	89	66	Incidence of 1%/yr	ND	ND	ND	ND	
Trout(?)	Trout processor	90	5	NA	ND	100% -	100% +	ND	
Shrimpmeal	Technician	91	1	NA	+	ND	ND	+	
Larva of silkworm	Sericulture	92	5519	0.2	100% of 9(?) +	1 of 1(?) +	P-K reaction	100% of 9 +	

Appendix B. Key references in occupational asthma—cont'd

Agent	Occupation or industry	Reference	Subjects (n)	Prevalence (%)	Skin test	Specific IgE	Other immunologic tests	Broncho-provocation test	Other evidence
Egg protein	Egg producer	93	188	7	34% +	29% +	ND	ND	PEFR, 7% +
Fish feed (*Echinodorus* larva)	Aquarium keeper	94	1	NA	+	+	ND	+	
Low–molecular-weight agents									
Red soft coral	Fisherman	95	74	9	2 of 2 +	ND	ND	ND	
Diisocyanates									
TDI	Polyurethane	96	112	12.5	3% +	0% +	0% + PCA	45% of 11 +	
	Plastics and varnish	97	26	28.0	ND	19% +	ND	100% +	
		98	195		ND	5% +	ND	70% of 17 +	
		99	91			ND	0% + specific IgG	ND	
MDI	Foundry	100	162†		ND	ND	ND	57% +	
		101	11		ND	27% +	36% + specific IgG	54.5% +	
		102	76	13.2	ND	3% +	7% + specific IgG	ND	
		103	26	27.0	4% +	4% +	15% + specific IgG	ND	
1,5-Naphthylene diisocyanate	Rubber manufacturer	104	3		ND	ND	ND	100% +	
Isophorone diisocyanate	Spray painter	105	1		ND	ND	ND	+	
Prepolymers of TDI	Floor varnisher	106	2	NA	ND	0% +	Specific IgG −	+	
Prepolymers of HDI	Spray painter	107	9	45	ND	33% +	56% +	+	
Combination of diisocyanates									
TDI, MDI, HDI, and PPI	Paint shop worker	108	51	11.8‡	ND	ND	ND	60% of 10 + to PPI	
TDI, MDI, and HDI	Various	109	24		ND	ND	ND	70% + to TDI, 33% + to MDI, 33% of 9 + to HDI	
		110	247†		60% of 53 +, 14% +	ND	ND		
	Paint shop worker	111	62		ND	15% +	47% + specific IgG	6% + to TDI, 16% to MDI, 24% to HDI	

Agent	Occupation	Reference	No.						Comments
TDI and MDI		112	28		ND	27% of 22 − TDI-HSA, 83% of 6 + MDI-HSA	ND	100% +	
Anhydrides									
Phthalic anhydride	Plastics	113	1		+	+	ND	+	
	Toolsetter or resin plant agent	114	3		ND	ND	ND	100% +	
	Production of resins	115	118	28	18% of 11 +	ND	ND	ND	
		116	60	14	ND	7% +	17% + specific IgG	100% of 1 +	
Trimellitic anhydride	Epoxy resins and plastics	117	4		100% +	75% +	100% + specific IgG	100% +	
Tetrachlorophthalic anhydride	Epoxy resins and plastics	118	5		ND	ND	ND	100% +	
Pyromellitic dianhydride	Epoxy adhesive	119	7		100% +	100% +	ND	100% +	
		120	7		ND	ND	ND	30% +	
Methyl tetrahydrophthalic anhydride	Curing agent	121	1		+	+	− specific IgG	ND	Improvement with removal
Hexahydrophthalic anhydride	Chemical worker	122	1	NA	ND	ND	ND	+	PEFR monitoring +
Himic anhydride	Manufacturer of flame retardant	123	20	35	ND	Evidence 40% of 7 +	Test RAST inhibition	ND	
Aliphatic amines									
Ethyleneamines									
Ethylenediamine	Shellac handler	124	7		100% +	ND	ND	100% +	
	Photographer	125	1		ND	ND	ND	+	
Hexamethylene tetramine	Lacquer handler	124	7		100% +	ND	ND	100% +	
Triethylene tetramine	Aircraft filter	114	1		ND	ND	ND	+	
Mixture of trimethylhexethylenediamine and isophorondiamine	Floor covering material salesman	126	1	NA	−	ND	ND	+	+ Bronchoalveolar lavage
Ethanolamines									
Monoethanolamine	Beauty culture	124	10	100% +	ND	ND	100% +		
Aminoethylethanolamine	Solderer	127	3		ND	ND	ND	100% +	
	Cable jointer	128	2		ND	ND	ND	+	

Continued.

Appendix B. Key references in occupational asthma—cont'd

Agent	Occupation or industry	Reference	Subjects (n)	Prevalence (%)	Skin test	Specific IgE	Other immunologic tests	Broncho-provocation test	Other evidence
Dimethylethanolamine	Spray painter	129	1		–	ND	ND	+	
Other									
3-(Dimethylamino)propylamine	Ski manufacturer	130	34	11.7	ND	ND	ND	ND	Cross-shift change in FEV1
Heterocyclic amines									
Piperazine hydrochloride	Chemist	131	2		50% +	ND	ND	+100%	
	Pharmaceutical	132	131	11.4	ND	ND	ND	100% of 1 +	
	Chemical plant	133	2		50% +	100% +	ND	ND	
N-Methylmorpholine		134	48	16.6§	ND	ND	ND	ND	
Aromatic amines									
Paraphenylene diamine	Fur dyeing	135	80	37.0	66% +	ND	ND	74% +	
Mixture of amines									
EPO 60	Mold maker	136	1	NA	ND	ND	ND	+	
Fluxes									
Colophony	Electronic worker	137	34		ND	ND	ND	100% +	
	Manufacture of solder flux	138	68 Low	4	ND	ND	ND	ND	
			14 Medium	21	ND	ND	ND	ND	
			6 High	21	ND	ND	ND	ND	
Zinc chloride and ammonium chloride flux	Metal jointer	139	2		ND	ND	ND	+	Changes in PC20
95% Alkylarul polyether alcohol + 5% polypropylene glycol	Electronic assembler	140	1		ND	ND	ND	+	
Wood dust or bark									
Western red cedar (Thuja plicata)	Carpentry	141	35		ND	ND	ND	ND	Improvement on removal
	Furniture making	142	1320	3.4	1.9% +	ND	ND	ND	
	Cabinetmaking or carpentry	143	22		100% –	ND	100% – precipitin	82% +	
	Sawmill worker	144	185		100% –	ND	ND	100% +	
		145	652	4.1	100% –	ND	ND	ND	
California redwood (Sequoia sempervirens)	Woodcarver	146	2		–	ND	– Precipitin	+	Questionnaire
	Carpenter	147	1		ND	ND	ND	+	

Wood (species)	Occupation	Ref.	No.			Immunology		Improvement on removal
Cedar of Lebanon (*Cedrus libani*)		148	6	17% +	ND	100% − precipitin	ND	ND
Cocabolla (*Dalbergia retusa*)		149	3	100% −	ND	ND	ND	ND
Iroko (*Chlorophora excelsa*)		150	1	+	ND	+ Precipitin	+	
English oak (*Quercus robur*)	Carpenter	151	1	ND	ND	ND	+	
Mahogany (*Shoreal* sp.)		152	1	−	ND	+ Precipitin	+	
Abiruana (*Pouteria*)		153	2	+	ND	− Precipitin	+	
African maple (*Triplochiton scleroxylon*)		154	2	+	+	Passive transfer	+	
Tanganyika aningre		155	3	100% +	100% −	100% − precipitin	100% +	
Central American walnut (*Juglans olanchana*)		156	1	−	−	− Precipitin	+	
Kejaat (*Pterocarpus angolensis*)		157	1	+	ND	ND	ND	
African zebrawood (*Microberlinia*)		158	1	+	+	ND	+	
Ramin (*Gonystylus bancanus*)	Woodworker	159	2	+	+	ND	+	
Quillaja bark	Factory to produce, saponin	160	1	ND	+	ND	+	
Fernambouc (*Caesalpinia echinata*)	Bow making	161	36	100% − (33.3)	ND	ND	100% of 1 +	
Ashwood (*Fraxinus americana*)	Sawmill worker	162	1	−	−	ND	+	
Pau Marfim (*Balfourodendron riedelianum*)	Woodworker	163	1	NA	+	ND	+	ND
Cabreuva (*Myyrocarpus fastigiatus* Fr. All.)	Parquet floor layer	164	1	NA	ND	ND	+	ND
Eastern white cedar (*Thuja occidentalis*)	Sawmill worker	165	1	ND	−	ND	+	PEFR recording
Ebony wood (*Diospyros crassiflora*)		166	1	−	ND	ND	+	

Continued.

Appendix B. Key references in occupational asthma—cont'd

Agent	Occupation or industry	Reference	Subjects (n)	Prevalence (%)	Skin test	Specific IgE	Other immunologic tests	Broncho-provocation test	Other evidence
Kotibe wood (Ne-sorgordonia pap-verifera)		167	1		+	ND	Passive transfer	+	
Cinnamon (Cinna-momum zeylani-cum)		168	40	22.5	ND	ND	ND	100% of 1 +	
?	Sawmills of eastern Canada and United States	169	11	ND	ND	ND	ND	+	PEFR monitoring
Metals									
Platinum	Platinum refinery	170	16		62% +	ND	ND	62% +	
		171	136	29	17% +	21% +	ND	ND	
Nickel	Metal plating	172	1		+	ND	− Precipitin	+	
		173	1		+	ND	− Precipitin	+	
		174	1		+	+	ND	+	
Cobalt	Hard-metal grinder	175	4		25% +	ND	ND	50% +	
	Diamond polisher	176	3		ND	ND	ND	100% +	
	Solderer	177	2		ND	ND	ND	+	
	Locksmith	178	1		ND	ND	ND	+	
Tungsten carbide	Grinder	179	1		ND	ND	ND	ND	Recovery on removal
Chromium	Printer	180	1		+	ND	ND	ND	
	Plater	181	1		+	ND	ND	ND	
Chromium and nickel	Welder	182	5		ND	ND	ND	100% of 2 +	
Cobalt and nickel	Tanner	183	1		−	+	ND	+	
		184	8		75% + to cobalt, 62% + to nickel	62% + to co-balt, 50% + to nickel	ND	100% + to both cobalt and nickel	
Drugs									
Penicillins and am-picillin	Pharmaceutical	185	4		100% −	ND	ND	75% +	
Penicillamine	Pharmaceutical	186	1		ND	−	ND	+	PEFR recording
Cephalosporins	Pharmaceutical	187	2		+	ND	ND	+	
	Pharmaceutical	188	91	7.7	71% +	ND	ND	ND	Improvement off work
Phenylglycine acid chloride	Pharmaceutical	189	24	29	37% +	37% +	Passive transfer	100% of 2 +	

Agent	Occupation	Ref	N						Comments
Psyllium	Laxative manufacturing	190	3		100% +	ND	ND	60% +	
	Pharmaceutical	191	130	4‡	9% of 120 +, 26% of 118 +	ND	ND	27% of 18 +	
	Nurse	192	5		80% +	100% +	ND	100% +	
	Health personnel	193	193	4‡	3% +, 12% of 162 +	ND	ND	26% of 15 +	
Methyldopa	Pharmaceutical	194	1		-	ND	ND	+	
Spiramycin	Pharmaceutical	195	1		+	ND	ND	+	
	Pharmaceutical	196	51	7.8‡	100% -	ND	ND	25% of 12 +	
	Pharmaceutical	197	2		ND	-	ND	+	
Salbutamol intermediate	Pharmaceutical	198	1		-	ND	ND	+	
Amprolium	Poultry feed mixer	199	1		ND	ND	ND	+	
Tetracycline	Pharmaceutical	200	1		ND	ND	ND	+	
	Pharmaceutical	201	1		+	ND	ND	+	
Isonicotinic acid hydrazide	Hospital pharmacy	202	1		+	+	ND	+	
Hydralazine	Pharmaceutical	203	1		-	-	- Specific IgG	+	
Tylosin tartrate	Pharmaceutical	204	1		ND	ND	ND	+	
Ipecacuanha	Pharmaceutical	205	42	47.6	52% of 13 +	66% of 18 -	ND	ND	
Cimetidine	Pharmaceutical	206	4		ND	ND	ND	25% +	
Opiate compounds	Pharmaceutical	207	39	26%	+	ND	ND	ND	PEFR, preshift and postshift FEV1
Chemicals									
Chloramine T	Chemical manufacturing	208	6		100% +	ND	66% + passive transfer	ND	
	Brewery	209	7		100% +	ND	ND	ND	Recovery with removal
	Janitorial/cleaning	210	5		100% of 4 +	ND	ND	100% of 3 +	
Polyvinylchloride									
Fumes	Meat wrapper	211	96	69.0	ND	ND	ND	27% of 11 +	
	Meat wrapper	212	3		ND	ND	ND	ND	History only
Powder	Manufacture of bottle caps	213	1		ND	ND	ND	+	PEFR recording
Ethylcyanoacrylate ester	Building airplane models	214	1		ND	ND	ND	+	
Organic phosphate insecticides	Chemical packaging plant	215	1		ND	ND	ND	ND	History only
Levafix brilliant yellow E36	Dye solution	216	1		+	ND	ND	+	
Drimaren brilliant yellow K-3GL	Textiles	216	1		+	ND	ND	+	

Continued.

Appendix B. Key references in occupational asthma—cont'd

Agent	Occupation or industry	Reference	Subjects (n)	Prevalence (%)	Skin test	Specific IgE	Other immunologic tests	Broncho-provocation test	Other evidence
Cibachrome brilliant scarlet 32	Textiles	216	1		+	ND	ND	+	
Drimaren brilliant blue K-BL	Textiles	216	1		+	ND	ND	+	
Reactive dyes	Reactive dye manufacture	217	309	25.2; 8% + black	7% + orange; 17% + black	17% + orange	ND	65% of 20 +	
Lanasol yellow 4G	Dyer	218	1	NA	+	ND	ND	+	
Persulfate salts and henna	Hairdresser	219	2		+	ND	ND	+	
	Hairdresser	220	2		+	ND	ND	100% of 4 +	
	Hairdresser	221	23	17.4	4% +	ND	ND	+	
	Hairdresser	222	1		−	ND	ND	+	
	Hairdresser	223	1		ND	ND	ND	+	
Azodicarbonamide (azobisformamide)	Plastics and rubber	224	151	18.5	ND	ND	ND	ND	Removal with improvement
	Plastic	225	2		ND	ND	ND	+	
	Plastics	226	4		ND	ND	ND	100% of 2 +	
Diazonium salt	Manufacture of photocopy paper	227	1		ND	ND	ND	+	
	Manufacture of fluorine polymer precursor	228	45	55.5	ND	20% +	ND	100% of 2	
Hexachlorophene (sterilizing agent)	Hospital staff	229	1		ND	ND	ND	+	
Formaldehyde	Hospital staff	230	28	29‡	ND	ND	ND	50% of 4 +	
	Various	231	15		ND	ND	ND	60% +	
	Various	232	230	5.2	ND	ND	ND	5% +	
Urea formaldehyde	Resin	233	2		−	ND	ND	+	
	Manufacture of foam	234	1		ND	ND	ND	+	
Freon	Refrigeration	235	1		ND	ND	ND	+	
Furfuryl alcohol (furan-based resin)	Foundry mold making	236	1		ND	ND	ND	+	
	Wool dye house	237	6		ND	83% +	100% +	ND	

Agent	Occupation/Source	Ref.	No.*	%					Method
Styrene	Plastics	238	2		−	ND	ND	+	
Glutaraldehyde	Hospital endoscopy unit	239	9	88.8	ND	ND	ND	ND	Questionnaire
Methyl methacrylate and cyanoacrylates	Adhesive	240	7		ND	ND	ND	86% +	PEFR 14% +
Iso-nonanyl oxy-benzene sulfonate	Nurse	241	1		ND	ND	ND	+	
	Laboratory technician	242	1		ND	ND	ND	+	
Chlorhexidine	Nurse	243	2		ND	ND	ND	+	
Tetraxzene	Detonator manufacture	244	1		ND	ND	ND	+	+ PEFR recording
Ethylene dioxide	Nurse	245	1	NA	ND	+	ND	+	Changes in PC20
Polyethylene	Paper packer	246	1	NA	ND	ND	ND	+	+ PEFR recording
Tetracholoroisophthalonitrile (fungicide)	Farmer	247	1	NA	ND	−	+ Patch test	+	+ FEV1 recording at work
Tributyl tin oxide (fungicide)	Venipuncture technician	248	1	NA	−	ND	ND	+	
Tall oil (pine resin)	Rubber tire manufacturer	249	1	NA	−	ND	− Patch test	+	+ PEFR recording
Synthetic material									
Plexiglass		250	1		ND	ND	ND	+	
Latex	Glove manufacture	251	81	6	11% +	ND	ND	ND	PEFR recording, preshift and postshift change in FEV1
Unidentified									
(?)	Respiratory therapist	252	194	18.7	ND	ND	ND	ND	Questionnaire
(?)	Mineral analysis laboratory worker	253	21	23.8§	ND	ND	ND	ND	Questionnaire, PC20
(?) Oil mists	Toolsetter	254	1		ND	ND	ND	+	PEFR recording
(?) Fluorine	Potroom worker	255	52		ND	ND	ND	ND	History
(?) Aluminum	Potroom worker	256	227	7.0	ND	ND	ND	ND	Questionnaire
	Potroom worker	257	35		ND	ND	ND	ND	History
	Potroom worker	258	57		ND	ND	ND	ND	History

Modified from Chan-Yeung M, Malo J-L. Compendium I. Table of the major inducers of occupational asthma. In Bernstein IL, Chan-Yeung M, Malo J-L, et al (editors): *Asthma in the workplace*, New York, 1993, Marcel Dekker. Also modified from Chan-Yeung M, Malo J-L. Etiologic agents in occupational asthma, *Eur Respir Rev* (in press).

*The number of subjects tested is not specified unless it did not include *all* subjects. All proportions including 3 or more as the denominator are expressed as a percentage.

†Subjects with symptoms.

‡Based on challenge data.

§Presence of airway hyperresponsiveness.

FEV1, Forced expiratory volume in 1 second; *HDI*, hexamethylene diisocyanate; *IgE*, immunoglobulin E; *IgG*, immunoglobulin G; *MDI*, diphenylmethane diisocyanate; *NA*, not applicable; *ND*, not done; *PCA*, passive cutaneous anaphylaxis; *PC20*, provocative concentration causing a fall of 20% in FEV1; *PEFR*, peak expiratory flow rate; *PPI*, polymethylene polyphenylisocyanate; *RAST*, radioallergosorbent test; *TDI*, toluene diisocyanate; +, positive; −, negative.

REFERENCES

1. Venables KM, Tee RD, Hawkins ER, et al: Laboratory animal allergy in a pharmaceutical company, *Br J Ind Med* 45:660-666, 1988.
2. Newman Taylor A, Longbottom JL, and Pepys J: Respiratory allergy to urine proteins of rats and mice, *Lancet* 847-849, 1977.
3. Mäntyjärvi J, Ylönen R, Taivainen A, et al: IgG and IgE antibody responses to cow dander and urine in farmers with cow-induced asthma, *Clin Exp Allergy* 22:83-90, 1992.
4. Bar-Sela S, Teichtahl H, and Lutsky I: Occupational asthma in poultry workers, *J Allergy Clin Immunol* 73:271-275, 1984.
5. Lutsky I, Teichtahl H, and Bar-Sela S: Occupational asthma due to poultry mites, *J Allergy Clin Immunol* 73:56-60, 1984.
6. Brennan NJ: Pig butcher's asthma—case report and review of the literature, *Ir Med J* 78:321-322, 1985.
7. Armentia A, Martin-Santos J, Subiza J, et al: Occupational asthma due to frogs, *Ann Allergy* 60:209-210, 1988.
8. Moneret-Vautrin DA, Pupil P, Courtine D, et al: Asthme professionnel aux protéines du lactosérum, *Rev Fr Allergol* 24:93-95, 1984.
9. Olaguibel JM, Hernandez D, Morales P, et al: Occupational asthma caused by inhalation of casein, *Allergy* 45:306-308, 1990.
10. El-Ansary EH, Gordon DJ, Tee RD, et al: Respiratory allergy to inhaled bat guano, *Lancet* 1:316-318, 1987.
11. Cuthbert OD, Jeffrey IG, McNeill HB, et al: Barn allergy among Scottish farmers, *Clin Allergy* 14:197-206, 1984.
12. Blainey AD, Topping MD, Ollier S, et al: Allergic respiratory disease in grain workers: the role of storage mites, *J Allergy Clin Immunol* 84:296-303, 1989.
13. Burge PS, Edge G, O'Brien IM, et al: Occupational asthma in a research centre breeding locusts, *Clin Allergy* 10:355-363, 1980.
14. Tee RD, Gordon DJ, Hawkins ER, et al: Occupational allergy to locusts: an investigation of the sources of the allergen, *J Allergy Clin Immunol* 81:517-525, 1988.
15. Gibbons HL, Dille JR, and Cowley RG: Inhalant allergy to the screwworm fly, *Arch Environ Health* 10:424-430, 1965.
16. Bagenstose AH, Mathews KP, Homburger HA, et al: Inhalant allergy due to crickets, *J Allergy Clin Immunol* 65:71-74, 1980.
17. Stevenson DD and Mathews KP: Occupational asthma following inhalation of moth particles, *J Allergy* 39:274-283, 1967.
18. Randolph H: Allergic reaction to dust of insect origin, *JAMA* 103:560-562, 1934.
19. Wittich FW: Allergic rhinitis and asthma due to sensitization to the Mexican bean weevil (*Zabrotes subfasciatus* Boh.), *J Allergy* 12:42-45, 1940.
20. Spieksma FTM, Vooren PH, Kramps JA, et al: Respiratory allergy to laboratory fruit flies (*Drosophila melanogaster), J Allergy Clin Immunol* 77:108-113, 1986.
21. Ostrom NK, Swanson MC, Agarwal MK, et al: Occupational allergy to honeybee-body dust in a honey-processing plant, *J Allergy Clin Immunol* 77:736-740, 1986.
22. Siracusa A, Verga A, Bacoccoli R, et al: l'Asma da bigattini (Larve della *mosca carnaria): studio clinico e immunologico, Med Lav* 80:489-497, 1989.
23. Schroeckenstein DC, Meier-Davis S, Graziano FM, et al: Occupational sensitivity to *Alphitobius diaperinus* (Panzer) (lesser mealworm), *J Allergy Clin Immunol* 82:1081-1088, 1988.
24. Lutsky I and Bar-Sela S: Northern fowl mite (*Ornithonyssus sylviarum*) in occupational asthma of poultry workers, *Lancet* 2:874-875, 1982.
25. Cuthbert OD, Brostoff J, Wraith DG, et al: "Barn allergy": asthma and rhinitis due to storage mites, *Clin Allergy* 9:229-236, 1979.
26. Granel-Tena C, Cistero-Bahima A, and Olive-Perez A: Allergens in asthma and baker's rhinitis, *Alergia* 32:69-73, 1985.
27. Michel FB, Guin JJ, Seignalet C, et al: Allergie à *Panonychus ulmi* (Koch), *Rev Fr Allergol* 17:93-97, 1977.
28. Meister W: Professional asthma owing to *Daphnia*-allergy, *Allerg Immunol* 24:191-193, 1978.
29. Axelsson IGK, Johansson SGO, and Zetterstrom O: Occupational allergy to weeping fig in plant keepers, *Allergy* 42:161-167, 1987.
30. Kaufman GL, Gandevia BH, Bellas TE, et al: Occupational allergy in an entomological research centre. I: Clinical aspects of reactions to the sheep blowfly *Lucilia cuprina, Br J Ind Med* 46:473-478, 1989.
31. Uragoda CG and Wijekoon PMB: Asthma in silk workers, *J Soc Occup Med* 41:140-142, 1991.
32. Chan-Yeung M, Schulzer M, MacLean L, et al: Epidemiologic health survey of grain elevator workers in British Columbia, *Am Rev Respir Dis* 121:329-338, 1980.
33. Williams N, Skoulas A, and Merriman JE: Exposure to grain dust. I. A survey of the effects, *JOM, J Occup Med* 6:319-329, 1964.
34. Skoulas A, Williams N, and Merriman JE: Exposure to grain dust. II. A clinical study of the effects, *JOM, J Occup Med* 6:359-372, 1964.
35. Chan-Yeung M, Wong R, and MacLean L: Respiratory abnormalities among grain elevator workers, *Chest* 75:461-467, 1979.
36. Musk AW, Venables KM, Crook B, et al: Respiratory symptoms, lung function, and sensitisation to flour in a British bakery, *Br J Ind Med* 46:636-642, 1989.
37. Block G, Tse KS, Kijek K, et al: Baker's asthma, *Clin Allergy* 13:359-370, 1983.
38. Sutton R, Skerritt JH, Baldo BA, et al: The diversity of allergens involved in bakers' asthma, *Clin Allergy* 14:93-107, 1984.
39. Valdivieso R, Quirce S, and Sainz T: Bronchial asthma caused by *Lathyrus sativus* flour, *Allergy* 43:536-539, 1988.
40. Picon SJ, Carmona JGB, and Sotillos MDMG: Occupational asthma caused by vetch (*Vicia sativa), J Allergy Clin Immunol* 88:135-136, 1991.
41. Ordman D: Buckwheat allergy, *S Afr Med J* 21:737-739, 1947.
42. Lachance P, Cartier A, Dolovich J, et al: Occupational asthma from reactivity to an alkaline hydrolysis derivative of gluten, *J Allergy Clin Immunol* 81:385-390, 1988.
43. Jones RN, Hughes JM, Lehrer SB, et al: Lung function consequences of exposure and hypersensitivity in workers who process green coffee beans, *Am Rev Respir Dis* 125:199-202, 1982.
44. Zuskin E, Valic F, and Kanceljak B: Immunological and respiratory changes in coffee workers, *Thorax* 36:9-13, 1981.
45. Osterman K, Johansson SGO, and Zetterstrom O: Diagnostic tests in allergy to green coffee, *Allergy* 40:336-343, 1985.
46. Panzani R and Johansson SGO: Results of skin test and RAST in allergy to a clinically potent allergen (castor bean), *Clin Allergy* 16:259-266, 1986.
47. Cartier A and Malo J-L: Occupational asthma due to tea dust, *Thorax* 45:203-206, 1990.
48. Blanc PD, Trainor WD, and Lim DT: Herbal tea asthma, *Br J Ind Med* 43:137-138, 1986.
49. Gleich GJ, Welsh PW, Yuninger JW, et al: Allergy to tobacco: an occupational hazard, *N Engl J Med* 302:617-619, 1980.
50. Lander F and Gravesen S: Respiratory disorders among tobacco workers, *Br J Ind Med* 45:500-502, 1988.
51. Newmark FM: Hops allergy and terpene sensitivity: an occupational disease, *Ann Allergy* 41:311-312, 1978.
52. Twiggs JT, Yuninger JW, Agarwal MK, et al: Occupational asthma in a florist caused by the dried plant, baby's breath, *J Allergy Clin Immunol* 69:474-477, 1982.
53. van Toorenenbergen AW and Dieges PH: Occupational allergy in horticulture: demonstration of immediate-type allergic reactivity to freesia and paprika plants, *Int Arch Allergy Appl Immunol* 75:44-47, 1984.
54. Symington IS, Kerr JW, and McLean DA: Type I allergy in mushroom soup processors, *Clin Allergy* 11:43-47, 1981.
55. Rubin JM and Duke MB: Unusual cause of bronchial asthma. Cacoon seed used for decorative purposes, *NY State J Med* 538-539, 1974.

56. Nemery B and Demedts M: Occupational asthma in a chicory grower, *Lancet* 1:672-673, 1989.

57. Kwaselow A, Rowe M, Sears-Ewald D, et al: Rose hips: a new occupational allergen, *J Allergy Clin Immunol* 85.704-708, 1990.

58. Bousquet OJ, Dhivert H, Clauzel AM, et al: Occupational allergy to sunflower pollen, *J Allergy Clin Immunol* 75:70-75, 1985.

59. Falleroni AE, Zeiss CR, and Levitz D: Occupational asthma secondary to inhalation of garlic dust, *J Allergy Clin Immunol* 68:156-160, 1981.

60. Lybarger JA, Gallagher JS, Pulver DW, et al: Occupational asthma induced by inhalation and ingestion of garlic, *J Allergy Clin Immunol* 69:448-454, 1982.

61. Catilina P, Chamoux A, Gabrillargues D, et al: Contribution à l'étude des asthmes d'origine professionnelle: l'asthme à la poudre de lycopode, *Arch Mal Prof* 49:143-148, 1988.

62. Charpin J and Blanc M: Une cause nouvelle d'allergie professionnelle chez les coiffeuses: l'allergie à la séricine, *Marseille Med* 104:169-170, 1967.

63. Zedda S: A case of bronchial asthma from inhalation of nacre dust, *Med Lav* 58:459-464, 1967.

64. Kraut A, Peng Z, Becker AB, et al: Christmas candy maker's asthma. IgG4-mediated pectin allergy, *Chest* 102:1605-1607, 1992.

65. Starr JC, Yunginger J, and Brahser GW: Immediate type I asthmatic response to henna following occupational exposure in hairdressers, *Ann Allergy* 48:98-99, 1982.

66. Côté J, Chan H, Brochu G, et al: Occupational asthma caused by exposure to *Neurospora* in a plywood factory worker, *Br J Ind Med* 48:279-282, 1991.

67. Juniper CP, How MJ, and Goodwin BFJ: *Bacillus subtilis* enzymes: a 7-year clinical, epidemiological and immunological study of an industrial allergen, *J Soc Occup Med* 27:3 12, 1977.

68. Franz T, McMurrain KD, Brooks S, et al: Clinical, immunologic, and physiologic observations in factory workers exposed to *B. subtilis* enzyme dust, *J Allergy* 47:170-179, 1971.

69. Colten HR, Polakoff PL, Weinstein SF, et al: Immediate hypersensitivity to hog trypsin resulting from industrial exposure, *N Engl J Med* 292:1050-1053, 1975.

70. Baur X, Konig G, Bencze K, et al: Clinical symptoms and results of skin test, RAST and bronchial provocation test in thirty-three papain workers: evidence for strong immunogenic potency and clinically relevant "proteolytic effects of airborne papain," *Clin Allergy* 12:9-17, 1982.

71. Cartier A, Malo J-L, Pineau L, et al: Occupational asthma due to pepsin, *J Allergy Clin Immunol* 73:574-577, 1984.

72. Wiessmann KJ and Baur X: Occupational lung disease following long-term inhalation of pancreatic extracts, *Eur J Respir Dis* 66:13-20, 1985.

73. Pauwels R, Devos M, Callens L, et al: Respiratory hazards from proteolytic enzymes, *Lancet* 1:669, 1978.

74. Cortona G, Beretta F, Traina G, et al: Preliminary investigation in a pharmaceutical industry: bromelin induced pathology, *Med Lav* 1:70-75, 1980.

75. Galleguillos F and Rodriguez JC: Asthma caused by bromelin inhalation, *Clin Allergy* 8:21-24, 1978.

76. Bernstein JA, Kraut A, Bernstein DI, et al: Occupational asthma induced by inhaled egg lysozyme, *Chest* 103:532-535, 1993.

77. Baur X, Fruhmann G, Haug B, et al: Role of *Aspergillus* amylase in baker's asthma, *Lancet* 1:43, 1986.

78. Birnbaum J, Latil F, Vervloet D, et al: Rôle de l'alpha-amylase dans l'asthme du boulanger, *Rev Mal Respir* 5:519-521, 1988.

79. Baur X, Weiss W, Sauer W, et al: Baking components as a contributory cause of baker's asthma, *Dtsch Med Wochenschr* 113:1275-1278, 1988.

80. Zachariae H, Høegh-Thomsen J, Witmeur O, et al: Detergent enzymes and occupational safety. Observations on sensitization during Esperase® production, *Allergy* 36:513-516, 1981.

81. Fowler PBS: Printers' asthma, *Lancet* 2:755-757, 1952.

82. Bohner CB, Sheldon JM, and Trenis JW: Sensitivity to gum acacia, with a report of ten cases of asthma in printers, *J Allergy* 12:290-294, 1941.

83. Gelfand HH: The allergenic properties of vegetable gums: a case of asthma due to tragacanth, *J Allergy* 14:203-219, 1943.

84. Feinberg SM and Schoenkerman BB: Karaya and related gums as causes of atopy, *Wis Med J* 39:734, 1940.

85. Malo J-L, Cartier A, L'Archevêque J, et al: Prevalence of occupational asthma and immunological sensitization to guar gum among employees at a carpet-manufacturing plant, *J Allergy Clin Immunol* 86:562-569, 1990.

86. Cartier A, Malo J-L, Forest F, et al: Occupational asthma in snow crab–processing workers, *J Allergy Clin Immunol* 74:261-269, 1984.

87. Gaddie J, Legge JS, Friend JAR, et al: Pulmonary hypersensitivity in prawn workers, *Lancet* 2:1350-1353, 1980.

88. Jyo T, Kohmoto K, Katsutani T, et al: Hoya (sea-squirt) asthma. In Frazier CA (editor): *Occupational asthma*, pp 209-228, London, 1980, Van Nostrand Reinhold.

89. Tomaszunas S, Weclawik Z, and Lewinski M: Allergic reactions to cuttlefish in deep-sea fishermen, *Lancet* 1:1116-1117, 1988.

90. Sherson D, Hansen I, and Sigsgaard T: Occupationally related respiratory symptoms in trout-processing workers, *Allergy* 44:336-341, 1989.

91. Carino M, Elia G, Molinini R, et al: Shrimpmeal asthma in the aquaculture industry, *Med Lav* 76:471-475, 1985.

92. Kobayashi S: Different aspects of occupational asthma in Japan. In Frazier CA (editor): *Occupational asthma*, pp 229-244, London, 1980, Van Nostrand Reinhold.

93. Blair Smith A, Bernstein DI, London MA, et al: Evaluation of occupational asthma from airborne egg protein exposure in multiple settings, *Chest* 98:398-404, 1990.

94. Resta O, Foschino-Barbaro MP, Carnimeo N, et al: Occupational asthma from fish-feed, *Med Lav* 3.234-236, 1982.

95. Onizuka R, Inoue K, and Kamiya H: Red soft coral–induced allergic symptoms observed in spiny lobster fishermen, *Aerugi* 39:339-347, 1990.

96. Butcher BT, Salvaggio JE, Weill H, et al: Toluene diisocyanate (TDI) pulmonary disease: immunologic and inhalation challenge studies, *J Allergy Clin Immunol* 58:89-100, 1976.

97. Butcher BT, O'Neil CE, Reed MA, et al: Radioallergosorbent testing of toluene diisocyanate–reactive individuals using *p*-tolyl isocyanate antigen, *J Allergy Clin Immunol* 66:213-216, 1980.

98. Baur X and Fruhmann G: Specific IgE antibodies in patients with isocyanate asthma, *Chest* 80:73S-76S, 1981.

99. Paggiaro PL, Filieri M, Loi AM, et al: Absence of IgG antibodies to TDI-HSA in a radioimmunological study, *Clin Allergy* 13:75-79, 1983.

100. Mapp CE, Boschetto P, Dal Vecchio L, et al: Occupational asthma due to isocyanates, *Eur Respir J* 1:273-279, 1988.

101. Zammit-Tabona M, Sherkin M, Kijek K, et al: Asthma caused by diphenylmethane diisocyanate in foundry workers. Clinical, bronchial provocation, and immunologic studies, *Am Rev Respir Dis* 128:226-230, 1983.

102. Tse KS, Johnson A, Chan H, et al: A study of serum antibody activity in workers with occupational exposure to diphenylmethane diisocyanate, *Allergy* 40:314-320, 1985.

103. Liss GM, Bernstein DI, Moller DR, et al: Pulmonary and immunologic evaluation of foundry workers exposed to methylene diphenyldiisocyanate (MDI), *J Allergy Clin Immunol* 82:55-61, 1988.

104. Harris MG, Burge PS, Samson M, et al: Isocyanate asthma: respiratory symptoms due to 1,5 naphthylene diisocyanate, *Thorax* 34:762-766, 1979.

105. Clarke CW and Aldons PM: Isophorone diisocyanate induced respiratory disease (IPDI), *Aust NZ J Med* 11:290-292, 1981.

106. Vandenplas O, Cartier A, Lesage J, et al: Occupational asthma caused by a prepolymer but not the monomer of toluene diisocyanate (TDI), *J Allergy Clin Immunol* 89:1183-1188, 1992.

107. Vandenplas O, Cartier A, Lesage J, et al: Prepolymers of hexamethylene diisocyanate (HDI) as a cause of occupational asthma, *J Allergy Clin Immunol* 91:850-861, 1993.

108. Séguin P, Allard A, Cartier A, et al: Prevalence of occupational asthma in spray painters exposed to several types of isocyanates, including polymethylene polyphenylisocyanates, *JOM, J Occup Med* 29:340-344, 1987.

109. O'Brien IM, Harries MG, Burge PS, et al: Toluene di-isocyanate–induced asthma. I. Reactions to TDI, MDI, HDI and histamine, *Clin Allergy* 9:1-6, 1979.

110. Baur X, Dewair M, and Fruhmann G: Detection of immunologically sensitized isocyanate workers by RAST and intracutaneous skin tests, *J Allergy Clin Immunol* 73:610-618, 1984.

111. Cartier A, Grammer L, Malo J-L, et al: Specific serum antibodies against isocyanates: association with occupational asthma, *J Allergy Clin Immunol* 84:507-514, 1989.

112. Pezzini A, Riviera A, Paggiaro P, et al: Specific IgE antibodies in twenty-eight workers with diisocyanate-induced bronchial asthma, *Clin Allergy* 14:453-461, 1984.

113. Maccia CA, Bernstein IL, Emmett EA, et al: In vitro demonstration of specific IgE in phthalic anhydride hypersensitivity, *Am Rev Respir Dis* 113:701-704, 1976.

114. Fawcett IW, Newman-Taylor AJ, and Pepys J: Asthma due to inhaled chemical agents—epoxy resin systems containing phthalic acid anhydride, trimellitic acid anhydride and triethylene tetramine, *Clin Allergy* 7:1-14, 1977.

115. Wernfors M, Nielsen J, Schutz A, et al: Phthalic anhydride–induced occupational asthma, *Int Arch Allergy Appl Immunol* 79:77-82, 1986.

116. Nielsen J, Welinder H, Schütz A, et al: Specific serum antibodies against phthalic anhydride in occupationally exposed subjects, *J Allergy Clin Immunol* 82:126-133, 1988.

117. Zeiss CR, Patterson R, Pruzansky JJ, et al: Trimellitic anhydride–induced airway syndromes: clinical and immunologic studies, *J Allergy Clin Immunol* 60:96-103, 1977.

118. Schlueter DP, Banaszak EF, Fink JN, et al: Occupational asthma due to tetrachlorophthalic anhydride, *JOM, J Occup Med* 20:183-187, 1978.

119. Howe W, Venables KM, Topping MD, et al: Tetrachlorophthalic anhydride asthma: evidence for specific IgE antibody, *J Allergy Clin Immunol* 71:5-11, 1983.

120. Meadway J: Asthma and atopy in workers with an epoxy adhesive, *Br J Dis Chest* 74:149-154, 1980.

121. Nielsen J, Welinder H, and Skerfving S: Allergic airway disease caused by methyl tetrahydrophthalic anhydride in epoxy resin, *Scand J Work Environ Health* 15:154-155, 1989.

122. Chee CBE, Lee HS, Cheong TH, et al: Occupational asthma due to hexahydrophthalic anhydride: a case report, *Br J Ind Med* 48:643-645, 1991.

123. Rosenman KD, Bernstein DI, O'Leary K, et al: Occupational asthma caused by himic anhydride, *Scand J Work Environ Health* 13:150-154, 1987.

124. Gelfand HH: Respiratory allergy due to chemical compounds encountered in the rubber, lacquer, shellac, and beauty culture industries, *J Allergy* 34:374-381, 1963.

125. Lam S and Chan-Yeung M: Ethylenediamine-induced asthma, *Am Rev Respir Dis* 121:151-155, 1980.

126. Aleva RM, Aalbers R, Koëter GH, et al: Occupational asthma caused by a hardener containing an aliphatic and cycloliphatic diamine, *Am Rev Respir Dis* 145:1217-1218, 1992.

127. Pepys J and Pickering CAC: Asthma due to inhaled chemical fumes—amino-ethil ethanolamine in aluminium soldering flux, *Clin Allergy* 2:197-204, 1972.

128. Sterling GM: Asthma due to aluminium soldering flux, *Thorax* 22:533-537, 1967.

129. Vallières M, Cockcroft DW, Taylor DM, et al: Dimethyl ethanolamine–induced asthma, *Am Rev Respir Dis* 115:867-871, 1977.

130. Sargent EV, Mitchell CA, and Brubaker RE: Respiratory effects of occupational exposure to an epoxy resin system, *Arch Environ Health* 31:236-240, 1976.

131. Pepys J, Pickering CAC, and Loudon HWG: Asthma due to inhaled chemical agents—piperazine dihydrochloride, *Clin Allergy* 2:189-196, 1972.

132. Hagmar L, Bellander T, Bergöö B, et al: Piperazine-induced occupational asthma, *JOM, J Occup Med* 24:193-197, 1982.

133. Welinder H, Hagmar L, and Gustavsson C: IgE antibodies against piperazine and N-methyl-piperazine in two asthmatic subjects, *Int Arch Allergy Appl Immunol* 79:259-262, 1986.

134. Belin L, Wass U, Audunsson G, et al: Amines: possible causative agents in the development of bronchial hyperreactivity in workers manufacturing polyurethanes from isocyanates, *Br J Ind Med* 40:251-257, 1983.

135. Silberman DE and Sorrell AH: Allergy in fur workers with special reference to paraphenylenediamine, *J Allergy* 30:11-18, 1959.

136. Lambourn EM, Hayes JP, McAllister WA, et al: Occupational asthma due to EPO 60, *Br J Ind Med* 49:294-295, 1992.

137. Burge PS, Harries MG, O'Brien I, et al: Bronchial provocation studies in workers exposed to the fumes of electronic soldering fluxes, *Clin Allergy* 10:137-149, 1980.

138. Burge PS, Edge G, Hawkins R, et al: Occupational asthma in a factory making flux-cored solder containing colophony, *Thorax* 36:828-834, 1981.

139. Weir DC, Robertson AS, Jones S, et al: Occupational asthma due to soft corrosive soldering fluxes containing zinc chloride and ammonium chloride, *Thorax* 44:220-223, 1989.

140. Stevens JJ: Asthma due to soldering flux: a polyether alcohol–polypropylene glycol mixture, *Ann Allergy* 36:419-422, 1976.

141. Milne J and Gandevia B: Occupational asthma and rhinitis due to western (Canadian) red cedar, *Med J Aust* 2:741-744, 1969.

142. Ishizaki T, Sluda T, Miyamoto T, et al: Occupational asthma from western red cedar dust *(Thuja plicata)* in furniture factory workers, *JOM, J Occup Med* 15:580-585, 1973.

143. Chan-Yeung M, Barton GM, MacLean L, et al: Occupational asthma and rhinitis due to western red cedar *(Thuja plicata)*, *Am Rev Respir Dis* 108:1094-1102, 1973.

144. Chan-Yeung M, Lam S, and Koener S: Clinical features and natural history of occupational asthma due to western red cedar *(Thuja plicata)*, *Am J Med* 72:411-415, 1982.

145. Chan-Yeung M, Vedal S, Kus J, et al: Symptoms, pulmonary function, and bronchial hyperreactivity in western red cedar workers compared with those in office workers, *Am Rev Respir Dis* 130:1038-1041, 1984.

146. Chan-Yeung M and Abboud R: Occupational asthma due to California redwood *(Sequoia sempervirens)* dusts, *Am Rev Respir Dis* 114:1027-1031, 1976.

147. doPico GA: Asthma due to dust from redwood *(Sequoia sempervirens)*, *Chest* 73:424-425, 1978.

148. Greenberg M: Respiratory symptoms following brief exposure to cedar of Lebanon *(Cedra libani)* dust, *Clin Allergy* 2:219-224, 1972.

149. Eaton KK: Respiratory allergy to exotic wood dust, *Clin Allergy* 3:307-310, 1973.

150. Pickering CAC, Batten JC, and Pepys J: Asthma due to inhaled wood dusts—western red cedar and iroko, *Clin Allergy* 2:213-218, 1972.

151. Azofra J and Olaguibel JM: Occupational asthma caused by iroko wood, *Allergy* 44:156-158, 1989.

152. Sosman AJ, Schlueter DP, Fink JN, et al: Hypersensitivity to wood dust, *N Engl J Med* 281:977-980, 1969.

153. Booth BH, Lefoldt RH, and Moffitt EM: Hypersensitivity to wood dust, *J Allergy Clin Immunol* 57:352-357, 1976.

154. Hinojosa M, Moneo I, Dominguez J, et al: Asthma caused by African maple *(Triplochiton scleroxylon)* wood dust, *J Allergy Clin Immunol* 74:782-786, 1984.

155. Paggiaro PL, Cantalupi R, Filieri M, et al: Bronchial asthma due to inhaled wood dust: *Tanganyika aningre, Clin Allergy* 11:605-610, 1981.

156. Bush RK and Clayton D: Asthma due to Central American walnut *(Juglans olanchana)* dust, *Clin Allergy* 13:389-394, 1983.

157. Ordman D: Wood dust as an inhalant allergen. Bronchial asthma caused by kejaat wood *(Pterocarpus angolensis), S Afr Med J* 23:973-975, 1949.

158. Bush RK, Yunginger JW, and Reed CE: Asthma due to African zebrawood *(Microberlinia)* dust, *Am Rev Respir Dis* 117:601-603, 1978.

159. Hinojosa M, Losada E, Moneo I, et al: Occupational asthma caused by African maple *(Obeche)* and ramin: evidence of cross reactivity between these two woods, *Clin Allergy* 16:145-153, 1986.

160. Raghuprasad PK, Brooks SM, Litwin A, et al: Quillaja bark (soap-bark)–induced asthma, *J Allergy Clin Immunol* 65:285-287, 1980.

161. Hausen BM and Herrmann B: Bow-makers disease: an occupational disease in the manufacture of wooden bows for string instruments, *Dtsch Med Wochenschr* 115:169-173, 1990.

162. Malo J-L and Cartier A: Occupational asthma caused by exposure to ash wood dust *(Fraxinus americana), Eur Respir J* 2:385-387, 1989.

163. Basomba A, Burches E, Almodovar A, et al: Occupational rhinitis and asthma caused by inhalation of *Balfourodendron riedelianum* (Pau Marfim) wood dust, *Allergy* 46:316-318, 1991.

164. Innocenti A, Romeo R, and Mariano A: Asthma and systemic toxic reaction due to cabreuva (*Myrocarpus fastigiatus* Fr. All.) wood dust, *Med Lav* 82:446-450, 1991.

165. Cartier A, Chan H, Malo J-L, et al: Occupational asthma caused by eastern white cedar *(Thuya occidentalis)* with demonstration that plicatic acid is present in this wood dust and is the causal agent, *J Allergy Clin Immunol* 77:639 645, 1986.

166. Maestrelli P, Marcer G, and Dal Vecchio L: Occupational asthma due to ebony wood *(Diospyros crassiflora)* dust, *Ann Allergy* 59:347-349, 1987.

167. Reques FG and Fernandez RP: Asthme professionnel à un bois exotique. *Nesorgordonia papaverifera* (danta ou kotibe), *Rev Mal Respir* 5:71 73, 1988.

168. Uragoda CG: Asthma and other symptoms in cinnamon workers, *Br J Ind Med* 41:224-227, 1984.

169. Malo J-L, Cartier A, and Boulet LP: Occupational asthma in saw-mills of eastern Canada and United States, *J Allergy Clin Immunol* 78:392-398, 1986.

170. Pepys J, Pickering CAC, and Hughes EG: Asthma due to inhaled chemical agents—complex salts of platinum, *Clin Allergy* 2:391 396, 1972.

171. Brooks SM, Baker DB, Gann PH, et al: Cold air challenge and platinum skin reactivity in platinum refinery workers, *Chest* 97:1401-1407, 1990.

172. McConnell LH, Fink JN, Schlueter DP, et al: Asthma caused by nickel sensitivity, *Ann Intern Med* 78:888-890, 1973.

173. Block GT and Yeung M: Asthma induced by nickel, *JAMA* 247:1600-1602, 1982.

174. Malo J-L, Cartier A, Doepner M, et al: Occupational asthma caused by nickel sulfate, *J Allergy Clin Immunol* 69:55-59, 1982.

175. Hartmann AL, Walter H, and Wuthrich B: Allergisches berufsasthma auf pektinase, ein pektolytisches enzym, *Schweiz Med Wochenschr* 113:265-267, 1983.

176. Gheysens B, Auxwerx J, Van Den Eeckhout A, et al: Cobalt-induced bronchial asthma in diamond polishers, *Chest* 88:740-744, 1985.

177. Malo J-L and Cartier A: Occupational asthma due to fumes of galvanized metal, *Chest* 92:375-377, 1987.

178. Vogelmeier C, König G, Bencze K, et al: Pulmonary involvement in zinc fume fever, *Chest* 92:946-949, 1987.

179. Bruckner HC: Extrinsic asthma in a tungsten carbide worker, *JOM, J Occup Med* 9:518-519, 1967.

180. Smith AR: Chrome poisoning with manifestations of sensitization, *JAMA* 94:95-98, 1931.

181. Joules H: Asthma from sensitization to chromium, *Lancet* 2:182-183, 1932.

182. Keskinen G, Kalliomaki PL, and Alanko K: Occupational asthma due to stainless steel welding fumes, *Clin Allergy* 10:151-159, 1980.

183. Novey HS, Habib M, and Wells ID: Asthma and IgE antibodies induced by chromium and nickel salts, *J Allergy Clin Immunol* 72:407-412, 1983.

184. Shirakawa T, Kusaka Y, Fujimura N, et al: Hard metal asthma: cross immunological and respiratory reactivity between cobalt and nickel, *Thorax* 45:267-271, 1990.

185. Davies RJ, Hendrick DJ, and Pepys J: Asthma due to inhaled chemical agents: ampicillin, bensyl penicillin, 6 amino penicillanic acid and related substances, *Clin Allergy* 4:227-247, 1974.

186. Lagier F, Cartier A, Dolovich J, et al: Occupational asthma in a pharmaceutical worker exposed to penicillamine, *Thorax* 44:157-158, 1989.

187. Coutts II, Dally MB, Newman-Taylor AJ, et al: Asthma in workers manufacturing cephalosporins, *Br Med J* 283:950, 1981.

188. Briatico-Vangosa G, Beretta F, Bianchi S, et al: Bronchial asthma due to 7-aminocephalosporanic acid (7-ACA) in workers employed in cephalosporine production, *Med Lav* 72:488-493, 1981.

189. Kammermeyer JK and Mathews KP: Hypersensitivity to phenylglycine acid chloride, *J Allergy Clin Immunol* 52:73-84, 1973.

190. Busse WW and Schoenwetter WF: Asthma from psyllium in laxative manufacture, *Ann Intern Med* 83:361-362, 1975.

191. Bardy JD, Malo J-L, Séguin P, et al: Occupational asthma and IgE sensitization in a pharmaceutical company processing psyllium, *Am Rev Respir Dis* 135:1033-1038, 1987.

192. Cartier A, Malo J-L, and Dolovich J: Occupational asthma in nurses handling psyllium, *Clin Allergy* 17:1-6, 1987.

193. Malo J-L, Cartier A, L'Archevêque J, et al: Prevalence of occupational asthma and immunologic sensitization to psyllium among health personnel in chronic care hospitals, *Am Rev Respir Dis* 142:1359-1366, 1990.

194. Harries MG, Newman Taylor A, Wooden J, et al: Bronchial asthma due to alpha-methyldopa, *Br Med J* 1461, 1979.

195. Davies RJ and Pepys J: Asthma due to inhaled chemical agents the macrolide antibiotic spiramycin, *Clin Allergy* 1.99-107, 1975.

196. Malo J-L and Cartier A: Occupational asthma in workers of a pharmaceutical company processing spiramycin, *Thorax* 43:371-377, 1988.

197. Moscato G, Naldi L, and Candura F: Bronchial asthma due to spiramycin and adipic acid, *Clin Allergy* 14:355-361, 1984.

198. Fawcett IW, Pepys J, and Erooga MA: Asthma due to "glycyl compound" powder—an intermediate in production of salbutamol, *Clin Allergy* 6:405-409, 1976.

199. Greene SA and Freedman S: Asthma due to inhaled chemical agents—amprolium hydrochloride, *Clin Allergy* 6:105-108, 1976.

200. Fawcett IW and Pepys J: Allergy to a tetracycline preparation, *Clin Allergy* 6:301 303, 1976.

201. Menon MPS and Das AK: Tetracycline asthma—a case report, *Clin Allergy* 7:285-290, 1977.

202. Asai S, Shimoda T, Hara K, et al: Occupational asthma caused by isonicotinic acid hydrazide (INH) inhalation, *J Allergy Clin Immunol* 80:578-582, 1987.

203. Perrin B, Malo J-L, Cartier A, et al: Occupational asthma in a pharmaceutical worker exposed to hydralazine, *Thorax* 45:980-981, 1990.

204. Lee HS, Wang YT, Yeo CT, et al: Occupational asthma due to tylosin tartrate, *Br J Ind Med* 46:498-499, 1989.

205. Luczynska CM, Marshall PE, Scarisbrick DA, et al: Occupational allergy due to inhalation of ipecacuanha dust, *Clin Allergy* 14:169-175, 1984.

206. Coutts II, Lozewicz S, Dally MB, et al: Respiratory symptoms related to work in a factory manufacturing cimetidine tablets, *Br Med J* 288:1418, 1984.

207. Biagini RE, Bernstein DM, Klincewicz SL, et al: Evaluation of cutaneous responses and lung function from exposure to opiate com-

pounds among ethical narcotics-manufacturing workers, *J Allergy Clin Immunol* 89:108-117, 1992.

208. Feinberg SM and Watrous RM: Atopy to simple chemical compounds—sulfonechloramides, *J Allergy* 16:209-220, 1945.

209. Bourne MS, Flindt MLH, and Walker JM: Asthma due to industrial use of chloramine, *Br Med J* 2:10-12, 1979.

210. Dijkman JG, Vooren PH, and Kramps JA: Occupational asthma due to inhalation of chloramine-T. 1. Clinical observations and inhalation-provocation studies, *Int Arch Allergy Appl Immunol* 64:422-427, 1981.

211. Andrasch RH, Bardana EJ, Koster F, et al: Clinical and bronchial provocation studies in patients with meatwrapper's asthma, *J Allergy Clin Immunol* 58:291-298, 1976.

212. Sokol WN, Aelony Y, and Beall GN: Meat-wrapper's asthma. A new syndrome?, *JAMA* 226:639-641, 1973.

213. Lee HS, Yap J, Wang YT, et al: Occupational asthma due to unheated polyvinylchloride resin dust, *Br J Ind Med* 46:820-822, 1989.

214. Kopp SK, McKay RT, Moller DR, et al: Asthma and rhinitis due to ethylcyanoacrylate instant glue, *Ann Intern Med* 102:613-615, 1985.

215. Weiner A: Bronchial asthma due to the organic phosphate insecticides, *Ann Allergy* 19:397-401, 1961.

216. Alanko K, Keskinen H, Byorksten F, et al: Immediate-type hypersensitivity to reactive dyes, *Clin Allergy* 8:25-31, 1978.

217. Park HS, Lee MK, Kim BO, et al: Clinical and immunologic evaluations of reactive dye-exposed workers, *J Allergy Clin Immunol* 87:639-649, 1991.

218. Romano C, Sulotto F, Pavan I, et al: A new case of occupational asthma from reactive dyes with severe anaphylactic response to the specific challenge, *Am J Ind Med* 21:209-216, 1992.

219. Pepys J, Hutchcroft BJ, and Breslin ABX: Asthma due to inhaled chemical agents—persulphate salts and henna in hairdressers, *Clin Allergy* 6:399-404, 1976.

220. Baur X, Fruhmann G, and Liebe VV: Occupational asthma and dermatitis after exposure to dusts of persulfate salts in two industrial workers, *Respiration* 38:144-150, 1979.

221. Blainey AD, Ollier S, Cundell D, et al: Occupational asthma in a hairdressing salon, *Thorax* 41:42-50, 1986.

222. Pankow W, Hein H, Bittner K, et al: Asthma in hairdressers induced by persulphate, *Pneumologie* 43:173-175, 1989.

223. Gamboa PM, de la Cuesta CG, García BE, et al: Late asthmatic reaction in a hairdresser, due to the inhalation of ammonium persulphate salts, *Allergol Immunopathol* 17:109-111, 1989.

224. Slovak AJM: Occupational asthma caused by a plastics blowing agent, azodicarbonamide, *Thorax* 36:906-909, 1981.

225. Malo J-L, Pineau L, and Cartier A: Occupational asthma due to azobisformamide, *Clin Allergy* 15:261-264, 1985.

226. Normand J-C, Grange F, Hernandez C, et al: Occupational asthma after exposure to azodicarbonamide: report of four cases, *Br J Ind Med* 46:60-62, 1989.

227. Graham V, Coe MJS, and Davies RJ: Occupational asthma after exposure to a diazonium salt, *Thorax* 36:950-951, 1981.

228. Luczynska CM, Hutchcroft BJ, Harrison MA, et al: Occupational asthma and specific IgE to diazonium salt intermediate used in the polymer industry, *J Allergy Clin Immunol* 85:1076-1082, 1990.

229. Nagy L and Orosz M: Occupational asthma due to hexachlorophene, *Thorax* 39:630-631, 1984.

230. Hendrick DJ and Lane DJ: Formalin asthma in hospital staff, *Br Med J* 1:607-608, 1975.

231. Burge PS, Harries MG, Lam WK, et al: Occupational asthma due to formaldehyde, *Thorax* 40:255-260, 1985.

232. Nordman H, Keskinen H, and Tuppurainen M: Formaldehyde asthma—rare or overlooked?, *J Allergy Clin Immunol* 75:91-99, 1985.

233. Cockcroft DW, Hoeppner VH, and Dolovich J: Occupational asthma caused by cedar urea formaldehyde particle board, *Chest* 82:49-53, 1982.

234. Frigas E, Filley WV, and Reed CE: Asthma induced by dust from urea-formaldehyde foam insulating material, *Chest* 79:706-707, 1981.

235. Malo J-L, Gagnon G, and Cartier A: Occupational asthma due to heated freon, *Thorax* 39:628-629, 1984.

236. Cockcroft DW, Cartier A, Jones G, et al: Asthma caused by occupational exposure to a furan-based binder system, *J Allergy Clin Immunol* 66:458-463, 1980.

237. Topping MD, Forster HW, Ide CW, et al: Respiratory allergy and specific immunoglobin E and immunoglobin G antibodies to reactive dyes used in the wool industry, *JOM, J Occup Med* 31:857-862, 1989.

238. Moscato G, Biscaldi G, Cottica D, et al: Occupational asthma due to styrene: two case reports, *JOM, J Occup Med* 29:957-960, 1987.

239. Jachuck SJ, Bound CL, Steel J, et al: Occupational hazard in hospital staff exposed to 2 per cent glutaraldehyde in an endoscopy unit, *J Soc Occup Med* 39:69-71, 1989.

240. Lozewicz S, Davison AG, Hopkirk A, et al: Occupational asthma due to methyl methacrylate and cyanoacrylates, *Thorax* 40:836-839, 1985.

241. Pickering CAC, Bainbridge D, Birtwistle IH, et al: Occupational asthma due to methyl methacrylate in an orthopaedic theatre sister, *Br Med J* 292:1362-1363, 1986.

242. Hendrick DJ, Connolly MJ, Stenton SC, et al: Occupational asthma due to sodium iso-nonanoyl oxybenzene sulphonate, a newly developed detergent ingredient, *Thorax* 43:501-502, 1988.

243. Waclawski ER, McAlpine LG, and Thomson NC: Occupational asthma in nurses caused by chlorhexidine and alcohol aerosols, *Br Med J* 298:929-930, 1989.

244. Burge PS, Hendy M, and Hodgson ES: Occupational asthma, rhinitis, and dermatitis due to tetrazene in a detonator manufacturer, *Thorax* 39:470-471, 1984.

245. Dugue P, Faraut C, Figueredo M, et al: Asthme professionnel à l'oxyde d'éthylène chez une infirmière, *Presse Med* 20:1455, 1991.

246. Gannon PFG, Sherwood Burge P, and Benfield CFA: Occupational asthma due to polyethylene shrink wrapping (paper wrapper's asthma), *Thorax* 47:759, 1992.

247. Honda I, Kohrogi H, Ando M, et al: Occupational asthma induced by the fungicide tetrachloroisophthalonitrile, *Thorax* 47:760-761, 1992.

248. Shelton D, Urch B, and Tarlo SM: Occupational asthma induced by a carpet fungicide–tributyl tin oxide, *J Allergy Clin Immunol* 90:274-275, 1992.

249. Tarlo SM: Occupational asthma induced by tall oil in the rubber tyre industry, *Clin Exp Allergy* 22:99-102, 1991.

250. Kennes B, Garcia-Herreros P, and Sierckx P: Asthma from Plexiglas powders, *Clin Allergy* 11:49-54, 1981.

251. Tarlo SM, Wong L, Roos J, et al: Occupational asthma caused by latex in a surgical glove manufacturing plant, *J Allergy Clin Immunol* 85:626-631, 1990.

252. Kern DG and Frumkin H: Asthma in respiratory therapists, *Ann Intern Med* 110:767-773, 1989.

253. Musk AW, Peach S, and Ryan G: Occupational asthma in a mineral analysis laboratory, *Br J Ind Med* 45:381-386, 1988.

254. Hendy MS, Beattie BE, and Burge PS: Occupational asthma due to an emulsified oil mist, *Br J Ind Med* 42:51-54, 1985.

255. Midttun O: Bronchial asthma in the aluminium industry, *Acta Allerg* 15:208-221, 1960.

256. Saric M, Godnic-Cvar J, Gonzi M, et al: The role of atopy in potroom workers' asthma, *Am J Ind Med* 9:239-242, 1986.

257. Wergeland E, Lund E, and Waage JE: Respiratory dysfunction after potroom asthma, *Am J Ind Med* 11:627-636, 1987.

258. O'Donnell TV, Welford B, and Coleman ED: Potroom asthma: New Zealand experience and follow-up, *Am J Ind Med* 14:43-49, 1989.

Appendix C

ABBREVIATIONS

ACGIH: American Conference of Governmental Industrial Hygienists
ACIP: Immunization Practices Advisory Committee
ACM: asbestos-containing material
ADA: U.S. Americans with Disabilities Act
AFL-CIO: American Federation of Labor and Congress of Industrial Organizations
AHA: American Hospital Association
AHR: airway hyperresponsiveness
AHU: air handling unit
AIDS: acquired immunodeficiency syndrome
ALA: American Lung Association
ALAPCO: Association of Local Air Pollution Control Officials
AM: alveolar macrophage
AMA: American Medical Association
ANSI: American National Standards Institute
APF: assigned protection factor
AQI: Air Quality Index
ARB: Air Resources Board
ARDS: adult respiratory distress syndrome
ASHRAE: American Society of Heating, Refrigerating, and Air-Conditioning Engineers
ATS: American Thoracic Society
ATSDR: Agency for Toxic Substances and Disease Registry

BACT: best available control technology
BAL: bronchoalveolar lavage
BCME: bis-chloromethyl ether
BED: biologically effective dose
BEIR: Biological Effects of Ionizing Radiation
BeLPT: beryllium lymphocyte proliferation test
BMR: basal metabolic rate
BPM: breaths per minute
BRI: building-related illness
BSC: biologic safety cabinets

CASAC: Clean Air Scientific Advisory Committee

CBD: chronic beryllium disease
CDC: U.S. Centers for Disease Control and Prevention
CERCLA: Comprehensive Environmental Response, Compensation, and Liability
CFR: U.S. Code of Federal Regulations
CGRP: calcitonin gene-related peptide
CHEMTREC: Chemical Transportation Emergency Center
CI: confidence interval
CMA: Canadian Medical Association
CMD: count medium diameters
CME: chloromethyl ether
CMME: chloromethyl methyl ether
CMN: Certificate of Medical Necessity
CMV: cytomegalovirus
CNSLD: chronic nonspecific lung disease
COPD: chronic obstructive pulmonary disease
COSH: coalition of occupational safety and health
CT: computerized tomography
CWP: coal workers' pneumoconiosis

DAN: Divers Alert Network
DCS: decompression sickness
DHHS: Department of Health and Human Services
DLCO: diffusing capacity of the lung for carbon monoxide
DMA: dimethylarsinic acid
DNA: deoxyribonucleic acid
DRDS: Division of Respiratory Disease Studies
DSHEFS: Division of Surveillance, Hazard Evaluation and Field Studies

EDXM: energy-dispersive x-ray spectroscopy using electron microscopy
EEC: European Economic Community
ELISA: enzyme-linked immunosorbent assay
EM: electron microscopy
EMR: electromagnetic radiation
EPA: U.S. Environmental Protection Agency
ETS: environmental tobacco smoke

FAA: Federal Aviation Administration
FAP: fused aluminosilicate particles
FCU: fan coil unit
FDA: Food and Drug Administration
FEC: forced expiratory capacity
FEF: forced expiratory flow
FEV1: forced expiratory volume in 1 second
FIP: Federal Implementation Plan
FLD: farmer's lung disease
FNA: fine needle aspiration
FRC: functional residual capacity
FREMEC: Frequent Traveler Medical Card
FVC: forced vital capacity

GDP: gross domestic product
GER: gas exchange region
GIP: giant cell interstitial pneumonitis
GM-CSF: granulocyte-monocyte colony-stimulating factor
GNB: gram-negative bacteria
Gus: upstream conductance

HAP: hazardous air pollutant
HAR: head airway region
HAST: hypoxic altitude simulation test
HCW: health care worker
HETA: health evaluation and technical assistance
HEPA: high-efficiency particulate air filter
HHE: health hazard evaluation
HHS: U.S. Department of Health and Human Services
HIV: human immunodeficiency virus
HMW: high molecular weight
HRCT: high-resolution computerized tomography
HVAC: heating, ventilation, and air-conditioning

IAH: immune adherence hemagglutination
IAQ: indoor air quality
IARC: International Agency for Research on Cancer
IC: integrated chip
ICOH: International Congress on Occupational Health
ICRP: International Commission on Radiological Protection
IDLH: immediately dangerous to life and health
IGF: insulinlike growth factor
ILO: International Labour Organization
IME: independent medical examination
IPPB: intermittent positive pressure breathing
ITRI: Inhalation Toxicology Research Institute
IUATLD: International Union against Tuberculosis and Lung Disease

JEM: job exposure matrix

LAA: laboratory animal allergy
LAER: lowest available emission rate
LDH: lactate dehydrogenase
LET: linear energy transfer
LMW: low molecular weight
LOX: liquid oxygen
LPS: lipopolysaccharide compound
LRSS: late respiratory systemic syndrome

MACT: maximum achievable control technology
MDI: methylene diphenyl diisocyanate
MMA: monomethylarsonic acid
MMAD: mass median aerodynamic diameter
MMWR: Morbidity and Mortality Weekly Report
MRI: magnetic resonance imaging
mRNA: messenger ribonucleic acid
MRP: medical removal protection
MS: mainstream smoke
MSA: Metropolitan Statistical Area
MSDS: material safety data sheets
MSHA: Mine Safety and Health Administration
MVV: maximal voluntary ventilation
MW: molecular weight

NAAQS: National Ambient Air Quality Standard
NADCA: National Air Duct Cleaners Association
NASA: National Aeronautics and Space Administration
NCI: National Cancer Institute
NCRP: National Committee on Radiation Protection and Measurements
NESCAUM: Northeast States for Coordinated Air Use Management
NHANES: National Health and Nutrition Examination Survey
NHDS: National Hospital Discharge Survey
NHIS: National Health Interview Survey
NIH: U.S. National Institutes of Health
NIOSH: U.S. National Institute for Occupational Safety and Health
NLM: National Library of Medicine
NMRD: nonmalignant respiratory disease
NOES: National Occupational Exposure Survey
NOHS: National Occupational Hazards Survey
NRC: U.S. Nuclear Regulatory Commission
NSBH: nonspecific bronchial hyperresponsiveness
NSCWP: National Study of Coal Workers' Pneumoconiosis
NSP: new source performance standards
NTP: National Toxicology Program
NVG: Nivagransvarde

OA: occupational asthma
ODC: ornithine decarboxylase
ODTS: organic dust toxic syndrome

OEP: olfactory evoked potential
OH⁻: hydroxyl radical
OR: odds ratio
OSHA: U.S. Occupational Safety and Health Administration
OSHAct: Occupational Safety and Health Act
OTA: U.S. Office of Technology Assessment

PA: plicatic acid
PA-HSA: plicatic acid-human serum albumin
PAH: polycyclic aromatic hydrocarbons
PAP: pulmonary aleveolar proteinosis
PAR%: population attributable risk percent
PCB: polychlorinated biphenyl
PCC: poison control center
PCE: tetrachloroethylene (perchlorethylene)
PCM: phase-contrast microscopy
PDGF: platelet-derived growth factor
PEEP: positive end-expiratory pressure
PEF: peak expiratory flow
PEFR: peak expiratory flow rate
PEL: permissible exposure limit
PFA: pulverized fluid ash
PFT: pulmonary function test
PM: particulate matter
PM$_{10}$: particulate matter <10 microns
PMF: progressive massive fibrosis
PMN: polymorphonuclear leukocyte
PMR: proportionate mortality ratio
PNL: Pacific Northwest Laboratory
PNP: Philadelphia Neoplasm Project
POPS: pulmonary overpressurization syndrome
PPD: purified protein derivative
PPE: personal protective equipment
PSD: prevention of significant deterioration
PSI: Pollutant Standards Index

RACT: reasonably available control technology
rad: radiation absorbed dose
RADS: reactive airways dysfunction syndrome
RAST: radioallergosorbent test
RCF: refractory ceramic fiber
RCI: retrospective cohort incidence
RCM: retrospective cohort mortality
REE: resting energy expenditure
REL: recommended exposure limit
rem: radiation equivalent in man
RNA: ribonucleic acid
RPE: relative perceived exertion
RR: rate ratio
RSP: respirable suspended particulates
RSV: respiratory syncytial virus

RTECS: Registry of Toxic Effects of Chemical Substances
RV: residual volume
RVH: right ventricular hypertrophy

SARA: U.S. Superfund Amendments and Reauthorization Act
SBS: sick building syndrome
SCBA: self-contained breathing apparatus
scuba: self-contained underwater breathing apparatus
SD: standard deviation
SEM: scanning electron microscopy
SENSOR: Sentinel Event Notification System for Occupational Risks
SEP: European Society of Pneumology
SI: Systeme International
SIDS: sudden infant death syndrome
SIP: State Implementation Plan
SIR: standardized incidence ratio
SMR: standardized mortality ratio
SOP: standard operating procedure
SS: sidestream smoke
SSI: Supplemental Security Income
STAPPA: State and Territorial Air Pollution Program Administrators
STEL: short-term exposure limit
SVOC: semivolatile organic compound
SWORD: Surveillance of Work-Related Occupational Respiratory Disease

TB: tuberculosis
TCE: trichloroethylene
TDI: toluene diisocyanate
TEAM: Total Exposure Assessment Methodology
TEM: transmission electron microscopy
TGV: Tarekgrandvarden
TLC: total lung capacity
TLV: threshold limit value
TMA: trimellitic anhydride
TM-HSA: trimellityl-human serum albumin
TNF: tumor necrosis factor
TNF-α: tumor necrosis factor-α
TSCA: Toxic Substances Control Act
TSP: total suspended particulates
TTP: transtracheal oxygen
TV: tidal volume
TVOC: total volatile organic compound
TWA: time-weighted average

UFFI: urea formaldehyde foam insulation
USC: United States Code

VAS: visual analog scales
VAV: variable air volume
VC: vital capacity

VGE: venous gas embolism
VO$_2$: oxygen consumption
VOC: volatile organic compound
VZIG: varicella immune globulin
VZV: varicella zoster virus

w$_R$: radiation weighting factor
w$_T$: organ weighting factor
WHO: World Health Organization
WL: working level
WLM: working level month

INDEX*

---

*Illustrations are indicated by italic page numbers. Tables are indicated by italic page numbers followed by *t*.